CURRENT
VETERINARY
THERAPY
XI

SMALL ANIMAL PRACTICE

EDITED BY

ROBERT W. KIRK, D.V.M.,
Dipl. A.C.V.I.M., A.C.V.D.

Professor of Medicine, Emeritus
New York State College of Veterinary Medicine
Cornell University
Ithaca, New York

and

JOHN D. BONAGURA, D.V.M.,
M.S., Dipl. A.C.V.I.M.
(Internal Medicine, Cardiology)

Professor, Department of Veterinary Clinical Sciences
College of Veterinary Medicine
The Ohio State University
Columbus, Ohio

Consulting Editors

CARL A. OSBORNE
Special Therapy

ROBERT J. MURTAUGH
Critical Care

GARY D. OSWEILER
Chemical and Physical Disorders

EDWARD B. BREITSCHWERDT
Infectious Diseases

MARK E. PETERSON
Endocrine and Metabolic Disorders

BRUCE R. MADEWELL
Hematology, Oncology, and Immunology

WILLIAM H. MILLER, Jr.
Dermatologic Diseases

DAVID C. TWEDT
Gastrointestinal Disorders

BRUCE W. KEENE
Cardiopulmonary Diseases

JEANNE A. BARSANTI
Urinary Disorders

VICKI N. MEYERS-WALLEN
Reproductive Disorders

JOE N. KORNEGAY
Neurologic and Neuromuscular Disorders

THOMAS J. KERN
Ophthalmologic Diseases

R. ERIC MILLER
Diseases of Caged Birds and Exotic Pets

ROBERT M. JACOBS and MARK G. PAPICH
Appendices

CURRENT VETERINARY THERAPY

XI

SMALL ANIMAL PRACTICE

W.B. SAUNDERS COMPANY
Harcourt Brace Jovanovich, Inc.

Philadelphia   London   Toronto   Montreal   Sydney   Tokyo

W. B. SAUNDERS COMPANY
Harcourt Brace Jovanovich, Inc.

The Curtis Center
Independence Square West
Philadelphia, Pennsylvania 19106

Library of Congress Cataloging-in-Publication Data

Current veterinary therapy. 1964/65—

Philadelphia, W. B. Saunders.

v. 26 cm.

"Small animal practice."

Editor: 1964/65- R. W. Kirk.

Key title: Current veterinary therapy, ISSN 0070–2218.

1. Veterinary medicine—Periodicals.   2. Pets—Diseases—
   Periodicals.   I. Kirk, Robert Warren, ed.
   [DNLM: W1 CU823]

SF745.C8   636.0896   64–10489
                               MARC-S

Library of Congress   [8308]

Editor: Linda E. Mills
Designer: W. B. Saunders Staff
Production Manager: Bill Preston
Manuscript Editor: W. B. Saunders Staff
Illustration Specialist: Brett MacNaughton
Indexer: Nancy Matthew

Kirk's Current Veterinary Therapy XI   ISBN 0–7216–3293–9

Last digit is the print number: 9   8   7   6   5   4   3   2   1

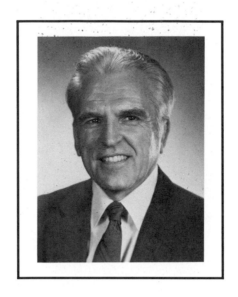

A Tribute to
ROBERT W. KIRK

The first edition of *Current Veterinary Therapy* was published in 1964. It was destined to become a best seller, as thousands of veterinarians throughout the world recognized it as an indispensable tool in their efforts to provide quality patient care. The first edition of *CVT* contained more than 200 chapters about the treatment and prevention of companion animal disorders and was written by 130 authorities in the field. Now, a quarter of a century later, there have been 11 editions of *Current Veterinary Therapy* containing more than 2750 chapters printed on more than 12,000 pages.

Who had the wisdom, insight, and energy to catalyze this scientific gem and to sustain its mission to provide life-giving information in a timely fashion? All who utilize this practitioners' bible know that it is a living legacy of Robert W. Kirk. With the assistance of his wife, Helen, a lamp of knowledge has been ignited whose light spreads diagnostic and therapeutic truths to all corners of the earth. When students, practicing veterinarians, and clinical teachers need an up-to-date source about the diagnosis, treatment, and prevention of companion animal diseases, the vast majority consult "Kirk."

If we were to ask Bob Kirk, "Of all the volumes of *Current Veterinary Therapy* that have been published, which one is the finest?" how would he answer? I invite all of you who have been helped by *Current Veterinary Therapy* to encourage him to say "The next one!" We need the wise and nurturing leadership of this special man to aid us in maintaining the unshakable principle that must guide our actions, that principle being that the welfare of our patients comes first—and last.

CARL A. OSBORNE, D.V.M., PH.D.

CONTRIBUTORS

SARAH K. ABOOD, D.V.M. Resident in Clinical Nutrition of Large and Small Animals; Graduate Student in Nutrition, The Ohio State University; Nutrition Support Service, The Ohio State University Veterinary Hospital, Columbus, Ohio
Section 1

NOHA ABOU-MADI, D.V.M., M.S. Resident in Zoological Medicine, University of Florida; Staff Veterinarian, Silver Springs, Inc., Gainesville, Florida
Section 14

LARRY G. ADAMS, D.V.M., PH.D., Dipl. A.C.V.I.M. Assistant Professor, Department of Veterinary Animal Sciences, School of Veterinary Medicine, Purdue University, West Lafayette, Indiana
Sections 1 and 10

TIMOTHY A. ALLEN, D.V.M., Dipl. A.C.V.I.M. Research Veterinarian, Mark Morris Associates, Topeka; Adjunct Clinical Professor, Kansas State University, Manhattan, Kansas
Section 1

DONNA WALTON ANGARANO, D.V.M., Dipl. A.C.V.D. Associate Professor, Department of Small Animal Surgery and Medicine, College of Veterinary Medicine, Auburn University, Auburn, Alabama
Section 7

M.J.G. APPEL, D.V.M., PH.D. Professor of Virology, New York State College of Veterinary Medicine, Cornell University, Ithaca, New York
Section 4

SUSI ARNOLD, D.V.M. Consultant, Small Animal Reproduction, Department of Reproduction,

Veterinary Medical Faculty of the University of Zurich, Zurich, Switzerland
Section 10

CLARKE E. ATKINS, D.V.M., Dipl. A.C.V.I.M. Associate Professor of Medicine/Cardiology, Department of Companion Animal and Special Species Medicine, School of Veterinary Medicine, North Carolina State University, Raleigh, North Carolina
Section 9

DAVID P. AUCOIN, D.V.M., Dipl. A.C.V.C.P. Research Associate Professor, School of Veterinary Medicine, North Carolina State University, Raleigh, North Carolina
Section 4

CLETA SUE BAILEY, D.V.M., PH.D., Dipl. A.C.V.I.M. (Neurology). Professor, Department of Surgery, School of Veterinary Medicine, University of California–Davis; Chief, Neurology/Neurosurgery Service, Veterinary Medical Teaching Hospital, University of California, Davis, California
Section 12

JEANNE A. BARSANTI, D.V.M., M.S., Dipl. A.C.V.I.M. (Internal Medicine). Professor, Department of Small Animal Medicine, College of Veterinary Medicine, University of Georgia; Internist, University of Georgia Veterinary Medical Teaching Hospital, Athens, Georgia
Section 10

OTA BARTA, M.V.DR., PH.D., Dipl. A.C.V.M. Professor, Virginia-Maryland Regional College of Veterinary Medicine, Virginia Polytechnic Institute and State University, Blacksburg, Virginia
Section 4

JOSEPH W. BARTGES, D.V.M. Veterinary Medical Associate, Department of Small Animal Clinical Sciences, College of Veterinary Medicine, University of Minnesota; Resident, Small Animal Medicine, Veterinary Teaching Hospital, University of Minnesota, St. Paul, Minnesota
Section 10

CATHERINE J. BATY, D.V.M. Resident, Small Animal Internal Medicine, School of Veterinary Medicine, North Carolina State University, Raleigh, North Carolina
Section 2

ELSA R. BECK, D.V.M., PH.D. Assistant Professor of Medical Physics (Adjunct), Oakland University, Rochester, Michigan; Senior Staff Investigator, Henry Ford Hospital, Detroit, Michigan
Section 6

RICHARD M. BEDNARSKI, D.V.M., M.S., Dipl. A.C.V.A. Associate Professor, College of Veterinary Medicine, The Ohio State University; Head of Anesthesiology, Veterinary Teaching Hospital, The Ohio State University, Columbus, Ohio
Section 1

BRUCE E. BELSHAW, D.V.M. Staff Member, Department of Clinical Sciences of Companion Animals, Faculty of Veterinary Medicine, University of Utrecht, Utrecht, The Netherlands
Section 5

CYNTHIA BESCH-WILLIFORD, D.V.M., PH.D., Dipl. A.C.L.A.M. Assistant Professor, Department of Veterinary Pathology; Associate Director, Research Animal Diagnostic and Investigative Laboratory, College of Veterinary Medicine, University of Missouri, Columbia, Missouri
Section 14

ROGER E. BRANNIAN, D.V.M. Teaching Assistant, Department of Veterinary Pathology, College of Veterinary Medicine, Iowa State University, Ames, Iowa
Section 14

EDWARD B. BREITSCHWERDT, D.V.M., Dipl. A.C.V.I.M. Professor of Medicine, College of Veterinary Medicine, North Carolina State University, Raleigh, North Carolina
Section 4

JANICE McINTOSH BRIGHT, Dipl. A.C.V.I.M. (Internal Medicine and Cardiology). Associate Professor of Internal Medicine and Cardiology, College of Veterinary Medicine, University of Tennessee, Knoxville, Tennessee
Section 9

RONALD M. BRIGHT, D.V.M., M.S., Dipl. A.C.V.S. Professor, Department of Urban Practice; Director of Surgical Services and Staff Surgeon, College of Veterinary Medicine, University of Tennessee, Knoxville, Tennessee
Section 8

SCOTT A. BROWN, V.M.D., PH.D., Dipl. A.C.V.I.M. (Internal Medicine). Assistant Professor of Physiology, Department of Small Animal Medicine, College of Veterinary Medicine, University of Georgia; Veterinary Teaching Hospital, University of Georgia, Athens, Georgia
Section 10

JAMES M. BUCHANAN, D.V.M., Dipl. A.C.V.I.M. Professor of Cardiology, School of Veterinary Medicine, University of Pennsylvania, Philadelphia, Pennsylvania
Section 9

C. A. TONY BUFFINGTON, D.V.M., Dipl. A.C.V.N. Assistant Professor, College of Veterinary Medicine, The Ohio State University; Chief, Nutrition Support Service, Veterinary Teaching Hospital, The Ohio State University, Columbus, Ohio
Section 1

THOMAS J. BURKE, D.V.M., M.S. Professor of Medicine, College of Veterinary Medicine, University of Illinois, Urbana; Consultant, Capitol Illini Veterinary Services, Ltd., Springfield; Research Associate, Lincoln Park Zoo, Chicago, Illinois
Section 14

MITCHELL BUSH, D.V.M., Dipl. A.C.Z.M. Chief, Department of Animal Health, National Zoological Park, Smithsonian Institution, Washington, D.C.
Section 14

P. A. BUSHBY, D.V.M., M.S., Dipl. A.C.V.S. Professor and Academic Program Director, College of Veterinary Medicine, Mississippi State University, Mississippi State, Mississippi
Section 1

MARTINE CACHIN, D.V.M. Institute of Animal Neurology, School of Veterinary Medicine, University of Bern, Bern, Switzerland
Section 12

CLAY A. CALVERT, D.V.M., Dipl. A.C.V.I.M. Associate Professor of Internal Medicine, College of Veterinary Medicine, University of Georgia, Athens, Georgia
Section 9

KAREN L. CAMPBELL, D.V.M., M.S., Dipl. A.C.V.I.M., A.C.V.D. Associate Professor, Department of Veterinary Clinical Medicine, College of Veterinary Medicine, University of Illinois; Veterinary Medical Teaching Hospital, Small Animal Clinic, University of Illinois, Urbana, Illinois
Sections 1 and 7

DIDIER N. CARLOTTI, D.V.M. Practitioner, Carbon-Blanc; Consultant at the Lyons Veterinary School; Veterinary Dermatology Clinic, Sainte Eulalie, France
Section 7

THOMAS L. CARSON, D.V.M., PH.D., Dipl. A.B.V.T. Professor of Veterinary Pathology/Toxicology, Veterinary Diagnostic Laboratory, College of Veterinary Medicine, Iowa State University, Ames, Iowa
Section 3

LESLIE J. CARTER, M.S. Critical Care Unit, Colorado State University Veterinary Teaching Hospital, Fort Collins, Colorado
Section 10

JONATHAN N. CHAMBERS, D.V.M., Dipl. A.C.V.S. Professor of Orthopedic Surgery, Department of Small Animal Medicine, College of Veterinary Medicine, University of Georgia; Chief of Staff, Small Animal Surgery, Veterinary Medical Teaching Hospital, College of Veterinary Medicine, University of Georgia, Athens, Georgia
Section 12

MARJORIE L. CHANDLER, M.S., D.V.M. Small Animal Resident, School of Veterinary Medicine, Colorado State University, Fort Collins, Colorado
Section 11

C. B. CHASTAIN, D.V.M., M.S., Dipl. A.C.V.I.M. Professor, College of Veterinary Medicine,

University of Missouri; Veterinary Teaching Hospital, University of Missouri, Columbia, Missouri
Section 5

DENNIS J. CHEW, D.V.M., Dipl. A.C.V.I.M. Professor of Internal Medicine, College of Veterinary Medicine, The Ohio State University; Attending, Veterinary Teaching Hospital, The Ohio State University, Columbus, Ohio
Section 10

SCOTT B. CITINO, D.V.M. Associate Veterinarian, National Zoological Park, Smithsonian Institution, Washington, D.C.
Section 14

GEOFFREY N. CLARK, D.V.M. Staff Surgeon, Animal Surgical Clinic of Seattle, Seattle, Washington
Section 2

SUSAN L. CLUBB, D.V.M. Agricultural Breeding and Research Center, Loxahatchee; Parrot Jungle and Gardens, Miami, Florida
Section 14

ELLEN C. CODNER, D.V.M., M.S., Dipl. A.C.V.I.M. (Internal Medicine). Assistant Professor, Department of Small Animal Clinical Sciences, Virginia-Maryland Regional College of Veterinary Medicine, Virginia Polytechnic Institute and State University; Small Animal Medicine, Veterinary Teaching Hospital, Virginia-Maryland Regional College of Veterinary Medicine, Virginia Polytechnic Institute and State University, Blacksburg, Virginia
Section 4

KEVIN T. CONCANNON, D.V.M. Clinical Instructor, Veterinary Medical Teaching Hospital, University of California, Davis, California
Section 2

PATRICK W. CONCANNON, PH.D. Senior Research Associate, New York State College of Veterinary Medicine, Cornell University, Ithaca, New York
Section 11

LINDA C. CORK, D.V.M., PH.D., Dipl. A.C.V.P. Professor, Division of Comparative Medicine and Department of Pathology, Johns Hopkins University School of Medicine, Baltimore, Maryland
Section 12

SUSAN M. COTTER, D.V.M., Dipl. A.C.V.I.M. Professor of Medicine, Section Head of Small Animal Medicine, Tufts University School of Veterinary Medicine, North Grafton, Massachusetts
Sections 2 and 6

C. GUILLERMO COUTO, D.V.M., Dipl. A.C.V.I.M. Associate Professor, Department of Veterinary Clinical Sciences, College of Veterinary Medicine, The Ohio State University; Chief, Oncology/Hematology Service, Veterinary Teaching Hospital, The Ohio State University, Columbus, Ohio
Sections 4 and 8

LARRY D. COWGILL, D.V.M., PH.D., Dipl. A.C.V.I.M. Associate Professor, Department of Medicine, School of Veterinary Medicine, University of California—Davis; Small Animal Medicine Service, Veterinary Medical Teaching Hospital, School of Veterinary Medicine, University of California, Davis, California
Section 6

GRAHAM J. CRAWSHAW, B. Vet. Med. Staff Veterinarian, Metropolitan Toronto Zoo, Toronto, Ontario
Section 14

DENNIS T. CROWE, JR., E.M.T., D.V.M., Dipl. A.C.V.S., A.C.V.E.C. Professor of Surgery and Director of Research, Veterinary Institute of Trauma, Emergency and Critical Care; Chief of Surgery, Animal Emergency Center, Milwaukee, Wisconsin; Formerly Associate Professor of Surgery and Chief, Emergency and Critical Care Service, College of Veterinary Medicine, University of Georgia, Athens, Georgia
Section 2

SHARON L. CROWELL-DAVIS, D.V.M., PH.D. Associate Professor, College of Veterinary Medicine, University of Georgia, Athens, Georgia
Section 12

PAUL A. CUDDON, B.V.SC., Dipl. A.C.V.I.M. (Neurology). Assistant Professor, University of Wisconsin School of Veterinary Medicine, Madison, Wisconsin
Section 12

J. F. CUMMINGS, D.V.M., PH.D. Professor of Anatomy, New York State College of Veterinary Medicine, Cornell University, Ithaca, New York
Section 12

PETER G. G. DARKE, B.V.SC. Senior Lecturer in Small Animal Medicine, University of Edinburgh, Edinburgh, Scotland
Section 9

DEBORAH J. DAVENPORT, D.V.M., M.S., Dipl. A.C.V.I.M. (Internal Medicine). Associate in Clinical Nutrition, Mark Morris Associates, Topeka; Adjunct Faculty, College of Veterinary Medicine, Kansas State University, Manhattan, Kansas
Section 2

MICHAEL DAVIDSON, D.V.M., Dipl. A.C.V.O. Assistant Professor of Ophthalmology, Department of Companion Animal and Special Species Medicine, School of Veterinary Medicine, North Carolina State University, Raleigh, North Carolina
Section 13

LAURA A. DeLELLIS, D.V.M., Dipl. A.C.V.I.M. (Cardiology). Staff Cardiologist, Michigan Veterinary Specialists, Bloomfield Hills, Michigan
Section 9

JOSEPH W. DENHART, D.V.M., M.S. Veterinary Research Manager, Lloyd Laboratories, Division of Vet-A-Mix Animal Health, Shenandoah, Iowa
Section 3

ROBERT C. DeNOVO, JR., D.V.M., M.S., Dipl. A.C.V.I.M. (Internal Medicine). Associate Professor of Medicine, Department of Urban Practice, College of Veterinary Medicine, University of Tennessee, Knoxville, Tennessee
Section 8

MARK W. DEWHIRST, D.V.M., PH.D. Associate Professor, Department of Radiation Oncology; Assistant Professor, Department of Pathology, Duke University Medical Center, Durham, North Carolina
Section 6

STEPHEN P. DiBARTOLA, D.V.M., Dipl. A.C.V.I.M. Professor of Medicine, Department of Veterinary Clinical Sciences, College of Veterinary Medicine, The Ohio State University; Small Animal Clinician, Veterinary Teaching Hospital, The Ohio State University, Columbus, Ohio
Section 10

KELLY J. DIEHL, D.V.M. Resident, Small Animal Medicine, Veterinary Teaching Hospital, Colorado State University, Fort Collins, Colorado
Section 5

THERESE M. DIERINGER, D.V.M., M.S. Staff Veterinarian, Central Veterinary Hospital, Upland, California
Section 10

DONNA S. DIMSKI, D.V.M., M.S., Dipl. A.C.V.I.M. Assistant Professor, Department of Veterinary Clinical Sciences, Louisiana State University; Veterinary Internist, Veterinary Teaching Hospital and Clinic, Louisiana State University, Baton Rouge, Louisiana
Section 8

SUSAN DONOGHUE, V.M.D., Dipl. A.C.V.N. Private Nutrition Practice, at Nutrition Support Services, Pembroke, Virginia
Section 11

DAVID C. DORMAN, D.V.M., PH.D., Dipl. A.B.V.T. Postdoctoral Fellow, Chemical Industry Institute of Toxicology, Research Triangle Park; Visiting Assistant Professor, College of Veterinary Medicine, North Carolina State University, Raleigh, North Carolina
Section 3

STEVEN W. DOW, D.V.M., M.S., Dipl. A.C.V.I.M. Special Assistant Professor, Department of Pathology, Colorado State University, Fort Collins, Colorado
Sections 4, 10, and 12

J. P. DUBEY, M.V.Sc., PH.D. U.S. Department of Agriculture, Beltsville, Maryland
Section 4

GENEVIEVE A. DUMONCEAUX, D.V.M. Clinic Veterinarian, Bolingbrook Animal Hospital, Ltd., and Naper-Ridge Animal Clinic, Naperville; Formerly Clinical Assistant Professor of Toxicology, University of Illinois, Urbana, Illinois
Section 3

JANICE A. DYE, D.V.M., M.S., Dipl. A.C.V.I.M. Postdoctoral Fellow, U.S. Environmental Protection Agency, Health Effects Research Laboratory, Research Triangle Park, North Carolina; Formerly, Department of Veterinary Clinical Medicine, College of Veterinary Medicine, University of Illinois, Urbana, Illinois
Section 9

DAVID A. DZANIS, D.V.M., PH.D., Dipl. A.C.V.N. U.S. Food and Drug Administration, Center for Veterinary Medicine, Rockville, Maryland
Section 1

ALICIA M. FAGGELLA, D.V.M. Director, Intensive Care Unit, Anesthesiology, Angell Memorial Animal Hospital, Boston, Massachusetts
Section 2

DANIEL A. FEENEY, D.V.M., M.S., Dipl. A.C.V.R. Professor of Radiology, College of Veterinary Medicine, University of Minnesota; Staff Radiologist, University of Minnesota Veterinary Teaching Hospital, St. Paul, Minnesota
Section 1

EDWARD C. FELDMAN, D.V.M., Dipl. A.C.V.I.M. Professor, Department of Veterinary Reproduction, School of Veterinary Medicine, University of California—Davis; Chief, Small Animal Internal Medicine Service, Veterinary Medicine Teaching Hospital, Davis, California
Section 5

LAWRENCE J. FELICE, PH.D. Associate Professor, Department of Veterinary Diagnostic Medicine, College of Veterinary Medicine, University of Minnesota, St. Paul, Minnesota
Section 10

PETER J. FELSBURG, V.M.D., PH.D. Professor of Immunology, Department of Veterinary Pathobiology, School of Veterinary Medicine, Purdue University, West Lafayette, Indiana
Sections 6 and 7

LUIS FERRER, D.V.M., PH.D. Associate Professor of Pathology, Department of Animal Pathology, Veterinary School, Universitat Autonoma de Barcelona, Barcelona, Spain
Section 4

MARTIN J. FETTMAN, D.V.M., Dipl. A.C.V.P. Department of Pathology, Colorado State University, Fort Collins, Colorado
Section 10

JAMES D. FIKES, D.V.M., M.S., Dipl. A.B.V.T. Postdoctoral Fellow, Department of Pathology, Michigan State University, East Lansing, Michigan
Section 10

DELMAR R. FINCO, D.V.M., PH.D., Dipl. A.C.V.I.M. Professor, Department of Physiology and Pharmacology, College of Veterinary Medicine, The University of Georgia, Athens, Georgia
Section 10

MARK R. FINKLER, D.V.M. Owner, Roanoke Animal Hospital, Roanoke, Virginia
Section 14

RICHARD E. FISH, D.V.M., PH.D., Dipl. A.C.L.A.M. Assistant Director, Office of Laboratory Animal Medicine; Assistant Professor, Department of Veterinary Biomedical Sciences, University of Missouri, Columbia, Missouri
Section 14

KEVEN FLAMMER, D.V.M. Associate Professor, College of Veterinary Medicine, North Carolina State University; Veterinary Teaching Hospital, College of Veterinary Medicine, North Carolina State University, Raleigh, North Carolina
Section 14

S. DRU FORRESTER, D.V.M., M.S., Dipl. A.C.V.I.M. (Internal Medicine). Assistant Professor, Department of Small Animal Clinical Sciences, Virginia-Maryland Regional College of Veterinary Medicine, Virginia Polytechnic Institute and State University; Small Animal Internist, Veterinary Teaching Hospital, Virginia Polytechnic Institute and State University, Blacksburg, Virginia
Section 10

THERESA W. FOSSUM, D.V.M., M.S., Dipl. A.C.V.S. Assistant Professor, Texas A&M University; Staff Surgeon, Texas Veterinary Medical Center, College of Veterinary Medicine, Texas A&M University, College Station, Texas
Section 9

MURRAY E. FOWLER, D.V.M., Dipl. A.B.V.T., A.C.V.I.M., A.C.Z.M. Professor Emeritus, School of Veterinary Medicine, University of California—Davis; Zoological Medicine Service, School of Veterinary Medicine, University of California, Davis, California
Section 14

JAMES G. FOX, D.V.M., Dipl. A.C.L.A.M. Professor and Director, Division of Comparative Medicine, Massachusetts Institute of Technology, Cambridge, Massachusetts
Section 14

PHILIP R. FOX, D.V.M., M.SC., Dipl. A.C.V.I.M. (Cardiology). Staff Cardiologist, Department of Medicine, and Chairman, Department of Clinic Services, The Animal Medical Center, New York, New York
Section 9

RONNA FULTON, D.V.M. Clinical Pathology Instructor, College of Veterinary Medicine and Biomedical Sciences, Colorado State University, Fort Collins, Colorado
Section 6

FRANCIS D. GALEY, D.V.M., PH.D., Dipl. A.B.V.T. Assistant Professor of Clinical Diagnostic Veterinary Toxicology, School of Veterinary Medicine, University of California, Davis, California
Section 3

PETER W. GASPER, D.V.M., PH.D. Associate Professor, Colorado State University; Co-Director, Marrow Transplant Laboratory, Pathology Department, College of Veterinary Medicine and Biomedical Sciences, Colorado State University, Fort Collins, Colorado
Section 6

LAUREL J. GERSHWIN, D.V.M., PH.D., Dipl. A.C.V.M. Professor of Immunology, School of Veterinary Medicine, University of California—Davis; Director, Clinical Immunology and Virology Laboratory, Veterinary Medical Teaching Hospital, University of California, Davis, California
Sections 1 and 6

URS GIGER, P.D. DR. Med. Vet. F.V.H., Dipl. A.C.V.I.M. Associate Professor of Medicine and Medical Genetics, School of Veterinary Medicine, University of Pennsylvania; Clinician, Veterinary Hospital of the University of Pennsylvania, Philadelphia, Pennsylvania
Section 6

ROBERT F. GILMOUR, JR., PH.D. Associate Professor of Physiology, New York State College of Veterinary Medicine, Cornell University, Ithaca, New York
Section 9

STEPHEN D. GILSON, D.V.M. Staff Surgeon, Sonora Veterinary Surgery and Oncology, Scottsdale, Arizona
Section 10

MARY B. GLAZE, D.V.M., M.S., Dipl. A.C.V.O. Associate Professor of Veterinary Ophthalmology, Department of Veterinary Clinical Sciences, School of Veterinary Medicine, Louisiana State University; Veterinary Teaching Hospital and Clinics, Louisiana State University, Baton Rouge, Louisiana
Section 13

NEIL T. GORMAN, B.V.Sc., Ph.D. Professor of Veterinary Surgery, University of Glasgow, Glasgow, Scotland
Section 6

WILLARD J. GOULD, D.V.M., Dipl. A.C.V.I.M. Assistant Professor, Department of Clinical Science, New York State College of Veterinary Medicine, Cornell University, Ithaca, New York
Section 14

IRA M. GOURLEY, D.V.M., Ph.D., Dipl. A.C.V.S. Professor, Department of Surgery, School of Veterinary Medicine, University of California, Davis, California
Section 10

GREGORY F. GRAUER, D.V.M., M.S., Dipl. A.C.V.I.M. Associate Professor, Department of Clinical Sciences, College of Veterinary Medicine and Biomedical Sciences, Colorado State University, Fort Collins, Colorado
Section 10

THOMAS K. GRAVES, D.V.M. Clinical Instructor, Department of Veterinary Clinical Sciences, College of Veterinary Medicine, The Ohio State University, Columbus, Ohio
Section 5

ROBERT A. GREEN, D.V.M., Ph.D., Dipl. A.C.V.P. Professor of Veterinary Pathology, Texas A&M University; Director of Veterinary Clinical Pathology Laboratory, Texas A&M Teaching Hospital, Texas A&M University, College Station, Texas
Section 10

CRAIG E. GREENE, D.V.M., M.S., Dipl. A.C.V.I.M. Professor, Department of Small Animal Medicine, College of Veterinary Medicine, University of Georgia; Veterinary Medical Teaching Hospital, University of Georgia, Athens, Georgia
Section 4

CLARE R. GREGORY, D.V.M., Dipl. A.C.V.S. Associate Professor, Department of Surgery, School of Veterinary Medicine, University of California—Davis; Chief, Small Animal Surgical Services, Veterinary Medical Teaching Hospital, University of California, Davis, California
Section 10

CRAIG E. GRIFFIN, D.V.M., Dipl. A.C.V.D. Director, Animal Dermatology Clinics, Garden Grove and San Diego, California
Section 7

W. GRANT GUILFORD, B.V.Sc., B.Phil., Dipl. A.C.V.I.M. Lecturer, Small Animal Medicine, Department of Veterinary Clinical Sciences. Massey University; Internist, Small Animal Clinic, Massey University, Palmerston North, New Zealand
Section 8

ELIZABETH A. HAHN, A.T.R. Clinical Oncology Research Technologist, Comparative Oncology Program, Purdue University, West Lafayette, Indiana
Section 6

KEVIN A. HAHN, D.V.M., Ph.D. Assistant Professor of Oncology, College of Veterinary Medicine, University of Tennessee, Knoxville, Tennessee
Section 6

ROBERT L. HAMLIN, D.V.M., Ph.D., Dipl. A.C.V.I.M. Professor of Veterinary Physiology and Pharmacology, College of Veterinary Medicine, The Ohio State University, Columbus, Ohio; Berwyn Veterinary Group, Berwyn, Illinois; Vienna Animal Hospital, Vienna, Virginia
Section 9

ALAN S. HAMMER, D.V.M. Assistant Professor, College of Veterinary Medicine, The Ohio State University, Columbus, Ohio
Sections 1 and 6

MICHAEL S. HAND, D.V.M., Ph.D., Dipl. A.C.V.N. Research Veterinarian, Mark Morris Associates, Topeka; Adjunct Professor, Anatomy and Physiology, Kansas State University, Manhattan; Adjunct Professor, Clinical Nutrition, College of Veterinary Medicine, North Carolina State University, Raleigh, North Carolina
Section 1

BERNIE HANSEN, D.V.M., M.S. Visiting Assistant Professor; Director of the Small Animal Intensive Care Unit, North Carolina State University, College of Veterinary Medicine, Raleigh, North Carolina
Section 2

ELIZABETH M. HARDIE, D.V.M., PH.D., Dipl. A.C.V.S. Associate Professor of Surgery, North Carolina State University, School of Veterinary Medicine, Raleigh, North Carolina
Section 2

ROBERT M. HARDY, D.V.M., M.S., Dipl. A.C.V.I.M. Professor of Internal Medicine, College of Veterinary Medicine, University of Minnesota; Staff Internist, University of Minnesota, Veterinary Teaching Hospital, St. Paul, Minnesota
Sections 1 and 8

NEIL K. HARPSTER, V.M.D., Dipl. A.C.V.I.M. (Cardiology). Clinical Associate Professor, Department of Medicine, Tufts University School of Veterinary Medicine, North Grafton; Director of Cardiology, Angell Memorial Animal Hospital, Boston, Massachusetts
Section 9

JAMES R. HARTKE, D.V.M. Resident in Pathology and Research Associate, Department of Veterinary Pathobiology, College of Veterinary Medicine, The Ohio State University, Columbus, Ohio
Section 6

ELEANOR C. HAWKINS, D.V.M. Dipl. A.C.V.I.M. Assistant Professor of Medicine, North Carolina State University College of Veterinary Medicine; Internist, Veterinary Teaching Hospital, North Carolina State University, Raleigh, North Carolina
Section 9

REBECCA L. HEGSTAD, PH.D. Endocrinology Laboratory, College of Veterinary Medicine, University of Minnesota, St. Paul, Minnesota
Section 11

PETER W. HELLYER, D.V.M., M.S., Dipl. A.C.V.A. Assistant Professor of Anesthesiology, North Carolina State University College of Veterinary Medicine, Raleigh, North Carolina
Section 9

ELIZABETH V. HILLYER, D.V.M. Staff Veterinarian, Rutherford Animal Hospital, Rutherford, New Jersey; Staff Veterinarian, Exotic Pet Medicine Service, The Animal Medical Center, New York, New York
Section 14

EDWARD A. HOOVER, D.V.M., PH.D., Dipl. A.C.V.P. Professor, Department of Pathology,

College of Veterinary Medicine and Biomedical Sciences, Colorado State University, Fort Collins, Colorado
Sections 4 and 12

JoGAYLE HOWARD, D.V.M., PH.D. Department of Animal Health, National Zoological Park, Washington, D.C.
Section 11

GILBERT JACOBS, D.V.M., Dipl. A.C.V.I.M. (Cardiology). Associate Professor of Medicine, College of Veterinary Medicine, University of Georgia; University of Georgia Veterinary Teaching Hospital, Athens, Georgia
Section 9

ROBERT M. JACOBS, D.V.M., PH.D., Dipl. A.C.V.P. Associate Professor of Pathology, Clinical Pathology Service Chief, Department of Pathology, Ontario Veterinary College, University of Guelph, Guelph, Ontario
Appendices

ELLIOTT R. JACOBSON, D.V.M., PH.D., Dipl. A.C.Z.M. Professor, Wildlife and Zoological Medicine, College of Veterinary Medicine, University of Florida; Professor and Clinician, Veterinary Medical Teaching Hospital, University of Florida, Gainesville, Florida
Section 14

OSWALD JARRETT, PH.D. Professor, University of Glasgow Veterinary School, Glasgow, Scotland
Section 6

PETER F. JEZYK, V.M.D., PH.D. Adjunct Associate Professor of Medicine in Medical Genetics, School of Veterinary Medicine, University of Pennsylvania, Philadelphia; Medical Director, Hatboro Animal Hospital, Hatboro, Pennsylvania
Section 1

CHERI A. JOHNSON, D.V.M., M.S., Dipl. A.C.V.I.M. Associate Professor, Department of Small Animal Clinical Sciences, College of Veterinary Medicine, Michigan State University, East Lansing, Michigan
Section 11

KENNETH H. JOHNSON, D.V.M., PH.D. Professor, Veterinary Pathology, Department of Veterinary Pathobiology, College of Veterinary Medicine, University of Minnesota, St. Paul, Minnesota
Section 1

LaRUE W. JOHNSON, D.V.M., PH.D. Associate Professor, College of Veterinary Medicine and Biomedical Sciences, Colorado State University; Colorado State University Veterinary Teaching Hospital, Fort Collins, Colorado
Section 14

SUSAN E. JOHNSON, D.V.M., M.S., Dipl. A.C.V.I.M. Associate Professor, Department of Veterinary Clinical Sciences, The Ohio State University; Internist, Veterinary Teaching Hospital, The Ohio State University, Columbus, Ohio
Section 8

SHIRLEY D. JOHNSTON, D.V.M., PH.D., Dipl. A.C.T. Associate Dean for Academic Affairs, University of Minnesota College of Veterinary Medicine, St. Paul, Minnesota
Section 11

BRENT D. JONES, D.V.M. Associate Professor, College of Veterinary Medicine, University of Missouri; Staff Gastroenterologist, Veterinary Teaching Hospital, University of Missouri, Columbia, Missouri
Section 8

RANDALL E. JUNGE, M.S., D.V.M. Associate Veterinarian, St. Louis Zoological Park, St. Louis; Adjunct Associate Professor, Department of Medicine and Surgery, University of Missouri College of Veterinary Medicine, Columbia, Missouri
Section 14

KATHLEEN M. KALAHER, D.V.M. Veterinary Practitioner, Baltimore, Maryland
Section 7

ANDREW J. KALLET, D.V.M., Dipl. A.C.V.I.M. Staff Internist, Madera Pet Hospital, Corte Madera, California
Section 5

RENEE L. KASWAN, D.V.M., M.S., Dipl. A.C.V.O. Associate Professor and Head of Ophthalmology, College of Veterinary Medicine, University of Georgia; Head of Ophthalmology, University of Georgia Veterinary Teaching Hospital, Athens, Georgia
Section 13

BRUCE W. KEENE, D.V.M., M.S., Dipl. A.C.V.I.M. (Cardiology). Associate Professor, North Carolina State University, School of Veterinary Medicine; Attending Cardiologist, Vet-

erinary Teaching Hospital, North Carolina State University, Raleigh, North Carolina
Section 9

E. T. KELLER, D.V.M., M.P.V.M. Resident in Oncology, Department of Medical Sciences, School of Veterinary Medicine, University of Wisconsin, Madison, Wisconsin
Section 6

ROBERT J. KEMPPAINEN, D.V.M., PH.D. Associate Professor and Director, Endocrine Diagnostic Laboratory, Auburn University College of Veterinary Medicine, Auburn, Alabama
Section 5

THOMAS J. KERN, D.V.M., Dipl. A.C.V.O. Associate Professor of Ophthalmology, New York State College of Veterinary Medicine, Cornell University; Veterinary Medical Teaching Hospital, Cornell University, Ithaca, New York
Section 13

PETER P. KINTZER, D.V.M., Dipl. A.C.V.I.M. Assistant to Director and Staff Veterinarian, Department of Laboratory Animal Medicine; Clinical Assistant Professor, Department of Medicine, Tufts University School of Veterinary Medicine, North Grafton, Massachusetts
Section 5

REBECCA KIRBY, D.V.M. Dipl. A.C.V.I.M., A.C.V.E.C.C. Director of Education, Veterinary Institute of Trauma, Emergency, and Critical Care, Milwaukee, Wisconsin
Section 2

SUSAN E. KIRSCHNER, D.V.M., Dipl. A.C.V.O. Staff Ophthalmologist, The Animal Medical Center, New York, New York
Section 13

BARBARA E. KITCHELL, D.V.M., Dipl. A.C.V.I.M. (Internal Medicine and Oncology). Postdoctoral Fellow, Department of Pathology, Stanford University School of Medicine, Stanford; Staff Oncologist, Special Veterinary Services, Berkeley Dog and Cat Hospital, Berkeley, California
Section 1

MARK D. KITTLESON, D.V.M., PH.D., Dipl. A.C.V.I.M. (Cardiology). Associate Professor, Department of Medicine, School of Veterinary Medicine, University of California, Davis, California
Section 9

GEORGE V. KOLLIAS, D.V.M., PH.D., Dipl. A.C.Z.M. Jay Hyman Professor of Wildlife Medicine, College of Veterinary Medicine, Cornell University, Ithaca, New York; Formerly Chief, Wildlife and Zoological Medicine, College of Veterinary Medicine, University of Florida, Gainesville, Florida
Section 14

ANITA M. KORE, D.V.M. Teaching Associate, Department of Veterinary Biosciences, College of Veterinary Medicine, University of Illinois, Urbana, Illinois
Section 3

JOE N. KORNEGAY, D.V.M., PH.D., Dipl. A.C.V.I.M. (Neurology). Professor of Neurology, Department of Companion Animal and Special Species Medicine, North Carolina State University College of Veterinary Medicine; Neurologist, Veterinary Teaching Hospital, North Carolina State University, Raleigh, North Carolina
Section 12

JAN P. KOVACIC, D.V.M. Assistant Professor, Veterinary Institute of Trauma, Emergency, and Critical Care; Director of Clinics, Animal Emergency Center, Milwaukee, Wisconsin
Section 2

SUSAN A. KRAEGEL, D.V.M., Dipl. A.C.V.I.M. Postdoctoral Fellow, Department of Surgery, School of Veterinary Medicine, University of California, Davis, California
Section 6

STEVEN KRAKOWKA, D.V.M., PH.D., Dipl. A.C.V.P. Professor, Department of Veterinary Pathobiology, College of Veterinary Medicine, The Ohio State University, Columbus, Ohio
Section 6

KARL H. KRAUS, D.V.M., M.S., Dipl. A.C.V.S., A.B.V.P. Assistant Professor, Tufts University School of Veterinary Medicine; Orthopedic Surgeon, Foster Hospital for Small Animals, North Grafton, Massachusetts
Section 2

ROBERT A. KROLL, D.V.M. Neurology Resident, Department of Veterinary Medicine and Surgery, College of Veterinary Medicine, University of Missouri; Veterinary Teaching Hospital, Columbia, Missouri
Section 12

STEPHEN A. KRUTH, D.V.M., Dipl. A.C.V.I.M. Associate Professor, Department of Clinical Studies, Ontario Veterinary College, University of Guelph; Internist, Veterinary Teaching Hospital, Ontario Veterinary College, University of Guelph, Guelph, Ontario
Section 4

CYNTHIA M. KUEHLER, M.S. Zoologist, Zoological Society of San Diego, San Diego, California
Section 14

KENNETH W. KWOCHKA, D.V.M., Dipl. A.C.V.D. Associate Professor of Dermatology, Department of Veterinary Clinical Sciences, College of Veterinary Medicine, The Ohio State University; Chief of Dermatology Service, Veterinary Teaching Hospital, The Ohio State University, Columbus, Ohio
Section 7

MARY ANNA LABATO, D.V.M. Clinical Assistant Professor, Department of Medicine, Tufts University School of Veterinary Medicine; Staff Clinician, Foster Hospital for Small Animals, Tufts University School of Veterinary Medicine, North Grafton, Massachusetts
Section 2

INDIA F. LANE, D.V.M. Resident in Small Animal Medicine, Department of Clinical Sciences, College of Veterinary Medicine and Biomedical Sciences, Colorado State University, Fort Collins, Colorado
Section 10

MICHAEL R. LAPPIN, D.V.M., Dipl. A.C.V.I.M. Assistant Professor, Department of Clinical Sciences, College of Veterinary Medicine and Biomedical Sciences, Colorado State University, Fort Collins, Colorado
Sections 4 and 10

GEORGE E. LEES, D.V.M., M.S., Dipl. A.C.V.I.M. Professor of Medicine, Department of Small Animal Medicine and Surgery, College of Veterinary Medicine, Texas A&M University; Small Animal Clinic, Texas Veterinary Medical Center, College of Veterinary Medicine, Texas A&M University, College Station, Texas
Section 10

MICHAEL S. LEIB, D.V.M., M.S., Dipl. A.C.V.I.M Associate Professor of Medicine, Virginia-Maryland Regional College of Veterinary Medicine, Virginia Polytechnic Institute

and State University; Staff Internist, Veterinary Teaching Hospital, Virginia-Maryland Regional College of Veterinary Medicine, Virginia Polytechnic Institute and State University, Blacksburg, Virginia
Section 8

CYNTHIA R. LEVEILLE, D.V.M. Postdoctoral Fellow, Department of Physiology, Tufts Medical School; Lecturer, School of Veterinary Medicine, Tufts University, North Grafton, Massachusetts
Section 2

DENISE M. LINDLEY, D.V.M., M.S., Dipl. A.C.V.O. Assistant Professor and Head, Comparative Ophthalmology, School of Veterinary Medicine, Purdue University, West Lafayette, Indiana; Staff Ophthalmologist, Animal Eye Consultants, Crestwood, Illinois
Section 13

MERYL P. LITTMAN, V.M.D., Dipl. A.C.V.I.M. Associate Professor of Medicine, University of Pennsylvania School of Veterinary Medicine, Philadelphia, Pennsylvania
Section 10

SI-KWANG LIU, D.V.M., PH.D. Senior Staff, The Animal Medical Center, New York, N.Y.; Visiting Professor of Cardiovascular Pathology, National Taiwan University, Taipei, Taiwan; Consultant, Pig Research Institute, Taiwan, Republic of China; Adjunct Professor, Cornell University Medical College; Scientific Fellow, New York Zoological Society, New York, New York
Section 9

DAVID H. LLOYD, B.Vet.Med., PH.D., F.R.C.V.S. Senior Lecturer in Medicine (Dermatology), Royal Veterinary College (University of London), North Mymms, Hertfordshire, United Kingdom
Section 7

W. EUGENE LLOYD, D.V.M., PH.D., Dipl. A.B.V.T. Shenandoah, Iowa
Section 3

MICHAEL R. LOOMIS, D.V.M., Dipl. A.C.Z.M. Director of Veterinary Services, North Carolina Zoological Park, Asheville, North Carolina
Section 14

JODY P. LULICH, D.V.M., PH.D., Dipl. A.C.V.I.M. Assistant Professor, Department of

Small Animal Clinical Sciences, College of Veterinary Medicine, University of Minnesota, St. Paul, Minnesota
Sections 1 and 10

JOHN H. LUMSDEN, D.V.M., M.SC., Dipl. A.C.V.P. Professor of Pathology, Ontario Veterinary College, University of Guelph, Guelph, Ontario
Appendices

RANDY C. LYNN, D.V.M. Agricultural Division, CIBA-GEIGY Corporation, Greensboro, North Carolina
Section 5

JOHN M. MACDONALD, D.V.M., Dipl. A.C.V.D. Associate Professor, Dermatology, College of Veterinary Medicine, Auburn University, Auburn, Alabama
Section 7

E. GREGORY MACEWEN, V.M.D., Dipl. A.C.V.I.M. (Oncology/Medicine). Professor of Medicine/Oncology, Department of Medical Science; Associate Dean for Clinical Affairs, School of Veterinary Medicine, University of Wisconsin; Affiliate Professor, Department of Veterinary Science, College of Agriculture and Life Sciences; Associate Member, Wisconsin Clinical Cancer Center; Department of Human Oncology, School of Medicine; Affiliate, Wisconsin Regional Primate Center; Affiliate, Institute on Aging; Affiliate, Department of Nutritional Sciences, University of Wisconsin, Madison, Wisconsin
Sections 5 and 6

BRUCE R. MADEWELL, V.M.D., Dipl. A.C.V.I.M. (Internal Medicine and Oncology). Professor, Department of Veterinary Surgery, University of California—Davis; Chief, Oncology Service, Veterinary Medical Teaching Hospital, University of California, Davis, California
Section 6

KENNETH V. MASON, M.V. SC. Director, Albert Animal Hospital, Springwood, Queensland, Australia
Section 7

LAWRENCE E. MATHES, PH.D. Associate Professor, The Ohio State University, Columbus, Ohio
Section 6

GUY NEAL MAULDIN, D.V.M., Dipl. A.C.V.I.M. (Internal Medicine and Oncology). Staff Oncologist, Donaldson-Atwood Cancer Clinic, The Animal Medical Center; Clinical Fellow, Memorial Sloan-Kettering Cancer Center; Research Fellow, Sloan-Kettering Institute, New York, New York
Section 5

DAVID M. McCLUGGAGE, D.V.M. Associate Veterinarian, All Pets Clinic and the Bird Hospital, Boulder, Colorado
Section 14

LEA B. McGOVERN, V.M.D. Center for Veterinary Medicine, U.S. Food and Drug Administration, Rockville, Maryland
Section 1

BRENDAN C. McKIERNAN, D.V.M., Dipl. A.C.V.I.M. Associate Professor of Medicine, Veterinary Medicine Teaching Hospital, College of Veterinary Medicine, University of Illinois, Urbana, Illinois
Section 9

LINDA MEDLEAU, D.V.M., M.S., Dipl. A.C.V.D. Associate Professor of Dermatology, Department of Small Animal Medicine, College of Veterinary Medicine, University of Georgia; Staff Dermatologist, University of Georgia Small Animal Teaching Hospital, Athens, Georgia; Dermatologist, South Carolina Dermatology Referral Service, Columbia, South Carolina
Section 7

SUSAN M. MERIC, D.V.M., Dipl. A.C.V.I.M. (Internal Medicine). Professor of Small Animal Medicine, Western College of Veterinary Medicine, University of Saskatchewan; Internist, Veterinary Teaching Hospital, Western College of Veterinary Medicine, University of Saskatchewan, Saskatoon, Saskatchewan
Section 12

VICKI N. MEYERS-WALLEN, V.M.D., PH.D., Dipl. A.C.T. Assistant Professor of Theriogenology, New York State College of Veterinary Medicine, Cornell University; Chief of Service, Small Animal Theriogenology, New York State College of Veterinary Medicine, Cornell University, Ithaca, New York
Section 11

MATTHEW W. MILLER, D.V.M. Dipl. A.C.V.I.M. (Cardiology). Assistant Professor, Texas A&M University; Staff Cardiologist, Texas Veterinary Medical Center, College of Veterinary Medicine, Texas A&M University, College Station, Texas
Section 9

MICHAEL S. MILLER, M.S., V.M.D., Dipl. A.B.V.P. Vice President, Cardiopet, Inc., Floral Park, New York; Consultant in Cardiology, A&A Veterinary Hospital, Franklin Square, New York
Section 9

R. ERIC MILLER, D.V.M., Dipl. A.C.Z.M. Adjunct Assistant Professor of Veterinary Medicine and Surgery, University of Missouri, Columbia; Associate Veterinarian, St. Louis Zoological Park, St. Louis, Missouri
Section 14 and Appendices

WILLIAM H. MILLER, JR., V.M.D., Dipl. A.C.V.D. Associate Professor of Medicine, New York State College of Veterinary Medicine, Cornell University, Ithaca, New York
Section 7

RUSSELL W. MITTEN, B.V.SC., D.V.R. Senior Lecturer in Small Animal Medicine, University of Melbourne School of Veterinary Science; Consultant, Small Animal Medicine, University of Melbourne Veterinary Clinic and Hospital, Melbourne, Australia
Section 9

LARS MOE, D.V.M., D.SC. Associate Professor, Department of Small Animal Clinical Sciences, Norwegian College of Veterinary Medicine, Oslo, Norway
Section 12

N. SYDNEY MOISE, D.V.M., M.S., Dipl. A.C.V.I.M. (Internal Medicine and Cardiology). Associate Professor of Medicine, New York State College of Veterinary Medicine, Cornell University, Ithaca, New York
Section 9

PAULA F. MOON, D.V.M. Research Fellow, Department of Anesthesiology, The University of Texas Medical Branch at Galveston, Galveston, Texas
Section 2

CARMEL T. MOONEY, M.V.B., M.Phil., M.R.C.V.S. Research Student, Department of Veterinary Medicine, University of Glasgow Veterinary School, Glasgow, Scotland
Section 5

ANTONY S. MOORE, B.V.Sc., M.V.Sc. Assistant Professor of Medicine, Tufts University School of Veterinary Medicine, North Grafton, Massachusetts
Section 6

KAREN A. MORIELLO, D.V.M., Dipl. A.C.V.D. Clinical Associate Professor of Dermatology, School of Veterinary Medicine, University of Wisconsin, Madison, Wisconsin
Section 7

WALLACE B. MORRISON, D.V.M., M.S., Dipl. A.C.V.I.M. (Internal Medicine). Associate Professor, Chief of Clinical Oncology, School of Veterinary Medicine, Purdue University; Veterinary Teaching Hospital, Purdue University, West Lafayette, Indiana
Section 9

CHRISTOPHER J. MURPHY, D.V.M., PH.D., Dipl. A.C.V.O. Assistant Professor, School of Veterinary Medicine, University of Wisconsin, Madison, Wisconsin
Section 13

ROBERT J. MURTAUGH, D.V.M., M.S., Dipl. A.C.V.I.M., A.C.V.E.C.C. Associate Professor, Department of Medicine, Tufts University School of Veterinary Medicine, North Grafton, Massachusetts
Section 2

LARRY A. NAGODE, D.V.M., PH.D. Associate Professor, Department of Veterinary Pathobiology, College of Veterinary Medicine, The Ohio State University; Consultant, Veterinary Teaching Hospital, The Ohio State University, Columbus, Ohio
Section 10

RICHARD W. NELSON, D.V.M., Dipl. A.C.V.I.M. Assistant Professor, Department of Medicine, School of Veterinary Medicine, University of California, Davis, California
Section 5

C. E. RHETT NICHOLS, D.V.M., Dipl. A.C.V.I.M. Associate Professor, College of Veterinary Medicine, Mississippi State University; Service Chief, Small Animal Medicine, Consultant (Endocrine), Veterinary Labs of America, Mississippi State, Mississippi
Section 5

EDWARD J. NOGA, M.S., D.V.M. Associate Professor of Aquatic Medicine, North Carolina State University College of Veterinary Medicine; Aquatic Animal Veterinarian, North Carolina State University Veterinary Teaching Hospital, Raleigh, North Carolina
Section 14

JAMES O. NOXON, D.V.M., Dipl. A.C.V.I.M. (Internal Medicine). Associate Professor, College of Veterinary Medicine, Iowa State University, Ames, Iowa
Section 7

JOYCE E. OBRADOVICH, D.V.M. Michigan Veterinary Specialists, Broomfield Hills, Michigan
Section 6

DENNIS P. O'BRIEN, D.V.M., PH.D., Dipl. A.C.V.I.M. (Neurology). Associate Professor of Neurology, Department of Veterinary Medicine and Surgery, College of Veterinary Medicine, University of Missouri; Staff Neurologist, Veterinary Teaching Hospital, University of Missouri, Columbia, Missouri
Section 12

TIMOTHY D. O'BRIEN, D.V.M., PH.D., Dipl. A.C.V.P. Associate Professor of Veterinary Pathology, College of Veterinary Medicine, University of Minnesota; Hospital Pathology Service, Lewis Hospital for Companion Animals, College of Veterinary Medicine, University of Minnesota, St. Paul, Minnesota
Section 1

LANELL OGDEN, D.V.M., Dipl. A.B.V.T. Assistant Professor, Toxicology Diagnostic Laboratory, Tuskegee University School of Veterinary Medicine, Tuskegee; Auburn University, College of Veterinary Medicine, Auburn, Alabama
Section 3

GREGORY K. OGILVIE, D.V.M., Dipl. A.C.V.I.M. (Internal Medicine and Oncology). Associate Professor of Oncology, Comparative Oncology Unit, Department of Clinical Sciences, College of Veterinary Medicine and Biomedical Sciences, Colorado State University; Medical Oncologist/Internist, Veterinary Teaching Hospital, Fort Collins, Colorado
Section 6

DEBORAH A. O'KEEFE, D.V.M., M.S., Dipl. A.C.V.I.M. (Oncology and Internal Medicine). Assistant Professor, Department of Veterinary Clinical Medicine, College of Veterinary Medicine, University of Illinois, Urbana, Illinois
Section 6

PATRICIA N. OLSON, D.V.M., Ph.D., Dipl. A.C.T. Clinical Associate Professor, College of Veterinary Medicine, University of Minnesota, St. Paul, Minnesota
Section 11

CARL A. OSBORNE, D.V.M., Ph.D., Dipl. A.C.V.I.M. Professor, Department of Small Animal Clinical Sciences, College of Veterinary Medicine, University of Minnesota, St. Paul, Minnesota
Sections 1 and 10

GARY D. OSWEILER, D.V.M., Ph.D., Dipl. A.B.V.T. Professor, Veterinary Pathology, Veterinary Diagnostic Laboratory, College of Veterinary Medicine, Iowa State University, Ames, Iowa
Section 3

CYNTHIA M. OTTO, D.V.M. Georgia Heart Association Research Fellow, Department of Small Animal Medicine, College of Veterinary Medicine, University of Georgia, Athens, Georgia
Section 2

KAREN OVERALL, V.M.D. Lecturer, Department of Clinical Studies, School of Veterinary Medicine, University of Pennsylvania; Clinician in Charge of Behavior Clinic, Veterinary Hospital, University of Pennsylvania, Philadelphia, Pennsylvania
Section 7

RODNEY L. PAGE, D.V.M., M.S., Dipl. A.C.V.I.M. (Oncology). Associate Professor of Medicine and Oncology, North Carolina State University School of Veterinary Medicine, Raleigh, North Carolina
Sections 6 and 9

LORI S. PALLEY, D.V.M. Postdoctoral Associate, Division of Comparative Medicine, Massachusetts Institute of Technology, Cambridge, Massachusetts
Section 14

DAVID PANCIERA, D.V.M., M.S., Dipl. A.C.V.I.M. (Internal Medicine). Assistant Professor of Medicine, School of Veterinary Medicine, University of Wisconsin; Assistant Professor of Medicine, University of Wisconsin Veterinary Teaching Hospital, Madison, Wisconsin
Section 9

RADA PANIĆ, D.V.M. Research Associate, New York State College of Veterinary Medicine, Cornell University, Ithaca; Veterinary Dermatology Consulting Service, New York, New York
Section 7

MARK G. PAPICH, D.V.M., M.S., Dipl. A.C.V.C.P. Departments of Veterinary Physiological Sciences and Veterinary Internal Medicine, Western College of Veterinary Medicine; Clinical Pharmacologist, Veterinary Teaching Hospital, Western College of Veterinary Medicine, Saskatoon, Saskatchewan
Appendices

MANON PARADIS, D.M.V., M.V.Sc., Dipl. A.C.V.D. Associate Professor of Medicine, Faculté de Médecine Vétérinaire, Université de Montréal, St. Hyacinthe, Québec
Section 7

MARK E. PETERSON, D.V.M., Dipl. A.C.V.I.M. Head, Division of Endocrinology, Department of Medicine, The Animal Medical Center, New York, New York
Section 5

TOM R. PHILLIPS, D.V.M., Ph.D. Assistant Member, The Scripps Research Institute, La Jolla, California
Section 4

PAUL DAVID PION, D.V.M., Dipl. A.C.V.I.M. (Cardiology). Postgraduate Researcher, University of California, Davis, California
Section 9

MICHAEL PODELL, M.S., D.V.M. Resident in Neurology, Department of Veterinary Clinical Sciences, College of Veterinary Medicine, The Ohio State University; Clinical Instructor, The Ohio State University Veterinary Hospital, Columbus, Ohio
Section 10

DAVID J. POLZIN, D.V.M., Ph.D., Dipl. A.C.V.I.M. Associate Professor, Internal Medicine, University of Minnesota, College of Veterinary Medicine, St. Paul, Minnesota
Sections 1 and 10

ERIC R. POPE, D.V.M., M.S., Dipl. A.C.V.S. Assistant Professor of Surgery, Department of Veterinary Medicine and Surgery, College of Veterinary Medicine, University of Missouri;

Veterinary Teaching Hospital, University of Missouri, Columbia, Missouri
Section 1

ROBERT H. POPPENGA, D.V.M., PH.D., Dipl. A.B.V.T. Assistant Professor of Veterinary Clinical Toxicology, Animal Health Diagnostic Laboratory and Department of Pathology, Michigan State University College of Veterinary Medicine, East Lansing, Michigan
Section 3

DEBORAH M. PRESCOTT, D.V.M., PH.D. Associate, Department of Radiation Oncology, Duke University Medical Center, Durham, North Carolina
Section 6

B. J. PURSWELL, D.V.M., PH.D., Dipl. A.C.T. Associate Professor, Virginia-Maryland Regional College of Veterinary Medicine, Virginia; Polytechnic Institute and State University, Blacksburg, Virginia
Section 11

KATHERINE QUESENBERRY, D.V.M. Service Head, Exotic Pet Service, Animal Medical Center, New York, New York
Section 14

JOHN F. RANDOLPH, D.V.M., Dipl. A.C.V.I.M. Associate Professor, Department of Clinical Sciences, New York State College of Veterinary Medicine, Cornell University; Small Animal Internist, Veterinary Teaching Hospital, Cornell University, Ithaca, New York
Section 5

PATRICK T. REDIG, D.V.M., PH.D. Associate Professor, Department of Small Animal Clinical Sciences, College of Veterinary Medicine, University of Minnesota; Director, The Raptor Center, St. Paul, Minnesota
Section 14

CRAIG R. REINEMEYER, D.V.M., PH.D. Associate Professor, College of Veterinary Medicine, University of Tennessee, Knoxville, Tennesee
Section 8

ROBERTA L. RELFORD, D.V.M., M.S. Veterinary Clinical Associate, Department of Small Animal Medicine and Surgery, College of Veterinary Medicine, Texas A&M University, College Station, Texas
Section 10

VIRGINIA T. RENTKO, V.M.D. Internal Medicine Resident, Tufts University, School of Veterinary Medicine; Staff, Foster Hospital for Small Animals, Tufts University, School of Veterinary Medicine, North Grafton, Massachusetts
Sections 2 and 4

KEITH P. RICHTER, D.V.M., Dipl. A.C.V.I.M. Internal Medicine Staff, Veterinary Specialty Hospital of San Diego, Rancho Santa Fe, California
Section 5

RONALD C. RIIS, M.T., D.V.M., M.S., Dipl. A.C.V.O. Associate Professor, New York State College of Veterinary Medicine, Cornell University, Ithaca, New York
Section 13

AD RIJNBERK, D.V.M., PH.D. Professor of Internal Medicine, Department of Clinical Sciences of Companion Animals, Faculty of Veterinary Medicine, University of Utrecht, Utrecht, The Netherlands
Section 5

KENITA S. ROGERS, D.V.M., M.S., Dipl. A.C.V.I.M. (Internal Medicine and Oncology). Assistant Professor of Oncology and Internal Medicine, Department of Small Animal Medicine and Surgery, College of Veterinary Medicine, Texas A&M University; Internist, Texas Veterinary Medical Center, Texas A&M University, College Station, Texas
Section 10

JENNIFER L. ROJKO, D.V.M., PH.D., Dipl. A.C.V.P. Associate Professor, College of Veterinary Medicine, The Ohio State University; Pathologist, The Ohio State University, Columbus, Ohio
Section 6

WAYNE S. ROSENKRANTZ, D.V.M., Dipl. A.C.V.D. Assistant Clinical Instructor for Summer Clinics, University of California, Davis, California
Section 7

LINDA A. ROSS, D.V.M., Dipl. A.C.V.I.M. Associate Professor, Department of Medicine, Tufts University, School of Veterinary Medicine; Chief of Staff, Tufts University, Foster Hospital for Small Animals, North Grafton, Massachusetts
Sections 4 and 5

EDMUND J. ROSSER, JR., D.V.M., Dipl. A.C.V.D. Associate Professor of Dermatology, Department of Small Animal Clinical Sciences, Veterinary Clinical Center, Michigan State University, East Lansing, Michigan
Section 7

PHILIP ROUDEBUSH, D.V.M., Dipl. A.C.V.I.M. Mark Morris Associates, Topeka, Kansas
Section 4

WILLIAM W. RUEHL, V.M.D., PH.D., Dipl. A.C.V.P. (Clinical Pathology). Assistant Professor, Department of Pathology, School of Medicine, Stanford University; Laboratory Director, Division of Laboratory Animal Medicine, School of Medicine, Stanford University, Stanford, California
Section 1

JOHN E. RUSH, D.V.M., M.S., Dipl. A.C.V.I.M. (Cardiology). Assistant Professor, Tufts University, School of Veterinary Medicine; Head Cardiologist and Co-Director of the Intensive Care Unit/Emergency Services, Foster Hospital for Small Animals, Tufts University, School of Veterinary Medicine, North Grafton, Massachusetts
Section 9

DAVID RUSLANDER, D.V.M. Resident, Small Animal Medicine, Tufts University, School of Veterinary Medicine, North Grayton, Massachusetts
Section 2

WILLIAM D. SAXON, D.V.M. Emergency/Critical Care Staff Member, Animal Care Center of Sonoma County, Rohnert Park, California
Section 2

MICHAEL SCHAER, D.V.M., Dipl. A.C.V.I.M. (Internal Medicine), A.C.V.E.C.C. Professor and Associate Chairman, College of Veterinary Medicine, University of Florida, Gainesville, Florida
Section 5

PAUL H. SCHERLIE, JR., D.V.M. Staff Ophthalmologist, Angell Memorial Animal Hospital, Boston, Massachusetts
Section 13

RONALD D. SCHULTZ, PH.D. Professor and Chairman, Department of Pathobiological Sciences, School of Veterinary Medicine, University of Wisconsin, Madison, Wisconsin
Section 4

DOROTHEA SCHWARTZ-PORSCHE, DR. Med. Vet. Professor of Small Animal Medicine, Free University of Berlin; Small Animal Clinic, Faculty of Veterinary Medicine, Free University of Berlin, Berlin, Germany
Section 12

DANNY W. SCOTT, D.V.M., Dipl. A.C.V.D. Professor of Medicine, New York State College of Veterinary Medicine, Cornell University, Ithaca, New York
Section 7

RANCE SELLON, D.V.M., Dipl. A.C.V.I.M. (Internal Medicine). Graduate Research Assistant, North Carolina State University; Resident, Internal Medicine, Veterinary Teaching Hospital, North Carolina State University, Raleigh, North Carolina
Section 4

DAVID F. SENIOR, B.V.Sc., Dipl. A.C.V.I.M. Associate Professor, Department of Small Animal Clinical Sciences, College of Veterinary Medicine, University of Florida; Chief, Small Animal Medicine, Veterinary Medical Teaching Hospital, University of Florida, Gainesville, Florida
Section 10

KEVIN SHANLEY, D.V.M., Dipl. A.C.V.D. Assistant Professor of Dermatology, School of Veterinary Medicine, University of Pennsylvania, Philadelphia, Pennsylvania
Section 7

G. DIANE SHELTON, D.V.M., PH.D., Dipl. A.C.V.I.M. Associate Clinical Professor, Department of Pathology, University of California, San Diego, School of Medicine, La Jolla, California
Sections 8 and 12

ROBERT G. SHERDING, D.V.M., Dipl. A.C.V.I.M. Professor and Head of Small Animal Medicine, Department of Veterinary Clinical Sciences, College of Veterinary Medicine, The Ohio State University, Columbus, Ohio
Section 8

DAVID SISSON, D.V.M., Dipl. A.C.V.I.M. (Cardiology). Associate Professor, College of Veterinary Medicine, University of Illinois; Director, Cardiology Service, Veterinary Medical Teaching Hospital, University of Illinois, Urbana, Illinois
Section 9

STEPHANIE L. SMEDES, D.V.M., Dipl. A.C.V.O. Ontario Veterinary College, University of Guelph, Guelph, Ontario
Section 13

CHARLES L. SMITH, M.D. Assistant Professor of Medicine, University of Minnesota Medical School at Hennepin County Medical Center; Staff Nephrologist, Hennepin County Medical Center, Minneapolis, Minnesota
Section 10

PATTI S. SNYDER, D.V.M., M.S., Dipl. A.C.V.I.M. (Internal Medicine). Assistant Professor, Internal Medicine/Cardiology, School of Veterinary Medicine, University of Wisconsin, Madison, Wisconsin
Section 9

D. C. SORJONEN, D.V.M., M.S., Dipl. A.C.V.I.M. (Neurology). Associate Professor, Neurology and Neurosurgery, College of Veterinary Medicine, Auburn University, Auburn, Alabama
Section 12

GARY L. STAMP, D.V.M., M.S., Dipl. A.B.V.P., A.C.V.E.C.C. Chief, Veterinary Medicine and Professional Programs Division, Headquarters U.S. Army Health Services Command, Fort Sam Houston, Texas
Section 2

ROBERT J. STARKEY, D.V.M. Med Vet—Specialty Practice, Columbus, Ohio
Section 10

JANE STEWART, B.V.M.S. Research Assistant, Department of Veterinary Surgery, University of Glasgow, Glasgow, Scotland
Section 6

ELIZABETH A. STONE, D.V.M., M.S., Dipl. A.C.V.S. Professor, College of Veterinary Medicine, North Carolina State University, Raleigh, North Carolina
Section 10

MICHAEL S. STONE, D.V.M. Staff Clinician, Department of Clinical Studies, Ontario Veterinary College, Guelph, Ontario
Section 6

TODD R. TAMS, D.V.M., Dipl. A.C.V.I.M. Executive Director and Staff Internist, West Los Angeles Veterinary Medical Group, West Los Angeles, California
Section 8

KEITH L. THODAY, B.Vet.Med., PH.D., D.V.D., M.R.C.V.S. Senior Lecturer in Veterinary Medicine, Department of Veterinary Clinical Studies, Royal (Dick) School of Veterinary Studies, University of Edinburgh, Edinburgh, Scotland
Section 5

WILLIAM P. THOMAS, D.V.M., Dipl. A.C.V.I.M. (Cardiology). Associate Professor, Department of Veterinary Medicine, School of Veterinary Medicine, University of California—Davis; Chief, Cardiology Service, Veterinary Medical Teaching Hospital, University of California, Davis, California
Section 9

DONALD E. THRALL, D.V.M., PH.D., Dipl. A.C.V.R. Professor of Radiology, College of Veterinary Medicine, North Carolina State University, Raleigh, North Carolina
Section 6

MARY ANNA THRALL, D.V.M., M.S., Dipl. A.C.V.P. Associate Professor, College of Veterinary Medicine and Biomedical Sciences, Colorado State University; Clinical Pathologist, Colorado State University, Veterinary Teaching Hospital, Fort Collins, Colorado
Section 6

LARRY P. TILLEY, D.V.M., Dipl. A.C.V.I.M. President, Cardiopet, Inc., New York, New York
Section 9

MARY B. TOMPKINS, D.V.M., PH.D. Associate Professor of Immunology, Department of Microbiology, Pathology and Parasitology, College of Veterinary Medicine, North Carolina State University, Raleigh, North Carolina
Section 6

WAYNE A. F. TOMPKINS, PH.D. Professor of Immunology, Department of Microbiology, Pathology, and Parasitology, College of Veterinary Medicine, North Carolina State University, Raleigh, North Carolina
Section 6

HAROLD L. TRAMMEL, Pharm.D. Operations Director, National Animal Poison Control Center, College of Veterinary Medicine, University of Illinois, Urbana, Illinois
Section 3

DAVID C. TWEDT, D.V.M., Dipl. A.C.V.I.M. Professor, Department of Clinical Sciences, College of Veterinary Medicine and Biomedical Sciences, Colorado State University; Small Animal Section Chief, Veterinary Teaching Hospital, Colorado State University, Fort Collins, Colorado
Section 8

LISA K. UNGER, C.V.T. Senior Veterinary Technician, Department of Small Animal Clinical Sciences, College of Veterinary Medicine, University of Minnesota, St. Paul, Minnesota
Section 10

SHELLY L. VADEN, D.V.M., Dipl. A.C.V.I.M. Graduate Research Assistant, Department of Anatomy, Physiologic Sciences and Radiology, College of Veterinary Medicine, North Carolina State University, Raleigh, North Carolina
Section 10

DAVID M. VAIL, D.V.M., M.S., Dipl. A.C.V.I.M. (Oncology). Assistant Professor, Department of Medical Sciences, School of Veterinary Medicine, University of Wisconsin, Madison, Wisconsin
Section 6

MARC VANDEVELDE, D.M.V. Professor and Chairman, Institute of Animal Neurology, School of Veterinary Medicine, University of Bern, Bern, Switzerland
Section 12

DEBORAH R. VAN PELT, D.V.M., M.S. Instructor, Emergency Medicine and Critical Care, College of Veterinary Medicine and Biomedical Sciences, Colorado State University; Instructor, Emergency Medicine and Critical Care, Colorado State University Veterinary Teaching Hospital, Fort Collins, Colorado
Section 2

WILLIAM VERNAU, B.Sc., B.V.M.S., D.V.Sc. Dipl. A.C.V.P. Veterinary Pathology Services, Sydney, Australia
Appendices

MICHAEL A. WALKER, D.V.M., Dipl. A.C.V.R. Professor of Radiology, Department of Large Animal Medicine and Surgery, College of Veterinary Medicine, Texas A&M University; Chief of Radiology, Texas Veterinary Medical Center, Texas A&M University, College Station, Texas
Section 10

MELISSA S. WALLACE, D.V.M. Associate Staff Veterinarian, Head of Nephrology, Endocrinology and Reproduction Service, Department of Medicine, The Animal Medical Center, New York, New York
Section 11

WENDY A. WARE, D.V.M., M.S., Dipl. A.C.V.I.M. (Cardiology). Associate Professor, Department of Veterinary Clinical Sciences, College of Veterinary Medicine, Iowa State University; Staff Cardiologist, Veterinary Teaching Hospital, Iowa State University, Ames, Iowa
Section 9

DOUGLAS J. WEISS, D.V.M., Ph.D., Dipl. A.C.V.P. Associate Professor, University of Minnesota College of Veterinary Medicine; Division Head, Clinical Laboratories, Veterinary Teaching Hospital, University of Minnesota, St. Paul, Minnesota
Section 6

STEVEN L. WHEELER, D.V.M., M.S., Dipl. A.C.V.I.M. Assistant Professor, Department of Clinical Sciences, College of Veterinary Medicine and Biomedical Sciences, Colorado State University; Assistant Head, Critical Care Unit, Veterinary Teaching Hospital, Colorado State University, Fort Collins, Colorado
Section 5

STEPHEN D. WHITE, D.V.M., Dipl. A.C.V.D. Associate Professor, College of Veterinary Medicine and Biomedical Sciences, Colorado State University; Dermatologist, Veterinary Teaching Hospital, Colorado State University, Fort Collins, Colorado
Section 7

DAVID A. WILKIE, D.V.M., M.S., Dipl. A.C.V.O. Assistant Professor, Department of Veterinary Clinical Sciences, College of Veterinary Medicine, The Ohio State University, Columbus, Ohio
Section 13

M. D. WILLARD, D.V.M., M.S., Dipl. A.C.V.I.M. Professor, Small Animal Medicine and Surgery, College of Veterinary Medicine, Texas A&M University; Clinican, Texas Veterinary Medical Center, Texas A&M University, College Station, Texas
Section 8

TON WILLEMSE, D.V.M., Ph.D., Dipl. Derm. R.N.V.A. Associate Professor of Veterinary Dermatology, University of Utrecht, Utrecht, The Netherlands
Section 7

DAVID A. WILLIAMS, Vet. M.B., Ph.D., M.R.C.V.S., Dipl. A.C.V.I.M. Associate Professor, Department of Clinical Studies, Kansas State University; Section Head, Small Animal Medicine, Veterinary Medical Teaching Hospital, College of Veterinary Medicine, Kansas State University, Manhattan, Kansas
Section 8

WAYNE E. WINGFIELD, M.S., D.V.M., Dipl. A.C.V.S., A.C.V.E.C.C. Professor, Department of Clinical Sciences, College of Veterinary Medicine and Biomedical Sciences, Colorado State University; Chief, Emergency Medicine/Critical Care, Veterinary Teaching Hospital, College of Veterinary Medicine and Biomedical Sciences, Colorado State University, Fort Collins, Colorado
Section 2

ALICE M. WOLF, D.V.M., Dipl. A.C.V.I.M. Associate Professor, Department of Small Animal Medicine and Surgery, College of Veteri-

nary Medicine, Texas A&M University; Veterinary Teaching Hospital, Texas A&M University, College Station, Texas
Sections 4, 8, and 11

DIANE W. YOUNG, Ph.D. Senior Research Fellow, Department of Physiology and Pharmacology, Auburn University College of Veterinary Medicine, Auburn, Alabama
Section 5

NORDIN S. ZEIDNER, D.V.M., Ph.D. Research Scientist, Department of Pathology, Colorado State University, Fort Collins, Colorado
Section 4

ELISABETH ZENGER, D.V.M., M.S. Lecturer, Department of Small Animal Medicine and Surgery, College of Veterinary Medicine, Texas A&M University; Lecturer, Texas Veterinary Medical Center, Texas A&M University, College Station, Texas
Section 4

CAROLE A. ZERBE, D.V.M., Ph.D. Assistant Professor, Department of Clinical Studies, School of Veterinary Medicine, University of Pennsylvania, Philadelphia, Pennsylvania
Section 5

PREFACE

This eleventh edition of Kirk's *Current Veterinary Therapy* is published in a time of continuing sophistication and specialization in veterinary practice. The small animal practitioner works in an information environment of increasing complexity. The veterinary student studies a multitude of animal diseases that include many recently discovered disorders. Technologic advances in medical diagnosis and treatment continue to be applied to our animal patients. Many of these advances are included in this edition of *Current Veterinary Therapy*.

This edition of *CVT*, including the appendices, is completely new. A section on critical care–emergency medicine has been added. The editors have totally updated the popular "Table of Common Drugs: Approximate Dosages" and have added columns that cross reference drugs to articles in both this and previous editions. The clinical pathology reference tables have been completely revised and extensively referenced for the reader who requires additional information. Many of the authors responded to the opportunity to annotate their references, and we hope that the reader will find this a helpful way to gain entry to the literature. As always, there are chapters that describe diagnoses and treatments ranging from the simple "Why didn't I think of that" variety to those experimental treatments that involve lasers, genetic engineering, and recent advances in biotechnology. We have expanded our authorship and received a number of excellent contributions from Europe and Australia. The expertise of these authors complements the excellence of our North American contributors. The consulting editors have constructed their sections with articles describing both readily applicable treatments and therapies so new that they are still considered experimental. A number of these newest therapeutic modalities may seem esoteric to some of us; nevertheless, medical therapy progresses, and eventually what is new and unrealistic may become accepted as a standard of care.

In keeping with our policy outlined in *Current Veterinary Therapy X*, we have made a conscious decision not to duplicate chapters if we still consider an article in a recent edition to be timely and accurate. There are two principal reasons for this decision. Veterinary medical information today is too extensive to fit into a single volume. Moreover, reprinting all chapters would cause an unnecessary expense to the reader. We believe that our readers will be best served by receiving a textbook that is updated frequently (every 3 years) and that doesn't waste page space.

Thus, not every medical problem can be discussed in each volume. This may be frustrating to the practitioner trying to discover the latest about a disorder that is not detailed in this edition. In an attempt to minimize this problem, we continue our practice of extensively cross-indexing information from this, the eleventh edition, with that in prior editions of *CVT*. If the reader first checks the index of this volume, he or she will be directed to the appropriate volume and page. What earlier editions of *Current Veterinary Therapy* could accomplish in a single edition, we hope to achieve by producing a "family" of complementary and cross-referenced volumes. In short, we want the reader to be assured that the editors and authors of *Current Veterinary Therapy* have done their best to keep the information current and available.

It is a great honor for me to be given the reins of *Current Veterinary Therapy*. I have attempted to follow the formula that Dr. Kirk initiated over 25 years ago. The most important part of his formula was the selection of outstanding authors who are actively working in an area relevant to veterinary practice. I am fortunate that so many excellent veterinarians and scientists have been willing to contribute to this book. I also have been lucky to work with an outstanding group of Consulting Editors, to whom I am most grateful for their expertise and hard work. Dr. Bob Kirk remains an active participant in the planning and editing of his textbook, and I have benefited greatly from his guidance.

Current Veterinary Therapy XI is a book for veterinary practitioners and students in veterinary medicine. I would be very grateful to receive any comments from you, our readers, including your concerns about possible errors or omissions as well as your ideas and comments. We appreciate your acceptance of this book, and Dr. Kirk and I hope that the volumes of *Current Veterinary Therapy* will continue to be a useful reference to you.

We appreciate the time and efforts of everyone who has participated in the production of this edition. The authors and section editors have made an outstanding effort to produce an informative, accurate, and useful textbook. The staff at W.B. Saunders has worked admirably to produce the best possible volume. I am particularly appreciative of Linda Mills, Veterinary Editor, Jody Murphy, our copy editor, and Bill Preston, who was production manager for this edition. I am also grateful to Franci Crowell, Lisa Kurtz, and my colleagues in the Department of Veterinary Clinical Sciences who helped me in Columbus during the planning and completion of this edition. My parents, Peter and Hazel, have always been a source of continued support, and I can never thank them enough.

JOHN D. BONAGURA, D.V.M.
Columbus, Ohio

CONTENTS

SECTION

8

GASTROINTESTINAL DISORDERS
David C. Twedt
Consulting Editor

SECTION

4

INFECTIOUS DISEASES
Edward B. Breitschwerdt
Consulting Editor

SECTION

5

ENDOCRINE AND METABOLIC DISORDERS
Mark E. Peterson
Consulting Editor

SECTION

6

HEMATOLOGY, ONCOLOGY, AND IMMUNOLOGY

Bruce R. Madewell
Consulting Editor

SECTION

7

DERMATOLOGIC DISEASES

William H. Miller, Jr.
Consulting Editor

SECTION

9

CARDIOPULMONARY DISEASES

Bruce W. Keene
Consulting Editor

SECTION

10

URINARY DISORDERS
Jeanne A. Barsanti
Consulting Editor

SECTION

11

REPRODUCTIVE DISORDERS

Vicki N. Meyers-Wallen
Consulting Editor

SECTION

12

NEUROLOGIC AND
NEUROMUSCULAR DISORDERS

Joe N. Kornegay
Consulting Editor

xl CONTENTS

NOTICE

Companion animal practice is an ever-changing field. Standard safety precautions must be followed, but as new research and clinical experience grow, changes in treatment and drug therapy become necessary or appropriate. The authors and editors of this work have carefully checked the generic and trade drug names and verified drug dosages to assure that dosage information is precise and in accord with standards accepted at the time of publication. Readers are advised, however, to check the product information currently provided by the manufacturer of each drug to be administered to be certain that changes have not been made in the recommended dose or in the contraindications for administration. This is of particular importance in regard to new or infrequently used drugs. Recommended dosages for animals are sometimes based on adjustments in the dosage that would be suitable for humans. Some of the drugs mentioned here have been given experimentally by the authors. Others have been used in dosages greater than those recommended by the manufacturer. In these kinds of cases, the authors have reported on their own considerable experience. It is the responsibility of those administering a drug, relying on their professional skill and experience, to determine the dosages, the best treatment for the patient, and whether the benefits of giving a drug justify the attendant risk. The editors cannot be responsible for misuse or misapplication of the material in this work.

THE PUBLISHER

Section

1

SPECIAL THERAPY

CARL A. OSBORNE

Consulting Editor

PROGNOSIS: GUIDELINES FOR SENTENCING PATIENTS

CARL A. OSBORNE,
and JODY P. LULICH
St. Paul, Minnesota

'Tis as dangerous to be sentenced by a physician as a judge.

Thomas Browne

DEFINITION

The word *prognosis* is derived from Greek words (*pro*, "before"; *gnosis*, "to know") and means a forecast of the probable outcome of abnormalities associated with one or more diseases. *Dorland's Medical Dictionary* defines prognosis as "a forecast as to the probable outcome of an attack of disease" or "the prospect as to recovery from a disease as indicated by the nature and symptoms of the case" (Taylor, 1988). Synonyms for the term prognosis include *prediction, foretelling,* and *forecast.* As with most aspects of patient care, prognosis requires judgment in the absence of certainty.

PROGNOSIS FROM THE CLIENT'S VIEWPOINT

From a client's point of view, the antemortem differentiation of potentially reversible from irreversible disease is usually the single most important question related to clinical assessment of disease. Clients typically ask, "Can you help, Doctor?" Our clients are concerned about the probability of recovery of their animals from disease states with or without therapy, the nature and cost of therapy, and whether recovery is likely to be partial or complete. The veterinarian's answers to these questions often profoundly influence the client's subsequent choice of alternatives. For some living beings, the prognosis is lifesaving; for others, it is a death sentence. It is therefore appropriate to ask, "How reliable are our prognoses?"

PROGNOSIS FROM THE VETERINARIAN'S VIEWPOINT

Forecasts of the outcome of problems associated with one or more diseases must, by definition, be based on recognition of the problems with the ultimate goal of obtaining a diagnosis. Although most veterinarians would agree that establishment of a specific diagnosis is an important component of patient management, the diagnosis is often a matter of opinion rather than of fact. If a specific diagnosis has been established on the basis of insufficient evidence, it may represent an overdiagnosis. In many situations, diagnosis of a clinical problem, or problems, does not represent unequivocal identification of the cause, or causes, of disease. The fact that clinical signs persist or undergo remission does not prove that our diagnosis and prognosis were correct.

Definition of the underlying cause of problems may lead to a more accurate forecast of the biologic process involved, and also to an assessment of the likelihood of various body compensatory mechanisms to overcome organ disease and organ failure. Likewise, detection of the cause or causes of disease is the only way to select specific (in contrast to supportive or symptomatic) therapy that is designed to halt progression, reverse the disease, or both (Table 1). Even when a specific diagnosis is established, however, formulation of a prognosis still requires judgment in the absence of certainty. In contrast to the situation confronting physicians, who often have large databases related to the biologic processes underlying many human illnesses, lack of information about the natural course of many diseases affecting animals forces veterinarians to rely on intuition. History confirms that prognoses guided primarily by intuition often result in erroneous conclusions. A vivid example is the former belief that canine and feline patients with renal failure characterized by a serum creatinine concentration greater than 5 mg/dl would not recover despite therapy. The needless euthanasia of countless numbers of patients resulted in a self-fulfilling prophecy. Even now, inaccurate prognoses remain a leading cause of life-threatening disease.

CONCEPTS INFLUENCING PROGNOSIS

Problem Definition

A *problem* can be defined as a situation that causes concern to the patient, to the owner, or to

Table 1. Types of Treatment

Type	Purpose	Examples
Specific	Eliminate, destroy, or modify the primary cause(s) of the disease process.	Antibiotics to eliminate bacterial infections. Antidotes to counteract toxins. Hormone replacement therapy.
Supportive	Modify or eliminate abnormalities that are secondary to primary disease.	Treatment designed to correct deficits and excesses in fluid, electrolyte, acid-base, endocrine, and nutrient balances caused by primary renal failure.
Symptomatic	Eliminate or suppress clinical signs.	Antiemetics to control vomiting. Glucocorticoids to control pruritus.

the veterinarian. In other words, a problem is anything that has required, does require, or may require health care management and that has significantly affected, or could significantly affect, a patient's well-being (Osborne, 1983). It may be (1) a historical finding; (2) a physical finding; (3) an abnormal laboratory, radiographic, or biopsy finding; (4) a syndrome; or (5) a diagnostic entity.

Problems must not be overstated through premature guessing of their cause. They should be stated at the level at which they are understood, and they should be described in such a way that their definition can be defended with reasonable certainty on the basis of current knowledge about the patient.

Depending on the knowledge, wisdom, and understanding of the diagnostician, and on the availability of medical data, the problems may be as unrefined as a clinical sign (e.g., persistent vomiting) or as refined as identification of the cause (e.g., diabetic ketoacidosis, acute nephrotoxic renal failure, or gastric foreign body).

Problems may be defined according to one of four levels of refinement (Osborne, 1983). Listed from the lowest to the highest level of refinement, problems may be defined as:

1. An unquantified clinical finding (e.g., vomiting, polydipsia, or depression). Further information is often required to verify the existence of such problems.

2. A reproducible diagnostic finding (e.g., palpable abdominal mass, proteinuria, leukocytosis, or hypercalcemia).

3. A pathophysiologic syndrome (e.g., renal failure, nephrotic syndrome, malabsorption syndrome, or congestive heart failure). Problem refinement of this degree requires integration of diagnostic information.

4. A diagnostic entity (e.g., pyelonephritis caused by staphylococci, congestive heart failure caused by *Dirofilaria immitis*, or osteogenic sarcoma of the femur with pulmonary metastases). In general, the greater the degree of problem refinement, the greater the likelihood that prognosis of the problems will be reliable.

In the process of defining problems, one must use care to avoid random mixing of observations with interpretations (Table 2). Observations and interpretations represent distinct facets of diagnosis and prognosis. Although observations are often correct, interpretations of observations are frequently erroneous. If misinterpretations are accepted as facts, the ultimate results may be misdiagnosis, misprognosis, and formulation of inappropriate or contraindicated therapy.

Reversibility

The definition of reversibility is of great clinical significance. The concept of reversibility may be applied to: (1) morphology, (2) the degree of organ dysfunction, and (3) the effect of specific, supportive, and symptomatic therapy on organ function (see Tables 1 and 2). Organ function "adequate" to sustain homeostasis is often not synonymous with "total" organ function. Even with irreversible organ lesions, signs of organ dysfunction do not develop when an adequate quantity of functional parenchyma (i.e., nephrons, hepatic lobules, and so forth) can maintain homeostasis. This concept is the basis

Table 2. Concepts That May Influence Prognosis

Observations vs. interpretations.
Possibilities vs. probabilities.
Level of problem refinement.*
Organ disease vs. organ failure.
Adequate vs. total organ function.
Age (in the context that advanced age is not synonymous with an unfavorable prognosis).
Nonprogressive disease vs. progressive, irreversible disease and dysfunction.
Clinical signs attributed directly to the underlying disease vs. clinical signs attributed to the body's compensatory responses to the disease.
Concomitant but etiologically unrelated diseases that influence body compensatory responses, selection of treatment, or both.
Short-term vs. long-term prognosis.
Specific vs. supportive or symptomatic treatment.
Disease-induced vs. treatment-induced illness.

*See text.

Table 3. *Definition of Prognostic Terms*

Term	Prediction of Recovery	
	Qualitative	*Quantitative*
Excellent	Highly probable	75–100%
Good	Probable	50–75%
Guarded	Unpredictable	50%
Poor	Improbable	25–50%
Grave	Highly improbable	0–25%

for distinguishing organ disease (such as cardiac valvular insufficiency) from organ failure (such as altered cardiac rate and rhythm, which may or may not occur as a consequence of valvular insufficiency). Similarly, if a patient has irreversible generalized organ lesions of sufficient magnitude to cause organ dysfunction, the polysystemic manifestations of organ failure may be minimized by supportive and symptomatic therapy (see Table 1). Irreversibility of morphologic changes in various organs is not synonymous with irreversibility of biochemical and clinical sequelae.

In addition, one must determine whether irreversible lesions or states of dysfunction are progressive or nonprogressive. Such knowledge should be encompassed in providing both a "short-term" prognosis and a "long-term" prognosis.

Recurrent Illness

Recurrence of signs related to various body systems and organs influences prognosis. Too often, however, the underlying cause of recurrent signs is not documented. This point is emphasized because tissues constituting various body systems and organs respond to different etiologic agents in only a limited number of ways. Recurrence of similar clinical signs may be associated with (1) a recurrent episode of the original disease induced by the same mechanism, or mechanisms; (2) late sequelae of the original disease; (3) onset of a different disease associated with clinical manifestations similar or identical to the original disorder; and (4) various combinations of these factors. These factors should be considered in forecasting the likelihood of additional episodes of recurrent illness with or without therapy.

RECOMMENDATIONS

To permit meaningful exchange of knowledge, every scientific discipline must define its terms. We recommend terminology that lends itself to quantification of the probability of a predicted outcome (Crow, 1985) (Table 3).

The prognosis for each problem affecting patients should also be consistently subcategorized according to predicted events in the immediate future (short-term prognosis), and according to the probability of resolution of morphologic and functional abnormalities in the distant future (long-term prognosis). For example, the short-term survival prognosis for subclinical glomerular amyloidosis characterized by proteinuria is good to excellent. However, the long-term survival prognosis of patients with glomerular amyloidosis has, to date, been poor to grave. In contrast, the short-term survival prognosis for postrenal azotemia caused by urethral obstruction with a urolith and and characterized by profound metabolic acidosis, severe hyperkalemia, and marked hypothermia may be guarded to poor. Removal of the urolith combined with appropriate supportive and symptomatic therapy, however, may be associated with good to excellent chances for long-term survival.

Other concepts that should be considered when formulating prognoses are summarized in Table 2. We emphasize the concept of aging and its relationship to prognosis. Aging is associated with a decline in total function (or functional "reserve") of several organs (e.g., the kidneys) and systems (e.g., the immune system). Thus, the short- and long-term prognoses for complete recovery of "aged" patients from a variety of metabolic, degenerative, neoplastic, traumatic, infectious, and toxic diseases may be less favorable than the prognoses of younger patients with similar disorders. This generality, however, should not be used as the primary basis for recommending "benign neglect" or euthanasia. Aged patients often regain and maintain adequate function of various organs and systems to sustain a good quality of life.

Once prognoses have been established, and a therapeutic plan has been formulated, follow-up evaluations of the course of the disease and its response to therapy (if any) are recommended. Clients should be informed in sufficient detail of the veterinarian's prediction of the progress of the case, so that they will be able to recognize deviations from the expected, and so that they will have some perspective of the significance of the deviations. Veterinarians should also convey to their clients that their opinions, judgments, diagnoses, and prognoses are not infallible, and that if significant changes from the expected are observed, the clients should call for help or return immediately for re-evaluation.

Clients must also be encouraged to consider their obligations to cooperate once a management decision is mutually agreed upon, to tell the truth, to respect promises, and to educate themselves sufficiently to deal with the information they receive. Lack of compliance with recommendations may be as detrimental to a predicted outcome as incorrect diagnoses or prescription of ineffective or contraindicated treatment.

References and Suggested Reading

Crow, S. E.: Usefulness of prognoses: Qualitative terms versus quantitative designations. J.A.V.M.A. 187:700, 1985.

Osborne, C. A.: The problem-oriented medical system: Improved knowledge, wisdom, and understanding of patient care. Vet. Clin. North Am. Small Anim. Pract. 13:745, 1983.

Taylor, E. J. (ed.): *Dorland's Illustrated Medical Dictionary*, 27th ed. Philadelphia: W. B. Saunders, 1988, p. 1361.

PROBLEM KNOWLEDGE COUPLER AS A DIAGNOSTIC TOOL

P. A. BUSHBY

Mississippi State, Mississippi

Problem Knowledge Coupler is a specific software system designed for computer-assisted diagnosis and patient management. The system consists of software and specific databases. The software program allows the veterinarian to assess information in each database. The software provides the user with a means of entering specific information regarding a clinical case and comparing that information with all information in a problem-specific database. Each database is structured to provide a comprehensive library of information relevant to a particular problem. The comparison of information specific to a particular patient with the library of information in the database provides the user with diagnostic and therapeutic information relevant to the patient (Bushby, 1988; Weed and Hertzberg, 1984).

THE SYSTEM

Databases

Databases for the Problem Knowledge Coupler system contain relevant information regarding specific problems. Each database is built to be problem-specific. For example, databases have been created

for canine cough, feline anemia, canine polyuria and polydipsia, and other clinical problems. Each database includes (1) a comprehensive list of diseases or conditions that can cause that problem; (2) all relevant historical, physical examination, laboratory, radiographic, and other ancillary diagnostic data for each disease or condition; and (3) relevant diagnostic or therapeutic recommendations for each disease or condition (Bushby, 1988; Zimny and Tandy, 1989).

Software

The Problem Knowledge Coupler software is the driver for this expert system designed for computer-assisted diagnosis. Although the system was originally designed for computer-assisted diagnosis and patient management in human medicine, it is easily adapted to veterinary medicine. The software, written to run on MS-DOS computers, creates user-friendly access to the databases. The software provides four basic functions: data entry, comparison to the database, presentation of results, and specific recommendations (Weed, 1985).

DATA ENTRY

The software presents the user with a menu of options. The precise content of the main menu depends on the specific database, but it usually includes information from the following sources: (1) history, (2) physical examination, (3) laboratory, and (4) radiographs. For each of the main menu options, the software presents a comprehensive list of relevant questions. All historical questions, all

---

Problem Knowledge Coupler databases have been developed on an experimental basis at several veterinary colleges. To date, acceptance of the Problem Knowledge Coupler system as a diagnostic tool has been limited. While the Problem Knowledge Coupler software is commercially available from PKC, Inc., 10 Mary St., So. Burlington, VT 05043, no Problem Knowledge Coupler databases are commercially available at present. PROVIDES is a commercially available system comparable to the Problem Knowledge Coupler system and is available from IMPROMED, Inc., 304 Ohio Street, Oshkosh, WI 54901-5827 (see CVT X, p. 2).

physical examination questions, all relevant laboratory data, and all relevant radiographic findings are presented to the user. A simple check-off method allows the user to enter specific findings pertinent to a clinical case. The software compiles all information entered and can provide the user with a list of all clinical findings entered for the patient. This list of clinical findings can be compared with the database, can be "saved to disk," and can be revised at any time for additional comparison with the database (Weed, 1985).

COMPARISON WITH THE DATABASE

The software allows a comparison between the clinical findings associated with a patient and the information available in the database. The system conducts a Boolean "or" search, which results in a thorough analysis of the clinical findings entered and the creation of a comprehensive list of "rule-outs" for the patient's problem. For example, in the canine cough program, if a veterinarian enters clinical findings of (1) fever, (2) diarrhea, and (3) peripheral lymphadenopathy for a patient, the system provides a list of all diseases or conditions that could cause any one of the three findings. The "rule-out" lists resulting from a Boolean "or" search are extensive and remind the user of all conditions that may be present. The length of the rule-out lists makes the specific means of presentation of the data important (Weed, 1985; Zimny and Tandy, 1989).

PRESENTATION OF RESULTS

Upon completion of the data entry and the comparison of patient clinical findings with the database, the system provides the user with a comprehensive list of diseases or conditions that could be causing the patient's problem. For each disease or condition listed, the system provides an indicator of the degree of congruence between the patient and the database. The "observed total" ratio is a measurement of the number of findings present in the patient that match a specific condition as compared with the number of findings present in the database for that condition. An observed total ratio of 17/22 would mean that the database contains 22 relevant clinical findings for a specific condition, and that the patient in question has 17 of those findings. This ratio indicates to the user a high level of congruence between the patient and the database. An observed/total ratio of 3/15 means that the database contains 15 relevant clinical findings for a specific condition and that the patient in question has only three of those 15 findings. Such a ratio indicates minimal congruence between the patient and the database.

The system is designed to list the rule-out entries in the order of those diseases or conditions with the most observed findings down to those with the least observed findings. The use of the observed/total ratio and the specific sequencing of rule-outs assist the user in prioritizing rule-outs when attempting to make a diagnosis.

In addition to providing a structured rule-out list, the system provides a complete analysis of the patient as compared with the database for every condition on the list. When the user selects the condition to be analyzed, the system provides a list of all findings entered for the patient that are expected for that condition and of all findings expected in the condition that were not entered for the patient. Review of this analysis can assist the veterinarian in the establishment of a specific diagnosis (Bushby, 1988; Weed and Hertzberg, 1984).

SPECIFIC RECOMMENDATIONS

For each condition in the rule-out list, the system also can provide a list of recommended diagnostic tests, therapeutic measures, and any comments relevant to diagnosis or therapy (Weed and Hertzberg, 1984).

THE DIAGNOSTIC PROCESS

Use of the Problem Knowledge Coupler system can aid in establishing a diagnosis of clinical prob-

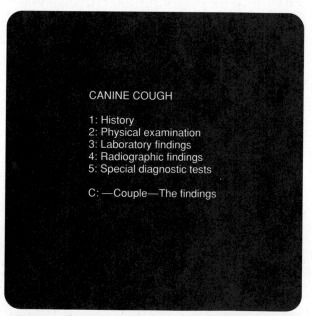

Figure 1. The main menu of the canine cough program of the Problem Knowledge Coupler presents the user with options of entering historical, physical examination, laboratory, radiographic, or other diagnostic information about a case. Upon selection of the history option, the user is taken to the first history question.

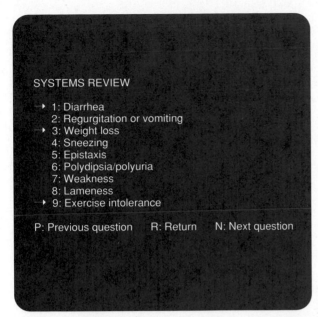

Figure 2. A historical question in the canine cough program. The arrow indicates that a finding has been selected, and this selection results in entry of that particular finding into the record for the patient. In this figure, diarrhea, weight loss, and exercise intolerance have been entered into the record. Each prompt is an on/off switch. Pressing the prompt (1) enters "diarrhea" into the record and inserts the arrow indicator in front of the term "diarrhea" on the screen. Pressing the prompt again deletes "diarrhea" from the record and removes the arrow indicator.

lems. The system does not alter the standard diagnostic process used in veterinary practice. The veterinarian still collects information about the patient, develops a rule-out list, and proceeds according to the elimination or confirmation of conditions on the rule-out list. The Problem Knowledge Coupler system aids this process by reminding the veterinarian of relevant historical questions to ask, relevant aspects of the physical examination, relevant laboratory and radiographic parameters that should be evaluated, and other relevant diagnostic procedures to consider. By responding to the computer-generated screens, the user creates a profile of the patient. That profile is compared with the database, resulting in development of a comprehensive rule-out list. This rule-out list may suggest conditions to be considered in pursuing a diagnosis that would not have been considered without use of the software. Then the system provides recommendations regarding specific diagnostic procedures for each condition on the rule-out list (Weed and Hertzberg, 1984; Zimny and Tandy, 1989).

A SAMPLE SESSION

When starting the programs, the user is presented with a main menu (Fig. 1). To proceed through a case in a normal sequence, the user

would press (1) on the keyboard to view the first screen of historical questions. The user selects, by pressing the prompt in front of the response, any response that applies to the patient. An arrow appears before each selected response. The bottom of the screen indicates navigational prompts, and by pressing (N), the user can move from one screen to the next. Pressing (P) allows the user to review the previous screen, and pressing (R) returns the user to the main menu.

Figure 2 represents a screen with select historical responses; Figure 3 represents a screen with select physical examination responses; Figure 4 represents a screen with select radiographic responses. After entering all available data for the patient, the user returns to the main menu and presses (C) to couple the responses (see Fig. 1). This action initiates the comparison with the database and presents the user with a list of all findings entered for the patient (Fig. 5). Pressing (C) provides the results in the form of the comprehensive rule-out list (Fig. 6). The program provides the user assistance in prioritizing rule-outs by displaying the observed/total ratio. Selecting the prompt in front of any of the conditions in the rule-out list provides the user with an analysis of the patient's problems in comparison with those expected for that disease. By selecting (1), the prompt in front of "Blastomycosis" (Fig. 6), the user sees the analysis of the patient's problems as compared with the database for blastomycosis. Displayed to the user is the list of findings in the patient that are consistent with a diagnosis of blastomycosis and a list of findings expected in blasto-

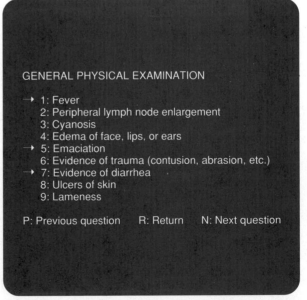

Figure 3. A physical examination question in the canine cough program. The arrow indicates that a finding has been selected. In this figure, the findings of fever, emaciation, and evidence of diarrhea have been entered into the record.

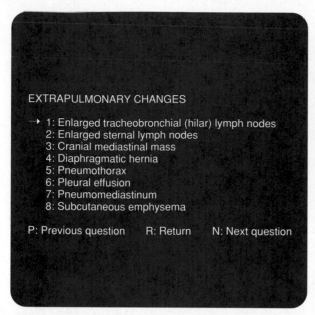

Figure 4. A radiographic examination question in the canine cough program. The arrow indicates that a finding has been selected. In this figure, the finding of enlarged tracheobronchial (hilar) lymph nodes has been entered into the record.

mycosis that were not entered for the patient (Fig. 7). Prompts at the bottom of the screen provide the user with a means of viewing additional information (N: Next), printing results (P: Print), viewing diagnostic or therapeutic options (O: Options), or returning to the rule-out list (R: Return). Selecting "O: Options" provides the user with recommenda-

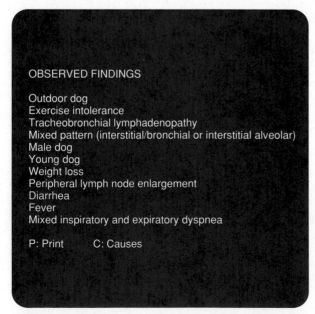

Figure 5. The list of observed findings for the patient. This list reveals all findings entered in the record for the patient. Pressing (C) provides the user with the list of possible causes ("rule-out" list) for the patient's problems.

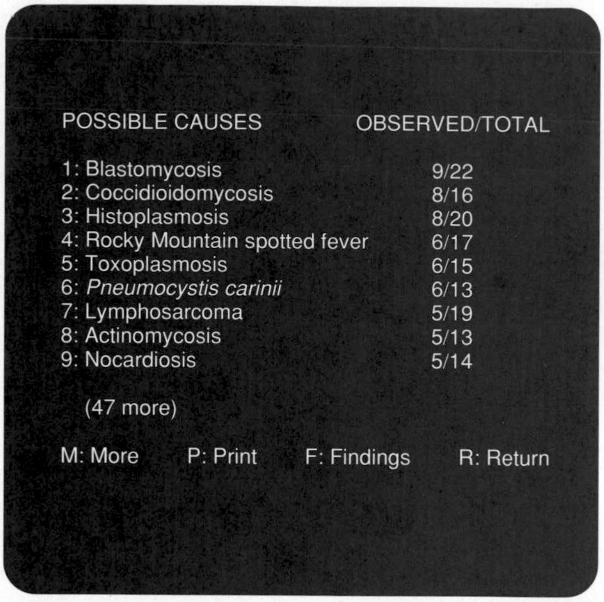

Figure 6. The initial screen of the rule-out list. This screen displays nine possibilities, and the "observed/total" ratio for each possibility. Pressing the prompt in front of any of the diseases reveals the detailed comparison of the patient with the database for that disease.

tions of specific diagnostic options for that disease (Fig. 8).

The Problem Knowledge Coupler system does not attempt to establish a diagnosis. This software can best be described as a sophisticated reminder system providing veterinary medical information applicable to patients with specific problems. The system reminds veterinarians of historical information to obtain, specific aspects of physical examination to perform, types of laboratory and radiographic parameters to select, and other diagnostic considerations for patients with specific problems. It then creates a comprehensive rule-out list to assist in establishing diagnostic considerations (Bushby, 1988; Weed and Hertzberg, 1984).

CONCLUSIONS

The Problem Knowledge Coupler system represents the first generation of computer-aided diagnostic tools. While the system has generated only limited interest in the veterinary profession, the concepts of computer-assisted diagnosis and patient management have been recognized in human medicine (Weed and Hertzberg, 1984; Zimny and Tandy, 1989). Veterinarians should explore the concepts of computer-assisted diagnosis and patient management, and should consider the potential value of such systems in their practice of veterinary medicine. As use of computer technology gains acceptance, the veterinary profession must deter-

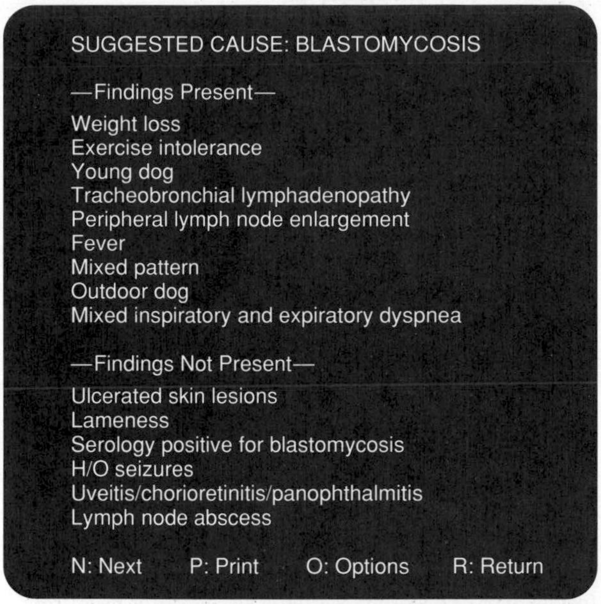

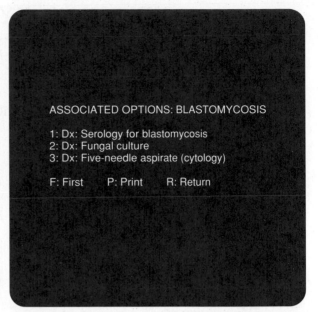

Figure 7. The first screen of the comparison of this patient with the database for blastomycosis. It contains the list of findings in this patient that are consistent with a diagnosis of blastomycosis as well as a list of findings expected in blastomycosis but not entered for the patient. Pressing (O: Options) from this screen provides the user with diagnostic and therapeutic options to be considered for blastomycosis. Pressing (R: Return) returns the user to the list of possible causes.

Figure 8. List of options to aid in establishing a diagnosis of blastomycosis.

mine which uses of computer technology are valuable and appropriate. The user of computer systems to manage financial information and reminder information in veterinary practice is well accepted. Computer systems that store, retrieve, and manipulate patient data are common in human medicine and are beginning to generate interest within the veterinary profession. The information that veterinarians deal with daily, but that has not yet been effectively computerized, is information regarding the hundreds of medical problems and thousands of diseases that occur in domestic and other animals. The value of computers in the management of information is unquestioned, but questions remain about which types of information should be processed by computer systems. The Problem Knowledge Coupler system represents a powerful example of both the management of basic medical information through use of the computer and the application of that information to specific patient problems.

References and Suggested Reading

Bushby, P. A.: The Problem Knowledge Coupler as information management and information processing tool. Can. Vet. J. 29:274, 1988.
A review of the use of the Problem Knowledge Coupler for information management in the diagnosis and treatment of patient problems.
Weed, L.: *Understanding and Using Problem Knowledge Couplers.* Burlington, VT: PKC Corporation, 1985, p. 3.
A user's manual for operation of the Problem Knowledge Coupler system.
Weed, L., and Hertzberg, R.: Problem solving: What's the best combination of man and machine? Comp. Med. Dig. 1:4, 1984.
A description of diagnostic and management Problem Knowledge Coupler systems and the value of the Problem Knowledge Coupler system in making clinical decisions for patient management.
Zimny, N. J., and Tandy, C. J.: Problem-knowledge coupling: A tool for physical therapy clinical practice. Phys. Ther. 69:155, 1989.
A discussion of the development, function, and philosophy of the Problem Knowledge Coupler system and its value in clinical decision making.

VETERINARY COMPUTED TOMOGRAPHY

DANIEL A. FEENEY,
and ROBERT M. HARDY

St. Paul, Minnesota

Advances in imaging technology have created a dilemma for progressive small animal practitioners. While trying to provide high-quality veterinary services, they must often choose between advanced and relatively costly imaging techniques that provide a high yield of diagnostic information and routine diagnostic techniques that are widely available and cost-effective, but less reliable. Over the past decade, computed tomography (CT) has become available to veterinarians for use in patient management. Because CT provides diagnostic information available by no other means, our goal is to provide insight into the applications of CT, to eliminate some of the mystique about how it works, and to provide information on where it can be obtained.

WHEN AND WHY IS CT A WORTHWHILE CONSIDERATION?

CT should generally not be the first diagnostic imaging procedure considered, because of associated cost and limited availability, particularly when compared with general radiography and two-dimensional, gray-scale ultrasonography. It should not be used only as a last resort, however. To facilitate a decision of when to use CT, one can consider the following questions. First, can available procedures adequately and predictably provide diagnostically useful information about the organ or organs involved in the disease under consideration? Second, what is the likelihood of the suspected disease being confidently considered or ruled out using less expensive and less sophisticated procedures? Third, does the cumulative cost of two or three less expensive and less predictable procedures approach or equal that of CT? Fourth, how does the client feel about the potential morbidity associated with invasive procedures (e.g., exploratory surgery) or about multiple imaging procedures likely to provide equivocal results? Clinical scenarios in which CT can provide needed information that is inaccessible or less definitive through use of other procedures are listed by anatomic region and summarized in Table 1.

Table 1. *Anatomic Regions Where Computed Tomography (CT) Is Applicable*

Head and Neck
Identification/characterization/staging of intracranial diseases (neoplasm, hydrocephalus, etc.)
Delineation/characterization of extraocular, periorbital processes (and some intraocular diseases if funduscopy and ultrasonography fail)
Identification of disease processes (e.g., abscess or neoplasm) in the region of the skull base foramina for cranial nerve deficits thought to arise in the extracranial compartment
Staging of nasal neoplasms (usually initially localized by survey radiography)
Staging of neck neoplasms, particularly of the thyroid and salivary gland

Spine and Pelvis
Confirmation/delineation of lumbosacral stenosis
Identification of laterally herniated disks
Identification of peripheral nerve neoplasms (such as those affecting spinal nerve roots and brachial plexus)
Identification of any gross (vs. microscopic) spinal cord lesion if myelography is not possible or is likely to provide equivocal results (e.g., complete obstruction)

Thorax
Identification of masses of the pericardium and base of the heart, which may elude detection by echocardiography
Characterization/staging of mediastinal diseases for specific regional therapy, such as surgery or radiotherapy (usually localized initially by survey radiography)
Identification of metastatic pulmonary nodules not detected by survey radiographs
Characterization/staging of pleural and chest wall masses even in presence of fluid

Abdomen
Characterization/staging of peritoneal or retroperitoneal disease for specific regional therapy such as surgery or radiotherapy (usually localized initially by survey radiography)
Search for metastatic disease or stage liver masses when information available via ultrasonography is inadequate
Predictable imaging of the pancreas and staging/characterization of pancreatic diseases
Clearest and most predictable method of identifying the normal adrenal glands and characterizing/staging their adrenal diseases

CT-Guided Biopsy
Situations in which fluoroscopy, and/or ultrasonography, or both are of limited value in identifying and localizing the lesion for biopsy. CT-guided techniques can be helpful because gas, bone, and so forth do not interfere with the CT image. The needle can be accurately directed to, and localized within, lesions.

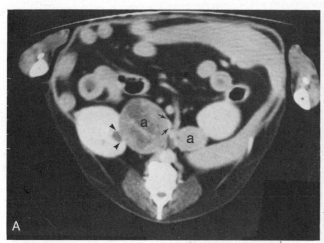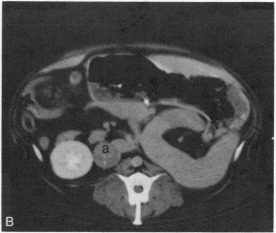

Figure 1. *A,* Contrast-enhanced transverse computed tomogram of a dog in which both the left and right adrenal glands (a) are enlarged. The left adrenal gland has a uniform density and is not invading the surrounding tissues or organs, whereas the right adrenal mass has nonuniform contrast enhancement and is invading both the right kidney (*arrowheads*) and the caudal vena cava (*arrows*). *B,* Transverse computed tomogram of another dog in which the right adrenal gland (a) is enlarged and contains foci of mineralization but does not invade regional structures. The right adrenal glands in both *A* and *B* are typical of those seen with invasive and noninvasive adrenal tumors, respectively. The left adrenal gland in *A* is typical of that seen with adrenal cortical hypertrophy.

Information gained from CT must be kept in perspective. First, specific morphologic or microbiologic diagnoses (such as identification of the tumor cell type or specific organism) are unlikely to be aided by CT. Although it is possible to rank the relative likelihood of infection versus neoplasia versus degeneration and hyperplasia, this ranking is based solely on the overall structural appearance and on the degree of contrast enhancement (defined in the next section). Second, because CT is a sophisticated, two-dimensional density analysis, it does not provide the same information about tissue as does diagnostic ultrasonography or magnetic resonance imaging (MRI).

CT is not a substitute for either structural or functional information provided by echocardiography; however, CT can provide more information about mediastinal and pleural diseases. Similarly, CT is not a practical substitute for ultrasonography of the liver, spleen, prostate gland, kidney, ovary, uterus, or testicles. It can, however, be used to identify these organs if ultrasonographic results are unsatisfactory. In our opinion, CT exceeds ultrasonography in detailed characterization of the retroperitoneal vasculature, the adrenal glands (particularly the normal glands), and the pancreas (Fig. 1). Neither CT nor ultrasonography is likely to pose a serious challenge to barium contrast radiographic procedures for practical and predictable identification of masses or of infiltrative diseases of the bowel or for the assessment of alimentary tract peristalsis. Some lesions of these organs can be identified using either CT or ultrasonography, depending on the expertise of the user and on the region imaged.

CT and MRI have provided the most predictable

and exacting methods of assessment of the brain (Fig. 2). Myelography is still the most practical method, however, of differentiating between extradural, intradural-extramedullary, and intramedullary lesions of the cervical through midlumbar spinal cord. Exceptions include situations involving (1) animals with a history of severe reactions to myelographic contrast agents, (2) technical problems with the myelogram, (3) nerve root neoplasms or laterally herniated disks not directly affecting the spinal cord, and (4) the lumbosacral region in general. In our opinion, myelography, vertebral venography, and epidurography are sufficiently unpredictable in detecting diseases such as lumbosacral stenosis or cauda equina syndrome that we recommend CT scanning if surgical intervention is being considered.

HOW DOES CT WORK?

The use of imaging to make a confident assessment of organ structure requires clear identification of the organ or region with limitation of the potential for interpretive errors. Lack of structural clarity (image contrast) and superimposition artifacts are among the more common causes of doubt and misinterpretation in diagnostic imaging. The goal of the continuous evolution of diagnostic techniques is to improve recognition of variations from normal without causing harm to the patient. In today's clinical environment, the decision regarding which imaging technique to use is influenced by a combination of potential information yield, cost, and patient risk. No one technique can replace all others

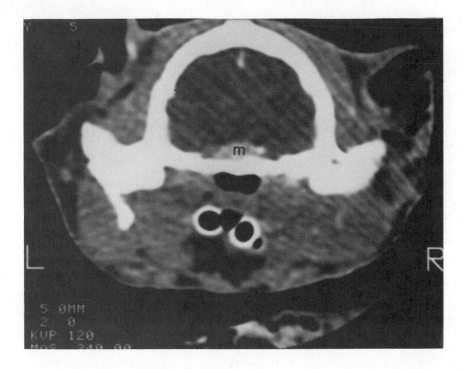

Figure 2. Contrast-enhanced computed tomogram obtained through the plane of the temporomandibular joints of an aging cat in which there is an enhancing hypothalamic mass (m), which was proved to be a neoplasm causing both acromegaly and increased circulating growth hormone concentration associated with insulin-resistant diabetes mellitus.

and general diagnostic radiology is unlikely to be replaced by either ultrasonography or CT. All techniques have limitations, however, including general radiography. The need for better image contrast and the need for elimination of superimposed (and potentially confusing) objects lead to the concept of tomography.

X-ray tomography or planigraphy is the radiographic process by which a planar image of a section through the body is made. By blurring or eliminating images of superimposed structures, tomographic imaging facilitates visualization of objects or organs. The result is improved radiographic contrast and improved object or organ clarity that are not possible when superimposed or adjacent objects are viewed by standard radiography, which produces "through and through" images. For example, the left kidney can be seen more clearly if, using tomography, the tail of the spleen (which commonly lies over it on a ventrodorsal radiographic view of the canine abdomen) is blurred out of the image. In x-ray tomography, the coordinated movements of the x-ray source (on one side of the patient) and the radiation detectors (on the opposite side of the patient) result in a blur of objects or organs outside the plane of focus, which is at the fulcrum between them. This tomographic process limits the non-blurred image to a slab of anatomy while reducing the influence caused by superimposed structures. The usual orientation of the movement of the tomographic tube and detector is parallel to the long axis of the patient. The images appear as blurred radiographs. Although still used in selected circumstances (e.g., nephrotomography in excretory urog-

raphy), noncomputed x-ray tomography has been virtually replaced by CT.

In *computed tomography*, coordinated movement between the x-ray tube and the radiation detectors (gas-filled chambers, crystals coupled to photomultiplier tubes, and so forth) is used, with the orientation of the combined movement of the x-ray source and detector perpendicular to the long axis of the patient (Fig. 3). The thickness of the plane or "slice" is governed by the width of the x-ray beam used to penetrate the region of interest (usually 1 to 10 mm). Each of these disklike "slices" is subdivided into smaller units of volume using the multiple converging vector approach (which is analogous to identifying the hub of a wheel by tracing the spokes). Through the use of complex mathematical and geometric processes (*algorithms*), the relative density and location of each subunit of volume can be determined. To obtain a perspective on the relative density of each of these volumetric subunits (*voxels*), the density determined for each of them with the aid of the algorithm is compared with that of water and converted to a CT number. These CT numbers can then be assigned one of numerous shades of gray in the picture subunits (*pixels*) to give a puzzle-like two-dimensional representation of each transverse slice.

Redistribution of shades of gray discernible by the human eye among these various relative densities using the CT number concept permits visual recognition of different densities beyond that of general film-based radiographic images. Because the "slices" are made up of numerical density equivalents of the volume subunits, images of planes

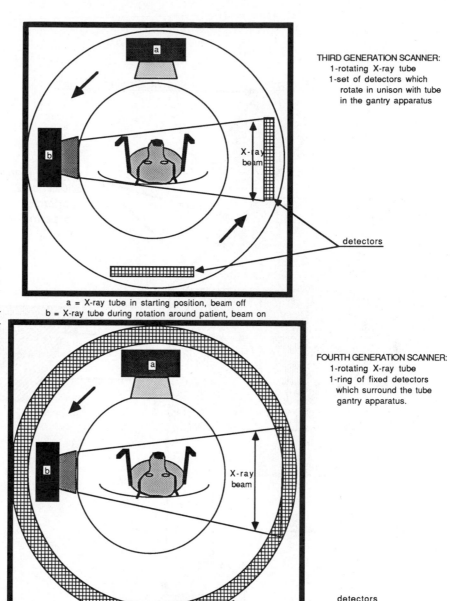

Figure 3. Diagram of third- and fourth-generation computed tomography (CT) scanners. (Reprinted with permission from Feeney, D. A., et al.: *Atlas of Correlative Imaging Anatomy of the Normal Dog: Ultrasound and Computed Tomography.* Philadelphia, W. B. Saunders, 1991, p. 337.)

other than the transverse (e.g., sagittal, dorsal, or oblique) can be produced through computer manipulation of data if the initial transverse slices were either contiguous or overlapping (Figs. 4 and 5). This latter manipulation provides the basis for the term "computed tomography." When first introduced and limited to the transverse or axial plane, CT was referred to as "computerized axial tomography" or "CAT" scanning.

Administration of contrast medium prior to CT scans is optional. Intravascular contrast medium facilitates differentiation of vessels from other structures (particularly masses and lymph nodes) viewed in the transverse plane. The subsequent distribution of contrast medium in tissues facilitates the evalua-

tion of normal organs such as kidneys and the identification of abnormalities such as brain tumors (which often become "enhanced" by contrast medium via a compromise in the otherwise impregnable blood brain barrier) (see Fig. 2). Oral *contrast enhancement* facilitates differentiation of the alimentary tract from other miscellaneous structures in the abdomen, including vessels.

CT imaging is basically a static or nondynamic imaging technique. Although rapid slicing sequences may provide some physiologic information about blood flow or even alimentary tract motility, the rate at which individual or sequential slices can be repeated is limited. Whereas rapid film-changing angiographic equipment can be used to obtain sev-

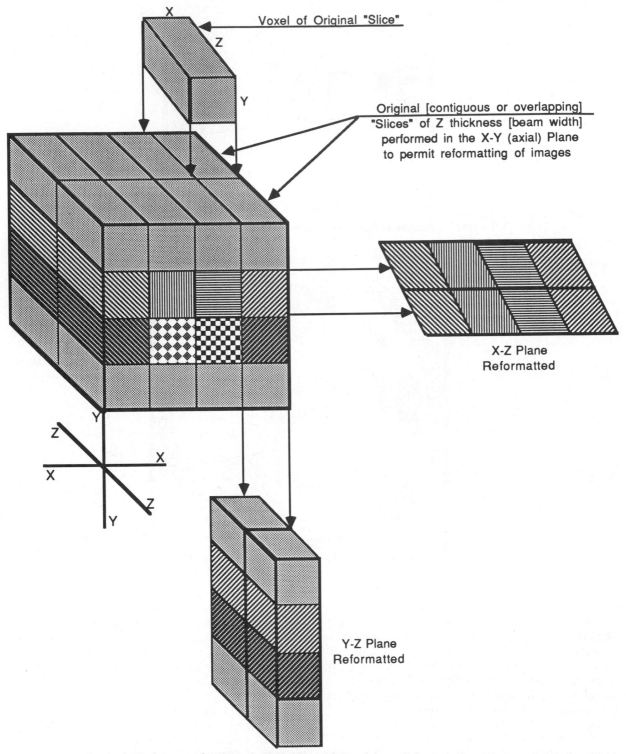

Voxel of Original "Slice"

Original [contiguous or overlapping]
"Slices" of Z thickness [beam width]
performed in the X-Y (axial) Plane
to permit reformatting of images

X-Z Plane
Reformatted

Y-Z Plane
Reformatted

Figure 4. Diagram of multiplanar two-dimensional reformatting of digitized density information from contiguous axial CT "slices." (Reprinted with permission from Feeney, D. A., et al.: *Atlas of Correlative Imaging Anatomy of the Normal Dog: Ultrasound and Computed Tomography.* Philadelphia, W. B. Saunders, 1991, p. 342.)

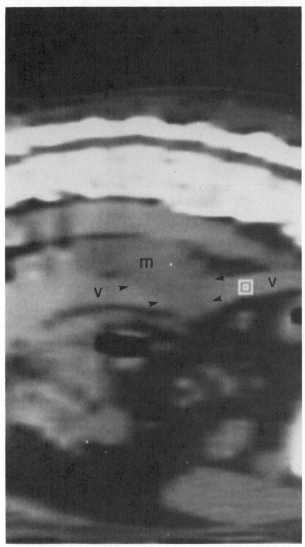

Figure 5. Sagittal (reformatted) computed tomogram of the right adrenal gland shown in Figure 1A. The reformatted plane is through the caudal vena cava (v), which has been distorted and invaded (*arrowheads*) by the right adrenal mass (m).

eral individual radiographic views per second, even the fastest general-use CT scanning equipment requires 1 to 2 sec per slice followed by a delay while the table moves. Cine CT can reduce the time required to obtain slices, but this equipment is rarely used, because of cost and space requirements. Therefore, CT scanning cannot be used as a substitute for the flow assessment capabilities of angiography or fluoroscopic dynamic studies.

WHAT KNOWLEDGE OF CT IS NECESSARY TO ADVISE CLIENTS?

When it becomes necessary to discuss the value of CT with clients, information summarized in the preceding section regarding why the procedure is justified and how it works should provide the necessary detail. Clients must be informed, however, that CT procedures require either deep sedation or general anesthesia to limit motion. When positioning a patient for scanning, the veterinarian should remember that metallic objects (e.g., ECG leads or metallic identification strips for esophageal stethoscopes as well as metallic orthopedic devices) create streak artifacts. For most CT scan procedures, the time during which the patient must be physically in the scanner ranges from 15 to 60 min, depending on the size of the area to be imaged. Clients may also be advised of the slight risks associated with administration of intravenous contrast media (Walter et al., 1986).

WHERE IS CT AVAILABLE?

A questionnaire about CT services was sent to representative diplomates of the American College of Veterinary Radiology and to representative neurologists of the American College of Veterinary Internal Medicine at English-speaking veterinary referral institutions in North America. These groups were considered the most likely to use or to know about availability of CT services in their institutions or referral areas. Results of the questionnaire are summarized in Table 2. Approximately 83% of the institutions surveyed offered CT services for their patients, often through a local human imaging center or hospital or through a mobile CT service. Most institutions responding performed an average of at least one CT scan per month; approximately 40% of the institutions performed more than three CT scans per month. Of the 27% of institutions that had on-site CT scanners, ten or more CT scans were performed per month.

The same questionnaire was sent to geographically representative neurologists and radiologists in private practice to sample the availability of CT services outside referral institutions and colleges. The private practice survey results are not in table form because a complete survey of licensed veterinary CT facilities assuring that all possible centers were found was not conducted. For further information about availability of CT scans in private practice, we suggest that individuals contact specialists in the area, particularly neurologists, radiologists, internists, and surgeons. For perspective, however, approximately 50% of the private practice radiologists and 86% of the private practice neurologists who responded to the questionnaire offered CT services to their patients, primarily through mobile CT services, human imaging centers, or hospital CT scanners. Overall, usually less than two CT scans per month were performed by these referral specialists. Of the private practice radiolo-

Table 2. Computed Tomography (CT) at English-Speaking North American Institutions

Respondents	Location	CT Services	CT Equipment Access*	CT Scans/ Month	Supervisor of Set-up and Protocol†	Multiplanar Reconstructions Made	Contact Person at Institution
Angell Memorial Hospital	Boston, MA	Yes	Local CT facility	3–5/month	AMH radiologist	No	Dr. M. McMillan
Animal Medical Center	New York, NY	Yes	On-site CT scanner	> 20/month	AMC radiologist	Yes	Dr. R. Burk
Auburn University (School of Veterinary Medicine)	Auburn, AL	Yes	On-site CT scanner	new venture	AUB neurologist	No	Dr. S. Simpson
University of California–Davis (School of Veterinary Medicine)	Davis, CA	Yes	On-site CT scanner	10–20/month	UCD radiologist	Yes	Dr. P. Koblik
Colorado State University (College of Veterinary Medicine)	Fort Collins, CO	Yes	On-site CT scanner	10–20/month	CSU radiologist or neurologist	Yes	Dr. R. Park
Cornell University (New York State College of Veterinary Medicine)	Ithaca, NY	No	—	—	—	—	—
University of Florida (College of Veterinary Medicine)	Gainesville, FL	No	—	—	—	—	—
University of Georgia (College of Veterinary Medicine)	Athens, GA	Yes	Mobile CT scanner	3–5/month	U-GA radiologist	Yes	Dr. B. Selcer
University of Guelph (Ontario Veterinary College)	Guelph, ON (Canada)	Yes	Local CT facility	New venture	Staff of CT facility	No	Dr. H. Dobson
University of Illinois (College of Veterinary Medicine)	Urbana, IL	Yes	Local CT facility	≤ 1/month	Staff of CT facility	No	Dr. J. Losonsky
Iowa State University (College of Veterinary Medicine)	Ames, IA	Yes	Local CT facility	≤ 1/month	ISU radiologist	No	Dr. E. Riedesel
Kansas State University (College of Veterinary Medicine)	Manhattan, KS	Yes	Local CT facility	≤ 1/month	KSU radiologist	No	Dr. C. Godshalk
Louisiana State University (School of Veterinary Medicine)	Baton Rouge, LA	No	—	—	—	—	—
Michigan State University (College of Veterinary Medicine)	East Lansing, MI	No	—	—	—	—	—
University of Minnesota (College of Veterinary Medicine)	St. Paul, MN	Yes	Mobile CT scanner	1–2/month	U-MN radiologist	Yes	Dr. D. Feeney
Mississippi State University (College of Veterinary Medicine)	Mississippi State, MS	Yes	Mobile CT scanner	1–2/month	MISS radiologist	No	Dr. G. Boring
University of Missouri (College of Veterinary Medicine)	Columbia, MO	Yes	Local CT facility	1–2/month	U-MO radiologist or neurologist	Yes	Drs. J. Lattimer or D. O'Brien

gists and neurologists who offered CT scans, however, approximately 38% used scanners installed in one of the referral practices where they performed their duties. This subgroup performed more than five CT scans per month.

In addition to questions about CT scanning, the institution-based and the private practice–based radiologists and neurologists were queried about utilization of MRI. Generation and applications of MRI imaging is beyond the scope of this discussion; nevertheless, more than any of the other imaging techniques, MRI produces images that most closely resemble computed tomograms. Instead of determining the density of the tissues as in CT scanning, however, MRI measures in the distribution, relative concentration, and degree of binding of hydrogen atoms in tissues. To date, most veterinary MRI has been focused on the central nervous system. This technique can be used to identify changes in signal intensity in tissue that are undetectable by either CT or myelography. About 20% of the private

practice radiologists, 53% of the veterinary institutions, and 86% of the private practice neurologists had access to MRI equipment. With the exception of the three institutions with MRI facilities on site, most institutions performed less than one MRI scan per month.

WHAT DOES CT COST?

While costs varied considerably among those responding to the survey, the majority of the prices for CT scanning of one region (e.g., head or lumbosacral spine) with a reasonable number of slices (up to 35 slices) range between $200 and $500. Some were $600. Some institutions and practices charged additional fees to perform the series with intravenous contrast medium. Costs varied among institutions and private practices. Among the private practice group, however, comments were made regarding charges for the time of the veterinarian

Table 2. *Computed Tomography (CT) at English-Speaking North American Institutions* Continued

Respondents	Location	CT Services	CT Equipment Access*	CT Scans/ Month	Supervisor of Set-up and Protocol†	Multiplanar Reconstruc-tions Made	Contact Person at Institution
North Carolina State University (School of Veterinary Medicine)	Raleigh, NC	Yes	On-site CT scanner	> 20/month	NCSU radiologist	No	Dr. D. Thrall
Ohio State University (College of Veterinary Medicine)	Columbus, OH	Yes	Local CT facility	6–10/month	OSU radiologist	No	Dr. M. Bailey
Oklahoma State University (College of Veterinary Medicine)	Stillwater, OK	Yes	Local CT facility	≤ 1/month	OSU radiologist	No	Drs. R. Bahr or G. Henry
University of Pennsylvania (School of Veterinary Medicine)	Philadelphia, PA	Yes	Local CT facility	6–10/month	Staff of CT facility	Yes	Dr. J. Wortman
University of Prince Edward Island (Atlantic Veterinary College)	Charlottetown, PEI (Canada)	Yes	Local CT facility	≤ 1/month	AVC internist	No	Dr. J. Miller
Purdue University (School of Veterinary Medicine)	West Lafayette, IN	Yes	Local CT facility	3–5/month	Purdue internist	No	Ms. C. Bretz
University of Saskatchewan (Western College of Veterinary Medicine)	Saskatoon, SK (Canada)	No	—	—	—	—	—
University of Tennessee (College of Veterinary Medicine)	Knoxville, TN	Yes	Mobile CT scanner	10–20/month	UTN radiologist or neurologist	Yes	Dr. R. Toal or R. Selcer
Texas A & M University (College of Veterinary Medicine)	College Station, TX	Yes	On-site CT scanner	10–20 month	TAM radiologist	Yes	Dr. Mike Walker
Tufts University (School of Veterinary Medicine)	North Grafton, MA	Yes	On-site CT scanner	10–20/month	Tufts radiologist	Yes	Dr. L. Kleine
Tuskegee Institute (School of Veterinary Medicine)	Tuskegee, AL	No response	—	—	—	—	—
Virginia-Maryland Regional College of Veterinary Medicine	Blacksburg, VA	Yes	Local CT facility	≤ 1/month	VAMRC radiologist	Yes	Dr. M. Moon
Washington State University (College of Veterinary Medicine)	Pullman, WA	Yes	On-site CT scanner	> 20/month	WSU radiologist	Yes	Dr. Dave Barbee
University of Wisconsin (School of Veterinary Medicine)	Madison, WI	Yes	Local CT facility	3–5/month	Staff of CT facility	No	Drs. P. Cuddon or B. Partington

For further information on availability of CT scans in private practice, individuals may inquire of specialists, particularly neurologists, radiologists, internists, or surgeons.

*On-site scanner, use of mobile CT imaging service at site, and patients taken to local CT scan center such as an imaging center or a hospital.
†Abbreviations are of institutions listed in first column.

in attendance, depending on where the scan was performed. In consideration of the costs of CT versus the cumulative bill of two or three conventional procedures (costing $100 each), CT scanning appears to be a cost-effective diagnostic technique.

References and Suggested Reading

Bailey, M. Q.: Use of x-ray computed tomography as an aid in localization of adrenal masses in the dog. J.A.V.M.A. 188:1046, 1986.

Berry, C. R., and Koblik, P. D.: Evaluation of survey radiography, linear tomography and computed tomography for detecting experimental lesions of the cribriform plate in dogs. Vet. Radiol. 31:146, 1990.

Feeney, D. A., Fletcher, T. F., and Hardy, R. M.: *Atlas of Correlative Imaging Anatomy of the Normal Dog: Ultrasound and Computed Tomography.* Philadelphia: W. B. Saunders, 1991, pp. 335–352.

Fike, J. R., LeCouteur, R. A., and Cann, C. E.: Anatomy of the canine brain using high-resolution computed tomography. Vet. Radiol 22:236, 1981.

Fike, J. R., LeCouteur, R. A., and Cann, C. E.: Anatomy of the canine orbital region: Multiplanar imaging by CT. Vet. Radiol. 25:32, 1984.

Fike, J. R., LeCouteur, R. A., Cann, C. E., and Pflugfelder, C. M.: Computerized tomography of brain tumors of the rostral and middle fossas in the dog. Am. J. Vet. Res. 42:275, 1981.

Fike, J. R., Druy, E. M., Zook, B. C., et al.: Canine anatomy as assessed by computed tomography. Am. J. Vet. Res. 41:1823, 1980.

Kaufman, H. H., Cohen, G., Glass, T. F., et al.: CT atlas of the dog brain. J. Comp. Assist. Tomogr. 5:529, 1981.

LeCouteur, R. A., Fike, J. R., Cann, C. E., and Pedroia, V. G.: Computed tomography of brain tumors in the caudal fossa of the dog. Vet. Radiol. 22:244, 1981.

LeCouteur, R. A., Fike, J. R., Scagliotti, R. H., and Cann, C. E.: Computed tomography of orbital tumors in the dog. J.A.V.M.A. 180:910, 1982.

Legrand, J. J., and Carlier, B.: Computerized tomography as a diagnostic aid in canine hydrocephalus. Rev. Med. Vet. 137:765, 1986.

Meuer, V. D.: Die Computer tomographie der Wirbelsaule zur Diagnose von Bandscheibenerkrankunger beim Hund. Kleinterpraxis 32:25, 1987.

Morgan, C. L.: *Basic Principles of Computed Tomography.* Baltimore: University Park Press, 1983.

Thrall, D. E., Robertson, I. D., McLeod, D. A., et al.: A comparison of radiographic and computed tomographic findings in 31 dogs with malignant nasal cavity tumors. Vet. Radiol. 30:59, 1989.

Turrel, J. M., Fike, J. R., LeCouteur, R. A., and Higgins, R. J.: Computed tomographic characteristics of primary brain tumors in 50 dogs. J.A.V.M.A. 188:851, 1986.

Voorhout, G.: X-ray computed tomography, nephrotomography and ultrasonography of the adrenal glands of healthy dogs. Am. J. Vet. Res. 51:625, 1990.

Voorhout, G., Stolp, R., Rijnberk, A., and van Waes, P. F.: Assessment of survey radiography and comparison with x-ray computed tomography for detecting hyperfunctioning adrenocortical tumors in dogs. J.A.V.M.A. 196:1799, 1990.

Walter, P. A., Feeney, D. A., and Johnston, G. A.: Diagnosis and treatment of adverse reactions to radiopaque contrast agents. *In* Kirk, R. W. (ed.): *Current Veterinary Therapy IX*. Philadelphia: W. B. Saunders, 1986, pp. 47–52.

Zook, B. C., Hitzelberg, R. A., and Bradley, E. W.: Cross-sectional anatomy of the beagle thorax. Vet. Radiol. 30:277, 1989.

Zook, B. C., Hitzelberg, R. A., Fike, J. R., and Bradley, E. W.: Anatomy of the beagle in cross-section: Head and neck. Am. J. Vet. Res. 42:844, 1981.

DIAGNOSIS OF INHERITED DISEASES IN SMALL ANIMALS

URS GIGER,
and PETER F. JEZYK
Philadelphia, Pennsylvania

The development and institution of diagnostic tests, therapeutic measures, and preventive strategies for acquired diseases caused by infections, nutritional imbalances, and intoxications have reduced morbidity and mortality in puppies and kittens. With these developments, the impact of another major group of diseases, namely, inherited defects, has become apparent. These diseases include anatomic malformations, susceptibility to infections and neoplastic diseases, and "inborn errors of metabolism." Inborn errors of metabolism include all biochemical disorders due to a genetically determined, specific defect in a protein molecule's structure or function, or both. Aside from the classic enzyme deficiencies, genetic defects in structural proteins, receptors, plasma and membrane transport proteins, and other proteins result in biochemical disturbances. Because genetic alterations are possible at any gene locus, inborn errors of metabolism constitute a large group of monogenic disorders. Although each individual disorder is seen only rarely, these errors as a group are responsible for a major proportion of all diseases encountered in humans and animals. More than 400 inherited disorders in dogs and cats have been described; several new defects are recognized each year. Furthermore, certain breeding practices in small animals, including inbreeding and the "popular sire effect," have led to an increased frequency of specific genetic defects in various breeds.

Animals may be screened for inherited disorders in two different ways. One method requires waiting until an animal is diseased and until a genetic cause is suspected before administering the laboratory tests to identify the disorder. The purpose of screening, however, is to test all animals for genetic diseases, which can be accomplished by physical and ophthalmologic examinations performed in conjunction with more specific laboratory tests. With simple and inexpensive screening tests, many genetic diseases can be detected before the animals develop clinical signs or are used for breeding. Discussion of a general approach toward detecting inherited diseases in small animals follows.

CLINICAL FEATURES

The patient's signalment is important, because certain inborn errors are known to occur in particular breeds. Typically, not all animals of a litter with inherited disease are affected, whereas full involvement of a litter is common with infectious diseases or intoxications. Related animals may have a history of a similar disorder. One might even speculate on the mode of inheritance depending on whether the parents are affected or whether clinical signs are recognized only in the males.

The onset of clinical signs usually occurs early in life, shortly after the maternal homeostatic system can no longer compensate for an endogenous defect. Some malformations occur *in utero*, however, while others, such as inherited eye diseases and Fanconi's syndrome, do not appear until adulthood. Animals affected with the same defect, however, develop clinical signs at about the same age.

Clinical manifestations of inborn errors are extremely variable and range from the benign to the debilitating and lethal. Although most conditions are chronic and progressive, they can be intermittent. Many inborn errors cause an isolated typical

This article was supported in part by a grant from the National Institutes of Health (RR02512).

sign, whereas others produce a characteristic overall pattern of anomalies or clinical syndrome. For instance, Kartagener's syndrome is the clinical triad of rhinitis, bronchiectasis, and situs inversus viscerum.

Most inborn errors cause relatively unspecific clinical signs, which may also be seen with acquired diseases (Table 1). A common presenting sign is failure to thrive. These animals lag behind healthy littermates in their development, and they do not gain weight at a normal rate. They are generally less active and attentive, do poorly, often "fade," and finally die. The well-known fading syndrome in puppies and kittens is commonly associated with inborn metabolic errors. This condition should not be confused with growth retardation, which refers to a proportionally stunted growth that may or may not be associated with other clinical signs.

Some disorders may cause specific clinical signs. Easy to recognize are malformations that involve any part of the skeleton and lead to disproportional dwarfism, gait abnormalities, or facial dysmorphism. These signs are typically seen with several of the lysosomal storage diseases. Some of these storage diseases also cause eye abnormalities owing to accumulation of material in the cornea, lens, or retina. Other inherited eye diseases may or may not be associated with systemic signs. Disorders affecting intermediary metabolism (e.g., those associated with hyperammonemia and organic acidemia) may cause severe vomiting, diarrhea, and anorexia. Many of these defects cause signs only when a concurrent problem, such as an infection, exists or in cases of increased catabolism caused by stress or fasting. Neurologic signs, including dementia and seizures, and hematologic disorders may also signal an inborn error of metabolism. Response to specific treatment (e.g., administration of clotting factors or a single vitamin) may further support the diagnosis of a particular defect, although effective treatment is available for only a few inborn disorders.

A certain percentage of neonatal deaths is accepted in the breeding of small animals; consequently, breeders often do not spend the time, effort, or money required to determine the cause of death in these animals. Repeated neonatal losses in related litters, however, should arouse suspicion of a genetic cause.

Table 1. *Typical Clinical Signs of Inborn Errors of Metabolism*

Neonatal death	Vomiting
Failure to thrive	Diarrhea
Growth retardation	Anorexia
Malformations	Neurologic signs
Eye abnormalities	Hematologic abnormalities

SCREENING TESTS

Inborn errors of metabolism may lead to the dysfunction of a biologic system or pathway either under normal conditions or during more demanding situations such as concurrent disease or stress, because most recognized errors affect catabolic pathways. Screening tests should allow detection of the failing system. Routine tests such as a complete blood cell count, chemistry screen, and urinalysis may reveal some specific metabolic problems, such as hyperlipidemia or inclusion bodies in white blood cells. Radiology or other imaging techniques may reveal skeletal malformations or cardiac anomalies. Gastrointestinal absorption, liver function, and renal clearance studies may more clearly define organ failure. Light microscopy, electron microscopy, or both, used with tissue biopsy from an affected dog or following the necropsy of a littermate or relative, may give the first clue to an inborn error. Light microscopic examination of tissue, together with cytology of white blood cells, has proved particularly useful in the diagnosis of storage diseases.

A complete ophthalmologic examination is a widely accepted screening test for inherited eye diseases. Some of these eye diseases do not cause visual impairment until the animal is several years old, and they cannot be recognized by examination before then. Cardiac examinations can be performed to detect many heart anomalies. Screening for inherited bleeding disorders, such as von Willebrand disease and hemophilia, is possible. Other less commonly used hematologic screening tests may reveal abnormal leukocytic or erythrocytic function, such as deficient bactericidal neutrophil activity or increased erythrocyte osmotic fragility. Karyotyping has been used to detect chromosomal abnormalities associated with sex development disorders and multiple malformations.

The Section of Medical Genetics at the School of Veterinary Medicine, University of Pennsylvania, has established a national metabolic screening laboratory to test for inborn errors of metabolism. Several hundred samples from animals with clinical signs suggestive of inborn errors are studied yearly.

Metabolic Screening

Disorders of intermediary metabolism typically produce a metabolic block in a biochemical pathway, leading to product deficiency, accumulation of substrates, and production of substances via alternative pathways (Figure 1). These disorders are often named according to the aberrant substance associated with the pathologic condition (e.g., cystinuria, porphyria, mucopolysaccharidosis) rather

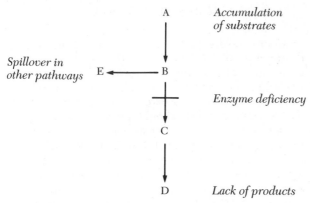

Figure 1. Metabolic consequences of enzyme deficiency.

than the truly defective (deficient) enzyme or cofactor.

The most useful test specimen for a suspected inherited metabolic disorder is a urine sample. It is the best specimen because most abnormal metabolites in blood are filtered through the glomerulus but fail to be reabsorbed by the renal tubules because of the lack of transport systems. In those disorders in which normal metabolites accumulate, the quantities of the metabolites usually exceed the renal threshold. As a consequence, the amounts of such compounds in a given volume of urine are often several times greater than those in blood. Defects in renal tubular transport also produce a drain of metabolites from blood into urine. Samples from normal littermates can be helpful for comparison. Plasma or serum samples are less useful for

metabolic screening but may be required to confirm or negate abnormal findings.

Urine samples can be collected by a free-catch method or by cystocentesis, and they are best kept frozen or refrigerated. Liquid samples should be sent on ice by overnight mail, to an appropriate laboratory.* Another approach is collection of urine, particularly from neonates or small animals, on a Whatman's 3-mm filter paper, which is then allowed to dry. The sample can then be shipped in an ₌envelope. This method limits some investigations, however. In any case, information regarding the animal's clinical appearance, history, medication, clinical features, and laboratory abnormalities should be included to help establish a specific diagnosis.

Figure 2 outlines the scheme of analysis currently used in our laboratory. For the most part, the tests are simple and inexpensive and are performed rapidly. We use essentially the same methods employed in human laboratories; however, interpretation of results involve marked species-related differences. Amino acids, organic acids, and carbohydrates are analyzed by a series of spot tests and one-dimensional paper chromatography. These tests are designed to screen for alterations in certain metabolic pathways; they are not in themselves diagnostic of any given disorder.

In the simple spot test used to screen for muco-

*One such laboratory is the Metabolic Screening Laboratory, Section of Medical Genetics, Veterinary Hospital of the University of Pennsylvania, 3850 Spruce Street, Philadelphia, PA 19104-6010.

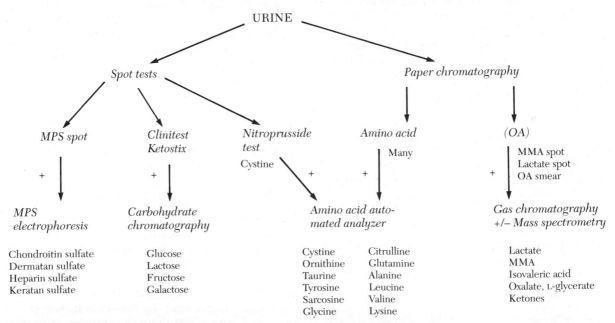

Figure 2. Metabolic screening of urine samples. Clinitest and Ketostix are products manufactured by Ames Company, Elkhart, IN. MMA, methylmalonic acid; OA, organic acid.

Table 2. *Abnormalities in Urinary Carbohydrates*

Urinary Carbohydrates	Name of Disorder	Species or Breed
Glucose	Diabetes mellitus	Dogs, cats
	Renal glucosuria	Norwegian elkhounds
	Fanconi's syndrome	Basenji, others
Lactose	Lactosuria	Nursing animals
Galactose	Liver disease	Dogs

polysaccharidosis, toluidine blue produces a metachromatic purple reaction with urinary glycosaminoglycosides (GAG). This stain can also be used to detect GAG storage in white blood cells or other tissue. To further characterize the type of mucopolysaccharidosis, cellulose acetate electrophoresis is used to separate urinary GAG into dermatan, heparin, and chondroitin sulfates. Very young, growing animals normally have some increased chondroitin sulfate in their urine, which may result in false-positive test results. Storage diseases other than mucopolysaccharidoses (e.g., alpha-mannosidosis, sphingolipidosis) are not detected by routine screening tests; they require histochemical analysis of tissue and determination of specific metabolites and enzyme. A large number of storage diseases have been recognized in small animals.

The copper reduction reaction (Clinitest, Ames Company) is used to screen urine for reducing substances, such as glucose. Glucosuria is confirmed by the specific glucose oxidase reaction (Clinistix, Ames Company). Positive reactions are further evaluated by paper chromatography. Inherited disorders that result in abnormal concentrations of urinary carbohydrates are listed in Table 2. Lactosuria is common in nursing animals, and ampicillin as well as drugs that are excreted as glucuronides can produce false-positive reactions. In contrast with humans, small animals rarely demonstrate positive

reactions for urine ketone bodies with the use of an acetone test (Acetest, Ames Company) except in cases of diabetic ketoacidosis—because of their resistance to fasting ketosis.

The cyanide nitroprusside reaction, which detects any compound containing a sulfhydryl group, is used to screen for cystinuria and homocystinuria. Cystinuria and other aminoacidurias (Table 3) can be detected by one-dimensional descending paper chromatography of urine, using a combination of butanol, acetic acid, and water as a solvent and a ninhydrin stain. Interpretation of these chromatograms is difficult because of the considerable diet-related variation in excretions. Therefore, specific or generalized abnormalities of urinary amino acid excretion, detected by paper chromatography, are confirmed by automated quantitative ion-exchange analysis. This technique is also used to detect taurine deficiency in cats. Cats and dogs usually have large amounts of methylated amino acids of tissue origin in their urine. A large amount of felinine excretion is normal in cats, but lack of felinine in urine is a nonspecific marker of a "sick" cat.

Ascending paper chromatography, similar to the technique used in analyzing amino acids, can identify urinary organic acids using a different stain. In cats, large amounts of hippurate are normally present. Increased lactic acid and increased methylmalonic acid are the two major abnormalities recognized by this technique (Table 4).

IDENTIFICATION OF A DEFECT

Although a combination of family history, clinical features, screening tests, and light microscopy of tissue may suggest a biochemical defect in a particular animal, more diagnostic studies are usually needed to identify or confirm a specific defect.

Table 3. *Abnormalities in Urinary Amino Acids in Small Animals With Typical Inborn Errors of Metabolism*

Urinary Amino Acids	Name of Disorder	Species or Breed
Increased		
Generalized	Fanconi's syndrome	Basenji and others
Cystine	Cystinuria	Basset, dachshund, Newfoundland
Ornithine	Ornithine aminotransferase deficiency (gyrate atrophy)	Domestic short-hair cats
Tyrosine	Tyrosine aminotransferase deficiency (tyrosinemia type II)	German shepherd
Citrulline	Argininosuccinate synthetase deficiency	Golden retriever, beagle
Sarcosine	Hypersarcosinemia	Portuguese water dogs
Alanine, glutamine	Portosystemic shunts Liver disease	Many breeds of dogs and cats
Glycine, alanine, protein	—	Sheltie, collie
Decreased		
Taurine	Taurine deficiency	Cats
Felinine	"Sick" cat	Cats

Table 4. Abnormalities in Urinary Organic Acids

Urinary Organic Acid	Name of Disorder	Species or Breed
Methylmalonic acid	Selective cobalamin intestinal malabsorption	Giant schnauzers
	Methylmalonic aciduria	Shar pei, Basset hound
Lactic acid	Lactic acidosis	Irish setter, Old English sheepdogs, other dogs and cats
	Fanconi's syndrome	Basenji, Norwegian elkhound
Isovaleric acid	Isovaleric aciduria	Siamese
Oxalate, L-glycerate	Primary hyperoxaluria	Cats, Tibetan spaniel

Inborn errors of metabolism result from a decrease in the functional activity of a protein, such as an enzyme or a receptor. Factors influencing the functional phenotype at the protein level include protein synthesis, post-translational processing, subcellular localization, stability, substrate affinity, cofactor binding and availability, and homeostatic regulators. The end result often may be reduced activity of an enzyme, commonly called "enzyme deficiency." Because most enzymes are present in abundant amounts, no major functional abnormalities are observed unless the enzyme activity is severely reduced, usually to less than 20% of normal value. Enzyme defects involving a rate-limiting step of a metabolic pathway are most apparent, particularly when that system is stressed. In a few instances, deficiency of one tissue-specific isoenzyme may lead to an abnormal or persistent expression of another isoenzyme, as is the case in pyruvate kinase deficiency. This finding complicates the diagnosis.

Despite lack of functional activity of a protein in a disorder, the dysfunctional protein may still be detected through immunologic techniques and is termed "cross-reacting material (CRM)." In this way, inherited defects can be divided into CRM positive and CRM negative (null mutation) disorders, depending upon the particular antibody used.

Most inborn errors of metabolism are inherited in an autosomal-recessive manner; therefore, affected animals are homozygous for the mutated gene. Clinically asymptomatic carriers or heterozygotic animals typically have about half-normal protein activity. Certain specific tests may therefore be used to detect carriers of genetic diseases. For instance, erythrocyte pyruvate kinase activity and phosphofructokinase activity are measured to detect carriers of hemolytic disorders in Basenjis and English springer spaniels, respectively. Similarly, the level of beta-galactosidase activity in white blood cells is used to identify carriers of GM_2 gangliosidosis in Portuguese water dogs. Also, specific clotting factor analysis can be used to find potential bleeders and asymptomatic carriers of clotting factor deficiencies.

In conclusion, inborn errors of metabolism represent a major group of disorders in small animals that are associated with a large variety of clinical signs. Simple and inexpensive screening tests may be used to recognize these diseases or to indicate the failing system. Special laboratory tests are usually required to make a definitive diagnosis. An accurate diagnosis can allow a prognosis, and, rarely, treatment can be given. In addition, genetic counseling can be provided to avoid further production of affected dogs.

References and Suggested Reading

Cohn, R. M. and Jezyk, P.: Metabolic screening. *In* Hicks, J. M., and Boeckx, R. L. (eds.): *Pediatric Clinical Chemistry*. Philadelphia: W. B. Saunders, 1984, p. 657.
A review of the methods used to screen for metabolic diseases in children.
Desnick, R. J., Patterson, D. F., and Scarpelli, D. F. (eds.): Animal models of inherited metabolic diseases. Prog. Clin. Biol. Res. Vol. 94, 1982.
A series of articles on inherited metabolic diseases in animals.
Harris, H. (ed.): *The Principles of Human Biochemical Genetics*, 3rd ed. Amsterdam: Elsevier, 1980.
A review of the principal concepts underlying human biochemical genetics and of human inherited enzyme defects.
Haskins, M. E., and Patterson, D. F.: Inherited metabolic diseases. *In* Holzworth, J. (ed.): *Diseases of the Cat*. Philadelphia: W. B. Saunders, 1987, p. 808.
A brief review of inherited metabolic diseases in cats.
Jezyk, P. F.: Metabolic diseases—an emerging area of veterinary pediatrics. Compend. Cont. Educ. Pract. Vet (Small Anim.). 6:1026, 1983.
A discussion of the veterinary approach to a young animal with an inherited metabolic disease.
Jezyk, P. F., Haskins, M. E., and Patterson, D. F.: Screening for inborn errors of metabolism in dogs and cats. Prog. Clin. Biol. Res. 94:93, 1982.
A further description of the metabolic screening test abnormalities in small animals.
McKusick, V. A. (ed.): *Mendelian Inheritance in Man: Catalogs of Autosomal Dominant, Autosomal Recessive, and X-Linked Phenotypes*, 8th ed. Baltimore: Johns Hopkins University Press, 1988.
A detailed description of all mendelian inherited diseases in man.
Scriver, C. R., Beaudet, A. L., Sly, W. S., and Valle, D. (eds.): *The Metabolic Basis of Inherited Diseases*, 6th ed. New York: McGraw-Hill, 1989.
A description of all inherited metabolic diseases in humans.
Valle, D. L., and Mitchell, G. A.: Inborn errors of metabolism in the molecular age. Prog. Med. Genet. 7:100, 1987.
A review of the techniques used in the molecular characterization of inborn errors.

DIAGNOSIS AND TREATMENT OF MIXED ACID-BASE DISORDERS

LARRY G. ADAMS,
and DAVID J. POLZIN
St. Paul, Minnesota

Coexistence of two or more primary acid-base disorders in the same patient is termed a *mixed acid-base disorder* or *disturbance*. Recognition of mixed acid-base disorders is often of considerable diagnostic and therapeutic value. The concept of mixed acid-base disorders requires an understanding of the concepts of acidosis, alkalosis, acidemia, and alkalemia. *Acidosis* and *alkalosis* are processes that tend to cause acid (acidosis) or base (alkalosis) to accumulate in the body. In contrast, *acidemia* and *alkalemia* refer to actual measured pH values of blood (Table 1). While a single determination of blood pH can be only acid, alkaline, or normal, the blood pH may reflect the net effect of one or more processes affecting acid-base balance. Thus, a patient may have several processes properly termed alkalosis, acidosis, or a combination of the two, but the net effect can be only acidemia, alkalemia, or normal blood pH.

PRIMARY ACID-BASE DISORDERS

The four primary acid-base disorders are metabolic acidosis, metabolic alkalosis, respiratory acidosis, and respiratory alkalosis. *Metabolic acidosis* is a process that causes nonvolatile acids to accumulate in the body, with nonvolatile acids defined as acids that cannot be eliminated through the lungs. Metabolic acidosis is characterized by a decrease in blood pH, a decrease in serum bicarbonate concentration, and compensatory hyperventilation resulting in a decrease in P_{CO_2}. *Metabolic alkalosis* is a process that causes alkali (usually bicarbonate) to accumulate in the body. Metabolic alkalosis is characterized by an increase in blood pH, an increase in serum bicarbonate concentration, and compensatory hypoventilation resulting in an increase in P_{CO_2}. *Respiratory acidosis* is a process that causes accumulation of carbon dioxide in the body. Respiratory acidosis is characterized by a decrease in blood pH, an increase in P_{CO_2}, and a variable compensatory increase in the serum bicarbonate concentration. *Respiratory alkalosis* is a process that causes increased elimination of carbon dioxide from the body. Respiratory alkalosis is characterized by an increase in blood pH, a decrease in P_{CO_2}, and a variable compensatory decrease in the serum bicarbonate concentration.

MIXED ACID-BASE DISORDERS

Causes

Mixed acid-base disturbances are often caused by concurrent development of two or more diseases that affect acid-base balance (e.g., metabolic acidosis due to renal failure and metabolic alkalosis due to gastric origin vomiting). Examples of conditions that are frequently associated with mixed acid-base disturbances include (1) cardiopulmonary arrest (respiratory acidosis, lactic acidosis from tissue hypoxia); (2) heat stroke (respiratory alkalosis due to thermo-

Table 1. Normal Arterial Blood-Gas Values†

	pH (units)	pO₂ (mm Hg)	pCO₂ (mm Hg)	HCO₃⁻ (mEq/L)	Base Excess (mEq/L)
Dogs					
Range	7.35–7.46	90–110	26–42	18–24	+1 to −3
Midpoint‡	7.41	100	34	21	−1
Cats					
Range	7.30–7.45	95–110	26–40	16.5–21	+1 to −5
Midpoint‡	7.38	103	33	19	−2

*Modified with permission from Hardy, R. M., and Robinson, E. P.: Treatment of alkalosis. *In* Kirk, R. W. (ed.): *Current Veterinary Therapy IX*. Philadelphia: W. B. Saunders, 1986, pp. 67–75.

†Normal values vary according to the laboratory used.

‡Midpoint of the normal range is presented. This value is used for the calculation of predicted compensatory changes from normal as discussed in the text.

regulatory panting, metabolic acidosis due to lactic acidosis and rhabdomyolysis); and (3) septic shock (metabolic acidosis due to lactic acidosis, respiratory alkalosis due to thermoregulatory panting).

Dogs with gastric dilatation–volvulus often sustain a variety of acid-base disturbances, including lactic acidosis, metabolic alkalosis, respiratory acidosis, respiratory alkalosis, and mixed disorders (Muir, 1982). The occurrence of lactic acidosis may be subsequent to reduced cardiac output, decreased effective circulating blood volume, and hypoxemia. Metabolic alkalosis may develop in association with sequestration of gastric acid accompanied by decreased effective circulating blood volume. Respiratory acidosis may occur if the gas-filled stomach impinges on the diaphragm, impairing ventilation. In some patients, however, hyperventilation due to pain or associated with sepsis may lead to respiratory alkalosis. Because these mechanisms occur independently, any of the mixed acid-base disturbances can potentially occur in dogs with gastric dilatation–volvulus.

Mixed acid-base disturbances may also be iatrogenic. Administration of narcotic analgesics or general anesthetics may promote respiratory acidosis by depressing pulmonary ventilation. Respiratory depression may be compounded by laryngospasm during endotracheal intubation. Together, these factors may induce significant respiratory acidosis. If the patient has pre-existing metabolic acidosis, the resultant mixed acid-base disorder can result in a dangerous reduction in blood pH. The treatment of metabolic acidosis prior to anesthesia or the selection of anesthetic protocols involving minimal respiratory depression, or both, may minimize or prevent development of mixed acid-base disorders in such patients. Administration of urine acidifiers (acidifying diets, ammonium chloride, D,L-methionine) to cats with undiagnosed renal failure or to cats remaining acidotic following relief of urinary tract obstruction is another common iatrogenic cause of mixed acid-base disorders.

Diagnosis

Mixed acid-base disorders are often suspected on the basis of medical history, physical examination, urinalysis, routine chemical analyses of serum, and serum electrolyte concentrations. Confirmation of mixed acid-base disorders requires blood gas analysis. The medical history frequently contains diagnostic clues prompting consideration of acid-base disorders. Previously diagnosed conditions, such as chronic renal failure, diabetes mellitus, chronic diarrhea, chronic vomiting, congestive heart failure, and hypoxemic cardiopulmonary diseases, are indications for further evaluation of the patient's acid-base status. Patients with such previously diagnosed conditions may be predisposed to development of mixed acid-base disorders if additional disturbances of acid-base balance occur. Likewise, history of recent drug intake (e.g., carbonic anhydrase inhibitors, diuretics, sodium bicarbonate, or urine acidifying agents) or toxin ingestion (e.g., ethylene glycol) may indicate evaluation of the patient's acid-base status.

Hyperventilation, hypoventilation, dyspnea, abnormal breathing sounds, or cyanosis of the mucous membranes are cardinal signs of respiratory disease, suggesting possible respiratory acid-base disorders. A uremic odor or ketones on the breath, dehydration, poor tissue perfusion (capillary refill), shock, congestive heart failure, urinary obstruction, and gastric dilatation–volvulus suggest possible metabolic acid-base disturbances.

Serum biochemical profiles and urinalyses often reveal metabolic diseases that may be associated with acid-base disorders (e.g., renal failure, diabetes mellitus, and hepatic disease).

SERUM ELECTROLYTE CONCENTRATIONS

Total carbon dioxide (CO_2) concentration is a commonly used estimate of serum bicarbonate (HCO_3) concentration. Total carbon dioxide concentration differs from serum bicarbonate concentration in that it also includes serum carbon dioxide and carbonic acid (H_2CO_3) (Polzin and Osborne, 1986). Although increased or decreased total carbon dioxide concentrations indicate disturbances of acid-base balance, changes in total carbon dioxide concentrations do not differentiate primary metabolic disorders from compensated respiratory disorders or mixed acid-base disorders. Therefore, blood gas analysis should be considered for patients with abnormal total carbon dioxide concentrations. For example, a total carbon dioxide concentration of 15 mEq/L could result from primary metabolic acidosis or be a compensatory response to chronic respiratory alkalosis. In addition, serum samples allowed to stand at room temperature in contact with room air may have spuriously decreased concentrations of serum total carbon dioxide because of volatilization of carbon dioxide.

The anion gap (AG) is defined as the difference between measured concentrations of serum cations (sodium [Na^+] and potassium [K^+]) and measured concentrations of serum anions (chloride [Cl^-] and bicarbonate [HCO_3^-]). The AG may be expressed by the following equation:

$$AG = ([Na^+] + [K^+]) - ([Cl^-] + [HCO_3^-])$$

Changes in AG usually result from changes in unmeasured anion concentrations (Polzin and Osborne, 1986). The most common unmeasured anions

Table 2. Calculations Used in Diagnosis of Mixed Acid-Base Disorders

$$\Delta AG = [AG]\text{Measured} - [AG]\text{Normal} = [AG]\text{Measured} - 18^*$$
$$\Delta HCO_3^- = [HCO_3^-]\text{Normal} - [HCO_3^-]\text{Measured} = 21^* - [HCO_3^-]\text{Measured}$$
$$\Delta Cl^- = [Cl^-]\text{Measured} - [Cl^-]\text{Normal} = [Cl^-] - 115^*$$

Expected Physiologic Compensation for Primary Acid-Base Disorders

Metabolic Acidosis
$$(Pa_{CO_2})\text{Expected} = \{Pa_{CO_2}\}\text{Normal} - \{([HCO_3^-]\text{Normal} - [HCO_3^-]\text{Measured}) \times 0.8\}$$

Metabolic Alkalosis
$$(Pa_{CO_2})\text{Expected} = \{([HCO_3^-]\text{Measured} - [HCO_3^-]\text{Normal}) \times 0.7\} + \{Pa_{CO_2}\}\text{Normal}$$

Acute Respiratory Acidosis
$$[HCO_3^-]\text{Expected} = \{([Pa_{CO_2}]\text{Measured} - [Pa_{CO_2}]\text{Normal}) \times 0.15\} + [HCO_3^-]\text{Normal}$$

Chronic Respiratory Acidosis
$$[HCO_3^-]\text{Expected} = \{([Pa_{CO_2}]\text{Measured} - [Pa_{CO_2}]\text{Normal}) \times 0.37\} + [HCO_3^-]\text{Normal}$$

Acute Respiratory Alkalosis
$$[HCO_3^-]\text{Expected} = [HCO_3^-]\text{Normal} - \{([Pa_{CO_2}]\text{Normal} - [Pa_{CO_2}]\text{Measured}) \times 0.2\}$$

Chronic Respiratory Alkalosis
$$[HCO_3^-]\text{Expected} = [HCO_3^-]\text{Normal} - \{([Pa_{CO_2}]\text{Normal} - [Pa_{CO_2}]\text{Measured}) \times 0.55\}$$

*The normal serum bicarbonate (HCO_3), chloride (Cl), and anion gap (AG) vary according to the laboratory used. The midpoint values from the normal ranges for each electrolyte are used for these calculations. Pa_{CO_2}, arterial carbon dioxide pressure.

in blood are those associated with various metabolic acids (e.g., lactate and beta-hydroxybutyrate). Therefore, an elevated AG is highly suggestive of metabolic acidosis (termed "high anion gap" metabolic acidosis) and is an indication for blood gas analysis. Not all metabolic acidoses, however, are associated with elevated AG. If the acid's anion is chloride (e.g., ammonium chloride), or if the anion is excreted in urine and replaced in serum by chloride, serum chloride concentration increases as serum bicarbonate decreases and AG remains normal. Such a disorder is termed "hyperchloremic metabolic acidosis." Thus, finding a normal AG does not rule out metabolic acidosis.

In patients with high anion gap metabolic acidosis, the increase in AG (ΔAG) approximates the decrease in serum bicarbonate concentration (ΔHCO_3^-) (Adams and Polzin, 1989; Polzin and Osborne, 1986). (Table 2 presents calculation of ΔAG and ΔHCO_3^-.) The parallelism of changes in ΔAG and ΔHCO_3^- provides a useful screening tool for mixed acid-base disorders. If ΔAG and ΔHCO_3^- are substantially different, a mixed acid-base disorder should be suspected. When the ΔAG exceeds the ΔHCO_3^-, a mixed disorder of high anion gap acidosis and metabolic alkalosis should be suspected. When the ΔHCO_3^- exceeds the ΔAG, a mixed disorder of high anion gap acidosis and hyperchloremic acidosis should be suspected.

Altered serum chloride concentrations can usually be attributed to changes in hydration or acid-base balance. Serum sodium and chloride concentrations parallel each other during changes in hydration. Serum sodium and chloride concentrations often diverge from one another with acid-base disorders (DuBose, 1983). Comparison of changes in serum chloride concentration with changes in serum so-

dium concentration may help detect mixed acid-base disorders. During hyperchloremic (normal anion gap) acidosis, increases in serum chloride concentration are typically not attended by similar increases in serum sodium concentration. Reduced serum chloride concentration without a proportionate reduction in serum sodium concentration is typical of metabolic alkalosis. Therefore, another useful calculation for detecting mixed acid-base disturbances is comparison of the change in serum chloride concentration against the change in serum bicarbonate concentration. In patients with hyperchloremic metabolic acidosis, ΔCl^- approximates ΔHCO_3^- (Adams and Polzin, 1989; DuBose, 1983) (see Table 2 for calculation of ΔCl^- and ΔHCO_3^-). Variations from this relationship suggest a mixed acid-base disorder. When ΔHCO_3^- exceeds ΔCl^-, a mixed disturbance of hyperchloremic acidosis and high anion gap metabolic acidosis should be suspected. When ΔCl^- exceeds ΔHCO_3^-, metabolic acidosis mixed with metabolic alkalosis should be suspected.

Changes in serum potassium concentration may prompt consideration of acid-base disorders. Serum potassium concentration typically increases with acidemia due to mineral acids, and it decreases with alkalemia. In human patients with acidemia due to mineral acids (e.g., renal failure), serum potassium increases approximately 0.6 mEq/L for each 0.10-unit decrease in blood pH; during alkalemia, these changes occur in the opposite direction (Bia and Thier, 1981; DuBose, 1983). Changes in serum potassium concentration appear to be greater with metabolic disorders than with respiratory disorders (Bia and Thier, 1981). Changes in serum potassium concentrations are less predictable in cases of acidemia resulting from organic acids (e.g., lactic aci-

Table 3. Compensatory Responses for Primary Acid-Base Disturbances*

Disturbance	Primary Change	Compensatory Response	Limits of Compensation
Metabolic Acidosis			
Human	For each 1 mEq/L $\downarrow$ in HCO_3^-	Pa_{CO_2} $\downarrow$ by 1.2 mm Hg	10 mmHg
Canine	For each 1 mEq/L $\downarrow$ in HCO_3^-	Pa_{CO_2} $\downarrow$ by 0.7–0.9 mm Hg	?
Metabolic Alkalosis			
Human	For each 1 mEq/L $\uparrow$ in HCO_3^-	Pa_{CO_2} $\uparrow$ by 0.6–0.7 mm Hg	55 mm Hg
Canine	For each 1 mEq/L $\uparrow$ in HCO_3^-	Pa_{CO_2} $\uparrow$ by 0.7 mm Hg	?
Acute Respiratory Acidosis			
Human	For each 1 mm Hg $\uparrow$ in Pa_{CO_2}	HCO_3^- $\uparrow$ by 0.1 mEq/L	30 mEq/L
Canine	For each 1 mm Hg $\uparrow$ in Pa_{CO_2}	HCO_3^- $\uparrow$ by 0.15 mEq/L	?
Chronic Respiratory Acidosis			
Human	For each 1 mm Hg $\uparrow$ in Pa_{CO_2}	HCO_3^- $\uparrow$ by 0.35 mEq/L	45 mEq/L
Canine	For each 1 mm Hg $\uparrow$ in Pa_{CO_2}	HCO_3^- $\uparrow$ by 0.34–0.39 mEq/L	?
Acute Respiratory Alkalosis			
Human	For each 1 mm Hg $\downarrow$ in Pa_{CO_2}	HCO_3^- $\downarrow$ by 0.2 mEq/L	18 mEq/L
Canine	For each 1 mm Hg $\downarrow$ in Pa_{CO_2}	HCO_3^- $\downarrow$ by 0.2 mEq/L	?
Chronic Respiratory Alkalosis			
Human	For each 1 mm Hg $\downarrow$ in Pa_{CO_2}	HCO_3^- $\downarrow$ by 0.5 mEq/L	12–15 mEq/L
Canine	For each 1 mm Hg $\downarrow$ in Pa_{CO_2}	HCO_3^- $\downarrow$ by 0.55 mEq/L	?

*Modified with permission from Adams, L. G., and Polzin, D. J.: Mixed acid-base disorders. Vet. Clin. North Am. Small Anim. Pract. 19:307, 1989.
HCO_3^-, serum bicarbonate concentration; Pa_{CO_2}, arterial carbon dioxide pressure.

dosis and ketoacidosis), and in cases of diseases associated with potassium depletion (e.g., renal tubular acidosis, diarrhea, and diabetes mellitus). When expected changes in serum potassium concentration do not occur, mixed acid-base disturbances should be considered.

BLOOD GAS ANALYSIS

Ideally, blood gas analysis should be performed on all patients with suspected acid-base disturbances. Arterial blood samples are preferred for blood gas analysis. The first step in evaluating blood gas data is the determination of whether the patient is acidemic, is alkalemic, or has a normal blood pH. The carbon dioxide partial pressure (PCO_2) and blood bicarbonate concentration should then be examined to determine the source of acidemia or alkalemia. If blood pH is within the normal range but PCO_2 and blood bicarbonate concentration are altered, one must determine whether the pH is to the alkaline side or to the acid side of the midpoint value in order to determine which change (PCO_2 or HCO_3^-) is the primary acid-base disorder. The data should then be examined to determine if normal physiologic compensation has occurred in response to the primary acid-base disorder. Mixed acid-base disorders are often identified through inappropriate compensatory responses to primary acid-base disorders. Expected compensatory responses for primary acid-base disorders can be estimated from information in Tables 2 and 3. If sufficient time has elapsed for compensation to develop, an inappro-

priate physiologic response suggests the likelihood of at least one additional primary acid-base disorder. For primary metabolic disorders, the appropriate compensatory PCO_2 should be calculated (see Tables 2 and 3). If measured PCO_2 differs substantially (>2 mm Hg) from calculated appropriate PCO_2, mixed metabolic and respiratory acid-base disturbance should be considered (Adams and Polzin, 1989). For primary respiratory disorders, the appropriate compensatory serum bicarbonate concentration should be calculated (see Tables 2 and 3). Estimation of the appropriate serum bicarbonate concentration requires one to ascertain from the history whether the respiratory disorder is acute or chronic. If measured serum bicarbonate concentration differs substantially (>2 mEq/L) from calculated serum bicarbonate concentration, mixed metabolic and respiratory acid-base disorders should be considered (Adams and Polzin, 1989).

Treatment

The primary goal in treatment of acid-base disorders is to minimize the physiologic impact of such disturbances. Therefore, determination of blood pH values by blood-gas analysis prior to initiation of treatment is essential. Mixed respiratory and metabolic acidosis or mixed respiratory and metabolic alkalosis causes additive changes in blood pH that may require more aggressive therapy than mixed disturbances that have neutralizing effects on blood pH. For example, blood pH may be normal or near normal in patients with mixed respiratory acidosis and metabolic alkalosis. Treatment should be directed at the underlying causes of respiratory acidosis and metabolic alkalosis in such patients. In contrast, patients with mixed metabolic and respiratory acidosis can have dangerous reductions in blood pH, requiring prompt therapy of the acid-base disorder in addition to the underlying cause.

The contribution of each acid-base disturbance to measured pH should be considered before, during, and after treatment. Anticipation of the impact of treatment and careful monitoring of the response of the patient are important. For example, in patients with mixed metabolic acidosis and respiratory alkalosis, correction of metabolic acidosis could result in unopposed respiratory alkalosis and alkalemia. Therefore, the respiratory alkalosis should be treated simultaneously.

Mixed respiratory and metabolic acidosis provides a particularly dramatic example of the potential adverse effects of inappropriate therapy. Treatment of the metabolic acidosis with sodium bicarbonate in such patients results in formation of carbonic acid, which disassociates into water and carbon dioxide. Patients with mixed metabolic and respiratory acidosis, however, cannot readily eliminate the carbon dioxide generated as a result of administration of bicarbonate. As a result, blood pH may remain unchanged, or even decline, subsequent to retention of carbon dioxide. Therefore, both metabolic and respiratory acidosis must be addressed simultaneously. A new agent for treatment of metabolic acidosis is Carbicarb (a mixture of sodium carbonate and sodium bicarbonate), which acts as a buffer without the net generation of carbon dioxide, thereby avoiding the problems with sodium bicarbonate in patients with mixed metabolic and respiratory acidosis (Bersin and Arieff, 1988; Sun et al., 1987). This product is not currently available commercially, however, and clinical use of the product in dogs or cats has not been reported.

References and Suggested Reading

Adams, L. G. and Polzin, D. J.: Mixed acid-base disorders. Vet. Clin. North Am. Sm. Anim. Pract. 19:307, 1989.
A review of etiology, diagnosis, and treatment of mixed acid-base disorders in dogs and cats, including a brief review of acid-base physiology and case examples.
Bersin, R. M., and Arieff, A.: Improved hemodynamic function during hypoxia with Carbicarb, a new agent for the management of acidosis. Circulation 77:227, 1988.
A study comparing carbicarb and sodium bicarbonate for treatment of induced hypoxic lactic acidosis in dogs.
Bia, M., and Thier, S. O.: Mixed acid-base disturbances: A clinical approach. Med. Clin. North Am. 65:347, 1981.
A review of a clinical approach to diagnosis and treatment of mixed acid-base disorders in humans.
DuBose, T. D.: Clinical approach to patients with acid-base disorders. Med. Clin. North Am. 67:799, 1983.
A review of etiology and diagnosis of simple and mixed acid-base disorders in humans.
Hardy, R. M., and Robinson, E. P.: Treatment of alkalosis. *In* Kirk, R. W. (ed.): *Current Veterinary Therapy IX.* Philadelphia: W. B. Saunders, 1986, p. 67.
A review of pathophysiology, diagnosis, and treatment of metabolic and respiratory alkalosis in dogs and cats, including case examples.
Muir, W. W.: Acid-base and electrolyte disturbances in dogs with gastric dilatation–volvulus. J.A.V.M.A. 181:229, 1982.
A prospective study of acid-base and electrolyte disturbances in dogs with gastric dilatation–volvulus.
Polzin, D. J., and Osborne, C. A.: Anion gap—diagnostic and therapeutic applications. *In* Kirk, R. W. (ed.): *Current Veterinary Therapy IX.* Philadelphia: W. B. Saunders, 1986, p. 52.
A review of clinical application of the anion gap in diagnosis of simple and mixed acid-base disorders in dogs and cats, including case examples.
Sun, J. H., Filley, G. F., Hord, K., et al.: Carbicarb: An effective substitute for $NaHCO_3$ for the treatment of acidosis. Surgery 102:835, 1987.
A study comparing Carbicarb and sodium bicarbonate for treatment of induced mixed metabolic and respiratory acidosis in rats.

RECENT ADVANCES IN INJECTABLE CHEMICAL RESTRAINT

RICHARD M. BEDNARSKI
Columbus, Ohio

Chemical restraint is often essential for many diagnostic and therapeutic procedures for small animals, because these animals can be fractious and uncooperative. Chemical restraint is even needed for seemingly docile animals that require procedures producing discomfort or pain, or procedures requiring lack of motion. The clinician should be familiar with several different restraint regimens because no one regimen is suitable for all animals or all situations. Familiarity with the pharmacody-

Table 1. Drugs and Manufacturers

Generic Drug(s)	Proprietary Drug	Manufacturer
Acepromazine maleate	Promace	Fort Dodge
Atipamezole	—	—
Buprenorphine hydrochloride	Buprenex	Norwich Eaton
Butorphanol tartrate	Torbugesic (10 mg/ml)	Fort Dodge
	Stadol (2 mg/ml)	Bristol Labs
	Torbutrol (0.5 mg/ml)	Fort Dodge
Diazepam	Valium	Roche-Products
	Diazepam	Elkins-Sinn (Multi-Source Products)
Fentanyl/droperidol	Innovar-Vet	Pitman-Moore
Ketamine hydrochloride	Ketaset	Fort Dodge
	Vetalar	Fort Dodge
Midazolam hydrochloride	Versed	Roche
Morphine sulfate	Morphine Sulfate Injection	Lilly
		Elkins-Sinn
		Wyeth-Ayerst
Nalmefene	Nalmefene	Key Pharmaceuticals
Naloxone hydrochloride	P/M Naloxone	Pitman-Moore
	Narcan	DuPont
Oxymorphone hydrochloride	P/M Oxymorphone	Pitman-Moore
	Numorphan	DuPont
Tiletamine hydrochloride/zolazepam hydrochloride	Telazol	A. H. Robins
Xylazine hydrochloride	Rompun	Haver
Yohimbine	Yobine	Lloyd Laboratories

namics of the restraint drugs allows the clinician to differentiate drug effects from disease effects. This chapter focuses on relatively new and useful techniques for short-term (<1-hr) chemical restraint of dogs and cats undergoing diagnostic or therapeutic procedures. Some chemical restraint drugs may be used alone, while others are more effective in combination. Combinations of two or more drugs are popular because of the theory that relatively small doses of two or more drugs synergize their desirable qualities and minimize their undesirable cardiopulmonary or central nervous system (CNS) effects observed when a "high" dose of only one drug is administered. Drugs and manufacturers are listed in Table 1.

SEDATIVES AND TRANQUILIZERS

Acepromazine Maleate

Acepromazine maleate is one of the most commonly used tranquilizers in veterinary medicine. It acts within the CNS at the thalamus, reticular formation, and brainstem and inhibits the neurotransmitters dopamine and norepinephrine. The CNS effects of acepromazine are fairly predictable; when used alone, acepromazine is excellent for calming nervous animals and reducing aggressive behavior. Acepromazine is commonly combined with opioids to produce short-term immobilization. Acepromazine is antiemetic, antihistaminic, and antidysrhythmic. It is an alpha-1 adrenergic receptor antagonist inducing dose-dependent vasodilation, which typically lowers blood pressure. Hypotension

can be induced with relatively low doses of acepromazine in dehydrated or hypovolemic animals (Table 2). This dose-related hypotension is not always predictable; 10 to 20 times the recommended dosage may not induce hypotension in healthy animals. Acepromazine-induced hypotension is readily reversible with infusion of a balanced electrolyte solution such as lactated Ringer's solution (20 to 80 ml/kg). Rarely, the alpha-1 agonist phenylephrine may be necessary to reverse the hypotension. Centrally induced bradycardia occurs occasionally, but heart rate typically is unchanged or is slightly lowered because of the calming effect of the drug. Heart rate can also increase as a reflex reaction to lowered blood pressure. Acepromazine causes a decrease in packed cell volume (PCV) as a result of sequestration of red cells in the spleen. It decreases platelet aggregation. Acepromazine is contraindicated in patients with epilepsy or other organically based seizure activity, but can attenuate drug-induced seizures (e.g., ketamine-induced seizures in dogs).

Alpha-2 Agonists—Xylazine Hydrochloride and Medetomidine

Medetomidine is not currently approved for use in the United States; however, its properties are similar to those of xylazine hydrochloride. Alpha-2 adrenergic receptor agonists act centrally by decreasing presynaptic release of, and blocking postsynaptic effects of, norepinephrine. Xylazine and medetomidine induce dose-dependent sedation,

Table 2. *Sedatives and Tranquilizers*

Drug	Dosage (mg/kg)*	Comments
Acepromazine maleate	0.025–0.2 IV, IM, SC (3–4 mg maximum)	Mild to moderate sedation of 1- to 2-hr duration.
Xylazine hydrochloride	0.3–2.2 IV, IM	Moderate to deep sedation, analgesia; 20 min to 1 hr.
Medetomidine	0.01–0.08 IV, IM	Similar effects to xylazine but 1- to 3-hr duration.
Diazepam	0.2–0.4 IV	Most useful when combined with other sedatives, opioids, or ketamine.
Midazolam hydrochloride	0.1–0.3 IV, IM, SC	Similar to diazepam but also useful by IM or SC route.

*In general, low dosages are used when these drugs are administered intravenously, and when they are given by any route to sick or debilitated patients.

muscle relaxation, and analgesia that can be profound at high dosages. The sedation can, however, be overridden; some dogs become aggressive upon arousal. Xylazine hydrochloride induces emesis in approximately 25% of dogs. In cats, it is an effective emetic, with the dose of 0.5 mg/kg IM producing emesis in most cats. Aerophagia can occur with subsequent bloating and respiratory compromise. Xylazine is associated with impaired thermoregulation for up to 12 h after cessation of sedation. Therefore, animals receiving the drug should not be exposed to extreme environmental temperatures. The alpha-2 agonists induce bradycardia and transient vasoconstriction. Cardiac output decreases, and the initial hypertension is replaced by hypotension. Bradycardia is reversible with an anticholinergic such as glycopyrrolate or atropine; however, such agents do not completely reverse the depression in cardiac output. Xylazine in low dosages is the sedative of choice for intradermal skin testing because it minimally interferes with the wheal-and-flare response. It is also the sedative of choice for performing cystometry because it minimally interferes with the detrusor reflex. Because of their receptor-specific mechanism of action, the effects of the alpha-2 agonists can be effectively antagonized by alpha-2 receptor antagonists (yohimbine, tolazoline, and atipamezole). Alpha-2 antagonists are effective in reversing all depressant effects attributable to stimulation of the alpha-2 receptor (see this volume, p. 194).

Benzodiazepines—Diazepam and Midazolam Hydrochloride

The benzodiazepines are not good sedatives for dogs and cats. Used alone, they are not suitable for chemical restraint except in sick or debilitated animals. They may be combined with opioids to produce moderate restraint, or with ketamine hydrochloride for short-term immobilization. The benzodiazepine-opioid combinations work well in geriatric or debilitated patients, whereas their effect in young healthy animals is unpredictable. Benzo-diazepine-opioid combinations produce less sedation and are shorter acting than acepromazine combined with the same opioid. Midazolam hydrochloride and diazepam are similarly acting drugs except that midazolam is slightly more potent. Midazolam is water-soluble and is suitable for intramuscular or subcutaneous administration; diazepam should be administered intravenously because it has a propylene glycol base and its absorption from the muscle is unpredictable. The benzodiazepines produce minimal cardiorespiratory depression and are therefore useful in compromised patients. Both drugs are effective appetite stimulants.

OPIOIDS AND NEUROLEPTANALGESICS

Opioids are excellent analgesics, but poor to moderate sedatives and muscle relaxants (Table 3). Opioid effects are due to activation of one or more endogenous opioid receptors within the central and peripheral nervous systems. In general, the opioid agonists, such as oxymorphone hydrochloride and morphine sulfate, induce excitement at higher dosages, particularly in the cat—an effect probably related to stimulation of opioid sigma-receptors. The most notable cardiovascular effect of the opioids, with the exception of meperidine hydrochloride, is bradycardia. This effect results from an increase in parasympathetic tone and is therefore readily reversible with anticholinergic agents. Even in patients with a compromised cardiovascular system, opioids such as oxymorphone minimally depress cardiac function, however, the opioid agonist meperidine does decrease cardiac contractility. Meperidine and morphine release histamine from mast cells and induce vasodilation; therefore, they should not be administered intravenously. Opioids induce dose-dependent respiratory depression, which is augmented by concurrent use of other anesthetic drugs. Because opioids obtund the cough reflex, they are not recommended for sedation during transtracheal lavage. Some opioids, such as butorphanol tartrate and buprenorphine hydrochloride, are agonists at some receptors and antagonists at

Table 3. *Opioids and Neuroleptanalgesics**

Drug(s)	Dosage (mg/kg)	Comments
Oxymorphone hydrochloride	0.05–0.1 IV, IM, SC	Excitement produced when used alone in young healthy dogs. Analgesia lasts 1 to 4 hr.
Morphine sulfate	0.2–0.6 IM, SC	Mild sedation produced when used alone. Analgesia lasts 1 to 4 hr.
Butorphanol tartrate	0.2–0.4 IV, IM, SC	Minimal sedation produced when used alone. Analgesia lasts 1 to 3 hr.
Fentanyl/droperidol (Innovar-Vet, Pitman-Moore)	1 ml/10–30 kg IV, IM	Excellent for aggressive dogs. Dose-dependent sedation produced, lasting 30 min to 1 hr.
Acepromazine maleate/oxymorphone hydrochloride	0.01/0.05–0.1 IV, IM	Can be combined in same syringe. Sedation lasts 15 min to 1 hr.
Acepromazine maleate/butorphanol tartrate	0.01/0.2 IV, IM	Can be combined in same syringe. Sedation lasts 15 min to 1 hr.
Acepromazine maleate/buprenorphine hydrochloride	0.03/0.0075–0.01 IV	Can be combined in same syringe. Moderate sedation lasts 2 to 3 hr.
Midazolam hydrochloride/oxymorphone hydrochloride	0.1–0.2/0.05–0.1 IV, IM	Can be combined in same syringe. Sedation lasts 15 to 40 min.
Midazolam hydrochloride/butorphanol tartrate	0.1–0.2/0.2 IV, IM	Can be combined in same syringe. Sedation lasts 15 to 40 min.

*In cats, lower-range dosages of opioids should be used.

others. The opioid agonist-antagonists produce less respiratory depression, and there is a ceiling on their respiratory depressant effects; higher doses are not associated with further increases in respiratory depression. The agonist-antagonists have low potential for addiction, and their purchase and use are therefore not subject to governmental regulation. Opioids often induce emesis several minutes following administration. They also induce gastrointestinal (GI) stasis, which is usually preceded by evacuation of the colon. This can be bothersome when performing procedures such as proctoscopy.

Opioids may be combined with acepromazine or the benzodiazepines to produce a state of analgesia, sedation, and muscle relaxation termed neuroleptanalgesia. Different combinations produce various degrees and durations of sedation, immobilization, and muscle relaxation. In general, benzodiazepine-opioid combinations produce less profound and shorter-acting effects than do acepromazine-opioid combinations. Neuroleptanalgesics are useful in the cat, provided that large opioid dosages are avoided.

The effects of opioids can be antagonized. Opioid agonists such as naloxone hydrochloride and nalmefene effectively reverse all opioid effects. Nal-

mefene has a relatively long duration of action but is not available for use in the United States.

CYCLOHEXYLAMINES AND COMBINATIONS

Ketamine hydrochloride

Ketamine hydrochloride is combined with other sedatives and tranquilizers for short-term immobilization because it induces poor muscle relaxation in dogs and cats as well as seizures in dogs (Table 4). In cats and in sick or debilitated dogs, relatively small dosages of ketamine, used alone, are useful for short-term immobilization. Notable effects of ketamine include increased salivation, maintenance of the swallowing reflex, minimal respiratory depression with occasional apneustic breathing, and eyes that remain open and require protection with a bland ocular lubricant. Ketamine supports cardiovascular function with increases in blood pressure, heart rate, and cardiac output in healthy animals. The increase in blood pressure and heart rate, however, may be detrimental in those patients with heart disease because of the associated increase in

Table 4. *Cyclohexylamines and Cyclohexylamine Combinations*

Drug(s)	Dosage (mg/kg)	Comments
Ketamine hydrochloride	2.0–10 IV, IM	Not useful when used alone in dogs. Useful restraint lasts 5 to 30 min.
Ketamine hydrochloride/diazepam or Ketamine hydrochloride/Midazolam hydrochloride	5.5/0.28 IV; (equivalent to 1 ml/9 kg of a 1/1 (v/v) mixture)	Diazepam and midazolam are equally effective in this combination. Useful restraint lasts 5 to 10 min.
Tiletamine hydrochloride/zolazepam hydrochloride (Telazol, A. H. Robins)	2.0–8.0 IV, IM	Limited shelf life after reconstitution. Useful restraint lasts 20 min to 1 hr.

v/v, volume of solute per volume of solution.

myocardial oxygen consumption. Ketamine is contraindicated in patients with head trauma, and in those with intracranial masses because it increases intracranial pressure.

Tiletamine Hydrochloride/Zolazepam Hydrochloride

Tiletamine hydrochloride/zolazepam hydrochloride (Telazol, A.H. Robbins) is a 1:1 (v/v) combination of tiletamine, a cyclohexylamine, and zolazepam, a benzodiazepine. The pharmacologic profile of tiletamine is similar to that of ketamine. Cardiovascular and respiratory function are fairly well maintained. Muscle relaxation is fair to good and comparable to that obtained with a ketamine/xylazine combination. Analgesia and sedation are more profound at higher doses. Because of its relatively mild cardiopulmonary effects, tiletamine/zolazepam can be useful for immobilization of intermediate duration in patients with cardiovascular disease. Notable side effects of tiletamine/zolazepam are prolonged recovery (hours) in cats and rough recovery in dogs, characterized by paddling and vocalization. These effects occur unpredictably, even after administration of small dosages. There is some evidence that the benzodiazepine antagonist flumazenil reduces these recovery-related side effects.

RECOMMENDATIONS

The choice of chemical restraint depends on the physical status of the patient, the duration and degree of immobilization required (see Tables 2 through 4), and the type of procedure to be performed. Short (<10-min) immobilization is accomplished with diazepam/ketamine or with one of the ultra–short-acting barbiturates (see *CVT X*, p. 63). Longer durations of sedation are accomplished with an alpha-2 agonist in healthy animals, with tiletam-ine-zolazepam, or with neuroleptanalgesia. Use of alpha-2 agonists should be avoided in animals with cardiovascular dysfunction (congestive heart failure or cardiomyopathy). Older animals and those that are sick and debilitated respond well to the benzodiazepine/opioid combinations. More profound neuroleptanalgesia is achieved with droperidol/fentanyl, or with acepromazine combined with oxymorphone, butorphanol, or buprenorphine. Droperidol/fentanyl and the acepromazine/opioid combinations produce good muscle relaxation for procedures such as ultrasonography. An advantage of using alpha-2 agonists or opioid combinations is the ability of specific receptor antagonists to reverse agonist action (Table 5). Relatively long-acting drugs such as the alpha-2 agonist medetomidine and the opioids oxymorphone and buprenorphine may require repeated antagonist administration because the antagonist half-life is shorter than that of the agonist. Nalmefene, an opioid antagonist, has a relatively long half-life and does not require repeated administration.

References and Suggested Reading

Bednarski, R. M., Muir, W. W., and Tracy, C. H.: The effects of tolazoline, doxapram, and Ro 15-1788 on the depressant action of Telazol. Vet. Med. 84:1016, 1989.
  A description of tiletamine/zolazepam anesthesia in the dog and cat and partial reversal with flumazenil (Ro 15-1788).
Copeland, V. S., Haskins, S. C., and Patz, J. D.: Oxymorphone: Cardiovascular, pulmonary, and behavioral effects in dogs. Am. J. Vet. Res. 48:1626, 1987.
  A description of behavioral and cardiopulmonary effects of oxymorphone in healthy dogs.
Dyson, D. H., Doherty, T., Anderson, G. I., et al.: Reversal of oxymorphone sedation by naloxone, nalmefene, and butorphanol. Vet. Surg. 19:398, 1990.
  A comparison of three different opioid reversal techniques in oxymorphone-sedated dogs.
Grandy, J. L., and Heath, R. B.: Cardiopulmonary and behavioral effects of fentanyl-droperidol in cats. J.A.V.M.A. 191:59, 1987.
  Description of fentanyl-droperidol (Innovar Vet, Pitman-Moore) in cats.
Haskins, S. C., and Patz, J. D.: Ketamine in hypovolemic dogs. Critical Care 18:625, 1990.
  A description of cardiopulmonary effects of ketamine given to dogs with hemorrhagic hypovolemia.
Ilkew, J. E., Suter, C., McNeal, D., et al.: Behavioral effects of midazolam following intravenous and intramuscular administration in healthy awake cats. Proceedings of the American College of Veterinary Anesthesiologists, Las Vegas, NV, 1990, p. 17.
  A description of the behavioral effects of midazolam in healthy cats.
Muir, W. W., Hubbell, J. A., and Skarda, R. T. (eds.): Handbook of Veterinary Anesthesia. St. Louis: C. V. Mosby, 1989.
  A reference source for sedation, neuroleptanalgesia, and other anesthetic techniques in domestic and exotic species.
Vähä-Vahe, A. T.: The clinical effectiveness of atipamezole as a medetomidine antagonist in the dog. J. Vet. Pharmacol. Ther. 13:198, 1990.
  Effectiveness of the alpha-2 agonist atipamezole for reversal of medetomidine sedation.
Vainio O, Vähä-Vahe, T., and Palmu, L.: Sedative and analgesic effects of medetomidine in dogs. J. Vet. Pharmacol. Ther. 12:225, 1989.
  Description of the sedative and analgesic effects of different dosages of medetomidine in dogs and comparison of medetomidine with xylazine.

Table 5. Antagonists

Drug	Dosage (mg/kg)
Alpha-2	
Yohimbine	0.1 IV, IM
Atipamezole	0.4–0.6 IM
Benzodiazepine	
Flumazenil	2.0–5.0 IV
Opioid	
Naloxone hydrochloride	.003–.01 IV, IM
Nalmefene	0.03 IV, IM

USE OF NASOGASTRIC TUBES: INDICATIONS, TECHNIQUE, AND COMPLICATIONS

SARAH K. ABOOD,
and C.A. TONY BUFFINGTON
Columbus, Ohio

INDICATIONS

Nutritional support is an important part of surgical and medical therapy. When animals are unable or unwilling to eat, nutrients should be provided unless a specific contraindication is present. We use the following criteria to evaluate for malnutrition: (1) recent weight loss of greater than 10% body weight; (2) decreased food intake or anorexia lasting longer than 1 week; (3) increased nutrient losses from vomiting, diarrhea, wounds, or burns; (4) increased nutrient needs due to trauma, surgery, infection, burns, or fever; (5) chronic disease processes; and (6) low serum albumin concentrations. Three or more of these criteria are sufficient to categorize a patient as malnourished.

Nutritional support as a component of therapy in small animal patients is often initiated as an afterthought, when animals do not recover as quickly as had been expected. The nutritional status of malnourished, anorexic, or critically ill animals should not be neglected. Tube feeding is an excellent means of providing short-term metabolic and immune system support to small animal patients.

Inappetent animals with functional gastrointestinal tracts and the ability to guard their airways are candidates for nutritional support via a nasogastric tube. Placement of a nasogastric tube is a simple procedure that allows nutritional support for extended periods of time. Nasogastric tubes are indicated for administration of liquid medications or other fluids, decompression of the stomach or esophagus, and diagnostic procedures such as contrast radiography. The technique does not usually require chemical restraint of the patient.

FEEDING TUBES

Polyvinyl chloride pediatric feeding tubes (Davol, Inc., C.R. Bard, Inc., Cranston, RI) are used for dogs and cats; they are the least expensive tubes and work well for intragastric feeding (Table 1).

Because polyvinyl chloride tubes may harden if they remain in the stomachs of dogs for prolonged periods, they should be changed about every 2 weeks. Polyurethane or silicone tubes are more expensive, but they are resistant to gastric acid and may be used for extended feeding. For dogs weighing greater than 15 kg, a No. 8 Fr. × 42 inch tube is used, supported by a 0.035-inch × 120 cm angiography guidewire (USCI Division, C.R. Bard, Inc., Tewksbury, MA). For dogs weighing 5 to 15 kg, a No. 5 Fr. × 36 inch tube is used, supported by a 0.025-inch × 100 cm angiography guidewire. A No. 5 Fr. × 36 inch tube is used without a guidewire for dogs weighing 2 to 5 kg and for most cats. Cats weighing between 6 and 10 kg can tolerate a No. 8 Fr. × 36 inch tube; a guidewire is not necessary.

A drop of mineral oil is placed in the tube before insertion of the guidewire to facilitate its easy removal. The length of tube to be inserted into the stomach is determined by measuring the distance from the tip of the nose to the caudal rib margin. This length is marked with a 5-cm strip of white tape, 1.25 cm in width, which is wrapped around the tube at a 45° angle. After 1½ turns, the tape is split longitudinally and adhered to itself over the tube, providing a small "butterfly" tab (Fig. 1).

Table 1. *Selection of Nasogastric Tubes*

Animal Size	Tube Diameter and Length	Use of Guidewire
Puppies/kittens	No. 3.5 Fr. × 15 in.	No
Cats < 10 lb	No. 5 Fr. × 36 in.	No
Cats > 10 lb	No. 5 or 8 Fr. × 36 in.	No
Dogs < 15 lb	No. 5 Fr. × 36 in.	Yes*
Dogs 15–30 lb	No. 5 Fr. × 36 in. or 8 Fr. × 42 in.	Yes*
Dogs > 30 lb	No. 8 Fr. × 42 in.	Yes†

*No. 5 Fr. × 36 inch tubes require use of a 0.025 inch × 100 cm angiography guidewire (USCI Division, C. R. Bard, Inc., Tewksbury, MA).

†No. 8 Fr. × 42 inch tubes require use of a 0.035 inch × 120 cm angiography guidewire.

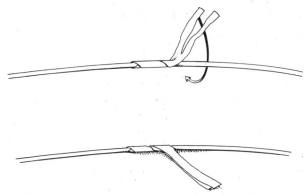

Figure 1. Schematic illustration of application of adhesive tape to a nasogastric tube, forming a "butterfly" tab. (Reprinted with permission from Abood, S. K., and Buffington, C. A.: Improved nasogastric intubation technique for nutritional support in dogs. J.A.V.M.A. 199:577, 1991.)

TECHNIQUE

Rarely is chemical restraint required for passage of a nasogastric tube, but a local anesthetic is necessary. One nostril is desensitized with a topical anesthetic, using 4 to 5 drops of 0.5 per cent proparacaine hydrochloride for cats (Ophthetic, Allergan) or 4 to 5 drops of 2 per cent lidocaine hydrochloride for dogs; then the head is tilted upward for a few seconds. Before passage, the tip of the tube should be lubricated with a water-soluble lubricant or 5% lidocaine ointment (E. Fougera & Co., Melville, NY).

To pass the tube in a cat, the animal's head is held in the normal angle of articulation, and the tip of the tube is directed in a caudoventral, medial direction (Crowe, 1986b; Ford, 1980). The tube should move with minimal resistance through the ventral meatus and oropharynx and into the esophagus. Manipulation of the external nares is not required, primarily because the anatomy of the head and skull does not vary among cats as it does in dogs.

Previously described techniques for nasogastric intubation of dogs have been difficult to perform because of their long, narrow nasal passages and extensive turbinate structures (Buffington, 1984; Crowe, 1986a & 1986b). We have developed a new technique that ensures successful passage of nasogastric tubes in dogs (Abood and Buffington, 1991). To avoid tracheal intubation, the animal's head should be held at the normal angle of articulation. The tip of the tube is directed in a caudoventral, medial direction (below the alar fold) into the ventrolateral aspect of the external nares. As soon as the tip is 2 to 3 cm inside the nostril (at the level of the median septum on the floor of the nasal cavity), the external nares are pushed dorsally (Fig. 2). This maneuver opens the ventral meatus and guides the tube into the oropharynx. Directing the tube below the alar fold while elevating the nasal planum increases the success rate of intubation, because this maneuver opens the ventral, and closes the dorsal, meatus.

Once the tube is passed to the level of the attached "butterfly" tape (see Fig. 1), the stylet or guidewire is removed, and the position of the tube in the stomach is confirmed. Placement is assessed by infusion of 3 to 5 ml of sterile physiologic solution through the tube. The animal is observed for coughing or gagging; if no reaction results, a small bolus of air (6 to 12 ml) is injected through the tube during auscultation for borborygmus in the cranial abdomen (the stethoscope is placed over the xiphoid). If any doubt exists about the location of the tube, survey lateral radiography may be used to evaluate its position because most nasogastric tubes are radiopaque. Alternatively, 1 ml of radiopaque dye (Novopaque, E-Z-EM, Inc., Westbury, NY) may be inserted into the tube prior to radiography.

Following confirmation of the tube's position, the tube is secured in place with either suture (3-0 Dermalon, Cyanamid, Montreal, Quebec) or glue (Super Glue, Loctite Corporation, Cleveland, OH).

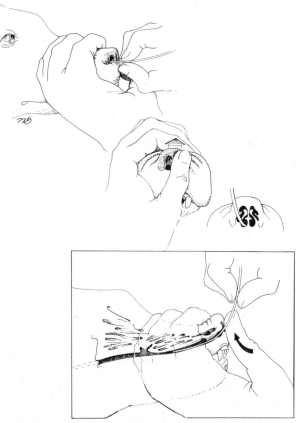

Figure 2. Schematic illustration of insertion of a nasogastric tube into the nostril of a dog. (Reprinted with permission from Abood, S. K., and Buffington, C. A.: Improved nasogastric intubation technique for nutritional support in dogs. J.A.V.M.A. 199:577, 1991.)

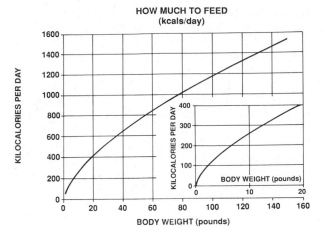

HOW MUCH TO FEED
(kcals/day)

Figure 3. Graph facilitating determination of canine and feline basal energy requirements. (Reprinted with permission from Abood, S. K., and Buffington, C. A.: Improved nasogastric intubation technique for nutritional support in dogs. J.A.V.M.A. 199:577, 1991.)

To meet basal needs: use graph

To meet needs of stress:
  1. mild stress   25% increase
  2. moderate stress   50% increase
  3. severe stress   100% increase

The tape tab that served as a marker for length can be sutured or glued to the skin, as close to the nostril as possible. Only 1 to 2 drops of glue are needed on the tape; once the glue is applied, the tape should be held to the skin. A second tape tab should be secured to the skin on the dorsal nasal midline (just between the eyes), again using suture or glue. In cats, and in some brachycephalic dogs, it may be easier to secure the second tape tab to the ipsilateral cheek or jowl. In these instances, suturing should be avoided; glue should be used. An Elizabethan collar or bucket should be placed on all patients to prevent inadvertent removal of the tube. During removal of tape tabs that have been glued, the glue should be *gently* teased away from hair with a scalpel blade.

COMPLICATIONS OF NASOGASTRIC TUBE PLACEMENT

Common complications of nasogastric tube placement include epistaxis, tracheal intubation, accidental tube removal by sneezing or vomiting, and lack of tolerance of the procedure requiring chemical restraint (Crowe, 1986a). Since instituting the technique described, we have not observed epistaxis in intubated patients. Tracheal intubation has occasionally occurred, but it has been identified by radiography and remedied before liquid feedings were begun. Displacement of the nasogastric tube out of the stomach due to sneezing, coughing, or

vomiting occurs occasionally. In this situation, the tubes are replaced, and the patient is reassessed. Feeding schedules continue uninterrupted in most of these patients. Animals are rarely unable to tolerate this procedure; only two patients (out of more than 60) required chemical restraint for nasogastric intubation in the past year.

FEEDING PROTOCOL

Feedings are initiated at rates calculated to achieve basal energy needs in the first 24 hr. Daily caloric needs are estimated by calculating the basal energy expenditure (BEE) (Abrams, 1977) (Fig. 3): BEE = 97 × body weight (kg)$^{0.655}$ According to the number and severity of clinical problems, basal energy needs are multiplied by 1.25, 1.5, or 2.0, as determined by an empirical assessment of the degree of stress (mild, moderate, or severe). Diets are fed full-strength (not diluted) on continuous (pump-infusion) or bolus (every 4 to 6 hr) feeding schedules. Advancement to higher goals (e.g., BEE × 1.5) is accomplished over another 24 to 48 hr. Animals with nasogastric feeding tubes in place should be offered fresh food before each bolus feeding, or periodically throughout the day if fed continuously.

Table 2 lists criteria used to monitor the feeding protocol. Patients should be weighed daily. The position of the tube should be checked at least once a day during continuous feeding and before each feeding during bolus feeding, by injection of 3 to 5 ml of water through the tube. Coughing or gagging should result if the tube is malpositioned. Flushing a small amount of water through the nasogastric tube before and after each bolus feeding clears it of residual food. The nasogastric tube should remain capped when not in use to prevent air from entering and filling the stomach. Blood glucose concentrations initially should be checked two to four times daily because of the high carbohydrate content of some liquid diets. To monitor the patient's nutritional status, we check daily body weight, serum albumin and total protein concentrations, urine and fecal output, and appetite for food and water. Although exceptions are encountered, most animals

Table 2. *Monitoring Protocol for Tube Feedings*

1. Weigh patient daily.
2. Check position of tubes during continuous feeding at least once a day, and check tubes before bolus feeding.
3. Check urine glucose (or blood glucose) concentrations 2 to 4 times daily initally, because of high carbohydrate content of some diets.
4. Perform other laboratory determinations as necessary (see text).

begin to eat even with the nasogastric tube in place. When the animal begins to eat half of its basal energy requirements (expressed in kilocalories per day), the amount of liquid diet can be decreased, and the patient can be weaned onto its normal diet. The goal of nutritional support is to bring the animal to a point at which it is eating the food it regularly eats in its own home.

The sizes of pediatric tubes that we use for nasogastric intubation and feeding require the use of liquid diets. Canned or prepared foods that are diluted and blended invariably clog the tube. Many types of liquid diets for enteral nutritional support of human patients are commercially available. There are also products recently made available for use in dogs and cats (Clinical Care Canine, Clinical Care Feline) (Pet-Ag., Inc., Elgin, IL). Criteria for choosing enteral diets for small animals include the nutrient profile, cost and availability of the product, ease of storage, and clinical response. In our hospital, we use commercial diets manufactured locally; they are easy to store and are well tolerated by our patients. The protein content of most liquid diets represents 17 to 22% of the total calories, which is adequate for most dogs (Schaeffer et al., 1989). For dogs with increased protein loss (or need), and for all cats, the protein content is too low. We routinely supplement this diet with a powdered whey protein (ProMod, Ross Laboratories, Columbus OH); 5 g of ProMod is added to 250 ml of liquid diet. Because cats have a relatively high requirement for arginine, 1 mg/kcal of arginine is added to their diets. Arginine can be purchased from hospital pharmacies, biochemical supply companies, or health-food stores. Recently, a high-protein liquid diet for human patients has been introduced that provides an amount of arginine (3 gm per can) adequate for cats (Impact, Sandoz, Minneapolis, MN); we do not add anything to this liquid diet when feeding it to our small animal patients.

COMPLICATIONS OF NASOGASTRIC TUBE FEEDING

Complications of tube feedings include obstruction or clogging, aspiration, vomiting, bloating, diarrhea, hyperglycemia and glucosuria, and hyperosmolar coma (Table 3). In our small animal intensive care unit, we closely monitor patients with nasogas-

Table 3. Complications of Nasogastric Tube Feeding

Problem	Treatment
Tube blocked	Flush with water.
	Replace tube if necessary.
Aspiration of stomach contents	Stop feeding.
Vomiting or bloating	Reduce flow rate or stop feeding.
Diarrhea	Reduce flow rate.
	Add fat or fiber.
	Dilute solution with water.
	Add antidiarrheal drug.
Hyperglycemia and glucosuria	Reduce flow rate.
	Administer insulin.
Hyperosmolar coma	Stop feeding.

tric tubes for vomiting, accidental tube removal, and the potential for aspiration or diarrhea. Placement of an Elizabethan collar almost always prevents animals from pulling out the tubes. Occasionally, however, an animal is able to cough or vomit up a nasogastric tube and bite through it. Vomiting is often associated with improper bolus feeding and usually resolves with adherence to the feeding protocol. Diarrhea can be managed by switching to a liquid diet with either a high-fat content (Pulmocare, Ross Laboratories, Columbus, OH) or a high-fiber content (Jevity, Ross Laboratories, Columbus, OH). In human hospitals, feeding tubes become blocked when medications in pill form are crushed and administered through the tube. We recommend that only liquids (diet formulas, fluids such as saline or lactated Ringer's solution, and liquid medications) be introduced into feeding tubes.

References and Suggested Reading

Abood, S. K., and Buffington, C. A.: Improved nasogastric intubation technique for nutritional support in dogs. J.A.V.M.A. 199:577, 1991.

Abrams, J. T.: The nutrition of the dog. *In* Rechcigl, M. (ed.): *CRC Handbook.* W. Palm Beach, FL: CRC Press, 1977, p. 1.

Buffington, C. A.: Anorexia. *In* Morris, M. (ed.): *Small Animal Clinical Nutrition,* 2nd ed. Topeka, KS: Mark Morris Associates, 1984, p. 1.

Crowe, D. T.: Clinical use of an indwelling nasogastric tube for enteral nutrition and fluid therapy in the dog and cat. J.A.A.H.A. 22:675, 1986a.

Crowe, D. T.: Enteral nutrition for critically ill or injured patients—part 1. Compendium 8:603, 1986b.

Ford, R. B.: Nasogastric intubation in the cat. Compendium 1:29, 1980.

Schaeffer, M. C., Rogers, Q. R., and Morris, J. G.: Protein in the nutrition of dogs and cats. *In* Burger, I. H. and Rivers, J. P. W. (eds.): *Nutrition of the Dog and Cat.* Cambridge: Cambridge University Press, 1989, p. 159.

THERAPEUTIC INDICATIONS
FOR DIETARY LIPIDS

KAREN L. CAMPBELL

Urbana, Illinois

The importance of dietary fatty acids for growth, reproduction, and maintenance of healthy skin was recognized more than 60 years ago. More recently, fatty acids have been shown to have important roles in inflammation and immune regulation. Veterinary pharmaceutical companies are now marketing various fatty acid combinations* as nutritional supplements to aid in the maintenance of healthy skin and in the management of inflammatory diseases of animals.

FATTY ACID METABOLISM

Fatty acids have a hydrocarbon "backbone" with a carboxyl acid group at one end and a methyl group at the other end. Unsaturated fatty acids contain one or more double bonds; the location of the double bonds is designated by counting back from the terminal methyl group. Additional double bonds are separated from the first by a single methylene group. If the first double bond is at the third carbon, the fatty acid belongs to the omega-3 (ω3) series; if the first double bond is at the sixth carbon, the fatty acid belongs to the omega-6 (ω6) series; and so forth. Naturally occurring fatty acids are in the ω3, ω6, ω7, and ω9 series.

Animals cannot synthesize ω3 and ω6 fatty acids *de novo*. In addition, animals lack enzymes to catalyze desaturations toward the methyl end. Consequently, animals *cannot* change one series of fatty acids to another. Fatty acids of the ω3 and ω6 series must exist in the diet to prevent clinical signs of fatty acid deficiency (i.e., they are essential fatty acids for animals).

Animals can elongate and desaturate fatty acids toward the carboxyl end (Fig. 1). The desaturase enzymes have the greatest affinity for ω3 fatty acids, a moderate affinity for ω6 fatty acids, and the least affinity for ω9 fatty acids. Thus, increasing the proportion of ω3 fatty acids in the diet decreases the metabolism of ω6 and ω9 fatty acids.

*Such products include DVM Derm Caps (DVM Pharmaceuticals, Inc., Miami, FL), Efamol Vet (Vet Kem, Division of Zoecon Corp., Dallas, TX), and Efa-Z Liquid (Allerderm, Inc., Hurst, TX).

FUNCTIONS OF FATTY ACIDS

Clinical signs associated with a dietary deficiency of ω3 and ω6 fatty acids include poor growth rates, weight loss, failure of ovulation and lactation, testicular degeneration, increased permeability of the skin and cell membranes, poor wound healing, increased susceptibility to infections, hair loss, and scaly dermatitis with hyperkeratosis and increased deoxyribonucleic acid (DNA) synthesis by keratinocytes.

Diets in which 1% or more of the calories are derived from linoleic acid and 0.3% of the calories are derived from arachidonic acid prevent clinical signs of essential fatty acid deficiency in normal dogs and cats. Improvements in skin and hair coat condition, growth, and feed efficiency occur when 2 to 3% of energy in the diet is derived from linoleic acid. Most commercial pet foods contain adequate levels of the essential fatty acids. To avoid oxidation of fatty acids, diets should not be stored longer than 6 months prior to feeding.

Fatty acids are incorporated into cell membrane phospholipids. These fatty acids maintain the integrity, fluidity, and permeability of cells. Three 20-carbon polyunsaturated fatty acids are found in cell membrane phospholipids: dihomo-γ-linolenic acid (ω6 series), arachidonic acid (ω6 series) and eicosapentanenoic acid (ω3 series). These 20-carbon polyunsaturated fatty acids are substrates for production of eicosanoids.

BIOSYNTHESIS AND FUNCTIONS OF EICOSANOIDS

Eicosanoids are produced in response to physical stimuli (e.g., trauma) or chemical stimuli (e.g., hormones). The first step in production of eicosanoids is the hydrolysis of polyunsaturated fatty acids from cell membranes. This hydrolysis is catalyzed by phospholipase A_2 or phospholipase C and diglyceride lipase. The liberated polyunsaturated fatty acid is then metabolized into the eicosanoids by either the cyclo-oxygenase or the lipoxygenase pathways. Dihomo-γ-linolenic acid is metabolized into the 1-series of prostaglandins and thromboxanes; it lacks the Δ5-desaturation required for lipoxygenase

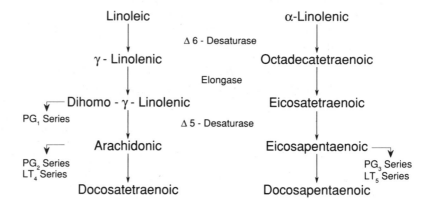

Figure 1. Metabolism of omega-3 (ω3) and omega-6 (ω6) fatty acids.

activity. Arachidonic acid is metabolized into the 2-series of prostaglandins and thromboxanes, and the 4-series of leukotrienes. Eicosapentaenoic acid is metabolized into the 3-series of prostaglandins and thromboxanes, and the 5-series of leukotrienes.

Eicosanoids are autacoids or local hormones (i.e., they are produced close to the site at which they are to exert a biologic effect and are then rapidly metabolized). One eicosanoid frequently predominates in a tissue as a result of (1) the availability of substrates, (2) the differing eicosanoid-synthesizing enzymes present and active, and (3) the differing rates of eicosanoid synthesis and metabolism. For example, prostaglandins E_1 (PGE_1) are highest in the kidney, prostaglandins D_2 (PGD_2) are highest in the brain, prostaglandins I_2 (PGI_2) are highest in the blood vessels, and thromboxane A_2 (TXA_2), is highest in the blood platelets.

Eicosanoids have numerous important physiologic functions (Table 1). Many of the effects are mediated via cyclic nucleotides (cyclic adenosine monophosphate [cAMP] and cyclic guanosine monophosphate [cGMP]). Eicosanoids derived from arachidonic acid are potent mediators of inflammation. Actions of PGE_2 include pyrexia, hyperalgesia, enhanced neutrophil chemotaxis, histamine release, vasodilation, increased vascular permeability, and increased DNA synthesis in keratinocytes. Actions of PGD_2 include vasodilation, hyperalgesia, and neutrophil chemotaxis. TXA_2 is a potent platelet aggregator and also causes vasoconstriction. Prostacyclin I_2 causes vasodilation and inhibits platelet aggregation. Leukotrienes C_4, D_4, and E_4 increase vascular permeability and function as the "slow-reacting substances of anaphylaxis." Actions of leukotriene B_4 include increased vascular permeability; neutrophil chemotaxis, adhesion, and degranulation with superoxide generation; and increased DNA synthesis in keratinocytes. Dihomo-γ-linolenic acid is metabolized into PGE_1 which is an inhibitor of phospholipase A_2 and may decrease the release of arachidonic acid from phospholipids.

Eicosanoids derived from eicosapentaenoic acid modulate inflammatory responses. TXA_3 is a weak platelet aggregator, while PGI_3 is an effective inhibitor of platelet aggregation, producing a net effect of a decrease in clot formation and a prolongation of bleeding times. Leukotriene B_5 is only one-tenth as potent as leukotriene B_4 in neutrophil chemotaxis. Diets high in eicospentaenoic acid also reduce plasma cholesterol and triglyceride concentrations and lower blood pressure (Schoene and Fiore, 1981).

USES OF FATTY ACID SUPPLEMENTATION

The Immune System

A complex network of mechanisms are involved in regulation of humoral and cell-mediated immune responses. Alterations in fatty acid concentrations in cell membrane phospholipids may change membrane fluidity and modify the mobility of cell surface receptors. Linoleic acid and arachidonic acid inhibit *in vitro* lymphocyte transformation responses to

Table 1. *Physiologic Functions of Eicosanoids*

Control of intrarenal blood flow
Control of blood pressure
Control of vascular tone
Regulation of neurotransmission
Regulation of cell differentiation and division
Regulation of the immune response
Initiation of parturition
Acceleration of luteolysis
Bronchoconstriction
Bronchodilation
Regulation of neuromuscular activity
Control of platelet aggregation
Regulation of natriuresis
Chemotaxis, adhesion, and degranulation of leukocytes
Regulation of body temperature

mitogens. Increased dietary intake of fatty acids enhances the incidence and growth of spontaneously occurring and chemically induced tumors. Low levels of fatty acids enhance cell-mediated immune responses. The effects of dietary fatty acids on the immune system may be mediated by eicosanoids; diets with high levels of $\omega3$ fatty acids decrease production of the 2-series of prostaglandins by the liver, brain, thymus, peripheral lymphocytes, and macrophages.

The Skin

The epidermis turns over rapidly (average 21 to 22 days in dogs) and thus depends on a continual source of polyunsaturated fatty acids. Both linoleic acid and arachidonic acid are essential fatty acids for the skin. Linoleic acid is the most active fatty acid in the maintenance of the cutaneous water permeability barrier, and arachidonic acid is important in the control of epidermal proliferation. Topical fatty acids are incorporated into epidermal structural lipids. Animals consuming low-fat diets and those with disorders of fat absorption, digestion, or metabolism may benefit from topical applications of $\omega6$ fatty acids (e.g., sunflower oil, safflower oil, or commercial products containing essential fatty acids*).

Burned skin contains reduced amounts of linoleic acid, which may be responsible for the high permeability of burned skin to water and other agents. Topical applications of linoleic acid may aid in the healing of burns. Further studies are needed, however, to determine the optimum usage of topical fatty acids in the management of burns and other cutaneous wounds.

Gamma-linolenic acid may be of benefit in treating disorders associated with decreased Δ6-desaturase activity. Humans and dogs with atopy may be deficient in Δ6-desaturase activity; their serum lipids have increased levels of linoleic acid with decreased levels of gamma-linoleic acid, dihomo-γ-linolenic acid, and arachidonic acid. Results of most, but not all, studies of humans with atopy have demonstrated a dose-dependent improvement in pruritus following dietary supplementation with evening primrose oil (contains gamma-linoleic acid). Dogs with experimental hypothyroidism (following bilateral thyroidectomy) have changes in serum and cutaneous fatty acid concentrations that suggest decreased Δ6-desaturase activity. Additional diseases may be associated with abnormalities in fatty acid metabolism. Studies of fatty acid metabolism in dogs with disorders of keratinization are needed to determine which, if any, fatty acid supplement

is most effective in nutritional management of these diseases.

The $\omega3$ fatty acids are ineffective in maintaining the cutaneous water permeability barrier and thus do not function as essential fatty acids for the skin. They may be useful, however, in the treatment of inflammatory skin diseases. Treatment of idiopathic seborrhea in four dogs with a supplement containing eicosapentaenoic acid* was associated with marked improvement (Miller, 1989). The same supplement was evaluated as an adjuvant for the treatment of canine atopy in three nonblinded studies. In a study of 93 dogs, Miller (1989) reported an excellent response in 17 dogs (18.3%) and a good response in 16 dogs (17.2%). Scott and Buerger (1988) found an excellent response in 11.1% of dogs studied and a moderate improvement in another 11.1%. Lloyd (1989) reported that in 33 atopic dogs treated with a supplement containing evening primrose oil (source of linoleic acid and gamma-linolenic acid) and eicosapentaenoic acid, 18% had an excellent response, and 76% had a good response. Results of Lloyd's study suggest that the decrease in skin inflammation was due to the evening primrose oil and not to eicosapentaenoic acid (dogs supplemented with evening primrose oil alone had no further improvement when supplemented with a mixture representing a 3:1 ratio of evening primrose oil to eicosapentaenoic acid). Additional controlled, double-blind studies are needed to determine the effectiveness of evening primrose oil and eicosapentaenoic acid in the management of atopy in dogs and cats.

Arthritis

Eicosanoids may function as primary mediators of inflammatory joint disease. Eicosanoids (e.g., PGE_2 leukotriene B_4, and 5-hydroxyeicosatetraenoic acid) increase vascular permeability, are chemotactic for macrophages and polymorphonuclear leukocytes, and mediate bone resorption. Double-blind crossover studies in humans with rheumatoid arthritis revealed a statistically significant improvement in joint tenderness and decreases in levels of leukotriene B_4 in joint fluid in patients receiving $\omega3$ supplements compared with controls. Miller (1989) reported improved gait, less pain, or both in six atopic dogs with symptomatic hip dysplasia that were given DVM Derm Caps.

Cardiovascular Diseases

Omega-3 fatty acid supplements may be useful in modifying platelet and vascular function. Humans

---

*An example of such a product is HyLyt efa Bath Oil Coat Conditioner (DVM Pharmaceuticals, Inc., Miami, FL).

*DVM Derm Caps (DVM Pharmaceuticals, Inc., Miami, FL).

fed diets high in eicosapentaenoic acid (e.g., salmon fillets and oil) have decreased plasma cholesterol (primarily very low density cholesterol) and triglyceride levels, reduced platelet counts, decreased platelet adhesion, and prolonged bleeding times. Humans with ischemic heart disease have low concentrations of linoleic acid in their plasma cholesterol esters. Low concentrations of polyunsaturated fatty acids in serum phospholipids is predictive of ischemic heart disease in humans. The relationship between low polyunsaturated fatty acids, presumed alterations in eicosanoid metabolism, and development of ischemic heart disease has yet to be elucidated. Omega-3 fatty acid supplements may benefit animals with diseases associated with increased risk of thromboembolism (e.g., feline cardiomyopathies, canine hyperadrenocorticism, canine dirofilariasis, or nephrotic syndrome). Omega-3 fatty acids may be useful in the management of hypertension in dogs. The blood pressure of strains of mice that develop hypertension spontaneously is lowered while they consume diets containing 4% menhaden oil. In addition, ω3 supplements may benefit miniature schnauzers with familial hyperlipidemia and hypertriglyceridemia.

SUMMARY

Great interest has developed in the potential use of fatty acids as "magic bullets" for the therapy of a multitude of disorders. Dietary manipulations can alter the amounts of arachidonic acid, dihomo-γ-linolenic acid, and eicosapentaenoic acid that: (1) are incorporated into cell membrane phospholipids and (2) compete as substrates in fatty acid metabolism and eicosanoid formation. Further studies are needed, however, to determine the dosage of ω3 fatty acid supplements required to obtain the desired anti-inflammatory or immune-mediatory effects without producing an ω6 fatty acid deficiency (i.e., studies need to determine the optimal ω3/ω6 ratio in the diet).

Bibliographies on the effectiveness of evening primrose oil and eicosapentaenoic acid are extensive and include almost all disorders. While there are champions of their use, placebo-controlled, double-blind studies are needed to evaluate the effectiveness of fatty acid supplements in the treatment of canine and feline diseases.

Inflammation is a complex process involving the eicosanoids, histamine, proteolytic enzymes, and other mediators. Thus, fatty acid supplements are expected to lessen, but not completely eliminate,

signs associated with inflammatory diseases. Eicosanoids have a role in almost all physiologic processes. The implications of altered eicosanoid metabolism for the whole animal must be carefully evaluated (e.g., amounts of high eicosapentaenoic acid may promote bleeding disorders, bronchoconstriction, and neoplasia).

References and Suggested Reading

Bonta, I. L., and Parnham, M. J.: Prostaglandins, essential fatty acids and cell-tissue interactions in immune-inflammation. Prog. Lipid Res. 20:617, 1981.
A review of the roles of essential fatty acids and prostaglandins in inflammatory and immune-mediated disorders.

Campbell, K. L.: Fatty acid supplementation and skin disease. Vet. Clin. North Am. Small Anim. Pract. 20:1475, 1990.
A review of the nomenclature, metabolism, and biologic functions of fatty acids and eicosanoids, including a discussion on the use of pharmacologic agents and dietary manipulations to alter eicosanoid production.

Goetzl, E. J.: Oxygenation products of arachidonic acid as mediators of hypersensitivity and inflammation. Med. Clin. North Am. 65:809, 1981.
A review of the metabolism of arachidonic acid and the biologic effects of the eicosanoids, including their roles in hypersensitivity and inflammatory diseases.

Horrobin, D. F.: Essential fatty acids in clinical dermatology. J. Am. Acad. Dermatol. 20:1045, 1989.
A review of the metabolism of fatty acids with an emphasis on the potential benefits of evening primrose oil in the management of a variety of conditions.

Lee, T. H., and Austen, K. F.: Arachidonic acid metabolism by the 5-lipoxygenase pathway, and the effects of alternative dietary fatty acids. Adv. Immunol. 39:145, 1986.
A review of the metabolism of arachidonic acid, the biologic effects of the leukotrienes, the modulation of eicosanoid production by the introduction of dietary alternative fatty acids, and the effects of eicosapentaenoic acid and dicosahexaenoic acid in human and animal studies.

Lloyd, D. H.: Essential fatty acids and skin disease. Journal of Small Animal Practice 30:207, 1989.
Results of dietary supplementation with evening primrose oil and fish oil in 16 dogs with atopic dermatitis.

Miller, W. H.: Fatty acid supplements as anti-inflammatory agents. In Kirk, R. W. (ed.): Current Veterinary Therapy X. Philadelphia: W. B. Saunders, 1989, p. 563.
Review of rationale for use of fatty acids as anti-inflammatory agents with results of use of DVM Derm Caps (DVM Pharmaceuticals, Inc., Miami, FL) in the treatment of eight atopic dogs, including six dogs with symptomatic hip dysplasia, and four dogs with idiopathic seborrhea.

Miller, W. H., Griffin, C. E., Scott, D. W., et al.: Clinical trial of DVM Derm Caps in the treatment of allergic disease in dogs: A nonblinded study. J. Am. Anim. Hosp. Assoc. 25:163, 1989.
Results of dietary supplementation with DVM Derm Caps in 93 dogs with atopic dermatitis.

Schoene, N. W., and Fiore, D.: Effect of a diet containing fish oil on blood pressure in spontaneously hypertensive rats. Prog. Lipid Res. 20:569, 1981.
A study of the effects of diets containing 5% corn oil or 1% corn oil plus 4% menhaden oil on three strains of rats (spontaneously hypertensive rats, stroke-prone spontaneously hypertensive rats, and Kyoto-Wistar normotensive controls). Blood pressures were monitored for 20 weeks.

Scott, D. W., and Buerger, R. G.: Nonsteroidal anti-inflammatory agents in the management of canine pruritus. J. Am. Anim. Hosp. Assoc. 24:425, 1988.
Results of medical management of pruritus in 45 dogs by administration of DVM Derm Caps, antihistamines, erythromycin, and acetylsalicylic acid.

CONDITIONALLY ESSENTIAL NUTRIENTS: ANTIOXIDANT NUTRIENTS AND GLUTAMINE

TIMOTHY A. ALLEN,
and MICHAEL S. HAND
Topeka, Kansas

The body contains thousands of organic compounds, but dietary intake of only a small number of organic and inorganic compounds is required to maintain homeostasis. These compounds are *essential*, because if they are not present in the diet, failure to grow or illness, or both, occur. The dietary essentiality of a compound indicates that it serves an indispensable physiologic function but cannot be synthesized endogenously. Many nutritionally *nonessential* compounds also serve an indispensable physiologic function, but if absent from the diet, they can normally be synthesized from nutritionally essential precursors at a sufficient rate to prevent untoward effects.

The classic approach to demonstrating dietary essentiality of a nutrient requires feeding purified diets containing all known required nutrients except the one under investigation. If the nutrient is essential, animals develop a deficiency syndrome manifested by reduced growth or by clinical signs and changes in tissue composition, physiologic function, or biochemical parameters. Certain amino acids, fatty acids, vitamins, and minerals are considered essential or indispensable in the dog and cat. If the nutrient is not essential, a deficiency syndrome does not develop when a diet devoid of the nutrient is fed.

To quantify the requirement for an essential nutrient, the required nutrient is incrementally replaced in the diet. The point at which signs of deficiency do not appear indicates the minimum requirement for that nutrient. The minimum amount of an essential nutrient required in the diet to prevent deficiency syndromes varies within a normal distribution among normal animals. The minimum amount of an essential nutrient required to prevent deficiency syndromes also varies with physiologic state. For example, requirements are increased in anabolic states such as growth, gestation, and lactation.

A *conditionally essential* nutrient is one that is indispensable because of a condition that has altered the normal homeostatic state (Chipponi et al., 1982).

The condition may alter the availability, metabolism, or excretion of the nutrient or may increase the requirement for a nutrient by increasing a specific metabolic process. The criteria for establishing a nutrient as conditionally essential are similar to those required for establishing a nutrient as essential. When establishing a nutrient as conditionally essential, however, one must understand the altered physiologic conditions that result in the requirement of an exogenous source of the nutrient. Ideally, to conclusively demonstrate conditional essentiality, the following criteria must be satisfied: (1) decreased tissue concentrations of the nutrient in the diseased state in the absence of exogenous supplementation, (2) altered physiologic function associated with decreased tissue concentrations, and (3) restoration of normal physiologic function by exogenous supplementation. Satisfying these criteria is usually difficult, however, because of extensive disease–nutrient and nutrient–nutrient interactions.

Accurate assessment of the micronutrient status of healthy and diseased animals can be difficult. The dietary requirement of a micronutrient can be defined as the intake required to maintain normal physiologic function. The body has the ability to store most micronutrients when dietary intake exceeds the absolute requirement. These stores prevent a deficiency state when intake is reduced. When net accretion remains less than the absolute requirement, however, progressive depletion occurs. During initial stages of progressive depletion, blood levels and corresponding physiologic functions remain normal. When the stores are exhausted, however, blood levels decrease and are associated with a corresponding decrease in physiologic function.

Following is a discussion of two different examples of conditionally essential nutrients. The first example reviews the role of antioxidant nutrients during increased free radical production. The second example outlines the function of glutamine in catabolic states.

40

ROLE OF ANTIOXIDANT NUTRIENTS IN IMMUNE SYSTEM FUNCTIONING

Many factors are known to affect the ability of individual animals to produce effective immune responses. One aspect that has been given increasing attention is nutritional status. Nutrients with recognized effects on the immune system include vitamins E and C, beta carotene, many of the B vitamins, protein, fat, and certain trace minerals, including selenium, iron, and zinc. Interactions have been demonstrated or suggested between vitamin E, selenium, beta carotene, and polyunsaturated fatty acids (Bendich and Olson, 1989). A common denominator of these interactions is likely to be prevention of free radical–mediated damage to polyunsaturated fats in cell membranes. Normal immune function requires a normal intact cell surface, because it is there that initiation of the immune response occurs.

Complex defense systems that protect against free-radical damage involve certain enzymes and the antioxidant nutrients vitamin E, beta carotene, and vitamin C. Vitamin E is considered the first line of defense against damage to cell membranes due to peroxidation (Rice and Kennedy, 1988). Glutathione peroxidate, which contains selenium, beta carotene, and vitamin C, also traps free radicals. Vitamin C is water-soluble, neutralizes free radicals in aqueous solution, and can also regenerate vitamin E.

Recent evidence indicates that dietary vitamin E, an antioxidant vitamin, influences immune system function and resistance to disease (Bendich and Olson, 1989). Intake of high levels of vitamin E optimize the immune response; vitamin E deficiency causes immunosuppression (Langweiler et al., 1981). The vitamin E requirement for normal immunologic function appears to be higher than the requirement for other physiologic functions. Results of studies indicate that vitamin E supplementation increases antigen-induced antibody production by lymphocytes and improves resistance to infectious diseases (Bendich et al., 1986).

Antioxidant nutrients protect the cell from free-radical injury. Free radicals have one or more pairs of unpaired electrons in their orbits (Floyd, 1990), and they are capable of damaging biologic systems through superoxide, hydrogen peroxide, and hydroxyl free-radical generation. These highly reactive derivatives of oxygen are both beneficial and detrimental to the immune response. Unstable free radicals, which are generated by immune cells to assist in destroying disease-causing organisms, can also damage cell surfaces in the process. If antioxidants, such as vitamin E, are not present, free radicals may cause a chain reaction (i.e., peroxidation of the polyunsaturated fatty acids in cell membranes). Besides protecting cells from free-radical damage, vitamin E also modulates synthesis of prostaglandins, which are important regulators of immune responses (Likoff et al., 1981). Because increased levels of prostaglandins may be immunosuppressive, the ability of vitamin E to prevent infection-induced increases in prostaglandin levels may be another way in which vitamin E enhances immune response.

ROLE OF ANTIOXIDANT NUTRIENTS IN CANCER PREVENTION AND TREATMENT

Recent epidemiologic studies of human populations have suggested an inverse relationship between the consumption of foods high in beta carotene and the development of several different tumor types (Bendich and Olson, 1989). Free-radical damage is thought to initiate and promote many cancers because free radicals damage nucleic acids. The lesions can be classified as deriving from either breaks in DNA strands or from products of nucleotide base modification; the latter may have serious consequences in terms of mutagenesis and carcinogenesis.

Beta carotene prevents certain types of experimentally induced tumors in animals. Beta carotene administration has been shown to prevent and treat oral carcinoma in the cheek pouch of the hamster (Shklar, 1982). *In vitro* research on the mechanisms by which beta carotene affects immune surveillance has been hampered because beta carotene is highly insoluble, and performance of *in vivo* studies in rodents has been difficult because rodents rapidly convert beta carotene to vitamin A. Other antioxidant nutrients, such as vitamin E, also may play a role in cancer prevention (Newberne and Saphakarn, 1983). In a study of induced colon cancer in mice, for example, animals supplemented with vitamin E had a reduced number of tumors, and those tumors that developed were less invasive.

GLUTAMINE AS A CONDITIONALLY ESSENTIAL NUTRIENT

Glutamine is a nonessential nutrient under normal conditions, but several unique properties of the amino acid suggest that it has a key role in several disease states (Souba, 1987). Glutamine is the most abundant amino acid in the body. It has the highest concentration in the plasma, and excluding taurine, it constitutes more than 50% of the free amino acid pool. This glycogenic amino acid is synthesized by a wide variety of tissues. Glutamine concentrations in whole blood and skeletal tissue decrease markedly after injury and other catabolic conditions.

Glutamine plays a key role in nitrogen metabolism because it has two amino moieties, an alpha amino group and an amide group. It acts as a nitrogen shuttle among various organs. Glutamine is also a precursor in the synthesis of nucleotides such as adenosine triphosphate (ATP), purines, pyrimidines, and other amino acids. Glutamine is rapidly consumed by rapidly dividing cells such as enterocytes, malignant cells, fibroblasts, and reticulocytes and has been shown to be a major oxidative fuel for these cells.

Fasting is associated with several adaptive changes in metabolism of glutamine. In the postabsorptive state, the liver, kidneys, and gut extract glutamine from the blood at similar rates. During the transition from the postabsorptive to the fasting states, the liver switches its balance of glutamine from net uptake to net release. The increase in hepatic glutamine production is associated with a simultaneous increase in the uptake of glutamine by the gut and kidneys.

Recent studies have demonstrated that the gastrointestinal tract actively metabolizes glutamine and that the metabolism of glutamine by enterocytes is an integral part of the intestine's role as a regulator of nitrogen balance in catabolic states (Souba et al., 1985). During starvation or prolonged malnutrition, the intestines are deprived of nutrients needed to maintain the high turnover rate of intestinal cells. Even if these nutrients are provided by the parenteral route, the intestines still atrophy. This observation suggests that intestinal function and structure are more greatly influenced by local nutrients in the intestinal lumen than by the systemic availability of the nutrients. Because the intestine preferentially uses glutamine as a major fuel source, addition of glutamine to parenteral or enteral critical care diets may enhance intestinal adaptation.

The signals that influence this local action of glutamine may be physical, chemical, hormonal, or neural. The physical presence of nutrients in the intestinal lumen may be sufficient to maintain structure and function, or absorbed nutrients may have biochemical effects. Luminally fed rats had greater intestinal mucosal mass and greater glucose absorption than either fasted rats or rats given an equivalent caloric intake parenterally (Souba et al., 1985). This observation suggests that luminal trophic factors increase glucose absorption by increasing mucosal mass. Support for the role of intraluminal glutamine is provided by studies that demonstrated increased subsequent absorption in experimental subjects compared with saline-infused controls.

The major site of glutamine production to support rapidly dividing cells appears to be skeletal muscle. Glutamine release from skeletal muscle is accelerated in various catabolic states, such as trauma, sepsis, and neoplasia. It has been proposed that glutamine flux in skeletal muscle may control the balance between catabolism and anabolism of muscle protein. Chronic glucocorticoid treatment causes skeletal muscle wasting. Trauma and neoplasia also result in muscle wasting; glucocorticoids may mediate this response. Glutamine accounts for approximately 25 to 30% of the total amino acid efflux during glucocorticoid-mediated muscle atrophy. The proportion of glutamine in muscle proteins cannot account for this amount of glutamine; therefore, increased biosynthesis of glutamine during muscle wasting is implied. Glutamine synthetase is the enzyme that catalyzes the ATP-dependent condensation of glutamic acid and ammonia to form glutamine. Glutamine synthetase in skeletal muscle is induced by glucocorticoids. Exercise can diminish glucocorticoid-mediated muscle wasting. A recent study demonstrated that exercise-induced muscle sparing was correlated with decreased activity of glutamine synthetase (Falduto et al., 1989). An alternative method of reducing glucocorticoid-mediated muscle wasting might be to provide exogenous glutamine in the form of stable dipeptides such as alanyl-glutamine.

CONCLUSIONS

The foregoing examples demonstrate that nutrients may have important roles in nutrition even though they do not satisfy the traditional definition of essentiality. Contemporary nutrition research is less concerned with absolute requirements than with optimal levels of various nutrients under various conditions. Although firm clinical recommendations regarding conditionally essential nutrients cannot be made at this time, future clinical studies are likely to indicate a need for micronutrient supplementation for specific clinical disorders.

References and Suggested Reading

Bendich, A.: Antioxidant nutrients and immune functions. *In* Bendich, A. et al.: *Antioxidant Nutrients and Immune Functions.* New York: Plenum Press, 1989, p. 1.
A chapter reviewing the role of free radicals and hence antioxidants in the function of the immune system.
Bendich, A., and Olson, J. A.: Biological actions of carotenoids. FASEB J. 3:1927, 1989.
A review of the biologic actions of carotenoids, including those distinct from their function as precursors of vitamin A.
Bendich, A., Gabriel, E., and Machlin, L. J.: Dietary vitamin E requirement for optimum immune responses in the rat. J. Nutr. 116:675, 1986.
A study in rats demonstrating that the vitamin E requirement for optimal T- and B-lymphocyte mitogen response is greater than the requirement for normal growth rate and prevention of myopathy.
Chipponi, J. X., Bleier, J. C., Santi, M. T., and Rudman, D.: Deficiencies of essential and conditionally essential nutrients. Am. J. Clin. Nutr. 35:1112, 1982.
A review of essential nutrients and examples of conditionally essential nutrients in human beings receiving total parenteral nutrition.
Falduto, M. T., Hickson, R. C., and Young, A. P.: Antagonism by glucocorticoids and exercise on expression of glutamine synthetase in skeletal muscle. FASEB J. 3:7673, 1989.
A study in rats demonstrating that exercise-induced muscle sparing is associated with decreased glutamine synthetase activity.

Floyd, R. A.: Role of oxygen free radicals in carcinogenesis and brain ischemia. FASEB J. 4:2587, 1990.
A review of oxygen free-radical reactions and the contribution of oxidative damage to aging, carcinogenesis, and stroke.

Langweiler, M., Schultz, R. D., and Sheffy, B. E.: Effect of vitamin E deficiency on the proliferative response of canine lymphocytes. Am. J. Vet. Res. 42:1681, 1981.

Likoff, R. D., Guptill, D. R., Lawrence, L. M., et al.: Vitamin E and aspirin depress prostaglandins in protection of chickens against *Escherichia coli* infection. Am. J. Clin. Nutr. 134:245, 1981.
A study demonstrating association between vitamin E and prostaglandin levels in chickens infected with E. coli.

Newberne, P. M., and Saphakarn, V.: Nutrition and cancer: A review with emphasis on the roles of vitamins C and E and selenium. Nutr. Cancer 5:107, 1983.
A general review of the potential role of several nutrients in the prevention of cancer.

Rice, D., and Kennedy, S.: Vitamin E: Function and effects of deficiency. Br. Vet. J. 144:482, 1988.
A review of control of lipid peroxidation by vitamin E and how seemingly diverse manifestations of vitamin E deficiency may be related.

Shklar, G.: Oral mucosal carcinogenesis in hamsters: Inhibition by vitamin E. J. Natl. Cancer Inst. 68:791, 1982.
A study demonstrating vitamin E inhibition of oral tumor induction in hamsters.

Souba, W. W.: Interorgan ammonia metabolism in health and disease: A surgeon's view. JPEN 11:569, 1987.
A review of the interorgan exchange of ammonia and the related metabolism of glutamine in normal and pathophysiologic states.

Souba, W. W., Smith, R. J., and Wilmore, D. W.: Glutamine metabolism by the intestinal tract. JPEN 9:608, 1985.
A review of selective metabolism of glutamine by the gut in normal and pathophysiologic states.

CURRENT CONCEPTS OF WOUND MANAGEMENT

ERIC R. POPE
Columbia, Missouri

Management of traumatic wounds is a major component of companion animal emergency medicine. Since there is considerable variability in the amount of local tissue damage, degree of wound contamination, and concomitant internal injuries, no single management protocol can be applied to all cases. But there are basic principles that can be used to select the most appropriate course of action regardless of the etiology. A thorough physical examination to rule out life-threatening internal injuries is the first priority. The goals of wound management are complete removal of devitalized tissue and foreign bodies and reduction of bacterial numbers to levels low enough to permit wound closure. Effective wound management practices result in faster patient recovery and decreased owner expense.

Most veterinarians have an almost irresistible urge to examine and probe a wound as soon as the patient is placed on the exam table. In most instances, though, complete examination of the wound is impossible, and the small amount of information gained by this procedure is not worth the risk of further contamination of the wound. If the wound is not covered with a bandage, it should be protected with a sterile dressing. The dressing can be applied with pressure to control hemorrhage.

GENERAL CONSIDERATIONS

All traumatic wounds contain bacteria. Many factors, such as the type and number of bacteria inoculated, time lapsed since wounding, presence of foreign bodies, and integrity of host defense mechanisms, determine whether or not contamination will progress to infection. In general, cleansing and debridement of the wound should be performed as soon as possible before bacterial multiplication reaches the infective level and tissue invasion occurs. Wounds associated with the classic signs of inflammation (redness, swelling, heat, and pain) are probably poor candidates for primary closure unless an *en bloc* excision of all damaged tissue can be performed.

The etiology of the wound can provide insight into the extent of damage to underlying tissues. With lacerations and penetrating injuries from low-velocity missiles and sharp objects, damage is usually confined to the area immediately adjacent to the path of the wounding agent. Minimal debridement of devitalized tissue along the path and wound lavage are all that is generally required prior to wound closure. This protocol is in sharp contrast to wounds caused by high-velocity missiles and animal bites, which often cause extensive damage to underlying tissues. Such damage can extend for considerable distance into the tissue surrounding the path of the wounding agent. Extensive debridement staged over several days may be necessary.

Although the use of local and regional anesthetics (e.g., ring blocks on the limbs) is often recommended, their effectiveness on wounds other than superficial lacerations is quite variable. In most instances, adequate inspection and treatment of deeper wounds requires general anesthesia. Epidural anesthesia is an excellent alternative for wounds involving the hindlimbs of patients considered to be poor anesthetic risks.

If bacterial culture and sensitivity testing are desired, specimens are collected by swabbing the wound before the wound is prepared for surgical debridement. It is imperative that the skin surrounding the wound be *widely* clipped and prepared before examination of the wound is begun because the size of the skin defect frequently belies the extent and severity of the damage to the deeper tissues. If the surrounding skin has not been adequately prepared, complete exploration and debridement of the wound may be impossible. The wound should be protected from further contamination by applying sterile gauze sponges, a water-miscible gel (e.g., K-Y Jelly, Johnson and Johnson), or both while the surrounding area is clipped. The sponges are replaced before the skin is prepared. Scrub soaps and strong antiseptics should not be placed directly in the wound.

WOUND DEBRIDEMENT

The keys to successful wound management are the debridement of devitalized tissue and foreign bodies and reduction of bacterial numbers to as close to zero as possible. These goals are generally best accomplished by a combination of surgical excision and copious wound lavage. In order to adequately inspect and debride a wound, it is often necessary to enlarge the original opening. Each tissue layer should be sequentially examined and debrided until the base of the wound is reached. Debriding and lavaging extensive wounds can be very time consuming, but failure to perform these procedures properly frequently leads to postoperative wound infection and dehiscence.

Assessing Tissue Viability

Assessment of tissue viability is often based on subjective criteria such as color and bleeding from the cut surface. These criteria are often imprecise, even in the hands of experienced surgeons. The following guidelines are offered:

SKIN. Color and bleeding are unreliable, especially following acute injury. Skin that is black or pearl white and has a leathery texture should be considered nonviable and excised. In areas where skin is not abundant, for example, on the limbs, and when large skin flaps have been avulsed, it is usually best to conserve as much skin as possible. Within a couple of days, the demarcation between viable and nonviable skin will become obvious and further debridement can be performed.

SUBCUTANEOUS FAT. Wide excision of damaged fat is indicated because of its poor blood supply. Subcutaneous tissue containing dirt or other small foreign bodies that are difficult to remove should be excised.

MUSCLE. Contraction following stimulation and bleeding are the most reliable indicators of viability. In general, large amounts of muscle can be debrided without interfering with function. Devitalized muscle quickly undergoes liquefaction necrosis, providing a good environment for bacterial growth.

BONE AND LIGAMENTS. Bone is often exposed in shearing injuries of the distal limbs. Small detached fragments should be removed. Foreign bodies embedded in the surface of the bone can be removed with curettes or a rongeur. Shearing injuries of the bones and ligaments of the distal limbs resulting in joint instability can be supported with splints or preferably with an external fixator. If possible, implants should not be placed in the wound until it contains only healthy tissue and is free of infection.

WOUND LAVAGE

Wound lavage is performed in conjunction with debridement to remove bacteria, loose debris, and blood clots. Large volumes applied under moderate pressure are most effective and result in the least number of complications. An efficient method of delivering the lavage solution is to attach an 18-gauge needle, 30-ml syringe, and three-way stopcock to a sterile intravenous administration set connected to a container of lavage solution. The stopcock is used to alternately fill the syringe and then deliver the fluid to the wound. The pressure generated with this setup is adequate to dislodge foreign bodies and bacteria without causing clinically significant additional tissue trauma or dissemination of bacteria deeper into the wound by separating normal tissue planes.

Selecting a particular lavage fluid is probably not as important as the quantity used. The addition of an antiseptic or antibiotic to the lavage solution may be helpful in killing residual bacteria remaining in the wound. My preference is to use a 0.05 to 0.1% chlorhexidine diacetate solution, prepared by diluting 1 part of the 2% stock solution with 40 or 20 parts sterile water, respectively. If other fluids, such as saline or lactated Ringer's solution, are used as the diluent, a precipitate will form within several hours. The effect of the precipitate on wound healing is unknown. However, I prefer to avoid placing solutions containing particulate matter into wounds. Chlorhexidine has a wide spectrum of activity, sustained residual activity, and, at these concentrations, minimal side effects. Although resistant bacterial strains exist, they are uncommonly encountered as primary pathogens. They tend to be selectively acquired through prolonged use of the antiseptic or poor wound management practices. If the wound is left open, lavage with the antiseptic solution is continued until evidence of infection (i.e., purulent exudate) is absent or until granulation tissue covers the wound. At this time only physiologic solutions such as saline or lactated Ringer's solution should be placed in the wound. The surface of the granulation tissue will become colonized by normal skin organisms, but the likelihood of promoting infection with highly resistant bacterial strains will be reduced.

DRAINS

Wound closure should be performed as soon as debridement is complete. The use of buried sutures should be minimized. Even the most inert sutures potentiate the development of infection. If dead space is present, the use of a closed suction drain should be considered. Closed suction drains reduce the incidence of ascending bacterial infection, keep the surrounding skin dry, and allow the clinician to monitor the volume and character of the drainage, important factors in deciding when to remove the drain. The drain should be thick walled so that it does not collapse under negative pressure and large enough so that it does not easily become obstructed with clots or tissue fragments. Drains for small areas can be made from butterfly catheters. Larger drains can be made economically from Silastic tubing. With either type, multiple fenestrations are cut in the buried portion with scissors. Suction should be applied as soon as possible to keep clots from forming in the tube. The catheter should be clamped when the collection device is changed to prevent fluid from being sucked back into the wound. Drains should always exit the site through a separate stab incision; they should be positioned so that they do not lie directly under the suture line. Antibiotic ointment can be placed on the incision line and around the tube exit site to prevent air leakage until a fibrin seal forms.

WOUND DRESSINGS

If complete debridement is impossible, if tissue of questionable viability is left in the wound, or if there is concern about infection, the wound should be covered with a bandage and not sutured. Wet-to-dry dressings can be used to mechanically debride devitalized tissue and to liquefy tenacious exudates. Wide-mesh gauze sponges should be used as the contact layer so that debris and exudate lifted from the wound by the capillary action of the bandage will become trapped in the gauze and removed with it when the bandage is changed. Bandages are changed once or twice daily depending on the condition of the wound and the amount of exudate produced. The secondary or intermediate layer of the bandage should be absorbent. If the outer layer of the bandage becomes wet, the bandage should be changed immediately. In many instances a delayed primary closure can be performed in 2 or 3 days.

ENZYMATIC AGENTS

Enzymatic debridement is most commonly employed as adjunctive therapy following incomplete surgical debridement but may be used as the primary treatment for selected wounds. In some instances complete surgical debridement is not possible because of the likelihood of damaging vital structures such as blood vessels and nerves. Enzymatic agents can be placed in these wounds to liquefy the devitalized tissue, enhancing its removal by wound lavage or entrapment in adherent dressings. The primary disadvantages of enzymatic debridement are the rather long time required to complete the debridement process, the potential of some products to cause additional tissue damage, and the expense of the products.

My primary indication for enzymatic therapy is treatment of superficial fight wounds which have formed an abscess and are being managed as open wounds following drainage and debridement. Enzymatic debridement could also be used in patients that are poor anesthetic risks for surgical debridement. One product containing trypsin, balsam of Peru, and castor oil (Granulex, Beecham Laboratories) is effective in liquefying exudate and debriding limited amounts of devitalized tissue and is safe and available in container sizes that are economical for dispensing to clients for home treatment.

CLASSIFICATION OF WOUND CLOSURE

Wound closure performed immediately after debriding and lavaging the wound is called a *primary closure*. If devitalized tissue, foreign bodies, or infection precludes immediate closure, the wound is allowed to remain open. Wounds converted to clean or clean-contaminated status in 2 to 5 days by repeated debridement and lavage can still be closed, but the closure is called a *delayed primary closure*. Closure of a wound after granulation tissue forms is called a *secondary closure*. Allowing a wound to heal completely as an open wound is called healing by *contraction and epithelialization* or *second-intention healing*.

References and Suggested Reading

Edlich, R. F., Thacker, J. G., Buchanan, L., et al: Modern concepts of treatment of traumatic wounds. Adv. Surg. 13:169, 1979.
A review of the pathophysiology of traumatic wounds and important considerations in their management.
Johnston, D. E.: Care of accidental wounds. Vet. Clin. North Am. Small Anim. Pract. 20:27, 1990.
A complete review of wound management from initial presentation to final resolution.
Lee, A. H., Swaim, S. F., and Henderson, R. H.: Surgical Drainage. Compend. Contin. Educ. Pract. Vet. 8:94, 1986.
The various types of drains and indications for their use are described.
Swaim, S. F.: Bandages and topical agents. Vet. Clin. North Am.: Small Anim. Pract. 20:47, 1990.
A useful guide for selecting the topical agents and bandage materials for different types of wounds.
Swaim, S. F., and Henderson, R. A.: *Small Animal Wound Management.* Philadelphia: Lea & Febiger, 1990, pp. 9–51.
The two chapters cited deal with evaluation and management of traumatic wounds.
Swaim, S. F., and Lee, A. H.: Topical wound medications: A review. J.A.V.M.A. 190:1588, 1987.
A review of the properties, indications, contraindications, and potential side effects of commonly used topical agents.

THERAPEUTIC APPLICATIONS OF MONOCLONAL ANTIBODIES

ALAN S. HAMMER

Columbus, Ohio

The hybridoma technology developed by Kohler and Milstein in the 1970's has revolutionized modern medicine and biologic research. One result of their work has been the development of technology that has increased our ability to produce uniform antibody directed against one or more specific antigens. The commercial production of these monoclonal antibodies holds great potential for the treatment of a variety of diseases.

Monoclonal antibodies are generated by the somatic fusion of antibody-producing cells from an immunized animal and immortal myeloma cells. The myeloma cells have been genetically altered with various drug selection markers such that only stable, fused hybridoma cells survive under selective conditions. The resultant colonies are then screened for production of a monoclonal antibody with the desired properties. While this is a difficult and slow process, once a stable hybridoma is selected, monoclonal antibody production can be increased to meet many requirements. Therapeutic applications of monoclonal antibodies range from the passive removal of toxic substances to active immunotherapy of cancer and use of immunoconjugates as cytotoxic agents.

REMOVAL OF DRUGS AND TOXINS

Most monoclonal antibodies used in medicine today are formulated for diagnostic purposes. Their ability to bind antigens *in vitro* allows for uniform identification of disease conditions (e.g., feline leukemia virus [FeLV] tests or occult heartworm tests).

This binding and removal or neutralization of antigens can also be used to treat various toxic conditions. One such situation is the use of monoclonal antibodies to treat septic shock (Tracey, 1987). Because gram-negative septic shock is mediated in part by tumor necrosis factor (TNF), administration of anti-TNF antibodies prior to gram-negative bacteremia or endotoxemia can prevent septic shock and organ failure. Clinical trials are ongoing in humans to evaluate the role of monoclonal antibodies in treating septic shock. Septic shock is commonly encountered in veterinary medicine in canine parvovirus infection, in canine pyometra, and in patients undergoing chemotherapy or immunosuppression. The availability of a monoclonal antibody against TNF may greatly improve survival rates in these patients. Other monoclonal antibodies have been developed to treat overdosage with drugs such as digoxin. (One of these is Digibind [Burroughs Wellcome], a Fab [Fragment, antigen binding] antibody.)

IMMUNOTHERAPY OF CANCER

A strong humoral response to tumor antigens is often poorly correlated with *in vivo* resistance to solid neoplasms. However, cells of hematopoietic origin may be more readily lysed by antibody-dependent cell-mediated cytotoxicity or by complement-mediated cytotoxicity (Fig. 1). Monoclonal antibodies developed against canine lymphoma have been shown to lyse cells of a lymphoma cell line *in vitro* by complement-mediated cytolysis and anti-

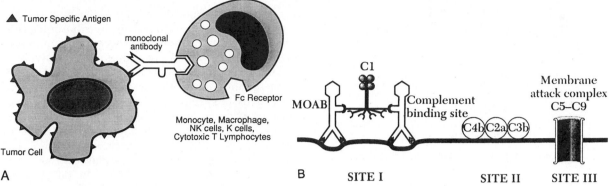

Figure 1. Mechanisms of humoral immunity against tumors. *A*, Antibody-dependent cell-mediated cytotoxicity. *B*, Complement-mediated cytotoxicity. MOAB, monoclonal antibodies.

body-dependent cell-mediated cytotoxicity in the presence of peripheral blood leukocytes, monocytes, and lymphocytes (Rosales, 1988).

Results of a clinical phase II trial using anti-canine lymphoma monoclonal antibody were recently presented (Jeglum, 1990). This trial was designed to evaluate the survival of dogs treated with combination chemotherapy followed by monoclonal antibody as a maintenance protocol. These survival times were compared with historical survival times of dogs treated with combination chemotherapy alone. Survival of dogs treated with chemotherapy and monoclonal antibody was significantly longer than dogs treated with chemotherapy alone (531 days versus 272 days). Toxicities reported include immediate pruritus, facial edema, dyspnea, diarrhea, and joint stiffness. Canine anti-mouse antibodies were demonstrated in these dogs. This monoclonal antibody is currently undergoing phase III trials at several veterinary institutions and is expected to be available commercially within the next year.

IMMUNOCONJUGATES

It has been almost 100 years since Paul Ehrlich coined the phrase "magic bullet" for therapy with drugs or toxins linked to target-specific carriers. He envisioned these agents to be highly effective and without side effects owing to nontarget cytotoxicity. With the advent of monoclonal antibodies and advances in understanding the structure and mechanisms of action of various toxins, we are coming closer to the fulfillment of that dream (Hertler, 1989).

Immunoconjugates is a more appropriate term for these "magic bullets," as a variety of agents have been attached to monoclonal antibodies to achieve the desired effect on the target cell. Common conjugates include plant, fungal, and bacterial toxins, chemotherapeutic agents, radioactive compounds, and photoactive compounds. Table 1 lists some of the conjugates currently undergoing investigation.

The common bacterial and plant toxins used in construction of immunoconjugates are enzymes of such potency that one molecule in the cytosol is believed to be lethal to the cell. Such highly toxic compounds are desirable for conjugation with monoclonal antibodies because even if weak binding or poor internalization occurs, a lethal event may still develop. The bacterial toxins (e.g., diphtheria toxin and *Pseudomonas* exotoxin-A) inactivate the elongation factor-2 by adenosine diphosphate (ADP)–ribosylation. Plant toxins (e.g., ricin, abrin, pokeweed antiviral protein, saporin, gelonin) enzymatically inactivate the 60S subunit of ribosomes. These toxic enzymes are capable of inactivating over 200 ribosomes or elongation factor-2 molecules per minute and can quickly halt protein synthesis leading to cell death.

Many plant toxins are composed of several components as indicated in Figure 2. The A chain of ricin toxin is the toxic portion. This is linked by acid-labile disulfide bonds to the B chain, which has a galactose-binding site and cell membrane translocating activity. Both A and B chains are glycosylated with oligosaccharide residues. Use of unmodified holotoxin bound to monoclonal antibod-

Table 1. *Compounds Linked to Monoclonal Antibodies as Immunoconjugates*

Plant toxins	Chemotherapeutic agents
Ricin	Daunomycin
Abrin	Doxorubicin
Modeccin	Mitomycin C
Pokeweed antiviral protein	Neocarzinostatin
Gelonin	Methotrexate
Saporin	Chlorambucil
Momordica toxin	*Radionuclides*
Bacterial toxins	Iodine-131
Diphtheria toxin	Yttrium-90
Pseudomonas exotoxin	Rhenium-186
Fungal toxins	*Photoactive substances*
Alpha-sarcin	Hematoporphyrin

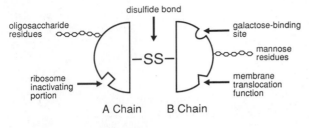

Ricin Holotoxin

Figure 2. Anatomy of a typical plant holotoxin.

ies can result in nonspecific toxicity owing to uptake by the reticuloendothelial cells secondary to binding to the carbohydrate residues and via the galactose-binding site on the B chain. Production of nonglycosylated ricin toxin with deletion of the galactose-binding site in the B chain by genetic engineering in *Escherichia coli* has resulted in a molecule closer to the ideal toxin.

Internalization of the constructed immunoconjugate and release of the toxic portion into the cytosol are vital steps in achieving cell death. The ideal target antigen would be exclusively located on the target cell, easily accessible to the immunoconjugate, and readily internalized. Once internalized, it should deliver the bound immunoconjugate to the Golgi compartment of the cell. The toxin should be

readily cleaved from the carrier antibody and translocated to the cytosol to act on the ribosomes (Fig. 3). Few immunoconjugates recognize tumor-associated antigens which are expressed exclusively on neoplastic tissue. Fortunately, the relative abundance of antigens on the target cells compared with normal tissues frequently allows for selective cytotoxicity when using immunoconjugates. Poor internalization of immunoconjugates may be the result of low antigen numbers or incorrect choice of antigen. Alpha-fetoprotein and various ovarian carcinoma antigens have been shown to be poorly internalized. Antibodies against the transferrin receptor have been shown to be readily internalized and deliver the endosome to a compartment from which the toxin can escape. Delivery of the endosome to a lysosome may cause acid or enzymatic destruction of the toxin before release into the cytosol.

Use of chemotherapeutic agents as immunoconjugates has increased the therapeutic index over the use of drug alone but is still subject to poor internalization and release from the endosome. Additionally, the number of molecules necessary for cell death is greater than that needed with potent toxins such as ricin or diphtheria toxin.

Use of radiolabeled immunoconjugates abrogates many of these difficulties. The immunoconjugate does not have to be internalized to cause cell death. If only a portion of the neoplastic cells possess the

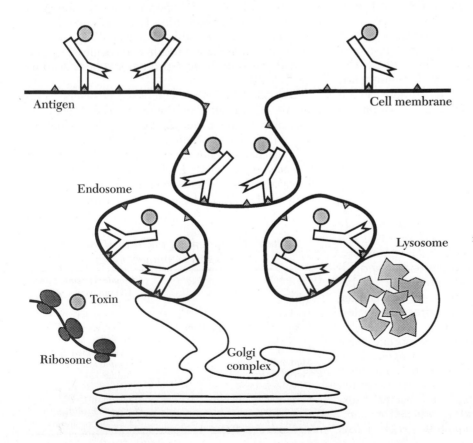

Figure 3. Internalization of an immunoconjugate.

Table 2. *Neoplastic Conditions in Human Patients Being Studied by Clinical Trials With Immunotoxins*

Melanoma
Colorectal carcinoma
Breast carcinoma
Chronic lymphocytic leukemia
Acute lymphoblastic (T-cell) leukemia
Ovarian carcinoma
B-cell lymphoma

target antigen, the "hand grenade" effect may still lead to death of neighboring cells lacking the antigen. Although the radiotherapeutic effect should be localized to the tumor cells, death of some normal cells may occur.

Additional difficulties in using immunoconjugates include nonspecific uptake by the reticuloendothelial system and formation of neutralizing patient anti-mouse antibodies. Side effects of infusion of ricin immunoconjugates in humans with melanoma included hypoalbuminemia, edema, malaise, fatigue, anorexia, and fever. More than 80% of these patients developed antibodies against the immunoconjugate, resulting in increased clearance and decreased efficacy. The ricin toxin portion of the immunoconjugate appears to be more immunogenic than the antibody portion. Concurrent use of cyclophosphamide in rats treated with ricin immunoconjugate decreased the formation of anti-ricin and anti-mouse antibodies. Efforts are now under way to "humanize" the monoclonal antibodies by substituting human constant regions in the molecule to decrease the immunogenicity of the immunoconjugate.

Many of the reported side effects of ricin immunotoxins is thought to be due to nonspecific binding via the Fc portion of the molecule. Additionally, it is thought that the large immunoconjugate may have difficulty in crossing the capillary to gain access to the target cell. Consequently, fragments of monoclonal antibodies have been used as the carrier portion; these fragments include $F(ab)_2$ and Fab'.

The first clinical application of immunotoxins was to deplete T cells from allogeneic marrow grafts to prevent graft-versus-host disease. Immunotoxins are being used or planned for use in clinical trials against a number of neoplastic conditions (Hertler, 1989) (Table 2). In addition, immunotoxins are used to purge bone marrow of neoplastic cells *ex vivo* prior to autologous bone marrow transplantation. Further work is ongoing to develop anti-idiotypic immunotoxins capable of selectively deleting clones of lymphoid cells causing autoimmune disease.

SUMMARY

As the difficulties in large-scale production of monoclonal antibodies are overcome, many more therapeutic uses for them will be discovered. Various manipulations of the antibody molecule itself, in addition to compounds conjugated to the molecule, will allow this novel treatment modality to flourish in the years to come.

References and Suggested Reading

Hertler, A. A., and Frankel, A. E.: Immunotoxins: A clinical review of their use in the treatment of malignancies. J. Clin. Oncol. 7:1932, 1989.
A review of the construction, clinical use, and obstacles involved in the application of immunotoxins.
Jeglum, K. A., Sorenmo, K., Steplewski, Z., et al.: Adjuvant immunotherapy of canine lymphoma with monoclonal antibody 231. Personal communication, ACVIM 1990 Synbiotics Conference.
Report on clinical trial in dogs with lymphoma following induction of chemotherapy.
Rosales, C., Jeglum, K. A., Obrocka, M., et al.: Cytolytic activity of murine anti-dog lymphoma monoclonal antibodies with canine effector cells and complement. Cell Immunol. 115:420, 1988.
In vitro work demonstrating ADCC and complement-mediated lysis of target cell line using monoclonal antibodies.
Tracey, K. J., Fong, Y., Hesse, D. G., et al.: Anti-cachectin/TNF monoclonal antibodies prevent septic shock during lethal bacteraemia. Nature 330:662, 1987.
Experimental work demonstrating protective effect of anti-TNF antibodies in baboons with E. coli bacteremia.

GENETIC ENGINEERING: THERAPY WITH RECOMBINANT DNA PRODUCTS

BARBARA E. KITCHELL,
and WILLIAM W. RUEHL
Stanford, California

The evolution of recombinant DNA technology represents one of the most significant advances in medical science in decades. The ability to understand this technology and to apply the products developed by genetic engineering will provide veterinarians with better diagnostic techniques, improved disease control, and more effective therapeutics.

PRINCIPLES OF MOLECULAR GENETICS

The fundamental information storage unit of the cell is the gene, which is composed of molecules of deoxyribonucleic acid (DNA). In turn, DNA molecules are long unbranched polymers composed of nucleotide subunits. The nucleotides consist of a sugar (deoxyribose), a phosphate group, and a purine or pyrimidine base. Chains of these nucleotides are linked by phosphodiester bonds joining the phosphate group at the 5′ carbon position of the sugar moiety with the 3′ position of the next residue in the chain. This pattern of polymerization results in a polarity of the DNA molecule which is recognized by the enzymes required to replicate DNA and to make messenger RNA, which codes for proteins made from the DNA template.

DNA exists in cells as a stable double helix. To form this double helix, the purine bases adenine and guanine form associations by their nitrogenous bases with the pyrimidine bases cytosine and thymine. These hydrogen bonds follow the Watson-Crick base-pairing rules of linking an adenine (A) residue with thymine (T), and guanine (G) with cytosine (C). In ribonucleic acid (RNA), the thymine is substituted by the base uracil, designated U. Thus, DNA exists as a double-stranded helix that resembles a winding staircase; the bases represent "steps" of the helical staircase, and the sugar-phosphate backbone constitutes the rail.

The sequence of nucleotide bases determines the information contained in the gene. DNA is transcribed to a single strand of messenger ribonucleic acid (mRNA) by RNA polymerase. The mRNA is then translated by ribosomes which read the ribonucleotide bases of the mRNA strand in triplets, with each triplet signifying an amino acid to be added to the growing peptide chain. Thus, a gene containing the DNA sequence TGC AGC TCC GGA CTC is transcribed to an mRNA strand that reflects the sequence of the DNA strand, except that U is substituted for T in the RNA (mRNA sequence: UGC AGC UCC GGA CUC). This mRNA strand is translated into the amino acid sequence cysteine (UGC), serine (AGC), serine (UCC), glycine (GGA), leucine (CUC) (Fig. 1). There are only 21 known naturally occurring amino acids, so that there are more triplet codons (4^3, or 64 total) available than there are amino acids to be encoded. The triplet codons predict unambiguously the amino acid sequence they encode, but it is more difficult to read "backward" from a known amino acid sequence to decipher the exact DNA sequence owing to "degeneracy" or redundancy of the code (that is, a given amino acid may be designated by more than one triplet codon). Another important fact is that the triplet genetic code is universal. Thus, a specific sequence of nucleotides encodes the same information for making a protein in bacteria, *Drosophila*, cabbages, cats, cattle, or human beings.

RECOMBINANT DNA TECHNOLOGY

Recombinant DNA technology combines enzymology, microbiology, and genetic approaches to create biologic systems that produce large quantities of specific products. This technology had its genesis in the discovery of ways to insert functional units of DNA, or genes, into special strains of bacteria, yeast, or eucaryotic cells. The host cell thus manufactures the protein molecules of interest according to the coding sequence specified by the foreign DNA. These mutant strains of organisms are cultivated to efficiently and economically produce quantities of the desired protein for diagnostic and therapeutic use.

50

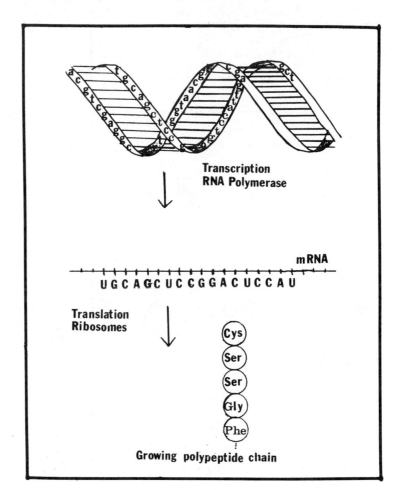

Transcription
RNA Polymerase

mRNA
UGCAGCUCCGGACUCCAU

Translation
Ribosomes

Cys
Ser
Ser
Gly
Phe

Growing polypeptide chain

Figure 1. Genomic deoxyribonucleic acid (DNA) is transcribed into single-stranded messenger ribonucleic acid (mRNA) by the enzyme RNA polymerase. Messenger RNA is translated by ribosomes in the cytoplasm into proteins. Messenger RNA is read as a triplet code, with 3 nucleotides designating the next amino acid to be added to the growing peptide chain.

There are several steps involved in making recombinant DNA (Fig. 2). First, the desired gene to be cloned must be isolated. In many cases, this involves fragmenting cellular DNA by means of bacterial enzymes called restriction endonucleases. Restriction endonucleases have the ability to recognize short nucleotide sequences and to cleave these specific sequences. These enzymes produced by bacteria prevent invasion by viruses, serving the bacteria as a sort of "intracellular immune system." Almost 200 useful restriction enzymes have been identified and named for the bacteria in which they were first discovered. For example, *Escherichia coli* elaborates an enzyme called Eco RI, which cuts DNA when it recognizes the sequence GAATTC. The resultant linear fragments can then be covalently attached to other DNA molecules, which have been cut by the same restriction enzyme, by using the cellular enzyme DNA ligase. Any two DNA molecules, no matter what their initial source, can be joined to create a new set of genetic instructions. This "recombination" of genetic material gives rise to the term "recombinant DNA."

Alternatively, it is possible to make DNA by first isolating messenger RNA from the cell. Since every cell of the body is identical at the DNA level, using genomic DNA as the starting material necessitates screening genes for approximately 200,000 proteins. The use of mRNA as a starting template limits the genes to be screened to a few hundred, or only those expressed in the differentiated cell from which the mRNA is collected. For example, in erythrocyte precursor cells, much of the protein made will be hemoglobin. The mRNA for hemoglobin will be abundant in these cells but nonexistent in other differentiated cells, such as epithelial cells, which do not make hemoglobin. It is possible to isolate all of the mRNA made in a cell, subject the mRNA to processing by a retroviral enzyme called reverse transcriptase ("reverse" because it transcribes the genetic code backward from RNA into DNA), and to produce complementary strands of DNA (cDNA). This cDNA is then inserted into an appropriate vector to create a cDNA "library" of all the genes expressed (actively making protein) by that cell.

The next step in making recombinant DNA is identification of desirable vectors for expression. Circular bacterial plasmids, which are extrachro-

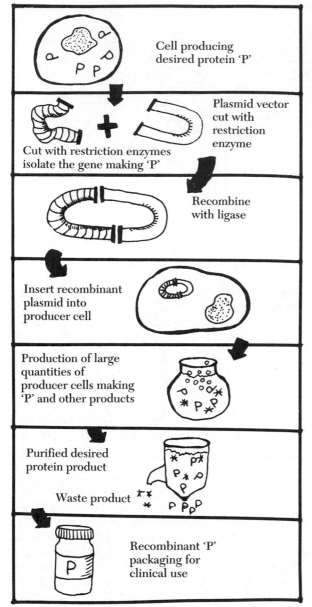

Cell producing desired protein 'P'

Plasmid vector cut with restriction enzyme

Cut with restriction enzymes isolate the gene making 'P'

Recombine with ligase

Insert recombinant plasmid into producer cell

Production of large quantities of producer cells making 'P' and other products

Purified desired protein product

Waste product

Recombinant 'P' packaging for clinical use

Figure 2. Recombinant DNA technology is used to splice or recombine a gene coding for a desired protein product into an expression vector, which allows the protein to be made in large quantities for therapeutic or diagnostic use.

mosomal genetic elements capable of replicating in bacteria independently of genomic replication, are the usual "expression vectors." These plasmids are isolated, cut with the same restriction enzymes used to prepare the target DNA for cloning, and mixed with the foreign DNA fragments. An enzyme called DNA ligase is used to join the plasmid DNA with target DNA, resulting in the production of closed circular DNA which can be introduced into suitable bacterial, yeast, or eucaryotic cells for expression of large amounts of the desired protein.

Genetically engineered bacteria must then be screened for colonies expressing the recombinant protein. This may be done by analyzing for biologic activity or structure of the protein or by assessing the sequence of DNA that has been inserted into the plasmid. In the latter case, the desired gene is sought by the use of DNA probes. Probes are short, single-stranded DNA molecules of known sequence labeled with a radioactive tracer or an enzyme. These probes will hybridize to complementary sequences in target DNA that has been denatured to single-strand form by heat treatment. A probe bound to target DNA can be detected by radiographic or enzymatic detection methods.

Commercial production and purification of recombinant DNA products has primarily involved traditional techniques of fermentation and protein chemistry. The recombinant product must be assessed for biologic activity because in some cases, the protein requires glycosylation (addition of carbohydrates) which cannot be accomplished by bacterial microorganisms. For proper glycosylation, some genes must be expressed in eucaryotic cells grown in cell culture.

RECOMBINANT DRUG PRODUCTS

Any protein made by a cell may be potentially made by recombinant DNA technology. Thus far, a number of peptide hormones and other intercellular signaling molecules such as interferons, growth factors, and cytokines have been produced and are either commercially available or are being evaluated in clinical trials. Also, proteins with enzyme activity, such as tissue plasminogen activator and superoxide dismutase, have been cloned (Table 1).

Structural proteins may also be made, as in the case of recombinant vaccines which express the surface antigen of viruses such as the gp70 envelope protein of feline leukemia virus (FeLV), the nucleocapsid of rabies virus, and the surface antigen of human hepatitis B virus. These recombinant vaccines offer advantages over traditional vaccines, such as lack of exposure to human tissue or blood products during production in the case of hepatitis vaccine and absence of potential for reversion to virulence of the vaccine in contrast to modified live virus vaccines.

Recombinant DNA products can be given as drugs to replace factors that the body cannot make for itself, such as insulin in the case of diabetes mellitus, coagulation factor VIII in hemophilia A, or surfactant to treat premature neonates. In other situations, the body may be capable of making a protein but may be helped by administration of a recombinant product in supraphysiologic levels. Recombinant immune system regulators such as interferons, interleukins, or tumor necrosis factor may thus play a role in the treatment of various infections

Table 1. List of Some Recombinant Therapeutic Agents*

Product Name	Human Indications	Potential Veterinary Indications
Erythropoietin	Dialysis anemia, anemia of AIDS, chemotherapy-induced anemia	Anemia of chronic renal failure, FeLV-associated anemia
Somatotropin	Growth hormone deficiency in children	Growth hormone deficiency
Human insulin	Diabetes mellitus	Refractory diabetes mellitus
Interferons: Alpha-2a, alpha-2b, and gamma	Various cancers, infectious disease	FeLV infection cancer, infectious disease
Granulocyte/macrophage colony stimulating factor	Adjuvant to chemotherapy, bone marrow transplant, sepsis, myelodysplasia	Chemotherapy effects, cyclic neutropenia, sepsis, myelodysplasia
Granulocyte colony stimulating factor	Chemotherapy effects, AIDS, leukemia, aplastic anemia	Chemotherapy effects, sepsis
Macrophage colony stimulating factor	Cancer therapy, bone marrow transplantation	Cancer therapy, bone marrow transplantation
Superoxide dismutase	Reperfusion injury of myocardial infarction, organ transplantation, oxygen toxicity of preterm infants	Reperfusion injury
Coagulation factor VIII	Hemophilia	Hemophilia
Epidermal growth factor	Corneal transplants, wound healing	Corneal injury, wound healing
Fibroblast growth factor	Chronic soft-tissue ulcers	Wound healing
Interleukin-2	Cancer immunotherapy	Cancer immunotherapy
Tumor necrosis factor	Cancer therapy	Cancer therapy
Tissue plasminogen activator	Myocardial infarction, stroke, pulmonary embolism, deep vein thrombosis	Saddle thrombus, pulmonary embolism
Feline leukemia vaccine (recombinant GP70)	None	FeLV prophylaxis
Rabies vaccine (recombinant)	None	Rabies prophylaxis

*Information provided by Pharmaceutical Manufacturers Association.
FeLV, feline leukemia virus.

or in the treatment of cancer. Recombinant drugs such as hematopoietic growth factors (granulocyte colony stimulating factor, granulocyte-macrophage colony stimulating factor, or erythropoietin) may prove useful in situations where these growth factors are deficient, as in certain aplastic anemias or erythropoietin deficiency secondary to renal failure, or where the body may need additional support in the rapid production of large numbers of blood cells, as in the case of bone marrow transplantation or overwhelming sepsis. Recombinant epidermal growth factor may prove useful for increasing the rate of healing of corneal injuries or burn wounds. Enzyme products such as tissue plasminogen activator could be helpful to promote dissolution of clots, such as in the case of saddle thrombi associated with cardiomyopathy in cats. Recombinant superoxide dismutase has been developed for use as a free radical scavenger to prevent reperfusion injuries in organ transplant and cardiac infarction patients.

One potential limiting factor of recombinant DNA proteins as drugs is their potential antigenicity. Since most products cloned to date have been of murine or human origin, the potential for utility in domestic animals depends on the homology of the amino acid sequence of the recombinant product with that of the treated species. Species differences in protein structure could result in total lack of effect of the recombinant product, transient therapeutic effect followed by antibody formation and subsequent loss of efficacy, anaphylactic reaction,

or even cross-reactive immune responses against the native protein in the treated species. An example of apparent immune reactivity to a human recombinant product that has been used in the dog is granulocyte colony stimulating factor (G-CSF) used in cyclic neutropenic collies and dogs with myelosuppression secondary to the administration of cancer chemotherapeutics. When the human recombinant G-CSF was administered, significant elevation in neutrophil numbers was observed for approximately 3 weeks of therapy. Subsequent administration had no therapeutic effect. However, when dogs were given a G-CSF product cloned from the canine gene, no antibodies were produced and leukocytosis persisted for extended periods. The canine G-CSF product was found to be efficacious and nonantigenic in cats as well. Some authors have suggested that antigenicity of recombinant products could be abrogated by simultaneous use of immune suppressive drugs, such as cyclosporin, with recombinant proteins.

FUTURE DIRECTIONS

Taking the theories of recombinant DNA technology further, one of the next steps is to add cloned genes to the genome of cells of the host so that the recombinant products can be made directly in the treated patient. An example of this approach used clinically is the introduction of functional copies of the tumor necrosis factor gene into a class of lymphocyte effector cells called tumor-infiltrating lymphocytes (TIL cells) derived from human patients with advanced melanoma. These engineered lymphocytes are given back to the patient from whom they were derived to induce a response against the melanoma.

Inactivation of genes that are expressed inappropriately or in excessive quantities is a more complicated task. For example, inactivation of oncogenes responsible for malignant transformation as treatment of cancer at the genetic level is being investigated in cell culture systems. One approach that may prove effective is the use of "antisense" oligonucleotides to decrease gene expression. The principle of antisense genetic modulation is that complementary single-stranded DNA may be able to hybridize with messenger RNA within the cell and block ribosomal attachment and translation of protein product (translation arrest). Antisense translation arrest has proved successful in decreasing replication and inducing phenotypic differentiation of neoplastic cells in culture. New techniques are being sought to directly attack aberrant or overexpressed genes in the chromosome by targeting toxic drugs, such as alkylating agents, to specific DNA sequences by using antisense delivery systems capable of binding chromosomal DNA. This type of antisense oligonucleotide would then induce gene inactivation in a highly specific manner. Antisense methodologies are being actively investigated as experimental treatment approaches to retroviral infections, such as human immunodeficiency virus or feline leukemia virus infection, or to inactivation of genes responsible for malignant transformation in cancer.

References and Suggested Reading

Black, W. J.: Drug products of recombinant DNA technology. Am. J. Hosp. Pharm. 46:1834, 1989.
A review of the steps in creating recombinant DNA molecules, examples of recombinant drug products, and a look at the future of this revolutionary biotechnology.

Dolnick, B. J.: Antisense agents in pharmacology. Biochem. Pharmacol. 40:671, 1990.
A review of the methodology, pitfalls, and potential utility of antisense oligonucleotides in pharmacology.

Lehn, P. M.: Gene therapy using bone marrow transplantation: A 1990 update. Bone Marrow Transplant 5:287, 1990.
A review of future current approaches and future potential uses for genetically engineered bone marrow transplants.

Lothrop, C. D., Warren, D. J., Souza, L. M., et al.: Correction of canine cyclic hematopoiesis with recombinant human granulocyte colony-stimulating factor. Blood 72:5624, 1988.
Human recombinant G-CSF transiently corrects cyclic neutropenia in grey collies.

Miller, A. D.: Progress toward human gene therapy. Blood 76:271, 1990.
A review of the state of the art in gene therapy in human medicine.

Murray, K.: Application of recombinant DNA techniques in the development of viral vaccines. Vaccine 6:164, 1988.
A review of recombinant genetic approaches to making third-generation vaccines.

Narang, S. A., Brousseau, R., and Georges, F.: Scope of DNA cloning and chemical methods in development of chemotherapeutic agents. Pharmacol. Ther. 26:163, 1984.
A comprehensive review of recombinant DNA methodology, laboratory techniques, and applications to therapeutic agents.

Rosenberg, S. A., Aebersold, P., Cornetta, K., et al.: Gene transfer into humans—Immunotherapy of patients with advanced melanoma, using tumor-infiltrating lymphocytes modified by retroviral gene transduction. N. Engl. J. Med. 323:570, 1990.
One of the first reports of clinical application of genetically engineered cells to treat human disease.

Obradovich, J. E., Ogilvie, G. K., Powers, B. E., et al.: Evaluation of recombinant canine granulocyte colony stimulating factor as an inducer of granulopoiesis: A pilot study. J. Vet. Intern. Med. 5:75, 1991.
Efficacy of canine recombinant G-CSF is demonstrated in the dog.

Watson, J. D., Hopkins, N. H., Roberts, J. W., et al.: *Molecular Biology of the Gene.* Menlo Park: Benjamin Cummings, 1987, p. 313.
This book is the bible of molecular biology and is must reading for a full understanding of the intricacies of the field. Chapter 11 (cited) is the recombinant DNA introductory chapter.

TREATMENT OF HYPERSENSITIVITY: GENERAL GUIDELINES

LAUREL J. GERSHWIN
Davis, California

DEFINITION AND CLINICAL SYNDROMES INVOLVED

Immune reactions that produce adverse effects on the patient are generally referred to as hypersensitivity reactions. Gell and Coombs are credited with defining the causative immunologic mechanisms responsible for these reactions and classifying them as types I to IV. The classic allergy is described by type I reactions: immunoglobulin E (IgE) is produced against an antigen, binds to mast cells, and, after contact with antigen, causes degranulation of mast cells with release of vasoactive mediators. Allergic inhalant dermatitis is an example of type I hypersensitivity. Type II reactions involve the cytotoxic reactions of immunoglobulins G and M (IgG and IgM) with cell surface antigens, as develops in transfusion reactions. Immune complexes interact with complement to create inflammation of the type III reaction. Antibodies involved in the immune complexes reaction may be autoantibodies, as in systemic lupus erythematosus. The classic delayed-type hypersensitivity reaction typified by a positive tuberculin skin test is caused by sensitized T lymphocytes reacting with antigen, resulting in influx of mononuclear cells. Contact allergy is a type IV hypersensitivity in which T lymphocytes respond to a variety of antigens, such as synthetic fibers, plastics, and metals.

This chapter will focus on type I hypersensitivities, including atopic allergy and anaphylaxis. Before considering modes of therapy, it is useful to understand the steps involved in sensitization and elicitation of the allergic reaction. Then points of therapeutic intervention can most easily be identified.

Small animal patients with allergy are atopic, that is, they have a genetic tendency to develop IgE antibodies against certain environmental antigens. These antigens, which include tree pollens, weeds, grasses, molds, and insect secretions, are collectively referred to as allergens. Food components can also elicit production of IgE antibodies. Before an allergen can cause signs of allergy, it must gain access to cells of the immune system by passing through the skin or mucous membranes. After penetrating these barriers, the allergen is processed by a macrophage or other antigen-presenting cell and presented to B and T lymphocytes. If the appropriate T-cell subset is stimulated, the event is followed by production of interleukin-4 (IL-4), a soluble factor that affects differentiation of B lymphocytes. Under the influence of IL-4, B cells develop into IgE-producing plasma cells that preferentially produce the IgE class of antibody. Another set of T lymphocytes—suppressor cells—has an important role. Suppressor cells modulate the IgE response and prevent large amounts of IgE from being produced. Diminished IgE-specific suppressor T-cell activity results in production of high levels of IgE and atopy.

Once allergen-specific IgE has been produced, it attaches to high-affinity receptors on mast cells located in the skin and along mucous membranes. At this point, the patient is poised for an allergic reaction. Re-exposure to the allergen that induced the production of the IgE antibodies cross-links IgE molecules on the mast cell, which triggers a complex series of biochemical events, including stimulation of phospholipid metabolism, membrane enzyme activation, and eventual degranulation with mediator release. The antigen-triggered bridging of IgE receptors on the mast cell causes a decrease in intracellular cyclic adenosine monophosphate (cAMP) concentrations and a change in the ratio of cAMP to cyclic guanosine monophosphate (cGMP). This acts as a second messenger system to stimulate degranulation. Simultaneous with degranulation there is stimulation of de novo synthesis of arachidonic acid metabolites of the cyclo-oxygenase (prostaglandins) and lipo-oxygenase pathways (leukotrienes). The process of IgE-triggered mast cell activation opens calcium channels in cell membranes. Once inside cells, calcium ions activate calcium-dependent intracellular enzymes. Fusion of perigranular membranes with the cytoplasmic membrane results in secretion of preformed mediators.

POINTS FOR POTENTIAL THERAPEUTIC INTERVENTION

Treatment of type I hypersensitivity can be targeted at any stage in the allergic reaction as illustrated in Figure 1.

DIAGNOSIS AND AVOIDANCE STRATEGIES

Before initiation of therapy it is necessary to establish a diagnosis of allergic disease and to determine the nature of the allergens involved. The medical history, including seasonal and environmental factors, is particularly important. The first step in diagnosis of allergy is to detect IgE antibodies specific for particular allergens. This is done by performing intradermal skin testing or in vitro testing using radioallergosorbent test (RAST) or enzyme-linked immunosorbent assay (ELISA) methods. The choice of allergens for skin testing may be influenced by the geographic locality of the patient. Tables are available (Baker, 1990) describing major weeds and their pollination patterns in each region of the U.S. Molds and dust are common environmental antigens that should also be included. Physician allergists may provide additional information about important weeds and other plants in the area as well as their pollination season. Although mixes of allergens are available, it is preferable to perform skin tests with individual allergens. Procedures for intradermal skin tests and their interpretation are described elsewhere (Baker, 1990; Halliwell and Gorman, 1989).

Once sensitization has occurred, prevention of re-exposure to the allergen, or allergens, is the best means of avoiding clinical signs of allergy. Avoidance therapy (see Fig. 1, step 4) simply prevents mast cell degranulation by preventing re-exposure

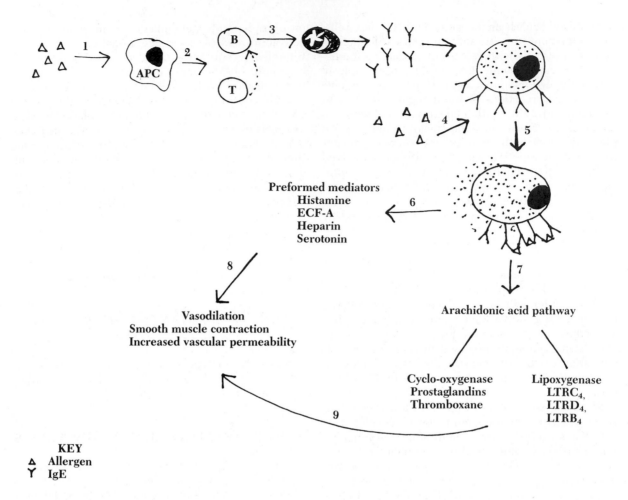

KEY
△ Allergen
Y IgE

Figure 1. Schematic diagram on the sensitization phase (1 through 3) and elicitation phase (4 through 9) of a typical Type 1 hypersensitivity reaction.

Sensitization phase:
1. Initial exposure to the allergen; processing by antigen presenting cells (APC).
2. Allergen stimulates B and T lymphocytes.
3. B lymphocytes differentiate into plasma cells making IgE, which binds to Fc receptors on mast cells and basophils.
Elicitation phase:
4. Re-exposure to the allergen; allergen binds to IgE on mast cells.
5. Mast cell degranulation.
6. Preformed mediators are released from mast cell granules.
7. Arachidonic acid metabolic pathways are triggered with production of leukotrienes and prostaglandins.
8. Preformed mediators cause immediate physiologic effects.
9. Leukotrienes (slow-reacting substance of anaphylaxis) cause a late-phase allergic reaction.

LTR, leukotriene. ECF-A, eosinophil chemotactic factor of anaphylaxis.

of sensitized cells to allergens. Some allergens, such as foods, can readily be avoided; others, such as inhaled pollens, are more difficult to avoid. It is possible to install air filters in the house to assist in minimizing exposure to house dust; this is commonly done for allergic human beings. Exposure to pollens can be limited by curtailing access to grass and fields, while exercising on cement with the aid of a leash. Avoidance is the only specific treatment available for food allergy; allergen immunotherapy is generally ineffective. The choices available for inhalant allergy include pharmacologic therapy, immunotherapy, or both.

IMMUNOTHERAPY

Immunotherapy, when effective, decreases production of specific IgE. Exactly how this occurs is still uncertain, but induction of suppressor T cells is thought to have a role (see Fig. 1, step 2). In addition, in most cases there is a concomitant increase in allergen-specific IgG, which serves as blocking antibodies (see Fig. 1, step 3).

Once specific allergy is documented, it is important that clients understand the need to comply fully with the injection program. Clients should be informed that immunotherapy may be ineffective in some patients. Immunotherapy is indicated in patients with proven IgE-mediated disease that are sufficiently young to benefit from therapy (i.e., it may not be worthwhile to desensitize an older dog). Immunotherapy is contraindicated in patients with autoimmune disease.

The choice of an immunotherapy regimen consists of allergen selection, dosage, and duration of treatment.

Allergen Selection

Allergens to be used in immunotherapy are chosen on the basis of skin tests or *in vitro* test results. Several companies now offer *in vitro* tests (RAST or ELISA) for allergen-specific IgE and immunotherapy vials containing the appropriate allergens. *In vitro* tests detect circulating IgE whereas skin tests detect mast cell–bound IgE. There may be some discrepancy when results of both tests are compared. This is related, at least in part, to the fact that IgE remains on mast cells for many weeks, while the serum half-life of IgE is just over 2 days. Most veterinary allergists consider results of skin tests as the most reliable criteria for formulating an immunotherapy program. However, when intradermal skin tests are not possible, *in vitro* tests may be considered. Inclusion of all allergens detected by positive skin tests into the immunotherapy regimen is the usual practice of veterinary allergists. Physicians also consider clinical symptoms when formulating the composition of the injection mixtures for human patients.

Dosage and Type of Preparation

There are two types of allergen preparations commercially available: an aqueous preparation and an alum-precipitated preparation. Adsorption of the allergen onto alum results in slower absorption of allergen and a more prolonged stimulation of the immune system. For low-dose immunotherapy, allergens are grouped; up to ten are placed in a single vial. Three vials are prepared; each one is tenfold more concentrated than the one before. Equal amounts of each allergen are placed into the vial. The quantity of allergen is expressed in terms of protein nitrogen units (PNU) so that a vial containing 7000 PNU of seven allergens would contain 1000 PNU of each allergen. Initial injections are given from the lower-dose vial. For high-dose im-

munotherapy, larger quantities of allergen are placed into each treatment vial (for example, vial 1, 10,000 PNU; vial 2, 20,000 PNU; and vial 3, 40,000 PNU).

Schedule and Duration of Treatment

A variety of schedules are used for immunotherapy (Baker 1990; Halliwell and Gorman, 1989; Reedy and Miller, 1989). After the initial treatment series, maintenance therapy schedules vary from weekly to every third week. The use of alum-adsorbed antigens prolongs the period between injections. Improvement is not immediate. For example, in one study, 25% of the patients improved within the first 3 months of therapy; another 25% improved by 6 months; by 1 year, a total of 75% improved (Reedy and Miller, 1989).

PHARMACOLOGIC INTERVENTION

When it is impractical to attempt desensitization, or during initial stages of immunotherapy, pharmacologic agents can be used to alleviate the clinical signs of allergy.

Agents That Inhibit Mediator Formation

Antiprostaglandins inhibit the cyclo-oxygenase pathway of arachidonic acid metabolism and prostaglandin synthesis (Fig. 1, step 9). Aspirin has anti-prostaglandin effects but often induces gastrointestinal irritation in dogs. Some authors do not recommend administration of aspirin to cats. The dosage of aspirin for dogs is 2.5 mg/kg t.i.d. Leukotrienes, important mediators of type 1 hypersensitivity, are not inhibited by aspirin.

Corticosteroids (see later) have been reported to interfere with replenishing histamine within mast cell granules. Corticosteroids apparently inhibit histidine decarboxylase, impairing the conversion of histidine to histamine.

Agents That Inhibit Mediator Release

Disodium cromoglycate (chromolyn) is a drug that prevents degranulation of mast cells even after re-exposure to allergen (see Fig. 1, step 5). Disodium cromoglycate must be administered to the patient for several weeks before the full beneficial effect occurs. Daily use during the allergy season is critical. It is available in powder form for inhalation by human patients with asthma, as a liquid effective in the treatment of allergic conjunctivitis, as a preparation designed for instillation into the nasal cavity, and as an oral preparation (not available currently in the United States). The oral preparation has been successful in treatment of cases of food allergy. Current uses in companion animals are limited to treatment of allergic rhinitis and conjunctivitis.

Mast cell membrane stabilization has also been attributed to corticosteroids, although there may be species differences (Adolphson, 1987).

The experimental drug CI-922 (Warner-Lambert/Parke-Davis) is a mediator-release inhibitor, known to be effective when given to ascaris-allergic dogs exposed to an aerosol of ascaris antigen. This drug inhibits antigen-induced leukotriene release when given 10 min before antigen challenge. The exact mechanism of action of this drug is unclear. It may exert its effect by altering metabolic pathways of arachadonic acid (Fig. 1, step 7).

Agents That Modulate Mediator Release

Theophylline and aminophylline modulate mediator release from mast cells by increasing intracellular concentrations of cAMP (see Fig. 1, step 5). Although theophylline only has a duration of action of up to 4 hr, there are several long-acting products available. The bronchodilatory effect of theophylline and aminophylline is of greatest use in patients with respiratory involvement (see later). However, the modulatory effects on mediator release must not be overlooked when designing a treatment regimen.

Agents That Interfere with Mediator Action

Antihistamines counteract the effects of histamine by competing with histamine for the H_1 or H_2 receptors on cells (see Fig. 1, step 8). In order for histamine to produce its effects, it must bind to H_1 receptors. If there is sufficient antihistamine available to cover these sites, histamine does not bind and cannot induce its effects (increased capillary permeability, smooth-muscle contraction, and so forth). However, the benefit of antihistamines is limited because they are ineffective in preventing the effects of the leukotrienes, chemotactic factors, prostaglandins, and other important mediators.

The most commonly used antihistamines are H_1 blockers. There are several different classes of antihistamines. These include alkylamines, ethanolamines, ethylenediamines, piperazine, piperidine, and phenothiazine. Terfenadine (Seldane, Marion Merrell Dow) is a relatively new antihistamine. It is used frequently in human medicine because its use is associated with minimal drowsiness. Terfenadine is a phenothiazine derivative. It has been used by veterinarians at a dose of 5 to 10 mg/kg b.i.d.

The antihistamine hydroxyzine (Atarax, Roerig) is a piperazine derivative that also induces mild tranquilization. This feature can be beneficial in dogs with extreme pruritus. It has been used at a dose of 2.2 mg/kg t.i.d.

There are a variety of other antihistamines available for use. Cyproheptadine (Periactin, Merck Sharp & Dohme), a piperidine, has an additional antiserotonin effect. Chlorpheniramine (Chlor-Trimeton, Schering-Plough Health Care), an alkylamine, is given in dosages of 2 to 8 mg b.i.d. Two antihistamines can be used simultaneously to increase effectiveness. Antihistamines can also be used in conjunction with corticosteroids. One veterinary allergist recommends initial use of an antihistamine in conjunction with corticosteroids, followed by gradual reduction and finally elimination of the corticosteroid while continuing with a maintenance dose of antihistamine (Baker, 1990).

Side effects of antihistamines include sedation, central nervous system (CNS) stimulation, and possible teratogenic effects if administered to pregnant animals.

Agents That Counteract Mediator Effects

Anaphylactic shock can be elicited by a variety of allergic insults, including reaction to immunotherapy, reaction to vaccines, reaction to drugs (particularly antibiotics), and reaction to insect stings (e.g., fire ants). Mediator release is rapid and massive; their effects must be reversed immediately to avoid a fatal outcome.

Beta-adrenergic stimulants, such as epinephrine and isoproterenol, cause smooth-muscle relaxation and decrease capillary permeability, thereby reversing the effects of the mediators (see Fig. 1). Epinephrine is the drug of choice for treatment of acute anaphylactic shock. It should be administered immediately and may be repeated if necessary to control clinical signs.

Theophylline, aminophylline, and ephedrine are also effective at the end-organ level where, by virtue of smooth muscle relaxation, they antagonize the effects of histamine and leukotrienes.

Corticosteroids: Multiple Sites of Action

Corticosteroids are well known for their anti-inflammatory effects. Accumulation of neutrophils in areas of inflammation is inhibited by corticosteroid-mediated reduction in chemotaxis, adherence to vascular endothelium, and capillary permeability. Stabilization of membranes is another benefit of corticosteroids that impairs mediator release from mast cells (see Fig. 1, step 5). Corticosteroids also inhibit synthesis of histamine within mast cell granules (see Fig. 1, step 6). Inhibition of the cyclo-oxygenase and lipoxygenase pathways of arachidonic acid metabolism decreases formation of prostaglandins and leukotrienes (see Fig. 1, step 7). Leukotrienes C4 and D4 are important mediators of the allergic reaction, particularly later phases of the reaction. Although administration of corticosteroids produces lymphopenia, there is debate as to their effectiveness in reducing antibody production. Generally, the dosages used to treat allergic disease do not suppress antibody formation. Thus, steroids do not "cure" the allergy, but they do effectively counteract several different levels of the allergic mechanism.

Both prednisone and prednisolone are synthetic analogues of endogenous corticosteroids and have short half-lives. Prednisolone is the active form of the drug, whereas prednisone must first be metabolized to prednisolone before it can be active. Longer-acting steroids, such as dexamethasone, are available but are more likely to cause adrenal suppression than prednisone or prednisolone. Corticosteroids can be quite effective when given on alternate days. Alternate-day therapy causes less adrenal suppression. Side effects of steroids can be numerous and have been reviewed (see CVT X, p. 54.)

The use of corticosteroids in treatment of type 1 hypersensitivity should be done judiciously. They should not be given, or they should be withdrawn for several weeks or more, before skin tests are performed. Then the smallest dose that will inhibit the clinical signs should be administered on an alternate-day schedule. When it is possible to stop the therapy, the drug should be withdrawn slowly by tapering the dose.

References and Suggested Reading

Adolphson, R. L., Finkel, M. P., and Robichaud, L. J.: CI-922—A novel, potent antiallergic compound—II. Activity in animal models of allergy. Int. J. Immunopharm. 9:51, 1987.
An experimental paper describing the effectiveness of a new mediator release inhibitor in dogs allergic to ascaris antigen.
Baker, E.: *Small Animal Allergy: A Practical Guide.* Philadelphia: Lea & Febiger, 1990, p. 72.
A well-written, concise, and practical source for the veterinarian who wants to begin an allergy practice.
Bevier, D. E.: Long-term management of atopic disease in the dog. Vet. Clin. North Am. Small Anim. Pract. 20:1487, 1990.
Contains detailed tables on drugs and dosages for pharmacologic therapy.
Halliwell, R. E. W., and Gorman, N. T.: *Veterinary Clinical Immunology.* Philadelphia: W. B. Saunders, 1989, pp. 232, 493.
A text containing basic immunology as well as descriptions of immunologic diseases and their therapy.
Reedy, L. M., and Miller, W. H.: *Allergic Skin Diseases of Dogs and Cats.* Philadelphia: W. B. Saunders, 1989.
Limited to dermatologic manifestations of allergy.

AMYLOID AND AMYLOIDOSIS

KENNETH H. JOHNSON,
and TIMOTHY D. O'BRIEN
St. Paul, Minnesota

DEFINITIONS

Amyloid consists of abnormal proteinaceous deposits within tissues. The disease condition, amyloidosis, is clinically significant because functional tissue components or cells, or both, are replaced by localized (i.e., organ- or tissue-limited) or systemic (multiple-organ) amyloid deposits. Thus, clinical signs associated with amyloidosis are directly related to the specific sites of amyloid deposition. Unfortunately, amyloid deposition is usually a progressive process with little or no likelihood of regression, and the efficacy of currently available treatment regimens is limited.

PATHOGENESIS OF AMYLOIDOSIS

Amyloid deposits in humans contain predominantly abnormal fibrillar proteins that can be derived from at least 15 different proteins (i.e., amyloid precursor proteins) normally found in blood or body tissues. To date, however, only three of these 15 protein precursors have been documented as a source of amyloid fibril formation in domestic animals. Different pathogenic mechanisms are likely to be involved in generation of amyloid fibrils from each different precursor molecule. Therefore, amyloidosis is not a single disease, nor does amyloid necessarily represent the same chemical substance in each case (Glenner, 1980).

Despite the variety of potential precursor proteins and pathogenic mechanisms involved in formation of various types of amyloid, all amyloid deposits have identical light and electron microscopic characteristics. All forms of amyloid are characterized by congophilia (red staining with bright field microscopy), green birefringence with polarized light, and characteristic ultrastructural fibrils that have amino acids arranged extensively in a beta pleated-sheet configuration. Each amyloid fibril is formed by polymerization of repeated peptides derived from either the entire precursor protein or a segment of the precursor protein.

The specific mechanisms resulting in formation of amyloid fibrils from different precursor proteins are incompletely understood, but it is clear that there is not a single underlying explanation that ties together all forms of amyloidosis. Normal proteins with a beta pleated-sheet conformation may be predisposed to amyloidogenesis if their tissue concentrations become abnormally elevated as a result of overproduction or decreased catabolism. Aberrant enzymatic processing of a normal protein may result in incompletely degraded peptide segments that are predisposed to self-aggregation (i.e., polymerization), and amyloid fibril formation. In addition, abnormal amino acid substitutions in some proteins predispose humans to an increased risk for amyloid formation. As a general rule, systemic forms of amyloidosis are derived from systemic protein precursors distributed throughout the blood vascular system, while organ-limited or localized forms of amyloidosis are associated with protein precursors normally or abnormally concentrated in localized sites.

The various forms of amyloidosis that affect humans and animals are most accurately classified on the basis of the chemical identity of the repetitive amyloid protein. The chemical identity of the amyloid protein can be determined by its isolation and purification, or by use of specific immunohistochemical (peroxidase-antiperoxidase) techniques (Fujihara et al., 1980). Immunohistochemical techniques, in which specific antisera to the different amyloid subunit proteins are used, are the most practical procedures for most diagnostic settings. In addition, sensitivity of the amyloid to oxidation by potassium permanganate (Wright et al., 1977) can be easily evaluated histochemically. Although less specific, the latter is a useful routine screening procedure for the tentative differentiation of so-called secondary amyloid (i.e., "reactive" or amyloid A [AA]) from other forms of amyloid.

CLINICOPATHOLOGIC FORMS OF SPONTANEOUS AMYLOIDOSIS IN DOGS AND CATS

The most common form of spontaneously occurring amyloidosis recognized in domestic animals is AA amyloidosis, (secondary or reactive amyloidosis). The precursor protein for this form of amyloid is an acute-phase reactant protein known as serum amyloid A (SAA). It is produced by the liver in response to a wide variety of persistent injurious stimuli (e.g., infection, inflammation, or neoplastic disease). SAA is synthesized as a 104–amino acid molecule; however, only the N-terminal part of the molecule (i.e., identified as protein AA, which commonly has 76 amino acids) is incorporated into amyloid fibrils. The normal function of SAA is unclear, as are the mechanisms accounting for transformation of this normal protein into amyloid fibrils.

Protein AA has been chemically and immunohistochemically identified as the major component of this systemic form of amyloidosis occurring in dogs (Westermark et al., 1985), cats (DiBartola et al., 1985; Johnson et al., 1989b), and other domestic animals, even though predisposing or concurrent diseases often are not apparent. Systemic AA amyloidosis in dogs is typically characterized by marked proteinuria and progressive renal disease because of extensive amyloid deposition within the renal glomerular mesangium and basement membranes. Thrombosis, especially within pulmonary vessels, occurs in a significant percentage (~40%) of dogs with renal amyloidosis (Slauson and Gribble, 1971). The pathogenesis of thrombosis associated with renal amyloidosis is multifactorial but includes the loss of low-molecular-weight anticlotting factors (e.g., antithrombin III) in the urine. Although systemic AA amyloidosis is relatively uncommon in cats as compared with dogs, a familial form frequently affects Abyssinian cats. Amyloid deposits in Abyssinian cats may be present in a number of tissues but predominate in the kidneys, leading to renal failure and death at a young age (DiBartola et al., 1986). Amyloid deposition in the kidneys of all breeds of cats involves the medullary interstitium more consistently and extensively than the glomeruli. Thus, proteinuria may or may not be a clinical feature of renal amyloidosis in cats.

An interesting form of familial systemic amyloidosis with some similarities to familial amyloidosis in Abyssinian cats was recently reported in 14 Chinese Shar pei dogs (DiBartola et al., 1990). This form of amyloidosis was diagnosed in relatively young Shar peis (mean age at the time of diagnosis was 4.1 yr), and it was associated with clinical signs of renal failure (e.g., polyuria, polydipsia, vomition, and dehydration). Based on its sensitivity to oxidation by potassium permanganate, the amyloid present in multiple organs was considered to be of protein AA origin. As in cats, renal medullary amyloid deposits were more consistently observed than glomerular deposits.

The immunoglobulin light chain–derived (amyloid L [AL]) form of amyloidosis (sometimes called primary amyloidosis) has recently been documented in a cat (Carothers et al., 1989), and it represents the first chemical confirmation of this form of amyloidosis in animals. The amyloid deposits in this case were systemic, involving the lymph nodes, spleen, and liver and were resistant to potassium permanganate oxidation. Amino acid sequence analysis of the purified amyloid protein from this cat confirmed a sequence corresponding with human immunoglobulin λ light chains. The precursor protein in this cat was derived from light chains of a monoclonal immunoglobulin, which was demonstrated as a globulin spike by serum electrophoresis and was produced by a large extramedullary plasmacytoma affecting the tarsus. Amyloid restricted to the interstitium of a localized plasmacytoma in a dog was also recently shown by immunohistochemistry to be of immunoglobulin λ light chain origin (Geisel et al., 1990). Systemic AL or primary amyloidosis develops in approximately 15% of human patients with multiple myeloma, where the repetitive amyloid protein may be derived from entire immunoglobulin light chains or from fragments of the variable immunoglobulin regions. In humans, immunoglobulin light chains with certain molecular characteristics (i.e., λ-VI light chains) are the most amyloidogenic. Amyloidosis has been reported in only a few cats and dogs with concurrent multiple myeloma; unfortunately, the type of amyloid affecting these patients was not characterized.

A third form of amyloid, observed in pancreatic islets of over 80% of aged diabetic cats (but not in the pancreatic islets of dogs), has recently been chemically characterized (Johnson et al., 1989a). This localized form of amyloid restricted to the pancreatic islets has been shown in diabetic cats and non–insulin-dependent (type 2) diabetic humans to be derived from a hitherto unknown hormone produced by islet beta cells. This hormone, identified as islet amyloid polypeptide (IAPP), is normally co-localized with insulin within beta-cell secretory vesicles and is co-secreted with insulin in response to hyperglycemia. In cats and humans, overproduction of IAPP due to as yet unknown factors appears to facilitate amyloidogenesis because the IAPP of these species normally incorporates a short amyloidogenic sequence. Overproduction of IAPP may also be significantly linked to the development of age-associated diabetes in cats and humans. The presence of IAPP-derived islet amyloid deposits in cats is predictive of a high probability (>90%) that the affected animals have either impaired glucose tolerance or overt diabetes mellitus.

Other clinicopathologic forms of amyloidosis, associated with protein precursors different from those discussed here, undoubtedly exist in dogs and cats. These conditions have unknown clinical significance, however, and their protein precursors have not been chemically characterized. For example, a prominent form of vascular amyloidosis (apparently not of protein AA origin, based on resistance to permanganate oxidation) occurs quite commonly within the hearts and lungs of aged dogs. Vascular amyloid and amyloid-containing plaques, similar to those seen in human patients with Alzheimer's disease, have also been observed in aged dogs, within the neuropil of the cerebral cortex.

DIAGNOSIS OF AMYLOIDOSIS

A definitive diagnosis of amyloidosis requires histologic evaluation of affected tissues obtained by biopsy or at necropsy examination. Congophilia and green birefringence in Congo red–stained sections examined with polarized light confirm the diagnosis of amyloidosis. AA amyloid can be tentatively identified by its sensitivity to oxidation, and thus its lack of Congophilia, following treatment with potassium permanganate. Using specific antibodies against different amyloid fibril proteins and the peroxidase-antiperoxidase technique on paraffin-embedded tissues, the specific biochemical form of amyloid can be determined. If these specific antisera are available, the chemical nature of amyloid deposits can also be determined at the ultrastructural level, using the protein A–gold labeling technique.

Subcutaneous abdominal fat aspirates or biopsies, directly stained with Congo red and examined by polarization microscopy, are effective (~90%) for the diagnosis of systemic amyloidosis in humans (Libbey et al., 1983). The effectiveness of this minimally invasive diagnostic procedure in animals has not been adequately evaluated. We have not found Congophilic deposits, however, in the subcutaneous fat of the few dogs we have studied that had multiple-organ amyloidosis.

Diagnostic radionuclide imaging of amyloid deposits, using labeled substances known to bind to amyloid (e.g., ^{123}I-labeled serum amyloid P [SAP] component; pyrophosphate or diphosphonate labeled with technetium-99m), has been used to diagnose, localize, and monitor systemic amyloidosis in humans (Hawkins et al., 1990). These procedures may be especially helpful in evaluation of the efficacy of therapeutic agents but apparently have not been used in animals.

TREATMENT OF AMYLOIDOSIS

In general, treatment of amyloidosis has not resulted in cure. Several preventative and therapeutic approaches, however, have been of some benefit to humans and laboratory animals. Aggressive management of underlying inflammatory diseases with antibiotic therapy reduces the probability of reactive systemic AA amyloidosis in animals and humans. In human cases of AL amyloidosis in which amyloid precursor proteins are produced by abnormal or neoplastic plasma cells, alkylating agents (such as melphalan) used in combination with corticosteroids reduced proliferation of neoplastic cells. Further deposition of amyloid was retarded by reducing the amount of amyloid precursor protein (Kyle et al., 1985). Colchicine blocks synthesis and secretion of SAA from hepatocytes in mice, thus inhibiting AA amyloidosis in the predeposition phase. Colchicine has also been effective in preventing development of AA amyloidosis in humans with familial Mediterranean fever. In addition to these approaches aimed at retarding deposition of amyloid in tissues, dimethyl sulfoxide (DMSO) has been occasionally effective in resorption of already formed amyloid deposits in mice and humans. DMSO, administered orally or by instillation at localized sites of amyloid deposition in humans, is also known to have anti-inflammatory properties, which could possibly reduce the stimulus for SAA production.

The efficacy of these therapeutic approaches in animals is difficult to evaluate because the number of reports documenting effects of treatment are limited, and also because adequately controlled studies are difficult to obtain. The results of therapy of four dogs given DMSO orally (300 mg/kg/day), and of one dog given three injections of DMSO per week (80 mg/kg SC) for 1 yr, have been reported (see *CVT X*, p. 1174). There was no evidence of clinical improvement in three of the four dogs given DMSO orally. No evidence of decreased amyloid deposition was found in the dogs that died. The dog given DMSO subcutaneously for 1 yr (followed by topical application for the rest of the animal's life) lived for 5 yr after the initial diagnosis of amyloidosis, but the extent of amyloid deposition at the time of death was not known. The therapeutic efficacy of DMSO in animals with amyloidosis re-

quires further study. Its unpleasant odor, however, makes long-term use objectionable to many owners.

References and Suggested Reading

Carothers, M. A., Johnson, G. C., DiBartola, S. P., et al.: Extramedullary plasmacytoma and immunoglobulin-associated amyloidosis in a cat. J.A.V.M.A. 195:1593, 1989.

DiBartola, S. P., Tarr, M. J., and Benson, M. D.: Tissue distribution of amyloid deposits in Abyssinian cats with familial amyloidosis. J. Comp. Pathol. 96:387, 1986.

DiBartola, S. P., Benson, M. D., Dwulet, F. E., and Cornacoff, J. B.: Isolation and characterization of amyloid protein AA in the Abyssinian cat. Lab. Invest. 52:485, 1985.

DiBartola, S. P., Tarr, M. J., Webb, D. M., et al.: Familial renal amyloidosis in Chinese Shar pei dogs. J.A.V.M.A. 197:483, 1990.

Fujihara, S., Balow, J. E., Costa, J. C., et al.: Identification and classification of amyloid in formalin-fixed, paraffin-embedded tissue sections by the unlabeled immunoperoxidase method. Lab. Invest. 43:358, 1980.

Geisel, O., Stiglmair-Herb, M., and Linke, R. P.: Myeloma associated with immunoglobulin lambda–light chain derived amyloid in a dog. Vet. Pathol. 27:374, 1990.

Glenner, G. G.: Amyloid deposits and amyloidosis: The β-fibrilloses. N. Engl. J. Med. 302:1283 and 1333, 1980.

Hawkins, P. N., Lavender, J. P., and Pepys, M. B.: Evaluation of systemic amyloidosis by scintigraphy with ^{123}I-labeled serum amyloid P component. N. Engl. J. Med. 323:508, 1990.

Johnson, K. H., O'Brien, T. D., Betsholtz, C., et al.: Islet amyloid, islet-amyloid polypeptide, and diabetes mellitus. N. Engl. J. Med. 321:513, 1989a.

Johnson, K. H., Sletten, K., Werdin, R. E., et al.: Amino acid sequence variations in protein AA of cats with high and low incidences of AA amyloidosis. Comp. Biochem. Physiol. B. 94:765, 1989b.

Kyle, R. A., Greipp, P. R., Garton, J. P., et al.: Primary systemic amyloidosis: Comparison of melphalan/prednisone versus colchicine. Am. J. Med. 79:708, 1985.

Libbey, C. A., Skinner, M., and Cohen, A. S.: Use of abdominal fat tissue aspirate in the diagnosis of systemic amyloidosis. Arch. Intern. Med. 143:1549, 1983.

Slauson, D. O., and Gribble, D. H.: Thrombosis complicating renal amyloidosis in dogs. Vet. Pathol. 8:352, 1971.

Westermark, P., Johnson, K. H., Sletten, K., et al.: AA-amyloidosis in dogs: Partial amino acid sequence of protein AA and immunohistochemical cross-reactivity with human and cow AA-amyloid. Comp. Biochem. Physiol. B. 82:211, 1985.

Wright, J. R., Calkins, E., and Humphrey, R. L.: Potassium permanganate reaction in amyloidosis: A histologic method to assist in differentiating forms of this disease. Lab. Invest. 36:274, 1977.

HOMEOPATHIC MEDICINE: FACT OR FICTION?

CARL A. OSBORNE
St. Paul, Minnesota

Recently, there has been renewed interest in homeopathy as a therapeutic modality in veterinary medicine. Homeopathy is derived from the Greek word *homeo;* which means "like," "resembling," "always the same," or "unchanging." *Pathos* is the

Greek term meaning "disease." Homeopathy is a system of therapeutics founded by Samuel Hahnemann in the early 1800's (Lee, 1983). It is based on a philosophy of treating various disease symptoms with "natural" drugs capable of producing comparable symptoms in healthy patients ("like cures like"). Homeopathic medicines are often (but not always) serially diluted by steps of 1:10 or 1:100 (so-called potentiations) with vigorous shaking (so-called succession) at each stage. The drugs are then administered in minute (sometimes 10^{-400}) and probably ineffective quantities (Fisher, 1986). The mode of action (if any) of remedies given at such extreme dilutions cannot be explained by contemporary scientific knowledge.

Homeopathy was a very popular modality throughout the 1800's and early 1900's. Perhaps its popularity can be attributed to the fact that most sick individuals fared better with homeopathic treatment than those who received care from physicians using more conventional methods of therapy. At that time, the pharmacopeia employed by orthodox medical professionals encompassed a large number of highly toxic materials, while those of the homeopath were likely to be harmless since they contained little or no active substance. Homeopaths were unlikely to do further harm with medicaments consisting essentially of water or sugar tablets. However, patients subjected to venesection, arsenic elixirs, and potions containing strychnine often fared poorly. Both animals and humans literally "died of the doctor," while homeopathy at least gave them the opportunity to die of the disease or to recover from it naturally (Smithcors, 1986).

Why has there been renewed interest in homeopathy? In part, it may be related to confusion between an idea (or hypothesis) and validation of the clinical application of that hypothesis. Too frequently the practice of medicine is based on empirical acceptance of a hypothesis as a result of experience or knowledge, without rigorous scientific testing. Hypotheses are then accepted as facts. Acceptance of the value of various therapeutic modalities is unconsciously reinforced by the fact that many diseases are self-limiting. In fact, the severity of many disorders declines within a day or two. In this situation, any form of treatment may appear to be beneficial as long as it is not overtly harmful. Just because a desired clinical response occurs coincidentally with the administration of a therapeutic agent does not demonstrate a cause-and-effect relationship.

The ability to understand the enormous conceptual difference between random clinical observations and results of controlled clinical trials should be a prerequisite for every reader of medical periodicals. Rational scientific treatment, rather than empirical therapy, emerged when clinical research changed from anecdotal documentation to prospective, randomized, controlled, double-blind studies. Randomized trials are not methods of discovery, but rather a means of validation. Empirical observations are extremely important. However, the therapist who accepts the results of uncontrolled studies in lieu of properly controlled ones may be responsible for the perpetuation of medical myths. Lacking acceptable evidence of therapeutic efficacy, the occasional dramatic result is vividly remembered, the failures are forgotten, and folklore therapy often becomes established.

I do not deny that some homeopathic preparations could be of therapeutic benefit. However, to date, there are very few published studies that provide reasonable evidence of their therapeutic efficacy. This is astounding when one considers the number of homeopathic substances that are prescribed. Based on available information, I conclude that the administration of most homeopathic veterinary remedies are an active form of doing nothing.

Since most diseases are self-limiting, who deserves the credit for their cure? The American Veterinary Medical Association (AVMA) has tactfully stated that "no scientific evidence presently exists to demonstrate safety or efficacy of homeopathy," and recommended that "judgment be withheld until suitable studies have been conducted" (AVMA, 1990). To those who champion the therapeutic value of homeopathy in veterinary medicine, the issue is clear: prove it!

References and Suggested Reading

American Veterinary Medical Association (AVMA): Guidelines on alternate therapies. *In* AVMA Directory. Schaumburg, IL: AVMA, 1990, p. 518.
Fisher, P.: Homeopathy: 200 years of non-animal methods. Alternatives to Laboratory Animals 14:24, 1986.
Lee, F.: Trends in homeopathy. Pharm. Int. 4:235, 1983.
Smithcors, J. F.: Veterinary homeopathy. Medical Heritage 2:261, 1986.

THE CVM'S ROLE
IN THE PRACTICE OF
SMALL ANIMAL MEDICINE

DAVID A. DZANIS,
LEA M. McGOVERN
Rockville, Maryland

The Center for Veterinary Medicine (CVM) of the U.S. Food and Drug Administration (FDA) is the federal government body with primary responsibility for ensuring the safety of animal feeds and drugs used in the United States. Congress gave the FDA the authority to promulgate regulations for these items under the Federal Food, Drug, and Cosmetic Act (FFDCA). These regulations are officially recorded in Title 21 of the Code of Federal Regulations (21 CFR). Regulations specifically pertaining to animal drugs and feeds are "codified" in Parts 500-599. (These regulations are available in public libraries or may be obtained directly from the Superintendent of Documents, U.S. Government Printing Office, Washington, D.C. 20402.)

Although largely involved in issues relating to food-producing animals, CVM activities have significant implications for the small animal practitioner. As CVM policies and procedures are constantly changing to reflect new knowledge and understanding of the field of veterinary medicine, practitioners should keep themselves informed of how these changes affect their practices.

ANIMAL DRUGS

Under Section 201(g)(1)(B) of the FFDCA, drugs are defined as "articles intended for use in the diagnosis, cure, mitigation, treatment, or prevention of disease in man or other animals." A drug used in animals is "unsafe" by definition unless it has prior sanction or is the subject of an approved New Animal Drug Application (NADA). A general determination of whether a drug is safe for use under specific prescribed conditions relies on, among other things, whether the conditions for use described in the proposed label are reasonably certain to be followed in practice. Another important factor affecting safety of drugs that are to be administered to food-producing animals is the prob-

able consumption of the drug or any substance that might form in food following use of such drug. The cumulative effect on man and on animals exposed to the drug is also of concern.

Animal Drug-Approval Process

The sale of drugs for use in non–food-producing animals in the United States requires premarket approval by CVM. This involves the submission of an NADA, which includes data sufficient to support the safety and efficacy of the product.

Safety studies include determination of the toxicologic profile of a drug to establish the margin of safety in relation to the therapeutic dose. This is accomplished by first conducting drug tolerance studies to determine the minimum toxic dose. A minimum of six animals per group are administered the drug at zero, one, three, and five times the proposed therapeutic dose for three times the recommended duration of treatment. Baseline and post-treatment results of comprehensive clinical hematologic, serum chemistry, urinalyses, and fecal examinations must be reported and evaluated. Another issue that must be addressed is the safety of the drug in breeding, pregnant, or lactating animals. However, unlike the requirements for drugs for food-producing animals, tissue residue studies are not required.

To provide substantial evidence that the drug is effective for the purpose or purposes indicated on the label, data from a minimum of two well-controlled studies are needed. A dose titration study using three nonzero drug levels is ordinarily relied on to determine an optimum dose/dosage regimen. The midlevel dose is identified as the most appropriate when bracketed by a lower dose that is less effective and a higher dose producing no greater beneficial results.

The second study required for demonstration of efficacy is a controlled clinical field trial designed to follow directions and conditions of use described on the label. Additional studies are needed if a

This article was written by Drs. Dzanis and McGovern in their private capacity. No official support or endorsement by the Food and Drug Administration is intended or should be inferred.

proposed product has more than one active ingredient. Results of component efficacy studies must prove that each active ingredient contributes to the overall efficacy of the product. Component efficacy studies include dose titration of individual ingredients, tests for an optimum combination (i.e., checking for noninterference and synergism), and verification of efficacy.

When NADA data are submitted, they must be accompanied by detailed information on the extent of experimental control and methods used to minimize bias on the part of the observers and the analysts of the data. Published articles from peer-reviewed publications may be used to support safety or efficacy, provided they contain information obtained in accordance with FDA standards. Abstracts or data summaries submitted without access to the raw data are considered to be inadequate to support the safety or efficacy of NADAs. There are also limits to the extent that data developed in foreign countries may be used to support the safety and efficacy of NADAs. When safety/efficacy studies are conducted, adequate methods of drug preparation, analysis, and control must be used to assure proper identification of the test substance. Standards of identity, strength, quality, purity, stability, and reproducibility must be sufficient to confirm that the drug tested is essentially the same formulation as that proposed for marketing.

Extra-Label Use of Animal Drugs

The Center has long recognized that situations occur in the practice of veterinary medicine when drug therapy at the dose and regimen recommended on the label is clinically ineffective and that conditions of disease exist for which there are no approved drugs for therapeutic use. Under these special circumstances, the extra-label use of FDA-approved drugs is permitted by an attending veterinarian. No other conditions, such as use for routine disease prevention or for production purposes (improvement in weight gain, feed efficiency) qualify as extra-label exceptions for drug use. Also, a lay person, whose training is not recognized by the scientific community as being sufficient to fully understand all the parameters of disease, toxicology, pharmacology, and drug interactions, is not permitted to use animal drugs other than as stated on the label or as prescribed by the attending veterinarian.

The extra-label use policy is intended to apply to the use of drugs in *food-producing* animals. Extreme caution must be exercised to assure that drugs are fully depleted from the animal's body and that no illegal residues occur in meat, milk, or eggs entering the food chain. While the issue is not directly addressed in the policy, CVM also has concern over potential safety risks of extra-label use

of drugs in non–food-producing animals. Considering our current litigious society, small animal practitioners should be aware of the possible ramifications of extra-label drug use and use their scientific knowledge, training, and experience before prescribing a drug in a manner not stated on the label. Also, practitioners should be aware that "policies" are not laws or regulations, and as such, they may be more readily updated to address changing needs or problems. The Center is currently engaged in redrafting the extra-label use policy in concert with the AVMA and others. Therefore, every veterinarian should keep informed as to the proper and legal use of animal drugs in the practice of veterinary medicine.

ANIMAL FEEDS

The term "food" is defined as "articles used for food or drink for man or other animals" under Section 201(f)(1) of the FFDCA. The common sense definition of a "food" dictates that the article offer nutriment, taste, or aroma. "Animal feed" is defined under Section 201(x) as "an article which is intended for use for food for animals other than man and which is intended for use as a substantial source of nutrients in the diet of the animal." There are specific federal regulations pertaining to the production and labeling of animal feeds, including pet foods. However, unlike drugs, animal feeds do not require premarket approval.

Disease-Related Claims on Pet Food Labels

A problem arises when a pet food label includes a claim that the product may be used for the prevention, treatment, or mitigation of disease. Historically, such a claim would serve to identify the intent to market the product as a drug. Furthermore, the product would be unsafe by definition, since it would not be the subject of an approved NADA. For example, a cat food on the market that claimed to prevent feline urological syndrome (FUS) would be considered a drug. Ordinarily, manufacturers of products that violate the law are subject to criminal or civil penalties as provided in the FFDCA under Section 301, Prohibited Acts, which can result in the removal of products from the market and the imposition of fines and imprisonment. The FDA's limited resources prevent regulatory actions against many of these products; the prevailing philosophy is to take action on the most egregious with the intent that resultant publicity will cause many firms and producers to voluntarily correct their product violations.

Despite this historical perspective, FDA and CVM recognize that the scientific knowledge of the relationship between diet and disease has reached a point where, in many instances, the scientific community generally believes that foods and ingredients play a major role in prevention and treatment of certain diseases and that claims to that effect on food labels should *not* render those products as drugs. For a number of years, the Center for Food Safety and Applied Nutrition (CFSAN) of the FDA has been investigating the feasibility of permitting health-related information ("health messages") on certain food labels. Under a CFSAN proposal, for example, the role of a high-fiber diet in the prevention of cardiovascular disease or cancer in man could be a suitable health message on appropriate breakfast cereal labels. Last year, Congress amended the FFDCA to incorporate the Nutrition Labeling and Education Act of 1990 (NLEA), which, among other things, sets forth by law the hows and whys whereby certain foods that claim to affect disease (cure, prevent, mitigate, etc.) are not regulated as drugs and do not require the submission of new drug applications.

It should be noted that neither CFSAN's earlier proposals nor the NLEA expressly included animal feeds. On the other hand, animal feeds were not expressly excluded either. Where specific regulations pertaining to animal feeds are not available, CVM often strives to follow the intent or spirit of the regulations promulgated for foods for human use. Therefore, with respect to health messages, CVM hopes to incorporate the appropriate aspects of the NLEA into its own activities with pet foods. Although the specific nutrients/diseases expressed in the document would not be suitable for pet food labels, the general concept would remain.

One aspect already initiated by CVM has been "gray area" claims on pet food labels. These are defined as claims that provide some useful health-related information but are distinct from drug claims or health messages in that they do not directly reference a disease or condition. For example, claims that a cat food might provide low dietary magnesium or produce acidic urine in cats consuming the product but that do not refer to FUS or similar disease terms may be acceptable provided sufficient data to assure safety are submitted and found acceptable by CVM. A number of companies have submitted data in relation to such claims.

Veterinary Medical Foods

Another aspect of the NLEA that may affect veterinary practice is the area of medical foods. Medical foods are defined as foods for oral or enteral use, designed for the dietary management of certain diseases or conditions, and limited to use under the direction of a physician. The NLEA specifically exempts medical foods from the nutritional and health message labeling requirements delineated in the Act. This creates a dilemma, since a product could be exempt from fulfilling any requirements for labeling (including the submission of data to support a health message) simply by meeting the category definition of a medical food. If anything, it would be even more prudent to require proof of safety and efficacy for medical foods than for foods with health messages. Therefore, FDA is actively exploring the feasibility of some form of premarket approval process for medical foods based on submission of scientific data.

The definition for medical foods cited above was in reference to foods for human consumption. However, it could also easily apply to the plethora of pet food products designed for dietary management of diseases in animals because they are "veterinary medical foods." While these products are often identified on the market by the label bearing the phrase "use only under the direction of a veterinarian" or similar wording, the original intent of this phrase was not for use on veterinary medical foods. This phrase was taken from the pet food regulations of the Association of American Feed Control Officials (AAFCO), a coalition of state regulatory officials responsible for registering animal feeds in their respective states. The original purpose of the pertinent regulation applied to labels for medicated pet foods (foods containing a drug, such as a heartworm control agent), not medical foods. A medicated pet food must undergo the same approval process required for new animal drugs.

However, veterinary medical foods, like all other nonmedicated pet foods, do not require the premarket submission of data to demonstrate safety and efficacy for their intended use. In fact, the present labels on many of these products lack sufficient feeding directions and assurances of nutritional adequacy. This appears contradictory, as the proper use and nutritional completeness of a diet takes on even greater importance when used for ill animals. The potential safety risks are especially significant when such products are obtained outside of the veterinary/client relationship.

In light of these facts, CVM is following the agency's lead in dealing with medical foods for humans and plans to implement a similar procedure for handling veterinary medical foods. CVM expects that products designed for dietary management of disease would be supported by data sufficient to prove safety and efficacy for their intended use. Also, the marketing or use of such products would be restricted to circumstances where there is adequate veterinary supervision.

CRITICAL CARE

ROBERT J. MURTAUGH

Consulting Editor

CLINICAL DECISIONS AND IATROGENESIS

ROBERT J. MURTAUGH

North Grafton, Massachusetts

Iatrogenesis can be defined as just what the doctor ordered, but did not intend. Iatrogenic illness results from diagnostic procedures, treatment, or other occurrences during hospitalization that are not a direct consequence of the animal's illness. Veterinary critical care clinicians are developing and using sophisticated diagnostic, monitoring, and treatment approaches in animal patients. In the context of clinical decision-making, clinicians must always be cognizant of the potential harm as well as the limitations of these interventions. Animals requiring high-intensity care (extensive monitoring and data collection, invasive procedures, multiple drug therapy) are the most likely to suffer iatrogenic complications.

LABELING

Many animals with different, specific illnesses present with similar clinical manifestations. The thought processes and investigation expended to uncover unknown factors usually cease once a diagnostic label is applied to these animals. Important aspects of an animal's illness may elude identification and continue to exert effects unabated, undiagnosed, and untreated unless these animals are reevaluated critically and perpetuation of erroneous "labeling" is prevented. For example, an animal spikes a fever and is evaluated for the development of bronchopneumonia. A tracheal wash is positive (neutrophilic inflammation), and pulmonary infiltrates on radiographs are detected. The animal is labeled as having fever attributable to bronchopneumonia, and the clinician fails to detect the septic thrombophlebitis (cause of problem) at a previous intravenous catheter site.

INTERVENTION VERSUS MANIPULATION

Therapeutic or diagnostic approaches applied to animals in critical care settings should have evidence to support their use. Scientific evidence that links a potential for effect on outcome with application of a technique or treatment should exist before clinicians implement that approach. If specific diagnostic or therapeutic approaches do not or

would not seem to affect outcome, the only possible results of their application are deleterious. Clinicians must distinguish between diagnostic or therapeutic interventions and diagnostic or therapeutic manipulations. Manipulations are moment-to-moment responses to abnormalities in physiologic variables ("attempts to re-establish normalcy") that often have potential only for a negative outcome. For example, the administration of many drugs to animals in critical care settings represent "manipulations." Drug-related iatrogenic occurrences are potentially prevalent and infrequently considered.

INFORMATIONAL OVERLOAD

Veterinary critical care clinicians have a vast array of potentially useful diagnostic tests from which to choose. The proper timing, sequence, and repetition of diagnostic testing compared with outcome criteria have not been studied. As with therapeutic approaches, a critical approach is required in evaluating the need for diagnostic testing. Insecurity, inexperience, tradition, fatigue, and training appear as some of the factors responsible for proliferation of testing in critical care settings. The quality of patient care is not diminished and may actually be enhanced by attempts to distinguish necessary from unnecessary testing. Significant harm can be associated with overzealous testing, including injury to the animal during repeated manipulations, information overload for the clinician, and economic hardship for an owner. Clinicians in critical care must concentrate efforts on thinking, assessing, and decision-making rather than on ordering, reacting, and intervening (Civetta, 1988). An ultimate effect in purifying, clarifying, distilling, and delineating information will be the elimination of misinterpretations, misdirections, and misadventures, i.e., iatrogenesis (Civetta, 1988).

One of the important issues faced in veterinary critical care medicine is the distinction between efforts that may return an animal to a good quality of life and ineffective efforts that only increase the risk for suffering and prolong dying. Diminishing unnecessary activity will decrease complications and have a salutary effect—additional time for patient

68

care and owner contact will fulfill the important goal of caring and decrease the sense of failure when clinicians are confronted with the death of our animal patients.

Reference and Suggested Reading

Civetta, J. M.: Iatrogenesis. *In* Civetta J. M., Taylor, R. W., Kirby, R. R., (eds.): *Critical Care*. Philadelphia: J. B. Lippincott, 1988, p. 1589.

ESTABLISHING A CRITICAL CARE PRACTICE

JAN P. KOVACIC
Milwaukee, Wisconsin

According to the Veterinary Emergency and Critical Care Society (VECCS), critical care is: "The care taken or required in response to a crisis. In medicine, a treatment of a patient with a life-threatening or potentially life-threatening illness or injury whose condition is likely to change on a moment-to-moment or hour-to-hour basis. Such patients require intense and often constant monitoring, reassessment, and treatment."

Throughout the veterinary community the interest in critical care practice is growing. Referrals by primary care practitioners to veterinary specialists and emergency clinics have improved the level of patient care and helped to solve patient, client, and practitioner-related problems in the delivery of veterinary medical care. The rise of the centralized 24-hour emergency and critical care referral center has further bridged the gap between quality patient care and logistics by providing the critically ill or seriously traumatized patient with needed continuous intensive care over an extended period.

Establishing a critical care practice places great demands on management, manpower, medical skills, and money. Problems are more often amplified than resolved in the process. It is not enough to open the hospital doors 24 hours a day and assume that the best interests of patient, client, and primary care practitioner are being met. The practice must be equipped to handle the diagnosis, treatment, and monitoring of the critically ill and unstable patient. Careful attention must be paid to the details of practice philosophy, personnel, and client relations.

PRACTICE PHILOSOPHY

Critical care must be founded on a practice philosophy committed to high-quality, diagnostic-oriented medical services. The standard of practice must meet or exceed that of every clinical facility in the area. Basic stabilization capabilities alone are not sufficient to encourage the ongoing referral of the most seriously ill patients from primary care clinicians. Clients want more than an empirical approach to the care of their pets; they want to know all the options available and are often willing to pursue diagnostic and therapeutic procedures in the face of a guarded to poor prognosis for their animals. These client expectations place great demands on the critical care clinician to maintain current knowledge and skills and to offer the best care available.

PERSONNEL

Doctors and staff in an intensive care practice must develop expertise in the field of emergency and critical care medicine and be recognized as experts. Only with this level of confidence can a primary care clinician transfer the most seriously ill patients (and most valued clients) into the hands of the referral facility. Sound business and medical practices are needed to attract, reward, and retain a medical staff capable of handling the personal and professional challenges that exist in a high-stress clinical setting. Skill and expertise cannot be developed in a vacuum; the medical staff needs to be encouraged and supported in its professional growth through in-house training and frequent opportunity for continuing education. The VECCS guidelines require that doctors and technicians receive, as a minimum, 16 hours a year of continuing education on emergency and critical care topics as one of the criteria for a facility to achieve the highest VECCS rating (VECCS, 1988).

CLIENT RELATIONS

The best measure of a critical care practice is the level of satisfaction among pet owners and referring doctors. This adds to day-to-day pressures but can also provide the opportunity to market medical services and to teach these clients about the availability of increasingly sophisticated medical capabilities. The singlemost valuable communications tool is the medical record. The medical record is the glue that holds together quality patient care during the course of multiple personnel changes and can be used to teach the pet owner and referring clinician about the scope of the critical care practice.

MONITORING

The greatest of the demands imposed by critical care patients on hospital staff is patient monitoring. By definition, the condition of the critical care patient is highly changeable and must be watched closely to anticipate problems and adjust therapy. In human patients, it has been demonstrated that "stat" bedside monitoring improves outcome, decreases overall medical costs, and shortens ICU stays (Chernow, 1990). Following is a list of current veterinary critical care monitoring techniques as well as human critical care techniques that are on the horizon for veterinary application.

PHYSICAL EXAMINATION. A thorough physical examination repeated at frequent intervals is still the best means of evaluating patient status.

BLOOD PRESSURE. Oscillometric blood pressure instruments (Dinamap, Critikon, Inc.) provide noninvasive evaluation of systolic, diastolic, and mean systemic arterial blood pressure. These results correlate well with direct arterial catheter measurements except in small patients or in low-flow states. Doppler blood flow detectors (Doppler BP Monitor, Park Electronics, Inc.) provide a noninvasive means of measuring systemic arterial blood pressure and provide an evaluation of regional blood flow.

ELECTROCARDIOGRAPHY. An ECG permits the assessment of cardiac electrical activity. Monitoring of the ST-segment can provide clues to changes in myocardial perfusion and oxygenation. Continuous cardiac monitoring, using telemetry if available, is recommended for patients at risk of developing potentially lethal cardiac arrhythmias or cardiac arrest.

RADIOGRAPHY. Serial radiographs of the thorax permit evaluation of the cardiac silhouette and lung fields. This monitoring is important for the critical care patient at high risk for cardiac disease, pulmonary edema, thromboembolism, or pneumonia.

ECHOCARDIOGRAPHY. Ultrasound evaluation of cardiac structure and function as well as pericardial and mediastinal structures yields valuable informa-tion. The addition of Doppler assessment provides information about flow dynamics and may have application in the noninvasive calculation of cardiac output.

BLOOD FLOW AND PERFUSION. Blood flow (as opposed to blood pressure) can be assessed using Doppler blood flow monitors, Doppler ultrasonography, or angiography.

CENTRAL VENOUS PRESSURE. Manometer measurement via a central venous catheter can be helpful in monitoring the patient's vascular fluid volume and the function of the pericardium and right side of the heart.

CARDIAC CATHETERIZATION. Cardiac catheterization using a Swan-Ganz catheter to measure pulmonary capillary wedge pressures is a useful technique for evaluating left ventricular preload and evaluating the cause of pulmonary edema.

CARDIAC OUTPUT. The Swan-Ganz thermodilution catheter permits measurement of cardiac output and the calculation of cardiac index (cardiac output per body surface area), systemic vascular resistance index, and pulmonary vascular resistance index.

MIXED VENOUS OXYGEN SATURATION. Pulmonary artery sampling using a Swan-Ganz catheter permits measurement of mixed venous oxygen saturation, a parameter being explored as an index of the balance between tissue oxygen demand and supply.

ARTERIAL BLOOD GAS. Arterial blood sampling using direct arterial puncture or arterial catheter yields measurement of Pa_{O_2}, Pa_{CO_2}, pH, HCO_3^-, and base excess, allowing assessment of the animal's oxygenation, respiratory, and acid-base status.

PULSE OXIMETRY. This technique permits noninvasive evaluation of the oxygen saturation of hemoglobin in the peripheral vasculature.

TRANSCUTANEOUS P_{O_2} AND P_{CO_2}. The usefulness of transcutaneous electrode measurement of P_{O_2} and P_{CO_2} and its applicability in animal patients are being explored as a means of estimating arterial oxygen and carbon dioxide levels without the need of arterial catheterization. These instruments measure oxygen tension at the dermal or conjunctival surface.

END-TIDAL CO_2. This monitor permits measurement of end-expiratory CO_2 which is useful in noninvasive assessment of trends in Pa_{CO_2}. The technique is most useful in intubated patients to optimize ventilator settings and to determine the appropriate time to begin weaning patients from ventilators (Hoffman, 1989). It is also valuable in the cardiopulmonary arrest patient during the resuscitation and postresuscitation period to help assess pulmonary circulation and pulmonary gas exchange.

PULMONARY COMPLIANCE. Compliance is the

Table 1. Equipment for a Critical Care Practice

General

CPR "crash" cart	IV stands–floor, ceiling, cage
MAST counterpressure pants or equivalent	IV bag compression device
Defibrillator with internal and external paddles	IV infusion pumps
Anesthesia machine with O_2	Feeding pumps
Isofluorane precision vaporizer	Fluid warmer
Halothane precision vaporizer	Microwave oven
Ventilator, volume-controlled with PEEP	Blood bank refrigerator and freezer
Anesthesia masks	Blood collection vacuum tank
Ambu bag	Autotransfusion equipment
Nonrebreathing system-Ayres, Baines	Wound suction drains
Endotracheal tubes	Wound suction reservoirs
Laryngoscope	Wash table
Oral speculum	Water blanket and heat pump
Flowmeter for nasal oxygen	Neonatal incubator
Oxygen cage	Ultrasonic instrument cleaner
Suction—surgical	Steam autoclave
Suction—thermotic	Ethylene oxide sterilizer
Thoracic suction drain system	Endoscope—flexible
Ultrasonic nebulizer	Cystoscope—rigid
Clippers and blades	X-ray machine 300 ma/125 KVP
Stretcher	Automatic processor
Gurney	X-ray film ID labeller
Exam lighting	X-ray film bin + cassette bin
Positioning bags or vac-packs	X-ray aprons, gloves
Walk-on scale	X-ray illuminators
Gram scale	X-ray spotlighter
Instrument tray–cold sterile	X-ray calipers
Stomach tubes	Fluoroscopic unit
Stomach pump	Ultrasound

Monitoring

Otoscope/Ophthalmoscope	Oscillometric BP monitor
Stethoscope	Direct arterial BP monitor
Esophageal stethoscope	Thermometers—mercury
CVP manometer	Thermometers—electronic
Electrocardiograph printer	Pulse oximeter
Electrocardiograph monitor	Oxygen sensors
Electrocardiograph telemetry	End-tidal CO_2 monitor
Doppler blood flow monitor	Respiratory monitor
	Tonometer-Tonopen or Schiotz

Laboratory

Microscope—cytologic	Hematology diluter
Differential hand counter	Chemistry analyzer
Hemacytometer	Glucometer
Centrifuge—serum	Electrolyte analyzer
Centrifuge—microhematocrit	Osmometer
Refractometer	Blood gas analyzer
Heat block	Coagulation analyzer
Hematology cell counter	Microbiology media
	Incubator

Surgical

Surgical lighting	Surgical staplers—auto
V-Top surgery table	Fascia staplers
Instrument table	Skin staplers
Surgical suction	Retractors—Balfour (sm, med, lg)
Electrosurgical unit—bipolar	Retractors—Gelpi
Head light—fiberoptic	Retractors—Senn
Major surgical packs	Retractors—Weitlanner
Minor surgical packs	Retractors—Army/Navy
Wound packs	Rongeurs—single action
Ophthalmic pack	Rongeurs—double action
Vascular cut-down pack	High speed drill—gas or electric
Vascular clamps	Bone pins, chuck, + pin cutter
Vascular ligating clips	External fixators

Table 2. *Supplies for Critical Care Practice*

Aerosol adhesive disolvent	Fluids—hypertonic saline 7.5%	Oxygen
Aluminum splint rods	Fluids—hyper. saline 7.5% in Dextran 70	Oxygen tubing
Autoclave rolls and pouches	Fluids—Intralipid 10% + 20%	Proparacaine
Autoclave cleaner	Fluids—Lactated Ringers	Paper towels
Bandage—abdominal pads	Fluids—Normasol R	Penlights—disposable
Bandage—gauze	Fluids—sterile water	Pressurized air—laboratory
Bandage—stretch gauze	Fluids—peritoneal dialysis	Rose Bengal stain
Bandage—cast padding	Fluids—saline for irrigation	Schirmer tear tests
Bandage—adhesive tape	Gas sterilizer ampules	Shampoo—general purpose
Bandage—conforming tape	Gas sterilizer bags	Shampoo—medicated
Bandage—Vetwrap	Gas sterilizer indicators	Silver nitrate applicators
Bleach	Gelatin cold packs	Soda lime
Blood administration sets	Halothane	Splints—plastic/aluminum
Blood collection sets (CPDA2)	Heimlich valves	Stockinette—tubular
Catheters—butterfly	Humidifier	Surgical blades—10, 11, 12, 15
Catheters—chest tube	Instrument cleaner	Surgical blades—beaver
Catheters—Foley	Instrument milk	Surgical suture—silk
Catheters—IV, outside needle	Isopropyl alcohol 70%	Surgical suture—Maxon
Catheters—IV, inside needle	Isofluorane	Surgical suture—PDS
Catheters—urinary, red rubber	IV fluid sets—adult	Surgical suture—Prolene
Catheters—polypropylene	IV fluid sets—pediatric	Surgical suture—Novafil
Catheters—urinary, tom cat	IV fluid sets—extension	Surgical suture—Ethilon
Catheters—TPN	IV fluid sets—"T" connector	Surgical suture—stainless steel
Catheters—peritoneal dialysis	IV fluid sets—secondary	Surgical suture—cassette
Catheters—peritoneal lavage	Kim wipes	Surgical suture needles
Chlorhexidine ointment	Lab—ACT tubes	Surgical wire—cerclage
Chlorhexidine scrub	Lab—glucose strips	Surgical sponges— 3 × 3 or 4 × 4
Chlorhexidine solution	Lab—azo strips	Surgical scrub brushes
Cleaners & Disinfectants	Lab—Diff Quick stain	Surgical sponge—Gelfoam
Connectors 5-in-1	Lab—new methylene blue stain	Surgical gloves
Cotton balls	Lab—Microfilaria microfilters	Surgical caps
Cotton-roll	Lab—sterilizing microfilters .2μ	Surgical masks
Dispensing vials—safety	Lab—blood collection tubes	Surgical gowns
Dispensing bottles—safety	Lab—slides and cover slips	Surgical drape material
Dispensing bottles—dropper	Lab—FeLV + FIV test kit	Swabs—cotton-tipped
ECG paper	Lab—formalin	Syringes—armed
ECG contact gel	Lab—fecal flotation solution	Syringes—unarmed
ECG contact patches	Lab—Gram's stain	Syringes—insulin
Elizabethan collars	Lab—hematocrit tubes	Syringes—catheter tipped
Endotracheal tubes	Lab—urine dipsticks	Syringes—bulb
Enemas	Lab—parvovirus test kit	Syringes—tuberculin
Exam gloves	Lab—boreliosis test kit	Telfa pads
Feeding tubes	Lab—thyroid test kit	Tincture of benzoin
Fluorescein strips	Litter—feline	Tongue depressor blades
Fluids—Dextran 70	Lubricant—clipper	Tracheostomy tubes
Fluids—Dextrose 5%	Lubricant—sterile surgical	Ultrasonic cleaner solution
Fluids—Dextrose 50%	Laparotomy sponges	Unopettes—WBC and platelet
Fluids—Dex 2.5% + 1/2LRS	Micronebulizer	Weck spears—ophthalmic
Fluids—Dex 2.5% + .9%NaCl	Muzzles—canine and feline	Xylocaine viscous
Fluids—Freeamine 3%	Mydriacyl	X-ray film
Fluids—Freeamine 8.5%	Nasal oxygen catheters	X-ray developer and fixer
Fluids—Hetastarch	Needles—hypodermic	
Fluids—normal saline .9%	Needles—spinal	

change in pulmonary volume per change in pulmonary airway pressure ($\Delta V/\Delta P$). This parameter is often evaluated subjectively in a ventilated patient by comparing thoracic expansion with ventilatory pressures. Pulmonary compliance can also be measured with a circumferential thoracic sensor that relates chest wall expansion to changes in thoracic volume.

CENTRAL NERVOUS SYSTEM (CNS). Serial neurologic exams have always been the principal means of CNS evaluation. For the stupor/coma patient,

this includes the assessment of level of consciousness, respiratory center function, pupillary and other brainstem reflexes, caloric testing, and spinal reflexes. Electroencephalography and brainstem auditory-evoked responses (BAER) can further define CNS status and establish both diagnosis and prognosis for brain function. The Glasgow Coma Score has been adapted for infants and may have applicability in animal patients for predicting outcome (Rubenstein and Hageman, 1988).

INTRACRANIAL PRESSURE. Intracranial pressure is

Table 3. Injectable Medications for a Critical Care Practice

Acepromazine	Dobutamine	Oxymorphone
Acetylcholine	Doxapram	Oxytocin
Acetylcysteine	Enalapril	2-PAM
ACTH gel	Ephedrine	Pancuronium bromide
Adriamycin	Epinephrine 1:1000	Penicillin—potassium
Amikacin	Ergonovine	Pentobarbital
Aminophyllin	Ethanol	Phenobarbital
Ampicillin	Euthanasia solution	Phentolamine
Antivenin-snakebite	Fentanyl	Phenylephrine
Atropine sulfate	Flunixin meglumine	Potassium chloride
BAL in oil	Furosemide	Prednisolone
Blood cells, packed	Gentamicin sulfate	Prednisolone sodium succinate
Blood plasma, frozen	Glucagon	Procainamide
Blood, whole in CPDA2	Glycopyrrolate	Prochlorperazine
Bretylium	Heparin	Propranolol
Bupivicaine .25%	Hypaque	Ranitidine
Bupivicaine .25% with	Innovar-Vet	Renografin
epinephrine	Insulin—NPH	Sodium bicarbonate
Butorphanol	Insulin—PZI	Stanozolol
Calcitonin	Insulin—regular	Succinyl choline
Calcium chloride 10%	Isometheptene	Terbutaline
Calcium gluconate 10%	Isoproterenol	Thiamine HCl
Calcium disodium EDTA	Ketamine	Thiamylal sodium
Cephalothin sodium	Lidocaine 2%	Ticarcillin
Cefotaxime sodium	Mannitol 20%	Ticarcillin + clavulinic acid
Cimetidine	4-methyl pyrozol	Trimethobenzamide
Demerol	Methylprednisolone sodium succinate	Trimethoprim + sulfa
Dexamethasone sodium phosphate	Metoclopromide	Tobramycin
Dexamethasone	Methcarbamol	Triethylperazine
Diazepam	Methylene blue	Verapamil
Digoxin	Midazolam	Vincristine
Diphenhydramine	Morphine sulfate	Vitamin B complex
Dipyrone	Naloxone	Vitamin K1
Dimethylsulfoxide	Nitroprusside sodium	Vitamin C
Dopamine	Norepinephrine	Xylazine

currently measured in human patients using invasive but relatively simple techniques. The technique uses a subarachnoid cranial bolt system, an intraventricular catheter, or an extradural fiberoptic sensor. Brainstem auditory-evoked responses may also have application in the serial assessment of intracranial pressure in animals with CNS dysfunction.

COMPUTED TOMOGRAPHY (CT). Veterinary access to CT technology is increasing through veterinary teaching hospitals, human hospitals, or mobile services available in larger cities. Veterinary radiologists and neurologists are available to interpret these studies and will be more accessible as digitized imaging and televideo capability is developed.

FLUID, ELECTROLYTE, AND KIDNEY ASSESSMENT. Homeostatic mechanisms can be disrupted by multiple organ system failure, by the long course of disease in the critical patient, and by therapeutic intervention. Serum electrolyte concentrations can drift dangerously. These concentrations need to be monitored serially and maintained within a physiologic range. Serial measurements of body weight as well as fluid intake and output are also important. Closed urine collection systems are easy to place, but not without patient risk for infection. Measured parameters of value include osmolality and concentrations of sodium, potassium, calcium, phosphorus, creatinine, and urea nitrogen in serum and urine. Fractional excretion of sodium and other electrolytes can also be calculated when indicated.

GLUCOSE. The high incidence of stress, sepsis, stupor/coma, and diabetes in critically ill animals makes monitoring blood glucose concentration a necessity.

LIVER. Hepatic function can be assessed by monitoring sulfobromophthalein excretion (BSP), prothrombin time (PT), partial thromboplastin time (PTT), and the serum concentration of bile acids, albumin, ammonia, and bilirubin. Measurements of serum alanine aminotransferase (ALT), aspartate aminotransferase (AST), and lactate dehydrogenase (LDH) activities help to evaluate hepatocellular injury or necrosis. Biliary function is monitored through measurement of serum alkaline phosphatase (SAP) and gamma-glutamyl transferase (GGT) activity and by ultrasonographic examination of the gallbladder and biliary tree.

COAGULATION. Coagulation processes are often altered in serious illness. In patients at risk for disseminated intravascular coagulopathy (DIC), early assessment is the key to successful therapy.

Table 4. Oral and Topical Medications for a Critical Care Practice

Oral

Acepromazine	Doxycycline
Allopurinol	Erythromycin
Aminophyllin	Furosemide
Amiodarone	Hydralazine
Amoxicillin	Hydrocodone
Amoxicillin + clavulinc acid	Imodium
Ampicillin	Keflex
Apomorphine	Lincomycin
Aspirin	Lomotil
Bethanechol	Metoclopramide
Butorphanol	Methcarbamol
Captopril	Metronidazole
Carbenicillin	Nifedipine
Cefadroxil	Omeprazole
Cephalexin	Phenobarbital
Charcoal, activated	Phenoxybenzamine
Chloramphenicol	Phenylbutazone
Cimetidine	Prednisolone
Cyclosporin	Prednisone
Cyclophosphamide	Primidone
D-Penicillamine	Procainamide
Danazol	Propranolol
Dichlorphenamide	Quinidine sulfate
Diltiazem	Ranitidine
Dexamethasone	Sucralfate
Dilantin	Trimethoprim + sulfa
Disopyramide	Tetracycline
Digoxin	Thyroxine
Digitoxin	Vitamin K1
DL-Methionine	Verapamil

Topical

Ophthalmic atropine	Otic antibiotics
Ophthalmic antibiotics	Otic antibiotic + steroid
Ophthalmic antibiotic + steroid	Flea & tick spray or powder
Ophthalmic artificial tears	Laxative paste
Ophthalmic pilocarpine	Minor wound lotion with steroid
Ophthalmic eye wash	Silver sulfadiazine cream
Otic cleanser	

Monitoring tests that aid in this assessment include platelet count, buccal bleeding time, activated clotting time, fibrinogen, fibrin split products, PT, and PTT. Antithrombin-3 assays are being used in human patients and are under development for use in veterinary patients.

INFECTION. The critically ill patient is at risk of overwhelming infection owing to a severely depressed immune system, invasive medical procedures, pre-existent infections, indiscriminate use of antibiotics, and exposure to nosocomial pathogens. Charting of body temperature patterns, frequent catheter evaluations, cytologic evaluation of body secretions, and serial hematologic examinations are valuable aids in determining early signs of infection in critically ill animals.

NUTRITION. Nutrition is commonly overlooked in the management of the critical care patient. Early nutritional support is vital to meeting the increased metabolic demands of the seriously ill or traumatized patient. Calculating dietary or parenteral nutritional requirements and then ensuring delivery of these nutrients is as important as maintaining hydration and monitoring other parameters (Crowe, 1986).

ARMAMENTARIUM

The rapidly changing demands of critical care practice make any list of practice armamentarium incomplete and soon outdated, requiring frequent review and revision. Tables 1 through 4 should serve as a guide for readiness in an intensive care environment.

References and Suggested Reading

APACHE III Study Design: Analytical plan for evaluation of severity and outcome. Crit. Care Med. 17:S169, 1989.

Chernow, B.: The bedside laboratory—A critical step forward in ICU care. Chest 97(5Suppl.):183S, 1990.

Crowe, D. T.: Enteral nutrition for critically ill or injured patients—Parts 1–3. Compendium on Continuing Education 8:603, 1986.

Hoffman, R. A., et al.: End-tidal carbon dioxide in critically ill patients during changes in mechanical ventilation. Am. Rev. Respir. Dis. 140:1265, 1989.

Kirby, R., and Stamp, G. (eds.): Critical care. Vet. Clin. North Am. 19:6, 1989.

Krentz, M. J.: Emergency care—Past, present, and future. Comp. Ther. 15:3, 1989.

Rubenstein, J., and Hageman, J.: Monitoring of critically ill infants and children. Crit. Care Clin. 4:621, 1988.

Runcie, C. J., et al.: Assessment of the critically ill patient. Br. J. Hosp. Med. 65:875, 1989.

Shoemaker, W., et al.: Textbook of Critical Care. Philadelphia: W. B. Saunders, 1989.

Veterinary Emergency and Critical Care Society Directory: Recommended definitions and guidelines for veterinary emergency service standards in the United States. San Antonio, TX, VECCS, 1988.

TRIAGE AND RESUSCITATION OF THE CATASTROPHIC TRAUMA PATIENT

GARY L. STAMP,
Fort Sam Houston, Texas

and DENNIS T. CROWE
Milwaukee, Wisconsin

Effective trauma management requires concomitant rapid diagnosis, monitoring, and therapy. Survival depends on many variables, including the type and severity of the trauma, interval from time of the incident until presentation for treatment, health status of the patient before injury, early recognition of life-threatening conditions, skill and preparedness of the veterinary staff, and willingness of owner and veterinarian to "do what is necessary" to sustain the patient's life.

PREPARATION

Practitioners must determine how and to what extent emergencies will be handled in their particular practices. What personnel and resources are to be committed to emergency care? Is there an emergency clinic accessible for referral? Is it open 24 hours a day or only after-hours, weekends, and holidays? Standards, guidelines, and definitions for various categories of emergency service have been developed and are available from the Veterinary Emergency and Critical Care Society (VECCS). Practitioners are obligated to clearly state the level of emergency care to be provided so as not to mislead owners of trauma victims.

Facility and Personnel

A room or specific portion of a large treatment area should be designated, organized, and equipped to allow assessment and treatment of life-threatening emergencies. Necessary life-saving equipment, instruments, and drugs should be located there and organized in a logical, consistent manner, each item always being maintained in the same location. A liberal use of wall charts specifying equipment uses/settings, protocols, and drug dosages/indications is very helpful. This emergency treatment area should have easy access to the operating room, surgical preparation area, and radiology.

Life-saving emergency care is best provided by a minimum of three individuals working as a team. Basic and advanced cardiac life support and emergency surgical interventions are compromised with a team of less than three. Training and practice are essential for the emergency team to function effectively. Timing and teamwork are critical elements in resuscitation of the emergency patient. Each member of the team (veterinarian, technician, receptionist, kennel attendant, etc.) must be trained to perform specific functions and be aware of his or her responsibilities in the resuscitation process.

The views expressed in this chapter are those of the authors and do not reflect the official policy or position of the Department of the Army, Department of Defense, or the United States government.

Individuals besides the veterinarian should be capable of performing a variety of emergency support procedures. A technician or nurse should be trained to place intravenous catheters (peripheral and central), obtain blood samples, give IV medication, administer general anesthesia, ventilate, perform closed chest CPR, assist in surgery, and monitor vital signs. Another assistant should capably record patient findings and treatment data, obtain diagnostic radiographs, and perform basic emergency laboratory tests. Someone must be designated to regulate, inventory, and stock the emergency drugs and maintain all emergency equipment in operable condition. A "readiness checklist" is recommended to ensure that everything is available when it is needed and that personnel are prepared (Crowe, 1989).

To further enhance efficiency and effective delivery of emergency care, it is advised that protocols be developed for the most serious and life-threatening problems, such as gastric dilatation volvulus (GDV), multiple systemic trauma, airway obstruction, cardiac arrest, etc. The protocols and guidelines should be discussed, revised, and practiced frequently to ensure that everyone involved knows what is expected and which skills are required of them. Algorithms are also helpful and can be incorporated into the various protocols or placed on wall charts.

EQUIPMENT AND DRUGS

The list of recommended emergency equipment and drugs will vary somewhat, depending on the level of emergency service being provided. The busy 24-hour full-service emergency clinic is expected to have on hand a much more comprehensive inventory of equipment and drugs than a routine, primarily outpatient small animal practice. Basic drugs considered essential for even the routine small animal practice (not specializing in emergencies) are listed in Table 1. The reader should consult other references for a more detailed list of emergency equipment and drugs (Crowe, 1989; Muir, 1990). The emergency drug list should be kept to a minimum and should include only those agents for which the clinician has a clear understanding of their use, mode of action, and interaction with other drugs.

Establishing instrument packs for specific conditions has proved quite helpful to emergency clinicians. Packs set up in advance with all the necessary items to treat specific life-threatening emergencies, such as GDV, pneumothorax, obstructed airway, or pericardial tamponade, can mean the difference between life and death. Precious time can be saved having the necessary materials and protocols immediately available as a unit.

Drugs (some in preloaded syringes) should be grouped logically as to general use, e.g., agents for CPR, cardiovascular support drugs, anesthetics and analgesics, and so forth. Intravenous fluids, whole blood, and oxygen with appropriate administration sets are essential. Drugs safely incorporated into standard intravenous solutions should be clearly marked. Bold instructional signs should be visible stating dosages, route and frequency of administration, and concentration. A numbering or color-coded system may be employed to facilitate organizing the emergency drug area, and a mobile crash cart can be used for those items best shared between the emergency treatment area, operating room, and other areas of the hospital.

TRIAGE, ASSESSMENT, AND RESUSCITATION

Patients with catastrophic injuries require simultaneous rapid assessment and treatment. To prevent death, the clinician must aggressively make decisions and perform life-saving procedures as necessary. A systematic and thorough approach should be used to ensure that no significant problem is overlooked. Such a routine approach or protocol would include initial assessment and triage, primary survey, resuscitation, secondary survey, and definitive care or referral as indicated.

Initial Assessment and Triage

Triage is the ranking of patients based on the severity of their injuries and the degree of urgency for treatment. Upon presentation to the hospital, initial assessment is made immediately by the first person who comes in contact with the owner and animal. With a quick scan of the patient and the client's brief comments about what happened, the animal's condition is tentatively classified and priorities are set for care.

The initial evaluation providing an overview of the patient will primarily consider the level of consciousness (LOC) and the presence of any life-threatening disruptions of physiologic functions, such as dyspnea, apnea, or major external hemorrhage. Patients with such serious problems are classified as catastrophic and are rushed to the emergency treatment area. Animals with historic or observed evidence of severe multiple trauma are also classified as catastrophic, considered to have life-threatening injury, and are immediately taken to the emergency treatment area. It is common for trauma to involve several regions of the body, and the distribution and severity of these multiple insults will determine the overall triage classification and urgency for treatment (Crowe, 1989). It is well

Table 1. *Selected Emergency Drugs*

Drug Name/Group	Use	Dosage/Route
Cardiovascular support		
Digoxin	Positive inotrope	.01–.02 mg/kg IV in 4 divided doses over 2 hr
Dobutamine	Positive inotrope; vasoconstriction at high doses	2–15 μg/kg/min in 5% dextrose IV constant rate infusion (Cat: 2.5–5.0 μg/kg/min)
Dopamine	Positive intrope and chronotrope; increase cardiac output and blood pressure	2–10 μg/kg/min in 5% dextrose IV constant rate infusion
Epinephrine*	Positive inotrope; stimulates heartbeat; increased BP early then may decrease	.1–.2 mg/kg IV .4 mg/kg IT (intratracheal)
Isoproterenol	Positive inotrope; may initiate heartbeat (causes peripheral vasodilation); not advised in CPR	.01–.04 μg/kg/min constant rate infusion in 5% dextrose (beware of hypotension; use only after fluid volume expansion)
Methoxamine	Increases arterial BP	.1–.2 μg/kg
Atropine sulfate	Parasympatholytic; (may correct bradycardia after rapid IV injection)	0.02–0.05 mg/kg IV
Bretylium	Chemical ventricular antifibrillatory agent (efficiency in animals undetermined)	10–50 mg/kg IV (dogs)
Lidocaine	Ventricular antiarrhythmic	1–2 mg/kg IV bolus up to 8 mg/kg in 10 min 40–80 μg/kg/min IV constant rate infusion (Cat: 0.25–1 mg/kg over 5 min)
Procainamide	Ventricular antiarrhythmic	5–20 mg/kg IV (2 mg/kg/minute boluses slowly). Cat: 3–8 mg/kg IM 25–50 μg/kg/min IV constant rate infusion
Propranolol	Antiarrhythmic for ventricular/superventricular arrhythmias; beta blocker	.04–.06 mg/kg IV slowly. Cat: .04–.06 mg/kg IV
Ventilation stimulants		
Doxapram	Stimulates respiratory centers	5–10 mg/kg IV
Methetharimide (Mikedimide)	Reverses barbituate respiratory depression	.4–.8 mg/kg IV
Miscellaneous		
Dexamethasone sodium phosphate	Increased cardiac output; stabilize lysosomal membranes; prevent reperfusion injury	5–8 mg/kg IV
Hypertonic NaCl (5–7.5%) (with dextran)	Reverse hypotension by expanding blood volume	3–6 ml/kg IV
Isotonic crystalloid fluids	Expand blood volume; treat hypotension	40–90 ml/kg/hr
Mannitol (20%)	Osmotic diuretic; prevent cerebral edema; prevents reperfusion injury (O_2 free radical scavenger)	1–2 gm/kg IV q 6 hr
Nalorphine	Narcotic antagonist	0.5–1 mg/kg IV
Naloxone	Narcotic antagonist	.04 mg/kg IV, IM, SC
Sodium bicarbonate	Treat metabolic acidosis (not recommended for first 5–10 min of CPR)	.5 mEq/kg q 5–10 min

*Dosages for epinephrine listed are higher than previous recommendations and are based on recent reports of improved results from CPR using this dosage. (Robello and Crowe, 1989.)

documented that long bone fractures and other external traumatic injuries are frequently accompanied by major pulmonary injuries as well (Spackman, 1984). Life-threatening complications, therefore, should be anticipated and ruled out in all but the mildest injuries.

During the hectic few moments of initial presentation, the very cursory examination is still performed in an orderly and routine manner, considering sequentially the ABCs of emergency care— Airway patency and patient alertness; Breathing performance; and Cardiovascular status. This initial assessment and triage phase may be considered phase I of the primary survey.

Occasionally, it may be necessary to triage many trauma patients at once. Not uncommonly in the busy emergency practice, several severely injured animals must be cared for simultaneously. The veterinarian and staff must rapidly assess, categorize, and set priorities for all patients present (incoming and hospitalized) according to injury type and severity, identifying those that are most life-threatening. Clinic staff preparedness and training will determine the efficiency and effectiveness of the care delivered.

Primary Survey

Following the initial assessment and subsequent triage, the primary survey is performed on the patient in the emergency treatment area. The goal of this survey (examination) is to instantly determine if a life-threatening condition is present and, if so, immediately perform the appropriate resuscitative procedure to sustain life. The primary survey should take less than 2 min and should optimally be performed with a team of at least three personnel. It is conducted to evaluate the ABCs, and the steps should be performed in the same sequence on every emergency patient.

AIRWAY PATENCY

The airway is examined; the examiner listens for breath sounds while palpating and visually inspecting the oral cavity, trachea, and larynx for abnormal position. Is there blockage or disruption of the airway? Carefully extending the head and neck may periodically relieve an upper airway obstruction. Blood, vomitus, or a foreign body can occlude the oropharynx and manual removal or suctioning may be necessary to clear it from the airway. Cricothyroidotomy, transtracheal catheterizations, or an emergency tracheostomy can provide an immediate but short-term open airway. Comatose or moribund patients can and should be intubated, but carefully to prevent further brain blood flow compromise. Further steps in the assessment should not be performed until a patent airway is secured.

BREATHING

Assess adequacy of ventilation by noting the presence, rate, depth, and quality of respirations, and mucous membrane color. Chest auscultation and palpation should be done to detect any abnormalities or injuries such as rib fractures, flail chest, or penetrating wounds. Flail chest and tension pneumothorax are considered life-threatening problems, and a thoracocentesis should be performed immediately if severe respiratory distress is observed. A tube thoracostomy may be placed later after completing the primary survey, but the initial thoracocentesis should be accomplished by using a 20–16 gauge needle (depending on patient size), intravenous extension tubing, three-way stop cock, and a 60-ml syringe (Wingfield, 1988). Supplemental oxygen via nasal catheter, mask, clear plastic bag over patient's head, or endotracheal tube is needed in most patients and can be administered at this time by an assistant while the clinician continues with other priorities. Positive pressure ventilation may be necessary in these patients to prevent or reverse hypoxemia and hypercarbia. In a conscious patient that remains dyspneic, a tracheostomy may be required.

Compromised respiratory function should be suspected in any trauma patient, especially those in which long bone fractures are identified. A study in dogs suffering motor vehicle trauma documented that thoracic injuries occur in 39% of all fracture cases and 58% of those had multiple thoracic injuries. Pulmonary contusions, pneumothorax, and fractured ribs were most commonly reported (Spackman, 1984).

CIRCULATION

Cardiovascular status is evaluated by determining the rate, rhythm, and quality of the femoral pulses (also carotid) and jugular venous pressure and pulses and by observing mucous membrane color, moisture, and capillary refill time (CRT). Failure to identify a pulse or heartbeat should activate the protocol for cardiac arrest, and cardiopulmonary resuscitation (CPR) should be initiated at once. Major external hemorrhage should be identified and controlled by direct pressure with a sterile dressing.

Regardless of the presence of active external hemorrhage, trauma-induced hypovolemic shock should be anticipated and corrective action taken. Using the team approach, several diagnostic and resuscitative procedures are performed simultaneously, including direct pressure hemorrhage control, placement of an intravenous catheter (preferably large-bore into central vein), preparation for rapid high-volume intravenous fluid or whole blood therapy, supplemental oxygen administration, and continued patient assessment.

Other catastrophic cardiovascular problems considered to be "show stoppers," unless identified and managed early, are pericardial tamponade and ventricular arrhythmias. Their presence may not be immediately evident during the primary survey, but one should have a heightened awareness of them as common sequelae to trauma.

LEVEL OF CONSCIOUSNESS (LOC) AND DISABILITY

The clinician assesses LOC and overall neurologic status during the first moments of the primary survey. The extent of neurologic malfunction continues to be evaluated concomitantly as the initial examination continues, and the primary survey concludes with a rapid examination of the head, spinal column, abdomen, and extremities. Is there evidence of specific central nervous system (CNS) trauma? Is there obvious spinal cord damage as manifested by gross vertebral column displacement or fractures? Are the pupils responsive? Dilated and fixed? Pinpoint? And of equal or unequal size? Preliminary neurologic findings and observations will be followed-up in the secondary survey but are factored into the initial prognosis and therapeutic plan. If the patient is unconscious, assume CNS damage and maintain the animal in lateral recumbency on a rigid backboard until a determination is made.

Obvious fractures are noted at this time, and if the situation allows, those below the stifle and elbow may be quickly splinted to prevent pain and additional soft-tissue injury. Fracture management may have to be delayed until after the catastrophic problems are under control.

Resuscitation Phase

Basic life-saving resuscitation is performed as needed during the primary survey. Depending on the findings and actions taken during that period, more definitive resuscitation procedures are implemented to continue to manage life-threatening problems. For example, transtracheal oxygen supplementation is replaced by laryngoscope-aided intubation, or peripheral vein intravenous catheterization is augmented by a jugular (cut-down) large-bore central catheter placement. Shock therapy is initiated in this phase. Resuscitation maneuvers are focused on obtaining physiologic stability of the patient, primarily of the respiratory and cardiovascular functions. These maneuvers have the best chance of succeeding if performed as early as possible during the "golden hour" of emergency care (Crowe, 1989; Eisenberg, 1988). This "golden hour" denotes the immediate period following trauma, generally considered to be an hour or less, during which effective treatment will ensure the best chance of patient survival.

Failures and problems in resuscitation of the seriously injured animal are frequent and frustrating. Great investment in time, effort, and money all too often are not positively rewarded. Why? In a review of human emergency fatalities, it was concluded that failures and treatment errors occurred not due to ignorance but because appropriate resuscitation was not applied expeditiously at the crucial moment. It further was shown that survival rates improved when an algorithmic approach was applied to the emergency treatment system (Shoemaker, 1989). A wall-mounted algorithm using a branch chain decision tree will enable the whole emergency care team to know the therapeutic strategies beforehand, thus encouraging a more orderly approach to resuscitation (Shoemaker, 1989).

When treating emergencies, one should be prepared and able to perform several resuscitation procedures to stabilize the injured patient (Table 2). For more detailed discussion of specific procedures, the reader is referred to other sections of this text and to the references listed at the end of this article (Crowe, 1989, 1990; Haskins, 1990a, 1990b; Wingfield, 1988).

Table 2. *Emergency Procedures*

Airway
Intubation using laryngoscope
Pharyngeal and tracheal suctioning
Slash (emergency) and elective tracheostomy
Foreign body dislodgement
Tracheal repair
Cricothyroidotomy
Percutaneous tracheal catheterization

Respiratory Support
Nasal oxygen catheterization
Transtracheal oxygen delivery
Positive-pressure ventilation
  Ambu bag
  Mechanical ventilator
Thoracentesis
Chest tube placement (intermittent and continuous drainage)
Thoracotomy
Flail chest stabilization

Cardiovascular Support
Open and closed chest CPR
Abdomen and hindlimb counterpressure
Peripheral and central vein percutaneous catheterization
Venous cut-down (peripheral and central vein)
Pericardial tamponade diagnosis and drainage
Intraosseous cannulation
Arterial blood pressure monitoring
Diagnostic peritoneal lavage
Central venous pressure measurement
Cardiac monitoring; ECG interpretation

Miscellaneous
Exploratory laparotomy, hemorrhage control
Gastric dilatation volvulus (GDV)
  Decompression
  Gastrocentesis
  Stomach tube
  Gastrostomy
Autotransfusion

AIRWAY RESUSCITATION MANAGEMENT

Severe airway obstructions are not common but, when present, are life-threatening. Locating the obstruction is the first priority. In addition to visual and digital examination of the upper airway structures, various breath sounds will also suggest the location of the obstruction. Obstructions in the oropharynx usually are "gurgly," while laryngeal and cranial tracheal obstructions are more stridorous or raspy. Caudal cervical or cranial thoracic obstructions will result in raspy breath sounds heard loudest near the thoracic inlet. Complete obstructions anywhere along the airway will usually be manifested by exaggerated inspiratory movements or apnea. Once the obstruction is located, rapid action is taken to either relieve or bypass the obstruction.

Oropharyngeal obstructions most commonly are vomitus, thick mucus/saliva, blood, or foreign bodies. The neck is carefully extended and a suctioning unit is used to remove any blood, vomitus, or saliva occluding the airway. Postural drainage by lowering the head may help when active nasal or oral bleeding is present. Tonsil or sponge forceps are used effectively to retrieve foreign bodies lodged craniad to the larynx. Foreign objects trapped in the larynx or lower trachea may be occasionally expelled by several rapid thoracic compressions.

If the obstruction is only partial, oxygen supplementation via a nasal catheter or face mask may adequately stabilize the animal. Nasal catheterization is the preferred technique as it allows freedom of movement, is more efficient on O_2 delivery, and less costly. Nasal O_2 flow rates are approximately 100 to 200 ml/kg/min. A detailed discussion of this technique is described elsewhere (Pasco, 1988).

When a more complete airway occlusion is present or the animal cannot be intubated, aggressive action should be taken to access the airway below the obstruction. Transtracheal oxygen, using a large-bore intravenous catheter as a cannula, may temporarily suffice, but more commonly, an emergency tracheostomy is required. A tracheostomy also is usually necessary when tracheal tears disrupt the continuity of the airway. The technique for this procedure should be mastered by all practitioners providing emergency service (Aron and Crowe, 1985).

Unconscious trauma patients should be intubated through the oropharynx if possible. This is most easily accomplished by using a laryngoscope with the patient in dorsal or right lateral recumbency. A tracheostomy should be performed if upper airway occlusion prevents passage of the tube or if the airway problem is caudal to the tube.

Ventilatory support is provided by manual ventilation with an Ambu bag or by a mechanical ventilator that is either volume or pressure limited. High-frequency jet ventilation with small tidal volumes and rapid rates may also be useful (see this volume, p. 98). A positive-pressure ventilation rate of 8 to 10 breaths per minute is usually adequate.

CARDIOPULMONARY RESUSCITATION (CPR)

CPR is administered to those trauma patients suffering cardiopulmonary arrest (CPA). CPA is the sudden disruption of respiratory and cardiovascular function which occurs as a result of either primary pulmonary failure or primary cardiovascular dysfunction. It is commonly felt that CPR is a useless therapeutic exercise, but in reality, a significant number of patients can be revived with CPR (Haskins, 1989). The major reasons for CPR failures include a delay in recognizing CPA and a delay in initiating CPR and associated resuscitation procedures (Shoemaker, 1989). A lack of staff preparedness and clinician reluctance frequently contribute to the delay in attempting CPR. Such delays result in the patient's being unresponsive and unsalvageable owing to irreversible cerebral damage.

Recent significant changes in CPR recommendations appear to have led to improved survival rates. It generally has now been concluded that:

1. Effective CPR is due to increased pressure obtained through the "thoracic pump mechanism."
2. Cats and small dogs (7 kg or less) should be placed in lateral recumbency while larger dogs should be in dorsal recumbency.
3. Simultaneous ventilation and chest compressions will maximize circulatory flow.
4. Chest compressions should be at a rate of 80 to 120/minute.
5. Open heart massage is much more effective than closed heart massage techniques. In many cases, closed chest CPR is a waste of valuable time and one should immediately institute open chest massage.
6. Emergency drug use during CPR is minimized and based on patient response and ECG pattern. Sodium bicarbonate and calcium agents are not recommended initially (Haskins, 1989; Muir, 1990).
7. The endotracheal route is, in the opinion of the authors, the preferred route of administration of most emergency drugs such as epinephrine, atropine, and lidocaine; IV route (central venous) is second choice; intracardiac route is not recommended (Robello and Crowe, 1989).
8. Cerebral resuscitation is a recognized goal of CPR.
9. Postresuscitation injury is being better defined and may be minimized with appropriate therapy. The most effective way to prevent this injury is CPR that establishes adequate cerebral blood flow. (For detailed discussions of CPR, see this volume, p. 112, and references listed at the end of this article [Haskins, 1989; Robello and Crowe, 1989; Safar, 1989].)

SHOCK THERAPY

Hypovolemic shock following trauma is a frequent occurrence and is due to an absolute or relative loss of circulating blood volume. In addition to controlling active external bleeding during the primary phase, one must aggressively act to restore blood volume by several means in the resuscitation phase.

The cornerstone of shock therapy remains vigorous, high-volume fluid replacement. This can only be accomplished by securing vascular access to a major vein, preferably the jugular. A 14- or 16-gauge catheter should be placed in the central vein percutaneously if possible but by venous cut-down if necessary. This will allow rapid delivery of large volumes of fluid, measurement of central venous pressure (CVP), and long-term catheter placement. A large-bore catheter for fluid delivery may also be placed into the intraosseous canal of the humerus or femur whenever venous access is a problem (see this volume, p. 107).

Initially an extracellular crystalloid replacement fluid such as lactated Ringer's solution should be administered. Approximately one blood volume of fluid (dogs, 90 ml/kg; cats 50 ml/kg) should be administered to restore vascular volume as rapidly as possible. An intravenous high-flow capacity (resuscitation) infusion pump or pressure infuser system can facilitate rapid fluid delivery. When crystalloid replacement is inadequate, one should consider using hypertonic saline, dextran, hetastarch, plasma, or whole blood (see *CVT X*, p. 37 and p. 316, for detailed discussion of fluid therapy). When pulmonary contusion is likely, colloids such as dextran, plasma, or hetastarch should be incorporated into the fluid therapy plan to minimize fluid accumulation in the bruised lung. Whole blood, plasma, or plasma substitutes should be administered to maintain a PCV of 20% or greater and a total protein of 3.5 gm/dl or greater (Haskins, 1990).

Cardiovascular support can be provided by employing other modalities, including external counterpressure to the rear limbs and abdomen or emergency surgery for hemorrhage control. This is a temporary measure until the circulation is stabilized. Sympathomimetics and other drugs may be administered in conjunction with fluids to improve cardiovascular performance and systemic arterial blood pressure (Haskins, 1990b; Schertel, 1989).

Monitoring procedures are initiated at this time (resuscitation phase) if patient stabilization allows. An ECG monitor is hooked-up, a base-line blood sample for PVC/total solids, glucose, ACT, and so forth is drawn from the initial catheterization, systemic arterial blood pressure monitoring is begun with a Doppler ultrasound instrument, and CVP measurements are recorded. A temporary problem list is established at this time as well as treatment and monitoring flow charts.

Secondary Survey

The secondary survey is begun after resuscitation and stabilization of the patient. It includes a thorough history, thorough physical examination, and noninvasive and invasive diagnostic tests. An in-depth history is obtained as the physical examination is performed. Here again the team approach is important as several functions require simultaneous management. The team remains prepared to focus on life-threatening problems if they re-appear.

This secondary examination generally follows the same course (ABCs) as the primary survey. The airway is more thoroughly examined, and the need for more definitive therapy is identified to be performed later. Patient deterioration or lack of re-

sponse may indicate that elective tracheotomy is needed. Laryngeal fractures or tracheal tears may require surgical treatment as soon as the animal is adequately stabilized or surgery may be required to achieve stabilization.

The respiratory system should be thoroughly and frequently evaluated as serious pulmonary dysfunction may not be apparent until hours after trauma. The development of tension pneumothorax, pleural hemorrhage, pulmonary contusions, and diaphragmatic hernias may not overtly compromise the patient for several hours. Breathing patterns, mucous membrane color, and blood gases (if possible) should be closely monitored.

Cardiovascular function remains a high priority and must be closely monitored to identify potential problems before they become life-threatening. Mucous membrane color and CRT, arterial blood pressure, CVP, and the electrocardiogram are repeatedly observed and findings recorded to identify trends that require treatment intervention. Particular attention is given to the ECG since severe cardiac dysrhythmias may not develop for 48 to 72 hours. Blunt chest trauma with myocardial contusion and focal ischemia can cause life-threatening ventricular tachyarrhythmias or electromechanical dissociation (EMD). Intravenous lidocaine by bolus at 2 mg/kg or constant-rate infusion (CRI) at 40 to 80 µg/kg/min is treatment of choice for ventricular tachycardia. Hypoxemia and electrolyte disturbances may also alter cardiac function, and treatment is directed at these complicating factors and at the underlying causes.

The abdomen is evaluated next by thorough palpation, visualization, and auscultation (for bowel sounds). The animal should be examined for signs of abdominal trauma, intra-abdominal hemorrhage, or organ displacement.

The remainder of the examination is conducted by systematically going over the animal from the tip of the nose to tip of the tail, examining in detail the head, spine, rib cage, pelvic canal, and extremities. An abbreviated neurologic examination is performed at this time.

Diagnostic procedures are necessary to complete the secondary survey in all but the very mild trauma cases. Care must be taken not to stress the animal into danger by performing procedures that provide low information yield for the risk involved. Radiographic evaluation, which can be extremely stressful, normally is required, but ultrasonographic examination should be used whenever possible, especially to evaluate the chest and abdomen. Ultrasound is very helpful in diagnosing pericardial tamponade, detecting free fluid, and evaluating soft-tissue problems. Abdominal paracentesis and peritoneal lavage should be performed when abdominal trauma is suspected. Bilateral thoracentesis is advised in trauma cases, and this diagnostic procedure is performed at this time (if not already done previously) to determine the presence of intrapleural air or fluid. Based on these findings, a decision is made about placing a thoracostomy tube and the need for further pulmonary diagnostic or treatment procedures.

Upon completion of the secondary survey, the temporary problem list is compiled and definitive medical and surgical priorities are established. As the situation moves from resuscitation (basic trauma life support—BTLS) to definitive care (advanced trauma life support—ATLS), the threats to the animal become sepsis, reperfusion injury, and multiple organ failure. Aggressive, timely resuscitation, and sound application of emergency medicine principles may prevent these complications and the untimely death of numerous trauma patients.

References and Suggested Reading

Aron, D. N., and Crowe, D. T.: Upper airway obstruction: General principles and selected conditions in the dog and cat. Vet. Clin. North Am. [Sm. Anim. Pract.] 15:891, 1985.
  A concise description and demonstration, through the use of figures, of tracheostomy techniques.
Crowe, D. T.: Symposium on critical care. Vet. Med. 84:34, 1989.
  A broad discussion on practical application of emergency and critical care principles and techniques.
Crowe, D. T.: Preparation for catastrophic surgical emergencies. Int. Vet. Emerg. Crit. Care. Proc., 1990, p. 269.
Eisenberg, M. S., and Copass, M. K.: Trauma. In Emergency Medical Therapy. Philadelphia: W. B. Saunders, 1988, p. 403.
  In-depth discussion of medical management of the human trauma patient with specific emphasis on resuscitation techniques and philosophy.
Haskins, S. C.: Cardiopulmonary resuscitation. In Kirk, R. W., (ed.): Current Veterinary Therapy X. Philadelphia: W. B. Saunders, 1989, p. 330.
  Review and update on CPR, incorporating new recommendations on drug uses and doses, CPR techniques, and postresuscitation monitoring and support.
Haskins, S. C.: Fluid, electrolyte, and acid-base therapy. Int. Vet. Emerg. Crit. Care Symp Proc., 1990a, p. 375.
  A review of fluid therapy principles, discussing traditional concepts plus recent recommendations on use of colloids, hypertonic saline, and sodium bicarbonate.
Haskins, S. C.: Shock update—What's new therapeutically. Int. Vet. Emerg. Crit. Care Proc., 1990b, p. 431.
Muir, W. W.: Emergency drugs: What's in? What's out? Am. Anim. Hosp. Assoc. Proceedings, 1990, p. 390.
  Concise presentation on emergency drugs used in the management of cardiopulmonary arrest.
Muir, W. W.: Reperfusion injury: Pathophysiology and treatment. Int. Vet. Emerg. Crit. Care Proc., 1990, p. 47.
Murtaugh, R. J., and Spaulding, G. L.: Initial management of respiratory emergencies. In Kirk, R. W., (ed.): Current Veterinary Therapy X. Philadelphia: W. B. Saunders, 1989, p. 195.
Pasco, P. J.: Oxygen and ventilatory support for the critical patient. Semin. Vet. Med. Surg. (Small Anim.) 3:202, 1988.
Robello, C. D., and Crowe, D. T.: Cardiopulmonary resuscitation: Current recommendations. Vet. Clin. North Am. Small Anim. Pract. 19:1127, 1989.
Safar, P.: Cardiopulmonary-cerebral resuscitation. In Shoemaker, W. C., Ayres, S., Grenvik, A., et al. (eds.): Textbook of Critical Care. Philadelphia: W. B. Saunders, 1989, p. 5.
  This is a comprehensive review article discussing the "state of the art" in human CPR, providing insight and basis for new techniques and procedures to be adopted by veterinary clinicians.
Schertel, E. R., and Muir, W. W.: Shock, pathophysiology, monitoring, and therapy. In Kirk, R. W., (ed.): Current Veterinary Therapy X. Philadelphia: W. B. Saunders, 1989, p. 316.
  Comprehensive article providing an update on the latest concepts, pathophysiology, and treatment of the various forms of shock.
Shoemaker, W. C.: Resuscitation in acute emergency conditions with clinical algorithms. In Shoemaker, W. C., Ayers, S., Grenvik, A., et al. (eds.): Textbook of Critical Care. Philadelphia: W. B. Saunders, 1989, p. 87.
  Thought-provoking article on how to better implement an emergency medicine program using algorithms.
Spackman, G. J. A., Caywood, D. D., Feeney, D. A., et al.: Thoracic wall and pulmonary trauma in dogs sustaining fractures as a result of motor vehicle accidents. J.A.V.M.A. 185:985, 1984.
  Retrospective study documenting the frequency with which thoracic trauma occurred simultaneously with long bone fractures.
Wingfield, W. E.: Treatment priorities in cases of multiple trauma. Semin. Vet. Med. Surg. (Small Anim.) 3:193, 1988.
  Review article discussing the diagnosis, management, and treatment of the severely injured trauma patient, focusing on life-threatening problems.

ANALGESICS IN CARDIAC, SURGICAL, AND INTENSIVE CARE PATIENTS

BERNIE HANSEN
Raleigh, North Carolina

The alleviation of pain in critically ill animals is a vital but daunting task. No other animal patients are more likely to experience pain associated with their care, and few are less able to tolerate it. These animals often have had debilitating and painful surgical procedures or suffer from painful disease. They may be cared for in a facility that is noisy and brightly illuminated 24 hours a day, disrupting circadian rhythms and their ability to sleep. In the course of their care they are moved, monitored, manipulated, palpated, aspirated, catheterized, and phlebotomized by people they do not know. They may be physiologically and behaviorally obtunded and incapable of showing "typical" pain behaviors or of mounting an observable physiologic response. Furthermore, overt evidence of beneficial responses to therapy may be difficult to find. The challenge is to recognize these needs and treat them in ways that enhance patient well-being, yet do not interfere with management of their disease.

Many of the metabolic and functional derangements characteristic of the stress response following surgical intervention or trauma are directly related to pain. This response may be important for the survival of an untreated injured animal; however, in many animals under direct veterinary care, it is probably maladaptive and deleterious. Pain and the stress response can contribute to anorexia, inability to sleep, tissue catabolism, muscle fatigue, and pulmonary, gastrointestinal, or urinary dysfunction. Consequences of these events include increased morbidity, distress, exhaustion, and prolonged convalescence.

A clinical axiom holds that postoperative pain in human patients is more easily controlled when it is pre-empted by analgesic therapy instituted before the patient becomes conscious of pain. Clinical studies in human patients confirm the validity of this observation (Tverskoy et al., 1990). The reasons for this phenomenon are not entirely understood; however, recent experimental evidence suggests that both the organization and function of the nervous system change following nociceptive stimulation. Consequences of this "wind-up" activity include neuronal hypersensitivity and enhanced ascending input to the brain, changes that may persist long after all nociceptive stimulation has ceased. The lesson from these findings is that it may be much easier to "prevent" pain, rather than try to suppress it once it is already present.

Potential barriers to the effective management of pain by clinicians include inappropriate attitudes, lack of knowledge about analgesic medications, and lack of skills in assessing pain and in applying therapeutic techniques. Animals in considerable distress may not be treated because caregivers assume that the pain should not be that severe or that the disease, injury, or surgical treatment was not traumatic enough to warrant therapy. Clinicians may withhold treatment because of concern about analgesic drug side effects or a belief that pain relief will mask the signs of underlying disease. In addition, pain relief may be relegated to a low priority during more heroic treatment efforts.

The experience of pain is complex, highly variable between patients, and very unpredictable. When severe, pain may result in physiologic distress and maladaptive behavior. Those behaviors that can be recognized by clinicians include restlessness, disruption of normal sleep, prolonged attempts to escape from pain, and reluctance to lie down. Any animal displaying maladaptive behavior or evidence of emotional distress merits some form of intervention, and therapy should never be withheld because one is uncertain whether pain is present.

GENERAL PRINCIPLES OF PAIN MANAGEMENT

Management of pain begins with the basic tenets of good patient care. For the surgical patient, this begins intraoperatively. Scrupulous regard for careful tissue handling, suture placement, and rapid completion of the surgical procedure are important considerations in order to minimize tissue trauma and subsequent postoperative pain.

Careful nursing care is not only essential to overall patient management but will help minimize discomfort and pain as well. Bandages and dressings should be inspected frequently and changed as needed to prevent irritation. Immobile animals should be maintained on blankets or mattresses and repositioned periodically. Urination and defecation should be assisted whenever necessary and patient hygiene maintained. Every effort should be made to provide for an environment conducive to rest and a normal sleep/wake cycle.

The animal's psychologic needs should be met. Apprehensive, fearful, anxious, or emotionally distressed animals may benefit dramatically from a few minutes of verbal and physical comforting by either the owner or clinician. Caregivers should routinely enter the animal's cage armed not with a needle but with comforting words. This approach will help prevent the learned avoidance and fear animals may develop when repeatedly given injections or subjected to painful manipulations. Alert animals with mild pain may benefit from simple distraction with a chew toy or by being placed near hubs of activity during the day. Animals with more severe apprehension or anxiety may benefit from the administration of anxiolytic drugs.

Local anesthetic administration should be considered for animals undergoing invasive diagnostic and therapeutic procedures, including intravenous catheterization when large-bore (14 to 20 gauge) catheters are used. Local anesthesia will often prevent struggling by the animal during the procedure and facilitate catheter placement. Lidocaine HCl 2% (0.1 to 0.5 ml) can be infiltrated subcutaneously and intradermally at the site of catheter entry. While the transient sting of subcutaneous lidocaine administration will cause pain responses from many animals, this brief event is often preferable to the sensation of a large-gauge catheter being forced through the skin. A eutectic mixture of local anesthetics (EMLA Cream, Astra Pharmaceuticals Ltd.)

Table 1. *Systemic Analgesics Used in the Intensive Care Unit*

Drug	Dose (mg/kg)	Route	Dose Interval (hr)*	Comments
Opioid agonists†				
Morphine	0.05–0.4 (dog)	IV	1–4	Observe cats for excitement.
	0.2 –1.0 (dog)	IM, SQ	2–6	
	0.05–0.2 (cat)	IM, SQ	2–6	
Oxymorphone	0.02–0.1 (dog)	IV	2–4	
	0.02–0.05 (cat)			
	0.05–0.2 (dog)	IM, SQ	2–6	
	0.05–0.1 (cat)			
Meperidine	1.0 –4.0 (dog)	IM	.5–1	Do not bolus IV.
Opioid agonist-antagonists				
Butorphanol	0.2 –1.0 (dog)	IM, IV, SQ	1–4	
	0.1 –0.4 (cat)	IM, IV, SQ	1–4	
Pentazocine	1.0 –3.0 (dog)	IM, IV	.5–3	
Nalbuphine	0.5 –1.5 (dog)	IM, IV	1–6	Inconsistent effectiveness.
Opioid partial agonist				
Buprenorphine	0.005–0.02 (dog)	IM, IV	4–12	Effects may be difficult to reverse.
	0.005–0.01 (cat)			
Nonsteroidal anti-inflammatory agents				
Aspirin	10 (dog)	PO	12	GI hemorrhage
	10 (cat)	PO	48	
Phenylbutazone	20 (dog)	PO	24	Do not exceed 800 mg/day.
Flunixin meglumine	0.5 –1.0 (dog)	IV	24	GI hemorrhage and renal ischemia. Avoid methoxyflurane.

*For continuous intravenous infusion, administer the first dose as a bolus and immediately begin infusion administration of the same dose over the anticipated dose interval. The infusion rate should be increased or decreased to achieve and maintain the desired effect.

†For the first intravenous dose, start with a low dose and then repeat it every 5–10 min to effect. Once effective analgesia is achieved, plan on repeating the total dose at regular intervals.

that provides effective, pain-free topical cutaneous anesthesia is available in Europe and will soon be available commercially in the U.S.

Drugs (including analgesics) should be administered intravenously through indwelling catheters whenever possible to minimize the number of injections the animal must endure, and blood samples should be drawn from these catheters, if possible, to avoid the pain and trauma of repeated phlebotomy.

Table 1 presents the systemic analgesics used in the intensive care unit.

PHARMACOLOGIC MANAGEMENT OF PAIN

Nonsteroidal Anti-Inflammatory Drugs (NSAIDs)

Prostaglandins are produced by most tissues and serve many physiologic functions. Prostaglandins are also liberated following cell injury or death, and these compounds mediate inflammation and enhance nociception following injury. Once liberated, prostaglandins sensitize C-fiber nociceptors and promote the hypersensitivity that follows inflammation. This phenomenon accounts in part for the tenderness of an area following injury and inflammation. Nonsteroidal anti-inflammatory drugs (NSAIDs) inhibit production of prostaglandins; hence, NSAIDs are most effective when adminis-

tered *before* surgical intervention and the onset of inflammation. These drugs are not effective at blocking sharp pain, and their role as analgesic agents for the treatment of acute injury and postoperative pain is limited. The use of NSAIDs is further limited by the fact that the analgesia produced is subject to a therapeutic ceiling effect, and higher dosages will not increase analgesia but will produce more side effects. Consequently, if NSAIDs are used in a critical care setting, it is typically in conjunction with other analgesic drugs. When used alone, the best use for these drugs may be for alleviation of pain of mild to moderate intensity associated with inflammation.

The NSAIDs have side effects that include gastric and duodenal ulceration and renal ischemia. These complications are much more likely in animals with poor visceral blood flow, as is seen in many critically ill animal patients with hemodynamic instability. Therefore, it may be best to delay therapy with any of these drugs until normal circulation is restored.

Opioid Analgesics

Opioid analgesics are the mainstay for management of acute pain. Commonly used opioid agonists include morphine, oxymorphone, and meperidine. These drugs are generally the most effective analgesics for the treatment of moderate to severe pain, particularly acute pain due to trauma and surgical procedures. Therapy with any of these drugs needs to be tailored to the individual animal. The response to these drugs varies with the individual animal and its level of consciousness, the degree of pain present and its source, and the presence of coexisting disease. All opioid drugs are characterized by dose-dependent analgesia as well as dose-dependent side effects. Side effects of concern for the critical care patient include respiratory depression, bradycardia, and hypotension.

Opioids must be used with caution in animals that cannot tolerate respiratory depression, including those with pre-existing central respiratory depression, metabolic acidosis, and pulmonary injury. This caution should not, however, be used as an excuse to withhold these drugs inappropriately. The vast majority of postoperative animal patients can tolerate the mild to moderate respiratory depression associated with therapeutic doses of these drugs with no adverse effect. There is no evidence for an additive effect promoting ventilatory failure associated with opioid administration in animals with pulmonary disease and an intact central respiratory drive. A painful patient with pulmonary disease or injury should not routinely be denied therapy with these drugs.

Animals with head injury accompanied by intracranial bleeding or edema are at particular risk from the respiratory depressant effects of opioids because hypercapnia increases cerebral blood flow. Therefore, if these drugs are used in patients with head injury, respiratory function must be monitored carefully. Monitoring variables include physical characteristics such as respiratory depth and rate, as well as more sophisticated tests, including arterial blood gases and end-tidal CO_2 concentration. Respirations should be controlled by mechanical ventilation if needed to maintain arterial P_{CO_2} at 25 to 35 mm Hg.

Respiratory depression and vasodilation may be beneficial to the dog with pulmonary edema, particularly edema due to heart failure. The vasodilation produced by morphine administration promotes blood pooling in peripheral veins and the liver, thereby unloading the pulmonary veins and reducing pulmonary venous pressure. Central respiratory depression may reduce the work of breathing in a patient that is anxious and struggling ineffectually to breath. This reduces the oxygen requirements of the chest muscles and diaphragm and lessens cardiac workload. Morphine may be administered at a dosage of 0.05 to 0.1 mg/kg intravenously and repeated every 5 to 10 min until the dog is mildly sedated and respirations have eased. Higher dosages are used if the patient requires tracheal intubation to control ventilation. The reduction of pulmonary venous pressure seen with morphine may not be observed following the administration of other opioid drugs. In fact, intravenous oxymorphone administration increases pulmonary venous pressure in normal dogs and may be contraindicated in dogs with cardiogenic pulmonary edema (Copland et al., 1987).

Morphine is the prototype opioid agonist and remains the standard of comparison for opioid drugs. Side effects associated with administration of this drug include histamine release, nausea and vomiting, and dysphoria, particularly when it is administered intravenously. These complications are infrequently observed and in general are not difficult to manage. Histamine release causes systemic hypotension and could worsen circulatory shock. For this reason oxymorphone (P-M Oxymorphone, Pitman-Moore) may be preferred in hypotensive animals. In either case, proper fluid therapy will usually prevent significant problems. Bradycardia is a side effect associated with the administration of all opioid agonists except meperidine and is commonly observed in animals under general anesthesia. Serious bradycardia appears to be relatively uncommon following opioid administration in the awake animal patient and will usually respond to the intravenous administration of 0.05 mg/kg of atropine.

The usefulness of meperidine is limited by its short duration of action. In addition, meperidine significantly depresses myocardial contractility and causes hypotension in both dogs and cats when administered intravenously. Despite those factors, meperidine can produce adequate analgesia when administered by continuous intravenous infusion (1 to 2 mg/kg/hr) to dogs that are hemodynamically stable.

The opioid agonist-antagonists include butorphanol, pentazocine, and nalbuphine. These drugs produce analgesia by agonist action at kappa opioid receptors, but are antagonists at μ receptors. If the central analgesic and sedative actions of μ agonists are therapeutically important for a particular animal, antagonism at these receptors by any of the agonist-antagonist drugs will reverse those effects and impair therapy. Therefore, the agonist-antagonists should not be administered simultaneously with the μ agonists in the morphine group. There is a ceiling effect on the analgesia and respiratory depression these drugs produce, and the risk of life-threatening hypoventilation is minimal. The therapeutic ceiling limits administration of these drugs to the treatment of mild to moderate pain. Butorphanol is unpredictable as a tranquilizer when given to alert animals, but most depressed dogs and cats are sedated by therapeutic doses. Butorphanol administration produces analgesia at dosages (0.4 to 1.0 mg/kg) that cause minimal cardiopulmonary depression (Raffe and Lipowitz, 1985).

The partial opioid agonist buprenorphine (Buprenex, Reckitt and Coleman Pharmaceuticals) binds avidly to μ receptors and appears to dissociate from these receptors very slowly. As a result, it has a relatively long duration of action, and its effects are not easily reversed with administration of naloxone. Mydriasis and agitation may be seen in some cats administered dosages above 0.02 mg/kg. Unless given with a tranquilizer, sedation is minimal.

Pain is only one of many internal and environmental stressors with which the critically ill or postsurgical animal must cope. Environmental events may disrupt sleep and engender anxiety and fear which, in turn, may intensify distress associated with pain. Therefore, alleviation of fear and anxiety by sedation may be beneficial. A state of calmness is in fact often used by clinicians as a clinical sign of adequate analgesia in animals. While an outwardly calm animal may still be experiencing significant pain, calmness may be associated with a relative absence of distress. Surgery is a physically exhausting event, and it may be advantageous to sleep for hours postoperatively. Since many major surgeries are not completed until near the end of a work day, overnight sedation is a reasonable therapeutic goal. Sedation is a common side effect of the opioid drugs, particularly when administered at higher dosages. This sedation may be very beneficial to ill animals in an intensive care environment, especially postoperatively. In many animals there appears to be an opioid dosage range characterized by the production of some subjective signs of adequate analgesia (reduced guarding, reduced muscle spasms, and others), but which is still accompanied by overt behavioral signs of anxiety or dysphoria, including restlessness and vocalization. These animals should be treated with either opioids alone at dosages high enough to produce sedation and sleep, or they should be treated with a combination of opioids *and anxiolytic drugs*. The addition of *low* doses of anxiolytic drugs such as acepromazine (0.03 to 0.05 mg/kg intravenously) or diazepam (0.1 to 0.3 mg/kg IV) to opioid therapy may be very helpful. In this situation, the opioid drug is given at regular fixed intervals (see later), and the anxiolytic drugs are given as needed and to effect.

LOCAL AND REGIONAL ANESTHESIA

Local anesthetic drugs useful in the critically ill animal patient include lidocaine and bupivacaine. The advantages of local and regional anesthesia include the potential for complete blockade of pain and a lack of cardiovascular and respiratory depression when these drugs are used correctly. Lidocaine has a short duration of action and is best suited for anesthesia for minor procedures where prolonged pain is not anticipated. The duration of action can be increased to over an hour by the use of a solution containing epinephrine at a dilution of 1:100,000.

Intravenous lidocaine 2% without epinephrine has been advocated as a systemic analgesic. Although it has been shown to have clinical benefit in human patients and will reduce anesthetic and opioid requirements (Cassuto et al., 1985), in our hands it does not appear effective as a sole agent. It may be administered at a dosage of 1–2 mg/kg followed by a continuous infusion at the rate of 25 to 40 μg/kg/min.

Bupivacaine has a longer duration of action than lidocaine and is better suited for relief of pain associated with surgical treatment or disease. Administration of bupivacaine with epinephrine 1:100,000 will provide local anesthesia for approximately 4 to 6 hr. For treatment of thoracic wall pain, bupivacaine 0.25% can be infiltrated near the proximal intercostal nerves along the caudal border of each rib. Several intercostal nerves on either side of an incision or lesion should be blocked. If administered intraoperatively for this purpose, 0.2 to 0.5 ml should be infiltrated close to the nerves as far dorsally as possible. Alternatively, undiluted bupivacaine 0.25% or 0.5% (up to a maximum of 2 mg/kg) can be administered through a chest tube into the affected side. The anesthetic effects will occur in areas where the drug pools; hence, it is important that the treated side be placed down (Riegler et al, 1989). Some animals appear uncomfortable during the infusion of the drug, but relief of pain may be rapid and lasts 4 to 6 hours.

All local anesthetics cause clinical signs of central nervous system and cardiovascular dysfunction when absorbed into the blood stream in sufficient quantity. Agitation and restlessness frequently precede the development of seizure activity. Depression and stupor may develop and are difficult to recognize in the seriously ill or postoperative patient. Cardiac arrhythmias and impaired cardiac contractility can occur with repeated high doses and are complications poorly tolerated by ill patients, especially cats. These complications can be prevented by careful dosing and by using solutions containing epinephrine to slow systemic absorption.

Methods of Administration

Analgesic administration on an "as needed" basis is the *least* desirable method of administering these drugs. This approach guarantees that the patient will experience pain. Many critically ill animal patients may be too weak to demonstrate overt pain behaviors and, as a result, will not be treated. Even after pain behaviors are identified, there will always be delays before effective therapeutic doses are administered. Anticipation of the potential for pain developing and early therapeutic intervention are desirable. Opioids and local anesthetics block the functional changes in the nervous system that follow nociception, and analgesic therapy should be initiated *preoperatively* when significant pain is anticipated. This approach may limit the neuronal hypersensitivity response and make subsequent management easier.

Appropriate single agent or combination analgesic drug administration should be individualized to each animal's particular circumstance. A particularly useful technique is to administer small, frequent (every 5 minutes) intravenous doses of opioid drugs and titrate administration to the desired effect. The animal's response to this cumulative dosing is evaluated, and subsequent therapy is planned based on factors such as the degree of pain, initial response to treatment, level of consciousness, and potential for complications. The total dosage is generally administered at intervals of 2 to 6 hours. This "fixed dose" schedule is subject to frequent review and is changed as needed. Table 1 summarizes dosage information for various systemic analgesics used in intensive care patients.

In the author's opinion, intravenous administration of opioid analgesics is preferred as this route of administration provides for rapid onset of action and enables the clinician to rapidly titrate therapy to meet the animal's needs. Additionally, in animals with poor peripheral circulation, intravenous administration ensures adequate distribution of the drug compared with subcutaneous administration and circumvents the necessity of using painful intramuscular injections to alleviate pain. If the animal cannot tolerate the more intense effects obtained with intravenous bolus administration of analgesics, these drugs may be administered as small frequent doses or as a constant infusion. Human patients demonstrate a fivefold dosage range for analgesic requirements following standardized surgical procedures. Our experience with dogs and cats has been similar. This tremendous interpatient variability requires individualization of therapy for optimal effect and an understanding that dosages of the opioid agonists should not be limited arbitrarily.

Future Trends

Improvements in patient care continue as clinicians recognize better methods to identify and manage pain in animal patients and discard the prejudices against analgesic drugs that currently limit their use. The continued development of new analgesic medications and methods of application will enhance our ability to effectively manage pain in many animals. A particularly exciting technique is the epidural administration of opioids (see this volume, p. 95). Preliminary experience suggests that chronic administration of these drugs through an indwelling epidural catheter is an effective technique for the management of pain in critically ill animals.

References and Suggested Reading

Bednarski, R. M.: Anesthesia and pain control. Vet. Clin. North Am. Sm. Anim. Pract. 19(6):1223, 1989.
A review of pharmacologic management of anesthesia and analgesia in the critical care patient.
Cassuto, J., Wallin, G., Högström, S., et al.: Inhibition of postoperative pain by continuous low-dose intravenous infusion of lidocaine. Anesth. Analg. 64:971, 1985.
A prospective study of the effects of intravenous lidocaine on postoperative pain following cholecystectomy in humans.
Copland, V. S., Haskins, S. C., and Patz, J. D.: Oxymorphone: Cardiovascular, pulmonary, and behavioral effects in dogs. Am. J. Vet. Res. 48(11):1626, 1987.
A study of the cardiopulmonary effects of oxymorphone in normal dogs.
Hansen, B. D.: Postoperative pain. *In:* Bojrab, M. J. (ed.): *Disease Mechanisms in Small Animal Surgery.* Philadelphia: Lea & Febiger (in press).
A review of the pathophysiology of postoperative pain, canine pain behavior, and principles of management.
Haskins, S. C.: Use of analgesics postoperatively and in a small animal intensive care setting. J. A. V. M. A. 191:1266, 1987.
A review of pain behaviors and analgesic therapy in critically ill dogs and cats.
Potthoff, A. P., and Carithers, R. W.: Pain and analgesia in dogs and cats. Compend. Contin. Educ. Pract. Vet. 11:887, 1989.
A review of the neuroanatomy of pain and selected analgesic agents.
Raffe, M. R., and Lipowitz, A. J.: Evaluation of butorphanol tartrate analgesia in the dog. Proceedings of the Second International Congress on Veterinary Anesthesia, p. 155, 1985.
An abstract showing the effects of different doses of butorphanol on experimental pain in dogs.
Riegler, F. X., VadeBoncouer, T. R., Pelligrino, D. A.: Interpleural anesthetics in the dog: Differential somatic neural blockade. Anesthesiology 71:744, 1989.
A study delineating the extent of thoracic wall anesthesia following interpleural bupivacaine in the dog.
Tverskoy, M., Cozacov, C., Ayache, M., et al.: Postoperative pain after inguinal herniorrhaphy with different types of anesthesia. Anesth. Analg. 70:29, 1990.
A prospective study showing the effect of preoperative local and spinal anesthesia on postoperative pain in humans.

ANESTHESIA FOR THE CRITICAL OR TRAUMA PATIENT

ALICIA M. FAGGELLA

Boston, Massachusetts

Companion animals suffering from severe life-threatening emergencies often require surgical intervention for diagnostic or therapeutic reasons. Although many anesthetic agents are available and numerous drug combinations possible, the key to a successful anesthetic outcome for the critical patient depends not only on the anesthetics selected but also the perioperative support administered. When selecting anesthetic techniques for the critical patient, the major body systems compromised must be identified and the function of all body systems must be considered to select the best agent(s) for use in that animal (Table 1). The age and physical status of the animal prior to the crisis as well as the presence of concomitant diseases must be considered in this evaluation.

All anesthetic agents have potential adverse effects. Healthy animals usually compensate for these side effects, but the metabolically or traumatically compromised animal may not. Analgesic, sedative, and anesthetic effects may be more profound than expected in these animals, and standard recommended dosages often need to be decreased by 25 to 75%. Opioids, dissociative agents, benzodiazepines, and inhalational anesthetic agents are the recommended anesthetic drugs for use in the critical patient. Thiobarbiturates have some indications for use, while phenothiazine tranquilizers (e.g., acepromazine [Prom Ace, Fort Dodge]) and alpha$_2$ agonist sedatives (e.g., xylazine [Rompun, Haver Lockhart]) have minimal or no indication for use in critically ill animals.

RESPIRATORY DISORDERS

Preoperative Evaluation and Stabilization

Respiratory compromise is a common clinical problem in the critically ill animal. Regardless of the etiology, the animal presented with respiratory distress requires immediate evaluation and stabilization. Establishment or maintenance of the airway and respiration should be the first concern, and diagnostics such as radiographs and blood gases may need to be delayed. Minimal restraint techniques and judicious sedative administration should be used in an effort to minimize an animal's stress and struggling, which may exacerbate respiratory dysfunction.

The respiratory system of animals with respiratory distress should be evaluated for injury or diseases of the upper and lower airway, thoracic wall, pleural space, and lung parenchyma. Evaluation of mucous membrane color; capillary refill time (CRT); respiratory rate, depth, and pattern; and chest auscultation and percussion are essential diagnostic procedures. If significant pneumothorax or pleural effusion is present or suspected, thoracentesis is indicated for diagnostic and therapeutic purposes.

Table 1. *Recommendations for Use of Selected Preanesthetic and Anesthetic Drugs in the Critical/Trauma Patient with Various Organ Dysfunction*

Drug	Respiratory	Cardiovascular	Acute Abdomen	Neurologic	Hepatic	Renal
Acepromazine	Yes	No	No	No	No	Yes—avoid hypotension.
Diazepam or Midazolam	Yes*	Yes*	Yes*	Yes*	Yes*	Yes*
Xylazine	No	No	No	No	No	No
Ketamine	Yes*	Yes*	Yes*	No	Yes—use with care in dogs.	No (cat) Yes (dog)
Tiletamine-zolazepam	?†	?†	Yes	No	Use with care.	No
Opioids	Yes—use with care.	Yes*	Yes*	Yes	Yes*	Yes*
Thiobarbiturates	Yes*	Variable‡	No	Yes*	Variable‡	Yes

*Author's preferred drugs.
†Manufacturer states is contraindicated in severe dysfunction.
‡Depends on extent or type of disease.

Table 2. *Preanesthetic Agents for Use in the Critical/Trauma Patient*†*

Drug		Dosage (mg/kg)	Route	Comments
Preanesthetics				
Morphine		1.1–2.2	IM	Dogs only
Oxymorphone		0.11–0.22	IM	
	Cats:	0.04–0.11	IM	Use with tranquilizer at higher doses
Meperidine		4–11	IM	Minimal sedation
	Cats:	2–6		
Butorphanol		0.2–0.4	IM, SC	Minimal sedation
Acepromazine		0.1 (max dose 3.0 mg)	IM, SC	May cause hypotension
Diazepam		0.22 (max dose 5.0 mg)	IV	Inconsistently absorbed IM/SC
Midazolam		0.1	IV, IM, SC	Variable effects
Ketamine	Cats:	6–11	IM	Can give IM to dogs if combined with midazolam
Tiletamine-zolazepam	Dogs:	6.6–10	IM	
	Cats:	9.5–11	IM	
Atropine		0.04	IM, SC	
Glycopyrolate		0.011	IM, SC	

*Adapted with permission from Faggella, A. M., and Raffe, M. R.: Anesthetic management of thoracotomy. Vet. Clin. North Am. Small Anim. Pract. 17:474, 1987.

†Doses often need to be decreased based on physical status of patient.

The absence of cyanosis in an animal does not rule out hypoxemia, and respiratory rate alone is not indicative of adequate ventilation but must be evaluated with respect to depth and effort.

Whenever possible, anesthetic procedures should be delayed until respiratory function has been stabilized. Supplemental oxygen administered through a nasal catheter or via an oxygen cage should be provided. Fluid therapy, administered to maintain intravascular volume and oxygen delivery, is an often overlooked, but vital approach to treatment prior to anesthetic induction of animals with respiratory compromise.

Anesthetic Techniques

PREMEDICATION

Premedication (Table 2) with an anticholinergic should be considered for animals with high vagal tone (brachycephalic breeds) or when vagally mediated bradycardia is anticipated. The routine use of anticholinergics is not recommended in the respiratory-compromised patient because while airway secretions are decreased, anticholinergic administration tends to make secretions more viscous and increases anatomic dead space (Muir, 1977).

The use of preanesthetic medications for tranquilization, sedation, analgesia, or restraint must be carefully considered (see this volume, p. 27). All anesthetic drugs depress respiration or potentiate the effects of other respiratory depressant drugs. The degree of respiratory depression varies with dosage and class of drugs used. Phenothiazine tranquilizers, such as acepromazine, cause little respiratory depression and can be administered if cardiovascular and metabolic function do not preclude their use. The benzodiazepine tranquilizers, such

as diazepam (Valium, Hoffman-LaRoche) and midazolam (Versed, Hoffman-LaRoche), have minimal effects on respiration but also have minimal, if any, tranquilizing effects except in depressed or debilitated animals (Bednarski, 1989). These drugs are much more effective when used in combination with opioid or dissociative drugs.

The opioid agonists and agonist/antagonists are respiratory depressants whose potency varies with dose and agent administered. Panting may be observed in animals following administration of some of the opioids, and frequently there is a decreased ventilatory response to increasing arterial carbon dioxide concentrations (Bednarski, 1989). Butorphanol (Torbugesic, Fort Dodge) or meperidine (Demerol, Wyeth-Ayerst) administration usually causes minimal respiratory depression and can be used safely alone or in combination with a tranquilizer for premedication of animals with respiratory dysfunction.

The dissociative anesthetic ketamine (Vetalar, Parke-Davis) produces a dose-dependent decrease in respiration following administration. This effect may be more pronounced when combined with other drugs or when respiratory compromise is present (Paddleford, 1981). An apneustic breathing pattern is often observed following ketamine administration.

Xylazine administration may cause respiratory depression when used alone or in combination with other drugs. This effect is greater if pre-existing respiratory disease is present (Paddleford, 1981).

ANESTHETIC INDUCTION AND MAINTENANCE

Anesthetic induction (Table 3) must be smooth and rapid so that control of the airway via endotra-

Table 3. Induction Techniques for Use in the Critical/Trauma Patient†

Drug	IV Dosage (mg/kg)	Comments
Thiamylal	Up to 17 8.8–13 after tranquilization 4.4–8.8 after opioid administration	Good for animals with respiratory compromise; avoid in cardiovascular disease.
Thiopental	Same as above	Same as above
Diazepam/midazolam plus thiamylal or thiopental	0.22 (maximum dose 5 mg)/0.11 8.8–13	Diazepam is protective against dysrhythmias; variable calming effect occurs with diazepam administration.
Thiamylal or thiopental plus lidocaine	Start with 4.4 and increase as needed 4.4 (maximum dose 8.8 mg/kg)	Thiobarbiturates and lidocaine may not be mixed. Give alternating incremental doses of drugs until intubation is possible.
Innovar-Vet	1 ml/18–27 kg	Preoxygenate; animals remain hyperresponsive to auditory stimuli; do not use on cats
Diazepam plus oxymorphone	0.22 (maximum dose 5 mg) 0.11–0.22	Same as above.
Midazolam plus oxymorphone	0.11 0.055–0.11	
Diazepam/midazolam plus butorphanol	0.22 (maximum dose 5 mg)/0.11 0.2–0.4	For dogs or cats; works well on depressed patients.
Diazepam/midazolam plus ketamine	0.22 (maximum dose 5 mg)/0.11 4.4–11	Maintains cardiovascular stability; transient tachycardia.
Tiletamine-zolazepam	Dog: 4.4–6.6 Cat: 4.4–8.8	

*Adapted with permission from Faggella, A. M., and Raffe, M.R.: Anesthetic management of thoracotomy. Vet Clin. North Am. Small Anim. Pract. 17:477, 1987.

†Doses often need to be decreased based on physical status of patient.

cheal intubation may be quickly established. Animals should be preoxygenated for 5 min prior to induction. If the animal is stable except for respiratory disease, the thiobarbiturates, although respiratory depressants, are excellent choices for rapid induction. These agents may be administered alone or preceded by intravenous administration of a benzodiazepine. This combination approach decreases the thiobarbiturate dose and the prevalence of thiobarbiturate-induced dysrhythmias. Ketamine administration, combined with a benzodiazepine, or tiletamine-zolazepam (Telazol, A. H. Robins) are also good induction techniques with a slightly slower onset than that observed with administration of the thiobarbiturates. Mask inductions using inhalation agents should be avoided as induction time is prolonged.

Once the animal is intubated, halothane (Fluothane, Wyeth-Ayerst) or isoflurane (Forane, Anaquest) may be used for anesthetic maintenance. Nitrous oxide administration is contraindicated in the presence of a pneumothorax as it will diffuse into the pleural space, worsening the pneumothorax. For other respiratory conditions, nitrous oxide should be used with care and should not be administered if cyanosis is present. Oxygenation of the blood should be monitored with a pulse oximeter or arterial blood gases. Hypoxia predisposes to cardiac dysrhythmias, which are often ventricular in origin. Intraoperatively the patient should have assisted or controlled ventilation established and the electrocardiogram (ECG), systemic arterial blood pressure, lung sounds, mucous membrane color, and CRT monitored. Crystalloid fluids should be administered at 10 to 20 ml/kg/hr intravenously, and administration should be adjusted based on the changes in cardiopulmonary status during the anesthetic procedure.

Postoperatively, the animal is extubated when minute volume is adequate. Cardiorespiratory parameters should be monitored closely, and oxygen supplementation along with intravenous fluid administration should continue for a minimum of 12 hr. Some patients may require post-operative ventilation (see this volume, p. 98). Postoperative administration of analgesic agents should be used post-thoracotomy to relieve pain and decrease the potential for hypoventilation (see this volume, p. 82). In the case of a lateral thoracotomy, intercostal nerve blocks may provide up to 6 hours of good postoperative analgesia. Using a 22-gauge, 1-inch needle, 0.25 to 1.0 ml of bupivicaine (Marcaine, Winthrop) may be injected below the transverse vertebral processes at the caudal aspect of the rib at the surgery site and the two ribs cranial and caudal to the surgical site. Intrapleural bupivicaine administration through a chest tube can be used in animals that have undergone a sternotomy. Systemic administration of opioids such as butorphanol, buprenorphine, or oxymorphone alone or in combination with a tranquilizer may also be used for analgesia (Table 4). Although opioid administration can produce respiratory depression, the analgesia provided may improve ventilation by decreasing the pain associated with chest expansion. Additionally, the opioid agonist/antagonist nalbuphine (Nubain,

Table 4. Analgesic Agents for Postoperative
Parenteral Administration*

Drug		Dosage IV, SC, IM	Estimated Duration of Action
Morphine†		0.2–0.4 mg/kg	2–5 hr
Oxymorphone	(Numorphan)	0.06–0.14 mg/kg	2–4 hr
Meperidine	(Demerol)	2–5 mg/kg	1–4 hr
Pentazocine	(Talwin)	2–4 mg/kg	1–2 hr
Butorphanol	(Torbutrol)	0.4 mg/kg	2–3 hr
Buprenorphine	(Buprenex)	0.01 mg/kg	6–12 hr

*Adapted with permission from Faggella, A. M., and Raffe, M. R.: Anesthetic management of thoracotomy. Vet. Clin. North Am. Small Anim. Pract. 17:491, 1987.
†Canine dose.

DuPont) may be used to reverse any untoward respiratory depression of pure opioid agonists while maintaining the analgesia (Magruder, 1982).

CARDIOVASCULAR DISORDERS

Preoperative Evaluation and Stabilization

Cardiovascular and hemodynamic dysfunction, whether due to shock, trauma, cardiac dysrhythmias, or congenital or acquired heart disease, is common in the critically ill animal and must be corrected or compensated for prior to anesthesia. To evaluate the degree of cardiovascular compromise, a physical examination should include evaluation of heart rate and rhythm, pulse quality, mucous membrane color, and CRT. A complete blood count (CBC), serum biochemical profile, ECG, chest radiographs, echocardiogram, systemic arterial blood pressure, and central venous pressure (CVP) should be evaluated in order to define cardiac and extracardiac causes of cardiovascular dysfunction.

The animal presented in shock, regardless of the etiology, has major hemodynamic instability and early intervention is required to prevent irreversible tissue damage. Fluid administration remains the backbone of shock therapy and needs to be pursued aggressively in septic and hypovolemic shock but must be used more judiciously in cardiogenic shock. Serial measurement of CVP (or pulmonary wedge pressure) may be helpful in monitoring fluid therapy. Replacement crystalloid fluids such as lactated Ringer's solution or 0.9% sodium chloride are most commonly used. The proper volume of fluid depends on the patient's needs, but initial loading dosages of 40 to 90 ml/kg IV in the dog and 20 to 60 ml/kg in the cat may be used over 20 to 30 min. Colloidal fluids such as dextran-40 (10 to 20 ml/kg/day IV, rate = 2 ml/kg/hr), hetastarch (20 ml/kg/day IV), or plasma (7.5 ml/kg IV, at rate of 4 to 6 ml/min) are recommended when total serum solids

are decreased (<3.5 mg/dl), fluid overload is anticipated, or when time is not available for administration of isotonic crystalloid fluids. Likewise, administration of hypertonic saline (7.5%, 4 ml/kg) may be useful in shock therapy, especially when combined with the administration of dextran for the purpose of prolonged effectiveness (see *CVT IX*, p. 313). Cardiovascular function is improved with the administration of hypertonic saline through osmotic effects, causing intravascular expansion from the interstitial and intracellular fluid spaces and possibly by a direct effect of the hypertonic saline increasing cardiac inotropy (Schertel, 1989).

Positive inotropic support with continuous intravenous infusions of dopamine (Intropin, DuPont) or dobutamine (Dobutrex, Eli Lilly) (Table 5) is often useful in improving cardiac function in an animal perioperatively. Care must be taken to ensure that the animal has had adequate intravascular volume expansion prior to using inotropic agents.

Cardiac dysrhythmias need to be controlled prior to anesthetizing an animal as persistence of dysrhythmias will interfere with cardiac filling and output and increase the workload (oxygen demand) of an already compromised heart. Generally, ventricular dysrhythmias are more harmful and dangerous than atrial dysrhythmias and paroxysmal, sustained, or multifocal dysrhythmias are more life-threatening than single, unifocal complexes. The presence of unifocal complexes preoperatively, however, may suggest the need for aggressive therapy to prevent more severe dysrhythmias during anesthesia. Lidocaine may be administered as a bolus (2 mg/kg IV) followed by a constant rate infusion (40 to 60 µg/kg/min IV). Cats are more sensitive to lidocaine administration (seizures), but lidocaine may be administered as a bolus of 0.22 to 0.66 mg/kg IV followed by a constant rate infusion (10 to 40 µg/kg/min IV).

Anesthetic Techniques

PREMEDICATION

The animal with cardiovascular dysfunction (see Table 2) may not tolerate even mild changes in heart rate or systemic arterial blood pressure. All anesthetic techniques should aim to maintain heart rate, cardiac output, and systemic arterial blood pressure while minimizing myocardial oxygen demand. Increased sympathetic influences on the myocardium should be avoided by minimizing the animal's anxiety and struggling. Anticholinergics should be administered only if bradyarrhythmias are present or if increased vagal effects are observed (e.g., after opioid administration) since these drugs may cause tachycardia and predispose to tachyarrhythmias.

Table 5. *Pharmacologic Support Agents for Intravenous Administration for the Animal with Cardiovascular Dysfunction**

Drug	Dosage (mg/kg IV)	Indications	Adverse Reactions
Lidocaine	1.1–2.2 dog 0.22–0.66 cat 30–80 μg/kg/min infusion	Ventricular tachycardia	Low safety margin in cats, seizures, heart block, asystole
Propranolol	0.07–0.18 dog 0.25 mg/1 ml saline, give 0.2 ml bolus to effect—cat	Supraventricular and ventricular tachycardia	Bradycardia, hypotension, bronchospasm
Isoproterenol	0.2–0.3 μg/kg/min infusion or 1 mg/500 ml to effect	Bradycardia, decreased myocardial contractility—low output states	Arrhythmias, tachycardia, hypotension, increased myocardial oxygen demand
Epinephrine (1 mg/ml)	22–33 μg/kg	Ventricular asystole inotropic effect	Do not use with inhalational agents
Dopamine	2–11 μg/kg/min to effect	Inotropic—increased output, increased renal blood flow	Tachycardia, arrhythmias, hypotension, vasoconstriction (at high dosage)
Dobutamine	2–10 μg/kg/min to effect	Inotropic—increased output	Tachycardia, arrhythmias, vasoconstriction (at high dose)
Phenylephrine	0.13	Hypotension due to peripheral vasodilation	Bradycardia, decreased cardiac output
Ephedrine	5.5–11 μg/kg	Hypotension due to decreased myocardial contractility	Tachycardia, arrhythmias, hypertension
Calcium (10%)	0.44–0.11 ml/kg	Inotropic	Cardiac arrest, tissue (brain) injury

*Reprinted with permission from Faggella, A. M., and Raffe, M.R.: Anesthetic management of thoracotomy. Vet. Clin. North Am. Small Anim. Pract. 17:482, 1987.

The necessity for premedication with other drugs should be evaluated based on the animal's physical status and attitude. If an animal is in shock, depressed, or debilitated, little anesthetic is required and premedication may not be necessary. However, if the animal is stable hemodynamically and premedication is needed, the opioids or benzodiazepines are the drugs of choice since these drugs produce minimal cardiovascular depression. Bradycardia may be observed following administration of some opioids, but this effect may be prevented or treated by concomitant administration of an anticholinergic drug. Phenothiazine tranquilizers and xylazine should not be used as these agents can produce profound, prolonged cardiovascular effects such as hypotension.

ANESTHETIC INDUCTION AND MAINTENANCE

Dogs requiring anesthesia while they are still cardiovascularly unstable can be induced with a neuroleptanalgesic combination (tranquilizer and opioid agent) or with a benzodiazepine-ketamine combination (see Table 3). The latter technique is also appropriate for use in cats. Neuroleptanalgesic techniques could include administration of fentanyl-droperidol (Innovar-Vet, Pitman Moore) or a benzodiazepine with oxymorphone or butorphanol. Induction is gradual, and intubation must be gentle as these animals are only heavily sedated, not anesthetized, and respond to stimulation of the larynx. All animals must be preoxygenated prior to

anesthetic induction as respiratory function is depressed with administration of these agents and needs to be supported.

Diazepam (or midazolam)-ketamine combinations provide rapid anesthetic induction, transient tachycardia, and maintenance of systemic arterial blood pressure and cardiac output. Transient apnea or apneustic breathing is often observed following administration of this drug combination, and ventilation should be supported.

Thiobarbiturate administration should be avoided in the animal with shock, volume depletion, hypoproteinemia, or cardiac dysrhythmias. However, the administration of IV lidocaine followed by thiopental has been shown to provide good cardiovascular stability in dogs with cardiopulmonary disease and does not produce the dysrhythmias seen with thiopental administration alone (Bjorling, 1984).

Mask induction with halothane or isoflurane either alone or preceded by an intravenous injection of a benzodiazepine is a reasonable alternative if the animal is depressed and only small quantities of an inhalational agent are needed. Gas anesthetics cause dose-related cardiovascular depression, including hypotension, and are not necessarily safe induction agents.

Isoflurane may be superior to halothane for anesthetic maintenance in these animals, although both agents can be used safely. Isoflurane administration is associated with fewer catecholamine-induced cardiac dysrhythmias. The heart rate remains stable and cardiac output is maintained with isoflurane administration in animals. Isoflurane does cause a dose-related decrease in systemic arterial blood pressure owing to peripheral vasodilation, but when administered at lower concentrations, these cardiovascular effects of isoflurane may be minimized (Eger, 1984).

During anesthetic procedures, the cardiovascular system of the animal should be supported with fluid administration and, if needed, inotropic or vasopressor support (see Table 4). Animals that received preoperative antiarrhythmic drugs should be maintained on these treatments during anesthesia. Intraoperative and postoperative monitoring should be done as described for animals with respiratory compromise, but urine output should be measured as well.

In the postoperative period, antiarrhythmic and inotropic support often needs to be continued. Analgesics should be administered to reduce postoperative pain (see this volume, p. 82). The opioid agonists-antagonists such as butorphanol and buprenorphine (Buprenex, Norwich Eaton) provide good analgesia with minimal sedation or depression of cardiopulmonary function (see Table 4). If respiratory depression occurs with buprenorphine, naloxone (Narcan, DuPont), a pure opioid antagonist, can be administered but has limited efficacy as a reversal agent (Gal, 1989).

ACUTE ABDOMEN

Preoperative Evaluation and Stabilization

Acute abdomen describes any number of surgical or medical emergencies that present as abdominal pain or distention (see this volume, p. 125). Although etiologies vary (gastric dilatation volvulus, gastrointestinal foreign body, abdominal mass), many animals with these conditions are presented in shock (hypovolemic or septic), and the treatment priority is to stabilize the cardiopulmonary system (see previous sections). A CBC, serum biochemical profile, urinalysis, arterial blood gas, abdominal radiographs, and possibly abdominocentesis are required in the evaluation of these animals. Before surgical intervention, the animal should receive treatment for shock and sepsis as well as have electrolyte and acid-base disturbances corrected.

Anesthetic Techniques

PREMEDICATION

Preanesthetic administration of an anticholinergic (see Table 2) should be used if bradycardia is present or anticipated. Preanesthetic medication for analgesia, sedation, or restraint, in the author's opinion, is usually unnecessary. However, if premedication is warranted, the administration of opioid agonists

is preferred. In all circumstances, the administration of acepromazine and xylazine should be avoided.

ANESTHETIC INDUCTION AND MAINTENANCE

The animal with an acute abdomen will benefit from preoxygenation prior to induction, and the preferable induction techniques involve administration of a neuroleptanalgesic (dogs) or benzodiazepine-dissociative combinations (dogs and cats) (see Table 3). In very depressed animals, an intravenous dose of a benzodiazepine is often enough to allow intubation.

Thiobarbiturates are not a good choice for induction of anesthesia in animals with an acute abdomen. These drugs have adverse cardiovascular effects associated with their administration, including hypotension and dysrhythmias. Animals with acute abdomen may have concomitant acidosis or hypoproteinemia which increases the amount of active thiobarbiturate available following administration, thereby increasing the likelihood of overdosage.

A mask induction with halothane or isoflurane is reserved for those animals requiring minimal administration of an anesthetic agent for induction. Mask inductions should be avoided if the animal is vomiting or if abdominal distention is compromising respiration. Many animals with acute abdomen fall into this category, and administration of injectable induction agents is preferred.

Halothane or isoflurane administration may be used to maintain anesthesia, although isoflurane is the preferred agent. Some animals have severe metabolic and cardiovascular compromise, and these animals cannot tolerate administration of typical anesthetic concentrations of inhalant agents. Intravenous fentanyl, oxymorphone, or butorphanol administration may be used to supplement low concentrations of inhalational agents in these situations. Morphine and meperidine administration should be avoided as these agents may cause hypotension and exacerbation of shock due to histamine release. Intraoperative treatment with fluids, inotropic drug administration, and ventilatory support may be required. These treatments and monitoring techniques should be used as previously described.

Postoperatively, these animals should be monitored closely. Cardiac dysrhythmias, particularly of ventricular origin, often appear 12 to 48 hours postsurgery. Renal function should be monitored and if adequate urine output is not observed in a normovolemic animal, mannitol administration is recommended (1 to 2 gm/kg IV). Persistent oliguria requires more aggressive therapy with hourly furosemide (Lasix, Horsch) administration (2 to 10 mg/

kg IV) and intravenous dopamine infusion (initially 1 to 4 µg/kg/min).

HEAD TRAUMA—CENTRAL NERVOUS SYSTEM (CNS) DISEASE

Preoperative Evaluation and Stabilization

The animal with head trauma that requires anesthetic management should have careful evaluation of the central nervous, cardiovascular, and respiratory systems. The use of corticosteroids in head trauma is controversial. Cerebral edema due to intracranial masses such as hematomas or tumors is often responsive to corticosteroids. Corticosteroid administration, however, has not been shown to be beneficial in global edema due to trauma and may be detrimental (Goodwin, 1989). If cerebral edema is suspected, mannitol (2 gm/kg IV) and Lasix (2 to 4 mg/kg IV) should be administered, provided cardiovascular status is stabilized. If vasogenic edema from hematoma formation is suspected, dexamethasone (2 to 3 mg/kg IV) may be administered.

Fluid therapy should be instituted to avoid hypovolemia, which will exacerbate cerebral ischemia, and fluid administration should be monitored closely to avoid overhydration, which may worsen cerebral edema. An isotonic fluid, such as normal saline, or a hypertonic saline solution are the fluids of choice in head trauma. Colloids may be used, but if the blood-brain barrier is damaged, cerebral edema will occur (Lam, 1989). Glucose-containing solutions should be avoided whenever cerebral ischemia is suspected because of the shift to anaerobic metabolism during ischemic events. The by-products of anaerobic metabolism (pyruvate and lactate) lead to acidosis, which increases cerebral injury (Lam, 1989).

Anesthetic Techniques

Most animals with head trauma are depressed, so preanesthetics are generally not required. But if required, the administration of benzodiazepines has the added benefit of an antiepileptic effect. Phenothiazine tranquilizers should be avoided as these drugs decrease seizure threshold. Dissociative drugs such as ketamine and tiletamine should not be used as these drugs increase cerebral blood flow and intracranial pressure and also have epileptogenic activity. Induction with thiobarbiturate administration remains one of the best techniques. If seizures have occurred or are anticipated, phenobarbital may be used preoperatively. Opioid administration has no direct effect on increasing intracranial pressure but does so secondarily to increased arterial carbon dioxide concentrations from respiratory depression (Paddleford, 1981). If ventilation is controlled, opioids may be used safely. Mask inductions are not generally recommended because high concentrations of inhalational agents may increase cerebral blood flow.

During anesthetic management of animals with head trauma, it is important to avoid increases in intracranial pressure. Therefore, hypercarbia and hypoxia should be avoided by controlling ventilation. Hyperventilation can be used to decrease intracranial pressure. Fluid overload, pain, or other causes of hypertension need to be avoided. Inhalational anesthetics (isoflurane or halothane) or narcotic administration (if ventilation is controlled) can be used for maintenance of anesthesia in the animal with head injury.

During anesthetic recovery, the animal should be excitement and pain free. The head of the animal should be elevated to avoid increasing intracranial pressure. Seizures should be controlled with diazepam or phenobarbital administration. Ventilation should be carefully monitored with arterial blood gases to avoid hypercarbia, and oxygen supplementation should be continued.

SUMMARY

The animal that has been severely traumatized or that is critically ill is an anesthetic challenge. The clinician must evaluate the entire animal and integrate all available information. Selection of an appropriate anesthetic regimen can only be made once the clinician has an understanding of the compromise to all body systems affected by the animal's illness or injury. There are not any perfect anesthetic agents, but proper selection and use of these drugs will provide safe and effective anesthesia.

References and Suggested Reading

Bednarski, R. M.: Anesthesia and pain control. The Vet. Clin. North Am. Small Anim. Pract. 19:1223, 1989.
Anesthetic management and pain control for the critical dog and cat are presented.

Bjorling, D. E., and Rawlings, C. A.: Induction of anesthesia with thiopental-lidocaine combination in dogs with cardiopulmonary disease. J. Am. Anim. Hosp. Assoc. 20:445, 1984.
Thiopental-lidocaine is a safe induction technique for dogs with cardiopulmonary disease.

Eger, E. I.: Isoflurane. Madison, WI: Anaquest BOC, Inc 1984.
A review of the physical and chemical properties of isoflurane and its effect on body systems.

Gal, T. J.: Naloxone reversal of buprenorphine-induced respiratory depression. Clin. Pharmacol. Ther. 45:66, 1989.
Naloxone has limited ability to displace buprenorphine bound to opioid receptors.

Goodwin, S. R.: The comatose child: Evaluation, treatment and prediction outcome. Annual refresher course lectures: American Society of Anesthesiologists, Section 173, 1989.
A review of the diagnosis and management of head injuries, especially the management of increased intracranial pressure.

Lam, A. M.: Management of the patient with a head injury. Annual refresher course lectures: American Society of Anesthesiologists, Section 103, 1989.
A discussion of the pathophysiology of head injury and anesthetic management.

Magruder, M. R., Delaney, R. D., and DiFazio, C. A.: Reversal of narcotic-induced respiratory depression with nalbuphine hydrochloride. Anesth. Rev. 9:34, 1982.
Nalbuphine reversed the respiratory depression but not the analgesia of narcotics in humans.

Muir, W. W.: Anesthesia for the dog with heart disease. In Kirk, R. W. (ed): Current Veterinary Therapy VI. Philadelphia: W. B. Saunders, 1977, p 388.
Anesthetic considerations and techniques are discussed.

Paddleford, R. R.: Preanesthetic medication for the critical patient. In Sattler, F. P., Knowles, R. P., and Whittick, W. G. (eds.): Veterinary Critical Care. Philadelphia: Lea & Febiger, 1981, p. 375.
Characteristics of commonly used preanesthetic agents and their use in the critical animal are discussed.

Schertel, E. R., and Muir, W. W.: Shock: Pathophysiology, monitoring, and therapy. In Kirk, R. W. (ed): Current Veterinary Therapy X. Philadelphia: W. B. Saunders, 1989, p. 316.
A review of shock and current trends in management.

EPIDURAL ANALGESIA

GEOFFREY N. CLARK

West Los Angeles, California

Effective pain relief is important for minimizing the stress response and improving the welfare of our animal patients. It is of particular concern to the veterinary surgeon and anesthetist in the perioperative period. Techniques for the relief of pain in small animal patients include the oral administration of analgesics (e.g., nonsteroidal anti-inflammatory drugs or corticosteroids), parenteral administration of opioids, and the regional use of local anesthetics. Perioperative pain relief often entirely depends on the analgesic properties of the preanesthetic drugs and the inhalational anesthetic agents administered, and these drugs may have minimal effects in the postoperative period (see this volume, p. 82).

An additional technique that may be used by veterinarians attempting to alleviate a patient's pain is epidural analgesia. Reluctance to use this technique may be due to the perceived relative ease of general anesthesia when compared with epidural injection. Once the technique has been learned, however, epidural analgesia can be used as a versatile method of providing pain relief in the perioperative period. Moreover, in certain situations, epidural analgesia may have significant advantages over general anesthesia.

The technique of epidural analgesia has been alternately described as spinal analgesia, lumbosacral analgesia, or caudal analgesia. For this discussion, epidural analgesia refers to the placement of an epidural agent into the epidural space, using an injection site located between the seventh lumbar vertebra and the sacrum. Although this technique may also be used in cats, this discussion focuses on the use of epidural analgesia in dogs.

Specific materials required for performing an epidural injection include an appropriate-size disposable spinal needle with stylet, a syringe containing the calculated dose of the analgesic agent, and sterile surgical gloves. The required size of the spinal needle varies with the size of the patient. A general guideline entails use of a 22-gauge, 1.5-inch (3.8-cm) spinal needle for small-breed dogs, a 20-gauge, 1.5-inch (3.8-cm) spinal needle for medium-breed dogs, and a 20-gauge, 2.5-inch (6.35-cm) spinal needle for large- or giant-breed dogs. The lumbosacral region is clipped, and an aseptic surgical scrub is performed, using povidone iodine or chlorhexidine. The epidural injection should be performed with the use of surgical gloves and sterile technique.

For many years, epidural analgesic agents were limited to the local anesthetics. More recently, a new choice for epidural analgesia has become available to veterinarians in the form of opioid preparations for epidural administration (spinal opioids). The administration of opioids into the epidural space represents an alternative technique for providing perioperative analgesia. Specific guidelines for the use of local anesthetics and spinal opioids are discussed later.

Epidural analgesia can be used as a primary anesthetic technique or as an adjunct to general anesthesia in procedures associated with a high degree of pain. In both instances, preanesthetic evaluation should include screening for evidence of clotting disorders or systemic infection, which are the two specific contraindications to epidural analgesia (Heath, 1986). During epidural analgesia, an intravenous catheter must be present, and fluids should be administered at a rate of at least 10 to 20 ml/kg of body weight per hour. Intraoperative patient monitoring is similar to that used for any anesthetized animal and should include electrocardiography, indirect blood pressure measurements, and temperature monitoring.

EPIDURAL INJECTION TECHNIQUE

The wings of the ilium and the dorsal spinal processes of the seventh lumbar vertebra and sacrum are used as anatomic landmarks in locating the lumbosacral space. The dog may be placed in either sternal or lateral recumbency for this procedure. The wings of the ilium are palpated with the thumb and middle finger of one hand and the index finger is directed caudally. The lumbosacral space is identified as a depression just caudal to the dorsal spinous process of the seventh lumbar vertebra. The spinal needle is inserted slowly, and the insertion is perpendicular to the skin, along the median axis. A distinct "popping" sensation is noted as the needle passes through the intervertebral ligament into the epidural space. A decreased resistance to the needle may be perceived as the needle is advanced further into the spinal canal. After the needle advances 0.25 to 1.0 cm into the canal (depending on the patient's size), the stylet is removed from the needle. If cerebrospinal fluid is obtained because of inadvertent subarachnoid puncture, then the needle must be removed and placement repeated. The anatomy of the canine spinal cord assures that this occurrence is unlikely at the level of the lumbosacral space. A syringe containing the appropriate volume of the analgesic agent is attached to the needle, and a slow injection is initiated. No resistance to injection should occur if the needle is in the epidural space. The complete injection requires 30 to 60 sec, because rapid injection of some local anesthetics may cause discomfort.

LOCAL ANESTHETICS

Several local anesthetics have been used as epidural analgesic agents. Lidocaine hydrochloride and mepivacaine hydrochloride are effective for brief procedures, such as cesarean sections, but these agents lack the duration of action necessary for lengthy orthopedic procedures. The local anesthetic of choice for epidural analgesia of long duration is bupivacaine hydrochloride. This drug is available as a 0.75% solution without epinephrine or preservatives. Bupivacaine provides 4.5 to 6 hr of surgical analgesia and greater muscle relaxation when compared with general anesthesia (Heath et al., 1989).

When epidural administration of bupivacaine is the primary anesthetic technique, it should be combined with light doses of sedation. The neuroleptanalgesics can be used quite effectively for this indication. Acepromazine maleate (0.025 to 0.05 mg/kg of body weight) can be combined with oxy-

Table 1. *Epidural Analgesia With Bupivacaine Hydrochloride**

Concentration: 0.75% solution
Dosage: 0.22 ml/kg (analgesia to level of L4)
        0.31 ml/kg (analgesia to level of T11–T13)
Rate of injection: 1 ml/4.5 kg/min
Latent period: 20–30 min
Duration of action: 4.5–6 hr
Neuroleptanalgesic dosages:
  Acepromazine maleate: 0.025–0.05 mg/kg (SC, IM, IV)
  Oxymorphone hydrochloride: 0.025–0.05 mg/kg (SC, IM, IV)

*Marcaine, Sterling-Winthrop Pharmaceuticals.
L4, fourth lumbar vertebra; T11–T13, eleventh to thirteenth thoracic vertebrae.

morphone hydrochloride (0.025 to 0.05 mg/kg) for lengthy procedures (see this volume, p. 27). Initial doses can be administered subcutaneously or intramuscularly. Additional sedation can be given as needed during surgery and the sedative agent may be titrated using small incremental doses administered intravenously. The addition of padding for patient comfort is recommended and may decrease the need for supplemental sedation (Heath et al., 1989). General guidelines for the epidural administration of bupivacaine are listed in Table 1.

The dosage of bupivacaine for epidural analgesia varies with the level of analgesia desired. For analgesia to the level of the fourth lumbar vertebra, 0.22 ml/kg of body weight is used, and a dosage of 0.31 ml/kg is effective to the level of the 11th to 13th thoracic vertebrae. These dosages can be reduced by 25% in pregnant or significantly obese animals (Heath, 1986). Rapid injection of bupivacaine is associated with patient discomfort. Therefore, slow delivery of the calculated dose is recommended, with a minimun injection time of 45 to 60 sec. After injection of bupivacaine, a latent period of 20 to 30 min occurs prior to maximum analgesia.

Position of the animal is important during this latent period because in exerting their effect, local anesthetics depend on gravity for proper distribution. In cases of unilateral hindlimb surgical procedures (e.g., femur fracture), the affected limb should remain in the ventral position. For bilateral effects, the patient should be placed in dorsal recumbency after injection of the local anesthetic. Loss of anal tone and decreased tail movement can be used as indicators of a successful injection. Reflex response to deep pinching of the hindlimb, or hindlimbs, can also be used to assess adequacy of the epidural analgesia.

Failure of the epidural injection to provide suitable surgical analgesia is often noticed during surgical preparation of the animal or during placement of the towel clamps. Lack of sedation must be distinguished from failure of the epidural injection. In one report detailing the use of bupivacaine in 636 dogs, failure of analgesia occurred in 12% of cases. This percentage includes cases in which anatomic factors (e.g., obesity) complicated the injection as well as cases in which the injection seemed to be satisfactory but resulted in inadequate analgesia (Heath et al., 1989). A similar percentage of analgesic failures has been reported in humans receiving epidural injections (Bromage, 1967).

SPINAL OPIOIDS

Another method of providing epidural analgesia is through the use of spinal opioids. This type of analgesia is an accepted method of pain relief in human beings and is becoming more popular in veterinary medicine. A variety of opioids have been given through this route in humans to provide effective postoperative, post-traumatic, and chronic pain relief. The opioids act by diffusion across the dural membrane into the cerebrospinal fluid, where they bind to opioid receptors in the spinal cord. In effect, the spinal opioids act via a selective blockade of pain without an associated sympathetic or motor blockade (Cousins and Mather, 1984). This selective action on spinal cord receptors is the feature that distinguishes the opioids from the local anesthetics, which act by an axonal membrane blockade, predominantly in the spinal nerve roots (Cousins and Mather, 1984). The most important clinical advantage to using the spinal opioids is that ambulation of the patient is not impaired, as it is with the epidural administration of local anesthetics.

The spinal opioids provide profound, long-lasting analgesia in selected surgical patients, but they do not completely block intraoperative pain. The analgesic effects of the opioids are best used as an adjunct to general anesthesia. In veterinary patients, epidural administration of morphine is the most commonly used form of spinal opioid analgesia. Epidural morphine administration has been documented to provide a significant reduction in the amount of halothane needed to produce general anesthesia in dogs (Valverde et al., 1989a). In addition, the administration of epidural morphine during the preoperative period appears to decrease the need for the administration of additional analgesics in the postoperative period. Side effects following administration of spinal opioids have been reported to occur in a small percentage of human patients, but these adverse effects are more common with intrathecal injections than with epidural injections (Cousins and Mather, 1984). In a report of more than 250 clinical cases in which epidural morphine was used in dogs, mild pruritus (in four dogs) was the only side effect observed, and the severity was of no clinical significance (Valverde et al., 1989b).

The speed of onset, duration of action, and analgesic potency vary among the different opioids. Meperidine hydrochloride, fentanyl citrate, and lo-

Table 2. *Epidural Analgesia With Morphine Sulfate**

Concentration: 1 mg/ml (10-ml ampules)
Dosage: 0.1 mg/kg
Rate of injection: Give entire dose in 30–60 sec
Latent period: 30–60 min
Duration of action: 10–23 hr

*Duramorph, Elkins-Sinn.

fentanil are all highly lipid-soluble opioids that produce analgesia of rapid onset and short duration. In contrast, morphine has low lipid solubility, which results in analgesia of slow onset and prolonged duration of action (Cousins and Mather, 1984). The low lipid solubility results in a latent period of 30 to 60 min before the peak effect of epidural morphine is achieved (Bromage et al., 1980). These properties of morphine can be used to an advantage in clinical patients. Epidural morphine is most effective when it is administered immediately after induction of general anesthesia. This approach allows the latent period to coincide with the presurgical preparation and should ensure that the peak analgesic effects are realized during surgical manipulation. The long duration of action also allows significant postoperative analgesia without the need for additional parenteral administration of analgesics. The analgesic effects of epidural morphine have been reported to last from 10 to 23 hr (Valverde et al., 1989b). The dosage for epidural morphine is 0.10 mg/kg of body weight, and the calculated dose should be administered slowly (Table 2).

In my experience, the administration of epidural morphine has proved to be an effective adjunct to general anesthesia. Its greatest application is in providing perioperative analgesia for patients undergoing hindlimb or pelvic orthopedic procedures. It is not unusual for a patient to manifest minimal or no pain for several hours after surgery when epidural morphine has been administered in the preoperative period. This effect reduces the requirement for systemic analgesics to be administered postoperatively. Epidural morphine administration does not appear to provide the same degree of postoperative analgesia for patients undergoing forelimb surgical procedures or thoracotomy.

The techniques of epidural analgesia should be considered as alternatives to general anesthesia in critical cases and for surgical procedures associated with significant perioperative pain. The availability of local anesthetics and spinal opioids allows effective perioperative analgesia in a large variety of surgical patients.

References and Suggested Reading

Bromage, P. R.: Physiology and pharmacology of epidural analgesia. Anesthesiology 28:592, 1967.
A comprehensive review of epidural analgesia in human patients.

Bromage, P. R., Camporesi, E., and Chestnut, D.: Epidural narcotics for postoperative analgesia. Anesth. Analg. 59:473, 1980.
  Pharmacology of spinal opioids and results of a study in human patients.
Cousins, M. J., and Mather, L. E.: Intrathecal and epidural administration of opioids. Anesthesiology 61:276, 1984.
  A comprehensive review of the pharmacokinetics and efficacy of spinal opioids.
Heath, R. B.: The practicality of epidural analgesia. Semin. Vet. Med. Surg. (Small Anim.) 1:245, 1986.
  A review of epidural analgesia techniques using local anesthetics.
Heath, R. B., Broadstone, R. V., Wright, M., and Grandy, J. L.: Using bupivacaine hydrochloride for lumbosacral epidural analgesia. Compend. Contin. Educ. Pract. Vet. 11:50, 1989.

  Results of a clinical study using epidural analgesia in dogs undergoing hindlimb or pelvic surgery.
Valverde, A., Dyson, D. H., and McDonell, W. N.: Epidural morphine reduces halothane MAC in the dog. Can. J. Anaesth. 36:629, 1989a.
  Results of a study measuring the effects of preoperative epidural morphine on general anesthesia requirements.
Valverde, A., Dyson, D. H., McDonell, W. N., and Pascoe, P. J.: Use of epidural morphine in the dog for pain relief. Vet. Comp. Orth. Traumatol. 2:55, 1989b.
  A review of the technique and results of a clinical trial using epidural morphine analgesia.

MECHANICAL VENTILATION

PAULA F. MOON,
and KEVIN T. CONCANNON
Davis, California

Mechanical ventilation, also called intermittent positive-pressure ventilation (IPPV), supports two aspects of pulmonary function: carbon dioxide elimination from the lungs and delivery of oxygen to the blood. Mechanical ventilation may be indicated for significant hypoxemia, in which the arterial partial pressure of oxygen (Pa_{O_2}) falls below 50 to 60 mm Hg, or for hypercarbia, in which the arterial partial pressure of carbon dioxide (Pa_{CO_2}) increases above 50 to 60 mm Hg. Oxygen supplementation via nasal insufflation or an oxygen-enriched environment should be attempted as the initial treatment in most hypoxemic patients. Because oxygen therapy is not palliative in many cases of pulmonary parenchymal disease, IPPV is indicated in these patients. Hypercarbia may be due to primary hypoventilation or to compensation for metabolic alkalosis. Assessment of the animal's acid-base status helps differentiate these two conditions. Another indication for IPPV is the decrease of intracranial pressure through a decrease of Pa_{CO_2}.

Even when IPPV is indicated, the clinician must also determine if IPPV is feasible, based on disease prognosis, patient acceptance, owner approval, and the available facilities. Specific indications for IPPV have been reviewed previously (Pascoe, 1983).

An understanding of the mechanical apparatus, its effects on normal physiologic processes, appropriate monitoring, and weaning methods is required for successful use of IPPV. Hemodynamically unstable patients and patients requiring long-term ventilatory support require additional considerations.

ARTIFICIAL VENTILATION

Despite their wide variety in design, all ventilators perform the same functions. A veterinarian who understands the different methods of accomplishing these functions should be able to operate any ventilator after minimal familiarization with the specific details of the machine.

Carbon Dioxide Elimination

Minute ventilation, a product of tidal volume and respiratory rate, is a main determinant of carbon dioxide elimination. The length of inspiration is a primary factor in determining tidal volume. Ventilators can terminate or limit inspiration when a preset airway pressure or period of time is reached, or when a chosen volume of gas is delivered to the patient. In pressure-limited ventilators such as the Mark 7 (Bird Corporation, Palm Springs, CA), increasing the inspiratory airway pressure results in larger tidal volumes. The relationship between a selected airway pressure and the resulting tidal volume is affected by pulmonary and chest wall compliance. Compliance is a measure of tissue elasticity and surface tension. As compliance decreases, the lungs and chest wall lose their ability to expand, and positive pressure applied to the patient must be increased to generate an equivalent tidal volume. The tidal volume in a time-limited ventilator (Small Animal Ventilator, North American Drager, Telford, PA) is determined not only by a preset inspiratory time, but also by gas flow rate. If flow rate remains constant, increasing the inspiratory time increases tidal volume. In volume-limited ventilators (Metomatic, Omeda, Atlanta, GA), inspiration is terminated after a preset volume of gas is expelled from the ventilator.

Each mechanism for terminating inspiration has advantages and disadvantages. Inadvertent disconnection of the patient from a single-circuit, pressure-limited ventilator may be signaled by a prolonged inspiration because the pressure limit now takes longer to be reached. In this same situation, a volume-limited ventilator would continue to cycle routinely unless it was fitted with an alarm. Many ventilators possess only one mechanism to limit inspiration, but others may be added as safety features. For instance, both time- and volume-limited ventilators are usually equipped with a pressure-relief valve to prevent excessive inspiratory pressures.

One of three different modes—assisted ventilation, controlled ventilation, or intermittent mandatory ventilation (IMV)—can be used to cycle the patient into inspiration. Respiratory rate is determined as follows: by the patient in assisted ventilation, by the clinician in controlled ventilation, and by both patient and clinician in IMV. In assisted ventilation, the negative pressure associated with a patient's respiratory effort triggers the inspiratory phase. The sensitivity on many machines is adjustable, and as it decreases, more negative pressure must be generated by the patient before the ventilator administers a breath. During controlled ventilation, the operator sets the respiratory rate, which is independent of any of the patient's efforts to breathe. IMV allows the patient to breathe spontaneously between mechanically delivered breaths with the amount of ventilatory assistance adjusted by the ventilator operator. Most ventilators can be set in different modes depending on patient needs.

As tidal volume or respiratory rate is increased, minute ventilation increases and Pa_{CO_2} drops. Although normal minute ventilation can be achieved by a variety of rate and tidal volume combinations, hypoventilation can result at the extremes of rate and volume. For example, a clinician's choice of a high rate and small volume promotes to-and-fro movement of gas in the large airways without any fresh gas reaching the alveoli.

Oxygen Delivery

Clinicians should attempt to achieve a minimum arterial oxygen tension (Pa_{O_2}) of 60 mm Hg. Hypoventilation should be corrected in a hypoxemic patient, since improving ventilation will often improve oxygenation. If hypoxemia persists, the clinician may choose to increase the inspired O_2 concentration, add positive expiratory pressure to the breathing circuit, or prolong the inspiratory time.

The relationship between inspired oxygen concentration and Pa_{O_2} is direct, and if the lungs are functioning normally, the Pa_{O_2} should be approximately five times the inspired oxygen percentage. Ventilators attached to anesthesia machines often deliver 100% oxygen, which may be detrimental during long-term therapy. With the addition of an air compressor and oxygen blender to the system, inspired oxygen concentration can be titrated to any desired level.

Positive expiratory pressure develops when exhalation continues to a predetermined positive pressure rather than to atmospheric pressure. The goal of its use is to provide an adequate Pa_{O_2} at the lowest possible inspired airway pressure and oxygen concentration. Blood passing through nonaerated lung units—intrapulmonary shunting—is a major cause of hypoxemia in many respiratory diseases. Positive expiratory pressure increases functional residual capacity, which prevents alveolar and small airway collapse between breaths and allows more lung units to participate in gas exchange. Positive expiratory pressure also increases alveolar volumes, resulting in a greater surface area for gas exchange.

Devices that provide positive expiratory pressure include specialized valves* that fit onto the exhalation side of the breathing circuit or dial-controlled mechanisms built into the ventilator. The valves utilize springs, ball deadweights, or magnets to maintain the positive pressure. Devices that use a restrictive orifice to generate pressure are not recommended because they increase the work of breathing excessively. Alternatively, the exhalation port of the breathing circuit can be connected to an open-ended tube, which is then placed perpendicularly under water. During expiration, the exhaled gas bubbles through the water and is vented to the atmosphere until lung pressure equals the pressure exerted by the weight of the water that is displaced from the tube. The amount of positive expiratory pressure is governed by the position of the tube under water. The pressure may be adjusted upward as necessary from a starting pressure of 2 to 5 cm H_2O. Adverse effects of positive expiratory pressure are similar to those of IPPV.

Lengthening the inspiratory time also prolongs alveolar inflation and improves gas exchange but does not prevent collapse during expiration. Depression of cardiac output associated with prolonged, high transpulmonary pressure limits the usefulness of this procedure, especially in hypovolemic and hypotensive patients.

---

*Such valves are manufactured by Boehringer Laboratories, Norristown, PA; Intertech-Ohio, Beaverton, OR; and Ambu, Hanover, MD.

ADVERSE EFFECTS OF MECHANICAL VENTILATION

In the normal canine lung, short-term inspiratory pressures of up to 50 cm H_2O do not cause damage (barotrauma) to the lungs. Elevated airway pressures are associated with an increase in pulmonary damage, but the incidence of barotrauma is more often related to underlying lung disease than to the inspiratory pressure. Even normal inspiratory pressures of 10 to 20 cm H_2O may cause pneumothorax or pneumomediastinum in patients with pulmonary disease. Therefore in patients at risk (e.g., those with pulmonary contusions or trauma, lung bullae or cysts, or postoperative lobectomies), ventilation may be maintained more safely with smaller tidal volumes and higher respiratory rates.

Positive-pressure ventilation tends to collapse intrathoracic vessels, which decreases both venous return to the heart and cardiac output. This effect is not significant in animals with normal hemodynamic compensatory capabilities. In hypovolemic or hypotensive patients, mechanical ventilation may improve respiratory function but decrease cardiac output, leading to progressive hypotension and inadequate tissue perfusion. Critical patients require low initial inspiratory pressures and gradual ventilator adjustments to assess the animal's compensatory ability. Volume loading followed by administration of inotropic and vasopressor agents may be required to maintain tissue perfusion in animals receiving IPPV.

Pulmonary oxygen toxicity is caused by oxidation of tissues and initially consists of interstitial edema, death of type I pneumocytes, and exudation of proteinaceous fluid into the small airways and alveoli. The later stages of toxicity result in fibroblastic proliferation and swelling of type II pneumocytes. The potential for oxygen toxicity increases as the inspired concentration and duration of therapy increase. Dogs developed pulmonary dysfunction within 24 hr and died within an average of 54 hr while breathing 100% oxygen (Smith et al., 1963). Exposure to oxygen concentrations of less than 50% did not result in clinical pulmonary dysfunction or failure. Maintaining the animal on the lowest oxygen concentration required to correct hypoxemia minimizes the chances for toxicity. Institution of positive expiratory pressure will often allow the inspired oxygen concentration to be decreased while adequate oxygenation is still maintained.

INITIATION OF MECHANICAL VENTILATION

In our description of the initiation of therapy, which is meant to familiarize the clinician with the process, we use a pressure-limited ventilator, the Bird ventilator. Basic controls on these machines include sensitivity, inspiratory pressure, inspiratory flow, and expiratory time; some models possess a positive expiratory pressure dial. A rebreathing bag may be placed on the patient port of the breathing circuit, and the following procedures may be carried out before patient connection. Troubles that become apparent can be managed more easily when one is not concerned about patient care in addition to ventilator adjustments.

The sensitivity is initially adjusted so that a negative pressure of 3 to 5 cm of water in the breathing circuit will trigger the ventilator to cycle into inspiration. Keeping the sensitivity high enough to permit the patient to trigger the ventilator may alert the clinician to changes in ventilatory drive. Next, the inspiratory pressure is set to 12 to 15 cm H_2O, which results in tidal volumes of 10 to 20 ml/kg in most normal cats and dogs. The operator should increase the inspiratory pressure as needed to obtain an adequate tidal volume in patients with decreased lung compliance. Some Bird models have an air-mix control that allows delivery of either 40% or 100% oxygen. Animals without respiratory disease often do well on room air, but increasing pulmonary dysfunction leads to the need for higher inspired oxygen concentrations.

Following connection of the patient to the ventilator, the machine is turned on by turning the inspiratory flow knob. The inspiratory flow is adjusted so that inspiration is approximately 1 sec. An initial respiratory rate of 8 to 10 with an adequate tidal volume should generate a minute ventilation of 150 to 200 ml/kg/min. Respiratory rate is adjusted by manipulating the expiratory time, which controls the time between breaths. The relationship between expiratory time and rate is reciprocal: an increase in expiratory time results in a decrease in rate. With several models of the Bird ventilator, pressure in the breathing circuit must reach atmospheric pressure for initiation of inspiration to occur during controlled ventilation. Therefore, these ventilators may cycle erratically, or not at all, with positive expiratory pressure applied to the circuit, because in such cases atmospheric pressure may not be reached.

MONITORING

Vigilant, continuous monitoring prevents respiratory or cardiovascular compromise and allows rapid adjustments in therapy in response to changing patient status. Hourly or more frequent evaluation of respiratory rate, chest-wall excursions, tidal volume, lung sounds, and ventilator settings is recommended. Monitoring need not be sophisticated because tidal volume can be measured by evaluation of chest wall excursions or with a respirometer, and lung sounds can be evaluated with a stethoscope.

Blood gas analysis that includes assessment of Pa_{O_2}, Pa_{CO_2}, pH, bicarbonate concentration, and base balance should be performed 10 to 15 min following any modification in ventilator settings or when the patient's condition changes. A flow chart of the results of blood gas analysis, along with concurrent ventilator settings, can illustrate trends that aid in decision making. For example, if an increasing airway pressure is needed to obtain the same tidal volume or blood gas values, compliance has probably decreased. Conscientious searching for trends is imperative because evaluation of the results of blood gas analysis or of clinical signs alone may not provide information on subtle life-threatening changes until the patient decompensates. Blood gas analysis performed every 6 hr is adequate in stable patients.

Pulse oximeters* measure the percentage of hemoglobin saturation and can be used when arterial blood gas analysis is not practical. At a Pa_{O_2} of 95 mm Hg, hemoglobin is nearly saturated ($\geq 97\%$), and for values higher than this Pa_{O_2} no additional information can be gained from the oximeter. When the saturation is 92%, the Pa_{O_2} is 60 mm Hg, and the clinician should be alerted to an ongoing hypoxemic event. As with arterial blood gas tensions, pulse oximetry does not give complete information on tissue oxygenation. An inadequate amount of oxygen may be carried to the tissues if an animal is anemic, even though the hemoglobin may be fully saturated. In our hands, IPPV monitoring by pulse oximeters has been limited by poor pulse detection caused by patient movement and by inconsistent results when the oximeter probe has not been placed on the tongue. Variable results have been reported when the probe has been placed on the upper lip or ear, or—in cats—on the toe. Vasoconstriction and poor perfusion at the probe site limit the oximeter's sensing capabilities in some critically ill patients.

Capnography allows continuous, breath-by-breath monitoring of patient carbon dioxide without requiring a blood sample.† The carbon dioxide concentration at the end of an expiration, the end-tidal carbon dioxide ($ETCO_2$), is similar to the Pa_{CO_2} and may be used to evaluate changes in Pa_{CO_2}. Increases in $ETCO_2$ can occur with increased carbon dioxide production, rebreathing, decreased alveolar minute ventilation, or pulmonary disease as the animal progresses toward failure. Positive expiratory pressure and certain diseases such as pulmonary

embolism may increase dead-space ventilation, leading to a significant gradient between the $ETCO_2$ and Pa_{CO_2}; therefore, arterial blood gases are necessary to provide periodic information on actual Pa_{CO_2} in these situations. The capnogram, graphically displaying the cyclic carbon dioxide wave form during inspiration and expiration, provides additional information, such as detection of rebreathing or a pulmonary embolic episode. Several books and review articles contain discussions of interpretation of the capnogram (Gravenstein et al., 1989; Paulus, 1989; Swedlow, 1986).

Monitoring of blood pressure, central venous pressure, and cardiac output is important in critically ill patients. Percutaneous placement of an arterial catheter in the dorsal metatarsal artery allows monitoring of direct blood pressure as well as access for arterial blood sampling. Indirect blood pressure measurements using Doppler or oscillometric techniques are useful when direct monitoring is not feasible. If blood pressure monitoring is unavailable, close attention to the patient's mucous membrane color, pulse quality, and heart rate may aid in evaluating cardiovascular function. Oxygen delivery to peripheral tissues can decrease in the face of a normal or rising Pa_{O_2} because of deleterious cardiovascular changes associated with IPPV. Whereas arterial oxygen tension provides information about inspired oxygen concentration and pulmonary function, mixed or jugular venous oxygen tension assesses tissue perfusion and oxygenation (Snyder, 1987). In unstable patients, even with appropriate cardiovascular support, a tradeoff must be maintained between achieving perfect ventilation and sustaining adequate tissue perfusion.

PATIENT CARE

Often, sedation may be necessary to minimize anxiety, induce tolerance of the monitoring equipment and ventilator apparatus, and facilitate patient handling (Table 1). The opioid agents oxymorphone and fentanyl usually provide adequate sedation for animals with normal lung function, such as those with postoperative thoracotomies or head trauma. Tranquilization may be supplemented by administration of a benzodiazepine such as diazepam. When opioids do not provide adequate sedation, when opioids must be given hourly for sedation (as frequently occurs in patients with severe pulmonary disease), or when long-term ventilatory support (lasting longer than 12 hr) is required, pentobarbital administration has been found to be a more successful means of providing necessary sedation. Paralysis may be required if the patient's own ventilation inhibits adequate controlled ventilation or if oxygen demand exceeds supply, because paralysis will decrease oxygen needs by decreasing the work

*Pulse oximeters are manufactured by Radiometer, Westlake, OH; Criticare Systems, Inc., Waukesha, WI; and Physio Control, Redmond, WA.

†Equipment used in capnography is available from Capnomac, Tewksbury, MA; Biochem, Waukesha, WI; and Gould, Cleveland, OH.

Table 1. Chemical Restraint for Mechanical Ventilation in the Dog

Drug	Dosage
Oxymorphone	Initial dose 0.2 mg/kg IV, then 0.05–0.10 mg/kg IV q 1–2 hr or less frequently as needed.
Oxymorphone plus	Same dosage for oxymorphone used alone.
Diazepam	Initial dose of 0.2–0.5 mg/kg IV, then 0.2 mg/kg IV q 1–2 hr alternately with oxymorphone.
Fentanyl	Loading dose of 10 μg/kg IV, then either 0.3–0.6 μg/kg/min IV infusion or 5–10 μg/kg IV q 30 min or less frequently as needed.
Fentanyl plus	Same dosage as for fentanyl used alone.
Diazepam	Same dosage as when used with oxymorphone, then 0.25–0.5 mg/kg/hr IV; or initial bolus, then repeat 0.2 mg/kg IV q 1 hr alternately with fentanyl.
Fentanyl plus	Same dosage as for fentanyl used alone.
Midazolam maleate	Loading dose of 0.2 mg/kg IV, then 0.1–0.6 mg/kg/hr IV infusion.
Pentobarbital	Loading dose of 1–5 mg/kg IV, then 1–4 mg/kg/hr IV infusion.
Atracurium plus adequate sedation using one of the foregoing combinations	Initial dose of 0.20 mg/kg IV, then 0.15 mg/kg IV as needed (approx. q 30 min); or initial dose, then 3–8 μg/kg/min IV infusion.

of breathing. Paralysis has the disadvantage, however, of not allowing spontaneous ventilation if accidental disconnection occurs, and it also necessitates monitoring of the extent of neuromuscular blockade.

Long-term ventilatory support is facilitated by placement of a tracheostomy cannula. Tracheostomy cannulas and endotracheal tubes interfere with the animal's mucociliary mechanisms for clearing airway secretions and with the ability to cough properly. Repositioning the patient every 2 to 4 hr improves gravity drainage of secretions from both lungs into the large airways, where they can be suctioned, and helps decrease atelectasis of the dependent lung. Atelectasis can also be decreased by providing six to eight deep breaths per hour.

Airway suctioning is mandatory when secretions are present in the respiratory tract. An initial protocol might include suctioning at least every 2 to 4 hr for the first 12 hr, with subsequent frequency based on the amount of secretions produced. The protocol must be individualized based on careful monitoring of the animal. Nebulization with sterile saline or increasing the humidity of the breathing circuit for 20 min prior to suctioning helps mobilize inspissated secretions. Alternatively, a small amount of sterile saline (0.5 to 4 ml) can be directly instilled into the patient's airway immediately prior to aspiration. The use of acetylcysteine as a mucolytic agent is not recommended because of its expense, its propensity to cause tracheal irritation and excessive mucus production, and its lack of demonstrated advantages over the use of saline alone. The suction catheter must be soft and pliable, and it must not exceed one half of the internal diameter of the tracheostomy cannula or endotracheal tube because larger catheters can result in severe hypoxemia and airway collapse. To avoid hypoxia during the suctioning procedure, the patient should be ventilated for 5 min with 100% oxygen prior to aspiration, and suctioning should be kept to a maximum of 5 to 10 sec. If the electrocardiogram is monitored during suctioning, hypoxia may be manifested as tachycardia, rhythm disturbances, or ST segment depression. With the use of sterile technique, the catheter is advanced into the trachea as far as possible without suction. As the catheter is slowly rotated out, suction is intermittently applied. This procedure is repeated up to three times, depending on the amount of secretions obtained; ventilation using 100% oxygen precedes each repetition. Several deep breaths of oxygen are given after the suctioning procedure to open up atelectatic areas produced by the subatmospheric pressure.

The tracheostomy cannula or endotracheal tube should be replaced with a clean tube every 24 to 48 hr or when dried secretions accumulate. The use of double-cannula tracheostomy tubes* maintains the airway when the inner tube is removed for cleaning. Before replacement, the inner cannula is cleansed and soaked in a 50:50 solution of sterile water and 3% hydrogen peroxide. To aid in the replacement of a single-cannula tracheostomy tube, stay sutures are placed in the trachea at the time of initial insertion and are used to elevate the stoma and ensure passage of the new tube into the lumen of the trachea. In either situation, the stoma and

---

*Double-cannula tracheostomy tubes are manufactured by Shiley Incorporated, Irvine, CA.

skin are cleaned two to three times daily with gauze or applicator sticks and the solution of hydrogen peroxide and water. Between cleanings, a light dressing of gauze should be placed under the flanges, encircling the tracheostomy cannula.

Nutrition is required for all patients receiving mechanical ventilation and should be provided using an appropriate technique (Armstrong and Lippert, 1988; Donoghue, 1989). Obtunded or anesthetized patients are at risk especially for passive regurgitation and aspiration pneumonia. If oral feeding is not feasible, other methods of enteral nutrition should be considered. Total parenteral nutrition is frequently required either when enteral nutrition is not tolerated by the patient or when the risk of aspiration is too high.

WEANING

The successful management of a ventilator patient involves not only the proper institution and maintenance of therapy but also the discontinuation of respiratory support. Weaning from long-term ventilatory support may require hours or days and is dictated by the patient's needs. A substantial number of patients who cannot be weaned from the ventilator have either irreversible lung disease or central nervous system disease.

A variety of methods are available for weaning animals from mechanical ventilation. Assisted ventilation might be used for animals with a presumed normal respiratory drive and gas exchange. Adequate ventilation in the assist mode does not necessarily imply that the patient will breathe adequately with spontaneous ventilation, because the ventilator still provides a modest amount of support. Alternatively, these patients may be extubated and placed on 30 to 50% oxygen via a face mask or nasal catheter. Other modes of weaning include synchronized intermittent mandatory ventilation (SIMV), pressure support ventilation, and use of a T-piece.

SIMV differs from IMV in that the ventilator breaths will occur only with the patient's initiation of inspiration. SIMV is used in an attempt to improve patient comfort and prevent the patient from "bucking" or fighting the ventilator. To wean the patient, the number of mechanical breaths is slowly decreased as the patient is monitored.

Pressure support ventilation (PSV) is a form of ventilatory support that is available on several new-generation, microprocessor-controlled ventilators. PSV is thought to provide improved patient comfort, better ventilator synchrony, and a balanced work load between machine and patient. The reader is referred to another article on the subject for a full description of PSV.*

---

*MacIntyre, N. R.: Respiratory function during pressure support ventilation. Chest 89:677, 1986.

Table 2. Indicators of Unsuccessful Weaning From Mechanical Ventilation*

Heart rate increased or decreased by >20 beats/min
Respiratory rate increased by >10 breaths/min
Decreased level of consciousness
Development of cardiac arrhythmia
Evidence of respiratory muscle fatigue (paradoxical breathing)
Anxiety unrelieved by reassurance
Desaturation below 90% as measured by pulse oximetry
Minute ventilation <150 ml/kg/min
$Pa_{O_2} < 50-60$ mm Hg
$Pa_{CO_2} > 50-60$ mm Hg

*Adapted with permission from Stone, A. M., and Bone, R. C.: Successful weaning from mechanical ventilation. Postgrad. Med. 86:317, 1989.

With a T-piece incorporating a one-way valve connected to the tracheostomy or endotracheal tube, the patient can breathe an enriched oxygen mixture from one side of the T and exhale through the other side. The inspired oxygen concentration should initially be 10% greater than what the patient was receiving while being mechanically ventilated.

The weaning trial is preceded by suctioning and tube care. Ventilatory support is decreased, and the patient closely observed for 30 min. This trial period can be shortened in patients who require a more conservative approach to discontinuation of ventilatory support. Criteria that indicate an unsuccessful weaning attempt are listed in Table 2. If no clinically apparent problems develop during the 30-min trial, an arterial blood gas measurement is obtained. Results demonstrating a Pa_{CO_2} greater than 50 mm Hg or a Pa_{O_2} less than 60 mm Hg indicate the need for continued ventilation therapy.

HIGH-FREQUENCY VENTILATION

High-frequency ventilation (HFV) describes three alternative methods of mechanical ventilation, all of which employ high respiratory rates and low tidal volumes. In high-frequency positive-pressure ventilation, conventional ventilatory apparatus with low compliance is used and provides respiratory rates of 60 to 120 breaths per minute. In high-frequency jet ventilation, high-pressure gas is forced through a jet nozzle; this method usually provides respiratory rates of 100 to 400 breaths per minute. High-frequency oscillation provides respiratory rates of 400 to 2400 breaths per minute and is produced by an oscillating diaphragm or piston. During the first two types of ventilation, inspiration is active and expiration is passive, whereas during high-frequency oscillation, both inspiration and exhalation are active.

The mechanism of gas exchange during HFV has not been fully determined but may include bulk gas flow as well as asymmetric inspiratory and expiratory gas flow patterns, redistribution of gas volumes between alveoli, radial molecular dispersion, molecular diffusion, and cardiogenic mixing.

HFV has potential advantages over conventional IPPV in that the maximum airway pressure is lower and the risks of cardiovascular depression and barotrauma may be lessened. Large fluctuations in intracranial pressure seen with IPPV do not occur with HFV, which suggests that HFV may benefit ventilated animals when increased intracranial pressure is to be avoided.

High-frequency jet ventilation has been used in selected veterinary cases such as laryngoscopy, bronchoscopy, and airway surgery, and as emergency ventilation during cardiopulmonary resuscitation when IPPV could not be instituted adequately. The use of positive expiratory pressure with HFV, similar to its use with IPPV, may be considered. Because HFV does not provide large tidal volumes, atelectasis does occur with its long-term use, and patients should be periodically sighed. Monitoring with these modes of ventilation must be as vigilant as with IPPV. High-frequency ventilation has been reported to cause decreased mucociliary transport, tracheobronchial damage, pneumothorax, pneumomediastinum and pneumoperitoneum from the jet stream, and alveolar overinflation from gas trapping due to inadequate exhalation times. The use of high-frequency ventilation in veterinary medicine has recently been reviewed (Bjorling, 1986).

References and Suggested Reading

Armstrong, P. J., and Lippert, A. C.: Selected aspects of enteral and parenteral nutritional support. Semin. Vet. Med. Surg. (Small Anim.) 3:216, 1988.

Bjorling, D. E.: High-frequency ventilation: A review. Vet. Surg. 15:399, 1986.

Donoghue, S.: Nutritional support of hospitalized patients. Vet. Clin. North Am. Small Anim. Pract. 19:475, 1989.

Dupris, Y. G.: *Ventilators: Theory and Clinical Application*. St. Louis: C. V. Mosby, 1986.
    Describes basic concepts of ventilator function and drive mechanisms and provides a detailed description of the specific ventilators available.

Gravenstein, J. S., Paulus, D. A., and Haynes, T. J.: *Capnography in Clinical Practice*. Boston: Butterworth, 1989.
    Explains basics of capnography, underlying physiology, and interpretation of common capnograms found in clinical practice.

Lenaghan, R., Silva, Y. J., and Walt, A. J.: Hemodynamic alterations associated with expansion rupture of the lung. Arch. Surg. 99:339, 1969.

Pascoe, P. J.: Short-term ventilatory support. In Kirk, R. W. (ed.): *Current Veterinary Therapy VIII*. Philadelphia: W. B. Saunders, p. 269, 1983.

Paulus, D. A.: Capnography. Int. Anesthesiol. Clin. 27:167, 1989.

Smith, C. W., Lehan, P. H., and Monks, J. J.: Cardiopulmonary manifestations with high O₂ tensions at atmospheric pressure. J. Appl. Physiol. 18:849, 1963.

Snyder, J. V.: *Oxygen Transport in the Critically Ill*. Chicago: Year Book, 1987.

Swedlow, D. B.: Capnometry and capnography: The anesthesia disaster early warning system. Semin. Anesth. 5:194, 1986.

TRANSFUSION THERAPY: RED BLOOD CELL SUBSTITUTES AND AUTOTRANSFUSION

VIRGINIA T. RENTKO,
and SUSAN M. COTTER
North Grafton, Massachusetts

RED BLOOD CELL SUBSTITUTES AND AUTOTRANSFUSION

Blood transfusions play an important role in veterinary medicine in the treatment of anemia and hemodynamic compromise due to surgery or trauma. Homologous blood products are used almost exclusively in animal patients. Insufficient availability and the risks of homologous blood have led to consideration of alternative sources such as autologous transfusion and development of blood substitutes. (For a discussion of homologous blood transfusions, see this volume, pp. 470 and 475.)

RED BLOOD CELL SUBSTITUTES OR OXYGEN-CARRYING SOLUTIONS

The advantage of blood over crystalloid or colloid solutions lies in its oxygen-carrying capacity. The development of an acellular oxygen-carrying solution has been a topic of research in human medicine for more than 50 years. Research efforts have inten-

Table 1. Comparison of Blood and Hemoglobin Solutions

	Fresh Whole Blood	Hemoglobin Solution
Oxygen transport	Excellent	Excellent, varies with preparation
Volume expansion	Excellent	Excellent
Time span of effectiveness	Normal red blood cell life span, 100–120 days	24–72 hr, depending on polymerization
Renal toxicity	None	Rare, depending on purification
Allergic reactions	None with autologous, uncommon with homologous	Rare
Disease transmission	Possible with homologous	Unlikely
Availability	Dependent on donor supply	Experimental
Blood typing/crossmatching	Important	Unnecessary

sified in the past decade with the increased recognition of diseases that can be transmitted by homologous blood transfusion, such as acquired immunodeficiency syndrome (AIDS) and hepatitis.

The ideal oxygen-carrying solution would load, transport, and deliver oxygen and remove carbon dioxide efficiently. This ideal solution would expand blood volume, be nontoxic, have minimal immunogenicity and appropriate intravascular persistence and viscosity, and be readily available at a reasonable cost (Table 1). The goal is to provide temporary oxygen-carrying capacity until additional red blood cells (RBCs) are available either by homologous transfusion or by regeneration. An oxygen-carrying solution would be especially useful in acute reversible anemia due to hemorrhage, hemolytic crisis, or parasites.

Current research focuses on several different approaches: (1) extraction and purification of hemoglobin from outdated human blood, (2) extraction and purification of hemoglobin of bovine blood, (3) cloning the human hemoglobin gene to make recombinant hemoglobin molecules, and (4) development of synthetic solutions of perfluorocarbons. Perfluorochemical compounds have limited usefulness owing to difficulties in solubilization, a low oxygen-carrying capacity at ambient oxygen pressure (room air), and in vivo accumulation in tissues containing large numbers of mononuclear cells and other phagocytes. The product does not produce any obvious adverse reactions but has been shown to lack efficacy in severe anemia (Gould et al., 1986).

The emphasis of research in recent years has shifted to hemoglobin solutions. Hemolyzed blood was tried first, but its usefulness was limited by a short half-life (20 to 30 min), increased oxygen affinity, complement activation with activation of the coagulation pathway, renal and coronary vasoconstriction, and renal tubular damage. The complement activation and vascular changes were caused by residual stromal elements in the solutions. Improvements in purification have increased the safety, and the removal of blood group antigens has eliminated the need for typing and crossmatching. Polymerization of the hemoglobin molecules

has increased the half-life to approximately 48 hr. Two approaches have been taken to improve oxygen availability to the tissues. In human hemoglobin solutions in which 2,3-diphosphoglycerate (2,3-DPG) is lost with RBC lysis, pyridoxal-5-phosphate is chemically bound to the hemoglobin to provide efficient unloading of oxygen. Bovine hemoglobin solution, antigenically similar to human hemoglobin, has been used because chloride ion performs the function of 2,3-DPG, resulting in a lower oxygen affinity than that achieved with human hemoglobin solutions, thereby improving oxygen delivery to the tissues. Bovine hemoglobin solutions are also free of the viruses that are of most concern in transfusions to humans and other species. This solution has been tested and used to replace large volumes of blood with minimal toxicity in animals of a variety of species. A limited number of clinical trials are under way in animals and humans.

AUTOTRANSFUSION

Autotransfusion is a procedure in which autologous blood is recovered and returned to the patient. The procedure has been used sporadically in human medicine for the past century and has been employed with increasing frequency in the past 10 years in both human and veterinary medicine. Autologous blood transfusions can be performed in three ways: (1) intraoperative blood salvage and reinfusion; (2) preoperative collection, storage, and transfusion during surgical procedures; and (3) immediate preoperative collection, with hemodilution by crystalloid solutions and retransfusion after most of the intraoperative blood loss has occurred.

Intraoperative blood salvage in human surgery currently uses mechanical cell washers, which are costly and require trained technicians for their operation. In veterinary medicine, blood is aspirated by syringe or via a gentle vacuum and readministered through a 170-μm filter. A simple method of collection and reinfusion of blood from the pleural or peritoneal cavity with a catheter, syringes, stopcocks, and extension tubing has been described (Crowe, 1980). Commercial autotransfusion devices vary in cost and complexity. Solcotrans (Solco Basle Inc., Rockland, MA) is a reasonably priced device in which pooled blood is suctioned directly into a sterile reservoir where it is mixed with an anticoagulant, and it can be reinfused from the same unit via filtered tubing. This device is nonmechanical and requires standard wall suction. Successful use of a similar device, Bard William Harvey H-4700 Series Cardiotomy Reservoir (C. R. Bard, Inc., Billerica, MA), has been reported (Niebauer, 1991). Intraoperative blood loss or traumatic bleeding into a body cavity is an instance in which blood can be salvaged for autologous transfusion. Blood in contact with pleural or peritoneal surfaces for longer than 1 hour becomes defibrinated and thombocytopenic as a result of platelet aggregation. Anticoagulation of the blood may be unnecessary under these circumstances. The RBCs have a normal life span after reinfusion and can provide adequate oxygen carrying capacity.

Blood that has been in contact with serosal surfaces for longer than 24 hours should not be used for autotransfusion. Microaggregates of white blood cells (WBCs) and platelets, lysis of red cells, and release of cellular components may elicit disseminated intravascular coagulation (DIC) after reinfusion.

Complications associated with hemolysis, coagulation, or contamination with bacteria, neoplastic cells, or particulate matter are primary concerns in the handling and reinfusion of salvaged blood. Microembolism from fat, protein, and microaggregates of WBCs and platelets, along with increased fibrin split products that predispose the patient to activation of the coagulation cascade and DIC, are additional potential complications associated with autotransfusions. For these reasons, the procedure of autotransfusion should be used only when there is major blood loss. Microaggregates and platelets may be removed with a 40-μm filter, but the filter often becomes clogged. Microaggregates appear to be a limited concern, and the use of such a fine filter seems unwarranted. Careful monitoring of suction pressure is key to minimizing trauma to the RBCs. Limiting the amount of suction and air aspirated with blood decreases turbulence in the blood and minimizes hemolysis. Transfusion of large amounts of hemolyzed blood decreases the oxygen-carrying capacity of the blood, and release of RBC stroma may precipitate DIC. The rate of reinfusion, varying from immediate, rapid administration to up to 4 hr, depends on the volume of blood collected and the severity of the anemia. The rate should be more rapid in patients with hemorrhagic shock and slower in these with cardiac or hepatic failure. The problems associated with collection and reinfusion of autologous blood can be minimized by using collection bottles with citrate, gentle aspiration of blood,

a collection of blood that does not contain bacteria or neoplastic cells, and a 170-μm filter for readministration of the blood.

In the traumatized animal patient with massive blood loss, blood salvage techniques provide an immediate source of large quantities of blood that may not be otherwise available. In addition, as the blood red cells are "fresh," the concentration of 2,3-DPG is normal and the oxygen-carrying capacity immediately after administration is better than that of stored homologous blood.

Preoperative blood collection for autologous transfusion is an option for elective surgical procedures such as mandibulectomy or maxillectomy, exploratory rhinotomy, and total hip replacement in which a large amount of blood loss is anticipated. Blood donation of up to a total of 20 to 30% of blood volume or 20 ml/kg weekly over a 2- to 3-week period preoperatively is easily tolerated and safe in animals with normal bone marrow function and iron stores and whose hematocrit is greater than 35%. Plasma volume is rapidly replaced within 72 hr. The technique of blood collection is reviewed by Authement and colleagues (1987). Administration of oral iron supplements to the animal is recommended during this time to achieve maximal RBC production after repeated phlebotomy. Administration of recombinant erythropoietin, Epogen (Amgen Corporation), is used currently to enhance maximal erythropoiesis in similar human patients. Recombinant human erythropoietin stimulates the bone marrow to make RBCs, causing a dose-dependent increase in RBC count, hemoglobin, and hematocrit (see this volume, p. 484).

With preoperative blood donation, the hematopoietic system of the patient is functioning maximally by the time surgical blood loss occurs, and this factor aids in rapid return of a normal RBC mass in the animal. This method of predeposit blood donation is contraindicated in patients with nonregenerative anemia or compromised cardiovascular status. The blood collected can be stored at 4°C for up to 21 days; when reinfused it will supply good oxygen-carrying capacity to the animal but will lack most coagulation factors and functional platelets.

Perioperative hemodilution as a source of autologous blood is an underutilized technique in veterinary medicine. Animals with normal hematocrits and adequate cardiovascular status scheduled for surgical procedures with significant expected blood loss may donate blood preoperatively. In these animals, up to one quarter of the blood volume can be collected with replacement by 3-ml crystalloid solutions per milliliter of blood removed. The resultant normovolemic anemia may actually increase oxygen delivery to tissues during anesthetic and surgical procedures by decreasing the viscosity of the blood and enhancing blood flow. The blood is stored at room temperature to preserve the platelet number and function. After the major operative blood loss ceases, or sooner if required, the predonated blood is reinfused. Reinfusion must occur within 6 hr of donation to avoid risks associated with bacterial contamination if the blood is stored at room temperature. The need for homologous blood is decreased in two ways: first, hemodilution results in decreased RBC loss associated with intraoperative bleeding, and second, the returned blood contains all coagulation factors and functional platelets.

In summary, the currently available procedures for autologous blood transfusions in veterinary medicine are blood salvage and reinfusion, preoperative donation, and perioperative hemodilution. In the future, alternative therapies for blood transfusions will include administration of blood-substitute oxygen-carrying solutions and recombinant erythropoietin.

References and Suggested Reading

Authement, J. M., Wolfsheimer, K. J, and Catchings, S.: Canine blood component therapy: Product preparation, storage and administration. J. Am. Anim. Hosp. Assoc. 23: 483, 1987.

Brzica, S. M., Pineda, A. A, and Taswell, H. F.: Autologous blood transfusion. Mayo Clin. Proc. 51: 723, 1976.

Cotter, S. M.: Comparative transfusion medicine. *In* Cotter, S. M. (ed.): *Advances in Veterinary Science and Comparative Medicine.* Orlando: Academic Press, 1991 (in press).

Crowe, D. T.: Autotransfusion in the trauma patient. Vet. Clin. North Am. [Small Anim. Pract.] 10:581, 1980.

DeVenuto, F., Friedman, H. I., Neville, J. R., et al.: Appraisal of hemoglobin solution as a blood substitute. Surg. Gynecol. Obstet. 149:417, 1979.

Gould, S. A., Rosen, A L., Sehgal, L. R., et al.: Fluosol-DA as a red-cell substitute in acute anemia. N. Engl. J. Med. 314:1653, 1986.

Niebauer, G. W.: Autotransfusion for intraoperative blood salvage: A new technique. Compendium Continuing Education 13:1105, 1991.

Saarela, E.: Autotransfusion: A review. Ann. Clin. Res. 13 (Suppl. 33):43, 1981.

Winslow, R. M.: Blood substitutes: current status. Transfusion 29:753, 1989.

Yawn, D. H.: Autologous blood salvage during elective surgery. Transfusion Science 10:107, 1989.

Zenoble, R. D., and Stone, E. A.: Autotransfusion in the dog. J.A.V.M.A. 172:141, 1978.

INTRAOSSEOUS RESUSCITATION TECHNIQUES AND APPLICATIONS

CYNTHIA M. OTTO,
Philadelphia, Pennsylvania

and DENNIS T. CROWE, Jr.
Milwaukee, Wisconsin

The ability to establish an intravenous catheter in an emergency situation often means the difference between life and death of a patient. This access is often difficult or impossible to attain for even the most experienced personnel in patients in a state of vascular collapse such as shock, and particularly in neonates, birds, or other small animals.

Alternative routes of drug administration for use when direct venous access is unattainable, particularly during cardiac arrest, have been described. Intratracheal epinephrine administration, for example, is an accepted method of administering a small quantity of drug rapidly. The intramuscular, intraperitoneal, and subcutaneous routes preclude the administration of fluids in large volumes and of many of the drugs used in resuscitation (e.g., cal-cium, sodium bicarbonate, and dopamine). When vascular collapse and poor peripheral circulation are encountered, substances administered intraperitoneally or subcutaneously are not absorbed sufficiently (if at all), and therefore may be inadequately available to support circulation and provide volume resuscitation.

Intraosseous infusions provide an alternative method of access to the circulatory system for rapid delivery of large volumes of fluids. With minimal experience, a veterinarian or technician can establish an intraosseous cannula in approximately 3 min from the time the skin is prepared to the time fluids or drugs can be delivered. The technique is relatively inexpensive because it can be performed using equipment routinely stocked in most veterinary hospitals.

INDICATIONS

Intraosseous infusions have been described for over 60 years, but only recently has there been a new focus on the intraosseous route for fluid and drug administration. Indications for the intraosseous route for administration of fluids and drugs in animals may include shock, cardiac arrest, severe burns, profound subcutaneous edema, severe obesity, and peripheral vascular thrombosis of vessels commonly used for catheterization (Hodge, 1985; Otto et al., 1989). Circulatory collapse leads to decreased blood flow, lowered systemic arterial blood pressure, and venous pooling of blood. Attending these changes are collapsed peripheral veins and poor venous return. While a cutdown technique can permit one to cannulate a collapsed peripheral vein, rapid fluid administration is hampered by vein fragility and by the sluggish column of blood between the access site and the heart. In contrast, the intraosseous cannula provides rapid access to the central compartment of the circulatory system through the capillary-rich bone marrow. The rigid support of bone surrounding the marrow prevents collapse of vessels during shock (Tocantins et al., 1941) and provides cannula stabilization, allowing easy administration and rapid delivery of blood, colloids, crystalloids, and drugs, even for patients in hypovolemic states (Hodge et al., 1987; Spivey et al., 1985). This route can be used as an interim therapy to expand the circulatory volume in hemodynamic failure (i.e., arrest or shock) until circulatory function is improved and an intravenous catheter can be placed. The uptake and distribution of fluids via the intraosseous route are inferior only to those achieved by the central venous route of administration, in which the tip of the catheter rests within the thoracic vena cava.

Drugs administered by the intraosseous route demonstrate efficacy and onset of action comparable to those of drugs administered by the peripheral intravenous route. The intraosseous route provides an excellent method of drug administration during cardiac arrest.

CONTRAINDICATIONS

Contraindications for the placement of intraosseous cannulas include skeletal abnormalities, skin and wound infections, and abscesses or fractures involving those tissues or bones involved in cannula placement. Sepsis is the only systemic disease that may be a contraindication for intraosseous cannula placement, because of the increased risk for the induction of septic osteomyelitis. In septic shock, however, the risk of initiating osteomyelitis must be weighed against the increased risk of mortality from inadequate fluid volume resuscitation.

TECHNIQUE

Equipment

Simple technology and minimal equipment are required for successful intraosseous infusions. The equipment necessary is the same as that needed for intravenous infusion with the exception of the intraosseous "catheter," a rigid cannula that can penetrate cortical bone. Ideally, the cannula should contain a stylet to prevent a core of bone from obstructing the lumen during insertion. Intraosseous cannulas are commercially available (Cooke Catheters, Bloomington, IN); however, an intraosseous infusion can be established using a standard hypodermic needle, a spinal needle, or a bone marrow needle as a cannula.

In cats, small exotic animals, birds, or young dogs, a 20- to 22-gauge, 1- to 1½-inch spinal needle works well; the stylet prevents obstruction of the lumen, and the needle is rigid enough to minimize bending during placement. Neonates have soft, spongy bones that can be penetrated with an 18- to 25-gauge hypodermic needle. If cortical bone obstructs the lumen of the needle, the needle can be withdrawn and a new, slightly larger, needle placed in the channel through the bone cortex.

Adult dogs (and some cats) have very dense cortical bone, and a small-gauge (20) hypodermic or spinal needle is likely to bend or break during placement. In these animals, a standard bone marrow needle provides relatively easy access. If such a needle is not available, a heavy-gauge K-wire or small intramedullary pin can be used to pre-drill a hole, and a hypodermic needle can then be guided through that hole into the marrow cavity. A needle slightly larger than the pre-drilled hole must be used, so that it is seated snugly in the bone, minimizing leakage around the cannula.

Choice and Preparation of Access Site

The most common sites for intraosseous cannula placement are the trochanteric fossa of the femur (Fig. 1); the flat medial surface of the proximal tibia, approximately 1 to 2 cm distal to the tibial tuberosity (Fig. 2); or the tibial tuberosity. In general, any bone containing a rich marrow cavity is a potential site for intraosseous cannula placement. The wing of the ileum, the ischium, the greater tubercle of the humerus, and the sternum are other possible sites.

In birds, the distal end of the ulna provides an excellent site for intraosseous cannula placement (Fig. 3). Pneumatic bones in birds *must* be avoided (Ritchie et al., 1990).

The decision regarding which site to use should be based on the ease of access and on the condition

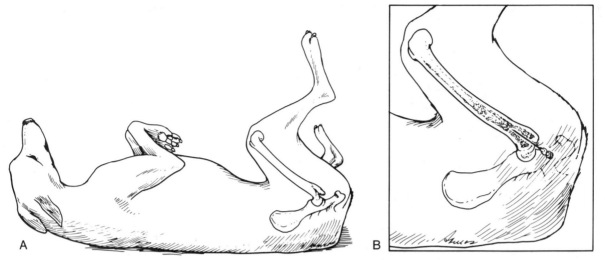

Figure 1. Patient positioning *(A)* and technique *(B)* for placement of a styleted needle used as an intraosseous cannula in the greater trochanter.

of the animal (e.g., one should avoid involving bones that have been traumatized and avoid entry into infected skin or bone). The tibia is more accessible in obese animals and allows easier stabilization of the cannula, especially in an animal undergoing seizures. The wing of the ilium represents the site with easiest access in animals that are orthopneic or that cannot be moved from sternal recumbency. In active animals, the trochanteric fossa of the femur is useful and does not limit mobility.

In neonates or small animals (less than about 7 kg) affected by hypovolemic shock, a single intraosseous line may be sufficient to supply fluids at shock doses (90 ml/kg). The administration rate can be increased by using the largest-bore needle possible for the insertion site and administering the fluids under pressurized flow. In larger animals, the use of two lines in separate bones or of pressurized flow, or both, may be required to deliver fluids for shock resuscitation. Often, once fluid resuscitation is started via the intraosseous cannula, the venous blood pressures are raised sufficiently to allow establishment of a conventional intravenous catheter. Low-volume resuscitative fluids such as hypertonic saline can be administered through an intraosseous cannula; however, the hypertonicity of this solution has been associated with lameness following infusion (Okrasinski, in press).

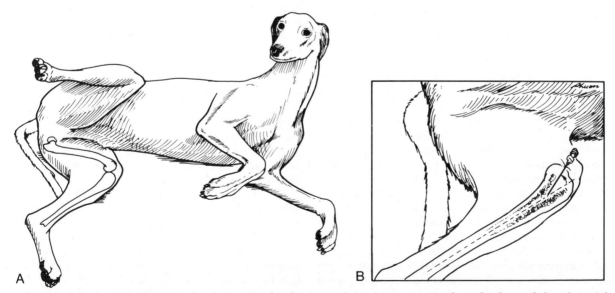

Figure 2. Patient positioning *(A)* and technique *(B)* for placement of an intraosseous cannula in the flat medial surface of the proximal tibia. The illustrations of Allison Lucas are gratefully acknowledged.

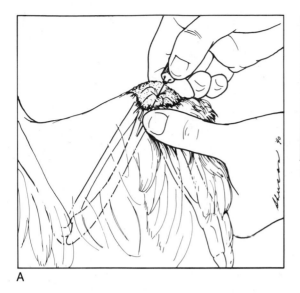

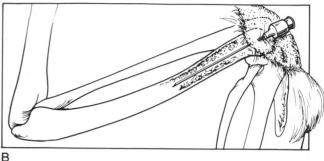

Figure 3. Positioning of birds (A) and technique (B) for placement of an intraosseous cannula in the ulna. The illustrations of Allison Lucas are gratefully acknowledged.

Aseptic technique must be used in preparing the access site. The area to be used should be clipped free of hair and be prepared with a surgical scrub. In *emergency* situations, the area should be clean of obvious dirt and debris. If an intraosseous cannula is placed under nonsterile conditions, it should be removed as soon as the animal is stable and either an aseptically placed intraosseous cannula or an intravenous catheter has been placed.

Cannula Placement

The skin and periosteum over the insertion site are infiltrated with 1% lidocaine (0.5% lidocaine should be used in neonates, geriatric patients, and cats). The appendage is properly positioned and the tip of a 20-gauge needle or scalpel blade is used to make a small incision over the insertion site to facilitate cannula placement and minimize bacterial contamination of the cannula. For placement in the medial tibia, the needle is directed distally into the bone, away from the proximal growth plate. For placement in the trochanteric fossa of the femur, the needle should be maneuvered off the medial aspect of the greater trochanter into the trochanteric fossa. To avoid damaging the sciatic nerve, the coxofemoral joint should remain in a neutral to slightly extended position, with the femur externally rotated, during placement of the cannula.

Following insertion of the cannula through the skin, pressure is applied to the needle along with firm rotation in 30° turns. This approach creates a small depression in the bone, which "seats" the needle. Once the needle has been seated, increasing pressure on the same rotation pattern drives the needle through the near cortex. As the needle passes through the cortex, a sudden loss of resistance is often detected. To test placement of the needle, the needle can be flicked with a finger. An appropriately placed needle is sufficiently stable in the bone so that it does not wobble when flicked. The limb should be moved and the hub of the needle observed. The hub of the needle should move with the limb without becoming dislodged.

If the needle is appropriately placed, a 10-ml syringe should be attached to the hub, and gentle suction should be applied. In most cases, bone marrow (fat, bone spicules, and blood) should be aspirated into the needle. In hypovolemic patients, aspirated bone marrow may not be visualized. In human patients, aspiration of marrow contents or high-pressure infusion creates an uncomfortable sensation, but transient constant infusion into the marrow is not reported to be painful. In animals, transient constant infusion is well tolerated.

Following confirmation of placement, if the cannula does not flush easily with heparinized saline, the needle should be rotated 90 to 180°, as the beveled edge of the needle may be positioned against the cortical bone, preventing flow. If fluid still does not flow freely, the needle should be gently withdrawn 1 to 2 mm, so that the tip is moved away from any corticocancellous intramedullary bone that may be obstructing flow. If impediment to free flow continues, a small amount of bone may be lodged in the lumen of the needle. Use of a woven wire stylet or forceful injection of heparinized saline with a tuberculin syringe should dislodge the obstruction.

The needle can be secured by suturing. The suture is placed in the periosteum near the cannula exit site. Following periosteal or fascial suture penetration, the suture is loosely tied to prevent skin irritation and ischemia. The suture is wrapped around the needle hub several times and tied tightly. Super Glue (Qualco Products Co., Fanwood, NJ) is applied to the hub of the needle to secure the suture further. Suturing of the cannula to a tape butterfly near the hub of the needle is an alternate method of securing the cannula. (Intraosseous catheters manufactured by Cooke Catheters have permanent butterflies for suturing.)

The entry site should be covered with triple antibiotic or antiseptic ointment and gauze. The needle should be protected from breaking or bending by application of a bulky wrap attached to the body. Use of a T-port extension set (Burron Medical, Inc., Bethlehem, PA 18018) to join the needle to the administration set or catheter plug minimizes bending and manipulation of the needle. In humans, this manipulation of intraosseous cannulas has been associated with discomfort, and we believe that this avoidable manipulation is also associated with a higher prevalence of infection and leakage of administered materials.

Once the cannula is placed securely, the substance to be infused can be connected to the needle by a standard intravenous administration set. If the cannula is to be used for intermittent injections, an intravenous catheter plug can be attached to flush heparinized saline into the needle. Either approach maintains continuous vascular access. The subcutaneous tissue must be observed for fluid extravasation following placement and institution of fluid administration. If more than one hole is placed through the cortex, extravasation of fluid into the subcutaneous tissue is likely to occur. In such a case, that bone should not be re-used for 12 to 24 hr. If extravasation is caused by leakage from a poorly created access channel, the needle should be removed and another bone chosen as the access site. A less desirable alternative involves insertion of a larger needle into the original access channel to prevent further leakage along the shaft of the needle at that access point in the cortical bone.

Maintenance of an intraosseous cannula that is not being used for continuous infusion is identical to that of an intravenous catheter; the cannula requires flushing every 6 hr with 0.5 to 1.0 ml of heparinized saline (2 to 10 units of heparin per milliliter of saline) to ensure patency. In neonates and cats, administration of heparinized saline containing benzyl alcohol as a preservative should be avoided.

COMPLICATIONS

The complications associated with intraosseous infusions in human patients are approximately the same as those associated with routine venous access. The most commonly reported complication of intraosseous infusion is infection. Long-term cannula placement (of several days' duration) and use of a cannula during sepsis are risk factors for osteomyelitis.

Fat and marrow embolism to the lungs may occur

with either gravitational or pressurized flow through intraosseous cannulas. Thus far, neither changes in pulmonary function nor the acute respiratory distress syndrome have been attributed to fat or marrow emboli occurring during intraosseous infusion in animals. Less frequently reported complications associated with intraosseous infusions include physeal damage from improperly directed cannulas and extravasation of fluids from puncture of both cortices. Evaluation of alterations in tibial growth plates in pigs following intraosseous infusions has shown no significant defects associated with placement of intraosseous cannulas (Brickman et al., 1988). Overzealous attempts at placing the cannula could result in fractures, particularly in young or osteoporotic animals, but such outcomes are rare.

COMMON CONCERNS

Some commonly asked questions regarding intraosseous resuscitation are enumerated as follows.

1. *How long does it take for fluids and drugs administered through an intraosseous cannula to be absorbed?* The intraosseous cannula sits within the vascular system; substances injected through it are delivered directly into the vascular system. The time required for drugs to take effect is the same regardless of whether they are given intravenously or intraosseously. In some instances, intraosseous administration is superior to *peripheral* intravenous administration (Spivey et al., 1985).

2. *How fast can fluids be administered intraosseously?* The bone is a rigid cavity and does not expand like a vein to accommodate increased flow; therefore, maximal flow rates are limited. Using large-bore needles (18-gauge) and pressurized flow facilitates fluid delivery. Experimental studies in calves (Shoor et al., 1979) and in hypovolemic puppies (Hodge et al., 1987) demonstrate that maximum pressurized flow rates are approximately 2 L/ hr. Clinical application of intraosseous therapy suggests that these rates may be lower in animal patients.

3. *What substances can be administered through an intraosseous cannula?* Any drug that can be administered intravenously can be infused through an intraosseous cannula. Clinical experience and pharmacokinetic trials have also demonstrated that drugs administered by the intraosseous route do not differ in efficacy, onset of action, or activity, even in hypovolemic states. Administration of hypertonic and alkaline solutions can be painful and can cause transient microscopic changes in bone marrow cellularity (Spivey et al., 1987). Vasosclerotic drugs, such as thiopental sodium, thiacetarsamide sodium, and many chemotherapeutic agents, must be administered with caution, and if there is any evidence of fluid extravasation associated with

the use of the cannula, intraosseous administration must be avoided.

4. *What happens to the bone marrow?* Changes in bone marrow that have been reported in association with intraosseous infusions are limited to transient decreases in cellularity. There are no reports of peripheral blood or radiographic changes in the bone (other than at the entry site for the cannula, which remodels rapidly).

5. *Should the intraosseous cannula replace the intravenous catheter?* For routine vascular access, the intravenous catheter should not be replaced by the intraosseous cannula. In neonates, birds, and exotics, however, the intraosseous route is the technique of choice. In animals in which a conventional intravenous catheter can be placed, the intravenous route is preferred over the intraosseous route because it provides greater patient comfort and sampling access. Although the complication rate associated with intraosseous catheters is approximately the same as that associated with intravenous catheters, the complications of the former may be more difficult to manage.

6. *How long can an intraosseous cannula be left in place?* Although there are no published reports of the recommended duration of intraosseous cannula placement, extrapolation from recommendations for intravenous catheter placement suggests that an intraosseous cannula can remain in place for up to 72 hr without complications, provided that aseptic technique, adequate fixation and bandaging, and routine cannula maintenance are employed.

Acknowledgment

The illustrations of Allison Lucas are gratefully acknowledged.

References and Suggested Reading

Brickman, K. R., Rega, P., Koltz, M., and Guiness, M.: Analysis of growth plate abnormalities following intraosseous infusion through the proximal tibial epiphysis in pigs. Ann. Emerg. Med. 17:121, 1988.

Hodge, D.: Intraosseous infusions: A review. Pediatr. Emerg. Care 1:215, 1985.

Hodge, D., Delgado-Paredes, C., and Fleisher, G.: Intraosseous infusion flow rates in hypovolemic "pediatric" dogs. Ann. Emerg. Med. 16:305, 1987.

Okrasinski, E. B., Krahwinkel, D. J., and Sanders, W. L.: Resuscitation of hemorrhagic shock by intraosseous infusions of hypertonic saline and dextrans. Vet. Surg. (in press).

Otto, C. M., Kaufman, G. M., and Crowe, D. T.: Intraosseous infusions of therapeutics. Compend. Cont. Ed. Vet. 11(4):421, 1989.

Ritchie, B., Otto, C. M., Latimer, K., Crowe, D. T.: Intraosseous infusions in birds. Comp. Cont. Ed. Pract. Vet. 12:55, 1990.

Shoor, P. M., Berryhill, R. E., and Beaumof, J. L.: Intraosseous infusion: Pressure-flow relationship and pharmacokinetics. J. Trauma 19:772, 1979.

Spivey, W. H., Lathers, C. M., Malone, D., et al.: Comparison of intraosseous, central and peripheral routes of administration of sodium bicarbonate during CPR in pigs. Ann. Emerg. Med. 14:1135, 1985.

Spivey, W. H., Unger, H. D., McNamara, R. M., et al.: The effect of intraosseous sodium bicarbonate on bone in swine. Ann. Emerg. Med. 16:773, 1987.

Tocantins, L. M., O'Neill, J. F., and Price, A. H.: Infusions of blood and other fluids via the bone marrow in traumatic shock and other forms of peripheral circulatory failure. Ann. Surg. 114:1085, 1941.

NEUROLOGIC MANAGEMENT FOLLOWING CARDIAC ARREST AND RESUSCITATION

DEBORAH R. VAN PELT,
and WAYNE E. WINGFIELD
Fort Collins, Colorado

One of the most frequent complications after cardiopulmonary arrest and resuscitation is the development of neurologic deficits. Unfortunately, return of spontaneous circulation (ROSC) does not ensure a neurologically intact patient. Many exciting new therapies are being evaluated to determine their effects on cerebral recovery after episodes of hypoxia. The effectiveness of many of these therapies, although promising, is still unproved and their use in clinical patients remains controversial. This article reviews the physiology of cerebral blood flow and metabolism, the pathophysiology of cerebral ischemia, and the forms of treatment that may help to preserve neurologic function after ROSC.

Table 1. *Factors Affecting Cerebral Blood Flow*

Cardiac output
Cerebrovascular resistance
  Cerebral metabolic requirement for oxygen
  Pa_{O_2}
  Pa_{CO_2}
  Cerebral perfusion pressure

CEREBRAL BLOOD FLOW AND METABOLISM

Consumption of energy by the brain depends on two factors: the energy necessary to maintain cellular integrity ("residual metabolism") and the energy needed for the generation of electrophysiologic signals and maintenance of neuronal function ("activation metabolism"). Normally, 45 to 50% of the oxygen consumed by the brain is necessary to maintain cellular integrity. The brain has limited stores of high-energy phosphates (adenosine triphosphate [ATP]), no oxygen stores, and minimal glucose reserves relative to its high rate of consumption. The brain is therefore very dependent on the circulation of blood for the continued substrate delivery required to maintain neuronal function and cellular integrity.

The carotid and vertebral arteries are the main sources of cerebral blood flow (CBF), which normally demands approximately 15% of the total cardiac output. Most vessels within the brain are "end arteries" (i.e., they lack collateral blood supply), making the brain extremely sensitive to the effects of hypoxia and the development of ischemia. The cerebrovascular resistance (CVR) is the main factor controlling CBF (Table 1). The CVR is in turn affected by changes in the cerebral metabolic requirement for oxygen ($CMRO_2$), the partial pressure of oxygen in arterial blood (Pa_{O_2}), the partial pressure of carbon dioxide in arterial blood (Pa_{CO_2}), and the cerebral perfusion pressure.

The $CMRO_2$ is mainly dependent on brain temperature and electrical activity. Hypothermia decreases oxygen requirements for both residual and activation metabolism. Profound depression of brain electrical activity, such as that seen with deep thiopental anesthesia, can decrease the $CMRO_2$ by as much as one-half, while seizure activity (the extreme of increased brain electrical activity) can markedly increase the $CMRO_2$. Under normal conditions, CBF and $CMRO_2$ are tightly coupled; as $CMRO_2$ increases or decreases, so does CBF. The mechanism of this coupling is thought to involve the local release of adenosine (Prough and Rogers, 1989).

Severe reduction Pa_{O_2} is associated with a dramatic increase in CBF; the latter increases substantially as Pa_{O_2} drops to below 50 to 60 mm Hg. Much of the change produced in CBF by changes in Pa_{O_2} also appears to be mediated by the local release of adenosine.

CBF is extremely sensitive to changes in Pa_{CO_2}. Increasing concentrations of carbon dioxide, within the cerebrospinal fluid (CSF) cause increased hydrogen ion concentration, a decrease in CVR, and a subsequent increase in CBF. Maximal vasodilation is thought to occur at Pa_{CO_2} values greater than 60 to 70 mm Hg. Because rapid changes in Pa_{CO_2} produce rapid changes in CBF and cerebral blood volume, acute hypocarbia (decreased Pa_{CO_2}) may be effective in temporarily reducing intracranial pressure.

The cerebral circulation has autoregulatory controls, in that constant blood flow is maintained in the face of changes in systemic arterial blood pressure. Little change in CBF occurs over a broad range of systemic arterial pressures (50 to 150 mm Hg), as CVR varies directly with cerebral perfusion pressure to maintain a constant CBF. Changes in intracranial pressure (normal = 5 to 10 mm Hg) therefore play a minimal role in the regulation of CBF.

PATHOPHYSIOLOGY OF ISCHEMIC BRAIN INJURY

Sudden circulatory arrest depletes the brain oxygen supply and causes subsequent unconsciousness within 10 to 15 secs. Exhaustion of brain glucose and ATP stores follows within 1 to 4 mins. Disruption of energy-dependent ionic gradients occurs, with acute increases in extracellular potassium concentration and intracellular concentrations of calcium, sodium, and chloride. Tissue edema occurs secondary to the loss of sodium/potassium ATPase activity and the accumulation of intracellular sodium and water .

It has been postulated that loss of calcium homeostasis plays a major role in the development of postarrest neurologic dysfunction (Fig. 1). Additional factors thought to be involved in the development of postischemic neurologic disease include oxygen-derived free radicals, prostaglandins, hyperglycemia, and the presence of incomplete ischemia. Detrimental effects of increased concentrations of intracellular calcium include neurotransmitter release, activation of phospholipase A_2 (with subsequent production of prostaglandins, endoperoxides and leukotrienes), protein phosphorylation, proteolysis, energy depletion, malfunction of calcium-regulated enzymes, and vasospasm of the cerebrovascular smooth muscle.

Changes in vascular smooth muscle tone secondary to an increase in intracellular calcium levels may contribute to the vascular changes observed after complete global ischemia and the re-establishment of spontaneous circulation. An initial period

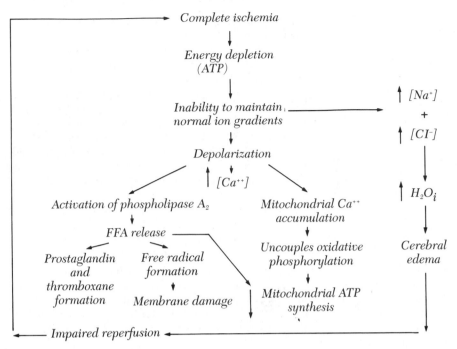

Figure 1. Role of calcium in ischemic injury. Energy depletion results in inability to maintain normal ion gradients, with subsequent development of cerebral edema and free-radical formation. ATP, adenosine triphosphate; $[Ca^{++}]_i$, intracellular calcium; $[Cl^-]_i$, intracellular chloride; FFA, free fatty acids; H_2O_i, intracellular water; $[Na^+]_i$, intracellular sodium.

of "reactive hyperemia" lasting 15 to 20 minutes occurs owing to a temporary decrease in vascular tone and blood viscosity as blood washes out of the microcirculation. A period of postischemic hypoperfusion ("no reflow") follows. Calcium activation of the contractile mechanism in the endothelial cells results in vasoconstriction, while aggregation of platelets and granulocytes also impedes CBF. Normal cerebral metabolic activity must proceed in the face of reduced CBF (30 to 50% of normal).

MANIFESTATIONS OF BRAIN ISCHEMIA

Constant monitoring of the patient's status during and immediately after cardiopulmonary resuscitation (CPR) allows prompt recognition of potentially treatable sequelae of cardiopulmonary arrest (CPA). Important clinical parameters to be assessed in these animals include the level of consciousness, voluntary and involuntary body movements, extraocular reflexes, pupil position, size and the presence of the pupillary light reflex, respiratory rate and pattern, and heart rate and rhythm. Acute changes or progressive deterioration in any of these parameters may indicate progressive neurologic disease.

The subcortical nuclei are extremely sensitive to hypoxia; ischemia to these areas may result in memory loss, movement disorders, weakness, and mild sensory deficits. Loss of the corneal reflex is indicative of herniation and brainstem compression. Bilateral pupillary constriction is typically an early response to cerebral hypoxia, while with complete cerebral ischemia, bilateral pupillary dilation oc-

curs. Persistent flaccid paralysis, cranial nerve areflexia, and complete unresponsiveness signal brain death.

Signs of neurologic injury may not be evident for up to 72 hr after resuscitation. The development of cerebral edema associated with compromised CBF can delay the onset of clinical signs. Transient restoration of near-normal mentation followed by gradual deterioration suggests the maturation of ischemic injuries or continuation of the processes responsible for cellular injury.

PATIENT MANAGEMENT AND POSTISCHEMIC THERAPY

Therapy directed toward maximizing neurologic recovery can be divided into three distinct phases. Therapy instituted *before* the ischemic insult is referred to as cerebral protection. Hypothermia has been found to be protective in the face of complete global ischemia, while barbiturate administration offers protection in the face of focal ischemia. Cerebral preservation refers to those forms of therapy initiated *during* the ischemic insult. The "gold standard" of cerebral preservation is the early initiation of CPR and rapid ROSC. The onset of cardiorespiratory arrest must be recognized quickly, and prompt and aggressive resuscitative measures instituted immediately. Simultaneous compression/ventilation and open-chest CPR may improve CBF better than conventional closed-chest CPR. Compression rates of 80 to 120/min are recommended to maximize CBF and cerebral oxygen delivery during CPR. Therapy directed at improving neurologic outcome *after* ROSC is referred to as cerebral resuscitation. With ROSC, prevention and limitation of secondary insults (such as hypotension, recurrence of CPA, hyperglycemia, and hypoxia) are the key strategies in optimizing CBF and neurologic outcome. This phase of therapy is controversial: many of the drug treatments proposed for use during this period are still clinically unproved.

Treatment aimed at cerebral resuscitation can be divided into two categories. Those therapies shown to be effective and universally accepted for postischemic encephalopathy include fluid therapy, hyperventilation, diuresis, and corticosteroid administration. Those therapies, as yet unproved but promising, include the administration of calcium channel blockers, iron chelators, and free radical scavengers.

Cerebral Resuscitation

TRADITIONAL THERAPY

CBF is encouraged by supporting systemic hemodynamics with the use of intravenous fluids. The goal of fluid therapy is to maximize cerebral oxygen delivery without taxing the cardiovascular system. Measurement of central venous pressure provides a reasonable estimate of the ability of the cardiovascular system to handle the delivered volume of fluids. Overzealous fluid administration is to be avoided because crystalloid fluids diffuse out of the vascular space into the interstitium, increasing the central nervous system interstitial fluid volume and intracranial pressure (ICP). It has been suggested that the administration of hypertonic fluids may decrease the prevalence of elevated ICP by temporarily retaining the administered fluids within the vasculature. However, studies in which hypertonic fluids were administered to dogs in the postischemic state failed to support this hypothesis consistently (Poole et al., 1986).

Control of the airway and support of the respiratory system is essential in animals after CPR. Ideally, endotracheal intubation and ventilatory support should be maintained in all patients until adequate spontaneous ventilatory efforts can be documented. In patients with inadequate ventilation or those developing pulmonary edema or aspiration, sedation or neuromuscular blockade may be necessary in order that mechanical ventilation (positive end-expiratory pressure may be instituted (see this volume, p. 98). The goal of ventilatory therapy is to maintain the Pa_{CO_2} between 25 and 35 mm Hg and Pa_{O_2} at 100 mm Hg, maximizing CBF and cerebral oxygenation. Moderate hyperventilation increases intracranial compliance but may not alter the long-term neurologic outcome (Bircher, 1989). This is probably because increased ICP may be an atypical problem after cardiac arrest.

Reduction of ICP and maintenance of cerebral perfusion pressure after CPR can be accomplished by means of diuresis. Mannitol, 1 to 2 gm/kg IV, acts as an osmotic diuretic and may prevent or decrease fatal brain swelling after ischemia. Mannitol administration may transiently increase cerebral blood volume, but once diuresis is accomplished, hypovolemia may be precipitated. An additional potential benefit of the use of mannitol is its ability to act as a free-radical scavenger. Furosemide, 1 to 2 mg/kg IV, functions as a loop diuretic, thereby facilitating sodium and chloride excretion by the kidneys, and as a weak carbonic anhydrase agonist. The carbonic anhydrase activity decreases sodium uptake by the brain, with a subsequent decrease in cerebral swelling. ICP is decreased without the transient increase in cerebral blood volume associated with mannitol administration.

Corticosteroid therapy has been proposed to preserve neurologic integrity by multiple mechanisms, including maintenance of membrane integrity, decreased prostaglandin and oxygen free-radical formation, stabilization of lysosomal membranes, and preservation of vascular integrity. Unfortunately, the success of corticosteroid administration in decreasing postischemic edema and improving survival in animals after CPR has not been documented consistently. Despite these conflicting results, the administration of a rapidly acting corticosteroid (dexamethasone sodium phosphate, 0.5 mg/kg IV) is recommended immediately after CPA.

EXPERIMENTAL THERAPIES

Sedative therapy, in the form of narcotic or barbiturate anesthesia, decreases both CBF and $CMRO_2$. This action apparently occurs as a result of these drugs causing cerebral vasoconstriction as well as decreased brain electrical activity (decreased activation metabolism). Despite the associated decrease in ICP, barbiturate loading has not improved the outcome of cases in which ICP was elevated secondary to head trauma or anoxic/ischemic injury after cardiac arrest or near-drowning (Prough and Rogers, 1989). The questionable efficacy and significant cardiovascular depression associated with barbiturate administration suggest that its routine use in the treatment of cerebral hypoxia cannot be recommended.

The detrimental effects of intracellular calcium accumulation during hypoxia suggest that calcium channel blockers could be potentially useful in the treatment of cerebral ischemia. These drugs appear to prevent calcium-induced vasospasm, calcium loading of the mitochondria, and activation of phospholipase A_2, thereby maintaining CBF and decreasing membrane damage and cytotoxicity. *In vivo* studies have shown that the ability of these drugs to improve neurologic recovery and inhibit calcium accumulation in the brain during postischemic reperfusion is extremely variable. This may be because several other routes of calcium entry into the cell are not blocked by the calcium channel blockers (Kochanek, 1988; Shapiro, 1985; Steen et al., 1985). The inconsistent effects on neurologic outcome, and the potential adverse side effects of hypotension and decreased myocardial contractility associated with administration of these drugs, suggest that further *in vivo* studies are warranted before calcium channel blockers can be recommended for the routine treatment of postischemic hypoxia of the central nervous system.

Iron chelators and free-radical scavengers show promise as drugs for the treatment of postischemic encephalopathy. Free iron is released by calcium-mediated mitochondrial injury and participates in the generation of oxygen-derived free radicals. Desferoxamine is an iron chelator that crosses the blood-brain barrier and promotes urinary iron excretion. Although administration of desferoxamine in dogs with complete global ischemia increased post-ischemic CBF, improvement in long-term survival and neurologic recovery has not been consistently demonstrated (Kochanek, 1988; Rosenthal et al., 1990). Free-radical scavengers such as superoxide dismutase and xanthine oxidase inhibitors such as allopurinol inhibit lipid peroxidation and subsequent membrane damage. Once again, administration of these drugs in postischemic situations has not convincingly improved neurologic outcome. It may be that antiradical therapy may achieve a favorable effect only if administered *before* reperfusion and reoxygenation (Kochanek, 1988; Safar, 1988).

Extracerebral Organ Support

Maintenance of adequate extracerebral organ function must not be overlooked in the postarrest patient. The cardiovascular system should be closely monitored in order to maintain blood pressure, normalize oxygen transport, correct hypovolemia, and prevent recurrent CPA. Venous blood gas determinations provide an assessment of the adequacy of tissue oxygenation, and measurement of central venous pressure and systemic arterial blood pressures helps to assess the need for fluid and pressor therapy.

The respiratory system must also be closely monitored (again, via the use of blood gases), and mechanical ventilation instituted if necessary. Maneuvers to prevent pulmonary atelectasis, such as elevation of the head and turning the patient from side to side every 3 to 4 hr, help to maintain adequate gas exchange.

Urinary output should be monitored and maintained at or above 1 ml/kg/hr. Appropriate measures (fluid therapy, diuresis, dopamine infusion) should be taken to maintain this minimal output.

If the animal is to be maintained on ventilatory support for several days or is unable to eat on its own for some other reason, nutritional support becomes an important consideration and may require the placement of a nasogastric or gastrostomy tube.

SUMMARY

Re-establishment or maintenance of normal neurologic function following cardiac arrest requires provision for adequate CBF and cerebral oxygenation. Effective CPR techniques that provide rapid return of spontaneous circulation and extracerebral organ support, including aggressive therapy directed toward the underlying disease that precipitated the cardiac arrest, provide the best hope of a successful neurologic recovery. Current recommendations in the treatment of cerebral hypoxia associated with CPA/CPR include the administration of intravenous fluids, diuretics, and corticosteroids and the initiation of hyperventilation. Therapies in which calcium-channel blockers, iron chelators, or free-radical scavengers are administered appear promising, but their benefits remain unproved.

References and Suggested Reading

Bircher, N. G: Neurologic management following cardiac arrest. Crit. Care Clin. 5:773, 1989.
Brain-oriented life support guidelines.
Kochanek, P. M.: Novel pharmacologic approaches to brain resuscitation after cardiorespiratory arrest in the pediatric patient. Crit. Care Clin. 4:661, 1988.
Describes mechanisms of cerebral injury, with emphasis on the role of calcium, oxygen free radicals, and prostaglandins.
Muir, W. W.: Brain hypoperfusion post-resuscitation. Vet. Clin. North Am. Small Anim. Pract. 19:1151, 1989.
Concise review of cerebral physiology, pathophysiology, and treatment modalities.
Poole, G. V., Jr., Johnson, J. C., Prough, D. S., et al.: Cerebral hemodynamics after hemorrhagic shock: Effects of the type of resuscitation fluid. Crit. Care Med. 14:629, 1986.
Compares cerebral resuscitation with lactated Ringer's solution vs. hetastarch and their effects on cerebral blood flow and oxygen delivery.
Prough, D. S., and Rogers, A. T.: Physiology and pharmacology of cerebral blood flow and metabolism. Crit. Care Clin. 5:713, 1989.
Describes physiologic regulation and pharmacologic manipulation of cerebral blood flow and metabolism.
Rosenthal, R. E., Marshall, G. H., Jr., and Shesser, R. F.: Prevention of cardiac arrest–induced neurologic injury and delayed mortality by a high molecular weight chelator of iron. (Abstract.) Ann. Emerg. Med. 19:468, 1990.
Evaluates use of an iron chelator in preserving neurologic function after cardiac arrest.
Safar, P.: Cerebral resuscitation after cardiac arrest: Summaries and suggestions. Am. J. Emerg. Med. 2:198, 1983.
Summary of a symposium dealing specifically with complete global ischemia and its treatment; provides a concise summary of many promising new therapies in the field of cerebral resuscitation.

Safar, P.: Resuscitation from clinical death: Pathophysiologic limits and therapeutic potentials. Crit. Care Clin. 16:923, 1988.
Describes the effects of CPR on cerebral blood flow and the pathophysiology of cerebral ischemia, and summarizes promising pharmacologic approaches to cerebral resuscitation.
Shapiro, H. M.: Post-cardiac arrest therapy: Calcium entry blockade and brain resuscitation. Anesthesiology 62:384, 1985.
Reviews calcium-related pathways activated by brain ischemia.

Steen, P. A., Gisvold, S. E., Milde, J. H., et al.: Nimodipine improves outcome when given after complete cerebral ischemia in patients. Anesthesiology 62:406, 1985.
Administration of nimodipine to monkeys after global ischemia results in improved neurologic function after resuscitation.

NUTRITIONAL MANAGEMENT OF THE CRITICAL CARE PATIENT

MARY ANNA LABATO

North Grafton, Massachusetts

Often, the medical and surgical needs of critical care or seriously ill patients are given attention while their nutritional needs are overlooked. Malnutrition often results, and the consequences may be disastrous. It is imperative to avoid becoming so involved with the medical and surgical management of the patient that nutritional support is forgotten. Critical care nutrition can be maintained in both institutional and small practices and, in some instances, may be continued at home by conscientious pet owners.

CONSEQUENCES OF MALNUTRITION

Starvation causes a gradual decrease in metabolic rate. The breakdown of body proteins is minimized because the animal's energy needs are provided primarily by the oxidation of fats. A loss of amino acids for glucose production occurs in the liver. Providing even small amounts of carbohydrates during starvation has a remarkable sparing action and avoids this otherwise obligatory loss. Protein-calorie malnutrition (PCM) is the progressive loss of lean body mass and adipose tissue due to inadequate intake or increased demand, or both, for protein and calories.

Carbohydrate, Fat, and Protein Metabolism

The body metabolizes carbohydrates as an immediate energy source. In addition, carbohydrate is stored as glycogen, a short-term reserve. Excess carbohydrate is converted into neutral fat, an animal's long-term energy reserve. The total energy reserve created by glycogenesis, representing approximately enough stored energy to meet an animal's needs for one day, is relatively small. To protect the glycogen reserve for emergencies when the source of glucose is temporarily depleted, the body manufactures glucose by utilizing hydrolytic products of lipids and protein.

Lipid is the chief stored energy substrate in the body. The amount of lipid stored in the body varies from animal to animal. In addition to being important as an energy reserve, lipid typically supplies a significant portion of routine dietary caloric intake. As an energy fuel, lipid supplies about 9 kcal/gm, more than twice the caloric output per gram of either carbohydrate or protein.

Relationship Between Protein and Energy

The protein content of a healthy animal is approximately 14 to 20% of lean body weight. Because amino acids are not stored in the body, the protein compartment must be maintained by daily intake. Depending on an animal's metabolic status, ingested protein may be used for protein synthesis; or if the body requires more energy than is obtained from carbohydrate and lipid intake, ingested protein may be used for energy. About one third of an animal's total body protein content is potentially available as an energy source in cases of extreme need. Another pathway by which ingested protein participates in body energy metabolism is lipo-

Portions of this article are reprinted with permission from Labato, M.A.: Nutritional intervention. Pet Veterinarian 2(3):31, 1990.

genesis. Ingested protein in excess of immediate energy and structural needs is stripped of nitrogen and converted to fatty acids for storage as triglycerides, initially through an intermediate step of conversion to glucose.

Once an animal's energy needs are met, ingested protein, in the form of amino acids, may be used for formation, replacement, growth, and repair; the maintenance of blood proteins (albumin, transferrin, fibrinogen, and antibodies); and the manufacture of enzymes. In a healthy animal, ingested protein must supply enough amino acids to maintain a constant level of body protein. To maintain lean body mass, the intake of protein must equal or exceed the breakdown of structural protein. The relationship between energy and protein requirements varies, depending on whether the patient is normal, nutritionally depleted, or hypermetabolic (as in sepsis, acute renal failure, fever, or burns). Hypermetabolic patients have a pronounced inefficiency in handling dietary protein.

Nitrogen Balance

Nitrogen balance may be neutral, positive, or negative. Neutral nitrogen balance indicates that protein synthesis is equal to protein degradation. Positive nitrogen balance indicates that protein synthesis exceeds protein degradation. This occurrence usually suggests tissue growth or rebuilding. Negative nitrogen balance is a sign of protein degradation exceeding protein synthesis. The most likely cause of this catabolic state is carbohydrate and lipid intake insufficient to meet the animal's energy requirements, which results in the diversion of protein from structural uses to energy supply. In addition, inadequate protein ingestion may arise from dietary problems and further contribute to a negative balance.

Starvation

During periods of starvation, body protein is split into amino acids, which can be (1) oxidized directly, (2) stripped of nitrogen and converted to glucose, or (3) re-assembled as protein to help maintain vital organs. The pattern of protein catabolism varies with the duration of starvation. Body protein is considered the final energy store because fat is utilized in preference to protein. Of the total protein content in the body, only a fraction (approximately one third) is available for energy production.

Response to Injury

The metabolic response to sepsis, trauma, or severe illness consists of hypermetabolism, hyper-

glycemia, glucose intolerance, and the use of skeletal proteins as energy substrate (Allen, 1989). Metabolic changes following severe injury, surgical intervention, and critical systemic illness differ markedly from those that occur following starvation. Pain, low–blood-flow states, acidosis, hypercapnia, and sepsis cause neuroendocrine activation, which results in the release of catecholamines, glucocorticoids, glucagon, antidiuretic hormone, and aldosterone. These counter-regulatory hormones cause the metabolic rate to increase in direct proportion to the severity of the stimulus. When the increase in metabolic rate is associated with a lack of nutritional intake, fat oxidation quickly achieves a maximum rate, and body protein is rapidly utilized in gluconeogenesis.

The administration of small amounts of carbohydrate, such as that provided by intravenous infusion of isotonic glucose solutions, has little, if any, sparing effect on body proteins during periods of PCM. There is some evidence that continued infusion of these glucose solutions, especially in amounts that exceed requirements to maintain blood glucose concentrations, further increases the metabolic rate and the release of insulin. As a consequence of the antilipolytic action of insulin in this circumstance, less use of endogenous fat stores occurs, and increased protein catabolism can occur in the absence of insulin resistance.

Adverse Effects of Protein-Calorie Malnutrition

A number of adverse consequences are associated with PCM. These include impaired cell-mediated immunity, increased susceptibility to infection (impaired humoral immunity), delayed wound and fracture healing, shock, increased prevalence of dehiscence, and poor tolerance to chemotherapy and radiation therapy (Wheeler and McGuire, 1989).

Inadequate food intake during a period of increased metabolic demand has adverse consequences involving several organ systems. Both depressed synthesis and increased degradation of skeletal muscle occur. Cardiac muscle is less able to use lactic acid. Electrophysiologic changes become apparent within a few days of PCM. In the pulmonary system, reduced lung elasticity develops. The kidney becomes a gluconeogenic organ under periods of nutritional stress. The kidney also becomes less able to respond to acid-base abnormalities. Pronounced effects may occur in the gastrointestinal tract. Gastric emptying and gastrointestinal transit times may be prolonged. The lack of local trophic and nutritional factors causes flattening of intestinal villi and reduced absorptive area. Carbohydrate digestion and fat digestion are impaired.

The immune system may be profoundly affected by PCM as revealed by impaired antibody and interferon synthesis, decreased T-lymphocyte numbers, decreased immunoglobulin A(IgA) production, and decreased inflammatory response. Leukocyte function may also be decreased because many leukocyte products (immunoglobulins, lymphokines, and bacteriocidal enzymes) are proteins. Deficiencies of individual amino acids lead to alterations in immune function similar to those described for PCM. Cell-mediated immunity may become impaired after only 3 to 5 days of anorexia accompanying PCM. Cell-mediated immunity is often compromised as indicated by decreased lymphocyte activation. The total lymphocyte count may be normal or decreased, but the proportion of T cells is often decreased with PCM. Atrophy of the thymus, spleen, and peripheral lymph nodes has been observed in clinical cases (Burkholder and Swecker, 1990). Although beta cells are responsible for immunoglobulin production, T-cell dysfunction in protein-deficient animals can result in decreased immunoglobulin production.

PCM affects humoral immunity. In most clinical cases, total serum immunoglobulin concentrations are normal or increased, yet these immunoglobulins bind antigen with less affinity than antibodies from normal individuals. Salivary, lacrimal, and mucosal secretory lgA levels have been shown to be decreased in PCM. Some researchers speculate that PCM prevents the formation of the secretory protein component of IgA or alters the number or type of leukocytes present in mucosal linings (Burkholder and Swecker, 1990).

Concentrations of complement proteins, as well as the bactericidal activity of neutrophils and monocytes, are decreased in PCM. The degree of compromise in complement opsonization and cytolytic activity is correlated with the severity of malnutrition. Transferrin concentrations may be decreased, allowing enhanced bacterial proliferation due to increased availability of iron.

Protein-Calorie Malnutrition and Surgical Patients

Nutritional status of surgical patients should be determined. Human patients with PCM have a higher incidence of infections, decreased wound healing, and dehiscence, resulting in prolonged hospitalizations. Nutritional assessment of the surgical patient should be based on the history, physical examination, laboratory data, and diagnosis (see this volume, p. 32). In the nutritional assessment, the presence of muscle wasting implies insufficient protein intake. Decreased muscle mass probably occurs prior to a decrease in serum protein concentrations because muscle wasting occurs as an energy-saving adaptation. Patients with muscle wasting, however, are poor surgical candidates because

their protein reserves have been used to maintain the higher-priority proteins (i.e., enzymes and plasma proteins). In such animals, nutritional support lasting 2 to 3 days is recommended, provided that surgical intervention can be safely postponed (Remillard and Martin, 1990).

Causes of Protein-Calorie Malnutrition

Causes of PCM include inadequate intake or absorption of nutrients, an increased metabolic demand for nutrients, or a combination of these conditions. Inadequate intake may be due to starvation, severe anorexia, or difficulties in prehension, mastication, or swallowing of food. Several gastrointestinal disorders may lead to PCM, namely, obstructive lesions, neoplastic lesions, and inflammatory bowel disease. Metabolic demand may be increased in the face of trauma, sepsis, burns, or severe illness.

Surgical manipulation results in at least a temporary metabolic disturbance. Complications seen after gastrointestinal surgery in animals include paralytic ileus, peritonitis, and leakage of gastrointestinal contents from anastomotic sites. These patients are nutritionally stressed and require some type of nutritional support.

Burns are an example of a severe nutritional stress. Extensive burns produce tissue necrosis and destruction that result in high metabolic demands, often complicated by sepsis. Skin damage leads to an outpouring of protein-rich fluid. Body heat is lost through water evaporation. The marked anabolic needs required for massive skin regeneration lead to increased energy expenditure.

Animals with malignancies suffer from cancer cachexia, which causes weight loss, protein deficiencies, and immunologic incompetence—conditions complicated by the administration of harsh chemicals and radiation. Cancer cachexia is a paraneoplastic syndrome of progressive weight loss that occurs even in the face of adequate nutritional intake. Human patients with this syndrome have a decreased quality of life, decreased response to treatment, and a decreased survival time when compared with individuals having the same malignancy without cancer cachexia syndrome (Ogilvie and Vail, 1990). There is evidence that nutritional support benefits these patients. Reported benefits include weight gain; increased response to and tolerance of radiation, surgery, and chemotherapy; increased thymic weight; improved immune responsiveness; and improved humoral and cell-mediated immunity (Ogilvie and Vail, 1990).

NUTRITIONAL SUPPORT

Specialized nutrition is the fulfillment of the animal's total daily caloric requirement to avoid or reverse PCM. Indications for nutritional support include (1) serum albumin level less than or equal to 1.5 gm/dl, (2) weight loss greater than 20%, (3) reduced or medically prohibited oral intake for more than 3 to 5 days, and (4) substantial or ongoing protein loss.

The immediate goals of nutritional support are maintenance of protein synthesis and stabilization of the patient's weight. Even obese animals may develop protein malnutrition while adequate energy is provided by large fat stores. The patient must be palpated carefully to detect decreased skeletal muscle mass. In PCM, death usually occurs with the loss of 40 to 50% of lean body weight, usually because of muscle failure (i.e., of the heart or diaphragm).

Clinical Indications

Protein loss is a primary indication for intervention. This loss may be the result of massive acute hemorrhage, chronic hemorrhage, severe and chronic diarrhea (infiltrative or inflammatory gastrointestinal disease), or excessive albuminuria.

Another clinical indication for nutritional support is difficulty in eating. This problem may be attributable to mandibular or maxillary fractures; palatal defects; oral, nasal, or esophageal surgical manipulations; stomatitis; or pharyngitis. A disorder that interferes with the prehension, mastication, or swallowing of food for longer than 3 days indicates the need for some form of nutritional support.

Nutritional intervention is indicated in certain neurologic disorders. Animals with head trauma present an excellent example. These patients may be in a semicomatose state for days, preventing their prehension or swallowing of food. As trauma victims, they are frequently in a hypermetabolic state, which represents the body's initial response to the insult. This hypermetabolic state is compounded by the inability to take in food and these animals require nutritional support. Oropharyngeal or cricopharyngeal dysphagia and megaesophagus are additional neurologic disorders that require nutritional intervention.

Animals with certain orthopedic problems may have difficulty eating or may be prevented from assuming a position in which they can reach the food without assistance. Nutritional support must therefore be considered in the treatment plans.

Assessing Nutritional Status

Assessment of the animal's nutritional state requires a complete evaluation of the clinical history, dietary history, physical examination, and laboratory evaluation (Allen, 1989). The clinician should determine the animal's home diet, the animal's hospital diet, the length of time the animal has been anorexic or unable to eat, and whether a change in weight has occurred, and if so, over what period of time. In addition, the clinician should ascertain whether any gastrointestinal problems, such as vomiting or diarrhea, are present, and whether the animal has received drugs that could influence nutrient intake or utilization, such as glucocorticosteroids or cancer chemotherapeutic agents. The clinician needs to determine the underlying disease process, to assess whether the animal is in hypermetabolic state, and to determine the expected duration of inadequate nutritional intake.

Indicators of Nutritional Stress

PROTEINS. Albumin is a relatively poor indicator of early protein malnutrition because serum concentrations change slowly; however, the serum albumin concentration is the best indicator for long-standing PCM. During protein malnutrition, the extracellular fluid compartment expands in relation to total body water. Combined with a decrease in albumin synthesis, this relative expansion of the extracellular fluid compartment leads to significant decreases in serum albumin concentrations. Conditions that can affect serum albumin concentrations include blood loss and hemodilution, overhydration, dehydration, and liver disease. These factors must be taken into consideration when the serum albumin concentration is interpreted (Crowe, 1985). Decreases in albumin concentrations denote prolonged negative nitrogen balance. In the dog, the serum half-life of albumin is 8.2 days. A serum albumin concentration of less than or equal to 1.5 gm/dl is a significant indication for supplementation.

Transferrin is a glycoprotein that transports iron. Transferrin has a shorter half-life and smaller body pool in comparison with albumin. Transferrin is considered to reflect more accurately acute changes in body protein content. Serum transferrin concentrations are best measured by radioimmunodiffusion, although an estimate can be obtained by measuring the total iron-binding capacity (Allen, 1989).

Additional serum proteins that may be indicators of protein-calorie balance are thyroxine-binding prealbumin (TBPA), retinol-binding protein, fibronectin, and somatomedin-C (Allen, 1989; Boosalis et al., 1989; Bounpane et al., 1989; Crowe, 1985; Labato, 1990).

IMMUNE FUNCTION. An animal's nutritional status can be evaluated by examining certain indices of the immune system. Examination of the total lymphocyte count is one of the most practical methods available. The current recommendation in human medicine is to perform total lymphocyte counts and intradermal skin testing. In humans, a lymphocyte count of less than 800/µl has been found to correlate well with severe immunologic incompetence of cells caused by protein depletion. In dogs and cats, a total lymphocyte count of less than 800/µl may also be used as an indicator of immune suppression (Crowe, 1985). The lymphocyte reduction due to malnutrition predominantly involves T cells (Allen, 1989; Crowe, 1985).

PHYSICAL MEASUREMENTS. Human nutritional status is often estimated by determination of fat reserves via skin fold measurement and of protein status via 24-hr urine creatinine excretion. These techniques have not been well standardized in veterinary medicine because of the size and shape variations in animal patients.

At this time, protein and immunologic parameters appear to offer the best methods for assessing and monitoring nutritional status in the veterinary patient. Values for some of these parameters, such as albumin concentration, total iron-binding capacity, and total lymphocyte counts, are easily obtained in a clinical setting.

DETERMINATION OF ENERGY REQUIREMENTS

Nutritional support does not equal administration of intravenous fluids with dextrose. It is impossible to meet the caloric requirement of a stressed animal with just 5% dextrose solution.

A number of different methods have been used to determine the energy needs of individual animals. As a general rule, the basal caloric requirements have been approximated so that a large-breed dog requires 40 kcal/kg/day, a medium-breed dog requires 50 kcal/kg/day, a small-breed dog requires 60 kcal/kg/day, and a cat requires 70 kcal/kg/day.

Another formula used to determine energy needs is based on the basal energy requirement (BER). The BER is the number of calories expended by an animal while awake and resting in a thermoneutral environment. The BER is determined using the following formula:

$$BER(kcal/24\ hr) = 70 \times BW(kg)^{0.75}$$

This formula is based on two parameters: 70 is a K factor for placental animals that is derived from specific core body temperature set points; the body weight (BW) raised to the power of 0.75 is an estimation of biologic size derived from the rate of oxygen consumption in relation to body size. If the animal is heavier than 2 kg, an alternate formula can be used:

$$BER = [30 \times BW(kg)] + 70$$

The maintenance energy requirement (MER) includes BER and the energy expended by normal animals in the process of obtaining and using food. In an ill animal, MER may also be referred to as the illness energy requirement (IER). The MER values of adult hospitalized patients are approximately 25% greater than their BER values. For an ill animal, the MER is computed as:

$$MER = BER \times stress\ factor$$

Stress factors are cage rest (1.25), postoperative periods (1.25 to 1.35), trauma or cancer (1.35 to 1.50), sepsis (1.50 to 1.70), and burns (1.7 to 2.0). In general, for an adult hospitalized cat without sepsis, the stress factor 1.4 should be used in determining MER. An average increase to the MER of 13% in energy expenditure is associated with each degree Celsius of fever (Crowe, 1985).

ROUTES OF NUTRITIONAL SUPPORT

The two main routes of nutritional support are the enteral and parenteral routes. A well-stated axiom is, "If the gut works, use it!" In other words, employ the enteral route whenever possible. Enteral nutritional support is physiologic and economical, and it entails few complications. It can easily be used in a busy clinical setting.

Enteral Routes

OROGASTRIC ROUTE. The advantage of orogastric feeding is that cost-efficient commercial pet foods or liquid diets may be used. The major disadvantage is patient stress, as larger dogs and cats may struggle excessively. Orogastric tube feedings can be performed in neonates and in many small dogs. Commercially available tubes with weighted tips (Travasorb Enteral Feeding Tube Placement Kits, Baxter Healthcare Corp; Kangaroo Weighted Tip Enteral Feeding Tube, Sherwood Medical) or fine-bore red rubber catheters (Bard Urological Catheter, Bard Urological Division, Bard, Inc.; Feeding Tube and Urethral Catheter, Sovereign, Monoject) may be employed.

NASOGASTRIC ROUTE. The nasogastric tube is well tolerated by both dogs and cats. Six to eight French polyurethane or polyvinyl chloride tubes are commonly used. Topical ophthalmic anesthetic or 2% lidocaine gel in the nostril aids in tube advancement. The head of the animal should be maintained in a neutral position to aid passage of the tube into the esophagus. Complications seen with the use of nasogastric tubes include dacryocystitis, nasal irritations, esophagitis, and vomiting (Armstrong et al., 1990) (see this volume, p. 32).

PHARYNGOSTOMY. Pharyngostomy tube feeding involves the surgical placement of a feeding tube through the pharynx and its passage into the lower esophagus (Armstrong, et al., 1990). The use of pharyngostomy or nasogastric feedings makes it difficult to determine when anorexia is resolving. The presence of a tube in the pharynx or esophagus may discourage some animals, especially cats, from eating voluntarily. Complications associated with pharyngostomy tubes have included potential airway occlusion, vomiting, mechanical irritation of the esophagus, gastroesophageal reflux, and aspiration pneumonia. Because of these limitations, the placement of pharyngostomy tubes has largely been superseded by the techniques of percutaneous tube gastrostomy (Armstrong and Lippert, 1988).

GASTROSTOMY. Gastrostomy tubes bypass the oral cavity, pharynx, and esophagus. Gastrostomy tubes may be placed through a left flank laparotomy or through a percutaneous approach using an endoscope. The advantages of a gastrostomy tube include an ability to initiate feeding shortly after the tube is introduced and the placement of food and medication directly into the stomach. Dogs and cats seem to tolerate gastrostomy tubes well, and animals can be sent home with the tube in place for long-term home care. Gastrostomy tubes have been left in place without problems for as long as 3 months. A silicone Foley urethral catheter (nos. 18 to 22 French for cats, and nos. 20 to 30 French for dogs) seems best for surigical placement. For percutaneous placement, a mushroom-tip urologic catheter (Bard Urological Division, Bard, Inc.) should be employed (Armstrong et al., 1990).

Complications associated with gastrostomy tubes have ranged from minor problems, such as the tube's becoming blocked or being chewed by the animal, to major problems, such as serious wound infection and peritonitis. In addition, gastric outflow tract obstruction may occur with overdistention of the balloon at the catheter tip. Vomiting and diarrhea are observed as common problems and are often secondary to diet formulations and the volumes instilled. Following long-term placement, excoriation of the skin around the gastrostomy tube is common.

JEJUNOSTOMY. Jejunostomy tube feeding requires a functional small intestine and a laparotomy for tube placement. Needle-catheter jejunostomy tubes are most frequently employed in cases of gastroparesis or proximal bowel resection. A 12- to 18-gauge intravenous catheter or a No. 5 French, 36-inch infant feeding tube is tunneled aborally through the antimesenteric border of the jejunum (Armstrong et al., 1990; Wheeler and McGuire, 1989). The ostomy site on the intestine is sutured to the parietal peritoneum/abdominal wall after the catheter has been tunneled through the body wall. The catheter is sutured to the skin. In addition, only elemental diets should be fed through jejunostomy tubes. Complications noted with jejunostomy tube feeding have included diarrhea, vomiting, hyperglycemia, electrolyte disturbances, hypoglycemia following withdrawal of the elemental diet, dislodgment or kinking of the catheter, and perforation of the intestine.

ENTERAL DIETS

The ideal tube-feeding diet is well tolerated, easily absorbed, and complete. In addition, it is inexpensive, has a long shelf life, is easy to use, and does not support rapid bacterial growth. Enteral diets for tube feeding may consist of canned cat or dog food that is mixed into a soupy gruel, baby food mixed into a gruel, or commercial liquid preparations. Vitamin-calorie supplement pastes (Nutrical, Evsco Pharmaceuticals) are not intended for total nutritional support.

Commercial enteral feeding preparations fall into two categories. The meal replacement formulations require some digestion (Osmolite, Ross; Osmolite HN, Ross; Ensure, Ross; CliniCare Canine and CliniCare Feline, PetAg, Inc.; Renal Care, PetAg. Inc.). The elemental formulations or monomeric diets do not require digestion (Peptamen, Baxter; Vivonex TEN, Norwich Eaton; Ensure Plus, Ross). The only liquid diets formulated for dogs and cats are CliniCare and Renal Care (PetAg, Inc.). The meal replacement formulations are composed of low-osmolarity, relatively inexpensive hydrolysates of protein, starches, and oligosaccharides. The elemental diets are low-residue, highly osmotic, and relatively expensive, and they are composed of amino acids, monosaccharides, disaccharides, and minimal fat. Peptamin (Baxter) is an exception in that it is a monomeric diet that is isotonic, containing primarily dipeptides, tripeptides, glucose, and medium-chain triglycerides.

ADMINISTRATION OF ENTERAL PRODUCTS

To avoid problems with abdominal cramping, vomiting, and diarrhea when using enteral products, the total requirement should not be administered on the first day. In cases of prolonged anorexia, one should start with 25% of the total daily volume requirement on day 1, increase to 50% on day 2, and increase to the full volume requirement on day 3. If the animal has been eating, one should start with one half of the daily total. Dilution of the liquid formulations with warm water (50:50) on the first day, with an increase to full concentration over

TPN Flow Sheet

Date: _____

Clinician: _____

STERILE GLOVES ONLY WHEN HANDLING LINE

Time						
Attitude/Edema/Cellulitis q.i.d.						
Temperature q.i.d.						
Resp. Rate/Auscult. q.i.d.						
Hr & Character q.i.d.						
Weight (same scale) t.i.d.						
Mucus Membranes q.i.d.						
Line/Daily Bandage Change s.i.d.						
Feces/Urine q.i.d.–walk						
Blood Ammonia EOD						
Blood Glucose t.i.d. (Day 1 q.i.d.)						
PCV/TSP/AZO s.i.d.						
CBC s.i.d.						
Blood Gases Twice Weekly						
Electrolytes s.i.d.						
Urine Specific Gravity q.i.d.						
Urine Glucose q.i.d.						
TPN/Fluid Rate						
Appetite						
Water Consumption						

Figure 1. Flow sheet for monitoring patients receiving total parenteral nutrition. (Reprinted with permission from Labato, M.A.: Nutritional intervention. Pet Veterinarian 2:31, 1990.)

the ensuing days, may aid in tolerance (see this volume, p. 32).

The total daily feeding volume should be divided and fed in four to six daily feedings. The exception to this approach is the use of jejunostomy tubes, in which a slow continuous infusion of diet is better tolerated. The fulfillment of additional maintenance fluid requirements may be needed in addition to those requirements met through enteral feedings.

Parenteral Route

Parenteral nutritional support, more commonly referred to as total parenteral nutrition (TPN), entails providing all necessary nutrients via administration through a central, peripheral, or portal vein. The goal of TPN is to prevent further deterioration in nutritional status until the animal can be returned to full enteral intake.

INDICATIONS FOR PARENTERAL NUTRITION. The indications for TPN include intestinal obstruction, extreme gastrointestinal resection, wasting diseases, burns, and trauma. In addition, TPN may be particularly beneficial in animals with severe pancreatitis, severe inflammatory bowel disease with protein-losing enteropathy, neurologic states (e.g., coma or semicoma), large open wounds or open abdomen in which significant protein loss is expected, and acute renal failure (Labato, 1990).

DETERMINATION OF NUTRITIONAL REQUIREMENTS. Although the BER and the MER are calculated as previously described (see the earlier section "Determination of Energy Requirements"), the administration of nutrients by the parenteral route requires certain modifications. When dogs are treated in our hospital, it is customary to supply the MER as nonprotein calories: 50 to 60% of the MER is supplied by 20% lipid solution (2 kcal/ml), and the remainder is supplied by 50% dextrose solution (1.7 kcal/ml). The daily protein requirement is compounded into the TPN solution and is determined using the following guidelines: adult dogs, 4 gm/kg; dogs with increased protien loss, 6 gm/kg; dogs with renal insufficiency 1.5 gm/kg; adult cats, 6 gm/kg; and cats with renal insufficiency, 3.5 gm/kg. Specialized amino acid formulations (RenAmin, Baxter; HepatAmine, Kendall McGaw) are available for use in animals with specific disease states (e.g., renal or hepatic failure), but in general these formulations are much more expensive than the basic mixtures.

Because they differ in metabolism from dogs, cats are particularly sensitive to overfeeding. In cats, an adjustment is made in formulating the nutritional requirement to avoid problems with overfeeding, such as glucose intolerance, lipidosis, and hyperammonemia. Thus, the calories supplied by protein (4 kcal/gm) are subtracted from the total calories needed, and the balance is provided as a 50:50 mixture of dextrose and lipid.

With TPN, the total daily caloric and protein requirement is provided intravenously by combining an amino acid solution, 50% dextrose, and a 20% lipid emulsion together in one receptacle. This process is referred to as "all-in-one" compounding. The resulting solution of nutrients is provided to the animal by continuous intravenous infusion, preferably using a variable-rate infusion pump. The resulting solution is hyperosmotic and an ideal medium for microbial growth. Strict aseptic technique in compounding, storage, and administration of the TPN solution is imperative, as is frequent supervision of the patient. The central venous catheter used for administration of TPN solution must be a "dedicated line" to minimize catheter-related problems.

The administration of TPN is not an emergency procedure, and an intensive care unit is not required, but close and careful observation is vital (Fig. 1). Total parenteral nutrition is best administered when 24-hr observation is available. If around-the-clock observation is not possible, then TPN can be administered over a 15-hr period. Care must be taken, however, to avoid wide fluctuations in the animal's blood glucose concentration and to avoid catheter occlusion when this approach is used.

Metabolic complications that can occur with TPN administration in animals include hyperglycemia, hypokalemia, hyperammonemia, and hypertriglyceridemia. Additional common complications are often catheter-related and include thrombophlebitis, edema, cellulitis, thromboembolism, sepsis, catheter occlusion, line disconnection or breakage, and an inability to recatheterize the animal.

References and Suggested Reading

Allen, T. A.: Specialized nutritional support. *In* Ettinger, S. J. (ed.): *Textbook of Veterinary Internal Medicine*, 3rd ed. Philadelphia: W. B. Saunders, 1989, pp. 450–455.
  A review of specialized nutritional support in the dog and cat.
Armstrong, P. J., and Lippert, A. C.: Selected aspects of enteral and parenteral nutritional support. Semin. Vet. Med. Surg. (Small Anim.) 3:216, 1988.
  A review of selected aspects of enteral and parenteral nutritional support.
Armstrong, P. J., Hand, M. S., and Frederick, G. S.: Enteral nutrition by tube. Vet. Clin. North Am. Small Anim. Pract. 20:237, 1990.
  A review article of enteral nutrition by tube feeding methods in the dog and cat.
Boosalis, M. G., Ott L., Pevine, A. S., et al.: Relationship of visceral proteins to nutritional status in chronic and acute stress. Crit. Care Med. 17:741, 1989.
  A review of the role of hypoalbuminemia in enteral nutrition in the critically ill patient.
Brinson, R. R., and Pitts, W. M.: Enteral nutrition in the critically ill patient: Role of hypoalbuminemia. Crit. Care Med. 17:367, 1989.
  A study of visceral protein levels in 78 critically ill patients to evaluate nutritional status in chronic and acute stress.
Buonpane, E. A., Brown, R. O., Boucher, B. A., et al.: Use of fibronectin and somatomedin-C as nutritional markers in the enteral nutrition support of traumatized patients. Crit. Care Med. 17:126, 1989.

A study of the use of fibronectin and somatomedin-C as nutritional markers in the enteral nutrition support of 12 traumatized patients.

Burkholder, W. J., and Swecker, W. S.: Nutritional influences on immunity. Semin. Vet. Med. Surg. (Small Anim.) 5:154, 1990.
A review of nutritional influences on the immune system.

Crowe, D. T.: Nutritional support for the seriously ill or injured patient: An overview. J. Vet. Emerg. Crit. Care 1:1, 1985.
A review of nutritional influences on immunity.

Donaghue, S.: Nutritional support of hospitalized patients. Vet. Clin. North Am. Small Anim. Pract. 19:475, 1989.
An overview of nutritional support for the seriously ill or injured patient.

Fischer, J. E., and Chance, W. T.: Total parenteral nutrition, glutamine, and tumor growth. J.P.E.N. 14:865, 1990.
A review of effective nutritional support for hospitalized dogs and cats.

Kaminski, M. V.: Enteral hyperalimentation. Surg. Gynecol. Obstet. 143:12, 1976.
A discussion of studies performed to evaluate the role of total parenteral nutrition and glutamine on tumor growth.

Labato, M. A.: Nutritional intervention. Pet Veterinarian 2:31, 1990.
A review of the procedures, complications, and therapeutic goals of enteral nutrition.

Lippert, A. C., and Armstrong, P. J.: Parenteral nutritional support. *In* Kirk, R. W. (ed.): *Current Veterinary Therapy X.* Philadelphia: W. B. Saunders, 1989, pp. 25–30.
An overview of indications and methods of nutritional support in the dog and cat.

Ogilvie, G. K., and Vail, D. M.: Nutrition and cancer: Recent developments. Vet. Clin. North Am. Small Anim. Pract. 20:969, 1990.
A discussion of the metabolic changes associated with cancer and cancer cachexia.

Remillard, R. L. and Martin, R. A.: Nutritional support in the surgical patient. Semin. Vet. Med. Surg. 5:197, 1990.
A discussion of nutritional support in the surgical patient.

Remillard, R. L., and Thatcher, C. D.: Parenteral nutritional support in the small animal patient. Vet. Clin. North Am. Small Anim. Pract. 19:1287, 1989.
A detailed discussion of parenteral nutritional support in the small animal patient, including indications, calculations and formulations.

Wheeler, S. L., and McGuire, B. H.: Enteral nutritional support. *In* Kirk, R. W. (ed.): *Current Veterinary Therapy X.* Philadelphia: W. B. Saunders, 1989, pp. 30–37.
A review of enteral nutritional support in the small animal patient.

THE ACUTE ABDOMEN

CYNTHIA R. LEVEILLE
North Grafton, Massachusetts

The acute abdomen is defined as the sudden onset of abdominal pain. Since this pain may originate from any intra-abdominal structure, the clinicopathologic manifestations of acute abdomen may be associated with gastrointestinal, urogenital, splenic, or peritoneal disease (Table 1). Animals with acute abdomen often present with life-threatening disease requiring immediate intervention. The decision whether this intervention should include both surgical and medical therapy can be a diagnostic challenge. Familiarity with the signalment clinical signs, laboratory abnormalities and radiographic and ultrasonographic manifestations associated with the common causes of acute abdomen can facilitate the proper diagnosis and treatment of these animals. This article focuses on the evaluation, treatment, and monitoring of the patient with acute abdominal pain.

PATIENT EVALUATION

Signalment is helpful diagnostically in evaluating the animal with acute abdomen. Gastric dilatation volvulus (GDV) is common in deep-chested, large-breed dogs such as Great Danes, German shepherds, Doberman pinschers, and Irish setters. Young German shepherd dogs are predisposed to mesenteric volvulus. The middle-aged, overweight female schnauzer with acute abdomen should be considered a suspect for pancreatitis. Ruptured splenic neoplasms are most common in the older, larger-breed dogs, especially German shepherds and golden retrievers. Hemorrhagic gastroenteritis (HGE) most often occurs in 2- to 4-year-old small-breed dogs. Dalmatians, schnauzers, dachshunds, and other breeds predisposed to the development of urinary calculi may present with acute abdomen associated with urethral obstruction from these calculi. Acute abdomen in cats is frequently associated with intestinal obstruction secondary to the ingestion of a linear foreign body and, in male cats, with urethral obstruction due to feline urologic syndrome (FUS). Young animals are more susceptible to viral enteritis and are more likely to develop intestinal obstruction or perforation due to ingested foreign bodies or intussusceptions. Older animals are more likely to develop acute abdomen as the result of abdominal neoplasia. Intussusceptions in older animals are often associated with an underlying intramural intestinal lesion. Pyometra and prostatitis should be considered as the source of abdominal pain in older intact female and male dogs, respectively.

HISTORY

Many animals with acute abdomen are presented without a lengthy history of clinical signs. Careful

Table 1. *Differential Diagnosis for the Acute Abdomen*

Gastrointestinal
  Acute pancreatitis
  Gastric dilatation/volvulus
  Mesenteric volvulus
  Infectious enteritis
  Hemorrhagic gastroenteritis syndrome
  Obstruction
    Foreign body
    Neoplasia
    Intussusception
  Acute hepatic failure
Urogenital
  Urethral or ureteral obstruction
  Bladder rupture
  Acute pyelonephritis or nephritis
  Pyometra
  Acute prostatitis
  Uterine or testicular torsion
  Renal artery thrombosis
Splenic
  Splenic torsion
  Ruptured spleen: neoplasia, trauma
Peritoneal
  Chemical peritonitis
    Bile
    Urine
    Hemoperitoneum
    Pancreatitis
  Septic peritonitis
    Ruptured viscus
    Perforated gastrointestinal ulcer
    Ruptured abscess: prostatic, hepatic
    Penetrating abdominal wound

questioning of owners, however, often reveals important historical information. Has the animal had exposure to specific toxins, garbage, or foreign objects? Is there a history of a recent high-fat meal? Is vaccination status current? Are other animals or people in the house sick? Have there been similar previous episodes, for example, of recurrent pancreatitis, prostatitis, FUS, or gastric dilatation? When was the dog last in estrus? What is the character of the stool and vomitus? Is the animal receiving any medications such as nonsteroidal anti-inflammatory agents or corticosteroids that may be associated with gastrointestinal ulceration or pancreatitis? Information concerning the onset and progression of the disease before admission of the animal is also important in considering the choice of diagnostic studies.

CLINICAL SIGNS

In addition to abdominal pain, animals with an acute abdomen have clinical signs related to the underlying etiology of their condition. GDV is characterized by nonproductive retching. Primary gastrointestinal disturbances may be associated with vomiting or diarrhea. The character of the vomitus may help to localize the site of a gastrointestinal lesion. Profuse vomiting of bile-containing fluid is associated with high intestinal obstructions, pancreatitis, and severe virus- or toxin-induced gastroenteritis. Vomiting may be projectile, with pyloric or high intestinal obstructions. Esophageal, gastric, or duodenal hemorrhage caused by gastrointestinal ulcers, severe gastroenteritis, or coagulation abnormalities is associated with hematemesis. This bloody vomitus generally has a coffee-ground appearance. The presence of diarrhea in addition to vomiting suggests more extensive involvement of the intestinal tract. Hemorrhagic diarrhea is associated with HGE, infectious enteritides (particularly parvovirus and salmonellosis), and occasionally pancreatitis. Abdominal distention is common in GDV and acute intestinal obstructive diseases such as mesenteric volvulus. Occasionally, dogs with intestinal obstruction assume a stretched or praying stance to relieve pressure on the abdominal organs. Some animals with acute abdomen present in acute collapse without a history of other relevant clinical signs.

PHYSICAL EXAMINATION

A rapid assessment of the cardiovascular status is essential in animals presented with an acute abdominal crisis. These animals may develop shock from acute blood loss, endotoxemia, sepsis, or hypovolemia secondary to vomiting, diarrhea, or sequestration of body fluids. Depression, tachycardia, pale mucous membranes, slow capillary refill, and poor peripheral pulses are findings on physical examination that indicate cardiovascular collapse. In these animals, treatment for shock should be initiated immediately while further diagnostic strategies are evolving.

A careful physical examination is important. Vital signs are recorded and re-evaluated often. Hydration status is quickly evaluated by assessing skin turgor and mucous membranes. Hyperthermia may be associated with infectious disease, sepsis, or pancreatitis. Hypothermia may develop in animals with shock, sepsis, or hypoglycemia. The base of the tongue is carefully examined for the presence of a linear foreign body in all vomiting animals.

Abdominal palpation is often the most important part of the evaluation of the animal with an acute abdomen. Localization of abdominal pain can narrow the differential diagnosis. Animals with pancreatitis often have pain in the cranial right quadrant of the abdomen. Cranial abdominal pain may also be present with perforated gastric or duodenal ulcers or with acute hepatic disease. Caudal abdominal pain may be found with pyometra, prostatitis or urethral obstruction. Peritonitis typically causes diffuse abdominal tenderness. Pain associated with intestinal foreign bodies, intussusceptions, and other causes of intestinal obstruction tends to be dull and poorly localized. Kidney pain may indicate acute renal injury, inflammation, or thrombosis. Abdominal palpation may reveal evidence of hollow organ distention in association with gastrointestinal or urogenital diseases such as GDV, mesenteric volvulus, pyometra, or urethral obstruction. Fluid-filled loops of bowel may be identified in cases of viral enteritis. Abdominal masses, organomegaly (e.g., a torsed spleen), intussusceptions, and intestinal foreign bodies may be palpated. Plicated loops of bowel are commonly palpated in animals with linear intestinal foreign bodies. The presence of ascites may be suspected from abdominal palpation and ballottement.

Abdominal auscultation may reveal increased borborygmus in cases of enteritis and recent-onset gastrointestinal obstruction, or decreased borborygmus associated with ileus in cases of peritonitis or prolonged gastrointestinal obstruction.

Rectal examination allows evaluation of feces for the presence of melena, frank blood, or foreign material. In male animals the prostate can be palpated for enlargement, symmetry, pain, and degree of mobility. The pelvic urethra can also be examined for evidence of calculi.

DATABASE

Many animals with acute abdomen are presented as emergencies. The minimal database that should be obtained in these patients includes packed cell volume (PCV), total plasma solids (TS), reagent test strip assays for blood urea nitrogen (BUN) (Azostix, Ames Co.) and glucose concentrations (Chemstrip bG, Boehringer Mannheim Corp), urine specific gravity, and abdominal radiographs. Four-quadrant abdominal paracentesis, diagnostic peritoneal lavage, or both may also be indicated. Samples of blood and urine should be submitted for a complete blood count, serum biochemical profile, and urinalysis.

LABORATORY FINDINGS

Polycythemia may be attributed to dehydration, especially when accompanied by an increase in TS. A markedly elevated PCV, often in conjunction with a normal to decreased TS, is characteristic of HGE. A decreased PCV and TS may indicate subacute or chronic blood loss. In the acute situation, however, a normal PCV does not exclude significant blood loss, because it takes several hours for compensatory fluid shifts to occur. Fragmentation anemia and thrombocytopenia are commonly encountered with splenic neoplasia and with the development of disseminated intravascular coagulation (DIC).

The character of the plasma in the centrifuged microhematocrit tube should be evaluated. Lipemic plasma may be seen with pancreatitis. Icteric plasma may accompany hepatobiliary disease (including extrahepatic biliary obstruction secondary to pancreatic inflammation) or hemolytic disease. Intravascular hemolysis of erythrocytes may result in reddish coloration of the plasma.

The BUN concentration may be elevated with dehydration, renal failure, urethral obstruction, or urinary bladder rupture. Differentiation between renal and prerenal or postrenal azotemia associated with acute abdomen can be aided by determination of urine specific gravity and serum osmolality, and by physical examination. Isosthenuria in the face of an elevated BUN concentration often suggests primary renal disease.

Alterations in blood glucose concentration are common in animals with acute abdomen. Hypoglycemia may accompany septic conditions. Hyperglycemia can be associated with pancreatitis and, especially in cats, with stress.

ABDOMINAL IMAGING

Abdominal radiography and ultrasound examination are essential parts of the initial diagnostic evaluation of the animal with acute abdomen (Table 2). Radiographic evaluations are especially important in animals in too much pain to allow systematic evaluation of the abdomen by palpation. Abdominal organs should be evaluated for changes in size, shape, and position. Distention of the gastrointestinal tract with gas, ingesta, or fluid may be associated with ileus or obstructive, neoplastic, or inflammatory gastrointestinal diseases. When GDV is suspected, the right lateral radiograph is the best view with which to evaluate the animal.

Intestinal obstruction is associated with radiographic findings of gaseous and/or fluid distention of bowel loops proximal to the site of obstruction. In evaluating intestinal distention on radiographs, a general rule of thumb is that the diameter of a segment of small intestine should not be greater than 50% of the average diameter of the remaining loops of small bowel. In animals with enteritis significant radiographic evidence of dilatation of bowel loops is usually not present. A generalized radiographic pattern of gaseous distention of small intestine can be associated with ileus accompanying severe gastrointestinal inflammation, peritonitis, or electrolyte abnormalities. If the generalized distention is marked, mesenteric volvulus should be considered.

Changes in the position of the bowel on radio-

Table 2. Abdominal Imaging of the Acute Abdomen

Etiology	Radiographic Changes	Ultrasonographic Changes
Pancreatitis	Increased soft-tissue opacity in right cranial abdomen	Diffuse to focal enlargement of pancreas with decreased echogenicity
	Widening of gastroduodenal angle	
	Gas accumulation in proximal duodenum and transverse colon	Dilation of main pancreatic duct
		Detection of pseudocysts and abscesses
Gastrointestinal obstruction	Nonuniform gaseous and/or fluid distention of bowel	Fluid accumulation within bowel proximal to obstruction
	Stacking of dilated loops of bowel with hairpin turns	Visualization of source of obstruction
	Identification of radiodense foreign bodies	
	Source of obstruction may be outlined by contrast material	
Intussusception	Visualization of cylindric mass	Multiple concentric ring pattern visualized on cross section of intussuscepted segment
	Coil spring pattern created by entrapment of gas or contrast material between walls of intussusceptum and intussuscipiens	
Linear foreign bodies	Accordion-like pleating of small bowel	Visualization of hyperechoic linear structure within lumen of bowel
	Bizarrely shaped luminal gas bubbles	
	Gathering of small bowel to midventral region of abdomen	
Splenic torsion	Marked splenomegaly	Diffusely enlarged hypoechoic spleen
Gastric dilatation/volvulus	Large distended stomach	
	Soft tissue incisura separating stomach into compartments	
	Pylorus shifted to left of midline and dorsal to fundus	
Gastrointestinal ulceration	Double-contrast gastrography best	Visualization of hyperechoic gas accumulation within ulcer crater
	Demonstration of ulcer crater as an outpouching of contrast material from gastric lumen	Localized thickening of gastric wall
	Pneumoperitoneum or signs of peritonitis with perforation	
Enteritis	Variable amount of fluid or gas distention of small bowel	Fluid accumulation within small bowel
Peritonitis	Regional or generalized loss of abdominal detail	Identification of free abdominal fluid

graphs may accompany obstructive intestinal lesions.

Plication of bowel loops with the accumulation of bizarrely shaped luminal gas bubbles is a radiographic pattern suggestive of a linear foreign body. Stacking of dilated loops of bowel with hairpin turns can be observed on radiographs of animals with small intestinal obstruction. Radiodense gastrointestinal foreign bodies may be visualized on survey radiographs. If radiolucent, foreign objects may occasionally be outlined on survey radiographs by a layer of gas within the intestinal lumen.

A radiographic upper gastrointestinal contrast study may be necessary to document obstructive gastrointestinal disease; for example, in the case of an upper gastrointestinal obstruction where vomiting by the animal may have relieved bowel distention and survey radiographs are nonconfirmatory.

An intussusception may result in an obstructive bowel pattern on radiographs, and may also be identified radiographically by the characteristic coil spring pattern. Ultrasonography is very useful to diagnose intussusception. Intussuceptions can be visualized ultrasonographically by identifying an excessive number of intestinal wall layers that correspond to the telescoping walls of the intussusceptum and intussuscipiens (Fig. 1).

Pancreatitis can be associated with characteristic radiographic and ultrasonographic changes, listed in Table 2.

A generalized loss of radiographic abdominal detail accompanies the presence of abdominal fluid. Although the presence of this fluid limits the diagnostic information that can be obtained by radiographic examination, it actually enhances the diagnostic capability of abdominal ultrasonography.

Gastric ulcers or neoplasia are difficult to identify on survey abdominal radiographs. Ultrasonographic evaluation of gastric mucosal lesions such as ulcers or tumors can often be enhanced by filling the stomach with water.

Splenomegaly may be detected and characterized by radiographic and ultrasonographic evaluation. For example, ultrasonographic examination of the spleen can help distinguish between focal splenic enlargement associated with splenic hemangiosarcoma and diffuse enlargement accompanying vascular engorgement.

Radiodense urinary calculi and distention of the bladder associated with urethral obstruction can be visualized on survey radiographs. Contrast radiographic studies are necessary to demonstrate radiolucent calculi and to verify urinary bladder or urethral rupture.

Prostatomegaly associated with prostatic inflammation, abscessation, or cyst formation can be dem-

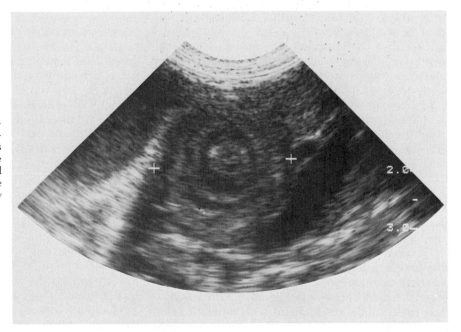

Figure 1. Cross-sectional ultrasonographic appearance of an intussusception in a dog. The cursors delineate the boundaries of the multiple concentric rings formed by the telescoping walls of the loops of bowel involved. Courtesy of Dr. Amy C. Tidwell.

onstrated radiographically and further characterized by ultrasound examination.

Pyometra may be suggested by the presence of an enlarged, fluid-filled tubular soft-tissue density between the colon and urinary bladder on radiographic or ultrasonographic examination.

ABDOMINOCENTESIS

Abdominocentesis is often indicated in the assessment of animals with acute abdomen. The indications for abdominocentesis include (1) palpable or ultrasonographically demonstrable abdominal fluid, (2) radiographic evidence of free gas or generalized decrease in radiographic abdominal detail, (3) penetrating abdominal wounds, and (4) suspected rupture of a hollow abdominal viscus. The presence of shock in a patient with acute abdomen is also an indication for performing abdominocentesis. A four-quadrant tap should be performed. If fluid is obtained, it should be analyzed by cytologic, biochemical, and microbiologic techniques.

If the fluid appears hemorrhagic, PCV and TS tests should be obtained on the fluid and compared with those on peripheral blood from the animal. If the PCV of the abdominal fluid is equal to or greater than that of the blood, significant hemorrhage is present and abdominal exploration should be considered. If the vital signs are stable or the abdominal fluid PCV is less than that of blood, medical therapy is administered and the patient monitored for clinical deterioration. If on repeated abdominocentesis a 5% increase in the abdominal fluid PCV is detected (e.g., if PCV of 6% has increased to 11%,

significant ongoing hemorrhage should be suspected.

Cytologic evaluation should be performed on stained slide preparations of the fluid. An increased number of neutrophils with the presence of intracellular bacteria on microscopic evaluation of the fluid indicates septic peritonitis and the need for abdominal exploration and drainage. A Gram's stain slide facilitates the identification of bacteria. In addition, classification of the organisms as either gram-positive or gram-negative facilitates the choice of appropriate empirical antibiotic therapy while culture results are pending.

Biochemical evaluation of the abdominal fluid can be performed. A BUN or creatinine concentration in the patient's abdominal fluid that is greater than comparative serum values suggests uroabdomen due to urinary tract rupture. Biliary tract rupture is accompanied by increased bilirubin concentration in the abdominal fluid. The detection of amylase or lipase activity in abdominal fluid is associated with pancreatitis, pancreatic trauma, or small bowel rupture or ischemia. This determination is especially useful in cats, in which serum activities of these enzymes are often normal in cases of pancreatitis.

DIAGNOSTIC PERITONEAL LAVAGE

Abdominocentesis with a needle is associated with significant numbers of false-negative results. This high inaccuracy rate is primarily due to the inability to obtain abdominal fluid. Experiments have shown that fluid volumes of 5 to 6 ml/kg must collect in the abdomen before abdominocentesis

will provide consistent results. Diagnostic peritoneal lavage, however, has been shown to have a
greater than 95% accuracy rate in determining the
need for surgical intervention in cases of acute
abdomen. Diagnostic peritoneal lavage is easily
performed by infusing 22 ml/kg of warm lactated
Ringer's solution into the peritoneal cavity through
a 14-gauge intravenous catheter (see CVT IX, p. 3).
After the fluid is distributed evenly by gently rolling
the animal, a sample of fluid is withdrawn for
analysis. On gross examination a clear, colorless
sample rules out peritoneal disease, a bloody sample
is associated with intra-abdominal hemorrhage, and
turbidity suggests peritonitis. If on cytologic examination the lavage fluid contains bacteria, vegetable
matter, or a white blood cell count in excess of 2000
cells/mm³, especially with degenerate neutrophils,
peritonitis is indicated and surgical intervention
warranted. Microbial cultures should be obtained
from the fluid sample. Lavage fluid with a PCV of
less than 5 indicates mild intra-abdominal hemorrhage. If the PCV is greater than 10, severe hemorrhage has occurred. To monitor ongoing hemorrhage, the lavage catheter can be kept in place and
sequential samples obtained for PCV determination.

Biochemical studies may also be conducted on
peritoneal lavage samples. An amylase activity in
the lavage fluid in excess of that detected in serum
indicates pancreatitis, pancreatic trauma, or small
bowel rupture. Uroabdomen is suggested by a lavage fluid creatinine concentration greater than that
in serum.

ANCILLARY DIAGNOSTIC TESTS

Leukocytosis, especially in conjunction with a left
shift, may indicate the presence of an infectious or
inflammatory disease or an ischemic bowel. Neutropenia is commonly seen in animals with viral enteritis or severe bacterial infection. Hyperamylasemia
or hyperlipasemia suggests acute pancreatitis. Increases in serum alanine aminotransferase or alkaline phosphatase activities indicate hepatobiliary
involvement. Abnormalities in serum electrolytes
may occur secondary to vomiting, diarrhea, bowel
ischemia, and urinary tract rupture or obstruction.

In the patient with hemoabdomen, hematemesis,
or melena, an activated clotting time measurement
can be made to screen quickly for coagulation
abnormalities. A full coagulation profile, including
determination of prothrombin time, (PT) partial
thromboplastin time (PTT), fibrin degradation products, platelet count, and fibrinogen, will clarify
abnormalities. DIC is a potential complication in
many conditions associated with acute abdomen and
should be suspected in the acutely ill, bleeding
patient with thrombocytopenia, hypofibrinogen-

emia, increased circulating fibrin degradation products, and prolonged PT or PTT.

Blood gas evaluation, when available, can be
helpful in managing the animal with an abdominal
crisis. Metabolic acidosis is the most common abnormality and can be associated with loss of bicarbonate-rich intestinal secretions, accumulation of
lactic acid associated with poor tissue perfusion, or
an inability to excrete hydrogen ions as in renal
failure and urinary tract rupture or obstruction.

THERAPY

Specific treatment for the patient with acute
abdomen depends on the cause, but certain principles of medical management are applicable regardless of etiology. In the animal with shock, fluid
replacement is the cornerstone of therapy. A large-
gauge intravenous catheter should be inserted and
crystalloid solutions, such as 0.9% saline or lactated
Ringer's solution, administered (60 to 90 ml/kg/hr).
The benefits of corticosteroid administration in animals with circulatory shock are controversial; if
used, these drugs should be administered at high
dosages as soon as possible and in physiologically
available forms. The most frequently used preparation is prednisolone sodium succinate (11 mg/kg
IV). Therapy with sodium bicarbonate is indicated
if metabolic acidosis is severe (e.g., blood pH less
than 7.1 to 7.2). The extracellular fluid bicarbonate
deficit is determined by the following formula:

$$\text{Base deficit} \times 0.3 \times \text{kg of body weight}$$

If blood gas evaluation is not available, the base
deficit for suspected mild, moderate, and severe
metabolic acidosis may be estimated at 5, 10, and
15, respectively. Sodium bicarbonate should be
administered intravenously at one half the calculated dose over 20 minutes followed by re-evaluation of the blood gases prior to additional therapy.
Intravenous antibiotic administration is indicated in
animals with bacterial peritonitis or sepsis. The
initial choice of antibiotics should be based on the
suspected source of infection and the results of
Gram's stains. Aerobic and anaerobic cultures
should be obtained to document infection and determine microbial antibiotic sensitivity before
choosing specific antimicrobial therapy.

Probably the most difficult and important therapeutic decision to be made is whether surgical
intervention is warranted. Some conditions require
immediate surgical treatment, others may be best
managed initially with medical therapy. Definite
indications for surgical intervention include the
presence of free abdominal gas on radiographs,
evidence of septic peritonitis on abdominal fluid
evaluation, and the presence of penetrating abdom-

inal or intestinal lessons. In addition, signs of complete small bowel obstruction, mesenteric volvulus, GDV, or severe ongoing abdominal hemorrhage are considered surgical emergencies.

Many conditions may ultimately require surgical treatment, but the animal may benefit from an initial period of medical stabilization. Animals with urinary tract rupture often have severe metabolic abnormalities. Hyperkalemia, metabolic acidosis, and uremia should be corrected in these patients by establishing percutaneous abdominal drainage and instituting diuresis before surgical intervention. A dog with a ruptured splenic tumor or splenic torsion may be stabilized by volume expansion with crystalloid administration and, if necessary, by blood transfusion. In animals with abdominal bleeding, the application of an abdominal pressure wrap to increase intra-abdominal pressure may help control ongoing hemorrhage. An animal in septic shock from a closed pyometra requires aggressive medical treatment and rapid surgical intervention, but in a nonseptic animal with an open pyometra, medical treatment may be sufficient initially. Biliary tract rupture results in slowly developing bile peritonitis that often can be easily overlooked and remain occult for 10 to 14 days. These patients generally are not surgical emergencies, but a high index of suspicion for this injury is necessary; the prognosis is poorer when diagnosis is delayed. Treatment involves open abdominal drainage.

Some animals with small bowel obstruction, especially if the obstruction is distal, may receive medical management and delayed surgical intervention. Linear foreign bodies caught at the base of the tongue may be cut and the animal monitored for passage of the materials. If significant intestinal plication exists, however, it is best to undertake rapid surgical intervention in view of the frequent occurrence of intestinal perforation with linear foreign bodies. Fever and discrete abdominal pain also may herald intestinal perforation.

Animals receiving extended medical therapy before surgical intervention must be carefully monitored for clinical deterioration that may necessitate immediate surgical treatment. In these animals, peripheral pulse quality, capillary refill time, rectal temperature, and mental status should be assessed frequently. The measurement of arterial blood pressure and central venous pressure provides an additional means of evaluating response to therapy.

Acute abdomen caused by pancreatitis, infectious and toxic gastroenteritis, HGE, fulminant hepatic failure, prostatitis, pyelonephritis and nonperforating gastrointestinal ulceration generally responds to medical management. If any of these conditions are suspected and the animal fails to respond to appropriate medical therapy, the diagnosis should be reconsidered and the animal re-evaluated by abdominal palpation, abdominal imaging techniques, and abdominocentesis. Protracted vomiting, continued abdominal pain, depression, persistent leukopenia, hypothermia, hyperthermia, or hypoglycemia in an animal should raise the clinician's index of suspicion for disease requiring additional medical therapy or possible surgical intervention.

Complications of medical conditions may develop and require surgical treatment. Young dogs with viral enteritis may respond to medical therapy and subsequently develop intussusceptions and recurrent clinical signs. In animals with acute pancreatitis that fail to improve or that deteriorate in condition (protracted vomiting, persistent fever, respiratory compromise from pulmonary edema, and the development of pleural and peritoneal effusion), surgical exploration for lavage and debridement of necrotic pancreatic and peripancreatic tissue should be considered. In addition, animals with pancreatitis should be monitored radiographically and ultrasonographically for the development of cranial abdominal masses, which suggest pancreatitic abscessation, a condition that warrants surgical intervention.

References and Suggested Reading

Crowe, D. T.: Diagnostic abdominal paracentesis techniques: Clinical evaluation in 129 dogs and cats. J. Am. Anim. Hosp. Assoc. 20:223, 1984.
A review that demonstrates the usefulness of diagnostic peritoneal lavage in evaluating animals with intra-abdominal injury or disease.
Kleine, L. J., and Lamb, C. R.: Comparative organ imaging: The gastrointestinal tract. Veterinary Radiology 30:133, 1989.
A review of radiography, ultrasonography, computed tomography, and nuclear scintigraphy in evaluating the gastrointestinal tract.
Macintire, D. K.: The acute abdomen—differential diagnosis and management. Semin. Vet. Med. Surg. (Small Anim.) 3:302, 1988.
An extensively referenced review article on the etiology of the acute abdomen.
Potts, J. R.: Acute pancreatitis. Surg. Clin. North Am. 68:281, 1988.
A review of acute pancreatitis in humans, with a discussion of when surgical intervention is warranted.
Strombeck, D. R., and Guilford, W. G.: *Small Animal Gastroenterology.* California: Stonegate Publishing, 1990.
A comprehensive textbook with chapters on the evaluation and management of gastrointestinal causes of acute abdominal pain.

HEMATEMESIS:
DIAGNOSIS AND TREATMENT

DEBORAH J. DAVENPORT

Topeka, Kansas

Hematemesis, the act of vomiting blood, is an uncommon clinical complaint in veterinary medicine. Despite its relative infrequency, hematemesis serves as an important marker of upper gastrointestinal disease. In addition, the condition can become an emergency requiring intensive therapy.

Hematemesis is manifested by flakes, streaks, or clots of fresh blood or by the presence of digested blood in the vomitus. Digested blood is most often described as "coffee grounds." Additional clinical findings in the dog or cat with hematemesis may include anorexia, diarrhea, melena, hematochezia, abdominal pain, pallor, tachypnea, tachycardia, systolic murmurs, weakness, or collapse.

It is often difficult for the pet owner to distinguish true from apparent hematemesis. Owners often assume that any blood coming from their pet's mouth was vomited. However, expectoration, sneezing, coughing, or regurgitation of blood due to disorders of the oropharnx, nasopharynx, airways, or esophagus can mimic hematemesis. In addition, orally administered iron or diathiazanine (Dizan) can stain vomitus and feces. Such dark staining can be interpreted by the owner as hematemesis. Occasionally dogs and cats will vomit blood ingested as uncooked meat or offal. A careful history and a thorough physical exam will allow the clinician to distinguish between true and apparent hematemesis (Table 1).

ETIOLOGY

Hematemesis is most often associated with gastric or duodenal erosions or ulcerations. However, other conditions can cause vomiting of blood. A variety of esophageal disorders can result in the delivery of blood to the stomach (Table 2). Esophageal conditions most likely to be associated with hematemesis or regurgitation of blood include esophagitis, esophageal foreign bodies, and neoplasia.

Occasionally animals suffering from coagulopathies will be presented with hematemesis, melena, or hematochezia. This finding is most common in dogs or cats with thrombocytopenia or platelet function disorders. Quantitative and qualitative platelet disorders are associated with the development of superficial hemorrhages. Owing to its enormous surface area, the gastrointestinal tract is prone to superficial mucosal hemorrhage. Anticoagulant rodenticide poisoning, disseminated intravascular coagulation, and congenital coagulation factor deficiencies may also lead to hematemesis. The potential for coagulopathies as a cause of hematemesis requires the veterinarian to perform routine coagulation tests on any animal with unexplained upper gastrointestinal hemorrhage.

Hematemesis developing after upper gastrointestinal surgery should be considered a surgical complication until proven otherwise. In the author's experience, postoperative gastrointestinal hemorrhage occurs most commonly following gastric resection necessitated by gastric dilatation-volvulus. As the use of gastrostomy tubes for nutritional support increases, there may be a parallel rise in the number of patients developing upper gastrointestinal hemorrhage following surgical or percutaneous endoscopic gastrostomy tube placement.

The prevalence of gastrointestinal ulcer disease in dogs and cats is low as compared with that reported in human patients. It is possible that an infrequent diagnosis of gastrointestinal ulceration is due to the lack of clinical signs in many cases. In experimental studies involving dogs, it has been demonstrated that extensive gastroduodenal ulceration may exist with only mild clinical signs (Dow, 1990).

Several metabolic disorders have been associated with the development of hematemesis and upper gastrointestinal ulceration. Uremia is frequently reported to result in diffuse gastrointestinal tract hemorrhage. Gastrointestinal erosions and ulcers are believed to result from the effects of uremic toxins on the gut mucosa. Additionally, increased circulating concentrations of gastrin have been identified in patients with uremia (Thornhill, 1983). Hypergastrinemia promotes hyperacidity and gastroduodenal ulceration.

Liver disease is a common cause of gastrointestinal ulcerations which may be manifested as hematemesis. The pathogenesis of mucosal ulceration associated with hepatopathies is multifactorial and associated coagulopathies may worsen clinical manifestations. Potential mechanisms include altered gastric blood flow due to portal hypertension, de-

Table 1. Etiologies of True Hematemesis Reported in Companion Animals

Coagulopathies
  Disseminated intravascular coagulation
  Anticoagulant rodenticide toxicity
  Thrombocytopenia
  Congenital or acquired coagulation factor deficiencies/defects
Heavy metal toxicity
  Arsenic
  Lead
  Zinc
Infectious disorders
  Gastrointestinal parasitism
  Viral gastroenteritis
  Bacterial gastroenteritis
Perioperative hemorrhage
  Gastric-dilatation volvulus
  Gastrectomy
  Gastrostomy
Gastric/duodenal erosions/ulcerations
  Infiltrative disease
    Neoplasia
    Inflammatory bowel disease
    Phycomycosis
  Metabolic disorders
    Renal disease
    Liver disease
    Hypoadrenocorticism
  Stress erosions/ulcerations
    Burns (Curling's ulcer)
    Neurologic disorders
      Head trauma (Cushing's ulcer)
      Spinal cord disorders
    Sepsis/septic shock
    Hypovolemic shock
    Multiple trauma
Drug administration
  Glucocorticoids
  Nonsteroidal anti-inflammatory agents
    Aspirin
    Indomethacin
    Phenylbutazone
    Naproxen
    Sulindac
    Ibuprofen
    Flunixin meglimine
    Meclofenamic acid
    Piroxicam
  Gastric/duodenal foreign bodies
  Neoplasia
    Mast cell tumor
    Gastrinoma (Zollinger-Ellison syndrome)
    Pancreatic polypeptide secreting tumor
    Basophilic leukemia
Hemorrhagic gastroenteritis
Esophageal disorders
  Esophagitis
  Esophageal neoplasia
  Esophageal foreign bodies

reported in dogs in conjunction with the use of a variety of nonsteroidal anti-inflammatory drugs (NSAIDs), including aspirin, indomethacin, naproxen, ibuprofen, phenylbutazone, flunixin, meglimine, piroxicam, and meclofenamic acid (Dow, 1990; Lipowitz, 1986; Wallace, 1990). The author has treated a perforating gastric ulcer in a dog receiving chronic sulindac administration. NSAIDs are most commonly administered for the relief of musculoskeletal pain; other indications include the treatment of ophthalmic disease and septic shock. The ulcerogenicity of NSAIDs is attributed to inhibition of the enzyme cyclo-oxygenase in the prostaglandin synthesis pathway, resulting in the loss of the gastric protective effects of prostacyclin and prostaglandin E.

The role of glucocorticoids in the development of gastric ulceration is controversial. Physiologic concentrations of glucocorticoid hormones are believed to be intrinsic to the maintenance of the gastric barrier to hyperacidity. However, in association with other disease conditions or the administration of other anti-inflammatory agents, glucocorticoid administration can have a potent ulcerogenic effect (Dillon, 1989; Dow, 1990).

A variety of infiltrative gastric and proximal intestinal disorders may be marked by hematemesis. Inflammatory bowel disease commonly presents as chronic recurrent vomiting, with or without hematemesis. In three dogs managed by the author, severe hematemesis was the primary presenting complaint in association with lymphocytic plasmacytic gastroenteritis.

Neoplastic infiltration of the bowel may also be associated with ulcer formation and hematemesis. This clinical presentation occurs most commonly in association with gastric adenocarcinoma in dogs and alimentary lymphosarcoma in cats. The granulomatous fungal disease phycomycosis (pythiosis) has also been associated with hematemesis (Miller, 1985).

Stress ulcerations are poorly defined entities in veterinary patients. However, gastroduodenal ulcerations have been noted in companion animals in conjunction with severe burns, heat stroke, multiple trauma, head injury, and spinal cord disorders. In addition, hypovolemic shock and sepsis may also be complicated by the development of gastrointestinal ulcers.

layed epithelial turnover, gastric hyperacidity, and hypergastrinemia. Recent experimental evidence suggests that hypergastrinemia is a less important mechanism than previously suspected (Booth, 1990).

Experimentally induced and spontaneous gastroduodenal ulcerations and hematemesis have been

Table 2. Potential Etiologies of Apparent Hematemesis

Oropharyngeal disease
Nasopharyngeal disease
Tracheobronchial disease
Pulmonary disease
Administration of hematinics
Administration of dithiazanine
Ingestion of blood

Gastrin-producing pancreatic tumors, histamine-producing tumors (mast cell tumors, basophilic leukemia), and a pancreatic polypeptide-producing pancreatic tumor have been associated with gastric or duodenal ulceration in dogs and cats. The induction of ulcers in these animals was believed to be due to persistent gastric hyperacidity stimulated by gastrin, histamine, or pancreatic polypeptide.

The ingestion of heavy metals has been associated with the development of hematemesis in the dog and the cat. Lead and arsenic exposures have been reported to cause hematemesis most frequently. However, in recent years hematemesis has been reported after the ingestion of zinc-containing coins and screws from portable kennels.

DIAGNOSIS

History, Signalment, Physical Examination

The patient history, signalment, and physical examination findings often are adequate to provide a diagnosis in the case of hematemesis. Owners should be questioned closely regarding the potential of toxin exposure (lead, arsenic, anticoagulant rodenticides) and foreign body ingestion (bones, coins, and other sources of zinc) by the animal. A history of NSAID administration provides a presumptive diagnosis of drug-induced gastrointestinal erosions or ulcerations. The veterinarian must be certain to query the owner specifically regarding the use of over-the-counter agents, such as aspirin and ibuprofen, as these agents often are administered without the knowledge of the veterinarian.

The signalment of the animal can provide useful information in formulating a differential diagnosis for hematemesis. The aged animal is likely to be suffering from metabolic or neoplastic conditions while the younger animal is likely to suffer from dietary indiscretion. The dachshund and miniature schnauzer are the breeds most commonly affected with hemorrhagic gastroenteritis. The Doberman pinscher and several terrier breeds (Bedlington, Skye, Cairn, and West Highland white) are known to have familial hepatopathies associated with hepatocellular copper accumulation. In addition, several canine breeds are recognized to have congenital renal disorders. All of the aforementioned conditions could result in animals manifesting hematemesis.

Routine physical examination findings may offer important information regarding the source of hematemesis. Animals presenting with hematemesis should be examined closely for cutaneous tumors. Any cutaneous or subcutaneous mass should be aspirated and the sample examined microscopically to include or exclude mast cell neoplasia as the cause of gastrointestinal hemorrhage. Splenomegaly

or hepatomegaly may be identified in animals with systemic mastocytosis or hepatic neoplasia. Assessment of kidney size and shape may be of assistance in determining the role of renal disease in the pathogenesis of suspected gastrointestinal erosions or ulcerations.

Laboratory Evaluation

Hematologic evaluations can be quite helpful in the diagnosis of hematemesis in animals. The hematocrit and hemogram are useful in assessing severity and chronicity of hematemesis. Inflammatory leukograms may be identified in animals with neoplasia, perforated gastrointestinal ulcers, inflammatory bowel disease, and phycomycosis. Extreme eosinophilia in the cat is suggestive of eosinophilic gastroenteritis or systemic mastocytosis. In the dog, eosinophilia and hematemesis may be indicative of parasitism or eosinophilic gastroenteritis. The identification of circulating mast cells is generally diagnostic for mast cell tumors.

Routine biochemical screening helps rule out metabolic causes of hematemesis. Renal disease, hepatopathies, and hypoadrenocorticism are often readily identified, but dogs with atypical hypoadrenocorticism may have normal serum biochemical findings.

Routine urinalysis is also useful in ruling out metabolic causes of hematemesis. In addition, the presence of macroscopic or microscopic hematuria in an animal with hematemesis would support a diagnosis of coagulopathy.

Fecal examinations for parasites and occult blood are important screening tests. Parasites are an unlikely cause of hematemesis in the adult animal but should be considered in the puppy or kitten. The accuracy of fecal occult blood testing has been confirmed in dogs consuming dry food diets (Dow, 1990; Gilson, 1990). Both the modified guaiac and orthotoluidine tests are sensitive and specific for the detection of occult blood in feces.

If the veterinarian is uncertain of the diagnosis after the completion of anamnesis, physical exam, and initial laboratory screening tests, coagulation testing (one-stage prothrombin time, activated partial thromboplastin time, platelet count, thrombin time, fibrinogen concentration, fibrin degradation products) should be evaluated before more invasive and expensive diagnostic tests are performed. If financial constraints exist, an activated clotting time test and a platelet count will suffice in most cases to rule out a bleeding disorder as the cause of upper gastrointestinal hemorrhage.

In some animals, a gastrin-secreting pancreatic tumor (Zollinger-Ellison syndrome) is the suspected diagnosis. In such cases, fasting serum gastrin concentrations and secretin or calcium challenge testing would be indicated. The diagnosis can then be confirmed by abdominal exploratory surgery. If a distinct mass cannot be identified at surgery, partial pancreatectomy is recommended. Histopathologic evaluation and immunocytochemical staining of the pancreatic tissue should be performed. Regional lymph nodes and liver should be biopsied.

Imaging

Imaging modalities such as survey and contrast radiography and ultrasonography offer the veterinarian noninvasive diagnostic techniques for the evaluation of hematemesis.

Radiography may be useful in the diagnosis of radiopaque foreign bodies and lead toxicity in animals. Abnormalities in renal size or shape may suggest renal insufficiency as the cause of gastrointestinal hemorrhage. Hepatosplenomegaly in the cat is suggestive of systemic mastocytosis or alimentary lymphosarcoma. The presence of free air in the abdomen is diagnostic for viscus rupture associated with a perforated gastrointestinal ulcer and serves as an indication for immediate exploratory surgery.

Contrast radiographic examinations may or may not be useful in the diagnosis of hematemesis. If gastrointestinal perforation is suspected, it is advisable to use organic iodide solutions (Gastrografin, Squibb & Sons) as contrast agents. Otherwise, barium sulfate is the contrast agent of choice for gastrointestinal studies because of its superior coating of the gastrointestinal mucosa. The best evaluation of the gastric mucosal surface is obtained with a double contrast study. In animals with gastritis, expected contrast radiographic findings include irregular rugal folds and flocculation of barium from increased mucus production. Malignancy- and non-malignancy-associated gastrointestinal ulcers in dogs and cats may be identified by contrast radiographic examinations. Ulcers appear as contrast material adherent to the mucosal surface, often with penetration of the contrast agent into a mucosal defect. Circumferential thickening of the gastric wall may be present in association with ulcerated neoplasms. A more complete description of roentgenographic findings in gastric and duodenal disease can be found in a recent review (Moon, 1986).

Ultrasonography is a useful diagnostic modality in the evaluation of animals with hematemesis. In the hands of a skilled operator, this noninvasive technique offers excellent assessment of size, shape, and texture of parenchymatous abdominal organs. Unfortunately, ultrasonography has only limited applicability in the direct examination of the gastrointestinal tract.

Endoscopy

Endoscopic examination is the most sensitive test for detection of gastroduodenal ulcerative disease.

Endoscopic evaluation by a skilled operator allows the identification of mucosal and submucosal hemorrhages, erosions, and ulcers. Most important, the procedures allows collection of multiple gastric and duodenal biopsies. In some animals with hematemesis, endoscopic examination may reveal no evidence of hemorrhage, erosion, or ulcers. Biopsies should still be collected from these animals as infiltrative disease may be present.

Contraindications to the endoscopic examination of the upper gastrointestinal tract in animals include lack of a skilled operator, suspected gut perforation, or cardiovascular instability of the animal.

TREATMENT

The first priority for the clinician in the management of hematemesis is to determine the status of the patient. Rapid assessment of the animal's attitude, mucous membrane color, and vital signs will determine if the dog or cat with hematemesis requires aggressive stabilization.

Animals with hematemesis in hemorrhagic shock should be aggressively treated with isotonic fluids, hypertonic saline, colloidal solutions, or blood components (see this volume, p. 0000). If blood or packed red blood cell (RBC) transfusion is necessary, typed, cross-matched blood components should be used. Stored whole blood is adequate for these treatments except in those animals with hematemesis complicated by coagulopathies. In such cases, the administration of fresh whole blood, fresh plasma, or fresh frozen plasma would be indicated to provide needed coagulation factors. The volume of whole blood needed for transfusion can be calculated using the formulas that follow

Feline:

$$\text{Volume} = \text{BW (kg)} \times 70 \times \frac{\text{PCV desired} - \text{PCV of recipient}}{\text{PCV of donor in anticoagulant}}$$

Canine:

$$\text{Volume} = \text{BW (kg)} \times 90 \times \frac{\text{PCV desired} - \text{PCV of recipient}}{\text{PCV of donor in anticoagulant}}$$

where BW and PCV are abbreviations for body weight and packed cell volume, respectively.

Plasma transfusion volumes range from 6 to 10 ml/kg and, owing to the short half-life of the coagulation factors, may need to be repeated every 6 to 12 hr until hemorrhage ceases. In the case of thrombocytopenia, fresh whole blood collected in plastic or platelet-rich plasma would be the blood component of choice for transfusion therapy.

Cessation of Bleeding

After achieving cardiovascular stabilization in the animal, the next goal of the clinician is to control further upper gastrointestinal hemorrhage. In most cases, hematemesis resolves spontaneously. Cessation can be aided by elimination of predisposing factors (i.e., nonsteroidal anti-inflammatory drug administration) and the application of conservative medical measures. The management of cases in which hematemesis does not cease spontaneously or recurs following appropriate medical therapy is controversial. The results of few controlled clinical studies in either human or veterinary medical patients are available.

The use of ice water lavage in the management of acute upper gastrointestinal hemorrhage has been recommended. Iced solutions are administered via an oro- or nasogastric tube at a rate of 10 to 20 ml/kg and are allowed to remain in the stomach for 15 to 30 min. The lavage is repeated until gastric bleeding ceases. The lavage procedure is often coupled with attempts at gastric mucosal vasoconstriction using norepinephrine diluted in the ice water solution (8 mg/500 ml). In experimental canine models of gastrointestinal hemorrhage, intraperitoneal lavage with iced saline improved survival by reducing gastric blood flow and hemorrhage. The potential for drastically decreasing the patient's core temperature is of concern with the use of this technique in small patients and animals with shock.

There are several reports in the human medical literature concerning the use of specialized endoscopic equipment for the control of gastric and duodenal hemorrhage. These techniques include the use of lasers, thermal cautery, electrocautery, and tissue glues aided by endoscopic visualization. These techniques are not currently employed in veterinary practice. However, the use of such instrumentation holds great promise for the noninvasive control of persistent upper gastrointestinal hemorrhage.

After initial control of hemorrhage has been accomplished, the animal may benefit from iron, copper, and B vitamin supplementation. The use of hematinics is indicated in those patients with nonregenerative, microcytic/hypochromic anemias attributable to iron deficiency. The administration of hematinics is probably not necessary in most animals that receive blood transfusions.

Ulcer Management

The mainstay of gastric and duodenal ulcer management is the control of acid production. "No acid, no ulcer" is considered to be true in man. However, there is no experimental or clinical evidence that the same mechanisms hold in spontaneous cases of gastrointestinal hemorrhage in animals. Anecdotal evidence suggests that reduction of acid production will aid in resolution of gastrointestinal ulceration, and experimental evidence exists that suggests con-

trol of acid production will decrease or block ulceration and gastrointestinal blood loss associated with the use of NSAIDs.

Antacid administration is the least expensive treatment available for decreasing gastric acidity. Antacid administration can be quite successful in reducing gastric acid production, but attaining efficacy requires administration every 2 to 4 hours. In addition, animals, particularly cats, dislike the taste of these medications, and this factor may decrease owner compliance.

The administration of anticholinergic agents will dispel gastric acid production through pharmacologic vagotomy. However, the administration of these drugs is associated with a number of side effects resulting from a decrease in autonomic innervation. Pirenzipin, an anticholinergic drug available in Europe and Canada, reduces gastric acid production at dosages less than those required for inducing anticholinergic side effects. This drug may prove useful in the treatment of gastrointestinal ulcers.

The H_2 receptor antagonist drugs reduce gastric acid production by blocking the effects of histamine on the gastric parietal cells. There are four H_2 receptor blocking agents available for use in the United States. Pharmacokinetic information for use of these agents in dogs is available for cimetidine (Tagamet, Smith Kline & French; 5 to 10 mg/kg every 6 to 8 hr PO, SQ, IV) and ranitidine (Zantac, Glaxo; 2 mg/kg every 8 to 12 hr PO, SQ, IM). The other two drugs, famotidine (Pepcid, Merck Sharp Dohme) and nizatidine (Axid, Lilly), have been used in dogs at dosages (5 mg/kg every 24 hr PO, SQ, IM; 5 mg/kg every 24 hr PO, respectively) extrapolated from usage in man. These agents have variable potency and half-lives in dogs. The pharmacokinetics of these agents in cats are not known.

Omeprazole (Losec, Merck Sharp Dohme) is a new gastrointestinal therapeutic agent that functions to reduce gastric acid secretion by blocking the proton pump within the parietal cell. This drug has been studied extensively in dogs and will inhibit gastric acid secretion in dogs for 24 hr following administration of a single dose (0.5 to 1.0 mg/kg PO).

Sucralfate (Carafate, Marion Laboratories; 0.25 to 1.0 gm PO every 6 to 8 hr) is a cytoprotective drug composed of a sulfated disaccharide (sucrose) and polyaluminum hydroxide. In an acid pH, the agent is extensively cross-polymerized to form a viscous gel that preferentially binds to and serves as a bandaid for the damaged mucosa. Because it requires an acid environment to fully dissociate, sucralfate administration should precede H_2 receptor antagonist administration by 30 min when these agents are used concomitantly.

Prostaglandin E2 analogues such as misoprostol (Cytotec, Searle) have recently become available for use in the prevention and therapy of gastrointestinal ulcers. Misoprostol is specifically recommended for the treatment and prevention of ulcers in human patients receiving NSAIDs, and the use of this drug in veterinary patients is limited at this time. The dosage of misoprostol (1 to 3 µg/kg every 6 to 8 hr PO) in dogs has been extrapolated from human dosage regimens and a dosage for cats has not been established. The side effects associated with the administration of misoprostol are dose-dependent and include diarrhea, nausea, and abortion in pregnant females.

Very rarely, surgical intervention will be necessary for the diagnosis or control of gastrointestinal hemorrhage. In the author's experience, surgical intervention has only been necessary for the management of animals with suspected perforations and obstructions or postoperative hemorrhage. The resection of an ulcer, the removal of a sharp foreign body, or the oversewing of a lesion may be indicated.

References and Suggested Reading

Booth, D. M.: Serum gastrin level in dogs with progressive liver disease. (Abstract.) Proc. 8th ACVIM Forum. Washington, D.C., 1990, p. 1124
Results of an experimental study of gastrin levels and gastrointestinal ulceration in pharmacologically induced canine liver disease.

Dillon, A. R.: Effects of glucocorticoids on the gastrointestinal system. *In* Kirk, R. W. (ed.): *Current Veterinary Therapy X.* Philadelphia: W. B. Saunders, 1989, p. 897.
A comprehensive review of the effects of glucocorticoid administration on the gastrointestinal tract of dogs and cats.

Dow, S. W., Rosychuk, R. A. W., McChesney, A. E., et al.: Effects of flunixin and flunixin plus prednisone on the gastrointestinal tract of dogs. Am. J. Vet. Res. 51:1131, 1990.
An experimental study of the ulcerogenic effects of flunixin alone and in combination with glucocorticoids on the gastrointestinal tract of dogs.

Gilson, S. D., Parker, B. B., and Twedt, D. C.: Evaluation of two commercial test kits for detection of occult blood in feces of dogs. Am. J. Vet. Res. 51:1385, 1990.
Results of an experimental study evaluating the efficacy of orthotoluidine and guaiac test kits for the detection of occult fecal blood in dogs consuming dry dog food.

Lipowitz, A. J., Boulay, J. P., and Klausner, J. S.: Serum salicylate concentrations and endoscopic evaluation of the gastric mucosa in dogs after oral administration of aspirin-containing products. Am. J. Vet. Res. 47:1586, 1986.
Experimental study of aspirin-induced gastrointestinal mucosal changes following aspirin administration in the dog.

Miller, R. I.: Gastrointestinal phycomycosis in 63 dogs. J.A.V.M.A. 186:473, 1985.
A retrospective clinical report of canine gastrointestinal phycomycosis (pythiosis).

Moon, M., and Myer, W.: Gastrointestinal contrast radiology in small animals. Semin. Vet. Med. Surg. 1:121, 1986.
A comprehensive review of gastrointestinal contrast radiography.

Thornhill, J. A.: Control of vomiting in the uremic patient. *In* Kirk, R. W. (ed.): *Current Veterinary Therapy VIII.* Philadelphia: W.B. Saunders, 1983, p. 1022.
A review of the pathophysiology and control of vomiting in the uremic dog and cat.

Wallace, M. S., Zawie, D. A., and Garvey, M. S.: Gastric ulceration in the dog secondary to the use of nonsteroidal antiinflammatory drugs. J. Am. Anim. Hosp. Assoc. 26:467, 1990.
Retrospective clinical review of NSAID-induced gastrointestinal ulcerations in dogs.

PULMONARY THROMBOEMBOLISM: DIAGNOSIS AND TREATMENT

CATHERINE J. BATY,
and ELIZABETH M. HARDIE
Raleigh, North Carolina

Thromboembolic disease has not been well characterized in veterinary medicine. At least two thromboembolic disease syndromes are generally recognized: aortic thromboembolism associated with cardiomyopathy in the cat and pulmonary thromboembolism (PTE) due to heartworm disease and treatment in the dog. These entities have been thoroughly described and will not be considered.

By definition, PTE refers to the formation of a clot (coagulation factors, platelets, fibrin, and cellular material) or embolus (fat, air, tumor fragment, hair, and so forth) at one site, followed by migration to another site in the pulmonary vasculature with associated vascular occlusion. Usually, this obstruction occurs within the smaller pulmonary arteries.

Conditions that predispose to venous thrombosis are classically described as Virchow's triad: (1) hypercoagulable state, (2) vascular stasis, and (3) disruption of vascular endothelium. Data from experimental studies suggest that the existence of a hypercoagulable state is the most important factor contributing to the development of thrombosis or thromboembolism. Many congenital hypercoagulable conditions have been identified in human patients (e.g., deficiencies of protein C, protein S, antithrombin III, and dysfibrinogenemia). These conditions have not been identified in the dog or cat.

Pulmonary thromboembolism is a significant clinical disease in dogs, and it is assuredly underdiagnosed, as it is in humans. There are no data available in veterinary literature to estimate the incidence of PTE, but it is estimated that 500,000 human patients per year suffer a pulmonary embolic event and that 50,000 of those die from the condition, approximately 10% within 1 hr of embolization.

Antemortem diagnosis of PTE is made in approximately 10 to 30% of human cases. Establishment of the diagnosis of PTE in human and veterinary medical patients is hindered by several important factors: occult presentation or clinical signs consistent with many other disease processes, relatively invasive or specialized diagnostic techniques required for diagnosis, and relatively low level of suspicion for the presence of PTE by clinicians.

Postmortem confirmation of the diagnosis is complicated by the rapid dissolution of thrombi. Experimental data from studies in dogs demonstrated substantial reduction, up to 50% of control, of embolic volume 3 hr after death (Moser et al., 1973).

DISEASES ASSOCIATED WITH PTE

Identification of those diseases or conditions in animals that predispose to PTE would be helpful. This knowledge forms the basis on which many diagnoses of PTE are made in humans. In humans, there is a strong correlation between the development of deep venous thrombosis (DVT) and PTE. The majority (approximately 90%) of thrombi resulting in PTE in humans originate from thrombosis of the deep veins of the lower extremities; the remainder are thought to originate within the right atrium and ventricle. Predisposing conditions for DVT identified in humans include polycythemia, dysproteinemia, obesity, pregnancy, and immobilization. Deep venous thrombosis occurs with increased frequency in humans following particular types of surgical intervention, especially orthopedic, pelvic, abdominal, or thoracic procedures. Armed with this knowledge, physicians can consider prophylactic anticoagulant therapy in people with conditions or undergoing procedures that carry a high risk for the development of DVT and can use less invasive imaging techniques to identify DVT in support of a diagnosis of PTE. If PTE develops as a postoperative complication, clinical signs may be expected to develop 8 to 12 days after surgery.

Deep venous thrombosis is not recognized as a significant disease entity in dogs or cats. It may be

an underdiagnosed condition in veterinary medicine, but it is also probably less prevalent in companion animals than humans. Differences in the postoperative care, health of patients prior to surgical procedures, posture, and prevalence of obesity may explain this difference in DVT prevalence.

Pulmonary thromboembolism in animals has been associated with hypothyroidism, pancreatitis, nephrotic syndrome, renal amyloidosis, disseminated intravascular coagulation, antithrombin III deficiency, hyperadrenocorticism, and immune-mediated hemolytic anemia (IMHA). Virchow's triad can be relied upon to deduce a mechanism for predisposition to PTE for most of the diseases listed, but the association of IMHA and PTE is less clear.

The association between IMHA and PTE in animals was documented in a retrospective study of 31 cases of IMHA; PTE was confirmed in ten of these cases (Klein et al., 1989). Variables associated with a statistically higher prevalence of PTE in these animals were hyperbilirubinemia, negative Coombs' test result, and use of an indwelling intravenous catheter. An increasing number of blood transfusions administered to these animals tended to be associated with a higher prevalence of PTE.

CLINICAL PRESENTATION

There are no pathognomonic clinical signs of PTE. Common symptoms and clinical signs identified in humans include chest pain, rales, apprehension, and cough. An acute onset of dyspnea is the most commonly described clinical sign in veterinary patients, and dyspnea is thought to occur in at least 80% of human patients with PTE. Tachypnea may be transient and occurs early in the course of the disease. Some individuals believe that the absence of tachypnea generally rules out PTE. Pulmonary thromboembolism should be considered in all animals with acute nonspecific cardiopulmonary signs. These animals may manifest other clinical signs attributable to the underlying disease.

In human patients, PTE is manifested in three different syndromes: (1) acute dyspnea with normal chest radiographs, (2) pulmonary hemorrhage or infarction, and (3) acute cor pulmonale. Infarction is relatively uncommon, while hemorrhage and acute cor pulmonale may be the result of disease progression.

ROUTINE DIAGNOSTIC STUDIES

As with clinical presentation, there are no specific laboratory findings that enable clinicians to diagnose PTE in animals. Changes in hematologic or serum biochemical findings are not reliably observed. Hypoxemia, as evidenced by a Pa_{O_2} less than 80 mm Hg, is common in PTE. However, it is estimated that approximately 10% of human patients with PTE have normal Pa_{O_2}.

Thoracic radiographs are frequently normal in animals or human patients with PTE, although pleural effusion, oligemia, or hemidiaphragm are observed. Unexpected differences in diameter of comparably located pulmonary vessels (e.g., right versus left hemithorax) may also be observed. The prevalence of pulmonary infiltrates may be higher in dogs than in humans. These conclusions are based on a retrospective radiographic study of 21 dogs with necropsy-confirmed PTE in which alveolar patterns were most commonly (10/21) observed (Fluckiger and Gomez, 1984).

Electrocardiography in animals with PTE may indicate right axis deviation or P-pulmonale, but these changes are neither sensitive nor specific for PTE.

DIAGNOSIS

The best approach for definitive diagnosis of PTE is controversial. The controversy centers on the question of when it is appropriate or necessary to perform a pulmonary arteriogram to confirm the diagnosis of PTE. A pulmonary arteriogram is the "gold standard" for diagnosis, but this procedure has potential complications and limitations. Arteriograms are invasive procedures, and in humans undergoing pulmonary arteriograms, the estimated morbidity and mortality are 4.0% and 0.2%, respectively. These complications would be expected to be higher in veterinary medicine as general anesthesia is usually required to perform pulmonary arteriograms in small animals (Koblik et al., 1989). Animals may be critically ill with cardiopulmonary disorders that preclude pulmonary arteriograms. Finally, angiography and the interpretation of arteriograms require specialized equipment and experienced, qualified personnel.

Pulmonary Scintigraphy

Scintigraphy is a noninvasive procedure that aids in, but cannot definitively confirm, the diagnosis of PTE. There are two types of nuclear medicine imaging procedures used in the diagnosis of PTE: ventilation and perfusion scans. The perfusion scan is done first because a normal study essentially rules out the diagnosis of clinically significant PTE. Ventilation scans may be done in cases where perfusion defects are observed. The combination of a normal ventilation scan and abnormal perfusion scan is consistent with the presence of PTE, and in some settings, this information is the basis on which therapy is initiated. However, this finding of an abnormal ventilation/perfusion scan is not synonymous with PTE.

Pulmonary perfusion scans are performed at some veterinary referral institutions. The procedure involves the injection of radionuclide-labelled, macroaggregated albumin into a peripheral vein of an animal; the particles are subsequently trapped in the pulmonary capillary bed. Immediate imaging of the animal with the use of a gamma camera demonstrates the extent of pulmonary blood flow. Perfusion defects are evaluated in terms of size, number, and location. As stated previously, the diagnosis of PTE is virtually excluded by the finding of a normal perfusion scan. Perfusion scans suffer from a lack of specificity because many other clinical conditions (pulmonary infiltrates, obstructive lung disease, pulmonary contusions, atelectasis) can cause perfusion defects.

Ventilation scans are performed in combination with perfusion scans to enhance diagnostic specificity. Radioactive inert gas such as xenon-133 or technetium-99m diethylene triamine pentacetate is inhaled by the animal while standard images are collected by the gamma camera. Normal ventilation scans in an animal show uniform distribution of radionuclide; uneven deposition or localized retention of radionuclide is observed in abnormally ventilated areas of the lung.

In most instances of PTE, an abnormal perfusion scan is accompanied by a normal ventilation scan; this combination is referred to as a ventilation/perfusion mismatch (V/Q mismatch).

Perfusion scans can be classified as normal, diagnostic, and nondiagnostic. In this scheme, abnormal perfusion scans are determined to be nondiagnostic if (1) radiographic infiltrates are present in the region corresponding to that of the perfusion defect or (2) the perfusion defect is small in size (subsegmental). If the perfusion scan is nondiagnostic, a pulmonary arteriogram is recommended. In cases of diagnostic perfusion scans, a ventilation scan may be undertaken. If a V/Q mismatch is observed, a high probability of PTE exists (approximately 90% based on several human studies). At this point, therapy is generally initiated without additional diagnostic evaluation. If there is a matching ventilation and perfusion defect, the scans are classified as nondiagnostic, and pulmonary arteriogram is recommended.

Pulmonary Angiography

Pulmonary arteriograms are indicated in those animals that require definitive confirmation or exclusion of diagnosis of PTE. Certainty in the diagnosis is required in critical, hemodynamically unstable animals suspected to have massive PTE, in animals with V/Q mismatch on scintigraphic evaluation in which anticoagulant therapy is contraindicated, and in animals known to have a disease that can mimic PTE. Pulmonary arteriograms are also indicated in most animals with nondiagnostic nuclear scans or when continued clinical suspicion does not correlate with findings from pulmonary ventilation and perfusion scans. Because the technique requires sedation or anesthesia and is invasive, there are greater risks and complications.

Two findings in pulmonary arteriograms are diagnostic for PTE: an intraluminal filling defect and sharp cutoff (i.e., occluded pulmonary artery). If either of these two abnormalities is demonstrated, the diagnosis is specific. Findings such as tortuous pulmonary arteries, decreased pulmonary perfusion, and delayed venous return to the left atrium may be observed but are nonspecific. Although a low number (5 to 10%) of false-negative results have been reported in the human medical literature, a negative pulmonary arteriogram of diagnostic quality essentially excludes clinically significant PTE.

PROGNOSIS

Presumably, as in humans, some animals die within hours of embolization, while others endure a chronic disease course. The majority of human deaths attributable to PTE occur in this acute population. In these cases, there is insufficient time for diagnostic confirmation, much less therapeutic approaches, to be implemented. Of those deaths in humans that occur after the first few hours following PTE (i.e., patients surviving acute disease), it is hypothesized that these deaths result from recurrent thromboembolism. The authors are unaware of any data in veterinary patients regarding the recurrence of PTE. In our experience, the prognosis for dogs with acute PTE is poor. If, however, the dog survives the acute episode, a guarded to fair prognosis may be expected. In all cases, the underlying cause of embolization must be considered in assessing long-term prognosis.

PROPHYLAXIS AND TREATMENT

Adequate guidelines for prophylaxis and treatment of PTE are unavailable for companion animals. The following guidelines for treatment of thromboembolic disease in the dog are based on clinical experience and extrapolation from human studies.

Prophylaxis

Prophylactic therapy is appropriate in the management of this disease syndrome owing to the prevalence of acute death, as well as the difficulty

of diagnosis and the potential complications of therapy associated with established PTE. Many studies have evaluated prophylactic options in various populations of human patients (e.g., orthopedic, gynecologic, urologic). The options available to reduce the prevalence of deep venous thrombosis (DVT) and PTE belong to two basic categories: the use of devices to modify blood flow and the administration of anticoagulant drugs. Since deep venous thrombosis (DVT) is not recognized as a significant risk factor for the development of PTE in companion animals, anticoagulant therapy would appear to be the more appropriate prophylactic option.

Low-dosage heparin administration has been documented to provide efficacious and safe prophylaxis in human patients with low to moderate risk of developing venous thrombosis. The standard regimen for low-dosage heparin administration in humans is 5000 U heparin subcutaneously every 8 to 12 hr, with therapy initiated prior to surgical intervention (or the time of risk) and continuing until the patient is ambulatory (or the risk is controlled). On this basis, a dog should receive approximately 70 U/kg of heparin every 8 to 12 hr. This low-dosage administration should not result in detectable changes in activated partial thromboplastin time (APTT) or activated coagulation time (ACT), and such monitoring is usually not required. This approach in human patients has resulted in a sharp reduction in the prevalence of PTE in all but the highest risk patients. Low-dosage heparinization is frequently not effective if initiated after surgical treatment, presumably because venous thrombosis develops intraoperatively. Significant hemorrhage has not been observed in surgical or postoperative patients treated in this manner.

Limited clinical experience has shown low-dosage heparin prophylaxis to be relatively safe in the dog, but additional experience and initiation of controlled prospective studies will be necessary to demonstrate efficacy. Since there are little data on which to estimate the natural prevalence of PTE in the dog, it is difficult to make a convincing argument for the need of prophylactic treatment. But considering the strong body of evidence justifying prophylaxis in humans, the apparent safety of low-dosage heparinization, and the clinical experience associated with the diagnosis and treatment of dogs with PTE, prophylactic therapy may be appropriate in many clinical situations. These situations include surgical patients believed to have increased risk of thrombosis (e.g., sepsis, neoplasia, prolonged recumbency) and animals with diseases associated with PTE (e.g., IMHA).

Treatment

The difficulty of providing a definitive diagnosis of PTE in the dog often causes many clinicians to decide to initiate empirical treatment based on clinical suspicion and evidence provided by nonspecific supporting data. If ventilation and perfusion scans are not available, treatment is usually indicated in animals with risk factors for PTE, a history of acute dyspnea with or without other cardiopulmonary signs, and supportive thoracic radiographs and blood gas analyses. It should be remembered that normal chest radiographs or normal blood gas analyses do not rule out a diagnosis of PTE. Ideally, pulmonary arteriograms should be performed in these cases.

TREATMENT IN HUMANS

Once the diagnosis of acute PTE is confirmed in human patients, high-dosage, intravenous, continuous-infusion heparin therapy is initiated. Heparin administration does not cause direct dissolution of existing thrombi, nor does it directly prevent acute embolism; heparin administration prevents thrombus growth and allows unopposed operation of the fibrinolytic system. In this way, heparinization contributes indirectly to thrombolytic resolution of the PTE. Acute embolization may still occur during heparinization owing to the presence of residual deep venous or cardiac thrombi. The clinical goal for heparinization is administration of heparin at a dosage that maintains the APTT at 1.5 times control values. Although monitoring of APTT is used to adjust heparin dosage, the results of this test are not a true measurement of the antithrombotic effect of heparin administration, nor is it entirely predictive of the potential for hemorrhagic complications. Loading doses in humans are usually 5000 to 15,000 U IV, followed by continuous intravenous infusion at 10 to 25 U/kg/hr. The initial high-dose bolus is aimed at preventing platelet aggregation and vasoconstriction associated with the release of platelet-derived vasoactive amines.

Human patients are usually maintained on intravenous heparin administration for at least a week. Anticoagulant therapy is frequently continued empirically for 6 months unless deep venous thrombi resolve in the interim. Subcutaneous heparin administration (10,000 U every 12 hr) is used in patients in whom warfarin therapy is contraindicated. Warfarin therapy is often instituted for chronic treatment.

HEPARIN THERAPY IN SMALL ANIMALS

Many veterinary clinicians have used heparin to treat PTE. Administration of an intravenous loading dose of heparin (100 to 200 U/kg) is recommended to achieve the desired antithrombotic effect as rapidly as possible. Intermittent subcutaneous administration of heparin (200 to 300 U/kg every 6 to 8 hours) should be initiated within 2 hours following the administration of the loading dose. If a dog is known or suspected to have antithrombin III deficiency (e.g., hepatic failure, glomerulonephropathy), it is necessary to administer fresh or fresh-frozen plasma (1 unit or dosage appropriate for severity of hypoalbuminemia) along with heparin administration. Initial doses of heparin may be mixed in with plasma or may be administered independently during plasma transfusion.

The subcutaneous administration of heparin should be adjusted to maintain the animal's APTT at least 1.5 times control values. Initially (usually 1 to 3 days), higher dosages of heparin (approximately 2 to 3 times normal dosage) may be required to achieve therapeutic goals. Different monitoring schemes have been recommended, but all of these schemes are complicated by the substantial differences in response to standard heparin dosages that exist between and within individual animals. The authors recommend that monitoring samples be obtained at 2 hours postinjection for an assessment of maximal anticoagulation or half-way between dose administration to assess a relative steady-state anticoagulation effect. One study in heparinized dogs (Green, 1980) showed that ACT can be used to monitor heparin therapy. Activated coagulation time monitoring is used by the authors when APTT values cannot be obtained.

WARFARIN

Warfarin is less commonly used as an anticoagulant by veterinary clinicians, but it can be used successfully in the dog. Warfarin therapy should be initiated in conjunction with heparin therapy as previously described. Recommended dosages for the dog are 0.1 mg/kg every 24 hr PO or 2 to 5 mg per dog every 24 hr PO, with individual dosages adjusted based on serial monitoring of the PT as described. If antithrombin III deficiency (or dysfunction) appears to be the underlying cause of PTE, warfarin administration is the treatment of choice (warfarin unlike heparin does not require the presence of antithrombin III to mediate its anticoagulant effect).

COMPLICATIONS

Bleeding is the most significant complication of anticoagulant therapy. Unfortunately, measurement of APTT, ACT, and PT does not reliably predict the likelihood of hemorrhage. Hemorrhage is estimated to occur in about 5% of human patients treated with warfarin or heparin, and certain factors are recognized to predispose to hemorrhage. These factors include age, coexistent disease, and potential for bleeding sites in the gastrointestinal tract or kidney. The administration of concurrent or recent therapies can aggravate bleeding tendencies, e.g., aspirin administration or blood transfusion (anticoagulant administration). Animals on anticoagulant therapy should be closely observed for signs of bleeding, and if bleeding occurs, those animals should be evaluated for underlying diseases and predisposing factors. A coagulation profile should be obtained in these animals in order to help define the bleeding tendency.

Heparin administration may induce thrombocytopenia, which, if severe, may necessitate interruption of heparin therapy. Administration of protamine may be used to reverse heparinization (1 mg of protamine for every 1 mg heparin administered during the last dose to the patient; administer protamine slowly IV in a 1% solution).

Hemorrhage in animals treated with warfarin may be managed in several ways, depending on its severity. Discontinuation of warfarin administration may be sufficient to control mild bleeding, while discontinuation and administration of fresh-frozen plasma or vitamin K_1 may be necessary in cases of significant hemorrhage. The effect of vitamin K_1 administration may preclude therapeutic oral anticoagulation for up to three weeks.

Warfarin administration is contraindicated in pregnant animals because the drug crosses the placenta and is teratogenic. Relative contraindications to warfarin administration are common due to drug interaction with frequently used drugs (e.g., tetracycline, thyroxine, barbiturates).

SUPPORTIVE CARE

Appropriate supportive therapy is indicated in all animals with PTE. Stable, hypoxemic animals may benefit most from the administration of oxygen therapy. Animals in cardiopulmonary distress due to PTE should be immediately treated with intravenous heparin and supplemented with oxygen. Mechanical ventilation may be necessary in some patients with severe dyspnea and hypoxemia; blood gas analyses can be used for guidance in these patients (see this volume, p. 98). Concomitant hypotension should be managed with the administration of crystalloids and appropriate pressor agents such as dopamine (5 to 15 μg/kg/min IV) administration. Echocardiographic evaluation of animals with PTE may be indicated to optimize cardiac therapy and to rule out the presence of thrombus in the right atrium or ventricle.

THROMBOLYTIC THERAPY

There are little data in veterinary literature to justify the use of thrombolytic agents in the treatment of PTE. Classically, thrombolytic agents have been considered as an option for treatment of patients with massive PTE and marked cardiopulmonary compromise. Although there is evidence that the administration of thrombolytics may hasten early thrombus resolution in human patients, improved survival has not been demonstrated. Any potential benefits from the administration of these drugs must be weighed against their significant expense and the increased risk of bleeding associated with their use.

References and Suggested Reading

Fluckiger, M. A., and Gomez, J. A.: Radiographic findings in dogs with spontaneous thrombosis or embolism. Vet. Radiol. 25:124, 1984.
A retrospective radiographic review of 21 dogs with pulmonary thrombosis or embolism.
Green, R. A.: Activated coagulation time in monitoring heparinized dogs. Am. J. Vet. Res. 41:1793, 1980.
Experimental study of IV and SQ heparin dosages monitored by ACT and APTT.
Hull, R. D., Coates, G., Raskob, G. E., et al.: Diagnosis of pulmonary embolism. In Colman, R. W., et al. (eds.): Hemostasis and Thrombosis, 2nd ed. Philadelphia: J. B. Lippincott, 1987, p. 1240.
Human review article.
Klein, M. K., Dow, S. W., and Rosychuk, R. A. W.: Pulmonary thromboembolism associated with immune-mediated hemolytic anemia in dogs: Ten cases (1982–1987). J.A.V.M.A. 195:246, 1989.
Retrospective study of 31 cases of IMHA; risk factors for PTE identified.
Koblik, P. D., Hornof, W., Harnagel, S. H., et al.: A comparison of pulmonary angiography, digital subtraction angiography, and 99 m Tc-DTCPA/MAA ventilation-perfusion scintigraphy for detection of experimental pulmonary emboli in the dog. Vet. Radiol. 30:159, 1989.
A comparison of imaging techniques in 18 dogs with experimental acute PTE.
Mohr, D. N., Ryu, J. H., Litin, S. C., et al.: Recent advances in the management of venous thromboembolism. Mayo Clin. Proc. 63:281, 1988.
Human review article.
Moser, K. M.: State of the art: Venous thromboembolism. Am. Rev. Respir. Dis. 141:235, 1990.
Human review article with particular focus on controversial aspects of diagnosis, prophylaxis, and treatment.
Moser, K. M., Guisan, M., Bartimmo, E. E., et al.: In vivo and post mortem dissolution rates of pulmonary emboli and venous thrombi in the dog. Circulation 48:170, 1973.
Experimental study in 87 dogs of post mortem and in vivo dissolution rates of induced thrombi.
Newman, G. E.: Pulmonary angiography in pulmonary embolic disease. J. Thorac. Imaging 4:28, 1989.
Human review article of applications of pulmonary angiography in PTE.
Rosenow, E. C., Osmundson, P. J., and Brown, M. L.: Pulmonary embolism. Mayo Clin. Proc. 56:161, 1981.
Human review article.

HEAT STROKE

DAVID RUSLANDER

North Grafton, Massachusetts

Heat stroke is a pathologic state caused by an excessive elevation in body temperature. A brief review of thermoregulation will aid in the understanding of heat stroke and its proper treatment. Body heat is produced from three main processes: basal metabolism, muscular activity, and the assimilation of food, known as oxidation. Body heat is dissipated by several means. Radiation of infrared heat waves accounts for the majority of heat loss from the body. Conduction is the exchange of heat between two objects in direct contact with one another. Convection is the removal of heat from the body by air currents. Evaporation of water or sweat cools the body by removing heat. A very small amount of heat is lost in association with excretion of feces and urine.

The thermoregulatory center is located in the preoptic region of the anterior hypothalamus. Thermoregulation is merely the balance between heat loss and heat production. Homeostatic mechanisms work to keep the body temperature within a very narrow range, called the set point. When an animal's body temperature decreases below this set point, heat-producing mechanisms are activated to raise the temperature. These heat-producing mechanisms include shivering, increased voluntary activity, increased catecholamine secretion, cutaneous vasoconstriction, postural changes, piloerection, and an increase in thyroxine production. The opposite effects occur when the temperature is elevated. Cutaneous vasodilation, increased respiration, panting, anorexia, postural changes, and sweating are some responses to an increased body temperature.

Hyperthermia is defined as an elevation in body temperature and can be divided into pyrogenic hyperthermia (hyperthermia due to fever) and nonpyrogenic hyperthermia. Fever is characterized by an increased body temperature attributable to a fully functional thermoregulatory mechanism. Exogenous pyrogens and endogenous pyrogens act on the anterior hypothalamus to raise the set point to a higher temperature. Nonpyrogenic hyperthermia occurs when the heat-dissipating mechanisms cannot compensate for the heat-producing mechanisms, leading to an increase in body temperature *above the set point*. Common causes of nonpyrogenic hyperthermia include heat stroke, excessive exercise, seizures, hypothalamic lesions, thyrotoxicosis,

and less commonly, malignant hyperthermia, a rare anesthetic complication.

Heat stroke is a complex pathologic state that results from direct thermal injury to body tissues exposed to excessive temperatures. The critical temperature associated with the consistent occurrence of enzyme alterations and cell membrane instability leading to multiple organ deterioration appears to be 109°F (43°C). Many factors predispose an animal to develop heat stroke, including lack of acclimatization, excessive environmental humidity, water deprivation, drug administration, obesity, underlying cardiovascular disease, exercise, central nervous system disease, and previous episodes of heat stroke. Brachycephalic breeds and dogs with upper airway disease such as laryngeal paralysis are extremely susceptible to the development of heat stroke. The overwhelming majority of heat stroke victims are dogs that have been confined in an automobile and left unattended, even for short periods of time.

PATHOPHYSIOLOGY

The multisystemic pathophysiologic processes of heat stroke are due to direct thermal effects. The central nervous system is often affected. Neuronal injury and cell death, the development of cerebral edema, and the occurrence of localized areas of intraparenchymal hemorrhage can lead to seizures, coma, and death. Signs of cerebellar dysfunction may also develop and remain permanent in animals that survive. Elevated temperatures in the hypothalamus may cause destruction and damage to the thermoregulatory centers, leading to an abnormally functioning hypothalamus and predisposition to subsequent hyperthermic episodes.

Hyperthermia leads to increased cardiac output and hypoxia due to increased metabolic demands, decreased systemic vascular resistance, and hypovolemia secondary to dehydration. Tachyarrhythmias and cardiogenic shock are common sequelae in heat stroke, most likely because of myocardial hemorrhage, ischemia, and necrosis.

Gastrointestinal effects of hyperthermia include ulceration secondary to ischemia and profuse bloody diarrhea. These conditions are often associated with the development of endotoxemia. These clinical signs occur initially and are not necessarily related to disseminated intravascular coagulation, which often develops later in the course of the disease process. Direct toxic thermal damage to the hepatic parenchyma may cause severe or fatal liver injury.

Some of the most profound and potentially life-threatening effects of hyperthermia occur in the kidney. Thermal injury to the kidney can lead to acute renal failure, especially in the severely dehydrated animal. Rhabdomyolysis is associated with muscle necrosis from thermal injury and is manifested by a dark, "machine oil"–colored urine. This occurrence may exacerbate the acute tubular necrosis via dehydration, hypoperfusion, and pigment deposition.

Hematologic abnormalities associated with heat stroke can include hemoconcentration secondary to dehydration, leukocytosis related to catecholamine secretion, anemia secondary to blood loss, and, most important, clotting abnormalities. Hyperthermic processes can cause direct destruction of clotting factors as well as a decrease in hepatic synthesis of these factors if severe liver damage occurs. The megakaryocytic cell lines appear to be especially sensitive to thermal injury, and thrombocytopenia is often seen. Thrombocytopenia associated with thermal damage to megakaryocytes will not become apparent for a few days and should not be confused with low platelet counts seen earlier in the disease process. This thrombocytopenia is most likely caused by a consumption of platelets secondary to gastrointestinal bleeding. Disseminated intravascular coagulation can manifest initially or within the first several days following heat stroke. Its development can be attributable to the previously mentioned coagulation defects, disruption of vascular endothelium, sludging of blood secondary to shock, and consumption of coagulation factors due to gastrointestinal bleeding.

Hyperthermia can have a profound effect on an animal's acid-base status and can lead to such derangements as respiratory alkalosis as a result of excessive panting and severe metabolic acidosis associated with excessive muscular activity and shock.

CLINICAL PRESENTATION

A diagnosis of nonpyrogenic hyperthermia should be considered when a dog presents with a body temperature higher than 106°F and no obvious evidence of infection. Fever or pyrogenic hyperthermia exists when there is an elevation in the hypothalamic set point; therefore a dog with a fever will not necessarily present with panting or hypersalivation, as these are heat-dissipating mechanisms. In contrast, an animal with heat stroke will present with extreme panting hypersalivation and darkened mucous membranes in an attempt to decrease the markedly elevated temperature.

Many animals, depending on the duration of the hyperthermic event, manifest shock with bloody vomitus and diarrhea as well as being stuporous or even comatose on initial presentation.

A thorough history should be obtained at some point to determine if there is an underlying cause for the animal's inability to dissipate heat. A history of a dog's being locked in a car for an hour on a hot afternoon would readily explain the circumstances. However, many dogs present as heat stroke victims without this history. These animals should be carefully evaluated for underlying disease such as laryngeal paralysis, upper airway disease, neurologic disease, cardiac disease, or some other precipitating cause.

EMERGENCY TREATMENT

The key to recovery from heat stroke lies in early recognition and treatment. Treatment should be instituted at home by the owners whenever possible. Following initial phone consultation, the dog should be sprayed with cold water *before* transporting it to the veterinary clinic. All the car windows should be left open on the way to the clinic, as this will help to increase convective heat losses from the dog.

On presentation at the clinic, the dog should be sprayed down with cold water or immersed in a cold water bath. Massaging the animal will help to increase blood flow, vasodilation, and cooling. An ice-water bath is usually not necessary and may actually decrease cooling of the animal because of vasoconstriction and decreased cutaneous blood flow. Furthermore, application of ice water may induce a shivering response, which is a heat-generating mechanism. Cold water enemas have been suggested as a means of decreasing body temperature, but this approach is often not necessary and inhibits temperature monitoring.

Isotonic fluids should be administered (90 ml/kg/hr, IV) to counteract cardiovascular shock. Corticosteroid administration has been advocated for its membrane-stabilizing effects, although there are no results of controlled studies supporting the efficacy of this treatment. Dogs may have severe upper airway obstruction requiring a tracheostomy, either as a cause (laryngeal paralysis) or as a result of the hyperthermia (laryngeal edema). Acetylpromazine (0.05 to 0.1 mg/kg IV or IM) can be used for its sedative effect to decrease shivering associated with the cold-water bath. Care should be exercised with the administration of acetylpromazine because many hyperthermic dogs may be epileptics, which is a contraindication to administration of this agent. Acetylpromazine should be used with care in the animal with shock because of the vasodilatory effects of the drug and the potential for creating a hypotensive crisis.

Administration of antipyretics such as aspirin and flunixin meglumine (Banamine, Schering) are *contraindicated* in a case of *nonpyrogenic* hyperthermia. These drugs decrease the hypothalamic set point via their antiprostaglandin effects. In heat stroke, the set point is normal; therefore attempts to decrease the set point will not lower body temperature. It must be remembered that the animal is being cooled via other means, and the potential exists for creating a hypothermic state with the administration of these drugs. Furthermore, administration of these drugs can have severe gastrointestinal side effects, especially in an animal that may have a compromised gastrointestinal tract and perfusion and coagulation defects. Aggressive efforts to lower body temperature should be discontinued when the animal's body temperature reaches 103°F (39°C), since further passive cooling will occur. Hypothermia can result from overzealous attempts to cool the animal.

EXTENDED TREATMENT AND MONITORING

Continued supportive care and careful monitoring of the heat stroke victim are imperative because sequelae often develop during the several days following the hyperthermic event. These animals should be maintained on intravenous fluid therapy, and careful attention should be paid to urine production by the animal because acute renal failure is a common sequela. Central venous pressures and serial thoracic auscultation can be followed as a means of ensuring adequate blood volume expansion if there is concern about urine production. An indwelling urinary catheter can be placed, and urine production can be closely monitored if renal function appears compromised. If there is concern over the possibility of acute renal failure, an intravenous dopamine infusion can be instituted (2 to 4 µg/kg/min) to increase renal blood flow. Furosemide can also be administered (2 mg/kg IV t.i.d. or q.i.d.) to increase urine production. Continuous electrocardiographic monitoring is an effective way of identifying any cardiac arrhythmias that may develop. Should cardiac arrhythmias develop, appropriate therapy should be instituted as soon as possible. Ventricular premature depolarizations and ventricular tachycardia should be treated with a lidocaine bolus initially (2 mg/kg IV), and if there is conversion to a normal sinus rhythm, an intravenous lidocaine infusion should be established (30 to 75 µg/kg/min). Treatment for metabolic acidosis should be instituted in all animals with a blood pH less than 7.1. Sodium bicarbonate (0.3 × body weight [kg] × base deficit IV) should be administered if this situation occurs, with 50% of the calculated dose administered as an intravenous bolus. If subsequent blood gas determinations indicate that the animal is not compensating and is still acidotic, the other 50% of the sodium bicarbonate should be given over the next 12 hours as a constant infusion. If disseminated intravascular coagulation is present, heparin therapy (50 to 100 units/kg SC q.i.d.) and fresh or fresh-frozen plasma transfusions may be required to prevent progression of the process.

Following resolution of the hyperthermia, diagnostic tests should be performed to identify and characterize any underlying disease process that may have precipitated the hyperthermic event as well as to identify sequelae associated with the hyperthermic episode. A complete blood count, serum biochemical profile, serial blood gas determinations, serial coagulation profiles, and a urinalysis should be performed on all animals that develop heat stroke. This approach will help identify underlying disease and establish baseline data for such parameters as Pa_{O_2}, serum creatinine, bicarbonate and electrolyte concentrations, and hepatic enzyme activities. Chest radiographs should be performed to identify animals with underlying cardiovascular disease and to evaluate pulmonary complications.

A serum biochemical profile, complete blood count, and coagulation profile should be obtained on the animal several days following the initial presentation in order to assess ongoing problems and identify sequelae associated with the liver, kidney, and coagulation systems. The length of hospitalization will depend on how quickly the animal responds and can range from several days to weeks if complications arise.

SUMMARY

The prognosis in heat stroke victims is variable and depends on the presence or absence of any underlying disease that may have precipitated the hyperthermia. In any case, the prognosis is guarded to poor, given the potential for life-threatening complications. Heat stroke victims often will have residual neurologic deficits and are predisposed to recurrent episodes of hyperthermia. Animals that recover are those whose temperatures are returned to normal early in the course of the disease, since the longer the animal remains hyperthermic, the greater is the damage that occurs to vital organ systems.

References and Suggested Reading

Curley, F., and Irwin, R.: Disorders of temperature control: Part I: Hyperthermia. J. Intensive Care Med. 1:5, 1986.

Provides an in-depth review of temperature regulation as well as pathogenesis and treatment of heat stroke in human patients.
Guyton, A.: Body temperature, temperature regulation and fever. *In* Guyton, A. (ed.): *Textbook of Medical Physiology*, 8th ed. Philadelphia: W. B. Saunders, 1991, pp. 797–807.
Provides an overview of temperature regulation in human beings.
Johnson, K.: Pathophysiology of heatstroke. Compend. Contin. Educ. Pract. Vet. 4:141, 1982.

Discusses the pathogenesis of heatstroke and its effects on the body systems.
Krum, S., and Osborn, C.: Heatstroke in the dog. A polysystemic disorder. J.A.V.M.A. 170:531–535, 1977.
Presents several case reports of heat stroke in dogs and discusses laboratory abnormalities as well as treatment.

TREATMENT OF ACUTE BURN INJURY AND SMOKE INHALATION

WILLIAM D. SAXON,
Modesto, California

and REBECCA KIRBY
Philadelphia, Pennsylvania

The causes of thermal injuries in small animals include direct contact with a heated surface or flames, scalds, chemical burns, and electric hair dryers. Smoke inhalation injury can occur alone or can accompany thermal injury and is most serious when an animal is in an enclosed space or is discovered to be unconscious at the scene of a fire. In humans, respiratory failure from inhalation is the leading cause of death during the initial 24 hr after a fire.

Much of the current knowledge concerning the pathophysiology and therapeutic management of burns is based on the results of animal studies. The mechanisms and therapeutic recommendations presented for small animals are derived from these animal studies and from therapeutic procedures used in domestic animals and humans.

CLASSIFICATION

Determining the severity of burn injury is important as a guide to initial resuscitation measures and prognosis. Burns are classified on the basis of degree or depth (Table 1) and percentage of total body surface area (TBSA) involved. TBSA can be rapidly estimated by employing the rule of nines. Using this rule, each forelimb accounts for 9% TBSA, each rear limb 18%, head and neck 9%, and dorsal and ventral thorax/abdomen each account for 18% of TBSA. TBSA can also be estimated by measuring the burned area in centimeters and using a chart converting body weight in kilograms to square meters.

The location of a burn is also considered when estimating severity. Small burns to the perineum, feet, eyes, ears, and face are considered severe injuries because of the potential loss of function and cosmetic appearance and the severity of associated pain.

Determination of the severity of thermal injury in animals is often difficult because the haircoat obscures complete visualization of the skin. Skin has a high specific heat and a low thermal conductivity, making it slow to overheat and slow to cool. Consequently, thermal damage can continue after the animal has been removed from the source of heat. Early accurate detection of the severity of a burn is difficult, making it best to overestimate rather than underestimate the extent of injuries.

BURN AND INHALATION PATHOPHYSIOLOGY

The classification, by Demling, of pathophysiologic changes into three groups according to time from onset of injury enables an appropriate understanding of the clinical progression and therapeutic requirements of the burn patient. Table 2 lists the anticipated pathophysiologic changes during each

Table 1. *Classification of Burns*

Classification	Skin Layer	Pain	Signs
Superficial	Epidermis	+ + +	Erythema; desquamation
Partial Superficial	Partial epidermis, mid-dermis	+ +	Erythema; subcutaneous edema
Deep	Total epidermis; partial dermis	+ +	Severe inflammation; dry surface; does not blanche
Full	Epidermis; dermis	−	Leathery (eschar); dry; anesthetic; blanched

period. Though a continuum, the early and later changes necessitate discussion separately.

RESUSCITATION PERIOD (0 TO 48 HOURS)

Microvasculature

A significant increase in microvascular permeability occurs throughout the body following severe burn injury. In burned tissue, the microvascular permeability changes are due to direct thermal injury causing vascular damage and to vasoactive substances (e.g., prostaglandins, leukotrienes, his-

Table 2. *Expected Pathophysiologic Changes in Burn Patients*

Resuscitation Period (0–48 hr)
Increased vascular permeability*
Decreased cardiac output
Decreased metabolic rate initially
Decreased immunity
Red blood cell hemolysis
Initiation of disseminated intravascular coagulation
Upper airway edema
Bronchospasms
Carbon monoxide intoxication
Wound/soft-tissue inflammation and edema
Corneal edema and ulceration

Early Postresuscitation Period (2–6 days)
Stabilization of microvasculature
Increased cardiac output
Increased metabolic rate
Decreased immunity
± Anemia
Increased bronchiolar edema/cellular debris
Pneumonia
Wound drying ± bacterial invasion
Improved upper airway disease

Inflammation, Infection, and Wound Closure Period (7 days–closure)
Intact microvasculature
Increased cardiac and urine output
Increased metabolic rate
Increased carbon dioxide production
Decreased immunity
Pneumonia, respiratory fatigue
Sepsis

*The most clinically significant early abnormality.

tamine, serotonin, kinins, and oxygen radicals) released from the damaged tissues. Within the burn wound the microcirculation becomes permeable to macromolecules 100 Angström radius or larger. Consequently, albumin and plasma water losses into the interstitium are substantial.

Edema of soft tissues in nonburn injured areas may be due to decreased plasma oncotic pressure and ease of water movement across microvascular membranes. Increased intracellular sodium concentration establishes an osmotic gradient for water movement from the vascular to the intracellular compartment. As much as 50% of total plasma water can be lost from the vascular compartment 2 to 3 hours after a 40% TBSA burn.

Hemodynamics

Cardiac output is significantly decreased following burn injury in an animal. This effect is attributed to hypovolemia and increased systemic vascular resistance (SVR) and pulmonary vascular resistance in response to high concentrations of circulating catecholamines. Depression of myocardial function is directly related to the severity of the burn, with the release of a myocardial depressant factor from burned tissue postulated as the etiology. Cardiac output returns to normal before restoration of plasma volume because of compensatory increases in heart rate and myocardial contractility. Consequently, central venous pressure and pulmonary capillary wedge pressure will remain low until plasma volume is restored.

Metabolism

Metabolic rate is decreased immediately after thermal injury because of decreased oxygen and nutrient delivery to cells. Poor perfusion, pain, and hypothermia stimulate increased circulating concentrations of stress hormones, such as catecholamines, glucagon, and glucocorticosteroids, which increase SVR, gluconeogenesis, and glycogenolysis. Shivering from hypothermia increases utilization of glucose and contributes to the rapid depletion of liver glycogen. Anaerobic metabolism and metabolic acidosis can result.

Immunologic/Hematologic Systems

Humoral and cell-mediated immunity are impaired in the early postburn period in patients with more than 20% TBSA burns. Mechanisms postulated include increased circulating cortisol concentration, suppression of lymphoid tissues, and release of immunosuppressive substances. Abnormalities in neutrophil, macrophage, and monocyte function; suppression of lymphocyte proliferation; loss of immunoglobulin G and fibronectin into the burn wound; and inhibition of complement and opsonin activity have been incriminated.

Abnormalities in red blood cells of animals with burn injury include hemolysis from direct thermal injury, passage through damaged microcirculation, and disseminated intravascular coagulation with resultant hemoglobinemia and hemoglobinuria; shortened circulating red blood cell lifespan; and depressed hematopoiesis. Coagulation abnormalities may be present, causing hypercoagulable states or excessive bleeding.

Pulmonary System

Damage to the respiratory tract occurs from both thermal and chemical mechanisms. High temperatures cause immediate injury to the upper airway mucosa. Unfiltered, heated particles cause mucosal congestion, hemorrhage, ulceration, and sloughing. Laryngospasm can result in suffocation.

Chemical injury to the respiratory tract is caused by inhalation of water- or lipid-soluble gases (e.g., carbon monoxide, sulfur dioxide, chlorine, nitrous oxide, hydrogen chloride, hydrogen cyanide, and aldehydes) that coat carbon particles and attach to the bronchi and alveoli. These toxic gases lead to hypoxemia by denaturing proteins, by decreasing oxygen binding to hemoglobin, and by impairing oxygen unloading from hemoglobin. Substances deposited deep within the respiratory tract result in immediate inactivation of ciliary movement and surfactant. The result is impaired clearance of bacteria and microatelectasis with resultant increase in small airway resistance and bronchospasms.

Inhalation injury immediately results in hypoxemia, hypercarbia, decreased cardiac output, and mixed metabolic and respiratory acidosis. Pulmonary shunting of blood and ventilation perfusion mismatching can be detected when the quotient of the arterial oxygen concentration divided by the fraction of inspired oxygen is less than 300 ($Pa_{O_2}/Fi_{O_2} < 300$). Fluid resuscitation for the treatment of shock contributes to the development of pulmonary edema during the latter part of this resuscitation period. Initial thoracic radiographs are usually normal. Burns to the chest wall cause pain and decrease chest wall compliance, leading to increased work of breathing and aggravation of diffuse microatelectasis from hypoventilation.

Wound

A zone of ischemia exists in the burn wound between the nonviable tissue and the viable deeper and adjacent tissue. This zone is composed of cells that have been reversibly damaged by heat, vasoactive substances, and ischemia. Loss of viability of cells in this zone can cause a superficial or partial-thickness wound to progress to a deep, full-thickness wound.

EARLY POSTRESUSCITATION PERIOD (2 TO 6 DAYS)

Microvasculature

Microvascular integrity is restored and the return of blood flow through the microcirculation of burned tissue results in resorption of edema fluid, osmotically active cell fragments, and proteins. This process augments plasma volume and should be considered when determining fluid requirements during this period in order to avoid volume overload.

Hemodynamics

Once adequate circulating blood volume has been restored, a hyperdynamic circulatory state develops characterized by increased heart rate, increased cardiac output, decreased myocardial depression, and decreased SVR. Urine output increases as the reabsorbed solute from burn-injured tissue causes an obligate solute diuresis.

Metabolism

A hypermetabolic state occurs, with metabolic rates increased three times above normal basal metabolic rates. Muscle catabolism and negative nitrogen balance are initiated and continue until wound closure. Weight loss occurs. Circulating catecholamine concentrations remain elevated, especially if pain and hypothermia are not controlled, and are partially responsible for propagating the catabolic state.

Immunologic/Hematologic Systems

In general, significant bacterial invasion of the burn wound does not occur unless initial debridement was inadequate. Immune dysfunction, however, continues until wound closure. Anemia may have developed as a consequence of hemolysis, decreased life span, and bone marrow suppression. Coagulation abnormalities may be present.

Pulmonary System

In the absence of inhalation injury, pulmonary function is usually normal during this period. Chest wall compliance may still be decreased. Upper airway edema resolves, but mucosal irritation persists and causes increased secretions and decreased mucociliary clearance. If inhalation injury has occurred, it progresses during this phase. Small airway obstruction occurs as heat-damaged mucosal cells lining bronchi and bronchioles slough into the lumen. This results in bronchial secretion and predisposes the lungs to bacterial invasion. During this stage, the animal may have a productive cough as well as an elevated respiratory rate and increased respiratory effort on physical examination, accompanied by an interstitial and bronchiolar pattern on thoracic radiographs.

Wounds

Early burn wound infection is usually caused by endogenous flora from the skin or gastrointestinal or respiratory systems. *Staphylococcus intermedius* and streptococci are first to colonize the wound, followed in several days by coliforms and *Pseudomonas* spp. Nosocomial infections with resistant organisms are potential hazards to animals with burn injury. Direct contact (hands of personnel) is the major route for spread of nosocomial infection, with air currents being a less common route of transmission.

PERIOD OF INFLAMMATION, INFECTION, AND WOUND HEALING (7 DAYS–WOUND CLOSURE)

Microvasculature

Unless sepsis has developed, the microvasculature remains intact.

Hemodynamics

Cardiac output and urine production remain elevated, since heart rate is increased and SVR is low. Hypovolemia associated with inadequate fluid administration should be differentiated from septic shock during this hyperdynamic phase, since elevated body temperature, increased heart rate, and decreased SVR may be observed with both conditions. Increased urine specific gravity and increased urine and plasma osmolality suggest hypovolemia. However, hypovolemia can present as a component of septic shock. Sepsis or septic shock should be strongly considered if a septic focus has been identified and increases in base deficit are measured.

Immunologic/Hematologic System

Impaired immunity may be the cause or result of sepsis. Abnormalities such as decreased plasma and tissue fibronectin concentrations have been observed in patients prior to the onset of sepsis. These abnormalities could be useful as predictive indexes in the early detection of sepsis.

Metabolism

The hypermetabolic state persists and its magnitude is directly proportional to the size of the burn wounds. Polymorphonuclear cells and macrophages in the wounds release chemical mediators of inflammation, such as interleukin-1, which are thought to initiate hypermetabolism. The metabolic rate will not return to normal until the wound is closed and inflammation resolves. Body temperature is elevated owing to resetting of the thermoregulatory center, and oxygen consumption and carbon dioxide production are increased. Persistent increases in circulating concentrations of stress hormones are partly responsible for the catabolism and increased gluconeogenesis during this phase.

Pulmonary System

Pulmonary function is often markedly abnormal during this period. Carbon dioxide production is increased by hypermetabolism, and often the hyperventilation that results increases the work of breathing and may lead to respiratory muscle fatigue. Pneumonia often becomes the major life-threatening problem in patients with inhalation injury. Lung defense mechanisms have been destroyed as a result of denuded mucosal surfaces, decreased mucociliary clearance and surfactant production, impaired alveolar macrophage function, and systemic immune dysfunction. Sepsis may result in concomitant development of the adult respiratory distress syndrome.

Table 3. *Resuscitation Therapy of Extensive Burn and Inhalation Injuries (0–48 hr)*

First Aid and Transport

1. Separate patient from offending burning agent. Do not attempt to neutralize acid or alkaline burns.
2. Remove collars and restrictive materials.
3. Flush and cool affected areas with copious amounts of cool water for several minutes, then cool only 10–20% of affected body surface area at a time.
4. Support breathing—extend neck and elevate head; provide mouth-to-nose resuscitation if necessary.
5. Wrap patient in clean (sterile if possible) sheet. Use additional blanket if necessary to avoid chilling.
6. *Avoid* owner placement of ointments to wound areas.
7. Transport quickly to critical care veterinary facility.

In-hospital Initial Resuscitation Therapy

1. Establish patent airway—intubate early if necessary.
2. Provide supplemental humidified oxygen, maintain ventilation.
3. Establish peripheral IV access through healthy tissue (consider intraosseous fluids if necessary).
4. Obtain samples for complete blood count, serum biochemical and coagulation profiles, arterial blood gas, urinalysis, carboxyhemoglobin determination, and blood typing and cross-match.
5. Administer balanced crystalloid solution. Treat shock and maintain adequate tissue perfusion. Estimated fluid needs—1–4 ml/kg % TBSA burn over 24-hour period.*
   (*Avoid* colloids, if possible, for first 6 hr of resuscitation.)
6. Remove collars and materials that may act as tourniquets.
7. Control pain.
8. Perform thorough physical examination.
9. Clip hair and estimate depth and extent of burns.
10. Clean wounds with copious flushing with water or saline.
11. Evaluate ocular involvement, stain corneas, and medicate.
12. Monitor electrocardiogram, urine output, arterial blood gases, blood pressure, central venous pressure, pulmonary capillary wedge pressure.
13. Add colloids to fluids 6–8 hr after burn (plasma, whole blood, hetastarch, or dextran).
14. *Avoid* prophylactic antibiotic administration—treat only identified bacterial infections (culture skin biopsy from wounds, urine, blood, sputum).
15. *Avoid* glucocorticosteroid administration.
16. Following stabilization, soak patient in tub with half strength providone-iodine solution for 20 min (if extensive deep burns) and rinse with water or saline. Debride burn wounds, cover with antibiotic burn ointment, such as silver sulfadiazine, and occlusive dressing.

*Formula extrapolated from dosage used for humans. Decrease volume 25–50% for cats.

TREATMENT

Guidelines for first aid and emergency room resuscitation of animals with moderate to severe burn and inhalation injuries are presented in Table 3. Once the animal has received initial resuscitative treatment, a thorough history is obtained to ascertain the cause of burn injury (thermal or chemical), the type of material burned, length of exposure, and any evidence of transient loss of consciousness in the animal that occurred prior to arrival at the emergency room.

TREATMENT DURING THE RESUSCITATION PERIOD

Fluid Therapy

The goal of fluid therapy is to maintain tissue perfusion. Intravenous fluids should be administered at a volume and rate sufficient to maintain adequate tissue perfusion. Crystalloids are recommended during the first 6 to 8 hr because the microcirculatory leakage is great and colloids and proteins will not be retained. However, patients that have life-threatening shock or life-threatening inhalation injury *may* benefit transiently from combination crystalloid-colloid or crystalloid-hypertonic saline infusion. Low-molecular-weight dextran (up to 20 ml/kg/day IV), hetastarch (up to 20 ml/kg/day), or 7.5% hypertonic saline (4 to 8 ml/kg IV) in combination with crystalloids may increase plasma volume, with less total volume administered. Side effects associated with these infusions can include cardiac arrhythmias, hypernatremia, decreased mean arterial pressure, coagulation abnormalities, and volume overload of the cardiovascular system once capillary membranes stabilize. If possible, it is best to wait until the vascular leak slows, usually within 6 to 12 hr after the burn, before plasma or colloids are administered.

Various formulas are used in human medicine to calculate the initial fluid requirements for the burn patient, and those formulas can serve as a guideline for treatment of the small animal patient. One such formula recommends 1 to 4 ml/kg × % TBSA burn during the first 24 hr, with a 25 to 50% reduction in this amount suggested for cats. The rate of fluid administration should be individualized for each patient, but guidelines are to administer one half of the calculated dose in the first 8 hr and the remainder over the next 16 hr.

Fluids should be administered through a peripheral catheter placed in nonburned tissue. If it is necessary to place a catheter through burn tissue, it should be removed and replaced at a different site every 24 hr. Intraosseous catheterization should be considered when no peripheral venous sites are available (see this volume, p. 107). An increased potential for sepsis and thromboembolism is reported in humans with central venous catheters. When central lines are required for monitoring, these catheters should be removed as soon as possible.

Urine production, heart rate, arterial and venous blood pressure, acid-base status, and venous oxygen tension should be serially monitored and used as indicators of tissue perfusion. Restoration of normal plasma volume during this period is difficult to achieve, resulting commonly in a less than "normal" urine output. The central venous pressure and pulmonary capillary wedge pressure typically remain low, even when cardiac output and perfusion are adequate. Overzealous attempts to normalize these parameters by restoring blood volume above what is necessary for adequate perfusion can accentuate tissue and pulmonary edema–related complications. Monitoring serum electrolyte concentrations is indicated because potassium released from heat damaged cells may cause significant hyperkalemia and cardiac arrhythmias.

Respiratory Therapy

The goals of respiratory therapy are (1) to treat carbon monoxide poisoning, (2) to prevent upper airway obstruction, and (3) to maintain small airway patency. Carbon monoxide poisoning is treated by increasing the percentage of inspired oxygen to 80 to 100% for at least 20 to 30 min. In the absence of significant upper airway injury, administering oxygen by mask, nasal cannula, or oxygen cage will suffice.

When facial deformity or severe laryngeal edema prevents orotracheal intubation, immediate tracheostomy is performed. Severe upper airway obstruction is best prevented by anticipation and early intubation in situations with evidence of mild, progressive obstruction. Placing a tracheostomy tube through burned tissue should be avoided to minimize the risk of wound and airway infection.

Strict asepsis is required during tube placement, tube cleaning, and pulmonary toilet (airway oxygenation, humidification, and suctioning). The tracheostomy tube with the largest appropriate internal diameter is selected to prevent occlusion from respiratory secretions.

Small airway patency and respiratory muscle support in the animal with mild respiratory compromise from smoke inhalation may be accomplished by bronchodilator administration (aminophylline, 6 to 10 mg/kg IV, IM, SC, PO every 8 hr for dogs; 4 to 8 mg/kg IM, SC, PO every 12 hr for cats) during the first 18 hr of injury. However, in the more severely compromised patient, intubation with intermittent positive pressure ventilation (IPPV) or positive end-expiratory pressure (PEEP) may be required (see this volume, p. 98). The prophylactic use of these measures in human patients with burn and inhalation injury has decreased deaths related to respiratory failure that develops during resuscitation. Clinicians should be aware of the decline in venous return and cardiac output associated with the use of IPPV and PEEP. Fluids, inotropic support (dobutamine, 5 to 10 μg/kg/min IV constant rate infusion [CRI]) and dopamine infusions (1 to 3 μg/kg/min IV CRI) may be necessary to maintain cardiac output and renal blood flow in animals receiving ventilatory support.

Antibiotic and corticosteroid administration is contraindicated during this phase of respiratory therapy because morbidity and mortality have been reported to be increased in human smoke inhalation patients that are given these medications. Chest radiographs, arterial blood gases, pulse oximetry, and pulmonary compliance should be serially monitored in animals experiencing moderate to severe respiratory compromise from smoke inhalation.

Wound Management

The goals of wound management are (1) to protect the zone of ischemia and (2) to prevent viable tissue from desiccation. Maintaining tissue viability in the zone of ischemia is accomplished by maintaining tissue perfusion and oxygen delivery to the burn wound. The use of cyclo-oxygenase inhibitors to block thromboxane A_2 mediated vasoconstriction is currently under investigation.

Aggressive cleansing of the wounds using copious lavage with water or saline along with wound debridement is performed at least once daily. Water-soluble antibiotic ointments, such as silver sulfadiazine, and sterile occlusive dressings are applied to prevent bacterial colonization and desiccation of the wound. Systemic antibiotic administration has a doubtful place in the early management of burn wounds. Ischemia and eschar prevent attainment of adequate tissue levels of these drugs. Local wound treatment is the key to preventing infection, and excessive use of antibiotics predisposes the animal to life-threatening nosocomial infections.

TREATMENT DURING THE POSTRESUSCITATION PHASE

Fluid Therapy

The goals of fluid therapy are (1) to restore plasma volume, (2) to provide nutrition, and (3) to maintain red cell mass. Edema fluid begins to be reabsorbed at this stage, and ongoing loss of free water and protein from the vascular space through the burn wound must be balanced with these fluid gains and fluid administration. Potassium loss in urine is increased, and potassium supplementation should be based on serial electrolyte measurements. Anemia and hypoproteinemia may progress, and transfusion of red cells, plasma, colloids, or whole blood may be necessary. Monitoring techniques during this phase are similar to those employed during early resuscitation. Urine output is expected to increase due to an obligate solute diuresis; consequently a urine output of 1 ml/kg/hr may reflect inadequate perfusion of the kidneys.

Respiratory Therapy

The goals of respiratory therapy are (1) to prevent pulmonary edema and (2) to treat inhalation injury. Iatrogenic pulmonary edema due to overzealous volume replacement should be avoided. Ventilatory support, supplemental humidified oxygen administration, PEEP, bronchial lavage and coupage, and administration of a bronchodilator may be necessary to treat bronchospasm and small airway obstruction. Water bath airway humidification (vaporization) is preferred over ultrasonic nebulization in order to avoid seeding the alveoli with bacteria. Physical parameters such as body temperature and respiratory rate and effort along with arterial blood gases, chest radiographs, transtracheal washings for culture and Gram's stain, and complete blood count should be serially monitored for indications of bacterial infection. Antibiotics should be selected and administered on the basis of results of Gram's stain or culture and sensitivity of transtracheal washings.

Nutrition

The goal of nutrition is to minimize negative nitrogen balance and catabolism. Maintaining the patient in a warmed 85 to 95° F environment will aid in maintaining body temperature and decrease the effects of stress hormones on catabolism and metabolic rate. Nutritional supplementation should begin within 48 hr after burn injury. Enteral feeding is preferred because it is a more physiologic approach to nutritional support and is associated with fewer complications than parenteral nutritional support. If enteral feeding is not possible because of craniofacial injury, prolonged ileus (which often accompanies severe burns up to 48 hr following the burn), or other conditions, parenteral nutrition should be administered (see this volume, p. 32).

Sufficient calories must be supplied as glucose and lipids to prevent amino acids from being catabolized for gluconeogenesis. Solutions with osmolalities of less than 600 mOsm/L (for example, 3% amino acid solution mixed with a 5 to 10% dextrose solution and a 10% lipid solution) can safely be administered through peripheral venous catheters. As the animal's fluid requirements are large during this period, a substantial proportion of caloric and protein requirements (up to 75%) can be provided using this mixture as the mainstay of volume administration. Serum osmolality, electrolytes, glucose, and triglycerides should be monitored and the

catheter site inspected daily for evidence of infection.

Wound Management

The goals of wound management are (1) to prevent and control infection and (2) to effect early wound closure. Strict isolation of severely burned patients and the use of sterile equipment, dressings, masks, gowns, and gloves are necessary to prevent and control infection. Lavage, debridement, and twice-daily application of water-soluble topical antibiotic ointments, such as silver sulfadiazine, are the primary approaches used for control and prevention of infection in deep wounds during this period.

Daily debridement of burned tissue is necessary until wound closure can be achieved. Biologic dressings or synthetic skin substitutes can be used to speed wound closure. Homografts and pig skin are examples of biologic dressings. Silicone polymers, polyurethane, or polyvinyl chloride polymers are used in the synthetic skin substitutes (Op-Site, Smith and Nephew; Biocclusive, Johnson & Johnson). These materials maintain a water layer on the surface of the wound that aids in re-epithelialization, clears surface bacteria, and minimizes fibrosis, inflammation, heat loss, and pain. These dressings and skin substitutes adhere best to burns with only moderate infection and minimal remaining eschar.

Early surgical closure of the burn wound is recommended. This approach in human patients has been shown to decrease morbidity, mortality, sepsis, catabolism, immune dysfunction, and length of hospital stay and to improve function and cosmetic appearance. Perioperative antibiotic administration is indicated to prevent surgically induced bacteremia or endotoxemia.

The decision to use systemic antibiotics should ideally be based on the results of quantitative culture of full-thickness biopsies of the burn wound. Bacterial counts higher than 10^5 gm of tissue indicate bacterial infection. The dosages for many antibiotics, especially aminoglycosides, are increased in burn patients owing to hypermetabolism and increased volume of distribution. Ideally, plasma peak and trough concentrations of antibiotics should be monitored to determine therapeutic dosages in individual animals.

TREATMENT DURING THE PERIOD OF INFLAMMATION, INFECTION, AND WOUND HEALING

Fluid Therapy

The goal of fluid therapy is volume replacement. Volume depletion in the animal must be avoided during this hyperdynamic state. Careful monitoring of hydration, perfusion, and central venous pressure may be required along with appropriate administration of crystalloids, red blood cells, plasma, colloids, or whole blood as needed.

Respiratory Therapy

The goals of respiratory therapy are (1) to prevent pneumonia and (2) to prevent sepsis. Owing to the presence of a hyperdynamic state, carbon dioxide production is increased. The resulting hyperventilation will increase the work of breathing and may further compromise respiratory function in patients with pneumonia or sepsis. Aggressive antibiotic administration based on cytologic and microbiologic evaluations of serial transtracheal washings, early wound closure to minimize immune dysfunction, and nutritional support to provide substrate for defense mechanisms are important considerations.

Nutrition

The goals of nutrition are (1) to maintain body weight and (2) to provide sufficient calories and protein to support animal during hypermetabolic state. The hypermetabolic state during this phase of burn injury is the most severe of any disease process and cannot be reversed until wound closure. The goal of nutritional therapy is to decrease protein loss and immune dysfunction and to support body weight until wound closure. Formulas for calculation of caloric requirements for the veterinary patient have been extrapolated from studies on human patients. One formula estimates daily caloric requirement as $(25 \times WT(kg)) \times (40 \times TBSA)$. It is estimated that daily protein losses may exceed 2 gm/kg/day. A calorie to nitrogen ratio of 100:1 (normal is 250:1) is recommended to offset this substantial protein loss.

Sixty per cent of the required calories should be administered as glucose and 40% as lipids in order to spare amino acids administered for anabolic purposes from being catabolized for gluconeogenesis. Lipids are used to provide more calories per gram of nutrient (i.e., 9 kcal/gm of fat versus 4 kcal/gm carbohydrate) and to decrease the production of carbon dioxide. Vitamin and mineral supplementation is indicated, especially of vitamins A and C, and zinc in order to offset losses into the burn wound. Overfeeding should be avoided, especially with respect to glucose, since that would cause increased carbon dioxide production and lead to fatty change within the liver. Serum osmolality, glucose, electrolytes, and triglycerides should be monitored and the catheter site inspected daily for signs of infection.

Wound Management

The goal of wound management is (1) to control infection and (2) to remove sloughing eschar. Gentle manipulation of any remaining devitalized tissue is indicated in order to prevent bacteremia/endotoxemia from occurring in association with an inflamed or infected wound. Surgical excision of this unhealthy tissue can be associated with excessive blood loss, the development of respiratory difficulty, and sepsis. Small areas of the wound should be excised in sequential fashion, and perioperative antibiotics (based on results of quantitative wound biopsy cultures) should be administered. Definitive surgical closure or grafting should be performed only on noninflamed tissue.

ANALGESICS FOR THE BURN PATIENT

The physiologic consequences of pain may significantly alter the course of disease owing to an increase in stress hormone release that can potentiate catabolism, hypermetabolism, glucose utilization, and immune dysfunction. In veterinary medicine, narcotic (oxymorphone, 0.02 to 0.06 mg/kg IV in dogs) and low-dosage ketamine (1 to 2 mg/kg IV) administration provide good somatic analgesia and have been recommended for use in burn patients. Narcotic agonist-antagonists, such as butorphanol (0.05 to 0.2 mg/kg IV every 2 to 6 hr or 0.2 to 0.4 mg/kg IM every 4 to 6 hr) and buprenorphine (0.005 to 0.03 mg/kg IV, IM, SC every 6 to 12 hr) may be especially useful because increasing the dosages of these drugs for analgesic support does not increase respiratory or central nervous system depression (i.e., ceiling effect). All analgesics should be administered intravenously when possible because intramuscular and subcutaneous absorption may be unpredictable in these animals (see this volume, p. 82).

PROGNOSIS

The prognosis for severe burn victims is related to the age and general health of the animal, burn size, the effectiveness of early resuscitative efforts, and the development of complications such as pulmonary dysfunction and sepsis. Previously, recommendations were to euthanize animals with burns in excess of 50% TBSA. However, it should be noted that improvements in resuscitation techniques and more aggressive early wound management have led to increased survival rates in human patients with burns in excess of 85% TBSA.

References and Suggested Reading

Demling, R. H.: Burns. N. Engl. J. Med. 313:1389, 1985.
   A review of pathophysiology and treatment of burns in man.
Demling, R. H.: Management of the burn patient. *In* Shoemaker, W. C.
   et al. (eds.): *Textbook of Critical Care.* Philadelphia: W. B. Saunders,
   1989, pp. 1301–1316.
   A review of pathophysiology and treatment of burns and smoke inha-
   lation in man.
Fox, S. M.: Management of thermal burns—Part I. Comp. Cont. Ed.
   7:631, 1985.
   A review of the pathophysiology and treatment of burns in the dog and
   cat.

Fox, S. M., Goring, R. L., and Probst, C. W.: Management of thermal
   burns—Part II. Comp. Cont. Ed. 8:439, 1985.
   A review of a series of dogs presenting with burns.
Mosley, S.: Inhalation injury: A review of the literature. Heart Lung 17:3,
   1988.
   A review of the pathophysiology and treatment of inhalation injury in
   man.
Onarheim, H., Missavage, A. E., Kramer, G. C., et al.: Effectiveness of
   hypertonic saline-dextran 70 for initial fluid resuscitation of major burns.
   J. Trauma 30:597, 1990.
   An experimental study of sheep with scald injuries and the results of
   resuscitation with hypertonic saline-dextran.

ACUTE MANAGEMENT OF OPEN FRACTURES, INCLUDING GUNSHOT, SHEARING, AND DEGLOVING WOUNDS

KARL H. KRAUS

North Grafton, Massachusetts

Open fractures are emergencies. Although the wounds are usually not a cause of death, immediate treatment decreases the incidence of infection and the loss of tissue. Conversely, if the treatment of these injuries is delayed, a contaminated wound can become infected, resulting in increased tissue loss, chronic osteomyelitis, or life-threatening bacterial infection.

The battlefield has been a laboratory for studying the treatment of massive trauma. Accounts of various methods of treatment have been recorded for more than 2000 years. Treatment protocols that have evolved and are now accepted include (1) early debridement, (2) copious lavage, (3) open wound management in most cases, and (4) judicious use of broad-spectrum antibiotics.

CLASSIFICATION OF OPEN FRACTURES

Open fractures are classified as types I, II, and III. The classification is based on the mechanism of injury and is related to the extent of tissue damage. The focus of this classification is the extent of tissue damage, which dictates the treatment required.

Open fractures occur when the patient and another object collide. There is a relative velocity between the objects related to kinetic energy by the equation:

$$\text{Kinetic energy} = \text{mass} \times \text{velocity}^2/2$$

The amount of energy imparted to tissues depends on the nature of the collision and the kinetic energy of the colliding objects. The more energy absorbed by tissues, the greater the tissue destruction. As is seen by the equation, doubling the mass of an object will double its kinetic energy; however, doubling the velocity of the object will quadruple its kinetic energy.

The relationship between impact velocity, kinetic energy, and tissue damage is best illustrated in gunshot wounds (Pavletic, 1986). In an acute study on the effects of gunshot wounds on pigs' colons using identical weight slugs, a low-velocity impact at 244 m/sec resulted in a 5 × 2 mm hole with no surrounding hemorrhage. When the impact velocity was increased to 503 m/sec, a 10-mm hole with hemorrhage extending 20 mm from the hole was the result. When the impact velocity was increased to 762 m/sec, the entire colon and part of the neighboring cecum were destroyed (Scott, 1983).

The treatment for these three injuries is very different. A sharp or small, slow-moving object passing through tissue causes minimal tissue disruption and minimal peripheral tissue necrosis. Unless the wound has been grossly contaminated with bacteria or foreign material, it is likely to heal without intervention. The presence of particulate matter within the wound greatly increases the possibility of infection and progressive tissue necrosis. With increased velocity of the projectile and consequently increased energy imparted to the tissues, there is increased necrosis of peripheral tissues. Many times the adjacent necrotic tissue can be resected to viable tissue that can be closed primarily. If large amounts of energy are imparted to tissue in a collision, tissue damage can be extensive. The viability of tissues is often difficult to assess initially, and tissues may regain or lose viability with time. These wounds must be treated with thorough, repeated debridement and left open so drainage can occur. Therefore, accurate classification of open wounds is imperative and dictates initial treatment.

TYPE I OPEN FRACTURES

These injuries occur when a bone is fractured and a fracture fragment is briefly forced out through the skin. The sharp fracture fragment lacerates tissue, without causing excessive tissue necrosis, leaving a communicating wound in the skin. The fracture is usually simple, suggesting minimal energy has been imparted to bone and surrounding soft tissues. Examples are an oblique fracture of the humerus or femur with a small laceration of the skin. The skin edges appear viable.

TYPE II OPEN FRACTURES

These injuries occur when an external force causes a fracture to a bone. As an external force imparts energy to bone through tissue, moderate tissue damage occurs. There is usually an area of laceration or devitalized skin of larger than 1 cm in length. Examples include fractures of the radius and ulna or tibia caused by trauma from an automobile or blunt object impact or a gunshot wound caused by a low-velocity missile (i.e., a handgun at long range). The impact leads to exposure of the bone and devitalization of a resectable amount of skin and underlying muscle and fascia.

TYPE III OPEN FRACTURES

These injuries occur when excessive energy has been imparted to bone and surrounding tissues, leading to physical or functional loss of a large amount of tissue. Physical loss of tissue includes shearing or degloving injuries. Functional loss of tissue includes devitalization owing to contusion or loss of vascular supply. Examples of this injury include shearing and degloving wounds to the distal extremities with fracture or bone loss, high-velocity gunshot wounds, short range shotgun injury, and blunt injury with fracture and impaction of particulate matter in the wound (lawn mower, crushing injury onto dirt or pavement).

An infected wound is always considered a type III open wound, even if the initial classification would have been type I or II, as infection will extend the amount of tissue necrosis.

ASSESSMENT OF TISSUE DAMAGE AND CONTAMINATION

Initially, damage to other organ systems may make thorough evaluation of the open fracture a secondary concern. In these cases, the wound can be quickly covered with a sterile bandage to prevent further contamination. If the wound has been covered by the owner, that bandage initially should be left in place. Splints and other means of support should be provided for unstable fractures whenever possible. Temporary stabilization of the fracture prevents further tissue trauma from movement of fracture fragments.

An open fracture should be assessed and classified as soon as possible. History, radiographic examination, and direct examination of the wound are used to assess an open fracture. A history should be taken with special concern for energy imparted to the tissues. Questions include the type of gun in a gunshot wound or the speed of a car and manner of impact in an automobile accident.

Radiographic examination, even if the radiographs are taken through bandage material or without perfect positioning, provides important information. Radiographic evidence of excessive tissue damage includes highly comminuted or segmental fractures, bone and tissue loss, the presence of a high-velocity bullet or fragments, and gross displacement of bone fragments.

The wound should be closely inspected, and this inspection should take place in a clean environment with all present wearing masks and caps. The inspector wears sterile gloves and uses sterile technique and instrumentation to prevent nosocomial infection. The animal should be given an analgesic and sedated to decrease pain and movement, facilitating the examination and preventing contamination of the wound (see this volume, p. 27). An opioid/tranquilizer combination is useful in these situations. With type I and II open fractures, the examination can be immediately followed by initial treatment. The wound can be gently probed with a hemostat to visualize underlying tissues for signs of devitalization and determine if the wound communicates with the fracture or is only a superficial laceration. The skin wound may need to be extended to facilitate initial inspection and debridement.

TREATMENT

If the wound is classified as a type I open fracture, the tissues are viable with minimal particulate matter contamination. The wound should be less than 6 hr old. In these cases, the wound is lavaged with 500 to 1000 ml of 0.9% saline or lactated Ringer's solution. Antibiotics or antiseptics should not be added to lavage solutions. The lavage should be allowed to exit the wound freely and should not be injected or allowed to dissect through tissue planes. If necessary, the edges of the skin wound are excised and the skin wound closed with nonabsorbable, monofilament sutures in a simple interrupted pattern. The wound should be covered and temporary external stabilization of the fracture applied whenever possible, pending definitive fracture repair.

If the wound is classified as a type II open fracture, there is devitalized tissue or some contamination. The wound is less than 6 hr old, and the examiner is confident that the wound is only contaminated and not yet infected. Since some debridement will be necessary, local or regional anesthesia, analgesia-tranquilization, or inhalation anesthetic will be needed. The wound should be thoroughly lavaged and debrided according to guidelines suggested for type III open wounds. The amount of lavage solution used for these wounds should be 2 L or greater. Lavage and debridement should be continued until all tissues are free of foreign matter and appear healthy and viable. If all tissues appear viable and *clearly* not infected, no foreign material is left in the wound, minimal hemorrhage is present, the wound is less than 6 hr old, and closure can be performed without tension, the wound may be closed. Deeper structures are apposed with monofilament, absorbable sutures and the skin apposed with monofilament nonabsorbable sutures. If nonviable tissue remains, substantial inflammation or hemorrhage is present or the wound is not easily closed, the wound should be left open (see the earlier section "Type III Open Fractures"). *If there is any question* about whether the wound can be safely closed, *the wound should be left open.*

If history, radiographs, or initial inspection reveal a type III open fracture, the wound will require meticulous attention. Treatment of the type III wound usually requires general anesthesia, but regional anesthesia such as caudal epidural anesthesia is a good choice for debridement of a caudal limb wound in a recently injured patient (see this volume, p. 95). Debridement of these severe or infected wounds should be performed under sterile conditions in a surgical suite, not in the nonsterile treatment area. Following induction of anesthesia, the wound should be covered with sterile, water-soluble lubricating jelly as this procedure will protect the wound from further contamination with hair or debris. The affected area is clipped and cleansed. The personnel involved should wear surgical caps, masks, and sterile gloves. Surgical scrub or skin preparation solutions should not be used in open wounds, as this application is injurious to tissues. The skin peripheral to the wound margins can be cleansed and the wound avoided. Following this preparation, the affected area is draped as it would be for a clean orthopedic procedure.

Debridement

Meticulous debridement is the single most important aspect in the treatment of open fractures. Failure to completely debride devitalized tissue leaves a substrate that supports bacterial colonization of the wound. Debridement of skin should be conservative in the distal limbs, but dead or severely devitalized skin should be removed. Skin should be excised until cut edges bleed and appear pink. If skin in a distal limb appears potentially viable, it should be retained and reassessed during a secondary debridement procedure 24 hr later. In the proximal limbs or trunk where secondary wound closure techniques are possible (e.g., axial pattern flaps), more aggressive debridement should be performed initially.

Fascia should be freely debrided as it is expendable and easily infected because of its relatively low vascularity. Exposed tendon and ligaments will become nonviable and should be debrided if not serving a supporting function. If major supportive tendons and ligaments (e.g., calcaneal tendon, collateral ligaments of the stifle) are exposed, they must be kept moist and covered as soon as possible with vascular soft tissue. If major tendons have been transected, the ends should be tagged with monofilament nonabsorbable suture to enable location for reanastomosis during subsequent secondary wound closure.

When debriding muscle, the four Cs (consistency, contractility, circulation, color) should be used to assess muscle viability. The consistency of muscle should be firm and resilient; nonviable muscle is friable. Viable muscle contracts when cut or pinched. Normal muscle has generous circulation and bleeds readily from capillaries when cut. The color of viable muscle is pink or bright red; dark red or cyanotic muscle is nonviable.

Bone fragments should be left when a supportive function or soft-tissue attachments are evident. Small pieces of bone without soft-tissue attachment should be removed. Nerves and blood vessels should be spared debridement.

Debridement must often be repeated daily for the first few days because tissues that initially appear viable subsequently may lose their blood supply. Even the most experienced surgeon cannot always determine the outcome of tissue viability during initial debridement.

Copious lavage is important in the treatment of any wound. Lavage serves to remove particulate matter, dilute bacterial contamination, restore viability to tissues, and delineate the extent of the wound. Sterile 0.9% saline or Ringer's solution should be used. The amount of lavage solution used in type III open wounds is rarely less than 3 to 5 L, and lavage should continue until the wound is free from all foreign matter and blood clots. Mechanical jet lavage systems have been designed specifically for wound irrigation, and other types of lavage systems have been adapted for use in wound management. An inexpensive, sterile, and effective apparatus for use in lavage is a 35-ml syringe with a 19-gauge needle. The stream intensity is easily controlled or varied for different purposes.

Dressings, Bandages, and Splints

Following debridement and lavage, a type III and most type II open fractures should be managed as open wounds and covered with "wet to dry" bandages. Gauze sponges moistened in sterile lavage solution are packed into the open wound covering all exposed tissue. The gauze sponges act as wicks, removing exudate from the wound. Additionally, the gauze interweaves with nonviable tissue and serves to further debride the wound when removed. The second layer of the bandage should be composed of an absorbable material such as cotton or cast padding that serves to remove and contain exudate produced from the wound. The third layer of the bandage is composed of a water-impermeable material that prevents moisture from entering the bandage and being carried to the wound.

If the fracture is distal to the elbow or stifle, the limb should be supported temporarily through application of an external coaptation device (Bartels, 1990). If the open fracture is proximal to the elbow or in the distal femur, a spica bandage is applied (Bartels, 1990). If the open fracture includes the proximal femur, a patch bandage is used. A patch bandage is either a "wet to dry" or occlusive bandage applied to an upper extremity or to the torso. It is held in place with either adherent tape or sutures.

In many cases debridement and definitive stabilization of the fracture are performed simultaneously. An unstable fracture will cause continued damage to surrounding tissues and prevent the migration of granulation tissue. An external fixation device is the most commonly used form of fixation for open fractures. This type of fixation allows open wound management with rigid stabilization of the bone fragments. Plate and screw fixation of open fractures provides rigid fixation; however, the required exposure involves additional tissue manipulation that can compromise blood supply to bone and permit extension of infection. The use of intramedullary pins should be avoided because this surgical approach provides less secure fixation and increases the potential for intramedullary spread of infection.

USE OF ANTIBIOTICS

Correct use of antimicrobials will decrease the infection rate in open fractures (Gustilo and Anderson, 1976); however, devitalized tissue will become infected despite aggressive antimicrobial therapy. Thorough debridement is the most important factor in the prevention of infection.

The goal of antimicrobial therapy in open fractures is to prevent infection of viable tissue by common bacteria found on skin and in soil. These wounds are contaminated initially with aerobic and anaerobic, gram-negative and gram-positive bacteria. A culture of these wounds, obtained at the onset of treatment, usually yields the infecting pathogen along with other bacteria. Contamination of a wound during hospitalization with resistant bacteria often occurs, and these organisms are not isolated with the initial culture.

Initial antimicrobial therapy should be with a broad-spectrum antimicrobial. The first-generation cephalosporins, specifically cephalothin, are recommended and have proved more effective in preventing infection when compared with penicillin/aminoglycoside combinations (Patzakis et al., 1974). Cephalothin should be administered for 3 days at a dose of 44 mg/kg every 6 to 8 hr intramuscularly or intravenously, with the initial dose administered intravenously. If after 3 days a wound infection is evident, a second culture should be obtained. Even though these cultures are obtained while an animal is receiving antibiotic treatment, they usually yield the infecting pathogen, which can then be specifically treated.

Open fractures caused by high-velocity gunshot wounds or bite wounds to the proximal limbs or trunk areas deserve special consideration. In these cases there is extensive tissue devitalization in areas that are difficult to thoroughly debride. These open fractures can become infected with aggressive anaerobic bacteria, including *Clostridium* spp. This complication occurs rapidly and may result in the loss of a limb by amputation or death of the animal within 24 hr. The clinical signs of this type of infection include the development of excessive edema, pain, and subcutaneous emphysema. The animal may or may not be febrile. The wound exudes a serosanguinous discharge if a route of drainage is present, and the exudate contains gram-positive rods. Hemolysis occurs to varying degrees and can result in decreased blood hemoglobin content and hemoglobinuria. Treatment for these infections involves aggressive debridement, which often entails limb amputation; open wound management; and antibiotic therapy with administration of penicillin G sodium, 20,000 IU/kg every 4 hr intravenously.

Open fractures are too often left untreated or are mistreated. With proper care of an open fracture, infection will be prevented and function preserved in most cases.

References and Suggested Reading

Bartels, K. E.: Splinting techniques for small animals. *In* Bojrab, M. J. (ed.): *Current Techniques in Small Animal Surgery*, 3rd ed. Philadelphia: Lea & Febiger, 1990.

Gustilo, R. B., and Anderson, J. T.: Prevention of infection in the treatment of one thousand and twenty-five open fractures of long bones. J. Bone Joint Surg. 58A:453, 1976.

Patzakis, M. J., Harvey, J. P., and Tyler, D.: The role of antibiotics in the management of open fractures. J. Bone Joint Surg. 56A:532, 1974.

Pavletic, M. M.: Gunshot wounds in veterinary medicine: Projectile ballistics—Part I. Comp. Cont. Ed. 8:47, 1986.

Pavletic, M. M.: Gunshot wounds in veterinary medicine: Projectile ballistics—Part II. Comp. Cont. Ed. 8:125, 1986.

Scott, R.: Pathology of injuries caused by high velocity missiles. Clin. Lab. Med. 3:273, 1983.

Section

3

CHEMICAL AND PHYSICAL DISORDERS

GARY D. OSWEILER
Consulting Editor

TAKING AND INTERPRETING A TOXICOLOGIC HISTORY

THOMAS L. CARSON

Ames, Iowa

History is a narrative of events and conditions as they exist prior to or concurrent with animal illness or death. Veterinarians evaluate this background information as an important component of any clinical evaluation. The history can be especially valuable in cases of potential animal poisoning. The clinician may need more background information either when a toxicosis is included in a differential diagnosis when a patient is presented or when the effects of a known product exposure may have to be evaluated. As clinicians, we recognize that certain management practices, circumstances, clinical syndromes, or sequences of clinical signs are more compatible with certain disease conditions than others. In a toxicologic history, we are looking for information about potential sources of toxicants, predisposing factors, situations compatible with potential exposure to toxicants, and the owner's description of clinical signs. To assist in the logical collection of this information, many veterinarians use a specific toxicologic history questionnaire as an important part of an overall clinical history-taking process. Using a standard form helps clinicians to be thorough and objective in their evaluation. The information in Table 1 may be used to develop such a questionnaire.

The technique used in taking a toxicologic history can also be important. Clients usually need to tell their account of what happened. It is important to listen carefully and then go back and inquire about areas that are less clear or items that you did not understand.

Animal poisoning cases are an interaction between the animal, the toxicant, its dosage, the environment, and the management circumstances. Information about all of these areas should be gathered in the history-taking process.

ANIMAL INFORMATION

An important starting point is to gather information about the animal. The value of routine animal information, such as species, breed, age, weight, sex, and physiologic condition (e.g., pregnant, lactating, or neutered), cannot be underestimated. For example, cats will be poisoned by a lower dose of

Table 1. *Areas of Information in a Toxicologic History**

Patient
  Species
  Breed
  Age
  Sex
  Weight
  Previous health status, including current medications and vaccination status
  Number of animals involved

Clinical Findings
  Clinical signs observed by client
  Time between exposure and onset of signs
  Duration of signs

Environment
  Housing and other accessible areas
  Geographic region
  Weather and season
  Plants, water
  Known toxicants

Product
  Trade names of product
  Generic ingredients and concentrations
  Formulation of the product (solid, liquid, or spray)
  Manufacturer's name

Exposure
  Amount of product to which animal was exposed
  Time since exposure
  Route of exposure
  Location of animal at time of exposure
  Source of product
  Intent of exposure (accidental, malicious, appropriate, or inappropriate)

Management
  Nutrition, when and how fed
  Sanitation
  Changes in location, food, water
  Medications, sprays, dips
  Human activity, occupation
  Unusual circumstances

*Modified with permission from Martinez, M. E., et al.: The toxicologic history. Vet. Tech. 10:292, 1989.

ethylene glycol than dogs. Some collies are poisoned by lower doses of ivermectin than other dogs, and smaller breeds of dogs are often more susceptible to problems simply because of their smaller size. Lactation may affect the rate of excretion of some compounds, and residues of a particular toxicant may appear in the animal's milk. Congenital and metabolic problems of some breeds, such as copper accumulation in the Bedlington terrier, may need to be differentiated from a toxicosis. Pre-existing medical conditions may either mimic the clinical signs of a toxicosis or predispose animals to the effects of poisons.

An account of the sequential clinical problem presented by the animal is particularly valuable. The client should be asked to describe in nonmedical terms the clinical signs demonstrated by the animal. It may sometimes be difficult to interpret an owner's description of clinical signs. For example, seizures and muscle tremors may look very similar to a client. Ask the client to describe specific symptoms that the animal showed rather than using general terms like "nervous symptoms." Try to determine which body systems are affected (e.g., gastrointestinal, nervous, neuromuscular) as well as the severity of specific clinical signs. Many commonly encountered toxicants produce characteristic clinical syndromes that may aid in their recognition. The client's description of the progression and the duration of clinical signs may also be helpful. For example, organophosphate poisoning is often acute in onset and progresses rapidly to severe clinical signs, whereas lead poisoning is usually more insidious and may involve changes in eating habits and personality over several days. Asking clients about the presence of specific clinical signs may help them remember information that they may not have considered to be significant but may be important as you evaluate the whole case.

ENVIRONMENTAL INFORMATION

The most important aspect of the environmental evaluation is to identify the physical area that the animal was in or had access to. For example, was it confined in a breeding kennel? Does it have access only to the house or to the backyard? Was it roaming or not? Did it have access to the neighbor's farm or vacant lot? The accessible environment may suggest a source of toxic material. Establish how long the animal was in the location. Was the animal recently acquired? What was the source of the animal? Rural animals may have access to different types of toxicants and infectious agents than urban animals. Other animals in the environment, whether of the same or different species, may be important as indicators of exposure to the same toxicant or as a source of infectious agents. For example, dogs and cats with access to swine have a higher potential risk of exposure to pseudorabies virus.

Weather conditions and season of the year may also be important. Most ethylene glycol poisoning occurs in late fall and early winter when permanent antifreeze is added to automobile radiators. Also, during cold weather unvented space heaters may produce carbon monoxide, or water sources may be frozen. Ventilation, air quality, and hygiene are especially important in confinement situations. The sources of water for the animal, either for drinking or play, as well as plants in the environment should be evaluated. Bluegreen algae in stagnant ponds and toxic house plants are examples of potential hazards. The geographic region may also be significant because metaldehyde and poisonous toads would be much more of a hazard near the Gulf Coast of the southern United States than in the upper Midwest.

The client may be very familiar with the physical environment of the animal but may not recognize certain potential toxicologic hazards that may be present. Questions about specific types or kinds of potentially toxic products should be asked. Are any rodenticides, garden materials, disinfectants, or medications (human or animal) accessible to the animal? The environment is often the source of the toxicant and so should be evaluated carefully and in great detail.

In some cases of unexplained animal toxicoses, a field investigation of the actual site of the affected animals may be helpful in discovering the source of the toxicant (Galey and Hall, 1990).

AGENT AND EXPOSURE

Some toxicologic cases are presented as an inquiry about a specific product to which the animal may have had access. In these circumstances it is most helpful for the client to provide the trade name (and ask them to spell it) of the product or medication. Information about the generic ingredients, the concentration, and the formulation (solid, liquid, powder, or spray) as well as the manufacturer's name should be recorded. Information about potential exposure to the animal should be clarified. The time since the exposure, the potential route of exposure (e.g., oral or dermal), and the approximate amount of the product that the animal was exposed to should be gathered. The intent of the exposure (i.e., was it accidental, malicious, or intentional—a dip, spray, or medication) should be established. This information will be helpful in calculating an approximate dosage of the product received by the animal and in evaluating the likelihood that poisoning will occur.

MANAGEMENT

By definition, small companion animals are involved with people. They share their lives and homes. Consequently, the activities of the people and their management practices can influence the health and potential toxicosis of these animals. A major part of management involves the nutritional aspect of the animals. Inquire about how and when they are fed and watered and the sanitation conditions under which they are kept. The daily activities of all animals should be reviewed, and any recent disturbance in their routine should be evaluated. The client should be asked about recent medications, sprays, dips, or other treatments received by the animal.

Changes in the animal's food, water, location, or other cultural practices that have occurred recently are often involved in toxicology cases. A movement to a different apartment, home, kennel, or other housing arrangement can influence animal behavior and perhaps make toxicants more available. Various activities of people or even their occupations or hobbies could be the source of a potential toxicant.

For example, the paint scraped off an old house may become a source of lead to the family pets. Unusual circumstances or unique events such as a wind storm, power outage, a neighborhood party, or even a burglary may be a clue to an animal's health problem and should not be overlooked.

A systematic approach to collecting historical data enables the veterinarian to collect the necessary information to evaluate potential poisoning. A complete and accurate history is then correlated with the clinical evaluation so that a differential diagnosis may be developed and appropriate therapy instituted.

Reference

Galey, F. D., and Hall, J. O.: Field investigation of small animal toxicoses. Vet. Clin. North Am.: Small Anim. Pract. 20(2):283, 1990.

COLLECTING AND USING TOXICOLOGIC INFORMATION AND RESOURCES

HAROLD L. TRAMMEL
Urbana, Illinois

and DAVID C. DORMAN
Research Triangle Park, North Carolina

The identification and interpretation of toxicologic information are critical to the management of animal poisonings. With adequate information resources and interpretation of the information in these resources, most veterinarians can successfully manage the more common animal poisonings. During 1988, the 100 most common poisons accounted for more than 50% of the total Illinois Animal Poison Information Center (IAPIC) call volume. The veterinarian prepared to deal with a small number of poisons can adequately manage a large percentage of animal poisoning cases.

Veterinary toxicology information resources available to the practicing veterinarian are limited. There is no single veterinary toxicology reference book or resource that covers the wide range of potential poisonings in animals. The veterinarian should develop a systematic approach to obtaining the information needed. Reference books are usually excellent initial sources of information because they compile information from a variety of sources into an easily used form. We recommend several cost-effective toxicology reference books for suggested additions to a veterinary practice library. Previous editions of *Current Veterinary Therapy* remain excellent toxicology resources for the practicing veterinarian and are highly recommended for inclusion in any veterinary library.

Because the information in reference books can become dated, the veterinarian should develop a personal information system that stores or files information from journals, product information sheets (e.g., packet inserts, advertisements), extension service publications, and reprints in order to maintain more current information. This system should also contain the names and telephone numbers of specialists or consultants. Having an organized system allows the rapid retrieval of toxicologic information. The information gained from continuing education seminars and personal experience should be collected and incorporated into the personal information system as well.

Most veterinarians eventually need to use telephone consultation services because of the magnitude of the poisoning problem and the limited resources that any one veterinarian will have available. These services include human and animal poison control centers and veterinary diagnostic laboratories.

SELECTION AND USE OF INFORMATION RESOURCES

The first step in the management of a poisoned animal is to obtain an adequate history to determine if the problem is a potential toxicologic case (see this volume, p. 160). This history-taking process is frequently enhanced by concomitant use of toxicology resources. Several questions can be used to help direct the veterinarian's search of the toxicologic information resources. What is the identity of the poison? What is the toxicity of the poison? What are the toxic effects of the poison? What is the time course of the poisoning? What diagnostic tests are available, if any? What treatments are indicated to manage the case? Because pesticides, pharmaceuticals, and household plants accounted for more than 70% of all small animal cases reported to the IAPIC during 1988, we will concentrate on these classes.

Identification of the Poison

The identity of the poison is important in managing a poisoning. It has been estimated that there are more than 30,000 species of plants of which more than 300 are significantly injurious to animals and humans. There are more than 300,000 household products, 50,000 prescription drugs, and more than 100,000 nonprescription drugs marketed in the United States. Obviously, accumulation of information concerning this range of products is beyond the capabilities of any individual veterinarian, and telephone consultation is needed. Fortunately, the identity of the poison is at least partially available in the majority of cases. In only 5% of the cases received by the IAPIC was it unable to identify the poison source. It should be noted that although the identity of the poison is important, treatment should be directed to the patient's needs. In other words: *treat the patient and not the poison.*

Positive identification of the poison in known cases of exposure can be difficult. A poison may be identified by trade/brand name (e.g., Dursban), generic name (e.g., chlorpyrifos), chemical name (e.g., *O,O*-diethyl *O*-(3, 5, 6-trichloro-2-pyridyl)-phosphorothioate), or classification (e.g., organophosphorous insecticide). Correct identification of the poison may be hampered by vague product labeling (e.g., incomplete ingredient listings, product repackaging), destroyed packaging and labels, a lack of information concerning the poison, and the diversity of potential poisons. Specific trade name information (e.g., d-Con Mouse Prufe II) may also be used to determine the concentration of the poison (e.g., 0.005% brodifacoum) in the formulated product.

Table 1 lists the relative merits of various reference books in identifying pesticides. If the needed information is not in these references, the veterinarian should consider calling a poison control center, pest control operator, garden supply store, or extension office for assistance. Table 2 shows the value of various reference books in identifying pharmaceuticals. Other sources include local pharmacies or veterinary drug wholesalers. Table 3 presents reference books useful in identifying plants. Local nurseries, extension agents, and florists can also help.

Toxicity of the Poison

The toxicity of a poison simply refers to the amount of poison capable of causing a toxic adverse effect. The importance of dose in the production of poisoning cannot be overstated. All compounds are potentially toxic, and it is the dose of the poison that determines effect. A partial list of various measures of toxicity includes the lethal dose, LD_{50}, low toxic dose, high toxic dose, therapeutic index, and margin of safety. The application of toxicity data to case management requires interpretation and is discussed in a later section.

Tables 1, 2, and 3 show the relative amount of toxicity data for pesticides, pharmaceuticals, and plants in various references. Poison control centers have available additional sources of toxicity data if these references do not have the needed information.

Toxic Effects of the Poison

Any adverse response following exposure to a poison may be considered to be a toxic effect. If the toxic effects stated to occur in a poisoning are not the effects seen in the animal being treated, further history-taking is indicated to verify the identity of the poison. As with toxicity data, interpretation of toxic effects is required and is also discussed later.

Reference books that show the toxic effects of

Table 1. Pesticide Toxicology Resources

Author	Title	Recommended*	Information Provided†				
			Identify	Toxicity	Effects	Diagnosis	Treatment
Beasley, 1990	Vet. Clin. North Am. Sm. Anim. Pract.	+ + +	+	+ +	+ + +	+ +	+ + +
Booth, 1988	Veterinary Pharmacology and Therapeutics	+ + +	+	+ +	+ +	+ +	+ +
Anonymous, 1990	Farm Chemicals Handbook	+ + +	+ + +	+ +	−	−	+
Goodman and Gilman, 1990	Pharmacological Basis of Therapeutics	+ +	−	−	+ +	−	+ +
Hayes, 1982	Pesticides Studied in Man	+	+ +	+ +	+ + +	+ +	+ +
Klassen, 1986	Casarett and Doull's Toxicology	+	+	+ +	+ + +	+ +	+
Osweiler, 1985	Clinical and Diagnostic Veterinary Toxicology	+ +	+ +	+ +	+ + +	+ + +	+ +
Thomson, 1990	Agricultural Chemicals	+	+ + +	+ +	—	—	—

*In the opinion of the authors. Key: + + + highly recommended, + + recommended, + specialized information.
†+ + + much information, + + moderate information, + some information, − limited or no information.

Table 2. Pharmaceutical Toxicology Resources

Author	Title	Recommended*	Information Provided†				
			Identify	Toxicity	Effects	Diagnosis	Treatment
Barnhart, 1990	PDR for Nonprescription Drugs	+	+ +	+	+	−	+
Barnhart, 1990	PDR for Prescription Drugs	+	+ +	+	+	−	+
Beasley, 1990	Vet. Clin. North Am. Sm. Anim. Pract.	+ + +	+	+	+ +	+ +	+ +
Booth, 1988	Veterinary Pharmacology and Therapeutics	+ + +	+ +	+ + +	+ + +	+ +	+ +
Goodman and Gilman, 1990	Pharmacological Basis of Therapeutics	+ +	+ +	+ +	+ +	+ +	+ +
McEvoy, 1990	AHFS Drug Information	+ + +	+ + +	+ +	+ + +	+ +	+ + +
McLaughlin, 1990	Veterinary Pharmaceuticals/ Biologicals	+ +	+ + +	+	+ +	−	+

*In the opinion of the authors. Key: + + + highly recommended, + + recommended, + specialized information.
†+ + + much information, + + moderate information, + some information, − limited or no information.

Table 3. Plant Toxicology Resources

Author	Title	Recommended*	Information Provided†				
			Identify	Toxicity	Effects	Diagnosis	Treatment
Fowler, 1981	Plant Poisoning in Small Animals	+ + +	+ + +	+ +	+ +	+ +	+ +
Klassen, 1986	Casarett and Doull's Toxicology	+	+	+	+	+	+
Lampe, 1988	AMA Handbook of Poisonous and Injurious Plants	+ + +	+ + +	+ +	+ +	+	+ +
Osweiler, 1985	Clinical and Diagnostic Veterinary Toxicology	+ +	+	+	+	+	+ +

*In the opinion of the authors. Key: + + + highly recommended, + + recommended, + specialized information.
†+ + + much information, + + moderate information, + some information.

pesticides, pharmaceuticals, and plants are presented in Tables 1, 2, and 3. Animal poison control centers collect clinical sign data for all cases received and frequently have more information about toxic effects in animals.

Diagnosis of Poisoning

A diagnosis of poisoning may be based on a history of exposure to a possible poison, demonstration of an adverse effect compatible with the poison, and the confirmation of exposure and absorption of the poison by chemical analysis. In certain cases, all of these aspects may not be available to the veterinarian. Correct sample collection and submission to veterinary diagnostic laboratories may increase the likelihood of diagnosis (see this volume, p. 168).

There is limited information in most reference texts on the diagnosis of pharmaceutical (see Table 2) and plant poisoning (see Table 3). More information is available on diagnosis of pesticide poisoning (see Table 1).

Treatment of Poisoning

Specific "antidotes" are generally not available for most poisons. Antidotal therapies are directed at either altering the toxicokinetics of the poison or antagonizing its pharmacologic effects. Treatment efficacy in the species of interest may not be predicted by studies performed in other species. For example, the use of the alcohol dehydrogenase inhibitor, 4-methylpyrazole, in the treatment of ethylene glycol toxicosis is an effective therapy in dogs but not cats. Additionally, these experimental studies may not parallel companion animal exposures (e.g., intraperitoneal exposure to rodent versus oral exposure in a companion animal). Parameters used experimentally to determine treatment efficacy may not be applicable in the actual toxic syndrome. The duration of treatment effect observed in an experimental study (e.g., survival to 24 hr) also may not correlate with the duration of the toxic syndrome. In considering these restrictions, the veterinarian must remember: *treat the patient and not the poison*.

The references providing treatment information for pesticide poisoning are given in Table 1. The references for pharmaceuticals and plants are in Table 2 and Table 3, respectively.

Consultative Resources

Poison control centers strive to be the most complete sources of up-to-date information on poisons and poisonings. Currently there is only one

Table 4. *Animal Poison Control Centers*

National Animal Poison Control Center
University of Illinois College of Veterinary Medicine
(800) 548–2423
$25 charge per case
(900) 680-0000
$2.75/min

animal-oriented poison control center (Table 4) and more than 70 human poison control centers in the United States. Both the human and the animal poison control centers can provide information concerning the identification of poisons, such as product formulation, trade name, generic name, scientific name (e.g., plants), or chemical name. Poison centers have access to a variety of resources, including medical libraries, reprint files, product material safety data, textbooks, manufacturers, and experts within toxicology. Most poison control centers have Poisindex (Micromedix Inc., Denver, CO), a computerized clinical toxicology information system updated quarterly.

An animal poison control center is usually a better resource for veterinarians because it is staffed by veterinarians trained in the diagnosis and management of animal poisonings and has little background in handling human cases. Human poison control center staffs are trained in the diagnosis and management of human poisonings and lack formal training and experience in veterinary medicine and veterinary toxicology.

Colleges of veterinary medicine and veterinary diagnostic laboratories often have specialists trained in veterinary toxicology. Veterinary toxicologists have experience and training in the use of specialized toxicology information resources and are another excellent resource available to the practitioner.

INTERPRETATION OF TOXICOLOGY DATA

Once the necessary data to manage the toxicologic case have been obtained, the veterinarian is faced with the need to interpret and apply these data to the specific poisoning case.

Toxicity Data

DOSE-RESPONSE RELATIONSHIPS

As mentioned earlier, all compounds are potentially toxic. It is the dose of the poison that determines its effect. A dose-response relationship is often used to explain this observation. Several assumptions are to be made when using this model, including (1) the response is due to the poison;

(2) the response is related to the dose; (3) there is a molecular or receptor site where the poison can interact; (4) the production and magnitude of the response are proportional to the concentration of poison at the site; and (5) the concentration at the site is a function of the administered dose. Toxicity data may be used to predict the magnitude of the response. If a large number of doses with a large number of animals per dose is used, a sigmoid dose-response curve is obtained. The slope of the dose-response curve correlates with the relative potency of the poison. Unfortunately, most toxicologic studies do not report the shape or slope of the dose-response curve.

THE LD_{50} AND OTHER MEASURES OF TOXICITY

The most commonly available form of toxicity data is the LD_{50}. The LD_{50} is defined as the dose of a poison that causes 50% mortality in a population. Neither the lowest lethal dose nor the toxic dose can be predicted from the median LD_{50}. Toxicity studies may not report the clinical signs observed during a study. Two poisons with similar LD_{50} may induce dissimilar clinical signs and target organ failures.

The slope (response/dose) of the dose-response curve, the time to death, clinical signs, and pathologic findings are all vital or even more critical than the LD_{50} in the evaluation of acute toxicity. Other, more meaningful terms to define toxicity include the highest nontoxic dose (the highest dose that does not result in hematologic, chemical, clinical, or pathologic drug-induced interactions), and the lethal dose (the lowest dose that causes poison-induced deaths in animals). Unfortunately, this information is infrequently reported.

The toxicity of a pharmaceutical agent may be defined by the therapeutic index. The therapeutic index is the ratio between the median lethal dose (LD_{50}) of the compound and the median therapeutically effective dose (ED_{50}). Another term, *the standard safety margin,* is also used to define the toxicity of pharmaceutical agents. The standard safety margin is defined as the ratio between the lethal dose for 1% of the population (LD_1) and the effective dose for 99% of the population (ED_{99}). Owing to the uncertainty of determining an effect for 1% of the population, this latter ratio is rarely determined.

LIMITATIONS OF TOXICITY DATA

The LD_{50} is a statistical estimate of lethality and is not a biologic constant. The LD_{50} depends on the number of animals used, biologic variability, formulation of the poison, and experimental variations.

In practice, the acute LD_{50} (exposure occurring within a 24-hr period) is most commonly determined in the rat or mouse. Experimental studies commonly involve the administration of the poison to healthy adult animals. These studies generally do not consider populations at special risk. For example, neonates and geriatric animals or animals with pre-existing disease states (e.g., liver failure) may have altered metabolic or excretory pathways and may be more sensitive to a poison. Similarly, animals with damaged skin (e.g., flea-bite dermatitis) may have increased sensitivity because of increased dermal absorption. These studies often involve single poison exposures that may not parallel the environmental exposure (e.g., a number of pesticides may be used within a given flea season). The role of additional poison exposures may alter the toxicity of a second poison. For these and other reasons, the use of the LD_{50} has fallen into disfavor as a measure of acute toxicity.

CLINICAL APPLICATIONS OF TOXICITY DATA

Under ideal circumstances, toxicity data would be available for (1) the correct formulation of the poison, (2) the species of interest, and (3) the appropriate route of exposure. This is rarely the case, however. Under most circumstances, the veterinarian must extrapolate toxicity data from one species to another. Difficulties in extrapolation arise because of differences between species in toxicokinetics (absorption, distribution, metabolism, and excretion) of the poison and qualitative or quantitative differences between target organs or receptors. For example, the sensitivity of cats to phenolic compounds is thought to be due in part to their relative inability to glucuronidate exogenous compounds.

Therefore, a tenfold variation in a poison's toxicity within a species is assumed. This tenfold difference will account for differences in toxicokinetics and organ sensitivity within members of the same species. For example, a possible tenfold range in lethal dose can be assumed for a given agent within one species. A similar tenfold variation between species is also assumed. This factor is used to account for potential differences in toxicokinetics and target organ sensitivity between species. Therefore, when no other data are available, a possible 100-fold variation in toxicity data is assumed when extrapolating from one species to the next. Once again, the veterinarian must remember: *treat the patient and not the poison.*

Clinical Signs and Responses to the Poison

TYPES OF TOXIC RESPONSES

Several types of toxic responses may occur following exposure to a poison. Chemical allergy is an adverse reaction to a chemical resulting from previous sensitization to the chemical or its structural analogues. Allergic reactions generally occur at low doses of chemicals and are dose-dependent; however, dose-response relationships are rarely obtained. Clinical signs of an allergic response vary among species and depend on the target organ for chemical allergies.

The type of clinical signs produced may be predicted by the mechanism of action for the poison. Therefore, similar classes of toxicants (e.g., carbamate and organophosphorus insecticides) that share a common mechanism of action (e.g., inhibition of acetylcholinesterase) will produce similar clinical signs (e.g., salivation, diarrhea, tremors, seizures). For many pharmaceutical agents, toxic effects are often an extension of their pharmacologic effects.

Species variations in the target organ (i.e., the organ most affected by the exposure) may also occur. For example, acetaminophen may produce acute liver failure in humans and dogs, whereas in the cat it produces cyanosis, methemoglobinemia, and facial and paw edema. Similarly, methanol produces blindness in humans, but dogs and cats are generally resistant to this effect because of alternate pathways of metabolism. Therefore, the toxicologist may not be able to predict adverse effects for a new compound in an exposed species.

TIME FRAME AND EXTENT OF THE TOXIC RESPONSES

Immediate toxic responses can be defined as those that occur or develop rapidly after a single administration of the poison, whereas delayed effects are those that occur after a lapse of time (e.g., tumor production). Some effects of a poison are considered reversible, whereas others are considered irreversible. If a poison produces pathologic injury to an organ, the ability of the organ to recover is generally dependent on the regenerative capacity of that organ. Long-term damage to an organ with the potential to regenerate or hypertrophy (e.g., the liver and kidney) is generally less than that observed in organs with little or no regenerative ability (e.g., cardiac muscle and brain).

The localization of the response is also important following exposure to a poison. Local effects are those that occur at the site of first contact between the poison and the animal (e.g., dermal burn from acid exposure). Systemic effects occur at a site distinct from the actual site of exposure to a poison. Systemic responses require poison absorption and distribution.

SUMMARY

A veterinarian needs to have quality toxicologic information immediately available. He or she must know how to use the resources and interpret the information contained in them. He or she must know the limitations of each resource and where to turn for additional information or consultation. At all times in managing a poisoned animal, the veterinarian must remember to *treat the patient and not the poison.*

References and Suggested Reading

Anonymous: *Farm Chemicals Handbook.* Willoughby, O. H.: Meister Publishing Company, 1991.
   Alphabetical index, fertilizer dictionary, pesticide dictionary, company trade names, product descriptions, precautions, chemistry, action/use, registration guidelines, safety guidelines (toxicity), and emergency guidelines. Highly recommended.
Barnhart, E. R.: *Physicians' Desk Reference for Nonprescription Drugs.* Oradell, NJ: Medical Economics Company, Inc., 1990.
   Descriptions, pictures, toxicity, and treatment. Limited to package inserts drug manufacturer chooses to have included.
Barnhart, E. R.: *Physicians' Desk Reference for Prescription Drugs.* Oradell, NJ: Medical Economics Company, Inc., 1991.
   Descriptions, pictures, toxicity, and treatment. Limited to package inserts drug manufacturer chooses to have included.
Beasley, V. R. (ed.): Toxicology of selected pesticides, drugs, and chemicals. Vet. Clin. North Am. Sm. Anim. Pract. 20:283, 1990.
   General veterinary toxicology, descriptions, diagnosis, toxicity, and therapeutics for common companion animal poisons. Highly recommended.
Booth, N. H., and McDonald, L. E.: *Veterinary Pharmacology and Therapeutics,* 6th ed. Ames, IA: Iowa State University Press, 1988.
   Therapy in animals, pharmacokinetics, toxicity, treatment, mechanism of action, uses and contraindications. Highly recommended.
Fowler, M. E.: *Plant Poisoning in Small Companion Animals.* St. Louis: Ralston Purina Company, 1981.
   Plant pictures and descriptions. Clinical signs and treatment of plant poisonings in animals. Highly recommended.
Goodman, L. S., Gilman, A. G., Rall, T. W., et al.: *Goodman and Gilman's The Pharmacological Basis of Therapeutics,* 8th ed. New York: Macmillan Publishing Company, 1990.
   Therapy in humans, pharmacokinetics, toxicity, treatment, mechanism of action, uses and contraindications. Recommended.
Hayes, W. J.: *Pesticides Studied in Man.* Baltimore: Williams & Wilkins, 1982.
   Identity, properties, uses, toxicity to laboratory animals, toxicity to man, basic findings, absorption, distribution, metabolism, excretion, mode of action, experimental exposure, therapeutic use, accidental poisoning, dosage response, laboratory findings, and treatment of poisoning. New edition in press which will be very expensive.
Klaassen, C. D., Amdur, M. O., and Doull, J.: *Casarett and Doull's Toxicology. The Basic Science of Poisons.* New York: Macmillan Publishing Company, 1986.
   Human-related toxicology of a wide range of substances using both systems affected and poison classification approaches. Definitions and descriptions for many fundamental toxicologic concepts.
Lampe, K. F., and McCann, M. A.: *AMA Handbook of Poisonous and Injurious Plants.* American Medical Association, Chicago, IL, 1988.
   Descriptions, pictures, toxic principles, clinical signs, and treatments. Highly recommended.
McEvoy, G. K. (ed.): *American Hospital Formulary Service Drug Information.* Bethesda: American Society of Hospital Pharmacists, Inc., 1991.
   Annual collection of drug monographs containing descriptions, acute and chronic toxicity, treatments, chemistry, pharmacology, mechanism of action, drug use, pharmacokinetics, adverse reactions, mutagenicity, and carcinogenicity. Highly recommended.
McLaughlin, D. M.: *Veterinary Pharmaceuticals and Biologicals.* Lenexa, KS: Veterinary Medicine Publishing Co., 1990.
   Product information, diets and nutritional supplements, and diagnostic aids and supplies. Information includes descriptions, labels, manufacturer, approved use, indications, contraindications, warnings, and preparations. Limited to package inserts drug manufacturer chooses to have included. Recommended.

Osweiler, G. D., Carson, T. L., Buck, W. B., et al.: *Clinical and Diagnostic Veterinary Toxicology*, 3rd ed. Dubuque: Kendall/Hunt Publishing Company, 1985.
General veterinary toxicology, descriptions, diagnosis, toxicity, definitions, and therapeutics for a wide range of common animal poisons (with heavy emphasis on large animal toxicologic problems). Recommended.

Thomson, W. T.: *Agricultural Chemicals*. Fresno: Thomson Publications, 1990.
Annual handbook covering descriptions, uses, precautions, and toxicity of insecticides, acaricides, and ovicides (Book I); herbicides (Book II); fumigants, growth regulators, repellents, and rodenticides (Book III); and fungicides (Book IV).

EFFECTIVE USE OF AN ANALYTICAL LABORATORY FOR TOXICOLOGY PROBLEMS

FRANCIS D. GALEY
Davis, California

Poisonings can present a real challenge for the small animal practitioner. Sudden or insidious onset of illnesses, nonspecificity of signs, and heightened client emotions regarding a pet contribute to the urgency of a situation. In such instances, it is incumbent upon the veterinary practitioner to deal with the case in a systematic and rational manner. This chapter presents an approach, or set of tools, for clinicians to use in tackling the diagnosis and initial disposition of a suspected animal poisoning.

Unfortunately, there is no "black box" into which a small sample can be placed for a "toxicity test." Potential toxicants (many of which have not even been characterized) are too numerous and chemically diverse to be able to develop such a test. Currently, there are so many potential toxicants that one could not even obtain sufficient tissue from the largest patient to screen for the chemicals for which we can test. Therefore, out of necessity, a toxicology diagnosis involves the piecing together of a diagnostic puzzle. The pieces of the puzzle come from a thorough environmental and clinical history, clinical findings, pathologic findings, chemical testing (when available), and, occasionally, bioassay. The analytical laboratory can be helpful in putting together this diagnostic puzzle. Practitioners are encouraged to consult the analytical laboratory if assistance in such cases is desired.

HISTORY

The type of case encountered by small animal toxicologists differs from those of their large animal colleagues. Small animal poisonings tend to involve fewer animals, less emphasis on production (more on the individual), and less information about the animal's potential environment (large animals are often kept in a known area, whereas dogs may roam freely). With that in mind, the basic, multifactorial approach can be applied to the toxicology diagnosis. That approach begins with a thorough environmental and clinical history (after implementation of any necessary life-supportive or decontamination procedures). (See this volume, pp. 160 and 162.)

Environmental History

An extensive environmental history is recorded to describe the spatial and time-related events surrounding onset of the syndrome under investigation. This description is obtained by tracing feed, water, events, and animals. Times and dates of events are organized temporally with clinical signs. Sources and times of purchase of feeds or ingredients are then documented. Recent exposure of animals to new items (e.g., toys), housing, or neighborhoods may also be important. For example, did signs of vomiting begin shortly after the neighbor flushed a radiator? Did a cat become lethargic and anorectic with lead toxicosis soon after the owner began restoring a house? Or did the bird die after exposure to a new zinc-alloy toy (or burning of a Teflon pan)?

It helps to obtain a description of a pet's neighborhood to identify industrial activities or angry neighbors. Weeds, ornamentals, and houseplants can be catalogued. A pet's usual haunts might subsequently be traced. During history-taking, a list of potential toxicants can be drawn up and their potential roles categorized. This is a good time to make suggestions that can prevent future problems. The list of potential hazards can be studied with the owner, and he or she can be instructed about how to obtain and bring samples to the practitioner for analyses. In particularly difficult cases, the veterinarian may wish to conduct a site visit to identify potential toxicants or other hazards. As potential toxic sources are located, samples can be obtained by the practitioner during the visit (Galey and Hall, 1990).

Samples of feed, water, or other sources should be obtained. If possible, split the samples and label both containers. One sample is held in reserve when the other is sent to a laboratory. The samples should be sent frozen unless otherwise requested. Potentially toxic plants should be identified. The owner will probably be able to identify many yard and house plants for the practitioner. If a plant needs to be identified, a potted plant can be taken to a plant store. Yard plants and hedges may need to be sampled (include stem, leaf, flower, and root if available). If rapid transport to a herbarium or diagnostic laboratory is possible, wrap the plant in a wet newspaper for transport. Otherwise, the plant can be pressed and dried in the fold of a newspaper underneath some books before shipment to a diagnostic laboratory. Regardless of the identification, evidence of consumption of the plant should be recorded if such evidence is available.

Clinical History

Signalment, addition or movement of animals, numbers of affected animals, time of onset, specificity, progression, severity, and outcome of clinical signs are all diagnostically useful to the toxicologist. Additionally, the species, age, breed, sex, and prior health status of animals all influence the effects of chemicals in animals. For example, cats are more sensitive than dogs to chlorpyrifos (an organophosphorus insecticide used for flea control in dogs). Acute toxicology cases may affect from one to all of a group of animals. If all animals are not affected, the reason(s) for the resistance or absence of exposure opportunity of some animals needs to be investigated. One animal may eat a plant in an isolated incident. On the other hand, an entire litter of cats may begin showing signs of organophosphorus toxicosis after exposure to chlorpyrifos.

The time of onset and progression of signs will vary depending on the toxicant and the associated magnitude of exposure. A high dose of strychnine can cause seizures and death within minutes to hours. A high dose of an anticoagulant rodenticide may take several days before having an effect. Multiple small doses of lead may eventually lead to dullness and anorexia in a cat. One high dose of lead may cause acute seizures. Often, signs such as vomiting, diarrhea, and seizures as observed in an organophosphorus insecticide case are nonspecific. Conversely, a dog exposed to fluoroacetate will suffer from seizures, including the specific sign of running in a straight line and barking.

Regardless of the specificity, the character of the signs can give the diagnostician a clue about which system(s) might be affected. Additionally, even nonspecific signs can be useful when considered with other diagnostic information.

CLINICAL FINDINGS

A thorough, systematic clinical examination of affected animals can yield additional information about affected organs. It is useful to monitor the progression and severity of clinical signs regularly. Once the initial examination is complete, nonspecific therapy, fluid volume replacement, and other measures can be instituted. If the signs and history suggest a diagnosis, the response of animals to a specific therapy can provide critical information about the syndrome (if such therapy is practical). For example, a dog with increased salivation, tremors, vomiting, diarrhea, and mild dyspnea may respond to atropine therapy, suggesting an acetylcholinesterase inhibitor or other cholinergic agent as the cause.

Clinical Laboratory Testing

Potentially useful clinical laboratory tests include hematology (e.g., characterization of anemia, identification of methemoglobinemia from acetaminophen toxicosis, or finding nucleated red blood cells in lead poisoning), serum chemistry (organ specificity such as liver or kidney), and chemical analysis for potential toxicants. Rapid tests are available for whole blood lead concentration, trace element concentration, and acetylcholinesterase activity determinations. From the live animal, whole blood, serum, urine, other body fluids, and gastrointestinal contents (e.g., vomitus) are potentially useful samples for testing (Table 1).

The human eye is perhaps the most valuable diagnostic tool. Visual examination of all samples prior to shipment to a laboratory can be valuable. If an owner calls with a complaint about a dog vomiting, ask to examine both the dog and the vomitus. That material may contain remains of toxic plants (e.g., oleander), pills, or metals (e.g., lead weights or zinc from galvanized bolts and pennies).

Table 1. *Samples That Might Be Needed for Chemical Analysis*†*

Sample	Amount	Condition	Examples
Antemortem			
Whole blood:	1–3 ml	EDTA anticoagulant	Lead, arsenic, selenium, acetylcholinesterase
Urine:	50 ml	Plastic screw-capped vial	Drugs, some metals
Serum:	5 ml	Remove from clot; special trace element tubes	Trace elements, drugs, ethylene glycol, electrolytes, botulinum
CSF:	1 ml	Clot tube	Sodium
GI contents:	500 gm	Obtain representative sample	Pesticides, plants, metals, feed-associated toxicants
Body fluids:	10–20 ml	Clot tubes	Anticoagulants
Hair:		Rarely useful, call laboratory Wash prior to sampling	Occasionally chronic selenosis
Postmortem			
Urine:	50 ml	Plastic screw-capped vial	Drugs, some metals
Serum:	20 ml	Remove from heart clot	Drugs, electrolytes
Liver:	250 gm	Plastic (wrap in aluminum foil for organics)	Pesticides, metals, botulinum
Kidney:	250 gm	Plastic (wrap in aluminum foil for organics)	Metals, 1080, calcium, ethylene glycol
Brain:	50%	Split sagittally, send half in formalin to pathologist, half frozen in plastic to analyst	Organochlorines, sodium, acetylcholinesterase
Fat:	250 gm	Foil inside plastic	Accumulated organochlorines
GI contents:	500 gm	Obtain representative sample	Pesticides and baits, plants, metals, feed-associated toxicants
Bone:	100 gm	1 long bone	Fluoride
Miscellaneous:		Injection sites, spleen	Some drugs
Environmental			
Baits, etc.	200 ml or gm	Clean mason jar (liquid), plastic	Unidentified chemicals
Feed	1 kg plus	Plastic sack, box; representative sample is imperative	Mycotoxins, feed additives, plants, pesticides, botulinum
Plants	Plant	Fresh or pressed and dried; send all plant parts	
Water	1 L	Clean mason jar, foil under lid for metals, plastic if organics	Metals, nitrates, pesticides, algae, salt, organics

*Adapted with permission from Galey, F. D.: Diagnostic toxicology for the equine practitioner. *In* Robinson, N. C. (ed.): *Current Therapy in Equine Medicine 3.* Philadelphia: W. B. Saunders (in press).

†All samples except blood and very dry samples should be submitted frozen. Sample amounts are optimum; call the laboratory regarding testing for smaller sized samples. When available, appropriate tissue samples should be properly fixed in formalin for histologic analysis as well. Do not submit material in syringes.

PATHOLOGY

Much like signs, pathologic lesions vary greatly in specificity. Arsenic toxicosis, occasionally anticoagulants, severe enteritis, caustic damage, some plants, and shock may all lead to a hemorrhagic gut. Conversely, other than ingestion of soluble oxalates, few compounds other than ethylene glycol will cause birefringent crystal formation in the renal tubules. Organophosphorus insecticides cause few, if any, gross or histologic lesions. Regardless of specificity, however, the lesions add another valuable component to the toxicologic diagnosis.

A complete postmortem examination is therefore critical to the toxicologic diagnosis. Before conducting that examination, the animal should be properly identified and the potential forensic nature of a case should be documented. The practitioner might want to consider referral of involved, unusual, or complicated postmortem examinations to a veterinary pathologist at a diagnostic laboratory. The examination should always be undertaken with an open mind and eyes. Diseases other than toxicosis should be carefully eliminated. Samples of organs for microbiologic examination should be obtained first to minimize contamination. After obtaining microbiologic samples, a urine sample should be obtained using a syringe and placed in a screw-capped plastic vial for possible toxicologic testing. All organs are examined in a systematic manner. Samples of the major organs need to be fixed for histopathologic study and frozen for toxicologic examination. Unless the clinician is sure of the diagnosis, adequate samples of all analytically important organs and gut contents (Table 1) can be obtained at this time. The samples can be labeled, frozen, and stored temporarily. Thus, the samples will be available if needed for analyses as suggested by pathology, histopathology, and negative microbiologic findings. It is much easier to mail a sample from the freezer than to reincarnate a sample after remains are no longer available.

ANALYTICAL CHEMISTRY

Analyses are available for several classes of toxicants, including heavy metals, organic residues (e.g., pesticides), drugs, and some natural toxicants (see Table 1). A diagnostic laboratory should be queried about available testing. Information regarding samples, sampling methods, storage, shipping, cost, and turnaround times can then be obtained. Analyses can involve a great deal of preparatory chemistry and often require significant amounts of material. Recommended sample sizes (see Table 1) cannot be obtained from some smaller animals. In those situations, fewer tests can be run, necessitating more cautious planning. In addition, smaller samples may compromise test sensitivity, because many tests require large quantities of specimen for extraction or digestion to recover even small amounts of a toxicant.

The best sample for toxicology analysis is often the source, gastrointestinal contents, or urine. The animal's body, especially the liver, will metabolize compounds, subsequently decreasing the concentration of the original chemical. Following that, compounds are concentrated and excreted in the urine and bile. In general, samples should be stored and shipped frozen. A written identification of the submitter, a history of the problem, and any pertinent chain of custody documentation should accompany the shipment. A description of unusual findings when the specimens were harvested is also useful. Pooled samples (e.g., liver and kidney or livers from two animals in the same bag) are unacceptable for toxicologic analysis because of potential cross-contamination. Likewise, formalin-fixed tissues are unacceptable for most analyses.

Heavy Metal Analyses

Most heavy metal analyses are done using spectroscopy. Samples are initially mixed with reagents (e.g., whole blood for lead) or digested (furnace or acid for other samples) to prepare them for analysis. Atomic absorption spectroscopy (AA) involves energization of electrons in metals using heat provided by a furnace or flame. This superheated material is in the path of a lamp emitting light at a wavelength specific for a given metal. The amount of light absorbed by the sample can then be related to the concentration of metal in the sample. This technique is used to quantify metals such as copper, zinc, and lead, among many others, in small quantities, for many different types of samples.

Another form of spectroscopy is inductively coupled plasma emission spectroscopy (ICP). This technique is based on the emission (versus absorption with AA) of superheated metal. Although ICP analysis is frequently not as sensitive as AA, it can quantify several metals in a sample in a single step (unlike AA, which can be used for only one metal at a time).

Organic Residue Analysis

Most organic residue analyses (e.g., insecticides, baits, solvents, and some natural toxins) involve some form of chromatography after organic or solid-phase extraction. Commonly, samples are first extracted into a solvent to begin removing them from their biologic matrices (e.g., liver). Following that, various solvents and columns are used to purify samples sufficiently to allow the chromatography to detect (sensitivity) and identify (specificity) toxicants at biologically relevant levels.

Chromatography takes advantage of the chemical characteristics of a chemical to separate it from its surroundings. To do this, a plate or column of a certain affinity (polarity, size, ionic character, or even immunoselectivity) is used to hold or separate compounds as they are moved through in a liquid (high-performance liquid chromatography) or gas (gas chromatography). The separated compounds are detected using instruments at the end of the column that identify characteristics of the compounds or their derivatives. Once a compound is located using one detector, a second test often may be run using a mass spectrometer as a detector for confirmation. Mass spectrometry is used to identify the molecular weight of a compound and its fragments. Gas chromatography with mass spectrometry detection can also be used as a screening tool to identify some compounds in forensic cases (Poppenga and Braselton, 1990).

Other Analyses

Many other analyses involving a variety of chromatographic and bench chemistry techniques are conducted in toxicology laboratories. For example, the activity of the enzyme acetylcholinesterase can be assayed on whole blood or brain. That assay is used to determine whether exposure to an inhibitor of that enzyme (e.g., an organophosphorus or carbamate insecticide) has occurred and if that exposure was physiologically significant. Serum cholinesterase can also be assayed, although that test can only suggest exposure, not the physiologic significance of the exposure (acetylcholinesterase in blood is associated with the red blood cell).

Other analyses might include screens for ionophore antibiotics, some plant toxins such as alkaloids or nitrates, mycotoxins, vitamin assays, baits, and other feed contaminants.

Interpretation of Analytical Results

Analytical chemistry, if properly done with appropriate quality control, usually generates very reliable numbers. Following that, the significance of the findings must be interpreted in light of the other pieces of the diagnostic puzzle, such as the history, clinical signs, and pathology. Generally, heavy metal analysis yields a number that can be compared with a known normal range for a given species of animal. If outside the range and if the syndrome is appropriate, a diagnosis might be suggested. Organic residue analysis may yield a quantity of a compound that may or may not be at a toxic level. Often such analyses merely confirm or suggest an exposure. The diagnostician must then correlate the level of toxicant with known effects. For example, a small amount of the organophosphorus insecticide chlorpyrifos might be found in a dog's gut or liver. It was known that the dog had been recently dipped for fleas in a product that contained the compound. That finding becomes more important, however, if it is correlated with typical signs of organophosphorus insecticide toxicosis (e.g., vomiting, diarrhea, and tremors with few postmortem lesions) and if the finding was also accompanied by a significant depression of whole blood and brain acetylcholinesterase.

BIOASSAY

Two general types of bioassay can be used. The first and most useful bioassay is simply to observe the response of an animal to treatment. An example might be the above-mentioned dog with chlorpyrifos toxicosis. That dog could have been given a test dose of atropine at a preanesthetic dose (around 0.02 mg/kg SC). If the dog did not respond with typical signs of atropinization, such as increased heart rate, mydriasis, and drying of the mucus membranes, an acetylcholinesterase inhibitor might be suspected. Such a finding would suggest that therapeutic doses of atropine might be needed to reverse the signs (from 0.2 to 0.5 mg/kg SC repeated based on the response and needs of the animal).

Another type of bioassay involves the administration, to a laboratory animal, of the source of an unknown toxicant or one for which no other alternative to bioassay exists. For example, the only reliable test for botulism involves administration of suspected material into mice and observing the response of the mice in the presence and absence of specific, antibotulinum antitoxins. Occasionally, a feed or plant suspected as being toxic might be fed in the laboratory to determine its potential toxicity.

SUMMARY

Often, at the end of the initial case investigation, the veterinarian will have a clue as to the identity, or at least the source, of the toxicant. Exposure to the materials should be quickly terminated. This can be done by denying the animal access to the toxicant, changing feed or water (if appropriate), and properly administering emetics or adsorbents (see this volume, p. 173). Once exposure to a toxicant has been terminated, animals can be treated. Treatment of toxicosis frequently centers on nonspecific supportive measures and therapy for clinical signs because many toxicants lack specific antidotes. Drugs should be carefully chosen to avoid compounds that are metabolized, excreted, or toxic to organs affected in a syndrome (e.g., avoid nonsteroidal anti-inflammatory agents such as banamine in dogs with pre-existing kidney or gastrointestinal damage). Once the final diagnosis is made, more specific treatments (if available) can be instituted and other remedies can be appropriately modified.

The tools presented here will assist the veterinary clinician in keeping the cool head and open mind needed for diagnosis and initial disposition of potential poisonings. If questions arise regarding a case, samples, or possible testing, veterinarians are encouraged to call a specialist in veterinary toxicology (such as a veterinary toxicologist certified by the American Board of Veterinary Toxicology) at a veterinary diagnostic laboratory.

References and Suggested Reading

Galey, F. D.: Diagnostic toxicology for the equine practitioner. In Robinson, N. E. (ed.): Current Therapy in Equine Medicine 3. Philadelphia: W. B. Saunders (in press).
Description of the use of an approach to diagnostic toxicology for the equine practitioner, including a table of appropriate samples for chemical analysis.

Galey, F. D., and Hall, J. O.: Field investigation of small animal toxicoses. Vet. Clin. North Am. Sm. Anim. Pract. 20:283, 1990.
A thorough approach to on-site investigation of a small animal toxicology problem is presented.

Osweiler, G. D., Carson, T. L., Buck, W. B., et al.: Diagnostic toxicology. In Clinical and Diagnostic Veterinary Toxicology, 3rd ed. Dubuque, IA: Kendall/Hunt Pub. Co., 1985, p. 44.
General information regarding the use and function of a diagnostic toxicology laboratory.

Poppenga, R. H., and Braselton, W. E.: Effective use of analytical laboratories for the diagnosis of toxicologic problems in small animal practice. Vet. Clin. North Am. Sm. Anim. Pract. 20:293, 1990.
Description of the use of a diagnostic laboratory for small animals with special emphasis on analytical methods and a description of extended screens that might be available.

ADSORBENT DETOXIFICATION THERAPY WITH ACTIVATED CHARCOAL

W. EUGENE LLOYD

Shenandoah, Iowa

Activated charcoal (AC) has been called the most important component in a historical "universal antidote," a combination of charcoal or burned toast, magnesium oxide, and tannic acid. The term antidote may be misleading, since AC does not directly counteract the effects of a poison and has little or no efficacy with some toxicants. The effectiveness of the "universal antidote" has been doubted, but finely ground AC is increasingly useful in the treatment of many intoxications in animals and humans. AC is administered orally and functions by adsorbing molecules of complex organic compounds, thereby preventing absorption of potential toxicants from the gastrointestinal tract and sequestering the toxicants to be eliminated with ingesta.

AC is usually manufactured by destructive distillation or heating wood or other organic substances anaerobically under relatively high temperatures, driving off organic compounds, and leaving the char, which is then ground. Adsorption of toxicants by AC is a surface-active phenomenon; therefore grinding into small particles increases the activity. One gram of activated charcoal, USP, contains approximately 15% water, has approximately 1500 m² surface area, and adsorbs 100 mg of strychnine sulfate in an aqueous medium. AC of larger particle size is often used to filter gases or water, but the activity is not suitable for detoxification therapy. Superfine meshes of AC should have greater adsorptive capacities than AC based on dry weights, but they may cost more than activated charcoal, U.S.P., and there are no standards of activity for superfine charcoal. The following discussions relate to activated charcoal, USP, which may hereafter be referred to as charcoal or AC.

USE

General Considerations

AC should normally be used as an oral adjunct to more direct antidotal or palliative therapy during treatment of poisoning in animals. If an oral emetic, such as syrup of ipecac, hydrogen peroxide, or apomorphine, is used, AC should not be administered until *after* emesis. Animals showing signs of acute intoxication should be treated with a more specific antidote initially. In case of intoxication with orally ingested cholinesterase inhibitors, the animal should be atropinized first, then administered AC. Dogs and cats affected with strychnine poisoning should be sedated or anesthetized before administering charcoal.

Specific Indications

Charcoal therapy has been proved to be effective in cases of intoxication with the following poisons: organophosphates (e.g., phorate), carbamates (e.g., carbofuran), chlorinated hydrocarbons, strychnine, ethylene glycol, and blister beetle. AC appears to reduce the gastrointestinal absorption of both inorganic and organic arsenicals and mercurial compounds. AC may be indicated in preventing and minimizing the effects of intoxication from almost any polycyclic organic compound, which includes most of the pesticides.

Other Indications

AC may assist in minimizing the effects of dermal toxicants, such as insecticide dips. The action is probably by adsorption of toxicants ingested during grooming by the animal and by sequestration of metabolites within the gut. Following the crude oil spill in Alaska in 1989, AC (ToxiBan, Vet-A-Mix Inc, Shenandoah, IA) administered orally to "oiled" sea otters following shampooing improved survivability of treated animals, probably by sequestering anthracenes and other polycyclic compounds.

Studies in humans have demonstrated that AC dramatically decreases serum concentrations of analgesics and anesthetics. The mechanism of this action is probably by adsorbing drugs excreted by the liver and preventing reabsorption from the gut. In fact, the metabolites excreted via the biliary route may be more actively adsorbed than the parent compound, thus minimizing enterohepatic recycling. There is evidence that AC may reduce the severity of most types of diarrhea and minimize intestinal gas formation.

DOSE

A general rule is to administer AC at a dose of at least 10 times the dose of the toxicant, if known. The usual practical dosage range of AC is 0.5 to 2.0 gm/kg body weight. If economically feasible, higher doses can generally be given without adverse effects. AC adsorbs many compounds, such as colloids, vitamins, phenolics, and normal constituents of foods and ingesta, as well as toxicants. Studies in our laboratories were conducted with bovine ruminal contents spiked with phorate and with canine stomach contents containing known quantities of strychnine. Analyses of the toxicants in the ingesta demonstrated that adsorption of the toxicants was not stoichiometric and that relative adsorption was curvilinear. Pragmatically, this means that 0.5 gm/kg will often be sufficient, and 2.0 gm/kg will not be expected to be four times better. The goal is to administer sufficient AC to adsorb enough potential poison to make the antidotal measures and normal recovery controllable. Administration of AC should reduce the need for continued specific antidotes, such as atropine, the oximes, sedatives, or anesthetics.

ADMINISTRATION

AC should normally be administered by stomach tube in an aqueous slurry. Acute oral intoxications will generally respond well to a single dose if used with more direct antidotes. In cases of dermal toxicoses or for reduction of absorbed toxicants with relatively slow plasma elimination rates, administration of charcoal at doses of 0.5 gm/kg every 12 hours for 2 days is probably beneficial.

Some veterinarians and medical doctors prefer to administer AC with other physical detoxifying agents, such as mineral oil, saline cathartics, or sorbitol. These agents may be efficacious, depending on the nature of the toxicant. Kaolin, another adsorbent, may be effective in alleviating the gastroenteritis associated with some toxicoses, as well as by its adsorbent actions.

CONTRAINDICATIONS

AC should not be administered with other oral drug therapy, since it may sequester the drug and lessen its effects. Of course, oral emetics should be given before charcoal. The therapeutic efficacy of most antibiotics, antibacterials, coccidiostats, analgesics, and sedatives will probably be significantly minimized if administered with AC. Animal owners should be reminded that charcoal administration will produce black feces.

References and Suggested Reading

Berg, M. J., Berlinger, W. G., Goldberg, M. J., et al.: Acceleration of the body clearance of phenobarbital by oral activated charcoal. N. Engl. J. Med. 307:642, 1982.
The half life (T½) of serum phenobarbital was reduced from 110 to 45 hours in men administered 180 gm activated charcoal (AC) per day in divided doses for 3 days.

Berlinger, A. G., Spector, R., Goldberg, M. J., et al.: Enhancement of theophylline clearance by oral activated charcoal. Clin. Pharmacol. Ther. 33:351, 1983.
The T½ of serum aminophylline was reduced from 6.4 to 3.3 hours in men administered 140 gm AC in divided doses over 12 hours.

Chin, L., Picchioni, A. L., and Gillespie, T.: Saline cathartics and saline cathartics plus activated charcoal as antidotal treatments. Clin. Toxicol. 18:865, 1981.
Na₂SO₄ (1.32 gm/kg) and AC (in adsorbent-to-drug ratio of 2:1 to 4:1) were more effective than AC alone in reducing the gastrointestinal absorption of aspirin, pentobarbital, and chloroquine in albino rats.

Goodman, L. S., and Gilman, A. G.: The Pharmacological Basis of Therapeutics. New York: Pergamon Press, 1990, p. 57.
The stomachs of poisoned individuals should be emptied of ingesta by the use of ipecac, apomorphine, or lavage, unless the risk of aspiration of volatile toxicants is high.

Grauer, G. F., Maziasz, T. J., and Hjelle, J. J.: The toxicokinetic approach to antidotal therapy: Toxicant absorption and distribution. Comp. Small Animal 10:1058, 1988.
Emetics, gastric lavage, and administration of AC and cathartics should be done as soon as possible in poisoned animals.

Jackson, J. E., Picchioni, A. L., and Chin, L.: Contraindications for activated charcoal use. Ann. Emerg. Med. 9:599, 1980.
AC should not be used in humans poisoned with caustics and is not effective in toxicoses from alcohols and N-acetylcysteine.

Johnson, J. B.: Why activated charcoal is nature's 'Black Magic.' American Druggist Aug. 26, 1980.
AC is effective in adsorbing most intestinal gases and toxins associated with diarrhea but should not be used continuously, since it may adsorb nutritional substances.

Levy, G.: Gastrointestinal clearance of drugs with activated charcoal. N. Engl. J. Med. 307:676, 1982.
AC is useful in reducing toxic serum concentrations of many drugs in individuals by adsorbing the conjugated drug and nonmetabolized drug in the intestinal tract, preventing enterohepatic recycling.

Matthews, D.: Saving oiled animals. Lamp 71:12, 1989.
AC (ToxiBan) administration and shampooing of marine animals with skin contaminated with crude oil decreased deaths.

Wurster, D. E., Burke, G. M., Berg, M. J., et al.: Phenobarbital adsorption from simulated intestinal fluid, U.S.P., and simulated gastric fluid, U.S.P., by two activated charcoals. Pharm. Res. 5:183, 1988.
Dried superfine activated charcoal adsorbed 2.6 to 3.1 times as much phenobarbital from gastrointestinal fluids as dried AC.

BROMETHALIN RODENTICIDE TOXICOSIS

DAVID C. DORMAN

Research Triangle Park, North Carolina

Bromethalin (N-methyl-2,4-dinitro-N-[2,4,6-tri-bromophenyl]-6-[trifluoromethyl] benzeneamine) was discovered in the mid-1970's following an extensive nonanticoagulant rodenticide development program by Eli Lilly and Company (Dreikorn and O'Doherty, 1984). Field trials have demonstrated its effectiveness against warfarin-resistant rats and mice. Bait acceptance is considered excellent, with no bait shyness observed in rodents during field trials. Since 1985, 0.01% bromethalin-containing rodenticides have been marketed under the trade names Vengeance (Roussel Bio Corporation), Assault (Purina Mills), and Trounce (Earth City Resources). These bromethalin rodenticides are pelleted, tan- or green-colored, grain-based products that contain 16 to 42.5 gm (0.57 to 1.5 oz) of bait in paper "place pack" envelopes. Vengeance is also available in bulk as loose pellets to commercial pest operators. Selective toxicity for bromethalin rodenticides has been proposed on the basis of greater relative consumption of the rodenticide by rodents versus larger animals (Jackson et al., 1982).

The accidental ingestion of bromethalin-based rodenticides by companion animals does, however, represent a new hazard to these animals. During 1988, the Illinois Animal Poison Information Center (IAPIC) received 189 case calls concerning bromethalin rodenticides. Of these calls, 11% were assessed as a toxicosis or suspected toxicosis by IAPIC veterinarians. Dogs were most commonly involved, representing 79% of bromethalin cases. Of these canine cases, 9% were assessed as toxicosis or suspected toxicosis. Cats were less frequently involved than dogs (11% of all cases); however, a higher percentage of cats had clinical signs compatible with poisoning (25% toxicosis or suspected toxicosis) at the time of the call.

ABSORPTION, DISTRIBUTION, METABOLISM, AND EXCRETION

Bromethalin is rapidly absorbed from the gastrointestinal tract. Peak plasma concentration occurs within 4 hr of ingestion, with a plasma excretion half-life of 5.6 days in the rat (VanLier and Cherry, 1988). Biliary excretion accounts for 5 to 25% of an orally administered dose given to rats. Urinary excretion of bromethalin by rats is minimal and accounts for less than 3% of an oral dose. A major route of bromethalin metabolism is by liver mixed-function oxygenases through N-demethylation to desmethylbromethalin (VanLier and Cherry, 1988).

MECHANISM OF ACTION

The presumed biochemical mechanism of action of bromethalin and its active metabolite, desmethylbromethalin, is uncoupling of oxidative phosphorylation. Uncoupling has been demonstrated in both isolated brain and liver mitochondria (VanLier and Cherry, 1988). Oxidative phosphorylation, which depends on the normal function of mitochondrial cytochromes, is the major mechanism for production of adenosine triphosphate (ATP) in the body. Uncoupling of oxidative phosphorylation, therefore, may result in a lack of adequate ATP concentrations such that insufficient energy is available for Na^+-K^+ ion channel pumps. The loss of ion pump activity may result in the development of cerebral and spinal cord edema. Bromethalin also induces cerebral lipid peroxidation damage, which may contribute to the production of clinical signs (Dorman 1991, unpublished observations).

TOXICITY

Reported LD_{50}s for technical grade bromethalin include 1.8 mg/kg in the cat, 2.0 mg/kg in the rat, 4.7 mg/kg in the dog, 13 mg/kg in rabbits, and greater than 1000 mg/kg in the guinea pig (VanLier and Cherry, 1988). The apparent lack of toxicity of bromethalin in guinea pigs may be the result of that species' relative deficiency in N-demethylase activity.

In comparison with other rodenticides, bromethalin is considerably more toxic to cats than the newer second-generation anticoagulants (e.g., brodifacoum). Oral LD_{50}s for the bait form of bromethalin are 36.5 gm/kg in the dog and 5.4 gm/kg in the cat (Dorman et al., 1990b; Dorman et al., 1990d). Minimal lethal doses of bromethalin bait for the dog and cat are 25 and 4.5 gm/kg, respectively.

Minimal toxic doses of bromethalin bait are 16.7 gm/kg in the dog and 4.5 gm/kg in the cat. It is possible that individual cats and dogs may develop severe clinical signs following exposures to even smaller doses, especially if ingested chronically. Some dogs and cats readily consume toxic doses of bromethalin rodenticides.

Secondary poisoning of nontarget animals has not been demonstrated. Dogs fed bromethalin-killed rats for 2 weeks did not develop signs of toxicosis (Jackson et al., 1982). Owing to the extreme sensitivity of the cat to bromethalin, however, it is possible that secondary poisonings may occur.

CLINICAL SIGNS

Bromethalin toxicosis in the dog and cat causes a variety of clinical signs. The primary target organ for bromethalin is the central nervous system (CNS), with clinical signs generally referable to that system. Frequent monitoring of the animal for the development of additional clinical signs is required. Bromethalin toxicosis in the dog is characterized by two distinct dose-dependent syndromes and is similar to that described in rats (Dorman et al., 1990b; VanLier and Cherry, 1988). Dogs given oral doses of bromethalin at or above the LD_{50} generally developed an acute syndrome in which clinical signs develop within 24 hr. This syndrome is characterized by severe muscle tremors, hyperthermia, extreme hyperexcitability, running fits, hyperesthesia, and focal motor or generalized seizures that appear to be precipitated by light or noise. Less common signs include abnormal postures (e.g., Schiff-Sherrington's phenomenon, forelimb extensor rigidity), loss of bark, anorexia, mild to severe CNS depression, semicoma, coma, resting or variable (positional) nystagmus, and anisocoria (Dorman et al., 1990b). Some lethally poisoned dogs have mild hyperglycemia. The high-dose syndrome observed in dogs has rarely been reported to the IAPIC.

More commonly, dogs are exposed to lower doses of bromethalin (i.e., less than an LD_{50} of bait), which results in a slower onset of signs developing within several days of ingestion. Commonly observed clinical signs in the delayed syndrome include hindlimb ataxia and paresis that often progresses to hindlimb paralysis, decreased conscious proprioception, loss of deep pain response, patellar hyper-reflexia, severe CNS depression, semicoma, anisocoria, vomiting, and fine muscle tremors (Dorman et al., 1990b).

The toxic syndrome observed in cats is similar to that seen in dogs given lower oral doses of bromethalin. The delayed syndrome in the cat is also characterized by a slow onset of clinical signs that develop within 3 to 7 days of ingestion. Commonly observed clinical signs in the cat include ataxia, vocalization, hindlimb paralysis, decreased conscious proprioception, loss of deep pain response, patellar hyper-reflexia, upper motor neuron bladder paralysis, CNS depression, semicoma, coma, decerebrate body posture, abdominal distention, anisocoria, and fine muscle tremors (Dorman et al., 1990d). Focal motor or generalized seizures may occur in the later stages of this syndrome. These signs are similar to those described in a recent case report of fatal bromethalin toxicosis in the cat (Martin and Johnson, 1989). Alterations in routine serum electrolytes and chemistries have not been reported in bromethalin-poisoned cats.

Some animals may recover from bromethalin toxicosis. Animals that display mild clinical signs (e.g., ataxia, depression) appear to recover within 1 to 2 weeks of ingestion. Animals with more severe clinical signs, including coma or paralysis, generally have a poor prognosis for recovery.

PATHOPHYSIOLOGY

Lesions are generally confined to the CNS. Gross evidence of cerebral edema may occur, but brain edema is generally mild. Spongy degeneration of brain, spinal cord, and optic nerve white matter occurs in lethally poisoned animals (Dorman et al., 1990a; VanLier and Cherry, 1988). This lesion has been characterized ultrastructurally as intramyelinic edema. The myelin lesion is generally not associated with an inflammatory response or neuronal cell death and may be reversible (VanLier and Cherry, 1988). Examination of cerebrospinal fluid from bromethalin-poisoned dogs generally revealed normal cytology, protein concentration, specific gravity, and cell count (Dorman et al., 1990b). As anticipated from the mechanism of action, clinical signs, and lesions, bromethalin toxicosis is associated with the development of increased cerebrospinal fluid pressure (CSFP) (Dorman et al., 1990b; VanLier and Cherry, 1988). The degree to which increased CSFP occurs in lethally poisoned dogs is not, however, as severe as that observed with other causes of cerebral edema. It is possible that the intramyelinic location of the edema may limit the extent of increased CSFP.

DIAGNOSIS

Currently, the diagnosis of bromethalin poisoning depends on (1) the presence of an exposure history to a potentially toxic dose of a bromethalin-based rodenticide, (2) the development of appropriate clinical signs, (3) the presence of diffuse white matter vacuolization in the CNS, and (4) analytic confirmation of bromethalin residues in tissues. Bromethalin has been detected in fat, liver, kidney, and brain tissues from lethally poisoned dogs (Dorman et al., 1990a). However, chemical confirmation of bromethalin residues is not widely available and may have limited clinical utility in cases in which a delay in presentation occurs.

Although not specific for bromethalin toxicosis, electroencephalographic abnormalities commonly occur in bromethalin-poisoned animals. Supportive findings may include spike and spike-and-wave activity (indicative of an irritative or seizure focus), marked voltage depression (indicative of cerebral hypoxia), and abnormal high voltage slow-wave activities (associated with cerebral edema formation) (Dorman et al., 1991).

TREATMENT

Treatment goals of the clinician are (1) to decrease bromethalin absorption, (2) to initiate specific therapies intended to minimize cerebral edema, and (3) to control seizures and severe muscle tremors. Other symptomatic therapies may also be required.

Detoxification procedures in the alert animal should be used for all recent (less than 2 hr) exposures to a potentially toxic dose of bromethalin. The animal should be fed a small meal, and an emetic should be administered. This should be immediately followed by the administration of activated charcoal (1 to 2 gm/kg PO) and a saline cathartic (sodium sulfate, 250 mg/kg in five to ten times as much water, PO). (See this volume, p. 173.) Magnesium sulfate as a cathartic is generally not recommended in order to avoid possible magnesium-induced depression in animals with compromised renal function. Repeated administration of activated charcoal is more effective than the administration of a single activated charcoal dose (Dorman et al., 1990b). Smaller subsequent doses of activated charcoal (0.5 to 1 gm/kg) and a saline cathartic (sodium sulfate, 125 mg/kg PO) should be given every 4 to 8 hr for at least 2 to 3 days to all animals that may have consumed a potentially toxic dose. The increased efficacy of repeated activated charcoal may be due to interference with the enterohepatic recirculation of bromethalin or its metabolites. Delayed deaths (15 to 19 days after dosing) have occurred in cats given bromethalin, even though they received treatment with repeated doses of activated charcoal (four total doses) (Dorman et al., 1990d).

Dexamethasone and osmotic diuretics have been reported to be effective in the treatment of bromethalin-induced cerebral edema in rats (VanLier and Cherry, 1988). The constant infusion of mannitol (250 mg/hr IV) or urea (300 mg/hr IV) or the daily administration of dexamethasone (0.75 mg/kg SC) resulted in reduced CSFP in sublethally dosed rats. If urea or mannitol infusion were discontinued, however, CSFP returned to preinfusion values.

Mannitol (250 mg/kg every 6 hr IV) and dexamethasone (2 mg/kg every 6 hr IV) may be given to dogs and cats for the control of cerebral edema. These therapies, however, have been ineffective at preventing the toxic syndrome or reversing the syndrome once it has developed (Dorman et al., 1990c, 1990d). Observed treatment failures with combined corticosteroid and mannitol therapy in both dogs and cats may indicate that in these species the toxic syndrome is not due to cerebral edema alone. Alternatively, it is possible that the intramyelinic location of the edema may limit the effectiveness of corticosteroid and mannitol therapy. Contraindications for the use of mannitol include renal disease, pulmonary edema, dehydration, and intracranial hemorrhage. Animals receiving mannitol therapy may become dehydrated during treatment. Rehydration of some animals is associated with a worsening of clinical signs possibly due to rebound cerebral and pulmonary edema. Maintenance of hydration is important and can be more safely accomplished through the administration of oral fluids.

Diazepam (1 to 2.0 mg/kg IV, as needed) or phenobarbital (5 to 15 mg/kg IV, as needed) may be given to abolish severe muscle tremors and seizures. Many animals recovering from bromethalin toxicosis exhibit prolonged anorexia and may require supplemental feeding to maintain caloric intake. Recumbent animals should be placed in padded cages to prevent decubital ulcers.

SUMMARY

Bromethalin rodenticides are neurotoxic to dogs and cats. The clinical syndrome is characterized by ataxia, vocalization, hindlimb paralysis, CNS depression, fine muscle tremors, and focal motor or generalized seizures. The production of cerebral edema may play a significant role in the development of clinical signs. Treatment should include (1) the repeated administration of activated charcoal and a saline cathartic to decrease bromethalin absorption, (2) mannitol and dexamethasone to reduce cerebral edema, (3) diazepam or phenobarbital to control seizures and severe muscle tremors, and (4) other supportive therapies, including supplemental feeding.

References and Suggested Reading

Dorman, D. C., Harlin, K. S., Simon, J., et al.: Diagnosis of bromethalin poisoning in the dog. J. Vet. Diagn. Invest. 2:123, 1990a.
  A review of the lesions and chemical residues associated with bromethalin toxicosis in the dog.
Dorman, D. C., Parker, A. J., and Buck, W. B.: Bromethalin toxicosis

in the dog. I: Clinical effects. J. Am. Assoc. Anim. Hosp. 26:589, 1990b.
Description of the clinical effects of bromethalin in the dog.
Dorman, D. C., Parker, A. J., and Buck, W. B.: Bromethalin toxicosis in the dog. II: Treatment of the Toxic Syndrome. J. Am. Assoc. Anim. Hosp. 26:595, 1990c.
Description of the use of activated charcoal and combined mannitol/dexamethasone therapy in lethal bromethalin toxicosis in the dog.
Dorman, D. C., Parker, A. J., Dye, J. A., et al.: Bromethalin neurotoxicosis in the cat. Prog. Vet. Neurol. 1:189, 1990d.
Description of the clinical effects of bromethalin and its treatment with activated charcoal and combined mannitol/dexamethasone therapy in the cat.
Dorman, D. C., Parker, A. J., and Buck, W. B.: Electroencephalographic changes associated with bromethalin toxicosis in the dog. Vet. Hum. Toxicol. 33:9, 1991.
Description of EEG changes associated with lethal bromethalin toxicosis in the dog.

Driekorn, B. A., and O'Doherty, G. O.: The discovery and development of bromethalin, an acute rodenticide with a unique mechanism of action. *In* Magee, P. S., Kohn, G. K., and Menn, J. J. (eds.): *Pesticide Synthesis Through Rational Approaches.* Washington: American Chemical Society, 1984, p. 45–63.
Review of the development of bromethalin-based rodenticides.
Jackson, W. B., Spaulding, S. R., VanLier, R. B. L., et al.: Bromethalin— A promising new rodenticide. Proc. Tenth Vertebrate Pest Conference, 10, 1982.
Review of the toxicity of bromethalin to rodents and nontarget species.
Martin, T., and Johnson, B.: A suspected case of bromethalin toxicity in a domestic cat. Vet. Hum. Toxicol. 3:239, 1989.
Case report of lethal bromethalin poisoning in a cat.
VanLier, R. B. L., and Cherry, L. D.: The toxicity and mechanism of action of bromethalin: A new single-feeding rodenticide. Fund. Appl. Toxicol. 11:664, 1988.
Review and description of the acute toxicity, mechanism of action, and treatment of bromethalin toxicosis in rodents.

HOUSEHOLD TOXICOSES IN EXOTIC ANIMALS AND PET BIRDS

GENEVIEVE A. DUMONCEAUX

Bolingbrook, Illinois

Exotic pets, especially birds, are becoming more popular in homes across the United States. As the popularity of exotic pets and birds increases, so does the incidence of risks to these animals from common items kept in homes. The National Animal Poison Control Center (NAPCC) receives several calls each year regarding various species of caged birds, ferrets, small rodents, rabbits, primates, reptiles, and other "nondomestic" pets. These calls primarily concern exposures to household items (Trammel et al., 1989).

INSECTICIDES

Commonly used household insecticides contain organophosphates, carbamates, pyrethrins, or combinations of these. They are often used in and around animal areas. Sometimes the uninformed owner may use them directly on the animal. Veterinarians occasionally recommend the use of these pesticides on and around the animal based on their familiarity with the use of these products on dogs and cats for external parasite control. However, tolerance to the toxic effects of these chemicals is not the same for all species. Whereas ferrets seem to tolerate the same pesticides used on cats, the author has encountered occasions in which rabbits have developed depression, tremors, seizures, or death after being sprayed or dipped with insecticides commonly recommended for cats.

Signs of intoxication by these chemicals are similar to those seen in domestic pets, for example, hypersalivation, vomiting (except rabbits and rodents), diarrhea, increased bronchial secretions, dyspnea, weakness, depression, anorexia, muscle tremors, seizures, respiratory or cardiac failure, and death. Not all of these signs occur in every animal (Osweiler et al., 1985).

Reptiles readily absorb chemicals through the skin and therefore are able to rapidly reach lethal systemic levels of insecticides. There have been incidents of snakes exhibiting signs of toxicosis within minutes of being sprayed with pyrethrin insecticides. Central nervous system (CNS) depression and muscle weakness have persisted for several days. In severe cases, reptiles have been reported to experience tremor or convulsions almost immediately after being sprayed, and some have died soon afterward. Therefore, the author does not advise the use of insecticidal sprays or liquids directly on reptiles to eliminate ectoparasites. Alternatives to using ectoparasiticides on reptiles are soaking the animal in warm fresh water (up to 48 hours with severe infestations) (Frye, 1981) along with manual removal of parasites. A small piece of a carbamate or pyrethrin flea collar or a 1-inch piece of a Vapona Pest Strip (Shell) can be placed in the enclosure out of direct contact with the animal to control parasites in the animal's environment. Silica gel powders in the enclosures have also been recommended for parasite control for snakes (Jacobson, 1986).

The feathers of birds can afford some degree of protection from skin exposure to insecticides. However, large ingestions are possible because birds preen themselves after being sprayed. Inhalation of aerosolized insecticides seems to be the more common route of toxin exposure in birds. Because of their highly efficient respiratory systems, birds are much more susceptible to gases and particles in the air than are other animals in the household. Respiratory distress has been reported as the major clinical sign of toxicosis in accidentally poisoned birds. Other signs may include incoordination, generalized weakness, seizures, gastrointestinal signs, and sometimes sudden death (Harrison and Harrison, 1986).

There have been reports over the past few years concerning reactions in rabbits, hamsters, gerbils, guinea pigs, and chinchillas after being sprayed or dipped with insecticides intended for use on dogs and cats. Signs reported range from depression, anorexia, and respiratory difficulty to seizures and death (NAPCC data base). Some toxicoses have occurred when the animal was left in the house during spraying of a room or fogging the house. Carbaryl and pyrethrin powders have been recommended for rabbits and rodents to treat ectoparasites on their bodies. Permethrin dust mixed into the bedding at weekly intervals has been shown to control several species of mites. These animals also may be dipped in 0.025% lindane solution as an initial treatment in severe mite infestations (Harkness et al., 1989). It is important to note that none of the commonly used pet insecticides is approved for use in animals other than dogs or cats.

Ferrets seem to tolerate the feline flea and tick formulations fairly well. These are primarily pyrethrin-based insecticides. Precautions should be observed as for cats. Use of organophosphate and carbamate insecticides should be avoided in ferrets because their sensitivity to these products has not been well established.

Ivermectin is an effective alternative to insecticides for exotic pets. An oral or topical dosage of 200 μg/kg, repeated in two weeks, is recommended to treat scaly face mites (*Knemidokoptes* sp.) in birds (Ritchie, 1990). This dose given SQ to small rodents has also been effective for mite treatment. Ivermectin should be avoided in turtles and tortoises.

Treatment

Treatment of insecticide intoxications is similar to that for domestic animals. If the exposure is topical, bathing with a mild detergent with warm water should be instituted as soon as signs are noted. If ingestion of the insecticide has occurred, emesis can be induced, provided the animal is not showing signs. Emesis is most effective within the first 1 to 1½ hr postingestion; however, emetics are not recommended in rabbits and rodents because these animals are incapable of vomiting. In birds, crop lavage may be more effective and reliable than emesis. After emesis or lavage is completed, USP grade activated charcoal should be given. A saline cathartic such as sorbitol or magnesium sulfate may be added to the charcoal slurry, but caution should be used in certain species such as birds and small rodents as their rapid gastrointestinal transit time predisposes them to dehydration and electrolyte imbalance following saline catharsis. Atropine may be an effective symptomatic measure (0.2 mg/kg initial dose) (Osweiler et al., 1985) except in some species of rabbits and rats that produce atropinase. Pralidoxime chloride is antidotal for organophosphate intoxications. The standard domestic small animal dose is 20 mg/kg IV or IM (Osweiler et al., 1985). This may be repeated q 12–24 h as needed for recovery.

RODENTICIDES

The common rodenticides on the market today contain anticoagulants, cholecalciferol, or bromethalin as the active ingredient. Each of these has very different mechanisms of action; therefore it is important to know which one is involved if an exposure has occurred. Rabbits, rodents, and ferrets may have a higher incidence of exposure to these baits than cats and dogs. This may be because when they are able to roam about on floors at home, they can easily get into crawl spaces and behind furniture and appliances where these baits are commonly placed. Their small body size also makes them more susceptible to intoxication from very small amounts.

Anticoagulant-based rodenticides can be treated with vitamin K_1 injections or oral dosing (see *CVTX*, p. 143). The recommended dose for small mammals is 1 to 10 mg/kg/day (Harkness et al., 1989). The upper end of this range should be used for the smallest mammals owing to their increased metabolic rates. For birds, the recommended vitamin K_1 dose is 2.5 to 5 mg/kg/day IM (McDonald, 1989). Baits containing warfarin require treatment with vitamin K_1 for 6 to 10 consecutive days. The longer acting baits containing bromadiolone, diphacinone, and brodifacoum require up to 30 consecutive days of treatment with K_1 (Murphy and Gerken, 1989). If the exposure is recent (within 6 hours), activated charcoal is helpful in minimizing the total dose of anticoagulant absorbed from the gastrointestinal tract.

Cholecalciferol- and bromethalin-based baits may have much more serious effects that are more difficult to treat. Toxic doses for nondomestic pets have not been established. Treatment should be as described for dogs and cats in the literature (Carson, 1989; Dorman, 1990) (see this volume, p. 175, and *CVT X*, pp. 147 and 148).

PLANTS

Many ornamental plants found in homes and yards are known to be toxic to domestic pets. Few documented cases of plant toxicoses in birds and smaller pets have been reported, however. The toxicity information for plants with regard to dogs and cats can be applied to smaller mammals, as well. The time frames for toxicoses may differ because of the more rapid gastrointestinal transit times of the smaller species.

Information from the NAPCC data base over the past several years indicates that the calcium oxalate–containing plants have been involved in a higher incidence of plant toxicoses and suspected toxicoses in these animals than have other ornamentals. This may be because of the popularity and prevalence of these plants in homes. It may also be a result in part of the relatively higher toxicity of these plants to these animals based on their smaller body weight.

The calcium oxalate–containing plants most often involved in toxicoses are dieffenbachia and the philodendrons. Signs most frequently reported are depression, anorexia, hypersalivation, head shaking, vocalizing, vomiting, and diarrhea. Renal failure may occur due to ingestion of plants containing soluble oxalic acids which precipitate in the kidneys as calcium oxalate, resulting in direct damage to these organs. Such plants include the begonia family (Begoniaceae), the goosefoot family (Chenopodiaceae), and the grape family (Vitaceae) (Frohne and Pfander, 1984).

Other plants to be avoided include oleander (cardiac glycosides), spurges (many contain volatile and irritating oils), and castor beans (toxalbumins). These plants are suspected to be toxic to larger domestic species (Frohne and Pfander, 1984; Harrison and Harrison, 1986). Treatment for plant toxicoses generally consists of activated charcoal and a saline cathartic (except in birds) along with symptomatic and supportive care.

Toxicoses can also occur with nontoxic plant species when the plant has been sprayed with insecticides; animals that chew on the plants are then directly exposed to the insecticide. This can provide a means of acute or chronic exposure to the animal. Animals at greatest risk include birds, rabbits, and ferrets. These animals particularly enjoy chewing on nearby plants. Hanging plants can be a danger to birds that are allowed to fly in the home.

It is commonly recommended that exotic pets, especially birds, should receive a wide variety of foods. These foods should include fruits, vegetables, pastas, and even some meats or high-quality dog foods that provide important nutrients. Although this is a good practice for keeping pets' diets nutritionally balanced and keeping the animals in optimal health, some types of food should be avoided in the diet.

A common food known to be toxic to birds and other animals is avocado (*Persea* spp.). There have been reports of toxicoses caused by avocado being fed to pet birds (Clipsham, 1987; Hargis et al., 1989). Previously, it was believed its toxicity was limited to the leaves, bark, and pit of the fruit. A recent study and the experience at NAPCC have shown that the fruit itself has the ability to cause toxicoses in birds (Hargis et al., 1989). Typical signs associated with avocado intoxications in birds include depression, ruffled feathers, increased respiratory rate, dyspnea, and death (Hargis et al., 1989). Lesions found in affected birds included subcutaneous edema and pectoral muscle edema. Some affected birds had slightly bulging pectoral muscles with pale streaks throughout (Hargis et al., 1989). Excess pericardial fluid has also been noted in birds that have succumbed to avocado toxicity (Hargis et al., 1989).

Problems associated with ingestion of avocado by a rabbit have also been reported (NAPCC data base, 1988 and 1989). Rabbits have been reported to develop mastitis after ingesting avocado leaves. Death has also resulted from such ingestions. Necropsy findings on affected rabbits revealed pulmonary congestion and diffuse edema (Craigmill et al., 1984).

The specific toxin responsible for the detrimental effects of avocado has not yet been identified. Based on clinical signs and necropsy findings, death is primarily due to respiratory distress. There is no specific treatment protocol outlined. Therapy is mainly directed at the clinical signs and instituting general supportive measures.

AIRBORNE TOXICANTS

One of the most lethal gases found in households is polytetrafluoroethylene (PTFE) gas. This gas is produced when nonstick-coated surfaces are overheated and the coating is broken down via pyrolysis. This results in the release of acidic gases and particulates. Pyrolysis of the coating occurs when treated surfaces are heated in excess of 260°C (over 530°F) (Wells, 1983). These temperatures can be reached when treated pans are left empty on a hot stove to overheat or with the PTFE-coated drip pans under the burner during normal use.

Mammals seem to be able to tolerate these vapors

with little consequence. In extreme cases of overheated surfaces, pet owners, as well as pets, will experience adverse effects from the gases, including dizziness, headaches, and nausea. Birds, however, are uniquely sensitive to the gases released in such situations, even when the overheating lasts only a few moments. This is because birds have such a highly efficient respiratory tract that the respiratory system extracts more of the toxic components from the air than does the typical mammalian lung. Often the intoxication occurs so rapidly that the pet bird is found dead in its cage before a problem is recognized.

Signs that have been reported in affected birds include noisy respiration, increased respiratory effort, rocking or bobbing movements, somnolence, eyelid blinking, ruffled feathers, and terminal convulsions. These signs are likely caused by hypoxemia as a result of the damaged respiratory tract (Wells, 1983). Observation of signs is uncommon, however, and the most common clinical feature is sudden death of the bird.

The most consistently reported lesion has been acute hemorrhagic pneumonitis. Necropsies may reveal severe abdominal visceral congestion and pulmonary congestion and hemorrhage. The lungs appear dark red and wet and may sink in formalin solution. The cut surfaces of the lungs ooze dark red to almost black blood. Major and minor airways are filled with hemorrhagic exudate. Loss of lining epithelium may be evident in some tertiary bronchi and air capillaries (Wells, 1983).

Treatment is difficult and often unrewarding. If signs are noticed in a bird prior to death, the bird should immediately be removed to fresh air. Transport to a veterinary hospital should not be delayed. The bird should be placed in an oxygen-rich environment. Fluids can be administered, and a broad-spectrum antibiotic is recommended to reduce secondary respiratory bacterial infections. Corticosteroids are also recommended to combat pulmonary edema and shock (Dumonceaux, 1989). The animal should be kept in a warm, dark environment with minimal handling until its condition stabilizes.

Aerosols in general should not be used in areas where birds are present. These products contain fluorocarbons and particulates that can cause considerable irritation to the respiratory tract. This can lead to bacterial infection and respiratory disease. Therefore, all birds and other pets should be removed from the area before aerosolized cleaners, disinfectants, or other such products are used. When disinfectants are used to clean food and water dishes and cages, these items must be rinsed thoroughly in clean fresh water before the animals are again exposed to the items. Gas leaks may also cause serious problems and should be checked for when pets develop sudden respiratory problems or depression of unknown etiology.

MISCELLANEOUS TOXICANTS

There are numerous household items that tend to attract pets. These include ink pens, markers, pencils, matches, and paints. Such items are easily held and chewed by small exotic pets. Although formulations of pens and markers vary depending on the manufacturer, the general formulation of ink pens often includes boric acid and xylene. Boric acid is well absorbed from the gastrointestinal tract, open wounds, and serous cavities. Gastrointestinal symptoms can be seen following all routes of exposure. Signs that may be noted after ingestion of toxic amounts of such inks are vomiting and diarrhea (which may become bloody), depression, anorexia, hypotension, renal failure with oliguria or anuria, and hypothermia or hyperthermia. Treatment should include expedient induction of emesis (except in rabbits and rodents) before signs develop. In the case of birds, crop lavage may be indicated, as is early treatment. This should be followed by administration of activated charcoal and a saline cathartic (no cathartics in birds). Fluids may help combat hypotension and preserve renal function. Renal function should be monitored closely, especially if the animal becomes symptomatic. Exposed eyes, skin, and oral cavity should be irrigated thoroughly (Rumack, 1990).

Xylene is a component of ink pens and markers of most types. This is a very volatile substance, and toxicosis usually occurs with repeated exposure by inhalation. Typical signs are upper respiratory tract irritation with increased noise, lacrimation, depression, respiratory distress, ataxia, muscle weakness, vomiting, diarrhea, and abdominal pain, especially after acute ingestions. Initial treatment consists of emesis followed by administration of activated charcoal and a cathartic if exposure has been by ingestion. If inhalation has occurred, the animal should be moved to fresh air. Oxygen may be necessary if respiratory difficulty is evident. Monitor fluid and electrolyte status closely, and give a balanced electrolyte solution as needed. Hypokalemia and acidosis may occur and can be corrected with potassium and bicarbonate supplementation. If significant respiratory irritation and difficulty are present, administer 100% humidified oxygen. Steroids may be indicated to control laryngeal (mammals) or pulmonary edema (Rumack, 1990).

Another frequently cited component of markers is ethylene glycol ethyl ether. High doses in animals produce renal injury, hematuria, and macrocytic anemia. More overt effects are immediate oral discomfort and conjunctival and corneal irritation (Rumack, 1990). Treatment is similar to that of ink pen ingestions.

Pencils are a particular favorite of many birds, as they are easily chewed apart and contain a soft inner core. Although lead was used in the manufacture of pencils several years ago, the current ingredient in the core is graphite. The components of pencils are considered to be nontoxic, and ingestions should be handled as a foreign body exposure (Rumack, 1990).

Birds and occasionally small mammals will chew the heads of matches. The most common ingredients in match heads are chlorates. These are potent oxidizing agents, and large exposure may result in hemolysis with methemoglobin formation. Chlorates are also directly nephrotoxic. Signs that have been reported with toxic ingestions are dyspnea, cyanosis, depression, nausea with vomiting and abdominal pain, seizures, and coma. Systemic effects include increases in serum glutamic oxalacetic transaminase and serum glutamic pyruvic transaminase values, hepatomegaly, acute renal insufficiency with oliguria or anuria, hyperkalemia, hemolysis, methemoglobinemia, and pallor. The clinically ill patient should be monitored for packed cell volume changes, renal function, and hemolytic problems. Treatment involves emesis initially, followed by activated charcoal and a cathartic. Alkaline diuresis may be of benefit to increase the elimination rate of the chlorate. Be sure that hydration and renal function are adequate. Methylene blue should be administered *slowly* to combat methemoglobinemia (Rumack, 1990). The dose recommended for domestic mammals is 5 to 15 mg/kg IV (Osweiler et al., 1985). Because methylene blue may induce methemoglobinemia in cats, ascorbic acid (250 to 500 mg, slow IV injection or subcutaneously) is recommended for this species (Osweiler et al., 1985).

Exotic pets have their own idiosyncrasies that occasionally preclude the typical treatment regimens for particular intoxications, for example, atropinase production by some rabbits and rodents and very rapid gastrointestinal transit times in several species. However, basic therapeutic guidelines for treatment of toxicoses in domestic animals can be used with these pets. This, combined with knowledge of the animal's physiology and having the proper dosages available, will enable practitioners to effectively treat these "nondomestic" pets for intoxications involving household items.

References and Suggested Reading

Carson, T. L.: Bromethalin poisoning. *In* Kirk, R. W. (ed.): *Current Veterinary Therapy X.* Philadelphia: W. B. Saunders, 1989, p. 147.
A review of the toxicity, clinical diagnosis, and treatment of bromethalin intoxication in small animals.
Clipsham, R.: Avocado toxicity. Bird Talk April/May, 1987.
A review of avocado toxicity in pet birds.
Craigmill, A. L., Eide, R. N., Shultz, T. A., et al.: Toxicity of avocado (*Persea americana* [Guatemalan var]) leaves: Review and preliminary report. Vet. Hum. Toxicol. 26:381, 1984.
A preliminary report of avocado toxicity in a breed of domestic goat.
Dorman, D. C.: Anticoagulant, cholecalciferol, and bromethalin-based rodenticides. *In* Beasley, V. R. (ed.): Vet. Clin. North Am. [Small Anim. Pract.] 20:339, 1990.
A review of the toxicologic and clinical effects and treatment for small animals with regard to three of the more common active ingredients in many of the rodenticides on the market today.
Dumonceaux, G. A.: Hazards of nonstick cookware in pet birds. National Animal Poison Information Network (NAPINet) Report: 2:2, 1989.
A summary of the toxicity, clinical effects, and treatment of PTFE intoxication in pet birds.
Frohne, D., and Pfander, H. J.: *A Colour Atlas of Poisonous Plants: A Handbook for Pharmacists, Doctors, Toxicologists, and Biologists.* Germany: Wolfe Publishing, 1984.
A text outlining the toxicologic aspects of several plant species.
Frye, F. L.: *Biomedical and Surgical Aspects of Captive Reptile Husbandry.* Melbourne: Krieger Publishing, 1981, p. 222.
A comprehensive text addressing the care and disease aspects and surgical techniques involving reptiles in captivity.
Hargis, A. M., Stauber, E., Casteel, S., et al.: Avocado (*Persea americana*) intoxication in caged birds. J.A.V.M.A. 194:64, 1989.
A report on the effects of avocado intoxication in pet birds.
Harkness, J. E., and Wagner, J. E.: *The Biology and Medicine of Rabbits and Rodents,* 3rd ed. Philadelphia: Lea & Febiger, 1989, pp. 58–113.
A comprehensive text on the care, management, and medical aspects of rodents and rabbits.
Harrison, G. J., and Harrison, L. R.: *Clinical Avian Medicine and Surgery.* Philadelphia: W. B. Saunders, 1986, p. 497.
A comprehensive text addressing the care, clinical diseases, and treatment of various types of birds.
Jacobson, E.: Parasitic diseases of reptiles. *In* Fowler, M. E. (ed.): *Zoo and Wild Animal Medicine,* 2nd ed. Philadelphia, W. B. Saunders, 1986, p. 162.
A summary of the diagnosis and treatment of the common parasitic diseases of captive reptiles.
McDonald, S. E.: Summary of medications for use in psittacine birds. J. Assoc. Avian Vet. 3:120, 1989.
Murphy, M. J., and Gerken, D. F.: The anticoagulant rodenticides. *In* Kirk, R. W.: *Current Veterinary Therapy X.* Philadelphia: W. B. Saunders, 1989, p. 143.
A review of the toxicities, clinical effects, and treatment of anticoagulant intoxications in domestic small animals.
Osweiler, G. D., Carson, T. L., Buck, W. B., et al.: *Clinical and Diagnostic Veterinary Toxicology,* 3rd ed. Dubuque, IA: Kendall/Hunt Publishing, 1985, p. 298.
A comprehensive text addressing the toxicologic and clinical aspects of several recognized biologic and manufactured toxins.
Personal Communication, Illinois Animal Poison Information Center Case Database, 1988–1990.
Ritchie, B. W.: Avian therapeutics. *In* Association Avian Veterinarians Proceedings, 1990, p. 415.
A summary of current commonly used avian therapeutic regimens, dosages, and routes of administration.
Rumack, B. H. (ed.): Poisindex Management. Denver: Micromedex, Inc. Spring, 1990.
A comprehensive information system covering many chemicals commonly encountered in commercial products.
Trammel, H. T., Dorman, D. C., Beasley, V. R., et al.: *Ninth Annual Report of the Illinois Animal Poison Information Center.* Dubuque, IA: Kendall/Hunt Publishing, 1989.
Wells, R. E.: Fatal toxicosis in pet birds caused by an overheated cooking pan lined with polytetrafluoroethylene. J.A.V.M.A. 182:1248, 1983.
A report on the effects of PTFE intoxication in pet birds.

COMMON TOXICOSES OF WATERFOWL, LOONS, AND RAPTORS

ROBERT H. POPPENGA

East Lansing, Michigan

Much interest is currently shown in the treatment and rehabilitation of ill or injured avian wildlife. Many of these birds are affected directly or indirectly by environmental contaminants present in their diets or natural habitats. It is important for veterinarians to be cognizant of common avian wildlife toxicants in order to effectively diagnose and treat individuals, to offer a prognosis for recovery and rehabilitation, and perhaps to investigate field outbreaks of suspected toxicoses. This article focuses on waterfowl such as ducks, geese, and swans; loons; and raptors such as eagles, hawks, and owls, because these groups of avian wildlife are commonly affected by various toxicants. Less common toxicants affecting these species are listed in Table 1. (See *CVT IX*, p. 719, for a discussion of the rehabilitation of oil-contaminated birds.) All applicable state and federal wildlife laws and regulations should be followed when handling or treating affected birds.

GENERAL COMMENTS ON THE DIAGNOSIS OF TOXICOSES

Knowledge of the ethology of waterfowl, loon, and raptor species is important for developing a differential list of possible toxicants for a given case. For example, puddle and bay diving ducks are particularly prone to ingesting lead shot during routine feeding, whereas teal, shovelers, wood ducks, whistling ducks, sea ducks, and mergansers ingest little or no shot because of specialization of feeding habits (Friend, 1987). Avian species for which fish or other birds constitute a major portion of their diet are more likely to be affected by toxicants such as organochlorine (OC) insecticides, polychlorinated biphenyls (PCBs), or methyl mercury, which are biomagnified through food webs.

One hindrance to field investigations of suspected avian toxicoses is the lack of suitable samples for laboratory evaluation. Avian carcasses may be quickly scavenged or decomposed. Rapid postmortem decomposition often precludes microbiologic and histologic evaluation. Fortunately, in many cases, chemical toxins can be detected in gastrointestinal contents or other tissues such as liver and brain for some time after death. However, freshly collected and properly stored specimens are crucial for proper interpretation of certain laboratory analytic results such as brain cholinesterase (ChE) activity in suspected organophosphate (OP) or carbamate (CA) insecticide toxicoses.

Tissues from affected birds often contain multiple toxicant residues, making interpretation of laboratory results difficult. It is not unusual for a single bird to contain several OC insecticides, PCBs, and one or more metals. In many cases, the potential for additive or synergistic toxicity and prospects for effective treatment and rehabilitation are not clear.

INSECTICIDES

Organochlorines

The OC insecticides include dichlorodiphenyltrichloroethane (DDT), aldrin, dieldrin, heptachlor, endrin, chlordane, methoxychlor, and lindane, among others. Because of their environmental persistence, biomagnification through wildlife food webs, and adverse affects such as eggshell thinning in certain avian wildlife species, most have been banned in the United States for use as agricultural insecticides for a number of years. However, continued use in less-developed countries contributes to the worldwide OC environmental contaminant burden. Although OC tissue residue concentrations have declined in many of the most severely affected avian species in the United States since discontinuation of their use, subpopulations of birds or individuals may still accumulate large body burdens. This is especially true of birds inhabiting areas that were heavily contaminated in the past. In particular, fish- or bird-eating raptors and fish-eating common loons may accumulate high tissue concentrations. The OCs most commonly detected in tissues include metabolites of DDT and heptachlor, dichlorodiphenyldichloroethylene (DDE) and heptachlor epoxide, respectively, and dieldrin.

Although acute exposure to a lethal concentration

Table 1. Other Waterfowl and Raptor Toxicants

Toxin	Source of Exposure	Acute Clinical Signs	Diagnosis	Treatment
Polychlorinated biphenyls (PCBs)	Diet, bioconcentration through contaminated food webs	Lethargy, ataxia, tremors, edema	Measurement of brain (>300 ppm), liver, or other tissue residues (>20,000 ppm); ppm expressed on a tissue fat basis; submit half the brain or minimum of 10 gm liver	Symptomatic and supportive
Mercury, primarily methyl mercury	Diet, bioconcentration through contaminated food webs or ingestion of treated seed grain	Weakness of the extremities, ataxia, inability to fly or walk, eyelid drooping, calmness, hypoactivity, hyporeactivity; may continue to eat	Histologic lesions in the central and peripheral nervous systems, elevated liver or kidney [Hg] (10–20 ppm); ppm expressed on a tissue wet weight basis; submit a minimum of 1 gm of each tissue Measurement of tissue [Se] may be necessary for proper assessment of [Hg]	Symptomatic and supportive
Selenium	Diet, bioconcentration through contaminated food webs	Emaciation, breast muscle atrophy, fibrin and fluid accumulations in the peritoneal cavity, feather loss on the head; embryotoxic and teratogenic	Gross postmortem examination, measurement of tissue [Se]; liver and kidney [Se] approach 100 ppm on a dry weight basis; submit a minimum of 1 gm of tissue	Symptomatic and supportive
Anticoagulant rodenticides	Secondary toxicosis from ingestion of poisoned prey	Weakness, labored breathing, coagulopathy	Gross postmortem examination, detection of anticoagulant in whole blood, liver, or other tissue; submit 1 ml of whole blood or 10 gm of liver	Vitamin K_1, the dosage regimen is empiric for avian species; a suggested regimen is 3–5 mg/kg in divided doses q 8 hr for a minimum of 3–4 weeks; initial doses may need to be given parenterally, with a switch to oral dose once bird is stabilized
Zinc phosphide	Ingestion of grain or pelleted bait Emetic action may be protective	Acute clinical signs other than emesis and diarrhea have not been described in avian wildlife; respiratory difficulties, hyperesthesia, and convulsions may be expected	Clinical signs, detection of phosphine gas in GI contents; GI samples should be collected, frozen, and analyzed as soon as possible after death	Symptomatic and supportive; decontamination of GI tract, although onset of toxicosis is probably too rapid for decontamination to be effective; gastric lavage with 5% sodium bicarbonate followed by activated charcoal as an aqueous suspension at 1–2 gm/kg PO
Strychnine	Secondary toxicosis in raptors from ingestion of poisoned prey	Hyperreactivity, stiffness, tetanic seizures with extensor rigidity	Clinical signs, detection of strychnine in GI contents; submit several gm of frozen GI contents	Control of seizures (diazepam); decontamination of GI tract; administration of activated charcoal as an aqueous suspension at 1–2 gm/kg PO
Aflatoxins	Ingestion of contaminated feedstuffs (peanuts, corn)	Apparent blindness, depression, hyporeactivity, weakness, inability to fly, extended head and neck with lowered eyelids, vigorous flapping of wings that subsides prior to death	At postmortem examination, hepatic lesions are most prominent on gross and histologic exam; detection of aflatoxins in feedstuffs or upper GI tract contents	Symptomatic and supportive

[ ], metal concentration; GI, gastrointestinal.

of an OC is possible, it is an infrequent occurrence. A more common scenario for intoxication involves the gradual accumulation of one or more OCs within the body during a period of time. Because OCs and their metabolites are extremely lipophilic, they are stored and concentrated in body fat. In a sense, storage in body fat can be regarded as a detoxification mechanism because body fat serves as a "sink" for OCs and prevents their accumulation to toxic concentrations in sensitive tissues such as the central nervous system. However, mobilization of storage fat as a result of an underlying disease or stress process causes rapid redistribution of OCs into other organs to maintain tissue equilibrium. When a critical concentration of one or more OCs is reached in the brain, acute toxicity occurs.

CLINICAL SIGNS AND POSTMORTEM FINDINGS

Signs of acute OC toxicosis are related to the overstimulation of the nervous system and include hypersensitivity, muscle fasciculations progressing to coarse tremors, jaw chomping, tonic-clonic convulsions, and hyperpyrexia. Postconvulsive depression may occur. Unusual behavior may be exhibited, such as tameness, irregular flight, and gait abnormalities.

No diagnostic gross or histologic lesions are associated with OC toxicosis. Grossly, most bird carcasses are found to be dehydrated and emaciated and to have little or no body fat. Little food is present in the gastrointestinal tract. Histologic lesions, if present, are nonspecific. Lesions in the liver may consist of nonzonal areas of fatty degeneration, necrosis, and hemorrhage. Pulmonary congestion and edema may be present, along with congestion of the kidneys and brain. It is emphasized that any disease process or stress that prompts rapid mobilization of body fat can precipitate acute OC toxicity. Therefore, gross and histologic lesions related to an underlying disease process also may be present.

DIAGNOSIS

The diagnosis of OC toxicosis is based on clinical signs and the demonstration of diagnostically significant OC tissue concentrations. Many veterinary diagnostic laboratories offer analytic screens that can detect one or more of the OC insecticides. The specimens of choice from a live bird include whole blood and plasma (2 ml). Frozen brain and liver (whole brain if possible and at least 5 to 10 gm liver) from dead birds should be submitted for analysis. Brain concentrations of OCs have traditionally been used to diagnose toxicoses. Diagnostically significant brain concentrations expressed on a tissue wet

weight basis for DDE, dieldrin, and heptachlor epoxide are considered to be 150, 5, and 8 ppm, respectively. However, detection of multiple OCs makes interpretation of laboratory results more difficult. Also, guidelines for interpretation of concentrations in whole blood, plasma, liver, or other tissues are less clear. OC concentrations are roughly equivalent in all tissues when they are expressed on a tissue fat basis. There is also a linear relationship between whole carcass concentrations expressed on a fat basis and brain concentrations expressed on a wet weight basis. Therefore, rough approximations of brain concentrations can be made based on knowledge of concentrations in the carcass or other tissues (Barbehenn and Reichel, 1981; Wiemeyer and Cromartie, 1981). The lowest OC concentrations expressed on a fat basis in the carcass (and by extrapolation other tissues) that approach a potentially lethal concentration in ospreys are reported to be 9200 ppm for DDE, 140 ppm for dieldrin, and 710 ppm for heptachlor epoxide. Unfortunately, the tissue:brain relationship is species- and chemical-specific, and data are not always available for making extrapolations in every case.

TREATMENT

Unfortunately, the prognosis for a symptomatic bird is poor. Therapy is largely symptomatic and supportive. Attempts should be made to control seizures. Diazepam at 0.6 mg/kg IM or IV may be tried. Anorectic, nonsymptomatic birds should be force-fed to halt fat mobilization. Any underlying disease process should be treated with appropriate medications.

Organophosphates and Carbamates

OP and CA insecticides have replaced the OCs and are the most commonly used agricultural insecticides in the United States. They are not environmentally stable and do not accumulate in food webs. However, they are considered to be more *acutely* toxic to avian wildlife species than the OCs. The OPs and CA are available in various formulations including liquids, wettable powders, and granules. Some of the more toxic chemicals are used as soil insecticides. These include phorate, terbufos, fonofos, and carbofuran. Moderately toxic OPs such as chlorpyrifos and diazinon are applied topically to crops and lawns, whereas others such as famphur and chlorpyrifos are used as livestock pour-on insecticides. There are regional differences in use patterns for these insecticides, and familiarity with such patterns may be of assistance in deciding which specific insecticides are likely to be involved in a suspected toxicosis. Fortunately, most veterinary diagnostic laboratories can screen for a large number of commonly used OPs and CAs.

Certain species of waterfowl are more likely to be exposed to lethal amounts of OPs and CAs as a result of ingestion of contaminated grain and forage. Also, available acute toxicity data indicate that waterfowl are much more sensitive to the toxic effects of some OPs and CAs than mammals (Smith, 1987).

Raptors can be secondarily poisoned after consuming small mammals or birds incapacitated or killed by OPs and CAs. There are several case reports of raptors being intoxicated after consuming birds that had been poisoned by contact with cattle treated with pour-on OP insecticides (Henny et al., 1987).

CLINICAL SIGNS AND POSTMORTEM FINDINGS

Toxicity results from the inhibition of acetylcholinesterase activity and resultant overstimulation of cholinergic receptors by acetylcholine. Clinical signs include ataxia, apparent flaccid paralysis or extensor rigidity of leg and wing muscles, inability to fly, bradycardia, and salivation. Diarrhea and miosis may also be seen.

In contrast to OC toxicosis, birds poisoned with OP or CA insecticides are generally in good physical condition and have food in the gastrointestinal tract. However, as with OC intoxication, no characteristic gross or histologic lesions are present on postmortem examination. Pulmonary congestion and an increase in bronchial secretions may be inconsistent findings.

DIAGNOSIS

The diagnosis of OP and CA toxicosis is based on clinical signs, measurement of depressed brain or plasma ChE activity, and detection of insecticide residues in gastrointestinal contents or tissues. A 20% depression of brain or plasma ChE activity below a normal range is considered to be indicative of exposure to an OP, whereas toxicosis is associated with a 50% or greater depression. However, interpretation of brain or plasma ChE activity can be difficult. Normal activity ranges are large within a given species, and the mean activity can be quite variable between species. Plasma ChE activity is more variable than brain activity and is influenced by physiologic variables. Brain ChE activity may increase with age to adulthood. Also, measured brain ChE activity increases as brain tissue decomposes. Thus, it is important to obtain tissue as soon after death as possible. It is particularly difficult to diagnose CA toxicoses based on ChE activity because of the spontaneous regeneration of enzyme activity within a sample over time. For these rea-

sons, a diagnosis of OP or CA toxicosis should not be based solely on measurement of ChE activity; gastrointestinal contents and liver should also be tested for the presence of an insecticide. One half of the brain cut midsagittally or 0.5 ml of plasma should be frozen and submitted for analysis. The suitability of using whole blood for ChE determinations has not been evaluated in birds. A compilation of brain ChE activities of several waterfowl and raptor species is available (Hill, 1988).

TREATMENT

Initial treatment should consist of administration of atropine in incremental doses to effect. Each dose of atropine may total 0.2 mg/kg or greater. One third of the dose is given IV, with the remainder given IM or SC. Atropine is repeated as necessary. Following atropinization, pralidoxime chloride (2-PAM) may be given IM or SC every 8 to 12 hours for a minimum of 48 hours. Clinical experience with the use of 2-PAM in avian species is limited, but doses up to 100 mg/kg have been used without adverse effects (Shlosberg, 1976). However, a generally recommended dose of pralidoxime in most species is 20 mg/kg. Atropine alone can be effective for treating toxicosis from cholinesterase-inhibiting insecticides. However, the combination of atropine and 2-PAM may substantially shorten the recovery period, particularly in cases of organophosphate toxicosis. The efficacy of 2-PAM in cases of carbamate toxicosis is questionable. In those cases in which the identity of the cholinesterase-inhibiting insecticide is not known, 2-PAM should be given.

It may be beneficial to remove any food material from the upper gastrointestinal tract physically or by lavage. Activated charcoal should be administered at 1 to 2 gm/kg in an aqueous slurry after gastrointestinal tract decontamination.

METALS

Lead

It has been estimated that more than a million waterfowl, primarily mallards and geese, die of lead poisoning each year. The major source of lead exposure for waterfowl is ingestion of lead shot. The toxicity of lead shot for waterfowl is variable and depends on factors such as age, sex, diet, and shot size. However, experimentally, death has occurred in ducks that ingested one number 6 shot. Fish-eating waterfowl such as the common loon have been poisoned after ingesting lead fishing sinkers. In addition, raptors are intoxicated by lead bullets or shot present in carcasses that they have consumed. Regurgitation of casts may lessen the occurrence of lead poisoning in raptors because ingested lead objects may be effectively eliminated from the upper gastrointestinal tract with the cast.

The incidence of lead poisoning in waterfowl will no doubt decline in the future as lead shot is replaced by steel shot. However, other bird species will remain at risk.

CLINICAL SIGNS AND POSTMORTEM FINDINGS

Clinical signs in affected birds include anorexia, lethargy, weakness, emaciation, muscle tremors, drooped wings, green diarrhea, ataxia, and impaired locomotion (Eisler, 1988). Affected birds may have lower than expected hematocrit and hemoglobin values, although dehydration at the time of blood collection may artificially elevate these values.

Gross postmortem findings include pulmonary edema; hydrothorax; hydropericardium; an enlarged, bile-filled gallbladder; an abnormal, bile-stained gizzard lining; esophageal impaction; and a pale, emaciated, dehydrated carcass. Histologic changes may include the presence of acid-fast inclusion bodies in proximal convoluted renal tubule cells, nephrosis, and myocardial and arterial fibrinoid necrosis. However, the occurrence of acid-fast inclusion bodies is species dependent, being more common in waterfowl than raptors.

DIAGNOSIS

The diagnosis of lead poisoning is based on characteristic clinical signs and postmortem lesions, demonstration of lead objects in the gastrointestinal tract, and elevated whole blood and tissue lead concentrations. However, the failure to demonstrate lead objects in the gastrointestinal tract does not rule out the possibility of lead poisoning.

Diagnostic whole blood, liver, and kidney lead concentrations on a tissue wet weight basis are reported to be greater than 0.2, 2, and 2 ppm, respectively, although concentrations in lead-intoxicated birds are likely to be much higher (Beyer et al., 1988). Kidney lead concentrations are generally higher than liver concentrations. Frozen samples of both tissues (1 gm) should be submitted for lead determinations. When submitting whole blood for analysis, the type of anticoagulant used for whole blood preservation is not critical, although it may be wise to consult with the analytic laboratory before collecting the sample. Depending on the analytic procedure used, as little as 100 μl of whole blood may be sufficient. Decreased red blood cell aminolevulinic acid dehydratase activity and increased free erythrocyte protoporphyrin concentrations have been reported to be sensitive indicators

of lead exposure in waterfowl, although these analyses may not be readily available.

TREATMENT

Chelation of lead with calcium disodium edetate (CaEDTA) has been successfully used to treat various avian species for lead intoxication. CaEDTA at 35 to 50 mg/kg IM every 8 hr for 5 days may be given between 5-day rest intervals until clinical improvement is noted. The efficacy of other chelating agents such as dimercaprol (BAL), alone or in combination with CaEDTA, has not been determined. Removal of lead shot or other lead fragments from the gastrointestinal tract is also critical for successful treatment. Removal of lead shot may be tried via lavage. Alternatively, surgical removal may be necessary. Follow-up whole blood lead concentrations should be determined periodically after cessation of treatment to see if additional chelation therapy is needed. Residual nervous system damage in recovered birds may prevent successful rehabilitation.

BIOTOXINS

Botulism

Nearly all avian species are affected by *Clostridium botulinum* toxin, although outbreaks in waterfowl, particularly ducks and geese, are most frequent. Cases in raptors such as peregrine falcons and bald eagles have been reported. Type C toxin is most commonly involved in outbreaks of avian botulism, with type E toxin less commonly implicated in sporadic die-offs of loons.

An anaerobic environment with fluctuating but shallow water levels, available animal protein source from dead invertebrate or vertebrate animals, and high ambient temperatures all are environmental factors necessary for optimal toxin production. The presence of vertebrate carcasses and high temperatures also permits the buildup of fly populations and toxin-containing maggots, which are subsequently ingested by ducks (Locke and Friend, 1987).

CLINICAL SIGNS AND POSTMORTEM LESIONS

Affected birds initially are not able to make a sustained flight, although they can usually walk and move on water with the aid of wings. The nictitating membrane becomes paralyzed and the eyes matted closed. Paralysis progresses to the point that leg muscles cannot be used, and the bird may move along its breast by flapping its wings. Greenish diarrhea may be noted, but constipation follows, and affected birds may have a plugged vent. Just before death, affected birds are unable to hold their heads up, resulting in a characteristic limberneck. Labored breathing, irregular pulse, and hypothermia ensue. Death is due to respiratory failure, drowning, starvation, lack of water, exposure, or predation. Postmortem lesions are not characteristic. Lesions associated with drowning may be all that are noted.

DIAGNOSIS

Diagnosis is based on the mouse protection test. Serum from a sick or freshly dead bird is injected into two groups of laboratory mice; one group is protected by type-specific antitoxin and the other is not. Characteristic signs of botulism in the unprotected mice are diagnostic of botulism. In lieu of serum, saline extracts of aseptically collected tissues such as liver may be used.

TREATMENT

Mildly affected birds in which paralysis has not progressed may recover with supportive care, shade, and fresh water. Antitoxin may be administered to individual birds, although such an approach is not practical in large outbreaks and the antitoxin may not be readily available. If used, antitoxin is administered at 0.5 to 1.0 ml IP.

Prevention is perhaps the best strategy for limiting mortality. Immediate removal of dead and decaying bird carcasses is mandatory to break the cycle of toxin production. If possible, lowering or raising water levels to dry out an area or to dilute the toxin may be tried. Dispersal of unaffected birds from localized areas can be attempted but may be of questionable value.

References and Suggested Reading

Barbehenn, K. R., and Reichel, W. L.: Organochlorine concentrations in bald eagles: Brain/body lipid relations and hazard evaluation. J. Toxicol. Environ. Health 8:325, 1981.

Beyer, W. N., Spann, J. W., Sileo, L., and Franson, J. C.: Lead poisoning in six captive avian species. Arch. Environ. Contam. Toxicol. 17:121, 1988.

Eisler, R.: Lead hazards to fish, wildlife, and invertebrates: A synoptic review. United States Department of the Interior, Fish and Wildlife Service, Biological Report 85(1.14), 1988, p. 55.

Friend, M.: Lead poisoning. In Friend, M. (ed.): *Field Guide to Wildlife Diseases: General Field Procedures and Diseases of Migratory Birds.* Washington, D.C.: United States Department of the Interior, 1987, p. 175.

Henny, C. J., Kolbe, E. J., Hill, E. F., et al.: Case histories of bald eagles and other raptors killed by organophosphorus insecticides topically applied to livestock. J. Wildl. Dis. 23:292, 1987.

Hill, E. F.: Brain cholinesterase activity of apparently normal wild birds. J. Wildl. Dis. 24:51, 1988.

Locke, L. N., and Friend, M.: Avian botulism. In Friend, M. (ed.): *Field Guide to Wildlife Diseases: General Field Procedures and Diseases of Migratory Birds.* Washington, DC: U.S. Department of the Interior, 1987, p. 83.

Shlosberg, A.: Treatment of monocrotophos-poisoned birds of prey with pralidoxime iodide. J.A.V.M.A. 169:989, 1976.

Smith, G. J.: Pesticide use and toxicology in relation to wildlife: Organophosphate and carbamate compounds. United States Department of the Interior, Fish and Wildlife Service, Resource Publication 170, 1987, p. 1.

Wiemeyer, S. N., and Cromartie, E.: Relationships between brain and carcass organochlorine residues in ospreys. Bull. Environ. Contam. Toxicol. 27:499, 1981.

FELINE CHLORPYRIFOS TOXICOSIS

JAMES D. FIKES
East Lansing, Michigan

Chlorpyrifos (0,0-diethyl-0-[3,5,6-trichloro-2-pyridyl] phosphorothioate) is one of the most widely used organophosphorus (OP) insecticides. More commonly identified by the trade name Dursban or Lorsban (Dow Chemical Co., Midland, MI), it has found widespread use in termite control and in agriculture as a corn rootworm insecticide and cattle parasiticide. Chlorpyrifos has excellent efficacy against fleas and has found wide acceptance and

application in flea control. For this purpose, chlorpyrifos is formulated for animal use as a dip, in a polymer-containing animal spray, in flea collars, and as over-the-counter and commercial preparations for household application. Except for flea collars, chlorpyrifos is *not approved* for use on cats. Cats nevertheless are frequently exposed to significant amounts of chlorpyrifos through the accidental or inappropriate use of these products. The product formulations most commonly associated with feline toxicosis are flea dips and other products for insect control in the home.

OP insecticides, including chlorpyrifos, are inhibitors of cholinesterase (ChE). Acetylcholinesterase (AChE) terminates the stimulatory effect of acetylcholine (ACh) by rapidly hydrolyzing ACh within the synaptic spaces of the nervous system. OP insecticides bind to the ChE enzyme, thereby inhibiting its normal hydrolytic activity. With AChE activity inhibited, ACh accumulates at the postsynaptic receptor site, producing prolonged stimulation of effector organs such as glandular tissue and smooth and skeletal muscle.

TOXICITY

Cats are relatively susceptible to acute chlorpyrifos toxicosis. The oral minimum lethal dose of chlorpyrifos in cats is between 10 and 40 mg/kg. The acute oral LD_{50} of chlorpyrifos is 118 to 245 mg/kg in rats, 504 mg/kg in guinea pigs, and approximately 2000 mg/kg in rabbits. A further indication of the sensitivity of cats to acute chlorpyrifos toxicosis is implied by data from the Illinois Animal Poison Information Center (IAPIC). In 1988, the IAPIC reported 168 calls about cats exposed to chlorpyrifos and 238 calls about dogs. Sixty-one per cent of the calls involving cats were assessed by IAPIC veterinarians as a toxicosis or suspected toxicosis, whereas only 28% of the calls involving dogs were similarly assessed.

A rather common exposure of dogs to chlorpyrifos is through the ingestion of the contents of small (less than 1 oz) plastic or metal ant and roach traps such as the Raid Roach Controller and Black Flag Ant Control System. These traps contain small amounts of chlorpyrifos at 0.3 to 0.5% and represent little threat to a healthy medium-sized (15 kg) or larger dog. Toxicosis in smaller dogs would be unexpected, but exposed dogs should be observed for signs of OP toxicosis.

CLINICAL SIGNS

Signs associated with chlorpyrifos toxicosis in cats are generally related to the nervous, gastrointestinal, and respiratory systems. However, these signs are somewhat different from the classically expected "SLUDD" signs produced by other OP insecticides. Onset is not uncommonly delayed 1 to 5 days following topical exposure. Oral exposure, either from direct ingestion or by grooming, may result in a more rapid onset. The predominant neurologic signs are tremors, especially of the muscles of the back, neck, and top of the head; ataxia; and seizures. Prominent nonspecific signs of mental depression

and anorexia occur frequently and, with tremors, may persist for 2 to 4 weeks. Other nonspecific signs related to AChE inhibition within the central nervous system include changes in personality, hyperesthesia, and hyperactivity. The most commonly described gastrointestinal signs include salivation, diarrhea, and vomiting. Pulmonary effects are related to bronchiolar constriction and hypersecretion, producing tachypnea or dyspnea. This occurrence can be life-threatening, especially in stressed animals. Although commonly reported during OP toxicosis, miosis is an inconsistent finding in chlorpyrifos toxicosis and probably with many other OPs. Mydriasis and miosis were reported to the IAPIC with equal frequency in chlorpyrifos-poisoned cats, illustrating how widely variable miosis can be in OP toxicosis, and it should *not* be relied on for diagnosis or monitoring the efficacy of treatment.

Experimentally, chlorpyrifos has been reported to produce delayed neuropathy in cats after intramuscular exposure. This is an infrequently observed syndrome associated with some OP compounds. The time to onset of hindlimb ataxia in the cats following chlorpyrifos exposure was approximately 19 days and was characterized by hindlimb hypermetria, waddling gait, and conscious proprioceptive deficits such as knuckling over.

DIAGNOSIS

The diagnosis of chlorpyrifos toxicosis is similar to that of other OP insecticide toxicoses. A history of exposure to a sufficient amount of the compound coupled with compatible clinical signs can serve as the basis for a tentative diagnosis of chlorpyrifos toxicosis. Further support in live animals is a marked reduction in whole blood or red blood cell ChE activity. Cats have low levels of red blood cell ChE activity, and feline plasma ChE is extremely sensitive to inhibition by OP insecticides. Clinically normal-appearing cats frequently have extremely low whole blood and plasma ChE activity after being exposed to an OP insecticide. Therefore, low whole blood or plasma ChE activity in an affected cat only verifies exposure and not necessarily toxicosis. In addition, extremely low ChE activity in an affected cat should not be given undue prognostic value, because many cats recover with appropriate treatment despite having almost total whole blood and plasma ChE inhibition.

At postmortem examination, brain tissue should be submitted for ChE activity. This is the most definitive diagnostic measure available for lethal OP toxicosis. Analysis of tissue for chlorpyrifos can be performed by many diagnostic laboratories but may be unrewarding because of relatively rapid metabolism and difficulty in interpreting the significance of tissue concentrations found. Chlorpyrifos is very lipophilic and may persist in adipose tissue. Chlorpyrifos has been identified in high concentrations in skin and subcutaneous tissue from a cat that died after topical chlorpyrifos exposure. Identification of chlorpyrifos in stomach or intestinal contents may also help to establish a diagnosis.

TREATMENT

Treatment of cats for chlorpyrifos toxicosis can be demanding and time-consuming. Animals are frequently not presented for treatment until 2 to 5 days after exposure. Redistribution of chlorpyrifos to adipose tissue, particularly subcutaneous fat following topical exposure, may create a depot that could slowly release insecticide, resulting in continued exposure. Treatment may therefore need to be continued for days to weeks, even when it is initiated within a few hours after exposure. In clinically affected animals, treatment with atropine or atropine and pralidoxime chloride before procedures such as bathing or feeding decreases the stress involved and may prevent triggering a respiratory crisis or seizures.

ATROPINE. Atropine sulfate (0.2 mg/kg) as needed is especially important to alleviate respiratory distress and occasional bradycardia. This dose is a guideline, and the amount required may vary with an animal's response. The initial dose should be divided, with one quarter given intravenously and the remainder given intramuscularly or subcutaneously. Atropine should be readministered as needed; however, it should not be given in excess. Long-term treatment with atropine may be necessary, and the lowest effective dose should be sought. Possible adverse signs associated with overatropinization include gut stasis, tachycardia, delirium, and hyperthermia. When considering the use of atropine, it should be remembered that animals do not die of constricted pupils or hypersalivation. Therefore, atropine therapy is used to control life-threatening signs such as dyspnea related to respiratory paralysis, bronchial hypersecretion, bronchospasms, or bradycardia. Atropine should not be given as a "reflex response" to all animals with an OP exposure. Atropine will not relieve nicotinic signs (tremors).

ENZYME REACTIVATORS. Pralidoxime chloride (Protopam chloride or 2-PAM chloride, Wyeth-Ayerst Laboratories, Philadelphia, PA 19101), 20 mg/kg every 12 hr, should be administered to relieve nicotinic signs such as tremors. The initial dose may be administered intramuscularly or slowly intravenously. Subsequent doses may be given intramuscularly or subcutaneously. Many OP insecticides, including chlorpyrifos, have a chemical structure that allows them to "age" once they are bound to the cholinesterase enzyme. Aging renders enzyme reactivators such as 2-PAM ineffective. Despite this potential limitation, 2-PAM therapy is still indicated, even if clinical signs have been present for an extended time. 2-PAM therapy should be continued until the animal is asymptomatic or discontinued if no improvement is seen after 24 to 36 hr following initiation of treatment. I have maintained cats on a once- or twice-a-day combined regimen of atropine and 2-PAM for up to 4 weeks in treating the persistent tremors associated with acute feline chlorpyrifos toxicosis.

SEIZURE CONTROL. If present, seizures should be controlled with diazepam (Valium, Hoffmann–LaRoche Inc., Nutley, NJ 07110), 2.5 to 5.0 mg/kg IV as needed. A barbiturate such as phenobarbital (6 mg/kg IV as needed) may be necessary.

TOPICAL EXPOSURE. Bathe topically exposed animals with a mild noninsecticidal shampoo or soap and water.

ACTIVATED CHARCOAL. If significant oral exposure is suspected, induce emesis and administer activated charcoal (0.5 to 1.0 gm/kg) with a saline or osmotic cathartic as soon as possible. Orally administered activated charcoal may help in some cases of topical exposures to some insecticides. The efficacy of oral activated charcoal after topical chlorpyrifos exposure has not been shown. Do not use a cathartic if diarrhea is present.

SUPPORTIVE CARE. Although listed last, supportive care may be the *most important* component of treatment for chlorpyrifos-poisoned cats. Cats should be monitored for hypo- and hyperthermia and treated accordingly. Cats frequently become hypokalemic during chlorpyrifos toxicosis, necessitating oral or parenteral potassium supplementation. Affected animals frequently have prolonged anorexia and mental depression requiring parenteral fluid, electrolyte, and nutritional support for days to weeks. Oral nutritional support may involve hand-feeding, tube-feeding, and even use of pharyngotomy tubes. However, with aggressive nursing care, many cats exhibiting signs of chlorpyrifos toxicosis of several days duration may be expected to survive and recover. Do not expose the animal to another ChE inhibitor such as OP or carbamate insecticides until the animal is fully recovered. Full recovery of AChE activity after excessive exposures may require weeks. If an insecticide is necessary, use a pyrethrin, first applying a small test dose. If no signs appear, use the insecticide as sparingly as possible.

References and Suggested Reading

Fikes, J. D., and Gerken, D. F.: Chlorpyrifos toxicosis in cats [Comments on the paper by S. B. Hooser et al.: Am. J. Vet. Res. 49:1371, 1988]. Adv. Small Anim. Med. Surg. 1:4, 1989.
Discussions of therapy for chlorpyrifos toxicosis in cats.

Fikes, J. D.: Chlorpyrifos toxicosis in cats and cattle. National Animal Poison Information Network Report 1:2, 1988.
Review of the clinical signs, diagnosis, and therapy of chlorpyrifos toxicosis in cats.

Fikes, J. D.: Organophosphorus and carbamate insecticides. Vet. Clin. North Am. Small Anim. Pract. 20:353, 1990.
Review of the mechanism of action, clinical signs, noncholinergic effects, diagnosis, and treatment of OP insecticide toxicosis in small animals.

Fikes, J. D., Zachary, J. F., Parker, A. J., et al.: Delayed neuropathy induced by chlorpyrifos: Studies in the cat. The Toxicologist 9:75, 1989.
Abstract describing experimental chlorpyrifos-induced delayed neuropathy in cats.

Hooser, S. B., Beasley, V. R., Sundberg, J. P., et al.: Toxicologic evaluation of chlorpyrifos in cats. Am. J. Vet. Res. 49:1371, 1988.
Toxicity data, clinical signs, and effects on cholinesterase activity, hematology, and serum biochemical values in cats following oral exposure to chlorpyrifos.

Jaggy, A., and Oliver, J. E.: Chlorpyrifos toxicosis in two cats. J. Vet. Intern. Med. 4:135, 1990.
Case reports of acute chlorpyrifos in cats with discussion of electrophysiologic alterations observed.

Meerdink, G. L.: Organophosphorus and carbamate insecticide poisoning. In Kirk, R. W. (ed.): Current Veterinary Therapy X. Philadelphia: W. B. Saunders, 1989, p. 135.
Review of the mechanism of action, clinical signs, diagnosis, and treatment of OP toxicosis.

Trammel, H. L., Dorman, D. C., Beasley, V. R., et al.: Tenth Annual Report of the Illinois Animal Poison Information Center. Dubuque: Kendall/Hunt Publishing, 1990.
Summary of clinical toxicologic assessments and clinical signs reported in association with inquiries concerning chlorpyrifos exposures.

IBUPROFEN

ANITA M. KORE
Urbana, Illinois

Ibuprofen is a nonsteroidal anti-inflammatory drug (NSAID) that has been available in an over-the-counter form in the United States since 1984. The National Animal Poison Control Center (NAPCC) has received 2260 calls concerning possible ibuprofen toxicity in dogs and cats since 1984, and ibuprofen has become the main generic drug generating calls to the NAPCC for both dogs and cats.

Ibuprofen is a propionic acid derivative within the carboxylic acid subcategory of NSAIDs. In human medicine, ibuprofen is used for the treatment of pain, dysmenorrhea, inflammation, and fever as well as other connective tissue, rheumatologic, and autoimmune diseases. Ibuprofen has a narrow margin of safety in dogs with repeated dosing and is therefore not commonly used therapeutically in veterinary medicine. Ibuprofen at 2.5 mg/kg PO every 12 hr has been used to reduce pain and inflammation in dogs, but 8 mg/kg PO every 24 hr for 30 days is likely to produce gastrointestinal irritation and hemorrhage (Conlon, 1988). The safety and efficacy of ibuprofen use in cats have not been established.

The most common form of ibuprofen is available without prescription as 200-mg tablets under a number of proprietary names (Advil, Whitehall; Medipren, McNeil; Midol, Upjohn; Motrin IB, Upjohn; Nuprin, Bristol-Myers; Pamprin IB, Chattem). Other over-the-counter forms available include a liquid suspension containing 100 mg ibuprofen per 5 ml (Advil Children's, Whitehall; Pediaprofen, McNeil) and a combination caplet containing 200 mg ibuprofen with 30 mg pseudoephedrine hydrochloride (CoAdvil Caplets, Whitehall). Ibuprofen tablets are also available in prescription strengths of 300, 400, 600, and 800 mg (Motrin, Upjohn; Rufen, Boots). New combinations and formulations of over-the-counter medications containing ibuprofen are likely to be introduced in the next few years.

Based on the calls received by the NAPCC, 46% of the cases displayed clinical signs consistent with ibuprofen toxicosis, 44% were asymptomatic at the time of the call, and 10% of the cases were classified as doubtful toxicoses or were informational calls about the use of ibuprofen in animals. Dogs ingesting ibuprofen constituted 80% of the call volume for ibuprofen, whereas cat exposures to ibuprofen contributed 17% of the calls. Accidental exposure to ibuprofen accounted for 83% of the calls, and administration by the animal's owner accounted for 10% of the calls.

MECHANISM OF ACTION

Ibuprofen possesses similar pharmacologic actions to other NSAIDs, although the exact mechanism of action for ibuprofen is not known. Ibuprofen is a reversible competitive inhibitor of the enzyme cyclo-oxygenase (prostaglandin synthetase), which blocks prostaglandin production, and thus diminishes the effects of prostaglandins. The anti-inflammatory and analgesic effects are thought to be due to the inhibition of synthesis or release of local prostaglandin mediators of inflammation. The antipyretic effect is postulated to be due to inhibition of prostaglandin synthesis in the hypothalamus, with heat dissipation increasing as a result of vasodilation and increased peripheral blood flow (see *CVT X*, p. 47).

Ibuprofen shares not only many therapeutic anti-inflammatory, antipyretic, and analgesic effects with other NSAIDs but also several adverse effects (see *CVT X*, p. 47). Gastrointestinal toxicity is thought to result from the inhibition of gastric prostaglandin synthesis. Prostaglandins are normally cytoprotective in the gastrointestinal tract by decreasing acid production, stimulating mucus and bicarbonate secretion by epithelial cells, and producing vasodilation in the gastric mucosa. Renal toxicity is postulated to result from inhibition of renal prostaglandin synthesis. Renal prostaglandins regulate renal blood flow, glomerular filtration rate, tubular ion transport, modulation of renin release, and water metabolism.

ABSORPTION, DISTRIBUTION, METABOLISM, AND EXCRETION

At pharmacologic doses in humans, ibuprofen is approximately 80% absorbed from the gastrointestinal tract, with peak plasma ibuprofen concentrations occurring 1 to 2 hr after ingestion. The presence of food in the stomach decreases the rate of absorption of ibuprofen and lowers the peak plasma concentration, although the extent of absorption is not affected. Ibuprofen is oxidized to two inactive metabolites by mixed-function oxidase enzymes in the liver. Excretion is mainly renal by glomerular filtration and tubular secretion of metabolites and glucuronide conjugates, with 50 to 60% of an oral dose being excreted within 24 hr. Less than 10% of an oral dose is excreted unchanged. Some biliary elimination of conjugates occurs. Ibuprofen is highly protein-bound (>90%), with the unbound drug being biologically active (McEvoy, 1990).

The pharmacokinetics and pharmacodynamics of ibuprofen at pharmacologic or toxic doses have not been determined in cats, and only limited information about dogs is available. In dogs, the plasma elimination half-life of ibuprofen at pharmacologic doses has been reported to be 2.5 hr. Compared with humans and rats, dogs are thought to be more predisposed to the toxic effects of NSAIDs because of their higher gastrointestinal absorption rates, their longer half-lives in dogs, and more prolonged high plasma drug concentrations (Spyridakis et al., 1986). Cats are thought to be more sensitive than dogs to the toxic effects of most NSAIDs, although the effects of ibuprofen have not been specifically studied in cats. Repeated doses of ibuprofen in both dogs and cats have been associated with more severe toxicoses than single acute exposures.

CLINICAL SIGNS

The clinical signs and course of ibuprofen toxicosis in dogs and cats vary with the dose of ibuprofen ingested, whether repeated doses of ibuprofen were administered, the age of the animal, the presence of concurrent medications or medical conditions, and many other factors. The most common clinical signs of ibuprofen toxicosis reported to the NAPCC include vomiting, depression, anorexia, diarrhea, and ataxia.

Based on the calls received by the NAPCC, dogs ingesting single ibuprofen doses less than 100 mg/kg and cats ingesting less than 50 mg/kg generally remain asymptomatic. Repeated doses of ibuprofen in both dogs and cats increase the likelihood of development of clinical signs. Other conditions that predispose animals to the development of clinical signs of toxicity to ibuprofen include pre-existing gastrointestinal disease, pre-existing renal disease or renal insufficiency, concurrent treatment with other NSAIDs, and general debilitation.

Acute ingestions of ibuprofen in excess of 100 mg/kg in dogs and greater than 50 mg/kg in cats have resulted in clinical signs of gastrointestinal irritation and hemorrhage. The onset of gastrointestinal upset is generally within the first 2 to 6 hr after ingestion, with the onset of gastrointestinal hemorrhage and ulceration occurring 12 hr to 4 days after ingestion. Common clinical signs of ibuprofen gastrointestinal toxicity include prolonged vomiting, anorexia, mild depression, hematemesis, and melena.

Acute ingestions of ibuprofen at doses greater than 300 mg/kg in both dogs and cats have resulted in clinical signs of acute renal failure in addition to gastrointestinal toxicosis. The onset of renal failure often occurs within the first 12 hr after a massive exposure to ibuprofen but may be delayed 3 to 5 days after exposure to ibuprofen at doses of approximately 300 mg/kg. Ibuprofen-induced acute renal failure is characterized by oliguria and azotemia initially, followed by either an oliguric or nonoliguric course.

Deaths of dogs and cats have been reported to the NAPCC after ingestions of greater than 600 mg/kg. Clinical signs in animals ingesting more than 600 mg/kg include severe depression, coma, seizures, metabolic acidosis, respiratory depression, and death. Clinical signs of gastrointestinal and renal toxicity are also present, and the time to onset of these clinical signs is usually shortened with increasing ibuprofen doses.

MANAGEMENT

Acute ingestion of massive amounts of ibuprofen is a commonly encountered problem in small animal practice. Management of acute ibuprofen poisoning involves detoxification measures in addition to supportive and symptomatic care.

Gastric emptying procedures may be of benefit if instituted soon after the ingestion. Induction of emesis should be followed by administration of activated charcoal and a saline cathartic. Ibuprofen tablets or capsules may occasionally form concretions in the gastrointestinal tract, causing slowed but very prolonged absorption. Adsorbents, cathartics, or lavage procedures consequently are sometimes of value even several hours after exposure (see this volume, p. 173, and *CVT X*, p. 116).

Symptomatic and supportive care is very important in cases of ibuprofen intoxication. Dogs consuming ibuprofen at doses in excess of 100 mg/kg and cats consuming ibuprofen at doses greater than 50 mg/kg should be monitored for the development of gastrointestinal irritation, ulceration, hemorrhage, or perforation. Gastrointestinal irritation, ulceration, and hemorrhage can be treated with antagonists of H_2 receptors such as cimetidine (Tagamet, SmithKline Beckman) and ranitidine (Zantac, Glaxo). Typical dosages for cimetidine are 5 to 10 mg/kg IV or PO every 6 to 12 hr in dogs and 5 mg/kg every 6 to 12 hr IV or PO in cats. Dosages for ranitidine are 2.2 to 4.4 mg/kg PO every 12 hr in dogs and 0.5 mg/kg IV or PO every 12 hr in cats. Sucralfate (Carafate, Marion) is also effective as a treatment for the gastropathy associated with ibuprofen. Dosages for sucralfate are 1 gm PO every 8 hr in dogs and 40 mg/kg PO every 8 hr in cats. If prolonged vomiting occurs, treatment with metoclopramide (Reglan, Robins) may be helpful. Dosages for metoclopramide are 0.2 to 0.4 mg/kg PO or SC every 6 to 8 hr for both dogs and cats. Mild gastrointestinal irritation may be treated symptomatically with nonabsorbable antacids such as magnesium or aluminum hydroxide. Antacid formulations containing bismuth subsalicylate should be avoided because they may further aggravate the gastritis.

Appropriate fluid therapy is needed to reverse dehydration caused by vomiting and to protect the kidneys from damage. Electrolyte abnormalities should be monitored with the administration of appropriate therapy as indicated. Whole blood should be given if loss of blood is significant. The animal should be monitored for the possibility of gastrointestinal perforation and development of peritonitis. Additional supportive care includes feeding the animal a high-quality, easily digestible diet frequently in small portions.

In general, acute renal failure resulting from NSAID administration has been considered reversible. Renal function should be monitored closely in animals consuming ibuprofen doses greater than 300 mg/kg. Correction of any dehydration secondary to gastrointestinal upset and maintenance fluid needs should be met using 0.45% saline and 2.5% dextrose IV. The animal's urine output should be monitored closely and fluid volumes adjusted accordingly to prevent the development of overhydration. The use of intravenous infusions of dopamine (Intropin, Du Pont Critical Care) at a dosage of 1 to 3 μg/kg/min or lower or dobutamine (Dobutrex, Lilly), at an initial dosage of 2.5 μg/kg/min may increase renal perfusion and minimize the degree of renal insufficiency. The animal should be monitored for the development of metabolic acidosis and hyperkalemia secondary to acute renal failure and corrections in the fluid therapy instituted as indicated. Peritoneal dialysis may be necessary if unresponsive oliguric or anuric renal failure has developed (see *CVT X*, p. 126).

Animals may occasionally develop seizures after ingesting large quantities of ibuprofen, and the use of diazepam (Valium, LaRoche) at doses of 0.5 to 1.5 mg/kg IV to abolish seizure activity is indicated. Mechanical ventilation is necessary in severely poisoned animals that develop respiratory depression.

Ibuprofen is highly protein-bound and extensively metabolized, and therefore forced alkaline diuresis, dialysis, or hemoperfusion is unlikely to enhance elimination of the drug. Since many of the NSAIDs undergo enterohepatic recirculation, repeated doses of activated charcoal may reduce the elimination half-life of ibuprofen.

References and Suggested Reading

Bailey, E. M.: Emergency and general treatment of poisonings. *In* Kirk, R. W. (ed.): *Current Veterinary Therapy X*. Philadelphia: W. B. Saunders, 1989, p. 116.
A review of decontamination and treatment procedures for animal toxicoses.

Conlon, P. D.: Nonsteroidal drugs used in the treatment of inflammation. Vet. Clin. North Am. Small Anim. Pract. 18:1115, 1988.
A review of the therapeutic uses of NSAIDs in veterinary medicine.

Grauer, G. F.: Toxicant-induced acute renal failure. *In* Kirk, R. W. (ed.): *Current Veterinary Therapy X*. Philadelphia: W. B. Saunders, 1989, p. 126.
A review of the mechanisms and management of toxicant-induced acute renal damage.

Kore, A. M.: Toxicology of nonsteroidal anti-inflammatory drugs. Vet. Clin. North Am. Small Anim. Pract. 20:419, 1990.
A review of the toxicity and mechanisms of action of NSAIDs and the management of NSAID poisonings.

McEvoy, G. K. (ed.): *AHFS Drug Information*. Bethesda, MD: American Society of Hospital Pharmacists, 1990, p. 1020.
A monograph of the pharmacology of ibuprofen in humans.

Rubin, S. I., and Papich, M. G.: Nonsteroidal anti-inflammatory drugs. *In* Kirk, R. W. (ed.): *Current Veterinary Therapy X*. Philadelphia: W. B. Saunders, 1989, p. 47.
A review of the pharmacology of nonsteroidal anti-inflammatory drugs.

Spyridakis, L. K., Bacia, J. J., Barsanti, J. A., et al.: Ibuprofen toxicosis in a dog. J.A.V.M.A. 188:918, 1986.
A case report of ibuprofen toxicosis in a dog.

Vale, J. A., and Meredith, T. J.: Acute poisoning due to non-steroidal anti-inflammatory drugs: Clinical features and management. Med. Toxicol. 1:12, 1986.
A review of NSAID poisonings and its clinical management in humans.

XYLAZINE REVERSAL WITH YOHIMBINE

JOSEPH W. DENHART

Shenandoah, Iowa

Xylazine (AnaSed, Lloyd Laboratories; Rompun, Mobay Corporation) is an alpha-2 agonist that, when injected into animals, stimulates centrally located alpha-2 adrenoceptors. It is used extensively in veterinary medicine as a sedative and an analgesic agent, as a restraining drug, or as a preanesthetic. Its action has resulted in xylazine's being used before many diagnostic and minor surgical procedures in dogs and cats. Xylazine affords good muscle relaxation, and this effect, along with the profound central nervous system depression it causes, usually results in recumbency. Its frequent side effects, other than the expected central nervous system (CNS) depression, involve the cardiovascular and respiratory systems. Bradycardia, initial hypertension followed by hypotension, cardiac arrhythmias, second-degree heart block, and respiratory depression are commonly associated with xylazine use in dogs, cats, and other animals. The hypotension, along with decreased cardiac contractility, cardiac output, and heart rate, may persist beyond the sedative period.

The development of a reversing agent that counteracts or antagonizes the effects of xylazine has made its use safer for the animal and more convenient for veterinary practitioners and for pet owners. Reversal with yohimbine (Yobine, Lloyd Laboratories) may expedite recovery and ambulation after the administration of xylazine for minor surgeries, wound repair, ear or teeth cleaning, biopsy, or diagnostic procedures such as radiography. The recumbency that occurs with xylazine may be reversed after a procedure is completed. The ability to return an animal that is alert with good motor control soon after a procedure is concluded can be an advantage to a busy practice and is appreciated by the client. Xylazine is frequently used as a preanesthetic agent for many general anesthesia procedures. If the level of general anesthesia becomes too deep, reversal of the xylazine portion of the anesthesia helps reduce the depth and duration of the sedation and effectively reduces the chances of anesthesia-related complications. The CNS depressant and other dose-dependent pharmacologic effects of xylazine, as well as patient hyperreactivity to xylazine, may be mitigated by a reversing agent.

PHARMACOLOGY

Yohimbine is a specific antidote for xylazine in instances of overdosing or in dogs that are hyperreactive to xylazine. An alpha-2 adrenergic receptor antagonist, yohimbine readily penetrates the blood-brain barrier and competitively blocks and displaces xylazine from the receptor sites, thereby antagonizing the effects of xylazine on the central nervous, cardiovascular, and respiratory systems. Yohimbine has many advantages as a reversal agent. There is little or no residual sedation or ataxia after its use as a reversing agent. Yohimbine rapidly reverses the duration and depth of xylazine-induced CNS depression. It effectively antagonizes the hypertension, hypotension, and bradycardia caused by xylazine. Thus, yohimbine is an excellent antidote for an overdose of xylazine. Yohimbine itself does not affect gastrointestinal motility, but it does prevent the prolonged gastrointestinal transit time effects caused by xylazine.

Description

Yohimbine is a botanical drug found in the *Corynanthe johimbe* K. Schum, Rubiaceae, and related trees. It is also found in the *Rauwolfia serpentina* plant. It is classed as an indolealkylamine alkaloid. Yohimbine is extracted, purified, and converted to the hydrochloride for animal use.

Mechanism of Action

Yohimbine produces a complex pattern of responses in the CNS at doses lower than those required to produce peripheral alpha-adrenergic blockade. It acts primarily by blocking central alpha-2 adrenoceptors, preventing the effects of alpha-2 agonists such as xylazine. Yohimbine also blocks peripheral 5-hydroxytryptamine (5-HT) receptors. It has little direct effect on smooth muscle.

CLINICAL EFFICACY

After the normal recommended dose of xylazine and regardless of the route of xylazine administra-

194

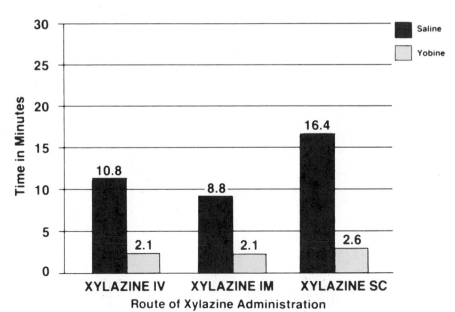

Figure 1. Mean arousal times after single intravenous doses of yohimbine (Yobine) in 187 xylazine-treated dogs. (Modified with permission from Yobine Technical Information Bulletin, 0789, Lloyd Laboratories, Shenandoah, IA.)

tion, a single intravenous dose of yohimbine significantly shortens the arousal time and time to walking in the dog. The reversal of the sedative effects of xylazine by yohimbine, as evidenced by dogs opening their eyes and lifting their heads in response to acoustic or touching stimuli, usually occurs within 1 to 3 min after injection of the reversal agent. A comparison of arousal times of yohimbine-treated dogs with the times in saline-injected controls after three different routes of xylazine injection is demonstrated in Figure 1. The average time it takes for a dog to be able to walk after yohimbine injection is usually 2 to 8 min. A comparison of the average walk times in 187 dogs given xylazine by three different routes and then injected with either yohimbine or sterile saline is illustrated in Figure 2.

Table 1 demonstrates the reduction from control values of the heart and respiratory rates by xylazine, and their subsequent increase after yohimbine administration. Analgesia, as determined by the animal's response to a needle prick, was measured on a scale of 1 to 3, 1 indicating no analgesia and 3 complete analgesia. The analgesia afforded by xylazine was not completely eliminated by yohimbine. This may be important clinically when some residual analgesia is preferred during the recovery period after a surgical procedure.

SAFETY AND SIDE EFFECTS

Because of yohimbine's action in the CNS, careful consideration should be given before it is administered to dogs with known or suspected CNS disorders. It should not be given to any animals that are epileptic or seizure prone. Rarely, a short-lasting seizure may occur following a high dose of yohim-

bine (five times the recommended dose). Occasionally a dog that has been given yohimbine becomes apprehensive and may appear confused. This is probably due to the rapid recovery from sedation and the CNS stimulation caused by the drug.

It should be emphasized that only the xylazine portion of an anesthetic regimen is reversed. If xylazine is used in combination with another anesthetic drug such as ketamine, following yohimbine reversal, the usual side effects that ketamine elicits in dogs may occur. The degree and extent of such side effects depend somewhat on the length of time that follows the initial injection of the ketamine: the longer the time span, the fewer are the ketamine-induced side effects. Rarely do any substantial side effects occur if a 30-min interval elapses between the ketamine injection and the yohimbine administration.

The safety of yohimbine use in pregnant bitches or in dogs intended for breeding purposes has not been determined.

No hematologic, serum biochemical, or urine measurements have been shown to be adversely affected by yohimbine injections.

DOSAGE AND ADMINISTRATION

The approved product contains 2 mg/ml yohimbine and is labeled to be used intravenously at the rate of 0.5 ml per 20 lb of body weight (0.11 mg/kg or 0.05 mg/lb) in dogs to reverse the sedative effects of xylazine. Although yohimbine is approved for use only in dogs, it has been used successfully in many other animals, including cats, birds, rabbits, chinchillas, and laboratory rats. Subcutaneous, intramuscular, and intraperitoneal routes result in more

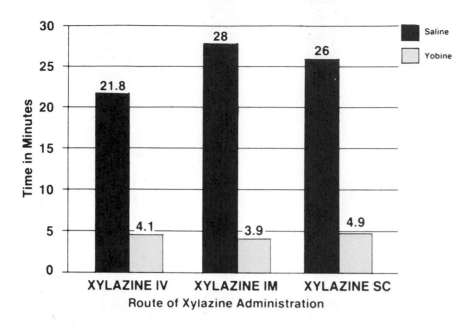

Figure 2. Mean walk times after single intravenous doses of yohimbine (Yobine) in 187 xylazine-treated dogs. (Modified with permission from Yobine Technical Information Bulletin, 0789, Lloyd Laboratories, Shenandoah, IA, 1989, p. 2.)

variation in response than that expected from the approved intravenous route. The pH of Yobine, the marketed product, is around 4.0, so some minor tissue irritation may be expected from extravascular routes of administration. The off-label use dose has varied considerably, depending on the species and the route of administration. The references and supplemental reading list should be consulted as an aid in determining dosage for a given species. Other than dogs, cats appear to be the animal in which yohimbine has been used most frequently in clinical practice. The dosage in cats appears to be the same as that in dogs (0.11 mg/kg or 0.05 mg/lb), or slightly lower. The dosage and technique of xylazine reversal depend on the individual patient circumstance, the anesthetic regimen, and the preference of the veterinary practitioner. An easy rule of thumb that has been used is to give the same milliliter amount of yohimbine (2 mg/ml) as was given intravenously of xylazine (20 mg/ml). This is an appropriate rule for both dogs and cats.

OTHER USES

In addition to yohimbine's value as an antagonist to alpha-2 agonists such as xylazine, it has been shown to counteract the CNS depression and bradycardia associated with amitraz (Mitaban, Upjohn) use in dogs (Hsu and Hopper, 1986). Yohimbine should be considered for use as an antidote for amitraz overdose or when untoward side effects are observed after amitraz use.

References and Suggested Reading

Degernes, L. A., Kreeger, T. J., Mandsager R. E., and Redig, P. T.: Ketamine-xylazine anesthesia in red-tailed hawks with antagonism by yohimbine. J. Wildl. Dis. 24:322, 1988.

Freed, D., and Baker, B.: Antagonism of xylazine hydrochloride sedation in raptors by yohimbine hydrochloride. J. Wildl. Dis. 25:136, 1989.

Hargett, C. E., Jr., Record, J. W., Carrier, M., Jr., et al.: Reversal of ketamine-xylazine anesthesia in the chinchilla by yohimbine. Lab. Anim. 18:41, 1989.

Hatch, R. C., Kitzman, J. V., Zahner, J. M., and Clark, J. D.: Antagonism of xylazine sedation with yohimbine, 4-aminopyridine, and doxapram in dogs. Am. J. Vet. Res. 46:371, 1985.

Hatch, R. C., Wilson, R. C., Jernigan, A. D., et al.: Reversal of thiopental-induced anesthesia by 4-aminopyridine, yohimbine, and doxapram in dogs pretreated with xylazine or acepromazine. Am. J. Vet. Res. 46:1473, 1985.

Hsu, W. H.: Antagonism of xylazine-induced CNS depression by yohimbine in cats. Calif. Vet. 7:19, 1983.

Hsu, W. H.: Effect of yohimbine on xylazine-induced central nervous system depression in dogs. J.A.V.M.A. 182:698, 1983.

Hsu, W. H.: Xylazine-pentobarbital anesthesia in dogs and its antagonism by yohimbine. Am. J. Vet. Res. 46:852, 1985.

Hsu, W. H., Bellin, S. I., Dellmann, H. D., and Hanson, C. E.: Xylazine-ketamine–induced anesthesia in rats and its antagonism by yohimbine. J.A.V.M.A. 189:1040, 1986.

Hsu, W. H., and Hopper, D. L.: Effect of yohimbine on amitraz-induced CNS depression and bradycardia in dogs. J. Toxicol. Environ. Health 18:423, 1986.

Hsu, W. H., and Lu, Z. X.: Effect of yohimbine on xylazine-ketamine anesthesia in cats. J.A.V.M.A. 185:886, 1984.

Hsu, W. H., Lu, Z. X., and Hembrough, F. B.: Effect of xylazine on heart rate and arterial blood pressure in conscious dogs, as influenced by atropine, 4-aminopyridine, doxapram, and yohimbine. J.A.V.M.A. 186:153, 1985.

Hsu, W. H., and McNeel, S. V.: Effect of yohimbine on xylazine-induced prolongation of gastrointestinal transit in dogs. J.A.V.M.A. 183:297, 1983.

Hsu, W. H., and Schaffer, D. D.: Effects of topical application of amitraz

Table 1. Yohimbine (Yobine) Efficacy in Xylazine-Treated Dogs Combining All Clinical Trial Test Sites (Mean Values for 187 Dogs)*

Parameter	Control	Xylazine	Yohimbine
Heart rate	115.6	53.0	95.5
Respiration	69.2	17.8	32.1
Analgesia (prick test)	1.0	2.8	1.9

*Adapted from Yobine Technical Information Bulletin, 0789, Lloyd Laboratories, Shenandoah, IA, 1989, p. 2.

on plasma glucose and insulin concentrations in dogs. Am. J. Vet. Res. 49:130, 1988.

Jensen, W. A.: Yohimbine for treatment of xylazine overdosing in a cat. J.A.V.M.A. 187:627, 1985.

Jernigan, A. D., Wilson, R. C., Booth, N. H., et al.: Comparative pharmacokinetics of yohimbine in steers, horses and dogs. Can J. Vet. Res. 52:172, 1988.

Klein, L. V., and Klide, A. M.: Central alpha-2 adrengeric and benzodiazepine agonists and their antagonists. J. Zoo Wildl. Med. 20:138, 1989.

Kreeger, T. J., Faggessa, A. M., Seal, U. S., et al.: Cardiovascular and behavioral responses of gray wolves to ketamine-xylazine immobilization and antagonism by yohimbine. J. Wildl. Dis. 23:463, 1987.

Kreeger, T. J., Mandsager, R. E., Seal, U. S., et al.: Physiological response of gray wolves to butorphanol-xylazine immobilization and antagonism by naloxone and yohimbine. J. Wildl. Dis. 25:89, 1989.

Kreeger, T. J., and Seal, U. S.: Immobilization of coyotes with xylazine hydrochloride–ketamine hydrochloride and antagonism by yohimbine hydrochloride. J. Wildl. Dis. 22:604, 1986.

Kreeger, T. J., Seal, U. S., Callahan, M., and Beckel, M.: Use of xylazine sedation with yohimbine antagonism in captive gray wolves. J. Wildl. Dis. 24:688, 1988.

Lipman, N. S., Phillips, P. A., and Newcomer, C. E.: Reversal of ketamine/xylazine anesthesia in the rabbit with yohimbine. Lab. Anim. Sci. 37:474, 1987.

Teare, J. A.: Antagonism of xylazine hydrochloride–ketamine hydrochloride immobilization in guineafowl (*Numida meleagris*) by yohimbine hydrochloride. J. Wildl. Dis. 23:301, 1987.

ZINC TOXICOSIS

LANELL OGDEN

Tuskegee, Alabama

Zinc is widely distributed in the environment, being found in foodstuffs, water, air, and living organisms. Seafood, meats, whole grains, dairy products, and nuts are rich sources of zinc, but little is found in green vegetables and fruits (Goyer, 1991). Zinc is extensively used to galvanize other metals, like iron, to prevent corrosion. Zinc oxide is widely used in the manufacture of paints, rubber products, cosmetics, textiles, pharmaceuticals, batteries, electrical equipment, soap, and printing inks. Zinc is capable of replacing many bivalent metals such as manganese, magnesium, iron, nickel, cobalt, copper, and cadmium in certain salts. Zinc forms stable complexes with side-chains of proteins, a property that is relevant to its specific biologic functions (Weast, 1989).

More than 200 zinc-containing enzymes and proteins function in catalytic, regulatory, and structural roles. Zinc is a component of many important enzymes such as alcohol dehydrogenase, carbonic anhydrase, lactic dehydrogenase, alkaline phosphatase, DNA and RNA polymerases, superoxide dismutase, thymidine kinase, and carboxypeptidase (Abdel-Mageed and Oehme, 1990). Zinc also has an important role in the proper functioning of taste and smell receptors of the tongue and nasal passages (Burch and Sullivan, 1976; Hambidge et al., 1986).

PHARMACOLOGY

Intestinal absorption of zinc is thought to be homeostatically controlled and is probably carrier-mediated (Goyer, 1991). About 20 to 30% of ingested zinc is absorbed. Absorption is affected by the form of zinc salt and the presence of agents that alter absorption of zinc. High levels of calcium, copper, and phytate in the diet inhibit absorption of zinc (Anke and Groppel, 1987). In the blood, about two thirds of zinc is bound to albumin and the remainder is complexed with $beta_2$-macroglobulin (Goyer, 1991). Circulating zinc distributes to various tissues, with greatest accumulation in the pancreas, liver, kidneys, spleen, and male reproductive organs. The principal route of excretion is via the feces, and significant amounts are excreted in sweat (Hambidge et al., 1986).

INCIDENCE

Zinc toxicosis has been reported in several mammalian species including humans, ferrets, cattle, sheep, horses, cats, and dogs (Latimer et al., 1989). Industrial workers who inhale zinc oxide are subject to zinc fume fever, which causes a mild to severe pulmonary inflammatory response and accompanying fever. Human and animal intoxications have been traced to accidental ingestion of excessive zinc from food and beverages stored in galvanized containers (Murphy, 1970). Studies of chronic ingestion of excessive zinc in animals reported evidence of poor growth and anemia (Hambidge et al., 1986).

Seven cases of zinc poisoning among dogs have been reported since 1984. The ten affected dogs represented various breeds, ages ranged from 4 months to 8 years, and both males and females were involved. Ferrets (Straube and Walden, 1981) and aviary birds (Reece et al., 1986) have reportedly been poisoned after ingesting zinc from galvanized wire. Skin ointment, metallic hardware, and pennies were identified as the sources of zinc. Ingestion was the primary route of exposure.

SOURCES

Many topical protectants contain approximately 20% zinc oxide, which is generally applied one to three times daily for a few days (Booth, 1988). Dogs and cats often lick treated wounds, obtaining sufficient amounts of zinc to induce emesis. In one case, a dog may have consumed ¾ lb of zinc oxide–containing ointment during a 4-day period (Breitschwerdt et al., 1986).

Three animals consumed zinc-containing plumbing nuts and transport cage nuts that lodged in the pyloric region of the stomach (Breitschwerdt et al., 1986; Torrance and Fulton, 1987). Stomach acidity provides an environment conducive to leaching of zinc from metallic objects and continuous absorption by the intestinal mucosa.

Ingestion of copper-clad zinc pennies was the second most common cause of zinc toxicosis in dogs in one report. Composition of the penny changed between 1982 and 1983 from approximately 95% copper and 4% zinc to 97% zinc and 2.5% copper, and the weight also changed from approximately 3.1 to 2.5 gm (Latimer et al., 1989; Meerdink et al., 1986; Ogden et al., 1988).

Several sources of zinc are capable of causing untoward effects in animals. Ingestion of the zinc-containing white powder found on galvanized wire cages reportedly caused toxicosis in aviary birds (Reece et al., 1986), ferrets (Straube and Walden, 1981), and farm animals (Pritchard et al., 1985). Lotions, shampoos, and wound-healing agents that contain zinc are also potential sources.

MECHANISM OF TOXICOSIS

The exact mechanism of zinc toxicosis is not understood. The hematopoietic effect of zinc is generally attributed to its antagonistic effect on copper and iron. Zinc induces the synthesis of a copper ligand in the mucosal cells, sequestering copper from the nutrient medium and making it unavailable for serosal transfer. Zinc has successfully been used in the treatment of Wilson's disease and in pyrrolidine alkaloid–induced hepatotoxicity. Zinc exerts an irritant effect, which may account for the gastrointestinal actions of the mineral (Hambidge et al., 1986).

CLINICAL MANIFESTATIONS

Zinc intoxication primarily affects the gastrointestinal, hematologic, and urinary systems. Vomiting has been the most common and consistent sign among all reported cases. Other effects commonly noted were anorexia, lethargy, depression, diarrhea, abdominal pain, and gastroenteric distress. A persistent pica occurred in one dog that selectively ingested pennies from among other coins and frequently licked brass objects (Ogden et al., 1988). The occurrence of pica is consistent with the concept that zinc affects the sense of taste (Burch and Sullivan, 1976).

Zinc poisoning has been associated with moderate to severe hemolytic anemia as well as an inflammatory leukogram (Torrance and Fulton, 1987; Latimer et al., 1989; Breitschwerdt et al., 1986).

The urinary system and other organ systems may also be affected in poisoned dogs. Azotemia, renal tubular changes, isosthenuria, hypercreatinemia, hyperphosphatemia, granular urinary casts, bilirubinuria, icterus, and elevated serum alkaline phosphatase levels were also reported (Breitschwerdt et al., 1986; Latimer et al., 1989; Torrance and Fulton, 1987).

PATHOLOGY

Most dogs recover from zinc poisoning; however, three dogs died during or after removal of a zinc-containing object. A liver biopsy of one dog revealed centrilobular hepatocytic vacuolation and cloudy swelling that progressed to centrilobular necrosis 5 days later. Mild alveolar emphysema, renal tubular casts, and pancreatic fibrosis were found at necropsy (Meerdink et al., 1986). Lesions reported in other cases were hemorrhagic gastritis (Hornfeldt and Koepke, 1984), gastric ulcers, and pancreatic fibrosis (Meerdink et al., 1986).

TOXICOLOGY

The oral dose of zinc required to induce poisoning is dependent on several factors, including the degree of intestinal absorption, the form of zinc salt, and the pH of the environment. The blood zinc levels were markedly elevated in all three reported cases of zinc poisoning in which blood was analyzed (Table 1). It appears that zinc levels rapidly decreased after removal of the source (Breitschwerdt et al., 1986; Meerdink et al., 1987; Torrance and Fulton, 1987), and two dogs recovered after treatment. Liver and kidney levels of zinc were elevated in four dogs, ferrets, and pet birds that were poisoned, compared with control levels of unexposed animals. The liver copper level was depressed in

Table 1. Zinc Concentrations Associated With Toxicosis

Reference	Tissue Analyzed	Detected Level (ppm)	Effects
Latimer et al., 1989	Serum	28.8	GI, H, S
Torrance and Fulton, 1987	Serum	32	GI, H, R, S
Meerdink et al., 1986	Whole blood	45	GI, H, R, D
	Liver	238	
Ogden et al., 1988	Liver	130	GI, R, D
	Kidney	175	
Breitschwerdt et al., 1986	Liver	369	GI, H, D, O
	Kidney	295	

D, death; GI, gastrointestinal; H, hematologic; O, other complications existed; R, renal; S, survival.

one case (Ogden et al., 1988). Hypocupremia has been associated with chronic high doses of zinc in humans (Hambidge et al., 1986).

DIAGNOSIS

A tentative diagnosis of zinc poisoning can be made on the basis of a history of exposure to zinc-containing substances accompanied by clinical manifestations of zinc poisoning. The consistent findings among zinc-intoxicated dogs were vomiting and anemia; abnormalities of the kidneys and liver may also occur. The presence of foreign objects (e.g., nuts, coins) in the gastrointestinal tract may be confirmed by radiography. The mere presence of a foreign object in the intestinal tract does not imply an elevated level of zinc in tissues. Determination of blood, liver, kidney, or pancreatic zinc levels is necessary to confirm a clinical diagnosis of zinc poisoning (see Table 1). Normal zinc levels in canine serum and liver are 0.7 to 2.0 µg/ml and 30 to 70 µg/g (wet weight), respectively (Fisher, 1977; Ogden et al., 1988; Torrance and Fulton, 1987). Tissue levels of zinc and other possible minerals such as iron and copper should be determined to define zinc toxicosis and mineral interactions more clearly. In addition, the source of zinc should be analyzed. Avoid contamination of blood samples with extraneous zinc, which may be present in traditional syringes, rubber grommets, and Vacutainer tubes (Division of Becton Dickinson & Co., Rutherford, NJ 07070). It is recommended to use special tubes for elemental analysis (royal blue top) and syringes that contain no rubber grommets. Tissue samples can be stored in clean plastic bags and frozen until analyzed (Minnick et al., 1982). Immune-mediated hemolytic anemia can be differentiated from toxicosis by a negative result on the Coombs test and confirmation of elevated tissue zinc levels.

THERAPY

Treatment of zinc toxicosis involves removing the source of zinc from the animal and providing sup-portive therapy. When foreign objects are present in the gastrointestinal tract, a gastrotomy or enterotomy may be indicated if endoscopy or emesis is contraindicated or ineffective. Supportive therapy such as fluids and blood transfusion may be necessary if dehydration, severe anemia, or acute renal failure exists. Chelation therapy has not been thoroughly investigated; however, zinc has been shown to have a high affinity for edetate calcium disodium (Brownie and Aronson, 1984; Domingo et al., 1988) as used in lead toxicosis. Dimercaprol (BAL) has been used successfully in human medicine to treat zinc intoxication (Murphy, 1970). Neither of these treatments has been documented for zinc toxicosis in dogs.

References and Suggested Reading

Abdel-Mageed, A., and Oehme, F. W.: A review of the biochemical roles, toxicity and interactions of zinc, copper, and iron, Part I. Zinc. Vet. Hum. Toxicol. 32:34, 1990.

Anke, M., and Groppel, B.: Toxic actions of essential trace elements. *In* Bratter, P. (ed.): *Trace Element-Analytical Chemistry in Medicine and Biology.* New York: Walter de Gruyter, 1987.

Booth, N. H.: Topical agents. *In* Booth, N. H. (ed.): *Veterinary Pharmacology and Therapeutics*, 6th ed. Iowa: Iowa State University Press, 1988.

Breitschwerdt, E. B., Armstrong, P. J., Robinette, C. L., et al.: Three cases of acute zinc toxicosis in dogs. Vet. Hum. Toxicol. 28:109, 1986.

Brownie, C. F., and Aronson, A. L.: Comparative effects of Ca-ethylenediaminetetra-acetic acid (EDTA), ZnEDTA, and ZnCaEDTA in mobilizing lead. Toxicol. Appl. Pharmacol. 75:167, 1984.

Burch, R. E., and Sullivan, J. F.: Diagnosis of zinc, copper, and manganese abnormalities in man. Symposium on Trace Elements. Med. Clin. North Am. 60:655, 1976.

Domingo, J. L., Llobet, J. M., Paternain, J. N., et al.: Acute zinc intoxication: Comparison of the antidotal efficacy of several chelating agents. Vet. Hum. Toxicol. 30:224, 1988.

Fisher, G. L.: Effects of disease on serum copper and zinc values in the beagle. Am. J. Vet. Res. 38:936, 1977.

Goyer, R. A.: Toxic effects of metals. *In* Klaasen, C. D. (ed.): *Casarett and Doull's Toxicology: The Basic Science of Poisons*, 4th ed. New York: Macmillan, 1991, p. 623.

Graham, T. W., Holmberg, C. A., Keen, C. L., et al.: A pathologic and toxicologic evaluation of veal calves fed large amounts of zinc. Vet. Pathol. 25:484, 1988.

Hambidge, K. M., Casey, C. E., and Krebs, N. F.: Zinc. *In* Mertz, W. (ed.): *Trace Elements in Human and Animal Nutrition*, 5th ed. Vol. 2. Orlando: Academic Press, 1986.

Hornfeldt, C. S., and Koepke, T. E.: A case report of suspected toxicity in a dog. Vet. Hum. Toxicol. 26:214, 1984.

Latimer, K. S., Jain, A. V., Inglesby, H. B., et al.: Zinc-induced hemolytic anemia caused by ingestion of pennies by a pup. J.A.V.M.A. 195:77, 1989.

Minnick, P. D., Braselton, W. E., Meerdink, G. L., et al.: Altered serum element concentrations due to laboratory usage of Vacutainer tubes. Vet. Hum. Toxicol. 24:413, 1982.

Murphy, J.: Intoxication following ingestion of elemental zinc. J.A.M.A. 212:2119, 1970.

Meerdink, G., Reed, R., Perry, D., et al.: Zinc poisoning from the ingestion of pennies. Proceedings of the American Association of Veterinary Laboratory Diagnosticians 29:141, 1986.

Ogden, L., Edwards, W. C., and Nail, N. A.: Zinc intoxication in a dog from the ingestion of copper-clad zinc pennies. Vet. Hum. Toxicol. 30:577, 1988.

Palmer, N.: Possible acute zinc toxicity in a dog. Can. Vet. J. 28:281, 1987.

Pritchard, G. C., Lewis, G., Wells, A. H., et al.: Zinc toxicity, copper deficiency and anemia in swill-fed pigs. Vet. Rec. 117:545, 1985.

Reece, R. L., Dickson, D. B., and Burrowes, P. J.: Zinc toxicosis (new wire disease) in aviary birds. Aust. Vet. J. 63:199, 1986.

Straube, E. F., and Walden, N. B.: Zinc poisoning in ferrets *(Mustella putoris furo)*. Lab. Anim. 15:45, 1981.

Torrance, A. G., and Fulton, R. B.: Zinc-induced hemolytic anemia in a dog. J.A.V.M.A. 191:443, 1987.

Weast, R. C. (ed.): *CRC Handbook of Chemistry and Physics*, 70th ed. Boca Raton, FL: CRC Press, 1989–1990, p. B42.

Section

4

INFECTIOUS DISEASES

EDWARD B.
BREITSCHWERDT
Consulting Editor

CANINE AND FELINE VACCINES

TOM R. PHILLIPS
La Jolla, California

and RONALD D. SCHULTZ
Madison, Wisconsin

Vaccination is a common procedure. Virtually every puppy or kitten that enters a veterinary hospital receives an initial series of vaccinations that continue, in the form of "boosters," for the duration of the animal's life. It is a testament to the overall quality of our commercial vaccines that few directly observable detrimental effects occur from immunization. Thus, it is no wonder that vaccination is frequently believed to be an innocuous procedure. However, it is important to recognize that although vaccination is an important weapon in preventing infectious disease, immunization, like any therapeutic procedure, does have limitations and can cause adverse reactions. This article describes potential problems associated with immunization, as well as when, where, and what type of vaccine should be used in various situations.

MODIFIED LIVE VACCINES, KILLED VACCINES, AND SUBUNIT VACCINES

Three types of vaccines are currently used in veterinary medicine: modified live (attenuated), killed (inactivated), and subunit vaccines. In modified live vaccines, the microorganisms are altered in such a way that they are no longer virulent to the majority of the host species yet retain the antigenic properties that induce a protective immune response. Modified live vaccines may be given locally or parenterally. Local administration of certain modified live vaccines to the mucous membranes of the eyes, nose, and mouth produces not only a strong systemic immunity but also a local immune response. Local immunity is important when the point of entry of the microorganism and the target organ of the disease are the same (e.g., feline calicivirus). An effective local immune response requires a live replicating vaccine and usually cannot be produced by noninfectious vaccines (killed or subunit). Some live vaccines are not fully attenuated and may require inoculation by an unusual route to produce immunity without causing disease (e.g., feline rhinotracheitis via a parenteral route). Care must be taken when immunizing with this type of vaccine, because aerosolization or environmental contamination may expose susceptible animals, resulting in the development of a mild form of the disease. Modified live vaccines must replicate after inoculation to produce enough antigen to induce an immune response. Thus, any inactivation of a modified live vaccine before or immediately after inoculation will result in vaccine failure. Because modified live vaccines replicate in the host, they more closely resemble virulent viral infections and generally produce a stronger and more durable protective immune response than the noninfectious vaccines (killed and subunit). Modified live vaccines may also induce interferon in the first few days after immunization, providing additional early protection against some virulent viral infections. However, this "better" immune response has a cost: a decrease in vaccine safety. Certain modified live vaccines can induce immunosuppression, may be shed into the environment, and may revert to virulence or cause vaccine-induced disease. Thus, even though modified live vaccines generally provide a better immune response that more closely resembles the natural infection, they are not always the best vaccine on all occasions or for all animals.

Killed vaccines are safer than modified live vaccines because they cannot replicate and are unable to cause infectious diseases. However, to induce a protective immune response, killed vaccines require a large antigenic dose, multiple immunizations, and often the use of adjuvants. These factors substantially increase the cost of inactivated vaccines and the probability of local and systemic vaccine reactions. Also, killed vaccines generally produce weaker immune responses with a shorter duration than the immune response produced by modified live vaccines.

Subunit vaccines are not infectious. Thus, subunit vaccines and killed vaccines have some of the same advantages and disadvantages. However, instead of containing the complete microorganism as found in the modified live and killed vaccines, the subunit vaccine theoretically contains only the components of the microorganism that are necessary to produce a protective immune response. The risk of developing an allergic reaction to nonessential vaccine elements is thus reduced. At present, subunit vaccines are not frequently used in veterinary medicine because of their higher cost and lack of proven efficacy. However, with the advent of recombinant DNA technology and the recent improvements in adjuvants, effective subunit vaccines may become more common (see this volume, p. 457).

PROPER USE, STORAGE, AND ADMINISTRATION

All vaccines should be stored according to the manufacturer's recommendations. Lyophilized products should be used immediately after reconstitution and not stored for prolonged periods in the reconstituted form. Modified live vaccines are particularly sensitive to improper storage. This type of vaccine relies on vaccine virus replication to generate enough antigen to induce an immune response. Thus, improper storage conditions may result in the inactivation of modified live vaccines and thus cause vaccine failures. Although modified live vaccines are more sensitive to improper storage, exposing killed and subunit vaccines to excessive heat or light may also result in reduced immunogenicity. To ensure proper immunization, careful attention should be given to the vaccine storage conditions.

It is important that a new needle and syringe be used to administer each vaccine. Reused syringes and needles may contain contaminants that inactivate the vaccine or interfere with immunization. Vaccines should only be administered at the manufacturer's recommended concentration and reconstituted using the diluent provided with the vaccine. Vaccine products from the same or different manufacturers should never be mixed together in one syringe unless specified in the package insert. Vaccine components from different products may interfere with or inactivate each other, resulting in improper immunization.

Adherence to the recommended route of administration is essential. A rabies vaccine labeled "for intramuscular inoculation only" should not be given subcutaneously. For successful immunization to occur, many modified live rabies vaccines require a well-innervated tissue (i.e., muscle). Nerves serve as a target for rabies virus replication. Viral replication is necessary for the production of enough antigen to induce a protective immune response. Thus, inoculation into the subcutaneous connective tissue (low in nerve endings) often leads to vaccine failure unless the vaccine is specifically approved for subcutaneous inoculation.

It is important for veterinarians to follow vaccine recommendations not only to ensure successful immunization but also to limit their liability should an adverse reaction or vaccine failure occur.

MATERNAL ANTIBODY

One of the most common problems associated with vaccination is maternal antibody interference with active immunization. Maternal immunity, a form of passive immunity, has a vital role for neonates. It helps to protect neonates during the critical transition from the protected uterine environment of the fetus to the hostile external environment of the newborn. This transition occurs not only at a time when a neonate's immune system is not fully developed but also when a neonate's immune system is naive to virtually all pathogens. Without the acquisition of maternal immunity, a neonate's chances of survival are greatly reduced. However, maternal immunity is not without its negative effects. Maternal antibody interference with immunization is the most common cause of vaccine failure, particularly in weanling and postweanling animals. It is generally believed that when this interference occurs maternal antibody binds to the vaccine in such a way that the vaccine is cleared from the body before it is able to stimulate an immune response. Because maternal antibody is acquired exogenously and is not actively being replaced, it is gradually depleted as the animal matures.

Maternal antibody is degraded at a *constant* rate. Its retention time in the animal is largely dependent on the class and quantity of antibody acquired at birth. The level of maternal immunity obtained at or around the time of birth is dependent on a number of factors: the immune state of the dam, the amount of colostrum produced, the immunoglobulin (antibody) content of the colostrum, the amount of colostrum ingested and absorbed, and the age of the neonate at the time of ingestion. These factors can cause substantial variation in the amount of maternal antibody that is transferred to newborn animals, even among littermates.

Because of these factors, it is difficult to accurately predict the level of maternal antibody for a specific puppy or kitten at the time of immunization. It is possible to obtain a serum sample from a given animal and determine the level of maternal antibody to each pathogen. From this information, the most appropriate immunization time for each agent can be determined. However, the cost and time requirements of such determinations would be prohibitive. The most successful and cost-effective approach to immunizing animals with unknown amounts of maternal antibody is based on multiple vaccinations, with the last immunization occurring at approximately 22 weeks of age for a puppy and approximately 16 weeks of age for a kitten.

By the time an animal reaches these ages, the vast majority (>95%) of animals no longer have levels of maternal antibody sufficient to interfere with active immunization. It is important to note that many of the previous puppy immunization schedules recommend that the last immunization in the series occur at 12 to 16 weeks of age. New information on maternal antibody to canine parvovirus demonstrates the need to extend the last immunization in the series to 20 to 22 weeks of age, so a greater percentage of puppies can be effectively immunized. As many as 20% of dogs at 18 weeks of age have enough maternal antibody to prevent successful canine parvovirus (CPV) immunization. Thus, it is important to recognize that unless the last immunization is given at 22 weeks of age or later that a certain percentage of the animals will remain unprotected until the next immunization, probably at the yearly booster vaccination. It is possible that under certain conditions, the level of maternal antibody at 20 weeks of age for a puppy and 14 weeks of age for a kitten may also interfere with the immunization of other canine and feline pathogens. Thus, for this reason, we recommend that the last immunization of the initial vaccination series occur at 22 weeks of age for puppies and 16 weeks of age for kittens. Various immunization programs have recommended initial vaccination ages of 6, 8, or 9 weeks with repeat immunizations at 2-, 3-, 4-, or 6-week intervals. The program that is correct for your practice largely depends on your philosophy and the incidence of disease within your community. Certainly, the more vaccinations an animal receives, within reason, the more likely it will become actively immunized at the earliest possible age and the less likely it will be susceptible when exposed to virulent agents. However, one must weigh the possible risk of infection versus the cost to the client and possible risks to the patient. We believe that a reasonable compromise for puppies would be three to four immunizations given at regular intervals between the ages of 6 and 22 weeks and for kittens two to three immunizations given at regular intervals between the ages of 6 and 16 weeks. Veterinarians frequently blame a vaccine failure on a "bad vaccine." However, it is more likely that the vast majority of vaccine failures, between the ages of 4 months and 1 year, occur as the result of giving the last vaccination when the maternal antibody levels are sufficient to prevent active immunization.

A substantial problem, especially for CPV, is that virulent virus is able to infect and cause severe disease in animals with levels of maternal antibody that prevent active immunization. There is a 2- to 5-week window of vulnerability when an animal can be infected with virulent virus but cannot be successfully immunized. This is of particular concern in some breeding kennels where the level of environmental contamination with CPV is so high that virtually every puppy born within the kennel contracts CPV disease before it can be successfully immunized. In kennels with this problem, the best solution, although often difficult to implement, is to totally remove the puppies from the kennel at 4 to 6 weeks of age and not allow them to return until they have completed their full immunization program, at approximately 6 months. It is important that these isolated puppies not have direct or indirect contact with persons or equipment from the contaminated kennel until their immunization program is complete, because CPV is very stable and can persist on fomites for weeks.

Maternal antibody interference with canine distemper virus (CDV) immunization is overcome by a unique approach: the development of heterotypic immunity. Heterotypic immunity is the production of an immune response to one microorganism by immunizing with a different but antigenically related microorganism. Measles virus (MV) is antigenically related to CDV. When MV is inoculated into a puppy with moderate levels of CDV maternal antibody, an immune response is produced that protects the puppy from CDV disease. It is important to realize, when considering the use of MV, that high levels of CDV maternal antibody will also prevent immunization with MV. For this reason, it is not advisable to vaccinate with MV before 6 weeks of age. MV vaccination should be given only once early in the immunization schedule. Multiple immunizations given to older animals may result in high MV maternal antibody titers, which will limit the effectiveness of MV as a heterotypic vaccine for the next generation. MV may be given alone or in combination with CDV vaccine. However, MV is more effective when inoculated alone. Another important and poorly understood aspect of MV vaccine is that MV should always be given *intramuscularly*.

MV vaccination does not prevent infection with CDV but does prevent the development of clinical CDV disease. This is accomplished by MV vaccination inducing a cross-reactive T-helper immunity to CDV. When MV-vaccinated dogs are exposed to CDV, through vaccination or virulent virus, they produce a rapid anamnestic antibody response to CDV. It is this rapid antibody response that prevents clinical CDV disease from developing.

VACCINATION AND IMMUNOSUPPRESSION

We recently reported that certain polyvalent vaccines cause immunosuppression, as measured by a significant decrease in an *in vitro* immune function assay, the lymphocyte blastogenesis test (Phillips et al., 1989). When the individual components of the immunosuppressive polyvalent vaccines were inoculated alone into dogs, the immunosuppression did not occur, leading us to believe that the suppression was caused by an interaction between two or more components of the vaccine. We were able to reproduce the suppression of the polyvalent vaccine by combined inoculations of the CDV component and the canine adenovirus type 1 (CAV-1) or canine adenovirus type 2 (CAV-2) components from various immunosuppressive polyvalent vaccines.

Although the degree of suppression induced by some of the polyvalent vaccines was significant (>80% suppression), it was transitory, persisting for 7 to 10 days. Generally, for immunosuppression to be clinically apparent, it must persist for weeks or months. Thus, vaccination by itself is unlikely to cause detectable adverse effects in an animal. However, under unusual circumstances, even this relatively short duration of lymphocyte suppression may become clinically important, especially if an animal is already in a partially immunosuppressed condition (e.g., nutritional deficiency). Also, it is possible that vaccine-induced immunosuppression may potentiate the severity of a concurrent disease or allow an inapparent infection to become evident.

It is important that results of our study not be misinterpreted. Our results do not suggest that polyvalent vaccines should not be used. All vaccines must be demonstrated safe and efficacious to be licensed. Polyvalent vaccines are efficacious and convenient for both veterinarians and clients. However, vaccination should not be viewed as an innocuous procedure and should be performed in accordance with a manufacturer's recommendations: that is, only *healthy, clinically normal* animals should be vaccinated. It should also be understood that adverse reactions can and will occur regardless of the type of vaccine used.

POLYVALENT VS. MONOVALENT VACCINES

Concern has been expressed about the frequent use of polyvalent vaccines in veterinary medicine. This concern primarily deals with the presumed problems of vaccine interference and antigen overload. Antigen overload occurs when the amount of antigen exceeds the ability of the immune system to respond, and vaccine interference occurs when the inoculation of one vaccine prevents the immune response to another vaccine. There is no scientific evidence that either problem occurs with the currently available canine or feline vaccines. However, as discussed earlier, some polyvalent vaccines have been shown to cause transitory immunosuppression and should be avoided when there is a high potential for concurrent immunosuppression. With monovalent vaccines, concerns about antigen overload, vaccine interference, and vaccine-induced immunosuppression are alleviated but at the expense of convenience and cost.

IMMUNIZATION OF HOSPITALIZED PATIENTS

All animals entering the hospital for elective procedures, boarding, or grooming should have a current vaccination history. If not, they should be immunized at least 10 days before admission. However, an acutely ill patient that requires immediate hospitalization but does not have a vaccination history, in most cases, should *not* be vaccinated for the following reasons: (1) vaccination is not likely to be effective until at least 3 to 7 days after immunization, (2) the immunosuppression of certain polyvalent vaccines may contribute to the current admitting illness, and (3) if the admitting illness has an immunosuppressive component, vaccination may not result in effective immunization or, worse, may result in postvaccinal disease (i.e., postvaccinal distemper encephalitis). Furthermore, if the animal has previously been immunized, it is likely that protective immunity remains. An exception to the foregoing counsel would be an outbreak of a new epizootic disease. In an epizootic outbreak, an acutely ill animal without a vaccination history should be immunized against the agent causing the disease, because the chances of exposure are greatly increased.

ANNUAL VACCINATIONS

A practice that was started many years ago and that lacks scientific validity or verification is annual revaccinations. Almost without exception there is no immunologic requirement for annual revaccination. Immunity to viruses persists for years or for the life of the animal. Successful vaccination to most bacterial pathogens produces an immunologic memory that remains for years, allowing an animal to develop a protective anamnestic (secondary) response when exposed to virulent organisms. Only the immune response to toxins requires boosters (e.g., tetanus toxin booster, in humans, is recommended once every 7 to 10 years), and no toxin vaccines are currently used for dogs or cats. Furthermore, revaccination with most viral vaccines fails to stimulate an anamnestic (secondary) response as a result of interference by existing antibody (similar to maternal antibody interference). The practice of annual vaccination in our opinion should be considered of questionable efficacy unless it is used as a mechanism to provide an annual physical examination or is required by law (i.e., certain states require annual revaccination for rabies).

IMMUNIZATION OF ANIMALS ON CORTICOSTEROIDS

The common use of glucocorticosteroids for various chronic inflammatory diseases raises a question about how affected animals should be immunized. It seems logical that suspected immunosuppressive agents should be avoided when attempting to induce a primary immune response. Interestingly, although glucocorticosteroids are frequently thought of as immunosuppressive agents, there are no data to suggest that they interfere with canine or feline immunization. On the contrary, the available studies suggest that they do not adversely affect immunization (Nara et al., 1979). However, if possible, prudence would suggest that glucocorticosteroid therapy gradually be reduced or eliminated a week before and for 2 weeks after primary vaccination. Animals with seasonal allergies should probably be vaccinated at the time of year when glucocorticosteroid therapy is not required. However, the available evidence suggests that vaccination will likely be successful whether the glucocorticosteroid dose is reduced or not.

VACCINE REACTIONS

It is common for an animal receiving its first immunization to have a mild vaccine reaction. At the site of inoculation, a local reaction consisting of a painful inoculation, pruritus, swelling, redness, or abscess formation can occur. These local reactions are more common with inactivated vaccines, because this type of vaccine often contains adjuvants (local irritants) and also a greater amount of antigen than the modified live vaccines. Mild systemic reactions occur, particularly with modified live vaccines, because these vaccines have virus that replicates after immunization. Vaccine virus replication may be viewed as a mild infection that can result in temperature elevation, decreased activity, or increased irritability.

It is important that pregnant animals not be inoculated with a modified live vaccine unless the vaccine has been approved for this use, because fetal resorptions, abortions, or birth defects may result. Inactivated vaccines have been reported to cause problems when given to pregnant dogs, possibly from the stress associated with vaccination or adverse reactions sometimes resulting from these products. Similarly, animals younger than 3 weeks should not receive a modified live vaccine, unless the vaccine has been shown to be safe at this early age.

An occasional dog develops an immune complex disease after being administered CAV-1 vaccine. This condition is called "blue eye," because the affected eye develops a bluish cast in the cornea. The blue is the result of corneal edema, occurring from the deposition of antigen-antibody complexes. This is an immune-mediated (type III hypersensitivity) reaction. The dog usually regains full vision in the affected eye. Because of this adverse reaction, we recommend that dogs be immunized only with CAV-2. CAV-2 vaccine does not appear to cause blue eye and effectively protects against both virulent CAV-1 and CAV-2.

On rare occasions, anaphylaxis (type I hypersensitivity) may occur after immunizations. Anaphylaxis usually develops within an hour after immunization, presenting as weakness, dyspnea, vomiting, mucous membrane pallor, collapse, or death. The vaccine component that is most commonly associated with this reaction is the leptospirosis bacterin, although any component of the vaccine can cause anaphylaxis. Animals that develop anaphylaxis should never be reimmunized with the same vaccine until the causative component has been identified. Problem animals should be observed at the veterinary clinic for 1 hr after immunization with all vaccines.

Incomplete vaccine attenuation or vaccination of an immunosuppressed host can result in modified live vaccines causing the disease they are designed to prevent. Examples of this problem are feline respiratory vaccines causing a mild upper respiratory tract disease after immunization and the development of postvaccinal encephalitis subsequent to canine distemper vaccination. An even more alarming example is vaccine induction of clinical rabies (Esh et al., 1982; Pedersen et al., 1978). The reasons why vaccines become virulent are not always known. However, it is important that veterinarians be familiar with these possible outcomes of immunization and give modified live vaccines only to approved animals that are in good general health and have no indication of immunosuppression.

Most infectious diseases of dogs and cats have been controlled through the use of conventional vaccines. Although not perfect, these vaccines are exceptionally safe and effective. The future challenge will be to continue to improve the safety and efficacy of our current vaccines and to develop new vaccine approaches for diseases that have thus far been resistant to immunization.

References and Suggested Reading

Esh, J. B., Cunningham, J. G., and Wiktor, T. J.: Vaccine-induced rabies in four cats. J.A.V.M.A. 180:1336, 1982.
Nara, P. L., Krakowka, S., and Powers, T. E.: Effects of prednisolone on the development of immune response to canine distemper virus in beagle pups. Am. J. Vet. Res. 40:1742, 1979.
Pedersen, N. C., Emmons, R. W., Selcer, R., et al.: Rabies vaccine virus infection in three dogs. J.A.V.M.A. 172:1092, 1978.
Phillips, T. R., Jensen, J. L., Rubino, M. J., et al.: Effects of vaccines on the canine immune system. Can. J. Vet. Res. 53:154, 1989.

RATIONAL USE OF
ANTIMICROBIAL DRUGS

DAVID P. AUCOIN

Raleigh, North Carolina

The correct diagnosis of a disease is the cornerstone of medical practice, but a definitive diagnosis frequently is elusive. Therapy is often used to validate a diagnosis. Antibiotics (antimicrobials) are the most commonly used group of drugs in veterinary medicine and are often used in therapeutic diagnostics. However, the basis on which antibiotics are selected, used, and monitored is often irrational. The common use of antimicrobials involves the axiom that antibiotics, even when given to a patient without a bacterial infection, are safe because the toxicity of most antimicrobials is small. A second axiom regards antibiotics as prophylactic since a "sick" animal might be more prone to develop secondary infections. These two axioms are tempered by a third stating that it is prudent to hold certain antimicrobials ("big guns") in reserve for nonresponding or very sick patients. These axioms are partially true: antimicrobials usually are safe, debilitated patients do develop secondary bacterial infections, and use of an inappropriate antibiotic can increase the probability of bacterial resistance. There are problems with this approach, however, and empiric therapy can be irrational and yield suboptimal results. In addition, when used in this manner, antimicrobials do not provide information that can be used in diagnostic decision making. This article addresses these points and provides a framework on which companion animal practitioners can develop a rational basis of antimicrobial use.

A STEP-BY-STEP METHOD FOR ANTIMICROBIAL SELECTION

Diagnosis of a microbial infection is based on clinical signs and laboratory tests that indicate presence of a pathogen. As will be seen, adherence to these criteria is absolutely necessary if antibiotic therapy is to be rational. When primary or secondary infection is diagnosed in a patient, the following questions should be answered:

1. What organ system is involved?
2. Is it an acute or chronic problem?
3. What pathogen is most likely present in that organ system?

4. What antibiotic is most likely efficacious against that pathogen?
5. How much antibiotic is required at the site of infection?
6. What dose and route of administration are most likely to achieve that concentration?

Site of Infection

Localization of a microbial infection is usually straightforward. The vast majority of microbial infections in companion animals are restricted to the skin, respiratory tract, and genitourinary tract. The gastrointestinal system is not a common site of bacterial infections, even though antibiotics are commonly used in treating gastrointestinal disorders. The vast majority of acute lower and upper gastrointestinal disorders are not caused by bacteria. Of course, organ systems may be affected by nonbacterial conditions in which an antibiotic may do little or nothing (e.g., feline urologic syndrome).

Acute Versus Chronic Problems

Monitoring a response to an antibiotic involves a set of realistic expectations. Monitoring the response to therapy depends to a large extent on the clinical signs exhibited by the patient. Acute infections often manifest readily observable clinical signs that appear suddenly and are just as likely to disappear rapidly if appropriately treated. Chronic infections present a greater challenge to practitioners. Bacterial colonization can alter the local environment. Mechanisms for this involve adherence to a mucosal surface, often using specific receptors, followed by secretion of a glycocalyx membrane that envelops the bacteria. This adhered and tissue-bound infection produces free-floating bacteria in an organ (e.g., urine); these are the organisms we culture. Antibiotic therapy directed against these free-floating organisms may be effective against this population, but the tissue infection may persist and will likely recur once antimicrobial therapy is discontinued.

Acute infections can be treated successfully in 5 to 10 days with the appropriate antibiotic. Response to therapy is monitored by a rapid change in clinical signs and inappropriate therapy, usually judged within 48 to 72 hr. If no response is noted within that time frame, the antibiotic is either incorrect or the diagnosis is wrong. It is illogical and irrational to treat an acute infection for weeks hoping that more prolonged exposure to therapy will be successful. Chronic infections, conversely, do require longer treatment, and the response is much harder to gauge. This is why it is critical to select the most appropriate antibiotic at the start of therapy rather than finish a 4-week course of an antibiotic only to find that it did not work. Culturing is helpful in determining an antibiotic's efficacy. If bacteria are still being cultured after 10 to 14 days of treatment, it is time to re-evaluate the therapy, the diagnosis, and the predisposing causes and not just continue treatment.

Identifying the Pathogen

Since 1987, the Clinical Microbiology Laboratory at North Carolina State University (NCSU) has had 14,327 requests for cultures. Forty-five per cent (6457) had no organisms isolated, and of the remaining 55% (7915), more than 148 different species of bacteria were isolated. All of the isolates, however, were not considered pathogens. In dogs, eight species accounted for the majority of bacteria cultured from infected sites. These species are listed in Table 1 along with the frequency of their occurrence. The two most commonly isolated species in dogs were *Escherichia coli* and *Staphyloccus intermedius,* which should not be surprising because they are common commensal organisms. From these data, it should be evident that bacteria have no significant role in many conditions and that once an infection is diagnosed, the number of possible pathogens is small, but predicting the exact isolate may be difficult. It is clear that the initial choice of antibiotics can be guided by data shown in Table 1 (see *CVTX,* p. 1204).

However, speculative therapy does not obviate obtaining a culture. Probabilities are useful only for making a rational initial choice of antibiotic. If the patient responds poorly to the initial treatment, a culture should be incubating to guide changes of antibiotic regimens.

In dogs, bacterial infections of the urinary tract predominate. At NCSU, more than three quarters of all urinary tract infections are due to five bacterial species. *E. coli* and other enterics are the major pathogens, accounting for approximately two thirds of all infections. *S. intermedius* is probably more frequently involved in initial episodes than our data would indicate.

Bacterial infections of the skin (including otitis externa) are the second most common bacterial infection of dogs. Superficial pyodermas are almost exclusively *S. intermedius.* Deep pyodermas, however, are often associated with enterics—most likely from secondary colonization. Cultures from cases of chronic otitis externa often yield *Pseudomonas aeruginosa,* an organism that may be very resistant following exposure to common aminoglycoside-containing ear medications. Chronic ear infections are unlikely to resolve with any antibiotic alone and require managing the cause of the inflammation and infection, a difficult task in many dogs.

Cultures from transtracheal washes or lavage may or may not represent true pathogens. Predicting the most likely pathogen involved in bronchial pneumonias often is difficult. A young dog that develops secondary pneumonia from tracheobronchitis while boarding is more likely to have a *Bordetella* infection than that same dog who 10 years later presents debilitated with cranial lung lobe consolidation. Appropriate management of these dogs requires that cultures be taken, by lavage if possible, and that four-quadrant antibiotic coverage be initiated (see the later section "Quinolones").

Choosing an Antibiotic

Table 2 lists the *in vitro* efficacy of the antibiotics most often used against the common canine pathogens. To be considered excellent, good, fair, or poor, an antibiotic must inhibit more than 90%, 75 to 90%, 50 to 75%, or less than 50% of the pathogens tested, respectively. *These guidelines should not be interpreted as predicting how successful the drugs will be in treating any given pathogen* in vivo, *but rather how well they performed* in vitro. The value of *in vitro* susceptibility testing is sometimes misunderstood.

Culturing in bacterial infections presents a different and more complex situation. A clinician may inappropriately perceive the information from the microbiologic report as a "yes and no" list of drugs to try. The susceptibility or resistance of the pathogen, the dose, or the route of drug administration to maximize the chances of success is not usually part of the interpretation. This information, however, is important and needs to be addressed if an optimal treatment regimen is to be developed.

Most *in vitro* susceptibility testing is performed by disk diffusion (Kirby-Bauer). The size of the zone of inhibition for a particular antibiotic is directly related to its concentration at that growth–no-growth border. The interpretation of whether that zone size indicates that an antibiotic is sensitive, resistant, or intermediate is unregulated in many veterinary laboratories. Other laboratories use the strict guidelines that have been developed for human pathogens by the National Committee for Clinical Laboratory Standards (NCCLS). Whether

Table 1. Bacterial Isolates from NCSU—Teaching Hospital

Site (No.)	Organism	% of Total	Site (No.)	Organism	% of Total
Urine	*Escherichia coli*	44	TTW	*E. coli*	29
683	*Proteus mirabilis*	11	87	*K. pneumoniae*	12
	Klebsiella pneumoniae	9		*S. intermedius*	10
	Staphylococcus intermedius	8		*Pasteurella multocida*	7
	Streptococcus faecalis	7		*P. mirabilis*	7
				Bordetella bronchiseptica	6
Ear	*S. intermedius*	24	Blood	*E. coli*	29
97	*P. aeruginosa*	16	28	*S. intermedius*	22
	P. mirabilis	15		*P. aeruginosa*	15
	S. faecalis	15		*K. pneumoniae*	11
	E. coli	10		*P. multocida*	9
Skin	*S. intermedius*	55	Bone	*S. intermedius*	23
52	*E. coli*	18	40	*K. pneumoniae*	18
	P. mirabilis	11		*E. coli*	15
	P. aeruginosa	7		*S. faecalis*	15
				P. mirabilis	13

No., number of specimen cultures; TTW, transtracheal wash.

or not these standards should be used in veterinary medicine misses the point. If a clinician knew how much antibiotic was needed to inhibit the growth of the pathogen *in vitro* and how much could be delivered by using a standard dosing range, the clinician could determine the susceptibility of the pathogen. This quantitative information is available in most national laboratories or in human hospitals. Determining the minimum inhibitory (MIC) or minimum bactericidal concentration (MBC) of an antibiotic against a given pathogen is similar to giving actual glucose concentrations on a serum chemistry panel rather than telling a clinician that the value is normal, high, or low. Similarly, the use of interpreted Kirby-Bauer susceptibility data does not give a clinician sufficient quantitative information regarding bacterial susceptibility to a given antibiotic.

Using MIC data is not more predictive of clinical success, just more informative for a clinician trying to decide which antibiotic to use.

The MIC breakpoint, or the maximum concentration at which an organism would be considered "sensitive," is given for each antibiotic in Table 2. These breakpoints are from the NCCLS. If an MIC is not available for a particular pathogen, then the chosen antibiotic should be dosed and delivered to obtain *at least* the breakpoint concentration at the site of infection. This does not apply to uncomplicated lower urinary tract infections, because urinary concentrations are often 10- to 100-fold higher than serum concentrations, and many "resistant" organisms can be overcome if enough antibiotic is present. However, it is important to keep in mind that the MIC merely reflects the degree of sensitiv-

Table 2. Antimicrobial in Vitro Efficacy

	Amox	Clav	Ceph	T/S	Gen	Amk	Chloro	Enro	Clin	Eryth
Gram-Negative Bacteria										
Escherichia coli	Poor	Good	Good	Good	Good	Excellent	Fair	Excellent	—	—
Proteus mirabilis	Good	Good	Good	Fair	Fair	Excellent	Good	Excellent	—	—
Klebsiella pneumoniae	Poor	Good	Good	Fair	Good	Excellent	Fair	Excellent	—	—
Pseudomonas aeruginosa	—	—	—	—	Good	Excellent	Poor	Excellent	—	—
Pasteurella multocida	Excellent	Excellent	Excellent	Excellent	Excellent	Excellent	Excellent	Excellent	—	—
Bordetella bronchiseptica	Excellent	Excellent	Excellent	Excellent	Excellent	Excellent	Excellent	Excellent	—	—
Gram-Positive Bacteria										
Staphylococcus intermedius	Poor	Excellent	Excellent	Good	—	—	Good	Excellent	Good	Good
Streptococcus faecalis	Excellent	Excellent	Good	Fair	—	—	Good	Fair	Fair	Fair

Amox, amoxicillin, ampicillin, breakpoint > 16 μg/ml (>1 μg/ml for staphylococci); Clav, amoxicillin + clavulanic acid (2:1), breakpoint > 16 μg/ml (>1 μg/ml for staphylococci); Ceph, cephalothin, cephalexin, cephradine, cefadroxil, breakpoint > 32 μg/ml; T/S: trimethoprim-potentiated sulfas, breakpoint > 4 μg/ml; Gen, gentamicin, breakpoint > 8 μg/ml; Amk, amikacin, breakpoint > 32 μg/ml; Chloro, chloramphenicol, breakpoint > 16 μg/ml; Enro, enrofloxacin, breakpoint > 2 μg/ml; Clin, clindamycin, lincomycin, breakpoint 4 μg/ml; Eryth, erythromycin, breakpoint > 8 μg/ml.

ity an organism has to an antibiotic. For example, an *E. coli* sensitive to ampicillin is sensitive at less than 4 μg/ml and its gram-negative breakpoint is greater than 16 μg/ml. In order to increase even moderately the percentage of susceptible isolates, concentrations of greater than 64 μg/ml must be achieved. Thus, an *E. coli* that required 64 μg/ml of ampicillin to be inhibited would be considered resistant if in the lung but could be successfully treated in the urine because ampicillin concentrations of greater than 250 μg/ml are achieved. Yet this MIC indicates that this organism has resistant mechanisms (most likely beta-lactamase production) and should be labeled as relatively insensitive. One can use MIC data in this fashion in selecting not only an effective antibiotic but the most sensitive one. An *E. coli* pneumonia with both a cephalothin MIC of 8 μg/ml and an ampicillin MIC of less than 0.5 μg/ml would be reported as sensitive. However, ampicillin would be expected to be more effective than cephalothin and would be the drug of choice. It is logical to assume that it would be easier to achieve the former MIC at the infection site, and choice of therapy should favor ampicillin.

Dose and Route of Administration

Determining a dose for an antibiotic is often just a matter of reading its label. Labeled dosages for most products, especially newer products, are effective in many cases. However, a single dose, rather than a dosing range, fails to allow a clinician the needed latitude in treating different infections. Treating a streptococcal infection with amoxicillin that has an MIC of 0.01 μg/ml versus an *E. coli* infection with an MIC of 4 μg/ml (or 400 times more resistant) would logically require different dosing. Similarly, if that *E. coli* infection were in bronchial tissue versus the urine, a higher dose would seem justified because amoxicillin accumulates 10- to 100-fold in the urine but less than 25% of plasma concentrations are achieved in bronchial tissues. Simple rules of thumb can assist a clinician in determining a dosing range. The labeled dose is a reasonable starting point. Many doses can be halved, doubled, or in some cases tripled. That gives a wide dosing range; however, drug toxicosis must be considered when using extralabel doses.

BETA-LACTAM ANTIBIOTICS

Beta-lactam antibiotics (i.e., penicillins, cephalosporins, amoxicillin, clavamox, and cefadroxil) have a dosing range of 10 to 30 mg/kg b.i.d. to t.i.d. At these dosages, peak serum concentrations range from 5 to 30 μg/ml when given orally and 50 to 500 μg/ml when given intravenously or intramuscularly.

An important point to be made is that response to a parenteral antibiotic does not mean that the response will persist when given orally. This is why determining the MIC is of more value than using a simple disk diffusion test. The efficacy of these drugs is more dependent on total drug exposure than on peak concentrations. In other words, the dose is more important than the frequency of dosing. This statement is not to be interpreted to mean that once a day at three times the dose is as effective as dosing three times a day. It means that the number of daily doses is less important than how much drug is delivered per day. As a family, these drugs are more potent (have lower MICs) against susceptible gram-positive organisms than gram-negative bacteria. They penetrate poorly into bronchial tissues, with peak concentrations a quarter of those achieved in blood, and they actively accumulate in the urine. Thus, treating a group D streptococcal urinary tract infection would require the lower dosing range twice a day and an *E. coli* pneumonia the highest.

AMINOGLYCOSIDES

Although their use has declined with the advent of the fluoroquinolone antibiotics, the aminoglycosides are still the drug of choice in many serious gram-negative infections. Like the beta-lactams, the efficacy of this family of antibiotics is dependent on peak concentration rather than total drug exposure. Therefore, the amount administered at each dose is very important. Too often a clinician is more concerned about potential toxicity than optimizing therapy. Toxicity is usually minimal or reversible if a patient is closely monitored. Risk factors for nephrotoxicity include pre-existing renal disease, prerenal azotemia, fever, and dehydration. Therefore, fluid therapy in a septic patient is important to minimize aminoglycoside toxicity. Gentamicin and tobramycin (especially effective against *P. aeruginosa*) are dosed at 2 to 4 mg/kg and amikacin at 4 to 8 mg/kg t.i.d. One should monitor for toxicity by monitoring the findings on urinalysis and the serum creatinine levels. It is critical that predosing renal function determinations be made so that a sample collected after 3 to 5 days of therapy can be compared. A 25% increase over baseline is reason to increase the interval to b.i.d. If the increase is greater than 50%, the drug should be stopped and another substituted. Do not decrease the amount of drug given to dogs at risk, but rather increase the interval to once or twice a day. These regimens will produce peak concentrations of 10 μg/ml (20 μg/ml for amikacin) and trough concentrations of less than 1μg/ml (2 μg/ml for amikacin). These have been both safe and effective doses in dogs at NCSU-College of Veterinary Medicine.

QUINOLONES

The advent of the newer fluorinated quinolones has been a major improvement in oral antimicrobial therapy. These drugs are the most potent known antibiotics against aerobic gram-negative bacteria. This potency translates into a high ratio of serum concentration to MIC during a given dosing interval. The efficacy of these drugs is best correlated with total drug exposure, like the beta-lactams. This guideline is especially helpful because the oral bioavailability of some quinolones in dogs is highly erratic. Ciprofloxacin is the most variable, with peak serum concentrations of 0.5 to 5.0 μg/ml following a 5- to 10-mg/kg dose. However, because the MIC_{90} for all the gram-negative bacteria, including *P. aeruginosa*, is less than 0.5 μg/ml, this is not a problem. Enrofloxacin, on the other hand, is more consistent and is absorbed faster and more completely than ciprofloxacin. Its dose is thus lower, with 2.5 to 5.0 mg/kg producing serum concentrations of 1 to 3 μg/ml. These drugs have less potency against gram-positive bacteria, although they have good efficacy against *Staphylococcus* species. They have little to no activity against anaerobic bacteria. Therefore, quinolones should not be considered broad-spectrum antibiotics. Actually, no monotherapy should be considered broad spectrum, because the connotation of the phrase implies complete coverage when all the term is intended to mean is that an antibiotic is effective against both gram-negative and gram-positive bacteria. A better term is *four-quadrant coverage*. Four-quadrant coverage implies coverage against aerobic and anaerobic gram-positive and gram-negative organisms. A quinolone combined with amoxicillin or clindamycin or an aminoglycoside combined with a beta-lactam antibiotic often provides true four-quadrant coverage.

References and Suggested Reading

Aronson, A. L., and Aucoin, D. P.: Antimicrobial drugs. *In* Ettinger, S. J. (ed.): *Textbook of Veterinary Internal Medicine*, 3rd ed. Philadelphia: W. B. Saunders, 1989, pp. 383–386.

Garvey, M. S., and Aucoin, D. P.: Therapeutic strategies involving antimicrobial treatment of disseminated bacterial infection in small animals. J.A.V.M.A. 185:1185, 1984.

Prescott, J. F., and Baggot, J. D.: Antimicrobial susceptibility testing and antimicrobial drug dosage. J.A.V.M.A. 187:363, 1985.

Prescott, J. F., and Baggot, J. D.: *Antimicrobial Therapy in Veterinary Medicine*. London: Blackwell Scientific, 1988.

FELINE ANTIVIRAL THERAPY

STEVEN W. DOW,
NORDIN S. ZEIDNER,
and EDWARD A. HOOVER
Fort Collins, Colorado

Viral infections are clearly the most important infectious diseases of cats, in terms of both morbidity and mortality. Despite the importance of viral disease in cats, few proven effective viral treatments are currently available. Most research efforts have been devoted to viral disease prevention through vaccination rather than to treatment of established disease. This situation has now begun to change, largely because of the tremendous increase in antiviral research triggered by the epidemic of acquired immunodeficiency syndrome (AIDS) in humans and the use of retrovirus-infected cats as models for evaluation of antiretroviral therapy.

Bacterial infections are generally simpler to treat than viral infections, because bacteria replicate extracellularly and possess features distinct from eukaryotic cells. By contrast, viruses are more intimately dependent on the host cell metabolic and replicative machinery for their survival and replication. Viruses have few distinct enzymatic or replicative functions that can be selectively inhibited. Virus latency and restricted replication further complicate design of effective treatments.

Many antiviral drugs, because they nonspecifically interfere with both viral and closely related host cell functions, are associated with serious adverse effects. Advances in our understanding of the molecular biology of viruses and virus-host interactions are likely to lead to the development of more specific and less toxic antiviral compounds.

In this article, we discuss feline viral diseases for which there are available data to make treatment recommendations. In addition, we have included the results of pertinent experimental studies of antiviral compounds in cats, particularly treatment of feline retroviral infections.

FELINE HERPESVIRUS INFECTION

Feline herpesvirus type I (feline viral rhinotracheitis [FVR]) is the most important cause of viral upper respiratory and ocular diseases in cats (Hoover, 1987). Infections occur primarily in kittens and in situations where many cats are housed together (boarding facilities, veterinary hospitals). FVR replication is temperature restricted, and viral effects are therefore largely confined to relatively cool mucosal surfaces, especially the nasopharynx, nasal turbinates, and conjunctiva. Infection with FVR induces epithelial cell necrosis at these sites; the inflammatory response is intensified by secondary bacterial infection. Clinical signs of infection include fever, sneezing, bilateral conjunctival hyperemia, serous oculonasal exudate, and depression and inappetence. Most cats recover within 1 to 2 weeks. Permanent injury to the nasal respiratory epithelium and turbinates may result when young kittens are infected. Ocular manifestations include conjunctivitis and keratitis, with development of dendritic corneal ulcers. FVR may establish latent infection in cats, resulting in a persistent carrier state. Virus shedding can be induced by natural stresses or administration of corticosteroids (Hoover, 1987).

Antiviral treatment of FVR has primarily been directed at management of the ocular manifestations of infection, particularly herpetic keratitis. Several antiviral compounds have been compared to determine their relative *in vitro* effectiveness against six feline herpesvirus strains (Nasisse et al., 1989). Trifluridine (a synthetic nucleoside that inhibits DNA synthesis) and idoxuridine (also a synthetic nucleoside) were found to be the most effective of five antiviral compounds evaluated. Use of both of these drugs is restricted to topical administration because both are toxic when administered systemically. Trifluridine is preferred over idoxuridine because of its greater corneal penetrability.

At present, recommended treatment for feline herpetic keratitis or conjunctivitis is one drop of trifluridine ophthalmic solution (Viroptic) administered hourly in the affected eye, or at least six times daily for 2 to 3 weeks. Treatment should not be extended beyond 3 weeks, as trifluridine may become toxic to the corneal epithelium. An alternative regimen is administration of idoxuridine (Stoxil) solution or ointment for 2 to 3 weeks.

Attempts to make a definitive diagnosis of herpesvirus infection should precede initiation of prolonged and costly treatment. Diagnosis is confirmed by immunofluorescent examination for the presence of FVR antigens in cells obtained by conjunctival or corneal scraping. Chlamydial infection should also be excluded by Giemsa's stain and cytologic examination of conjunctival scrapings in any cat with severe conjunctivitis.

At present, an effective treatment for systemic FVR infection in cats has not been reported. Acyclovir, a synthetic nucleoside that selectively inhibits herpesvirus DNA polymerase, shows the most promise for this use in cats. The drug has fewer side effects than other antiherpes drugs when given systemically to humans and has been safely administered intravenously to cats. However, compared with several other antiviral compounds, acyclovir was found to be relatively ineffective *in vitro* against feline herpesviruses (Nasisse et al., 1989). Gancyclovir, another nucleoside analogue, may prove more effective than acylovir for systemic administration. Use of these drugs systemically in cats awaits results from controlled clinical or experimental trials.

FELINE INFECTIOUS PERITONITIS VIRUS

Although many coronavirus strains may infect cats, most induce inapparent or mild infections of the gastrointestinal or respiratory tracts. However, several strains (the feline infectious peritonitis viruses [FIPV]) are associated with severe and almost invariably fatal disease in cats (Pedersen, 1987; Scott, 1989). FIPV initially infects epithelial cells in the oropharynx and upper respiratory tract. Once an antiviral antibody response develops, the virus-antibody complexes appear to be engulfed by circulating monocytes and distributed to perivascular areas throughout the body. The primary lesion in feline infectious peritonitis (FIP) is antibody mediated and complement dependent and consists of perivascular inflammation. As the disease progresses, exudation of protein-rich fluid may occur, but pyogranulomatous lesions more commonly develop, characteristic of the noneffusive form of FIP.

Despite numerous investigations, an effective treatment for clinical FIP has not been found. Studies have shown that prior immunization with a nonvirulent or cross-sensitizing strain of FIP may enhance disease susceptibility and accelerate disease progression. For this reason, humoral immune responses to FIPV have been implicated in the pathogenesis of the disease, and immunosuppression has been proposed as a means to slow or reverse the disease. However, little experimental or clinical data are available to support this contention (Scott, 1989). In fact, generalized immunosuppression actually seems to increase susceptibility to FIP, as evidenced by the frequent development of fulminant FIP in cats that have been immunocompromised as a result of feline leukemia virus (FeLV) infection. Because FIPV preferentially infects monocytes, treatments designed to enhance monocyte antiviral function seem more logical, and immunomodulators have shown some benefit in early trials, although data from controlled clinical trials have not been published.

Ribavirin (a broad-spectrum triazole nucleoside that inhibits viral protein synthesis) in combination with recombinant human alpha-interferon (a glycoprotein that inhibits viral synthesis, assembly, and release) has been shown to inhibit FIPV replication in cell culture (Weiss and Oostrom-Ram, 1989). The combination appeared to be synergistic *in vitro*, which may allow ribavirin to be effective at lower doses *in vivo*. Ribavirin at high doses is toxic to cats, leading to weight loss, bone marrow suppression, and evidence of hepatic dysfunction (Povey, 1978). However, human recombinant alpha-interferon apparently does not induce adverse effects in cats when given systemically at therapeutic dosages. Therefore, the combination of low-dose ribavirin plus interferon offers some promise for the short-term treatment of cats with FIP.

FELINE LEUKEMIA VIRUS

FeLV has long been associated with the development of lymphocytic and myelocytic leukemias, lymphosarcoma, and aplastic anemia in cats (Hardy and McClelland, 1977). Of equal or greater significance, however, are the immunosuppressive properties associated with this virus (Hardy, 1980). Immunodeficiency disease is the most frequently occurring FeLV-related cause of death in pet cats, and it has been estimated that 83% of persistently infected animals die within 3.5 years of initial diagnosis, usually of secondary opportunistic infections (Hardy, 1980). A naturally occurring isolate of FeLV (FeLV-FAIDS) that induces a high incidence of immunodeficiency syndrome in infected specific pathogen-free cats has been characterized (Hoover et al., 1987).

Central to the issue of FeLV-induced immune impairment is the effect of persistent and high levels of antigenemia on both humoral and cellular immunity (Hardy, 1982). *In vitro*, FeLV-associated antigen has been shown to depress lymphocyte response to free antigen and mitogens, impair secretion of cytokines such as interleukin-2 (IL-2) as well as gamma- and alpha-interferon, and directly suppress bone marrow progenitor colony growth and neutrophil function (Engelman et al., 1985; Hebrebrand et al., 1979; Lafrado et al., 1987; Orosz et al., 1985; Trainin et al., 1983; Wellman et al., 1984; Yasuda et al., 1987). *In vivo*, high levels of virus-specific circulating antigen in persistently viremic animals induce elevated levels of circulating immune complexes and associated immune complex–mediated disease. Clinically, persistent antigenemia has been associated with hypocomplemen-

temia, suppression of the humoral immune response to soluble antigen, and direct impairment of gamma-interferon production and IL-2 secretion, the latter directly correlated with the stage of disease (Day et al., 1980; Koblinsky et al., 1979; Liu et al., 1984; Pardi et al., 1991; Tompkins et al., 1989). Thus, any proposed therapy of FeLV viremia or FeLV-induced disease should be directed at decreasing circulating antigen and reversing associated immune suppression.

Investigators developing experimental antiretroviral chemotherapy have focused their attention on nucleoside analogues, compounds that selectively bind to virus-specific reverse transcriptase, thereby inhibiting the formation of proviral DNA, an essential initial step in the retrovirus life cycle (Richman, 1990). Although the majority of these compounds have been developed for retrovirus-induced AIDS in humans, preclinical studies have documented the ability of many of these analogues to inhibit the infectivity of a diverse group of mammalian and avian retroviruses (Dahlberg et al., 1987; Frank et al., 1987; Olsen et al., 1987; Ruprecht et al., 1986).

The drug 3′-azido-3′-deoxythymidine, or azidothymidine (AZT) (Retrovir, Burroughs Wellcome), has been shown to inhibit FeLV replication *in vitro* at concentrations ranging from 0.005 to 5 μg/ml (Tavares et al., 1987; Zeidner et al., 1990b). Oral administration of this drug at 20 mg/kg resulted in peak plasma concentrations of 3 μg/ml 2 hr postadministration and a plasma half-life of 1.6 hr (Zeidner et al., 1990a) (Fig. 1). AZT given orally or by subcutaneous injection at either 20 or 10 mg/kg prevented the development of persistent viremia and resultant progression to clinical disease if given within 72 hr of exposure to FeLV (Tavares et al., 1987; Zeidner et al., 1990b). However, a delay in treatment to as late as 28 days after virus inoculation reduced effectiveness to only marginal and transient suppression of FeLV antigenemia (Tavares et al., 1987). Treatment of persistently viremic animals given AZT orally at 20 mg/kg t.i.d. had no significant effect on circulating antigenemia (Haschek et al., 1990; Zeidner et al., 1990b). Toxicity associated with AZT included transient anorexia and weight loss and a regenerative macrocytic anemia that was dose dependent (Haschek et al., 1990; Zeidner et al., 1990a,b).

Alpha-interferon has been shown to block the terminal stages of virus maturation and budding from cellular membranes (Fig. 2) (Poli et al., 1989). Combination therapy using AZT and alpha-2b interferon (IntronA, Schering) at concentrations of interferon ranging from 500 to 1000 units/ml acts synergistically to block FeLV-FAIDS infectivity *in vitro* (Fig. 3) (Zeidner et al., 1990b). Delivered subcutaneously, the plasma half-life of alpha-2b interferon in cats was 2.9 hr, plasma levels of 1000 units/ml could be maintained for as long as 10 hr,

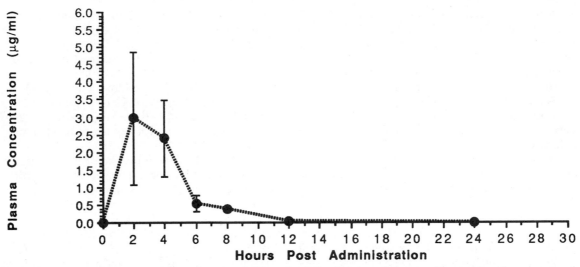

Figure 1. Pharmacokinetics of azidothymidine (AZT) (20 mg/kg PO) administered to cats. (Reprinted with permission from Zeidner, N. S., et al.: Zidovudine in combination with alpha interferon and interleukin-2 as prophylactic therapy for FeLV-induced immunodeficiency syndrome (FeLV-FAIDS). J. Acquir. Immune Defic. Syndr. 3:787, 1990.)

and clinical toxicity was not observed with daily delivery of this agent during a 12-week treatment period (Zeidner et al., 1990a). Delivery of interferon at 1.0 to 1.6 × 10⁵ units/kg once daily in combination with AZT at 10 to 20 mg/kg t.i.d. proved effective in completely aborting experimental FeLV-FAIDS infection when given immediately after virus exposure (Zeidner et al., 1990b). Latent provirus could not be reactivated in these animals, and systemic viremia or secondary opportunistic infections were not apparent during a 285-day observation period (Zeidner et al., 1990b). In contrast, cats receiving either AZT alone, AZT in combination with IL-2, or interferon alone were unable to resist

the development of persistent viremia, and a significant number of these cats developed secondary opportunistic infections during this same period (Zeidner et al., 1990b). In cats persistently infected with FeLV-FAIDS (Zeidner et al., 1990a), alpha-2b interferon given during a 12-week period with or without AZT induced a significant reduction in circulating antigen. However, this effective antiviral activity could be maintained only for a period of 7 weeks, because cats developed antibodies to interferon that were dose dependent, neutralizing, and specific for exogenously delivered alpha-2b interferon (Zeidner et al., 1990a). The antiviral activity of alpha-interferon appears to be dose dependent,

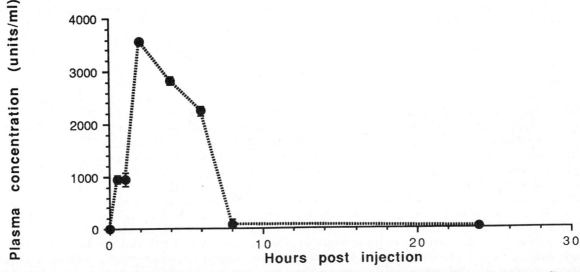

Figure 2. Pharmacokinetics of alpha interferon (2b) (1.6 million units/kg) delivered by subcutaneous injection to cats. (Reprinted with permission from Zeidner, N. S., et al.: Alpha interferon (2b) in combination with zidovudine for the treatment of presymptomatic feline leukemia virus–induced immunodeficiency syndrome. Antimicrob. Agents Chemother. 34:1749, 1990.)

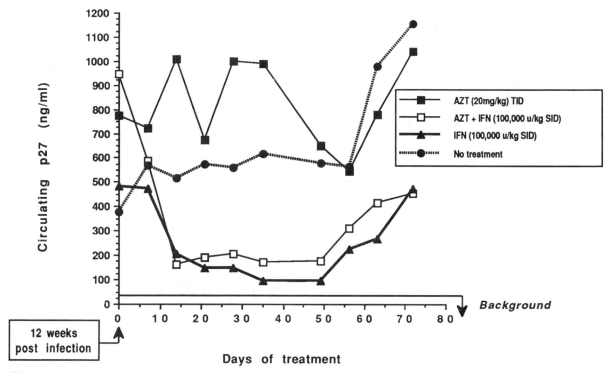

Figure 3. Treatment of early asymptomatic FeLV-FAIDS infection utilizing AZT and alpha interferon (2b) (IFN). (Reprinted with permission from Zeidner, N. S., et al.: Alpha interferon (2b) in combination with zidovudine for the treatment of presymptomatic feline leukemia virus–induced immunodeficiency syndrome. Antimicrob. Agents Chemother. 34:1749, 1990.)

because lower doses (10^4 units/kg) had significantly less effect on circulating viremia and extremely low doses given orally (5 units per cat daily for 7 days biweekly) could not prevent the development of persistent viremia or associated disease in experimentally inoculated cats (Cummins et al., 1988; Zeidner et al., 1990a). Nevertheless, the relative lack of clinical toxicity associated with alpha-interferon indicates that this agent offers promise in developing therapies to reduce FeLV antigenic load. Current research efforts are directed at combined therapy regimens using AZT, alpha-interferon, and immune cell transfer to reduce levels of virus replication in FeLV-infected cats.

A second nucleoside analogue, 2',3'-dideoxycytidine (ddC), has also been used in an attempt to prophylactically block the onset of persistent viremia in cats (Polas et al., 1990; Zeidner et al., 1989). Although concentrations ranging from 1 to 10 μg/ml of this agent were effective in inhibiting virus replication *in vitro*, persistent FeLV infection could not be prevented even if delivery was instituted 48 hr before experimental inoculation of virus and delivered either by continuous intravenous infusion or by sustained-release subcutaneous implantation (Polas et al., 1990; Zeidner et al., 1989). Delivery of ddC by subcutaneous sustained-release implantation (increasing the half-life of this drug 18-fold) in combination with either alpha-2b interferon or alpha-interferon plus human recombinant tumor

necrosis factor could only delay the onset of FeLV-FAIDS viremia relative to placebo-treated control cats (Zeidner et al., 1989). Significant amplification of virus replication was noted when therapy was discontinued (Polas et al., 1990; Zeidner et al., 1989).

Initial *in vitro* data suggest that other nucleoside analogues, 2',3'-dideoxyadenosine (ddA) and 2',3'-dideoxyinosine (ddI) also have inhibitory effects on FeLV replication at concentrations ranging from 10 to 100 μM (Tavares et al., 1989). Results of *in vivo* studies using these compounds against FeLV have not yet been reported.

Phosphonylmethoxyethyl nucleoside derivatives such as 9-(2-phosphonomethoxyethyl adenine) (PMEA) have also been evaluated for activity against FeLV. These drugs may prove valuable because of their broad spectrum of antiviral activity (DNA as well as RNA viruses) and relatively low toxicity (De Clercq et al., 1987). PMEA produced 50% inhibition of FeLV replication and FeLV-FAIDS–induced cytopathicity in T lymphoid cells at concentrations ranging from 0.5 to 3.0 μg/ml. PMEA delivered subcutaneously in divided doses at 6.25 mg/kg/day enabled cats to resist infection with FeLV-FAIDS (Hoover et al., 1990). Treated cats remained aviremic throughout a 16-week observation period, latent virus was not detected in bone marrow progenitor cells, and these cats completely resisted a second challenge with FeLV-FAIDS 9 weeks after cessation of initial therapy (Hoover et al., 1991). Significant clinical toxicity (anemia, leukopenia, diarrhea) was observed with doses of PMEA greater than 10 mg/kg (Hoover et al., 1991).

Suramin, a polyionic dye originally used in therapy of human filarial and protozoal disease, has been shown to be a potent inhibitor of retroviral reverse transcriptase (De Clercq, 1979). Initial studies used intravenous delivery of suramin every 7 to 10 days throughout a 42 to 70-day treatment period. Although a transient decrease in the levels of infectious virus was noted in two cats, a long-term antiviral effect or enhancement of antiviral immunity was not observed in this study (Cogan et al., 1986).

FELINE IMMUNODEFICIENCY VIRUS

Feline immunodeficiency virus (FIV) is a lentivirus of domestic cats that has been associated with several important disease syndromes, including immunodeficiency, cytopenias, opportunistic infections, gingivitis and stomatitis, neoplasia, and neurologic disease (Dow et al., 1990; Pedersen et al., 1987). The virus infects primarily T lymphocytes and mature tissue macrophages. Infection is presumed to be lifelong and is characterized by a persistent, long-lasting antibody response and restricted low-level virus production. In general, FIV infection is slow to induce disease, and most cats have been infected for years before they develop clinical signs of infection.

The tremendous research effort currently directed at developing an effective treatment for human immunodeficiency virus (HIV) infection in humans will undoubtedly have an immediate impact on the treatment of FIV-infected cats. At present, AZT, an inhibitor of the retroviral reverse transcriptase enzyme, is the only drug licensed for treatment of HIV-infected individuals. In vitro, AZT has been shown to inhibit FIV replication (North et al., 1989). PMEA also has been reported to inhibit FIV replication in vitro (Egberink et al., 1990; Hoover et al., 1991) and to produce clinical improvement in two FIV-infected cats treated for 21 days at 2.5 mg/kg b.i.d. (Egberink et al., 1990). However, both AZT and PMEA induce bone marrow suppression and anemia in cats after administration for several weeks; use of these two drugs therefore appears limited to cats without anemia or serious leukopenia. Other treatments currently under investigation for FIV infection include other nucleoside analogues, specific viral enzyme inhibitors, and recombinant interferons.

References and Suggested Reading

Cogan, D. C., Cotter, S. M., and Kitchen, L. W.: Effect of suramin on serum viral replication in feline leukemia virus–infected pet cats. Am. J. Vet. Res. 47:2230, 1986.

Cummins, J. M., Tompkins, M. B., Olsen, R. G., et al.: Oral use of human alpha interferon in cats. J. Biol. Response Mod. 7:513, 1988.

Dahlberg, J. E., Mitsuya, H., Blam, S. B., et al.: Broad spectrum antiretroviral activity of 2',3'-dideoxynucleosides. Proc. Natl. Acad. Sci. U.S.A. 84:2469, 1987.

Day, N. K., O'Reilly-Felice, C., Hardy, W. D., et al.: Circulating immune complexes associated with naturally occurring lymphosarcoma in pet cats. J. Immunol. 126:2363, 1980.

De Clercq, E.: Suramin: A potent inhibitor of the reverse transcriptase of RNA tumor viruses. Cancer Lett. 8:9, 1979.

De Clercq, E., Sakuma, T., Baba, M., et al.: Antiviral activity of phosphonylmethoxyalkyl derivatives of purine and pyrimidines. Antiviral Res. 8:261, 1987.

Dow, S. W., Poss, M. L., and Hoover, E. A.: Feline immunodeficiency virus: A neurotropic lentivirus. J. Acquir. Immune Defic. Syndr. 3:658, 1990.

Egberink, H., Borst, M., Niphuis, H., et al.: Suppression of feline immunodeficiency virus infection in vivo by 9-(2-phosphonomethoxy-ethyl)adenine. Proc. Natl. Acad. Sci. U.S.A. 87:3087, 1990.

Engelman, R. W., Fulton, R. W., Good, R. A., et al.: Suppression of gamma interferon production by inactivated feline leukemia virus. Science 227:1368, 1985.

Frank, K. B., McKernan, P. A., Smith, R. A., et al.: Visna virus as an in vitro model for human immunodeficiency virus and inhibition by ribavirin, phosphonoformate, and 2',3'-dideoxynucleosides. Antimicrob. Agents Chemother. 31:1369, 1987.

Gilden, R. V., and Oroszian, S.: Structural and immunologic relationships among mammalian C-type viruses. J.A.V.M.A. 158:1099, 1971.

Hardy, W. D.: The virology, immunology and epidemiology of the feline leukemia virus. In Hardy, W. D., Essex, M., and McClelland, A. J. (eds.): Feline Leukemia Virus. Developments in Cancer Research. Vol. 4. Amsterdam: Elsevier, 1980, pp. 33–79.

Hardy, W. D.: Immunopathology induced by the feline leukemia virus. Springer Semin. Immunopathol. 5:75, 1982.

Hardy, W. D., and McClelland, A. J.: Feline leukemia virus: Its related disease and control. Vet. Clin. North Am. 7:93, 1977.

Haschek, W. M., Weigel, R. M., Scherba, G., et al.: Zidovudine toxicity to cats infected with feline leukemia virus. Fundam. Appl. Toxicol. 14:764, 1990.

Hebrebrand, L. C., Olsen, R. G., Mathes, L. E., et al.: Inhibition of human lymphocyte mitogen and antigen response by a 15,000 dalton protein from feline leukemia virus. Cancer Res. 39:443, 1979.

Hoover, E. A.: Viral respiratory diseases and chlamydiosis. In Holzworth, J. (ed.): Diseases of the Cat. Philadelphia: W. B. Saunders, 1987, pp. 214–237.

Hoover, E. A., Ebner, J. P., Zeidner, N. S., et al.: Early therapy of feline leukemia virus infection (FeLV-FAIDS) with 9-(2-phosphonyl-methoxyethyl)adenine (PMEA). Antiviral Res. (in press).

Hoover, E. A., Mullins, J. I., Quackenbush, S. L., et al.: Experimental transmission and pathogenesis of immunodeficiency syndrome in cats. Blood 70:1880, 1987.

Koblinsky, L., Hardy, W. D., and Day, N. K.: Hypocomplementemia associated with naturally occurring lymphosarcoma in pet cats. J. Immunol. 122:2139, 1979.

Lafrado, L. J., Lewis, M. G., Mathes, L. E., et al.: Suppression of in vitro neutrophil function by feline leukemia virus (FeLV) and purified FeLV-p15e. J. Gen. Virol. 68:507, 1987.

Liu, W. T., Good, R. A., Trang, L. Q., et al.: Remission of leukemia and loss of feline leukemia virus in cats injected with staphylococcus protein A: Association with increased circulating interferon and complement-dependent cytotoxic antibody. Proc. Natl. Acad. Sci. U.S.A. 81:6471, 1984.

Nasisse, M. P., Guy, J. S., Davidson, M. G., et al.: In vitro susceptibility of feline herpesvirus-1 to vidarabine, idoxuridine, trifluridine, acyclovir, or bromovinyldeoxuridine. Am. J. Vet. Res. 50:158, 1989.

North, T. W., North, G. L., and Pedersen, N. C.: Feline immunodeficiency virus, a model for reverse transcriptase targeted chemotherapy for acquired immunodeficiency syndrome. Antimicrob. Agents Chemother. 33:915, 1989.

Olsen, J. C., Furman, P., Fyfe, J. A., et al.: 3'-azido-3'-deoxythymidine inhibits the replication of avian leukosis virus. J. Virol. 61:2800, 1987.

Orosz, C. G., Zinn, N. E., Olsen, R. G., et al.: Retrovirus-mediated immunosuppression, Part II. FeLV-UV alters in vitro murine T lymphocyte behavior by reversibly impairing lymphokine secretion. J. Immunol. 135:583, 1985.

Pardi, D., Hoover, E. A., Quackenbush, S. L., et al.: Defective humoral immunity in FeLV-induced immunodeficiency. Vet. Immunol. Immunopathol (in press).

Pedersen, N. C.: Coronavirus diseases (coronavirus enteritis, feline infectious peritonitis). In Holzworth, J. (ed.): Diseases of the Cat. Philadelphia: W. B. Saunders, 1987, pp. 193–213.

Pedersen, N. C., Ho, E. W., Brown, M. L., et al.: Isolation of a T-lymphotropic virus from cats with an immunodeficiency-like syndrome. Science 235:790, 1987.

Polas, P. J., Swenson, C. L., Sams, R., et al.: *In vitro* and *in vivo* evidence that the antiviral activity of 2′,3′-dideoxycytidine is target cell dependent in a feline retrovirus animal model. Antimicrob. Agents Chemother. 34:1414, 1990.

Poli, G., Orenstein, J. M., Kinter, A., et al.: Interferon-α but not AZT suppresses HIV expression in chronically infected cell lines. Science 244:575, 1989.

Povey, R. C.: Effect of orally administered ribavirin on experimental feline calicivirus infection in cats. Am. J. Vet. Res. 39:1337, 1978.

Richman, D. D.: HIV and other human retroviruses. *In* Galasso, G. J., Whitley, R. J., and Merigan, T. C. (eds.): *Antiviral Agents and Viral Diseases of Man*. Vol. 3. New York: Raven Press, 1990, pp. 581–646.

Ruprecht, R. M., O'Brien, L. G., Rossoni, L. D., et al.: Suppression of mouse viraemia and retroviral disease by 3′-azido-3′-deoxythymidine. Nature 323:467, 1986.

Scott, F. W.: Feline infectious peritonitis and other feline coronaviruses. *In* Kirk, R. W. (ed.): *Current Veterinary Therapy IX*. Philadelphia: W. B. Saunders, 1989, pp. 1059–1062.

Tavares, L., Roneker, C., Johnston, K., et al.: 3′-azido-3′-deoxythymidine in feline leukemia virus infected cats: A model for therapy and prophylaxis of AIDS. Cancer Res. 47:3190, 1987.

Tavares, L., Roneker, C., Postie, L., et al.: Testing of nucleoside analogues in cats infected with feline leukemia virus: A model. Intervirology 30:26, 1989.

Tompkins, M. B., Ogilvie, G. K., Gast, A. M., et al.: Interleukin-2 suppression in cats naturally infected with feline leukemia virus. J. Biol. Response Mod. 8:86, 1989.

Trainin, Z., Wernicke, D., Essex, M.: Suppression of the humoral antibody response in natural retrovirus infections. Science 220:858, 1983.

Weiss, R. C., and Oostrom-Ram, T.: Inhibitory effects of ribavirin alone or combined with human interferon alpha on feline infectious peritonitis virus replication *in vitro*. Vet. Microbiol. 20:255, 1989.

Wellman, M. L., Kociba, G. J., Lewis, M. G., et al.: Inhibition of erythroid colony-forming cells by a $M_r 15,000$ protein of feline leukemia virus. Cancer Res. 44:1527, 1984.

Yasuda, M., Good, R. A., and Day, N. K.: Influence of inactivated feline retrovirus on feline alpha interferon and immunoglobulin production. Clin. Exp. Immunol. 69:240, 1987.

Zeidner, N. S., Myles, M. H., Mathiason-Dubard, C., et al.: Alpha interferon (2b) in combination with zidovudine for the treatment of presymptomatic feline leukemia virus–induced immunodeficiency syndrome. Antimicrob. Agents Chemother. 34:1749, 1990a.

Zeidner, N. S., Rose, L. M., Mathiason-DuBard, C., et al.: Zidovudine in combination with alpha interferon and interleukin-2 as prophylactic therapy for FeLV-induced immunodeficiency syndrome (FeLV-FAIDS). J. Acquir. Immune Defic. Syndr. 3:787, 1990b.

Zeidner, N. S., Strobel, J. D., Perigo, N. A., et al.: Treatment of FeLV-induced immunodeficiency syndrome (FeLV-FAIDS) with controlled release capsular implantation of 2′,3′-dideoxycytidine. Antiviral Res. 11:147, 1989.

IMMUNOADJUVANT THERAPY

OTA BARTA

Blacksburg, Virginia

The goal of immunoadjuvant therapy is to strengthen the immune defense mechanisms of an animal nonspecifically. Immunoadjuvant therapy is thus distinguished from immunotherapy, which increases the amount of specific antibodies and specifically sensitized lymphocytes through vaccination or by administration of a hyperimmune serum.

Immunoadjuvant therapy is used in cases requiring an increase or optimization of the immune response. It is also called *nonspecific immunotherapy, immunostimulation, immunologic enhancement, augmenting of the immune response,* or *immunopharmacology.*

Agents used to achieve an increase or optimization of immune responses are commonly called *biologic response modifiers* (BRM), but also *immunomodulators, immunoaugmentors, immunoadjuvants, immunorestoratives, immunostimulators,* or *immunopotentiators.* BRM may be biologic products of animal cells or microorganisms or synthetic chemical compounds. BRM include both the augmenting and suppressing biologics or drugs, because optimization of the immune response may sometimes require an increase and at other times a suppression of the immune response. Some authors also include vaccines and biopreparations of tumor-associated antigens on the list of BRM, but these are rather agents of specific immunotherapy.

A list of more commonly used BRM is presented in Table 1. The following discussion is limited to those BRM that were tested in dogs and cats. This does not mean that other BRM would be ineffective; it only reflects the fact that they were insufficiently used to evaluate their potential for small animal clinicians' use.

BRM have been reviewed in more detail in various publications and books listed as references. All BRM were found effective on lymphocytes or monocytes *in vitro*. Their clinical use, however, may differ, because (1) the immune system is very complex and agents used *in vivo* may affect factors not included in *in vitro* systems, (2) the agents used are degraded or metabolized faster *in vivo* than *in vitro*, and (3) the immune system is very conservative—it tends to preserve the existing status and resist changes induced from outside. The studies done on animals so far have brought both satisfaction and disappointment.

***Table 1.** Biologic Response Modifiers and Biologics Most Commonly Used in Immunotherapy*

Immunomodulating Agents

Bacillus Calmette-Guérin (BCG): Attenuated live bacteria of *Mycobacterium bovis;* a potent inducer of cytokines

Bestatin: Immunomodulating dipeptide from *Streptomyces olivoreticuli;* increases tumoricidal activity of mononuclear phagocytes

Cimetidine (Tagamet; Smith Kline & French): Histamine H_2 receptor antagonist; restores cell-mediated immunity suppressed by histamine

Corynebacterium parvum (see *Propionibacterium acnes*)

Diethylcarbamazine (*N,N*,-diethyl-4-methyl-1-piperazine carboxamide [DE]): Used for treatment of filariasis; affects T cells

Endotoxin: Lipopolysaccharide of bacterial origin; activates B cells and complement

Equimune (Vetrepharm): Mycobacterial cell wall fraction

Glucans: Polysaccharides composed of D-glucose; derived from bacterial cell wall

Immunoregulin (*P. acnes;* ImmunoVet): Stimulates macrophages and interferon production; enhances resistance to viral infections

Isoprinosine: Synthetic inosine–containing complex; suppresses viral ribonucleic acid (RNA), augments RNA and messenger RNA (mRNA) synthesis in lymphocytes; augments both humoral and cell-mediated immunity

Lentinan: Neutral polysaccharide from mushroom *Lentinus edodes*

Levamisole: Phenylimidazothiazole; anthelmintic stimulating interferon production and T-cell function

Levan: Polysaccharide compound of D-fructose

Maleic anhydride-divinyl ether (MVE-2): Activates macrophages; nephrotoxic in dogs

Muramyl dipeptide (MDP): Peptidoglycan of bacterial cell wall

Muramyl tripeptide (MTP): Peptidoglycan of bacterial cell wall

Nocardia rubra cell wall skeleton

Promodulin: L-thiazolidine-4-carboxylic acid (Linworth Research)

Propionibacterium acnes (previously *Corynebacterium parvum*): Killed bacteria with immunomodulating properties

Prostaglandin inhibitors (aspirin, indomethacin)

Protein A (*Staphylococcal* protein A, SpA): Binds IgG, activates complement

Prosorba: SpA covalently bound to silica

Regressin (Ragland Research, Summit Hill Laboratories, and Vetrepharm): Mycobacterial cell wall immunostimulant

Ribogen: Mycobacterial cell wall preparation

Sodium diethylthiocarbamate (DTC): Nontoxic compound preventing trauma-induced immunosuppression; increases T-cell–associated events and natural killer (NK) activity

Tuftsin (leukokinin): Tetrapeptide derived from gamma-globulin; stimulates endocytosis by neutrophils

Interferons and Interferon Inducers

Brucella spp.–derived interferon-alpha (leukocyte-derived, 18–20 kd), beta (fibroblast or epithelial cell–derived, 22–30 kd), or gamma (T-cell–derived, 40–50 kd): Inhibition of viral replication, modulation of cytocidal activities of macrophages and NK cells

Polynucleotides:

    Polyinosinic-polycytidylic acid (poly IC)

    Polyadenylic-polyuridylic acid (poly AU)

    Poly IC adsorbed onto poly L-lysine and carboxymethylcellulose (poly ICLC)

Tilorones: Synthetic compounds inducing interferon production in animals

Viruses

Cytokines (Lymphokines and Monokines)

Antigrowth factor

Lymphokines, interleukins 1 through 10 (at the time of this writing, and the list is still growing): Products of lymphocytes and some other cells; control maturation and various functions of lymphocytes and other blood and reticuloendothelial cells

Tumor necrosis factor (TNF): Monokine released from activated macrophages; tumoricidal in presence of interferon-gamma

Thymic Extracts*

Thymic factors (thymic factor X, thymostimulin, thymopentin, thymulin, thymic hormonal factor, and others)

Thymosin, alpha$_1$, alpha$_2$, beta

Thymosin, fraction 5

Monoclonal Antibodies†

Anti–growth-promoting factor

Anti-T cell

Anti-T suppressor cell

Antitumor antigen

Miscellaneous BRM and Approaches

Allogenic immunization

Bone marrow transplantation

Effector cell transfer or induction (macrophages, lymphokine-activated killer [LAK] cells, NK cells, T-cytotoxic cells)

Passive immunotherapy with gamma globulin, whole plasma, or immune serum globulin

Plasmapheresis and extracorporeal treatment of plasma

Virus oncolysates of cells

---

*All induce surface markers on prothymocytes and receptors on lymphocytes or augment some form of cellular immune functions.

†Used to depress immune functions of given cells or factors.

USE OF IMMUNOADJUVANT THERAPY

Immunoadjuvant therapy represents only *adjunct* treatment that improves the immune status of the animal but that, with the exception of bone marrow transplant, cannot replace the basic defect or deficiency of the animal. Thus, disappointing results are usually reported when immunoadjuvant therapy is used in severely debilitated or immunologically incompetent animals.

Immunoadjuvant therapy was successful in animals with temporarily suppressed immune functions, when proper doses and regimen were used for several weeks. The success was often increased when combinations of various BRM and other drugs or specific vaccines were used. In many cases, the same BRM can act as a stimulator at some concentrations and as an inhibitor at other concentrations. The pathways of the action of BRM are often unknown or very complicated, involving various cells or cofactors. The same dose may have different results in different animals. Therefore, BRM should always be used cautiously and with the consent of an animal's owner.

Immunoadjuvant therapy may be *indicated* when any of the following are present:

1. Temporary physiologic, pathologic, or environmentally induced suppression of immune function.
2. Suppression of immune functions caused by infection.
3. A need for improving or increasing the existing immune potential (e.g., in old or very young animals, overwhelming infections, or tumor elimination).
4. Dysfunction of the immune system (e.g., in autoimmune diseases).

BIOLOGIC RESPONSE MODIFIERS TESTED IN DOGS AND CATS

Examples of more recent clinical experiments in using immunotherapy in canine and feline patients are given in Table 2. The following discussion summarizes the present knowledge.

Levamisole

Levamisole, the levo-isomer of 2,3,5,6-tetrahydro-6-phenylimidazo-(2,1-b)-thiazole, was originally developed as a broad-spectrum anthelmintic for cattle, sheep, and swine. Renoux and Renoux detected its effect on immune responses in 1971. The exact mechanisms of immunomodulating action are unknown. Levamisole stimulates phagocytosis and intracellular killing by macrophages and granulocytes and increases DNA synthesis in mitogen-stimulated lymphocytes. The drug yielded very disappointing results in dogs and cats when used in treatment of tumors, pyoderma, and *Dirofilaria immitis* infections (administered daily or every other day in doses from 2.2 to 24 mg/kg PO). In all clinical tests in dogs and cats, levamisole had very little or no effect. The side effects of peroral administrations were mild, but they increased with increasing doses and were particularly severe when intravenous administration was tested. They included gastrointestinal and liver disorders, lethargy, neurotoxicity, and agranulocytosis. Thus, levamisole cannot be recommended for use for immunomodulation in dogs and cats.

Propionibacterium acnes

Propionibacterium acnes (formerly *Corynebacterium parvum*) is available as a killed bacterial vaccine commercially produced with concentrations around 10^9 bacteria per milliliter (Immunoregulin, ImmunoVet). *P. acnes* stimulates mainly macrophage activity. The preparation should be repeatedly administered intraperitoneally or intravenously for several weeks. The doses used in clinical tests ranged from 0.2 to 0.5 mg/kg IP, and a single treatment intralesionally was also tested in tumors. The results of treatment of feline infectious peritonitis (FIP) and various tumors in dogs or cats were disappointing. On the other hand, improved remission from chronic recurrent canine pyoderma was noticed when a dose of 0.03 to 0.07 ml/kg was used twice weekly for 10 weeks combined with antibiotics (Becker et al., 1989). Extended survival time and temporary suppression of disease signs were reported in cats with FIP *only* when *P. acnes* treatment was combined with recombinant human interferon-alpha treatment (Weiss et al., 1990). No protection against lethal doses of FIP virus was observed with this combination of treatment. Repeated use of *P. acnes* in toxicity testing led to the development of side effects such as vomiting, anorexia, malaise, increased water consumption, acidosis, fever, and hepatitis (Leifer et al., 1987).

Muramyl Peptides

Muramyl dipeptide (MDP; N-acetylmuramyl-L-alanyl-D-isoglutamine) was found to be the minimal structure capable of replacing whole killed bacteria in complete Freund's adjuvant. Muramyl tripeptide (MTP-PE; N-acetylmuramyl-L-alanyl-D-isoglutaminyl-L-alanine-1'-2'-dipalmitoyl-sn-glycerol-3'-hydroxy-phosphoryloxy-ethylamide), MDP, and related compounds activate macrophages. These agents cause fever, increase antibody response,

Table 2. *Recent Uses of Immunotherapy in Dogs and Cats*

Material	Dose and Route	Species	Disease	Effect	Reference
Levamisole hydrochloride	5 mg/kg PO, Mon, Wed, Fri, continuously	Feline	Mammary gland tumor	No significant effect on survival or recurrence	MacEwen et al., 1984
Levamisole hydrochloride	5–20 mg/kg PO twice daily for 14 days	Canine	*Dirofilaria immitis*	>10 mg/kg decreased number of microfilariae; no effect on adult; toxic at 20 mg/kg	Carlisle et al., 1984
Levamisole hydrochloride	12–24 mg/kg/day PO for 3 days	Canine	*D. immitis*	Short time decrease number of microfilariae; no effect on adult or number of larvae in mosquitoes fed on the dogs	Barriga and Andujar, 1988
Levamisole hydrochloride	5 mg/kg, Mon, Wed, Fri, continuously	Canine	Mammary gland cancer	No effect on survival or cancer-free survival	MacEwen et al., 1985a
Levamisole hydrochloride	5 mg/kg, Mon, Wed, Fri, continuously	Canine	Lymphosarcoma	No effect on remission or survival	MacEwen et al., 1985b
BCG and *Corynebacterium parvum* (*Propionibacterium acnes*)	1 mg = 10^7 living bacteria; 10^9 killed bacteria intralesionally, single dose	Canine	Mammary gland tumor	No effect on survival rate	Parodi et al., 1983
C. parvum (*P. acnes*)	1–2 × 10^9 units intralesionally, single dose	Canine and feline	Various tumors	No effect	Misdorp, 1987
P. acnes	0.03–0.07 ml/kg/ twice/wk for 2 wk, once/wk for 10 wk	Canine	Pyoderma	Doubling the number of complete remissions of pyoderma	Becker et al., 1989
Immunoregulin (*P. acnes*)	0.4–4 mg IP twice/wk for 2 wk, once/wk for wk 3 and 4	Feline	Feline infectious peritonitis 0.6 or 200 LD_{100}	No effect	Weiss et al., 1990
Immunoregulin and rHuIFN-alpha	4 mg IP twice/wk for 2 wk, once/wk for wk 3 and 4 10^6 U/kg/day IM for 8 days, alternate days for 3 wk	Feline	Feline infectious peritonitis 0.6 and 200 LD_{100}	Extended survival time and temporary suppressed disease signs; no protection against lethal doses	Weiss et al., 1990
Protein A and prednisolone sodium succinate	6.6 µg/kg IP twice/wk for 10 wk, 2.2 mg/kg PO b.i.d. for several wk	Feline	FeLV-related hemolysis and secondary bone marrow depression	Normalization of red blood cell counts, enzyme-linked immunosorbent assay for FeLV negative, IFA of peripheral lymphocytes and bone marrow negative	Hitt and McCaw, 1988
Muramyl tripeptide in liposomes	2 mg/m² IV twice/wk for 8 wk after amputation	Canine	Osteosarcoma	Extended survival time	MacEwen et al., 1989
Diethylcarbamazine	10 mg/kg/day for 30 days	Feline	FeLV infection	Extended survival time, decreased serum infectivity, increased serum antibody to FOCMA	Kitchen and Cotter, 1988
rHuIFN-alpha	0.5–5 U/kg/day PO	Feline	FeLV-related diseases	Prevented development of fatal diseases	Cummins et al., 1988

IFA = Immunofluorescent antibody test.
FOCMA = Feline oncornavirus–associated cell membrane antigen.

regulate T-cell activity, increase production of prostaglandin E_2 and enhance slow-wave sleep; these effects are similar to the biologic activities of interleukin-1 (IL-1), a cytokine produced by macrophages. The lipophilic derivatives of muramyl peptides encapsulated in liposomes were found to be more effective than water-soluble derivatives. MTP-PE administered intravenously increased the survival time of canine tumor patients after surgical removal of tumors, as a study of 14 cases indicated. The need for repeated slow intravenous administration of this drug is a disadvantage. The dose of 2 mg/m² of liposome-encapsulated MTP was used with success and without noticeable side effects (MacEwen et al., 1989). Many of the experiments showing effects of muramyl peptide compounds in laboratory animals have not yet been repeated in dogs or cats.

Diethylcarbamazine, a drug originally used to treat filariasis, has shown promising results in a report of 35 cats with feline leukemia virus (FeLV) infection at a dosage of 10 mg/kg PO daily for 4 weeks: the infectivity of serum decreased, whereas the serum antibody increased and the survival of the treated cats was prolonged (Kitchen and Cotter, 1988). Peroral administration of the drug has great advantages. The treatment is continued for several weeks.

Cytokines

Interferons (IFN) are produced by various body cells: IFN-alpha is produced by leukocytes, IFN-beta by fibroblasts and epithelial cells, and IFN-gamma by T cells. IFN of canine or feline origin are not commercially available so far, but the cross-species reactivity of IFN-alpha was demonstrated *in vitro* and *in vivo* (Tompkins and Tompkins, 1990) (see this volume, p. 461). The use of human recombinant IFN-alpha at low doses (0.01 to 0.1 U/ml) increased production of IL-1 and IL-2 by canine cells cultivated *in vitro* but had no effect on blastogenesis of cultured lymphocytes. Interestingly, the activity of natural killer cells was enhanced only with higher doses (10² U/ml), which inhibited B-cell differentiation (Krakowka et al., 1988). A single intramuscular treatment of healthy cats with 10² or 10⁴ U/kg significantly enhanced responses of lymphocyte to concanavalin A (T-cell stimulator) *in vitro*, whereas higher doses (10⁶ U/kg) significantly suppressed the same. The effect on B cells was insignificant (Weiss and Oostrom-Ram, 1990). Single or repeated doses of human IFN were tested in cats with FIP or FeLV with mixed results. One report suggested retarded development of disease following experimental infection of cats with FeLV; an unorthodox peroral treatment with recombinant human IFN-alpha was used (Cummins et al., 1988). Indications for a broader clinical use of IFN in cats and dogs still require more experimental use and studies.

Cytokines of human or recombinant human and canine origin were tested in dogs and cats (reviewed by Tompkins and Tompkins, 1990). For example, canine granulocyte/monocyte-colony stimulating factor (GM-CSF) induced neutrophilic leukocytosis

and monocytosis in healthy dogs. Neutrophilia was also observed after injections of recombinant human IL-1 in experimental dogs (see this volume, p. 466). Recombinant human IL-2 induced eosinophilia in experimental cats. Recombinant human tumor necrosis factor (TNF) or IL-2 in various combinations, however, did not bring improvement in postoperative treatment of various tumors in dogs. Recombinant human IL-4 was found to be a potent mitogen for feline T cells.

Cytokine Inducers

In addition to direct injections of cytokines to animals, one may induce formation of autologous cytokines by stimulating an animal with cytokine inducers using products of *Serratia marcescens* or bacillus Calmette-Guérin (BCG), another IFN inducer. BCG, however, at a dose of 10⁷ living bacteria intralesionally, did not produce a noticeable effect on canine mammary tumors (Parodi et al., 1983).

Staphylococcal Antigens and Phages

Use of extracorporeal immunoadsorption of plasma on *Staphylococcus aureus*, Cowan I strain, was reported in 1984 as an effective treatment of various tumors in cats (Jones et al., 1984). This treatment is suggested to remove circulating immune complexes from plasma and may have other ill-defined effects on the immune function. However, the need for sterile laboratory treatment of plasma limits the use of extracorporeal immunoadsorption to specialized hospitals.

Staphage Lysate (Delmont Laboratories) is a bacteriologically sterile vaccine containing components of *S. aureus* bacteriophage and culture medium ingredients. It is treated neither by heat nor with preservatives. The recommended dosages are 1 ml SC (regardless of weight) in weekly intervals for at least 12 weeks in combination with antibiotics. When pyoderma is cleared, the Staphage Lysate is recommended to be used in 10- to 14-day intervals.

Protein A, derived from *S. aureus*, Cowan I strain, binds specifically to immunoglobulin G and therefore has been used for treatment of diseases in which high levels of circulating immune complexes contribute to the pathogenesis of signs. Protein A is also suggested to activate complement via the alternate pathway. Use of intravenous injections of protein A seems to be a promising technique; it was reported to be effective (at 6.6 μg/kg twice weekly in combination with prednisolone) in the treatment of immune-mediated hemolysis and bone marrow depression associated with FeLV infections (Hitt and McCaw, 1988). Dosages of 60 up to 600 μg/kg/week IV for several weeks were reported to be effective in decreasing the size of various carcinomas, lymphomas, and sarcomas in dogs. This treatment, however, had increasingly severe toxic side effects at doses greater than 400 mg/kg/week (Bowles et al., 1984).

Histamine Receptor Antagonist

Cimetidine (Tagamet, Smith Kline & French Laboratories) is an antagonist for H_2 histamine receptor on cells. Because histamine suppresses various aspects of cellular immunity, cimetidine augments it. Cimetidine was used in conjunction with antibiotics in treatment of canine recurrent pyoderma at a dosage of 3 to 4 mg/kg PO twice daily until pyoderma cleared and for a minimum of 12 weeks thereafter.

FUTURE TRENDS

We have only begun to understand the ways by which one may affect and improve the immune responses of the body. The clinical uses of BRM were in many cases less successful than anticipated from the results of *in vitro* testing. More testing must be done in experimental and clinical situations with combinations of various BRM, vaccines, monoclonal antibodies, and other drugs to achieve better treatment efficacy.

Practically all BRM of cellular origin are administered at toxic or nearly toxic levels to produce a therapeutic effect. Their use in combination or in addition to other treatments often lowers the necessary doses to subtoxic levels. Therefore, we may expect that only medications including various combinations of BRM will be usable in treatment of animal diseases associated with immunologic suppression or deficiency.

We may expect cytokines to become an important adjuvant to vaccines. So far, IL-1, IL-2, and IFN-alpha have shown the most promise in this connection. Species cross-reactivity of cytokines was demonstrated *in vitro*, but the *in vivo* use of cytokines from other species produces generally disappointing results. Consequently, production of species-specific recombinant cytokines seems to be essential for their future therapeutic or vaccine adjuvant use.

The route of administration and the cost limit a broader use of most BRM. Production of cytokines is relatively expensive, and they are usually administered parenterally.

The diseases that will be treated by immunoadjuvant therapy include those that either compromise the immune system or that thrive when the immune system is depressed. They include various types of immunosuppressions (temporary decrease of immune functions) and immunodeficiencies (permanent or long-lasting depression of immune functions), cancerous diseases, and many viral and some bacterial infections.

References and Suggested Reading

Bardana, E. J.: Recent developments in immunomodulatory therapy. J. Allergy Clin. Immunol. 75:423, 1985.
A review on immunomodulation in experimental animals and humans before 1985.

Barriga, O. O., and Andujar, F.: Limited efficacy of levamisole against adults of *Dirofilaria immitis* in a dog. J.A.V.M.A. 192:1743, 1988.
A temporary drop in microfilarial counts in a dog was detected after use of subtoxic doses of levamisole, which had no effect on adult worms.

Barta, O. (ed.): *MHC, Differentiation Antigens, and Cytokines in Animals and Birds.* Blacksburg: BAR-LAB, 1990.
A multiauthor review of the existing knowledge including cytokines.

Becker, A. M., Janik, T. A., Smith, E. K., et al.: *Propionibacterium acnes* immunotherapy in chronic recurrent canine pyoderma: An adjunct to antibiotic therapy. J. Vet. Intern. Med. 3:26, 1989.
The addition of Propionibacterium acnes to the treatment with antibiotics improved the treatment results from 38 to 80% of significant improvements or complete remissions.

Bowles, C. A., Messerschmidt, G., and Deisseroth, A. B.: Experience with *Staphylococcus aureus* and protein A treatment of canine malignancies. J. Biol. Response Mod. 3:260, 1984.
Results with treating canine malignancies with staphylococcal protein A.

Carlisle, C. H., Atwell, R. B., and Robinson, S.: The effectiveness of levamisole hydrochloride against the microfilaria of *Dirofilaria immitis.* Austral. Vet. J. 61:282, 1984.
Subtoxic doses of levamisole resulted in a temporary decrease in microfilarial counts but had no effect on the adult worms.

Cummins, J. M., Tompkins, M. B., Olsen, R. G., et al.: Oral use of human alpha interferon in cats. J. Biol. Response Mod. 7:513, 1988.
Report on the effect of oral administration of IFN-alpha in cats.

Fudenberg, H. H., Whitten, H. D., and Ambrogi, F. (eds.): *Immunomodulation. New Frontiers and Advances.* New York: Plenum, 1984.
A multiauthor review on the progress in immunomodulation before 1984.

Gilman, S. C., and Rogers, T. J. (eds.): *Immunopharmacology.* Caldwell, NJ: Telford Press, 1989.
A textbook on immunopharmacology.

Grassi-Gialdroni, G., and Grassi, C.: Bacterial products as immunomodulating agents. Int. Arch. Allergy Appl. Immunol. 76(suppl. 1):119, 1985.
A review on immunomodulating agents of bacterial origin.

Hitt, M. E., and McCaw, D. L.: FeLV infection, hemolytic anemia and hypocellular bone marrow in a cat: Treatment with protein A and prednisone. Can. Vet. J. 29:737, 1988.
A study on the use of protein A in treating FeLV-associated diseases.

Jacobsen, K. L., and Rockwood, G. A.: Interferons. Their origin and action. J. Vet. Intern. Med. 2:47, 1988.
A general review of interferons and their action.

Jones, F. R., Grant, C. K., and Snyder, H. W.: Lymphosarcoma and persistent feline leukemia virus infection of pet cats: A system to study responses during extracorporeal treatments. J. Biol. Response Mod. 3:286, 1984.
Reported success of extracorporeal immunoadsorption of plasma on Staphylococcus aureus, Cowan I strain in treating lymphosarcoma.

Kitchen, L. W., and Cotter, S. M.: Effect of diethylcarbamazine on serum antibody to feline oncornavirus-associated cell membrane antigen in feline leukemia virus infected cats. J. Clin. Lab. Immunol. 25:101, 1988.
Report on decreases of infectivity, increases of antibody, and survival time in cats treated with diethylcarbamazine.

Krakowka, S., Cummins, J. M., and Ringler, S. S.: The effect of human interferon-alpha upon *in vitro* canine immune responses. Vet. Immunol. Immunopathol. 19:185, 1988.
Report on IL-1 and IL-2 production, blastogenic response, and NK activity after exposure of canine lymphocytes to human IFN-alpha in vitro.

Leifer, C. E., Page, R. L., Matus, R. E., et al.: Proliferative glomerulonephritis and chronic active hepatitis with cirrhosis associated with *Corynebacterium parvum* immunotherapy in a dog. J.A.V.M.A. 190:78, 1987.
Case report on the side effects of C. parvum immunotherapy.

MacEwen, E. G.: Approaches to cancer therapy using biological response modifiers. Vet. Clin. North Am. Small Anim. Pract. 15:667, 1985.
A review on immunotherapy in cancer.

MacEwen, E. G., Harvey, H. J., Patnaik, A. K., et al.: Evaluation of effects of levamisole and surgery on canine mammary cancer. J. Biol. Response Mod. 4:418, 1985a.

No effect was found of levamisole treatment on the survival of dogs with mammary tumors.

MacEwen, E. G., Hayes A. A., Mooney, S., et al.: Evaluation of effect of levamisole on feline mammary cancer. J. Biol. Response Mod. 3:541, 1984.

No significant effect was detected on survival or recurrence of mammary gland tumors in cats treated with levamisole.

MacEwen, E. G., Hayes, A. A., Mooney, S., et al.: Levamisole as adjuvant to chemotherapy for canine lymphosarcoma. J. Biol. Response Mod. 4:427, 1985b.

No effect of levamisole treatment was found on the remission or survival of dogs with lymphosarcoma.

MacEwen, E. G., Kurzman, I. D., Rosenthal, R. C., et al.: Therapy for osteosarcoma in dogs with intravenous injections of liposome-encapsulated muramyl tripeptide. J. Natl. Cancer Inst. 81:935, 1989.

Report on 14 cases of osteosarcoma treated with liposome/muramyl tripeptide.

Misdorp, W.: Incomplete surgery, local immunostimulation, and recurrence of some tumor types in dogs and cats. Vet. Q. 9:279, 1987.

Intralesion administration of Corynebacterium parvum (Propionibacterium acnes) *had no effect on various tumors.*

Mulcahy, G., and Quinn, P. J.: A review of immunomodulators and their application in veterinary medicine. J. Vet. Pharmacol. Ther. 9:119, 1986.

A general review of immunomodulators with a brief section on veterinary application.

Oldham, R. K., and Samlley, R. V.: Immunotherapy: The old and the new. J. Biol. Response Mod. 2:1, 1983.

A review on immunotherapy experience before 1983.

Parodi, A. L., Misdorp, W., Mialot, J. P., et al.: Intratumoral BCG and Corynebacterium parvum therapy of canine mammary tumours before radical mastectomy. Cancer Immunol. Immunother. 15:172, 1983.

Report on unsuccessful treatments of mammary tumors in dogs.

Renoux, G., and Renoux, M.: Effet immunostimulant d'un imidothiazole sur l'immunisation des souris par *Brucella abortus.* Compte Rendu Acad. Sci. (Paris) 269 D:1467, 1971.

Rutten, V. P., Misdorp, W., Gauthier, A. Z., et al.: Immunological aspects of mammary tumors in dogs and cats: A survey including own studies and pertinent literature. Vet. Immunol. Immunopathol. 26:211, 1990.

Circulating immune complexes play a negative role in the generation of effective antitumor immune response.

Tompkins, M. B., Tompkins, W. A. F.: Cytokines in the immunoregulatory network: Potential for therapy in the canine and feline species. *In* Barta, O. (ed.): *MHC, Differentiation Antigens, and Cytokines in Animals and Birds.* Blacksburg: BAR-LAB, 1990, p 81.

A review of cytokines and their use in cats and dogs.

Weiss, R. C.: Immunotherapy for feline leukemia, using staphylococcal protein A or heterologous interferons: Immunopharmacologic action and potential use. J.A.V.M.A. 192:681, 1988.

A review of experience in the use of human IFN and protein A in cats with leukemia.

Weiss, R. C., Cox, N. R., and Oostrom-Ram, T.: Effect of interferon or *Propionibacterium acnes* on the course of experimentally induced feline infectious peritonitis in specific-pathogen-free and random source cats. Am. J. Vet. Res. 51:726, 1990.

Extended survival time reported in interferon and P. acnes treated cats with feline infectious peritonitis.

Weiss, R. C., and Oostrom-Ram, T.: Effect of recombinant human interferon-alpha *in vitro* and *in vivo* on mitogen-induced lymphocyte blastogenesis in cats. Vet. Immunol. Immunopathol. 24:147, 1990.

Report on the effect of human interferon on cat lymphocytes.

PATTERNS OF INFECTION ASSOCIATED WITH IMMUNODEFICIENCY

C. GUILLERMO COUTO

Columbus, Ohio

Recurrent episodes of bacterial and fungal infections and infections with atypical or opportunistic organisms have been recognized in dogs and cats for several decades. However, the pathogenesis of these disorders was not completely understood until the past 10 to 15 years, when basic and applied small animal immunology underwent explosive development. It is now evident that dogs and cats suffer from both congenital and acquired immunodeficiency disorders leading to repeated episodes of fever and infection. Congenital immunodeficiencies appear to be more common in dogs, whereas acquired immunodeficiency syndromes seem to be more common in cats. This article reviews the clinical and laboratory evaluation of dogs and cats with recurrent and atypical infections, as well as the clinical management of the affected patients.

It is currently known that a host defends itself from invading organisms by diverse complex mechanisms (Table 1); all these mechanisms are interrelated. Failure of one or more of these mechanisms to protect the host often leads to the development of infectious disorders that are uncommonly encountered in healthy animals. Depending on the magnitude of the immunodeficiency, these infectious episodes can be severe enough to be life-threatening. In general, the causative organisms and sites of infection are determined by the nature of the defect (Table 2); this phenomenon aids in the selection of diagnostic tests (Johnston, 1984).

Infections in immunocompromised hosts are usually due to one or more of the following organisms: the normal host's bacterial or fungal (or, rarely, viral) flora (e.g., gram-negative bacterial sepsis in neutropenic dogs and cats; candidiasis in dogs with protracted neutropenia after cancer chemotherapy);

Table 1. *Host Defense Mechanisms**

Nonimmunologic Barriers
  Skin and mucous membranes
  Mucociliary apparatus of the respiratory tract
  Microbiologic flora
Immunologic System
  Phagocytic system
    Adhesion
    Migration
    Phagocytosis
    Killing
  Humoral immunity
    Circulating antibodies
    Mucosal antibodies (IgA)
    Complement
  Cellular immunity
    Effector lymphocytes
    Natural killer cells

---

*Modified with permission from Johnston, R. B.: Recurrent bacterial infections in children. N. Engl. J. Med. 310:1237, 1984.

opportunistic organisms (e.g., *Pneumocystis carinii* in dogs with a suspected cell-mediated immunologic defect); pathogens that also occasionally infect immunocompetent animals (e.g., *Toxoplasma gondii* infection in cats infected with feline leukemia virus [FeLV] or feline immunodeficiency virus [FIV] infected cats); or viruses in modified live vaccines (MLV) (e.g., distemper or parvoviral enteritis after using MLV in immunocompromised dogs). Also, immunocompromised patients commonly acquire infections while hospitalized (i.e., nosocomial infections).

CLASSIFICATION OF IMMUNODEFICIENCY SYNDROMES IN DOGS AND CATS

According to the age of onset, immunodeficiency syndromes can be classified as either *congenital* or *acquired* (Tables 3 and 4). Both types of immunodeficiencies have been described in dogs and cats (Greene, 1990) (see this volume, p. 448).

CLINICAL MANIFESTATIONS OF IMMUNODEFICIENCY

As discussed earlier, the type of immunologic defect determines the pattern of infection (i.e., type of organism and site) (see Table 2). Therefore, there are two main clinical manifestations of immunodeficiency: *localized* and *systemic*. Localized infections are usually due to defects in nonimmunologic mechanisms, such as integumentary and mucosal barriers (e.g., urinary bladder diverticuli, neoplasm, or lithiasis leading to recurrent lower urinary tract infections), alterations in the microbiologic flora (e.g., chronic use of antibiotics leading to proliferation of pathogenic organisms), or outflow obstruction (e.g.,

neoplasm in a bronchus leading to secondary pneumonia). Localized recurrent infections occasionally are secondary to systemic immunodeficiencies (e.g., recurrent respiratory tract infections or giardiasis in dogs with IgA deficiency).

Systemic immunodeficiencies usually lead to multifocal or systemic infections with various microorganisms (see Table 2). It is not uncommon to evaluate a patient who has experienced repeated episodes of pneumonia, diarrhea, and pyoderma, either singly or in combination, as a result of a clinically significant immune defect.

LABORATORY EVALUATION OF PATIENTS WITH RECURRENT INFECTIONS

When dealing with a patient with recurrent episodes of infection, clinicians must ask: How many infectious episodes are too many? Unfortunately, there is no clinical rule of thumb to determine when a patient should be evaluated aggressively, so clinicians should exercise their clinical judgment. The following guidelines established for children with recurrent infections may be beneficial for such dogs and cats (Johnston, 1984):

1. Two or more episodes of bacterial infection in the same location (e.g., upper respiratory tract infection, pneumonia, urinary tract infection) should suggest the possibility of an abnormality in a mucosal (cutaneous) barrier, such as ciliary dyskinesia, nasopharyngeal polyps, or urinary bladder diverticuli.

2. Two or more serious episodes of deep pyoderma should suggest the possibility of neutropenia or of a neutrophil function defect; these patients may also have respiratory tract infections coexisting with the pyoderma.

3. Two or more episodes of septicemia may suggest neutropenia, a neutrophil function defect, defects in humoral immunity, or asplenia.

4. Two episodes of bacterial pneumonia within a year should raise the suspicion of a defect in host defense mechanisms.

5. Recurrent or protracted diarrhea or upper respiratory tract infections may suggest a selective IgA deficiency, particularly when coccidia or giardiae are identified as the cause.

6. A single infection with certain intracellular parasites such as *P. carinii* or the development of listeriosis, chronic mucocutaneous candidiasis, or aspergillosis should suggest the possibility of a cell-mediated immunologic defect.

Physical findings in patients with recurrent infections are quite variable and depend on the immunologic defect and the type of organism involved. Three physical findings suggestive of immunodeficiency are oculocutaneous albinism and bleeding tendencies in Persian cats with Chédiak-Higashi syndrome, broad facial features due to skeletal deformity in cats with mucopolysaccharidoses, and

Table 2. *Patterns of Infection in Immunocompromised Dogs and Cats**

Mechanism	Abnormality	Organisms	Sites/Types
Nonimmunologic System			
Skin and mucosae	Diverticuli, lithiasis	Pyogenic, enteric, yeast	Recurrent, same location
Mucociliary flow	Ciliary dyskinesia, bronchial mass	Same	Same
Microbiologic flora	Chronic antibiotic treatment	Same	Same
Phagocytic System			
Adhesion/migration	Adhesive protein defect, defects in migration	Staphylococci, enterics	Skin and respiratory tract
Phagocytosis	Neutropenia	Staphylococci, enterics, yeast	Skin and respiratory tract, diarrhea
	Asplenia/hyposplenia	Pyogenic	Septicemia
	Cell defect	Staphylococci, enterics	Skin and respiratory tract
Killing	Cell defect	Staphylococci, enteric, Candida, aspergillus?	Skin and reticuloendothelium, abscesses
Humoral System			
Circulating Igs	Hypogammaglobulinemia, selective Ig deficiency (except IgA)	Pyogenic, less common enteric	Any site (local or systemic)
Mucosal antibody	IgA deficiency	Pyogenic, enterics?	Respiratory tract, giardiasis, diarrhea, UTI?
Complement	Deficiency	Pyogenic	Bacteremia, meningitis, pyoderma
Cellular Immunity	T-lymphocyte defects	Viruses, fungi, protozoa, bacteria	Any site (local or systemic)
Combined Immunodeficiency		Viruses, fungi, protozoa,	Any site (local or systemic)

*Modified with permission from Johnston, R. B.: Recurrent bacterial infections in children. N. Engl. J. Med. 310:1237, 1984.
Ig, immunoglobulin; ?, not documented in small animals; UTI, urinary tract infection.

Table 3. *Classification of Congenital Immunodeficiency Syndromes in Dogs and Cats*

Disorder	Species	Breed
Phagocytic System		
Cyclic hematopoiesis	D	Gray collie
Neutropenia (B_{12} malabsorption)	D	Giant schnauzer
Adhesive protein deficiency	D	Irish setters
Defective bactericidal capacity	D	Doberman pinscher
Defective bactericidal capacity?	D	Weimaraners
Ciliary dyskinesia	D	English pointer
Chédiak-Higashi syndrome	C	Persian cat
Pelger-Huët syndrome	D	Foxhound, basenji
	C	DSH
Mucopolysaccharidosis	C	Siamese, DSH
Neutrophil granulation defect	C	Birman
Humoral System		
Complement deficiency	D	Brittany spaniel
Selective IgA deficiency	D	Shar pei, beagle, Weimaraner, Airedale?, German shepherd?
Transient hypogammaglobulinemia?	D?	Samoyed?
Selective IgM deficiency?	D?	Doberman pinscher?
Cellular System		
Thymic atrophy/hypoplasia	D	Weimaraner
	C	Burmese cat
Pneumocystosis	D	Dachshund
Lethal acrodermatitis	D	Bull terrier
Systemic aspergillosis?	D	German shepherd
Combined Immune Defects		
Combined immunodeficiency	D	Basset hound

C, cat; D, dog; DSH, domestic short-hair cat; ?, not well documented.

Table 4. *Classification of Acquired Immunodeficiency Syndromes in Dogs and Cats*

Cause	Defect/Mechanism
Infectious Diseases	
Feline panleukopenia	Neutropenia
Feline leukemia virus	Neutropenia, PMN dysfunction, CMI deficiency
Feline immunodeficiency virus	Neutropenia, PMN dysfunction?, CMI deficiency
Canine parvovirus	Neutropenia, CMI deficiency
Canine distemper virus	CMI deficiency
Ehrlichia canis	Neutropenia, CMI deficiency
Demodex canis	CMI deficiency
Bacteremia/septicemia	Neutropenia, PMN dysfunction. asplenia/hyposplenism
Metabolic Disorders	
Diabetes mellitus	PMN dysfunction?
Hyperadrenocorticism	PMN dysfunction?, CMI deficiency, decreased serum immunoglobulin concentration?
Hypophosphatemia	PMN dysfunction?
Uremia (chronic renal failure)	PMN dysfunction
Burns	PMN dysfunction, barrier destruction
Malnutrition	CMI deficiency, PMN dysfunction?
Intestinal lymphangiectasia	Lymphopenia, CMI deficiency?
Malignancy	Neutropenia, PMN dysfunction?, CMI deficiency?
Drug Therapy	
Cancer chemotherapy	Neutropenia, PMN dysfunction?, CMI deficiency
Estrogen	Neutropenia
Anticonvulsants	Neutropenia
Antithyroid drugs	Neutropenia
Some antibiotics	Neutropenia, PMN dysfunction?
Corticosteroids	CMI deficiency, PMN dysfunction?, decreased I. levels
Other	
Immune-mediated neutropenia	Decreased PMN numbers
Cyclic neutropenia	Decreased PMN numbers
Splenectomy	PMN dysfunction?

PMN, neutrophil; CMI, cell-mediated immunity; ?, not well documented.

situs inversus in dogs with ciliary dyskinesia (Kartagener's syndrome).

Routine hematologic and serum biochemical evaluation of patients with suspected immunodeficiency is usually unrevealing. Most hematologic and serum biochemical abnormalities are nonspecific and are secondary to the infectious processes rather than to the primary immune defect. Certain changes, however, may suggest an underlying immune defect, including neutropenia (in infectious or drug-induced disorders, cyclic neutropenia, congenital cobalamine malabsorption in giant schnauzers), marked neutrophilia (i.e., $\geq 100,000$ cells/μl) (in setters with neutrophil adhesive protein deficiency), abnormal polymorphonuclear leukocyte granulation (in Chédiak-Higashi syndrome in Persian cats and abnormal neutrophil granulation of Birman cats), marked neutrophilic pseudo–left shift (in Pelger-Huët anomaly), lymphopenia (in lymphangiectasia), or hypoglobulinemia (in selective immunoglobulin deficiencies).

If a patient appears to be actively infected, collection of appropriate samples for microbiologic analysis is imperative. Samples for bacterial and fungal cultures should be collected from the suspected (or confirmed) septic focus before instituting antimicrobial therapy; if a septic focus cannot be identified, urine and blood cultures should be obtained. Samples for serology (e.g., FeLV, FIV, ehrlichiosis, fungal diseases) should also be submitted if any of those disorders are considered likely (Couto and Giger, 1989).

With the recent advances in veterinary clinical immunology, several diagnostic laboratories now offer various tests for the evaluation of presumed or confirmed immunodeficient patients. Table 2 provides guidelines to order specific tests based on the pattern of infection, and Table 5 lists immunologic tests available for evaluation of dogs and cats with such clinical signs (also see this volume, p. 441).

Overall, the humoral arm of the immune system is relatively easy to evaluate, whereas the phagocytic and cellular arms are more difficult. The difficulty stems from the fact that for most neutrophil function and cell-mediated immunity studies, fresh blood samples are required (i.e., the patient should be the container for the blood), therefore limiting the availability of these tests for private practitioners. Moreover, phagocytic and cell-mediated immunity studies are mainly limited to teaching and research institutions, whereas most com-

Table 5. *Laboratory Evaluation of Dogs and Cats With Recurrent Infections**

Suspected Abnormality	Screening Test	Confirmatory Test
Mucocutaneous Barrier†		
Phagocytic Defect		
Neutropenia	CBC	Bone marrow, other hematologic evaluation
Abnormal chemotaxis	None	Leukocyte migration
Abnormal phagocytosis	None	Bacterial killing, chemiluminescence, flow cytometry
Abnormal killing	NBT	Bacterial killing
Humoral Defect		
Antibody deficiency	SPE, SPIE	Ig concentrations, response to immunizations
Mucosal antibody deficiency	None	Secretory Ig concentration
Complement deficiency	None	Complement determination
Cellular Defect	CBC	Lymphocyte blastogenesis, B- and T-cell subsets

*Modified with permission from Johnston, R. B.: Recurrent bacterial infections in children. N. Engl. J. Med. 310:1237, 1984.
†As indicated by specific location and type of infection.
CBC, complete blood count; NBT, nitroblue tetrazolium test; SPE, serum protein electrophoresis; SPIE, serum protein immunoelectrophoresis.

mercial veterinary diagnostic laboratories perform serum protein electrophoresis and radial immunodiffusion for serum immunoglobulin concentrations.

MANAGEMENT OF PATIENTS WITH RECURRENT INFECTIONS

In general, dogs and cats with suspected immunodeficiency and recurrent or atypical infections should be treated aggressively, because if the immune defect is severe, overwhelming sepsis leading to death is common. Immediately after sample collection, empiric antimicrobial treatment should be instituted, until results of antimicrobial sensitivity tests are available. Overall, antimicrobial treatment should be based on the results of *in vitro* chemosensitivity assays; however, as discussed later, empiric antibiotic therapy also constitutes a viable alternative treatment.

If the clinical findings are suggestive of a severe bacterial infection or of septicemia (e.g., fever or hypothermia, prolonged capillary refill time, tachycardia), aggressive antibiotic treatment should be initiated immediately (i.e., before results of microbial culture and sensitivity tests become available). In our clinic, we use a combination of gentamicin (2.2 mg/kg IV t.i.d.); (or amikacin, 6.7 mg/kg IV

t.i.d.) and cephalothin (Keflin; 20 mg/kg IV t.i.d.). Aminoglycoside therapy should not be initiated if a patient is hypoperfused, because renal hypoperfusion potentiates nephotoxicity. If the clinical signs do not subside within 24 to 48 hr, we substitute moxalactam (Moxam; 15 to 20 mg/kg IV t.i.d.) for the cephalothin, because this drug is extremely active against *Klebsiella*, a common nosocomial organism. If the infection is judged to be mild (and bacterial), sulfadiazine-trimethoprim (Tribrissen; 13 to 20 mg/kg PO b.i.d.) or enrofloxacin (Baytril; 2.3 mg/kg PO b.i.d.) is recommended.

Antifungal therapy should only be instituted if a diagnosis of fungal disease has been confirmed or if the clinical features strongly suggest a mycosis but microbiologic confirmation cannot be obtained; clinicians should be mindful that antifungal therapy is usually quite toxic, and its cost is high.

References and Suggested Reading

Couto, C. G., and Giger, U.: Congenital and acquired neutrophil function abnormalities in dogs. *In* Kirk, R. W. (ed.): *Current Veterinary Therapy* X. Philadelphia: W. B. Saunders, 1989, p. 521.
Greene, C. E.: Immunodeficiency and infectious disease. *In* Greene, C. E. (ed.): *Infectious Diseases of the Dog and Cat.* Philadelphia: W. B. Saunders, 1990, p. 55.
Johnston, R. B.: Recurrent bacterial infections in children. N. Engl. J. Med. 310:1237, 1984.

INFECTIOUS PNEUMONIA

PHILIP ROUDEBUSH

Topeka, Kansas

Along with the gastrointestinal tract, the respiratory tract constitutes a major interface between the environment and the internal tissues of the organism. During normal ventilation or as a result of aspiration, infectious agents may be deposited on mucosal surfaces of airways or may penetrate into the lung parenchyma. Inhaled or aspirated infectious agents encounter a highly integrated defense system that is designed to prevent infection and invasion of host tissues. The integrated system of host defense includes mechanical, phagocytic, and immune mechanisms of resistance. Infectious agents enter the lungs less commonly by the hematogenous route. Whether or not a respiratory tract infection develops depends on the complex interplay of many factors: size, inoculation site, and virulence of the organism versus resistance of the host.

INTEGRATED PULMONARY DEFENSE SYSTEMS

Mechanical Defenses

Mechanical defenses include aerodynamic filtration, airway reflexes, epithelial barriers, and transport mechanisms. These mechanical defenses operate continuously and are nonspecific in that they require no prior exposure of the host to the infectious agent for effective action.

Aerodynamic filtration includes impaction and inertial deposition primarily in the upper airways and sedimentation in the lower airways. Humidification of inhaled air enhances the mechanical defenses by adsorbing noxious gases, preventing dehydration of the epithelial barrier, and forming hygroscopic particles around foreign particulates, thus improving inertial deposition. The complex nasal passages and upper airways of dogs and cats form an imposing aerodynamic barrier to infectious agents. Inspired air is subjected to considerable turbulence in the nasal passages and acute directional changes in flow through the pharynx, larynx, and trachea. Immunologically active tissue (e.g., tonsil) is often found in areas where deposition is likely. As air proceeds to the lung periphery, flow rates decrease rapidly and sedimentation occurs on epithelial barriers as a result of gravitational forces or brownian motion.

Airway reflexes that form part of the integrated defense system include sneeze, cough, and bronchospasm. Cough is a normal physiologic mechanism by which excessive secretions and foreign material are removed from the major airways. A cough that increases in frequency or severity, develops suddenly, or is associated with other respiratory problems is considered a clinical sign of disease.

Epithelial barriers include the epithelial cells and mucus that limit particle penetration. Nonspecific soluble factors in airway secretions that have antimicrobial activity include protease inhibitors, lactoferrin, and lysozyme.

Transport mechanisms include the mucociliary escalator, which moves particulates cephalad, and interstitial lymphohematogenous drainage, which clears particulates centripetally to immunologic tissue. The interstitial lymphohematogenous pathway is a two-edged sword in that it may serve to sequester and disseminate infective organisms (e.g., systemic fungi) and thus be an important contributor to the pathogenic evolution of some infectious respiratory diseases.

Phagocytic Defenses

Infective agents that penetrate mechanical barriers are ingested, inactivated, and removed by phagocytic cells. Ongoing phagocytic activity is fundamentally nonspecific. However, the efficiency of phagocytosis is markedly enhanced by specific antibody and immune activation. In this context, phagocytic defenses provide a vital link between nonspecific mechanical defenses and the antigen-specific immune mechanisms that defend the lungs.

The functions of polymorphonuclear leukocytes and pulmonary macrophages in phagocytic defense are highly integrated and perhaps synergistic. Some aerosolized gram-positive bacteria such as *Staphylococcus* species are cleared by alveolar macrophages alone, whereas gram-negative bacteria such as *Pseudomonas aeruginosa* and *Klebsiella pneumoniae* require both leukocytes and alveolar macrophages for effective clearance.

Immune Defenses

Immunologic mechanisms act to amplify, direct, and augment the nonspecific defenses. Mechanical

228

and phagocytic defenses can be overwhelmed either quantitatively, by the inhalation, aspiration, or hematogenous spread of massive numbers of organisms, or qualitatively, by the deposition of highly virulent organisms that are resistant to nonspecific antimicrobial defenses. Antibody and cellular immune mechanisms constitute the specific mechanisms of respiratory defense. Local humoral immunity is primarily accomplished by immunoglobulin A (IgA) in the upper portions of the respiratory tract and immunoglobulin G (IgG) in the lungs.

Collections of lymphocytes and macrophages, lymphoid aggregates, and nodules are part of a comprehensive mucosal immune system (mucosa-associated lymphoid tissue [MALT]) that includes the cervix, mammary glands, salivary glands, lacrimal glands, gut, and lungs. Submucosal lymphoid nodules located directly subjacent to bronchial mucosa of conducting airways have been called *bronchus-associated lymphoid tissue* (BALT). There is considerable species variation with respect to BALT; rats and rabbits always have BALT, dogs and cats do not have BALT, and the presence and size of BALT in some species (pig) seem dependent on microbial stimulation. BALT does not appear to be a constitutive structure like Peyer's patches, tonsils, or lymph nodes. Tracheobronchial lymph nodes are important in pulmonary immune responses because they contain both antigen-processing cells (macrophages) and the full spectrum of antigen-reactive T and B lymphocytes that are required to mount immune responses to infectious agents entering the lungs.

NORMAL MICROBIAL FLORA IN LOWER RESPIRATORY TRACT

The normal tracheobronchial tree and lung are not continuously sterile. Studies using guarded culture swabs or samples of the lower trachea of clinically healthy dogs have found bacteria in 40 to 50% of samples (Table 1). In one study, aerobic bacteria were isolated from 37% of lung samples, whereas only 10% of dogs examined had no growth from cultures of multiple samples of their lung tissue

Table 1. Bacterial Isolates From Trachea and Lungs of Healthy Dogs

Staphylococcus (coagulase positive and negative)
Streptococcus (alpha and nonhemolytic)
Pasteurella multocida
Klebsiella pneumoniae
Enterobacter aerogenes
Acinetobacter
Moraxella
Corynebacterium

(Lindsey and Pierce, 1978). Most of the bacteria cultured from the trachea and lungs are identical to those found in the pharynx of those same dogs.

These data support the concept that oropharyngeal bacteria are frequently aspirated and may be present for an unknown interval in the normal tracheobronchial tree and lung. This microbial population has the potential to cause or complicate respiratory infection and clouds interpretation of airway and lung cultures.

PREDISPOSING FACTORS

Clinical Conditions

In general, infections with the major respiratory viruses are short-lived, self-terminating events. However, respiratory virus infections have been found to alter bacterial colonization patterns, increase bacterial adherence to respiratory epithelium, and reduce mucociliary clearance and phagocytosis. This impairment of host defenses by the virus may allow resident bacteria to invade the lower respiratory tract, resulting in secondary infection.

Clinical conditions that predispose an animal to bacterial pneumonia include pre-existing viral, mycoplasmal, or fungal respiratory infections; regurgitation, dysphagia, and vomiting; reduced levels of consciousness (stupor, coma, anesthesia); severe metabolic disorders (uremia, diabetes mellitus, hyperadrenocorticism); thoracic trauma or surgery; immunosuppressive therapy (anticancer chemotherapeutic agents, glucocorticoids); therapy with certain drugs (aspirin, digoxin); and functional or anatomic disorders (tracheal hypoplasia, primary ciliary dyskinesia). The most common cause of hematogenous pneumonia is probably intravenous catheter-associated bacteremia, especially in patients with severe underlying disease. All of these conditions overwhelm the existing integrated defense mechanisms or adversely affect defense function.

Parasitic and fungal infections of the respiratory tract primarily occur in young adult animals with significant environmental exposure to these pathogens. Endemic areas for systemic fungi are well documented, whereas exposure to respiratory parasites and their intermediate or transport hosts is more variable.

Malnutrition

Protein-calorie malnutrition has profound adverse effects on systemic and pulmonary defense systems (see this volume, p. 117). Systemic effects of protein-calorie malnutrition include delayed cutaneous hypersensitivity, impaired T-lymphocyte transformation, impaired immunoglobulin turnover, and mild decreases in blood phagocyte function. Malnutrition impairs pulmonary clearance of both aerosolized bacteria and viruses. Protein-calorie malnutrition specifically impairs macrophage recruitment to the lungs in response to organisms whose clearance requires normal cell-mediated immunity (Martin et al., 1983). Alveolar macrophage activation by T lymphocytes is abnormal, and macrophages fail to accumulate in lungs of malnourished animals. Malnutrition may reduce the absolute numbers of T cells or T-cell subpopulations, impair T-cell proliferation, or impair lymphokine production in response to antigenic stimulation. Subclinical malnutrition may be an important factor predisposing critical care patients or patients with prolonged anorexia to infectious pneumonia.

Immunodeficiency

Because immune defenses are an essential part of the integrated pulmonary defense system, immunodeficiencies frequently result in respiratory tract infections. Defects in phagocytic function often result in infections with pyogenic bacteria; defects in humoral immunity or complement often result in encapsulated pyogenic bacterial infections; and defects in cell-mediated immunity encourage infections with viruses, fungi, protozoa, *Mycobacteria*, and *Pneumocystis carinii* (Greene, 1990). Host defense failure syndromes involving defects in neutrophil function, complement, and cell-mediated immunity predispose to more generalized infections, including pneumonia, whereas defects of humoral immunity often result in pneumonia.

PHAGOCYTE DYSFUNCTION

Abnormal neutrophil chemotaxis, adherence, phagocytosis, or bacterial killing predisposes animals to pneumonia. Congenital abnormalities in neutrophil function should be suspected in neonate or juvenile animals with recurrent pneumonia, whereas acquired deficiencies in neutrophil function may occur in adults.

Impaired phagocyte chemotaxis occurs with feline leukemia virus infection, aspirin treatment, and severe hypophosphatemia (phosphorus < 1 mg/dl). Phagocyte adherence defects may accompany poorly regulated diabetes mellitus and aspirin therapy. Phagocytosis is also depressed with severe hypophosphatemia. Impaired bactericidal function has been reported in closely related Doberman pinschers with chronic rhinitis and pneumonia and in cats with feline leukemia virus infection.

Pneumonia is a sequela of acquired neutropenia due to malignancy, cancer chemotherapy, and feline leukemia virus infection. Two commonly used drugs may contribute to bacterial pneumonia. Digoxin blunts the influx of neutrophils into the lungs by inhibiting pluripotential hematopoietic stem cells and granulocyte progenitor cells. Aspirin impairs recruitment of granulocytes by inhibiting adherence and depressing chemotaxis and spontaneous mobility. Aspirin also impairs the nonspecific defense system by reducing both lung mucociliary clearance and tracheal mucociliary transport rate. These effects on the respiratory defense system may be shared by other nonsteroidal anti-inflammatory drugs.

COMPLEMENT DEFICIENCY

Deficiency of C′ 3 is inherited as an autosomal recessive trait. Affected dogs are deficient in hemolytic, opsonic, and chemotactic activities, with a large percentage of animals developing serious bacterial infections, including pneumonia.

B-LYMPHOCYTE DYSFUNCTION

Stimulation of secretory IgA is of primary importance in preventing viral infections of the respiratory and gastrointestinal tract and inhibiting bacterial adherence to mucosal surfaces. Selective IgA deficiency is the most common primary immunodeficiency disease in human beings. Absent or markedly reduced levels of serum and secretory IgA result in respiratory and gastrointestinal tract infections and an increased incidence of allergies and autoimmune diseases.

Selective IgA deficiency has been reported in beagles with recurrent bordetellosis, canine parainfluenza virus infections, otitis externa, pyoderma, and viral enteritis. Sharpei puppies with chronic respiratory tract infections and skin disease were also found to be IgA-deficient. Young dogs suffering from recurrent respiratory tract infections and pyoderma should be tested for IgA levels.

T-LYMPHOCYTE AND COMBINED IMMUNODEFICIENCY

Selected deficiencies in cell-mediated immune function and combined T-cell and B-cell dysfunction have been poorly documented in animals. Concurrent abnormalities in cell-mediated immune function and growth hormone metabolism resulted in wasting disease, unthriftiness, retarded growth, and suppurative pneumonia in one group of inbred weimaraners. A group of miniature dachshunds with *P. carinii* pneumonia were not studied immunologically, but combined immunodeficiency was strongly suspected. Animals with combined immunodeficiency often die of overwhelming viral infections during the neonatal period.

ACUTE PNEUMONIAS

Etiopathogenesis

VIRAL PNEUMONIA

Viral infections that frequently result in pneumonia include canine distemper virus, canine adenovirus, and feline calicivirus. Canine distemper virus infects epithelial tissues throughout the body, including the respiratory tract. Interstitial pneumonia develops as part of the distemper syndrome but is frequently complicated by secondary bacterial pneumonia. Canine adenovirus is frequently implicated in infectious tracheobronchitis but can also cause severe bronchiolitis and subsequent complications with bacterial pneumonia. Feline calicivirus has distinct tropism for alveolar pneumocytes in gas exchange portions of the lungs. Pathogenic strains of calicivirus can cause acute death in kittens and severe signs in older cats by producing a multifocal exudative pneumonia affecting terminal bronchioles, alveolar ducts, and alveoli. Alveolar macrophages and pneumocytes infected with the virus elaborate a neutrophil chemotactic factor that results in massive influx of polymorphonuclear cells into the gas exchange units.

BACTERIAL PNEUMONIA

Bacterial pneumonia is more common in dogs than in cats (Roudebush, 1990). *Bordetella bronchiseptica* and *Streptococcus zooepidemicus* appear to be the principal primary pathogens of canine pneumonia. Most isolates in dogs with pneumonia are thought to be opportunistic invaders, the most common of which are staphylococci, streptococci, *Escherichia coli*, *Pasteurella multocida*, and *Klebsiella pneumoniae* (Table 2). A single bacterial

Table 2. *Most Common Isolates From Dogs With Suspected Bacterial Pneumonia*

Bacterial Organism	% of Dogs
Bordetella bronchiseptica	7–22
Escherichia coli	17–29
Klebsiella	10–15
Pasteurella	7–34
Pseudomonas	6–34
Staphylococcus	9–20
Streptococcus	15–27
Others	17–35

Table 3. *Number of Bacterial Isolates per Positive Sample From Dogs With Suspected Bacterial Pneumonia*

Number of Bacteria	% of Dogs
1	58–60
2	22–23
3	11–16
>4	2–7

pathogen is isolated in the majority of cases, but mixed infections are common (Table 3). Gram-negative isolates predominate in both single and mixed infections.

Bacterial pathogens in feline pneumonia are poorly documented. *B. bronchiseptica* and *Pasteurella* are reported most frequently.

RICKETTSIAL PNEUMONIA

The two major rickettsial agents in dogs, *Rickettsia rickettsii* and *Ehrlichia canis*, can cause pulmonary lesions. Rocky Mountain spotted fever (RMSF) results in respiratory signs more commonly than ehrlichiosis. In one study, 73% of RMSF cases showed evidence of pneumonitis, dyspnea, or cough.

PROTOZOAL PNEUMONIA

Toxoplasmosis can occur in both dogs and cats, though cats are the definitive host for the organism. Immunodeficiency syndromes such as feline leukemia virus or canine distemper virus infection predispose an animal to clinical disease, including pneumonia. One report documented that 9 of 12 cats with acute toxoplasmosis had pulmonary signs.

PARASITIC PNEUMONIA

Dogs and cats are often infected by parasites that reproduce in the trachea, bronchi, and pulmonary parenchyma. These parasitic infections must be differentiated from parasites whose larval forms only migrate through the respiratory system and parasites that migrate aberrantly into the respiratory system.

The severity of clinical manifestations is quite variable, from asymptomatic to acute, fatal infections. This broad range of clinical syndromes depends largely on the number of organisms that infect the respiratory tract, the site of predilection within the respiratory system by the particular parasite, and the nature of a host's response to the adult parasite, ova, or larvae.

Four respiratory parasites are of clinical and practical importance in dogs and cats: *Filaroides (Oslerus) osleri, Aelurostrongylus abstrussus, Capillaria aerophila*, and *Paragonimus kellicotti*. Feline aelurostrongylosis and paragonimiasis in both dogs and cats can cause severe, acute pneumonia. Other primary parasitic respiratory infections occur but are considered uncommon and sporadic.

Clinical Findings and Diagnosis

Historical findings and clinical signs of acute pneumonia include cough, fever, dyspnea, anorexia, serous or mucopurulent nasal discharge, depression, and dehydration. Auscultation usually reveals abnormal breath sounds including increased intensity or bronchial breath sounds, crackles, and wheezes.

Diagnosis of acute pneumonia is confirmed by hematologic findings, thoracic radiographs, and microbiologic, parasitic, and cytologic examination of material from the tracheobronchial tree, lungs, or feces (Zinkl, 1986). A neutrophilic leukocytosis with a left shift is frequently (but not invariably) found in patients with bacterial pneumonia. Fecal evaluation for parasites should include a direct smear, flotation, sediment examination, and Baermann's technique. Arterial blood gas values correlate well with the degree of physiologic disruption in patients with pneumonia and are a sensitive monitor of a patient's progress during treatment. Thoracic radiographs reveal an interstitial pattern with viral and rickettsial pneumonia, whereas bacterial pneumonia results in an alveolar pattern characterized by increased pulmonary densities in which margins are indistinct and in which air bronchograms or consolidation may be seen (Kneller, 1986). A patchy or lobar alveolar pattern will be present in a cranial ventral lung lobe distribution with bacterial pneumonia.

The definitive method of establishing a diagnosis is to obtain aspirates, washings, or brushings for microbiologic and cytologic examinations. Procedures that bypass the oropharynx such as transtracheal aspiration, bronchoscopy, or fine-needle lung aspiration are recommended to obtain these specimens (McKiernan, 1989; Roudebush, 1983). Blood cultures may be helpful in identifying the etiologic agent causing bacterial pneumonia.

Treatment Principles

Unlike treatment of upper respiratory tract infections, therapy for pneumonia must be aggressive, and systemically effective antimicrobials or antiparasitics must be used. Drug penetration into consolidated lung tissue is more effective systemically than by topical means.

ANTIMICROBIALS

Oral and parenteral antibacterials are the principal therapy for bacterial pneumonia. It is unrealistic to expect any single antibacterial to be routinely effective against the wide variety of organisms causing bacterial pneumonia. The most important criterion for selection of an antibacterial agent is identification of the bacterial organism. Substantially more patients recover if antibacterial therapy is administered according to culture results and *in vitro* susceptibility testing than if empirically administered (see this volume, p. 207).

Initial choices of antibacterials can be based on the shape of bacteria noted on airway or lung cytologic preparations (Table 4). Cocci are usually staphylococci or streptococci. Rods are usually members of the family Enterobacteriaceae, which are the most unpredictable with respect to antibacterial agents. Levels of antibacterials in airway secretions after oral or parenteral administration are much lower than serum levels. Therefore, systemic antibacterials should be administered in high doses for long periods so that maximum concentrations are reached in lung tissue and airway secretions.

ANTIPARASITICS

The most successful mode of therapy for respiratory parasites is use of the drugs levamisole, thiabendazole, albendazole, fenbendazole, invermectin, and praziquantel. Documented drug efficacies are listed in Table 5. Benzimidazoles both kill

Table 4. *Antimicrobial Therapy for Infectious Pneumonia*

Gram-positive cocci	Ampicillin, amoxicillin, chloramphenicol, gentamicin, trimethoprim-sulfonamide, first-generation cephalosporin
Gram-negative rods	Amikacin, chloramphenicol, gentamicin, trimethoprim-sulfonamide, fluroquinolones
Bordetella	Amikacin, chloramphenicol, tetracycline, gentamicin, kanamycin
Anaerobes	Ampicillin, amoxicillin, penicillin, second- or third-generation cephalosporins, clindamycin
Rickettsia	Chloramphenicol, doxycycline, imidocarb dipropionate, minocycline, tetracycline
Toxoplasma	Clindamycin, pyrimethamine, sulfonamides
Fungi	Amphotericin B, intraconazole, ketoconazole

Table 5. *Drug Efficacies for Respiratory Parasites*

	Aelurostrongylus	Capillaria	Filaroides	Paragonimus
Albendazole	x	x	x	x
Fenbendazole	x	x	x	x
Ivermectin	x	x	x	
Levamisole	x	x	x	
Praziquantel				x
Thiabendazole			x	

helminths and cause temporary suppression of egg production by female worms that survive treatment. Results of fecal examination for eggs or larvae may be negative for several weeks after treatment. Fecal examinations should be repeated in 6 to 8 weeks to further evaluate benzimidazole therapy.

HYDRATION

Maintenance of normal systemic hydration is an important therapeutic objective in patients with pneumonia. Dehydration hinders mucociliary clearance and secretion mobilization because normal respiratory secretions are more than 90% water.

AEROSOLS

The goal of aerosol therapy is to mobilize secretions by adding water to the mucociliary blanket. A nebulizer that produces particles between 0.5 and 3.0 μm must be used to ensure that water is deposited in the lower airways. Water vaporizers or humidifiers are inadequate for this purpose. The animal is placed in an enclosed chamber and a bland aerosol (normal saline) is nebulized into the chamber. The animal should be treated several times daily for 30 to 45 min per treatment. Because bronchoconstriction often develops, pretreatment with bronchodilators is recommended.

Nebulization with bland aerosols has subjectively resulted in more rapid resolution of cases of canine bronchopneumonia when used in conjunction with physiotherapy and systemic antibacterials. Physiotherapy should always be used immediately after aerosolization to enhance secretion clearance. Physiotherapy methods include mild forced exercise, chest wall coupage, tracheal manipulation to encourage cough, and postural drainage. Although aerosol administration of nonabsorbable antibacterials such as aminoglycosides substantially reduces the number of bacteria in airways, routine intratracheal or aerosol administration of antibacterials is not recommended with current techniques available for animals.

SUPPORTIVE MEASURES

Animals with severe tachypnea, dyspnea, or marked hypoxemia (Pa_{O_2} < 60mm Hg) require oxygen therapy. The early period of highest mortality with pneumonia corresponds to the period of greatest hypoxemia. Drugs such as antitussives and antihistamines that inhabit mucokinesis and exudate removal from the airways are contraindicated.

CHRONIC PNEUMONIAS

Etiopathogenesis

VIRAL PNEUMONIA

The common clinical picture of feline infectious peritonitis (coronavirus) is pleural effusion or ascites. However, feline infectious peritonitis can involve the pulmonary parenchyma, resulting in pyogranulomatous pneumonia. This noneffusive form of the disease is rarely encountered but represents a unique immunopathologic response of cats to infection with coronavirus.

BACTERIAL PNEUMONIA

Bacterial pneumonia usually presents as an acute clinical condition. However, several chronic sequelae to bacterial pneumonia are important.

Bronchiectasis is pathologically defined as an abnormal and permanent dilation of subsegmental airways. The affected airways become tortuous and flabby and are usually partially obstructed by purulent or viscid exudates. Peripheral airways are inflamed and sometimes filled with secretions because of the more proximal obstruction. Focal bronchiectasis most often results from foreign body aspiration. Diffuse bronchiectasis often occurs subsequent to aspiration or inhalation injury, bordetellosis in puppies, primary ciliary dyskinesia, or chronic bronchitis. Abnormal host defense may have a role in many cases of bronchiectasis but has received little attention in veterinary medicine. Humoral immunodeficiency, usually panhypogammaglobulinemia, is frequently associated with bronchiectasis in humans. Selective IgA deficiency is the most common immunodeficiency but is usually associated with chronic upper airway infections rather than bronchiectasis.

A "vicious cycle" hypothesis for the pathogenesis of bronchiectasis has been proposed (Barker and Bardana, 1988). In this hypothesis, damaging insults to the bronchial tree may compromise the first-line bronchial defense mechanism of mucociliary clearance and predispose to microbial colonization of the bronchial tree. A host's inflammatory response to these microorganisms fails to eliminate microbial colonists, resulting in damage to host lung tissue in the process. This damage is likely to reduce mucociliary clearance further and lead to increasing microbial colonization and progressive lung damage. Immunohistologic evidence suggests that a significant cell-mediated immune response develops in inflamed areas of bronchiectatic lung. This could be responsible, at least in part, for progressive lung damage, either by the emergence of a cytotoxic lymphocyte population or by the activation of macrophages.

Hypergammaglobulinemia and autoantibodies have also been detected in human patients with bronchiectasis of unknown etiology. More than 73% of people in one study had panhypergammaglobulinemia with a high prevalence of rheumatoid factors (52%) and antinuclear antibodies (19%). Increased levels of circulating immune complexes have also been reported in people with bronchiectasis.

Chronic bronchitis is a heterogenous syndrome characterized by chronic inflammation and excessive mucus production in the bronchial tree, resulting in chronic or recurrent cough. The airways in patients with chronic bronchitis are characterized by goblet cell metaplasia, smooth-muscle hypertrophy, submucosal gland hypertrophy, and airway wall fibrosis and inflammation. Airway mucosal and luminal inflammation correlates with volume of mucus production, implying that neutrophils may have a pathogenetic role in chronic bronchitis. Potential causes that may incite or perpetuate the disease include ciliary dysfunction, chronic exposure to inhaled irritants (smoke, pollen, air pollutants), allergy, and chronic bronchial infection, especially with B. bronchiseptica.

A pulmonary abscess is a necrotic area of lung parenchyma containing purulent material usually produced by pyogenic infection. Pulmonary abscesses are uncommon in dogs and cats. Most arise from aspiration of oropharyngeal or gastric contents and are termed primary lung abscess. Secondary lung abscess results from a primary underlying process such as bronchial obstruction, septic or heartworm thromboemboli, paragonimiasis, foreign body, bullous emphysema, tuberculous cavities, or neoplasia. Obligate anaerobic bacteria are identified more frequently than aerobes, but mixed infections are common.

Mycobacterial infections causing tuberculosis are uncommon today. A recent report described dogs that had intimate association with humans who had tuberculosis. Pulmonary lesions of tuberculosis include pleural effusion, tracheobronchial lymphadomegaly, and interstitial granulomatous pneumonia. Systemic signs of fever, weight loss, anorexia, uveitis, generalized lymphadomegaly and hepatosplenomegaly are most common.

PROTOZOAL PNEUMONIA

Pulmonary signs occur in approximately one fourth of cats with chronic toxoplasmosis. Chronic disease generally affects the nervous system, muscles, and eyes. In dogs, the disease often occurs concurrently with canine distemper.

P. carinii is a protozoal organism that causes pulmonary disease in immunocompromised patients. Increased awareness of this disease has occurred as a result of complications in people with immunodeficiency virus infection (AIDS) and those receiving intense immunosuppressive therapy. P. carinii is a saprophyte of low virulence that inhabits the mammalian respiratory tract. Most reports of clinical pneumonia are linked with documented or suspected immunodeficiency in the host. In general, Pneumocystis infections in dogs and cats are thought to be latent or subclinical. The organism has been found in the lungs of cats, but no clinical disease was reported. Most canine cases have been in dachshunds that were less than 6 months old and that had suspected congenital immunodeficiency. The typical clinical history in dogs is gradual weight loss and respiratory difficulty.

PARASITIC PNEUMONIA

The clinical signs and lesions of feline aelurostrongylosis depend to a great extent on the number of parasites involved and the response of the individual cat to the adult parasites, eggs, and larvae. The parasites and larvae can stimulate an intense granulomatous inflammatory response consisting of mononuclear cells and eosinophils, which may develop as nodules throughout the lungs, especially in the subpleural region. On the other hand, many cats show little or no clinical disease due to infection. Typical signs of clinical aelurostongylosis include a chronic, harsh, nonproductive cough, as well as dyspnea, tachypnea, anorexia, fever, and lethargy. These signs may be quite progressive and severe. The most dangerous period is 6 to 13 weeks after infection, when great numbers of eggs and larvae are deposited in the pulmonary parenchyma.

Clinical signs of paragonimiasis in dogs and cats vary with the number of parasites infecting the host and a host's reaction to the adults and ova. Experimentally inoculated cats have been clinically normal despite radiographic evidence of lesions. This may also occur in natural infection. Typical clinical signs of paragonimiasis include chronic productive cough, respiratory distress, acute dyspnea associated with pneumothorax, hemoptysis, ptyalism, and systemic signs such as anorexia, lethargy, and weight loss. The pathologic features of paragonimiasis consist of parasitic cysts or cavities (pneumatocysts) and an intense eosinophilic inflammatory response to both the adults and ova. Pneumothorax occurs frequently as a result of communication of the pneumatocyst with the pleural space.

FUNGAL PNEUMONIA

The organisms that cause systemic or deep mycotic infections are endemic in large areas of North America. Mycotic pneumonias are common in dogs and cats because of fungi's wide environmental distribution and their use of airborne spores for reproduction.

Pulmonary lesions are reported in one fourth to one half of feline cases of cryptococcosis, although the upper respiratory tract, central nervous system, eyes, skin, and lymph nodes are the most common sites of infection. Cryptococcal pneumonia may represent direct infection of the lungs from environmental sources or merely an extension of the infection from primary sites in the upper airways. *Cryptococcus* is an opportunistic fungus that usually causes disease in immunosuppressed cats. Feline leukemia virus infection, malignancy, chronic glucocorticoid administration, and malnutrition are commonly associated with feline cryptococcosis. Pneumonia and tracheobronchial lymphadomegaly are rare clinical presentations in canine cryptococcosis. Most dogs with cryptococcal lung lesions are not diagnosed antemortem, but approximately 50% of reported cases had respiratory lesions.

The pathophysiology of pulmonary histoplasmosis, blastomycosis, and coccidioidomycosis are so similar that they are discussed together here. In general, the immunopathologic response of a host determines the extent and severity of the lesions. After exposure to the spores, a self-limited acute pulmonary infection often occurs in which the organisms initially reproduce but are later eliminated by the cell-mediated immune response. Transient fever and cough signal the acute pneumonia, but these clinical signs are often indistinguishable from those of viral or bacterial tracheobronchitis. An animal may initially recover from the acute pneumonia, but the organisms remain quiescent in the lungs. Endogenous reactivation of this infective focus may occur at a later time.

With an inadequate host response during the acute pneumonia, the organisms continue to proliferate, and massive granulomatous or pyogranulomatous inflammation results in interstitial and alveolar flooding. Progressive pulmonary infection ensues, with or without extrapulmonary involvement. Progressive pulmonary infection is recognized as chronic cough, wheezing, tachypnea, dyspnea, anorexia, weight loss, fever, and death.

The second major pathophysiologic pathway is noted in animals that do not initially exhibit clinical signs of acute pneumonia. In one group of animals, multiplication of the organisms is restricted by cell-mediated immune mechanisms, and the organisms are destroyed before clinical signs develop. This subclinical form of infection may be very common. A smaller group of animals has an insidious onset of chronic pulmonary or extrapulmonary disease. Chronic pulmonary fungal infections usually result in granulomatous or pyogranulomatous interstitial pneumonia, tracheobronchial lymphadomegaly, and rarely pleural effusion.

Immunopathogenesis

Granulomatous inflammation is manifested in chronic inflammatory diseases that often result in tissue destruction. The common histopathologic feature of granulomatous inflammation, infiltrating mononuclear leukocytes, is observed in various granulomatous disease caused by infectious agents (tuberculosis, histoplasmosis), as well as noninfectious (silicosis, berylliosis) and unknown agents. A granuloma has classically been defined as a chronic, focal immune reaction characterized by mononuclear phagocytes. However, granulomatous inflammation demonstrates wider heterogeneity with regard to the cellular infiltrate. Hypersensitivity-type (immunologic) granulomas involve a delayed-type, antigen-specific immunologic response induced by a plethora of infectious agents including bacteria, viruses, fungi, and helminths. At the onset of pulmonary granulomatous inflammation, monocytes and macrophages become activated and synthesize various potent mediators (cytokines).

Mononuclear phagocytic cells are crucial in maintaining a granulomatous lesion by exerting a strong influence on neighboring immune and nonimmune cells. The local or systemic production of macrophage-derived mediators may stimulate and regulate lymphocyte responses, recruit and activate inflammatory cells, prime the host for a systemic immune response, and alter the activity of fibroblasts. Future therapeutic intervention will undoubtedly target the pharmacologic regulation of specific cytokines. By selectively removing specific cytokines from the mediator "cocktail," hypersensitivity and inflammatory reactions may be reduced or controlled.

Clinical Findings and Diagnosis

Historical findings, clinical signs, and diagnostic protocols for chronic pneumonias are similar to those outlined for acute pneumonia. Bronchoscopy is essential in the evaluation of chronic bronchitis and bronchiectasis. Serologic tests can also be added for the evaluation of patients suspected of having mycotic infection.

Complete evaluation of patients with chronic or recurrent pulmonary infections should include assessment of the respiratory defense mechanisms. This is especially important in young dogs and cats with recurrent disease but should also encompass adults with severe infectious disease, such as mycotic pneumonia (Degen and Breitschwerdt, 1986). Ciliary function can be assessed with nasal biopsies and mucociliary clearance studies. Phagocytic defenses are assessed with cell bioassay studies of neutrophil or macrophage chemotaxis, phagocytosis, and bacterial killing. Complement activity is most commonly measured by a 50% hemolytic complement (CH_{50}) assay. Humoral immune defenses are assessed by protein electrophoresis and quantitation of immunoglobulins by immunoelectrophoresis or radial immunodiffusion. Cell-mediated immune function is usually screened with *in vitro* lymphocyte responses to mitogens. Intradermal mitogen stimulation tests can be used as a rapid method for *in vivo* assessment of cell-mediated immunity. Skin-fold thickness and skin biopsy samples for assessment of cellular responses are obtained 24 hr after intradermal injection of a mitogen such as phytohemagglutinin P. This technique was successful is estimating the survival of dogs with canine distemper and should be evaluated more widely in animals with chronic or recurrent infectious diseases (see this volume, p. 441).

Treatment Principles

Treatment of animals with chronic infectious pneumonia is similar to that outlined for acute pneumonia. Animals with documented abnormalities in the respiratory defense mechanisms should warrant aggressive and long-term therapy with antimicrobials and supportive care.

References and Suggested Reading

Barker, A. F., and Bardana, E. J.: Bronchiectasis: Update of an orphan disease. Am. Rev. Respir. Dis. 137:969, 1988.
  A review of the etiology, pathology, host-insult pathogenesis, prognosis, and suggested evaluation of human patients with bronchiectasis.
Degen, M. A., and Breitschwerdt, E. B.: Canine and feline immunodeficiency, Part II. Comp. Cont. Ed. Pract. Vet. 8:379, 1986.
  Offers suggestions for diagnostic evaluation of immunodeficient patients and covers therapeutic considerations in treating them.
Greene, C. E.: Immunodeficiency and infectious disease. *In* Greene, C. E. (ed.): *Infectious Diseases of the Dog and Cat.* Philadelphia: W. B. Saunders, 1990, p. 55.
  Review of immunodeficiencies and how they relate to infectious diseases in dogs and cats.
Kneller, S. K.: Thoracic radiography. *In* Kirk, R. W. (ed.): *Current Veterinary Therapy IX.* Philadelphia: W. B. Saunders, 1986, p. 250.
  Review of positioning and technique, gross pulmonary anatomy, and roentgen signs of the thorax, with helpful explanatory diagrams.
Lindsey, J. O., and Pierce, A. K.: An examination of the microbiologic flora of normal lung of the dog. Am. Rev. Respir. Dis. 117:501, 1978.
  Describes culture results from the pharynx, trachea, and lungs of healthy adult dogs.
Martin, T. R., Altman, L. C., and Alvares, O. F.: The effects of severe protein-calorie malnutrition on antibacterial defense mechanisms in the rat lung. Am. Rev. Respir. Dis. 128:1013, 1983.
  Discusses mechanisms that may underlie the pathogenesis of pulmonary infections associated with malnutrition.
McKiernan, B. C.: Bronchoscopy in the small animal patient. *In* Kirk, R. W. (ed.): *Current Veterinary Therapy X.* Philadelphia: W. B. Saunders, 1989, p. 219.
  Review of equipment, indications, contraindications, technique, and normal and abnormal findings during bronchoscopy of dogs and cats.
Roudebush, P.: Diagnostics for respiratory disease. *In* Kirk, R. W. (ed.): *Current Veterinary Therapy VIII.* Philadelphia: W. B. Saunders, 1983, p. 222.
  Reviews ancillary diagnostic techniques such as transtracheal aspiration, thoracocentesis, endoscopy, and fine-needle lung aspiration.
Roudebush, P. Bacterial infections of the respiratory system. *In* Greene, C. E. (ed.): *Infectious Diseases of the Dog and Cat.* Philadelphia: W. B. Saunders, 1990, p. 114.
  Comprehensive review of normal respiratory tract flora, upper respiratory tract bacterial infections (rhinitis, sinusitis), lower respiratory tract infections (pneumonia), and pleural infections.
Zinkl, J. G.: Cytology of respiratory tract disease. Semin. Vet. Med. Surg. (Small Anim.) 1:302, 1986.
  Comprehensive review that discusses sampling techniques, sample preparation, normal cellular elements, inflammation, neoplasia, agents, and pleural effusion.

INFECTIOUS DIARRHEA IN THE DOG AND CAT

STEPHEN A. KRUTH

Guelph, Ontario

One of the most common presenting complaints in small animal practice is diarrhea. Many cases resolve spontaneously within a few days or with only supportive therapy. A large proportion of these cases are probably due to dietary indiscretion or are of viral origin. Animals with chronic diarrhea may pose difficult diagnostic and management challenges. A specific diagnosis may not be reached, and the animal is treated for "nonspecific" diarrhea. Management usually includes feeding a low-fat, easily digested diet and may include gastrointestinal motility–modifying drugs and intestinal absorbents/protectants. Antibiotics are often included in the therapeutic protocol. Unfortunately, the prevalence of infectious agents causing simple, hemorrhagic, or chronic diarrhea in dogs and cats is not known. Little is known about the role of infectious agents as a cause of diarrhea in companion animals, especially compared with what is known about their role in humans and livestock.

The health of the gastrointestinal system depends on interactions between the normal gastrointestinal flora, nonspecific mechanisms that moderate bacterial numbers, and the gastrointestinal immune system. Many disease processes (e.g., allergy, neoplasia), as well as clinical interventions (e.g., administration of antibiotics and chemotherapeutic drugs), can potentially disrupt these systems. These perturbations lead to abnormal intestinal function and the clinical sign of diarrhea, even without exposure to specific pathogens.

The definition of an enteric pathogen is at times difficult. Many normal animals carry *Salmonella*, *Campylobacter*, and *Giardia*, and it may be difficult to induce diarrhea experimentally in healthy animals with organisms such as canine coronavirus, *Clostridium perfringens,* or *Isospora.* Simple exposure to these potential "pathogens" is not sufficient to cause diarrhea; perturbations of the complex intestinal environment are also necessary. In many cases, dietary factors, microbial interactions, immunosuppression, and therapeutic interventions are probably cofactors in the establishment of enteric infections.

The goals of this article are to review the ecology and immunology of the gastrointestinal system, to present a general approach to the diagnosis and management of a dog or cat with infectious diarrhea, and to catalogue known and suspected gastrointestinal pathogens of dogs and cats.

NORMAL ENTERIC FLORA

The normal enteric flora is acquired both from the body of the mother and from the environment shortly after birth and is established by a few weeks of age. The enteric microbial population is tremendously complex, with environmental requirements ranging from aerobic through obligate anaerobic conditions. In humans, more than 400 bacterial species may live within an individual's colon. The type, number, and location of organisms within the gut are surprisingly stable. If disrupted, the normal bacterial population usually re-establishes itself quickly after removal of the disruptive influence.

Resident and pathogenic bacteria sometimes attach to the gut epithelium to establish residence. Adherence is mediated by bacterial fimbriae and pili, which bind to receptors on epithelial cells. The location of organisms within the gut is partially determined by the specificity of these structures.

In healthy individuals, the stomach and small bowel contain relatively small numbers of gram-positive aerobes or facultative anaerobes, which are derived primarily from the oropharynx. Coliforms may be transiently present but are not normally resident. The ileum is a zone of transition from these relatively sparse populations of aerobic flora to the dense anaerobic populations found in the colon. The ileocecal valve is an anatomic barrier that limits colonic residents from colonizing the small intestine. The colon has an extremely dense population of anaerobes such as *Bacteroides*, clostridia, anaerobic lactobacilli, spirochetes, and yeasts. A numerically minor population of aerobic and facultative anaerobic gram-positive organisms such as *Streptococcus* are also present. The facultatively anaerobic gram-negative Enterobacteriaceae population includes *Escherichia coli, Enterobacter,* and *Klebsiella.* The Enterobacteriaceae are clinically significant as potential pathogens in other organ systems.

This complex bacterial population is a determinant of normal gut morphology and function. Bacteria are involved in the metabolism of cholesterol and bile acids and the degradation of protein. They influence gut motility as well as the gastrointestinal immune system.

Several nonspecific mechanisms regulate the normal type and number of flora; these mechanisms also serve as defenses against colonization by pathogens. The most important are postprandial and interdigestive motility patterns, which move ingesta through the gut. Alterations in motility can significantly affect bacterial populations. Ileus secondary to drugs or disease can lead to a bloom of bacteria in the small bowel. This overgrowth of normal aerobes or anaerobes can in itself cause diarrhea. Bacteria may directly damage the mucosal brush border, leading to decreased secretion of enzymes and maldigestion. Bacterial deconjugation of bile acids may result in deficiencies in fat absorption. Deconjugated bile acids are secretagogues, which induce fluid and electrolyte loss. Hydroxylated fatty acids are produced by bacteria from unabsorbed fats. They have detergent effects and further damage the brush border. Commonly used drugs, such as parasympatholytics, can alter gastrointestinal motility and can potentially disrupt the numbers and location of normal flora (Willard, 1989).

Gastric acidity kills many organisms and is another mechanism that limits normal flora numbers in the small intestine and protects the gut from colonization by pathogens. Achlorhydria is associated with bacterial overgrowth, and the administration of drugs that neutralize gastric pH can potentially disrupt the normal flora. Other nonspecific mechanisms that regulate normal flora include the bacteriostatic action of bile and the steric interference of lysozyme. Intestinal mucus aids in the mechanical process of removing organisms, as does epithelial cell turnover.

The normal colonic flora deters colonization by pathogens by preventing their attachment by steric hindrance. Other interactions include the mutual competition for essential nutrient substrates, the induction of low local pH and oxidation-reduction potentials, the metabolism of toxins, and the inhibition of bacterial translocation (the passage of bacteria from the lumen into the mesenteric lymph nodes). The normal residents produce colicins and free bile acids that inhibit bacterial growth in the colon. Short-chain fatty acids, especially acetic and butyric acids, are secreted by obligate anaerobes. The combination of fatty acids, low pH, and low oxidation-reduction potentials inhibits the growth of Enterobacteriaceae. The normal flora also has indirect effects that are potentially protective, including the enhancement of local antibody production and the stimulation of peristalsis. The normal flora may potentially complicate the medical management of bacterial infections by conferring antibiotic resistance to pathogens through the transfer of plasmids.

GASTROINTESTINAL IMMUNE SYSTEM

The gastrointestinal immune system is part of the common mucosal immune system, which includes bronchial-associated lymphoid tissue and lymphoid tissue in the female reproductive tract and mammary glands. The local immune system of the gut is centered around the gut-associated lymphoid tissue (GALT), which is a major peripheral lymphoid organ. The primary functions of the GALT are to prevent the adherence of microorganisms and parasites and to neutralize bacterial toxins. The GALT is organized into isolated lymphoid follicles, Peyer's patches, diffuse lymphoid cells in the lamina propria, intraepithelial lymphocytes, and the mesenteric lymph nodes. Nonlymphoid cells involved in the immune response include macrophages, eosinophils, and mast cells. Little is known about the GALT of dogs and cats, and the following information is generalized from studies of other species.

Isolated lymphoid follicles are abundant in the intestinal mucosa and are scattered throughout the length of the intestine. In the terminal small intestine, aggregates of follicles form Peyer's patches. These are specialized aggregates of lymphoid tissue that are compartmentalized into B-cell follicles and interfollicular areas that primarily contain helper T lymphocytes. Peyer's patches are sampling sites for intestinal antigens and play a major part in the initiation of the intestinal immune response. They give rise to immunoglobulin A (IgA) and immunoglobulin E (IgE)–secreting B cells, IgA-specific helper T cells, immunoglobulin G (IgG)–specific suppressor T cells, precursors of intraepithelial lymphocytes, and mucosal mast cells. Peyer's patches are covered by the follicle-associated epithelium (FAE), which characteristically contains cuboidal epithelial cells and reduced numbers of goblet cells. The epithelial cells are called M (membranous) cells, with the role of antigen uptake from the luminal environment. Cells in contact with the FAE include helper T cells, macrophages, and dendritic cells, which are responsible for antigen processing and presentation. M cells may also act as the portal of entry for some viruses.

Although B cells become committed to the IgA class in Peyer's patches, they do not mature into antibody-secreting cells until they have completed a systemic migration. Lymphocytes leave Peyer's patches then migrate through afferent lymphatics to the mesenteric lymph nodes, thoracic duct, and systemic circulation and eventually return to the lamina propria. Some of these cells travel to other areas of the mucosal immune system, allowing integration of the immune response. One benefit of lymphocyte migration is that antigen specificity of colostral IgA reflects the antigenic exposure that the B cells had in the maternal gut.

B lymphocytes and plasma cells are scattered

throughout the lamina propria. Seventy to 90 per cent of these cells secrete a dimer of IgA that is complexed to a glycoprotein called secretory component (SC). Secretory IgA (sIgA) is transported through the epithelial cells and is associated with the luminal side of the gut epithelium. It is also found in high levels in bile. In addition to providing the mechanism for transporting the IgA dimer, SC appears to stabilize sIgA against proteolysis at the brush border. Secretory IgA inhibits microorganism and parasite attachment, neutralizes toxins, limits replication and mucosal penetration of viruses, and restricts the absorption of food antigens. IgA does not activate the complement cascade, does not significantly participate in antibody-dependent cell-mediated cytotoxic reactions, and is not an opsonizing antibody. Because the intestinal mucosa is continuously exposed to a broad array of antigenic material with the potential of activating mucosal inflammatory reactions, it seems appropriate that IgA does not have these functions.

Fifteen to 20 per cent of B cells in the lamina propria secrete IgM. IgE-positive lymphocytes are variably present. IgE may be a potent mediator of antibody-dependent cell cytotoxicity and is thought to have a role in the host response to metazoan parasites, whereas abnormal IgE responses appear to be associated with allergic intestinal disorders. There is a paucity of IgG-secreting cells in the gut. Approximately 25% to 40% of lamina propria T cells have markers characteristic of helper cells. A smaller percentage have markers consistent with cytotoxic and suppressor functions. The suppressor cells appear to limit systemic IgG responses to dietary antigens. Also, there appears to be antigenic similarity between the epithelial cell surfaces and the associated normal flora; thus, normal animals do not develop an immune response to their resident flora. Intraepithelial lymphocytes are primarily T cells; their function has not been determined.

Cell-mediated cytotoxic responses are probably important in the gut; however, they are poorly understood. Cytotoxic T cells may play a major part in the defense against viruses, intracellular bacteria, and fungi. Natural killer (NK) cells may have a role in tumor cell surveillance. Antibody-dependent cytotoxic activity has also been demonstrated in the gut.

Live, inactivated, and subunit oral vaccines against *Salmonella typhi*, *Vibrio cholerae*, *Shigella*, and rotavirus are under development for use in humans. Kennel-specific oral *E. coli* vaccines have been shown to significantly decrease morbidity and mortality in high-risk kennels. The development of effective vaccines against enteric pathogens and oral vaccines for systemic pathogens will require a better understanding of the GALT physiology in dogs and cats. The gastrointestinal immune system and vaccination against enteric bacterial diseases in humans have been reviewed elsewhere (Hone and Hackett, 1989).

CONSEQUENCES OF INFECTION

For a pathogen to cause diarrhea, it must be ingested in sufficient numbers so that a minimum population survives gastric acidity and other nonspecific protective mechanisms. Bacterial pathogens must then compete with normal flora, attach to the appropriate receptors on epithelial cells, and survive the effects of local immunity. Antibiotic-induced changes in resident flora have been shown to facilitate infection with *Salmonella* and presumably other organisms, and motility-modifying drugs that increase gastrointestinal transit time increase the time that pathogens have to attach to the mucosa. The consequences of infection with an enteric pathogen then vary considerably.

Enteric viral infection causes direct damage to the epithelial cells. The location of the absorptive complex to which viruses attach varies. Some viruses (e.g., canine parvovirus [CPV]) damage rapidly dividing crypt cells, resulting in decreased replacement of absorptive apical cells and hence decreased absorption. Other viruses (e.g., canine coronavirus [CCV]) damage the apical epithelial cells directly. Villus atrophy may result.

Bacterial and protozoal pathogens may cause diarrhea through the elaboration of enterotoxins, by invasion of the lamina propria, or by both mechanisms. Enterotoxins can cause diarrhea through several mechanisms. Cytotoxic enterotoxins affect intracellular enzyme systems and induce secretory diarrhea without morphologic damage to the enterocyte. The enterotoxins of enterotoxigenic *E. coli* (ETEC) are relatively well characterized and serve as models of enterotoxigenic enteritis in dogs and cats. The heat-labile toxin (LT) binds to GM-1 monosialoganglioside receptors on the epithelial cell. This leads to inhibition of guanosine triphosphate–binding protein, which is a regulator of adenyl cyclase (AC). AC activity increases, leading to increased levels of cyclic adenosine monophosphate (cAMP), which causes an increased secretion of chloride and decreased absorption of sodium. Water is lost into the gut lumen along with electrolytes. A heat-stable toxin (ST) has also been described; it induces a secretory diarrhea through alterations in cyclic guanosine monophosphate (cGMP).

The calcium-binding protein calmodulin is present in high levels in the intestinal epithelium and mediates calcium-dependent inhibition of sodium and chloride transport in addition to stimulating adenylate cyclase. Alterations in mucosal calmodulin levels appear to be important in secretory diarrhea and may be involved in the cAMP/cGMP mechanisms. Enterotoxigenic infections usually affect the small intestine, cause secretory diarrhea, and may be associated with severe dehydration.

Enteropathogenic *E. coli* (EPEC) do not produce LT or ST, nor are they invasive. Some of these strains attach to the surfaces of intestinal epithelial cells and efface microvilli, resulting in characteristic histologic and ultrastructural lesions. These strains are called *attaching and effacing E. coli.* Enteritis associated with these organisms has been reported in cats.

Other enterotoxins such as Vero (Shiga-like) toxins (also secreted by *E. coli*) and those secreted by *Clostridium perfringens* types A and C and *Campylobacter* are cytotoxic. These cause structural damage to the intestinal epithelial cells, leading to malabsorptive diarrhea.

Some bacteria and protozoa, such as enteroinvasive *E. coli* (EIEC), *Salmonella*, and *Entamoeba histolytica*, breech the epithelium and invade the underlying tissues, causing inflammation and exudative diarrhea. These organisms often affect the colon.

Diarrhea occurs when the colonic absorptive capacity is exceeded. Water, sodium, chloride, potassium, bicarbonate, and possibly protein, blood, and neutrophils are lost into the intestinal lumen. The outcome of infection depends on the dose and strain of infecting organism, the degree of fluid and electrolyte loss, the magnitude of physical damage to the epithelium, and the effectiveness of the local immune response. Healing of the epithelium is rapid once the infection is controlled.

DIAGNOSIS OF INFECTIOUS DIARRHEA

A history of exposure and lack of vaccination in a young dog combined with demonstration of the virus is highly suggestive of parvoviral diarrhea. In most cases, however, the specific diagnosis of infectious diarrhea is difficult. Demonstration of bacterial or viral pathogens does not always verify the diagnosis, because these organisms can often be recovered from significant percentages of the normal population. The presumptive diagnosis rests on the association of clinical signs, the isolation of an organism (and possibly demonstrating that it is an enterotoxic or invasive strain), and response to specific therapy.

Infectious diarrhea may be acute or chronic. It is probably most common in dogs and cats less than 1 year of age, especially those living in crowded, unsanitary conditions. Other risk factors include hospitalization, illness, and surgery. Animals that are immunosuppressed by corticosteroids or chemotherapy are also at risk. Retrovirus-induced immunosuppression in cats is an important risk factor. The recent description of feline immunodeficiency virus (FIV) suggests that many enteric infections

with organisms such as *Cryptosporidium, Mycobacterium,* and *Candida* are not primary events.

As for any other medical problem, the history and physical examination are extremely important. Vaccine and antiparasitic drug administration history should be obtained, as well as history of exposure to other animals and travel to areas endemic for histoplasmosis (Ohio, Mississippi, Missouri river regions), pythiosis (Gulf of Mexico), or salmon disease complex (northwestern California to southwestern Washington). Vomiting and other signs should be identified. The duration and magnitude of signs, as well as response to any therapy, help a clinician determine the severity of the illness.

The physical examination should include an assessment of hydration by evaluation of mucous membranes, tissue turgor, and body weight. Fever may be associated with some viral enteropathies, such as parvoviral enteritis, as well as with infection with invasive bacteria. Lymphadenopathy occurs with rickettsial infections in dogs, and fine-needle aspiration of enlarged nodes may be useful for demonstrating the organisms within the cytoplasm of monocyte-macrophage cells. Findings on abdominal palpation may be normal or may reveal fluid and gas-filled loops of bowel. *Pythium* may cause thickening of the intestinal wall, often resulting in stricture. A thickened, irregular rectal wall is suggestive of chronic transmural granulomatous proctitis/colitis. Gross inspection of the stool may reveal blood or mucus. Bloody stool is suggestive of inflammatory, infectious, or neoplastic disease. The presence of blood indicates that the epithelial surface has been damaged and that the animal may be at risk for sepsis with organisms originating from normal enteric flora. No characteristics of stool are pathognomonic for any specific infectious agent.

Clinicians should attempt to localize the diarrhea to the small or large bowel. Viruses and enterotoxigenic bacteria often affect the small bowel, whereas invasive organisms tend to affect the colon, resulting in increased frequency of stool, tenesmus, mucus, and frank blood in the stool.

Multiple fecal examinations should be performed. Direct or saline smears are used to identify protozoal trophozoite motility, and stained smears are used to examine trophozoite morphology. The zinc sulfate centrifugation technique is preferable for demonstrating *Giardia* cysts, whereas Sheather's sugar centrifugation technique is used to demonstrate *Toxoplasma* and *Cryptosporidium* cysts. Spirochetes are normal intestinal flora and may be present in large numbers in diarrheic stool. New methylene blue can be used to stain colonic mucus or stool for the presence of fecal neutrophils and macrophages. A positive smear is suggestive of invasive colonic disease or CPV enteritis.

Depending on the severity of signs, the minimum database may include a complete blood count

(CBC), serum biochemistry panel, urinalysis, and blood gas analysis. Leukocytosis is consistent with loss of the integrity of the mucosal surface and the potential for sepsis. The findings of blood in the stool, fever, and leukocytosis are of special concern. Neutropenia may be associated with CPV infection. Many nonspecific CBC findings, including eosinophilia, can be associated with diarrhea of infectious or noninfectious origin. The serum biochemistry panel is useful for identifying electrolyte abnormalities, dehydration (blood urea nitrogen [BUN], creatinine, total proteins), significant protein loss, and many systemic disorders associated with vomiting and diarrhea. Urinalysis assists in evaluation of azotemia and helps localize protein loss by ruling out proteinuria. Cats with chronic diarrhea should be evaluated for feline leukemia virus (FeLV) p27 antigen and FIV antibody level. Abdominal radiography may be included in the workup; however, diarrhea of infectious etiology does not have any specific radiographic pattern. CPV enteritis may be associated with ileus.

Most viral enteropathies resolve within a few days, and virus identification tests are usually of academic interest in such instances. If CPV is a rule-out, an enzyme-linked immunosorbent assay (ELISA) (CITE Parvo Test, IDEXX Corp.) can be performed on stool as an in-house test. This assay appears to have a high positive predictive value. The test result should be positive for virus when a dog begins showing clinical signs and remains positive for several days. The result then becomes negative when local antibody excess binds virus. A strong positive reaction is associated with clinical cases of parvovirus, whereas recent vaccination with modified live parvovirus vaccines gives a faint reaction, if any.

The main indication for virus identification is an outbreak of diarrhea in a kennel or community. Electron microscopy and cell culture are used to identify and isolate viruses. Because there is a large degree of variation in techniques between laboratories, clinicians should consult with a local laboratory to determine which samples should be submitted. The presence of virus in stool does not always mean that it is the causal agent. Various viruses have been recovered from dogs with normal stools, and Koch's postulate has not been fulfilled for many of these viruses (e.g., rotavirus, herpesvirus, calicivirus, parainfluenza virus).

Diagnosis of bacterial enteritis is also problematic. Isolation of a potential pathogen from the stool is only suggestive of causation, because many of these organisms have been isolated from the stools of normal dogs. Bacterial isolation should be attempted in cases of chronic diarrhea or in acute diarrheas when a bacterial etiology may be of zoonotic importance, such as *Campylobacter*. The bacteria associated with enteritis often have both specific media and atmospheric requirements, and clinicians should specifically request the isolation of enteric pathogens when submitting stool samples. As for viral isolation, clinicians should consult a local laboratory for specific sample requirements.

Identification of enterotoxigenic bacterial infection is based on rabbit ileal loop or suckling mouse models or on tissue culture assays. The genes for *E. coli* LT, ST, and VT have been cloned, and DNA probes have been developed. These may be available in the future for the identification of ETEC infection directly from stool samples.

The diagnosis of giardiasis may be difficult, because trophozoites and cysts are shed intermittently. Evaluation of aspirated duodenal contents, obtained either through endoscopy or by aspiration of the duodenum at laparotomy, may be necessary. A simple, inexpensive peroral string test (Entero-Test, HDC Corp., Mountain View, CA) that samples duodenal contents in awake dogs has been described (Hall et al., 1988).

Rectal scrapings, colonoscopy, and biopsy may be diagnostic of histoplasmosis, and biopsies of the small bowel may be diagnostic of cryptosporidiosis and phycomycosis.

PRINCIPLES OF MANAGEMENT

The management of infectious diarrhea should include supportive care (fluid and electrolyte therapy), symptomatic care (administration of drugs that may decrease the frequency of diarrhea), specific therapy directed against the organism, and identification of infection of zoonotic importance.

Infectious diarrhea, especially when caused by enterotoxigenic organisms, may be associated with clinically significant losses of water, sodium, chloride, potassium, and bicarbonate. Intravenous fluid and electrolyte support should be given to animals with moderate to severe losses. Fluid deficits, maintenance requirements, and ongoing losses should be replaced with a balanced electrolyte solution (lactated Ringer's; Plasmalyte 148 [Baxter Corp., Toronto, Ontario]), usually supplemented with potassium chloride (20 mEq/L if the serum potassium level is within the normal range and the fluids are given at a maintenance rate over 24 hr). Glucose-containing solutions may be required in septic patients, especially in neonates, who may develop hypoglycemia. Oral rehydration therapy is a realistic option for animals with mild to moderate deficits and an intact mucosa (nonhemorrhagic diarrhea) when frequent vomiting is not present. Oral rehydration is based on the principle that glucose facilitates enteric sodium absorption and that water is passively absorbed with sodium. Oral fluid therapy has been reviewed elsewhere (Zenger and Willard, 1989).

The utility of symptomatic therapy is controversial. Motility-modifying drugs such as the synthetic opiates diphenoxylate (Lomotil, Searle) or loperamide (Imodium A-D, McNeil Consumer) decrease the frequency of diarrhea. However, studies of humans with various pathogens suggest that the use of these drugs increases the duration of clinical signs by decreasing the rate of clearance of organisms and toxins. Loperamide is the drug of choice because it has greater potency, quicker onset of activity, longer duration, and fewer side effects than diphenoxylate; it is available as an over-the-counter liquid preparation. In dogs and cats, a dose of 0.1 to 0.2 mg/kg PO every 6 to 8 hr, not to exceed 0.6 mg/kg/day, appears to be safe and effective (Johnson, 1989). In healthy humans, the primary effect of loperamide is on motor function. It may also have an antisecretory action by altering mucosal prostaglandin E_2 levels, calmodulin-mediated calcium-dependent inhibition of sodium chloride transport, and AC activity. Loperamide is also a potent inhibitor of colonic mucus secretion. It is not clear which factor is more significant in various types of diarrhea. Other calmodulin antagonists may decrease secretion without affecting motility, and several investigational drugs are under development.

The utility of intestinal protectants has not been determined. Kaolin, pectin, attapulgite, and bentonite appear to have limited efficacy. Charcoal and cholestyramine may have some benefit by binding toxins. An interesting review of the use of intestinal absorbents has been published (Wilcke and Turner, 1987).

Bismuth subsalicylate (BSS, Pepto-Bismol, Norwich Eaton Pharmaceuticals) may have beneficial activity in infectious enteritis. The mechanism of action of BSS is complex. Salicylate is readily absorbed and may have a role in inhibiting prostaglandin-mediated inflammation, enterotoxin-induced secretion, and abnormal motility. Also, bismuth salts have antibacterial effects. *In vitro* studies have shown that BSS inhibits the growth of *E. coli, Salmonella, Campylobacter, Clostridium difficile,* and *Bacteroides fragilis* at levels that should be achieved in the gastrointestinal tract. In a randomized double-blind placebo-controlled trial in children with acute diarrhea, it was shown that those receiving BSS had a significantly lower stool weight and improved stool consistency, lower number of stools, decreased need for intravenous fluids, and a shorter hospital stay. Other studies suggest that BSS is not as effective as loperamide. In dogs and cats, 1 mg/kg PO divided into four to eight equal daily doses appears to be safe (Papich et al., 1987). Other nonsteroidal anti-inflammatory drugs (NSAIDs) have been shown to interfere with enterotoxin-associated intestinal hypersecretion in humans, apparently by blocking the production of cAMP. However, many NSAIDs are toxic to dogs and cats and are not recommended.

Elevated levels of circulating plasma endotoxin (lipopolysaccaride [LPS]) have been found in dogs with hemorrhagic enteritis due to various causes. Therapy of endotoxemia with polyvalent equine hyperimmune serum containing anti-LPS IgG has been described. Anti-LPS IgG binds LPS, opsonizes bacteria, and has bactericidal effects via complement activation (Wessels et al., 1987). The utility of anti-LPS serum therapy remains to be determined.

Specific therapy with antimicrobial drugs depends on identification of the causative agent. In addition to demonstrating a specific pathogen, the major indication for antibiotic therapy is evidence of significant damage to the mucosa (increased fecal leukocytes, melena or hematochezia, leukocytosis, fever, positive blood culture, shock) such that bacterial entry into the portal circulation is likely. The goal of therapy is to control bacteremia caused by enteric organisms, primarily anaerobes and Enterobacteriaceae. Parenteral therapy is indicated, and an aminoglycoside and penicillin combination (e.g., gentamicin, 2 mg/kg IV every 8 hr, and ampicillin, 5 to 10 mg/kg IV every 6 hr) is usually recommended. Less nephrotoxic alternatives are enrofloxacin (Baytril, Haver; 5 mg/kg IV every 12 hr) and metronidazole (8 to 15 mg/kg IV every 8 hr).

The indiscriminate use of antibiotics in animals with diarrhea has several consequences. First, disruption of normal flora (usually anaerobes) may allow potential pathogens (usually gram-negative anaerobes) to colonize the gut. This concern is justifiable based on experience in humans; however, the magnitude of risk for veterinary patients is not known. Second, the induction of bacterial resistance to antibiotics may be significant, both for the individual animal and potentially for the community. Antibiotic resistance is mediated by extrachromosomal plasmids. Plasmids confer resistance to multiple antibiotics and are transmitted between bacteria by conjugation. Several studies have demonstrated the presence of antibiotic-resistant plasmids in the normal flora of dogs. The clinical significance of plasmid induction is resistance of bacteria to commonly used antibiotics (Hirsh, 1989).

Several pathogens have zoonotic significance. The most important organism is probably *Campylobacter*, which may be acquired by children from puppies and kittens with diarrhea (see *CVI X*, p. 944). Evidence suggests that the infection can also be transmitted from humans to pets. *Salmonella, Yersinia, Mycobacterium,* and *Cryptosporidium* may also be of zoonotic importance. It is still not clear if *Giardia* isolated from dogs and cats is infectious for humans, but it should probably be considered as having zoonotic potential. If a pathogen of zoonotic importance is identified, owners should be advised to notify their physician if they or family members have enteric signs.

CURRENT ISSUES

Canine Parvovirus

Despite widespread vaccination, diarrhea caused by CPV-2 is still common. Doberman pinschers, Rottweilers, and pit bull terriers appear to be at increased risk (Glickman et al., 1985). Practitioners are concerned about the efficacy of vaccines and the development of new strains of parvovirus. Minor genetic and antigenic changes occurred in the virus (CPV-2a) around 1981; however, these changes are not significant with respect to the canine immune response. Vaccines using the original canine virus are effective in inducing immunity to the current street strains of virus. CPV-2a may be more virulent and have a shorter incubation period (4 to 5 days, rather than 6 to 8 days). Sudden collapse and shock have been reported in addition to diarrhea, anorexia, lymphopenia, and weight loss (Carmichael and Parrish, 1989).

Maternal antibody levels can persist for 18 weeks or longer in some puppies and may interfere with immunization at a level that is lower than that required to protect the puppy from challenge. Puppies receiving the last vaccine at 16 weeks of age may not be adequately immunized (see this volume, p. 202). In areas or kennels where CPV disease is endemic, bitches can be vaccinated with a modified live virus vaccine 2 to 4 weeks before breeding; if already pregnant, they can be given two doses of inactivated vaccine 3 to 4 weeks apart in the last trimester. This regimen ensures high colostral immunoglobulin levels, which will optimize protection while puppies are still in the kennel and at risk for exposure. Vaccination can begin at 6 to 8 weeks of age but should be repeated at 3- to 4-week intervals through 20 weeks of age, followed by annual vaccination. Because CPV-2 is extremely hardy, it is important to emphasize to owners that puppies should not be taken out of their home environment until the vaccination protocol is completed.

Some dogs have been shown to have transient decreases in lymphocyte blastogenesis following vaccination. This suppression of the cellular immune response may be associated with a lowered ability to mount an appropriate humoral response, as shown by lower canine distemper virus antibody titers in these dogs when vaccinated concurrently (Mastro et al., 1986). Epidemiologic evidence suggests that modified live virus CPV vaccines are immunosuppressive and that killed virus products are safer (Brenner et al., 1989). These concerns have not yet been resolved, and vaccination with modified live virus vaccines is still advocated by many because they may be more effective in the presence of maternal antibody, may induce immunity of longer duration, and may decrease the amount of virulent virus shed after challenge.

Table 1. *Viruses and Rickettsiae Associated With Enteritis in Dogs and Cats*

Organism	Species Affected	Review Reference
Viruses thought to be primary enteric pathogens		
Canine parvovirus-2	D	Pollock, 1984a
Canine coronavirus	D	Pollock and Carmichael, 1990
Feline enteric coronavirus	C	Pedersen et al., 1981
Viruses occasionally isolated from diarrheic stools		
Rotavirus	D, C	McGuire and Castro, 1982
Astrovirus	D, C	Harbour et al., 1987
Herpesvirus	D	Evermann et al., 1982
Calicivirus	D	Evermann et al., 1985
Parainfluenza virus	D	Macartney et al., 1985
Viruses causing systemic disease in which diarrhea may occur		
Feline panleukopenia virus	C	Pollock, 1984b
Canine distemper	D	Greene and Appel, 1990
Feline coronavirus (FIP)	C	Barlough and Stoddart, 1988
Feline leukemia virus	C	Reinacher, 1987
Feline immunodeficiency virus	C	Pedersen et al., 1989
Rickettsia		
Rickettsia rickettsii	D	Hibler and Greene, 1985
Neorickettsia helminthoeca and Neorickettsia elokominica	D	Hibler and Greene, 1986

D, dogs; C, cats.

In a retrospective study of 98 dogs with parvoviral enteritis, *E. coli* was isolated from the liver or lungs of 88 dogs (90%). Pulmonary lesions compatible with adult respiratory distress syndrome (ARDS) were found in 64 dogs (69%). Gram-negative sepsis and endotoxemia are recognized as predisposing factors for ARDS. The investigators concluded that *E. coli* septicemia and pulmonary disease are common complications in fatal CPV infection (Turk et al., 1990). These findings emphasize the need for bactericidal antibiotic therapy in this condition.

Canine Coronavirus

The clinical importance of CCV is not clear. Experimental infection may be associated with mild enteritis; however, it is difficult to induce diarrhea with this virus in many normal dogs. Laboratories performing virus isolation find the prevalence of coronavirus enteritis to be low, especially compared with CPV. In one study, stools from dogs with diarrhea were tested for CCV and CPV. Overall results were that 477 of 772 samples (62%) were positive for CPV, 216 of 714 samples (30%) were

Table 2. *Bacteria Associated With Diarrhea in Dogs and Cats*

Organism	Species Affected	Review Reference
Campylobacter	D, C	Dillon et al., 1987
Salmonella	D, C	Uhaa et al., 1988
Yersinia pseudotuberculosis	C	Pedersen, 1988
and *enterocolitica*	D	Papageorges et al., 1983
Escherichia coli	D, C	
ETEC, EIEC,		Abaas et al., 1989
EPEC		Broes et al., 1988
Mycobacterium	C	Pedersen, 1988
Clostridium perfringens	D	Kruth et al., 1989
Enterococcus durans	D	Collins et al., 1988

D, dogs; C, cats.

positive for CCV, and 110 of 585 samples (19%) were positive for both viruses. Marked regional variations throughout North America were reported (Evermann et al., 1989).

Concerns regarding mixed CPV and CCV infections have been raised because of the potential synergy between the viruses. Coronavirus infects villus epithelial cells. During recovery from CCV infection, crypt cells divide rapidly to repair the villus epithelium. These rapidly dividing cells are more likely to become infected with CPV. Experimentally, infection with CPV after infection with CCV is more severe than either infection alone. Some investigators suggest that this is an indication for CCV vaccination (Appel, 1988). The overall clinical importance of CCV and CCV vaccines remains to be determined.

Feline Immunodeficiency Virus

Chronic diarrhea has been described in cats infected with FIV. The organisms involved are pri-

Table 3. *Pythium, Algal, and Fungal Enteritis in Dogs and Cats*

Organism	Species Affected	Review Reference
Oömycosis		
Pythium insidiosum	D	Miller, 1985
Zygomycosis		
Basidiobolus,	D, C	Miller, 1985
Conidiobolus,		
Absidia, Rhizopus,		
Rhizomucor,		
Mortierella		
Aspergillus	C	Ossent, 1987
Candida	D, C	Anderson and Pidgeon, 1987
Histoplasma capsulatum	D, C	Clinkenbeard et al., 1989a, b
Algal		
Prototheca	D	Migaki et al., 1982

Table 4. *Protozoa Associated with Diarrhea in Dogs and Cats*

Organism	Species Affected	Review Reference
Isospora	D, C	Kirkpatrick and Dubey, 1987
Cryptosporidium	D, C	Moore et al., 1988
Giardia	D, C	Kirkpatrick, 1986

marily resident flora that are normally controlled by cell-mediated immunity. Cats presenting with chronic diarrhea, especially mature cats that roam freely, should be evaluated for FIV. The CITE FIV ELISA antibody (IDEXX Corporation, Portland, ME) is available as an in-house assay. The CITE Combo product tests for both FIV antibody and FeLV p27 antigen. In the presence of clinical signs, the positive predictive value of these tests is high.

Clostridium perfringens

Infection with multiple serotypes of *C. perfringens* has been described as being associated with outbreaks of nosocomial diarrhea in dogs in a veterinary teaching hospital. Metronidazole (10 to 15 mg/kg PO q 8 hr for 5 days) was given if the diarrhea was severe or lasted longer than 3 days. *C. perfringens* enterotoxin has also been identified in stools of dogs with acute and chronic diarrhea. Some of these animals appeared to be responsive to antibiotic therapy. The true significance of these findings is not known.

SPECIFIC PATHOGENS

Tables 1 through 4 list organisms that have been associated with diarrhea in dogs and cats. The prevalence of these infections is not known. Readers are directed to the appropriate reference, which details diagnosis and management.

References and Suggested Reading

Abaas, S., Franklin, A., Kuhn, I., et al.: Cytotoxin activity of Vero cells among *Escherichia coli* strains associated with diarrhea in cats. Am. J. Vet. Res. 50:1294, 1989.

Anderson, P. G., and Pidgeon, G.: Candidiasis in a dog with parvoviral enteritis. J. Am. Anim. Hosp. Assoc. 23:27, 1987.

Appel, M. J. G.: Does canine coronavirus augment the effects of subsequent parvovirus infection? Vet. Med. 83:360, 1988.

Barlough, J. E., and Stoddart, C. A.: Cats and coronaviruses. J.A.V.M.A. 193:796, 1988.

Brenner, J., Markus, R., Klopfer-Orgad, U., et al.: The possible enhancement of parvovirus vaccination on the mortality rate of disease dogs. J. Vet. Med. B36:547, 1989.

Broes, A., Drolet, R., Jacques, M., et al.: Natural infection with an attaching and effacing *Escherichia coli* in a diarrheic puppy. Can. J. Vet. Res. 52:280, 1988.

Carmichael, L. E., and Parrish, C. R.: Clinical significance of antigenic variation in canine parvovirus. *In* Kirk, R. W. (ed.): *Current Veterinary Therapy X.* Philadelphia: W. B. Saunders, 1989, p. 1076.

Clinkenbeard, K. D., Wolf, A. M., Cowell, R. L., et al.: Feline disseminated histoplasmosis. Comp. Cont. Ed. Pract. Vet. 11:1223, 1989a.

Clinkenbeard, K. D., Wolf, A. M., Cowell, R. L., et al.: Canine disseminated histoplasmosis. Comp. Cont. Ed. Pract. Vet. 11: 1347, 1989b.

Collins, J. E., Bergeland, M. E., Lindeman, C. J., et al.: *Enterococcus (Streptococcus) durans* adherence in the small instestine of a diarrheic pup. Vet. Pathol. 25: 396, 1988.

Dillon, A. R., Bossinger. T. R., and Blevins, W. T.: Campylobacter enteritis in dogs and cats. Comp. Cont. Ed. Pract. Vet. 9:1176, 1987.

Evermann, J. F., McKeirnan, A. J., Euguster, A. K., et al.: Update on canine coronavirus infections and interactions with other enteric pathogens of the dog. Comp. Anim. Pract. 19:6, 1989.

Evermann, J. F., McKeirnan, A. J., Ott, R. L., et al.: Diarrheal condition in dogs associated with viruses antigenically related to feline herpesvirus. Cornell Vet. 72:285, 1982.

Evermann, J. F., McKeirnan, A. J., Smith, A. W., et al.: Isolation and identification of caliciviruses from dogs with enteric infections. Am. J. Vet. Res. 46:218, 1985.

Glickman, L. T., Domanski, L. M., Patronek, G. J., et al.: Breed-related risk factors for canine parvovirus enteritis. J.A.V.M.A. 187:589, 1985.

Greene, C. E., and Appel, M. J.: Canine distemper. *In* Greene, C. E. (ed.): *Infectious Diseases of the Dog and Cat.* Philadelphia: W. B. Saunders, 1990, p. 226.

Hall, E. J., Rutgers, H. C., and Batt, R. M.: Evaluation of the peroral string test in the diagnosis of canine giardiasis. J. Small Anim. Pract. 29:177, 1988.

Harbour, D. A., Ashley, C. R., Williams, P. D., et al.: Natural and experimental astrovirus infection of cats. Vet. Rec. 120:555, 1987.

Hibler, S. C., and Greene, C. E.: Rickettsial infections in dogs, Part I. Rocky Mountain spotted fever and *Coxiella* infections. Comp. Cont. Ed. Pract. Vet. 7:856, 1985.

Hibler, S. C., and Greene, C. E.: Rickettsial infections in dogs, Part III. Salmon disease complex and haemobartonellosis. Comp. Cont. Ed. Pract. Vet. 8:251, 1986.

Hirsh D. C.: Clinical and public health significance of antimicrobial-resistant enteric bacterial infections. *In* Kirk, R. W. (ed.): *Current Veterinary Therapy X.* Philadelphia: W. B. Saunders, 1989, p. 1096.

Hone, D., and Hackett, J.: Vaccination against enteric bacterial diseases. Rev. Infect. Dis. 11: 853, 1989.

Johnson, S. E.: Loperamide: A novel antidiarrheal drug. Comp. Cont. Ed. Pract. Vet. 11:1373, 1989.

Kirkpatrick, C. E.: Feline giardiasis: A review. J. Small Anim. Pract. 27:69, 1986.

Kirkpatrick, C. E., and Dubey, J. P.: Enteric coccidial infections. Vet. Clin. North Am. Small Anim. Pract. 17:1405, 1987.

Kruth, S. A., Prescott, J. F., Welch, M. K., et al.: Nosocomial diarrhea associated with enterotoxigenic *Clostridium perfringens* infection in dogs. J.A.V.M.A. 195:331, 1989.

Macartney, L., Cornwell, H. J. C., McCandlish, I. A. P., et al.: Isolation of a novel paramyxovirus from a dog with enteric disease. Vet. Rec. 117:205, 1985.

Mastro, J. M., Axthelm, M., Mathes, L. E., et al.: Repeated suppression

of lymphocyte blastogenesis following vaccinations of CPV-immune dogs with modified-live CPV vaccines. Vet. Microbiol. 12:201, 1986.

McGuire, S. J., and Castro, A. E.: Evaluation of a commercial immunoassay for rapid diagnosis or rotavirus in fecal specimens from domestic species. Am. Assoc. Vet. Lab. Diagn. 25th Annual Proceedings, 375, 1982.

Migaki, G., Font, R. L., Sauer, R. M., et al.: Canine prototothecosis: Review of the literature and report of an additional case. J.A.V.M.A. 181:794, 1982.

Miller, R. I.: Gastrointestinal phycomycosis in 63 dogs. J.A.V.M.A. 186:473, 1985.

Moore, J. A., Blagburn, B. L., and Lindsay, D. S.: Cryptosporidiosis in animals including humans. Comp. Cont. Ed. Pract. Vet. 10:275, 1988.

Ossent, P.: Systemic aspergillosis and mucormycosis in 23 cats. Vet. Rec. 120:330, 1987.

Papageorges, M., Higgins, R., and Gosselin, Y.: *Yersinia enterocolitica* enteritis in two dogs. J.A.V.M.A. 182:618, 1983.

Papich, M. G., Davis, C. A., and Davis, L. E.: Absorption of salicylate from an antidiarrheal preparation in dogs and cats. J. Am. Anim. Hosp. Assoc. 23:221, 1987.

Pedersen, N. C.: *Feline Infectious Diseases.* Goleta, CA: American Veterinary Publications, 1988, pp. 172, 189.

Pedersen, N. C., Boyle, J. F., Floyd, K., et al.: An enteric coronavirus infection of cats and its relationship to feline infectious peritonitis. Am. J. Vet. Res. 42:368, 1981.

Pedersen, N. C., Yamamoto, J. K., Ishida, T., et al.: Feline immunodeficiency virus infection. Vet. Immunol. Immunopathol. 21:111, 1989.

Pollock, R. V. H.: The parvoviruses, Part I. Feline panleukopenia virus and mink enteritis virus. Comp. Cont. Ed. Pract. Vet. 6:227, 1984a.

Pollock, R. V. H.: The parvoviruses, Part II. Canine parvoviruses. Comp. Cont. Ed. Pract. Vet. 6:653, 1984b.

Pollock, R. V. H., and Carmichael, L. E.: Canine viral enteritis. *In* Greene, C. E. (ed.): *Infectious Diseases of the Dog and Cat.* Philadelphia: W. B. Saunders, 1990, p. 281.

Reinacher, M.: Feline leukemia virus–associated enteritis: A condition with features of feline panleukopenia. Vet. Pathol. 24:1, 1987.

Turk, J., Miller, M., Brown, T., et al.: Coliform septicemia and pulmonary disease associated with canine parvoviral enteritis: 88 cases (1987–1988). J.A.V.M.A. 196:771, 1990.

Uhaa, I. J., Hird, D. W., Hirsh, D. C., et al.: Case-control study of risk factors associated with nosocomial *Salmonella krefeld* infection in dogs. Am. J. Vet. Res. 49: 1501, 1988.

Wessels, B. C., Gaffin, S. L., and Wells, M. T.: Circulating plasma endotoxin (lipopolysaccharide) concentrations in healthy and hemorrhagic enteric dogs: Antiendotoxin immunotherapy in hemorrhagic enteric endotoxemia. J. Am. Anim. Hosp. Assoc. 23:291, 1987.

Wilcke, J. R., and Turner, J. C: The use of adsorbents to treat gastrointestinal problems in small animals. Semin. Vet. Med. Surg. (Small Anim.) 2:266, 1987.

Willard, M. D.: Chronic intestinal bacterial overgrowth. *In* Kirk, R. W. (ed.): *Current Veterinary Therapy X.* Philadelphia: W. B. Saunders, 1989, p. 933.

Zenger, E., and Willard, M. D.: Oral rehydration therapy in companion animals. Comp. Anim. Pract. 19:6, 1989.

INFECTIOUS POLYARTHRITIS IN THE DOG AND CAT

ELLEN C. CODNER

Blacksburg, Virginia

The etiology of joint disease in dogs and cats is diverse and includes both noninflammatory (degenerative, traumatic, and neoplastic) and inflammatory processes (Table 1). Noninflammatory joint disorders often cause an increased volume of synovial fluid, but cytologic analysis of the fluid reveals normal or nearly normal findings. In contrast, inflammatory joint disease is characterized by inflammatory changes in the synovial membrane and synovial fluid and is frequently accompanied by systemic signs of illness such as fever, depression, anorexia, leukocytosis, and hyperfibrinogenemia. Synovial fluid analysis demonstrates increased numbers of white blood cells with a greater proportion of neutrophils (Table 2).

Inflammatory polyarthritis can be further subdivided into infectious and noninfectious (immune-mediated) diseases (see Table 1). Because synovial fluid analysis and radiographic findings are similar for many infectious and noninfectious inflammatory arthritides, the diagnosis of infectious polyarthritis usually relies on microscopic identification or culture of organisms from synovial fluid or synovial membrane.

Infectious agents have also been associated with immune-mediated arthritis (Table 3). Because the offending organism cannot be recovered from involved joints, the disease is likely the result of deposition of immune complexes within the synovium, leading to a sterile synovitis. Changes in the synovial fluid and synovial membrane are identical to those due to other causes of immune-mediated polyarthritis (systemic lupus erythematosus, enteropathic/hepatopathic arthritis, drug-induced polyarthritis, and idiopathic polyarthritis). Diagnosis and successful treatment depend on identifying and eliminating the underlying infectious process.

Although infectious polyarthritis is uncommon, accurate diagnosis is particularly important, because immunosuppressive therapy may exacerbate the disease. When an infectious agent is suspected but cannot be documented, a trial course of tetracycline may be warranted in some cases, before immunosuppressive drug therapy. This article discusses the diagnostic features of bacterial, mycoplasmal, fungal, rickettsial, spirochetal, protozoal, and viral arthritis. The association of systemic infection with development of immune-mediated polyarthritis is also addressed.

BACTERIAL ARTHRITIS

Septic arthritis occurs more often in medium and large breeds of dogs than in smaller dogs, and males are more commonly affected than females. The pattern of joint disease is usually monarticular or pauciarticular (fewer than five joints) and most frequently involves larger, proximal joints (shoulder, elbow, carpus, hip, and stifle). These clinical features help differentiate bacterial arthritis from immune-mediated arthritis, which typically presents as a polyarthritis (more than five joints) involving predominantly distal joints in small breeds of dogs.

Bacteria may gain access to the joint through penetrating wounds, by extension of infection from adjacent bone or soft tissue, or by hematogenous

Table 1. *Classification of Arthropathies*

Noninflammatory joint disease
  Degenerative
  Traumatic
  Neoplastic
Inflammatory joint disease (arthritis)
  Infectious arthritis
    Bacterial
    Bacterial L-forms
    Mycoplasmal
    Rickettsial (granulocytic ehrlichiosis)
    Spirochetal (*Borrelia*)
    Fungal
    Protozoal (*Leishmania*)
    Viral
  Noninfectious arthritis (immune mediated)
    Nonerosive (nondeforming) arthritis
      Idiopathic polyarthritis
      Systemic lupus erythematosus
      Arthritis associated with chronic infectious diseases
      Arthritis associated with malignant neoplasia
      Drug-induced polyarthritis
      Enteropathic/hepatopathic arthritis
      Plasmacytic-lymphocytic synovitis
    Erosive (deforming) arthritis
      Rheumatoid arthritis
      Polyarthritis of greyhounds
      Feline progressive polyarthritis

Table 2. *Synovial Fluid Characteristics in Various Types of Canine Arthritis**

Condition	Nucleated Cells/mm³	Differential (%)	
		Mononuclear	*Neutrophilic*
Normal	250–3000	94–100	0–6
Degenerative joint disease	1000–5000	88–100	0–12
Plasmacytic-lymphocytic synovitis	5000–20,000	60–90	10–40
Rheumatoid arthritis	8000–38,000	20–80	20–80
Nonerosive arthritis (all types)	4400–371,000	5–85	15–95
Septic arthritis	4300–267,000	1–57	43–99

*Modified with permission from Pedersen, N. C., and Pool, R.: Canine joint disease. Vet. Clin. North Am. Small Anim. Pract. 8:465, 1978; and Bennett, D., and Taylor, D. J.: Bacterial infective arthritis in the dog. J. Small Anim. Pract. 29:207, 1988.

spread. The source of infection frequently cannot be identified. Trauma, degenerative joint disease, treatment with corticosteroids, or other immunosuppressive factors may predispose the joints to infection. Common sources of systemic infection include cystitis, pyelonephritis, prostatitis, pyoderma, peritonitis, and pneumonia. Resulting septicemia often causes bacterial endocarditis or diskospondylitis associated with septic arthritis. Bacterial septicemia and subsequent joint abscessation occur in puppies and kittens secondary to umbilical vein infection (omphalophlebitis) or streptococcal pharyngitis; they may also originate from uterine or mammary gland infection in the queen or bitch.

The onset of clinical signs can be sudden or gradual. A more gradual onset has been associated with milder degrees of lameness and less severe pathologic changes. Septic arthritis often causes pain on palpation or manipulation of the joint and is frequently accompanied by swelling of overlying soft tissue, muscle atrophy, and regional lymphadenopathy. Redness of the skin, crepitus, reduced joint motion, and edema of the limb distal to the infected joint can be present. Systemic signs including fever, lethargy, and anorexia are uncommon

Table 3. *Chronic Infectious Diseases Associated With Immune-Mediated Arthritis*

Bacterial
  Subacute bacterial endocarditis
  Diskospondylitis
  Actinomycotic granulomas (migrating grass awn)
  Pyometra, vaginitis
  Urinary tract infection
  Periodontitis
  Deep pyoderma
  Chronic salmonellosis
  Chronic otitis externa/media
Fungal
  Coccidioidomycosis
Parasitic
  Dirofilariasis
Viral?
  Feline leukemia virus/feline syncytium-forming virus (chronic progressive polyarthritis of cats)

except in cases of sepsis or endocarditis. Hematologic data do not consistently show evidence of inflammation. Low-grade anemia, mild thrombocytopenia, elevated levels of hepatic enzymes, and hyperglobulinemia have been reported in some dogs. Low titers for antinuclear antibody and rheumatoid factor are occasionally present.

Radiographic changes vary with stage of disease. Changes associated with concurrent orthopedic diseases may be superimposed. Some joints show no obvious radiographic changes, even though inflammation is apparent on synovial fluid analysis. Early radiographic findings in bacterial arthritis are limited to soft-tissue changes and are nonspecific. These signs include joint capsule thickening and distention with displacement of adjacent fascial planes, slight widening of the joint space due to effusion, and in the stifle, loss of the intra-articular fat pad. Similar radiographic findings involving soft tissues occur with traumatic joint disease and nonerosive, immune-mediated arthritis. Chronic, persistent cases of bacterial arthritis may exhibit radiographic changes involving bone, similar to those seen with rheumatoid arthritis or degenerative joint disease. These signs are destruction of articular cartilage and subchondral bone with increased or irregular joint spaces, discrete bone erosions or generalized mineral loss, periosteal new bone, osteosclerosis, and osteophyte production. In severe infection, fibrosis and bony ankylosis may occur.

Histologic evaluation of the synovial membrane is consistent with nonspecific inflammation. In some cases there is widespread neutrophilic infiltration with microabscessation, and in others, a more chronic, mononuclear cell infiltrate of lymphocytes and plasma cells predominates. In view of these nonspecific findings, the trauma and risk of surgery associated with synovial membrane biopsy are probably not justified for routine diagnostic purposes, unless the joint is to be surgically explored for some other reason. Synovial membrane biopsy may be helpful if the diagnosis remains elusive or response to treatment is unsatisfactory.

Synovial fluid analysis shows characteristics of inflammatory joint disease. The fluid typically contains increased numbers of white blood cells and an increased percentage of neutrophils, has decreased viscosity, and frequently clots on exposure to air. Neutrophil numbers are usually high, but values for both relative and absolute neutrophil counts overlap those in synovial fluid from nonseptic inflamed joints (see Table 2). Synovial fluid from septic joints is frequently hemorrhagic; however, acute trauma and coagulopathies also produce hemarthrosis. Acute septic arthritis often causes degenerative and toxic changes in neutrophils, although vacuolization sometimes occurs in rheumatoid arthritis and nonerosive immune-mediated arthritis. When sample volume is adequate, protein and glucose content can be determined. Excessive protein concentration (4 to 5 gm/dl) and a very low ratio of synovial fluid glucose to blood glucose (less than 0.5) suggest bacterial infection (Werner, 1979).

Septic arthritis is diagnosed by finding microorganisms in synovial fluid with Gram's stain or by culturing organisms from synovial fluid or synovial membrane. Samples should be submitted for both aerobic and anaerobic culture, as well as for culture of *Mycoplasma*. Reports differ on the likelihood of obtaining positive cultures from infected joints. Pedersen and Pool (1978) state that organisms can be cultured from most infected joints if proper samples and culture media are used. Others report that synovial fluid culture yields false-negative results in 50% of cases (Montgomery et al., 1989) and that culture of the synovial membrane is more sensitive than culture of synovial fluid (Bennett and Taylor, 1988). A study of experimentally infected joints found that cultures of either synovial fluid or synovial membrane yield positive results in only 50% of joints, whereas positive cultures were consistently obtained when synovial fluid was incubated in blood culture medium 24 hr before culturing (Montgomery et al., 1989). Hopper (1989) recommends using broth enrichment media such as thioglycolate to enhance recovery of organisms. If bacteria cannot be cultured from the joint, positive isolation from blood or urine should be considered diagnostic.

Organisms commonly isolated from infected joints include staphylococci, streptococci, coliforms, and anaerobes. *Erysipelothrix, Pasteurella, Salmonella, Pseudomonas, Proteus, Nocardia, Corynebacterium,* and *Brucella* have been isolated less frequently. The significance of culturing diphtheroid-like organisms is uncertain, and in humans a positive culture is regarded as evidence for secondary invaders or media contamination (Bennett and Taylor, 1988). *Pasteurella,* which normally inhabits a queen's oral cavity, is the usual offending organism in kittens with omphalophlebitis and secondary arthritis. Degenerative or toxic changes in neutrophils in the synovial fluid may suggest the presence of organisms (staphylococci and some coliforms) that cause rapid destruction of articular cartilage (Pedersen et al., 1989).

The *treatment* of bacterial arthritis depends on identification of the organism and determination of antibiotic sensitivities. Systemic treatment is usually effective, because most antibiotics penetrate the vascular bed of inflamed joints. Bactericidal antibiotics are preferred and should be continued long term (minimum 6 to 8 weeks) and for at least 2 weeks after complete clinical resolution. With concurrent bacterial endocarditis, antibiotic therapy may be required for a longer period. In monarticular disease with marked articular damage, surgical debridement, drainage, and lavage may be of benefit. Gentamicin-impregnated polymethyl methacrylate beads have been surgically implanted for long-term treatment of arthritis caused by highly resistant *Escherichia coli* organisms. Effective local concentration of the antibiotic was provided without causing systemic toxic effects.

In some cases of bacterial arthritis, lameness and joint inflammation persist after long-term antibiotic therapy and initial improvement. Inability to culture bacteria and subsequent response to corticosteroids suggest that immune-mediated inflammation may be directed against nonviable bacterial fragments in the joint (Bennett and Taylor, 1988). A similar phenomenon has been described in humans, particularly with staphylococcal infections, and in pigs with *Erysipelothrix* infections.

The prognosis in bacterial arthritis depends on the amount of joint damage at the time of diagnosis. Systemic antibiotic therapy is generally successful, providing that early diagnosis is made and articular damage is not rapidly progressive. In a study of 57 canine cases, 56% made a complete recovery, 32% remained slightly lame, and 12% responded poorly with severe residual lameness (Bennett and Taylor, 1988).

Bacterial L-Forms

L-forms are cell wall–deficient bacteria that morphologically resemble mycoplasmas. Formation of L-forms is aided by the use of cell wall–damaging antibiotics and by host immune responses. A bacterial L-form has been associated with a distinct disease syndrome of cats characterized by multiple subcutaneous abscesses and, in some cases, an erosive polyarthritis (Carro et al., 1989). The abscesses typically fistulate and spread to other parts of the body. Joints become infected by either local extension or hematogenous seeding. Affected joints are swollen, painful, and crepitant. With time, they drain purulent material. Radiographic abnormalities include periarticular soft-tissue swelling and periosteal proliferation. In severe cases, damage occurs to the articular cartilage and subchondral bone. Cats often develop signs of systemic illness (anorexia, fever, depression, mature neutrophilia, lymphocytosis, and mild anemia). Microbiologic cultures and special stains fail to identify aerobic or anaerobic bacteria, mycobacteria, mycoplasmas, or fungi. Diagnosis is difficult because these organisms are hard to demonstrate by light microscopy and are also difficult to culture using bacterial or mycoplasmal media. The disease is progressive and unresponsive to most broad-spectrum antibiotics but can be successfully treated with tetracycline. Transmission of the disease among cats has presumably occurred through penetrating wounds or by the use of contaminated ointment for wound treatment. Immunosuppressive factors have not been identified. A bacterial L-form was incriminated in this syndrome by experimental transmission of the disease with organisms propagated in special L-form broth and by electron microscopic appearance of the organism recovered from an experimentally infected animal.

An L-form of *Nocardia asteroides* was isolated from a dog with progressive polyarthritis that was unresponsive to antibiotics and immunosuppressive drugs (Buchanan et al., 1983). Bacterial L-forms have been intermittently identified in various disease processes in both humans and animals, but their significance is unclear because they occur in both normal and diseased individuals.

Mycoplasmal Arthritis

Mycoplasma organisms are normal inhabitants of the conjunctival membrane, respiratory passages, and urogenital tract of dogs and cats. When host defenses are compromised, the organism may cause localized disease and occasionally spread systemically. Isolated cases of mycoplasma polyarthritis have been reported in immunocompromised dogs and cats, and pathogenicity of the organism has been confirmed by experimental reproduction of the disease and recovery of the organism. In a case report of a young greyhound with nonerosive polyarthritis caused by *Mycoplasma*, predisposing factors were not identified. The significance of this one isolate in the syndrome of polyarthritis of greyhounds remains to be determined.

Mycoplasmas cause an inflammatory, nonerosive polyarthritis. Affected animals exhibit signs of systemic illness in addition to painful, swollen joints. Synovial fluid contains elevated numbers of nondegenerate neutrophils. Radiographs show no significant bony lesions. Specialized media are necessary to culture the organism and thereby diagnose mycoplasmal arthritis. Because mycoplasmas are fragile organisms, care must be taken in transporting the specimen to the laboratory. The ability to recover the organism depends on several factors, including the type of mycoplasma and the stage of infection. Susceptibility testing to antimicrobial agents is not routinely available for mycoplasmas. They are generally susceptible to the newer quinolones, tylosin, erythromycin, lincomycin, tetracycline, chloramphenicol, and aminoglycosides. It is necessary to treat for an extended period of time.

Rickettsial Arthritis

Nonerosive polyarthritis has been associated with a granulocytic strain of canine ehrlichiosis (Stockham et al., 1986). Most dogs are febrile and present with acute lameness involving several joints (carpus, tarsus, elbow, stifle). Other clinical signs usually associated with canine ehrlichiosis (anorexia, weight loss, hemorrhage, lymphadenopathy) are not typically encountered. Hematologic abnormalities occur in some dogs and include mild thrombocytopenia, mild anemia, and variable neutrophil counts. Synovial fluid analysis indicates inflammation (30,000 to 50,000 cells/μl, 60 to 80% nondegenerate neutrophils, 4.5 mg protein/dl). Radiographic findings are limited to soft-tissue changes (joint effusion). The diagnosis of ehrlichiosis has been made by identifying *Ehrlichia* morulae in 1 to 2% of neutrophils, either in the peripheral blood or in the synovial fluid (Cowell et al., 1988). *Ehrlichia* morulae are also occasionally found in blood eosinophils and monocytes. This is in contrast to typical (monocytic) *Ehrlichia canis* infections, in which morulae are usually found only during the acute phase of infection and are generally present in lymphocytes, less frequently in monocytes, and rarely in neutrophils. In many but not all of the polyarthritis cases, serologic titers are positive to *E. canis* and are negative to *Ehrlichia equi*, *Ehrlichia sennetsu*, and *Ehrlichia risticii*. Whether the causative agent is actually *E. canis* or some other strain of *Ehrlichia* with cross-reactivity remains to be determined. Polyarthritic dogs respond rapidly to tetracycline therapy.

Borrelial Arthritis

Lyme disease has been diagnosed with increasing frequency during the past decade, although Koch's postulates have not been satisfied for this disease. The pathogenesis of the clinical syndrome is poorly understood. Spirochetes are detected within organs that are not inflamed, despite elevated specific antibody titers. When clinical signs occur, an inflammatory process is often present and is thought to be related to persistence of the organism causing immune complex deposition (Greene, 1990). (For additional information, see this volume, pp. 256 and 260.)

Disease manifestations in dogs have been predominantly characterized on the basis of questionable serologic evidence. Most affected dogs are young adults that have been exposed to ticks for at least one spring-to-autumn season. An acute onset of lameness that is frequently shifting and episodic is the primary clinical manifestation that has been reported for canine borreliosis. Fever and anorexia are noted in about 50% of suspected cases. A nonerosive arthritis affects one or more joints (carpus, digits, shoulder, elbow, tarsus, and stifle), with the carpus being most commonly involved. Radiographs of affected joints show normal findings. Examination of joint fluid reveals an inflammatory response (mean cell count in one series was 46,300/mm^3 with 80% neutrophils).

Spirochetes are rarely identified or isolated from synovial fluid, synovial membrane, or blood culture. Visualization of the organism requires darkfield or phase microscopy. A special medium (modified Kelly's) is required to grow Borrelia. Because nonpathogenic spirochetes exist, isolated organisms must be positively identified with monoclonal antibodies. However, isolation of Borrelia burgdorferi in tissues may be an incidental finding and probably should be surrounded by an inflammatory process to be considered significant.

Because of the difficulty in culturing or visualizing B. burgdorferi, serology is the most practical laboratory aid in diagnosis. Serologic results must be interpreted with great caution, however, because the frequency of subclinical infection is high in endemic areas. In naturally infected dogs, there is considerable overlap between antibody titers of dogs with presumed clinical infection and those with subclinical infection. Dogs in endemic areas can be asymptomatic and have titers as high as 1:8192. The mean titer in subclinically affected dogs is 1:285, but 42% have titers of 1:512 or greater, a cutoff value that has been used by some to support clinical infection. Titers of clinically affected dogs have ranged from 1:512 to 1:16,384, with a mean titer of 1:2700 (Kornblatt et al., 1985). Seropositive rates are lower in cats than in dogs in endemic areas. B. burgdorferi has not been isolated from cats, and no appreciable difference in seropositivity has been found between groups of cats with and without lameness (Magnarelli et al., 1990). Because inapparent infection may be the cause of high titers, it is important to rule out other potential causes of arthritis before diagnosing borreliosis.

No therapeutic regimen has been systematically tested in dogs, but rapid response to tetracycline is reported. Other antibiotics recommended for human borreliosis include doxycycline, minocycline, penicillin, ampicillin, amoxicillin, ceftriaxone, and cefotaxime. Glucocorticoids may interfere with response to antibiotics and cause recrudescence of spirochetemia.

FUNGAL ARTHRITIS

Fungal arthritis is uncommon in dogs and cats. Inhalation of spores and subsequent hematogenous dissemination of the organisms to bones and joints is considered a likely mechanism of infection, especially when pulmonary disease is present. Foreign body penetration or trauma to the joint can create portals of entry for the organisms in some cases. Depending on geographic location, species, and immunocompetence, the most likely encountered organisms are Coccidioides, Cryptococcus, and Blastomyces. Sporothrix and Aspergillus have been identified in isolated cases.

Fungal arthritis is frequently accompanied by subcutaneous infection or osteomyelitis and is usually monarticular or pauciarticular. Radiographic findings include soft-tissue swelling, osteopenia (osteoproduction in coccidioidomycosis), and periosteal proliferation. These radiographic changes can be confused with those seen in rheumatoid arthritis. In most instances, synovial fluid analysis indicates inflammation. Histologic evaluation typically reveals pyogranulomatous inflammation.

Ideally, the diagnosis of fungal arthritis is made by identifying the organisms with special stains in synovial fluid, tissue exudates or aspirates, or in histologic sections of involved tissues. When organisms cannot be identified, the diagnosis can be aided by serologic tests and confirmed by isolating the organism in culture using Sabouraud's medium. When blastomycosis is suspected, culture is not routinely attempted because of public health considerations.

Commonly used antifungal drugs include amphotericin B, ketoconazole, and more recently itraconazole and fluconazole. Response to therapy is variable.

PROTOZOAL ARTHRITIS

Visceral leishmaniasis is a chronic systemic disorder caused by Leishmania protozoans (Slappendel and Greene, 1990). Endemic areas include the Mediterranean region, Africa, Asia, and South and Central America and are extending into Mexico. Isolated foci of infection have been found in Texas, Oklahoma, and Ohio. The organism parasitizes macrophages throughout the reticuloendothelial system. Commonly observed clinical signs include weight loss, lethargy, skin lesions, lymphadenopathy, lameness, and splenomegaly. Hyperglobulinemia, hypoalbuminemia, elevated hepatic enzymes, and azotemia are frequent clinical pathologic abnormalities (see this volume, p. 266).

A diagnosis of leishmaniasis can be made by identification of the organism in macrophages, especially in lymph node or bone marrow aspirates. The kinetoplast, a perinuclear organelle, is a characteristic morphologic feature and is easily seen under light microscopy. In one dog presented for an intermittent, shifting leg lameness, organisms were identified in occasional macrophages in synovial fluid, even though the synovial fluid showed a normal cell count and differential. Radiographs of affected joints showed normal findings. In other cases, numerous organisms have been seen within synovial membrane macrophages.

Leishmaniasis in dogs is resistant to therapy. Relapses usually occur in a few months to a year after therapy and should be treated with another course of antimonial drug. At present, meglumine antimonate and sodium stibogluconate are considered the most effective drugs for the treatment of canine leishmaniasis.

VIRAL ARTHRITIS

Natural calicivirus infection can produce a transient polyarthritis in kittens 8 to 14 weeks of age (Pedersen et al., 1983). Affected kittens usually demonstrate stiffness, lameness, and fever and recover after 2 to 4 days. The joint fluid shows an increased number of macrophages, some of which contain phagocytosed neutrophils. Several strains of calicivirus have been recovered from the blood during the acute phase of illness, and the disease can be reproduced by feeding tissue culture–propagated virus to susceptible kittens.

A transient polyarthritis has been uncommonly observed 5 to 7 days after vaccination in both dogs and cats. The postvaccinal reaction is usually associated with multivalent live virus vaccines and is generally self-limiting. Corticosteroid therapy has been used if symptoms persist for more than 5 days (Pedersen et al., 1989).

IMMUNE-MEDIATED ARTHRITIS ASSOCIATED WITH CHRONIC INFECTIOUS DISEASES

Nonseptic, nonerosive (immune-mediated) polyarthritis is relatively common in dogs and also occurs in cats. The disease probably results from immune complex deposition within the synovium leading to a sterile synovitis. The inciting antigen can be derived from a diverse group of underlying diseases, including various chronic infections, systemic lupus erythematosus, neoplasia, drug hypersensitivity, and chronic gastrointestinal or liver disease. When an underlying antigenic stimulus cannot be identified, the disease is termed idiopathic polyarthritis.

Chronic infectious diseases that have been associated with immune-mediated polyarthritis are listed in Table 3 and include bacterial, fungal, parasitic, and possibly viral diseases. The clinical signs of immune-mediated polyarthritis may be limited to those of polyarthritis or complicated by those of the associated primary disease. The joint disease tends to be intermittent and has a predilection for small distal joints, the carpus and tarsus in particular. Monarticular disease most frequently involves the elbow joint. Radiographic findings are either nonexistent or limited to periarticular soft-tissue swelling, and there is no evidence of cartilage loss or osteolysis. Normal or increased quantities of synovial fluid contain increased numbers of leukocytes, most of which are nondegenerate neutrophils. Cultures of synovial fluid are negative for aerobic and anaerobic bacteria, mycoplasmas, and fungi. Cytologic study of synovial fluid and histologic evaluation of synovial membrane fail to reveal an etiologic agent, and abnormal findings are consistent with an inflammatory process. Results of immunologic tests for antinuclear antibody and rheumatoid factor are usually negative, but low titers are occasionally obtained. Routine hematologic, biochemical, and urine analyses may reveal abnormalities related to the primary underlying disease. Microorganisms can usually be identified by culture or histologic examination of the primary infectious foci. In some obscure infections, culture of blood or urine may reveal an etiologic agent. Serologic findings (occult heartworm, fungal) may give supportive evidence in some cases.

Treatment is directed at the primary underlying disease process. If the infectious disease is eliminated, the immune-mediated polyarthritis usually subsides gradually over a period of several weeks. Residual lameness has been treated with corticosteroids and rarely with combination immunosuppressive therapy.

References and Suggested Reading

Bennett, D., and Taylor, D. J.: Bacterial infective arthritis in the dog. J. Small Anim. Pract. 29:207, 1988.
A retrospective study of the clinical findings in 58 cases of bacterial arthritis in dogs.
Brown, A., and Bennett, D.: Gentamicin-impregnated polymethylmethacrylate beads for the treatment of septic arthritis. Vet. Rec. 123:625, 1988.
Case study describing the surgical use of antibiotic-impregnated beads for local treatment of a resistant infection involving the stifle joint.
Buchanan, A. M., Beaman, B. L., Pedersen, N. C., et al.: *Nocardia asteroides* recovery from a dog with steroid- and antibiotic-unresponsive idiopathic polyarthritis. J. Clin. Microbiol. 18:702, 1983.
Case report of polyarthritis in a dog from which an L-form of N. asteroides was isolated.
Carro, T., Pedersen, N. C., Beaman, B. L., et al.: Subcutaneous abscesses and arthritis caused by a probable bacterial L-form in cats. J.A.V.M.A. 194:1583, 1989.
Case study of three naturally infected cats from one household and experimental transmission of the infectious agent, characterized as a bacterial L-form.
Cowell, R. L., Tyler, R. D., Clinkenbeard, K. D., et al.: Ehrlichiosis and polyarthritis in three dogs. J.A.V.M.A. 192: 1093, 1988.

Three case reports of canine granulocytic ehrlichiosis in dogs presenting with acute lameness.

Greene, R. T.: Lyme borreliosis. *In* Greene, C. E. (ed.): *Infectious Diseases of the Dog and Cat.* Philadelphia: W. B. Saunders, 1990, p. 508.

A comprehensive review of canine borreliosis including etiopathogenesis, clinical findings, and therapeutic management.

Hopper, P. E.: Immune-mediated nonerosive arthritis in the dog. *In* Kirk, R. W. (ed.): *Current Veterinary Therapy X.* Philadelphia: W. B. Saunders, 1989, p. 543.

A review of nonerosive immune-mediated arthritis in the dog including clinicopathologic findings, differential diagnosis, and treatment.

Kornblatt, A. N., Urband, P. H., and Steere, A. C.: Arthritis caused by *Borrelia burgdorferi* in dogs. J.A.V.M.A. 186:960, 1985.

A comparison of antibody titers to B. burgdorferi *in 34 dogs with arthritis and in 43 normal dogs from an area endemic for human Lyme disease, and a clinical description of those dogs with suspected borrelio arthritis.*

Magnarelli, L. A., Anderson, J. F., Levine, H. R., et al.: Tick parasitism and antibodies to *Borrelia burgdorferi* in cats. J.A.V.M.A. 197:63, 1990.

A serologic survey of 71 cats from the Connecticut area for antibodies to B. burgdorferi *and comparison of clinical information in 34 of the tested cats.*

Montgomery, R. D., Long, I. R., Milton, J. L., et al.: Comparison of aerobic culturette, synovial membrane biopsy, and blood culture medium in detection of canine bacterial arthritis. Vet. Surg. 18:300, 1989.

A comparison of three culture techniques using synovial fluid and synovial membrane from experimentally infected joints.

Pedersen, N. C., Laliberte, L., and Ekman, S.: A transient febrile, "limping" syndrome of kittens caused by two different strains of feline calicivirus. Feline Pract. 13:26, 1983.

Calicivirus isolation from naturally infected lame kittens and experimental transmission of the clinical syndrome.

Pedersen, N. C., and Pool, R.: Canine joint disease. Vet. Clin. North Am. Small Anim. Pract. 8:465, 1978.

A review of noninflammatory and inflammatory joint disease in dogs.

Pedersen, N. C., Wind, A., Morgan, J. P., et al.: Joint diseases of dogs and cats. *In* Ettinger, S. J. (ed.): *Textbook of Veterinary Internal Medicine.* Philadelphia: W. B. Saunders, 1989, p. 2362.

A comprehensive review of inflammatory and noninflammatory joint diseases of dogs and cats, emphasizing etiology, pathogenesis, and clinical findings.

Slappendel, R. J., and Greene, C. E.: Leishmaniasis. *In* Green, C. E. (ed.): *Infectious Diseases of the Dog and Cat.* Philadelphia: W. B. Saunders, 1990, p. 769.

A comprehensive review of leishmaniasis including etiopathogenesis, clinicopathologic findings, therapy, and prevention.

Stockham, S. L., Schmidt, D. A., Tyler, J. W., et al.: Polyarthritis associated with canine granulocytic ehrlichiosis. Vet. Clin. Pathol. 15: 8, 1986.

Clinical findings in nine dogs with naturally occurring granulocytic ehrlichiosis and in two dogs experimentally infected.

Werner, L. L.: Arthrocentesis and joint fluid analysis: Diagnostic application in joint diseases of small animals. Comp. Cont. Ed. Pract. Vet. 1:855, 1979.

A review of the causes of joint disease, the technique of arthrocentesis, and interpretation of joint fluid analysis.

LABORATORY DIAGNOSIS OF TICK-TRANSMITTED DISEASES IN THE DOG

EDWARD B. BREITSCHWERDT

Raleigh, North Carolina

Tick-transmitted diseases are typically limited to the geographic region in which infectious ticks reside. However, the frequent transport of dogs within our society and the chronic insidious course of diseases such as ehrlichiosis and potentially borreliosis suggest that previous geographic history should be pursued, even in nonendemic regions, as is routinely done for potential systemic mycotic infections. Because different tick species are responsible for the transmission of the various pathogens, increased familiarity with species identification of ticks is also of clinical relevance.

The history, clinical findings, and results of standard clinicopathologic testing can be similar among the various tick-transmitted diseases, as well as other infectious and noninfectious disease processes. For example, diagnostic differentiation of Rocky Mountain spotted fever (RMSF), acute ehrlichiosis, gram-negative sepsis, or acute pancreati-

tis, solely on the basis of historical and clinicopathologic abnormalities, can be extremely difficult. Familiarity with the temporal course and idiosyncrasies of these diseases greatly facilitates initial diagnostic and therapeutic impressions; however, confirmation of the diagnosis requires cytologic demonstration of the organism (*Ehrlichia morula*), serologic testing, or culture of the organism. Because of the difficulty and potential danger associated with culturing rickettsiae and spirochetes, this means of diagnosis is generally limited to academic and research institutions.

Although an important adjunct to the diagnosis of tick-transmitted diseases, serologic testing is fraught with problems related to accurate interpretation. When interpreting a serologic result, it is important to know the sensitivity and specificity of the testing procedure, the degree of cross-reactivity with other infectious agents, the prevalence of a given disease in the area, the immunoglobulin being detected by the test, and the reliability of the laboratory performing the test.

In general, serologic tests for infectious diseases detect either immunoglobulin M (IgM) antibodies, immunoglobulin G (IgG) antibodies, or both IgM and IgG antibodies, depending on the conjugate used in the testing procedure. If the test detects only IgG antibodies to the offending organism, a dog will generally remain seronegative during the initial 3- to 4-week period following the onset of illness. Therefore, documentation of seroconversion, generally defined as a fourfold increase in antibody titer for diagnostic purposes, is required to confirm a diagnosis. A serum sample obtained during the early acute illness and a second serum sample obtained approximately 3 weeks after the onset of illness must be evaluated. A single elevated antibody titer does not differentiate active versus past infection. IgM antibodies are generally detectable approximately 7 to 10 days after the onset of illness; however, various factors, including increased variability among individual dogs in mounting an IgM response, the influence of early treatment, and an increased propensity for cross-reactivity with other infectious agents, limit the utility of detecting only IgM antibodies in many instances. The absence of a measurable antibody titer does not eliminate the possibility of a specific infectious disease, because rarely dogs fail to mount a humoral immune response.

Specific considerations for the serodiagnosis of each important tick-transmitted disease are considered separately in the pages that follow.

BABESIOSIS

Canine babesiosis is caused by *Babesia canis* or *Babesia gibsoni*. The indirect fluorescent antibody test is currently recommended for serodiagnosis of patent or occult parasitemia in dogs. Because of cross-reactivity between *B. canis* and *B. gibsoni*, demonstration of the organism in a blood smear is necessary for species differentiation, which is important in the selection of an effective chemotherapeutic agent. In most laboratories, an IgG antibody titer of greater than 1:40 is considered positive for either organism. Serologic evaluation is not useful for diagnosis of babesiosis in puppies and very young dogs because they are often incapable of mounting a detectable immunofluorescent antibody (IFA) titer. Although specific instances have been documented, the extent to which *Babesia* organisms cause disease but are not detected during blood film examination is unknown. Because of the relatively high seroprevalence of *Babesia* in the Southeast, it is probable that strains of *Babesia* indigenous to the United States do not induce serious patho-

genicity in immunocompetent, nonstressed adult dogs. In contrast, babesiosis in puppies can cause severe hemolytic anemia and death and can be misdiagnosed as hookworm anemia. Documentation of seroconversion should be used when babesiosis is suspected without evidence of parasitemia.

BORRELIOSIS

Serodiagnosis of canine borreliosis is controversial. The high prevalence of antibodies (50 to 90% seropositivity) to *Borrelia burgdorferi* in dogs in Lyme-disease endemic regions invalidates the use of a single antibody titer to support a clinical diagnosis of canine borreliosis. Recent identification of an infectious but nonpathogenic *B. burgdorferi* isolate may help to explain the high degree of seropositivity in healthy dogs (Anderson et al., 1990). Both indirect IFA assays and enzyme-linked immunosorbent assays (ELISA) have been used to detect *B. burgdorferi* antibodies, with the ELISA test being favored because of increased sensitivity and less variable results. Cross-reactivity with other spirochetes, particularly *Borrelia hermsii*, may also contribute to the seroepidemiologic prevalence of antibodies to *B. burgdorferi* and further complicates the use of serologic findings for confirming a clinical diagnosis. One study (Magnarelli et al., 1990), comparing lame and healthy dogs living in tick-infested areas of New York and Connecticut, found no difference in the prevalence of seropositivity among the two groups when tested several times during periods up to 15 months in duration. Additionally, treatment of lame dogs with tetracycline or amoxicillin caused little or no change in antibody titer in convalescent serum obtained 2 or more months after the initial sample collection. A diagnostically significant increase or decrease in antibody titer was reported in 4 of 40 antibiotic-treated dogs, thereby supporting a potential causal role for *B. burgdorferi* in the disease process. Current antibody detection techniques document previous exposure to *B. burgdorferi* or, if seronegative, the lack of humoral evidence of exposure to the organism. Documentation of seroconversion or a significant decrease in antibody titer following antibiotic treatment is supportive of a diagnosis of canine Lyme disease (see this volume, p. 256).

EHRLICHIOSIS

Canine ehrlichiosis is characterized by an acute phase, a subclinical carrier state that can last from months to years, and a chronic disease phase. Serologic testing for *Ehrlichia canis* by IFA is not beneficial during acute disease, unless acute and convalescent antibody titers are compared. Experimentally, immunoglobulin A (IgA) and immunoglobulin M (IgM) antibodies are detectable 7 days post inoculation, whereas IgG antibodies become detectable in most dogs by day 21 after inoculation. The antibody titer peaks approximately 80 days after inoculation and remains positive until the dog is treated with a rickettsiostatic or rickettsiocidal antibiotic. After treatment, the titer progressively declines and generally becomes negative in 6 to 9 months. Infection with *E. canis* does not imply protective immunity; therefore, subsequent exposure to infected ticks will result in disease, generally of decreased severity. Some dogs become asymptomatic but maintain high *E. canis* titers for years after treatment with antibiotics. Clinically, these dogs are assumed to have eliminated the rickettsiae if the hyperglobulinemia resolves progressively following treatment. Infrequently, a dog maintains a high antibody titer, and a hematologic abnormality such as thrombocytopenia persists for years, despite antimicrobial therapy. It is unclear whether these dogs are chronically infected with *E. canis* or if the persistent abnormalities are mediated through altered immunoregulation induced by the infection. There is similar serologic cross-reactivity between the neutrophilic (potentially another species of *Ehrlichia*) and monocytic strains of *E. canis* and lesser cross-reactivity with *E. equi*, *E. sennetsu*, and *E. risticii*. The extent to which serologic cross-reactivity complicates the diagnosis of canine ehrlichiosis in various geographic regions requires additional clarification.

INFECTIOUS CYCLIC THROMBOCYTOPENIA

Infectious cyclic thrombocytopenia of dogs is caused by *E. platys*, which is serologically distinct from other ehrlichiae. Presumed to be tick transmitted, this organism infects platelets and causes cyclic thrombocytopenia at 1- to 2-week intervals. Seroprevalence studies suggest that exposure to *E. platys* is frequent in thrombocytopenic and *E. canis*–infected dogs in the southeastern United States. Although experimental inoculation of *E. platys* does not induce clinical illness, it is probable that chronic infection with the organism complicates the diagnostic and therapeutic management of other infectious and noninfectious diseases. An IFA titer of 1:100 or greater is considered positive for *E. platys*. Treatment with tetracycline is recommended even if the dog is asymptomatic.

ROCKY MOUNTAIN SPOTTED FEVER

RMSF is caused by *R. rickettsii*, a member of the spotted fever group of rickettsiae. The organism causes a spectrum of clinicopathologic abnormalities that mimic many other diseases. RMSF is clinically indistinguishable from acute ehrlichiosis, thereby necessitating serologic testing to differentiate these diseases. The kinetics of the IgM and IgG antibody response following experimental inoculation of *R. rickettsii* are similar to ehrlichiosis. IgM antibodies are first detected by IFA on postinoculation day 9, peak by postinoculation day 20, and are no longer detectable by postinoculation day 80. IgG antibodies are generally detectable between postinoculation days 22 and 28, peak by day 42, and decrease gradually during the next 6 to 9 months. Because canine RMSF is an acute disease of 5 to 14 days' duration, serodiagnosis requires documentation of a fourfold increase in antibody titer between acute and convalescent samples. Sole detection of IgM antibodies to facilitate early diagnosis of RMSF in dogs has not proved useful because of poor diagnostic specificity. Considering the lack of clinical and serologic response to challenge inoculation of *R. rickettsii* 3 years after experimental RMSF, immunity following natural infection is probably lifelong. Therefore, recurrent bouts of tick fever should not be attributed to recurrent RMSF. Another factor that necessitates evaluation of acute and convalescent serum for diagnosis of RMSF is the extensive cross-reactivity between *R. rickettsii* and other presumably nonpathogenic spotted fever group rickettsiae, most notably *Rickettsia rhipicephali* and *Rickettsia montana*. Because the prevalence of nonpathogenic spotted fever group rickettsiae in ticks is much greater than the prevalence of *R. rickettsii*, the likelihood of canine exposure to these organisms in the environment is much greater. In clinical terms, this means that many dogs tested for RMSF during the summer will have low but diagnostically significant ($\geq$ 1:64) titers to *R. rickettsii* that represent cross-reacting antibodies to common nonpathogenic rickettsiae.

Table 1 illustrates the complexities of serologic confirmation of tick-transmitted diseases and the importance of evaluating acute and convalescent serologic results in dogs in which RMSF is suspected. These dogs, selected from our hospital patient population, were evaluated for lameness. Cytologic examination of synovial fluid documented neutrophilic inflammatory polyarthritis for which one of the differential diagnoses was RMSF. Final diagnoses included ehrlichiosis, systemic lupus erythematosus, immune-mediated polyarthritis, drug-induced polyarthritis, and RMSF. Because of previous exposure to spotted fever group rickettsiae, several dogs with serologic confirmation of other diseases had acute-phase *R. rickettsii* titers of 1:64 or greater. These dogs did not seroconvert, in contrast to dogs one and two, in which RMSF was confirmed by documenting seroconversion. Also, as illustrated by these cases, thrombocytopenia, a fre-

Table 1. *Selected Laboratory and Serologic Findings From Acutely Lame Dogs in Which Inflammatory Polyarthritis Was Diagnosed*

Patient Number	Platelet Count	Neutrophil Count (/μl)	Band Neutrophils (/μl)	Rickettsia rickettsii Titers Acute	Rickettsia rickettsii Titers Convalescent	Borrelia burgdorferi Titer	Ehrlichia canis Titer	Antinuclear Antibody Titer	Blood Cultures	Diagnosis
1	115,000	13,035	1815	Neg	1:2048	Neg	Neg	Neg	Neg	RMSF
2	128,000	10,664	0	1:16	1:8192	ND	Neg	Neg	Neg	RMSF
3	52,000	17,200	0	1:256	1:256	1:64	1:320	Neg	Neg	Ehrlichiosis
4	94,000	21,336	0	1:256	1:128	Neg	Neg	Neg	Neg	Immune-mediated polyarthritis
5	221,000	30,960	0	1:256	1:128	Neg	Neg	Neg	Neg	Immune-mediated polyarthritis
6	158,000	16,647	0	1:32	Neg	1:128	Neg	Neg	Neg	Immune-mediated polyarthritis
7	4000	12,672	0	Neg	ND	ND	Neg	1:600	Neg	Systemic lupus erythematosus
8	160,000	5940	0	Neg	Neg	Neg	Neg	1:80	ND	Systemic lupus erythematosus
9	287,000	11,242	154	1:16	1:16	Neg	Neg	1:20	ND	Trimethoprim/ sulfadiazine polyarthritis

ND, not done; RMSF, Rocky Mountain spotted fever.

quent finding in *R. rickettsii* polyarthritis, occurs in association with other infectious and noninfectious diseases.

In recent years, there has been enhanced awareness of the importance of ticks in the transmission of infectious agents to dogs and people. Because of transovarial or trans-stadial transmission of infectious agents as well as other factors, tick-transmitted diseases generally occur in focal geographic clusters of varying size and infective density. Therefore, because environmental exposure to *B. burgdorferi*, *E. canis*, and *R. rickettsii* is frequently similar for people and their pets, accurate diagnosis of canine infection with these agents also has potentially important implications for human health. Diagnosis of canine infection can serve as a harbinger of human disease or facilitate appropriate tick control practices that could prevent subsequent infection in humans.

References and Suggested Reading

Anderson, J. F., Barthold, S. W., and Magnarelli, L. A.: Infectious but nonpathogenic isolate of *Borrelia burgdorferi*. J. Clin. Microb. 28:2693, 1990.
A report describing an isolate of B. burgdorferi *that is not pathogenic in experimental models of borreliosis.*
Breitschwerdt, E. B., Malone, J. B., MacWilliams, P., et al.: Babesiosis in the greyhound. J.A.V.M.A. 182:978, 1983.
A report describing clinical and serologic findings in greyhound kennels in the southeastern United States.
Breitschwerdt, E. B., Moncol, D. J., and Corbett, W. T.: Antibodies to spotted fever group rickettsiae in North Carolina dogs. Am. J. Vet. Res. 48:1436, 1987.
A report describing extensive antibody cross-reactivity in canine serum to spotted fever group rickettsiae.
Breitschwerdt, E. B., Levy, M. G., Davidson, M. G., et al.: Kinetics of IgM and IgG responses to experimental and naturally-occurring *Rickettsia rickettsii* infection. Am. J. Vet. Res. 51:1312, 1990.
A study describing the IgM and IgG serologic response in experimental canine Rocky Mountain spotted fever.
French, T. W., and Harvey, J. W.: Serologic diagnosis of infectious cyclic thrombocytopenia in dogs using an indirect fluorescent antibody test. Am. J. Vet. Res. 44:2407, 1983.
A study describing the IgG serologic response to Ehrlichia platys *infection in dogs.*
Greene, R. T., Levine, J. F., Breitschwerdt, E. B., et al.: Clinical and serologic evaluation of experimental canine *Borrelia burgdorferi* infection. Am. J. Vet. Res. 49:752, 1988.
A study describing the IgM and IgG serologic response in experimental canine borreliosis.
Greene, R. T.: An update on the serodiagnosis of canine Lyme borreliosis. J. Vet. Intern. Med. 4:167, 1990.
A review of factors influencing the serologic diagnosis of canine borreliosis.
Hoskins, J. D., Breitschwerdt, E. B., Gaunt, S. D., et al.: Antibodies to *Ehrlichia canis*, *Ehrlichia platys* and spotted fever group rickettsiae in Louisiana dogs. J. Vet. Intern. Med. 2:55 1988.
A serologic study of thrombocytopenic dogs illustrating the importance of tick-transmitted pathogens in this patient population.
Levy, M. G., Breitschwerdt, E. B., and Moncol, D. J.: Antibodies to *Babesia canis* in North Carolina dogs. Am. J. Vet. Res. 48:339, 1987.
A study that describes the seroprevalence of Babesia canis *in stray and pet dogs in North Carolina.*
Magnarelli, L. A., Anderson, J. F., and Suhreier, A. B.: Persistence of antibodies to *Borrelia burgdorferi* in dogs of New York and Connecticut. J.A.V.M.A. 196:1064, 1990.
A study that describes sequential serologic results in healthy, lame, treated, and untreated dogs in a Lyme-endemic region.
Ristic, M., Huxsoll, D. L., Weisiger, R. M., et al.: Serological diagnosis of tropical canine pancytopenia by indirect immunofluorescence. Infect. Immun. 6:226, 1972.
A study that provides the basis for serologic diagnosis of ehrlichiosis.

CANINE LYME DISEASE: TOWARD SATISFYING KOCH'S POSTULATES

M.J.G. APPEL

Ithaca, New York

Lyme disease has received extensive media coverage in the past decade. Much of the available information about Lyme disease in dogs has been deduced from our knowledge of Lyme disease in humans: the etiologic agent, epizootiology, clinical signs, immune response, diagnosis, treatment, prevention, and control.* Apart from a few case reports and serologic surveys, there is little documented information about the disease in dogs. Many unsuccessful attempts have been made to experimentally reproduce the disease in dogs, but only a few negative studies have been reported (Burgess, 1986; Greene et al., 1988a). One of Koch's postulates, therefore, had by and large not been fulfilled.†

It is extremely difficult to isolate the causative organism from blood or urine, and so positive serologic findings are usually the only indication of infection in dogs. However, in endemic areas, more than 50% of dogs may become seropositive without showing any clinical signs. It is not known whether the serologic response in symptomatic and asymptomatic dogs can be differentiated. For these reasons, concern has been voiced that canine borreliosis may not be a disease at all but only an immunologic response to an organism that may not be pathogenic for dogs (Frank, 1989).

Strong evidence for the existence of Lyme disease in dogs comes from the personal experience of veterinarians in areas of endemic human disease: the sudden onset of severe depression with acutely swollen, hot, and painful joints and total reluctance to move. Prompt response to antibiotic therapy and positive serologic findings in many animals are field evidence of an emerging syndrome that had not been encountered before Lyme disease in humans became a problem during the past 15 years.

The difficulties in satisfying Koch's postulates, therefore, may be due to the lack of knowledge of the pathogenesis of Lyme disease in dogs. A research group of the Fort Dodge Company has claimed that they were able to reproduce lameness and fever in dogs after inoculation with *Borrelia burgdorferi* organisms. These dogs were used as controls for another group of dogs that were protected by a vaccine that has now been marketed. If these results can be confirmed independently, we may be able to learn about the pathogenesis of Lyme disease in dogs.

What do we know about the disease today?

HISTORY

Lyme disease—under different names—has been known in Europe for about 100 years. It became a new disease entity on this continent when, in 1975, an unexplained cluster of cases of joint disease resembling juvenile rheumatoid arthritis suddenly appeared in children in Lyme, Connecticut. The deer tick *Ixodes dammini* was found to be the vector of the pathogen causing the disease. The detection of spirochetes in these ticks happened by coincidence. Dr. Willy Burgdorfer of the Rocky Mountain Laboratory in Hamilton, Montana, was searching for *Rickettsia rickettsii*, the causative agent of Rocky Mountain spotted fever, and found spirochetes in the midgut of 60% of *I. dammini* ticks from endemic areas. *Borrelia* was isolated, found to be the causative agent of Lyme disease, and named *Borrelia burgdorferi* in honor of the scientist (reviewed by Appel, 1990.)

ETIOLOGY

A spirochete of the genus *Borrelia* (*B. burgdorferi*) causes Lyme disease. Organisms of the genera *Leptospira* and *Treponema* (the causative agent of syphilis) are related pathogenic spirochetes with different structures and vectors.

---

*The author wishes to thank Drs. Allan, Baldwin, Fish, Jacobson, Lissman, Olsen, Post, Shin, Spielman, and Travis, as well as Eric Shaw, M.S., for informative discussions and Dr. Summers for reading the manuscript.

†However, during the past months (and after this original manuscript was written), we have repeatedly reproduced clinical Lyme disease in dogs. Recurrent, severe lameness due to arthritis, fever, and depression developed in dogs we exposed to *Borrelia burgdorferi*–infected ticks (*Ixodes dammini*, nymphs or adult ticks). The incubation period ranged from 2 to 5 months.

EPIZOOTIOLOGY

Hard-shell ticks of the genus *Ixodes* (*I. dammini* in the Northeast, *Ixodes pacificus* in the West and Midwest, *Ixodes scapularis* in the southern United States, *Ixodes ricinus* in Europe, and *Ixodes persulcatus* in Asia) transmit *B. burgdorferi*.

Most available information is on *I. dammini*. It requires three hosts and four developmental stages to complete its 2-year life cycle. Larvae that emerge from eggs in the spring feed predominantly on white-footed mice (*Peromyscus leucopus*) in the northeastern United States. In areas where Lyme disease is enzootic, a high percentage of mice are persistently infected with *B. burgdorferi*, and the tick larvae become infected during a 2-day feeding period. Infection in ticks persists during all stages. The larvae drop off and enter a resting stage until the following spring, when they molt into the nymphal stage.

During spring and early summer, the nymphs attach themselves to a new host, predominantly again white-footed mice, although hosts can include a wide variety of wild and domestic animals and humans. During a 3- to 4-day feeding period, spirochetes are transmitted to the host. Nymphs drop off and molt into the adult stage toward the end of summer.

During fall and early winter, adult ticks can be found on vegetation about 1 m above the ground, where they attach to deer and other mammals, including dogs. During a 5- to 7-day feeding period, ticks transmit spirochetes to the host. Infected adult ticks are probably an important source of infection in dogs, whereas infected nymphs appear to be the main source of infection in humans.

Male ticks tend to stay on the host after mating and die. Female ticks drop off and survive the winter on the ground. The following spring, a female tick lays between 2000 and 4000 eggs, thus completing the 2-year life cycle.

In addition to tick bites, blood and urine of infected animals are potential sources of *B. burgdorferi* that could infect dogs. However, the agent is present in very low concentrations in blood and urine, if at all, and it deteriorates rapidly (reviewed by Appel, 1990).

CLINICAL SIGNS

Dogs seldom display the early skin rash (erythema chronicum migrans) at the site of a tick bite that is a telltale sign in humans. The rash has been seen in some dogs in the groin or other hairless areas (Appel, 1990).

First signs in dogs are sudden lameness and evidence of severe pain. Joints, usually bilateral and predominantly carpal, become swollen, hot, and painful when touched. Severe depression, total reluctance to move, and sometimes fever or swollen lymph nodes are early signs. Signs of pain in the head and neck regions and muscle pain are not uncommon (reviewed by Appel, 1990).

In contrast to human Lyme disease, in which three different stages of the disease are common, with chronic arthritis appearing months to years after infection as the final stage, the disease in dogs most often appears to be acute. Treatment with antibiotics usually cures the disease. Nevertheless, second-stage signs such as carditis (with complete heart block), kidney involvement, and neurologic signs have been claimed (Levy and Durray, 1988; Lissman, personal communication, Magnarelli et al., 1987).

IMMUNE RESPONSE

Antibody to *B. burgdorferi* antigens can be detected in dog sera by 8 to 10 days after inoculation with the organism. The timing of antibody production after natural exposure is not known. Antibody in human serum is usually not found until 3 weeks after the onset of a skin rash. Both IgM and IgG can persist for at least 9 months in naturally infected dogs.

The relationship between immune response and clinical disease in dogs is completely unknown. More than 50% of dogs in endemic areas have antibody to *B. burgdorferi* antigens and remain asymptomatic.

It was suggested that immune responses to surface proteins of the spirochetes may determine persistence or elimination of the organism. Experimentally exposed asymptomatic dogs produced antibodies to one of two surface proteins (OSpA), whereas naturally exposed dogs did not (Greene et al., 1988b). In human Lyme disease, serologic differentiation between the different stages of disease and asymptomatic infection appears feasible by immunoblot analysis of IgM and IgG to different polypeptides of *B. burgdorferi*.

Tests for cellular immune responses in dogs with Lyme diseases have not been developed. Specific T-lymphocyte responses to *B. burgdorferi* are detectable early in the course of human infection, often before a measurable humoral immune response develops.

DIAGNOSIS

The diagnosis of Lyme disease in dogs often is difficult. Clinical signs may be nonspecific; there are many causes of lameness and pain. Serologic findings alone are useless, because more than 50% of seropositive dogs remain asymptomatic whereas dogs with acute signs of Lyme disease may be seronegative. Testing 3 to 4 weeks later, however, may reveal seroconversion.

The diagnosis of Lyme disease in dogs should be based on a combination of history (recent exposure to an enzootic area or detection of ticks on dogs) with clinical signs, serologic test results, and prompt response to antibiotic therapy.

Attempts to demonstrate or culture the spirochetes from blood, urine, synovia, or skin are usually unsuccessful.

Interpretation of serologic results is difficult. Although most infected dogs with acute lameness and pain have high levels of antibodies to *B. burgdorferi* antigens, some dogs in the early phase of the disease may be seronegative. A fourfold rise in antibody titer 2 to 4 weeks later may confirm the diagnosis.

Two techniques have been used predominantly in the past decade to detect serum antibody to *B. burgdorferi* antigens: the indirect fluorescent antibody (IFA) test and the enzyme-linked immunosorbent assay (ELISA). It is now generally agreed that the ELISA is more sensitive and specific than the IFA test. These tests, however, are not standardized among laboratories. Titers reported from different centers may vary greatly.

Commercial test kits are now available for detecting *B. burgdorferi* antibody in dog sera.

Although strain differences of *B. burgdorferi* are known to occur within the United States and worldwide, the antigens commonly used for serologic testing sufficiently cover the different strains.

Exposure to other *Borrelia* species must be considered; several *Borrelia* species that cause relapsing fever in humans are present in the United States, and antibodies to these spirochetes react in Lyme disease tests. It is not known whether dogs become infected with these agents. They would not be expected in the Northeast but may be a source of confusion in other states. Some cross-reaction would also be expected with *Treponema* species. Cross-reaction with antibodies to *Leptospira* organisms is minimal.

For differential diagnosis, a hemogram (findings expected to be normal in Lyme disease), serum biochemical panel, urinalysis, and serologic study may suggest other infectious diseases such as Rocky Mountain spotted fever or *Ehrlichia canis* infection. Immune-mediated diseases should be ruled out by testing for antinuclear antibodies, lupus erythematosus preparations, and rheumatoid arthritis factor. Radiographs and analysis of synovia or synovial fluid might help to diagnose lameness due to different causes (see this volume, p. 246).

Response to antibiotic therapy within 2 or 3 days is a useful diagnostic criterion in acute cases.

TREATMENT

Antibiotics are the treatment of choice for Lyme disease in dogs as well as in humans. The efficacy of different antibiotics in dogs with the disease is unknown, and conclusions have been drawn from treatment of humans. The tetracyclines, including tetracycline hydrochloride, doxycycline, and minocycline, all are effective in dogs and are similar in their activity against *B. burgdorferi*. Among the beta-lactam antibiotics, penicillin, ampicillin, amoxicillin, ceftriaxone sodium, and cefotaxime all are effective (Luft et al., 1989).

Ceftriaxone sodium is most active and enters synovia and cerebrospinal fluid, but it is expensive and must be administered parenterally. It is often used in chronic cases of Lyme disease in humans in which other antibiotics have failed. Amoxicillin and ampicillin are more effective than penicillin. Amoxicillin is better absorbed than ampicillin. Erythromycin is active *in vitro*; however, it has *limited* effect *in vivo*. Tetracycline has a more rapid action than the penicillins; however, it has various side effects in young animals. Doxycycline has lipophilic properties that allow penetration into tissue. The antibiotics can be used at normally recommended doses.

How long should a patient with Lyme disease be treated? A period of 10 to 14 days is most commonly used by veterinarians; the range employed is from a single-treatment regimen to 28 days of therapy. The durations of therapy have been arbitrarily chosen without data. Because *B. burgdorferi* may persist if not eliminated, treatment for 3 to 4 weeks appears advisable. If dogs do not respond to an antibiotic within a week to 10 days, the antibiotic should be changed.

The use of anti-inflammatory drugs to reduce joint swelling and pain in dogs with Lyme disease is debatable. The diagnostic value of antibiotic treatment, which is usually effective within a few days, would be greatly influenced by anti-inflammatory drugs.

Should antibiotic treatment be initiated after ticks (*Ixodes*) are found on dogs in areas where Lyme disease is enzootic? In humans, only one of 35 tick bites results in transmission of *Borrelia* because ticks are usually removed before infection takes place. Antibiotic treatment in asymptomatic humans, therefore, is not recommended.

The infection rate in dogs is unknown but may be high, because tick exposure is more frequent and ticks are removed later than in humans. A high percentage of dogs become asymptomatically infected. The question of treatment, therefore, is debatable, especially in areas where daily exposure of dogs to ticks can be anticipated. Because infection occurs only after engorgement of ticks, it may be advisable to initiate treatment of dogs with engorged ticks. Most veterinarians initiate treatment only after the onset of clinical signs.

Should antibiotic treatment be indicated after seroconversion? The answer for humans is yes, because chronic infections can be harmful for years. Because chronic infection in dogs is rare and asymptomatic infections are common, the answer is uncertain. Chronic infection with disease can occur, however, and failure to initiate treatment after seroconversion may be considered malpractice.

PREVENTION AND CONTROL

A vaccine for the prevention of Lyme disease in dogs produced by Fort Dodge Laboratories was licensed conditionally in the spring of 1990. The vaccine is a bacterin that resembles the bacterin found to induce protection in hamsters (Johnson et al., 1986).

The vaccine has been shown by the company to be safe and efficacious when administered to dogs infected in the laboratory. Nonvaccinated control dogs developed fever and lameness for a few days by 4 to 5 weeks after inoculation with *B. burgdorferi* organisms. No lameness and less fever were encountered in vaccinated and challenged dogs. These results would indicate protection from disease but not from infection.

Several questions have been raised about the use of the vaccine. For example, if Lyme disease is an immune-mediated disease, could the vaccine induce disease in previously exposed dogs? Also, the exact method of challenge is still considered proprietary data by the company and cannot yet be confirmed by other laboratories. It is therefore difficult to arrive at a conclusion regarding the safety and efficacy of this bacterin.

Use of the vaccine in the field for a year or more should produce sufficient data for a clearer evaluation. Use of the vaccine should be *restricted to endemic areas*, unless dog owners plan to travel into endemic areas with their dog. Once a dog is vaccinated, positive serologic findings cannot be differentiated from the same findings in a dog after natural exposure.

Besides vaccination, reducing the risk of tick exposure appears to be the best approach. Attempts to reduce the population of primary hosts for ticks are not practical because other hosts are readily available.

Selective chemical control of ticks is more promising. The spraying of wooded areas with acaricides is not advisable for environmental reasons. Boston-based Eco Health, Inc., however, has developed a different approach: biodegradable tubes containing permethrin-treated cotton batting (Damminix) are dispersed in infected areas. The cotton is used by white-footed mice for nesting material. *I. dammini* larvae and nymphs are exposed to the acaricide-covered nesting material and are killed.

With individual dogs and cats, the use of acaricide sprays and daily removal of ticks are the best approaches. A newly designed tweezer (Tick Solution*) especially for tick removal has reached the market.

PUBLIC HEALTH ASPECTS

Humans become infected with the Lyme disease agent *B. burgdorferi* through the bite of an infected tick. It has been speculated that dogs can carry home loosely attached infected ticks, which then attach to humans and induce infection.

Blood and urine of animals are potential sources of *B. burgdorferi* and could be infective for humans, although the agent is present in very low concentrations. *Borrelia* organisms deteriorate quickly in urine, and there is currently no evidence that humans have become infected after contact with dogs.

The nonprofit, national Lyme Borreliosis Foundation (LBF) is a central coordinator of information and support on Lyme disease and related disorders. It is devoted to the prevention and treatment of, and education in all aspects of the disease. LBF is headquartered in Tolland, CT, and can be contacted by calling (203) 871-2900.

References and Suggested Reading

Appel, M. J. G.: Lyme disease in dogs and cats. Comp. Cont. Ed. Pract. Vet. 12:617, 1990.

Burgess, E. C.: Experimental inoculation of dogs with *Borrelia burgdorferi*. Zentralbl. Bakteriol. Microbiol. Hyg. A263:49, 1986.

Frank, J. C.: Taking a hard look at *Borrelia burgdorferi*. J.A.V.M.A. 194:1521, 1989.

Greene, R. T., Levine, J. F., Breitschwerdt, E. B., et al.: Clinical and serological evaluations of induced *Borrelia burgdorferi* infection in dogs. Am. J. Vet. Res. 49:752, 1988a.

Greene, R. T., Walker, R. L., Nicholson, W. L., et al.: Immunoblot analysis of immunoglobulin G response to the Lyme disease agent (*Borrelia burgdorferi*) in experimentally and naturally exposed dogs. J. Clin. Microbiol. 26:648, 1988b.

Johnson, R. C., Kodner, C., and Russell, M.: Notes: Active immunization of hamsters against experimental infection with *Borrelia burgdorferi*. Infect. Immun. 54:897, 1986.

Levy, S. A., and Durray, P. H.: Complete heart block in a dog seropositive for *Borrelia burgdorferi*. J. Vet. Intern. Med. 2:138, 1988.

Luft, B. J., Gorevic, P. D., Halperin, J. J., et al.: A perspective on the treatment of Lyme borreliosis. Rev. Infect. Dis. 2 (suppl. 6):S1518, 1989.

Magnarelli, L. A., Anderson, J. F., Schreier, A. B., et al.: Clinical and serologic studies of canine borreliosis. J.A.V.M.A. 191:1089, 1987.

*Tick Solution is available from Instruments of Sweden, P.O. Box 10810, Waterbury, CT, or by calling 800-955-TICK.

CANINE LEPTOSPIROSIS

VIRGINIA T. RENTKO
and LINDA A. ROSS
North Grafton, Massachusetts

Leptospirosis is a zoonotic disease affecting many species of animals worldwide. Leptospires are aquatic spirochetes and consist of two species: *Leptospira biflexa*, which is a saprophyte, and *L. interrogans*, which is pathogenic. *L. interrogans* is subdivided into serovars on the basis of differing surface antigens. These antigens form the basis for many diagnostic serologic tests for leptospirosis as well as the immunogenic properties of bacterins. Although the surface antigens of different serovars are distinct, they do share some epitopes with other serovars. This property is responsible for the cross-reactions that occur with certain serologic tests.

EPIZOOTIOLOGY

Canine leptospirosis has been considered an uncommon disease during the past 30 years as a result of vaccination and limited exposure of pets to wildlife reservoirs. Dogs are considered to be a maintenance host for infection by serovars *icterohaemorrhagiae*, *canicola*, and *grippotyphosa*. Infection in a maintenance host is characterized by high susceptibility, chronic renal infection with urinary shedding, and efficient transmission to other dogs. In contrast, infection in an incidental host is marked by low susceptibility, a short renal phase, severe pathogenic effect, a strong antibody response, and poor transmission. Dogs are an incidental host for infection with serovars *autumnalis*, *australis*, *tarassovi*, *ballum*, *bataviae*, and *bratislava* (Ellis, 1986; Greene and Shotts, 1990; Hanson, 1982). Serologic surveys in cats suggest that infection occurs in this species, but clinical disease is rare.

The epidemiology of canine leptospirosis appears to be changing. Serovars *icterohaemorrhagiae* and *canicola* were reported as the primary pathogens in canine leptospirosis as recently as 1984 (Greene, 1984). However, in 1990, serovar *grippotyphosa* was noted as an important pathogen in dogs, and evidence now suggests that serovar *pomona* may also be a common canine pathogen (Rentko et al., 1991).

The epizootiology of leptospirosis is complex. Environmental survivability is poor, but optimal conditions include wetness, moderate temperatures, and mildly alkaline soil. These conditions occur most commonly in the autumn months and,

to a lesser extent, in the spring. The organisms are transmitted through the urine and, rarely, venereally. Other potential means of transmission include transplacental, through bite wounds, and by ingestion of infected meat. Rats have been reported to be important in transmitting serovars *icterohaemorrhagiae* and *canicola* among the canine population. Other common wildlife reservoirs include raccoons, skunks, and opossums. The migration of these species into suburban areas may provide a source of exposure of serovars *grippotyphosa* and *pomona* for dogs.

Infection occurs after leptospires penetrate mucous membranes or abraded skin. The leptospiremic phase of infection lasts for 4 to 12 days, depending on the virulence of the organism and the response of the host. Nonspecific signs such as fever, depression, anorexia, and generalized pain occur during this time. Vasculitis, thrombocytopenia, and a coagulopathy may develop. Within a few days, the leptospires colonize the renal tubular epithelial cells, azotemia develops, and signs of uremia become evident. The liver may be variably affected, and the degree of icterus often reflects the severity of disease. Other systems may be involved. Meningitis, uveitis, and abortion have been reported in association with acute infection.

Leptospiral infections may be peracute, subacute, or chronic. Peracute infections are associated with massive leptospiremia. Death usually occurs early in the course of the disease as a result of dehydration, vasculitis, and disseminated intravascular coagulation before organ failure has developed. Subacute infections are characterized by acute renal failure and hepatitis with cholestasis. Chronic and subclinical infections occur commonly and are manifested by nonspecific signs such as fever, anterior uveitis, signs of chronic active hepatitis, or chronic interstitial nephritis.

The clinical syndrome appears to vary depending on the serovar causing the infection. Acute hepatic failure may occur as a result of infection with serovars *icterohaemorrhagiae* and *grippotyphosa* and results in icterus, progressive elevations in liver enzymes, and gastrointestinal signs. Renal failure may be the primary clinical syndrome, as reported in a retrospective survey of dogs with clinical signs and serologic evidence of infection with serovars *grippotyphosa* and *pomona* (Rentko et al., 1991).

When icterus occurred in these dogs, it was mild, and elevations of liver enzymes were mild and transient. Hemolysis, which occurs in cattle infected with serovar *pomona*, was not encountered. This presentation is in contrast to the classic clinical picture involving both renal and hepatic disease.

CLINICAL PRESENTATION

The history of most dogs with leptospirosis includes lethargy, depression, anorexia, vomiting, and fever. Reluctance to move or stiffness, polyuria and polydipsia, weight loss, posterior paresis, diarrhea, cough, nasal discharge, and labored breathing have also been reported. Most abnormalities found on physical examination are nonspecific and reflect the systemic nature of the disease. Abdominal pain and myalgia are common signs. Vomiting and diarrhea attributable to uremia also occur. Respiratory signs may be present as the result of uremic pneumonitis or pulmonary edema secondary to leptospiral toxins or vasculitis.

Hematologic abnormalities include leukocytosis, lymphopenia, and monocytosis. Thrombocytopenia, thought to be due to platelet aggregation, occurs early in the disease. It may be associated with vasculitis or disseminated intravascular coagulation or may occur as the sole abnormality of coagulation. Serum chemistry assays often reveal azotemia and elevations in levels of hepatic enzymes (alanine aminotransferase, aspartate aminotransferase, serum alkaline phosphatase, lactate dehydrogenase, total bilirubin) due to hepatocellular necrosis and intrahepatic cholestasis. Electrolyte abnormalities reflect gastrointestinal disturbances and acute renal dysfunction and may include hyponatremia, hypochloremia, hypokalemia or hyperkalemia, and hyperphosphatemia. Urinalysis usually reveals an active sediment containing erythrocytes, leukocytes, and granular casts and reflects renal tubular damage, characterized by isosthenuria, proteinuria, and glucosuria.

DIAGNOSIS

Diagnosis of leptospirosis is based on correlation of clinical signs, laboratory findings, and serologic test results. Dogs with acute renal disease should be suspected of having leptospirosis. Titers should be determined and therapy instituted early in the clinical course in these dogs, with or without evidence of hepatic disease. Differential diagnoses include infectious nephritis and toxic nephritis due to ethylene glycol or heavy metals. If hepatic disease is present, toxic or infectious hepatitis should be ruled out. The key to diagnosis and successful management of canine leptospirosis is early recog-

nition as a result of a high index of suspicion of any patient with acute renal disease, and aggressive supportive care along with leptospirocidal antibiotics.

The microscopic agglutination test (MAT) is the standard, most frequently used serologic test. In this test, the patient's serum is serially diluted and exposed to live leptospires in a liquid medium. Agglutination of 50% of the organisms is the end point at which the serum titer is read. The serum titer is often negative early in the disease, and a convalescent titer should be measured in 2 to 3 weeks. Although a fourfold increase in serum titer is the most accurate serologic method for diagnosis, single high titers with compatible clinical signs are considered adequate. Dogs with prior infections may also have moderately high MAT titers. Evaluation of the convalescent titer helps distinguish a recent infection from a prior one, in that the convalescent titer from a past infection would remain unchanged from the acute titer.

Agglutination titers do not correlate with protection. Animals in the incubation stage of the disease or chronic carriers with localized infections may have a low titer or no titer at all (Hanson, 1982). Administration of antibiotics early in the disease can also blunt the agglutination titer. Vaccination usually induces low, transient titers (less than 1:200) for 1 to 3 months, although titers as high as 1:800 have been reported (Hanson, 1982). Conversely, vaccinated dogs may have no agglutination titer but can still be protected. Perhaps the most important potential shortcoming of the MAT is the possibility that vaccination may considerably reduce the MAT response to natural infection but be ineffective in preventing chronic leptospirosis, thus interfering with serodiagnosis of a chronic carrier animal. Another limitation of the test is that it may not distinguish serovars within a serogroup as a result of cross-reactions. Cross-reactivity may occur also between serogroups.

Use of an enzyme-linked immunosorbent assay (ELISA) to measure immunoglobulin M (IgM) and immunoglobulin G (IgG) antileptospiral antibodies has addressed several shortcomings of the MAT. The combination of the IgM and IgG ELISA tests may help to distinguish natural infections from vaccinal responses. IgM titers are high within 1 to 2 weeks of infection, when the MAT may still be negative. IgG titers increase 2 to 3 weeks after infection. A recently vaccinated dog would be expected to have high MAT and IgG titers and a low IgM titer.

Several other tests are useful in the diagnosis of canine leptospirosis. The microcapsular agglutination test (MCAT) is another method for diagnosing leptospirosis in which the titer parallels the IgM response to infection. This test is therefore effective in detecting recent infections and has the advantage of high specificity. Direct visualization of leptospires by darkfield microscopy of urine or tissue homogenates may be helpful in reaching a diagnosis if the sample is fresh and a large number of leptospires are present. Silver staining of leptospires in fixed tissue may yield false-negative results and therefore is an unreliable screening technique. Isolation is the ideal method for diagnosis, but it is time-consuming, expensive, and tedious. New, sensitive laboratory techniques using deoxyribonucleic acid (DNA) hybridization to detect organisms will revolutionize the diagnosis of leptospirosis when they become available clinically. The major advantage of the use of DNA probes over immunologic assays is the lack of interference with the assay by constituents of urine or serum. It is important to know which diagnostic test is performed by the laboratory so that accurate interpretation of the test can be made with respect to the stage of infection.

THERAPY

The clinical presentation dictates the plan for management of the patient. A dog may present with signs of acute renal failure and associated oliguria, anuria, or polyuria. Because the renal effects of leptospirosis may be reversible, aggressive management is indicated in oliguric patients to re-establish circulatory fluid volume, systemic blood pressure, and renal perfusion. Once a dog is hydrated, urine flow should be 2 to 5 ml/kg/hr. If urine production is not sufficient, specific therapy to restore urine production should be instituted. Diuretics are the first step in such therapy. It should be noted that diuretics used alone are not likely to improve glomerular filtration rate (GFR) or renal blood flow. The increase in urine flow is due to tubular effects of the diuretic. Their benefit lies in the fact that they facilitate management of patients so that intravenous diuresis can be continued. Furosemide (Lasix, Hoechst-Roussel; 2.2 mg/kg IV) should increase urine production within 30 min of administration. The dose may be doubled or tripled at hourly intervals, to effect. Mannitol (20%) (Astra Pharmaceutical; 0.5 to 1.0 gm/kg over 20 min) causes an osmotic diuresis within 1 hr of administration (Ross, 1989). Careful attention must be paid to the state of hydration of the animal. Overhydration in an oliguric patient is worsened by the osmotic effects of mannitol. The use of a vasodilator, dopamine (Inotropin, Elkins-Sinn), will improve glomerular filtration rate and renal blood flow. Furosemide (1 mg/kg infused over the first 4 hr) and dopamine (2 to 5 µg/kg/min) in a continuous intravenous infusion promote diuresis and support renal blood flow (Kirby, 1989). Patient monitoring should include measurement of urine output, central venous pressure, packed cell volume, total solids, and blood

pressure to assess volume overload and hemodilution. If diuretic therapy and vasodilator therapy are ineffective in increasing urine output, peritoneal dialysis may be necessary (Thornhill, 1983).

Thrombocytopenia and decreased production of clotting factors due to hepatic disease may result in a bleeding disorder, as may disseminated intravascular coagulation. Clinicians should be alerted to the early recognition and prompt treatment of complications such as disseminated intravascular coagulation, hepatoencephalopathy, and acid-base disorders. Treatment with fresh whole blood or blood components may be indicated based on the presence of petechiae or ecchymoses and evaluation of coagulation (platelet count, fibrinogen, fibrin split products, prothrombin time, and partial thromboplastin time) (see *CVT X*, p. 451).

Leptospirocidal antibiotic therapy is indicated in dogs in which the clinical presentation suggests leptospirosis. Prompt use of antibiotics shortens the duration of the illness and urine shedding and reduces renal and hepatic damage (Baldwin and Atkins, 1987). Two phases of therapy are necessary. Procaine penicillin G (40,000 units/kg IM or SC every 24 hr or a divided dose every 12 hr) is the antibiotic of choice for leptospiremia. The dose or dosing interval of the drug needs to be adjusted if an animal is in renal failure. A rough clinical approximation to dosage alterations can be obtained by dividing the dose by the serum creatinine concentration or by multiplying the interval in hours by the serum creatinine concentration. Penicillin should be used for 14 days or until azotemia resolves. Tetracycline (5 to 10 mg/kg IV every 12 hr) and chloramphenicol (50 mg/kg IV every 8 hr) have also been used with variable efficacy in the treatment of leptospiremia. Dihydrostreptomycin (10 to 15 mg/kg IM every 12 hr for 14 days) is the drug of choice to eliminate the organism from renal tubular cells and the carrier state. Because of its nephrotoxicity, use of dihydrostreptomycin should be delayed until azotemia resolves. Doxycycline (5 mg/kg PO loading dose, then 2.5 mg/kg in 12 hr PO, then 2.5 mg/kg every 24 hr PO) has been used in all phases of treatment. Because of the current questionable availability of dihydrostreptomycin, doxycycline may be an acceptable alternative therapy once an animal can tolerate oral medications. Unlike other tetracyclines, the dose of doxycycline does not need to be adjusted for renal failure because it is primarily excreted in the feces. Hospitalized patients suspected of having leptospirosis should be isolated to avoid exposure of other animals. Areas contaminated with infected urine should be washed and disinfected with an iodine-based solution. Because leptospirosis is a zoonotic disease, animal care personnel should wear gloves and practice meticulous hygiene in handling blood, urine, and tissues of infected dogs. Likewise, the owners should be made aware of the human health hazard and potential urinary shedding of organisms for up to 3 months after infection.

VACCINATION

Commercial bacterins for canine leptospirosis are derived from chemically inactivated cell cultures of serovars *canicola* and *icterohaemorrhagiae*. Bacterins protect against clinical disease but do not ensure protection against infection and development of the renal carrier state. In addition, protective antibodies are serovar specific. Although some evidence suggests cross-immunity in animals that recover from infection, this does not appear to be true for bacterins. Vaccinated dogs may therefore be infected and develop clinical disease when exposed to nontraditional serovars such as *pomona* and *grippotyphosa*. This problem may partially explain the resurgence of canine leptospirosis as a more common clinical disease in recent years.

Initial immunization for canine leptospirosis requires three to four injections 3 weeks apart. Annual boosters are recommended, but dogs in endemic areas may need to be vaccinated more frequently to maintain protective IgG antibodies.

References and Suggested Reading

Baldwin, C. J., and Atkins, C. E.: Leptospirosis in dogs. Comp. Cont. Ed. Pract. Vet. 9:499, 1987.

A review of the clinical presentation, laboratory findings, and pathology of canine leptospirosis.
Broughton, E. S., and Scarnell, J.: Prevention of renal carriage of leptospirosis in dogs by vaccination. Vet. Rec. 117:307, 1985.
Results of vaccinal protection and serologic response to vaccination against canine leptospirosis.
Ellis, W. A.: Leptospirosis. J. Small Anim. Pract. 27:683, 1986.
A review of leptospirosis in humans and domestic animals.
Greene, C. E.: Leptospirosis. *In* Greene, C. E. (ed.): *Clinical Microbiology and Infectious Disease of the Dog and Cat.* Philadelphia: W. B. Saunders, 1984, p. 588.
Greene, C. E., and Shotts, E. B.: Leptospirosis. *In* Greene, C. E. (ed.): *Infectious Diseases of the Dog and Cat.* Philadelphia: W. B. Saunders, 1990, p. 498.
A complete review of canine leptospirosis.
Hanson, L. E.: Leptospirosis in domestic animals: The public health perspective. J.A.V.M.A. 181:1505, 1982.
A review of the clinical signs, diagnosis, and control measures of leptospirosis in domestic animals.
Kirby, R.: Acute renal failure as a complication in the critically ill animal. Vet. Clin. North Am. Small Anim. Pract. 19:1189, 1989.
A review of the pathophysiology and therapy of acute renal failure.
Navarro, C. E., Kociba, G. J., and Kowalski, J. J.: Serum biochemical changes in dogs with experimental *Leptospira interrogans* serovar icterohaemorrhagiae infection. Am. J. Vet. Res. 42: 1125, 1981.
Report of serum biochemical changes caused by infection with Leptospira interrogans serovar icterohaemorrhagiae.
Rentko, V. T., Clark, N., and Ross, L. A.: Canine leptospirosis: A retrospective study of 17 cases. J. Vet. Intern. Med. (in press).
A retrospective review of canine leptospirosis as primarily a renal syndrome.
Ross, L. A.: Fluid therapy for acute and chronic renal failure. Vet. Clin. North Am. Small Anim. Pract 19:343, 1989.
A review of the treatment of renal failure with attention to electrolyte and water balances and fluid therapy.
Thornhill, J. A.: Continuous ambulatory peritoneal dialysis. *In* Kirk, R. W. (ed.): *Current Veterinary Therapy VIII.* Philadelphia: W. B. Saunders, 1983, p. 1028.
Review of indications and procedure of peritoneal dialysis.

NEOSPORA CANINUM INFECTIONS

J. P. DUBEY

Beltsville, Maryland

Neospora caninum is a recently recognized fatal protozoan parasite of dogs and other animals. Until 1988, it was misdiagnosed as *Toxoplasma gondii* (Dubey, 1990; Dubey et al., 1988a, 1988b).

Bjerkås and colleagues (1984) first found a *Neospora*-like parasite in Norway in a litter of dogs with neuromuscular disease. They distinguished it structurally and antigenically from the closely related parasite *T. gondii*. Dubey and associates (1988a) found a similar parasite in ten dogs from the United States, distinguished it from *T. gondii*, and named the canine parasite *N. caninum*. Dubey and collaborators (1988b) isolated *N. caninum* in cell cultures and in mice inoculated with tissues from paralyzed dogs and induced neosporosis in dogs inoculated experimentally.

STRUCTURE AND LIFE CYCLE

The complete life cycle of *N. caninum* is not known. Although *N. caninum* appears structurally to be a coccidian, its sexual stages and the definitive

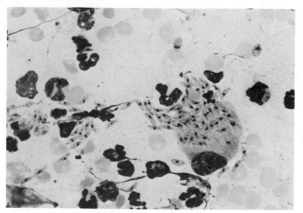

Figure 1. *Neospora caninum* tachyzoites in a smear. (Methanol fixed, Giemsa's stain; × 750.)

host are not known. The terminology used to describe the life cycle is the same as that used for *T. gondii*. Tachyzoites and tissue cysts are the only known stages.

Tachyzoites, approximately 6 × 3 μm in size, divide into two zoites by endodyogeny (Fig. 1). Individual tachyzoites are ovoid, lunate, or globular and contain one or two nuclei. A host cell may contain a few or many tachyzoites. In infected animals, tachyzoites are found within neural cells, macrophages, polymorphonuclear cells, spinal fluid, myocytes, dermal cells, and many other types of cells.

Tachyzoites are located within the host cell cytoplasm with or without a parasitophorous vacuole (Dubey et al., 1988a). Tachyzoites have organelles commonly found in zoites of *T. gondii*, including apical complex and conoid organelles, rhoptries, micronemes, and mitochondria. Unlike *T. gondii*, *N. caninum* may have more than 12 rhoptries in the tachyzoites, some of them extending to the posterior end of the tachyzoite. The micronemes are numerous and may be arranged perpendicular to the plasmalemma.

Tissue cysts are found only in the brain and spinal cord (Fig. 2). They may be round or elongated and up to 110 μm long. The cyst wall is 1 to 4 μm thick and encloses slender (7 × 1.5 μm) bradyzoites. The cyst wall and enclosed bradyzoites are variably stained with periodic acid–Schiff reagents.

The source of *N. caninum* infection is not known. Tachyzoites and tissue cysts of *N. caninum* are infectious orally; thus carnivores may become infected by ingesting infected tissues. Transplacental transmission is the only proven route of infection (Dubey and Lindsay, 1989a, 1989b). *N. caninum* has been experimentally transmitted transplacentally in cats, dogs, and sheep. *N. caninum* can be transmitted from a subclinically infected dam to a fetus, and more than one litter may be infected by the same dam.

HOST RANGE AND DISTRIBUTION

Naturally occurring disease in dogs has been found in Norway, Sweden, France, the United States, England, Canada, and Australia. An *N. caninum*-like parasite was found in tissues of neonatal calves in the United States, England, and Australia. It was also found in the central nervous system (CNS) of a week-old lamb born paralyzed and in an aborted equine fetus (Dubey, 1990). Experimentally, *N. caninum* is infectious to sheep, cats, dogs, mice, gerbils, and rats.

PATHOGENESIS

N. caninum is an intracellular parasite that can rapidly kill host cells by active multiplications of tachyzoites. Although the presence of toxic products liberated by *N. caninum* has not been ruled out, *N. caninum* appears to be a primary pathogen in dogs because there has been no evidence of concurrent undermining disease thus far (Dubey et al., 1988a). The cause of hyperextension of limbs is not known. The presence of severe mononuclear infiltrations in spinal nerves and the CNS with relatively few *N. caninum* suggests immune-mediated disease. Tissue cysts apparently do not cause host reaction, but cyst rupture does. The cause of tissue cyst rupture is not known. The administration of *corticosteroids can aggravate* acute and chronic neosporosis in experimentally infected animals. The transmission of *N. caninum* from a chronically infected dog to its fetus suggests recurrent parasitemia in the dam. Breed and sex susceptibility of neosporosis in dogs is not known, although most described cases were in pedigreed dogs, mostly retrievers.

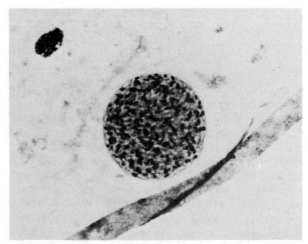

Figure 2. A tissue cyst of *N. caninum* in a smear from the brain of a dog. (Methanol fixed, Giemsa's stain; × 750.)

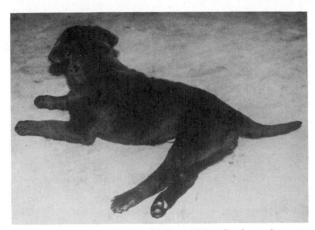

Figure 3. A naturally infected dog with hindlimb paralysis. *N. caninum* was isolated from the tissues of this dog.

NEOSPOROSIS IN DOGS

Clinical Signs

Both pups and older dogs are affected. The most severe infections have been encountered in young dogs with ascending paralysis (Cummings et al., 1988). The pelvic limbs are more severely affected (Fig. 3). The rigid contraction of the muscles of the affected limbs may be permanent. Cervical weakness, dysphagia, and death can develop with time. Dogs with hindlimb paralysis may be otherwise alert and survive for months with hand-feeding and care (Hay et al., 1990). Skin sores and muscle atrophy may develop. The disease may be localized or generalized. Older dogs may have clinical signs of multifocal CNS involvement, polymyositis, myocarditis, dermatitis, or multifocal dissemination. In neonatally infected pups, clinical signs may not be apparent until pups are 5 weeks old, and not all pups in a litter may be diseased. In neonatally infected animals, ascending paralysis is the main clinical sign. Subclinical infection may be activated during immunosuppression.

The frequency of clinical disease in a subclinically infected population is not known. In one report, 29 of 39 dogs from four litters in one household developed paralysis of limbs (Dubey et al., 1990).

Lesions

Multifocal streaks of necrosis and mineralization in muscles of the body, particularly in the diaphragm, and malacia in the CNS are the most important gross lesions. Microscopic lesions consist of necrosis followed by inflammation. Nonsuppurative encephalomyelitis, myocarditis, hepatitis, and myositis are the predominant microscopic lesions. The meningoencephalomyelitis is characterized by polyradiculoneuritis, ganglionitis, axonal degeneration, and glial nodulation, in both gray and white matter. The muscle lesions may range from focal necrosis of myocytes to severe myositis involving virtually all skeletal muscles.

Diagnosis

Ascending limb paralysis in young dogs, particularly involving littermates, should arouse suspicion of neosporosis. It is likely that most cases of neosporosis polyradiculoneuritis described in the literature were misdiagnosed as toxoplasmosis. Hematologic and biochemical findings vary depending on the organ system involved, but in dogs with hindlimb paralysis, values may be normal. *N. caninum* may be found in cerebrospinal fluid and in biopsy tissue. Inoculation of cell cultures may help in the isolation of the parasite from biopsy tissue (Hay et al., 1990).

Clinically, *neosporosis resembles toxoplasmosis*. However, the two parasites can be distinguished structurally and immunologically. Tissue cysts of *N. caninum* have 1- to 4-μm-thick cyst walls, whereas tissue cysts of *T. gondii* have cyst walls thinner than 0.5 μm. *N. caninum* tachyzoites have numerous rhoptries, whereas, in *T. gondii*, rhoptries are few. However, it must be remembered that the structure of *N. caninum* and *T. gondii* varies with the stage of the parasite and divisional state, and it is not always possible to distinguish *N. caninum* from *T. gondii* structurally. For example, organelles in dividing tachyzoites (either *T. gondii* or *N. caninum*) are fewer than those in nondividing organisms. Antigenically, *N. caninum* antiserum does not react with *T. gondii* and vice versa. An indirect fluorescent antibody test and an immunoperoxidase test that can aid in distinguishing *N. caninum* from *T. gondii* (Dubey et al., 1988b; Lindsay and Dubey, 1989) are available.

Treatment

Because neosporosis has been recognized only recently, little is known of treatment in naturally infected dogs. However, drugs used for therapy of toxoplasmosis should be tried early in the course of infection. In a dog, treatment with clindamycin was effective in treating polymyositis considered due to *T. gondii* but probably due to neosporosis (Greene et al., 1985; Dubey et al., 1990). Clindamycin, however, did not reverse CNS deficit and paralysis in a dog with a marked muscle contracture (Hay et al., 1990). Tribrissen (Coopers), containing sulfadiazine and trimethoprim, and pyrimethamine (Daraprim, Wellcome), given orally, dramatically improved the clinical condition of a dog with mild hindlimb paresis thought to be due to neosporosis (McGlennon et al., 1990). Sulfadiazine was found to be effective in treating neosporosis in experimentally infected mice (Lindsay and Dubey, 1990).

NEOSPOROSIS IN CATS

There is yet no report of *N. caninum* infection in cats. However, cats were susceptible to experimental *N. caninum* infection (Dubey and Lindsay, 1989b; Dubey et al., 1990c). The disease was most severe in prenatally and neonatally infected cats. Polymyositis, encephalitis, and hepatitis were the main lesions in 3-day-old kittens inoculated with *N. caninum*. Adult cats inoculated with *N. caninum* developed mild myositis, but infected littermates given corticosteroids developed fatal generalized neosporosis (Dubey et al., 1990c).

PUBLIC HEALTH SIGNIFICANCE

There is as yet no report of *N. caninum* infection in humans. However, *N. caninum* appears to have a wide host range. Its greatest economic importance is in cattle. It is now considered a major cause of abortion in dairy cattle in certain parts of the United States.

References and Suggested Reading

Bjerkås, I., Mohn, S. F., and Presthus, J.: Unidentified cyst-forming sporozoan causing encephalomyelitis and myositis in dogs. Z. Parasitenk 70:271, 1984.
First report of suspected neosporosis in littermate dogs.

Cummings, J. F., de Lahunta, A., Suter, M. M., et al.: Canine protozoan polyradiculoneuritis. Acta Neuropathol. 76:46, 1988.
Describes neuroanatomic findings in a pup.

Dubey, J. P.: *Neospora caninum*: A look at a new *Toxoplasma*-like parasite of dogs and other animals. Comp. Cont. Ed. Pract. Vet. 12:653, 1990.
General review of the problem including gross and microscopic lesions with color photographs.

Dubey, J. P., Carpenter, J. L., Speer, C. A., et al.: Newly recognized fatal protozoan disease of dogs. J.A.V.M.A. 192:1269, 1988a.
Original description of Neospora caninum *and retrospective study 1945–1987.*

Dubey, J. P., Greene, C. E., and Lappin, M. R.: Toxoplasmosis and neosporosis. *In* Greene, C. E. (ed.): *Infectious Diseases of the Dog and Cat.* Philadelphia: W. B. Saunders, 1990a, p. 818.
Review paper.

Dubey, J. P., Hattel, A. L., Lindsay, D. S., et al.: Neonatal *Neospora caninum* infection in dogs: Isolation of the causative agent and experimental transmission. J.A.V.M.A. 193:1259, 1988b.
First isolation of N. caninum *in the laboratory, clinical description in littermate pups.*

Dubey, J. P., Koestner, A., and Piper, R. C.: Repeated transplacental transmission of neosporosis in dogs. J.A.V.M.A. 197:857, 1990b.
Retrospective study 1957–1959, outbreak of congenital neosporosis in one breeding establishment.

Dubey, J. P., and Lindsay, D. S.: Transplacental transmission of *Neospora caninum* infections in dogs. Am. J. Vet. Res. 50:1578, 1989a.
Experimental transmission from bitch to pups.

Dubey, J. P., and Lindsay, D. S.: Transplacental *Neospora caninum* infection in cats. J. Parasitol. 75:765, 1989b.
Experimental transmission in cats.

Dubey, J. P., Lindsay, D. S., and Lipscomb, T. P.: Neosporosis in cats. Vet. Pathol. 27:335, 1990c.
Effect of corticosteroids on neosporosis in cats.

Greene, C. E., Cook, J. R., and Mahaffey, E. A.: Clindamycin for treatment of *Toxoplasma* polymyositis in a dog. J.A.V.M.A. 187:631, 1985.
Successful treatment in a naturally infected dog.

Hay, W. H., Shell, L. G., Lindsay, D. S., et al.: Diagnosis and treatment failure of *Neospora caninum* in a dog. J.A.V.M.A. 197: 87, 1990.
Clinical history, diagnosis, and treatment failure.

Lindsay, D. S., and Dubey, J. P.: Immunohistochemical diagnosis of *Neospora caninum* in tissue sections. Am. J. Vet. Res. 50:1981, 1989.
Differentiation from other related protozoan infections.

Lindsay, D. S., and Dubey, J. P.: Effects of sulfadiazine and amprolium on *Neospora caninum* (Protozoa: Apicomplexa) infections in mice. J. Parasitol. 76:177, 1990.
Experimental treatment in mice.

McGlennon, N. J., Jefferies, A. R., and Casas, C.: Polyradiculoneuritis polymyositis due to a *Toxoplasma*-like protozoan: Diagnosis and treatment. J. Small Anim. Pract. 31:102, 1990.
Treatment of a naturally infected dog.

LEISHMANIASIS

LUIS FERRER
Barcelona, Spain

Canine leishmaniasis (CL) is a disease caused by a protozoan of the genus *Leishmania*. It is a serious systemic illness that is difficult to diagnose because of the diversity of clinical presentations; moreover, it is hard to cure. CL is very common in some parts of the world. Leishmaniasis has the additional importance of being a zoonosis in which dogs are considered to be the chief reservoir of the parasite. The majority of the information contained in this article refers to canine leishmaniasis as found in Europe and Africa. The bulk of the data and statements, however, is equally valid for canine leishmaniasis as occurs in Asia and the United States (see this volume, p. 271).

ETIOLOGY AND TRANSMISSION

Leishmania is a genus of protozoa belonging to the order Kinetoplastida and the family Trypanosomatidae. In common with the remaining members of this order, the leishmaniads possess a kinetoplast—a modified mitochondrium with abundant deoxyribonucleic acid (DNA)—associated with a basal body from which a single flagellum arises. The life cycle of *Leishmania* has two distinct stages: the amastigote and the promastigote. The parasite is present as the amastigote in the vertebrate host. These are oval bodies, 2 to 5 μm in diameter, containing the central kinetoplast and nucleus but no flagellum. The promastigote is the stage present in the insect vector. It is a fusiform element, 10 to 15 μm long, with one long (20 μm) flagellum. This form is also the one found in laboratory cultures.

The classification of the genus *Leishmania* and the nomenclature of the various species and serotypes are extremely complex and confusing. The two methods of classification most frequently used at present are isoenzyme electrophoretic analysis and analysis of the kinetoplast DNA by means of restriction enzymes. Populations of parasites with identical isoenzymes are called *zymodemes*. The populations of leishmania with mitochondrial DNA of similar characteristics are known as *schizodemes*. The populations of *Leishmania* that are found in the Mediterranean geographic area and that are responsible for canine leishmaniasis and part of the human leishmaniasis are known as *Leishmania infantum*.

The leishmaniads are dixenic parasites that complete their life cycle in two hosts: a vertebrate belonging to various orders (*Carnivora, Rodentia, Edentata*) that acts as the reservoir, and an insect of the subfamily Phlebotominae, the phlebotomine sand fly, which acts as the vector. The cycle begins when a female fly feeds on an infected vertebrate host and ingests a small number of amastigotes. The amastigotes multiply in the gut of the sand fly and become flagellated promastigotes, which migrate to the esophagus and pharynx of the insect attracted by chemotaxic substances in the fly's crop. A small number of promastigotes become lodged in the proboscis of the fly, and these are then responsible for transmission of the parasite to a fresh vertebrate host. The duration of the complete cycle in the sand fly varies from between 4 and 20 days. The promastigotes introduced into the skin of the new host rapidly undergo phagocytosis by cutaneous macrophages. The interaction between the macrophage and the leishmania is extremely complex, but it would seem that a glycolipid and a glycoprotein on the protozoal surface link to different receptors of the macrophage membrane, initiating endocytosis. Opsonization with immunoglobulins and complement could also, according to some researchers, aid penetration. The increased temperature (35°C), together with other factors, causes the promastigotes to transform into amastigotes in the interior of the lysosomes, where they actively begin to multiply.

All types of leishmaniasis in animals and humans are transmitted by the bite of the sand fly. Although direct transmission by contact with inflammatory secretions or following blood transfusions has been reported, these routes of transmission should be considered exceptional, and they play no part in the epidemiology of leishmaniasis. The sand fly is widely distributed throughout the world and may be found between the parallels 50° N and 40° S. These insects have little tendency to roam and complete their life cycle in a diameter of less than 1 km. They move at dawn and dusk in search of food, and it is then that the females, the only bloodsuckers, take blood from vertebrates. In view of the low tendency of the sand fly to roam, the appearance of canine leishmaniasis in a nonendemic area can be explained only by the arrival of infected animals from endemic zones. If sand flies are found in the area, a focus of leishmaniasis may be established.

PATHOGENESIS

The parasites, introduced by a sand fly into the skin of a dog, multiply rapidly in the macrophages and eventually burst the cell to then undergo phagocytosis by other macrophages. The mechanisms by which the amastigotes overcome the defensive systems of the macrophage are not completely understood. The amastigotes, whether in the interior of the macrophages or free swimming, distribute themselves throughout the entire organism, with preference for the hematopoietic organs, particularly the bone marrow, where they continue to multiply. The leishmaniads later migrate from these multiplication points to other organs, particularly the skin, liver, pancreas, kidneys, adrenal glands, digestive tract, eyes, testes, bone, and joints. Parasites have been encountered in nearly all organs, with the exception of the central nervous system. This dissemination lasts for weeks or months and continues into the advanced phases of the disease unless treatment is begun.

The parasite causes serious lesions by means of two main pathogenic mechanisms: (1) the production of nonsuppurative inflammatory lesions, and (2) the production of circulating immune complexes that deposit in the renal glomeruli, blood vessels, and joints. The chronic inflammatory granulomas are responsible for the cutaneous manifestations of the disease and for the hepatic, enteric, and osseous lesions and part of the ocular and renal lesions. The immune complex deposits are responsible for the frequent development of serious glomerulonephritis, for some of the ocular lesions, and for vasculitis. Other less important or still undefined pathogenic mechanisms also participate in canine leishmaniasis. The anemia present in the majority of the animals is nonregenerative and is probably due to chronic disease. The formation of autoantibodies capable of producing tissue lesions and destruction of erythrocytes has been demonstrated in laboratory animals and humans. Their formation has not been definitely demonstrated in dogs, but in our experience more than 30% of dogs infected with leishmaniasis show a positive antinuclear antibody (ANA) titer, and 10% have a positive result on Coombs' test, although we cannot define the significance of these findings. In a small number of cases, amyloid is deposited in different organs, although these fibrils are rarely the main cause of the clinical symptoms.

The immunology of leishmaniasis is also a highly complex subject and is not well understood. Although the majority of infected animals show considerable polyclonal hypergammaglobulinemia, the great majority of the antibodies produced are nonspecific for leishmania and lack protective value. This hypergammaglobulinemia is a reflection of a polyclonal stimulation of B lymphocytes. There is no correlation between the antibody titer measured by immunofluorescent assay (IFA) or enzyme-linked immunosorbent assay (ELISA) and the intensity of the hypergammaglobulinemia. It has been demonstrated in laboratory animals that T lymphocytes are the most effective means of defense against parasites of the genus *Leishmania*.

CLINICAL ASPECTS

The clinical features of CL vary widely. This is doubtless a consequence of the numerous pathogenic mechanisms participating in the disease process and of the diversity of immune responses in an individual host. CL is found equally in males and females, without predilection for any breed, although some practitioners consider it more common in the large and giant breeds. This is probably because these animals spend more time outdoors, where they are exposed to the sand fly. The period of incubation of the disease is quite variable, ranging from 3 months to several years; thus, CL is rarely found in animals less than 6 months of age.

Dogs infected with leishmaniasis usually present for treatment with one or more of these main clinical features: (1) skin lesions, (2) loss of weight or poor appetite, (3) local or generalized lymphadenopathy, (4) ocular lesions, (5) chronic diarrhea, (6) renal failure, (7) liver failure, (8) epistaxis, (9) anemia, and (10) lameness, sometimes with visible swelling

of the joint. The signs invariably show a slow, progressive evolution, with little or no response to antibiotics or glucocorticoids. When a dog demonstrates several of the signs (e.g., skin lesions, weight loss, lymphadenopathy, and uveitis), clinical diagnosis is easy. If the animal presents with only one sign or lesion, however, the clinical diagnosis becomes more difficult.

Skin abnormalities are the most usual manifestation of CL. Several dermatologic entities associated with this disease have been described (Ferrer et al., 1988a), although they are all chronic, nonpruritic disorders, and the lesions almost always show a symmetric distribution. The most frequent symptom is alopecia with intense, dry desquamation (dry seborrhea), usually commencing on the head and extending to the rest of the body. Other animals develop chronic ulceration, located particularly on the head and limbs, that is neither pruritic nor painful. With much less frequency, the animals present with sterile pustular dermatosis or multiple skin nodules. Boxers seem especially susceptible to this latter form. Leishmaniasis occasionally causes the appearance of nodules or tumors in the skin or mucous membranes (nose, mouth). These nodules are accumulations of inflammatory cells with numerous parasites and may easily be mistaken for neoplasms.

Weight loss and poor appetite are present, to a greater or lesser degree, in the majority of cases, and a clear atrophy of the facial muscles is occasionally noted.

The ocular lesions vary widely. The most common is blepharitis, in association with the facial dermatitis, although it is not rare to encounter a serous bilateral keratoconjunctivitis. These lesions are caused by parasites in the eye. In some dogs, uveitis, generally bilateral, may also be observed and is associated with corneal edema or the formation of synechiae. Granulomatous uveitis, with numerous amastigotes present within macrophages, or lymphoplasmacellular uveitis, with absence of parasites, can be encountered. In the latter case, the uveitis is possibly immune mediated (Roze, 1986). One investigator (Slappendel, 1988) has observed uveitis more frequently in dogs undergoing treatment and has suggested that iridocyclitis in CL is an allergic manifestation similar to post–kala-azar leishmaniasis in humans.

A small number of animals (less than 5%) suffer chronic large-bowel diarrhea with melena. Endoscopic examination reveals ulcerative colitis, and a biopsy specimen shows a granulomatous inflammation of the intestinal mucosa with numerous parasites.

In CL it is common to find a glomerulonephritis caused by immune complexes. The clinical signs provoked by this lesion are those of proteinuria, which progresses to renal failure when the renal lesion deteriorates. This progressive renal failure often causes the death of the affected animals. Liver failure occurs in a small percentage of dogs (<5%) as a result of chronic hepatitis caused by the presence of parasites in the liver. Affected animals manifest vomiting, polyuria and polydipsia, poor appetite, and weight loss. A liver biopsy specimen reveals periportal inflammatory infiltrates formed by macrophages filled with parasites and "piecemeal" and "bridging" necroses, lesions characteristic of chronic active hepatitis.

Approximately 10% of dogs infected with leishmaniasis have episodes of nosebleed. Although the cause of this bleeding is not fully understood, it would seem to result from inflammatory and ulcerative lesions of the nasal mucosa rather than from disorders of clotting mechanisms. Despite the finding of subnormal platelet counts in many animals, these are rarely low enough to explain a nosebleed.

CLINICAL LABORATORY TESTS

The results of blood and urine tests in dogs with leishmaniasis show great variation. The majority of animals have constant polyclonal hyperproteinemia. In some advanced stages of the disease, the total protein exceeds 10 gm/dl. According to our data, anemia is found in about 60% of dogs. Some animals show leukocytosis (15%), whereas others have leukopenia (20%). More than 50% of the dogs are thrombocytopenic, in some cases very severely. In the animals with renal lesions, it is also usual to find increased plasma urea and creatinine values, proteinuria, and hematuria. The alanine aminotransferase and aspartate aminotransferase values are elevated in dogs with hepatic involvement, and a decrement in plasma albumin values is occasionally noted.

DIAGNOSIS

The most reliable diagnostic test for leishmaniasis is direct observation of the parasite. For this purpose, it is very useful to make a bone marrow puncture (iliac crest, femur, or rib) and stain the smear by the May-Grünwald–Giemsa or Diff-Quik method. The parasites appear as oval basophilic bodies in the cytoplasm of the macrophages (Fig. 1). Detection of one single parasitized cell is pathognomonic. Fine-needle aspiration of a lymph node is also useful. The cytologic picture in the nodes is of reactive hyperplasia: lymphocytes, lymphoblasts, plasma cells, and parasitized macrophages. The disadvantage of these methods is that it is sometimes impossible to detect the parasite in infected animals. The problem occurs more frequently in the lymph nodes than with bone marrow

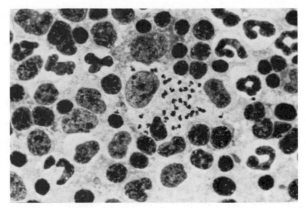

Figure 1. Bone marrow smear shows numerous amastigotes of *Leishmania* in the cytoplasm of a macrophage. (May-Grünwald–Giemsa.)

aspiration. A skin biopsy is also very useful when skin lesions are present, and extremely sensitive immunocytochemical techniques have been described for detecting the parasite in tissue slices (Ferrer et al., 1988b). Serologic methods are also very helpful in the diagnosis of leishmaniasis, most commonly indirect immunofluorescence and ELISA. It is always necessary to inquire in the laboratory concerning the lowest titer at which a result may be considered positive because this varies according to the method used and the laboratory. The result of a serologic test should be interpreted in conjunction with the clinical picture. A clearly positive result in an animal with a classic picture of leishmaniasis may suffice to establish the diagnosis. In contrast, in view of the imperfect state of our knowledge of the pathogenesis of the disease and of the kinetics of antibodies in leishmaniasis, caution should be exercised when interpreting a positive or doubtful serologic test result in a dog with no lesions or with lesions incompatible with the diagnosis. Direct observation of the parasite should be attempted in all doubtful cases, either by repeating the aspiration or by biopsy.

TREATMENT

The treatment of leishmaniasis is one of the aspects of this complex disease most subject to discussion. It is necessary to determine whether the health legislation of the country concerned permits treatment, because euthanasia of infected dogs is obligatory in some countries. It is then necessary to consider whether the patient's condition will allow treatment with any chance of success. A dog in an advanced stage of hepatic or renal failure due to irreversible lesions should not be treated because the possibility of a cure is nonexistent.

If a practitioner decides to treat an animal, the drugs of choice are the pentavalent antimony derivatives, particularly *N*-methylglucamine antimonate (meglumine antimonate [Glucantime, Rhodia]). Although the mechanism of action is not fully understood, it would seem that antimony blocks the metabolism of the parasite, inhibiting adenosine triphosphate synthesis and killing the leishmania. Meglumine antimonate contains 28.3% antimony. No extensive and rigorous studies of the kinetics of meglumine in dogs exist, and only partial data are available. The product is administered parenterally (intramuscularly). Tissue distribution is widespread, and excretion is mainly urinary. The half-life ranges from 24 to 48 hours. The most usual dose regimen includes two or three treatment periods of 15 injections of 100 mg/kg/day, separated by injection-free intervals of 10 days. In the majority of cases, the symptoms and lesions disappear in the course of treatment, but *relapses* occur in more than 75% of animals during the following 2 years; these are treated in the same way. Complete cure is uncommon in our experience, and the scant data published support this conclusion (Mancianti et al., 1988). Published experimental results seem to indicate that the administration of liposome-encapsulated meglumine antimonate may have greater effectiveness in the treatment of CL, but data on the effectiveness of this treatment in cases of spontaneous disease are not available.

Although a great deal of experimental work has been carried out, at present there is no effective vaccine against CL. Some experiments directed at immunizing the host against the *Leishmania* receptor responsible for entry into the macrophages are giving encouraging results.

PUBLIC HEALTH ASPECTS

It is obvious that CL is a zoonosis and that dogs act as a reservoir of the parasite for human beings. In the regions of Europe where canine leishmaniasis is endemic, cases of human leishmaniasis, of both the visceral and the cutaneous types, are frequent. It is nevertheless also true that the annual incidence is low; in Spain, between 100 and 200 cases of human leishmaniasis are diagnosed yearly, compared with 8000 cases in dogs. Immunocompetent humans probably have considerable resistance to the species/zymodemes of *Leishmania* encountered in Europe. This opinion is supported by the higher incidence of visceral leishmaniasis in very young children and in patients with acquired immunodeficiency syndrome.

Control of CL is nevertheless desirable if the incidence of human leishmaniasis is to be reduced. Eradication of the disease is difficult in view of the extent of the incubation period, the presence of symptom-free infected animals, and the existence of other hosts. In endemic countries it is possible only to control the infection—that is, reduce its annual incidence among the canine population. Sacrifice of dogs diagnosed as having CL as the only method of control is not adequate, for the reasons cited earlier. In order to initiate a program of control, it is necessary to combat the insect vectors (sand flies), control stray and homeless dogs, and determine the part played by other possible hosts in the area (Marsden, 1984).

References and Suggested Reading

Chang, K. P., Fong, D., and Bray, R. S.: Biology of *Leishmania* and leishmaniasis. *In* Chang, K. P., and Bray, R. S. (eds.): *Leishmaniasis.* Amsterdam: Elsevier Science, 1985, p. 1.
Extensive review of the biology of leishmaniads and general concepts about human and animal leishmaniasis.

Chapman, W. L., Hanson, W. L., Alving, C. R., et al.: Antileishmanial activity of liposome-encapsulated meglumine antimoniate in the dog. Am. J. Vet. Res. 45:1028, 1984.
Results of treatment with liposome-encapsulated meglumine antimoniate in dogs with experimental infection with Leishmania donovani.

Ferrer, L., Rabanal, R., Fondevila, D., et al.: Skin lesions in canine leishmaniasis. J. Small Anim. Pract. 29:381, 1988a.
Clinical and histopathologic description of the most common lesions in canine leishmaniasis.

Ferrer, L., Rabanal, R., Domingo, M., et al.: Identification of leishmania amastigotes in canine tissues by immunoperoxidase staining. Res. Vet. Sci. 44:194, 1988b.
Description of a highly specific method for the histopathologic diagnosis of leishmaniasis.

Mancianti, E., Gramiccia, M., Gradoni, L., et al.: Studies on canine leishmaniasis control, Part I. Evolution of infection of different clinical forms of canine leishmaniasis following antimonial treatment. Trans. R. Soc. Trop. Med. Hyg. 82:566, 1988.
One of the few published reports of the evolution of spontaneous cases after treatment with meglumine antimoniate.

Marsden, P.: Selective primary health care: Strategies for control of disease in the developing world, Part XIV. Leishmaniasis. Rev. Infect. Dis. 6:736, 1984.
Description of the human health problem of leishmaniasis and of the main strategies of control.

Roze, M.: Manifestations oculaires de la leishmaniose canine. Rec. Med. Vet. 162:19, 1986.
Description of the clinical aspect and possible pathogenesis of the ocular lesions present in canine leishmaniasis.

Russell, D. G., and Talamas-Rohana, P.: *Leishmania* and the macrophage: A marriage of inconvenience. Immunol. Today 10:328, 1989.
Discussion of the attachment of mechanisms of Leishmania *promastigotes to macrophages.*

Scott, P., Pearce, E., Natovitz, P., et al.: Vaccination against cutaneous leishmaniasis in a murine model, Part I. Induction of protective immunity with a soluble extract of promastigotes. J. Immunol. 139:221, 1987.
Demonstration of the induction of immunity in mice after vaccination with a soluble extract of promastigotes.

Slappendel, R. J.: Canine leishmaniasis. Vet. Q. 10:1, 1988.
A review based on 95 cases of leishmaniasis diagnosed in the Netherlands.

LEISHMANIASIS IN THE UNITED STATES

RANCE SELLON

Raleigh, North Carolina

Though considered primarily a disease of the Old World and Central and South America, leishmaniasis endemic to the United States is emerging as an important disease in humans and animals. Numerous reports of human cutaneous leishmaniasis from the south central area of Texas have conclusively established this state as a focus of autochthonous human leishmaniasis. The first case of endemic visceral leishmaniasis in a dog was reported in Oklahoma in 1980. Since then, endemic visceral leishmaniasis has been reported in dogs in Ohio and Texas. Cutaneous leishmaniasis has been reported in a cat in Texas. Another focus of endemic visceral leishmaniasis in a kennel of dogs in Michigan is currently under investigation (Lengerich, E., personal communication, Centers for Disease Control, Atlanta, GA, 1990). In Texas, sand flies of the genus *Lutzomyia* may be important in the transmission of leishmanial organisms. The role of vectors other than phlebotomine sand flies in the transmission of the disease in the United States is not known.

In reports originating from the United States, fever, anorexia, weight loss, and hematochezia are typical clinical signs of canine visceral leishmaniasis. Consistent hematologic abnormalities have included anemia, neutrophilic leukocytosis, hypoalbuminemia, and hyperglobulinemia (also see this volume, p. 266).

In contrast to the standard European practice of treating dogs with leishmaniasis, dogs in the United States have not consistently been treated. Pentavalent antimonial compounds, the therapy of choice for canine leishmaniasis, are not approved for use in the United States. There has been little experience with drugs other than the preferred antimonial compounds. An apparent positive therapeutic response was observed in one dog treated with diminazene aceturate and ketoconazole. These and other drugs should be investigated to determine therapeutic efficacy. Treatment of dogs infected with *Leishmania* presents a dilemma to veterinarians and public health officials because of the zoonotic potential of the disease. Infected dogs may serve as a reservoir for human or other animal infections and may contribute to the establishment of a disease that is not yet widespread. The fact that relapses may occur following treatment underscores the complexity of the treatment dilemma. Until such time that safe, effective treatments for leishmaniasis are established, euthanasia of infected animals appears warranted to diminish the potential establishment of zoonotic focuses of disease.

References and Suggested Reading

Anderson, D. C., Buckner, R. G., Glenn, B. L., et al.: Endemic canine leishmaniasis. Vet. Pathol. 17:94, 1980.
A case report that establishes Oklahoma as the first reported focus of endemic canine leishmaniasis in the United States.
Craig, T. M., Barton, C. L., Mercer, S. H., et al.: Dermal leishmaniasis in a Texas cat. Am. J. Trop. Med. Hyg. 35:1100, 1986.
A report of an autochthonous case of cutaneous leishmaniasis in Texas.
Gustafson, T. L., Reed, C. M., McGreevy, P. B., et al.: Human cutaneous leishmaniasis acquired in Texas. Am. J. Trop. Med. Hyg. 34:58, 1985.
A description of cutaneous leishmaniasis in four people, further establishing Texas as a focus of endemic human leishmaniasis.
Sellon, R. K., Menard, M. M., Meuten, D. J., et al.: Endemic visceral leishmaniasis in a dog from Texas. J. Vet. Intern. Med. (in press).
A case report that identifies Texas as a focus of endemic leishmaniasis: a dog that responded positively to treatment with diminazene aceturate and ketoconazole.
Swenson, C. L., Silverman, J., Stromberg, P. C., et al.: Visceral leishmaniasis in an English foxhound from an Ohio research colony. J.A.V.M.A. 193:1089, 1988.
A case report that establishes Ohio as another focus of endemic canine leishmaniasis.

AN UPDATE ON FELINE RETROVIRUS INFECTIONS

ELISABETH ZENGER
and ALICE M. WOLF
College Station, Texas

Retroviruses consist of a ribonucleic acid (RNA) genome that contains three genes in a series that codes for core protein (GAG), the enzyme reverse transcriptase (POL), and envelope protein (ENV). Additionally, long terminal repeat segments contain signals for starting, stopping, and enhancing gene expression. The name *retro* derives from reverse transcriptase, which is found within the virions of all members of this family. This enzyme allows viral RNA to serve as a template for production of double-stranded deoxyribonucleic acid (DNA) that is inserted into the host's genome as a provirus. The fusion of viral and cellular genetic material ensures long-term survival of the virus in the host. In the presence of a sufficiently strong immune system, the viral genes may remain latent indefinitely. Studies now suggest that most cats that apparently recover from retroviral infections are in fact latently infected with virus. Potential problems that the presence of the provirus may create in the host cell, whether or not viral proteins are produced, include disruption of normal cellular genes, production of excessive quantities of normal cell gene products, difficulty in immune eradication, malignant transformation, antiproliferative disease such as bone marrow dyscrasias, and immunodeficiency. The family Retroviridae consists of three subfamilies: Spumavirinae, Oncovirinae, and Lentivirinae.

SUBFAMILY SPUMAVIRINAE

Spumavirinae have been found in several animal species including humans, monkeys, cattle, hamsters, California sea lions, and wild and domestic cats. They induce persistent infection without evident pathogenesis in their natural hosts. Feline syncytium-forming virus (FeSFV) has not been thought to be involved in any illness, except that its infection has been statistically linked to chronic progressive polyarthritis. There seems also to be a statistical linkage between feline immunodeficiency virus (FIV) and FeSFV; 74% of FeSFV-infected cats were coinfected with FIV, compared with 38% FIV infection rate in cats that were not infected with FeSFV (Yamamoto et al., 1989). Furthermore, a statistically significant higher FeSFV infection rate is noted in diseased cats than in healthy cats (Mochizuki et al., 1989).

SUBFAMILY ONCOVIRINAE

Feline oncoviruses may be endogenous, exogenous replication–competent (feline leukemia virus [FeLV]), or exogenous replication–defective (feline sarcoma viruses [FeSV]), producing no pathologic effects, leukemia, or sarcoma, respectively. RD114 and CCC are endogenous oncoviruses present in all cat cells. Because the genes are repressed, these viruses do not replicate or cause any known disease. There is evidence that endogenous retroviral elements may combine with FeLV to create highly virulent strains of FeLV (i.e., FeLV subgroup B).

FeLV is probably the most important retrovirus of cats. FeLV-associated diseases are second only to trauma as the leading cause of death in pet cats in the United States. Factors relating to pathogenicity are mediated by the genetic information coded by ENV. Isolates (subgroups A, B, and C) can be differentiated according to their interference properties that are attributed to factors present in the gp70 region of ENV. Subgroup A is found in all cats with FeLV; B is associated with a higher rate of malignancies and immunosuppressive disorders and arises as a consequence of recombination of A envelope sequences with endogenous retroviral sequences; C, which is derived from A by mutation, is rarely isolated in nature and causes aplastic anemia.

FeLV virions are released from infected cells by budding. When the host cell membrane is assembling and associated with viral antigen, it is considered transformed. Feline oncornavirus cell membrane antigen (FOCMA) is an FeLV-induced antigen found on the cell membranes of transformed cells. The host recognizes this transformation and produces anti-FOCMA antibodies. High FOCMA antibody levels protect cats from malignancies but not from other FeLV-related disease. In fact, cats with FOCMA antibody have a significantly higher prevalence of disease than cats without FOCMA antibody (Swenson et al., 1990).

Virus-neutralizing antibody (VNA) blocks adsorption of FeLV onto the host cell. Most immunocompetent cats develop VNA and prevent proliferation before marrow or epithelial infection occurs. VNA protects against infection and immunosuppressive diseases but not malignancies.

Three major syndromes occur with FeLV infection: (1) proliferation, (2) degeneration (e.g., degeneration of progenitor or blast cells resulting in anemia, leukopenia, and/or thrombocytopenia), and (3) immunosuppression. Other syndromes that are not well characterized include neurologic and reproductive disorders.

Immunodeficiency due to FeLV

An extensive review of feline acquired immunodeficiency syndrome induced by FeLV (FeLV-FAIDS) can be found elsewhere (see *CVT IX*, p. 436). Following is a summary of the important points regarding immunodeficiency due to FeLV as well as the most recent information on the pathogenesis. The three basic mechanisms by which FeLV may cause immunodeficiency are (1) lymphopenia and granulocytopenia, (2) envelope protein p15E interference with cellular functions of lymphocytes and neutrophils, and (3) formation of immune complexes. Envelope protein p15E is responsible for most of the immunosuppression encountered in FeLV infections. The profound depression in cell-mediated immunity apparently affects T cells and particularly T helpers and T suppressors most severely. The failure of T-helper cells probably leads to ineffective humoral surveillance of FOCMA-bearing preneoplastic or neoplastic cells. Immunosuppression is favored by high levels of viremia, which ensures that T cells are exposed to p15E. However, cats need not be viremic to suffer the immunosuppressive effects of FeLV exposure.

The hydrophobic envelope protein p15E inserts itself into the plasma membrane of T cells and alters intracellular messages influenced by the cyclic nucleotide systems. Envelope protein p15E has been shown to cause depressed lymphocyte blastogenesis through altered production and reception of T-cell growth regulatory factors, decreased FOCMA antibody response and tumor enhancement, blocked conversion of immunoglobulin M (IgM) to immunoglobulin G (IgG), and inhibition of cyclic nucleotide accumulation in lymphocytes and neutrophils.

FeLV-induced lymphocyte depletion is primarily due to antibody-dependent cytotoxicity against FOCMA. Thymic atrophy, paracortical lymphoid depletion in lymph nodes, and persistent lymphopenia can result. This might explain why cats with high FOCMA antibody titers are protected against FeLV-associated neoplastic diseases but have a higher incidence of other FeLV-associated diseases.

FeLV-Induced Anemia

Anemia due to FeLV may be primary or secondary. Primary anemias are classified as erythroblastosis (i.e., abnormal maturation of red blood cell precursors) and pure red blood cell aplasia or pancytopenia. Anemias that are secondary to the effects of FeLV infection include those due to myelophthisic disease, to hemolytic (i.e., Coombs'-positive) anemias, and to infections (e.g., *Hemobartonella felis*). The importance of differentiating primary from secondary FeLV-associated anemias lies in the fact that secondary anemias can often be treated successfully whereas primary anemias cannot.

FeLV-Associated Oncogenesis

There are two major types of oncogenic retroviruses: chronic leukemia viruses (e.g., FeLV) and acute transforming viruses (e.g., FeSV). The former replicate to high titers and cause myeloproliferative disease or lymphosarcoma (LSA) after long latent periods. The acute transforming viruses possess oncogenes and induce tumors shortly after infection. An estimated 30% of all feline tumors are LSAs due to FeLV. Approximately 33% of cats with LSA are FeLV negative by enzyme-linked immunosorbent assay (ELISA) and indirect immunofluorescent assay (IFA), but evidence exists that FeLV causes the majority of these LSAs. Cats with FeLV-negative LSA have the same exposure to FeLV as do cats that develop FeLV-positive LSA. Although not an absolute requirement for lymphomagenesis, viremia increases the probability of the transforming event and decreases the latent period before it.

Feline sarcoma viruses are strong oncogenic viruses that arise by recombination between FeLV and cat cellular genes. Ten FeSVs that contain seven distinct oncogenes have been identified. FeSVs cause multifocal subcutaneous fibrosarcomas that are highly anaplastic, grow rapidly, and frequently metastasize. One strain induces melanosarcomas as well as fibrosarcomas. Experimental infection of species other than cats with FeSVs demonstrated that fibrosarcomas can be induced in a wide range of different mammals, including primates.

Miscellaneous Effects of Feline Leukemia Virus

Infertility, stillbirths, abortions, and "fading kittens" may occur in viremic and nonviremic FeLV-infected cats. Seventy per cent of cats with a history of fetal death, abortion, or infertility are FeLV-positive. Many immune-mediated disorders have been attributed to FeLV infection. These include glomerulonephritis, polyarthritis, ulcerative mucocutaneous disorders, systemic lupus erythematosus-like syndrome, and immune-mediated hemolytic anemia and thrombocytopenia. Neurologic disorders described in cats with FeLV infection include urinary incontinence, anisocoria, myelopathy, and peripheral neuropathy. Other miscellaneous associations with FeLV infection include enteritis, seborrheic dermatitis, eosinophilic granuloma complex, cutaneous horns, multiple cartilaginous exostosis, and persistent cystitis.

Feline Leukemia Virus Testing

The immunodiagnosis of FeLV has been described elsewhere (see *CVT IX*, p. 448). As we learn more about the pathogenesis of FeLV, we can better interpret what the test results mean in an individual cat. The most commonly used tests for detection of FeLV infection are ELISA and IFA. Both test for p27, the major viral core protein produced in the cytoplasm of infected cells, but they detect the antigen in different forms and therefore detect infection at different stages. To better understand test results, it is important to review the stages of FeLV infection (Hosie and Jarrett, 1990).

Stage 1 occurs soon after exposure of a susceptible cat to virulent FeLV via the oropharyngeal route. Local oropharyngeal lymphoid tissue is affected. If infection is not aborted at this stage by nonspecific immune mechanisms (e.g., neutrophils), it progresses to stage 2, infection of small numbers of circulating lymphocytes and monocytes. These cells disseminate the virus to systemic lymphoid tissues (stage 3). The vast majority of cats are able to mount an immune response by this time and do not allow the infection to progress to stage 4, bone marrow infection. Stage 4 seems to be the point of no return; once bone marrow infection is established, persistent FeLV infection is almost inevitable. Stage 5 occurs with appearance of infected neutrophils and platelets released from the bone marrow. Stage 6 follows when systemic epithelial tissues (e.g., salivary and tear glands, urinary bladder) are infected. At this stage, a cat is shedding virus and is a source of infection for other cats.

The ELISA antigen test for FeLV detects soluble FeLV core protein p27 in body fluids. Cats in stages 2 through 6 have positive results on a serum ELISA test. The sensitivity of the serum ELISA tests is close to 100%, but specificity varies. A healthy cat with a positive FeLV result on ELISA should be retested in 6 to 8 weeks because of the likelihood that an immune response will be mounted before bone marrow infection occurs. It is important to remember that even if a cat reverts to a negative status, there is a possibility of latent FeLV infection. Antimouse reactivity, which is present in 0.35% of cats, may cause false-positive serum ELISA results, though most commercially available test kits have been modified so as not to react to antimouse antibodies (Lopez and Jacobson, 1989). FeLV is not present in saliva or tears until infection is well established (e.g., stage 6). Tears correlate better with blood test results than does saliva (approximately 80% correlation) and may be more specific than some blood tests.

The FeLV IFA test detects p27 within white blood cells and platelets in circulation. A positive FeLV result on IFA indicates that the cat has reached stage 4. The IFA is very specific (approximately 99% correlation with viral isolation) but less sensitive than the ELISA. False-negative results may occur in leukopenic or thrombocytopenic cats.

Positive FeLV results on ELISA coincident with negative IFA results are discordant. There may be a valid biologic reason for this, or these results may be due to laboratory errors. Cats in stage 2 or 3 may have an early infection or may be immune carriers that have developed a well-localized infection in peripheral tissue. These discordant cats may not be shedding virus in their secretions, but it is advisable to treat them as potentially infectious. Approximately 50% of these discordant cats will develop FeLV-related disease. Also, one of the test results may be false as a result of the presence of antimouse antibody (ELISA), or neutropenia, or thrombocytopenia (IFA).

Vaccination for FeLV

Various approaches have been considered for vaccinating cats against FeLV, including inactivated vaccines as well as subunit and synthetic peptide vaccines. A panel discussion on the efficacy and safety of the widely used subunit vaccine against FeLV can be found elsewhere (see this volume, p. 457; also see *CVT X*, p. 1052). Several new FeLV vaccines have become available in the past few years, but FeLV vaccination remains controversial.

The first commercially available vaccine against FeLV (Leukocell, SmithKline Beecham) contained specific FeLV proteins and FOCMA. Vaccination with Leukocell reduced expected incidence density and cumulative incidence of persistent viremia among vaccinated cats. Leukocell 2 is said to have enhanced quantities of protective antigen in a form more accessible to a cat's immune system. Trials using Leukocell 2 indicate that this vaccine may be more effective than the older vaccine.

At least four additional FeLV vaccines are currently available. VacSyn/FeLV (Synbiotics), Fevaxyn FeLV (Solvay), and Fel-O-Vax (Fort Dodge) are killed vaccines having advertised protection rates of close to 90%. Leucogen (Virbac) is an FeLV vaccine that has been in use in France since 1988 and has now become available in the United States as GenetiVac (Pitman-Moore). It contains sequences of gp70 of type A FeLV manufactured by recombinant technology. Little information is currently available on these vaccines other than proprietary data.

Researchers in the Netherlands (Weijer et al., 1989) have described the induction of a protective immune response in cats against FeLV infection using a novel structure for the antigenic presentation of membrane proteins: the immunostimulating complex (ISCOM). ISCOM containing the gp70/85 of FeLV induced VNA in cats and protected against oronasal challenge with the virus. These experiments indicate that an FeLV ISCOM candidate vaccine is effective in inducing anti-FeLV antibodies and protects cats against FeLV under field conditions.

Treatment of Retroviral Infections

Since the discovery of the human immunodeficiency virus (HIV), major research efforts have been directed at finding ways to minimize or eliminate the effects of retroviral infections. Strategies to eliminate these viruses would generally apply for all retroviral infections, although FeLV has been used for the majority of trials in cats. Regrettably, symptomatic and supportive therapy are still our best means of prolonging the lives of cats with illness caused by retroviral infections.

The most promising antiretroviral drugs thus far have been those affecting reverse transcriptase (e.g., suramin, 3'azido3'deoxythymidine [AZT], dideoxycytidine [DDC]), and 9-(2-phosphonylmethoxyethyl) adenine [PMEA]). Although these agents have been shown to inhibit replication of FeLV *in vivo*, the effects are transient and toxicity has been a problem. These drugs generally are not effective in reversing persistent viremia. Alpha-interferon inhibits viral replication *in vitro* but has not been shown to have any *in vivo* antiviral effect. Some cats have become virus negative after whole-body irradiation and bone marrow transplantation (see this volume, p. 211).

Removal of circulating immune complexes and reversal of FeLV expression in viremic FeLV-infected cats have been successful through extracorporeal immunoadsorption (i.e., plasmapheresis) with staphylococcal protein A (SPA). SPA functions primarily by binding immune complexes; additional properties include interferon induction and T- and B-cell mitogenesis. In persistently infected cats, SPA immunoadsorption has cleared FeLV viremia and enhanced antiviral antibody titers. SPA given

by injection neither reversed FeLV viremia nor resulted in consistent improvement in humoral immune responses to FeLV antigens but did induce a proliferative response in bone marrow granulocytic lineage (Lafrado et al., 1990).

SUBFAMILY LENTIVIRINAE

FIV was discovered in 1986 in a California cattery. Early information on FIV infection from that cattery and on experimentally infected cats is described elsewhere (see *CVT X*, p. 530). Since its isolation, FIV has been found in every region and country in which testing has taken place. Prevalence varies but may be as high as 14% in cats of ill health and as low as 1.2% in cats in low-risk groups in the United States and Canada. A significant association has been found between FIV infection and FeLV seropositivity. As previously mentioned, there is also a pronounced linkage between FIV and FeSFV.

FIV is similar to HIV and simian immunodeficiency virus (SIV) in morphology and protein structure but differs antigenically and in species specificity. Phylogenetic tree analyses of gene-encoded protein sequences demonstrate that FIV is more closely related to ungulate lentiviruses, equine infectious anemia, and visna than to the primate lentiviruses HIV and SIV. Features of lentiviruses in general include species specificity, lifelong infection, and slowly progressive diseases.

Risk factors associated with FIV infection relate to the route of transmission. The virus is present in saliva, blood, and cerebrospinal fluid but it is fragile in the environment. Biting is the only proven method of natural transmission. Casual contact is not believed to be an important method of transmission. FIV has not been demonstrated to be present *in utero* or in milk. Male cats are twice as likely as females to be infected with FIV. The incidence of FIV infection is higher in domestic cats than in pure breeds, and the incidence is almost zero in catteries. Free-roaming cats are more likely to be infected than housed cats. The age range reported is 2 months to 18 years; the mean/median age is 5 years or more.

Table 1 summarizes the major characteristics of FIV in comparison with those of FeLV.

Clinical Syndromes Associated With FIV Infection

Experimental infection of cats with FIV has induced a biphasic illness with acute and chronic syndromes. The acute phase starts 4 to 6 weeks post infection and is characterized by fever lasting

Table 1. Comparison of Feline Leukemia Virus (FeLV) and Feline Immunodeficiency Virus (FIV)

	FeLV	FIV
Age predilection	1–5 years	5–12 years
Sex predilection	Equal	Males > females
Route of transmission	Saliva, urine, feces, *in utero*, lactogenic	Bites
Signs	Immunosuppression	Immunosuppression
	Lymphosarcoma and myeloproliferative disease	Miscellaneous tumors
		Gastrointestinal signs
		Respiratory signs
	Neurologic signs	Neurologic signs
Diagnosis	Antigen tests	Antibody tests
Treatment	Supportive	Supportive
Prevention	Avoid casual contact	Avoid fighting
	Vaccination	No vaccine

several days, leukopenia for 4 to 9 weeks, and lymphadenopathy that may last 1 to 9 months. Occasional complications during the acute phase included sepsis, cellulitis, anemia, diarrhea, and myeloproliferative disease. There is a profound suppression of the T-helper to T-suppressor ratio during the acute phase. After the acute phase, cases progress to the asymptomatic phase, during which signs of illness are not observed for a period ranging from months to years. The chronic phase of FIV infection then ensues and is characterized by immunodeficiency, tumors, or neurologic signs.

FIV is cytotoxic for T lymphocytes and thereby induces a progressive immunodeficiency syndrome. The mechanism of FIV-induced immunodeficiency is yet unknown; however, FIV-infected cats have deficient lymphocyte blastogenic function. Chronic gingivitis, stomatitis, and periodontitis have been reported to be the most common signs of FIV in cats, but recent epidemiologic surveys may dispute this. Nevertheless, *chronic disease* and *opportunistic infections* are the hallmark of the chronic phase of FIV infection. Chronic diarrhea, sinusitis, pneumonia, skin disease, and other signs have been reported. Intraocular disease attributed to FIV infection has included anterior plasmacytic lymphocytic uveitis, glaucoma, and pars planitis.

The incidence of toxoplasmosis seems to be high in FIV-infected cats. Witt and colleagues (1989) reported that 57% of cats infected with FIV were coinfected with *Toxoplasma gondii*. A high *Toxoplasma* titer may represent a specific B-cell response to reactivation of latent *Toxoplasma* infection secondary to FIV immunodeficiency, or cats infected with FIV may have increased *Toxoplasma* titers as part of a general nonspecific polyclonal B-cell activation as is typically encountered in HIV. Lappin (1990) described a delayed antibody shift with *T. gondii*/FIV coinfection. IgM is not detected by latex agglutination and indirect hemagglutination tests, so active *Toxoplasma* infection may be missed. *T.*

gondii is the most common cause of opportunistic cerebral infection in persons with acquired immunodeficiency syndrome.

All retroviruses are to various degrees neuroinvasive and neurovirulent. Dementia, aggression, and convulsions have been reported in FIV-infected cats. Neuropathologic lesions in experimental and naturally infected cats have included perivascular mononuclear cell infiltrates and both glial nodules and diffuse gliosis (Dow et al., 1990).

The association between FIV and neoplasia deserves further investigation. In one report, 11 of 49 cats with FIV infection had neoplastic diseases (Hopper et al., 1989), and the incidence of unusual tumors (i.e., hepatic myelolipoma) was high. Others have found a significant correlation between FIV infection and lymphoproliferative malignancies (Shelton et al., 1990).

Cofactors are believed to be important in a cat's progression from the asymptomatic to the chronic phase of FIV. Concurrent viral, parasitic, or bacterial infections are suspected of being important cofactors. Cats naturally coinfected with FeLV and FIV die earlier than cats with FIV infection alone. Experimentally coinfected cats developed much more severe illness than cats with either FeLV or FIV alone.

Diagnosis of FIV Infection

Diagnosis of FIV infection is generally based on the detection of antibody because of the limited expression of lentiviral antigens. Experimentally infected cats become antibody positive 2 to 6 weeks following infection. Following infection, antibodies develop first to p24 and subsequently to p17, p55, and gp120 as detected by Western blot analysis. Positive Western blots correlate well with viral isolation but 20 to 30% false-positive results have been reported to occur with ELISA testing owing to the presence of nonspecific cross-reacting antibodies (Hosie and Jarrett, 1990). False-negative results may occur when the cat is in terminal AIDS, as reported in one study in which seven of 46 cats (15%) had chronic diseases and FIV infection based on viral isolation but had negative results on FIV ELISA antibody testing. Colostral antibodies disappeared by 10 weeks of age in kittens born to FIV-infected queens.

References and Suggested Reading

Dow, S. W., Poss, M. L., and Hoover, E. A.: Feline immunodeficiency virus: A neurotropic lentivirus. J. Acquir. Immune Defic. Syndr. 3:658, 1990.
Report of an investigation into the neurotropism of FIV in naturally and experimentally infected cats.
Hopper, C. D., Sparkes, A. H., Gruffydd-Jones, T. J., et al.: Clinical

and laboratory findings in cats infected with feline immunodeficiency virus. Vet. Rec. 125: 341, 1989.
Report on the clinical and laboratory findings in naturally infected FIV-positive cats.

Hosie, M. J., and Jarrett, O.: Serological responses of cats to feline immunodeficiency virus. J. Acquir. Immune Defic. Syndr. 4:215, 1990.

Lafrado, L. J., Mathes, L. E., Zack, P. M., et al.: Biological effects of staphylococcal protein A immunotherapy in cats with induced feline leukemia virus infection. Am. J. Vet. Res. 51:482, 1990.
Report of the biologic effects of staphylococcal protein A immunotherapy in control cats and FeLV-infected viremic and nonviremic cats.

Lappin, M. R.: Clinical toxoplasmosis in cats coinfected with feline immunodeficiency virus. Proceedings of the Eighth Annual Veterinary Medical Forum, 1990, pp. 805–808.
Overview of the biology and clinical diagnosis of feline toxoplasmosis and report of clinical feline toxoplasmosis in feline immunodeficiency virus–infected cats.

Lopez, N. A., and Jacobson, R. H.: False-positive reactions associated with anti-mouse activity in serotests for feline leukemia virus antigen. J.A.V.M.A. 195:741, 1989.
A report on the false-positive reactions that were observed in commercial test kits designed to detect FeLV infections.

Mochizuki, M., Kawaji, I., Ogawa, H., et al.: Seroepizootiologic survey of feline syncytial virus infections in domestic cats. Jpn. J. Vet. Sci. 51:649, 1989.
Report of the results of serologic analysis of cat serum for FeSFV in Japan.

Shelton, G. H., Grant, C. K., Cotter, S. M., et al.: Feline immunodefi-ciency virus and feline leukemia virus infections and their relationships to lymphoid malignancies in cats: A retrospective study (1968–1988). J. Acquir. Immune Defic. Syndr. 3:623, 1990.
Retrospective serologic investigation of the relationship between lymphoid malignancies and retrovirus infection in cats in Boston, Los Angeles, New York, and Seattle.

Swenson, C. L., Kociba, G. J., Mathes, L. E., et al.: Prevalence of disease in nonviremic cats previously exposed to feline leukemia virus. J.A.V.M.A. 196:1049, 1990.
Report of the prevalence of disease in nonviremic cats previously exposed to FeLV.

Weijer, K., Uytdehaag, F. G. C. M., and Osterhaus, A. D. M. E.: Control of feline leukemia virus. Vet. Immunol. Immunopathol. 21:69, 1989.
Overview of control of FeLV including epidemiologic measures, preexposure immunoprophylaxis, and postexposure treatment.

Witt, C. J., Moench, T. R., Gittelsohn, A. M., et al.: Epidemiologic observations on feline immunodeficiency virus and *Toxoplasma gondii* coinfection in cats in Baltimore, Md. J.A.V.M.A. 194:229, 1989.
Report of the results of a seroepidemiologic survey of the prevalence of FIV infection and T. gondii/FIV coinfection in a diverse population of cats.

Yamamoto, J. K., Hansen, H., Ho, F. W., et al.: Epidemiological and clinical aspects of feline immunodeficiency virus infection in cats from the continental United States and Canada and possible mode of transmission. J.A.V.M.A. 194:213, 1989.
Report of the epidemiologic features of FIV in the United States and Canada, including major clinical manifestations.

CANINE ZOONOSES

CRAIG E. GREENE

Athens, Georgia

Of the household pets, dogs usually share the strongest emotional bond with their owners. As a result, they come into close contact with family members, often eating and sleeping in the same dwelling. Under such circumstances, the chance of interspecies infection is possible. However, infections are more likely to be transmitted between family members in the household than to or from family dogs. Nevertheless, certain infections in dogs require public health awareness. The following summary of each of the diseases describes newly recognized or established zoonoses that could be transmitted from people to dogs or for which dogs act as a sentinel for human infection. Aspects of the human illness are emphasized in the discussion. Table 1 outlines the other major known North American canine zoonotic diseases.

EHRLICHIOSIS

Human infection with an organism closely related serologically to *Ehrlichia canis* has been described. Most cases have been reported from the south central and southern portions of the United States and have involved people recently exposed to ticks in the outdoors during recreational or occupational activities. Clinical findings that mimic those of spotted fever have included fever, headache, myalgia, ocular pain, and gastrointestinal signs. Petechial hemorrhages have occurred in only 20% of cases. Hematologic abnormalities have included anemia, leukopenia, and thrombocytopenia. Diagnosis has been made using immunofluorescent procedures employing *E. canis* as the test antigen. The organism has been visualized on rare occasions as an inclusion in granulocytes. A fourfold rise in titer has been used to confirm active infection. Tetracycline is effective in treatment of infected humans, as in dogs. Dogs are probably not the source of infection in people, but both may become infected by exposure to the same ticks. *Rhipicephalus sanguineus* is probably not the responsible vector.

LYME BORRELIOSIS

Lyme borreliosis is a multisystemic, tick-borne, spirochetal disease caused by *Borrelia burgdorferi* and is transmitted by various species of ixodid ticks.

Text continued on page 282

Table 1. Zoonoses of Dogs

Disease (agent)	Synonyms	Geographic Distribution	Source of Infection	Affected Vertebrates	Clinical Signs
Viral Diseases					
Pseudorabies (herpesvirus)	Mad itch, Aujeszky's disease	Cosmopolitan	Direct contact	Humans,* dogs, pigs	*Human:* Transient severe pruritus *Dog:* Encephalitis
Rabies (rhabdovirus)	Hydrophobia	Cosmopolitan	Animal bite, inhalation	Humans, dogs, cats, all mammals	*Human:* Progressive neurologic disorder and death *Dog:* As in humans
Venezuelan equine encephalitis (VEE virus,† togavirus)	Sleeping sickness	North and South America	Mosquito vector	Horses, dogs, occasionally humans	*Human:* Encephalitis *Dog:* Depression, fever, aggressive behavior (encephalitis not reported)
Rickettsial Diseases					
Rocky Mountain spotted fever (*Rickettsia rickettsii* and other spotted fever group rickettsiae)	Sao Paulo typhus, Choix fever, pinta fever, others	North and South America, worldwide	Tick vector	Humans, rodents, small mammals, dogs	*Human:* Fever, rash, malaise, central nervous system signs, myocarditis, interstitial pneumonia *Dog:* Fever, malaise, petechial hemorrhages, lymphadenopathy, abdominal pain, limb edema, nystagmus
Q fever (*Coxiella burnetii*)	Abattoir fever, query fever, Balkan grippe	Cosmopolitan	Milk, airborne, tick-borne?	Humans, dogs, ruminants, many mammals	*Human:* Headache, chills, recurrent fever, malaise, myalgia, pneumonitis, rash *Dog:* Encephalitis
Bacterial Diseases					
Brucellosis (*Brucella canis*)	None	Cosmopolitan	Exposure to aborted canine fetuses, placenta, vaginal discharges, or urine	Humans, dogs, possibly foxes	*Human:* Asymptomatic, intermittent fever and malaise *Dog:* Asymptomatic, abortions, generalized lymphadenopathy, orchitis, scrotal dermatitis, bacteremia, diskospondylitis
DF-2 infection (*Capnocytophaga canimorsus*)	None	Uncommon	Dog bite‡	Humans and unknown other hosts	*Human:* Septicemia, meningitis, bacterial endocarditis *Dog:* None
Leptospirosis (*Leptospira* spp.)	Fort Bragg fever, Weil's disease, Stuttgart's disease, canecutter's disease, swineherd's disease, harvest fever	Cosmopolitan	Direct contact with urine or urine-contaminated water, oral ingestion of contaminated meat, bite from infected animal	Humans, dogs, occasionally cats, most mammals	*Human:* Malaise, fever, myalgia, jaundice, hemolysis, hepatitis, acute nephritis, uveitis, aseptic meningitis *Dog:* As in humans
Pasteurellosis (*Pasteurella multocida* and other species)	None	Cosmopolitan	Animal bite	Humans, dogs, cats, and most mammals	*Human:* Skin abscesses and ulcers, osteomyelitis, sinusitis, pleuritis, leptomeningitis, arthritis, lymphadenopathy *Dog:* As in humans and also otitis media
Tuberculosis (*Mycobacterium tuberculosis*, M. bovis)	None	Cosmopolitan	Inhalation	Humans, dogs, cats, ruminants, rodents, primates, horses	*Human:* Pulmonary granulomas, generalized debilitation, ulcerative dermatitis, meningitis, lymphadenopathy, osteoarthritis *Dog:* As in humans
Yersiniosis (*Yersinia enterocolitica*)	None	Cosmopolitan	Ingestion, contact, fecal contamination	Humans, dogs, cats, primates, pigs, poultry, beavers	*Human:* Severe gastroenteritis *Dog:* Asymptomatic to mild diarrhea
(*Y. pseudo-tuberculosis*)	None	Europe, Australia, occasional reports in North America	Ingestion, inhalation, dog bite	Humans, dogs, cats, other mammals, and birds	*Human:* Lymphadenopathy, ileitis, arthralgia, septicemia, cutaneous swellings *Dog:* Anemia and gastroenteritis
Fungal Diseases					
Dermatophytoses (*Microsporum canis,§ Trichophyton mentagrophytes*)	Ringworm, favus	Cosmopolitan	Direct contact with infected animal, soil	Humans, dogs, cats, and many mammals	*Human:* Erythematous circular alopecic lesions with raised borders, hyperkeratosis *Dog:* As in humans
Coccidioidomycosis (*Coccidioides immitis*)	San Joaquin Valley fever, valley fever, desert fever	Areas of hot, dry climate—southwestern United States, Central and South America	Soil organism	Humans, dogs, cats, most mammals	*Human:* As for blastomycosis *Dog:* As in humans

Table 1. *Zoonoses of Dogs* Continued

Disease (agent)	Synonyms	Geographic Distribution	Source of Infection	Affected Vertebrates	Clinical Signs
Fungal Diseases *Continued*					
Dermatophilosis (*Dermatophilus congolensis*)	Cutaneous streptotrichosis, lumpy wool disease	Cosmopolitan	Commensal organism on skin of normal animals; mechanical transmission by flies; soil reservoir uncertain	Humans, dogs, cats, horses, ruminants	*Human:* Exudative dermatitis *Dog:* As in humans, also subcutaneous abscesses
Histoplasmosis (*Histoplasma capsulatum*)	Cave sickness, Darling's disease	Cosmopolitan; in United States, endemic to Mississippi and Ohio River valleys and bordering regions	Soil organism, associated with bird and bat guano	Humans, dogs, cats, most mammals	*Human:* Asymptomatic, mild to severe pneumonia, lymphadenopathy; occasionally can become disseminated *Dog:* Mild to severe pneumonia, hepatomegaly, diarrhea, weight loss, lymphadenopathy; occasionally may become disseminated
(*H. duboisii*)	None	Africa	As above	As above	
Rhinosporidiosis (*Rhinosporidium seeberi*)	None	Cosmopolitan, but endemic to tropical regions	Unknown; seems to be associated with water	Humans, dogs, cows, horses, goats, poultry	*Human:* Pink polypoidal lesions on mucous membranes, nares, nasopharynx, soft palate; rarely on skin *Dog:* As in humans
Sporotrichosis (*Sporothrix schenckii*)	Rose grower's disease	Cosmopolitan	Soil organism	Humans, dogs, cats, rodents, ruminants, primates	*Human:* Cutaneous lesions— circular alopecic plaques that may ulcerate; subcutaneous and lymphatic lesions— nodules that ulcerate and spread along lymphatic chains; can disseminate *Dog:* As in humans
Oömycosis (*Pythium insidiosum*)	Phycomycosis	Cosmopolitan	Subtropical regions; ingestion of spore-contaminated water	Humans, dogs, horses, cattle	*Human:* Cutaneous— proliferative ulcerated and draining lesions usually on extremities; gastrointestinal— granulomatous mass or infiltrate of stomach, bowel, or parenchymatous organ *Dog:* As in humans
Zygomycosis (Many fungi of the orders Mucorales or Entomophthorales: *Rhizopus, Mucor, Mortierella, Absidia, Conidiobolus, Basidobolus*, others)	Mucormycosis, phycomycosis	Cosmopolitan	Ubiquitous organisms found in soil and vegetation	Humans, dogs, horses, cows, primates, seals	*Human:* Rhinocerebral signs‖; nasal, pulmonary, and gastrointestinal granulomas; occasionally disseminated *Dog:* As in humans
Protothecosis (*Prototheca wickerhamii* and *P. zopfii*)	None	Cosmopolitan	Ubiquitous organisms probably acquired from soil or water	Humans, dogs, cats, ruminants, bats, beaver	*Human:* Cutaneous lesions; may become systemic with signs reflecting organ system affected *Dog:* Granulomatous skin lesions; may become systemic and cause gastrointestinal or nervous system signs
Protozoal Diseases					
Amebiasis (*Entamoeba histolytica*)	Amebic dysentery	Cosmopolitan	Fecal contamination	Humans, dogs, cats, primates, rodents, pigs, and reptiles	*Human:* Asymptomatic, severe gastroenteritis with ulceration; may become systemic and invade liver, lungs, and skin *Dog:* As in humans
Balantidiasis (*Balantidium coli*)	None	Cosmopolitan	Fecal contamination	Humans, pigs, and occasionally dogs	*Human:* Asymptomatic, severe gastroenteritis with ulceration *Dog:* Asymptomatic, chronic gastroenteritis
Giardiasis (*Giardia lamblia, G. duodenalis*, and other *Giardia*)	None	Cosmopolitan	Fecal contamination	Humans, dogs, cats, rodents, birds, and many mammals	*Human:* Asymptomatic, chronic diarrhea, malabsorption, steatorrhea *Dog:* As in humans
Babesiosis (*Babesia*)	Piroplasmosis	Cosmopolitan	Tick vector	Humans, dogs, cats, many carnivores and herbivores	*Human:* Malaise, arthralgia, myalgia, hemolytic anemia, hepatosplenomegaly *Dog:* Malaise, fever, anemia, icterus, splenomegaly

Table continued on following page

Table 1. Zoonoses of Dogs Continued

Disease (agent)	Synonyms	Geographic Distribution	Source of Infection	Affected Vertebrates	Clinical Signs
Protozoal Diseases Continued					
Chagas' disease (*Trypanosoma cruzi*)	American trypanosomiasis	South America, Southeast and Southwest Asia	Reduviid bug vector; rarely direct contact?	Humans, dogs, cats, rodents, and primates	*Human:* Asymptomatic, chagoma, fever, lymphadenopathy, nervous system signs, cardiac arrhythmias, watery diarrhea, megaesophagus *Dog:* As in humans
Leishmaniasis (*Leishmania tropica*)	Cutaneous leishmaniasis, Oriental sore, Bagdad boil, Aleppo button	North Africa, Middle East	Sand flies serve as intermediate hosts	Humans, dogs, cats, rodents, bears	*Human:* Papule at site of bite, pruritus, ulcerations of skin, lymphadenopathy *Dog:* Pruritus, lymphadenopathy
(*L. braziliensis*)	Mucocutaneous leishmaniasis, espundia, uta, chiclero ulcer, forest yaws	South America	As above, rarely direct contact	Humans, dogs, cats, rodents	*Human:* Ulceration of oral and nasal mucosa and cutaneous regions *Dog:* Ulcerations of mucous membranes and cutaneous regions
(*L. donovani*)	Visceral leishmaniasis, kala-azar, Dumdum fever	Asia, Africa, South America, Mediterranean region	As above, rarely direct contact	Humans, dogs, jackals, rodents	*Human:* Abdominal swelling, hepatosplenomegaly, fever, ascites, dermal ulceration *Dog:* Ulcerative skin lesions, alopecia, cachexia, ocular lesions
Coccidiosis (*Isospora canis*, *I. neorivolta*, *I. ohioensis*, *I. burrowsi*)	None	Cosmopolitan	Fecal contamination	Humans and Canidae	*Human:* Asymptomatic, monozoic cyst in lymph nodes *Dog:* Asymptomatic, enteritis
Toxoplasmosis (*Toxoplasma gondii*)	None	Cosmopolitan	Soil, raw meat, cat feces, transplacental transmission	Humans, dogs, cats, over 350 species of vertebrates	*Human:* Asymptomatic, abortions, stillbirths, congenital defects, encephalitis, myositis, retinochoroiditis, pneumonia, enteritis, myocarditis, lymphadenopathy *Dog:* As in humans
Helminthic Diseases **Trematoid Infection** Nanophyetus infection (*Nanophyetus salmincola*)	None	Pacific Northwest, Russia	Snails are first intermediate hosts, and fish are second intermediate hosts	Canidae, occasionally humans are definitive hosts	*Human:* Asymptomatic *Dog:* Superficial to hemorrhagic enteritis if fluke is infected with *Neorickettsia helminthoeca*
Paragonimiasis (*Paragonimus westermani*)	Lung fluke	Asia	Snails are first intermediate hosts, and freshwater crabs or crayfish are second intermediate hosts	Humans, dogs, cats, most carnivores are definitive hosts	*Human:* Asymptomatic, coughing, hemoptysis, dyspnea, possibly nervous system signs *Dog:* As in humans
(*P. kellicotti*)	Endemic hemoptysis	North America	As above	As above	As above
Schistosomiasis (*Schistosoma japonicum*)	Katayma's disease, Oriental blood fluke, Yangtze River fever, world scourge, bilharziasis	Far East	Snails are first intermediate hosts, and free-swimming cercariae are second intermediate hosts	Humans, dogs, cats, and most mammals are definitive hosts	*Human:* Malaise, fever, urticaria, bloody diarrhea, neurologic signs, hepatitis; can cause primary liver carcinoma; signs reflect organ system affected *Dog:* As in humans
(*S. mansoni*)	World scourge, bilharziasis	Africa, Near East, Central and South America	As above	As above	As above
(*S. rodaini*)	World scourge, bilharziasis	Africa	As above	As above	As above
Cestoid Infection Coenuriasis (*Multiceps multiceps*)	None	Cosmopolitan	Herbivores and occasionally humans are intermediate hosts	Canidae are definitive hosts	*Human:* Nervous system signs, usually forebrain *Dog:* None
(*M. serialis*)		As above	Rodents and occasionally humans are definitive hosts	As above	*Human:* Nervous system signs *Dog:* None

Table 1. Zoonoses of Dogs Continued

Disease (agent)	Synonyms	Geographic Distribution	Source of Infection	Affected Vertebrates	Clinical Signs
Cestoid Infection Continued					
Echinococcosis (*Echinococcus granulosus*)	Hydatid disease, unilocular echinococcosis	Cosmopolitan	Domestic herbivores, occasionally wild herbivores or humans are intermediate hosts	Canidae are definitive hosts	*Human:* Signs variable, associated with organ system of cyst involvement *Dog:* Asymptomatic, moderate enteritis
Dipylidiasis (*Dipylidium caninum*)	None	Cosmopolitan	Fleas or biting lice are intermediate hosts	Dogs, cats, occasionally humans are definitive hosts	*Human:* Asymptomatic, mild intestinal disturbance *Dog:* Asymptomatic, anal pruritus
Nematoid Infection					
Trichinosis (*Trichinella spiralis*)	Trichinelliasis	Cosmopolitan	Most mammals, especially pigs and bears, are intermediate hosts	Humans, dogs, cats, and most mammals and some birds are definitive hosts	*Human:* Adult parasites cause severe enteritis; larvae cause fascial edema, myalgia, arthralgia, meningitis, encephalitis, myocarditis *Dog:* Asymptomatic, anorexia, diarrhea, malaise, fever
Dioctophyma infection (*Dioctophyma renale*)	Giant kidney worm	Cosmopolitan	Annelid worms are the first intermediate hosts, and crayfish or fish are the second intermediate hosts	Humans, dogs, cats, seals, wild carnivores, some herbivores are definitive hosts	*Human:* Asymptomatic, peritonitis, renal failure, cystitis *Dog:* As in humans
Dirofilariasis (*Dirofilaria immitis*)	Heartworm disease	Cosmopolitan	Mosquitos are intermediate hosts	Canidae, cats, occasionally humans are definitive hosts	*Human:* "Coin" lesions in lungs, pulmonary infarction, ectopic migrations *Dog:* Asymptomatic, lethargy, dyspnea, hemoglobinuria, right heart failure
Cutaneous larva migrans (*Ancylostoma caninum, A. braziliense, Uncinaria stenocephala*)	Creeping eruption	Cosmopolitan	Soil¶	Humans, Canidae, Felidae	*Human:* Clinical signs caused by larva; linear cutaneous eruptions, serpiginous tunnels, erythema; rarely matures in intestinal tract *Dog:* Clinical signs caused by adults; weakness, melena, anemia
Strongyloidiasis (*Strongyloides stercoralis*)	Threadworms	Cosmopolitan	Soil¶	Humans, Canidae, Felidae	*Human:* Asymptomatic, red wheals at site of penetration, pneumonia, diarrhea with steatorrhea, ulcerative colitis, melena *Dog:* Asymptomatic, severe diarrhea, rarely dermatitis or pneumonia
Visceral larval migrans (*Toxocara canis, T. cati,* and *Toxascaris leonina* have been incriminated)	None	Cosmopolitan	Soil¶	Humans, Canidae, Felidae	*Human:* Asymptomatic, larvae cause pneumonia, myositis, arthralgia, hepatomegaly, splenomegaly, abdominal and chest pain, nervous system signs, uveitis, endophthalmitis *Dog:* Asymptomatic, adult forms cause potbelly, unthriftiness, intestinal obstruction
Miscellaneous Arthropodic Diseases					
Sarcoptic mange (*Sarcoptes scabiei*)	Scabies	Cosmopolitan	Direct contact	Humans, Canidae, cats	*Human:* Transient papuloeruptive dermatitis, pruritus *Dog:* As in humans
Tunga infestation (*Tunga penetrans*)	Sand flea, chigoe	Southern United States, South America, Africa	Soil	Humans, dogs, pigs, many mammals	*Human:* Nodules on soles of feet that become confluent and ulcerate *Dog:* As in humans

*Very poor documentation for human pseudorabies infection; it is doubtful whether humans can become infected from dogs or pigs.

†Dogs have seroconverted after exposure to St. Louis encephalitis virus with no clinical signs observed.

‡DF-2 infections have not always been proved to be caused by a dog bite. DF-2 is a commensal of the dog's mouth; most cases have been in immunosuppressed or splenectomized patients.

§*Microsporum canis* has also been called *M. felineum, M. lanosum,* and *M. equinum.*

‖This form of zygomycosis most commonly afflicts patients with poorly controlled diabetes mellitus. All forms of zygomycosis are usually encountered in debilitated patients.

¶Contaminated by feces from infected dogs.

Ixodes ricinus is the three-host tick that is primarily responsible for transmitting the disease in the endemic regions of the midwestern and northeastern United States and in Europe. Other insect vectors have been found to harbor the organism but are not considered to be responsible for maintenance of the disease in nature. Their role, however, as transport hosts for human and animal infection should not be overlooked. Infection in experimental animals has occurred presumably through urinary contamination of mucous membranes. Whether such transmission occurs between people and infected pets is uncertain.

The spectrum of clinical signs in infected people includes dermatologic, orthopedic, cardiac, and neurologic manifestations. Localized or generalized inflammatory dermatosis, suppurative polyarthritis, myocarditis, and meningoencephalitis are responsible for the clinical signs. Predominant acute manifestations include fever, headache, vomiting, myalgia, arthralgia, and regional lymphadenomegaly. Tick exposure may be apparent in the history, although the vectors are often overlooked because of their small size. The characteristic dermatologic lesion at the site of a tick bite is an expanding, nonpainful erythematous lesion known as *erythema chronica migrans* (ECM). The lesion lasts 1 to 2 weeks.

Arthritis is the principal chronic clinical finding in a majority of untreated patients. Syncope or heart failure may develop as a late manifestation of cardiac arrhythmias. Neurologic manifestations such as headache, photophobia, behavioral changes, and cranial nerve or other lower motor neuron deficits develop in people with untreated borreliosis.

Diagnosis of borreliosis in people as in dogs involves screening of serum antibody titers for IgG and in some cases IgM (see this volume, p. 252). Interpretation of single antibody measurements can be confusing because of the persistence of antibodies following initial exposure. Methods involving organism detection with immunoassay or nucleic acid procedures may offer hope in more specific recognition of the disease.

Treatment of people and pets is similar and involves antimicrobial therapy with tetracycline, penicillin derivatives, and erythromycin. Ceftriaxone has been used to help eliminate the infection in resistant cases of arthritis or meningoencephalitis. Prevention and tick avoidance are the primary ways to minimize human infection. People might become infected by handling or removing ticks brought into the household on their pets. The available vaccine for canine borreliosis reduces the prevalence of spirochetemia and spirocheturia in experimentally infected dogs. The vaccine may be of benefit in reducing the chance of this urinary spread, although its significance has not been determined.

CAMPYLOBACTERIOSIS AND SALMONELLOSIS

Campylobacteriosis and salmonellosis are the most common enteric bacterial infections that can be transmitted from dogs to people. Human health risks from contaminated food or water sources are probably much greater than the chance of acquiring such infections from contact with feces from infected pets. In fact, under most circumstances, dogs are of minimal health risks for such infections unless they have diarrheic stools. In such cases, small children and immunosuppressed individuals are at greatest risk. Of increasing concern is the risk of humans' contracting antibiotic-resistant strains of these bacteria because of the extensive use of antimicrobials in their pets.

Isolation of the organisms from the stools of dogs is the definitive means of determining the carrier state. Mere isolation of the organism does not signify that it is the cause of diarrhea in a dog; however, it indicates the potential human health risk. Fecal samples for *Salmonella* isolation must be cultured on special media containing selective inhibitors for other commensal flora. Similarly, culture conditions for *Campylobacter* are unique, requiring special media and higher than usual temperatures.

Therapy for infections with these organisms involves the same drugs in human and animal patients. Because campylobacteriosis in people is much more severe than in animals, even subclinically affected animals should be treated. Drugs of choice in descending order include erythromycin, chloramphenicol, and quinolones. Appropriate therapy for salmonellosis varies according to the type and severity of clinical illness. For septicemic animals, parenteral fluids and antimicrobials are essential and are usually given intravenously. For gastroenteritis, treatment may merely prolong the carrier state. Uncomplicated *Salmonella* gastroenteritis should not, therefore, be treated unless the animal is diarrheic and unless children or immunosuppressed people are in the household. Antimicrobials usually effective against *Salmonella* include chloramphenicol, trimethoprim-sulfonamides, and amoxicillin. Aminoglycosides should be given parenterally or orally depending on whether systemic or intestinal infection, respectively, is involved. Quinolones that are also effective against *Salmonella* should be used only in limited circumstances because of the risk of inducing bacterial resistance.

GROUP A STREPTOCOCCAL INFECTIONS

Humans are the main natural reservoir hosts of group A streptococcal infections. *Streptococcus pyogenes* is the primary group A organism that is responsible for causing tonsillitis, pharyngitis, otitis, superficial pyoderma, and systemic bacteremia, usually in young children. The sites of localization of group A streptococci in asymptomatic people are the caudal aspects of the pharynx and tonsillar region. Most infections are associated with direct or close contact between susceptible people. Some harbor the infection as inapparent carriers. In households where recurrent infections occur in children, school or day-care contacts are usually responsible. Nevertheless, pediatricians commonly blame close contact with household pets as a source of infection. Group G streptococci are much more commonly isolated from the throats of dogs and are the principal organism found in disease states. In households where group A streptococcal infections develop in children, the isolation rate of these human pathogens from the dogs is increased. The frequency of isolation is 1 to 10% in unaffected households, whereas the rate in households with infected pets may be 30% or higher. Because the animals are clinically asymptomatic, antimicrobial treatment should be concurrent with that of other family members to reduce the chance of reinfection in the household. The antimicrobial spectrum for group A strains is the same in dogs and people. Penicillins, erythromycin, and chloramphenicol can be used. For resistant cases or when recurrent infections develop, first-generation cephalosporins can be used.

BLASTOMYCOSIS

The systemic mycoses are usually acquired from exposure to organisms in the soil under appropriate circumstances. There is no danger of aerosol transmission of the organism from infected pets. Infection of a dog in a household merely indicates the possibility that *common environmental exposure* may exist. However, penetrating wounds from sharp objects contaminated with the organism in dogs' tissues have produced infections in people. Care must be taken to wear gloves during diagnostic procedures or necropsy of affected animals. Cultivation of the organism in the laboratory produces mycelial forms of the organism that are highly infectious. Culture should be undertaken only by an experienced diagnostic laboratory.

GIARDIASIS

Giardia are anaerobic intestinal protozoa that affect dogs and many mammalian species, including humans, and avian species. Giardiasis is ubiquitous, and most infections are asymptomatic. Immature and immunodeficient animals are most predisposed to clinical illness. Congregations of animals and poor sanitary practices heighten the increased frequency and severity of infections.

Giardiasis is an extremely common disease in people. Most infections are probably acquired from drinking contaminated municipal water supplies. Infants and children in day-care facilities have a particularly high rate of infection. Some biochemical and cross-infection studies suggest that the organism is not host specific. However, other cross-infection studies between humans and dogs or cats have not yielded conclusive evidence of interspecies infection. Pet ownership is not of epidemiologic significance in the prevalence of human infections; however, it seems logical to treat diarrheic infected animals.

Diarrhea is the principal clinical sign in pups and results in weight loss if it continues. The stool has often been characterized as being pale and greasy. Fever and vomiting are rare. These same manifestations are noted in affected people.

Detection of *Giardia* cysts is most accurate by the zinc sulfate flotation procedure. Examination of direct smears of freshly collected feces may be valuable in that trophozoites, when present, show a characteristic darting motion.

Drugs such as metronidazole are the first choice in the management of giardiasis. Quinacrine or furazolidone can be used as an alternative.

CRYPTOSPORIDIOSIS

Cryptosporidium is an extremely small (4 to 8 μm diameter) coccidium that primarily inhabits the digestive system of vertebrates. Ileal infections are most common. Resistant oocysts are spread by the fecal-oral route. Contamination of feed or drinking water is most common. As with many protozoa, cryptosporidia are opportunists, clinically affecting the young or immunosuppressed. Naturally occurring cryptosporidiosis has been described in young pups, those with concurrent distemper infection, and rarely in adult dogs. People may be similarly affected, with diarrhea being the main clinical sign. In most people, the illness is transient or subclinical; however, people with acquired immunodeficiency syndrome show protracted and severe diarrhea.

Diagnosis is made by isolating oocysts with the Sheather's flotation test and negative staining with acid-fast methods.

Treatment for this disease is symptomatic. Drugs such as spiramycin have not been curative.

Cryptosporidial infections in people have been recognized with increasing frequency in the past decade. Animal handlers, medical personnel, people in developing countries, and children in day-care facilities have had the highest prevalence of infections. *Cryptosporidium* cysts resist routine disinfectants, and only steam heat or concentrated

(50%) ammonia has been effective in their eradication.

References and Suggested Reading

Acha, P. N., and Szyfres, B.: *Zoonoses and Communicable Diseases Common to Man and Animals*. Washington, DC, Pan American Health Organization, World Health Organization, 1987.

Greene, C. E. (ed.): *Clinical Microbiology and Infectious Diseases of the Dog and Cat*. Philadelphia, W. B. Saunders, 1984.

Greene, C. E. (ed.): *Infectious Diseases of the Dog and Cat*. Philadelphia, W. B. Saunders, 1990.

FELINE ZOONOSES

MICHAEL R. LAPPIN

Fort Collins, Colorado

A zoonosis is a disease of animals that can be transmitted to humans. Cats are gaining in popularity as pets; it has been estimated that there are at least 54 million pet cats in the United States. Thus, the potential for feline zoonoses is increasing. Table 1 lists the feline zoonoses recognized in the Americas. Many of the feline zoonoses occur more frequently in veterinary personnel because of their direct contact with cats and the potential for exposure to infected body tissues or fluids. The following is an update on several of the more important or emerging feline-associated human illnesses that occur in the United States. The emphasis of the discussion is on the role that cats have in the transmission to humans and on the disease in humans.

DISEASES ASSOCIATED WITH BITE WOUNDS, SCRATCHES, OR EXUDATE CONTACT

Cat-Scratch Disease

Cat-scratch disease (cat-scratch fever, benign nonbacterial lymphadenitis) is caused by a gram-negative bacillus that has been isolated from lymph nodes and other tissues of humans showing various clinical signs such as lymphadenopathy, fever, malaise, weight loss, myalgia, headache, conjunctivitis, skin eruptions, and arthralgia (see *CVT X*, p. 1099). Similar bacteria have been found in the lymph nodes of cats, although cats do not appear to be clinically affected. Although the majority of afflicted humans have had a history of exposure to cats (bites, scratches, or kissing), other sources of infection have included scratches from other species including dogs, squirrels, and goats and wounds induced by crab claws, barbed wire, and plant material.

Men younger than 21 years have been infected most frequently, and the disease is reported most commonly in the cooler months in temperate climates. The incubation period appears to be approximately 3 weeks, and multiple family members are involved approximately 5% of the time. The diagnosis is made by combining documentation of exposure (history of cat contact or wounds) with characteristic histopathologic changes in lymph nodes, a positive skin test result, documentation of an increasing antibody titer, or exclusion of other common etiologies of lymphadenopathy. Most cases are self-limiting but may take several months to resolve completely. The bacterium is susceptible to several antibiotics *in vitro*, including the aminoglycosides.

Feline Plague

Yersinia pestis is a gram-negative coccobacillus that induces plague in cats and humans. This infectious agent is found most commonly in mid- and far-western states (majority of the human cases have been from California, Arizona, and New Mexico) (see *CVT X*, p. 1088). Rodents are the natural hosts for this bacterium and maintain the organism in the environment. Cats are most commonly infected by ingesting bacteremic rodents or lagomorphs or by being bitten by *Yersinia*-infected rodent fleas. Although the majority of humans are infected by rodent flea bites, cases of transmission by exposure to wild animals and infected domestic cats have been documented. Exposure can be from inhalation of respiratory secretions of cats with pneumonic plague or by contaminating mucous membranes or skin wounds with secretions or exudates. Thus, veterinary care personnel are at increased risk.

Bubonic, septicemic, or pneumonic plague can develop in cats and humans. Suppurative lymph-

Table 1. Feline Zoonoses

Disease (Agent)	Synonyms	Geographic Distribution (Human Occurrence)	Source of Infection	Affected Vertebrates	Clinical Signs
Viral					
Cowpox (poxvirus)	—	Cosmopolitan (rare)	Direct contact	Humans, horses, cats, cows	Human: Papulovesicular skin lesions Cat: Circumscribed, ulcerative, and pruritic skin lesions, mild conjunctivitis
Rabies (rhabdovirus)	Hydrophobia	Cosmopolitan (rare)	Animal bite, inhalation, ingestion, live virus vaccines (cats)	Humans, cats, dogs, all mammals	Human: Progressive neurologic disorder and death Cat: As in humans
Bacterial					
Anthrax (*Bacillus anthracis*)	Woolsorter's disease, ragpicker's disease, milzbrand, splenic fever	Cosmopolitan (rare)	Wounds, inhalation, or ingestion	Humans, cats, dogs, and most mammals	Human: Cutaneous ulcer with necrotic center, pneumonia, bloody diarrhea, hematemesis, occasionally central nervous system signs from meningitis Cat: Subacute to chronic; carbuncular lesions of jowl and tongue; swelling of lips, head, and throat; severe gastroenteritis
Campylobacter infection (*Campylobacter jejuni*)	—	Cosmopolitan (rare)	Fecal contamination	Humans, dogs, cats, others	Human: Subclinical; bacteremia, gastroenteritis, myalgia, arthralgia Cat: Subclinical; mild to severe gastroenteritis; diarrhea, occasionally containing blood
Cat-scratch disease (gram-negative bacillus)	Cat-scratch fever, benign nonbacterial lymphadenitis	Cosmopolitan; more common in temperate climates	Bite wounds and scratches	Humans	Human: Fever, lymphadenomegaly, malaise, headache, anorexia, encephalitis Cat: Subclinical
DF-2 infection (*Capnocytophaga canimorsus*)	—	Uncommon (rare)	Bite wounds, possibly scratches	Humans	Human: Septicemia, meningitis, bacterial endocarditis Cat: Subclinical
Diphtheria (*Corynebacterium diphtheriae*)	—	Cosmopolitan (rare)	Inhalation, contact with secretions	Humans, cats	Human: Fever, pharyngitis, diphtheric membrane, cervical lymphadenopathy, myocarditis Cat: Subclinical; membrane covering lower larynx and upper trachea, enlarged kidneys with fatty degeneration, occasionally paralysis
Leptospirosis (*Leptospira*)	Fort Bragg fever, Weil's disease, Stuttgart's disease, canecutter's disease, swineherd's disease	Cosmopolitan (rare)	Direct contact with urine, oral ingestion of contaminated meat, bite by infected animal	Humans, dogs, rarely cats, most mammals	Human: Malaise, fever, chills, myalgia, jaundice, hemolysis, hepatitis, acute nephritis, uveitis, aseptic meningitis Cat: Fever, icterus, nephritis
Listeriosis (*Listeria monocytogenes*)	Tiger River disease	Cosmopolitan (rare)	Vertical transmission—human carriers; isolated from soil, water, vegetation, and silage	Humans, cats, dogs, ruminants, rodents	Human: Abortions, stillbirths, neonatal death, septicemia, meningoencephalitis, uveitis, lymphadenopathy Cat: Subclinical intestinal carrier
Lyme disease (*Borrelia burgdorferi*)	—	Northeastern, midwestern, and southern states; California (common)	*Ixodes* tick bites; urine of infected cats or dogs?	Humans, dogs, rarely cats	Human: Skin rash, fever, arthralgia, central nervous system disease, cardiac arrhythmias, arthritis Cat: Fever, arthralgia, arthritis; clinical syndrome milder than in dogs
Plague (*Yersinia pestis*)	Sylvatic plague, black plague, bubonic plague	Cosmopolitan; Arizona, New Mexico (rare)	Flea contact, exudate contact (feline abscessed lymph nodes)	Humans, cats, dogs, rodents, lagomorphs, bats	Human: Bubonic, septicemic, pneumonic forms Cat: Fever, respiratory disease, and suppuration of cervical lymph nodes

Table continued on following page

Table 1. Feline Zoonoses Continued

Disease (Agent)	Synonyms	Geographic Distribution (Human Occurrence)	Source of Infection	Affected Vertebrates	Clinical Signs
Bacterial Continued					
Salmonellosis (*Salmonella*)	—	Cosmopolitan (common)	Fecal contamination	Humans, cats, dogs, most mammals, birds, and reptiles	Human: Subclinical; gastroenteritis, localized abscesses, septicemia Cat: Fever, malaise, gastrointestinal signs in approximately 50%
Shigellosis (*Shigella* spp.)	—	Cosmopolitan (common)	Fecal contamination	Humans, dogs, cats, most mammals	Human: Subclinical; gastroenteritis Cat: Subclinical; questionable zoonosis in cats
Streptococcal infection (*Streptococcus* group A)	—	Cosmopolitan (common)	Aerosol	Humans, dogs, cats	Human: Pharyngitis, sinusitis Cat: Asymptomatic; pharyngitis, sinusitis
Tularemia (*Francisella tularensis*)	Rabbit fever, deerfly fever, O'Hara's disease, lemming fever, Pahvant Valley fever	Cosmopolitan (rare)	Handling infected carcasses, blood-sucking arthropods, ingestion or contact with infected meat or water, cat bites or scratches, inhalation	Humans, dogs, cats, other vertebrates, and invertebrates	Human: Ulceroglandular, oculoglandular, glandular, pneumonic, or typhoidal (dependent on route of infection) Cat: Fever, depression, anorexia, icterus, pneumonitis, death
Yersinia infection (*Yersinia enterocolitica*)	—	Cosmopolitan (rare)	Fecal contamination	Humans, cats, dogs, primates, pigs, poultry, beavers	Human: Severe gastroenteritis Cat: Subclinical; possibly gastroenteritis (rare)
(*Y. pseudo-tuberculosis*)	—	North America (rare)	Ingestion, inhalation	Humans, cats, dogs, other mammals, and birds	Human: Lymphadenopathy, ileitis, arthralgia, septicemia, cutaneous swellings Cat: Anorexia, gastroenteritis, abdominal pain, icterus
Miscellaneous bacteria (*Bacteroides, Fusobacterium, Actinomyces, Nocardia, Pasteurella,* and others)	—	Cosmopolitan (common)	Bite wounds, contamination by oral fluids	Humans, cats, multiple vertebrates	Human: Abscess at bite wound, bacteremia Cat: Abscess at bite wound, pyothorax, bacteremia
Rickettsial and Chlamydial					
Q fever (*Coxiella burnetii*)	Abattoir fever, gray fever, Balkan grippe	Cosmopolitan; Nova Scotia (rare)	Milk, airborne (contact with aborted fetus), tick-borne?	Humans, cats, dogs, ruminants, other mammals	Human: Fever, malaise, headache, pneumonitis, hepatomegaly, valvular endocarditis Cat: Subclinical fever, anorexia
Chlamydiosis (*Chlamydia psittaci*)	—	Cosmopolitan (common)	Direct contact with ocular discharge	Humans, cats, other vertebrates	Human: Conjunctivitis Cat: Conjunctivitis, mild pneumonitis
Fungal					
Blastomycosis (*Blastomyces dermatitidis*)	—	Cosmopolitan (rare)	Soil organism, dog bite wounds (cat?)	Humans, dogs, cats	Human: Pneumonia, cutaneous granulomas, osteomyelitis, uveitis, meningitis Cat: Cutaneous, uveitis, respiratory, central nervous system disease
Dermatophytoses (*Microsporum canis, Trichophyton mentagrophytes*)	Ringworm	Cosmopolitan (common)	Soil, direct contact with infected animal	Humans, dogs, cats, and many mammals	Human: Circular, raised erythematous lesions, hyperkeratosis, alopecia Cat: As in humans; subclinical, miliary dermatitis
Sporotrichosis (*Sporothrix schenckii*)	Rose grower's disease	Cosmopolitan (rare)	Soil organism, contact with exudate from cats	Humans, cats, dogs, ruminants, rodents, primates	Human: Cutaneous lesions that spread along lymphatics Cat: Cutaneous lesions that spread along lymphatics

Table 1. *Feline Zoonoses* Continued

Disease (Agent)	Synonyms	Geographic Distribution (Human Occurrence)	Source of Infection	Affected Vertebrates	Clinical Signs
Helminths					
Cutaneous larval migrans (*Ancylostoma braziliense, Uncinaria stenocephala*)	Creeping eruption	Cosmopolitan (rare)	Soil	Humans, cats, dogs	Human: Linear cutaneous eruptions Cat: Gastroenteritis
Visceral larval migrans (*Toxocara cati, Toxascaris leonina*)	—	Cosmopolitan (10% of humans seropositive)	Egg ingestion, fecal-oral contact, fomites	Humans, cats, dogs (*Toxascaris*)	Human: Asymptomatic; pneumonitis, myositis, arthralgia, hepatosplenomegaly, uveitis, central nervous system disease, endophthalmitis Cat: Subclinical; unthriftiness, gastroenteritis, intestinal obstruction
Cestodes					
Dipylidiasis (*Dipylidium caninum*)	—	Cosmopolitan in areas with fleas (common)	Ingestion of flea (intermediate host)	Definitive: humans, cats, dogs Intermediate: fleas and biting lice	Human: Diarrhea and pruritus ani Cat: Subclinical; pruritus ani
Echinococcosis (*Echinococcus multilocularis*)	Hydatid disease, alveolar echinococcosis	North America (rare)	Ingestion of eggs	Definitive: cats and dogs Intermediate: small rodents and occasionally humans	Human: Cystic disease of liver, brain, or lung Cat: Subclinical; moderate enteritis
Protozoan					
Amebiasis (*Entamoeba histolytica*)	Amebic dysentery	Cosmopolitan (common)	Ingestion of cysts, rarely trophozoites (fecal contamination)	Humans, cats, dogs, primates, rodents, pigs, reptiles	Human: Subclinical; severe gastroenteritis with ulceration, occasionally polysystemic Cat: Ulcerative colitis •
Cryptosporidiosis (*Cryptosporidium*)	—	Cosmopolitan (common)	Ingestion of oocysts (fecal contamination)	Humans, cats, dogs, many mammals and birds	Human: Immunocompetent: acute, self-limiting gastroenteritis; immunodeficient: chronic, severe diarrhea Cat: As for humans
Giardiasis (*Giardia* spp.)	—	Cosmopolitan (common)	Ingestion of cysts, rarely trophozoites (fecal contamination)	Humans, cats, dogs, rodents, birds, and many mammals	Human: Subclinical; chronic diarrhea Cat: Subclinical; acute, chronic, or intermittent diarrhea with or without weight loss, and steatorrhea
Toxoplasmosis (*Toxoplasma gondii*)	—	Cosmopolitan (common)	Fecal contamination (oocysts), intermediate host ingestion, transplacental transmission	Humans, cats, dogs, almost all vertebrates	Human: Immunocompetent: subclinical; malaise, fever, lymphadenopathy, stillbirth, congenital defects; Immunodeficient: as above except more severe encephalitis, myositis, pneumonia, retinochoroiditis, death Cat: As for humans
Trichomoniasis (*Pentatrichomonas hominis*)	—	Cosmopolitan (rare)	Ingestion of trophozoites, fecal contamination (rare)	Humans, cats, dogs	Human: Subclinical; mild enteritis Cat: Subclinical; mild enteritis
Ectoparasites					
Cheyletiella infestation (*Cheyletiella*)	Walking dandruff	Cosmopolitan (rare)	Direct contact	Humans, cats, dogs, rabbits, and some wild mammals	Human: Pruritic skin disease with erythema and wheals Cat: As for humans
Sarcoptic mange (*Sarcoptes scabiei*)	Scabies	Cosmopolitan (common)	Direct contact	Humans, dogs, cats	Human: Transient, pruritic papuloeruptive skin disease Cat: As for humans

adenitis (buboes) of the cervical and submandibular lymph nodes is the most common clinical manifestation. Each form has accompanying fever, headache, weakness, and malaise. Untreated pneumonic plague is considered 100% fatal in infected humans. Exudates from cats with lymphadenomegaly should be examined cytologically for large numbers of the characteristic bipolar rods. Culture of exudates, the tonsillar area, and saliva, as well as documented rising antibody titers, can confirm the diagnosis. Felines with suppurative lymphadenitis should be considered plague suspects and extreme caution exercised when handling exudates or treating draining wounds. Aminoglycosides, chloramphenicol, and tetracyclines can be used successfully for the treatment of plague.

Tularemia

Tularemia is caused by *Francisella tularensis*, which is a gram-negative bacillus found throughout the continental United States. Human tularemia occurs most commonly following tick exposure and less commonly from contact with infected animals (rabbits). Exposure of humans through cat bites can occur. Cats are infected most frequently by tick bites or by ingesting infected rabbits or rodents. Infected cats develop generalized lymphadenopathy and abscess formation in organs such as the liver and spleen, leading to fever, anorexia, icterus, and death. Clinical signs in humans are dependent on the route of exposure. Ulceroglandular (inoculation of extremities), oculoglandular (inoculation of the conjunctiva), glandular (unknown inoculation site), oropharyngeal or pneumonic (inoculation by inhalation), and typhoidal (inoculation by ingestion) forms have been described.

The organism is not often recognized in exudates or lymph node aspirates from infected cats. Cultures and rising antibody titers can be used to confirm the diagnosis in cats and humans. As with plague, contact with oral secretions and exudates from clinically ill cats should be avoided. Streptomycin and gentamicin are the drugs most commonly used in humans. Tetracycline and chloramphenicol can be used in cases not requiring hospitalization but may be associated with relapses.

Miscellaneous Bacteria

A multitude of aerobic and anaerobic bacteria colonize the mouths of healthy and clinically ill cats. Many of these bacteria cause clinical signs of disease in humans if they are inoculated through the skin or mucous membranes via bite or scratch wounds. In immunocompetent individuals, the majority of the bacteria associated with cat bites or scratch wounds lead only to local infection. Immunocompromised humans or individuals exposed to *Pasteurella* or *Capnocytophaga* (DF-2 and DF-2-like) more consistently develop systemic clinical illness. Generally, local cellulitis is noted initially, followed by evidence of deeper tissue infection. Bacteremia and the associated clinical signs of fever, malaise, and weakness are common, and death can occur from either of these two genera. Fatal disease is most commonly associated with concurrent immunosuppression. Polyarthritis, osteomyelitis, meningitis, and endocarditis are common with persistent infections. The diagnosis is confirmed by bacterial culture. Treatment includes local wound drainage and systemic antibiotic therapy. Penicillin derivatives are very effective against most *Pasteurella* infections. Penicillins, cephalosporins, and other antibiotics are effective *in vitro* against *Capnocytophaga*. Immediate, thorough washing of all bite wounds and scratches is imperative. Soaking the wounds in aqueous organic iodine solutions may be helpful. Irrigation of the wound with isotonic fluids delivered by intermittent high-pressure pulsations is reportedly the most effective way to dislodge bacteria.

Induction of *Mycobacterium* (atypical mycobacteriosis) infection in humans following bites or scratch wounds induced by infected cats or by contamination by exudates from infected cats has not been documented but potentially could occur.

Fungal Agents

Although many systemic fungal agents infect both humans and cats, only *Sporothrix schenckii* has been shown to infect humans after direct exposure to infected cats. *Blastomyces dermatitidis* has been transmitted to humans by bites from infected dogs. Both of these organisms are cosmopolitan in distribution, and the soil is thought to be the natural reservoir. *Blastomyces* infection in cats is rare compared with its incidence in dogs, but dyspnea, draining skin lesions, and weight loss are common clinical findings. *Sporothrix* infection in cats can be cutaneolymphatic, cutaneous, or disseminated. The cutaneolymphatic and cutaneous forms commonly are ulcerated and may be a source of infection of humans. Cats commonly produce large numbers of the organism in feces, tissues, and exudates. Veterinary care personnel thus are at high risk when treating infected cats. The clinical disease in humans is similar to that in cats. Ketoconazole and potassium iodide are used for treatment.

DISEASES ASSOCIATED WITH DIRECT FECAL-ORAL CONTACT OR FOMITES

Parasites

VISCERAL AND OCULAR LARVA MIGRANS

Visceral larva migrans in humans can be associated with the feline parasite *Toxocara cati* or *Toxascaris leonina*. These common roundworms pass eggs in feces. The eggs become infectious after approximately 2 weeks and can survive in the environment for months. Dogs cause more environmental contamination with parasite eggs than cats. However, areas such as children's sandboxes may be an important source of infection because of defecation habits of cats. It is extremely unlikely that human infection would develop after direct contact with cats, because the eggs are not immediately infectious and cats are usually fastidious and do not leave feces contaminating skin surfaces for long periods.

Cats can be subclinically affected or may develop poor coats, poor weight gain, and gastrointestinal signs. Because of their habit of geophagia, children are more commonly infected. Following ingestion of infectious eggs, larvae penetrate the intestinal wall and migrate through the tissues. Eosinophilic granulomatous reactions involving the skin, lungs, central nervous system, and eyes then occur, potentially leading to clinical signs of disease. Clinical signs and abnormalities on physical examination include skin rash, fever, failure to thrive, central nervous system signs, cough, pulmonary infiltrates, and hepatosplenomegaly. Peripheral eosinophilia is common. Ocular larva migrans most commonly involves the retina and can cause reduced vision and strabismus. Uveitis and endophthalmitis can also occur. Visceral larva migrans is most common in children between 1 and 4 years of age, whereas ocular larva migrans is most common in older children. Seroprevalence studies suggest that approximately 10% of humans are exposed; however, clinical disease is unusual. Diagnosis in humans is confirmed by biopsy or can be presumed in cases with classic clinical manifestations, eosinophilia, and positive serology. Treatment has been attempted with several drugs including diethylcarbamazine and mebendazole. Prevention revolves around control of animal excrement in human environments. All puppies and kittens should be routinely treated with an anthelmintic such as pyrantel pamoate two times, 21 days apart, during their initial vaccination period.

CUTANEOUS LARVA MIGRANS

Ancylostoma braziliense and *Uncinaria stenocephala* are hookworms that infect cats in the United States and have been associated with cutaneous larva migrans. Cats are either subclinically ill or show nonspecific signs such as a poor coat, poor weight gain, or gastroenteritis. After the passage of hookworm eggs into the environment in feces, infectious larvae are released, potentially infecting humans through skin penetration. These larvae cannot penetrate the dermoepidermal junction and so usually die in the epidermis. Clinical signs are related to migration of the larvae, resulting in an erythematous, pruritic cutaneous tunnel. Clinical signs usually resolve within several weeks. Topical thiabendazole solutions may speed resolution. Prevention is as described for visceral larva migrans.

ENTERIC PROTOZOANS

Cats can be infected by *Entamoeba histolytica* (amebic dysentery), *Cryptosporidium* (coccidia), *Giardia* (flagellate), and *Pentatrichomonas hominis* (flagellate). Each of these parasites has been associated with human illness. Cats do not readily form cysts after infection by *Entamoeba* or *Pentatrichomonas*, suggesting that the risk of transmission to humans is low. The incidence of human *Giardia* and *Cryptosporidium* infections resulting from exposure to infected cats is unknown. Each of these agents can be subclinical or can cause gastrointestinal disease in cats or humans. The severity of disease is much greater in immunocompromised individuals. *Cryptosporidium* can cause severe secretory diarrhea, dehydration, and death in patients with the acquired immunodeficiency syndrome (AIDS). Cats immunocompromised by feline leukemia virus infection, feline immunodeficiency virus infection, or drug therapy are more likely to develop clinical disease and possibly shed greater numbers of the organisms, increasing the zoonotic potential. A combination of direct fecal examination and flotation techniques is used for diagnosis. *Cryptosporidium* is most commonly found using sugar solution centrifugation and staining procedures such as acid-fast stain. *Entamoeba*, *Giardia*, and *Pentatrichomonas* generally respond to metronidazole. There is currently no drug of choice for *Cryptosporidium*; however, spiramycin (macrolide antibiotic) has controlled the clinical signs in some AIDS victims. Prevention of human infection with these parasites involves controlling exposure to and treatment of infected cats.

Bacterial Diseases

Salmonella, *Campylobacter jejuni*, *Escherichia coli*, and *Yersinia enterocolitica* all infect cats and can cause disease in humans. Gastroenteritis can occur in both species. Subclinical infection by *Sal-*

monella is common in cats. Approximately 50% of clinically affected cats do not have gastroenteritis. These cats can have fever, depression, weakness, hypothermia, and rarely cardiovascular collapse and death. *In utero* infection occasionally occurs and may result in abortion, stillbirth, and weak kittens.

Y. enterocolitica is probably a commensal agent in cats. Humans are an atypical host and develop fever, abdominal pain, and bacteremia after infection. Diagnosis is based on culturing the organism from feces. Several antibiotics can be effective, including chloramphenicol, tetracycline, cephalosporins, and trimethoprim-sulfonamides. As for all the enteric bacterial zoonoses, prevention is based on sanitation and control of exposure to feces.

MISCELLANEOUS AGENTS

Q Fever

Coxiella burnetii is a rickettsial agent found throughout the world, including North America. Infection of cats most commonly occurs after tick exposure, ingestion of contaminated carcasses, or aerosolization from a contaminated environment. Human illness associated with direct contact with infected cats is primarily associated with aerosol exposure to the organism passed by parturient or aborting cats. Clinical signs are unusual in infected cats. Humans commonly develop fever, malaise, headache, pneumonitis, hepatomegaly, and valvular endocarditis. Tetracycline derivatives are usually effective therapeutic agents. Gloves and masks should always be worn when handling parturient or aborting cats.

Toxoplasmosis

Toxoplasma gondii is a tissue protozoan that is one of the most ubiquitous parasites known. Most seroprevalence studies performed in the United States suggest that at least 30% of cats and humans have previously been exposed to this protozoan (see *CTV X*, p. 1112). Cats are the definitive hosts of the organism and are the only species known to complete the enteroepithelial cycle (sexual phase). The enteroepithelial cycle results in the passage of unsporulated oocysts in feces. These oocysts sporulate in the environment in the presence of oxygen (1 to 3 days depending on temperature and humidity) and then are infectious to most mammals, birds, fish, and reptiles. Infectious oocysts survive in the environment for months to years. After exposure, cats and all other hosts develop an extraintestinal cycle that ultimately leads to the formation of tissue cysts containing the organism. In immunocompe-

tent individuals, these cysts can be quiescent in tissue for years.

Humans are most commonly infected with toxoplasmosis by ingesting sporulated oocysts, by ingesting tissue cysts, or transplacentally. In immunocompetent individuals, clinical signs generally do not occur. Self-limiting fever, lymphadenopathy, and malaise occur in some individuals. Transplacental infection (primary exposure of the mother resulting in fetal infection) during the first two trimesters commonly leads to infection of at least 50% of the fetuses, with severe clinical disease in at least 10%. Clinical manifestations include stillbirth, hydrocephalus, hepatosplenomegaly, and retinochoroiditis. Many babies develop recurrent ocular or neurologic disease later in life. The organism in tissue cysts can be reactivated by immunosuppression, leading to dissemination and severe clinical illness. This has been associated with drug-induced immunosuppression as well as with AIDS. It has been estimated that approximately 10% of the AIDS victims diagnosed by 1991 will suffer from toxoplasmic encephalitis.

The role of cats in the human zoonosis is primarily related to the production of oocysts and perpetuating the disease in the environment. However, individual cats generally only shed oocysts once in their life, and the oocyst-shedding period usually has a duration from days to several weeks. Infection due to direct contact with oocyst-shedding cats is extremely unlikely. Because oocysts have to sporulate to be infectious, fresh fecal contact cannot cause infection. Cats are very fastidious and usually do not allow feces to remain on their skin long enough to lead to oocyst sporulation. Because of the short oocyst-shedding period and the failure of most cats to repeat oocyst shedding on repeated exposure, it is *not* recommended that pet cats be removed from the home environment of pregnant or immunosuppressed individuals. To avoid oocyst induction of infection, high-risk individuals should not feed their cats undercooked meats or allow them to hunt; should clean the litter box daily, with incineration or flushing of feces, and should clean the litter pan with scalding water; should wear gloves when working with soil; should always keep the children's sandbox covered; should always boil water for drinking that has been obtained from the general environment; and should control potential paratenic hosts such as cockroaches and earthworms. It has been shown that it is unlikely that cats with toxoplasmosis will shed oocysts a second time after the administration of clinical doses of glucocorticoids. Humans are very likely to be infected after the ingestion of tissue cysts in undercooked meats. In the United States, pork products have the highest incidence of *Toxoplasma* cysts. Meats should be cooked to at least 66°C (150°F). Gloves should be worn when handling raw meats (including field dressing) for cooking, or hands should be cleansed thoroughly. Freezing meat at $-20°C$ for several days greatly reduces tissue cyst viability.

Sugar solution centrifugation works well for the demonstration of oocysts in feces but is only positive for short periods. Accurate serologic testing of cats for prediction of when primary exposure (and resultant oocyst shedding) occurred still is not available. The assessment of both *T. gondii*–specific immunoglobulin M (IgM) and immunoglobulin G (IgG) antibody titers can aid in the documentation of exposure to *T. gondii* and clinical illness due to toxoplasmosis but is not accurate enough to predict the oocyst-shedding period. Subclinically ill cats usually have detectable IgM titers by 2 weeks after inoculation; these titers are usually negative by 12 weeks after inoculation. Thus, a positive titer can predict recent infection. However, clinically ill cats often have persistent IgM titers for months, long after the oocyst-shedding period has ended, rendering the IgM assay inaccurate for predicting when the oocyst-shedding period had occurred.

A number of drugs have anti-*Toxoplasma* effects *in vitro*. Clindamycin hydrochloride is commonly used for the treatment of clinically ill cats and humans.

References and Suggested Reading

Elliot, D.L., and Tolle, S.W., Goldberg, L., et al.: Pet-associated illness. J. Am. Anim. Hosp. Assoc. 22:387, 1986.

Greene, C.E. (ed.): *Clinical Microbiology and Infectious Diseases of the Dog and Cat.* Philadelphia: W. B. Saunders, 1984.

Greene, C.E. (ed.): *Infectious Diseases of the Dog and Cat,* 2nd ed. Philadelphia: W. B. Saunders, 1990.

Pedersen, N.C.: *Feline Infectious Diseases.* Goleta, CA: American Veterinary Publications, 1988.

Section
5

ENDOCRINE AND METABOLIC DISORDERS

MARK E. PETERSON
Consulting Editor

ENDOCRINE AND METABOLIC CAUSES OF POLYURIA AND POLYDIPSIA

C. E. RHETT NICHOLS

Mississippi State, Mississippi

Various endocrine and metabolic disturbances account for the majority of polyuria and polydipsia disorders. The etiology of the polyuria in most cases involves either interference with the normal action of antidiuretic hormone (ADH) and its renal tubular receptors, a reduction in renal medullary interstitial hypertonicity (partial or total medullary washout), renal tubular cell dysfunction, or the presence of excess solute (usually either glucose or urea) in the renal tubules. Reversal of the polyuria and polydipsia is dependent on the treatability of the underlying endocrine and metabolic disturbance.

PHYSIOLOGY OF WATER BALANCE

ADH release and action, renal medullary hypertonicity, and renal tubular function all are important variables in the control of water balance. Interference with any of these variables affects urine concentration and may cause polyuria and polydipsia.

ADH has a fundamental role in the regulation of water balance. The primary effect of ADH is to conserve body fluids by reducing the rate of urine production. This antidiuretic action is achieved by promoting the reabsorption of solute-free water in the distal tubules and collecting ducts of the kidneys. The combination of ADH release and thirst mechanism ensures the maintenance of normal water and osmotic concentration of body fluids.

ADH is formed in the supraoptic and paraventricular nuclei of the hypothalamus and stored in the posterior lobe of the pituitary. Probably the most important stimulus for ADH secretion under physiologic conditions is the influence of plasma osmolality on hypothalamic receptors. At plasma osmolalities below a certain minimum or threshold level, plasma ADH is suppressed to low or undetectable levels. Above this point, plasma ADH increases dramatically in direct proportion to increases in plasma osmolality. In humans, a change in plasma osmolality of only 1% is sufficient to evoke a significant change in ADH secretion.

The secretion of ADH can also be affected by changes in blood volume or pressure, nausea, hypoglycemia, the renin-angiotensin system, and nonspecific factors such as pain, emotion, and physical exercise. In addition, a large number of drugs, hormones, and metabolic disturbances have been implicated in the alteration of ADH secretion or the effects of ADH at the level of the renal tubule.

ADH exerts its effect by binding to specific receptors on the renal tubular cell. ADH-sensitive adenylate cyclase is then stimulated, resulting in the generation of cyclic adenosine monophosphate (cAMP) within the cell. These intracellular events increase the number of aqueous channels on the luminal membrane. The net effect is free-water absorption and the formation of concentrated urine.

Two other important factors necessary for the regulation of water balance are the presence of "adequate" renal function and a hypertonic renal medullary interstitium. First, at least one third of the nephrons in both kidneys must be functional; if two thirds of the nephron mass is lost, the kidneys lose their ability to concentrate urine. Second, increased medullary hypertonicity is the driving force for passive water reabsorption in the distal tubule and collecting duct; a reduction in medullary solute concentration results in dilute urine and excessive water loss even in the presence of excessive ADH secretion.

ROUTINE LABORATORY EVALUATION OF POLYURIA AND POLYDIPSIA

A practical approach to the problem of water balance is to rule out the common causes of polyuria and polydipsia, which include the many causes of acquired nephrogenic diabetes insipidus (DI) (see later). Recommended initial diagnostic tests include a complete blood count (CBC), serum chemical profile with electrolytes, and complete urinalysis with culture and sensitivity test results obtained by cystocentesis. The more common causes of polyuria

293

and polydipsia, in most instances, have specific and obvious abnormalities associated with the serum biochemical and electrolyte profile and urinalysis. On the other hand, routine blood work is generally unremarkable in dogs and cats with central DI, primary nephrogenic DI, and primary polydipsia (compulsive water drinking). When abnormalities are present, they are usually secondary to dehydration from water restriction by the pet owner. Such abnormalities may include a slightly increased hematocrit or hypernatremia.

The urinalysis is a key in establishing the presence of a polyuric state. Urine specific gravity less than 1.030 in dogs and 1.035 in cats frequently suggests a concentrating defect and hence supports the complaint of polyuria. Most dogs with DI, for example, have a water diuresis (urine specific gravity <1.007). Results of the urinalysis may also be important diagnostically. Persistent glycosuria is diagnostic of primary renal glycosuria or, more commonly, diabetes mellitus. Significant proteinuria (urine protein:creatinine ratio >1), the presence of an inactive urine sediment, and urine of low specific gravity are highly suggestive of either "occult" pyelonephritis or hyperadrenocorticism with secondary glomerulonephritis or amyloidosis. An active urine sediment (pyuria, hematuria, or bacteriuria) clearly is indicative of urinary tract inflammation or infection and possibly pyelonephritis.

The direction of a diagnostic workup, especially in those cases with a normal serum chemistry profile, many times can be based on urine specific gravity or osmolality. For example, animals with a urine specific gravity of greater than 1.030 and without glycosuria are probably not polyuric and therefore need no further workup, at least for polyuria and polydipsia. Animals with a urine specific gravity in the isosthenuric range (1.008 to 1.012) or greater (but <1.030) and a normal blood urea nitrogen (BUN) and serum creatinine level may have early renal insufficiency or one of the many causes of acquired nephrogenic DI. Performing a water deprivation test as a diagnostic tool in the presence of unsuspected renal insufficiency could induce overt renal failure. To avoid this complication, a sensible approach is first to evaluate renal size or architecture with abdominal radiography or preferably with renal ultrasonography. Decreased renal size or ultrasonographic changes described as diminished corticomedullary architecture are characteristic of chronic kidney disease. If radiographic or ultrasonographic results are equivocal, a creatinine clearance test may be indicated. Animals with normal radiographic or ultrasonographic results or, alternatively, animals with a urine specific gravity less than 1.007 and normal results on blood work usually do not have renal tubular disease (pyelonephritis is one major exception) and are generally safe candidates for a water deprivation test.

CAUSES OF POLYURIA AND POLYDIPSIA

Diabetes Insipidus

Diabetes insipidus (DI) is a disorder of water metabolism characterized by polyuria, a urine of low specific gravity or osmolality (so-called insipid or tasteless urine), and polydipsia. DI can result from any of three basic defects (Robertson, 1988). The most common is *renal insensitivity to ADH*. This defect is most often caused by various renal, endocrine, and metabolic disorders. These disorders include hyperadrenocorticism, hypokalemia, hypercalcemia, chronic renal failure, liver disease, and pyometra. This type of DI is referred to as *acquired* or *secondary nephrogenic DI*. Congenital or primary nephrogenic DI appears to be rare in veterinary medicine. The second type of DI is caused by excessive intake of water. It can result from a defect in the thirst mechanism (dipsogenic DI) or it may be a manifestation of a behavioral problem, in which case it is often referred to as *primary polydipsia, psychogenic polydipsia,* or *compulsive water drinking*. The third type of DI results from a primary deficiency in secretion of ADH. It can also be caused by a wide variety of disorders and is variously referred to as *neurogenic, cranial, ADH-responsive,* or *central DI*.

Central DI is characterized by an absolute or relative lack of circulating ADH and is classified as primary (idiopathic) or secondary in nature. The idiopathic forms of central DI are the most common in veterinary medicine. Secondary central DI usually develops after head trauma or neoplasia. Although hypothalamic or pituitary tumors have been reported as potential causes of central DI, head trauma in small animals appears to be the most common cause of transient or permanent central DI in this second category.

Findings on the physical examination of most dogs or cats with central DI are unremarkable despite owner complaints of polyuria, polydipsia, nocturia, and incontinence. In general, the only laboratory abnormality is urine of low specific gravity. A practical diagnostic approach (because central DI is uncommon) is to rule out more common causes of polyuria and polydipsia that may present with normal findings on blood studies, such as hyperadrenocorticism or pyelonephritis. Specific tests used to confirm the diagnosis of central DI include the modified water deprivation test and the ADH trial (see *CVT X*, p. 973).

The most effective treatment of ADH deficiency (central DI) is hormone replacement. Standard therapy in veterinary medicine has long been the parenteral administration of vasopressin tannate in oil (Pitressin Tannate in Oil, Parke-Davis). This agent is a partially purified preparation of ADH in repository form. Unfortunately, this product is no longer available from the manufacturer.

A synthetic ADH analogue, desmopressin (1-desamino-8-D-arginine vasopressin, DDAVP, Rorer Laboratories), is available for use and now appears to be the treatment of choice in central DI, at least in human patients (Kosman, 1978). DDAVP is available as both a sterile aqueous solution for subcutaneous injection (cartons of 10 dose ampules, each containing 4 μg in 1 ml) and as an aqueous solution intended for intranasal use (100 μg/ml, 2.5 ml per vial). Intranasal administration of DDAVP to dogs and cats may be difficult, but the medication is also effective when placed into the conjunctival sac. Recommended initial dosages of the two DDAVP preparations are 1 to 2 μg SC and 1 to 2 drops intraconjunctivally, respectively, administered once or twice daily. The daily dose should gradually be adjusted as needed to control signs of polyuria and polydipsia. A rare side effect is water intoxication with resultant hyponatremia. Although the duration of action of DDAVP is usually less than 24 hr, a single daily treatment may provide an adequate degree of control of water intake. The major drawback of use of either DDAVP preparation is its considerable expense (at least $80 to $100 a month for most animals).

If the degree of polyuria remains unacceptable to the owner after initial treatment with ADH, the additional use of nonhormonal therapy can be considered. The use of chlorothiazide diuretics (hydrochlorothiazide) or the oral sulfonylurea hypoglycemic agent chlorpropamide (Diabinese, Pfizer) may effectively reduce polyuria in some cases of central DI; potential side effects of these drugs include hypokalemia and hypoglycemia, respectively (Schwartz-Porsche, 1980).

Hyperadrenocorticism

Hyperadrenocorticism (Cushing's syndrome) is one of the most common endocrine causes of polyuria and polydipsia in middle-aged and older dogs. Cushing's syndrome appears to be rare in cats. The polyuria associated with hyperadrenocorticism is most likely related to the interference of cortisol with the action of ADH on the renal collecting ducts. The "classic" Cushing's case presents with a potbellied appearance; a history of polyuria, polydipsia, and polyphagia; and serum biochemical elevations of serum alkaline phosphatase, alanine aminotranferase, and cholesterol. Unfortunately, some with hyperadrenocorticism may have absolutely normal blood findings and a normal physical appearance. Specific diagnostic testing may include the adrenocorticotropic hormone (ACTH) stimulation test, low- and high-dose dexamethasone

suppression tests, ACTH determinations, urine cortisol:creatinine ratio, and computed tomography (CT) scanning where available (see *CVT X*, pp. 961 and 1024).

All dogs with hyperadrenocorticism should be carefully screened for concurrent overt or subclinical illness such as urinary tract infection, diabetes mellitus, glomerulonephritis, and hypertension. A thorough workup should include a CBC, serum biochemical profile, chest and abdominal radiographs, a complete urinalysis including urine culture and sensitivity test results obtained by cystocentesis, and blood pressure measurements if available. The success or failure of the medical management of the hyperadrenocorticism and the associated polyuria and polydipsia may depend on the recognition and modification of the many related problems that develop with this disorder.

The cause of hyperadrenocorticism determines treatment. Pituitary-dependent hyperadrenocorticism can be treated surgically with bilateral adrenalectomy or hypophysectomy, or, more commonly, it can be managed medically with the adrenocorticolytic agent o,p'-DDD (Lysodren, Bristol-Myers) (see this volume, p. 345, and *CVT X*, p. 1024) or the cortisol synthesis inhibitor ketoconazole (Nizoral, Janssen Pharmaceutical) (see this volume, p. 349), or with radiation (see this volume, p. 319, and *CVT X*, p. 1031). Unilateral adrenocortical tumors should be surgically removed because of metastatic potential, although medical therapy has been used with some success (see *CVT X*, p. 1034). Most dogs with pituitary-dependent hyperadrenocorticism (the most common type of Cushing's disease) respond to medical therapy with o,p'-DDD with a reduction in polyuria and polydipsia within 5 to 16 days. The average time of response is 11 days (Feldman and Nelson, 1987). Treatment failure should be expected after 14 to 21 days without response. Reasons for apparent failure include an undiagnosed tumor (adrenal tumors are relatively resistant to the cytotoxic effects of o,p'-DDD), poor drug potency, an incorrect diagnosis, a rare case of pituitary-dependent hyperadrenocorticism that requires 30 to 60 days of o,p'-DDD therapy, concurrent anticonvulsant therapy (many anticonvulsants increase the metabolism of o,p'-DDD), and iatrogenic hyperadrenocorticism in dogs. Some hyperadrenal dogs, despite correct diagnosis and appropriate therapy with o,p'-DDD, remain polyuric and polydipsic. This frustrating problem may be explained by concurrent urinary tract infection or renal disease, medullary washout, concurrent psychogenic polydipsia or central DI, or any combination of these. Regardless of the treatment chosen, hyperadrenocorticism cannot be treated easily, inexpensively, or without close monitoring and follow-up.

Hypoadrenocorticism

Polyuria, although not a common complaint of owners, is frequently associated with hypoadrenocorticism. Despite normal kidney function and severe hypovolemia, the urine specific gravity in most dogs with hypoadrenocorticism is less than 1.030. It is likely that chronic sodium wasting secondary to hypoaldosteronism results in renal medullary washout and decreased concentrating ability with resultant polyuria. In addition, hypercalcemia (usually mild but at times more than 15 mg/dl) is present in approximately 20% of the cases and may also contribute to the polyuria and polydipsia. Diagnostically, hypoadrenocorticism that presents with azotemia and a urine-concentrating defect can be difficult to differentiate from primary renal failure. Definitive diagnosis of hypoadrenocorticism is based on an inadequate or absent response to ACTH stimulation.

The treatment of hypoadrenocorticism is directed toward correcting hypotension and hypovolemia, improving vascular integrity by providing an immediate source of glucocorticoid, and correcting electrolyte imbalance and acidosis if present. The vast majority of dogs in hypoadrenal crisis with hyperkalemia can be treated successfully by rapid intravenous administration of 0.9% sodium chloride. Some dogs may require the addition of glucose if hypoglycemia (an uncommon complication of hypoadrenocorticism) is suspected or known to be present. The polyuria and polydipsia of hypoadrenocorticism are reversible with chronic mineralocorticoid administration. Once a patient is stabilized and eating without vomiting, oral mineralocorticoid therapy (fludrocortisone acetate) can be initiated. Fludrocortisone acetate (Florinef, Squibb) must be administered daily for the control of hypoadrenocorticism. The average dosage for most dogs is about 20 μg/kg/day. An alternative to daily oral mineralocorticoid administration is the long-acting injectable mineralocorticoid preparation desoxycorticosterone pivalate (Percorten, Ciba-Geigy) (see this volume, p. 353). Desoxycorticosterone pivalate is given every 25 days at a dose of 1 to 2 mg/kg, IM. Desoxycorticosterone pivalate is not yet approved by the Food and Drug Administration for veterinary use; however, this drug can be obtained along with owner waiver forms from the manufacturer. Rarely, oral sodium chloride supplementation may be needed in addition to mineralocorticoid administration to normalize a "washed-out" renal medullary interstitium.

Hyperthyroidism

Hyperthyroidism (thyrotoxicosis) is a multisystemic disorder resulting from excessive circulating concentrations of the two thyroid hormones thyroxine (T_4) and triiodothyronine (T_3). Feline hyperthyroidism, although first documented in the past decade, has become the most common endocrine disorder of middle-aged to old cats and is one of the most frequently diagnosed disorders in small animal practice. In most cats with hyperthyroidism, functional thyroid adenomatous hyperplasia (or adenoma) involving one or both thyroid lobes is responsible for the thyroid oversecretion. Thyroid carcinoma only very rarely causes hyperthyroidism in cats, with a prevalence of approximately 1 to 2% Canine hyperthyroidism, on the other hand, is almost always associated with thyroid adenocarcinoma; however, this disorder is uncommon and will not be discussed here (see this volume, p. 319).

Polyuria and polydipsia are frequent clinical signs in cats with hyperthyroidism. The exact cause of these signs is unknown. The hyperthyroid state may impair urine-concentrating ability by increasing total renal blood flow and thereby decreasing renal medullary solute concentration. In addition, concurrent primary renal disease contributes to polyuria and polydipsia in some cats with hyperthyroidism. Alternatively, in cats with normal concentrating ability, a hypothalamic disturbance caused by thyrotoxicosis may produce compulsive polydipsia with secondary polyuria.

Increased basal serum thyroid concentrations are the gold standard for the diagnosis of hyperthyroidism. Resting serum concentrations of both T_3 and T_4 are above the normal range in the vast majority of cats with hyperthyroidism. Cats with mild hyperthyroidism or hyperthyroid cats with severe concurrent nonthyroidal illness (e.g., diabetes mellitus, liver disease, renal failure, or other chronic disease) may occasionally have normal or high-normal serum thyroid hormone concentrations at the time of initial evaluation. In cases such as these, a T_3 suppression test, thyroid-stimulating hormone (TSH) stimulation test, or repeating serum thyroid hormone concentrations at a later date may be necessary to definitively diagnose the hyperthyroid state (Graves and Peterson, 1990) (see this volume, p. 334).

Treatment options for feline hyperthyroidism include surgical thyroidectomy, radioactive iodine (^{131}I), or chronic administration of an antithyroid drug (usually methimazole). Antithyroid drug therapy is also extremely useful as a short-term treatment in the preparation of hyperthyroid cats before thyroidectomy. The treatment of choice for an individual cats depends on several factors, including the age of the cat, the presence of associated cardiovascular disease or other major medical problems, the availability of a skilled surgeon or nuclear medicine facilities, and an owner's willingness to accept the form of treatment advised.

Hypokalemia

Hypokalemia is seldom of clinical importance until serum potassium levels decline below 3.5 mEq/L. Hypokalemia occurs as a result of factors that influence the transcellular distribution of potassium or total body potassium. Common causes include (1) overzealous administration of fluids devoid of or low in potassium (this is especially common in the treatment of diabetic ketoacidosis); (2) potassium loss from the gastrointestinal tract during severe vomiting or diarrhea (e.g., parvovirus gastroenteritis); (3) urinary loss (e.g., renal tubular acidosis, potassium-losing nephropathy in cats, polyuric renal failure); and (4) alkalosis, both respiratory and metabolic. Hypokalemia may cause a nephropathy that manifests as an inability to concentrate urine (Dow and LeCouteur, 1989). The degree of concentration impairment is a function of the duration and severity of the potassium deficit. Hypokalemia can impair renal tubular cell transport functions and therefore may disturb the accumulation of solute in the renal medulla. Hypokalemia may also affect the release of ADH. The nephropathy of potassium depletion can be readily corrected by restoring normal serum potassium levels, providing irreversible tubular damage has not occurred.

The treatment of established or anticipated potassium deficiency requires evaluation of several factors, including the type of potassium salt to be supplemented, the route of replacement, the quantity and rate of potassium administration, and correction of the primary disease process that caused this electrolyte disturbance.

Potassium should be supplemented orally whenever possible, because this is the safest route of administration. For example, mild hypokalemia may be treated conservatively with foods having high potassium content, such as meats, nuts, bananas, citrus juices, or vegetables, or by commercially available oral potassium preparations (Tumil-K, Daniels Pharmaceutical).

An anorexic or vomiting patient with moderate or severe hypokalemia (<3 mEq/L) usually requires parenterally administered potassium in the form of potassium chloride. Potassium can be administered subcutaneously or slowly intravenously after being diluted in parenteral fluids. The maximum rate of intravenous potassium administration should not exceed 0.5 mEq/kg/hr. However, in cats with severe hypokalemic nephropathy, oral supplementation of potassium has been recommended to avoid dilutional effects of intravenous fluids and further loss of potassium from diuresis (Dow and LeCouteur, 1989). A hypokalemic dog or cat often requires 3 to 5 mEq/kg of potassium per day to correct existing potassium deficits.

Hypercalcemia

Polyuria and polydipsia are early signs associated with hypercalcemia. Several conditions are commonly associated with hypercalcemia in dogs and cats: paraneoplastic syndromes (e.g., lymphosarcoma, multiple myeloma, and apocrine gland adenocarcinoma), hypoadrenocorticism, and primary renal failure. It is also common in young, growing animals (nonpathologic). Primary hyperparathyroidism, a common cause of hypercalcemia in humans, is uncommon in veterinary medicine (see CVT X, p. 985).

Hypercalcemia in mature animals is often an indication of underlying malignant neoplasia (see CVT X, p. 988). The tumor is thought to produce physiologically active substances that stimulate bone resorption or alter calcium excretion by the kidneys. Hypercalcemia impairs renal concentrating ability, thereby causing primary polyuria. Proposed mechanisms for the inability to form urine of high specific gravity include (1) damage to ADH receptors in the collecting tubule, (2) decreased transport of sodium and chloride into the renal medullary interstitium due to inactivation of sodium-potassium adenosine triphosphatase, and (3) late in the disease process, mineralization of renal tubular cells.

Hypercalcemia should be regarded as a medical emergency because of its effects on the kidneys. The decision for aggressive medical therapy is based on the severity of clinical signs, renal function, electrocardiographic (ECG) changes, and neurologic abnormalities. When the product of the serum calcium and phosphate levels is less than 60, there is usually no urgent requirement for lowering the calcium level because the risk for soft-tissue mineralization is low. However, when dehydration, renal dysfunction, cardiac arrhythmias, or severe neurologic disease exists, the need for medical therapy is imperative. A serum calcium level greater than 15 mg/dl in association with stupor or coma and renal insufficiency (hypercalcemic crisis) requires immediate treatment.

Therapy of acute symptomatic hypercalcemia begins with volume expansion, which alone may be adequate in mild to moderate hypercalcemia. Intravenous infusion of 0.9% sodium chloride causes natriuresis and increases calcium excretion in the urine. An adjunct to therapy, once hydration has been established, is a loop diuretic such as furosemide, which serves to potentiate calciuria by inhibiting sodium and calcium transport at the ascending loop of Henle. The dose of furosemide is 2 to 4 mg/kg in dogs and 1 to 2 mg/kg in cats. In addition, glucocorticoids may be given (prednisolone, 1 to 2 mg/kg PO b.i.d.) in suspected cases of lymphoproliferative disease or multiple myeloma. Glucocorticoids have a direct toxic effect on some cancer cells, limit bone resorption, decrease intestinal calcium absorption, and enhance renal excretion of calcium. Additional therapy depends on the severity of clinical signs. In most instances, the addition of mithramycin or calcitonin (both agents decrease bone absorption by inhibiting osteoclasts) to saline-furosemide infusion enhances therapy for emergency situations. Rarely is the immediate reduction of serum calcium levels by infusion of the calcium chelator sodium ethylenediamenetetra-acetic acid required.

Pyelonephritis

Pyelonephritis (infection and inflammation of the renal pelvis) can destroy the countercurrent mechanism in the renal medulla with resultant dilute urine, polyuria, and polydipsia. Early signs of pyelonephritis may include fever, tenderness in the area of the kidneys, and leukocytosis. Typical signs of renal failure may also be exhibited. Urine sediment examination may show white blood cells, red blood cells, bacteria, and occasionally white blood cell casts; however, in some cases the urine sediment may be absolutely normal. Suspicion of pyelonephritis should be raised if a urinary tract infection cannot be cleared after proper antibiotic therapy based on urine culture and sensitivity results obtained by cystocentesis. Patients that have hyperadrenocorticism or diabetes mellitus and that remain persistently polyuric despite appropriate medical management to lower cortisol or glucose levels, respectively, into the normal range are also suspected of having upper urinary tract infection. Pyelonephritis is best diagnosed by contrast dye studies of the kidneys, renal biopsy, and renal ultrasonography in conjunction with urine sediment examination and urine culture and sensitivity test results. Long-term antibiotic therapy, up to 6 weeks or longer in most cases, is the treatment of choice.

Pyometra

Pyometra is commonly associated with marked impairment of renal concentration ability. A proposed mechanism for the polyuria suggests renal tubular insensitivity to the action of ADH as a result of tubular damage caused by *Escherichia coli* endotoxins. Tubular immune complex injury may also have a role. Successful treatment of pyometra involves surgery or the administration of prostaglandin ($PGF_2\alpha$). Generally, normal urine concentration ability returns within days to weeks after successful elimination of the pyometra, providing irreversible renal tubular damage has not occurred (see *CVT X*, p. 1034).

Chronic Liver Disease

Chronic liver disease is frequently associated with polyuria and polydipsia. Inadequate metabolism of adrenal corticosteroids may result in a relative state of cortisol excess with resultant polyuria and polydipsia. Liver disease may also impair metabolism of aldosterone and ammonia. Sodium retention secondary to hyperaldosteronism may result in polydipsia. Decreased urea formation from ammonia may lead to decreased renal medullary hypertonicity and subsequent hyposthenuria. Finally, the hypokalemia that often accompanies chronic liver disease can further impair renal concentrating ability.

The cause of the liver disease determines treatment. Common reversible hepatopathies include "hyperthyroid hepatopathy" and hepatic lipidosis in cats, vacuolar hepatopathy from hyperadrenocorticism in dogs, and portal vein anomalies in both dogs and cats. Liver disease of inflammatory and neoplastic origin is generally irreversible.

Diabetes Mellitus

Diabetes mellitus is a common cause of polyuria and polydipsia in both dogs and cats. The high concentration of glucose in the renal tubular fluid exceeds the glucose transport ability of the tubules and creates an osmotic diuresis and secondary polydipsia.

The cause of diabetes in most dogs and cats is not known. However, it is well documented that diabetes can develop in association with other conditions, including pancreatitis, Cushing's syndrome, estrus, acromegaly, and prolonged administration of glucocorticoids or progesterone-like drugs.

The diagnosis of overt diabetes mellitus is based on the finding of persistent fasting hyperglycemia (usually >200 mg/dl). The diagnosis of diabetes should never be established solely on the basis of single or even multiple urine glucose determinations, because certain proximal tubular disorders can cause renal glycosuria. Most diabetic dogs and cats have both marked hyperglycemia and glycosuria.

Proper treatment is based on the severity of the disorder and recognition of any underlying condition that may predispose to the diabetic state. Regular (crystalline zinc) or Semilente insulin is used in conjunction with fluid and electrolyte replacement therapy to treat ketoacidotic and nonketotic hyperosmolar syndromes (see this volume, p. 359). These short-acting insulins have a relatively rapid onset of action and a relatively short duration of action (5 to 8 hr) (see this volume, p. 356). They can be administered intravenously, intramuscularly, or subcutaneously. Neutral Protamine Hagedorn (NPH) and Lente insulins are intermediate-acting formulations that are commonly used in the long-term management of uncomplicated diabetes in dogs and cats. These insulin types should be given subcutaneously, once or preferably twice daily. Protamine zinc insulin (PZI) and Ultralente insulins are long-acting formulations that are administered by the subcutaneous route once or twice daily. These insulin preparations appear to be most useful in treatment of those animals that owners cannot give two insulin injections per day. They are the insulin preparations of choice in cats. Generally, the dose of insulin in dogs should start at 0.25 U/kg per administration, whereas the dose of insulin in cats should start at 0.5 to 1 U per cat per administration (see this volume, p. 364).

Oral hypoglycemic agents, although commonly used for treatment of non–insulin-dependent (type II) diabetes mellitus in humans, have not been widely evaluated in diabetic dogs and cats. Preliminary results indicate that they may be effective in some obese, nonketotic diabetic cats (Wallace and Kirk, 1990). Two sulfonylureas have been used for the treatment of canine and feline diabetes mellitus. Glipizide (Glucotrol) has been given at a dosage of 0.25 to 0.5 mg/kg b.i.d., whereas glibenclamide (DiaBeta, Micronase) is administered at a dosage of 0.2 mg/kg/day. These drugs have several antidiabetic actions, including the acute stimulation of insulin secretion by B cells, chronic enhancement of muscle and adipose tissue carbohydrate transport, a direct effect on the liver to decrease hepatic glucose output, and the potentiation of insulin action on the liver. The signs of uncomplicated diabetes mellitus (i.e., polyuria and polydipsia, polyphagia, and weight loss) should resolve with proper insulin therapy. In addition, urine glucose testing should be negative for glycosuria during most of the day. A diabetic dog or cat may occasionally have persistent morning glycosuria (1 to 2%) or continued polyuria, polydipsia, or polyphagia despite insulin therapy. These signs indicate a potential problem with the insulin therapy, and an investigation should be undertaken to determine its cause.

An effort to eliminate the simple or obvious causes of poor diabetic control should be made before expensive, sophisticated, or time-consuming studies are performed (see CVT X, p. 1012). A thorough review of the owner's injection method is extremely important. Lack of satisfactory response to therapy may involve improper insulin administration by the owner, inadequate mixing of insulin before withdrawal into the syringe, use of outdated insulin, inactivated insulin from improper storage, or outdated urine glucose strips. Once these obvious potential problems are ruled out in a problematic case of diabetes, the following measures are recommended. Ensure that all female dogs are spayed (not important in diabetic regulation of cats). If the patient is currently on a single dose of intermediate-

acting insulin, the dose should be divided into two daily injections. Finally, blood glucose determinations at 1- to 2-hr intervals for 10 to 24 hr usually are of great help in defining the problem. Common disturbances that may be identified using serial blood glucose determinations include insulin-induced hyperglycemia (Somogyi's overswing), rapid metabolism of insulin, and insulin resistance secondary to acromegaly, Cushing's syndrome, or the administration of glucocorticoids or progestogens.

Primary Renal Glycosuria

Two distinct disorders of normoglycemic glycosuria or primary renal glycosuria are recognized in dogs. Primary renal glycosuria has been recognized in Norwegian elkhounds, Scottish terriers, and mixed breeds. The primary tubular defect, thought to be hereditary in Norwegian elkhounds, prevents normal reabsorption of filtered glucose. The high concentration of glucose in the tubular fluid creates an osmotic diuresis and a secondary polydipsia. A second syndrome, similar to Fanconi's syndrome in humans, has been described in Basenjis, Norwegian elkhounds, Shetland sheepdogs, and schnauzers (see CVT X, p. 1163). The onset of signs occurs between 1 and 6 years of age, with glycosuria and moderate weight loss being noted in addition to polyuria and polydipsia. This syndrome is associated with defects in tubular reabsorption of water, phosphate, sodium, potassium, bicarbonate, uric acid, and amino acids, as well as glucose. The serum chemistry profiles are initially normal in most cases; however, many affected dogs develop chronic renal insufficiency or die of acute renal failure within 90 days of diagnosis. The diagnosis of primary renal glycosuria is made by the presence of clinical signs, glycosuria without hyperglycemia, and aminoaciduria if present (made by paper chromatography). Treatment is directed at slowing the progression of any underlying renal disease. Careful screening for urinary tract infection and hypertension and periodic monitoring for progressive azotemia are recommended, especially in patients with the disorder resembling Fanconi's syndrome. Depending on the case, the therapeutic use of low-protein diets, antihypertensive agents, antibiotics, and intestinal phosphate binders may be indicated.

Chronic Renal Failure

Chronic renal failure, regardless of etiology, is usually characterized by polyuria with the loss of fluid and electrolytes. As more nephrons become nonfunctional there is a compensatory increase in glomerular filtration rate per surviving nephron, with a resultant increase in the amount of fluid presented to the distal tubules. Increased tubular flow rate causes less urea, sodium, and other substances to be reabsorbed. The result is an osmotic diuresis that is further complicated by a reduced renal medullary concentration gradient.

The workup of patients with chronic renal failure should include a careful search for curable causes (e.g., hypokalemia, hypercalcemia, urinary tract obstruction, pyelonephritis, renoliths) and remediable aggravators (e.g., congestive heart failure, hypertension, urinary tract infection or partial obstruction) of azotemia. In general, chronic renal failure and the associated polyuria and polydipsia are irreversible. Therapy is typically directed toward slowing the progression of the renal disease and alleviating uremic symptoms (see *CVT X*, pp. 1166, 1195, and 1198). An approach to retard the progression of chronic renal failure would include (1) identification and control of hypertension with a low-salt diet, diuretics, or vasodilators, (2) treatment of urinary tract infection, (3) limiting dietary protein, and (4) control of hyperphosphatemia with a low-protein diet or intestinal phosphate binders. Therapy to alleviate uremic symptoms would include dietary protein restriction, histamine H_2 blockers for uremic gastritis, anabolic steroids for muscle wasting and anemia, human recombinant erythropoietin for anemia, calcitriol to maintain serum calcium, and subcutaneous fluid therapy.

Postobstructive Diuresis

Postobstructive diuresis occurs after the relief of urinary tract obstruction. This syndrome is most commonly encountered after relieving a urethral obstruction in male cats with feline urologic syndrome. The elevated BUN level resulting from reduced glomerular filtration rate (postrenal azotemia) creates an osmotic diuresis. In addition, prolonged urinary tract obstruction may create a tubular defect (usually transient), which further impairs sodium and water reabsorption. Postobstructive diuresis is usually self-limiting; however, aggressive fluid therapy is occasionally necessary to match the increased urine output. For example, in some cases, the urine output can be as high as 10 to 20 ml/kg/hr post obstruction. After a few days, the volume of fluid therapy should be slowly reduced because it may perpetuate the polyuria.

Renal Medullary Washout

Many human medical nephrologists believe that renal medullary solute washout can occur to some degree with any polyuric disorder. Water and osmotic diuresis increase tubular flow rates and volumes and decrease the amount of sodium and urea

that the medullary interstitium is able to reabsorb. Decreased medullary hypertonicity causes urine concentration to decrease even in the presence of excessive ADH. Osmotic diuresis also causes an increase in medullary blood flow, reducing the hypertonicity of the medullary interstitium even further. Ordinarily, very sluggish blood flow through the vasa recta (the blood supply to the renal medulla) allows the formation of a hypertonic medullary interstitium.

Medullary washout could be caused by any of the polyuric endocrine or metabolic disorders already mentioned or could attend the prolonged use of diuretics. It has also been associated with abnormalities in circulation such as hyperviscosity syndromes, renal lymphatic obstruction, systemic vasculitis, and hypertension.

Renal medullary washout may cause diagnostic confusion during a workup for polyuria and polydipsia. When medullary washout has occurred secondary to compulsive water drinking or central DI, the patient will be unable to respond to a water deprivation test or to ADH administration. If medullary washout is suspected, the treatment is to limit water intake gradually without producing dehydration and to supplement the diet with sodium chloride for several days.

Primary Polydipsia
(Compulsive Water Drinking)

Primary polydipsia is usually encountered in young, hyperactive dogs that are underexercised or exposed to some type of stress. With complete water deprivation, these animals can usually concentrate their urine greater than 1.025 unless severe medullary washout exists. Treatment may include tranquilization, behavioral modification, or severe water restriction but in many cases is not very successful.

References and Suggested Reading

Dow, S. W., and LeCouteur, R. A.: Hypokalemic polymyopathy of cats. *In* Kirk, R. W. (ed.): *Current Veterinary Therapy X.* Philadelphia: W. B. Saunders, 1989, p. 812.
Complete discussion of hypokalemic nephropathy in cats including etiology, diagnosis, and treatment.
Feldman, E. C., and Nelson, R. W.: Hyperadrenocorticism. *In* Feldman, E. C., and Nelson, R. W. (eds.): *Canine and Feline Endocrinology and Reproduction.* Philadelphia: W. B. Saunders, 1987, pp. 137–194.
A current and thorough review of clinical endocrinology in dogs and cats.
Graves, T., and Peterson, M. E.: Diagnosis of occult hyperthyroidism in cats. *In* Nichols, R. (ed): *Problems in Veterinary Medicine: Endocrinology.* Vol. 2. Philadelphia: J. B. Lippincott, 1990, p. 683.
The use of the T_3 suppression test and the TSH stimulation test are discussed in relation to the diagnosis of early and "occult" hyperthyroidism.
Kosman, M. E.: Evaluation of a new antidiuretic agent desmopressin acetate DDAVP. J.A.M.A. 240: 1896, 1978.
General discussion of DDAVP.

Robertson, G. L.: Differential diagnosis of polyuria and polydipsia. Annu. Rev. Med. 39:425, 1988.
An excellent review of primary polyuria and polydipsia in humans.
Schwartz-Porsche, D.: Diabetes insipidus. *In* Kirk, R. W. (ed.): *Current Veterinary Therapy VII.* Philadelphia: W. B. Saunders, 1980, p. 1005.
A good review of diabetes insipidus in dogs.

Wallace, M. S., and Kirk, C. A.: The diagnosis and treatment of insulin-dependent and non-insulin dependent diabetes mellitus in the dog and cat. *In* Nichols, R. (ed): *Problems in Veterinary Medicine: Endocrinology.* Vol. 2. Philadelphia: J. B. Lippincott, 1990, p. 573.
Problems associated with the treatment of diabetes mellitus are addressed.

ENDOCRINE AND METABOLIC CAUSES OF WEAKNESS

MICHAEL SCHAER

Gainesville, Florida

Weakness refers to a specific loss of strength in voluntary muscle movement, usually typified as an inability to complete a specific and familiar act. Weakness as a clinical disorder can be subdivided into lassitude, fatigue, and generalized muscle weakness (asthenia) with variable degrees of consciousness ranging from alert to marked mental depression, depending on the particular etiology.

Weakness can be clinically classified into two main subtypes, continuous or episodic. The continuous form is a persistent loss of muscle strength that may or may not progress over a period of time, whereas episodic weakness typically has periods of normalcy or near normalcy alternating with overt signs of asthenia. Although several causes of weakness characterize a specific type, in some types such as hypoglycemia and hypocalcemia, episodic signs eventually become continuous. Although weakness has various causes, this chapter dwells on the metabolic and endocrine etiologies. Table 1 lists the main clinical features and treatments pertaining to the several electrolyte disorders that are mentioned in this and the following sections.

Any major metabolic dysfunction that leads to obvious illness can make an animal weak. This is typically shown with advanced liver and renal failure, in which weakness is one of many other clinical signs. Of the various metabolic causes, serum electrolyte abnormalities occur commonly and are frequent concomitant disorders with major organ dysfunction. For this reason, the section describing metabolic causes of weakness addresses several serum electrolyte disorders involving deficiencies and excesses in potassium, calcium, magnesium, and sodium ions. In general, most serum electrolyte imbalances do not cause noticeable asthenia until severe excess or depletion states occur. At that particular time, the weakness is usually of the continuous type.

METABOLIC CAUSES OF WEAKNESS

Hypokalemia and Hyperkalemia

Hypokalemia in dogs and cats is seldom of clinical importance until the serum level declines below 3 mEq/L (normal 3.5 to 5.5 mEq/L). Pathophysiologically, hypokalemia increases the cellular resting membrane potential, resulting in a larger difference between the resting and threshold potential necessary for an action potential and muscle contraction. This is clinically characterized as difficulty in stimulating muscles to contract, thus producing the clinical signs of muscle weakness and impaired cardiac conduction.

Hyperkalemia increases the resting membrane potential almost to threshold, thus producing a weaker action potential when threshold is reached, the result being muscle weakness and disturbed cardiac excitation and conduction. Hyperkalemia is seldom of clinical importance until the serum level exceeds 7 mEq/L; beyond this amount, severe life-threatening cardiac conduction abnormalities begin to develop.

In general, severe hypokalemia (serum potassium < 2.5 mEq/L) and marked hyperkalemia (serum potassium > 7 mEq/L) cause continuous weakness, except in the rare clinical disorders of familial periodic hypokalemia and hyperkalemia.

Hypocalcemia and Hypercalcemia

Tetany is the cardinal manifestation of hypocalcemia; it expresses the excessive irritability of the

Table 1. The Clinical Features of Serum Electrolyte Disorders in Dogs and Cats

Disorder	Primary Causes	History and Physical Signs	Electrocardiographic Changes	Other Distinguishing Diagnostic Features	Treatment
Hypokalemia	Redistribution Metabolic alkalosis Insulin administration Potassium depletion Renal Gastrointestinal	Signs of the primary disorders Mainly muscle weakness when serum K^+ < 2.5 mEq/L Hypovolemia is frequently present Common with use of kaliuretic drugs (furosemide)	Depressed ST segment Flattened T wave Extreme changes include AV blocks; ectopic, reentrant, and atrial and ventricular arrhythmias Note: The ECG changes do not always reflect the degree of hypokalemia.	Metabolic alkalosis commonly occurs with pyloric outflow obstruction. Commonly occurs when treatment for diabetic ketoacidosis is inadequately supplemented with potassium.	Correct the primary underlying cause and reverse any alkalosis. Correct dehydration with 0.9% NaCl. Do not use alkalinizing solutions. Correct moderate to severe hypokalemia (serum K < 3 mEq/L) with a slow intravenous infusion of potassium chloride: 3–10 mEq/kg body weight over a 24-hr period. Oral potassium-containing elixirs can be used in the absence of vomiting at a dosage of 1–1.5 mEq/kg/day, divided.
Hyperkalemia	Redistribution Metabolic acidosis Hyperkalemic periodic paralysis Potassium loading Endogenous Exogenous Reduced excretion Acute renal failure Hypoadrenocorticism Potassium-sparing diuretics	Signs of the primary disorder Mainly muscle weakness at serum levels > 7 mEq/L Irregular cardiac rhythm	Tall or deeply deflected T waves Lengthened P-R interval with short P-wave amplitude Widened QRS complex Bradycardia Atrial standstill Sine waves Cardiac arrest	Metabolic acidosis common Azotemia common with renal impairment Hyponatremia frequent with adrenocortical insufficiency	Correct underlying cause and reverse. Give isotonic 0.9% NaCl IV. Monitor urine output. Life-threatening myocardial toxic signs warrant any combination of the following therapies: Calcium gluconate 10%—1 ml/kg IV over 5–10 min. Sodium bicarbonate—1–2 mEq/kg IV Insulin-glucose—¼–½ U of regular crystalline insulin per kg body weight along with 2 gm dextrose/each unit of insulin added to the 0.9% NaCl infusion.
Hypocalcemia	Primary hypoparathyroidism Surgical removal of parathyroid glands Acute hyperphosphatemia Paraparturient eclampsia	Tetany Seizures Mental depression Weakness	Prolonged Q-T interval ECG not always reliable for detection	Hyperphosphatemia and low plasma PTH levels in primary ↓ PTH Eclampsia occurs proximal to parturition History usually of strong diagnostic assistance	Acute: 10% calcium gluconate at starting dose of 1–1.5 ml/kg IV administered over 5–10 min. Additional amounts can be given pending response. Maintenance (in-hospital): 10% calcium gluconate at 5 ml/kg distributed over 24 hr by vein. This amount can also be given in 2 divided SC injections, each diluted in 100 ml 0.9% NaCl. Home maintenance: see CVT IX, p. 93.

Disorder	Causes	Clinical Signs	ECG	Comments	Treatment
Hypercalcemia	Malignant tumors Primary hyperparathyroidism Hypervitaminosis D	Presence of primary extraparathyroid tumor Anorexia, vomiting Constipation Weakness Mental depression Polydipsia/polyuria	Shortened Q-T interval ECG not always reliable for detection	Renal failure Nephrocalcinosis Hypophosphatemia with primary ↑ PTH or hypercalcemia of malignancy Elevated serum PTH levels with primary hyperparathyroidism	Intravenous 0.9% NaCl with brisk diuresis. Can promote diuresis with furosemide. Prednisone: 1 mg/kg/day divided when not due to primary hyperparathyroidism. Calcitonin: 4 U/kg IV initially, followed by 4–8 U/kg SC once or twice daily.
Hypomagnesemia	Obligatory renal losses during dietary restriction Intestinal malabsorption Prolonged parenteral nutrition without Mg^{2+} supplementation	Apathy, depression, ataxia, neuromuscular irritability Anorexia, nausea	Wide T waves and QRS complexes Prolonged P-R and Q-T intervals Severe arrhythmias occur with digitalis toxicity	Frequently coexists with hypokalemia Hypocalcemia commonly coexists with chronic hypomagnesemia Uncommonly recognized in small animal practice	Treat cause. Manage specific disorder. Mild hypomagnesemia (1.1–1.4 mEq/L): use oxide or hydroxide salts orally at approximate dosage of 1–2 mEq/kg/day. Severe (< 1.1 mEq/L): use 50% magnesium sulfate solution at 0.2 mg/kg IV dose q 4–8 hr.
Hypermagnesemia	An uncommon clinical problem Usually iatrogenic when Mg^{2+} salts used to treat renal failure patients	Lethargy Severe muscle weakness Depressed deep-tendon reflexes Hypotension	Sinus bradycardia Increased P-R and Q-T intervals Heart block	History often denotes treatment with Mg $(OH)_2$-containing antacids	Avoid Mg^{2+}-containing antacids in patients in renal failure. Calcium gluconate 10%: acute—1–1.5 ml/kg IV. Maintain with 5 ml/kg IV over 24 hr. Insulin-dextrose: see the earlier entry "Hyperkalemia."
Hyponatremia (true)	Gastrointestinal loss Hypoadrenocorticism Diuretic induced Hypotonic fluid administration Inappropriate ADH secretion	Clinical signs more common in acute disorder Lethargy, nausea, weakness Seizures (usually with rapid-onset hyponatremia) Coma	None	Signs characteristic of underlying disorder; i.e., Addison's disease	Hypertonic (3%) saline infusion seldom necessary. True hyponatremia best corrected with 0.9% saline. Inappropriate ADH syndrome best treated with water restriction. Specific treatment for primary disorder.
Hypernatremia	Pure water loss Hypotonic losses from vomiting and diarrhea Water deprivation Excess salt gain with water loss	Depression, lethargy Weakness Muscle rigidity Tremors Seizures Coma	None	Might commonly occur in patient with diabetes insipidus that is water deprived	Correct hypovolemia with 0.9% saline IV. Correct serum Na^+ level slowly over a 48-hr period. After restoration of euvolemia, can use 0.45% saline and D_5W solution by slow IV infusions. Correct underlying disorder.

ADH, antidiuretic hormone; AV, atrioventricular; ECG, electrocardiogram; K, potassium; Mg^{2+}, magnesium; Mg^{2+} $(OH)_2$, magnesium hydroxide; NaCl, sodium chloride; PTH, parathyroid hormone; ↑ PTH, hyperparathyroidism; ↓ PTH, hypoparathyroidism.

motor nervous system. Hypocalcemia (< 9 mg/dl; normal 9 to 12 mg/dl or 2.25 to 3.0 mmol/L) increases the membrane threshold potentials, thereby reducing the difference between the resting and threshold potentials and making the membrane more excitable. Severe hypocalcemia (serum calcium < 5 mg/dl or 1.25 mmol/L) produces life-threatening tetany or seizures if it progresses without prompt diagnosis and treatment.

Complications associated with high serum calcium levels (hypercalcemia) occur at amounts in excess of 15 mg/dl (> 3.75 mmol/L). The consequences are several and involve many organ systems, including the central nervous system (CNS), heart, and kidneys. The main adverse clinical effects of hypercalcemia include marked mental depression; weakness; cardiac tachyarrhythmias; anorexia, nausea, vomiting, and abdominal pain; renal calculi, nephrocalcinosis, and renal failure. The pathophysiology of hypercalcemia rests on the deleterious effect of increased serum concentrations of ionized calcium on the integrity of cellular function, causing alterations in cell membrane permeability and cell membrane calcium pump activity. The weakness is brought about by hypercalcemia-induced decreased cell membrane permeability of neuromuscular tissues, thereby depressing the excitability of these tissues by lowering the threshold potential. A primary neuropathy as found in primary hyperparathyroidism is probably a major contributing cause of the muscle weakness (Turken et al., 1989).

Hypomagnesemia and Hypermagnesemia

Magnesium is predominantly an intracellular cation, and normal blood levels are between 1.4 and 2.0 mEq/L. Hypomagnesemia (serum level < 1.4 mEq/L) is frequently accompanied by low serum calcium levels because of the ability of chronic hypomagnesemia to inhibit the release of parathyroid hormone from the parathyroid glands (Kassirer et al., 1989). Although moderate to severe magnesium deficiency is rare, its assessment should be considered in disease states characterized by gastrointestinal malabsorption and renal disorders with high urine output.

Hypermagnesemia decreases impulse transmission across neuromuscular junctions. This curare-like effect results from presynaptic inhibition of acetylcholine release, decreased postsynaptic membrane responsiveness, and an increase in the threshold for axonal excitation (Kassirer et al., 1989).

Hyponatremia and Hypernatremia

The pathophysiologic effects of hyponatremia and hypernatremia are closely associated with their effects on plasma tonicity. Hyponatremia is frequently caused by water excess and causes plasma hypo-osmolality, and hypernatremia is commonly caused by water depletion, resulting in hyperosmolar states. The weakness associated with these conditions is primarily due to the adverse osmolar effects on the brain.

Hyponatremia (serum sodium < 137 mEq/L; normal 140 to 155 mEq/L) can be spurious or real depending on the etiology. Several different types based on effects on plasma volume and osmolality are described. *Euosmolar* hyponatremia, as occurs in hyperlipidemia, and *hyperosmolar* hyponatremia, as found in marked hyperglycemia, are spurious clinical laboratory phenomena that do not represent true sodium loss from the body. *Hypervolemic, hypo-osmolar* hyponatremia can be dilutional and is associated with severe heart failure, cirrhosis, and nephrotic syndrome, although it does not represent a true sodium depletion state. *Hypovolemic, hypo-osmolar* (gastrointestinal losses, adrenal insufficiency, and diuretic therapy) hyponatremia, on the other hand, clearly results in a true sodium loss from the body. *Euvolemic, hypo-osmolar* hyponatremia as caused by the syndrome of inappropriate antidiuretic hormone (ADH) and myxedema is actually a water excess state. Severe hyponatremia (serum sodium < 120 mEq/L) exerts its main effects on the CNS, where it causes cellular overhydration, brain edema, and an increase in intracranial pressure.

Hypernatremia (serum sodium > 155 to 160 mEq/L) invariably signifies the presence of a hyperosmolar state. The overwhelming majority of patients with hypernatremia are frankly hypovolemic, and hypernatremia is a consequence of a deficit of water disproportional to any deficit of sodium (e.g., hypodipsia). The major clinical manifestations of hypernatremia involve the CNS and vary depending on the rapidity with which hyperosmolality develops. Acute-onset hypernatremia (serum sodium > 170 mEq/L) is most detrimental and is characterized by an osmotic shift of water out of the intracellular department, causing a marked increase in the permeability (or rupture) of capillaries in the brain and subarachnoid space.

ENDOCRINE CAUSES OF WEAKNESS

The main clinical features and therapeutic principles of the several endocrine disorders discussed next are listed in Table 2.

Diabetes Mellitus

Weakness in a diabetic animal is characteristically continuous and progressive. It usually does not occur until the decompensating stages of ketoacidosis or diabetic neuropathy ensue. The former is due to the catabolic effects of insulin deficiency, causing proteolysis, hypokalemia, hypophosphatemia, and hypovolemia.

Diabetic neuropathy consists of several structural, functional, and metabolic abnormalities (Bays and Pfeifer, 1988). Some of these include abnormal myelin production, nerve conduction defects, myoinisitol deficiency, sorbitol polyol pathway stimulation, reduction in nerve sodium-potassium–adenosine triphosphatase, increased peripheral nerve glycosylation, and nerve hypoxia. In dogs, the primary signs include muscle weakness, decreased conscious proprioception, and depressed limb reflexes. In cats, the typical sign is rear limb plantar posturing in addition to rear limb weakness. Signs predictably diminish over several weeks after improved blood glucose control.

Hyperadrenocorticism

The weakness associated with Cushing's disease and syndrome is mainly due to the adverse effects of glucocorticoid hormone excess. Muscle wasting occurs as a result of increased catabolic rate and inhibition of myofibrillar proteins. Type II muscle fibers are more sensitivie to the glucocorticoid effects than type I fibers (Shelton and Cardinet, 1987). Impaired insulin action can also contribute to the muscle atrophy.

In dogs with Cushing's disease, a rare form of pseudomyotonia characterized by persistent muscle contraction after a voluntary effort can develop. Pelvic limb stiffness and proximal appendicular muscle enlargement are typical.

Weakness in Cushing's disease might also be associated with a large pituitary macroadenoma causing pressure on the brain's motor tracts. Other signs include dementia, circling, and hyperventilation.

The muscle weakness associated with hyperadrenocorticism is often reversible if treatment is provided early in the course of the disease. Protracted and chronic weakness in the more advanced cases and weakness associated with large macroadenomas offer a very guarded prognosis.

Hypoadrenocorticism

Canine and feline Addison's disease is commonly accompanied by muscle weakness resulting primarily from the combined effects of glucocorticoid deficiency and hyperkalemia (see the earlier section "Hyperkalemia"). Hypoglycemia can also contribute to the weakness, but this biochemical abnormality is found in less than 20% of addisonian dogs and cats.

Hypotension also strongly contributes to a patient's overall constitutional malaise. Fortunately, treatment for Addison's disease offers a patient an excellent prognosis.

Hypothyroidism

Neuromuscular dysfunction in hypothyroid dogs is characterized by weakness, stiffness, decreased conscious proprioception, and muscle wasting (Bichsel et al., 1988; Feldman and Nelson, 1987). Physiologic complications of hypothyroidism include impaired energy metabolism and reduced protein turnover, leading to restricted repair and replacement of muscle proteins (Shelton and Cardinet, 1987). Myopathic changes include type II muscle fiber atrophy, hypertrophy of type I fibers, and the absence of degenerative or inflammatory changes.

Peripheral nerve dysfunction results from mucinous deposits in and around nerve fibers. Clinically affected patients show hyporeflexia and dysfunction of cranial nerves VII and VIII. Treatment brings about remarkable clinical improvement (see this volume, p. 330).

Hyperthyroidism

Muscle weakness can occur in cats with advanced thyrotoxicosis and may be related to an impaired ability of thyrotoxic muscle to phosphorylate creatine (Ingbar, 1985). Metabolic changes include decreased synthesis and especially degradation of protein. This situation is well illustrated by the emaciation that commonly occurs in chronically affected cats.

The weakness of hyperthyroidism can also be associated with cardiac malfunction, in which impaired output can result from myocardial dysfunction or various conduction and rhythm disturbances. The cardiac disease and generalized weakness can normalize after euthyroidism is re-established.

Hypoparathyroidism

The signs associated with primary hypoparathyroidism result from abnormally low serum calcium levels. The weakness caused by hypocalcemia has already been discussed (see the earlier section "Hypocalcemia").

Hyperparathyroidism

The syndrome of neuromuscular disease in primary hyperparathyroidism consists of rapid tiring,

Table 2. *The Common Clinical Characteristics of Endocrine Causes of Weakness in Dogs and Cats*

Disorder	Primary Causes	History and Physical Signs	Characteristic Diagnostic Findings	General Treatment Measures
Diabetes mellitus	Hypoinsulinemia Peripheral insulin antagonism	Polydipsia Polyuria Polyphagia (rare) Weight loss, lethargy, vomiting, inappetence, weakness, and dehydration with ketoacidosis	Sustained hyperglycemia Glycosuria With ketoacidosis: ketonemia, ketonuria, normo- or hypokalemia, normo- or hyponatremia, normo- or hypophosphatemia, hypobicarbonatemia, azotemia, elevated liver enzymes	Provide NPH, protamine zinc (or ultralente) insulin in clinically compensated patients. In sick ketoacidotic patients: Rehydrate and provide maintenance fluids with lactated Ringers' or 0.9% saline solutions. Correct serum electrolyte deficiencies, especially hypokalemia (KCl 3–10 mEq/kg/24 hr.) Begin regular crystalline insulin at ½ U/kg SC and titrate subsequent doses as needed q 6–8 hr. Avoid using $NaHCO_3$ until blood pH < 7.0–7.1.
Hyperadrenocorticism	Pituitary dependent (85% of endogenous cases) Adrenal tumor Iatrogenic	Polydipsia Polyuria Polyphagia Muscle wasting Dermatologic changes: alopecia, hyperpigmentation, calcinosis cutis Muscle weakness (moderate to late stage)	Eosinopenia Lymphopenia Elevated liver enzymes Endogenous Cushing's: ACTH-induced hyperresponsive cortisol secretion Resistant cortisol suppression to low-dose dexamethasone Exogenous: hyporesponsive cortisol secretion to ACTH stimulation	Endogenous O,p'DDD (dog): (1) load at 50 mg/kg/day with prednisone 0.3 mg/kg/day for first 7–10 days. (2) maintain at 25 mg/kg every 3 days. Bilateral adrenalectomy for cats Unilateral adrenalectomy for adrenal tumor in both dogs and cats Exogenous: Discontinue glucocorticoid treatment
Hypoadrenocorticism	Primary idiopathic most common O,p'-DDD induced cortical ablation Exogenous glucocorticoid use	Inappetence Lethargy Weight loss Mental depression Bradycardia and weak pulses with hyperkalemic crisis Muscle weakness	With primary Addison's: Hyponatremia Hypochloremia Hyperkalemia (see previous section) Azotemia Hyporesponsive cortisol secretion to ACTH stimulation ECG abnormalities (see the earlier entry "Hyperkalemia")	Rehydrate and maintain hydration with 0.9% saline. Administer prednisone sodium hemisuccinate or dexamethasone at *initial* dose 5–10 mg/kg and 2–5 mg/kg, respectively. Give fludrocortisone acetate (Florinef, Squibb) orally at 0.1 mg/10 kg/day. Chronic maintenance: (a) fludrocortisone acetate at 0.1–1.0 mg/day or (b) desoxycorticosterone pivalate 1–2 mg/kg q 25–30 days with prednisone 0.3 mg/kg/day.
Hypothyroidism	Primary—idiopathic or autoimmune Secondary—(pituitary) rare Tertiary (hypothalamic) rare	Weight gain Mental dullness Lethargy Poor reproductive performance Dermatologic changes: alopecia, hyperpigmentation, dull coat Muscle weakness—in advanced cases	Hypercholesterolemia Low serum T_3 and T_4 Inadequate response to TSH stimulation	Levothyroxine, 0.02 mg/kg b.i.d. Rarely require triiodothyronine supplementation.

Condition	Etiology	Clinical Signs	Laboratory/Diagnostic Findings	Treatment
Hyperthyroidism	In cats: usually adenomatous hyperplasia Rarely due to thyroid adenocarcinoma in dogs and cats	Weight loss Increased appetite ± Loose stools ± Shortness of breath Occasionally polydipsia and polyuria Unkempt coat occasionally Palpable thyroid gland enlargement(s) Elevated heart rate Weakness in advanced cases	Increased serum T_3 and T_4 levels Elevated SGPT (ALT) and serum alkaline phosphatase Increase uptake with radionuclide scan Sometimes cardiomegaly on radiographs	Methimazole: initial, 5 mg b.i.d.–t.i.d. until euthyroid. Propranolol (for tachycardia): 2.5–5 mg b.i.d.–t.i.d. Radioiodine ^{131}I treatment. Surgical removal of affected thyroid glands.
Hypoparathyroidism	Idiopathic or immune destruction In cats: removal or ischemic dysfunction associated with thyroidectomy procedure	See the earlier entry "Hypocalcemia."	Hypocalcemia ± Hyperphosphatemia	See the earlier entry "Hypocalcemia"
Primary hyperparathyroidism	Parathyroid adenoma most common Parathyroid adenocarcinoma rare	See the earlier entry "Hypercalcemia."	Hypercalcemia Hypophosphatemia initially Azotemia and hyperphosphatemia with secondary renal failure Elevated serum parathormone levels Isosthenuria	See the earlier entry "Hypercalcemia" See CVT IX, p. 93.
Hypoglycemia	Iatrogenic insulin overdose Functional pancreatic B-cell tumor Sepsis Extrapancreatic cancer Decreased glycogen reserves (puppies and kittens)	Signs are intermittent or continuous depending on cause (see text) Weakness Depressed consciousness Behavioral changes Seizures	Hypoglycemia Relative hyperinsulinemia with pancreatic B-cell tumor Others as related to sepsis or extrapancreatic cancer	Treat cause For insulinoma: administer diazoxide at initial dose of 10 mg/kg/day, divided. prednisone: ¼–½ mg/kg/day, divided. feed frequent small meals surgical tumor removal For hypoglycemic emergency, give dextrose 50%: 1 ml/kg IV push.
Pheochromocytoma	Primary adrenal medullary tumor most common. Has been reported in a cat subsequent to writing this chapter. Rarely, other foci of neurectoderm	*Episodic:* Weakness Shortness of breath Anxiety Tachycardia Cutaneous flushing Hypertension	Elevated plasma catecholamine levels Elevated urinary catecholamine and catecholamine metabolite levels Radiographic abnormalities Electrocardiographic tachyarrhythmias	Reduce hypertension with phenoxybenzamine at 0.2–1.5 mg/kg b.i.d. Treat tachyarrhythmias with propranolol at 0.2–2.0 mg/kg t.i.d. It is essential to give phenoxybenzamine before administering propranolol. Surgical tumor removal, if possible.

ACTH, adrenocorticotropic hormone; ALT, alanine aminotransferase; KCl, potassium chloride; $NaHCO_3$, sodium bicarbonate; SGPT, serum glutamic-pyruvic transaminase; TSH, thyroid-stimulating hormone.

symmetric muscle weakness, and muscle atrophy. These myopathic features are associated with neurologic signs such as hyper-reflexia, gait abnormalities, shivering, trembling, and twitching that can progress to stupor, coma, or seizures with extreme hypercalcemia. Electromyograms show characteristic small polyphasic potentials, and atrophy of type II muscle fibers as seen on examination of muscle tissue from affected dogs and humans (Feldman and Nelson, 1987; Turken et al., 1989). The clinical and electromyographic findings are reversible after successful parathyroid surgery.

The main biochemical basis for the neuromuscular findings of primary hyperparathyroidism remains unknown. Although hypercalcemia is thought to have a primary role, there might also be a contribution by parathyroid hormone (see the earlier section "Hypercalcemia").

Hypoglycemia

Unlike the continuous weakness that characterizes the majority of the disorders discussed earlier, weakness associated with hypoglycemia is frequently episodic, although it too can be persistent and progressive depending on the cause. Weakness is primarily due to central nervous system dysfunction caused by the brain's requirement for continuous glucose supply in lieu of its lack of adequate glycogen stores. When inadequate glucose is available for neuronal oxidative phosphorylation, a decline in energy-rich compounds such as adenosine triphosphate (ATP) ensues. These energy-deprived neurons undergo cellular changes typical of hypoxia (pseudolaminar necrosis), resulting in neuronal death.

There are several causes of hypoglycemia in dogs and cats, each with its own characteristic clinical presentation. For example, the progressive form of continuous weakness and mental depression in a food-deprived hypoglycemic puppy contrasts with the usual episodic manifestations of weakness and altered consciousness in an adult dog with a functional pancreatic B-cell adenocarcinoma. (Certain other malignant tumors are capable of causing marked asthenia unassociated with hypoglycemia as a result of paraneoplastic effects; this particular weakness is characteristically continuous and progressive.)

A peripheral polyneuropathy of vague pathogenesis associated with pancreatic B-cell tumors has been described in dogs and humans (Braund et al., 1987). One hypothesis speculates that subsequent to hyperinsulinism, peripheral nerves may develop metabolic defects that render them incapable of utilizing fatty acids and amino acids. Because these nerves would then be dependent on glucose as their sole source of energy, hypoglycemia would have deleterious effects similar to those noted in the central nervous system. The neuropathy might also represent a paraneoplastic effect of the malignant tumor.

Pheochromocytoma

Pheochromocytoma in dogs usually originates from the adrenal medulla. Weakness can be caused by (1) the adverse cardiac effects resulting from hypersecretion of the catecholamine hormones epinephrine and norepinephrine and (2) the hemodynamic impairment associated with tumor invading the posterior vena cava. In the former, the weakness is typically episodic, whereas in the latter, the weakness is continuous and progressive.

The weakness associated with catecholamine excess can be due to the combined effects of cardiac arrhythmias, congestive heart failure, and hypertension. Atrial fibrillation, premature ventricular contractions, and ventricular tachycardias are the most common rhythm disturbances. The cardiac conduction abnormalities can be episodic, coinciding with tumor catecholamine secretion.

The signs associated with pheochromocytoma are reversible if the tumor can be resected before advanced cardiac pathology or tumor invasion into the caudal vena cava has occurred. Unfortunately, this neoplasm often evades clinical suspicion and is diagnosed during postmortem examination.

References and Suggested Reading

Bays, H. E., and Pfeifer, M. A.: Peripheral diabetic neuropathy. Med. Clin. North Am. 72:1439, 1988.
A contemporary description of the pathogenesis, signs, and management of diabetic neuropathy in humans.

Bichsel, P., Jacobs, G., and Oliver, J. E., Jr. Neurologic manifestations associated with hypothyroidism in four dogs. J.A.V.M.A. 192:1745, 1988.
A clinical report describing signs of peripheral and CNS disease associated with canine hypothyroidism.

Braund, K. G., Steiss, J. E., Amling, K. A., et al.: Insulinoma and subclinical peripheral neuropathy in two dogs. J. Vet. Intern. Med. 1:86, 1987.
A detailed clinical and pathologic description and review of pancreatic B-cell tumor-associated peripheral neuropathy.

Feldman, E. C., and Nelson, R. W.: *Canine and Feline Endocrinology and Reproduction.* Philadelphia: W. B. Saunders, 1987.
An informative clinical text describing the various endocrinologic disorders in dogs and cats.

Ingbar, S. H.: The thyroid gland. In Wilson, J. D., and Foster, D. W. (eds): *Williams' Textbook of Endocrinology.* Philadelphia: W. B. Saunders, 1985, p. 746.
A detailed review of thyroid physiology, pathophysiology, and clinical disorders in man.

Kassirer, J. P., Hricik, D. E., and Cohen, J. J: *Repairing Body Fluids—Principles and Practice.* Philadelphia: W. B. Saunders, 1989.
A practical and informative text describing disorders of fluid, electrolyte, and acid-base physiology.

Kruger, J. M., Osborne, C. A., and Polzin, D. J: Treatment of hypercalcemia. In Kirk, R. W. (ed.): *Current Veterinary Therapy IX.* Philadelphia: W. B. Saunders, 1986, p.75.
A current review of the diagnosis and treatment of hypercalcemic disorders in dogs and cats.

Russo, E. A, and Lees, G. E.: Treatment of hypocalcemia. *In* Kirk, R. W. (ed.): *Current Veterinary Therapy IX*. Philadelphia: W. B. Saunders, 1986, p. 91.
  A thorough description of treating hypocalcemia in dogs and cats.
Schaer, M. (ed.): Fluid and electrolyte disorders. Vet. Clin. North Am. Small Anim. Pract. 19:203, 1989.
  A current source of information describing fluid and electrolyte disorders in dogs and cats.
Shelton, D. G., and Cardinet, G. H. III: Pathophysiologic basis of canine muscle disorders. J. Vet. Intern. Med. 1:36, 1987.

A current review of the primary myopathies and metabolic muscle disorders in dogs.
Turken, S. A., Cafferty, M., Silverberg, S. J. et al.: Neuromuscular involvement in mild asymptomatic primary hyperparathyroidism. Am. J. Med. 87:553, 1989.
  A study of the neuromuscular abnormalities associated with primary hyperparathyroidism in humans.

ENDOCRINE HYPERTENSION

LINDA A. ROSS

North Grafton, Massachusetts

Hypertension in dogs and cats has received little attention in the veterinary clinical literature until recently. The incidence of primary, or essential, hypertension is low (less than 1%), but secondary hypertension occurs in association with a number of diseases, many of which are endocrine disorders. The incidence of hypertension in humans with these disorders can be as high as 98% (Kuchel, 1983). The incidence of hypertension in small animals with each of the corresponding endocrine disorders is not known. However, the incidence in those disorders that has been determined has proved similar to that reported in humans (Table 1). Because endocrine disorders are common in small animal practice, it behooves the clinician to be aware of the existence and clinical consequences of and therapy for the hypertension that may be associated with them.

The pathogenesis of secondary hypertension is complex and varies with the primary disease process. The factors resulting in increased blood pressure in association with endocrine disorders are discussed below.

The clinical consequences of hypertension depend on the severity and duration of the increase in blood pressure. Sustained hypertension results in pathologic lesions in small arteries and arterioles that consist of hypertrophy and hyperplasia of the tunica media, loss of the internal elastic lamina, and fibrinoid necrosis. These vascular lesions may lead to pathologic conditions in several organs. Neurologic abnormalities, including seizures and dementia may be associated with intracerebral hemorrhage. The latter occurs following ruptures of the pathologically weakened arterial or arteriolar walls. Ocular lesions, including dilated, tortuous retinal arteries, "cotton-wool" retinal lesions, and retinal hemorrhages, exudates, and detachments, have also been associated with vascular pathology.

Hypertension has been associated with renal disease in several ways. Sustained increases in blood pressure have been associated with glomerular proliferation and glomerulosclerosis. It has also been suggested that systemic hypertension may contribute to glomerular hyperfiltration in the presence of renal insufficiency, and thereby hasten the progression of renal failure.

Hypertension can cause left ventricular hypertrophy and cardiomegaly. Although rarely a cause of heart failure, hypertensive heart disease can contribute to decompensation in dogs and cats with pre-existent heart disease.

Arterial blood pressure can be measured by direct or indirect methods (see this volume, p. 834). A number of studies have shown good correlation between the two methods as long as attention is paid to careful technique (Ross, 1989). Direct blood pressure measurement involves the placement of a needle or catheter into a peripheral artery, usually the femoral. Indirect measurements are made by occluding a peripheral artery with an inflatable cuff and, during deflation of the cuff, determining the pressure at which blood flow returns by palpatory, auscultatory, or oscillometric methods. The upper

Table 1. *Endocrine Disorders Associated With Hypertension*

Hyperadrenocorticism
Hyperthyroidism
Hypothyroidism*
Pheochromocytoma
Acromegaly*
Hyperparathyroidism*
Diabetes mellitus*
Pregnancy*

*Not yet documented in dogs or cats.

limits of normal blood pressure are considered to be 160/90 in dogs and 190/140 in cats (systolic/diastolic).

ENDOCRINE DISORDERS ASSOCIATED WITH HYPERTENSION

Hyperadrenocorticism

Hyperadrenocorticism has been associated with hypertension in up to 84% of affected humans (Hamet, 1983). Several studies have documented a substantial incidence of hypertension in dogs with hyperadrenocorticism. One study found that nine of 11 dogs (82%) with spontaneous hyperadrenocorticism had elevations in both systolic and diastolic blood pressure; one additional dog had an elevated systolic pressure (Scott, 1979). In another report, eight of 14 affected dogs (59%) were hypertensive (Kallet and Cowgill, 1982). The criteria for diagnosis of hyperadrenocorticism were not stated, nor was the number of dogs having pituitary-dependent disease as opposed to adrenal tumors.

In humans there appear to be several mechanisms by which hyperadrenocorticism causes hypertension. Elevated levels of glucocorticoids increase the production of angiotensinogen, which leads to angiotensin-mediated vasoconstriction. They also increase the sensitivity of the cardiovascular system to catecholamines (Hamet, 1983). Volume expansion due to increased renal sodium reabsorption and secondary water retention may contribute to elevations in blood pressure (Feldman and Nelson, 1987; Hamet, 1983).

Hyperthyroidism

Hyperthyroidism is the most common endocrine disorder in cats. In humans with hyperthyroidism the incidence of hypertension is approximately 50%, the elevation usually occurring in the systolic phase (Hamet, 1983). One veterinary study of hyperthyroid cats found that 34 of 39 (87%) had increased systolic and/or diastolic blood pressure (Kobayashi et al., 1990). There are several mechanisms by which elevated circulating levels of thyroxine (T_4) and triiodothyronine (T_3) cause increased arterial pressure. Hyperthyroidism appears to induce an increase in the number of beta-adrenergic receptors in the heart, which enhances the cardiac response to catecholamines. Thyroid hormones have a direct inotropic and chronotropic effect that appears to be mediated by a thyroid hormone–specific adenylate cyclase-adenosine monophosphate (cAMP) system. These effects result in tachycardia, increased stroke volume, and a high cardiac output, which contribute to the increases in blood pressure.

Hypothyroidism

Approximately 50% of people with hypothyroidism have hypertension (Hamet, 1983). The mechanism for the increase in blood pressure is not clear but may be related to the presence of myxedema or atherosclerosis, which results in decreased vascular compliance. The incidence of hypertension in dogs and cats with hypothyroidism has not been reported, although there is one clinical case report of a dog with hypertension and hypothyroidism (Gwin, 1978).

Pheochromocytoma

Pheochromocytomas cause hypertension by the secretion of catecholamines that originate from chromaffin cells of the tumor. The increase in blood pressure may be severe, and signs referable to hypertension may be the presenting clinical complaint. Hypertension occurs in 98% of people with pheochromocytomas, although it is paroxysmal in 50% (Kuchel, 1983). One study of dogs with pheochromocytomas found hypertension in 50% of those animals in which blood pressure was determined (Twedt and Wheeler, 1984). Another report of 39 dogs with pheochromocytomas described a similar incidence (Feldman and Nelson, 1987).

Acromegaly

Acromegaly (elevated circulating levels of growth hormone) in humans is associated with hypertension in 23% to 40% of cases. The mechanism for the increase in blood pressure may be an increase in exchangeable sodium and extracellular fluid (ECF) volume. Acromegaly may cause diabetes mellitus, and the resultant vascular lesions may also play a role in the pathogenesis of hypertension (Hamet, 1983). In dogs, acromegaly most commonly occurs in association with progestogen administration and presents clinically as conformational abnormalities or upper airway stridor. In cats, acromegaly is usually due to pituitary neoplasia and is associated with insulin-resistant diabetes mellitus. The incidence of hypertension in dogs and cats with acromegaly has not been reported, although the apparent high incidence of cardiomyopathy and congestive heart failure in affected cats could be partly related to increased blood pressure (Peterson, et al., 1990).

Hyperparathyroidism

Primary hyperparathyroidism in people is associated with hypertension in 33 to 70% of patients

(Hamet, 1983). The exact mechanism is not known but probably involves the associated hypercalcemia and its effect on smooth muscle contractility. Elevated levels of parathyroid hormone may directly affect plasma renin activity and sodium excretion. The incidence of hypertension in animals with primary hyperparathyroidism has not been reported, although it is interesting to speculate that secondary hyperparathyroidism could be involved in the pathogenesis of hypertension in animals with renal failure.

Diabetes Mellitus

In people, systemic hypertension occurs with both type I and type II diabetes mellitus (Brenner and Anderson, 1990). Estimates of the incidence of hypertension in human diabetics range from 40% to 80% (Sowers and Zemel, 1990), and most of these are due to primary (essential) hypertension. However, the incidence of hypertension is higher in the diabetic population than in nondiabetics, suggesting that secondary hypertension also occurs (Sowers and Zemel, 1990).

The underlying pathophysiologic mechanisms that initiate and sustain increases in blood pressure in diabetics are poorly understood. It is known that the prevalence and severity of hypertension in people with diabetes are related to the duration of disease. It has been suggested that the nephropathy that frequently develops in diabetics may be responsible for this increase (Sowers and Zemel, 1990). Others have suggested that it is the hypertension that contributes to the nephropathy (Brenner and Anderson, 1990).

Although diabetes mellitus is a common disorder in dogs and cats, the incidence of hypertension in this disease has not been reported. Glomerular lesions attributed to diabetic nephropathy have been reported in diabetic dogs (Feldman and Nelson, 1987); it is possible that hypertension in these animals may have contributed to the renal lesions.

Pregnancy

In normal women, mean blood pressure decreases early in pregnancy; after midtrimester, it gradually returns to normal levels near term. Preeclampsia is a condition that occurs after the 20th week of gestation, characterized by hypertension, proteinuria, edema, and occasional coagulation abnormalities. A characteristic and almost pathognomonic renal lesion termed *glomerular endotheliosis* occurs in affected women. The mechanism by which hypertension develops in preeclampsia is not well understood but appears to be multifactorial (Lind-

heimer and Katz, 1983). Hypertension in association with pregnancy in animals has not been documented.

THERAPY

Because endocrine hypertension is secondary to the pathophysiologic changes induced by the primary endocrinopathy, the first and most efficacious therapy is diagnosis and treatment of the endocrine disorder. In humans, correction of the underlying disorder frequently restores normal blood pressure. Information in animals is limited, but existing data suggest a similar situation. Seven cats with hyperthyroidism and hypertension were re-evaluated 2 to 4 months after being rendered euthyroid by surgical thyroidectomy or administration of radioactive iodine. All cats showed a significant decrease in systolic pressure into the normal range after therapy. Diastolic pressure did not decrease significantly, but only three of the cats had pretreatment diastolic pressures that exceeded the normal range (Kobayashi et al., 1990).

If blood pressure does not return to normal after treatment of the underlying endocrine disease, or if the disease cannot be or is not being treated, antihypertensive therapy should be instituted. Because data in animals with spontaneous disease are almost nonexistent, the following recommendations are extrapolated from those for humans with the same disorders.

If the animal has an endocrinopathy for which the hypertension-producing mechanism is known, specific therapy can be instituted. The hypertension in cats with hyperthyroidism is most appropriately treated with beta-adrenergic antagonists such as propranolol. Animals with hypertension due to a pheochromocytoma are best treated with an alpha-antagonist to counteract the effects of increased levels of catecholamines. Oral phenoxybenzamine at a dosage of 0.2 to 1.5 mg/kg every 12 hr may be used in animals that are not showing clinical abnormalities referable to hypertension. Some animals with pheochromocytomas present in a hypertensive crisis. This is defined as a severe increase in blood pressure associated with clinical signs such as tachyarrhythmias, in which blood pressure must be rapidly lowered to prevent extensive end-organ damage or death. Phentolamine is an alpha-antagonist and the drug of choice in these situations administered as an initial IV bolus of 0.02 to 0.1 mg/kg, followed by IV infusion to maintain the reduction in blood pressure. Other drugs that may be used in hypertensive crisis include sodium nitroprusside administered as a constant IV infusion at a rate of 0.5 to 3 μg/kg/min, and acepromazine as an IV bolus of 0.05 to 0.1 mg/kg body weight. In the presence of tachyarrhythmias associated with pheochromocytomas, an alpha-antagonist must be given before betablocker administration to prevent a hypertensive crisis.

In cases of diabetes mellitus, it has been suggested that antihypertensive therapy with angiotensin-converting enzyme (ACE) inhibitors such as captopril or enalapril may be more beneficial in slowing glomerular injury than other classes of drugs. In humans, captopril when added to an existing antihypertensive regimen in doses that did not further reduce systemic blood pressure reduced proteinuria. This has been attributed to the efferent arteriolar dilation that occurs with ACE inhibitors, reduction in mean glomerular capillary pressure, and therefore reduced glomerular hyperfiltration (Brenner and Anderson, 1990). The use of ACE inhibitors for antihypertensive therapy in diabetic dogs and cats may therefore be appropriate.

Other antihypertensive therapy should be started in a stepwise fashion. After institution of each drug or treatment regimen blood pressure is monitored at 1- to 2-week intervals. If reduction to normal levels is not achieved within 2 to 4 weeks, the drug constituting the next step of therapy is added to or substituted for the drug currently being administered.

Dietary sodium restriction lowers total body sodium, reduces ECF volume, and is the first step in antihypertensive therapy. It may be effective in animals with acromegaly and hypothyroidism, in which volume expansion has been implicated as a cause of hypertension. It is recommended that sodium intake be restricted to 0.1 to 0.3% of the diet (10 to 40 mg/kg of body weight) for dogs; data are not available for cats.

Diuretics constitute the next step in therapy. As with dietary sodium restriction, they contract the ECF volume. Thiazide diuretics such as chlorothiazide or hydrochlorothiazide can be administered. Furosemide may be tried if thiazides are ineffective.

Beta-adrenergic antagonists represent the next step in therapy. The mechanism by which these drugs reduce blood pressure in disorders other than hyperthyroidism is not entirely known. Propranolol is the most commonly used agent in this class and can also be administered in conjunction with diuretics; it should be used with caution in animals with pre-existing cardiac or pulmonary disease because it can cause bradycardia, decreased cardiac output, and bronchospasm.

Vasodilators represent the next class of antihypertensive drugs. They may be used as the sole pharmacologic agent or may be given in conjunction with diuretics and beta-adrenergic antagonists. Prazosin is an alpha-adrenergic receptor antagonist that causes dilation of both arterioles and veins. It is a potent and effective antihypertensive agent in dogs and cats, administered at a dosage of 0.25 to 2 mg PO every 8 hr. Calcium channel blocking agents such as verapamil or diltiazem (0.5 to 1.5 mg/kg PO every 8 hours) cause arteriolar dilation by inhibiting calcium transport through slow channels in smooth muscle cell membranes. They may be considered for antihypertensive therapy in an animal with hyperparathyroidism and hypercalcemia.

ACE inhibitors are an additional class of pharmacologic agents. They act by inhibiting the conversion of angiotensin I to angiotensin II, resulting in arteriolar dilation and venodilation. Aldosterone secretion is also suppressed, which results in increased sodium excretion. Drugs in this class include captopril (0.5 to 2 mg/kg PO every 8 hr) and enalapril (0.25 to 0.5 mg/kg PO every 12 to 24 hr). They may be used for hypertension refractory to other drugs, or for disorders that may involve alterations of the renin-angiotensin-aldosterone system, such as hyperadrenocorticism.

References and Suggested Reading

Brenner, B. M., and Anderson S.: Glomerular function in diabetes mellitus. Adv. Nephrol. 19:135, 1990.
A discussion of the pathophysiology and therapy of the glomerular lesions in diabetic nephropathy with an emphasis on the role of glomerular hyperfiltration.
Feldman, E. C., and Nelson, R. W.: *Canine and Feline Endocrinology and Reproduction.* Philadelphia: W. B. Saunders, 1987.
A complete discussion of the normal physiology of the endocrine and reproductive systems, as well as the pathophysiology, clinical signs, diagnosis, and therapy of associated disorders.
Gwin, R. M.: Hypertensive retinopathy associated with hypothyroidism, hypercholesterolemia and renal failure in a dog. J. Am. Anim. Hosp. Assoc. 14:200, 1978.
A clinical case report; title is descriptive.
Hamet, P: Endocrine hypertension: Cushing's syndrome, acromegaly, hyperparathyroidism, thyrotoxicosis, and hypothyroidism. *In* Genest, J. (ed.): *Hypertension,* 2nd ed. New York: McGraw-Hill, 1983, p. 964.
A comprehensive discussion of the incidence and pathophysiology of hypertension in various endocrine disorders in humans.
Kallet, A, and Cowgill, L. D.: Hypertensive states in the dog. (Abstract.) *In* ACVIM Scientific Proceedings, Salt Lake City, 1982, p. 79.
A report of blood pressure in normal dogs and dogs with renal failure or hyperadrenocorticism.
Kobayashi, D. L., Peterson, M. E., Graves TK, et al.: Hypertension in cats with chronic renal failure or hyperthyroidism. J. Vet. Intern. Med. 4:58, 1990.
A study of the incidence of hypertension in cats with spontaneous chronic renal failure or hyperthyroidism.
Kuchel, O.: Adrenal medulla: Pheochromocytoma. *In* Genest, J. (ed.): *Hypertension,* 2nd ed. New York: McGraw-Hill, 1983, p. 947.
A comprehensive discussion of the hypertension associated with pheochromocytomas in people.
Lindheimer, M. D., and Katz, A. I.: Hypertension and pregnancy. *In* Genest, J. (ed.): *Hypertension,* 2nd ed. New York: McGraw-Hill, 1983, p. 889.
A discussion of blood pressure in normal pregnancy in women, and the classification, pathophysiology, and management of hypertension in pregnancy.
Peterson, M. E., Taylor, R. S., Greco, D. S., et al.: Acromegaly in 14 cats. J. Vet. Intern. Med. 4:192, 1990.
A description of the clinical characteristics, diagnosis, and therapy of spontaneous acromegaly in 14 cats.
Ross, L. A.: Hypertensive disease. *In* Ettinger, S. J. (ed.): *Textbook of Veterinary Internal Medicine,* 3rd ed. Philadelphia: W. B. Saunders, 1989, pp. 2047–2056.
A review of the pathophysiology, causes, consequences, and therapy of hypertension in the dog and cat.
Scott, D. W.: Hyperadrenocorticoidism (hyperadrenocorticoidism, hyper

adrenocorticalism, Cushing's disease, Cushing syndrome). Vet. Clin. North Am. Small Anim. Pract. 9:3, 1979.
An early description of the epidemiology, clinical signs, diagnosis, and therapy of canine hyperadrenocorticism.
Sowers, J. R., and Zemel, M. B.: Clinical implications of hypertension in the diabetic patient. Am. J. Hypertens. 3:415, 1990.

A discussion of the epidemiology, cardiovascular risks, pathophysiology, and therapy of hypertension in people with diabetes mellitus.
Twedt, D. C., and Wheeler, S. L.: Pheochromocytoma in the dog. Vet. Clin. North Am. Small Anim. Pract. 14:767, 1984.
A comprehensive review of canine pheochromocytoma.

OBESITY

E. GREGORY MacEWEN
Madison, Wisconsin

Obesity is defined as an excess of body fat. By using body fat alone as an index, obesity has classically been defined as weight 20 to 25% in excess of ideal body weight. It is estimated that between 25 and 44% of pet dogs are obese. Prevalence information on cats is lacking. A study in 1972 reported 6 to 12% of pet cats to be obese (Edney, 1972). It is more likely that the percentage of obese cats is much higher.

Although the exact pathogenesis of obesity is unknown, most studies suggest that obesity results from an imbalance between energy intake and energy output; that balance is controlled by neurologic, physiologic, metabolic, and hormonal factors. The body requires energy to do work such as maintaining normal muscular and neural polarization, contracting muscles, controlling body temperatures, and carrying out basic metabolic functions. This is called *basal metabolic energy* or *resting energy requirement*. Factors influencing resting energy requirement are fat-free body mass, age, sex, thyroid hormones, and genetics (breed). Evidence gathered from studies of humans also suggests that certain individuals have chronically subnormal energy expenditure as a major perturbation leading to a positive energy balance, with obesity developing. Approximately 60 to 75% of energy expended by a dog is for resting energy requirement. Diet-induced thermogenesis is the heat produced for food utilization. Protein has the highest thermogenic effect and fat the lowest. Approximately 1% of the energy expended is associated with meal-induced thermogenesis. The remaining energy expenditure (approximately 30%) is due to physical activity. Surplus energy that is not required for immediate needs is stored as fatty acids in fat tissue. Fatty acids are the most efficient way to conserve surplus energy because they can store 2.25 times more energy per unit mass than can proteins or carbohydrates (Brown, 1989).

Fat tissue (white fat) can be stored throughout the body in almost limitless quantities. Obesity results when there is an excess in body stores. Brown adipose tissue constitutes a very small percentage of the total body fat. It functions primarily in the generation of heat to maintain body temperature. Brown adipose tissue is an effector organ of the sympathetic nervous system and is involved in the regulation of body temperature by way of adaptive thermogenesis. Hypothalamic regulation of brown adipose tissue thermogenesis is related primarily to thermal balance and second only to energy balance. The role of brown adipose tissue in either nonshivering or diet-induced thermogenesis in larger animals is much less clear. Although brown adipose tissue is present in very small quantities, it is well vascularized and innervated and rich in mitochondria (hence the brown color), whose electron transport system can be readily but controllably uncoupled from adenosine triphosphate (ATP) formation through a specific ion conductance pathway mediated by a protein, the uncoupling protein (thermogenin) (Stock and Rothwell, 1989). Suppression of thermogenesis in brown adipose tissue occurs in exercise, hyperthyroidism, pregnancy, lactation, and during the stable hyperthermia of fever, acute lateral hypothalmic lesions, and high levels of glucocorticoids. The heat produced from brown adipose tissue following ingestion of a meal helps to control appetite. Defects in brown fat in some genetically defined mice have demonstrated that obesity can be related to hyperphagia.

Diet-induced thermogenesis is an adaptive phenomenon that would allow an animal to overeat a low-protein diet, achieving enough nitrogen for growth and development and dissipating the excess calories without acquiring the adverse effects of the increased fuel storage as fat. This effect is reduced in obese individuals by as much as 40 to 50%. Weight loss worsens the reduction in diet-induced thermogenesis because with weight loss lean body mass is lost along with fat, altering the normal thermogenic response to food ingestion (James, 1983). Aging also reduces diet-induced thermogenesis.

ETIOLOGY

The primary environmental factor associated with obesity is overfeeding. In humans, overfeeding early in life results in adipocyte proliferation, leading to what is called hyperplastic-hypertrophic obesity, whereas overfeeding later in life results in only hypertrophic obesity. Although this effect has not been studied in dogs or cats, a similar phenomenon may exist. Most animals seem to have stable weight. Factors such as boredom, idleness, nervousness, and conditioning are likely to contribute to overeating in dogs. The ability for an animal to maintain a stable weight by controlling food intake is called the set-point. It has been postulated that the set-point is determined by the hypothalamus; however, regulatory signals may arise from the fat cells themselves.

In mature animals, body weight increases 1 gm for each 7 to 9 kcal ingested in excess. Therefore, if a dog or cat consumes 1% more calories than needed, it will be almost 25% overweight by middle age (Lewis et al., 1987).

Body weights are usually stable for prolonged periods, indicating that energy expenditure varies about the same mean as energy intake, even though appreciable deviation from energy balance occurs from day to day. The steady state of weight maintenance requires not only that energy expenditure and energy intake be commensurate but also that protein, carbohydrate, and fat balances be maintained. Changes in food intake exert control over the energy balance to a far greater extent than alterations in energy expenditure. Carbohydrate and fat together provide the bulk of energy substances used for ATP generation. Weight maintenance is determined mainly by metabolism of carbohydrates and fats. Studies in ad libitum fed mice show that carbohydrate balance is much more closely regulated than fat balance and that carbohydrate oxidation is positively correlated with variation in food intake whereas fat oxidation is negatively correlated.

The type of diet can also contribute to overfeeding. Fat increases caloric density in the diet. Less energy is lost through diet-induced thermogenesis with a high-fat diet than with an equal-calorie diet containing more carbohydrate and proteins. In high-fat diets, only 3% of the energy content is lost when it is stored as body fat, compared with 23% with carbohydrate and protein. Therefore, high-fat diets can induce obesity more efficiently without increased caloric intake.

Genetics is also thought to play a part in obesity.

Some breeds are particularly prone to developing obesity. Those considered more at risk are the beagle, Cairn terrier, dachshund, Bassett hound, golden retriever, cocker spaniel, and Labrador retriever (Edney and Smith, 1986). In humans, children born to obese parents have a greater chance of becoming obese even if they are not raised in the same household.

One explanation about why certain breeds of dogs may be prone to obesity has been derived from the observation that certain human populations (most notably the Pima Indians) who have experienced extended periods of famine have decreased metabolic rates, ultimately enhancing survival. This has been coined the thrifty gene hypothesis.

Another factor contributing to the development of obesity has been termed adaptive hyperlipogenesis (Vasselli et al., 1983), defined as the enhanced production and storage of lipid from calories consumed by the refeeding of weight-reduced obese individuals. Two mechanisms have been suggested: increased adipose tissue lipoprotein lipase (LPL) activity, which may take place during the period of caloric restriction itself, and increased glucose uptake into adipose tissue during refeeding, possibly as a result of increased insulin binding. LPL may influence a feedback mechanism; the increase in enzyme might be a regulatory mechanism counteracting weight loss. With weight loss, the increase in LPL activity may enhance lipid storage, therefore making weight loss more difficult.

LPL hydrolyzes the triglycerides of circulating triglyceride-rich lipoprotein into free fatty acids and may instigate a signal from adipose tissue to the central nervous system that stimulates food consumption. Long-term overfeeding may induce a perpetual state of activation of the LPL protein.

Fat cell hypertrophy, as may develop when lost body weight is rapidly regained or in response to highly palatable diets, may ultimately trigger fat cell hyperplasia and thereby produce a more long-term stimulus to weight gain. Adipocytes tend to fill with lipids when adequate levels of lipid substrate are continuously available. The term ratchet effect has been used to denote the concept that body fat and thus body weight can always increase but cannot decrease (except under extreme conditions) below a minimum level set by the total number of adipocytes in combination with their tendency to remain lipid filled (Vasselli et al., 1983). Various hormones, including insulin, 17-beta-estradiol, and some prostaglandins, have been shown to influence the conversion of precursor cells to lipid-filled cells.

An endocrine basis for obesity has long been sought. Neutering approximately doubles the incidence of obesity in dogs and cats of both sexes. This weight gain is frequently attributed to a decrease in energy expenditure with either no change or an increase in food intake. Estrogen has been shown to depress food intake in several animal species. Aging may cause further weight gain because it results in a reduction in energy expenditure.

Obesity is also associated with various endocrine abnormalities such as hypopituitarism, hypothyroidism, hyperadrenocorticism, and hyperinsulinemia. One hormone that may be associated with obesity is the adrenal steroid dehydroepiandrosterone (DHEA) and its metabolite, DHEA-sulfate (DHEAS).

DHEA is the major secretory product of the adrenal gland, and serum concentrations of its sulfate ester, DHEAS, are the most abundant of any steroid except for cholesterol. Although DHEA is the main precursor of placental estrogen and may be converted to active androgens and estrogens in peripheral tissues, there is no obvious biologic role for either DHEA or DHEAS in normal animals. DHEA is derived from metabolism of pregnenolone following its hydroxylation to 17-beta-hydroxypregnenolone and cleavage of the C17 side-chain.

DHEAS represents more than 99% of the circulating steroid with less than 1% as free DHEA. Plasma concentrations of DHEAS in humans peak at around 50 to 100 μg/dl at 20 to 30 years of age and decline thereafter (Orentreich et al., 1984). On the average, it is estimated that the decrease in DHEA production is approximately 20% for every decade after age 25 and that by the age of 85 to 90 years, production remains constant at 5%.

A number of studies have demonstrated that DHEA administered to obese rodents results in significant weight loss without reduction in food intake (Gordon et al., 1987). Studies of humans have shown that as obese people lose weight, their urinary excretion of DHEA increases. The converse is also true: weight gain is associated with a decrease in urinary excretion of DHEA. In a recent study of nonobese normal men, DHEA administration resulted in a 31% reduction in mean percentage of body fat, with no weight loss (Nestler et al., 1988).

By far the most common hormonal abnormality observed in obesity is hyperinsulinemia; basal insulin secretion as well as glucose-induced insulin secretion is excessive in most experimental models of obesity. The development of obesity induces insulin resistance, which tends to reduce the rate of glucose oxidation relative to that of fat. The development of insulin resistance thus enhances the effect that the enlargement of the adipose tissue mass exerts on promoting the oxidation of fat relative to that of glucose. This observation, together with the knowledge that insulin is the major stimulus of triglyceride synthesis and an inhibitor of lipolysis in adipose tissue, suggests that excessive insulin secretion may be an underlying cause of obesity in some animals. The most common view of the relationship between insulin and obesity is that the hyperinsulinemia of obese individuals is a consequence rather than a cause of obesity; it is considered to be the result of increased insulin secretion in response to excessive caloric intake or insulin resistance (Stern and Haffner, 1986).

A number of theories have been proposed to explain the insulin resistance noted with obesity (Amatruda et al., 1985). The major alteration appears to be a postreceptor defect resulting in a decrease in insulin sensitivity or insulin responsiveness. With hyperphagia or obesity, there is an increase in plasma free fatty acids from the diet or by augmented hepatic production, resulting in an alteration of the receptor.

Several other hormones are now recognized to be sensitive to the level of energy intake and energy balance and also to dietary composition, specifically the carbohydrate content of the diet. Diet-induced alterations in thyroid hormone metabolism, sympathetic nervous system factors, and changes in glucagon can all play a part in metabolic adaptations (Danforth, 1989). For example, during complete fasting in humans, thyroxin (T_4) decreases as do T_4-binding proteins. Triiodothyronine (T_3) decreases, and reverse T_3 (rT_3) increases as a result of decreased plasma clearance. Free rT_3 also increases with fasting. In rodent studies, carbohydrate and to a limited degree protein increase T_3 generated *in vivo*, but fat does not. Overfeeding produces changes in the circulatory concentrations of T_3 and rT_3 that are opposite to those found during fasting and underfeeding.

METABOLIC AND CLINICAL COMPLICATIONS OF OBESITY

Because obesity tends to develop gradually, many owners do not present their animal for the primary problem of obesity. They may present their animal for a problem that is unrelated or associated with obesity. It is important to keep in mind that nearly one third of the owners of obese dogs do not even realize that their dogs are overweight. It is imperative to make your clients aware that they have an obese animal and that the condition requires attention.

Obesity can have a profound effect on reducing life span. In addition, other problems have been associated with obesity:

1. Joint and locomotion problems. It has been reported that 24% of obese dogs have serious joint problems. These include arthritis, herniated intervertebral disks, and ruptured anterior cruciate ligaments.

2. Respiratory difficulties. Small and miniature breeds are particularly affected.

3. Hypertension. A recent canine study sup-

ports an association between obesity, blood pressure, and hyperinsulinemia.

4. Decreased hepatic function as a result of a fatty liver. In cats, obesity may have a role in feline hepatic lipidosis.

5. Potential reproductive problems. It has been reported that the incidence of reproductive problems was 64% higher in dogs that were overweight.

6. Diabetes mellitus. Obesity results in an increase in fasting insulin levels and increased insulin secretion in response to glucose, potentially making an animal prone to the development of diabetes.

7. Heat intolerance due to excessive subcutaneous fat.

8. Increased surgical and anesthetic risk. Excessive fat alters drug kinetics and may influence anesthesia management. Obesity may compromise pulmonary function.

9. Possible lower resistance to infectious diseases, especially viral diseases.

10. Impaired gastrointestinal function resulting in an increase in constipation and flatulence.

11. Hypercholesterolemia and hypertriglyceridemia.

12. Increased risk of cancer development.

ASSESSMENT OF OBESITY

Obesity is difficult to determine and measure. In most studies, dogs are judged to be obese on the basis of clinical observation and by palpation of the amount of adipose tissue over the thorax, back, and pelvic region. Dogs whose ribs are easily discernible in outline beneath the skin are considered to be thin. Dogs with rib outlines just faintly discernible by the eye or easily palpated are considered normal. Dogs whose rib outlines are not discernible by eye or on palpation of the thorax have an obvious layer of fat and are considered obese. Further assessment of the extent or degree of obesity can be made on certain conformational characteristics, such as a pendulous abdomen with excessive intra-abdominal fat and localized fat deposits lateral to the iliac crest. The degree of obesity can also be estimated by using standard breed tables with corresponding ideal body weight ranges (Lewis et al., 1987).

Quantitative assessment of the degree of obesity can be very difficult. No objective techniques have been devised to determine adiposity in dogs. In humans, hydrostatic weighing, measurement of skinfold thickness, and bioelectrical impedance testing are relatively simple and reliable methods to determine percentage of body fat and lean body mass. None of these procedures has been found to be reliable in dogs. One method that may provide some quantitative method to determine body fat content uses ultrasound to measure subcutaneous fat (Wilkinson and McEwan, 1990).

DIAGNOSTIC EVALUATIONS

Once an animal has been determined to be obese, it is important to evaluate that animal for a potential underlying medical or hormonal abnormality that may be associated with the development of obesity or that may be a consequence of the obesity. The two major causes of obesity are *hypothyroidism* and *hyperadrenocorticism*. A complete physical examination should be performed to rule out conditions that may be mistaken for obesity. These conditions include organomegaly (especially liver or spleen enlargement), ascites, and peripheral edema. Routine laboratory diagnostic tests should include a complete blood count, chemistry profile (including serum cholesterol), and urinalysis.

MANAGEMENT

The most effective way to manage obesity in dogs and cats involves simple calorie restriction. Although exercise seems to be quite important in treating and controlling obesity, it is difficult to get owners to exercise their dogs adequately. Obtaining clients' cooperation is essential for treating an obese animal. Clients must be convinced that their animals have an obesity problem and must be willing to work with you on correcting it. Once clients agree to participate and cooperate, the next step is to set goals for the animal's weight reduction program. In setting up goals, it is important to inform the owner that this program will probably take at least 4 to 8 months to achieve desired weight loss. If an animal is 20 to 25% overweight, it may take 5 to 7 weeks to reduce it to normal weight. Overweight of 25 to 35% may take 7 to 16 weeks, and 30 to 50% overweight may take 16 to 36 weeks. It is important to inform owners that some dogs may not lose any weight at all, even with calorie restriction. This is especially true of dogs 50 to 100% overweight. A suitable goal to follow is a percentage reduction method—that is, a 2 to 3% weight loss per week for at least the first 6 weeks and possibly a 2% weight loss thereafter.

Next reduce the caloric intake to about 60% for dogs and 66% for cats for maintaining *optimum* or ideal body weight (Table 1). Although any degree of calorie restriction may be used, these levels seem to be the best. Greater calorie restriction results in little increase in rate of weight loss yet increases the risk of potential detrimental effects and encourages begging by the animal. Less severe restriction results in a such slow rate of weight loss that many owners become discouraged. Advise owners to feed obese dogs three to four times a day. Increases in feeding cause increased energy loss through diet-induced thermogenesis. Heat production associated with food intake also tends to have an appetite-suppressing effect.

Instruct clients to keep pets out of the room when

Table 1. *Calorie Requirements for Maintenance and Weight Reduction**

Optimum Body Weight (kg)	kcal/kg Body Weight/day Needed for†		Present Weight (lb)	kcal/lb Body Weight/day Needed for†	
	Maintenance	*Weight Reduction*		*Maintenance*	*Weight Reduction*
Dog:			Dog:		
3	110	70	6	50	30
6	85	55	12	40	25
10	75	50	20	35	22
20†	70	45	50†	30	20
Cat:			Cat:		
2.5–5.5	65	40	6–12	30	20

*Reprinted with permission from Lewis, L.D., Morris M.L., and Hard, M.S.: Obesity. In Small Animal Clinical Nutrition III. Topeka: Mark Morris, 1987, Ch. 6, pp. 1–39.

†Interpolation between these values will give the approximate amount needed for a dog of any size.

preparing food or eating to prevent begging and the temptation to offer snacks.

It is also recommended that obese animals be changed to a weight reduction diet rather than just restrict the animal's regular diet. For example, Prescription Diet r/d (Hill's Pet Products) is a high-fiber diet with low total kilocalories. When a high-fiber low-calorie-dense diet such as this is fed, the caloric intake is reduced by 45% even though the same amount of food is eaten.

Regardless of the diet used, make it very clear that the animal must be fed only the specific amount of foods prescribed. If the clients feel that they cannot resist giving treats, have them give either their pet a nugget of the dry form of the high-fiber restricted calorie food. Treats may be high-calorie foods that are frequently overlooked in determining an animal's total caloric intake or as a reason why weight loss is not occurring.

Try to get the owner to weigh the animal every 2 weeks and keep a chart or graph of the progress of the weight loss program. The animal should be weighed at the same time each day, preferably the first thing in the morning before eating.

Once the weight goal has been reached, the animal should be fed the correct number of calories to maintain optimum weight. It is important that clients continue to weigh their animals on a frequent basis and monitor the weight closely. If an animal resumes its previous diet and is allowed to increase food intake, it may reset its set-point and again gain weight.

Establish a recheck program with the client to examine and evaluate the animal at monthly intervals. If clients know they will be bringing their pets back, they are able to make a more consistent effort at maintaining the new regimen.

Some veterinarians have advocated starvation as a method of reducing weight. During starvation, there initially is a rapid loss of fluid as the body adjusts to using stored fat. Much of the weight loss occurring during this initial period is not adipose tissue, and weight is regained when feeding is reinstituted. After the first few weeks of starvation,

weight loss is due primarily to utilization of adipose tissue, which is relatively anhydrous, and weight loss slows as a result. Starvation results in a more rapid weight loss than dietary restriction, but after about 7 weeks, the percentages of reduction using restriction versus starvation are very similar. Other problems associated with starvation include protein loss, magnesium depletion, increased risk of hypotension, altered intestinal absorption, and some liver abnormalities. In cats, severe calorie restriction may predispose cats to the syndrome of idiopathic hepatic lipidosis (see *CVT X*, p. 869). In other animals such as humans and rodents, ketone bodies can be a problem, but dogs have a more efficient peripheral utilization of ketone bodies and thus do not become ketotic. Other problems with starvation include the fact that clients have an aversion to starving their pets, and starvation procedures must usually be done in a hospital situation at significant cost. Starvation is also viewed by some as inhumane. Furthermore, if clients are not involved in the weight reduction program, obesity may be expected to redevelop when the animal goes home.

Although a number of *pharmacologic agents* are available to treat obesity in humans, these have not been thoroughly tested in canine obesity studies. During the past few years, phenethanolamines have been studied as a new class of antiobesity agents. In animal studies, these agents have reduced body fat by stimulating lipolysis and thermogenesis through their stereospecific beta-adrenergic agonist activity, which is mediated by cyclic adenosine monophosphate.

We have recently reported on a study using the *experimental hormone DHEA* (Kurzman et al., 1990). Nineteen euthyroid obese dogs were treated with DHEA at a dose range of 30 to 60 mg/kg PO daily for a 3-month period. Thirteen of the 19 dogs (68%) lost weight while on DHEA. Because of the wide variation in size of the obese dogs in this study (weight range from 7 to 51 kg), weight loss was recorded for each dog as a percentage of total body weight. The mean weight lost for the 13 dogs was

3% of total body weight per month. All dogs except one maintained their normal food intake. Six normal adult nonobese dogs were also given DHEA at the same dose and for the same 3-month period. None of these dogs lost weight or reduced their food intake (Kurzman et al., 1990).

The most marked change observed during DHEA therapy was the alteration in serum cholesterol levels. The mean cholesterol for the obese dogs declined from 226 mg/dl before treatment to 173 mg/dl after treatment, a reduction of 23% ($P <$ 0.0005). These values in nonobese dogs decreased from a mean of 128 mg/dl to 89 mg/dl, a reduction of 30% ($P < 0.02$). These results include three obese dogs that did not show a reduction in serum cholesterol, although they did lose weight. The reduction in serum cholesterol for the remaining 16 obese dogs did not correlate with the amount of weight lost. Mean serum triglyceride levels also decreased in the obese dogs by 28% and increased by 46% in the nonobese dogs during DHEA therapy; however, because of the great variance in the triglyceride concentrations for each group, these alterations were not statistically significant.

More recent studies in our laboratory further indicate that DHEA has both antiobesity and hypocholesterolemic activity in dogs. We are currently conducting a prospective randomized double-blind study evaluating euthyroid spontaneously obese dogs fed a low-calorie high-fiber reducing diet (Hill's r/d). Thirteen dogs have been treated with DHEA (60 mg/kg PO daily), and 10 have been treated with a placebo. Of the dogs evaluated, the mean total body weight lost for dogs receiving DHEA was 3.69 ± 0.75 kg, compared with 2.38 ± 0.66 kg for those given a placebo. The percentage of excess body weight lost for the DHEA groups was 65.7 ± 9.1 versus 31.4 ± 6.6 for the placebo ($P < 0.02$). The percentage of excess body weight lost per month for the DHEA group was 15.0 ± 2.8 versus 8.2 ± 2.1 for the placebo group ($P = 0.069$). In the dogs given DHEA, the serum cholesterol level showed a 44% reduction, from a mean of 279 mg/dl to a mean of 160 mg/dl ($P = 0.0001$). The group given the placebo showed no significant change from a pretreatment mean cholesterol of 349 mg/dl to a post-treatment mean of 304 mg/dl. Although these results are preliminary, they indicate that when combined with a low-calorie high-fiber diet, DHEA enhances the loss of excess body weight when compared with just diet modification alone (Mac-Ewen and Kurzman, 1991). Unfortunately, DHEA is not available commercially and is still considered an investigational drug.

In conclusion, a weight reduction program should be instituted for all dogs and cats that are more than 20 to 25% above their optimal weight. Weight reduction will (1) decrease health problems, (2) decrease future health care costs, (3) improve ap-

pearance, and (4) increase an animal's enjoyment and length of life. The most effective means of treating obesity is through total calorie restriction. The use of high-fiber low-calorie diets such as Hill's Prescription Diet Canine r/d and Hill's Prescription Diet Feline r/d are most effective. Special diets prepared at home can serve equally well.

References and Suggested Reading

Amatruda, J. M., Livingston, J. N., and Lockwood, D. H.: Cellular mechanisms in selected states of insulin resistance: Human obesity, glucocorticoid excess and chronic renal failure. Diabetes Metab. Rev. 1:293, 1985.
A good review of the mechanism of insulin resistance in obesity.
Brown, R. G.: Dealing with canine obesity. Can. Vet. J. 30:973, 1989.
A concise review of canine obesity.
Danforth, E., Jr.: Hormonal adaptations to energy balance and imbalance and the regulation of energy expenditure. *In* Lardy, H., and Stratman, F. (eds.): *Hormones, Thermogenesis, and Obesity.* New York: Elsevier Science, 1989, pp. 19–32.
A good review of the influence of thyroid hormones and thermogenesis.
Edney, A. T. B.: Current trends in small animal nutrition. Vet. Annu. 195:195, 1972.
An older review of canine and feline obesity.
Edney, A. T. B., and Smith, P. M.: Study of obesity in dogs visiting veterinary practices in the United Kingdom. Vet. Rec. 100:391, 1986.
A study providing some important epidemiologic information on canine obesity.
Gordon, G. B., Shantz, L. M., and Talalay, P.: Modulation of growth, differentiation and carcinogenesis by dehydroepiandrosterone. Adv. Enzyme Regul. 26:355, 1987.
An excellent study of the antiobesity activity of DHEA in rodent models.
James, W. P. T.: Energy requirement and obesity. Lancet, p. 386–389, 1983.
A review of energy requirement and brown adipose tissue in obesity.
Kurzman, I. D., MacEwen, E. G., and Haffa, A. L. M.: Reduction in body weight and cholesterol in spontaneously obese dogs by dehydroepiandrosterone. Int. J. Obes. 14:95, 1990.
A clinical study of 19 obese dogs showing weight loss without a reduction in caloric intake in 70% of the dogs treated.
Lewis, L. D., Morris, M. L., and Hard, M. S.: Obesity. *In Small Animal Clinical Nutrition III.* Topeka: Mark Morris, 1987, Ch. 6, pp. 1–39.
An excellent chapter on the etiology, assessment, complications, and management of canine and feline obesity.
MacEwen, E. G., and Kurzman, E. G.: Obesity in the dog: Role of the adrenal steroid dehydroepiandrosterone. J. Nutr. (in press).
Nestler, J. E., Barlascini, C. O., Clove, J. N., et al.: Dehydroepiandrosterone reduces serum low density lipoprotein levels and body fat but does not alter insulin sensitivity in normal men. J. Clin. Endocrinol. Metab. 86:57, 1988.
A clinical study to evaluate DHEA in normal adult males.
Orentreich, N., Brind, J. L., and Rizer, R. L.: Age changes and sex differences in serum dehydroepiandrosterone sulfate concentrations through adulthood. J. Clin. Endocrinol. Metab. 59:551, 1984.
Cross-sectional study of blood levels in a large population of humans.
Stern, M. P., and Haffner, S. M.: Body fat distribution and hyperinsulinemia as risk factors for diabetes and cardiovascular disease. Arteriosclerosis 6:123, 1986.
An excellent review of the relationship between hyperinsulinemia and obesity.
Stock, M. J., and Rothwell, N. J.: The role of brown adipose tissue in adaptive diet-induced thermogenesis in humans. Lardy, H., and Stratman, F. (eds.): *Thermogenesis and Obesity.* New York: Elsevier Science, 1989, pp. 95–116.
A good review of brown adipose tissue and obesity.
Vasselli, J. R., Cleary, M. P., and Van Itallie, T. B.: Modern concepts of obesity. Nutr. Rev. 41:361, 1983.
A comprehensive review of new concepts related to obesity.
Wilkinson, M. J., and McEwan, N. A.: The use of ultrasound in the measurement of subcutaneous fat and prediction of total body weight in dogs. J. Nutr. (in press).
An experimental study of dogs to correlate ultrasound with fat thickness and total body fat.

RADIATION THERAPY FOR ENDOCRINE NEOPLASIA

GUY NEAL MAULDIN
New York, New York

Tumors arising from endocrine tissues cause a wide variety of paraneoplastic syndromes, primarily because of their autonomous production of polypeptide hormones, such as adrenocorticotropic hormone (ACTH), and the thyroid hormones (Morrison, 1984). Aberrant hormone production can result in severe systemic disease. Complete surgical resection is the preferred treatment for these tumors and the resolution of these associated disorders; however, variations in the biologic behavior of endocrine neoplasia often result in tumors that cannot be completely excised. Therefore, radiation therapy plays an important role in the treatment of unresectable endocrine neoplasia, both primary and metastatic. Radiation may be delivered either by an external source, such as cobalt-60 (^{60}Co), or by radionuclide therapy, such as iodine-131 (^{131}I). Because radiation therapy requires referral to a hospital, with suitable equipment and trained personnel, specific details of therapy are not discussed here (see *CVT X*, p. 1031). This article advises the practicing veterinarian of alternative methods of therapy for endocrine disorders and reviews the current states of radiation therapy in the treatment of these conditions.

PITUITARY TUMORS

Pituitary adenomas and, less frequently, adenocarcinomas have been described in dogs and cats. ACTH is the hormone most frequently produced by pituitary tumors in dogs; both ACTH and growth hormone production have been reported in cats with pituitary tumors. Surgical resection of these tumors is extremely difficult and dangerous and should be attempted only by a highly skilled surgeon. Radiotherapy has been used successfully to treat pituitary tumors in companion animals. Megavoltage external beam therapy, such as ^{60}Co, is the preferred type of radiation treatment for neoplasms located deep within the central nervous system (CNS).

In dogs, the most common secretory pituitary tumors are corticotropic and result in pituitary-dependent hyperadrenocorticism (PDH). Medical management of pituitary-dependent hyperadreno-

corticism has been well described (see *CVT X*, p. 1024). Animals that do not tolerate or respond to medical treatment may benefit from radiotherapy. Clinical signs associated with PDH, such as polyuria/polydipsia, polyphagia, and integumentary changes, might not resolve until several months after treatment is completed. ACTH and TSH stimulation tests can be used to monitor pituitary function after treatment, and they should be performed at least once yearly. Hormonal replacement therapy should be initiated if necessary, but panhypopituitarism seems to be an uncommon sequela to pituitary irradiation in companion animals.

Pituitary tumors in cats may be either corticotropic or somatotropic. The excessive production of growth hormone may result in a wide variety of systemic effects, including acromegaly and peripheral insulin resistance. *Acromegaly* is most frequently characterized by clinical signs related to the anabolic changes induced by somatomedins (Peterson et al., 1990). These signs include proliferation of bone and connective tissue with resultant inspiratory stridor, conformational changes, visceral enlargement, and, occasionally, cardiomyopathy. Excessive levels of growth hormone also cause peripheral insulin resistance that may lead to diabetes mellitus. Cats with diabetes due to excessive growth hormone may be extremely difficult to regulate with exogenous insulin administration. Few reports of medical management of hypersomatotropism in cats are available. At present, radiotherapy may be the only effective therapy that can be offered these cats, although clinical data are scant at this time.

Neurologic deficits might be observed in animals with large or invasive pituitary tumors. Tumors greater than 1 cm in diameter, classified as macrotumors, can be either adenomas or adenocarcinomas. Antemortem diagnosis of a macrotumor can be accomplished only with advanced imaging techniques, such as computed tomography or magnetic resonance imaging. While these tumors may not be secretory, many of the animals with neurologic deficits caused by a pituitary mass have previously developed PDH. Unfortunately, there is no way to predict which animals with PDH subsequently will develop signs referable to the CNS. Irradiation of pituitary tumors might be indicated to decrease tumor mass and peritumoral edema, in order to improve neurologic function and increase survival.

Our *current recommendations* for the use of radiotherapy in animals with *pituitary* tumors are:

1. As primary treatment in patients with PDH that are unresponsive to medical management, even if no neurologic signs are present.

2. As primary treatment in patients with macrotumors and mild to moderate neurologic deficits.

3. As primary treatment in cats with clinical signs of acromegaly, including poorly regulated diabetes mellitus, with evidence of a pituitary mass on CT scan.

4. As primary treatment in any dog with an identified pituitary macrotumor regardless of the development of PDH or neurologic signs. Alternatively, these patients can be monitored closely and not treated; however, any change in neurologic status, no matter how slight, warrants re-evaluation for radiotherapy.

Animals with pituitary tumors and severe neurologic deficits have a grave prognosis, and treatment should be initiated only after extensive client education (Mauldin and Burk, 1990). The prognosis for cats with acromegaly treated with radiotherapy is not known at present.

THYROID TUMORS

Secretory thyroid tumors have been well documented in companion animals. In cats, tumors resulting in hyperthyroidism are usually adenomas or adenomatous hyperplasia, whereas secretory thyroid tumors in dogs are most often adenocarcinomas (Peterson, et al., 1989; Turrel et al., 1984). There is extensive veterinary literature covering the surgical and medical management of thyroid neoplasms (see this volume, pp. 334 and 388, and *CVT X*, p. 1002). Malignant thyroid tumors in companion animals, especially dogs, are usually highly invasive, and resection is frequently difficult, if not impossible.

Radionuclide therapy using ^{131}I is the preferred method of radiotherapy for hyperfunctional thyroid neoplasms, and such treatment is available at a number of veterinary teaching hospitals and referral centers. Radioiodine therapy can control both primary and metastatic tumors. In dogs and cats with thyroid carcinoma, tumor control is best achieved with a combination of aggressive surgical resection and postoperative radiation therapy. Ablation of thyroid tissue can be accomplished with very high doses of radioiodine, but the risk of severe radiation toxicity increases substantially at higher doses. Severe radiation toxicity is rarely encountered at the doses of radioiodine commonly used to treat companion animals. Unfortunately, in many cases these doses may not be adequate to achieve tumor control. Animals treated with ^{131}I must be hospitalized in radiation isolation facilities, and proper collection and disposal of all waste materials is necessary.

The prognosis for dogs with *hyperfunctional* thyroid tumors is guarded. Treatment of these tumors with radioiodine is possible but may require high doses of ^{131}I to achieve a clinical response and may pose a significant risk both to the patient and to the people around that patient. Severe bone marrow suppression with life-threatening leukopenia can develop following high doses of radioiodine. Acute radiation pneumonitis is seen in some patients with pulmonary metastases after ^{131}I treatment, especially if ablative doses are used. These animals also emit clinically significant levels of radiation. Thus, serious consideration should be given to the potential for life-threatening toxicity and to human radiation exposure before this form of radiation therapy is advised or pursued in dogs with hypersecretory thyroid carcinoma.

The situation in cats is completely different. Hyperthyroid cats with thyroid adenomas or adenomatous hyperplasia respond very well to ^{131}I treatment. Relatively small doses of radioiodine (< 5 mCi) are required to control the hyperthyroidism, and there is minimal danger for either the patient or its handlers. Radionuclide therapy is a very good choice in those patients that are neither responsive to medical management nor good surgical candidates.

Nonfunctional thyroid tumors in dogs are usually malignant, highly invasive tumors that frequently metastasize. Approximately one third of the dogs have clinically detectable pulmonary metastasis at the time of diagnosis (Harari et al., 1986). Complications of local invasion, including development of arteriovenous fistulas, also can be observed. Nonsecretory thyroid tumors should *not* be treated with ^{131}I therapy, as there is no differential absorption of the radioiodine by the neoplastic thyroid tissue. Thyroid neoplasias are also fairly resistant to the dosages of external beam radiation that can be safely delivered to the affected animal. Surgical cytoreduction may be of benefit, but the surgery may be difficult and distant metastasis is likely. These relatively radiation-resistant aggressive tumors require innovative treatments to achieve adequate control. Several veterinary cancer centers are currently investigating protocols incorporating radiotherapy and chemotherapy, including doxorubicin, cisplatin, and various alkylating agents. Responses have been seen in both primary and metastatic lesions to a protocol incorporating megavoltage radiotherapy and low-dose doxorubicin. Clinical trials of this protocol are ongoing at The Animal Medical Center. The ideal therapy for nonsecretory thyroid tumors has not been defined, and the practicing veterinarian is advised to consult an oncologist or cancer specialist when formulating therapy.

APOCRINE GLAND ADENOCARCINOMA OF THE ANAL SAC (ApGA)

Although the anal sac is not usually considered an endocrine organ, tumors arising from the apocrine glands of this structure have the ability to cause humoral hypercalcemia. Tumor extracts obtained from hypercalcemic dogs with ApGA demonstrate potent adenyl cyclase–stimulating activity, beta-transforming growth factor–like activity, and bone-resorbing activity similar to that seen with parathyroid hormone (PTH). A PTH-like polypeptide, isolated from ApGA, is thought to be the cause of hypercalcemia in these animals (Weir et al., 1988). Approximately 90% of the animals with ApGA will have paraneoplastic hypercalcemia.

ApGA is a very aggressive tumor, highly invasive, and metastasis to the lymph nodes in the sublumbar region is not uncommonly observed at the time of diagnosis. Metastasis to liver, spleen, and lung is also possible but usually occurs later in the disease process. As with functional thyroid tumors, surgical excision is recommended, although it may result in fecal incontinence in those animals affected with large infiltrating tumors. Complete surgical resection of the primary tumor and nodal metastases must be accomplished if hypercalcemia is to resolve. External beam radiation (e.g., ^{60}Co) of the affected anal sac and regional lymph nodes is recommended in animals that have incomplete surgical resection. Local tumor control and resolution of hypercalcemia have been achieved in animals treated solely with radiation or using a combination of radiation with surgery. Radiotherapy is not a consideration in animals with distant metastases; therefore, thoracic radiographs and abdominal ultrasound, with emphasis directed to the liver and spleen, should be performed prior to treating these animals with radiotherapy.

Acute radiation toxicity is rare. However, approximately 30% of the dogs treated with radiotherapy for ApGA have developed rectal stricture 9 to 12 months after the completion of radiotherapy. Some of these rectal strictures have been severe, necessitating surgical correction. Because of this potentially serious sequelae, we currently recommend radiotherapy only for animals with residual disease or persistent hypercalcemia and with no evidence of distant metastases. The overall quality of life for these animals has been acceptable to most owners.

FUTURE CONSIDERATIONS

Radiotherapy can play a vital role in the treatment of some forms of endocrine neoplasia. Investigational protocols have proven the feasibility of intraoperative pancreatic irradiation in the dog, and new methods for the diagnosis and treatment of pheochromocytoma have recently been described in the human literature. At present, the scope of our experience is very limited; however, as our diagnostic ability and clinical expertise grow, radiotherapy will very likely play an increasingly important role in the treatment of endocrine neoplasia in companion animals.

References and Suggested Reading

Harari, J., Patterson, J. S., and Rosenthal, R. C.: Clinical and pathologic features of thyroid tumors in 26 dogs. J.A.V.M.A. 188:1160, 1986.
A description of the clinical presentation and biologic behavior of thyroid carcinoma in the dog.
Mauldin, G. N., and Burk, R. L.: The use of diagnostic computerized tomography and radiation therapy in canine and feline hyperadrenocorticism. *In* Nichols, R., (ed.): *Problems in Veterinary Medicine.* Philadelphia: J. B. Lippincott, 4:557, 1990.
A review of recent advances in the diagnosis and treatment of pituitary-dependent hyperadrenocorticism.
Morrison, W. B.: The clinical relevance of APUD cells. Comp. Cont. Ed. Pract. Vet. 6:884, 1984.
A discussion of the characteristics, properties, and syndromes associated with Amine Precursor Uptake and Decarboxylation cells (APUD cells).
Peterson, M. E., Taylor, S., Greco, D. S., et al.: Acromegaly in 14 cats. J. Vet. Intern. Med. 4:192, 1990.
A description of the clinical syndrome associated with chronic growth hormone hypersecretion in cats.
Peterson, M. E., Kintzer, P. P., Hurley, J. R., et al.: Radioactive iodine treatment of a functional thyroid carcinoma-producing hyperthyroidism in a dog. J. Vet. Intern. Med. 3:20, 1989.
A case report of a dog with a hyperfunctional thyroid carcinoma and pulmonary metastases treated with radioactive iodine.
Turrel, J. M., Feldman, E. C., Hays, M., et al.: Radioactive iodine therapy in cats with hyperthyroidism. J.A.V.M.A. 184:554, 1984.
A case study of 11 cats with hypersecretory thyroid tumors treated with radioactive iodine.
Weir, E. C., Centrella, M., Matus, R. E., et al.: Adenylate cyclase-stimulating, bone-resorbing and beta-TGF-like activities in canine apocrine cell adenocarcinoma of the anal sac. Calcif. Tissue Int. 43:359, 1988.
A discussion of the biologic behavior of apocrine cell adenocarcinoma of the anal sac and of the factors involved in humoral hypercalcemia of malignancy seen with this tumor type.

ACROMEGALY
(GROWTH HORMONE EXCESS)
SYNDROMES IN DOGS AND CATS

John F. Randolph
Ithaca, New York

and Mark E. Peterson
New York, New York

Excess production of growth hormone (GH), also called somatotropin, causes overgrowth of bone, connective tissue, and viscera as a consequence of cellular hypertrophy and hyperplasia. Growth hormone excess in humans may result in the clinical syndromes of giantism or acromegaly. Giantism develops when GH hypersecretion occurs before closure of the epiphyses, whereas acromegaly results if hypersomatotropism occurs after epiphyseal closure. In acromegaly, the increase in bone length is limited to the membranous bones (e.g., nose, mandible, and portions of the vertebrae) because the long bones cannot grow longitudinally once the epiphyses have fused. In dogs and cats, giantism has not been documented, but acromegaly syndromes do occur.

Growth hormone is normally synthesized by the somatotrophs of the anterior pituitary gland. The secretion of GH is episodic and controlled by two hypothalamic hormones: GH-releasing hormone (which stimulates production and secretion of GH) and somatostatin (which inhibits secretion of GH). Growth hormone exerts its effects both directly and indirectly through the elaboration of somatomedin C (also known as insulin-like growth factor I [IGF-I]). The indirect actions of GH, mediated by somatomedin C/IGF-I, are anabolic and include increased protein synthesis and soft-tissue and skeletal growth. In contrast, the direct effects of GH are predominantly catabolic (e.g., lipolysis and restricted cellular glucose transport).

Assays for plasma GH in the dog and cat have allowed confirmation of the diagnosis of acromegaly in these species. Although the syndrome of acromegaly shares many common clinical and laboratory features in the dog and cat, the disorder also has unique characteristic findings for each species (Table 1).

ETIOLOGY

In dogs, acromegaly is most often caused by endogenous or exogenous progestogens that induce

Table 1. Manifestations of Acromegaly in 14 Cats and 22 Dogs

	Cat (n = 14)* No. (%)	Dog (n = 22)† No. (%)
Polyuria/polydipsia	14 (100)	12 (55)
Hyperglycemia (>10 mmol/L)	14 (100)	6 (27)
Increased alkaline phosphatase	1 (7)	12/18 (67)
Inspiratory stridor	0 (0)	19 (86)
Erythrocytosis	5 (36)	0 (0)
Anemia	0 (0)	7/20 (35)
Arthropathy	6 (43)	Rare

*Data from Peterson, M. E., et al.: Acromegaly in fourteen cats. J. Vet. Intern. Med. 4:192, 1990.
†Data from Eigenmann, J. E., and Venker-van Haagen, A. J.: Progestogen-induced and spontaneous canine acromegaly due to reversible growth hormone overproduction: Clinical picture and pathogenesis. J. Am. Anim. Hosp. Assoc. 17:813, 1981.

hyperplasia and hypertrophy of the pituitary somatotrophs with subsequent GH overproduction. Older intact female dogs may spontaneously develop acromegaly because of the increased progesterone concentrations characteristic of diestrus. Attempts to suppress estrus with long-term progestogens (such as medroxyprogesterone acetate) may also lead to acromegaly. Although it may take longer to develop the clinical features of acromegaly, initial increases in GH concentrations occur after 9 weeks of treatment with medroxyprogesterone acetate at 10 mg/kg every 3 weeks (Eigenmann and Rijnberk, 1981) and after 8 months at 75 mg/kg every 3 months (Concannon et al., 1980).

In contrast, progestogens in cats do not seem to stimulate GH hypersecretion. Instead, the predominant cause of acromegaly in cats, as in humans, is a GH-secreting tumor of the pituitary gland. In a recent review of 14 cats with acromegaly in which ten cats were ultimately subjected to necropsy examinations, all ten cats had a large pituitary adenoma (Peterson et al., 1990). The association

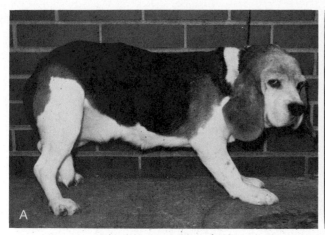
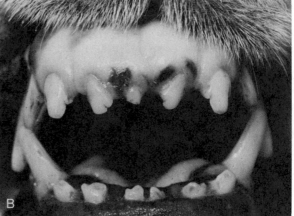

Figure 1. Intact female beagle with naturally occurring progesterone-induced acromegaly. A, Note the enlarged head and paws, and redundant skinfolds. B, Note the widened interdental spaces. (Courtesy of P. Concannon, Ithaca, New York.)

between acromegaly and pituitary tumors has also been reported in the dog, but very infrequently.

In humans, ectopic production of GH or GH-releasing hormone by extrapituitary neoplasms has also been associated with acromegaly.

SIGNALMENT

In humans, dogs, and cats, naturally occurring acromegaly is a disease of middle to old age. Yet, in contrast to humans in which acromegaly has no sex predilection, most acromegalic cats (93%) are male, whereas all acromegalic dogs are female. The female predisposition for canine acromegaly is understandable based on progesterone's stimulation of GH production in that species. The reason for the strong male sex predilection for feline acromegaly remains unknown. There is no apparent breed predilection for either feline or canine acromegaly.

CLINICAL SIGNS

Growth hormone overproduction in humans leads to thicker skull and mandible, broader hands and feet, and progressive increase in soft-tissue growth. Facial alterations in humans include large nose, thick lips, prominent skinfolds, macroglossia, prognathism, and widened interdental spaces of the mandible. Many of these same changes occur in acromegalic dogs and cats, but as in humans, the changes develop so insidiously that they are frequently overlooked. Both dogs and cats with acromegaly have been reported to show mandibular enlargement resulting in prognathism, widened interdental spaces, thickening of the bony ridges of the skull, large paws, and soft-tissue swelling of the head and neck (Fig. 1).

Most dogs and cats with acromegaly have an increase in body size and weight and enlargement of various organs (e.g., liver, kidneys, heart). The increase in weight is usually not due to increase fat depots, but rather results from the soft-tissue and bony overgrowth. Growth hormone acts to accelerate mobilization of fatty acids from adipose tissue and so uses up fat stores. In fact, some acromegalic animals lose weight. On physical examination, the acromegalic animal may have a pot-bellied appearance with palpable organomegaly. The skin feels thick and puffy from dermal and epidermal hyperplasia with excessive accumulation of dermal collagen and mucopolysaccharides (Scott and Concannon, 1983). The haircoat may be long and thick, or coarse. The toenails tend to grow rapidly.

Respiratory System

In dogs with acromegaly, the soft-tissue proliferation in the oropharyngeal region may be so profound that many dogs (86% in one study [Table 1]), suffer from panting, exercise intolerance, and inspiratory stridor due to compression of the upper airway. Inspiratory stridor due to upper airway narrowing is not seen in cats with acromegaly; however, dyspnea may develop in acromegalic cats as a result of pulmonary edema or pleural effusion from GH-induced cardiac failure.

Cardiovascular System

Cardiovascular manifestations of acromegaly in cats include systolic murmur, cardiomegaly, and occasionally congestive heart failure. Cardiac murmurs were detected in 9 of 14 acromegalic cats, while radiographic evidence of heart enlargement was seen in 12 (Peterson et al., 1990). Echocardiography most frequently demonstrated left ventricular and septal hypertrophy, but electrocardiography was normal in all cats. Cardiac enlargement develops as a result of GH-directed hypertrophy of individual cardiac muscle cells and increased interstitial fibrous tissue. In some acromegalic humans, hypertension also plays a role in myocardial hypertrophy. Unfortunately, blood pressure determinations were not performed routinely on cats with acromegaly. Congestive heart failure characterized by pulmonary edema, pleural effusion, or ascites developed in about half of the acromegalic cats. The cause of the myocardial failure is uncertain but may be related to increased collagen formation within the heart muscle.

Endocrine System

Some dogs and all cats with acromegaly have had concomitant insulin-resistant diabetes mellitus. Even in the absence of overt diabetes mellitus, acromegalic dogs may demonstrate carbohydrate intolerance (Eigenmann et al., 1983). Excess GH causes insulin antagonism by inducing a postreceptor (i.e., distal to insulin binding) defect in glucose transport. This postreceptor defect in insulin action may lead to hyperinsulinemia and subsequent down-regulation of insulin receptors (Muggeo et al., 1979). These abnormalities in insulin binding and action result in hyperglycemia and glucosuria and the accompanying clinical signs of polyuria, polydipsia, and polyphagia. Because of the GH-mediated insulin resistance, large doses of insulin (> 2.2 U/kg/day) are frequently needed to control the sustained hyperglycemia. Despite the poorly regulated diabetic state of most acromegalic cats and the usual promotion of ketogenesis by GH, ketosis rarely develops in cats.

Enlargement of endocrine glands (e.g., thyroid, parathyroid, adrenal) is also observed in acromegalic cats as a result of the growth-promoting effects of GH. However, basal T_4 and T_3 concentrations and results of ACTH stimulation and dexamethasone suppression tests are normal in all cats tested (Peterson et al., 1990). In contrast, low cortisol concentrations may develop in dogs in which acromegaly is created by chronic administration of progestogens. The intrinsic glucocorticoid-like activity of these progestogens probably suppresses ACTH secretion, causing the secondary hypoadrenocorticism (Concannon et al., 1980).

Skeletal System

In humans with acromegaly, joint disorders are common. Initially, excess GH causes proliferation of cartilage and soft tissue, resulting in widening of the joint space and bone remodeling. Later in the disease, as a result of the distorted joint architecture, features of the more typical degenerative arthropathy develop. However, the initial histologic changes of the articular cartilage in human acromegalic arthropathy are unique and distinct from degenerative joint disease.

Degenerative articular changes, such as osteophyte formation, have been demonstrated radiographically in the weight-bearing joints of six acromegalic cats. Surprisingly, only half of these arthritic cats showed any signs of joint discomfort. Dogs seem less likely than cats to develop joint problems in acromegaly. In fact, in one study, adult dogs treated with bovine growth hormone showed minimal to no histologic or biochemical changes in their articular cartilage (Mankin et al., 1978).

Other skeletal changes observed in dogs and cats with acromegaly include mandibular enlargement (prognathism), spondylosis deformans, and hyperostosis of the skull.

Nervous System

Peripheral neuropathies, reported in acromegalic humans, have been attributed to nerve entrapment and damage by exuberant soft-tissue overgrowth. A plantigrade stance caused by a tibial motor neuropathy was seen in one acromegalic cat (Morrison et al., 1989). However, this peripheral neuropathy was probably attributable to the concurrent diabetes mellitus since the posture resolved with reduction in the blood glucose concentration despite progression of the acromegaly.

Central neurologic signs (e.g., circling, seizures, behavioral changes) may be caused by expansion of the pituitary tumor in feline or human acromegaly.

Urinary System

The kidneys hypertrophy in response to GH excess, and glomerular filtration rate and renal plasma flow increase. The altered renal hemodynamics may be related to GH-mediated renal hypertrophy and vasodilation, and retention of sodium with its attendant volume expansion. As feline acromegaly progresses, renal failure develops in about 50% of the cats. All acromegalic cats that developed renal failure had persistent proteinuria with urine specific gravities of 1.015 to 1.025 (Peterson et al., 1990). Histologically, the kidneys of these cats were characterized by mesangial thickening of the glomeruli. These histologic changes may result from the glomerulosclerosis associated with unregulated diabetes mellitus or GH-mediated glomerular hyperfiltration.

Reproductive System

In dogs with progesterone-induced acromegaly, pyometra, mucometra, and mammary gland nodules may also develop. Seemingly, high circulating concentrations of progesterone alone could result in these conditions. In one study, however, the development of mammary gland nodules correlated more with increased GH levels superimposed on increased progesterone concentrations (Concannon et al., 1980).

ROUTINE LABORATORY TESTS

Clinicopathologic abnormalities on routine laboratory testing of dogs and cats with acromegaly are variable. By far the most striking abnormality reported in all cats and some dogs with acromegaly is severe *hyperglycemia* and *glucosuria*. Less frequent increases in cholesterol, alanine aminotransferase, and serum alkaline phosphatase may be related to the diabetic state. However, even in many acromegalic dogs without diabetes, serum alkaline phosphatase activity was increased. Possible causes for the increased serum alkaline phosphatase activity in these dogs include isoenzyme induction by the glucocorticoid-like properties of progesterone, bone isoenzyme increase associated with GH-accelerated turnover of bone, or hepatic lipidosis associated with GH-stimulated mobilization of fat from adipose tissue (Feldman and Nelson, 1987).

About 50% of acromegalic cats are mildly to moderately hyperproteinemic. Serum electrophoresis shows a normal pattern of protein distribution (Peterson and Randolph, 1989). The cause of the hyperproteinemia is unknown. Acromegalic dogs and cats are hyperphosphatemic secondary to increased renal tubular reabsorption of phosphorus by GH.

The hemogram may reveal a stress leukogram, anemia (dogs), or mild erythrocytosis (cats). The erythrocytosis in cats is caused by GH-stimulated erythropoiesis. The reason that some dogs with hypersomatotropism develop anemia is uncertain.

RADIOLOGY

Radiography in acromegalic animals reveals visceral enlargement (e.g., cardiomegaly, hepatomegaly, renomegaly), soft-tissue proliferation (oropharyngeal region, head, and limbs), and bony changes (e.g., spondylosis, hyperostosis of the calvarium, periarticular periosteal reaction).

Nuclear imaging and computerized tomography are helpful in identifying a possible pituitary tumor.

DIAGNOSIS

A diagnosis of acromegaly should be suspected in bitches receiving progestogens and intact female dogs that develop diabetes mellitus or laryngeal stridor due to soft-tissue overgrowth. A diagnosis of acromegaly should be suspected in all cats with insulin-resistant diabetes mellitus. Confirmation of the diagnosis requires demonstration of increased circulating GH concentrations. However, GH concentrations may be mildly increased in a variety of diseases in humans. Furthermore, GH concentrations in some acromegalic humans may be normal since GH secretion remains pulsatile in acromegaly.

Since hyperglycemia is a potent suppressor of GH secretion, demonstration of increased GH concentration with profound hyperglycemia is considered supportive of acromegaly. When acromegaly is suspected in nonhyperglycemic humans, a glucose suppression test is performed. Following administration of a glucose load (1 gm/kg PO or IV), GH concentration will decline to less than 5 ng/ml within 60 minutes in a normal patient, while the GH concentration will not decrease in an acromegalic human. Similar results occur following glucose infusion in dogs (Eigenmann et al., 1983). Alternatively, an integrated 24-hr GH value determined by frequent sampling throughout the day may be more indicative of GH hypersecretion than a solitary determination.

Unfortunately, the limited availability of veterinary laboratories performing feline and canine GH radioimmunoassays prevents the routine use of GH determinations in the diagnosis of acromegaly in dogs and cats. Instead, the presumptive diagnosis of feline acromegaly is made based on characteristic clinical and laboratory features, radiographic documentation of a pituitary mass, and normal results on thyroid and adrenal testing. Most cases of canine acromegaly are tentatively diagnosed based on characteristic clinical and laboratory findings, exposure to a progesterone source and improvement in clinical signs following withdrawal of progesterone, and no evidence of spontaneous hyperadrenocorticism on adrenal testing.

Indirect evaluation of GH concentration may also be performed by measurement of somatomedin C/IGF-I. In humans, somatomedin C/IGF-I is increased in acromegaly. Similarly, dogs with acromegaly have increased somatomedin C/IGF-I concentrations. Comparable studies in cats are not available.

TREATMENT

Progesterone-Induced Acromegaly

Treatment for dogs with progesterone-induced acromegaly is ovariohysterectomy or discontinuation of progestogen drugs. The GH levels will normalize (rapidly following ovariohysterectomy and more slowly following withdrawal of progestogen drugs) accompanied by resolution of the soft-tissue proliferation and signs of respiratory stridor; however, the skeletal changes may persist. The insulin requirement for GH-induced diabetes mellitus will also decline, but the reversibility of the diabetes depends on the insulin reserve of the pancreatic beta islet cells.

GH-Secreting Pituitary Tumor

In humans with GH-secreting pituitary tumors, there are three approaches to management: surgery, radiation, or pharmacologic therapy.

Surgery has not yet been attempted for the correction of feline acromegaly. The surgical procedure for hypophysectomy has been performed in the dog, but the technique has not been applied to the sporadic case of canine acromegaly attributable to a somatotroph adenoma. Since surgical excision of the tumor would probably necessitate hypophysectomy, deficiencies of pituitary hormones should be expected postoperatively. Prior to surgical intervention, precise localization of the pituitary tumor by nuclear imaging or computerized tomography is essential since neoplastic extension into the hypothalamus would preclude surgery.

Cobalt irradiation (total dose of 4800 centiGray divided equally in 12 treatments during 4 weeks) has shown variable results in two acromegalic cats (Peterson et al., 1990). In one, no effect was seen on tumor size or GH concentration, while in the other the tumor shrunk with subsequent reduction in GH concentration. These changes were noted within 2 months of radiation treatment, but only lasted for 6 months before relapse. Unfortunately, only few veterinary institutions offer this modality. In humans undergoing radiation treatment of pituitary tumors, side effects include lethargy, cranial neuropathies, and hypopituitarism.

In humans with acromegaly, pharmacologic management has included dopamine agonists and long-acting somatostatin analogues. Dopaminergic agents (e.g., bromocriptine) cause a reduction in GH concentration in many acromegalic humans but have not been evaluated for treatment of acromegalic cats. In humans and dogs, side effects (vomiting and depression) from bromocriptine are frequent. Long-acting somatostatin analogues (SMS 201-995 [octreotide]) inhibit GH secretion in 90% of human patients with acromegaly. No reduction in GH concentration was observed in four acromegalic cats following subcutaneous dosages of SMS 201-995 ranging from 10 to 60 µg/day for 2 to 4 weeks, or even as high as 200 µg/day for 4 days. The ineffectiveness of SMS 201-995 in acromegalic cats may indicate inability to bind to feline somatostatin receptors, failure to inhibit GH secretion in cats, or the refractoriness of feline somatotroph adenomas.

Concurrent Conditions

Most of the disorders resulting from GH excess are best treated by removing the progesterone source (dogs) or reducing the GH concentration (cats). So far, attempts at decreasing the GH concentrations in cats by hypophysectomy, irradiation, and medical management are either unproven or unsuccessful. Therefore, symptomatic treatment of GH-related disorders should be undertaken in the initial management of acromegalic dogs and the long-term care of acromegalic cats.

The inspiratory stridor seen in acromegalic dogs should respond to cage rest, cooling, and oxygen therapy. If the inspiratory dyspnea is severe, emergency tracheostomy may be necessary. The congestive heart failure accompanying acromegaly in some cats appears initially responsive to furosemide treatment. The diabetes mellitus of acromegaly is usually best controlled by adjusting insulin type and dosages. Most acromegalic cats require NPH or PZI insulin twice daily. In some cats, combinations of short-acting insulin (regular insulin) with NPH insulin help control hyperglycemia.

Major causes of death in acromegalic humans are hypertension, diabetes, pneumonia, and cancer. Cats with acromegaly ultimately succumb to euthanasia, congestive heart failure, renal failure, or neurologic sequelae of an expanding pituitary tumor. Yet, despite the widespread effects of uncontrolled GH production, median survival of acromegalic cats is almost 2 years.

References and Suggested Reading

Concannon, P., Altszuler, N., Hampshire, J., et al.: Growth hormone, prolactin, and cortisol in dogs developing mammary nodules and an acromegaly-like appearance during treatment with medroxyprogesterone acetate. Endocrinology 106:1173, 1980.
Results of treatment with medroxyprogesterone acetate in dogs that developed acromegaly and mammary nodules.
Eigenmann, J. E., Eigenmann, R. Y., Rijnberk, A., et al.: Progesterone-controlled growth hormone overproduction and naturally occurring canine diabetes and acromegaly. Acta Endocrinol. 104:167, 1983.
Progestogen induced and spontaneous hypersomatotropism is reported in 21 dogs that developed diabetes mellitus and/or acromegaly.
Eigenmann, J. E., and Rijnberk, A.: Influence of medroxyprogesterone acetate (Provera) on plasma growth hormone levels and on carbohydrate metabolism. Acta Endocrinol. 98:599, 1981.
Results of treatment with medroxyprogesterone acetate in six dogs that developed hypersomatotropism and mild glucose intolerance.
Eigenmann, J. E., and Venker-van Haagen, A. J.: Progestogen-induced and spontaneous canine acromegaly due to reversible growth hormone overproduction: Clinical picture and pathogenesis. J. Am. Anim. Hosp. Assoc. 17:813, 1981.
Progestogen-induced and spontaneous hypersomatotropism that reversed with ovariohysterectomy and discontinuation of progestogen drugs is reported in 22 dogs.
Feldman, E. C., and Nelson, R. W.: Growth hormone. *In* Feldman,

E. C., and Nelson, R. W. (eds.): *Canine and Feline Endocrinology and Reproduction.* Philadelphia: W. B. Saunders, 1987, p. 29.
  A review of the causes, clinical features, diagnosis, and treatment of disorders of growth hormone production in the dog and cat.
Mankin, H. J., Thrasher, A. Z., Weinberg, E. H., et al.: Dissociation between the effect of bovine growth hormone in articular cartilage and in bone of the adult dog. J. Bone Joint Surg. [Am.] 60:1071, 1978.
  Study of effects of bovine growth hormone on bone and articular cartilage in adult dogs.
Morrison, S. A., Randolph, J. F., and Lothrop, C. D.: Hypersomatotropism and insulin resistant diabetes mellitus in a cat. J.A.V.M.A. 194:91, 1989.
  Case report of unsuccessful treatment of acromegalic diabetic cat with large doses of SMS 201-995.
Muggeo, M., Bar, R. S., Roth, J., et al.: The insulin resistance of acromegaly: Evidence for two alterations in the insulin receptor on circulating monocytes. J. Clin. Endocrinol. Metab. 48:17, 1979.
  Results of studies of insulin binding to insulin receptors on circulating monocytes in 11 acromegalic humans.
Peterson, M. E., and Randolph, J. F.: Endocrine diseases. *In* Scherding, R. G., (ed.): *The Cat Diseases and Clinical Management.* New York: Churchill Livingstone, 1989, p. 1095.
  A review of the causes, clinical features, diagnosis, and treatment of endocrine diseases of cats.
Peterson, M. E., Taylor, R. S., Greco, D. S., et al.: Acromegaly in fourteen cats. J. Vet. Intern. Med. 4:192, 1990.
  A retrospective summary of the historical and clinical signs and laboratory and pathologic findings in 14 cats with acromegaly.
Scott, D. W., and Concannon, P. W.: Gross and microscopic changes in the skin of dogs with progestagen-induced acromegaly and elevated growth hormone levels. J. Am. Anim. Hosp. Assoc. 19:523, 1983.

CANINE TRIIODOTHYRONINE AUTOANTIBODIES

ROBERT J. KEMPPAINEN
and DIANE W. YOUNG
Auburn, Alabama

Autoantibodies to triiodothyronine (T_3) are relatively uncommon in dogs, but their occasional occurrence can confuse the clinical evaluation of patients that have these immunoglobulins in circulation. The T_3 autoantibodies produce an artifact when serum or plasma T_3 concentrations are measured by radioimmunoassay (RIA), often resulting in an elevated apparent concentration of T_3 in affected dogs. Not uncommonly these values will be markedly increased, causing the clinician to consider the possibility that the dog has hyperthyroidism. In our experience, thyroxine (T_4) concentrations in these dogs are usually in the normal range or are low. Aside from these effects on measurement of circulating T_3 concentrations, neither the clinical significance nor the possible prognostic relevance associated with the presence of the autoantibodies is clear at present.

PREVALENCE AND RECOGNITION

In a study based on samples sent to our endocrine diagnostic lab, T_3 autoantibodies were present in less than 1% of all canine samples submitted by veterinarians for thyroid hormone measurement

(Young et al., 1985). Whether this represents an estimate of the actual frequency in the general population is not known, since the majority of samples were submitted because of suspicion of a thyroid disorder (usually hypothyroidism). Based on this small population of affected dogs, there is a suggestion that the autoantibodies occurs more frequently in females. The possible presence of T_3 autoantibodies was suggested in each sample, based on the measurement of an apparent T_3 concentration greater than our established normal range, or upon the finding of a low T_4 value with a T_3 concentration in the high normal range. Apparent T_3 concentrations (as generated by computer extrapolation) as great as 230 nmol/L (our normal range for serum T_3: 0.7 to 2.3 nmol/L) have been reported from our lab.

INTERFERENCE WITH THE RADIOIMMUNOASSAY FOR T_3

Radioimmunoassays involve a competition reaction where unlabeled hormone competes with radiolabeled hormone for limited binding sites on a specific antibody. Remarkably, T_3 autoantibodies have an equal or greater affinity for T_3 than do commercial RIA antibodies. Consequently, in the presence of the T_3 autoantibodies, less of the radiolabeled T_3 is available to bind the RIA antibody. The apparent T_3 concentration is then artifactually

Reprinted with permission from Young, D. W., et al.: Characterization of canine triiodothyronine (T_3) autoantibodies and their effect on total T_3 in canine serum. Proc. Soc. Exp. Biol. Med. 188:219, 1988.

elevated or lowered, depending on the method used to separate free T_3 from T_3 bound to antibody (either RIA antibody or T_3 autoantibodies). In solid phase separation assays, the presence of T_3 autoantibodies cause an artifactual elevation in the concentration of T_3. In assays employing charcoal to separate bound from free hormone, the apparent T_3 concentration is low (often not detectable). Assays using second antibody separation may yield either high or low values, depending on whether the second antibody is capable of binding to the autoantibodies. Because most veterinary endocrine diagnostic laboratories currently use solid-phase RIA for T_3, results from samples submitted from most dogs with T_3 autoantibodies indicate high apparent T_3 concentrations. However, some diagnostic labs employ other types of T_3 assays, so low results are also possible. As mentioned previously, these high or low T_3 concentrations are an artifact caused by the fact that T_3 autoantibodies compete with RIA antibodies for binding labeled T_3. Procedures capable of measuring the true T_3 concentrations (see later) have shown that the concentration of this hormone varies from below the normal range to values approximately four times greater than the upper limit of normal (Young et al., 1988).

GENERAL CHARACTERISTICS

The belief that the T_3 binding factor in serum from these dogs is an autoantibody is supported by the fact that the majority of binding is associated with the immunoglobulin G fraction of serum proteins (Rajatanavin et al., 1989; Young et al., 1985, 1988). Further, the binding activity exhibits relative resistance to heat inactivation, is not affected by addition of chemicals that block T_3 binding to thyroxine-binding globulin, and exhibits high binding affinities characteristic of such autoantibodies described in humans (Young et al., 1985, 1988). Although the identity of the antigenic stimulus for the antoantibody production is not known, it is possible that thyroglobulin, the storage protein containing T_3 and T_4 within thyroidal colloid, serves this role. Canine T_3 autoantibodies show the highest affinity for T_3, a tenfold lower affinity for purified canine thyroglobulin and, surprisingly, an additional tenfold lower affinity for T_4 (Young et al., 1990). Autoantibodies to thyroglobulin occur frequently in dogs with hypothyroidism (Haines et al., 1984). These thyroglobulin autoantibodies are distinct from T_3 autoantibodies, because they display different specificities for ligand binding (Young et al., 1990). It is interesting to note, however, that thyroglobulin autoantibodies have been identified in the serum of all dogs tested who have T_3 autoantibodies (Rajatanavin et al., 1989; Young et al., 1990). The converse is not true, that is, thyroglobulin autoantibodies

Table 1. *Results of Thyrotropin-Stimulating Hormone (TSH) Stimulation Tests in 12 Dogs With T_3 Autoantibodies*

Hypothyroid Responses			Euthyroid Responses		
Dog No.	Pre-TSH T_4	Post-TSH T_4	Dog No.	Pre-TSH T_4	Post-TSH T_4
1.	8	11	8.	33	122
2.	5	4	9.	19	54
3.	6	5	10.	33	53
4.	19	23	11.	44	103
5.	6	20	12.	17	62
6.	6	8			
7.	14	14			

T_4 concentrations in nmol/L. Auburn University Endocrine Diagnostic Laboratory normal values for TSH stimulation test: pre-TSH T_4, 20 to 55 nmol/L; post-TSH T_4, >45 nmol/L.

occur in dogs that do not concurrently display T_3 autoantibodies. If thyroglobulin is the antigenic source for T_3 autoantibodies, something unique to its chemical structure or presentation to the immune system must account for the fact that autoantibodies against T_3 occur with much greater frequency in dogs than do autoantibodies to T_4. We have observed canine T_4 autoantibodies in only two dogs during the past 8 years.

ASSOCIATION WITH HYPOTHYROIDISM

In our experience, dogs with T_3 autoantibodies can have serum T_4 concentrations that are either in the normal or below normal range (our normal range for serum T_4: 20 to 55 nmol/L). Slightly greater than one half of the dogs with T_3 autoantibodies have had serum T_4 concentrations below the normal range. We have obtained results of serum T_4 concentrations in response to thyrotropin (TSH) stimulation in several dogs with T_3 autoantibodies (Table 1). Nine of the 12 dogs tested had resting T_4 concentrations below the normal range, and 7 of 12 had responses to TSH that we considered consistent with hypothyroidism. Two dogs that showed normal responses to TSH had resting serum T_4 concentrations below the normal range. Based on the results in this small group of dogs and observations in other dogs that we have studied, it appears that the presence of T_3 autoantibodies is associated with hypothyroidism in about 60% of dogs presenting with T_3 autoantibody activity. However, a significant percentage of dogs with T_3 autoantibodies appear to have normal thyroid function, based on their responses to exogenous TSH. We have developed an accurate assay to measure total T_3 concentrations in dogs with T_3 autoantibodies and have found that actual concentrations of T_3 are usually above the normal range in such dogs presenting with normal concentrations of T_4 (Young et al., 1988) (Table 2).

Table 2. *Thyroid Hormone Concentrations in 18 Dogs With T₃ Autoantibodies**

Group	Total T$_4$	Apparent† Total T$_3$	Actual‡ Total T$_3$	T$_3$ Not Bound to T$_3$ Autoantibodies
Dogs with normal T$_4$ (n = 7)	24 ± 2	7.1 ± 4.5	5.8 ± 2.4	2.2 ± 2.2
Dogs with low T$_4$ (n = 11)	5 ± 3	20.8 ± 27	1.5 ± 1.0	0.2 ± 0.4

*Reprinted with permission from Young, D. W., et al.: Characterization of canine triiodothyronine (T$_3$) autoantibodies and their effect on total T$_3$ in canine serum. Proc. Soc. Exp. Biol. Med. 188:219, 1988.

†Apparent total T$_3$ concentration determined using an unmodified, solid phase RIA for T$_3$. Several values represented computer extrapolated estimates.

‡Actual total T$_3$ concentration using a modified assay that eliminates the effect of the T$_3$ autoantibodies.

Values are mean ± SD. Normal values: T$_4$, 20 to 55 nmol/L; T$_3$, 0.7 to 2.3 nmol/L.

Estimation of the concentration of T$_3$ not bound to the autoantibodies (which is equivalent to total T$_3$ in normal dogs) in these dogs gives a value for this hormone within the normal range (Table 2). Thus it appears that mechanisms exist whereby, in the presence of T$_3$ autoantibodies, a functioning thyroid can increase peripheral T$_3$ concentrations to compensate for binding to autoantibodies and thus provide adequate levels of this hormone to target tissues. In contrast, dogs presenting with low T$_4$ concentrations and T$_3$ autoantibodies uniformly had calculated available T$_3$ concentrations (i.e., T$_3$ not bound to T$_3$ autoantibodies) below the normal range (Table 2).

RECOMMENDED THERAPY

The likelihood of hypothyroidism is high for a dog presenting with clinical signs of the disease, low serum T$_4$ concentrations, and T$_3$ autoantibodies. We have found that such dogs respond as well to standard L-thyroxine replacement therapy as do hypothyroid dogs that do not have T$_3$ autoantibodies. There is no evidence that the autoantibodies inhibit the tissue response to thyroid hormone replacement therapy, nor does it appear that the dose of L-thyroxine need be raised (our recommended dosage for L-thyroxine; 20 µg/kg, every 12 hours or every 24 hours, PO). In all other dogs with T$_3$ autoantibodies (T$_4$ concentrations in the normal or borderline low range), we recommend performing a TSH stimulation test to obtain more definitive information about thyroid function. No treatment is recommended if the T$_4$ response to TSH is normal. Instead, we advise periodic (every 1 to 2 months) re-evaluation of resting T$_4$ concentrations and, if possible, repeated TSH stimulation tests at 6-month intervals. Hypothyroidism would be associated with low resting T$_4$ concentrations and a reduced to absent increase in serum T$_4$ concentrations after TSH stimulation.

PROGNOSIS

A key and as yet, unanswered, question is whether a dog with T$_3$ autoantibodies and apparently normal thyroid function (normal resting T$_4$ concentration, normal response to TSH) will eventually develop hypothyroidism. Based on the fairly high frequency of concurrent T$_3$ autoantibodies and hypothyroidism and the uniform presence of thyroglobulin autoantibodies in dogs with T$_3$ autoantibodies, we believe that dogs with T$_3$ autoantibodies have sustained some "leakage" of thyroidal thyroglobulin which has initiated an autoimmune response to various epitopes on the thyroglobulin molecule. Consequently, we feel that it is likely that the presence of these autoantibodies signals or participates in causing thyroidal damage, eventually leading to hypothyroidism. However, we have not had the opportunity to study an adequate number of dogs with T$_3$ autoantibodies over time to present this theory as anything more than speculation. Nevertheless, the presence of T$_3$ autoantibodies should serve as a signal to the clinician that a dog presenting with this immunoglobulin should, for the remainder of its life, remain at potential risk for development of hypothyroidism. We do *not* recommend treating such dogs with immunosuppressive drugs to attempt to stop the progression of such an attack because of the questionable efficacy of such treatment and the possibility of side effects more deleterious than those occurring in hypothyroidism.

References and Suggested Reading

Chastain, C. B., Young, D. W., and Kemppainen, R. J.: Anti-triiodothyronine antibodies associated with hypothyroidism and lymphocytic thyroiditis in a dog. J.A.V.M.A. 194:531, 1989.
A case report describing a dog with concurrent T$_3$ autoantibodies and hypothyroidism.
Rajatanavin, R., Fang, S-L., Pino, S., et al.: Thyroid hormone antibodies and Hashimoto's thyroiditis in mongrel dogs. Endocrinology 124:2535, 1989.
Examination of thyroid hormone concentrations and thyroid hormone binding in 19 dogs with T$_3$ autoantibodies.
Haines, D. M., Lording, P. M., and Penhale, W. J.: The detection of canine autoantibodies to thyroid antigens by enzyme-linked immunosorbent assay, hemagglutination and indirect fluorescence. Can. J. Comp. Med. 48:262, 1984.
A comparison of methods to detect circulating autoantibodies to thyroid antigens in dogs with hypothyroidism.
Young, D. W., Haines, D. M., and Kemppainen, R. J.: The relationship between autoantibodies to triiodothyronine (T$_3$) and thyroglobulin (Tg) in the dog. Autoimmunity, 9:41, 1991.
Comparison of the frequency of occurrence and co-occurence of autoantibodies to T$_3$ and thyroglobulin in dogs.
Young, D. W., Kemppainen, R. J., and Sartin, J. L.: Characterization of

canine triiodothyronine (T$_3$) autoantibodies and their effect on total T$_3$ in canine serum. Proc. Soc. Exp. Biol. Med. 188:219, 1988.
Description of the biochemical characteristics of T$_3$ autoantibodies in dogs, including affinity determination and development of a method to measure T$_3$ concentrations in these patients.

Young D. W., Sartin, J. L., and Kemppainen, R. J.: Abnormal canine triiodothyronine-binding factor characterized as a possible triiodothyronine autoantibody. Am. J. Vet. Res. 46:1346, 1985.
Initial description of the T$_3$ autoantibody phenomenon in dogs illustrating that the factor is an immunoglobulin.

UNUSUAL MANIFESTATIONS OF HYPOTHYROIDISM IN DOGS

C. B. CHASTAIN
Columbia, Missouri

Hypothyroidism is the most commonly diagnosed endocrinopathy in the dog. Primary hypothyroidism is the cause in more than 96% of the cases, usually the result of lymphocytic thyroiditis or idiopathic thyroid atrophy.

Hypothyroidism is particularly a risk for middle-aged dogs, 4 to 10 years of age, of mid-size to large breeds. The golden retriever, Doberman pinscher, Irish setter, miniature schnauzer, dachshund, cocker spaniel, Airedale terrier, Great Dane, and Old English sheepdog are especially susceptible. German shepherd dogs and mongrels have a relatively low risk.

TYPICAL MANIFESTATIONS

Severe primary hypothyroidism affects practically every organ of the body and is easily recognized. Common clinical signs are alopecia with or without hyperpigmentation, physical lethargy, mental dullness, dry flaky haircoat, cold intolerance, slow heart rate, infertility, constipation, and weight gain. Myxedema of the skin may be evident on the head, particularly over the eyes. Laboratory findings often include hypercholesterolemia, hypertriglyceridemia, and normochromic normocytic anemia. Serum creatine kinase (CK) is occasionally elevated. Oligospermia may occur in hypothyroid male dogs.

Not all dogs with hypothyroidism have classical clinical signs and laboratory findings. The first reason can be the presentation in an early developmental stage of the disease. The development of thyroid hormone deficiency of primary origin is slow and insidious. The clinical signs and laboratory findings of mild to moderate hypothyroidism are nonspecific. They are mild and incomplete manifestations of the complete spectrum of problems that occur with severe hypothyroidism.

The second reason for atypical manifestations of hypothyroidism is idiopathic. In some animals atypical manifestations may be the result of an individual variation in the location and number of thyroid hormone receptors or a variation among cells in the intracellular action of thyroid hormones. In other animals common manifestations may have gone unnoticed until a sign of severe hypothyroidism, not typically seen, is the presenting complaint.

UNUSUAL MANIFESTATIONS

Myopathy and Neuropathy

Severe hypothyroidism can cause pseudomyotonia and profound muscle weakness. Some dogs exhibit slow, stiff locomotion described by owners as muscle cramps. Affected dogs usually have elevated serum CK values and hypercholesterolemia. Other, more characteristic signs of hypothyroidism are present but may be overshadowed by the degree of muscular weakness.

The most common finding in affected dogs is a metabolic dysfunction in type II fibers leading to type II fiber atrophy (Braund et al., 1981) However, myopathic findings in dogs with hypothyroidism and neuromuscular abnormalities are inconsistent and vary with the severity of hormone deficiency. Additional findings can be bizarre high frequency discharges on electromyography and a type I myofiber atrophy with an excessive accumulation of glycogen in type I fibers (Indrieri et al., 1987).

Dogs with hypothyroidism occasionally have central or peripheral nerve disturbances. The clinical signs can be dragging of the front feet, hearing impairment, head tilt, circling, or nystagmus. Electromyography may reveal fibrillation potentials and positive sharp waves. Motor nerve velocity can be slowed. Lesions in affected dogs include segmental demyelination, peripheral nerve entrapment from myxedema in surrounding soft tissue, and central nervous system (CNS) vascular accidents resulting from atherosclerosis (Bichsel et al., 1988).

Impaired Mental State

An impaired mental state resulting from associated atherosclerosis, cerebral myxedema, or a hypothalamic or hypophyseal tumor can be a presenting sign of hypothyroidism. Atherosclerosis can lead to cerebral infarction, seizures, disorientation, coma, circling to one side, head tilt, and amaurosis (Liu et al., 1986). Moderate to severe atherosclerosis has been observed in related hypothyroid beagles and sporadically in other breeds. Serum triglycerides are generally elevated and serum-cholesterol levels usually exceed 400 mg/dl. Other effects of atherosclerosis such as hypertension, retinopathy, and renal failure may also be present.

The most dangerous sequela of severe hypothyroidism is myxedema coma. Most recognized cases have involved Doberman pinschers (Kelly and Hill, 1984). Associated mortalities are high. Severe hypothyroidism can cause an obtunded mental state, stupor, and then coma. Myxedema coma is further characterized by hypothermia, usually without shivering; hypoventilation; hypotension; and bradycardia, in addition to signs of classic hypothyroidism such as alopecia or seborrhea. Laboratory findings may include hypoxia, hypercarbia, dilutional hyponatremia, hypocortisolemia, and hypoglycemia.

Precipitating factors of myxedema coma are respiratory depressant drugs, infectious diseases (especially respiratory), heart failure, decreased blood volume (diuretics or vasodilators), and exposure to a cold environment.

The treatment of myxedema stupor or coma must begin before the results of measuring serum tetraiodothyronine (T_4) levels are received. Treatment consists of intravenous L-thyroxine, mechanical respiratory support, intravenous administration of glucocorticoids, broad-spectrum antibiotics, and passive rewarming with blankets. If thyroxine for injection is not available, L-thyroxine can be dissolved in tap water and administered by gastric tube. Fluid administration, respiratory depressant drugs, diuretics, vasopressors, and active attempts to warm should be avoided or used sparingly with caution until L-thyroxine has been administered and a response noted.

Hypothalamic or hypophyseal tumors can cause tertiary or secondary hypothyroidism, respectively. An altered mental state caused by intracranial compression can accompany or overshadow signs of hypothyroidism in such cases.

Stunted Growth

Thyroid hormones are essential for normal musculoskeletal growth. Untreated congenital or juvenile-onset hypothyroidism will result in stunted physical growth.

Most dogs with congenital hypothyroidism probably die before weaning. The two most common causes include thyroid dysgenesis and dyshormonogenesis. Other forms of dyshormonogenesis, serum transport abnormalities, congenital thyroid-stimulating hormone (TSH) deficiency, goitrogens, and severe iodine deficiency are also possible causes. If the condition is mild or the puppy is reared by hand, it can survive.

Goitrous congenital cretinism has been reported in a German shepherd dog and St. Bernard crossbred pup. Nongoitrous congenital cretinism from apparent thyroidal dysgenesis has been reported in a German shepherd dog and Alaskan malamute crossbred pup and Scottish deerhounds. Nongoitrous congenital or juvenile cretinism from unestablished causes has also been reported in a bull mastiff and in giant schnauzers.

Clinical signs may go unnoticed until the period after weaning, when impaired growth and maturation of the skeletal and nervous systems become obvious. Severe congenital hypothyroidism causes short-legged dwarfism and subnormal mentality. Other physical signs can include short-broad skull, shortened mandible, protruding tongue, lateral strabismus, exophthalmus, alopecia, hypothermia, bradycardia, muscular weakness, delayed dental eruption, and (depending on the cause) goiter.

Suggestive laboratory findings can include hypercholesterolemia, nonregenerative anemia, elevated serum CK levels, impaired secretion of growth hormone, and hypoglycemia. Thyroid dysgenesis is made evident by abnormal findings in a thyroid scan. A defect in organification is substantiated by abnormal findings in a perchlorate discharge test.

Radiographic evidence of epiphyseal dysgenesis (ragged epiphyses with few foci of calcification) is pathognomonic for congenital hypothyroidism. Other radiographic findings include delayed epiphyseal closure, shortened vertebral bodies, deformities of the open cranial suture joints, kyphosis, and degenerative arthritis.

Although administration of thyroid hormones can promote significant physical growth after prolonged cretinism, treatment must be begun in the first few weeks of life to preserve normal intelligence and behavior.

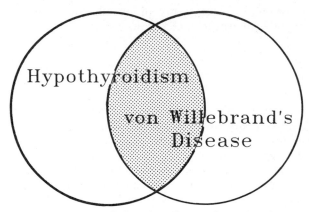

Figure 1. Dogs with hypothyroidism and von Willebrand's disease can have both diseases concurrently. Those that do (shown in the overlapping shaded area) have an increased risk for severe bleeding and will benefit from thyroid hormone supplementation.

Bleeding

A relationship between bleeding tendencies, particularly von Willebrand's disease (vWD), and hypothyroidism has been proposed. Thyroxine amplifies the production of factor VIII and factor VIII-related antigen. Laboratory changes that resemble vWD can occur in hypothyroidism in man, but bleeding is mild (Dalton et al., 1987). However, untreated hypothyroidism can make vWD more severe, perhaps by converting a subclinical bleeding tendency into a clinical problem. Most of the canine breeds at high risk for hypothyroidism are also at high risk for vWD, so that hypothyroidism concurrent with vWD is not surprising. However, most hypothyroid dogs do not have a clinical bleeding tendency, and not all dogs with vWD are hypothyroid (Fig. 1). Those that are not hypothyroid should *not* be given thyroid hormone for vWD because the detrimental effects of unnecessary thyroid hormone administration are too serious in euthyroid dogs and because it is an unnecessary expense for the owner.

Other Signs of Endocrinopathy

Other endocrine gland dysfunctions concurrent with hypothyroidism can mask the presence of hypothyroidism (Table 1). For example, in myxedema coma there can be impaired secretion of adrenocorticotropic hormone (secondary hypoadrenocorticism) and enhanced secretion of antidiuretic hormone (SIADH—the syndrome of inappropriate ADH).

INAPPROPRIATE GALACTORRHEA AND ANESTRUS

Hyperprolactinemia apparently occurs in dogs with severe hypothyroidism and is likely caused by an excess of thyrotropin-releasing hormone (TRH) and deficient concentrations of hypothalamic dopamine as documented in human patients. The resulting hyperprolactinemia may cause inappropriate galactorrhea, consisting of a serous, milky, or hemorrhage-like discharge from the nipples in at least 25% of hypothyroid, sexually intact bitches. Galactorrhea induced by hypothyroidism depends on the mammae's being previously primed for lactation. This phenomenon must be differentiated from other possible causes of galactorrhea, particularly pregnancy, pseudocyesis, and mammary trauma.

Hyperprolactinemia may also be at least partially responsible for infertility in dogs with severe hypothyroidism. Prolactin may interfere with gonadotropin-releasing hormone (GnRH) or directly interfere with gonadal production of steroids.

SECONDARY AND TERTIARY HYPOTHYROIDISM

Secondary and tertiary hypothyroidism are rare in dogs. In juvenile dogs, secondary hypothyroidism can result from a cystic Rathke's pouch, producing compression of the hypophysis. Pituitary dwarfism from cystic Rathke's pouch is inheritable in German shepherd dogs and Carelian bear-dogs. Congenital secondary or tertiary hypothyroidism has been reported in giant schnauzers. In adult dogs, secondary hypothyroidism is usually caused by adenohypophyseal adenomas.

Clinical signs of secondary hypothyroidism in juvenile dogs may be accompanied by multiple adenohypophyseal hormone deficiencies. Growth hormone deficiency is always concurrent and is due to compression of the hypophysis or is secondary to the deficiency of thyroxine's required permissive effect on growth hormone secretion, or both. Hypophyseal compression from enlarging cysts may cause secondary hypogonadism or secondary hypoadrenocorticism.

Clinical signs suggestive of adult-onset canine secondary hypothyroidism are indications of hypothyroidism concomitant with signs of intracranial disease. Adenohypophyseal hormone deficiencies, in addition to TSH deficiency and progressive neurologic abnormalities, are to be expected. Clinical signs may include stumbling, head pressing, brady-

Table 1. *Other Endocrine Diseases Present in Some Hypothyroid Dogs*

Addison's-like disease
Syndrome of inappropriate antidiuretic hormone
Hyperprolactinemia
Diabetes mellitus
Hypoparathyroidism

cardia, episodic blindness, and behavioral changes, in addition to signs of mild hypothyroidism. Suggestive laboratory abnormalities are hypercholesterolemia or hyposthenuria (diabetes insipidus).

The diagnosis of secondary or tertiary hypothyroidism can be confirmed by showing the lack of colloid vacuoles in biopsies of the thyroid, along with radiographic or computed tomography (CT) evidence of adenohypophyseal enlargement. Typically, baseline serum T_4 levels are low and become normal or near normal after 3 to 8 days of injections of thyroid-stimulating hormone. Images produced by thyroid scans will also increase in size following the administration of TSH for 3 days, if secondary or tertiary hypothyroidism is present. Repeated TSH injections in cases of primary hypothyroidism do not significantly alter serum T_4 levels or thyroid scan images.

AUTOIMMUNE POLYENDOCRINOPATHIES

Dogs with hypothyroidism caused by lymphocytic thyroiditis can concurrently develop hypoadrenocorticism, hypoparathyroidism, primary hypogonadism, or diabetes mellitus. These concurrent endocrinopathies often represent autoimmune (lymphocytic) destruction of multiple endocrine glands. Dogs with hypoadrenocorticism or diabetes mellitus have been reported to have a greater incidence of antithyroglobulin antibodies than the general canine population.

Hypothyroidism and hypoadrenocorticism have been reported in a dog with antibodies demonstrated against thyroid microsomes and adrenocortical cells (Bowen et al., 1986). This is identical to type II autoimmune polyglandular syndrome of humans (Schmidt's syndrome).

QUESTIONABLE MANIFESTATIONS OF HYPOTHYROIDISM

Physical findings are important initial clues to the possibility of hypothyroidism. Some, such as hypothermia without shivering, have a relatively reliable association with hypothyroidism. Some other physical abnormalities that have become linked with hypothyroidism have an as yet unsubstantiated or a refuted association with thyroid disease (Table 2). Often, the reason for these questionable associations is confusion between hypothyroidism and physiologic adaptations to illness or starvation (the euthyroid sick syndrome).

The myth that obesity is often caused by hypothyroidism dies hard. Although 60% of hypothyroid dogs have been reported to have weight gain or obesity, weight gain and obesity are not synonymous. Obesity is a body weight that is 15% or more

Table 2. *Physical Abnormalities with a Questionable Association with Hypothyroidism*

> Obesity
> Horner's syndrome
> Facial paralysis
> Megaesophagus
> Laryngeal paralysis
> Dilated cardiomyopathy
> Diarrhea

above the optimum range. Modest weight gains do occur with hypothyroidism, but hypothyroidism is not a common cause of obesity. The incidence of obesity in the general population of pet dogs in affluent societies is 25%, or more. The incidence of hypothyroidism is less than 1% (see this volume, p. 313). Furthermore, the incidence of obesity in hypothyroid dogs does not exceed the incidence of obesity in the general population.

Since hypothyroidism can cause neuropathies and myopathies, hypothyroidism has been associated with the development of certain neuromuscular disease syndromes, including Horner's syndrome, facial paralysis, megaesophagus, and laryngeal paralysis. It has also been associated with dilated cardiomyopathy. However, when a TSH stimulation test has been used as the criterion for diagnosis, no relationship has been demonstrated between hypothyroidism and Horner's syndrome or facial paralysis (Kern et al., 1989). No data have been presented to support the proposal that megaesophagus is associated with hypothyroidism. Although some dogs with laryngeal paralysis evaluated by TSH stimulation have been interpreted as having hypothyroidism, hypothyroidism has not been established as a triggering factor. In some Doberman pinschers with dilated cardiomyopathy, baseline serum T_4 levels are abnormally low; however, most have had normal responses to TSH stimulation.

Hypothyroidism can cause constipation due to decreased electrical and motor activity of the digestive tract. There is no explanation why diarrhea could occur from hypothyroidism, but diarrhea is a potential cause for euthyroid sick syndrome.

References and Suggested Reading

Bichsel, P., Jacobs, G., and Oliver, J. E.: Neurologic manifestations associated with hypothyroidism in four dogs. J.A.V.M.A. 192:1745, 1988.
Four hypothyroid dogs are described with neurologic deficits caused by apparent segmental demyelination, axonopathy, or atherosclerotic vascular disease.
Bowen, D., Schaer, M., and Riley, W.: Autoimmune polyglandular syndrome in a dog: A case report. J. Am. Anim. Hosp. Assoc. 22:649, 1986.
A nine-year-old, neutered female weimaraner presented in myxedema stupor and having autoimmune thyroiditis and adrenalitis is described.

Braund, K. G., Dillon, A. R., August, J. R., et al.: Hypothyroid myopathy in two dogs. Vet. Pathol. 18:589, 1981.
Two dogs, plus two more in an addendum, with hypothyroid myopathy were studied with histologic, histochemical, and morphometric techniques.

Buckrell, B. C., and Johnson, W.: Anestrus and spontaneous galactorrhea in a hypothyroid bitch. Can. Vet. J. 27:204, 1986.
A 30-month-old Chesapeake Bay retriever with hypothyroid-induced anestrus and galactorrhea is described and compared with previous reports.

Chastain, C. B., and Ganjam, V. K.: *Clinical Endocrinology of Companion Animals.* Philadelphia: Lea & Febiger, 1986, p. 135.
Chapter on hypothyroidism reviews all aspects of hypothyroidism in dogs, including unusual manifestations.

Dalton, R. G., Dewar, M. S., Savidge, G. F., et al.: Hypothyroidism as a cause of acquired von Willebrand's disease. Lancet 1:1007, 1987.
Laboratory changes that resemble spontaneous von Willebrand's disease in man can occur from hypothyroidism, but bleeding is rare.

Indrieri, R. J., Whalen, L. R., Cardinet, G. H., et al.: Neuromuscular abnormalities associated with hypothyroidism and lymphocytic thyroiditis in three dogs. J.A.V.M.A. 190:544, 1987.
Electrophysiologic, serum biochemical, and muscle biopsy findings in three hypothyroid dogs are reported.

Kelly, M. J., and Hill, J. R.: Canine myxedema coma and stupor. Comp. Cont. Ed. Pract. Vet. 6:1049, 1984.
Two Doberman pinscher dogs with myxedema coma or stupor are described and compared with previous reports.

Kern, T. J., Aromando, M. C., and Erb, H. N.: Horner's syndrome in dogs and cats: 100 cases (1975–1985). J.A.V.M.A. 195:369, 1989.
When a TSH stimulation test was used as the criterion for diagnosis of hypothyroidism, there was not a relationship between hypothyroidism and Horner's syndrome.

Liu, S., Tilley, L. P., Tappe, J. P., et al.: Clinical and pathologic findings in dogs with atherosclerosis: 21 cases (1970–1983). J.A.V.M.A. 189:227, 1986.
At least five of 21 dogs with atherosclerosis had hypothyroidism and neurologic deficits caused, at least in part, by cerebral infarction.

OCCULT HYPERTHYROIDISM IN CATS

THOMAS K. GRAVES
Columbus, Ohio

and MARK E. PETERSON
New York, New York

Recent advances in diagnostic testing for hyperthyroidism in cats have made it possible for veterinarians to confirm a diagnosis much earlier in the course of the disease than was previously possible (Graves and Peterson, 1990). The appearance of mild clinical signs of hyperthyroidism in the face of normal or equivocally abnormal basal serum thyroid hormone concentrations can be referred to as occult hyperthyroidism. Clinical signs of this condition are often subtle, but most cats should be treated before more severe signs develop, thus avoiding the complications (e.g., cardiac disease) caused by inevitable progression of disease. Traditional treatment regimens for hyperthyroidism in cats include administration of antithyroid drugs, surgical thyroidectomy, and radioiodine therapy (Peterson, 1989). While each of these therapeutic modalities may be of use in the treatment of occult hyperthyroidism, traditional regimens should be re-evaluated and modified to fit the severity of the disease.

DIAGNOSIS OF OCCULT HYPERTHYROIDISM

Basal Total Thyroid Hormone Determinations

The finding of high serum concentrations of total thyroxine (T_4) or triiodothyronine (T_3) is strong evidence in support of a diagnosis of hyperthyroidism in cats. We have demonstrated, however, that serum concentrations of T_4 and T_3 can fluctuate in and out of the normal range over a period of days in some cats with mild or even moderate hyperthyroidism (Peterson et al., 1987). This fluctuation may explain the finding of normal or high normal serum concentrations of T_4 and T_3 in some cats with clinical hyperthyroidism. Therefore, it is advisable to repeat the basal T_4 determination when a single normal or high normal test result is found in a cat suspected of having hyperthyroidism. Since there is greater variation over a period of days than over a period of hours, we suggest that a second serum T_4 determination be made 1 to 2 weeks later. If the result is again in the normal to high normal range, a T_3 suppression test or thyrotropin-releasing hormone (TRH) stimulation test is recommended.

Triiodothyronine (T_3) Suppression Test

Thyroid suppression testing has been used for many years to evaluate human patients in whom a diagnosis of hyperthyroidism could not be established with simpler tests such as basal serum T_4 and T_3 determinations. Inhibition of pituitary thyroid-stimulating hormone (TSH) secretion by high circulating concentrations of thyroid hormone is a characteristic feature of normal pituitary-thyroid regulation. Normally, administration of thyroid hormone decreases pituitary secretion of TSH, which results in reduced endogenous thyroid secretion; this can be detected by a fall in the percent thyroid radioiodine (^{131}I or ^{123}I) uptake value or, when exogenous T_3 is given, a decrease in serum T_4 concentrations. In contrast, when thyroid function is autonomous, that is, relatively independent of normal TSH secretion, administration of thyroid hormone has little or no effect on thyroid function, because TSH secretion has already been suppressed to a great extent. This is invariably true when clinical hyperthyroidism is present, whatever the cause.

Methods of determining radioactive iodine uptake and assays for TSH are not readily available for use in cats. Serum T_4 and T_3 assays are widely available, however, and we have developed a protocol for a T_3 suppression test in cats in which serum thyroid hormone concentrations alone are determined (Peterson et al., 1990). To perform the T_3 suppression test in cats, a blood sample is drawn for determination of basal serum concentrations of total T_4 and T_3. This blood sample should be centrifuged and the serum removed and kept refrigerated or frozen. The owners are instructed to administer T_3 orally (liothyronine; Cytomel, Smith Kline & French Laboratories) on the following morning at a dosage of 25 μg three times daily for 2 days. On the morning of the third day, a seventh 25-μg dose of liothyronine is given, and the cat is returned to the veterinary clinic for blood sampling (for serum T_4 and T_3 determinations) 2 to 4 hours after drug administration. Both the basal (day 1) and post-liothyronine serum samples should be submitted to the laboratory together to eliminate the effect of interassay variation in hormone concentrations.

When the T_3 suppression test is performed in normal cats, there is a marked fall in serum T_4 concentrations after exogenous T_3 administration. In contrast, when the test is performed on cats with hyperthyroidism, even on cats with only slightly high or high normal resting serum T_4 concentrations, minimal, if any, suppression of serum T_4 concentrations is seen. In our study of 77 cats with hyperthyroidism and 66 cats that were either clinically normal or had a variety of nonthyroidal diseases, we found that the post-liothyronine serum T_4 values were most valuable in distinguishing between the two groups of cats (Peterson et al., 1990). All of the hyperthyroid cats had post-liothyronine T_4 concentrations of greater than 20 nmol/L (approximately 1.5 μg/dl), whereas the post-liothyronine T_4 concentrations in the nonhyperthyroid cats were all below 20 nmol/L. Serum T_3 concentrations, as part of the T_3 suppression test, are not useful in the diagnosis of hyperthyroidism per se. However, these pre- and post-liothyronine serum T_3 determinations can be used to monitor owner compliance in giving the drug. In our study, serum T_3 increased in both normal cats and cats with hyperthyroidism after administration of liothyronine. If inadequate T_4 suppression is found, but serum T_3 values do not increase after treatment with liothyronine, problems with owner compliance should be suspected and the test result considered questionable. Failure to measure serum T_3 concentrations in such a situation could result in the erroneous diagnosis of hyperthyroidism. This reliance on owner compliance in giving liothyronine and on the willingness of the cat to swallow the pill may be the main disadvantage of the T_3 suppression test for use in cats.

Thyrotropin-Releasing Hormone (TRH) Stimulation Test

Over the last few years, the thyrotropin-releasing hormone (TRH) stimulation test has been widely used as a means of diagnosing hyperthyroidism in humans and has generally replaced the T_3 suppression test. This is a provocative test of the hypothalamic-pituitary axis and involves administration of exogenous TRH. In clinically normal subjects, intravenous administration of TRH is followed by a prompt increase in serum TSH concentrations within 15 to 30 minutes, whereas the TSH response to TRH is blunted or totally absent in patients with hyperthyroidism. The reason for the lack of response is again the fact that TSH secretion is chronically suppressed to a great extent in patients with hyperthyroidism.

Unfortunately, a valid homologous TSH assay for use in cats is not yet available; therefore, application of the TRH stimulation test in cats requires measurement of serum T_4 concentrations, a less sensitive means of assessing the pituitary-thyroid axis after TRH administration. However, the serum T_4 response to TRH stimulation clearly differentiates most normal cats from cats with mild hyperthyroidism. In normal cats, intravenous administration of TRH at the dosage of 0.1 mg/kg generally causes a twofold or greater increase in serum T_4 concentrations over basal values at 4 hours. In contrast, serum T_4 concentrations in cats with mild hyperthyroidism generally increase little, if at all, after administration of TRH. In the 21 cats with hyperthyroidism we have tested, only one had a serum T_4 increase of greater than 60%, the lower limit of normal response (Peterson, 1991). Serum T_3 determinations are less helpful in separating normal from hyperthyroid cats, because of the greater variability in both groups.

The advantages of the TRH response test over the T_3 suppression test include the shorter time needed to perform the test (4 hours versus 3 days) and the fact that the TRH test is not dependent on the owner's ability to administer oral medication. The major disadvantage of the TRH stimulation test in cats is that transient side effects (e.g., salivation, vomiting, tachypnea, and defecation) almost invariably occur immediately after administration of the TRH (Peterson, 1991). Further studies need to be done to confirm the ability of the TRH test to reliably differentiate normal cats and cats with nonthyroidal diseases from cats with mild hyperthyroidism.

TREATMENT OF OCCULT HYPERTHYROIDISM

When managing a cat with confirmed occult hyperthyroidism, one must first decide whether or not to treat the condition. If a cat has noticeable clinical signs of the disease (e.g., weight loss and hyperexcitability), some form of treatment should be initiated. On the other hand, if clinical signs are very mild or if none have been noticed by the owner, one may elect to delay treatment until the disease progresses. In such cases, close observation and monitoring by both owner and veterinarian is recommended, with complete physical examinations performed (body weight and heart rate recorded) and serum T_4 concentrations repeated at 3-month intervals.

In addition to the severity of hyperthyroidism, factors such as the age of the cat, concurrent disease, economic constraints of the client, and availability of facilities all enter into the decision and determine not only whether or not to treat but which form of treatment should be used. For example, it is probably not advisable to treat occult hyperthyroidism in an old cat with concurrent nonthyroidal disease (e.g., chronic renal failure). Such a cat will likely succumb to the effects of the concurrent nonthyroidal disease before the hyperthyroidism becomes life-threatening. If one does decide that treatment of hyperthyroidism is needed in a cat with concurrent disease, a conservative approach is generally recommended (i.e., antithyroid drug medical treatment), at least initially. On the other hand, a young or middle-aged cat with mild hyperthyroidism that is in relatively good health and free from nonthyroidal disease is best treated definitively (i.e., with surgery or radioactive iodine) early in the course of disease before serious complications associated with chronic hyperthyroidism, such as heart failure, develop.

Antithyroid Drugs

Antithyroid drugs are useful in preparing cats for thyroidectomy and in the long-term treatment of hyperthyroidism. These drugs block thyroid hormone synthesis but do not cure the underlying disease, because they do not destroy adenomatous thyroid tissue. Methimazole (Tapazole, Eli Lily) in the United States and carbimazole (Neo-Mercazole, Nicholas) in Europe are the antithyroid drugs of choice for treatment of hyperthyroidism (see this volume, p. 338). These drugs are relatively inexpensive and are effective in lowering circulating thyroid hormone concentrations in cats. However, treatment has been associated with a number of side effects, mostly transient, including vomiting, anorexia, lethargy, and various blood dyscrasias (Peterson et al., 1988). The most common reason for failure of long-term treatment with antithyroid drugs is a lapse in owner compliance in administering the drug or unwillingness of the cat to take it.

In cats with occult hyperthyroidism, chronic use of antithyroid drugs is recommended primarily in old cats and cats that have one or more nonthyroidal diseases. We do not generally recommend treatment in young cats or cats that do not have obvious clinical signs of hyperthyroidism, since the drugs do not cure the disease. The goal of drug therapy in cats with occult hyperthyroidism is to lower serum thyroid hormone concentrations into the low normal range (i.e., 10 to 25 nmol/L). This can usually be accomplished with relatively low doses of methimazole (or carbimazole), i.e., 5 to 7.5 mg/day administered in single or divided doses. Serum T_4 concentrations should be determined at 2- to 3-week intervals during initial treatment and the dosage of the antithyroid drug adjusted to achieve the desired concentration of circulating thyroid hormone. In addition, we recommend that complete blood counts (including platelet counts) be monitored every 2 to 3 weeks during the first 3 months of drug therapy.

Surgical Thyroidectomy

The use of surgical thyroidectomy as a treatment for occult hyperthyroidism presents advantages as well as problems. One advantage is that this mode of treatment is usually curative. The surgery itself is relatively simple in the hands of an experienced surgeon and is associated with few side effects or complications. The most serious complication is postoperative hypocalcemia due to damage or removal of the parathyroid glands; this is obviously a danger only when a bilateral thyroidectomy is performed.

Because cats with occult hyperthyroidism have mild disease, preoperative preparation with an antithyroid drug or beta-adrenergic blocking agent (e.g., propranolol) is less important than in cats with moderate to severe hyperthyroidism. Nevertheless, we still recommend preoperative preparation for 1 to 2 weeks to decrease the cardiac and metabolic complications associated with hyperthyroidism, at least in cats that can be given medication orally.

Surgical thyroidectomy in cats with occult hyperthyroidism may be problematic. In general, cats with occult hyperthyroidism have smaller adenomatous thyroid glands than do cats with more overt disease, making it difficult to visually distinguish between a normal and adenomatous thyroid tissue. In cats with both lobes involved, one lobe may be obviously large and the other lobe only slightly large and easily mistaken as normal. Preoperative thyroid imaging is helpful in defining the extent of thyroid lobe involvement in these cases, but thyroid imaging is not readily available to many private practitioners. If thyroid imaging is not feasible, we recommend removal of the obviously large thyroid lobe with preservation of the associated external parathyroid gland in all cats with suspected unilateral thyroid gland involvement.

It can also be more difficult to identify, and therefore preserve, the external parathyroid glands in cats with mild hyperthyroidism compared with cats with more severe hyperthyroidism. The primary reason for this is that the external parathyroid glands tend to be embedded (and therefore hidden) in adipose tissue, because these cats do not have the extent of weight loss that generally develops with more severe hyperthyroidism.

Because of these difficulties, one may elect to use antithyroid drugs to control thyroid hormone concentrations and allow the thyroid tissue to gradually enlarge before surgery is considered. Again, antithyroid drugs, while they interfere with thyroid hormone synthesis, will not stop the progressive growth of adenomatous thyroid gland tissue.

Radioiodine Therapy

As in overt hyperthyroidism, radioiodine therapy is a good option for treating occult hyperthyroidism in many cats, especially younger cats without associated nonthyroidal disease. None of the disadvantages of surgery in cats with overt hyperthyroidism pertain to the use of radioiodine. If the disease is treated in its early, mild stages, it can usually be cured with a single injection of a relatively small dose, often less than 3 mCi, of ^{131}I. With this treatment modality anesthesia is not required, but a period of hospitalization is (generally less than 2 weeks). Again, as with surgery, this form of treatment may not be appropriate in old cats with concurrent nonthyroidal disease. Also, radioiodine therapy is less widely available than the other treatment modalities.

References and Suggested Reading

Graves, T. K., and Peterson, M. E.: Diagnosis of occult hyperthyroidism in cats. *In Problems in Veterinary Medicine—Endocrinology.* Philadelphia: J. B. Lippincott, 1990, pp. 683–692.
A review of tests useful for diagnosis of cats with early mild hyperthyroidism.

Peterson, M. E.: Treatment of feline hyperthyroidism. *In Kirk RW (ed.): Current Veterinary Therapy X.* Philadelphia: W. B. Saunders, 1989, pp. 1002–1008.
A review of treatment options available for hyperthyroidism in cats.

Peterson, M. E.: Use of a thyrotropin-releasing hormone (TRH) stimulation test as an aid in the diagnosis of mild hyperthyroidism in cats. J. Vet. Intern. Med. 5:129, 1991 (abstract).
Study of the evaluation of a TRH stimulation test for diagnosis of cats with occult hyperthyroidism.

Peterson, M. E., Graves, T. K., and Cavanagh, I.: Serum thyroid hormone concentrations fluctuate in cats with hyperthyroidism. J. Vet. Intern. Med. 1:142–146, 1987.
This study documents that considerable fluctuation in serum T_4 and T_3 concentrations can occur over a period of days in cats with hyperthyroidism.

Peterson, M. E., Graves, T. K., and Gamble, D. A.: Triiodothyronine (T_3) suppression test: An aid in the diagnosis of mild hyperthyroidism in cats. J. Vet. Intern. Med. 4:233–238, 1990.
Study of the evaluation of a T_3 suppression test for diagnosis of cats with occult hyperthyroidism.

Peterson, M. E., Kintzer, P. P., and Hurvitz, A. H.: Methimazole treatment of 262 cats with hyperthyroidism. J. Vet. Intern. Med. 2:150–157, 1988.
A large study that evaluated the efficacy and safety of methimazole in cats with hyperthyroidism.

MEDICAL MANAGEMENT OF FELINE HYPERTHYROIDISM

KEITH L. THODAY
and CARMEL T. MOONEY
Edinburgh, Scotland

Since its first description in 1979, hyperthyroidism (thyrotoxicosis) has emerged as the most common endocrine disorder of the domestic cat. The usual cause is functional adenomatous hyperplasia (or adenoma), a benign change involving thyroid tissue. Functional thyroid carcinoma is the cause of feline hyperthyroidism in only 1 to 2% of cases. The condition, therefore, carries a favorable prognosis with effective therapy.

The treatment of feline hyperthyroidism is directed at controlling the excessive production of the metabolically active thyroid hormones L-thyroxine (T_4) and L-triiodothyronine (T_3). Spontaneous or drug-assisted remissions have not been described.

While antithyroid drugs may be used in the long term to manage feline hyperthyroidism, medical treatment is usually also essential to control the disorder in preparation for surgical thyroidectomy. With the exception of the beta-adrenoceptor blocking drugs, combining antithyroid medical therapy with radioactive iodine therapy appears to be contraindicated as antithyroid agents may reduce the radiosensitivity of thyroid tissue.

The use of antithyroid drugs in the long-term management of feline hyperthyroidism is becoming increasingly popular. Such treatment may be particularly recommended when unrelated medical conditions increase surgical risks, owners refuse surgery, and nuclear medicine facilities are unavailable. Long-term medical management has a number of advantages and disadvantages over surgical or radioiodine therapy. Advantages include the absence of perioperative complications, including life-threatening cardiac arrhythmias, hemorrhage, or laryngeal spasm, and postsurgical hypoparathyroidism, voice changes, Horner's syndrome, and permanent hypothyroidism. The drugs are inexpensive, and administration requires no advanced skills, training, or isolation facilities. However, chronic therapy requires daily drug administration and regular hematologic and biochemical determinations to ensure efficacy and monitoring for adverse reactions, with potential difficulties with owner compli-

The authors' investigations described in this article were supported by grants from the British Small Animal Veterinary Association's Clinical Studies Trust Fund.

338

Table 1. *Drugs Used in the Management of Hyperthyroidism*

Drug	Main Indications for Use
Thioureylenes	
Thioglyoxalines	
Methimazole	Preoperative preparation
Carbimazole	Long-term medical management
Pyrimidines	
*Propylthiouracil	
Stable iodine	
Iodine and potassium iodide (Lugol's solution)	Preoperative preparation (in combination with other agents)
Potassium iodide	
†Potassium iodate	
Beta-adrenoceptor blocking drugs	
Propranolol	Thyrotoxic crises
†Other related drugs	Preoperative preparation (in combination with other agents)
	Preparation for, and subsequent to, radioactive iodine therapy
	Intraoperative arrhythmias
Oral cholecystographic contrast media	
‡Calcium ipodate	Currently experimental
†Sodium ipodate	
Sedatives	
†Phenobarbital	Where sedation is required

*No longer recommended for clinical use.
†Use not yet reported in feline hyperthyroidism.
‡Use currently experimental in cats.

ance and cost. As medical management does not remove thyroid tissue, it should not be used alone to treat uncommon cases of hyperfunctional thyroid carcinoma.

A number of classes of pharmacologic agents may be employed in the management of feline hyperthyroidism. These and possible indications for their use are summarized in Table 1. Each agent has specific site(s) of action (Fig. 1), although these have generally been extrapolated from human and laboratory animal studies as such investigations in cats have yet to be reported. Currently, neither ipodate nor phenobarbital has been employed in the naturally occurring feline disease.

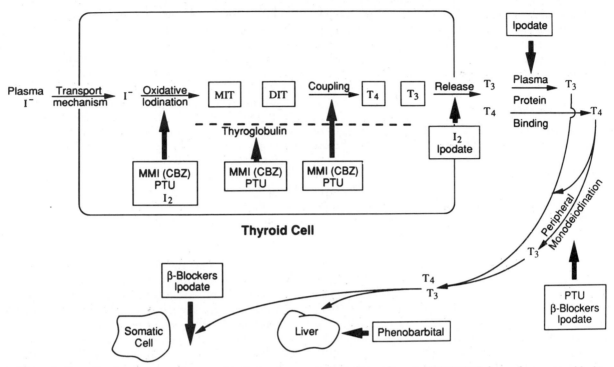

Figure 1. Sites of action of various drugs used in the management of hyperthyroidism. β-BLOCKERS: beta-adrenoceptor blocking drugs; CBZ: carbimazole; DIT: diiodotyrosine; I⁻: iodide; I₂: stable iodine; MIT: monoiodotyrosine; MMI: methimazole; PTU: propylthiouracil; T₃: L-triiodothyronine; T₄: L-thyroxine. (Modified from Solomon, D. H.: Treatment of Graves' hyperthyroidism. *In* Ingbar, S. H., and Braverman, L. E. (eds.): *Werner's The Thyroid. A Fundamental and Clinical Text,* 5th ed. Philadelphia: J. B. Lippincott, 1986, p. 988.)

CURRENT METHODS OF MANAGEMENT

Thioureylenes

The thionamides are a family of compounds that share antithyroid activity. Those used to manage feline hyperthyroidism are all thioureylenes, the currently recommended drugs being the thioglyoxalines methimazole (Tapazole, Eli Lilly) and carbimazole (Neo-Mercazole, Nicholas). Methimazole is available in the U.S.A and carbimazole in Europe, where they were respectively first synthesized and marketed. Propylthiouracil, a pyrimidine, is widely available and was the first thioureylene to be used in cats. However, because of the incidence of severe hematologic complications, it is no longer recommended for the management of feline hyperthyroidism.

MECHANISM OF ACTION

The thioureylenes are actively concentrated by the thyroid gland. Subsequently, they interfere with the synthesis of thyroid hormones by inhibition of thyroid peroxidase catalyzed reactions at various sites blocking the oxidation of iodide, the iodination of tyrosyl residues in thyroglobulin, and the coupling of mono or diiodotyrosines to form T_3 and T_4. In addition, they may further prevent the coupling reaction by binding to thyroglobulin, thereby altering its structure. The thioureylenes do not inhibit iodide transport and thus do not affect the thyroid gland's ability to trap iodide, nor do they block the release of preformed hormone. Methimazole and carbimazole, unlike propylthiouracil, do not inhibit the peripheral deiodination of T_4 to T_3.

METHIMAZOLE AND CARBIMAZOLE

Carbimazole was originally developed for use in human medicine with the intention of obtaining a drug with a duration of action longer than that of methimazole. Although carbimazole itself has inherent antithyroid activity *in vitro*, it was later found to be rapidly and completely converted to methimazole both *in vitro* (at alkaline pH and by serum contact) and *in vivo* such that only methimazole accumulates in the thyroid gland, by which it exerts its effects. On the basis of conversion of carbimazole to methimazole, the dose equivalent is 10 mg carbimazole to 6.1 mg methimazole. Nevertheless, in humans, carbimazole and methimazole are equally effective in 10 mg doses, which may reflect a less pronounced interindividual variation in absorption or, since the thyroid gland actively concentrates the thioglyoxalines, a similar intrathyroidal concentration of methimazole despite a lower plasma concentration after carbimazole administration (Marchant et al., 1978).

Therapeutic Indications

A 3-year evaluation of the efficacy and safety of methimazole in 262 cats has been reported (Peterson et al., 1988). We have investigated the use of carbimazole in a series of 47 thyrotoxic cats, for preoperative preparation in 39 and for long-term treatment in 8 cats. Overall, it is clear that carbimazole and methimazole can be considered the antithyroid drugs of choice both for preoperative and long-term medical management of feline hyperthyroidism.

PREOPERATIVE PREPARATION. Methimazole should initially be administered orally at a dosage of 10 to 15 mg/day in divided doses every 8 to 12 hours, according to the severity of the hyperthyroid state. At this dosage, serum T_4 concentrations decrease to within or below the reference range within 2 to 3 weeks of treatment in most cats, when serum T_4 concentrations and complete blood and platelet counts should be determined to monitor both efficacy and the possible development of adverse reactions. If only a marginal decrease in serum T_4 concentration results, the initial dosage should be gradually increased in 5 mg increments once lack of owner compliance or difficulties in administering the medication have been eliminated as a concern. A small number of cats with extremely elevated pretreatment serum T_4 concentrations and large thyroid nodules may require 25 to 30 mg/day together with a longer treatment period before achieving euthyroidism.

We have used carbimazole in 39 hospitalized cats in preparation for surgical thyroidectomy. In 34 cats given carbimazole at an oral dosage of 5 mg every 8 hours, carbimazole induced euthyroidism in 31 of the cats (91%) in 3 to 15 days (mean, 5.7 days). In three of these 34 cats (9%), this regimen had little effect on serum T_4 concentrations (one cat) or an initial decrease followed by apparent "resistance" (two). In humans, true resistance to methimazole or carbimazole effectively does not occur, and these cats might have responded to an increased dosage. In 5 cats in which the 15 mg daily dose was given in three divided doses within a 12-hour period, euthyroidism was produced in only one of the cats treated. The importance of regular 8 hourly doses of carbimazole during initial treatment is therefore stressed. Clinical evidence of euthyroidism tends to lag behind biochemical changes but is generally apparent after 2 weeks. Serum T_4 and T_3 concentrations are determined at this time to confirm euthyroidism.

Elevations in serum concentrations of alanine aminotransferase (ALT) and alkaline phosphatase (AP) commonly occur in feline hyperthyroidism. We have found that the concentrations of these enzymes decrease significantly as euthyroidism is achieved using carbimazole. The progressive decrease in AP and ALT concentrations may be used as a nonspecific indicator of therapeutic efficacy which may be measured in-house by many veterinary practitioners during the initial 2-week carbimazole treatment period.

When methimazole or carbimazole is administered preoperatively, surgery can be performed once the animal is euthyroid. However, currently, at the 2-week reinspection period, we dispense potassium iodide to be administered together with carbimazole, for a further 10 days prior to thyroidectomy to reduce the friability and vascularity of the thyroid gland (discussed later). In cases where serum T_4 concentrations are depressed below the reference range, the surgical risks do not appear to be increased. The transient effect of antithyroid drugs in blocking thyroid hormone synthesis necessitates administration of the drug on the morning of surgery.

LONG-TERM MEDICAL MANAGEMENT. Feline hyperthyroidism may be effectively managed by long-term use of the thioglyoxalines. Once euthyroidism is achieved with methimazole, the daily drug dosage should be reduced by 2.5 to 5 mg decrements and further determinations of serum T_4 concentrations carried out at 2- to 3-week intervals. The aim of therapy is to administer the lowest possible dosage that effectively maintains the serum T_4 concentration toward the low end of the reference range. Only a small minority of cases can be controlled using daily dosages between 2.5 and 5 mg, rarely are doses in excess of 15 mg/day required, and most cats are maintained on a daily dosage of 7.5 to 10 mg. Serum thyroid hormone concentrations should be determined at intervals of 3 months and the methimazole dosage adjusted accordingly.

Divided doses of methimazole, given every 8 or 12 hours, tend to be most effective in maintaining euthyroidism. In humans, the plasma half-life of methimazole is approximately 4 to 6 hours, but the intrathyroidal residence time (where the drug exerts its effect) is approximately 20 hours. Therefore, in cases where owners have difficulty in administering the drug two or three times daily, once daily dosing may be effective. The frequency of administration cannot be reduced further or the serum T_4 concentration will again increase into the thyrotoxic range.

Our experience with chronic carbimazole therapy in eight cats suggests that a consistent dose of 5 mg administered twice daily is necessary to maintain euthyroidism. Once daily dosing appears to be inadequate and may be related to the lower plasma concentration of methimazole achieved after carbimazole administration. The greatest problem associated with chronic treatment is poor owner compliance in regularly administering the drug. As with methimazole therapy, serum thyroid hormone concentrations and carbimazole dosage adjustments, where necessary, are carried out every 3 months.

Chronic treatment with methimazole or carbimazole may also result in serum T_4 concentrations below the reference range. Clinical signs suggestive of hypothyroidism (Thoday, 1990) have not been observed. The serum T_3 concentrations in these cases usually remain within the reference range. Since T_3 is the more metabolically active of the two hormones, the animal remains clinically euthyroid. In the face of a low serum T_4 concentration, there may be increased extrathyroidal production of T_3 from T_4 or preferential T_3 production by the thyroid gland itself. Normal serum T_3 concentrations probably prevent the development of clinical signs of hypothyroidism.

Adverse Effects

Side effects associated with thioglyoxaline administration tend to occur within the *first 3 months* of therapy. The most serious reactions are associated with hematologic abnormalities, and complete blood and platelet counts are therefore recommended every 2 to 3 weeks, at least for the first 3 months of treatment. Adverse reactions can potentially occur at any time after this period, but it is usually sufficient to monitor complete hematologic parameters only when they are suspected clinically.

Reported adverse effects of methimazole therapy are summarized in Table 2. Mild reactions develop in approximately 15% of cases (Peterson et al., 1988) and include anorexia, vomiting, and lethargy. These signs are transient and only rarely necessitate discontinuing the drug. Should self-induced excoriations of the head and neck occur, the drug should be stopped and glucocorticoids administered. Hepatic toxicity, suggestive of both hepatocellular and cholestatic abnormalities, and characterized by marked increases in serum concentrations of ALT, AP, and total bilirubin with associated anorexia, vomiting, and lethargy, is a rare complication. Clinical improvement results within days once the drug is discontinued. Rechallenge with the drug will induce recurrence of the signs.

Mild hematologic abnormalities also appear to be common with methimazole therapy, occurring in 16% of cases. These reactions, which include eosinophilia, lymphocytosis, and transient leukopenia with a normal differential count, are not associated with any clinical effects. More serious hematologic reactions develop in approximately 4% of cats and include thrombocytopenia (platelet count $< 75,000/mm^3$ [$< 75,000 \times 10^9/L$]) and agranulocytosis (severe leukopenia with a total granulocyte

Table 2. *Clinical Side Effects and Hematologic and Immunologic Abnormalities Associated with Methimazole Treatment in 262 Cats with Hyperthyroidism***

Sign	No. (%) of Cats	Time When Signs Develop (Days)	
		Range	*Median*
Anorexia	29 (11.1)	1–78	18.0
Vomiting	28 (10.7)	7–60	15.0
Lethargy	23 (8.8)	1–60	21.0
Excoriations	6 (2.3)	6–40	19.0
Bleeding	6 (2.3)	15–50	22.5
Hepatopathy	4 (1.5)	15–60	41.0
Thrombocytopenia	7 (2.7)	14–90	24.0
Agranulocytosis	4 (1.5)	26–95	62.5
Leukopenia	12 (4.7)	10–41	23.0
Eosinophilia	30 (11.3)	12–490	21.0
Lymphocytosis	19 (7.2)	14–90	18.5
Antinuclear antibodies†	52 (21.8)	10–870	46.0
Positive Coombs' test†	3 (1.9)	45–60	50.0

*Reprinted with permission from Peterson, M. E.: Treatment of feline hyperthyroidism. *In* Kirk, R. W. (ed.): *Current Veterinary Therapy X: Small Animal Practice.* Philadelphia: W.B. Saunders, 1989, p. 1003. Originally modified from data in Peterson, M. E., et al.: Methimazole treatment of 262 cats with hyperthyroidism. J. Vet. Intern. Med. 2:150, 1988.

†Antinuclear antibodies determined in 239 cats and direct antiglobulin (Coombs') tests performed in 160 cats.

count $< 250/mm^3$ [$< 250 \times 10^9/L$]). Concomitant thrombocytopenia and agranulocytosis may occur. Overt bleeding (epistaxis, oral hemorrhage) usually signals the development of thrombocytopenia, although occasionally this is noted on routine blood counts in the absence of clinical signs. Agranulocytosis predisposes to severe bacterial infection, pyrexia, and systemic toxicity. These reactions resolve within approximately 5 days once the drug is withdrawn and supportive therapy administered. Rechallenge with the drug induces the same reactions. Although a positive direct Coombs' test develops in a small number of treated cats, immune-mediated anemia, a common adverse reaction to propylthiouracil therapy, has not yet been described with methimazole.

A potentially serious complication is the development of serum antinuclear antibody (ANA). Approximately 50% of cats treated for longer than 6 months develop serum ANA, and most of these are receiving doses of 15 mg/day or more. Although clinical signs of a lupus-like syndrome have not been observed, the daily dosage should be reduced to the lowest one that maintains euthyroidism, when the ANA titer will become negative in most cats.

Adverse reactions associated with carbimazole therapy appear to be less common than with methimazole. Mild side effects (vomiting, with or without associated anorexia and depression, or hematologic evidence of lymphocytosis or leukopenia) develop in approximately 15% of cases, but withdrawal of the drug is not usually required. These reactions generally occur within the first 2 weeks of therapy. To date, serious adverse reactions have not been noted, although only a small number of cats have been treated chronically. However, adverse reactions in human patients are considered by many authors to occur less frequently with carbimazole than with methimazole. As the drugs are equipotent *in vivo*, this may reflect lower plasma methimazole concentrations after carbimazole therapy because the incidence of all types of adverse reaction in man are partially dose-related (Solomon, 1986). It is possible that carbimazole may prove to be a better tolerated drug than methimazole in cats. However, we still recommend complete blood and platelet counts every 2 weeks for the first 3 months of therapy and withdrawal of the drug should any serious adverse reactions be noted. Obviously, carbimazole should not be reintroduced nor methimazole be substituted, and an alternative form of therapy (surgery or radioactive iodine) should be sought. A further advantage of carbimazole, at least in humans, is that it is tasteless, whereas methimazole has a bitter taste.

Stable Iodine

MECHANISM OF ACTION

Stable iodine (^{127}I) was the earliest agent used effectively to treat human thyrotoxicosis. Large doses result in a dramatic decrease in the rate of thyroid hormone synthesis (the Wolff-Chaikoff effect), which may involve reduced peroxidase catalyzed organification of iodide. The rate of thyroid hormone release is also markedly reduced as a result of inhibition of thyroglobulin endocytosis, colloid accumulates in the follicular lumina, and the size of the follicular cells and the vascularity of the gland are decreased. However, the effects of stable iodine are inconsistent and short-lived, and escape from inhibition may occur. Thus, iodine should not be used as the sole method of therapy for feline thyrotoxicosis.

THERAPEUTIC INDICATIONS

Stable iodine may be administered orally as potassium iodide with or without iodine, or intravenously as sodium iodide. Oral iodine is generally given in aqueous solution (distilled water) either as a saturated solution of potassium iodide (SSKI; 100 gm potassium iodide per 100 ml solution, yielding a concentration of 50 mg iodide per drop), in dilute solution (SSKI diluted to produce 10 mg potassium iodide per ml), or as Lugol's solution (5 gm iodine

with 10 gm potassium iodide per 100 ml of solution, yielding a concentration of 6 mg iodine per drop).

Pharmaceutical preparations of both potassium iodide and iodine are currently unavailable in the UK and, where required, Analar grades of chemical reagents are used. However, potassium iodate (170 mg tablets yielding 100 mg free iodine; Cambridge Self-Care Diagnostics) is the currently preferred iodine preparation in human medicine in the UK because of its longer shelf-life. We have only early experience of its use in cats.

PREOPERATIVE PREPARATION

Iodine as the sole preoperative therapy for feline hyperthyroidism is contraindicated because of the potential for enrichment of hormone stores within the gland, with subsequent release and exacerbation of the clinical signs. Initially, methimazole or carbimazole should be used to induce euthyroidism with potassium iodide (30 to 100 mg/day in single or up to three equally divided doses) added for 10 to 14 days before surgery. Stable iodine may have additive effects with methimazole or carbimazole in lowering plasma thyroid hormone concentrations but, more important, it markedly reduces the vascularity and friability of the thyroid gland induced by the antithyroid drugs and adenomatous hyperplasia *per se*. The result is firmer and less hemorrhagic tissue, more easily manipulated at the time of surgery, and readily appreciated by palpation of the goiter before and at the conclusion of iodine administration. Iodine preparations should not be given for more than 14 days as these effects may subsequently be overriden. Potassium iodide may also be used in combination with propranolol in preparation for thyroidectomy, when administration of the two drugs may be begun simultaneously (discussed later).

ADVERSE EFFECTS

SSKI may cause salivation, lack of appetite, or anorexia, purportedly as a result of its unpleasant, brassy taste. This may be prevented by administering the solution in a gelatin capsule or, as is our usual procedure, by giving potassium iodide in dilute (10 mg/ml) solution.

Beta-Adrenoceptor Blocking Drugs

For many years, the similarity between the manifestations of sympathetic hyperactivity and hyperthyroidism has been evident to physicians. The development of the beta-adrenoceptor blocking group of drugs opened another chapter in the management of human hyperthyroidism. Only the use of propranolol (Inderal, ICI Pharmaceuticals) has been reported in the management of feline hyperthyroidism.

MECHANISM OF ACTION

The specific mechanism of action of the beta-adrenoceptor blocking drugs in ameliorating the signs of hyperthyroidism remains unclear. Currently, it is believed that an excess of thyroid hormones causes an increase in the number of beta-adrenoceptors and that many of the signs of hyperthyroidism are due to subsequently enhanced catecholamine action. Thyroid hormones do not change receptor affinity for beta-adrenoagonists or antagonists, and therefore, beta-adrenoceptor blocking drugs are highly effective in eliminating such actions (Solomon, 1986).

Propranolol is a nonselective $beta_1$- and $beta_2$-adrenoceptor blocking drug which effectively reverses the signs of feline hyperthyroidism. While it has no effect on the thyroid gland, like most other such drugs in humans, it inhibits the peripheral monodeiodination of T_4 to T_3. However, even with high dosage regimens, serum T_3 concentrations fall by only 30%, serum T_4 concentrations are usually unaffected, euthyroidism is not restored, and such effects are adjunctive to its other actions in hyperthyroidism. Propranolol does not alter the serum basal and post-thyrotropin (TSH) concentrations of T_4, T_3, and reverse triiodothyronine (rT_3) in healthy dogs (Center et al., 1984), but such studies have not been reported in cats.

THERAPEUTIC INDICATIONS

Propranolol results in the symptomatic control of many aspects of feline hyperthyroidism. It partially corrects the elevation in metabolic rate, heat intolerance and fever, and diarrhea and steatorrhea are reduced. Most obviously, many of the cardiovascular (tachycardia, prominent precordial impulse, and strength of the femoral pulse), respiratory (polypnea), and neurologic (increased activity, restlessness, irritability) manifestations of thyrotoxicosis are rapidly reversed.

Although propranolol has been used as the sole preoperative treatment for feline hyperthyroidism, this is far from ideal as symptomatic relief may be incomplete and plasma thyroid hormone concentrations remain elevated. Thus, propranolol should be restricted to an *adjunctive role* in combination with other agents where rapid control of the signs of hyperthyroidism is desirable before surgery or radioiodine therapy or, occasionally, used alone in cats that cannot tolerate other drug treatments. Its use in selected cases may significantly improve the management of the severely symptomatic patient and, in thyrotoxic crisis, may be life-saving.

PREOPERATIVE PREPARATION

Propranolol is *not* required for the preoperative preparation of most hyperthyroid cats. However, it may be given in conjunction with methimazole or carbimazole to promote symptomatic relief in severely thyrotoxic individuals until the patient reaches a euthyroid state.

Propranolol should be administered at an initial oral dosage of 2.5 mg every 8 hours for 3 days. If the resting heart rate does not decrease below 200 beats/minute and polypnea and excitability are not controlled, the 8 hourly dosage should be increased to 5.0 mg. This causes resolution of these signs in most hyperthyroid cats. However, in humans, there are great individual variations in the oral bioavailability of propranolol, and the plasma concentrations may vary by as much as 20-fold on the same dosage schedule. Therefore, consideration must be given to further increases in the doses of propranolol in cats in which symptoms do not resolve. As serum T_4 and T_3 concentrations return to their respective reference ranges as a result of the methimazole or carbimazole therapy, propranolol administration may be discontinued.

Recently, it has been reported that a combination of potassium iodide and propranolol is considerably more effective in inducing euthyroidism in humans with Graves' disease than either drug alone. A secondary rise or "escape" of thyroid hormones was seen in only 20% of patients. The authors suggested that there may be a previously unrecognized synergism between the drugs and that the combination may be the optimum preoperative preparation for thyrotoxic humans (Feek et al., 1980). We have carried out a preliminary investigation into this drug regimen in the preoperative preparation of six hyperthyroid cats using a combination of 10 mg aqueous potassium iodide and 2.5 mg propranolol, each administered orally three times daily for a minimum of 7 days. The treatment was effective in slowing the resting heart rate to below 200 beats/minute in all cases, decreasing serum T_4 and T_3 concentrations in five cats but into their respective reference ranges in only one. We are currently carrying out further studies to determine whether this may be an acceptable method of preoperative preparation of hyperthyroid cats.

Occasionally, propranolol is used alone for the preoperative management of hyperthyroidism. Its major advantage over other agents is the short time required for surgical preparation (although individuals remain hyperthyroid, a marked disadvantage), and it may be helpful where rapid thyroidectomy is required. Propranolol therapy also helps prevent arrhythmias, which may develop during anesthesia in animals not rendered euthyroid before surgery, and is thus of value in animals that cannot tolerate the thioglyoxalines. In these circumstances, it should be administered on the morning of, and for 2 to 3 days after, surgery to allow elevated plasma thyroid hormone concentrations to fall to reference or subreference ranges.

An additional beneficial action of propranolol is that, like iodine, it may decrease thyroid vascularity, facilitating surgical removal and diminishing operative blood loss.

Radioactive Iodine Therapy

Propranolol may also be used in conjunction with ^{131}I therapy of feline hyperthyroidism. In this situation, it provides pretreatment relief from the effects of thyrotoxicosis and from the effects of thyroid hormone release, which may be associated with radiation thyroiditis, should this complicate treatment. The latter may be of particular importance in animals with related or unrelated cardiac disease where the release of thyroid hormones is more likely to cause acute adverse effects. The dosage regimen for propranolol in association with radio-iodine therapy is as described earlier.

ADVERSE EFFECTS

The adverse effects of propranolol administration are of two types: those directly related to beta-adrenoceptor blockade, and idiosyncratic, idiopathic reactions.

Effects related to beta-adrenoceptor blockade include bronchospasm, decreased cardiac output and contractility, hypotension, bradyarrhythmias, and hypoglycemia. Propranolol therapy is, therefore, contraindicated in hyperthyroid cats with asthma or uncontrolled congestive cardiac failure. In the latter, even when cardiac function has been improved, propranolol should still be administered with caution because of its depressive effects on myocardial function. It should also be used with care in hyperthyroid cats with concurrent diabetes mellitus that are receiving insulin therapy. It should be noted that beta-adrenoceptor blocking drugs may also be deleterious during anesthetic emergencies and that some surgeons prefer to use these drugs only if intraoperative arrhythmias develop.

In humans, selective beta$_1$-adrenoceptor blocking drugs, e.g., atenolol (Tenormin, Stuart), which are less prone to cause adverse effects mediated by blockage of beta$_2$-adrenoceptors, are now used more frequently in the management of thyrotoxicosis. Atenolol has a longer duration of action, resulting in increased patient compliance. The use of selective beta$_1$-adrenoceptor blocking drugs has not been reported in the management of feline hyperthyroidism.

Idiosyncratic reactions to propranolol in humans (rash, fever, agranulocytosis, thrombocytopenia) are poorly documented in cats.

OTHER DRUGS AFFECTING THYROID FUNCTION

A number of other drugs are employed in primary and secondary roles in the management of human thyrotoxicosis. Of particular interest are the oral cholecystographic contrast media and phenobarbital, which may prove to have a place in the management of feline hyperthyroidism.

Oral Cholecystographic Contrast Media

A number of oral cholecystographic contrast media have been shown to affect thyroid function in humans. The most potent of these are sodium ipodate (Biloptin, Schering), and calcium ipodate (Solu-Biloptin, Schering). When hyperthyroid patients are treated with ipodate, there is a rapid and marked decrease in serum T$_3$ concentrations and a less marked but significant decrease in serum T$_4$ concentrations. These biochemical changes are maintained with continuing drug administration and are associated with dramatic clinical improvement (Wu et al., 1982).

Ipodate appears to exert its effects at a number of sites. Initially, there is a sharp drop in peripheral conversion of T$_4$ to T$_3$ with a subsequent slower and less marked decrease in the secretion of thyroid hormones from the gland owing to iodine released as the ipodate is metabolized. In addition, ipodate may interfere with the binding of thyroid hormones to plasma proteins and to cellular receptors.

Currently, the use of ipodate in human thyrotoxicosis is experimental, but it may have considerable potential in the management of thyrotoxic crisis, preparation for surgery and as adjunctive therapy after radioactive iodine administration. No associated toxic reactions have been reported.

The effects of calcium ipodate administered to cats made hyperthyroid by T$_4$ administration have been described by Ferguson et al. (1988). At an oral dosage of 15 mg/kg twice daily, the serum T$_3$ concentration and T$_3$/T$_4$ ratio were significantly reduced and the weight gain significantly increased in the ipodate treated cats when compared with controls. The drug was well tolerated with few (unspecified) clinical or hematologic adverse reactions. Further studies are required to investigate the possible value of ipodate in the management of naturally occurring feline hyperthyroidism.

Phenobarbital

Phenobarbital enhances biliary clearance of T_4 as a result of drug-induced stimulation of hepatic metabolism and bile flow. It may also increase the rate of peripheral turnover of thyroid hormones, reducing plasma concentrations. Its use in human thyrotoxicosis is adjunctive to other therapeutic measures, but it may have a place in the management of feline hyperthyroidism where sedation is desirable.

References and Suggested Reading

Center, S. A., Mitchell, J., Nachreiner, R. F., et al.: Effects of propranolol on thyroid function in the dog. Am. J. Vet. Res. 45: 109, 1984.
A study documenting the lack of effects of propranolol on basal and post-TSH serum T_4, T_3, and rT_3 concentrations in six euthyroid beagles.

Feek C. M., Sawers, J. S. A., Irvine, W. J., et al.: Combination of potassium iodide and propranolol in preparation of patients with Graves' disease for thyroid surgery. N. Engl. J. Med. 16: 883, 1980.
A prospective study of the effects of a combination of potassium iodide and propranolol on serum T_4, T_3, and rT_3 concentrations in 10 patients with Graves' disease.

Ferguson D. C., Jacobs G. J., and Hoenig, M.: Ipodate as an alternative medical treatment for feline hyperthyroidism. Proc. Am. Coll. Vet. Intern. Med. 718, 1988.
A study of the effect of calcium ipodate on the clinical signs and serum T_4 and T_3 concentrations of three healthy cats made hyperthyroid with exogenous T_4.

Marchant, B., Lees, J. F. H., and Alexander, W. D.: Antithyroid drugs. Pharmacol. Ther. Part B. Gen. Syst. Pharmacol. 3:305, 1978.
A pharmacologic review of antithyroid drugs used in human medicine.

Peterson, M. E., Kintzer, P. P., and Hurvitz, A. I.: Methimazole treatment of 262 cats with hyperthyroidism. J. Vet. Intern. Med. 2:150, 1988.
A comprehensive study on the efficacy of, and adverse reactions to, methimazole therapy in hyperthyroid cats.

Solomon D. H.: Treatment of Graves' hyperthyroidism. *In* Ingbar, S. H., and Braverman, L. E. (eds.): *Werner's The Thyroid. A Fundamental and Clinical Text,* 5th ed. Philadelphia: J. B. Lippincott, 1986, p. 987.
An overview of current concepts in the management of human thyrotoxicosis.

Thoday, K. L.: Clinical features of experimentally induced hypothyroidism in cats. *In* von Tscharner, C., and Halliwell, R. E. W. (eds.): *Advances in Veterinary Dermatology,* Vol. 1. London: Ballière Tindall, 1990, p.482.
A report on the progressive clinical changes occurring in two cats made hypothyroid with radioactive iodine.

Wu, S-Y., Shyh, T-P., Chopra, I. J., et al.: Comparison of sodium ipodate (Oragrafin) and propylthiouracil in early treatment of hyperthyroidism. J. Clin. Endocrinol. Metab. 54:630, 1982.
A prospective study of the effects of sodium ipodate and propylthiouracil on the clinical signs and serum thyroid hormone concentrations of 12 patients with Graves' disease.

o,p'-DDD TREATMENT OF CANINE HYPERADRENOCORTICISM: AN ALTERNATIVE PROTOCOL

AD RIJNBERK
and BRUCE E. BELSHAW
Utrecht, The Netherlands

It is now almost 20 years since Schechter et al. (1973) introduced o,p'-DDD for the treatment of pituitary-dependent hyperadrenocorticism. In recent years, the use of o,p'-DDD has also been recommended for the treatment of hyperadrenocorticism due to adrenocortical neoplasia (Kintzer and Peterson, 1989). This article deals with the treatment of pituitary-dependent hyperadrenocorticism, with which the most experience has been gained, and with the treatment of hyperfunctioning adrenocortical tumor.

PITUITARY-DEPENDENT HYPERADRENOCORTICISM

From the beginning of its use in dogs, the aim of the o,p'-DDD treatment has been the selective destruction of the adrenal cortices, i.e., destruction of the zona fasciculata and zona reticularis, while sparing the zona glomerulosa. In this approach the glucocorticoid overproduction is usually corrected without inducing mineralocorticoid deficiency. Protocols for this purpose consist of an initial induction phase designed to gain control of the disorder and a lifelong maintenance phase to prevent recurrence (Feldman et al., 1989). In order to reduce the side effects associated with the glucocorticoid withdrawal, some authors (Lubberink, 1980; Peterson, 1986) advise glucocorticoid supplementation during the initial phase. The effectiveness of treatment is assessed by owners' observations, physical changes, laboratory data, and, most commonly, results of ACTH-stimulation tests.

Despite these measures, mineralocorticoid production is affected in about 5% of the dogs to the extent that iatrogenic hypoadrenocorticism occurs, while in about 50% of cases there is recurrence of the disease (Peterson, 1983; Kintzer and Peterson, 1989). The favorable results of inadvertently induced hypoadrenocorticism and the very low incidence of problems in lifelong substitution therapy in dogs with spontaneous adrenocortical insufficiency prompted us to introduce a treatment schedule that is aimed at the complete destruction of the adrenal cortices, with substitution therapy for the ensuing adrenocortical insufficiency (Rijnberk and Belshaw, 1988). This is an alternative to the traditional method (Peterson, 1991).

Treatment Schedule

o,p'-DDD (Lysodren, Bristol-Myers) is given for 25 days in a dose of 50 to 75 mg/kg daily and up to 100 mg/kg daily for toy breeds. Dividing the daily dose into 3 or 4 approximately equal and equally spaced portions, with food, minimizes neurologic complications and ensures good intestinal absorption (Watson et al., 1987).

Lifelong cortisone substitution is begun on the third day of o,p'-DDD administration in a temporarily high dose of 2 mg/kg, divided twice daily. This is continued until 1 week after the o,p'-DDD therapy. Thereafter the dose is 1 mg/kg, in two equal portions or two thirds in the morning and one third in the evening.

Lifelong substitution for mineralocorticoid deficiency with fludrocortisone and NaCl is begun on the third day of o,p'-DDD therapy. Fludrocortisone is given in a dose of 0.0125 mg/kg of body weight. NaCl is usually given in dose of 0.1 mg/kg per day, divided over two or three meals, often as tablets or capsules. A summary of the treatment schedule is given in Table 1.

During the first month the owner is requested to report by telephone at least once each week and as often as questions or problems arise. The owner is also instructed very clearly to stop o,p'-DDD administration when partial or complete inappetance develops but, with equal emphasis, to continue adrenocortical hormone substitution and to contact the veterinarian, who may increase the cortisone

Table 1. *Summary of Treatment Schedule*

Treatment protocol
50–75 mg o,p'-DDD/kg/day (divided into three or four portions, with food) is given for 25 days.
On the third day, supplementation begins:
   Cortisone, 2 mg/kg/day
   Fludrocortisone, 0.0125 mg/kg/day
   Sodium chloride, 0.1 gm/kg/day
   All doses are divided into at least two administrations.
After 25–30 days, control examination:
   Cortisone is reduced to 1 mg/kg/day.
   Fludrocortisone or salt is adjusted according to the results of measurements of Na and K in plasma.

substitution temporarily. When a reduction in appetite is neglected and the o,p'-DDD treatment is continued the dog may start to vomit, refuse substitution therapy, and develop a hypoadrenocorticoid crisis. However, with good instructions, this is rare and usually the o,p'-DDD administration can be resumed after 4 to 5 days without further problems.

Follow-up

The first follow-up examination is made about 1 week after completion of the o,p'-DDD therapy, and if there are no complications, the replacement dose of cortisone is then reduced to 1 mg/kg. Plasma Na and K are measured at this examination to ascertain that the doses of fludrocortisone and salt are correct. Subsequent follow-up examinations are made once every 5 to 6 months.* Adjustments of the doses for fludrocortisone and salt are carried out as follows:

- Slight elevations or decreases of Na in combination with normal K are corrected by adjusting the dose of salt alone.
- If Na is low and K is high, or the reverse, only the dose of fludrocortisone is changed.
- If Na is normal and K is abnormal, the dose of fludrocortisone is changed. In 2 to 3 weeks, Na and K are checked again to decide whether to change the dose of salt as well.

Temporary Use of Injections

The owner should be provided with a vial of cortisone or hydrocortisone acetate suspension (25 mg/ml) and a vial of deoxycorticosterone acetate

---

Editor's comment: I would recommend that one also perform a follow-up ACTH stimulation test after this 25-day period of treatment. Some dogs with hyperadrenocorticism, particularly dogs with functional adrenal tumors, require a more prolonged induction time for adrenal destruction.

(DOCA) (1 mg/ml),* with suitable syringes and needles, and should be taught how to give subcutaneous injections. The injectable medications should be kept in the refrigerator. Some owners prefer to have these injections given by their veterinarian.

The injections are started whenever the dog cannot be given or cannot retain the oral cortisone, fludrocortisone, and salt. They are also used in place of the oral medications in connection with anesthesia, surgery, or trauma. In all of these situations, the dose of the injectable cortisone or hydrocortisone acetate is double the oral maintenance dose of cortisone, i.e., 2 mg/kg/day, divided twice daily, and the dose of DOCA to replace the fludrocortisone and salt is 0.1 mg/kg subcutaneously daily.

The injectable medications should definitely be started when two successive oral doses have been missed. It is emphasized to the owners that it is far easier to begin the injections to prevent a crisis, than it is to have to undertake the emergency treatment measures, including intravenous saline infusions, because these precautionary steps have been ignored or delayed too long. If there is any doubt about the dog's response to the injectable medication or if the client has any trouble administering it, the dog should be re-examined.

Recurrence

Owners who have observed the entire cycle of the insidious development of the disease and the recovery following o,p'-DDD treatment usually notice recurrence in a very early stage.

The first sign is usually an increased appetite, sometimes in combination with recurrence of polyuria. Omitting the cortisone substitution may ameliorate the signs temporarily, but the recurrence of hyperadrenocorticism should be investigated by measurements of the urinary corticoid/creatinine ratio (Rijnberk et al., 1988; Rijnberk and Mol, 1989). Two morning urine samples are collected at an interval of 4 to 5 days, each time omitting the cortisone and fludrocortisone administration on the preceding evening.†

Urinary corticoid/creatinine ratios exceeding the

---

*In the U.S. and other countries where DOCA is not available, it is advisable to inject double the dose of hydrocortisone indicated below. Its intrinsic mineralocorticoid effect will enable the animal to cope with the deficiency.

†*Editor's comment:* ACTH stimulation tests, performed at 6-month intervals, or sooner if clinical signs of hyperadrenocorticism develop, can also be used to check for recurrence of disease. If a rise in serum concentrations of basal or post-ACTH stimulated cortisol is detected, I would recommend reinstituting another 25-day course of daily o,p'-DDD treatment. Cortisol concentrations can rise months before recurrence of clinical signs in some dogs.

upper limit of the reference range indicate glucocorticoid excess, and o,p'-DDD therapy is then repeated in the same dose for 25 days, followed by once weekly administration of o,p'-DDD for 5 to 6 weeks. Substitution with cortisone, fludrocortisone, and NaCl is carried out as in the first course.

Comment

In our experience the treatment aimed at the complete destruction of the adrenal cortices has some advantage over lifelong maintenance therapy with o,p'-DDD. The disease is not merely suppressed, but stopped completely soon after the initiation of the treatment, although relapses do occur in about one third of the cases within 1 year. In other cases the recovery may last for 5 years or longer.

Lifelong substitution therapy is provided for the resulting primary hypoadrenocorticism, all but eliminating the risk of sudden, unexpected adrenocortical insufficiency. Concurrent diabetes mellitus is more easily managed. When employing generic drugs, on average, the total cost of medication in The Netherlands is less than in animals that are on maintenance therapy with o,p'-DDD.

We have developed instructions for owners that seem to contribute substantially to the adherence to the protocol by both the owner and the veterinarian. Also, in our experience, hesitations and reservations of practitioners with regard to this protocol are more easily overcome. Therefore, this text is given below:

Instructions for Owners

Your dog has Cushing's disease. The signs result from an excessive production of the hormone cortisol by the adrenal cortex. The aim of treatment with o,p'-DDD is to completely destroy the cortex of both adrenal glands. The normal requirement for the hormones they produce is then provided by lifelong administration of replacement hormone tablets. It is very important that the instructions for the replacement hormone be followed carefully and completely, for deficiency of these hormones can result in a life-threatening crisis.

As initial treatment your dog receives _____ tablets of o,p'-DDD _____ times daily for 25 days. For good absorption and to prevent vomiting, the tablets should always be given with food. For the first 2 days only the o,p'-DDD is given. On the third day the replacement of the adrenocortical hormones is begun, with the administration of cortisone, fludrocortisone, and ordinary salt. To allow a more gradual change from the excessive hormone production, the dose of cortisone is kept higher than the normal requirement until 1 week after the end of the o,p'-DDD therapy.

The replacement treatment during the first month consists of:

Cortisone acetate:

_____ × daily _____ tablets of _____ mg

Fludrocortisone acetate:

_____ daily _____ tablets of _____ mg

Salt: _____ × daily _____ gram

The first follow-up is 1 month after the beginning of the o,p'-DDD therapy. At this time the dose of cortisone is usually reduced by one-half. Results of a blood examination will be used to determine whether the doses of fludrocortisone and salt need to be changed. After this, follow-up examinations are usually made once every 5 or 6 months. Their purpose is to be certain that the recovery continues satisfactorily and to be certain that the replacement doses of fludrocortisone and salt are correct. Sometimes, in spite of the destructive action of o,p'-DDD on the adrenal cortex, signs of the disease reappear. This can occur after several months or even after 4 to 5 years. It is then necessary to repeat the treatment with o,p'-DDD.

The first signs of recovery often appear during the course of o,p'-DDD therapy. The excessive thirst and hunger disappear and the dog's endurance returns. The recovery of the coat takes longer, but once this begins, after about 2 months, a very thick coat usually develops. The recovery of the skin and coat may be preceded by a short period of excessive dandruff and some itching. You can relieve this by giving the dog a thorough washing once or twice a week with an ordinary shampoo for people, but take care to rinse the dog well after shampooing.

Complications: With the above treatment instructions, most dogs recover without complications. There can be complications associated with the o,p'-DDD or the replacement therapy. If you notify the veterinarian in time, problems can usually be resolved without difficulty.

In the beginning of treatment there may be mild side effects from o,p'-DDD, such as nausea, incoordination, or slight disorientation. These signs usually disappear if you omit one or two doses of o,p'-DDD and then resume administration but spread more widely over the day. If the dog refuses to eat or eats almost nothing, stop the o,p'-DDD completely, but be sure to continue the replacement medications and notify the veterinarian.

A deficiency in replacement medications can lead to a life-threatening crisis, and emergency treatment may be required. It is far better to contact the veterinarian before a crisis occurs. The first warning is often loss of appetite. Many dogs with Cushing's disease have an excessive appetite, and a decrease in appetite is an expected sign of recovery from the disease. However, an almost complete refusal to eat should be recognized as a warning. You should stop o,p'-DDD immediately, continue the replacement medications, and obtain the veterinarian's advice promptly.

Special Circumstances in Replacement Therapy. It is extremely important to give the replacement medications without interruption. Yet there may be situations in which your dog cannot or will not take anything orally or cannot retain the medications because of vomiting. If for any reason your dog cannot take or retain the tablets and salt for two times in succession, injectable medications should be started. This applies, for example, when your dog is brought to the veterinarian for a treatment that requires anesthesia. Then:

- The cortisone tablets are replaced by subcutaneous injections of hydrocortisone acetate (25 mg/ml) in a dose of _____ ml twice daily. The hydrocortisone injections are continued until the dog can again swallow and retain the cortisone tablets.
- The fludrocortisone tablets and salt are replaced by subcutaneous injections of DOCA (1 mg/ml) in a dose of ml once daily. In countries, such as the U.S., where DOCA is unavailable, it is advised to administer double the dose of hydrocortisone. The salt is not needed when DOCA injections are used. The DOCA injections are continued until the dog can again swallow and also retain the fludrocortisone and salt.

If you take your dog on vacation or on a trip away from home for more than 1 or 2 days, also take the injectable medications, syringes, and needles, and this instruction sheet, for not all veterinarians will have these medications at hand. If you leave the dog in the care of someone else, also make provision for the possible need for the injections, even if you have not yet had to use them yourself.

In cases of anesthesia, severe physical stress, or injury, the dose of cortisone should be doubled for 1 or 2 days. With these exceptions, the dose of cortisone remains unchanged for life, while the doses of fludrocortisone and salt may have to be adjusted by the veterinarian.

HYPERADRENOCORTICISM DUE TO ADRENOCORTICAL TUMOR

The use of o,p'-DDD has been recommended only recently for dogs with hyperadrenocorticism due to adrenocortical tumor (Kintzer and Peterson, 1989). In our experience, treatment with the recommended dose of at least 50 mg/kg for about 10 days was not very satisfactory, for the results were unpredictable. In some cases there was no improvement, and in others, there was a rapid decrease in hormone production.

Therefore we also tried the protocol described above in dogs with hyperfunctioning adrenocortical tumors. This has given satisfactory results, including complete disappearance of the ultrasonographically visualized tumor. These results were obtained in a limited number of cases, and more follow-up is needed before this protocol can be recommended for general use. In these follow-up studies, periodic measurements of urinary corticoid/creatinine ratios may prove to be useful.

These results might even suggest that it may be possible to treat all dogs with hyperadrenocorticism according to this protocol, irrespective of whether the disease is pituitary-dependent. This would also remove the need to differentiate between pituitary-dependent hyperadrenocorticism and hyperadrenocorticism due to adrenocortical tumor. However, the differential diagnosis is still desirable, for in dogs with resectable adrenocortical tumor, surgery can result in complete recovery without continuing medication.

References and Suggested Reading

Feldman, E. C., Bruyette, D. S., and Nelson, R. W.: Therapy for spontaneous canine hyperadrenocorticism. *In* Kirk, R. W. (ed.): *Current Veterinary Therapy X.* Philadelphia: W. B. Saunders, 1989, pp. 1024–1031.
A current review of standard treatment of hyperadrenocorticism in dogs.

Kintzer, P. P., and Peterson, M. E.: Mitotane (o,p′-DDD) treatment of cortisol-secreting adrenocortical neoplasia. *In* Kirk, R. W. (ed.): *Current Veterinary Therapy X.* Philadelphia: W. B. Saunders, 1989, pp. 1034–1037.
Method for treatment of adrenocortical neoplasia with o,p′-DDD.

Lubberink, A.A.M.E.: Therapy for spontaneous hyperadrenocorticism. *In* Kirk, R. W. (ed.): *Current Veterinary Therapy VII.* Philadelphia: W. B. Saunders, 1980, pp. 979–983.
Review of treatment methods for hyperadrenocorticism in dogs.

Peterson, M.E.: O,p′-DDD (mitotane) treatment of canine pituitary-dependent hyperadrenocorticism. J.A.V.M.A. 182:527–528, 1983.
Review of the standard treatment protocol for hyperadrenocorticism in dogs.

Peterson, M. E.: Canine hyperadrenocorticism. *In* Kirk, R. W. (ed.): *Current Veterinary Therapy XI.* Philadelphia: W. B. Saunders, 1986, pp. 963–972.
Review of treatment methods for hyperadrenocorticism in dogs.

Peterson, M. E.: Pituitary-dependent hyperadrenocorticism in the dog: Standard maintenance o,p′-DDD treatment. Vet. Med. Rep. 3:65–69, 1991.
Outlines the advantages of the standard o,p′-DDD treatment protocol.

Rijnberk, A., and Belshaw, B. E.: An alternative protocol for the medical management of canine pituitary-dependent hyperadrenocorticism. Vet. Rec. 122:486–488, 1988.
Outlines advantages of the alternative o,p′-DDD treatment protocol.

Rijnberk, A., and Mol, J. A.: Adrenocortical function. *In* Kaneko, J. F. (ed.): *Clinical Biochemistry of Domestic Animals,* 4th ed. San Diego: Academic Press, 1989, pp. 610–629.

Rijnberk, A., van Wees, A., and Mol, J. A.: Assessment of two tests for the diagnosis of canine hyperadrenocorticism. Vet. Rec. 122:178–180, 1988.
Compares the value of the low-dose dexamethasone suppression test to the urinary corticoid/creatinine ratio for the diagnosis of hyperadrenocorticism in dogs.

Schechter, R. D., Stabenfeldt, G. H., Gribble, D. H., et al.: Treatment of Cushing's syndrome in the dog with an adrenocorticolytic agent (o,p′-DDD). J.A.V.M.A. 162:629–639, 1973.
First paper in the veterinary literature describing use of o,p′-DDD for treatment of hyperadrenocorticism.

Teske, E., Rothuizen, J., de Bruijne, J. J., et al.: Corticosteroid-induced alkaline phosphatase isoenzyme in the diagnosis of canine hypercorticism. Vet. Rec. 125:12–14, 1989.
Evaluation of the heat inactivation test for alkaline phosphatase as a screening test for hyperadrenocorticism in dogs.

Watson, A. D. J., Rijnberk, A., and Moolenaar, A. J.: Systemic availability of o,p′-DDD in normal dogs, fasted and fed, and in dogs with hyperadrenocorticism. Res. Vet. Sci. 43:160–165, 1987.
Study showing that o,p′-DDD is better absorbed when administered with food.

USE OF KETOCONAZOLE FOR CONTROL OF CANINE HYPERADRENOCORTICISM

EDWARD C. FELDMAN
and RICHARD W. NELSON
Davis, California

Several therapeutic options are available for treating naturally occurring hyperadrenocorticism (Cushing's syndrome) in the dog. Approximately 80 to 85% of dogs with Cushing's syndrome have pituitary-dependent disease (PDH). The available options for treating PDH include o,p′-DDD, ketoconazole, hypophysectomy, and bilateral adrenalectomy. Cobalt teletherapy may be recommended if a pituitary macroadenoma is present (see this volume, p. 319). The remaining 15 to 20% of dogs with Cushing's syndrome have functional adrenocortical tumors (AT), of which approximately 50% are benign. The most commonly recommended therapy for these dogs is surgical removal of the tumor. If surgery is not allowed by an owner, or if metastatic disease is present, o,p′-DDD or ketoconazole may provide short- or, in some dogs, long-term relief of clinical signs.

Regardless of the therapeutic option chosen, excellent rapport must be established between the veterinarian and owner for successful long-term management of these animals. Time spent explaining pathophysiology in lay terms is well worth the effort to improve client understanding and to establish a good basis for future communications. The surgical and medical options should be discussed in detail, including what is expected of the owner. The goal is to return these dogs to a normal endocrine state, but this is not always possible. All potential complications should be discussed. These dogs may have endocrine excesses or deficiencies after treatment, and the prepared owner can accept these setbacks.

Ketoconazole (Nizoral, Janssen) is an imidazole derivative that has antifungal properties. Its antifungal activity is linked to the inhibition of ergosterol synthesis and to interference with other membrane lipids. In addition to its antifungal activity, ketocon-

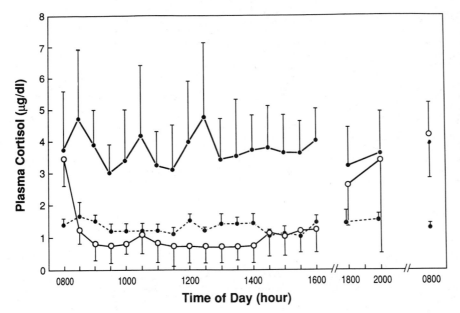

Figure 1. Mean (±SD) plasma cortisol concentrations every 30 min from 0800 through 1600 hr and again at 1800, 2000, and 0800 hr (the following day) from eight dogs with hyperadrenocorticism (five with PDH, three with adrenocortical tumor) prior to treatment (●——●) and after a single dose of ketoconazole (15 mg/kg) immediately after obtaining the 0800-hr blood sample (○——○). Plasma cortisol concentrations from 15 healthy, untreated control dogs are included (●----●). Ketoconazole caused significant (*P* <0.05) reductions in plasma cortisol concentration from 0830 through 1600 hr. (Reprinted with permission from Feldman E. C., et al.: Plasma cortisol response to ketoconazole administration in dogs with hyperadrenocorticism. J.A.V.M.A. 197:71, 1990.)

azole has been shown to interfere with gonadal and adrenal steroid synthesis both *in vitro* and *in vivo* through inhibition of cytochrome P-450–dependent enzymes. The drug is an enzyme blocker, active for 8 to 16 hr after oral administration. It is not a cytotoxic drug and does not damage tissue, in contrast to a drug such as o,p'-DDD (Mitotane, Lysodren). As an enzyme blocker, dosage requirements remain static and do not reduce with time, as is common with cytotoxic drug therapy.

We have evaluated the use of this drug in dogs with PDH as well as those with hyperadrenocorticism secondary to AT. Most of these ketoconazole-treated dogs have shown a rapid reduction in plasma cortisol concentrations (Fig. 1) and a reduction in adrenocortical responsiveness to ACTH (Fig. 2). In dogs treated for more than 2 months, there has been significant improvement in their clinical condition as evidenced by a reduction in water intake, urine production, appetite, weight, and regrowth of hair.

INDICATIONS

Ketoconazole, with its low incidence of toxicity, reversible inhibition of adrenal steroidogenesis, and negligible effects on mineralocorticoid production, promises to be an attractive (albeit expensive) alternative in the management of canine hyperadrenocorticism. Ketoconazole is useful in the following circumstances: (1) medical management of those dogs that have malignant AT and for whom surgical intervention is not an option; (2) medical management for dogs with AT if an owner refuses surgery; (3) as a short-term test therapy to provide evidence

for or against a diagnosis of hyperadrenocorticism in dogs with vague test results; and (4) as primary therapy in dogs that cannot be treated with o,p'-DDD because of drug sensitivity.

TREATMENT PROTOCOL

Our recommendations are to use ketoconazole at an initial dosage of 5 mg/kg, PO, given every 12 hr for 7 days. This initial low dose is used merely to evaluate dogs for side effects such as acute hepatitis or gastritis. Although there have been no such reports for dogs, ketoconazole can cause hepatopathy in people. This may result in anorexia, lethargy, jaundice, and abnormal liver enzyme activities. If no ill effects are observed, the dosage should be increased to 10 mg/kg (every 12 hr) for 14 days, and an ACTH stimulation test should be performed at that time. If an owner does not see improvement in the pet's condition, or if normal or exaggerated response to exogenous ACTH is observed, increase the ketoconazole dosage to 15 mg/kg (every 12 hr) and again monitor the dog with at least a history, physical examination, and an ACTH stimulation test following 14 additional days of therapy. It is important that a dog receive ketoconazole on evaluation days, just as it receives the drug on other days. Hormone testing (specifically, the ACTH stimulation test) should begin 1 to 3 hours following drug administration. One cannot evaluate the effectiveness of an enzyme blocker if the patient has not been given the drug. We do not believe that a basal cortisol concentration is of benefit in evaluating therapy. If financial constraints preclude submission of the routine pre- and post-ACTH plasma samples

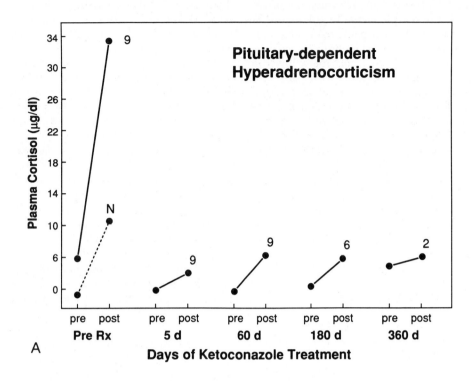

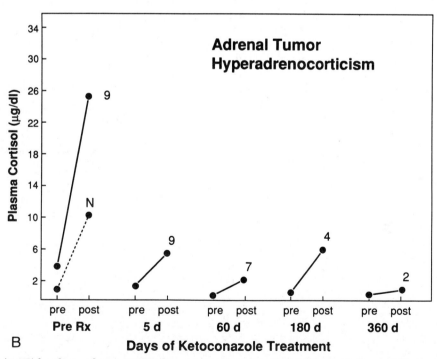

Figure 2. Mean (± SD) baseline and post-ACTH plasma cortisol concentrations in dogs with hyperadrenocorticism before and at 5, 60, 180, and 360 days during ketoconazole administration. After initiation of ketoconazole treatment (15 mg/kg every 12 hr), all baseline (pre) and post-ACTH (post) plasma cortisol concentrations were significantly ($P < 0.05$) less than the pretreatment values. Test results from 15 control dogs (N) are included (●----●). *A*, Values in dogs with PDH. Numbers at each time point indicate number of dogs being tested at that time; Rx = ketoconazole treatment. *B*, Values in dogs with adrenocortical tumor. Numbers at each time point indicate number of dogs being tested at that time; Rx = ketoconazole treatment. (Reprinted with permission from Feldman, E. C., et al.: Plasma cortisol response to ketoconazole administration in dogs with hyperadrenocorticism. J.A.V.M.A. 197:71, 1990.)

for cortisol assay, veterinarians are encouraged to submit a post-ACTH sample because this result is of greater value than a basal hormone concentration. The goals in therapy are obvious clinical improvement and a post-ACTH plasma cortisol below the reference range for that laboratory (Fig. 2). The normal post-ACTH plasma cortisol concentration reference range for the Pituitary Function Laboratory (University of California, Davis) is 150 to 450 nmol/L (5.5 to 16 μg/dl), and the goal in therapy, therefore, is a plasma cortisol concentration of less than 150 nmol/L. It would be unusual to observe clinical improvement without a low post-ACTH plasma cortisol concentration. Several of our dogs have required dosages in excess of 15 mg/kg b.i.d. (15 to 20 mg/kg b.i.d.), but this is not common. Complete response to 10 mg/kg, b.i.d., would also not be common.

COMPLICATIONS

It must be emphasized that 8 of 43 (20%) dogs with hyperadrenocorticism have demonstrated absolutely no response to ketoconazole. Failure to absorb the drug is one explanation for this frustrating lack of effect. It is possible, although not proven, that absorption would be improved by dissolving the tablet (200 mg) with a few drops of 1N hydrochloric acid and then neutralizing the pH with an adequate volume of water. The solution will be pale pink and should be administered soon after the tablet is dissolved and the mixture diluted.

The most common clinical signs associated with ketoconazole *overdosage* would be those resulting from cortisol deficiency. These signs would include weakness, inappetence, vomiting, diarrhea, abdominal pain, and shivering. We have not observed electrolyte disturbances suggestive of mineralocorticoid deficiency, although monitoring serum sodium and potassium concentrations is strongly encouraged. Treatment includes discontinuation of the ketoconazole plus glucocorticoid administration. Other supportive medications, such as IV fluids, should be used as needed. Response to such treatment is rapid. These dogs can usually be given lower dosages of ketoconazole following several days of being completely stable.

In conclusion, ketoconazole can be an effective therapeutic drug for dogs with PDH or AT. The pathway of cortisol synthesis can be inhibited by this enzyme blocker, regardless of the cause for excess cortisol secretion. Ketoconazole has been effective quickly (within 30 min of first administration), over a period of weeks, as well as for periods of greater than 18 months in several dogs. The major limitations in using ketoconazole are (1) the need for continuing b.i.d. administration; (2) expense; and (3) the failure of some dogs to respond.

References and Suggested Reading

Feldman, E. C., Bruyette, D. S., Nelson, R. W., et al.: Plasma cortisol response to ketoconazole administration in dogs with hyperadrenocorticism. J. A. V. M. A. 197:71, 1990.
  The results of ketoconazole treatment in dogs with hyperadrenocorticism.
Pont, A., Williams, P. L., Loose, D. S., et al.: Ketoconazole blocks adrenal steroid synthesis. Ann. Intern. Med. 97:370, 1982.
  One of the first papers describing the effects of ketoconazole on steroid synthesis.
Sonino, N.: The use of ketoconazole as an inhibitor of steroid production. N. Engl. J. Med. 317:812, 1987.
  This is a review paper on the use of ketoconazole in people.
Willard, M. D., Nachreiner, R., McDonald, R., et al.: Ketoconazole-induced changes in selected canine hormone concentrations. Am. J. Vet. Res. 47:2504, 1986.
  This is the first paper in the veterinary literature describing the effects of ketoconazole on healthy dogs.

DESOXYCORTICOSTERONE PIVALATE (DOCP) TREATMENT OF CANINE AND FELINE HYPOADRENOCORTICISM

EDWARD C. FELDMAN
RICHARD W. NELSON
Davis, California

and RANDY C. LYNN
Greensboro, North Carolina

Adrenocortical insufficiency (hypoadrenocorticism) results from deficient adrenal production of glucocorticoids and mineralocorticoids. Destruction of the adrenal cortex as a result of immune-mediated inflammation is, perhaps, the most frequent cause of this uncommon syndrome (primary adrenocortical insufficiency, Addison's disease). Among the other causes of adrenocortical destruction are hemorrhage, cancer, granulomatous diseases, and the use of o,p'DDD, an adrenocorticolytic drug. Deficient pituitary ACTH production (secondary adrenocortical insufficiency) may impair glucocorticoid synthesis and secretion but would not likely result in mineralocorticoid deficiencies.

CLINICAL FEATURES AND DIAGNOSIS

Hypoadrenocorticism is a fairly uncommon endocrine disorder in the dog and is rare in the cat. The disorder develops most frequently in dogs 1 to 7 years of age, although puppies and older dogs with the syndrome have been described. Typical of immune-mediated disorders in dogs, 80 to 85% of hypoadrenocorticism cases are diagnosed in females and castrated males. There also may exist familial or genetic predispositions to the development of hypoadrenocorticism in several breeds, including standard poodles, Labrador retrievers, and Portugese water spaniels.

This work represents the results of a multi-center trial. In addition to the authors, participants included Michael Bernstein, Boston, MA; Roger A. Bradley and Kimberly Ann Robertson, San Jose, CA; Maynard R. Clark, Lafayette, CA; James Gent, Springfield, OR; Ingrid B. Hardy, San Carlos, CA; Roger K. Johnson and Michael A. Paul, Walnut Creek, CA; Mitchell Kornet, Hicksville, NY; Mark J. Miller, Midland, TX; J. Catherine R. Scott-Moncrieff, West Lafayette, IN; Guy T. Newton, Fort Worth, TX; Mark E. Peterson and Rhett Nichols, New York City, NY; James C. Preuter and J. Lynn Turner, Bedford Heights, OH; Rod A.W. Rosychuk, Ft. Collins, CO; Elaine Salinger, San Bruno, CA; Michael Schaer, Gainesville, FL; and Sherri Speede, Portland, OR.

The problems observed by owners of dogs with hypoadrenocorticism include depression, lethargy, inappetence or anorexia, weakness, vomiting, diarrhea, weight loss, shaking or shivering, and polydipsia/polyuria. It should be emphasized that the severity of each sign is quite variable. Additionally, some dogs have numerous signs while others have only one or two. Depression (obtundation), weakness, and dehydration have been the most common abnormalities noted on the physical examination of dogs with hypoadrenocorticism. Bradycardia, weak femoral pulses, hypothermia, emaciation, and melena are also described, but these are less frequent findings.

At the time of diagnosis, dogs with hypoadrenocorticism often have a normocytic, normochromic, nonregenerative anemia, which can be masked by dehydration. The percentages of eosinophils and lymphocytes present on a complete blood count exceed those usually found in stressed or ill dogs. Prerenal azotemia (increased blood urea nitrogen concentration) due to hypovolemia is common. This azotemia may be confusing because these dogs often have a urine specific gravity less than 1.020 owing to renal medullary washout caused by renal sodium losses. Thus, primary renal disease is a major differential in the diagnosis of hypoadrenocorticism. Hypoglycemia is an unusual feature of this disease and, when present, may cause central nervous system signs of extreme weakness, depression, or convulsions. Mild to moderate hypercalcemia has been described in about one third of dogs with untreated hypoadrenocorticism. Hypercalcemia is observed usually in the extremely ill hypoadrenal dogs, and its severity is typically in direct proportion to the severity of dehydration or serum electrolyte abnormalities. Hypercalcemia does not occur in all dogs suffering a hypoadrenal crisis but, when present, may confuse a veterinarian unaware of this association. Hypoadrenal crisis may result in mild to moderate acidosis.

Among the classic laboratory abnormalities asso-

353

ciated with hypoadrenocorticism are the changes in serum electrolyte concentrations, including hyponatremia, hyperkalemia, and hypochloremia. This pattern is a direct result of mineralocorticoid (aldosterone) deficiency, which results in a loss of sodium and chloride into the urine and the simultaneous failure of the kidneys to excrete potassium. Most untreated, ill, hypoadrenal dogs have a sodium:potassium ratio less than 20, but this highlighted feature is not present in every case and, when present, is not pathognomonic for the disease. Normal serum electrolyte concentrations have been observed in approximately 10% of dogs with primary hypoadrenocorticism. Further, the hyperkalemia and hyponatremia associated with this endocrinopathy have also been observed in dogs and cats with renal failure, acidosis, and severe gastrointestinal or hepatic disease.

Measurement of plasma or serum cortisol concentrations before and following the administration of exogenous ACTH (ACTH stimulation test) is the most reliable means of confirming or refuting the diagnosis of adrenocortical insufficiency. Either animal extract ACTH gel or synthetic ACTH can be used in assessing adrenocortical reserve in dogs and cats. Dogs and cats with adrenocortical failure have post-ACTH plasma cortisol concentrations unequivocally less than normal values, and they are usually quite similar to or below the low or low-normal baseline concentration. This excellent test, however, cannot distinguish dogs with primary hypoadrenocorticism from those with secondary adrenocortical insufficiency resulting from a pituitary disorder or chronic corticosteroid administration. Assessment of aldosterone concentrations before and after ACTH administration is a study that can further support a diagnosis, although its value is academic in most situations. Measurement of plasma endogenous ACTH concentrations, while interesting and occasionally helpful, is also usually academic.

TREATMENT

History

The history of treating people who were afflicted with hypoadrenocorticism was dismal until the rather recent past. It wasn't until the 1920's that the existence of a hormone controlling serum electrolyte concentrations was recognized. This was a major step forward in appreciating the pathophysiology of this uniformly fatal disease. In the late 1930's, successful synthesis of desoxycorticosterone was described, a landmark in providing a pharmacologic basis for the treatment of afflicted individuals. Desoxycorticosterone administered daily, by injection, replaced the use of crude animal extracts

of adrenal tissue. The cumbersome need for frequent injections was somewhat relieved when the trimethylacetate (pivalate) ester of desoxycorticosterone was synthesized in the 1950's. This new material had a 20- to 30-day duration of action, providing a good deal of stability to what had been a rather fragile population. Desoxycorticosterone pivalate (DOCP) remained a cornerstone in the management of hypoadrenocorticism until the 1960's, when an oral mineralocorticoid (fludrocortisone acetate) was developed and marketed. People choosing between monthly IM injections or taking a pill once every 24 to 48 hr invariably chose the latter. Over a period of several years, the use of DOCP diminished, until 1987 when production of the drug was halted.

Soon after the efficacy of DOCP had been demonstrated for the management of people with hypoadrenocorticism, similar efficacy was described for a dog with the naturally occurring disease. This was a logical progression, since the animal models used in establishing the actions and safety of DOCP were adrenalectomized dogs. The common use of DOCP in hypoadrenal people by medical doctors was parallelled by its use in hypoadrenal dogs by veterinarians. However, while many people with hypoadrenocorticism readily switched to oral therapy in the late 1960's and 1970's, a significant percentage of veterinarians and their clients chose injectable therapy for the management of dogs with naturally occurring or iatrogenic hypoadrenocorticism. The authors, beginning in late 1989, directed a nationwide, multi-center trial of DOCP in hypoadrenal dogs. This chapter is based on our experience with this large trial in dogs, completed in early 1990. At the time of writing, the drug is not approved for veterinary use.

Maintenance Therapy

DOCP is formulated as an aqueous suspension containing 25 mg/ml. The initial dose of DOCP is 2.2 mg/kg, IM, every 25 days. This drug is mineralocorticoid and provides little or no glucocorticoid activity. Therefore, it is also recommended that prednisone or prednisolone be administered to these dogs at an initial dose of 0.2 mg/kg orally, daily. Dogs so treated are receiving two drugs that must be individualized in dose to the needs of the patient. When a dog is declared stable and healthy by both owner and veterinarian, slow reduction in glucocorticoid dosage should be attempted. This dose reduction is suggested to minimize polydipsia/polyuria and other glucocorticoid side effects. Fully one half of our patients receive no glucocorticoid medication, although their owners have the drug available for emergency use. Ten per cent of our dogs receive daily glucocorticoids while the balance receive prednisone every second or third day.

More than 50% of the treated dogs remain on 2.2 mg/kg, DOCP, every 25 days. However, the veterinarian and owner must expect subtle or significant variation in the needs of an individual dog. To assure that DOCP is providing its expected activity and to assess duration of action, it is recommended that serum sodium, potassium, and blood urea nitrogen (BUN) concentrations be monitored approximately 2 weeks after administration as well as at the time of injection for the initial 2 to 3 months of therapy. Normal parameters at 2 weeks indicate that the dosage is adequate, but they do not provide information on duration of action. DOCP treatment alternatives arise if normal parameters are demonstrated on the day of injection: (1) progressively lower the dosage of DOCP by 0.2 mg/kg at each subsequent injection to define the lowest efficacious dose for an individual, or (2) maintain the dosage but prolong the interval between injections. Veterinarians participating in the drug trial used both alternatives. Approximately 15% of the dogs currently receive 1.1 mg/kg of DOCP, and another 30% receive less than 2.2 but more than 1.1 mg/kg of DOCP at each injection. Of equal or greater interest to most owners is attempting to prolong the interval between injections, with a goal of one injection per month. However, only 20% of these dogs currently receive the drug on a monthly basis, and 5% need to receive their DOCP every 3 weeks. These results demonstrate the need for tailoring the medication to the requirements of the individual dog.

Most dogs receiving DOCP for more than 6 months require 1.5 to 2.2 mg/kg every 25 to 30 days. The need for frequent monitoring of serum electrolyte concentrations cannot be overemphasized. The maximum acceptable period between assessments should be 3 to 4 months. It is recommended that periodic blood samples for electrolytes and BUN be obtained at the time of injection, to assess and ensure that the medication has the desired duration as well as effect. Many of our owners have been taught to administer the DOCP themselves; thus, these rechecks also serve indirectly to monitor the injection technique of the owner. When dogs are brought to us on the day they are due for their injection (the ideal time for an examination), we have owners administer the DOCP in our presence, further helping us to assess their skill as well as the results of our history, physical examination, and blood tests.

One of the dogs we treated with DOCP did not respond as well as it did to oral fludrocortisone acetate therapy, and another dog suffered an acute relapse despite DOCP therapy. Therefore, due caution is warranted. No treatment is 100% reliable,

and this is true of DOCP. The hypoadrenal dog can become ill or have a relapse at any time. Owners should be instructed that excess concern is preferable to complete confidence in any treatment provided to a pet with hypoadrenocorticism.

To date we are aware of five hypoadrenal cats being treated with DOCP. They have responded well to the medication. Further observation of these and additional cats will be necessary before recommendations are made regarding the long-term care of feline hypoadrenocorticism.

Therapy in Addisonian Crisis

Crisis, with respect to hypoadrenocorticism, refers to an animal in critical condition owing to hypovolemia, hyperkalemia, hyponatremia, and the various other abnormalities associated with this acute severe syndrome. Treatment traditionally involves the use of intravenous fluids, glucocorticoid and mineralocorticoid replacement, and bicarbonate, glucose, or other medications as required by the patient. Until recently, mineralocorticoid therapy consisted of desoxycorticosterone acetate (DOCA), a mineralocorticoid with approximately 24 hr of effect. DOCA is no longer commercially available. DOCP is not intended for use in the hypoadrenal crisis. However, we have successfully used DOCP in several crisis situations. The disadvantage of DOCP would be its prolonged duration of action prior to confirmation of the diagnosis. However, we are not aware of worrisome side effects should DOCP be administered to dogs that do not have hypoadrenocorticism. Such dogs could be prone to sodium and, therefore, fluid retention, which in turn could result in hypertension. Additionally, hypokalemia could also occur, especially if the dog or cat is anorexic. Atrial natriuretic factor, however, should prevent volume overload and hypertension in dogs overdosed with mineralocorticoid medication.

References and Suggested Reading

Feldman, E. C., and Nelson, R. W.: *Canine and Feline Endocrinology and Reproduction.* Philadelphia: W. B. Saunders, 1987.
   This reference provides general information on a series of dogs with hypoadrenocorticism.
Peterson, M. E., Greco, D. S., and Orth, D. N.: Primary hypoadrenocorticism in ten cats. J. Vet. Intern. Med. 3:55, 1989.
   This reference provides the first and largest series of studies on cats with hypoadrenocorticism.
Shaker, E., Hurvitz, A. I., and Peterson, M. E.: Hypoadrenocorticism in a family of Standard Poodles. J.A.V.M.A. 192:1091, 1988.
   Report on familial hypoadrenocorticism.
Willard, M. D., Schall, W. D., McCaw, D. E., et al.: Canine hypoadrenocorticism: Report of 37 cases and review of 39 previously reported cases. J.A.V.M.A. 180:59, 1982.
   This is an excellent review of this syndrome in dogs.

INSULIN
AND INSULIN
SYRINGES

MARK E. PETERSON
New York, New York

Insulin was discovered in 1921, and the pharmaceutical industry has since made great strides in improving its purity and stability, modifying its duration of action, and producing it from different sources. Until recently, all insulin came from beef or pork pancreas, and its purity and strength were not reliable. Today there are more than 40 insulin preparations available in the United States, including human insulin, which is genetically engineered by recombinant DNA technology (Table 1). Today's insulins are extremely pure, with human insulin being the purest and pork insulin a close second. But even the beef and beef-pork insulins are far more pure than they were just a decade ago.

The fact that there are so many different insulin preparations available tends to make the veterinarian's role in treating diabetics confusing. In addition, an increasing number of improved insulin syringes are also now available, confusing the issue further.

All mammalian insulin is structurally similar, containing 51 amino acids in two polypeptide chains, the 21-amino acid A-chain and the 30-amino acid B-chain (Smith, 1972). Until recently, most commercial insulins produced in the United States were beef-pork combinations composed largely of beef insulin, since beef pancreata far outnumber pork pancreata as a by-product of the meat-packing industry. Beef-pork insulin preparations contain a mixture of 70% beef and 30% pork insulin. Recently, human insulin has become available and is the insulin of choice in the treatment of human diabetes. Pork insulin is close to human insulin in structure, differing by only one amino acid in the B-chain, and beef insulin differs by three amino acids. Pork insulin is identical to the insulin of dogs in its amino acid structure. Cat insulin, which differs from pork and dog insulin by four amino acids, is most similar to beef insulin, differing only in one position, amino acid 18 of the A-chain (Hallden et al., 1986).

In human diabetic patients, human insulin is generally preferred, especially in individuals who develop allergies or immune resistance to animal-derived insulin preparations. Most diabetic cats and dogs are still successfully treated with beef-pork insulin, which is the least expensive preparation available. Although insulin antibodies do develop in some dogs and cats treated with beef-pork combinations, the development of insulin resistance secondary to these antibodies appears to be rare. If insulin resistance secondary to the development of insulin antibodies is suspected in a diabetic dog or cat, however, a change in insulin type may be warranted. Because dog and pork insulin are identical in structure, pork insulin is the most appropriate for use in dogs with insulin resistance. Since human insulin differs from dog insulin in only one position, human preparations might also be used in dogs with insulin resistance and, since they are so widely available, may be easiest to obtain. However, since cat insulin differs considerably from those of human and pork, these insulins may not be helpful in the treatment of cats with insulin resistance. Although the sole use of beef insulin has not been reported in cats with insulin resistance, beef insulin may be the preparation of choice because of its similarity to cat insulin.

If a change in insulin is contemplated, it is important to realize that different types and brands of insulin have different pharmacologic properties. For example, pork insulin has a shorter duration of action than does beef-pork insulin in dogs, as does human insulin in humans. Thus, choosing pork over beef-pork insulin may necessitate more frequent injections in some dogs.

Insulin is available in short-, intermediate-, and long-acting preparations that are usually injected separately but may be mixed together in the same syringe. Short-acting preparations include regular and Semilente insulins. Intermediate-acting preparations include neutral protamine Hagedorn (NPH) and Lente insulins. Long-acting preparations include protamine zinc insulin (PZI; no longer manufactured in the United States) and Ultralente insulin. Although not commonly used in animals, insulin preparations with a predetermined proportion of NPH mixed with regular insulin (e.g., 70% NPH to 30% regular) are also commercially available. Confusion can result if one does not realize that different companies have adopted different

Table 1. Insulins*

Product	Manufacturer	Form	Strength
Rapid-acting			
Iletin I Regular	Lilly	Beef/Pork	U-40, U-100
Iletin II Regular	Lilly	Beef	U-100
Iletin II Regular	Lilly	Pork	U-100, U-500
Purified Pork R (Regular)	Novo Nordisk	Pork	U-100
Velosulin (Regular)	Novo Nordisk	Pork	U-100
Regular	Novo Nordisk	Pork	U-100
Iletin I Semilente	Lilly	Beef/Pork	U-40, U-100
Semilente	Novo Nordisk	Beef	U-100
Humulin Regular	Lilly	Human	U-100
Novolin R (Regular)	Novo Nordisk	Human	U-100
Novolin R Penfill (Regular)	Novo Nordisk	Human	U-100
Velosulin Human (Regular)	Novo Nordisk	Human	U-100
Intermediate-acting			
Iletin II Lente	Lilly	Beef	U-100
Iletin II NPH	Lilly	Beef	U-100
Iletin II Lente	Lilly	Pork	U-100
Iletin II NPH	Lilly	Pork	U-100
Insulatard NPH	Novo Nordisk	Pork	U-100
Purified Pork Lente	Novo Nordisk	Pork	U-100
Purified Pork N (NPH)	Novo Nordisk	Pork	U-100
Lente	Novo Nordisk	Beef	U-100
Iletin I Lente	Lilly	Beef/Pork	U-40, U-100
Iletin I NPH	Lilly	Beef/Pork	U-40, U-100
NPH	Novo Nordisk	Beef	U-100
Humulin L (Lente)	Lilly	Human	U-100
Humulin N (NPH)	Lilly	Human	U-100
Insulatard Human NPH	Novo Nordisk	Human	U-100
Novolin L (Lente)	Novo Nordisk	Human	U-100
Novolin N (NPH)	Novo Nordisk	Human	U-100
Novolin N Penfill (NPH)	Novo Nordisk	Human	U-100
Long-acting			
Iletin I PZI	Lilly	Beef/Pork	U-40, U-100
Iletin I Ultralente	Lilly	Beef/Pork	U-40, U-100
Ultralente	Novo Nordisk	Beef	U-100
Humulin U (Ultralente)	Lilly	Human	U-100
Iletin II PZI	Lilly	Beef	U-100
Iletin II PZI	Lilly	Pork	U-100
Mixtures			
Mixtard	Novo Nordisk	Pork	U-100
Mixtard Human 70/30	Novo Nordisk	Human	U-100
Novolin 70/30	Novo Nordisk	Human	U-100
Novolin 70/30 Penfill	Novo Nordisk	Human	U-100
Humulin 70/30	Lilly	Human	U-100

*As of 12/90, manufacture of all U-40 insulins and all PZI was discontinued in the United States.

names for the same short-, intermediate-, and long-acting forms of insulin or their mixtures (Table 1).

Insulin is commercially available in concentrations of 40, 100, and 500 U/ml (designated U-40, U-100, and U-500). One unit of insulin equals approximately 36 µg of insulin. U-40 insulin is widely favored by many veterinarians for use in diabetic dogs and cats, because a small dose can be more easily measured than with U-100 insulin. However, in the United States, U-100 insulin has replaced U-40 insulin (no longer manufactured in the United States) as the most commonly used in human patients. U-40 insulin is still widely available in other parts of the world, including Europe and Latin America. The U-500 concentration, the only insulin that requires a prescription, is indicated only in rare cases of insulin resistance when an insulin dosage of hundreds of units per day is required.

Whatever insulin preparation is used, it is critical that owners purchase the correct syringe to match the concentration of insulin to be administered. In other words, one must use U-40 syringes with U-40 insulin, and U-100 syringes with U-100 insulin. If U-100 insulin were to be inadvertently drawn with a U-40 syringe, the dose would be more than twice what it should be.

Over the past few years, insulin syringes have become smaller and the needles have sharper points and special coatings that work to make injections less painful. As before, the syringes are marked in insulin units, but there may be some differences in

Table 2. *Insulin Syringes*

Name and Manufacturer	Insulin	Needle Gauge	Needle Size	Packaging
1-ml syringes				
B-D Microfine IV	U-100	28G	½″	100 (10 packs of 10)
B-D Microfine	U-100	27G	⅝″	100 (10 packs of 10)
B-D Microfine IV	U-40	28G	½″	100 (10 packs of 10)
Can-Am E-Z Ject	U-100	27G	½″	100 (individually wrapped)
Can-Am E-Z-Ject	U-100	28G	½″	100 (individually wrapped)
Monoject Ultra Comfort 28	U-100	28G	½″	100 or 30 (individually wrapped)
Pharma-Plast	U-100	28G	½″	100 (10 packs of 10)
Terumo	U-100	29G	½″	100 (individually wrapped)
Terumo	U-100	27G	½″	100 (individually wrapped)
¼-ml syringes				
Terumo	U-100	29G	½″	100 (individually wrapped)
½-ml syringes				
B-D Microfine IV	U-100	28G	½″	100 (10 packs of 10)
Can-Am E-Z-Ject	U-50	28G	½″	100 (individually wrapped)
Monoject Ultra Comfort 28	U-100	28G	½″	100 or 30 (individually wrapped)
Pharma-Plast	U-100	28G	½″	100 (10 packs of 10)
Terumo	U-100	29G	½″	100 (individually wrapped)
Terumo	U-100	27G	½″	100 (individually wrapped)
³⁄₁₀-ml syringes				
B-D Microfine IV	U-100	28G	½″	100 (10 packs of 10)

the way units are indicated, depending on the size of the syringe and the manufacturer. Hard-to-read syringes may be a problem for visually impaired owners.

In general, there are four different insulin syringes available (Table 2). U-100 insulin syringes are manufactured with a 0.3-, 0.5-, and 1-ml capacity, whereas only one U-40 insulin syringe is available with a 1-ml capacity (B-D Microfine IV, Table 2). The smaller-sized syringes are designed for patients that require a smaller dosage of U-100 insulin. For example, the 0.3-ml syringes are designed for patients that require less than 30 U of insulin per injection. These syringes make it easy to accurately draw up a small dosage of U-100 insulin without the need for dilution of the insulin preparation. In dogs and cats that require very small dosages of insulin, the U-100 insulin preparations can be diluted with saline or pH-adjusted diluents obtained from the manufacturer. Special care must be taken to ensure that the correct dose of the diluted insulin is administered with an ordi-

nary insulin syringe. For example, if a 1:10 dilution of insulin is prepared, a full 1-ml, U-100 insulin syringe will hold only 10 units, a full 0.5-ml syringe will hold only 5 units, and a full 0.3-ml syringe will hold only 3 units.

References and Suggested Reading

Hallden, G., Gafvelin, G., Mutt, V., et al.: Characterization of cat insulin. Arch. Biochem. Biophys. 247:20, 1986.
  Description of the isolation and characterization of the insulin amino acid structure in cats.

Neubauer, H., and Schone, H.: The immunogenicity of different insulins in several animal species. Diabetes 27:8, 1978.
  Because the insulins of dogs and pigs have identical amino acid sequences, no antigenicity of porcine insulin in dogs could be observed.

Smith, L.: Amino acid sequences of insulins. Diabetes 21 (suppl. 2):457, 1972.
  A review of the amino acid sequence of insulin in a variety of species, including the human, pig, cattle, and dog.

Position Statement of the American Diabetes Association. Insulin administration. Diabetes Care 13:28, 1990.
  Reviews the current recommendations of the American Diabetes Association concerning use of insulin and insulin syringes.

PATHOGENESIS AND MANAGEMENT OF DIABETIC KETOACIDOSIS

KELLY J. DIEHL
and STEVEN L. WHEELER

Fort Collins, Colorado

Diabetic ketoacidosis (DKA) is one of the most common endocrinopathics encountered in the emergency setting. Although the pathogenesis of diabetic ketoacidosis is becoming well understood, DKA remains a diagnostic and therapeutic challenge. Accurate diagnosis and prompt appropriate therapy are essential for a favorable outcome. (See *CVT X*, pp. 1008 and 1012). The pathogenesis and management of diabetic ketoacidosis will be reviewed.

PATHOGENESIS

DKA is characterized by concurrent hyperglycemia, acidosis, and ketosis. Diabetic ketoacidosis results from the metabolic derangements secondary to absolute or relative insulin deficiency and excessive secretion of counter-regulatory hormones. It is the interplay of these two events that leads to the development of ketoacidosis. Studies in humans show that withdrawal of insulin alone will not cause ketosis in the unstressed diabetic. Similarly, increases in counter-regulatory hormones without concurrent insulin deficiency do not lead to ketosis.

Insulin is normally released in response to elevations of blood glucose. Insulin acts on the liver to increase the rate of glucose uptake from the portal blood, stimulates glycogen synthesis, and inhibits gluconeogenesis and glycogenolysis. In muscle, insulin also stimulates glucose uptake from the blood, inhibits proteolysis, and stimulates protein synthesis. Insulin enhances glucose and lipoprotein uptake by fat cells, as well as stimulating lipogenesis and inhibiting lipolysis.

Insulin action is opposed by counter-regulatory hormones: glucagon, the catecholamines, cortisol, and growth hormone. Glucagon directly opposes most actions of insulin and is understandably the most important of the counter-regulatory hormones in the pathogenesis of DKA. Cortisol and catecholamine levels are increased in DKA owing to stress-induced stimulation of the sympathoadrenal axis. Glucagon stimulates hepatic glucose production by accelerating glycogenolysis and gluconeogenesis and also enhances hepatic ketone production. The remaining counter-regulatory hormones, the catecholamines, cortisol, and growth hormone, are also antagonistic to insulin. Catecholamines increase blood glucose by stimulating hepatic glycogenolysis and gluconeogenesis. Catecholamines also stimulate lipolysis, thereby providing fatty acids for ketogenesis. Cortisol and growth hormone depress peripheral glucose utilization and increase hepatic gluconeogenesis. The net result of insulin deficiency and counter-regulatory hormone excess is hyperglycemia and ketosis (Fig. 1).

Hyperglycemia in diabetic patients occurs secondary to glucose overproduction and decreased peripheral utilization. The increased ratio of glucagon to insulin in the portal blood is thought to be the primary cause of glucose overproduction in diabetic ketoacidosis. Hyperglycemia causes an osmotic diuresis leading to dehydration and electrolyte depletion. Hyperglycemia can also lead to hyperosmolality.

Glucagon excess appears to be the major stimulus in promoting hepatic ketogenesis. An increased ratio of glucagon to insulin in the portal blood favors hepatic ketogenesis over triglyceride formation. Acetoacetate and beta-hydroxybutyrate are the primary ketones formed and exist in equilibrium, with acetoacetate predominating in reduced conditions and beta-hydroxybutyrate predominating in oxidized conditions. The rate of ketone production is proportional to the amount of free fatty acid delivered to the liver; therefore, not only is ketone production enhanced by glucagon excess but it is further driven by increased concentrations of free fatty acids delivered to the liver secondary to insulin deficiency. Metabolic acidosis with an increased anion gap ensues when the buffering systems of the body are overwhelmed by the increasing levels of ketoacids.

DIAGNOSIS

Diagnosis of diabetic ketoacidosis is based on the identification of acidosis, hyperglycemia, and keto-

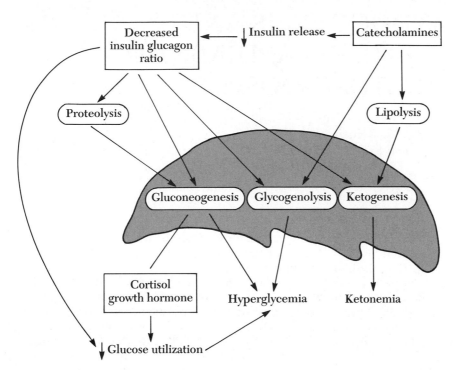

Figure 1. The effects of increased counter-regulatory hormones and insulin deficiency on glucose, protein, and lipid metabolism are illustrated. The end results are hyperglycemia and ketonemia. Refer to text for complete discussion of the mechanisms of the altered metabolism.

sis. Animals with diabetic ketoacidosis usual present with nonspecific signs, including anorexia, depression, vomiting, and diarrhea. Classic signs of diabetes such as polyuria/polydipsia, polyphagia, and weight loss may precede the signs of acute illness. Physical examination findings often reveal dehydration, hepatomegaly, cataracts, Kussmaul-type respirations, and a "fruity" odor of the breath. However, since many other diseases can cause similar signs, diagnosis is usually made by detecting ketones and glucose in the urine in conjunction with the history and physical examination findings. Fever may be present but is not a consistent finding, even with concurrent infection. If an increased rectal temperature is detected, pancreatitis and infection should be suspected and appropriate diagnostic and therapeutic measures started.

The suggested minimum database for the ketoacidotic patient includes urinalysis, blood glucose, sodium, potassium, BUN and creatinine, serum osmolality, lead II ECG strip, anion gap, and blood gas analysis. These tests are critical for immediate patient assessment and formulation of a treatment protocol. Further diagnostic tests can be performed as dictated by patient status after initial treatment is begun. Urine should be collected via cystocentesis whenever possible. A free-catch sample is acceptable, but urinary catheterization is not recommended since these patients are immunocompromised and are predisposed to urinary tract infections. Unless urine output is questionable and renal disease is suspected, placement of indwelling urinary catheters is likewise discouraged.

Special reagent strips are commonly employed to detect glucose and ketones in urine. One failing of these reagent strips is their relative inability to detect beta-hydroxybutyrate. The ratio of beta-hydroxybutyrate to acetoacetate is approximately 3:1 in the diabetic ketoacidotic but can be as high as 8:1 in severely dehydrated patients. Therefore, significant ketosis may exist with a negative or only weakly positive nitroprusside test or urine ketone reaction. One method to circumvent this problem is to add a few drops of hydrogen peroxide to the urine specimen, which will oxidize beta-hydroxybutyrate to acetoacetate. The acetoacetate will give a positive nitroprusside reaction if urinary ketone levels are significant. In human diabetics, increases in serum acetoacetate also interfere with measurement of serum creatinine, leading to facetious elevations. For this reason, BUN may be preferred over creatinine for evaluating renal function in DKA.

TREATMENT

The therapeutic goals in the treatment of diabetic ketoacidosis are correction of hypovolemia, normalization of electrolyte imbalances, reversal of acidemia and hyperglycemia, and treatment of identifiable precipitating causes. Although the specific management of diabetic ketoacidosis remains controversial, the cornerstones of therapy are fluid support, electrolyte supplementation, and insulin administration.

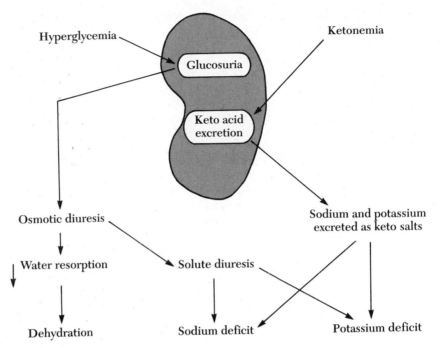

Figure 2. Development of electrolyte abnormalities secondary to hyperglycemia and ketonemia. Total body depletion of sodium and potassium results from both an osmotic diuresis and ketosalt formation.

Fluids

Fluid losses in diabetic ketoacidosis are secondary to the osmotic diuresis induced by hyperglycemia. Vomiting, pyrexia, decreased fluid intake, and hyperventilation also contribute to fluid loss. Restoration of intravascular volume is the most important aspect of therapy for DKA. Since most diabetic ketoacidotic patients are in a state of hypertonic dehydration, ultimately, free water must be given to reverse this abnormality. Fluid therapy continues to be a subject of debate, but most reviews suggest 0.9% saline for immediate volume expansion, followed by 0.45% saline when the patient's vascular status is stable. If the patient presents in shock, colloids appear to be the fluid of choice for initial volume expansion. One recent review recommends that fluid therapy be based on a corrected serum sodium concentration. For each 100 mg/dl of plasma glucose over 100 mg/dl, 2.75 mEq/L is added to the measured serum sodium. If the corrected sodium concentration is less than 140 mEq, then 0.9% saline is administered. If the corrected sodium concentration is greater than 160 mEq, 0.45% saline is used for fluid replacement. Ringer's solution has also been advocated for fluid replacement when serum sodium levels are 140 to 160 mEq/L. Fluid therapy alone will lower serum blood glucose levels in three ways. First, fluids increase urine flow, which enhances renal glucose excretion. Second, fluids decrease the concentration of counter-regulatory hormones, especially catecholamines. Finally, improved peripheral glucose utilization secondary to cellular rehydration may also contribute

to decreases in blood glucose levels. Human studies have demonstrated that large fluid volumes administered rapidly to diabetic ketoacidotic patients for volume replacement may not be indicated. Metabolic recovery was quicker in patients receiving lower fluid infusion rates than higher rates. High fluid rates have been implicated in the development of cerebral edema in humans. Cerebral edema has not yet been identified as a significant problem in veterinary patients but should be considered during initial volume replacement. For this reason, volume deficits should be replaced over a relatively long period, 24 to 48 hr. Total fluid volume to be replaced equals maintenance requirements (60 mL/kg/day) plus 80% of fluid deficits (% dehydration $\times$ body weight$_{kg}$ $\times$ 1000 mL/kg) plus ongoing fluid losses (i.e., gastrointestinal). Ongoing fluid losses should be replaced as they occur. The patient should be weighed frequently.

Electrolytes

The osmotic diuresis resulting from hyperglycemia leads to loss of electrolytes as well as free water. Serum hyperosmolality and acidosis also cause shifts in electrolytes, especially potassium, from the intracellular to extracellular space. The result is depletion of total body sodium, potassium, and phosphate. Despite total body deficits, measured serum levels may be decreased, normal, or increased initially because of extracellular shifts of electrolytes (Fig. 2).

Fluid replacement with 0.9% saline is usually

adequate to replace sodium losses (see discussion above of fluid choice). Even though initial serum potassium may be normal, or even increased, total body depletion of potassium is present in all patients with diabetic ketoacidosis secondary to acidosis, urinary losses, and hyperglycemia. Serum levels of potassium will drop during therapy as potassium moves back into the intracellular space and continues to be lost in the urine. If hyperkalemia is present initially, potassium replacement is withheld until fluid therapy has been instituted. Within 2 to 4 hr after starting fluid therapy, potassium concentrations will drop considerably in most patients. It is imperative that the patient be closely monitored during this period and the potassium levels checked and supplementation provided as needed. Those patients with normal or decreased potassium concentrations on presentation should be supplemented immediately. If electrolyte determination is not available, a crude estimate of potassium concentration can be made by running a lead II ECG strip. Electrocardiographic changes associated with progressive hyperkalemia include peaking of the T wave, widening of the QRS complex, decreased P-wave amplitude, and atrial standstill. Ultimately, ventricular fibrillation can occur with profound hyperkalemia. Conversely, hypokalemia can cause a progressive depression of the ST segment and decreased amplitude of the T wave. Prolongation of the QT interval is the most consistent change seen caused by hypokalemia. Atrial and ventricular premature contractions can occur in hypokalemic patients. The most prominent ECG changes are seen when the serum potassium level drops below 2.5 mEq/L. Although ECG changes can be helpful in monitoring therapy, they do not replace measurement of serum potassium levels. In practice settings where immediate potassium levels are not available, potassium should be administered at 0.1 to 0.2 mEq/kg/hr with the rate of supplementation not to exceed 0.5 mEq/kg/hr, provided the patient is not oliguric and a lead II ECG does not show any signs of hyperkalemia.

Phosphate depletion also occurs in the ketoacidotic patient. Phosphate shifts out of cells in response to acidosis and is lost in the urine secondary to osmotic diuresis. Fluid and insulin therapy causes an intracellular shift of phosphorus and can lead to hypophosphatemia. Normal serum phosphate concentrations are necessary for (1) adequate levels of red blood cell 2,3-diphosphoglycerate, which ensures adequate tissue oxygenation, (2) proper cardiac and respiratory muscle function, and (3) formation of energy-dependent intermediates such as ATP. Several studies have shown that phosphate supplementation has no beneficial effect and may exacerbate hypophosphatemia because of increased urinary phosphorus excretion. No definitive studies have been conducted in veterinary medicine, but

Table 1. Guidelines for Regular Insulin Therapy

Route	Dose	Monitoring
IM	0.25 U/kg initially, then 0.1 U/kg q 1 hr for animals > 10 kg 2 U initially, then 1 U q 1 hr for animals < 10 kg but > 3 kg 1 U initially, then 1 U q 1 hr for animals < 3 kg	blood glucose q 1 hr
IV	2.2 U/kg/day for dogs and 1.1 U/kg/day for cats given as a constant-rate infusion	blood glucose q 1 hr
SC	0.5 U/kg q 6 hr; adjust dose according to blood glucose	blood glucose q 3–6 hr

phosphorus supplementation is probably necessary only in patients with severe hypophosphatemia (< 1 mg/dl). Since insulin acts to move phosphorus intracellularly, hypophosphatemia is most commonly observed after initiating insulin therapy. Phosphate can be administered at a rate of 0.01 to 0.03 mmol/kg/hr for 6 hr and then rechecked. If potassium phosphate is used, this source of potassium must be calculated into the patient's potassium requirements.

Insulin

Insulin therapy is necessary for treatment of ketoacidosis and hyperglycemia. Insulin enhances peripheral glucose uptake, decreases mobilization of free fatty acids from tissues, opposes the actions of glucagon, and lowers blood glucagon levels.

Since the early 1970's, the trend in human medicine has been toward low-dose insulin regimens. It has been demonstrated in people that low-dose insulin therapy is as effective in treating DKA as high-dose therapy and causes fewer adverse side effects, such as hypoglycemia and hypokalemia. Even though some degree of insulin resistance exists in all diabetic ketoacidotic patients secondary to acidosis and hypersecretion of counter-regulatory hormones, low-dose insulin generally is sufficient to provide maximal effects on lipid and carbohydrate metabolism.

Only regular insulin should be used in the emergency treatment of diabetic ketoacidosis. The onset of the longer-acting insulin preparations precludes their use in the initial management of DKA. Regular insulin can be administered intravenously, subcutaneously, or intramuscularly (Table 1). Intravenous infusion is the recommended route of administration for the initial treatment of DKA in humans. Since insulin will absorb to plastic and glassware, 50 ml of the fluid/insulin mixture can be flushed through the intravenous tubing and discarded before starting the infusion. Patients on IV insulin infusion require close monitoring to avoid hypoglycemia.

Many veterinary practices may not yet have the equipment (e.g., infusion pumps, etc.) nor the personnel to practically and safely infuse IV insulin. Intramuscular insulin administration is an effective alternative to IV infusion and, in the authors' opinion, is the optimum method of insulin therapy in DKA. Regular insulin can also be given subcutaneously; however, poor tissue perfusion can inhibit absorption initially, and subsequent insulin doses may be resorbed quickly once the patient is rehydrated, promoting a rapid decrease in blood glucose. Subcutaneous insulin therapy is therefore not recommended initially in the treatment of DKA. Blood glucose should be monitored hourly if the IV or IM protocol is used. Once the blood glucose concentration declines to 250 mg/dl, 5% dextrose should be added to the fluids to prevent hypoglycemia. In most cases, hydration status will have improved, and regular insulin can now be administered by the subcutaneous route (Table 1). Although blood glucose levels decrease within 4 to 8 hours of starting fluid and insulin therapy, ketonemia may take up to 48 hr to resolve and insulin is necessary to prevent further synthesis of ketoacids. Although high concentrations of glucose theoretically should stimulate more rapid ketoacid metabolism, prospective human studies have not shown any difference between 5% and 10% dextrose solutions in rapidity of patient recovery. Once the acidosis is resolved and the animal is eating and drinking, fluids can be discontinued and therapy with a longer-acting insulin preparation started.

Bicarbonate

Treatment of DKA with bicarbonate remains controversial. Two prospective human studies did not find any significant difference in clinical course in patients given bicarbonate versus those patients not treated with bicarbonate. Fluid and insulin therapy is usually adequate to reverse even severe acidosis. Although acidosis decreases cardiac performance and perpetuates electrolyte shifts to the extracellular space (particularly potassium and phosphorus), bicarbonate administration does not enhance resolution of ketosis. Increased hemoglobin oxygen affinity secondary to bicarbonate administration can decrease peripheral oxygen delivery, especially in hypovolemic patients. Rapid correction of acidemia can also result in cerebrospinal fluid acidosis with subsequent central nervous system (CNS) signs such as depression and coma. Once treatment for DKA is initiated, ketoacids are metabolized, generating bicarbonate. Additional exogenous bicarbonate can lead to an iatrogenic metabolic alkalosis. Bicarbonate is not recommended, in our opinion, unless serum HCO_3 (or total CO_2) is less than or equal to 5 mEq/L. The dose of bicarbonate to be used equals $0.3 \times$ body weight in kg $\times$ base excess. One third of the dose is given over 15 min and the remainder over the next 12 hr in the patient's fluids.

OTHER THERAPEUTIC CONSIDERATIONS

In all cases of DKA, there is a precipitating event that must be identified and treated. Infection is a common predisposing factor, but any systemic illness can lead to DKA. Bronchial, blood, and urine cultures may be warranted in these patients. Many older patients with DKA may also have concurrent renal and/or cardiac disease. Fluids must be delivered cautiously to these patients, particularly when large volumes are being administered.

Hyperosmolar diabetes mellitus (HDM) is a syndrome characterized by marked hyperglycemia, hyperosmolarity, and CNS depression. Ketoacidosis is usually not a feature of HDM. Hyperosmolar diabetic coma can clinically resemble DKA but has a more insidious onset. The two must be distinguished from each other since the therapy for HDM differs somewhat from that for DKA. Severe CNS signs, marked hyperglycemia, hyperosmolarity, and lack of ketoacidosis suggest HDM rather than DKA. For further information on management of HDM, see Wheeler (1988), and Kitabchi and Murphy (1988).

References and Suggested Reading

Chastain, C. B., and Nichols, C. S.: Low-dose intramuscular insulin therapy for diabetic ketoacidosis in dogs. J.A.V.M.A. 178:561, 1981.
Description of intramuscular insulin therapy regimen in dogs.
Feldman, E. C., and Nelson, R. W.: *Canine and Feline Endocrinology and Reproduction.* Philadelphia: W. B. Saunders, 1987, p. 274.
An in-depth review of the pathogenesis and treatment of diabetic ketoacidosis in dogs and cats.
Foster, D. W., and McGarry, J. D.: The metabolic derangements and treatment of diabetic ketoacidosis. N. Engl. J. Med. 309:159, 1983.
A review of the pathophysiology and treatment of diabetic ketoacidosis in humans.
Israel, R. S.: Diabetic ketoacidosis. Emerg. Med. Clin. North Am. 7:859, 1989.
A review of current emergency therapy for diabetic ketoacidosis in humans.
Kitabchi, A. E., and Murphy, M. B.: Diabetic ketoacidosis and hyperosmolar hyperglycemic nonketotic coma. Med. Clin. North Am. 72:1545, 1988.
An extensive review of the pathogenesis and treatment of diabetic ketoacidosis and hyperosmolar hyperglycemic nonketotic coma in humans.
Krane, E. J.: Diabetic ketoacidosis. Pediat. Clin. North Am. 34:935, 1987.
A review of the treatment of pediatric and adolescent diabetic ketoacidosis.
Wheeler, S. L.: Emergency management of the diabetic patient. Semin. Vet. Med. Surg. 3:265, 1988.
A review of the pathogenesis and treatment of both diabetic ketoacidosis and hyperosmolar hyperglycemic nonketotic coma in small animals.
Willard, M. D., Zerbe, C. A., Schall, W. D., et al.: Severe hypophosphatemia associated with diabetes mellitus in six dogs and one cat. J.A.V.M.A. 190:1007, 1987.
A retrospective review of the clinical presentation, clinical course, and treatment of severe hypophosphatemia secondary to diabetes mellitus in small animals.

TREATMENT OF FELINE DIABETES MELLITUS

RICHARD W. NELSON
and EDWARD C. FELDMAN
Davis, California

Insulin-dependent diabetes mellitus (IDDM; type I diabetes) is the most common clinically recognized form of diabetes mellitus in cats. IDDM is characterized by hypoinsulinemia and minimal to no increase in endogenous insulin secretion during an insulin response test. Common histopathologic abnormalities include islet-specific amyloidosis and beta-cell vacuolation/degeneration. Loss of beta-cell function is irreversible in IDDM, and lifelong insulin therapy is mandatory to maintain glycemic control of the diabetic state.

Non–insulin-dependent diabetes mellitus (NIDDM; type II diabetes) has been diagnosed in approximately 20% of our diabetic cats. Carbohydrate intolerance in these cats is believed to develop secondary to impaired insulin secretion by the beta cells, insulin resistance in insulin-responsive tissues, and accelerated hepatic glucose production. Beta cells have the ability to secrete insulin; however, the secretory response to stimulants is delayed and the total amount of insulin secreted abnormal. Obesity and partial loss of beta-cell mass and function by islet-specific amyloid deposition may play a part in some cats with NIDDM.

Because the beta cells maintain some insulin secretory function in cats with NIDDM, hyperglycemia tends to be mild, ketoacidosis uncommon, and the necessity for insulin therapy variable in these cats. For many of these cats, insulin requirements wax and wane. Some diabetic cats may never require insulin therapy once the initial bout of insulin-requiring diabetes mellitus has dissipated, whereas others become permanently insulin dependent.

GOALS OF THERAPY

The primary goal of therapy for both forms of diabetes mellitus is the elimination of clinical signs (i.e., polydipsia, polyuria, polyphagia, and weight loss) that occur secondary to hyperglycemia and glucosuria. This can be accomplished by maintaining blood glucose concentrations close to normal (i.e., 100 mg/dl) through insulin therapy, diet, exercise, or oral hypoglycemic medications. Avoid-

ance or control of concurrent illness is also invaluable. The therapeutic regimen that is ultimately successful depends, in part, on the number of functional beta cells in the pancreas at the time of diagnosis and whether the underlying etiology is progressive.

Veterinarians must balance the possible benefits of "tight" glucose control obtainable with insulin therapy against the risks of inducing hypoglycemia. For some diabetic cats with beta-cell secretory capabilities, correction of obesity, dietary therapy, and oral hypoglycemic drugs are effective in minimizing clinical signs, despite failing to obtain tight control. Hypoglycemia is most likely to occur with overzealous insulin therapy, especially in cats with NIDDM.

DIETARY THERAPY

Dietary therapy has an important role in the successful management of diabetes mellitus. Dietary therapy should correct obesity, maintain consistency in the timing and caloric content of the meals, and furnish a diet that minimizes postprandial fluctuations in blood glucose.

Diabetic cats should be fed a diet high in fiber and complex carbohydrates at a caloric intake designed to correct obesity. Diets containing increased amounts of fiber help promote weight loss, slow glucose absorption from the intestinal tract, reduce postprandial fluctuations in blood glucose, and enhance control of hyperglycemia. The diets likely to be most effective for the correction of excess body weight and improvement of glycemic control are those that contain the most fiber and digestible complex carbohydrates on a dry matter basis (Table 1).

In insulin-responsive tissues, obesity causes insulin resistance that is reversible after correction of the obese state. In obese cats, weight reduction should be gradual, requiring 2 to 4 months to obtain the targeted body weight. Gradual weight reduction minimizes development of the hepatic lipidosis syndrome. The beneficial effects associated with correction of obesity and the feeding of diets containing

Table 1. *Fiber and Digestible Complex Carbohydrate Content of Some of the Commercially Available High-Fiber Cat Foods*

	Crude Fiber	Digestible Complex Carbohydrates
Prescription Diet R/D		
Canned	28	24
Dry	19	30
Prescription Diet W/D		
Canned	12	22
Dry	10	37
Science Diet Maintenance		
Light		
Canned	7	25
Dry	7	39
Iams Less Active		
Dry	2	41

Values listed as per cent dry matter.

increased fiber are often observed before the targeted body weight is reached. In some cats with NIDDM, feeding a high-fiber diet at a caloric intake designed to achieve ideal body weight may eliminate the need for insulin therapy.

Diets containing increased fiber content should be fed with caution to thin diabetic cats. High-fiber diets have a low caloric density, which can interfere with weight gain and may cause further weight loss. For these cats, weight gain usually requires establishment of glycemic control through insulin therapy and feeding a calorie-dense, low-fiber diet. Once normal body weight has been attained, a diet containing an increased fiber content can gradually replace the prior diet.

Diabetic cats should be fed multiple small meals during the day to help minimize the hyperglycemic effect of each meal, thereby helping to control fluctuations in blood glucose. Cats that are "nibblers" should be allowed free access to food. "Gluttonous" cats should be fed several equal-sized meals at defined times during the day. Most cats receiving insulin once daily are fed at the time of injection and approximately 10 hr later. Cats on twice-daily insulin are fed equal-sized meals at the time of each insulin injection.

ORAL HYPOGLYCEMIC DRUGS

Sulfonylureas are the only oral hypoglycemic drugs approved for use in the United States (Table 2). The primary effect of sulfonylureas is to stimulate secretion of preformed insulin from the pancreas. Functional beta cells must exist for sulfonylureas to be effective. Sulfonylureas are relatively ineffective as the sole form of therapy in improving glycemic control in humans with IDDM or severe NIDDM.

With chronic administration, sulfonylureas de-

crease hepatic glucose production, partially reverse the postbinding defect in insulin action, and increase the number of cellular insulin receptors. It is controversial whether these actions are a direct effect of the sulfonylureas or secondary to sulfonylurea-induced increased insulin secretion.

In healthy cats, the second-generation sulfonylurea glipizide (Glucotrol, Roerig Division, Pfizer) stimulates insulin secretion within 10 min of oral administration. Glipizide has been efficacious in improving glycemic control (i.e., maintaining blood glucose concentration < 200 mg/dl) in some of our diabetic cats with NIDDM when used in conjunction with dietary therapy and correction of obesity. Other diabetic cats have shown clinical improvement (i.e., increased activity, reduction in polyuria/polydipsia, gain in body weight) despite fasting blood glucose concentrations between 200 and 400 mg/dl. Several diabetic cats have been successfully treated for longer than 18 months.

We are currently evaluating the glipizide dose of 2.5 to 5.0 mg given two to three times a day, in conjunction with a meal, to those diabetic cats shown to have some insulin secretory capacity (i.e., serum insulin concentration > 120 pM/L) on an insulin response test (e.g., glucose tolerance test or glucagon tolerance test). Vomiting and hepatic enzyme alterations have been the primary adverse reactions, occurring in approximately 10% of our cats. Among the adverse reactions following chronic administration of glipizide in humans are bone marrow depression and blood dyscrasias. These problems have not been identified in our cats. Nevertheless, periodic evaluation of a hemogram and serum biochemical panel is indicated in any cat on long-term glipizide therapy.

INSULIN THERAPY: SHOULD IT BE INITIATED?

The identification of NIDDM in cats raises questions concerning the need for insulin therapy in this species. Glycemic control can be maintained in some cats with NIDDM with dietary therapy and oral hypoglycemic drugs. Cats with little or no

Table 2. *Oral Sulfonylurea Drugs Currently Available in the United States**

Generic Name	Trade Name	Relative Potency
Tolbutamide	Orinase	1
Acetohexamide	Dymelor	2.5
Tolazamide	Tolinase	5
Chlorpropamide	Diabinese	6
Glipizide	Glucotrol	100
Glyburide	Micronase, DiaBeta	150

*Reprinted with permission from Nelson, R. W.: Feline diabetes mellitus. Vet. Med. Rep. 3:4, 1991.

insulin reserve, however, require insulin therapy. Unfortunately, at the time of a cat's initial presentation, veterinarians cannot easily differentiate between a cat with IDDM and one with NIDDM. Therefore, the therapeutic approach should be based on the severity of clinical signs, the presence or absence of ketoacidosis, the general health of the cat, and ideally, the results of an insulin response test. If clinical signs are mild in a cat that is obese and nonketotic, a conservative therapeutic approach relying on dietary therapy and oral hypoglycemic drugs may be tried. Response to therapy can be monitored at home by measuring urine glucose concentrations whenever possible. In addition, weekly in-hospital evaluations, consisting of fasting and six to eight postprandial (hourly) glucose concentrations, should be considered. During the initial 1 to 2 months of oral therapy, if blood glucose concentrations decrease to less than 200 mg/dl, insulin therapy may not be indicated. Conversely, if hyperglycemia and glucosuria persist, ketoacidosis develops, or the cat becomes ill, then insulin therapy should be initiated.

An alternative approach is to initiate insulin therapy in conjunction with dietary therapy once the diagnosis of diabetes is established. This is especially important if ketoacidosis is present or the cat is thin, in poor condition, or ill. NIDDM should be suspected if, during subsequent evaluations of insulin therapy, the blood glucose is consistently < 200 mg/dl, insulin requirements seem nominal for the body weight of the cat, or the cat seems exquisitely sensitive to the glycemic effects of insulin. For these cats, attempts should be made to reduce the insulin dose and possibly discontinue insulin therapy while continuing appropriate dietary therapy.

INITIAL INSULIN THERAPY

Protamine zinc (PZI) and Ultralente insulin are the insulins of choice for initial regulation of diabetes in cats. The antigenicity of exogenous insulin preparations and the potential for insulin resistance due to insulin antibody formation in cats are conjecture at this time. As such, we initially use beef/pork insulin in diabetic cats and reserve other insulins (e.g., purified pork insulin, recombinant human insulin) for those cats having problems with insulin activity (i.e., insulin resistance).

In cats, we begin insulin therapy with Ultralente insulin as a single morning injection. Diabetic cats can usually be controlled with doses of 0.2 to 1.0 U of Ultralente insulin per kilogram of body weight. The average cat is started on 1 to 3 U of Ultralente as a single morning injection.

ADJUSTMENTS IN INSULIN THERAPY

Assessment of insulin therapy is mandatory during regulation of diabetes in cats. It is necessary to monitor the status of glycemic control in cats apparently doing well in the home environment as well as to re-establish glycemic control when clinical manifestations of hyperglycemia or hypoglycemia have developed. When assessing glycemic control, the insulin and feeding schedule used by the owner should be monitored and blood glucose concentrations measured every 1 to 2 hr throughout the day. This practice allows clinicians to determine the time of peak insulin effect, the duration of effect, and the degree of fluctuation in blood glucose concentrations. The dose of insulin, type of insulin, frequency of administration, and time of feeding may be altered depending on the results of the blood glucose measurements. There is no substitute for assessing multiple glucose concentrations, whether for the first check or after years of therapy. Serial glucose concentrations are far from perfect, but they represent the most accurate method of assessing diabetes in cats.

The ideal goal of insulin therapy is to maintain blood glucose concentrations between 100 and 250 mg/dl throughout each 24-hr period. If using glucose test strips, the blood glucose level should remain greater than 80 mg/dl. Blood glucose concentrations falling outside of this range are an indication for a change in insulin therapy, especially if a cat has clinical signs of hyperglycemia or hypoglycemia.

Lack of insulin effect, short duration of insulin effect, and hypoglycemia are the most common problems encountered in diabetic cats. Hypoglycemia is usually a result of overzealous insulin doses, often in conjunction with inappropriate monitoring of blood glucose concentrations or a failure to recognize NIDDM in a cat.

Lack of insulin effect can be due to inappropriate insulin administration technique, insulin underdose, falsely increased blood glucose concentrations associated with severe stress during the blood sampling procedure, and insulin resistance. There is no insulin dose that clearly differentiates insulin resistance from insulin underdose. Clinicians should suspect insulin resistance when insulin doses exceeding 6 U of long-acting insulin per cat are administered once or twice a day with minimal improvement in glycemic control. If insulin resistance is suspected, a diagnostic evaluation is warranted to identify the underlying cause (Table 3). Some cats, however, require large amounts of insulin without an obvious explanation for the relative insulin ineffectiveness.

Short duration of insulin action is common with the use of NPH, PZI, and even Ultralente insulin in cats. More than 75% of our diabetic cats require

Table 3. *Differential Diagnoses for Apparent Insulin Resistance in Cats*

Problems in insulin administration
Inactive or outdated insulin
Post-Somogyi's effect
Diestrus or pregnancy
Hyperadrenocorticism
Acromegaly
Infection
Administration of diabetogenic medications
Glucocorticoids
Megestrol acetate
Poor insulin absorption (esp. Ultralente)
Anti-insulin antibodies (?)

insulin twice a day to maintain some semblance of glycemic control. In diabetic cats, clinical signs of hyperglycemia, especially weight loss, usually develop when the duration of insulin action is less than 14 to 16 hr. The duration of insulin action is roughly defined as the time from the insulin injection until the blood glucose level exceeds 250 mg/dl. Assessment of the duration of insulin effect should not be done until an acceptable glucose nadir (i.e., > 80 but < 150 mg/dl) is established. Assessment of duration of insulin effect may not be valid when the glucose nadir is less than 80 mg/dl because of the potential for Somogyi's effect or if it is greater than 150 mg/dl because the dose is inadequate.

Determining the duration of effect is not a problem when a 24-hr blood glucose curve is obtained. Many practitioners, however, obtain only a 10- to 14-hr "abbreviated" curve. When generating an abbreviated serial glucose curve, it is important to obtain at least one blood glucose concentration 2 to 3 hr after the early evening meal. Classically, the abbreviated glucose curve in a cat with short duration of insulin action demonstrates the highest blood glucose concentration at the first blood sampling in the morning; blood glucose concentrations decline throughout the day; the glucose nadir occurs at the time of the early evening meal; and subsequent postprandial blood glucose concentrations increase. The severity of the clinical signs, magnitude of the morning hyperglycemia, and time of the blood glucose nadir allow assumptions to be made about the duration of action of the insulin.

The duration of insulin effect dictates any changes needed to establish glycemic control. If the effect of PZI or Ultralente insulin is 12 hr or less, equal doses of PZI or Ultralente insulin are given twice a day at approximately 12-hr intervals. If the effect of PZI or Ultralente insulin is greater than 12 hr and the cat is doing well at home, a change in frequency of administration may not be warranted. If the effect of PZI or Ultralente insulin is greater than 12 hr and the owner reports clinical signs of hyperglycemia, administration of PZI or Ultralente insulin twice a day at 12-hr intervals may be required. A reduction in the insulin dose may also be necessary to prevent hypoglycemia. The blood glucose concentration should be monitored closely for 5 to 7 days after initiating twice-daily insulin therapy. If the blood glucose concentration continues to decrease at the time of each insulin injection, the insulin dose must be modified.

References and Suggested Reading

Gerich, J. E.: Oral hypoglycemic agents. N. Engl. J. Med. 321:1231, 1989.
A complete discussion of the use of oral hypoglycemic agents for the treatment of diabetes mellitus in humans is presented in this manuscript.
Johnson, K. H., O'Brien, T. D., Betsholtz, C., et al.: Islet amyloid, islet-amyloid polypeptide, and diabetes mellitus. N.Engl. J. Med. 321: 513, 1989.
The role of islet-specific amyloidosis in the development of diabetes mellitus in cats and the implications for human type II diabetes mellitus is the emphasis of this manuscript.
Nelson, R. W.: Feline diabetes mellitus. Vet. Med. Rep. 3:4, 1991.
The etiology, diagnosis, and treatment of feline diabetes mellitus are summarized in this manuscript.
Nelson, R. W.: *Textbook of Veterinary Internal Medicine.* Philadelphia: W. B. Saunders, 1989, p. 1676.
A complete discussion of canine and feline diabetes mellitus is presented.
Nelson, R. W., and Lewis, L. D.: Nutritional management of diabetes mellitus. Semin. Vet. Med. Surg. 5:178, 1990.
Dietary therapy for canine and feline diabetes mellitus is emphasized.
Nelson, R. W., Himsel, C. A., Feldman, E. C., et al.: Glucose tolerance and insulin response in normal-weight and obese cats. Am. J. Vet. Res. 51:1357, 1990.
This manuscript documents the effect of obesity on glucose tolerance in cats.
Wallace, M. S., Peterson, M. E., and Nichols, C. E.: Absorption kinetics of regular, isophane, and protamine zinc insulin in normal cats. Domest. Anim. Endocrinol. 7: 509, 1990.
This manuscript documents the pharmacokinetic properties, including duration of effect, of commonly used insulins in cats.

ISLET CELL TUMORS SECRETING INSULIN, PANCREATIC POLYPEPTIDE, GASTRIN, OR GLUCAGON

CAROLE A. ZERBE

Auburn, Alabana

TYPES OF ISLET CELL TUMORS

Normal pancreatic islets contain four cell types: A cells secrete glucagon; B cells secrete insulin; D cells secrete somatostatin; and F (or P) cells secrete pancreatic polypeptide. Islet cell tumors that secrete excessive amounts of glucagon, insulin, and pancreatic polypeptide have been documented in small animals. In addition, some islet cell tumors secrete other hormones, including gastrin and adrenocorticotropic hormone (ACTH), which are not normally produced by the pancreas. Islet cell tumors that secrete excessive gastrin have been described in small animals.

The most frequently reported functional islet cell tumor of small animals is the insulin-secreting beta-cell tumor (insulinoma), followed by the much less common gastrin-secreting tumor (gastrinoma). A pancreatic polypeptide-secreting tumor (pancreatic peptidoma) has been documented in one dog, whereas the existence of a glucagon-secreting tumor (glucagonoma) in dogs remains controversial.

Even though islet cell tumors contain and secrete many peptide hormones, the clinical syndrome associated with islet cell tumors is generally related to excessive secretion of only one hormone. Thus, the four islet cell tumors listed earlier are associated with distinct clinical syndromes that involve differing treatments and prognoses. The distinct clinical syndrome, as well as diagnosis and management of insulinoma, gastrinoma, pancreatic peptidoma, and glucagonoma, are discussed separately here.

INSULINOMA

Islet cell tumors that primarily contain and secrete insulin are known as *insulinomas*. Excessive insulin secretion by the tumor interferes with glucose homeostasis and ultimately results in hypoglycemia (see *CVT IX*, p. 987, or other general texts for a discussion of the pathophysiology of insulinomas and hypoglycemia).

Clinical Features

SIGNALMENT

Insulin-secreting tumors usually occur in middle-aged to older medium to large breeds of dogs. There is no apparent sex predilection. Insulinomas, which appear to be very rare in cats, occur in middle-aged to old animals. Two of three reported cats were male Siamese, and one was a female Persian.

CLINICAL SIGNS

Seizures are by far the most common clinical abnormality occurring in dogs with insulinoma. These seizures include grand mal and focal facial seizures or status epilepticus. Other common clinical signs are generalized weakness, collapse or fainting, posterior paresis, depression or lethargy, and ataxia. Most dogs exhibit more than one of these clinical findings, with the frequency and severity of clinical signs generally increasing as the disease progresses. A study of 73 dogs with insulinoma found no significant difference in survival in regard to duration of clinical signs, nor was there a correlation between duration of clinical signs and clinical stage of disease.

Laboratory Findings

With the exception of hypoglycemia, which is found about 90% of the time at initial examination, results of the hemogram, urinalysis, and biochemical profile are usually unremarkable. Hypoalbuminemia, hypophosphatemia, hypokalemia, and increases in alkaline phosphatase and alanine aminotransferase have occasionally been reported; however, these findings are not specific nor helpful in achieving a definitive diagnosis.

Diagnostic Tests

The finding of fasting hypoglycemia is not specific for insulin-secreting tumors. Measurement of serum insulin concentration is necessary to support a diagnosis of insulinoma. Gross and histopathologic findings are also important to the diagnosis (and treatment) of insulinoma.

The best screening test for an insulin-secreting tumor is demonstration of excessive insulin secretion at a time when hypoglycemia is present (see *CVT X*, p. 961). To document hyperinsulinemia, an animal should be fed a normal meal early in the day (8:00 AM) then fasted for the remainder of the study. Glucose should be monitored with Chemstrip bG test strips at hourly intervals. When glucose concentration is about 60 mg/dl, a blood sample should be obtained for glucose and insulin measurement. The animal is then fed small meals during the next several hours.

In most affected dogs, hypoglycemia occurs within 8 or 10 hr of fasting, but an occasional dog may require more than 24 hr before developing low blood glucose concentration. If fasting beyond this 8- to 10- hr period is necessary, it is recommended that the dog be fed at 5:00 PM, 8:30 PM, and midnight. Then the animal should be fasted and blood glucose monitored beginning at 8:00 AM the following morning.

In normal animals, insulin levels fall as blood glucose decreases. However, in animals with insulinoma, insulin secretion generally remains high despite hypoglycemia. Thus, a serum insulin concentration greater than the normal range measured in a sample with a serum glucose of less than about 60 mg/dl is consistent with the presence of an insulin-secreting pancreatic tumor. An insulin concentration in the mid to upper range of normal measured during hypoglycemia is suggestive but not diagnostic of an insulin-secreting pancreatic tumor, and the test should be repeated. The amended insulin-to-glucose ratio is probably not a useful manipulation of insulin and glucose values for diagnosis of insulin-secreting tumors.

Insulin measurement is important not only for diagnosis but also for prognosis. Dogs with higher preoperative serum insulin concentrations have significantly shorter survival times than dogs with lower insulin values before tumor excision.

Pathologic Abnormalities: Necropsy or Surgery Findings

All dogs with insulin-secreting tumors had beta-cell tumors of the pancreas. Tumors may be located in the left lobe (44%), right lobe (35%), or body (14%) of the pancreas. Tumors are usually solitary, but multiple masses may occur, or rarely there is a diffuse islet cell tumor with no discrete nodule. There does not appear to be a difference in survival in relation to tumor location within the pancreas.

Metastasis occurs in approximately 40% of dogs. The liver or regional lymph nodes are the most common sites of metastasis. Local metastasis to the duodenum, mesentary, omentum, and spleen also occurs. Distant metastasis (other than to the liver) is rare.

Treatment

Management of insulinoma should be directed at specific treatment of the tumor, reduction of insulin secretion, and correction of hypoglycemia.

TREATMENT OF THE TUMOR

Surgical resection of pancreatic tumor (and metastatic tumor masses) should be the first approach to treatment. Exploratory laparotomy and tumor removal allow for confirmation of diagnosis, reduction of tumor mass(es) and subsequently insulin-secreting capacity, as well as prognostic information based on clinical stage of tumor. Dogs classified as clinical stage III (distant metastasis of neoplasm) have a significantly shorter survival time than dogs in clinical stages I (tumor confined to the pancreas) and II (tumor confined to the pancreas and regional lymph nodes).

A complete inspection of the abdominal contents at surgery is imperative, because metastasis is common. Particular attention should be given to the pancreas, which should be both visually and digitally inspected. Care must be taken in palpation of the pancreas, because severe life-threatening pancreatitis can occur following manipulation. If metastasis is considered too extensive for excision, the tumor should be debulked and a partial pancreatectomy performed to obtain tissue for biopsy and to decrease tumor burden. Euthanasia is not recommended, because many dogs will do well with medical therapy.

Administration of a 5% dextrose solution before, during, and immediately after surgery is helpful in preventing hypoglycemia. Blood glucose levels should be monitored during surgery so that the rate of fluid therapy can be adjusted if hypoglycemia develops. It is also important to provide adequate fluid therapy, which ensures good circulation through the pancreatic microvasculature and minimizes the development of pancreatitis after manipulation of the pancreas. It is recommended that fluids be given at two times the maintenance rate during and for 24 to 48 hr after surgery.

Postoperative recovery is routine in many cases, but complications including pancreatitis, hyperglycemia, overt diabetes mellitus, and hypoglycemia occur. Regardless of the extent of surgical manipulation, patients should be managed as though they had pancreatitis for 48 to 72 hr following surgery. Fluid therapy should be continued after surgery, and the animal should be given nothing by mouth. First water and then bland food can usually be offered by the third day, provided that vomiting has not occurred.

Blood glucose concentrations may be low, normal, or high after surgery. Hypoglycemia is usually found in those patients in which metastasis has occurred and tumor removal was incomplete. Hyperglycemia occurs in approximately 20% of dogs and is usually mild and transient, lasting from days to months. However, a few dogs require long-term insulin therapy.

MEDICAL THERAPY OF HYPOGLYCEMIA

If widespread metastasis is present or if hypoglycemia recurs after surgery, medical methods of controlling hypoglycemia are necessary. Medical management includes dietary alteration and use of drugs that inhibit insulin secretion or that antagonize the effects of insulin.

Frequent feedings (three to six times daily) of small amounts of a diet high in proteins, fats, and complex carbohydrates should be the first medical therapy attempted. Exercise should also be limited. However, because of the malignant nature of insulinoma in dogs, this therapy alone is not usually effective in long-term management.

When dietary treatment fails to control hypoglycemia, prednisolone, a short-acting glucocorticoid, is added to the treatment regimen. Prednisolone inhibits the action of insulin in peripheral tissues and stimulates hepatic glycogenolysis, both of which increase blood glucose concentration. It does not decrease tumor mass or block insulin production.

The initial dose of prednisolone is 0.5 to 1 mg/kg, divided, twice daily. The amount should then be decreased to the minimum effective dose. If hypoglycemia is not controlled, however, the dose should be increased gradually until control is achieved. Iatrogenic Cushing's syndrome develops in dogs undergoing long-term treatment or treatment with high doses.

Diazoxide is a benzothiadiazide diuretic that inhibits insulin secretion by blocking calcium mobilization. It also stimulates hepatic gluconegenesis and glycogenolysis through stimulation of the beta-adrenergic system as well as by decreasing peripheral glucose utilization. Diazoxide is initially administered at 10 mg/kg, divided, twice daily and given with meals. The dose may be increased to 60 mg/kg as needed to control the clinical signs associated with hypoglycemia. Care should be taken to avoid

causing hyperglycemia and diabetes mellitus. However, the most common complications of diazoxide therapy are anorexia, vomiting, and diarrhea. Tachycardia, bone marrow suppression, aplastic anemia, thrombocytopenia, and electrolyte and fluid retention may also occur. Concurrent administration of thiazide diuretics (hydrochlorothiazide, 2 to 4 mg/kg) reportedly may enhance the hyperglycemic effects of diazoxide.

Sandostatin (Octreotide, Sandoz) is a somatostatin analogue that has been effective in the treatment of about 50% of persons and two of five dogs with insulinoma. Somatostatin inhibits insulin synthesis and secretion. It presumably is not effective in some patients because their tumor cells do not express somatostatin receptors. The initial dose of sandostatin in dogs was 10 to 20 μg two to three times daily. Two dogs became refractory after 1 to 2 weeks of therapy. A dose as high as 40 μg three times daily was used unsuccessfully in one dog after it became refractory to lower doses. An attempt should be made to withdraw sandostatin after amelioration of clinical signs, and this was successfully accomplished in a dog subsequently maintained on prednisolone for more than 1 year.

Prognosis

Insulinoma in dogs is highly malignant, and there is already gross evidence of metastasis at the time of diagnosis in 36% of all dogs reported. The long-term prognosis thus is guarded to grave. Many dogs do well with medical and surgical management of tumor and hypoglycemia, however. One dog is reportedly alive longer than 60 months after the initial diagnostic surgical procedure. Age, degree of hyperinsulinemia, and clinical stage of tumor appear to be important prognostic indicators. Younger dogs have shorter survival times than older dogs. Dogs with higher serum insulin concentrations have shorter survival times than dogs with lower insulin concentrations. Dogs with clinical stage I have a significantly longer disease-free interval than dogs in clinical stages II and III.

GASTRINOMA

Islet cell tumors that secrete excessive amounts of gastrin are referred to as *gastrinoma* or *Zollinger-Ellison syndrome*. Gastrin is not normally found in the pancreas but is secreted by G cells located in the gastric mucosa and duodenal mucosa. The principal biologic activity of gastrin is stimulation of hydrochloric acid secretion by gastric parietal cells, but it also exerts trophic effects on the mucosa of the gastrointestinal tract.

In addition to gastrin receptors, parietal cells also

Table 1. Incidence of Historic and Clinical Signs of Gastrinoma in 17 Dogs and 2 Cats

Sign	No. of Animals	(%)
Vomiting	17/19	(89)
Weight loss	17/19	(89)
Anorexia	14/19	(82)
Diarrhea	14/19	(74)
Lethargy/depression	12/19	(63)
Polydipsia	5/18	(28)
Melena	5/19	(26)
Abdominal pain	3/19	(16)
Hematemesis	3/19	(16)
Hematochezia	2/19	(11)
Fever	2/19	(11)
Obstipation (alternating with diarrhea)	1/19	(6)
Ravenous appetite	1/19	(6)
Abdominal mass	1/19	(6)
Tachycardia	1/19	(6)

have distinct receptors for histamine and acetylcholine. Gastric acid output is a function of these three secretagogues that have various degrees of synergism with each other. Therapeutic control of gastric acid secretion can be achieved by use of specific receptor antagonists.

Clinical Features

SIGNALMENT

Gastrinomas usually develop in middle-aged dogs. There is no breed predilection. Females are more often affected (69%) than males (31%). Of the two cats reported, both were 12 years old and neutered. One cat was a female domestic short-hair, and the other was a male European short-hair.

CLINICAL SIGNS

Vomiting and weight loss are the most frequently observed clinical features of gastrin-secreting tumors (Table 1). Depression, lethargy, anorexia, and intermittent diarrhea are also common. The duration of clinical signs varied from 2 weeks to 2 years. Discounting the cat with a history of intermittent vomiting for 2 years, the average duration of clinical signs was 8.3 weeks.

Laboratory Findings

COMPLETE BLOOD COUNT

Regenerative anemia is present in 44% of the dogs and cats with gastrinoma and results from gastrointestinal blood loss. Leukocytosis (44%), neu-

trophilia (30%), and increased band cells (11%) also occur and probably reflect gastrointestinal inflammation.

SERUM BIOCHEMISTRY

The most common biochemical abnormalities of dogs and cats with gastrinoma include hyperglycemia, hypoalbuminemia, hypocalcemia, hypokalemia, and increased levels of serum alkaline phosphatase, but these biochemical changes occurred infrequently.

OTHER LABORATORY FINDINGS

Survey abdominal radiographs usually appear normal unless ulcer perforation caused peritonitis. Contrast upper gastrointestinal studies may show evidence of a plaquelike defect in the stomach or duodenum consistent with ulceration, prominent rugal folds, small-intestinal mucosal scalloping consistent with gastritis, or complete pyloric obstruction or a thickened pyloric antrum.

Gastroesophageal endoscopy may show esophageal inflammation or ulceration, thickened gastric rugae, gastric ulceration or hemorrhage, excessive liquid in the stomach, duodenal ulceration, or a hypertrophied pyloric antrum.

Diagnostic Tests

Diagnostic tests for gastrinoma include evaluation of fasting gastrin concentration, basal gastric acid secretion, or provocative tests such as secretin and calcium challenge. Gross and histopathologic findings are also important to the diagnosis of gastrinoma.

BASAL GASTRIN CONCENTRATION

The most reliable screening test for a gastrinoma is measurement of fasting serum gastrin concentrations. Dogs and cats with gastrinoma had serum gastrin concentrations that varied from 3.5 to 100 times the highest value reported for the respective normal range. However, hypergastrinemia alone is not diagnostic of gastrinoma and may be increased in dogs with renal failure, gastric outlet obstruction, chronic gastritis, liver disease, and small-intestinal resection. Thus, *provocative testing* is usually necessary to confirm a diagnosis of gastrinoma. Only when very high fasting levels ($>$ 10 times normal) occur with increased gastric acidity is a diagnosis of gastrinoma considered in persons without provocative testing. Too few small animal cases have been diagnosed to allow for such a statement in veterinary patients. I recommend provocative testing be performed in dogs and cats whenever possible, especially if gastrin levels are increased less than 10-fold.

SECRETIN CHALLENGE TEST

Experience with secretin challenge testing in dogs is limited. It has been performed in three dogs with gastrinoma and one dog with a pancreatic peptidoma. The test has not been used in cats with gastrinoma. This is the preferred test in humans because it is reliable and easy to do. However, my experience has been that secretin is expensive ($80 to $200 per 75-unit vial) and not always readily available. In patients with gastrinoma, secretin should cause an increase in gastrin concentrations, whereas gastrin in normal individuals may remain unchanged or may be slightly increased or decreased after secretin administration. Samples should be collected before and 2, 5, 15, and 30 min after an intravenous bolus of secretin administered at a dose of 2 to 4 units/kg. It is crucial to obtain blood samples at the 2- and 5-min time points after secretin infusion because the maximum (diagnostic) response usually occurs in that time frame. A diagnostic response in humans is a twofold or greater rise in gastrin. Although similar criteria have not been established for dogs, two dogs with gastrinoma had greater than a twofold increase, whereas one dog only had a 1.4-fold increase in gastrin within 5 min of secretin administration.

CALCIUM CHALLENGE TEST

Experience with the calcium challenge test in small animals is limited to two dogs with gastrinoma and one dog with a pancreatic peptidoma. As with secretin challenge, patients with gastrinoma should experience an increase in gastrin levels whereas normal patients should experience no change or minimal change in gastrin levels. The source of calcium is usually calcium gluconate, which is administered as a 1-min infusion (2 mg/kg) or as an intravenous infusion over several hours (5 mg/kg/hr). Serum samples are collected before and at 15, 30, 60, 90, and 120 min after administration. Maximum gastrin concentrations occurred 60 min after calcium bolus in two dogs with gastrinoma. Both dogs had greater than a twofold response to calcium. In one dog, the calcium but not the secretin challenge test was diagnostic of gastrinoma. A combined secretin-calcium stimulation test has been shown to be superior and effective for diagnosis of gastrinoma in humans when the secretin

Table 2. *Incidence of Gross Pathology Findings (Surgical or Necropsy) of Gastrinoma in 17 Dogs and 2 Cats*

Pathology	No. of Animals	(%)
Tumor location		
Pancreas	18/18	(100)
Left lobe	1/13	(8)
Body	5/13	(38)
Right lobe	8/13	(62)
Liver	11/18	(61)
Lymph node	5/18	(28)
Other (spleen, peritoneum, mesentery)	4/18	(22)
Gastrointestinal ulceration	17/19	(89)
Esophagus	4/18	(22)
Stomach	8/18	(44)
Duodenum	13/16	(81)
Jejunum	1/15	(7)
Perforated ulcers	4/18	(22)
Miscellaneous		
Gastric hypertrophy	1/15	(73)
C-cell increase	4/8	(50)
Adrenocortical hyperplasia	2/9	(22)

challenge test alone fails. A 1-min infusion of 2 mg/kg of calcium gluconate, together with an intravenous bolus of 2 units/kg of secretin, generally causes a twofold increase in gastrin in humans.

BASAL GASTRIC ACID SECRETION

Measurement of basal gastric acid secretion is commonly done in humans as an aid to the diagnosis of gastrinoma. Gastric acid secretion was measured in only three dogs with gastrinoma, however. An orogastric aspiration technique for evaluation of pentagastrin-stimulated gastric acid analysis and reference values for volume, pH, hydrogen ion output, and hydrochloric acid output in healthy anesthetized dogs has been reported.

Pathologic Abnormalities: Necropsy or Surgery Findings

All animals with gastrinoma had an islet cell tumor of the pancreas (Table 2). Tumors occurred most commonly in the right lobe and body of the pancreas, with only one report of a tumor in the left lobe. Most dogs and cats had solitary nodules in the pancreas, but multiple masses were found in 3 of 11 animals. It is important to remember that tumors may be small and can easily be missed during surgical exploration, as happened in one dog.

At the time of diagnosis, the tumor had metastasized in 72% of the cases (Table 2). The liver was the most common site of metastasis (61%), with lymph node a distant second. Other sites of metastasis included the mesentery, spleen, peritoneum, omentum, and serosal surface of the duodenum and jejunum.

Light microscopic appearance of gastrinoma may be consistent with an islet cell tumor but is not specific for gastrinoma. Ideally, at the time of surgery (or necropsy), portions of the tumor should be frozen (for immunocytochemistry and hormone extraction) and fixed in formalin or Bouin's solution (for routine histopathology and immunocytochemistry) and glutaraldehyde (for electron microscopy).

Gastrointestinal ulceration was present in 89% of dogs and cats with gastrinoma (see Table 2). Duodenal ulceration occurred most commonly, followed in descending order by gastric, esophageal, and jejunal ulceration. Duodenal and esophageal ulcers perforated before admission or during hospitalization in four dogs.

Treatment Aims

The management of gastrinoma should be directed at specific treatment of the tumor, controlling gastric acid hypersecretion, treatment of gastrointestinal ulceration, and correcting fluid, electrolyte, and acid-base imbalances that are associated with persistent vomiting.

TREATMENT OF THE TUMOR

Treatment specific for the tumor generally consists of surgical resection. Exploratory laparotomy and tumor removal allow for confirmation of diagnosis, reduction of tumor mass and subsequently gastrin-secreting capacity, as well as prognostic information. The reader is referred to the insulinoma section of this article for a specific discussion of pancreatic surgery. In gastrinoma patients, care should also be taken to neutralize gastric acidity and reduce the possibility of gastroesophogeal reflux. Because most gastrin-secreting tumors are located within the right lobe and body of the pancreas, I recommend that partial pancreatectomy of the right lobe be performed if a specific tumor nodule cannot be located.

If metastasis is considered too extensive for excision, the tumor should be debulked and a partial pancreatectomy performed to obtain tissue for biopsy and to decrease tumor burden. I do not recommend euthanasia even with widespread metastasis because of the potential for successful medical management.

Chemotherapy has not been used as an adjunct to surgery in dogs and cats with gastrinoma. Sandostatin, a somatostatin analogue, has been used successfully for treatment of gastrinoma in humans and one dog. Somatostatin inhibits serum gastrin levels as well as parietal cell hydrogen secretion, which is probably independent of the effect on gastrin levels. In addition, regression of liver metastasis has been reported after sandostatin therapy in persons with gastrinoma. One dog with gastrinoma that failed to respond to traditional medical therapy had a good response to sandostatin. The animal was managed effectively for more than 10 months with 10 to 20 µg three times daily of sandostatin, as well as sucralfate and cimetidine.

CONTROLLING GASTRIC ACID HYPERSECRETION

Because of the difficulty in finding and removing all of the tumor masses, gastric acidity usually remains increased and specific therapy aimed at controlling gastric acidity is necessary. The therapeutic agents used for reducing gastric acid secretion include anticholinergics, histamine blockers (H_2), proton pump inhibitors, and somatostatin analogues (see *CVT X*, p. 911). Two anticholinergic agents, isopropamide iodide (Darbid, Smith Kline & French) and propantheline (Pro-Banthine, Searle) reduce basal and stimulated gastric acid secretion by blocking the acetylcholine receptor on parietal cells. These are often used in combination with H_2 antagonists.

Cimetidine (Tagamet, Smith Kline & French) and ranitidine (Zantac, Glaxo) are H_2 antagonists used in small animal practice. These drugs block the histamine receptors on gastric parietal cells. They are potent inhibitors of both secretory volume and hydrogen concentration. Cimetidine appears to be effective in controlling clinical signs associated with gastrinoma in dogs and one cat. The recommended dose of cimetidine for dogs is 5 to 10 mg/kg PO, SC, or IV every 4 to 6 hr. Gastrinoma patients may require a higher dose to control gastric acidity. Ranitidine is more potent, has a longer duration of action than cimetidine, and fails to inhibit hepatic microsomal enzymes. For this reason, it may allow for decreased frequency of administration and thus improved owner compliance. The dose of ranitidine is 2 mg/kg PO or IV every 8 hr.

Nizatidine (Axid, Lilly) and famotidine (Pepcid, Merck, Sharp & Dohme) are also H_2 antagonists, but their use in small animal patients is limited, and doses have not been established. Nizatidine, which is similar in potency to ranitidine, may have the advantage of requiring only twice-daily administration. Famotidine is more potent than either cimetidine or ranitidine.

Omeprazole (Losec, Merck Sharp & Dohme), a proton pump inhibitor, is a potent inhibitor of gastric acid secretion and has a long duration of action in dogs. Although it appears to be very effective in the treatment of gastrinoma in humans, it has not been available clinically for use in dogs. Furthermore, in experimental animals, chronic suppression of acid secretion has caused hypergastrinemia that has been associated with mucosal cell hyperplasia, rugal hypertrophy, and development of carcinoids. A preliminary report concluded that there was no difference in the healing times of mechanically induced ulcers in dogs treated with omeprazole (2 μmol/kg PO) once daily versus cimetidine (10 mg/kg PO) three times daily.

Sandostatin, discussed earlier, is also a potent antisecretory drug. It reduces gastric acidity by direct inhibition of gastric acid secretion, as well as its effects on reducing gastrin concentrations.

TREATMENT OF GASTROINTESTINAL ULCERATION

Treatment of gastrointestinal ulceration consists of reducing gastric acidity (discussed earlier) and use of coating agents to protect and promote ulcer healing. Sucralfate (Carafate, Marion) is a complex of sulfated sucrose and aluminum hydroxide that when ingested reacts with gastric acid to form an adherent and protective complex with proteins at the base of the ulcer. It also inactivates pepsin, absorbs bile acids, and increases mucus and bicarbonate secretion. It does not inhibit gastric acid secretion. It is available as a 1-gm tablet. Recommended doses are 1 gm every 8 hr for larger dogs, 0.5 gm every 8 hr for smaller dogs, and 0.5 to 0.25 gm every 8 to 12 hr for cats. Because sucralfate may bind to other drugs that are administered orally, its administration should be separated from that of other drugs by at least 2 hr. In addition, because sucralfate requires an acid environment in order to bind to the ulcer crater, H₂ antagonists should not be given at the same time as sucralfate. The only reported side effect of sucralfate in small animals is constipation.

Perforated ulcers are life-threatening and should receive immediate surgical attention.

Prognosis

Gastrinoma in cats and dogs appears to be highly malignant, with gross evidence of metastasis at the time of diagnosis in 76% of all animals reported. The long-term prognosis is grave. Ten of 19 animals with gastrinoma died or were euthanized without the benefit of therapy because diagnosis was made postmortem. Animals that were treated received surgical or medical therapy or both. Survival after treatment ranged from 1 week to 18 months (average 4.8 months). It is more difficult to ascertain the disease-free interval, but it would appear to be 0 days to 12 months. However, several animals were diagnosed as having gastrinoma before the availability of H₂ antagonists. In many cases, the disease was very advanced and animals were in poor condition, having perforated ulcers or electrolyte and acid-base imbalances. I believe that with heightened degree of suspicion of gastrinoma, the availability of antisecretory drugs such as H₂ antagonists, omeprazole, and sandostatin, as well as experience with previous cases, we may gain a significant increase in short-term survival time.

PANCREATIC PEPTIDOMA

Pancreatic polypeptide (PP) is the second most common hormone identified by immunocytochemistry within canine pancreatic endocrine tumors (77% of 52 dogs). However, excessive plasma PP concentration has been documented in only one dog. In that case, the PP levels were thought to contribute to the dog's clinical abnormalities.

The clinical syndrome of chronic vomiting and hypertrophic gastritis, duodenal ulceration, pancreatic adenocarcinoma, and fasting hypergastrinemia in this dog were highly suggestive of gastrinoma. However, this dog had normal gastrin concentrations in response to both calcium and secretin, and no immunocytochemical staining of gastrin was noted in the pancreatic tumor and its metastases. The dog also failed to respond to cimetidine. For these reasons, a gastrin-secreting tumor was thought to be an unlikely cause of the clinical signs in this case.

In contrast, immunocytochemistry revealed very intense staining of the pancreatic tumor and its metastases for PP. Plasma PP levels were also extremely high (637,000 pg/ml; normal dogs < 155 pg/ml). The investigators propose that the very high PP levels may have contributed to the dog's gastrointestinal ulceration and vomiting because PP decreases pancreatic bicarbonate secretion and mildly increases gastric acid secretion. The tumor also contained and secreted insulin, which led to significant hypoglycemia.

GLUCAGONOMA

Glucagonoma is a very rare syndrome in humans. A presumptive diagnosis of glucagonoma has been made in two dogs. Persons with glucagonoma have a characteristic skin rash referred to as *necrolytic migratory erythema* (NME). They also develop mild diabetes mellitus, venous thromboses, depression, anorexia, weight loss, glossitis or stomatitis, diarrhea, and normocytic normochromic anemia. The skin rash results from hypoaminoacidemia rather than the hyperglucagonemia itself, whereas diabetes mellitus results from the glycogenolytic and gluconeogenic actions of glucagon. The diagnosis of glucagonoma is confirmed by finding elevated plasma glucagon concentrations and pancreatic islet cell tumor.

In 1986, a similar syndrome of NME and diabetes mellitus was described in four dogs. Glucagonoma was suggested as a possible cause of the clinical abnormalities, but its presence could not be documented. Gross has described the presence of glucagon in islet cell tumors of two dogs that had similar clinical signs as those described earlier. The dogs were an 11-year-old male fox terrier and a 9-year-old female Labrador retriever. They intially presented with erythematous, ulcerative, crusting dermatitis and later developed a nonketoacidotic diabetes mellitus. Skin biopsy findings were consistent with NME, and pancreatic tumors were found during exploratory laparotomy. Both dogs died or were euthanized 3 days after surgery. Plasma glucagon concentrations were not determined.

The presence of diabetes mellitus, NME, and a pancreatic islet cell tumor containing glucagon is very suggestive of a glucagonoma. However, the presence of glucagon in islet cell tumors is not specific for glucagonomas and has been documented in 26 of 70 dogs (37%) with insulinoma or gastrinoma.

In persons with glucagonoma, plasma glucagon concentration is usually increased 5 to 10 times above normal. Plasma glucagon concentration was assayed in only one dog with NME. Provocative testing, which may be necessary in humans if glucagon concentrations are normal, has not been performed on any dog. Care must be taken to use a glucagon assay that has been validated for use in dogs. I am not currently aware of a validated assay.

As with other islet cell tumors, surgical resection of the pancreatic tumor is the treatment of choice.

It is important to note that the presence of NME in dogs has been documented with diabetes mellitus and hepatic cirrhosis as well as pancreatic tumor. The cutaneous syndrome has been referred to as *diabetic dermatopathy and hepatocutaneous syndrome*. One investigator proposes the descriptive term *superficial necrolytic dermatitis*. Regardless of the term applied to this cutaneous syndrome, it is apparent that the majority of dogs do not have a glucagonoma. Of the 17 reported descriptions of this cutaneous syndrome, only two dogs had pancreatic tumors (described earlier). The majority of dogs had liver disease.

References and Suggested Reading

Caywood, D. D., Klausner, J. S., O'Leary, T. P., et al.: Pancreatic insulin-secreting neoplasms: Clinical, diagnostic, and prognostic features in 73 dogs. J. Am. Anim. Hosp. Assoc. 24:577, 1988.
  A retrospective study of clinical, diagnostic, and prognostic features of insulinoma in 73 dogs.
Gross, T. L., O'Brien, T. D., Davies, A. P., et al.: Glucagon-producing pancreatic endocrine tumors in two dogs with superficial necrolytic dermatitis. J.A.V.M.A. 197:1619, 1990.
  A case report of two dogs with a presumptive diagnosis of glucagonoma.
Happé, R. P., van der Gaag, I., Lamers, C. B. H. W., et al.: Zollinger-Ellison syndrome in three dogs. Vet. Pathol. 17:177, 1980.
  A report of gastrinoma in three dogs.
Johnson, S. E.: Pancreatic APUDomas. Semin. Vet. Med. Surg. 4: 202, 1989.
  A discussion of insulinomas, gastrinomas, pancreatic peptidomas, and glucagonomas in small animal patients.
Zerbe, C. A., Boosinger, T. R., Grabau, J. H., et al.: Pancreatic polypeptide and insulin-secreting tumor in a dog with duodenal ulcers and hypertrophic gastritis. J. Vet. Intern. Med. 3:178, 1989.
  A case report of excessive secretion of insulin and pancreatic polypeptide by an islet cell tumor in a dog with clinical signs resembling those of gastrinoma.

HYPOPARATHYROIDISM AND OTHER CAUSES OF HYPOCALCEMIA IN CATS

MARK E. PETERSON

New York, New York

HYPOPARATHYROIDISM

Hypoparathyroidism is a metabolic disorder characterized by hypocalcemia and hyperphosphatemia and either transient or permanent parathyroid hormone insufficiency. In cats, the most common cause of hypoparathyroidism is iatrogenic injury or removal of the parathyroid glands during thyroidectomy for treatment of hyperthyroidism (Flanders et al., 1987; Welches et al., 1989). Spontaneous (idiopathic) hypoparathyroidism appears to be relatively rare in cats, with only six cases reported (Peterson et al., 1991; Forbes et al., 1990).

Hypocalcemia is responsible for the main clinical manifestations of hypoparathyroidism because it increases the excitability of both the central and peripheral nervous systems. Classic peripheral neuromuscular signs include muscle tremors, twitches, and tetany. Generalized convulsions, resembling those of an idiopathic seizure disorder, are the predominant central nervous system manifestations of hypoparathyroidism.

Diagnosis of Hypoparathyroidism

Diagnosis of hypoparathyroidism is made on the basis of history, clinical signs, laboratory evidence of hypocalcemia and hyperphosphatemia, and exclusion of other causes of hypocalcemia (e.g., hypoproteinemia, malabsorption, pancreatitis, and renal failure).

After bilateral thyroidectomy for treatment of hyperthyroidism, development of iatrogenic hypoparathyroidism should be *anticipated*. The serum calcium level should be monitored daily until it normalizes. A mild degree of suppression of the serum calcium level appears to be a nonspecific response to surgery and requires no treatment. However, if severe hypocalcemia and accompanying signs of heightened neuromuscular excitability develop, treatment with vitamin D and calcium is indicated. In most cats that require treatment for iatrogenic hypoparathyroidism, severe life-threatening hypocalcemia usually develops within 3 days after surgery (Flanders et al., 1987; Welches et al., 1989).

If idiopathic hypoparathyroidism is suspected, the disorder can be confirmed by histologic examination of parathyroid gland tissue and documentation of parathyroid atrophy or destruction. At surgery, a unilateral thyroidectomy should be performed to ensure that adequate parathyroid tissue is available for examination, because the parathyroid glands are not visible in cats with hypoparathyroidism. In contrast to cats with iatrogenic hypoparathyroidism, which have a rapid onset of signs, clinical signs may occur intermittently in cats with the idiopathic form of the disorder. In one report of five cats with idiopathic hypoparathyroidism, one cat had signs of hypocalcemia 6 months before diagnosis, suggesting a physiologic adaptation to severe hypocalcemia (Peterson et al., 1991). Such adaptation to long-standing hypocalcemia is well recognized in humans and dogs with primary hypoparathyroidism.

Treatment of Hypoparathyroidism

The treatment protocols for both iatrogenic and spontaneous hypoparathyroidism are the same—that is, administration of calcium supplements and vitamin D. Although many parenterally administered calcium preparations are available, calcium gluconate is preferred for intravenous use. Oral calcium supplements are available as gluconate, lactate, chloride, carbonate, and glubionate salts. Because of the big differences in calcium content between the calcium salts, the most common mistake is prescribing in terms of weight of salt rather than quantity of elemental calcium. The relatively small tablet size and high elemental calcium content (40%) of calcium carbonate (e.g., Tums tablets) make it preferred for oral use in cats.

The three main vitamin D preparations available include vitamin D_2, dihydrotachysterol, and 1,25-dihydroxyvitamin D. Although all vitamin D preparations raise serum calcium concentrations primarily by increasing the gastrointestinal absorption of calcium, there are important differences between the doses of these three preparations needed to achieve normocalcemia in cats with hypoparathyroidism, as well as differences in the times of maximal onset of effect and duration of action. Dihydrotachysterol is generally preferred over vitamin D_2 for use in cats, because it raises serum calcium levels more rapidly and its effects are dissipated more quickly when the drug is discontinued (if hypercalcemia develops). Dihydrotachysterol is available as 0.125-mg, 0.2-mg, and 0.4-mg tablets or capsules and as an oral solution containing 0.25 mg/ml of vitamin D. The latter is convenient for long-term treatment of hypoparathyroid cats. Although 1,25-dihydroxyvitamin D (Calcitrol) offers the advantage of a rapid onset of action (1 to 4 days) and short half-life (<1 day), the drug is expensive, and the potency of available capsule sizes (0.25 and 0.5 µg), designed for use in human patients, is not well formulated for a cat's small body size.

ACUTE HYPOCALCEMIA

Hypocalcemic tetany or convulsions are indications for the immediate intravenous administration of 10% calcium gluconate (1.0 to 1.5 ml/kg), which should be slowly infused over a 10- to 20-min period. Electrocardiographic monitoring is advisable during this infusion; if bradycardia, premature ventricular complexes, or shortening of the Q-T interval develops, the intravenous injection should be slowed or temporarily discontinued.

Once tetany or convulsions are controlled, intravenous administration of calcium should be continued as a slow infusion of 60 to 90 mg/kg/day of elemental calcium (i.e., 2.5 ml/kg of 10% calcium gluconate added to fluids and administered every 6 to 8 hr). Serum calcium concentration should be determined once to twice daily. One should adjust the rate of calcium administration to maintain normal serum calcium concentrations and continue the infusion for as long as necessary to prevent recurrence of hypocalcemia. Although this continuous calcium infusion will maintain normocalcemia, its effects are short-lived; hypocalcemia will recur within hours of stopping the infusion unless other treatment is given. Therefore, oral calcium and vitamin D should be initiated as soon as oral medication can be tolerated.

During initial treatment, large doses of vitamin D should be administered concomitantly with oral and intravenous calcium supplementation. Use of a loading dose of dihydrotachysterol shortens the time needed to maintain normocalcemia. I have found that by administering dihydrotachysterol at a dosage of 0.125 to 0.25 mg/day for 2 to 3 days, then 0.08 to 0.125 mg/day for 2 to 3 days, and finally 0.05 mg/day, stable serum calcium concentrations (8.5 to 9.5 mg/dl) can usually be achieved within a week.

During this initial period, oral calcium supplements that provide 50 to 100 mg/kg/day of elemental calcium (e.g., one to two Tums tablets) should be administered in three to four divided daily doses. Inasmuch as many affected cats are not eating, oral calcium supplementation is an important part of the protocol to ensure that sufficient calcium is available for increased intestinal absorption by the vitamin D, this being the only way that vitamin D acts to raise blood calcium. The doses of calcium and vitamin D described here are effective in most cats, but it is important to realize that higher doses may be needed in some patients.

After normal serum calcium concentrations are maintained for 1 or 2 days by the combined oral and parenteral administration of calcium and vitamin D, the dose of intravenous calcium should be reduced and finally discontinued. It may be necessary, however, to reinstate the calcium infusion for an additional 24 to 48 hours if the serum calcium concentration again declines to less than 7 mg/dl. Serum calcium should be determined once to twice daily during this initial treatment period until concentrations have stabilized in the low-normal range.

MAINTENANCE TREATMENT

The long-term treatment of hypoparathyroidism requires administration of a maintenance dose of a vitamin D preparation together with adequate dietary or supplemental calcium intake. In contrast to initial treatment, in which control of signs of hypocalcemia is paramount, the aim of long-term treatment is to maintain serum calcium concentrations within the low-normal range (8.0 to 9.5 mg/dl). This concentration is high enough to control signs of hypocalcemia while minimizing the risk of overt hypercalcemia from vitamin D overdose. In the absence of parathyroid hormone, renal tubular resorption of calcium is abnormally low, and much of the calcium absorbed from the gastrointestinal tract is lost in the urine. If serum calcium concentration is normalized to concentrations of 10 to 11 mg/dl with vitamin D and calcium administration, urine calcium excretion may be dangerously high, leading to nephrocalcinosis and deterioration of renal function.

The ingestion of adequate amounts of calcium is an important component of the treatment regimen for hypoparathyroidism, because vitamin D (whatever preparation is used) raises serum calcium concentrations by promoting intestinal absorption. Although cats given a well-balanced commercial diet may not require an additional source of calcium, it is advisable to supplement the diet with approximately 25 mg/kg/day of elemental calcium to ensure adequate calcium for vitamin D action. Additional calcium can be provided by supplementing the diet with appropriate amounts of calcium-rich foods. For example, ½ cup of milk contains 150 mg elemental calcium, 1 tablespoon cottage cheese 25 mg, and ¼ cup yogurt 70 mg. Alternatively, if a cat cannot obtain the desired amount of calcium by dietary means because of lactose intolerance or distaste for foods rich in calcium, calcium supplements (e.g., approximately one half of a Tums tablet daily) can be given in three to four divided doses. Whatever regimen is used, it is important that the amount of daily calcium supplementation be consistent; a dramatic change in calcium ingestion can cause hyper- or hypocalcemia.

Vitamin D maintenance therapy must be strictly individualized, with dose adjustments based on frequent determinations of serum calcium concentrations. When dihydrotachysterol is used, the serum calcium level should be monitored weekly after initial stabilization, and the dose should be adjusted by 15 to 20% increments until a dose is found that maintains serum calcium concentration in the low-normal range. Thereafter, calcium should be measured every 1 to 2 months and further dose adjustments made as needed. Small dose changes can be achieved most readily by use of the oral solution of dihydrotachysterol, measured with a tuberculin syringe. The daily dose of dihydrotachysterol can be administered either directly into the cat's mouth or placed in a small gelatin capsule (to avoid the aftertaste that bothers some cats).

The main complication associated with treatment of hypoparathyroidism is hypercalcemia, which develops as a consequence of overtreatment with calcium and vitamin D. Owners should frequently be reminded of the clinical signs of hypercalcemia (i.e., anorexia, lethargy, polyuria, and polydipsia) so that prompt treatment can be initiated to prevent hypercalcemic nephropathy and soft-tissue calcification. If high serum calcium concentrations develop during the course of treatment, calcium and vitamin D treatment should be temporarily discontinued. In addition, diuresis induced by saline and furosemide administration may be indicated if severe hypercalcemia is present. Once normocalcemia has been restored, vitamin D administration should be reinstituted at a lower maintenance dose (approximately 20% less than that previously administered). In cats with hypoparathyroidism that may be transient (e.g., after thyroidectomy), however, vitamin D and calcium treatment should be reinstated only if significant hypocalcemia (<8 mg/dl) again develops.

In cats with iatrogenic hypoparathyroidism, recovery of parathyroid function may occur weeks to months after surgery. After 2 to 3 months of treatment, one should attempt to taper the dose of vitamin D and wean the cat from medication. This can be safely accomplished by first reducing the vitamin D dose by 25 to 50% and monitoring calcium concentration at weekly intervals. If the serum calcium concentration remains within the normal range, gradual dose reduction is continued until the vitamin D preparation is finally stopped completely.

PHOSPHATE ENEMA TOXICITY

Hypertonic sodium phosphate (e.g., Fleet) enemas may cause severe biochemical abnormalities, especially when administered to dehydrated cats with colonic atony and mucosal disruption. Colonic absorption of sodium and phosphate from the enema solution, as well as transfer of intravascular water to the colonic lumen (because of the hypertonicity of the solution), causes hypernatremia and hyperphosphatemia (Jorgenson et al., 1985). Hyperphosphatemia leads to precipitation of serum calcium with resultant hypocalcemia. Clinical signs of phosphate enema toxicosis resulting from these electrolyte and fluid alterations include shock and neuromuscular irritability. Treatment consists of volume expansion by intravenous administration of an electrolyte-poor solution (e.g., 5% dextrose in water), as well as treatment of hypocalcemia (as described in the earlier section on acute hypocalcemia of hypoparathyroidism).

RENAL FAILURE

Because chronic renal failure is so common in cats, it represents a well-recognized cause of hypocalcemia. The hypocalcemia associated with renal failure, however, is rarely if ever clinically significant (i.e., muscle tremors, twitches, tetany, or convulsions do not develop). In addition, most cats with chronic renal failure have normal serum calcium concentrations.

HYPOPROTEINEMIA

Cats with hypoalbuminemia may be hypocalcemic because of a decrease in the protein-bound fraction of calcium, but the ionized calcium fraction remains normal and clinical signs of hypocalcemia do not develop. Management of these cases should be directed at determining the underlying cause of the hypoproteinemia rather than at treatment of the associated hypocalcemia.

PANCREATITIS

Hypocalcemia in cats with pancreatitis is often mild and subclinical. The exact mechanism of hypocalcemia in these cats is unknown, but the traditional theory is that the pancreatic enzyme lipase, on release into the abdominal cavity by the diseased pancreas, saponifies peripancreatic fat, causing calcium to be precipitated in the form of insoluble soaps. Research now suggests that hypocalcemia may be, at least in part, the result of an acute shift of calcium into soft tissues, especially muscle (Bhattacharya et al., 1985).

PUERPERAL TETANY

Puerperal tetany (eclampsia) is an acute, life-threatening disease caused by an extreme decrease in circulating calcium concentrations in a lactating queen (Bjerkas, 1974). Unlike in dogs, this disorder is extremely rare in cats. The severe hypocalcemia associated with eclampsia develops during the nursing period (several days to several weeks postpartum). The pathophysiology of puerperal tetany remains poorly understood but appears to result from an imbalance between the rate of inflow (e.g., bone resorption, gastrointestinal absorption) and outflow (e.g., mammary gland) of calcium from the extracellular calcium pool. Treatment consists of slow intravenous administration of calcium (e.g., 1.0 to 1.5 ml/kg of 10% calcium gluconate slowly infused over 10 to 20 min) and removal of the kittens from the queen.

References and Suggested Reading

Bhattacharya, S. K., Luther, R. W., Pate, J. W., et al.: Soft tissue calcium and magnesium content in acute pancreatitis in the dog: Calcium accumulation, a mechanism for hypocalcemia in acute pancreatitis. J. Lab. Clin. Med. 105:422, 1985.
The calcium content of muscle, liver, and pancreas increased significantly after induction of experimental pancreatitis in dogs, suggesting that hypocalcemia may be due to a shift in calcium uptake into tissues.

Bjerkas, E.: Eclampsia in the cat. J. Small Anim. Pract. 15:411, 1974.
Severe hypocalcemia and associated neuromuscular signs developed in a 1-year-old female cat 1 month postpartum but resolved after intravenous calcium administration and weaning of the kittens.

Flanders, J. A., Harvey, H. J., and Erb, H. N.: Feline thyroidectomy: A comparison of postoperative hypocalcemia associated with three different surgical techniques. Vet. Surg. 16:362, 1987.
Of 41 hyperthyroid cats that had bilateral thyroidectomy, postoperative hypocalcemia (not always associated with clinical signs) developed in 82% treated with an extracapsular technique, 36% treated with an intracapsular technique, and 11% treated with two separate thyroidectomies performed 3 to 4 weeks apart.

Forbes, S., Nelson, R. W., and Guptill, L.: Primary hypoparathyroidism in a cat. J.A.V.M.A. 196:1285, 1990.
Clinical signs, laboratory findings, and results of treatment are described in a 1-year old cat with spontaneous primary hypoparathyroidism.

Jorgenson, L. S., Center, S. A., and Randolph, J. F.: Electrolyte abnormalities induced by hypertonic phosphate enemas in two cats. J.A.V.M.A. 187:1367, 1985.
Two cats that developed hypocalcemia, hypernatremia, and hyperphosphatemia after administration of a phosphate enema are described.

Peterson, M. E., James, K. M., Wallace, M., et al.: Idiopathic hypoparathyroidism in five cats. J. Vet. Intern. Med. 5:47, 1991.
The historic and clinical signs, laboratory findings, and results of treatment with calcium and vitamin D are reported in five young to middle-aged cats with idiopathic hypoparathyroidism.

Welches, C., Scavelli, T., Matthiesen, D., et al.: Three techniques of bilateral thyroidectomy in cats: Prevalence of problems after surgery according to technique. Vet. Surg. 18:392, 1989.
Of 106 hyperthyroid cats, postoperative hypocalcemia developed in 22% treated with the original intracapsular technique, 33% treated with a modified intracapsular technique, and 23% treated with a modified intracapsular technique, but clinical signs only developed in cats with severe hypocalcemia.

PRIMARY HYPERPARATHYROIDISM IN THE CAT

KEITH P. RICHTER,
Rancho Santa Fe, California

ANDREW J. KALLET,
Corte Madera, California

and EDWARD C. FELDMAN
Davis, California

Primary hyperparathyroidism is a disorder resulting from the autonomous secretion of parathyroid hormone (PTH) by one or more parathyroid glands, resulting in hypercalcemia. Though relatively rare, the disease is well documented in dogs. This endocrinopathy has been described in cats, but few reports detail clinical findings. Seven cats with parathyroid adenomas were identified among 3145 feline necropsies in one report (Patnaik, et al., 1975), and nine cats with 10 parathyroid tumors (nine adenomas and one carcinoma) were observed in a survey of 3248 feline tumors (Carpenter et al., 1987). Of the nine cats in this latter report, six had serum calcium and phosphorus determinations performed antemortem, only two of which demonstrated hypercalcemia. The clinical findings of seven cats with primary hyperparathyroidism were described by Kallet and colleagues (in press). This report summarizes our experience with these seven cats.

PATHOPHYSIOLOGY

Serum concentration of calcium is dependent on several factors, including intestinal absorption, calcium deposition and resorption from bone, and renal clearance. These factors are controlled primarily by activity of PTH, calcitonin, and vitamin D. PTH release is controlled by a unique feedback control mechanism dependent on the concentration of ionized serum calcium (and to a lesser extent serum magnesium). Increases in serum calcium concentration lower serum PTH concentration, whereas decreases in serum calcium concentration increase serum PTH concentration. Blood phosphorus level has no direct regulatory effect on the

concentration of PTH, although phosphorus can indirectly affect PTH concentration by altering serum calcium concentration. Biologic effects of PTH include (1) increase in blood calcium, (2) decrease in blood phosphorus, (3) increase in urinary excretion of phosphorus (decreased tubular reabsorption), (4) decrease in urinary excretion of calcium (increases tubular reabsorption), (5) increase in skeletal remodeling and calcium release from bone, (6) mobilization of calcium from bone by increasing osteocytic osteolysis and numbers of osteoclasts on bone surfaces, and (7) increase in active vitamin D formation by the kidneys (and therefore an indirect increase in intestinal absorption of calcium). Primary hyperparathyroidism results from the autonomous secretion of PTH, and therefore these biologic effects are accentuated, with changes associated with hypercalcemia predominating.

CLINICAL FINDINGS IN CATS WITH PRIMARY HYPERPARATHYROIDISM

The clinical features of feline hyperparathyroidism are summarized in Table 1, and a comparison with canine hyperparathyroidism is summarized in Table 2. The seven cats with primary hyperparathyroidism were 8 to 15 years of age (mean 12.9 years). There seemed to be a predisposition in Siamese and female cats. Clinical signs were nonspecific, including anorexia, lethargy, vomiting, weakness, and weight loss. Dogs with hypercalcemia commonly exhibit polydipsia and polyuria, a problem observed in only approximately one third of cats with primary hyperparathyroidism. Some of these cats with primary hyperparathyroidism were asymp-

Table 1. *Clinical, Laboratory, and Histopathologic Findings in Seven Cats With Primary Hyperparathyroidism*

Finding	No. (%) of Cats
Anorexia	4 (57)
Lethargy	4 (57)
Vomiting	2 (29)
Polyuria/polydipsia	2 (29)
Weakness	1 (14)
Weight loss	1 (14)
Obtunded/tremors	1 (14)
Asymptomatic	1 (14)
Palpable cervical mass	4 (57)
Parathyroid adenoma	2 (29)
Cervical cyst	2 (29)
Hypercalcemia	7 (100)
Hypophosphatemia	2 (29)
Normophosphatemia	4 (57)
Mild azotemia	4 (57)
Mild increased SGPT (alanine aminotransferase) activity	3 (43)
Mild increased serum alkaline phosphatase activity	2 (29)
Isosthenuria	3 (43)
Urinary tract calculi/bacteriuria	0 (0)
Solitary parathyroid adenoma	5 (71)
Bilateral parathyroid cystadenomas	1 (14)
Parathyroid carcinoma	1 (14)

SGPT, serum glutamic-pyruvic transaminase.

tomatic, and the duration of clinical signs varied from a few days to several months before veterinary examination.

Physical examination findings in cats with primary hyperparathyroidism were usually unremarkable, with the exception of a palpable cervical mass in four cats (two of these represented a parathyroid adenoma; two were unrelated cysts). The palpable masses ranged in size from 1 to 3 cm in diameter.

The most consistent laboratory abnormality in the cats with primary hyperparathyroidism was persistent hypercalcemia, present in all the cats. The mean serum calcium concentration in these cats with primary hyperparathyroidism was 15.8 mg/dl and varied between 13.3 and 22.8 mg/dl (reference range 8.8 to 11.0 mg/dl). The serum phosphorus concentration was normal or slightly below normal. Four of the cats had mild azotemia. Isosthenuria was noted in three of the cats. Urinary tract calculi and bacteriuria were not encountered in cats with primary hyperparathyroidism, as opposed to dogs with primary hyperparathyroidism, in which approximately 40 to 50% have urinary tract calculi or bacteriuria (Berger and Feldman, 1987; Feldman, 1989). Other laboratory findings were noncontributory, including serum thyroxine concentration, findings on hemograms, and results of feline leukemia virus testing.

Pathologic evaluation of seven cats with primary hyperparathyroidism revealed a solitary parathyroid adenoma in five cats, bilateral parathyroid cystadenomas in one cat, and a parathyroid carcinoma in one cat.

DIAGNOSTIC EVALUATION

Feline primary hyperparathyroidism should be suspected in any cat that has persistent hypercalcemia. The diagnostic evaluation should attempt to rule out other causes of hypercalcemia in the cat. Other disorders associated with hypercalcemia in cats (in order of relative frequency) include (1) lymphosarcoma, (2) vitamin D-containing rodenticide ingestion, (3) myeloproliferative diseases (lymphocytic leukemia, erythroleukemia, multiple myeloma), (4) chronic renal failure, and (5) squamous cell carcinoma. Spurious causes of hypercalcemia should also be ruled out, including laboratory error, lipemia, hemolysis, hemoconcentration, and hyperalbuminemia.

A complete history should be obtained to rule out vitamin D–containing rodenticide ingestion. A careful physical examination should be repeated, paying particular attention to peripheral lymph nodes (looking for lymphosarcoma) and any other findings suggesting the presence of other types of neoplasia. The ventral neck should be carefully palpated, because approximately one third of cats with primary hyperparathyroidism in our series had a palpable parathyroid mass. Laboratory evaluation should include a complete blood count (looking for evidence of myeloproliferative diseases) and serum chemistry profile (looking for evidence of chronic renal failure, multiple myeloma, or hepatic neoplasia). Thoracic radiographs should be obtained to rule out the presence of a mediastinal mass or other evidence of neoplasia. Other tests to look for disorders resulting in hypercalcemia may include bone marrow aspirate/biopsy, lymph node aspirate/biopsy, and abdominal ultrasonography. If all these diagnostic efforts fail to identify a cause of hypercalcemia, surgical exploration of the neck to look

Table 2. *Comparison of Primary Hyperparathyroidism in the Dog and Cat*

Feature	Dog	Cat
Older animals	Always	Always
Nonspecific and mild signs	Usually	Usually
Long-standing and persistent hypercalcemia	Always	Always
Polyuria/polydipsia	Common	Infrequent
Normophosphatemia	Common	Common
Bacteriuria/calculi	Common	Absent
Parathyroid adenoma	Common	Common
Parathyroid carcinoma	Rare	Rare
Postoperative hypocalcemia	Common	Infrequent
Prognosis	Excellent	Excellent

for a functional parathyroid tumor should be considered. Finally, the measurement of serum PTH may be helpful to suggest the presence of primary hyperparathyroidism before surgical exploration of the neck, but a validated assay for feline PTH is not currently available.

TREATMENT

Surgical exploration of the thyroid/parathyroid area should be performed. Parathyroid tumors have been visible as a distinct nodule separate from the associated thyroid and larger than normal parathyroid glands. Extirpation can be accomplished by blunt dissection. After surgery, serum calcium concentrations have decreased into reference limits during the initial 24 hr following adenoma or cystadenoma removal in all cats. Postoperative complications were minimal. Two of six cats that underwent surgery developed asymptomatic transient hypocalcemia, and one of six cats developed transient Horner's syndrome and a persistent harsh meow. Hypocalcemia can be easily managed by temporary oral administration of vitamin D-containing products (dihydrotachysterol or 1,25-dihydroxyvitamin D_3), but because postoperative hypocalcemia is not a major clinical problem, prophylactic postsurgical vitamin D therapy is not recommended. This contrasts to findings in dogs with primary hyperparathyroidism, in which approximately 60% develop postsurgical hypocalcemia (Berger and Feldman, 1987; Feldman, 1989). As with dogs, postoperative hypocalcemia was noted in the two cats with the highest preoperative serum calcium concentration. Recurrence of hypercalcemia associated with the development of parathyroid carcinoma was observed in one cat that had a parathyroid adenoma surgically removed 569 days previously.

CONCLUSION

Primary hyperparathyroidism should be considered as a differential diagnosis in all middle-aged to older cats with hypercalcemia. If a thorough diagnostic evaluation rules out other causes, surgical exploration of the parathyroid gland area should be considered. Surgical removal of a solitary parathyroid adenoma or bilateral cystadenomas resulted in resolution of hypercalcemia in all cases in which it was attempted. Primary hyperparathyroidism in cats treated by parathyroid adenoma removal has an excellent prognosis.

References and Suggested Reading

Berger, B., and Feldman, E. C.: Primary hyperparathyroidism in dogs: 21 cases (1976–1986). J.A.V.M.A. 191:350, 1987.
  A retrospective review of 21 dogs with primary hyperparathyroidism.
Carpenter, J. L., Andrews, L. K., and Holzworth, J.: Tumors and tumor-like lesions: Tumors of the parathyroid gland. *In* Holzworth, J. (ed.): *Diseases of the Cat: Medicine and Surgery.* Philadelphia: W. B. Saunders, 1987, pp. 548–550.
  A retrospective review of pathologic findings in the parathyroid glands of cats.
Feldman, E. C.: Canine primary hyperparathyroidism. *In* Kirk, R. W. (ed.): *Current Veterinary Therapy X.* Philadelphia: W. B. Saunders, 1989, pp. 985–987.
  A review of the syndrome of primary hyperparathyroidism in dogs.
Kallet A. J., Richter K. P., Feldman E. C., et al.: Primary hyperparathyroidism in seven cats. J.A.V.M.A. (in press).
  A retrospective review of the clinical findings and outcome of seven cats with primary hyperparathyroidism.
Klausner, J. S., Ford, W. V., Hayden, D. W., et al.: Hypercalcemia in two cats with squamous cell carcinomas. J.A.V.M.A. 196:103, 1990.
  A report on two cats with squamous cell carcinomas that developed hypercalcemia.
Moore F. M., Kudish M., Richter K., et al.: Hypercalcemia associated with rodenticide poisoning in three cats. J.A.V.M.A. 193:1099, 1988.
  A report on three cats that ingested a vitamin D-containing rodenticide that developed hypercalcemia.
Patnaik A. K., Liu S. K., Hurvitz A. I., et al.: Nonhematopoetic neoplasms in the cat. J. Natl. Cancer Inst. 54:855, 1975.
  A retrospective review of neoplasia in cats.

POLYENDOCRINE GLAND FAILURE SYNDROMES IN DOGS

PETER P. KINTZER

North Grafton, Massachusetts

Polyendocrine gland failure is characterized by the occurrence of two or more hormone-deficient states in the same animal. These disorders can include primary hypothyroidism, primary hypoadrenocorticism (Addison's disease), insulin-dependent diabetes mellitus, hypoparathyroidism, and possibly hypogonadism. The occurrence of primary hypothyroidism and primary hypoadrenocorticism is the most common association reported in dogs, but any combination of these diseases is possible. That these disorders result from an autoimmune process is increasingly apparent, although for some disorders, this is not as well documented in dogs as it has been in human patients. The terms *polyendocrine gland failure, polyglandular failure syndrome, autoimmune polyglandular syndrome, organ-specific autoimmunity, and Schmidt's syndrome* all have been used to describe the association of multiple autoimmune endocrine disorders.

ETIOPATHOGENESIS

Although there is reasonably strong evidence for the autoimmune nature of polyendocrine gland failure as well as isolated endocrine gland failure, little work has been done to elucidate the underlying mechanisms of this autoimmunity in dogs. In humans, there is strong support for familial or genetic predisposition (Eisenbarth and Rassi, 1983). An association with specific major histocompatibility antigens has been described for one polyendocrine failure syndrome in humans. Genetic susceptibility alone is not sufficient, however, and environmental factors or triggers also appear to be necessary. Viral infections and certain drugs have been implicated in some autoimmune endocrine disorders in humans, but in general these environmental factors are poorly described (Neufeld et al., 1980).

Both cell-mediated and humoral processes appear to be responsible for immune-mediated destruction of the target tissues. Cell-mediated immune destruction is evidenced by a characteristic lymphoplasmacytic infiltration of the affected glands (thyroiditis, adrenalitis, insulitis) and is a relatively common pathologic finding in cases of canine primary hypoadrenocorticism, primary hypothyroidism, and insulin-dependent diabetes mellitus if histologic examination of affected tissue is not delayed. Fibrosis and atrophy may be the only remaining histologic abnormalities in long-standing cases. Circulating autoantibodies specific to the involved glands may be present, although they too may be absent by the time the process has progressed to marked destruction and overt glandular tissue failure.

The immune-mediated destruction is a slow process. Clinical manifestations of hormonal deficiency become evident only after a certain critical amount of tissue has been destroyed. It follows that autoantibodies may be present before clinically apparent disease. This phenomenon is well illustrated by insulin-dependent diabetes mellitus in humans; the presence of islet cell autoantibodies may precede the development of glucose intolerance and overt diabetes mellitus by years (Eisenbarth and Rassi, 1983). In fact, the autoantibodies may no longer be detectable by the time overt beta-cell failure is present. This type of process has not been well documented in dogs. Nonetheless, an example of the progressive nature of glandular destruction is the clinical observation that in many dogs with hypoadrenocorticism the replacement dose of mineralocorticoid must be periodically increased during the first year or so of therapy. This is attributed to the continuing immune-mediated destruction of the adrenal cortex. Circulating autoantibodies to the corresponding target organ have been demonstrated in some cases of primary hypothyroidism, primary hypoadrenocorticism, and insulin-dependent diabetes mellitus in dogs. The inability to demonstrate the presence of autoantibodies does not rule out an autoimmune process. Sufficient normal tissue to generate a measurable antibody response may no longer remain by the time clinical disease is apparent.

DIAGNOSIS

Although polyendocrine gland failure syndromes are diagnosed infrequently, the occurrence of unrecognized subclinical disease is undoubtedly higher. In human insulin-dependent diabetic patients, for example, concurrent subclinical involvement of other endocrine glands, as evidenced by the presence of organ-specific autoantibodies, is much higher than the incidence of overt glandular failure. In some studies, 20% of insulin-dependent diabetic persons were found also to have chronic thyroiditis (Neufeld et al., 1980). Because not all develop thyroid failure, the incidence of hypothyroidism is much lower. Similar results have been found in studies of primary hypothyroidism and Addison's disease in humans. Such studies have not been reported in dogs, but similar results could be expected.

A high index of suspicion is paramount for the recognition of polyendocrine gland failure syndromes. The hormone deficiencies may be noted simultaneously, or a second (or more) deficiency may occur at a later date, complicating the management of a previously well-controlled case. Concurrent primary hypothyroidism and primary hypoadrenocorticism probably represent the most frequently recognized polyendocrine failure state in dogs. It should be suspected whenever clinical signs or clinicopathologic abnormalities of both diseases are present or when appropriate therapy for one of the disorders fails to result in adequate clinical improvement. Hypoglycemic episodes and a decreasing insulin requirement can be the first indications of the development of thyroid or adrenal insufficiency in a diabetic patient. A decline in the amount of mineralocorticoid replacement needed may herald the onset of thyroid failure in a dog with primary hypoadrenocorticism. Similarly, the recurrence of unexplained lethargy, weakness, or anorexia in a well-controlled addisonian patient may signal the development of hypothyroidism. The presence of hypocalcemia in a dog with a known hormone deficiency should prompt investigation for hypoparathyroidism with serum parathyroid hormone levels.

Diagnosis of the component diseases in a case of polyendocrine failure is confirmed by routine serum biochemistry and electrolyte determinations and standard endocrine diagnostic tests (see *CVT X*, p. 961). As previously mentioned, autoantibodies to the specific endocrine target organ can be detected using special laboratory studies in some dogs with hormone-deficient states. Measurements of most canine autoantibodies are not readily available, and there can be problems with test specificity and sensitivity. Despite these limitations, determination of autoantibody titers may be useful in selected cases to identify dogs at risk of developing additional disorders. Early recognition may avert subsequent morbidity and mortality. For example, an adrenal crisis precipitated by a stressful event such as surgery can be avoided if subclinical adrenal insufficiency is recognized beforehand.

TREATMENT

Treatment of polyendocrine failure is directed at replacing the deficient hormones, not at the underlying immune disorder. Such replacement therapy is usually not complicated provided the diseases are recognized at an early stage. Should diagnosis not occur until late in the course of the disease—once events such as ketoacidosis, adrenal crisis, myxedema coma, and tetanic seizures have occurred—treatment will be substantially more difficult and morbidity and mortality higher. The hormone replacement doses for polyendocrine gland failure are identical to those used for treatment of isolated deficiencies (see the relevant articles in this volume and in *CVT X*). A few precautions must be exercised, however. In cases of concurrent hypothyroidism and hypoadrenocorticism, replacement of thyroxine without previous treatment of the adrenal insufficiency can precipitate an adrenal crisis. Replacement of thyroxine increases the metabolic rate and therefore the need for endogenous steroids, possibly taxing the failing adrenal glands. Likewise, thyroxine replacement without previous or simultaneous administration of calcium and vitamin D can precipitate tetany in a dog with concurrent hypothyroidism and hypoparathyroidism. Gradual introduction of thyroid hormone replacement is recommended in dogs with diabetes, hypoadrenocorticism, or hypoparathyroidism in which concurrent or subsequent thyroid failure is diagnosed. Divided-dose protocols are recommended, and the amount administered should be increased in 25% increments over a period of 4 to 8 weeks until the desired dose is achieved. Because thyroid hormone increases the metabolism of all administered hormones (including itself), the doses should be reassessed by both clinical and laboratory determinations after the induction period of thyroid hormone replacement. Insulin requirements will likely increase after adrenal steroid or thyroid hormone replacement in diabetic dogs. Careful monitoring both at home and by periodic determinations of blood glucose curves is necessary until insulin requirements have once again stabilized.

With early diagnosis and treatment, the *prognosis* in most cases of polyendocrine gland failure is good. Hormonal replacement therapy is adequate in most cases, although regulation of some cases of diabetes can prove frustrating. The key to the early recognition of polyendocrine gland failure syndromes is a high index of suspicion.

References and Suggested Reading

Bowen, D., Schaer, M., and Riley, W.: Autoimmune polyglandular syndrome in a dog. J. Am. Anim. Hosp. Assoc. 22:649, 1986.
    A case report of concurrent hypoadrenocorticism and hypothyroidism.
Eigenmann, J. E., van deer Haage, M. H., and Rijnberk, A.: Polyendo-

crinopathy in two canine littermates: Simultaneous occurrence of carbohydrate intolerance and hypothyroidism. J. Am. Anim. Hosp. Assoc. 20:143, 1984.
Concurrent carbohydrate intolerance and hypothyroidism as a manifestation of polyglandular autoimmunity.

Eisenbarth, G. S., and Rassi, N.: Polyglandular failure syndromes. *In* Davies, T. F. (ed.): *Autoimmune Endocrine Disease.* New York: John Wiley & Sons, 1983, p. 193.
A review of the clinical aspects and immunogenetics of human polyglandular failure.

Hargis, A. M., Stephens, L. C., Benjamin, S. A., et al.: Relationship of hypothyroidism to diabetes mellitus, renal amyloidosis, and thrombosis in purebred beagles. Am. J. Vet. Res. 42:1077, 1981.
A report of concurrent diabetes mellitus and hypothyroidism.

Neufeld, M., MacLaren, N., and Blizzard, R.: Autoimmune polyglandular syndromes. Pediatr. Ann. 9:154, 1980.
A review of the various polyglandular syndromes in human patients.

Section

6

HEMATOLOGY, ONCOLOGY, AND IMMUNOLOGY

BRUCE R. MADEWELL
Consulting Editor

GENETIC DETERMINANTS OF CANCER

BRUCE R. MADEWELL

Davis, California

Cancer is a genetically determined disease. Tumorigenesis is a multistep process in which multiple genetic events govern the initiation, promotion, and progression of neoplastic disease (Weinberg, 1989). Oncogenes are the most thoroughly studied of the genetic determinants of cancer, and more than 50 have been identified. By definition, oncogenes are genes capable of inducing neoplastic transformation. Other genes associated with cancer are the tumor suppressor genes. These genes are a diverse group that share the property that their expression inhibits the cancer phenotype. Metastasis is distinct from tumorigenesis, and there are data to show that it is also regulated at the genetic level by the activation or inactivation of specific genes.

Other genes influence susceptibility to cancer, the progression of disease within the tumor-bearing host, and even treatment response. For example, because immunologic response to tumors involves recognition of class I and class II major histocompatibility antigens, genes controlling expression of these antigens may influence the host immune response to the neoplasm. From a treatment perspective, expression of the multidrug resistance gene (*mdr1*) confers multidrug resistance on the cell. This is the ability to withstand exposure to lethal doses of many structurally unrelated antineoplastic agents.

The purpose of this article is to provide an overview of some of the genetic determinants associated with the development and behavior of neoplasms. It is anticipated that as our understanding of cancer expands on a molecular level, new strategies will be developed for early diagnosis, for more accurate prognosis, and ultimately for cancer treatment through innovative biotechnologies.

ONCOGENES

Proto-oncogenes are normal constituents of the genome. They are well-conserved genes found in all vertebrate species and are presumed to represent a subset of a larger group of genes that have important regulatory roles in cell growth and differentiation (Studzinski, 1989). The proteins encoded by proto-oncogenes have been classified by function into four groups—namely, growth factors, growth factor receptors, cytoplasmic proteins (i.e., protein kinases or guanosine triphosphate [GTP]-binding proteins), and nuclear (DNA-binding) proteins (Table 1). Proto-oncogenes may also be classified by the location of their encoded products: secretory proteins, cell surface proteins, cytoplasmic proteins, and nuclear proteins. Although proto-oncogenes are normal cellular genes involved in the control of cell proliferation and differentiation, when activated by specific genetic alterations, they become oncogenes that contribute to the initiation or maintenance of malignancy.

Virally altered or activated proto-oncogenes (oncogenes) lead to abnormal cellular proliferation and tumor formation. Oncogenes contribute to tumor formation as a result of either constitutional activation that prevents them from following regulatory signals or structural changes that incapacitate their

Table 1. *Oncogene Families Categorized by Function of Gene Product*

GTP-binding (signal transducing) proteins and protein kinases	
c-*src*	protein tyrosine kinase
c-*fes/fps*	protein tyrosine kinase
c-*abl*	protein tyrosine kinase
c-Ha-*ras*	GTP-binding, GTPase
c-Ki-*ras*	GTP-binding, GTPase
c-*raf*	serine, threonine kinase
c-*fgr*	protein tyrosine kinase
Nuclear (DNA-binding) proteins	
c-*myc*	DNA binding
c-*myb*	?
c-*jun*	transcription factor
c-*fos*	transcription factor
c-*ski*	transcription factor
Growth factors	
c-*sis*	PDGF
hst	factor related (?)
int-2	fibroblast growth factor
Growth factor receptors	
c-*erb*B	EGF receptor
c-*fms*	CSF-1 receptor
c-*erb*A	thyroid hormone receptor

CSF, colony-stimulating factor; DNA, deoxyribonuclease; EGF, epidermal growth factor; GTP, guanosine triphosphate; GTPase, guanosine triphosphatase; PDGF, platelet-derived growth factor.

normal signaling function. Proto-oncogenes become activated by a number of mechanisms, including those that are discussed next.

Translocation

Proto-oncogenes may be activated by translocation with or without fusion into another locus. This is a common mechanism in human hematopoietic neoplasms; proto-oncogenes situated at the breaking point are activated as a result of the translocation. For example, in Burkitt's lymphoma, c-*myc* is placed by translocation under the influence of immunoglobulin promoters and enhancers, and in most cases of follicular lymphoma, *bc12* is similarly activated. Most patients with chronic myelogenous leukemia have translocation of the c-*abl* gene in the Philadelphia chromosome (Renan, 1990). This translocation results in the juxtaposition of a strong transcription enhancer with a growth-related gene. The encoded hybrid fusion protein has kinase activity that is thought to have a role in cellular transformation.

Amplification

Proto-oncogenes may also be inappropriately amplified or overamplified in neoplasms. Oncogene amplification is a process by which tumor cells make multiple copies of oncogenes and subsequently large amounts of a gene product important in the process of transformation. For example, in human breast cancer, c-*myc*, c-*erb*B-2 (also known as HER-2/*neu*) oncogene amplifications occur consistently in association with advanced neoplasms, and those oncogene amplifications are associated with a poor prognosis.

Mutation

Mutation is another mechanism of proto-oncogene activation resulting in altered protein products. Mutations in *ras* oncogenes occur with high frequency and predictability in some types of neoplasms at codons 12, 13, and 61, conferring transforming properties to the *ras* p21 proteins.

Additional mechanisms of activation exist in some tumors. Mechanisms of activation of oncogenes associated with *retrovirus* infections include transduction and insertional mutagenesis.

Transduction

Transduction by a retrovirus was the first mechanism discovered to be capable of activating *onc*

genes. Retroviruses synthesize a double-stranded copy of their RNA that integrates as the proviral form into host cellular DNA. Recombination between viral and host DNA may transduce an adjacent growth-related gene into the viral DNA. The virus may then re-enter other cells as a rapidly transforming oncogenic virus (Studzinski, 1989). The resultant combination of viral and cellular material may have enhanced tumorigenesis potential as a result of fusion of the proto-oncogenes with viral coding sequences or as a result of damage of the transduced gene by mutations, deletions, or substitutions compared with its normal cellular counterpart. For example, the viral *fms* protein is homologous to the receptor for colony-stimulating factor (CSF-1). The viral *fms* is truncated at the carboxy terminus, and the truncation appears to cause constitutive activation of the growth stimulatory protein kinase activity of the molecule.

Insertional Mutagenesis

In insertional mutagenesis, slowly transforming retroviruses integrate into cellular DNA. As a consequence, normal cellular proto-oncogenes are modified by being placed under the control of strong retrovirus transcriptional signals in the long terminal repeat of the viral DNA. For example, the putative *onc* gene *int*-1 (a member of the fibroblast growth factor family) shows enhanced transcription in mouse mammary tumor virus-induced mammary carcinomas as a consequence of viral integration in its vicinity.

TUMOR SUPPRESSOR GENES

Neoplasms may also be associated with or result from deletions or mutations in recessive oncogenes or tumor suppressor genes. In tumor suppressor genes, it is their loss or inactivation that is oncogenic (Sager, 1989). Although dominant oncogenes are identified by their positive role in the transformation of host cells, tumor suppressors have an essentially negative effect, blocking transformation and driving cells toward normalcy. When they become homozygously inactivated by a deletion or point mutation, tumors can arise. At present, only a few such tumor suppressor genes have been cloned and sequenced, but evidence suggesting their existence is persuasive.

Most thoroughly studied of the tumor suppressor genes are the retinoblastoma (*Rb*) and p53 genes. Clinical evidence for the presence of growth-restraining genes comes from studies of human tumors such as retinoblastoma in which loss of specific DNA sequences results in the development of neoplasia. The concept of tumor suppressor genes evolved from epidemiologic studies of retinoblastoma (Knudson, 1971). It was subsequently determined that in human familial retinoblastoma, affected individuals inherit one normal and one defective allele of the *Rb* gene (i.e., they are heterozygous for the defect). In tumor cells arising in such individuals, however, the normal gene is lost (by somatic mutation or some other chromosomal alteration affecting the normal allele), and the tumors are homozygous for the defect. It has been proposed, therefore, that the normal allele acts as a tumor suppressor gene and that its loss precipitates tumor formation. The *Rb* gene product is expressed in all tissues and appears to have a role within the cell in the regulation of expression of other genes, but its precise function is still not understood. Loss of *Rb* gene activity is now reported in various human neoplasms, including retinoblastoma and those neoplasms arising as secondary malignancies not only in patients with the hereditary form of retinoblastoma but also in patients with diverse other neoplasms derived from the lung, breast, and urinary bladder.

The second tumor suppressor gene to be recognized was p53 (human 17p13 region), and it also acts negatively to block transformation. Protein p53 may have dual roles; it appears to act as a tumor suppressor in its normal form and as an oncoprotein that directly promotes tumor growth in its mutant form. Inactivating mutations of p53 have been associated with osteosarcomas, soft-tissue sarcomas, brain tumors, leukemias, and carcinomas of the lung and breast. The presence of p53 mutations in the sporadic forms of various human neoplasms suggests that these genetic alterations are an important step in the transformation of diverse cells. More recently, germline p53 mutations have been described in some cancer-prone families; thus two tumor suppressor genes (*Rb* and p53) that manifest somatic and germline mutations have now been identified (Maulkin et al., 1990). It is anticipated that the development of molecular diagnostic tests to identify carriers of these mutations will allow new tools for screening members of highly cancer-prone families.

METASTASIS GENES

Considerable effort has been made in recent years to define the biochemical mechanisms governing tumor invasion and metastasis (Liotta and Kohn, 1990). Metastasizing cells must progress through multiple steps while overcoming host defences during the process of establishing a replicating colony at a distant site. It is suspected that each discrete step of the metastatic process is regulated by permanent changes in the DNA or transient changes at the RNA level of different genes. For example,

the major histocompatibility genes have been shown to affect the metastatic process. Transfection of oncogenes such as *ras, mos, raf, src, fes,* and *fms* can increase the metastatic potential *in vivo* of tumor cells. Amplification of the c-*erb*B-2 oncogene has been correlated with metastases in human breast carcinomas (Slamon et al., 1987), whereas N-*myc* amplification has been associated with metastasis in neuroblastomas. The mechanism by which these amplified genes relate to tumor aggressiveness is unknown. A number of investigators have identified genes that are specifically expressed in metastatic cells. One gene that has been isolated is expressed in metastatic cells, and its gene product has a high degree of homology to a calcium-binding family.

Analogous to the oncogenc/anti-oncogene model of tumor progression, metastasis is probably governed by both metastasis-promoting and -suppressing genes. A candidate metastasis suppressor gene, *nm23*, has been identified. Analogous to the anti-oncogene *Rb*, the function of the gene appears to be suppression of the metastatic phenotype. Levels of mRNA transcribed from the *nm23* gene were decreased in highly metastatic tumor cells in four rodent models of metastasis. In human patients with breast cancer, *nm23* levels in tumor tissues were directly correlated with the presence of metastasis (Steeg et al., 1988). We have found preliminary evidence of decreased transcription of *nm23* in metastatic cells compared with the primary tumor in matched samples from dogs.

MULTISTEP TUMORIGENESIS

There is no evidence that the activation of a single oncogene or inactivation of a single tumor suppressor gene can change a normal diploid cell into a tumor cell *in vivo*. Tumorigenesis is a multistep process in which multiple genetic events govern the initiation, promotion, and progression of human (and animal) tumors (Weinberg, 1989; Vogelstein et al., 1988). Each step in multistep tumorigenesis represents a physiologic barrier that must be overcome for a cell to progress further toward the end point of malignancy. Tumor progression is thought to occur when variant cells that have selective growth characteristics arise within a cell population. For example, some of the genetic events controlling colon cancer have been identified. In that disease, tumorigenesis proceeds through a series of genetic aberrations leading to unlimited proliferative capacity (induction of immortality), oncogene activation, and inactivation of tumor suppressor genes. Data also suggest that the human colorectal model of multistep tumorigenesis is applicable to other tumor types such as those affecting the lung, breast, bladder, and brain.

CLINICAL APPLICATIONS

Diagnosis, Classification, and Prognosis

Determining alterations in oncogenes and tumor suppressor genes in neoplasms may eventually be useful for the establishment of new diagnostic classifications, the development of tests for predicting cancer susceptibility, and the introduction of novel therapeutic strategies. From the diagnostic perspective, improved nosologic definition in some neoplasms might be obtained by molecular analyses. For example, the immunoglobulin gene and the T-cell receptor gene might be used for diagnosis of undifferentiated lymphoid tumors and to determine whether they are of T- or B-cell origin (Bignon et al., 1988; Renan, 1990). These studies could also be used to determine the clonality of neoplasms of lymphoid lineage.

Identification of tumor-specific translocations already assists in the accurate diagnosis of hematopoietic tumors in humans, including the c-*myc* rearrangement in Burkitt's lymphoma, the *bcr-abl* hybrid in chronic myelogenous leukemia, the *bcl*-1 oncogene translocation in chronic lymphocytic leukemia and some lymphomas, and the *bcl*-2 translocation in follicular lymphomas.

Detection of N-*myc* oncogene amplification may assist in the categorization of neuroblastoma. For some neoplasms, differences in proto-oncogene expression between closely related tumors may reflect unique biologic features of the precise cell or origin of the neoplasm, and it has been possible to distinguish genetically distinct forms of colon cancer on the basis of c-*myc* expression.

Alterations in oncogenes and tumor suppressor genes may also be used for assessment of prognosis. Although there are few data showing oncogene perturbations in animal neoplasms of veterinary importance at this time, the methodologies to establish those data are now available for veterinary application (Madewell et al., 1989). For example, in human patients with breast cancer, overexpression of the HER-2/*neu* oncogene has been shown to correlate with a poor prognosis. Other associations with poor clinical outcome include amplification of the N-*myc* oncogene in neuroblastoma and small-cell lung cancer, c-Ki-*ras* mutations in myelodysplasia, and the Philadelphia chromosome translocation involving the *abl* oncogene in acute lymphoid leukemia. Prognosis is also determined by the chemosensitivity of neoplasms, and measurement of multidrug-resistant (*mdr1*) gene expression in tumor specimens may assist in determining treatment regimens.

Another application of molecular genetics for cancer patients is the detection of those patients with residual disease after treatment. Molecular diagnosis allows detection of minimal residual disease and vastly improves the crude limits of detecting residual disease as offered by cytologic and cytogenetic methods of detection. These detection methods exploit the high sensitivity of *in situ* hybridization or polymerase chain reaction to detect a genetic disease marker, such as the *bcr-abl* translocation in human patients with chronic myelogenous leukemia.

Molecular genetic studies may also be used for early detection of cancer. Genetic markers may allow detection of preneoplastic lesions, such as the presence of *ras* mutations in preneoplastic colonic adenomas or in myelodysplastic syndromes. Similarly, *Rb* gene sequencing can be used to predict the probability of retinoblastomas in fetuses of affected families.

Treatment

Gene therapy is a novel technique under consideration for the treatment of genetic diseases. Gene therapy is defined as the transfer of genetic material into the cells of an organism to treat disease. Gene *replacement* therapy involves precise replacement of a defective gene in the cells of an affected organ. More practically, in gene *addition* therapy, genes are added to correct a disease. Somatic gene therapy introduces the gene only into the somatic cells and not into the germline; it is unlikely that somatic gene therapy would raise the ethical objections of germline therapy. The method for gene transfer currently involves the use of retroviral vectors to insert an unarranged copy of a gene into a host cell genome, ensuring its presence in all progeny of the infected cell (Miller, 1990). The immediate prospects for gene therapy include those genetically determined diseases characterized by the loss of a critical enzyme due to a single gene abnormality. An example of this is human severe combined immunodeficiency resulting from deficiency of the enzyme adenosine deaminase. Gene therapy for multigenetic diseases, such as most neoplasms, will require more precise, concerted gene expression for correction (Kohn et al., 1989). A possible application of gene transfer therapy to patients with malignant disease is to restore functional expression of revelant tumor suppressor genes that have been rendered inactive as the result of mutations affecting the expression of both alleles of the wild-type gene. For somatic gene therapy to be accomplished, it is important that the candidate disease have a consistent and severe phenotype (i.e., most neoplasms), that the gene to be introduced has been cloned, that the expression of the gene product not require too precise regulation or high levels of expression, and that there be a suitable delivery system for implantation of the genetically modified cells.

Selective inhibition of oncogene expression also

has therapeutic potential. One method would be the use of monoclonal antibodies directed at oncogene-encoded proteins. Another method is the use of drugs that interfere with gene expression. For example, mithramycin, a guanine-cytosine (G-C) specific binding drug, selectively inhibits c-*myc* expression perhaps by preventing regulatory protein binding to G-C–rich regions in the c-*myc* promoter.

The most provocative strategy to prevent oncogene activity is to transfer "antisense" (complementary) messages into cells. Antisense strategy is attractive because it is based on the simple molecular recognition code of base pairing by hydrogen bonds between complementary bases (i.e., the interaction is very specific). Such antisense messages may be used to shut off inappropriately expressed oncogenes in malignancies or viral genes in virus-induced neoplasms. Much of the emphasis in this regard has focused on the use of synthetic oligonucleotides (oligoribo- or oligodeoxyribonucleotides), short nucleotide sequences formulated to exert some regulatory function. The cytoplasmic location of messenger RNA (mRNA) provides a target readily accessible to antisense oligonucleotides entering the cell. Thus, much of the work in this area has focused on mRNA as a target (Rothenberg et al., 1989). Cellular proto-oncogenes represent attractive targets for oligonucleotide therapy in the treatment of cancer. Because of the pivotal role of oncogenes in the pathogenesis of some neoplasms, therapy could be targeted at those oncogene-expressing malignant cells while sparing normal cells that lack oncogene expression. For example, an oligonucleotide complementary to the mutated region of a *ras* oncogene could discriminate between the mutated and normal allele, thus specifically inhibiting the expression of that oncogene.

SUMMARY

Molecular genetics has been introduced to the diagnostic laboratory and is already influencing the clinical management of human cancer patients. Cancer is now recognized as an end result of a series of genetic perturbations that cumulatively influence primary tumor growth, tissue invasion, and metastasis. The critical study of molecular genetics in animal and human patients with cancer is quickly leading not only to new perspectives regarding tumor biology but also to new phenotypic characterizations of neoplasms that influence diagnosis, treatment, and prognosis. The advent of rapid and

precise genetic measurements derived from studies of small clinically procured specimens in animals will soon profoundly influence our management of tumor-bearing patients.

References and Suggested Reading

Bignon, Y. J., Dastugue, B., and Plagne, R.: Molecular biology diagnosis in oncology. Biomed. Pharmacother. 42:653, 1988.
  An overview of the applications of molecular biology in cancer diagnosis.
Knudson, A. G.: Mutation and cancer: Statistical study of retinoblastoma. Proc. Natl. Acad. Sci. U.S.A. 68:820, 1971.
  A seminal study proposing that a defect in one allele of a suppressor gene causes a cancer predisposition.
Kohn, D. B., Anderson, W. F., and Blaese, R. M.: Gene therapy for genetic diseases. Cancer Invest. 1:179, 1989.
  Description of the basic techniques for transferring genes into human cells.
Liotta, L. A., and Kohn, E.: Cancer invasion and metastases. J.A.M.A. 263:1123, 1990.
  An overview of the role of genes in cancer invasion and metastasis.
Madewell, B. R., Gumerlock, P. H., Saunders, K. A., et al.: Canine and bovine *ras* family expression detected and discriminated by use of polymerase chain reaction. Anticancer Res. 9:1743, 1989.
  A strategy for detection of proto-oncogenes in animal tissues using polymerase chain reaction technology.
Maulkin, D., Li, F. P., Strong, L. C., et al.: Germ line p53 mutations in a familial syndrome of breast cancer, sarcomas, and other neoplasms. Science 250:1233, 1990.
  Data showing the association of both somatic and germline p53 alterations with neoplasms in some cancer-prone families.
Miller, A. D.: Progress toward human gene therapy. Blood 76:271, 1990.
  Gene therapy strategies for treatment of human diseases.
Renan, M. J.: Cancer genes: Current status, future prospects, and applications in radiotherapy/oncology. Radiother. Oncol. 19:197, 1990.
  Review article on the genetic basis of cancer.
Rothenberg, M., Johnson, G., and Laughlin, C.: Oligodeoxynucleotides as anti-sense inhibitors of gene expression: Therapeutic implications. J. Natl. Cancer Inst. 81:1539, 1989.
  A commentary on the development of oligonucleotides as potential therapeutic agents.
Sager, R.: Tumor suppressor genes: The puzzle and the promise. Science 246:1406, 1989.
  Critical analysis of the tumor suppressor gene literature.
Slamon, D. J., Clark, G. M., Wong, S. G., et al.: Human breast cancer: Correlation of relapse and survival with amplification of the HER-2/*neu* oncogene. Science 235:177, 1987.
  A study illustrating the clinical application of oncogene profiles.
Steeg, P. S., Bevilacqua, G., Kopper, L., et al.: Evidence for a novel gene associated with low metastatic potential. J. Natl. Cancer Inst. 80:200, 1988.
  One of the earliest descriptions of the putative metastasis suppressor gene, nm23.
Studzinski, G. P.: Oncogenes, growth, and the cell cycle: An overview. Cell Tissue Kinet. 22:405, 1989.
  An overview of the role of oncogenes in the cell cycle.
Tronick, S. R., and Aaronson, S. A.: Oncogenes. *In* Cossman, J. (ed.): *Molecular Genetics in Cancer Diagnosis.* New York: Elsevier, 1990, p. 29.
  A survey of viral oncogenes and the role of oncogenes in the development of human neoplasms.
Vogelstein, B., Fearson, E. R., Hamilton, S. R., et al.: Genetic alterations during colorectal-tumor development. N. Engl. J. Med. 319:525, 1988.
  A genetic model of common malignancies, in which neoplasms develop by a stepwise accumulation of mutations affecting both oncogenes and tumor suppressor genes.
Weinberg, R. A.: Oncogenes, antioncogenes, and the molecular bases of multistep carcinogenesis. Cancer Res. 49:3713, 1989.
  An analysis of the multistep basis of tumorigenesis.

EPIRUBICIN (4'-EPI-DOXORUBICIN) CHEMOTHERAPY

KEVIN A. HAHN
and ELIZABETH A. HAHN
West Lafayette, Indiana

4'-EPI-DOXORUBICIN

Anthracycline antibiotics, including epirubicin (4'-epi-doxorubicin, Epirubicin, Farmitalia Carlo Erba), are a subfamily of quinones with antitumor activity. These compounds contain a planar anthraquinone nucleus with a side-chain moiety that determines the specific antitumor activity. Many anthracyclines have demonstrated severe dose-related and clinically limiting toxicities, including cardiotoxicity. Consequently, the emphasis of anthracycline analogue research has become directed toward understanding the mechanism(s) and the biochemical origin(s) of antitumor activity while minimizing toxicity through structural modifications. Common anthracyclines used in human oncologic therapy include doxorubicin, (Adriamycin, Adria Laboratories), daunorubicin (Cerubidine, Wyeth Laboratories), and epirubicin. All are biologic products, or structural analogues, from *Streptomyces peucetus* var *caesius* (Oki, 1988).

Epirubicin is a stereoisomer of doxorubicin. The hydroxyl group on the 4' carbon of the amino sugar side-chain moiety of the anthraquinone nucleus is epimerized (equatorial instead of axial). Extensive clinical trials in humans (Cammagi et al., 1988), preclinical trials in normal animals (Ganzina, 1983), and preliminary results from a multi-institutional veterinary oncology clinical trial in dogs with multicentric malignant lymphoma have demonstrated epirubicin to have equivalent antitumor activity to doxorubicin and lesser systemic toxicity at similar and equipotent therapeutic doses.

PHARMACOKINETICS

Epirubicin is supplied in 10-mg and 50-mg rubber disk-capped vials as a sterile red-orange lyophilized powder. The drug is reconstituted in sterile saline or in sterile water for a concentration of 2 mg/ml and administered by intravenous injection through a patent catheter. Epirubicin should be refrigerated at 4°C (40°F) until reconstituted; the remaining drug is stable for 24 hr at room temperature and should be protected from exposure to sunlight (Ganzina, 1983).

Clinical pharmacokinetic studies in humans suggest that no clear relationship exists between epirubicin plasma levels and systemic toxicity or therapeutic response (Cersosimo and Hong, 1986). Epirubicin, administered intravenously, has a triphasic distribution and elimination pattern that is similar to doxorubicin (Cammagi et al., 1988; Cersosimo and Hong, 1986). The first phase lasts 3 to 5 min and represents the rapid tissue distribution of the drug to the liver, lungs, heart, kidneys, and spleen. Epirubicin, like doxorubicin, does not cross the blood-brain barrier. The second phase, release of the drug back into the vascular compartment, lasts approximately 3 hr. The third phase, metabolism and elimination, is biliary and is proportional to the plasma flow to the liver.

The tissue distribution in humans is similar between epirubicin and doxorubicin; however, the concentration of epirubicin is lower in the heart, spleen, and kidneys than that of doxorubicin. Plasma levels of epirubicin in humans are significantly lower than plasma levels of doxorubicin; the terminal half-life of epirubicin is 30 to 40 hr, compared with 43 to 70 hr for doxorubicin (Ganzina, 1983). In four dogs with malignant lymphoma treated with epirubicin, the plasma concentration of epirubicin peaked within 1 hr after administration, diminished rapidly, and was undetectable 8 hr after administration.

Following epirubicin administration in humans, epirubicin, doxorubicin, doxorubicin metabolites, and two additional metabolites may be detected in the plasma. An additional metabolic pathway appears to provide more efficient elimination of epirubicin than doxorubicin. Conjugation with glucuronic acid takes place at the hydroxyl group in the 4' position of the aminosugar. The resultant glucuronides, 40% of the inactive epirubicin metabolites, are more water soluble than doxorubicin glucuronide metabolites. The equatorial orientation of the 4'-hydroxyl group makes epirubicin a good substrate for D-glucuronyl transferase; consequently, doxorubicin is not an appropriate substrate (Arcamone and Penco, 1988). In dogs (n = 4), 90 to 95% of the administered dose of epirubicin can be detected in the urine within 4 hr after administration.

ANTITUMOR ACTIVITY

Epirubicin has three probable mechanisms of antitumor action. First, the enzymatic reduction of the anthraquinone nucleus by xanthine oxidase, cytochrome P-450 reductase, cytochrome b_5 reductase, and the reduced form of nicotinamide-adenine dinucleotide (NADH) dehydrogenase begins a free-radical production cascade that is cytotoxic (Myers et al., 1988). Second, the anthraquinone nucleus and the glycosidic side-chain possess a unique stereochemical orientation that allows the compound to intercalate into the minor groove of B-type double-helical DNA (Myers et al., 1988). The lethal event is due to an irreversible conformational change within the DNA structure, preventing topoisomerase II, DNA-polymerase-a, and RNA-polymerase from physically interacting with DNA for the initiation of replication. The optimal fit and antitumor activity can be modified proportionally by the addition, removal, or epimerization of the side-chain sugar moiety bound to the anthraquinone nucleus. For example, 3'-epi-daunorubicin has reduced activity and DNA-binding affinity, whereas 4'-epi-daunorubicin and 4'-epi-doxorubicin have similar antitumor efficacy and show higher affinity compared with their respective parent drug (Myers et al., 1988). Third, epirubicin alters many membrane functions, including lectin-induced cell agglutination, ion transport, membrane fluidity, lipid membrane organization, and membrane morphology. Of these inhibitory functions, the most critical appears to be the high affinity of anthracyclines to bind to membrane phospholipids, resulting in the disruption of membrane fluidity (Myers et al., 1988).

Epirubicin has demonstrated *in vitro* cytotoxicity against human mammary carcinoma, leukemia, lung carcinoma, colon carcinoma, metastatic lung carcinoma, and some doxorubicin-resistant cell lines (Grandi et al., 1988). As a single agent in humans, epirubicin has been most effective (complete remission and partial remission >70%) for non-Hodgkin's lymphoma (Casazza et al., 1978). It has also shown single-agent efficacy against breast, ovarian, pancreatic, lung, gastric, bladder, thyroid, hepatic, colorectal, and cervical neoplasms as well as soft-tissue sarcomas, melanoma, leukemia, and head and neck carcinomas.

The antitumor activity of epirubicin in dogs is known only for malignant lymphoma. The short-term clinical response in dogs with stage IIIA to VB malignant lymphoma receiving either a cumulative dose of 60 mg/m² epirubicin (n = 51 dogs) or doxorubicin (n = 48 dogs) (30 mg/m² IV once every 3 weeks) was prospectively evaluated. All dogs were clinically staged before and 6 weeks after the initiation of chemotherapy. Of 51 epirubicin-treated dogs, 37 achieved complete remission, 4 achieved partial remission, 3 maintained a stable response, and 7 showed no clinical response. Of 48 doxorubicin-treated dogs, 30 achieved complete remission, 5 achieved partial remission, 4 maintained a stable response, and 9 showed no clinical response. Longevity of response (remission length and survival time) is pending completion of this multi-institutional clinical trial.

ADVERSE EFFECTS

Hematologic Toxicity

The acute dose-limiting toxicity associated with epirubicin is myelosuppression. Leukopenia and thrombocytopenia are predictable and reversible within 3 weeks in almost all instances. Hematologic toxicity was evaluated in eight dogs with multicentric malignant lymphoma receiving either 30 mg/m² IV epirubicin or doxorubicin in the treatment of stage IIIA to VB malignant lymphoma (Richardson et al., 1988). The nadir of 21 daily white blood cell (WBC) counts occurred between day 6 and day 10 for epirubicin and between day 7 and day 10 for doxorubicin. The mean WBC count per mm³ at nadir was 2700 in dogs given epirubicin and 3600 in dogs given doxorubicin. The nadir of 21 daily platelet counts occurred between day 2 and day 10 for epirubicin and between day 3 and day 8 for doxorubicin. The mean platelet count per mm³ at nadir was 185,000 in dogs given epirubicin and 144,500 in dogs given doxorubicin.

Gastrointestinal Toxicity

Vomiting, diarrhea, and pancreatitis developed in 10 of 48 dogs receiving doxorubicin and 7 of 51 dogs receiving epirubicin. The 10 dogs with epirubicin gastrointestinal toxicity required immediate medical attention (intravenous fluid, antiemetic, antibiotic therapy). The severity of epirubicin gastrointestinal toxicity appeared to be independent of clinical stage; however, our observations are preliminary.

Cardiotoxicity

Anthracycline-induced cardiotoxicity has been quantitatively measured histopathologically for various analogues (Grandi et al., 1988). All 4'-anthracycline analogues have had significantly fewer or absent cardiac lesions when compared with doxorubicin. The reason for anthracycline cardiotoxicity is not clearly established in human or veterinary medicine. The generation of reactive oxygen species, in particular hydrogen peroxide, superoxide anion radicals (O_2^-), and hydroxyl anion radicals (OH), produces peroxidative injury to membrane lipids and DNA. Such damage could be particularly serious in cardiac tissues because of lowered concentrations of the detoxifying enzymes superoxide dismutase, catalase, and glutathione peroxidase.

Anthracyclines, including epirubicin, have been clinically associated with two forms of cardiac toxicity. Acute effects, characterized by electrocardiographic arrhythmias, occur in an average of 15% of humans who receive the drug (Cersosimo and Hong, 1986). Abnormalities include transient atrial and ventricular arrhythmias, premature atrial or ventricular contractions, and atrioventricular junctional premature beats. Chronic anthracycline therapy can result in congestive heart failure and death. In comparing the myocardial function of humans before and during therapy with either doxorubicin or epirubicin, greater than 10% decline in left ventricular ejection fraction from pretreatment values occurred only after a cumulative dose of 850 mg/m² of epirubicin compared with a cumulative dose of 360 mg/m² of doxorubicin (Young, 1984). The minimum cumulative dose of epirubicin associated with a decline in myocardial function was 200 mg/m². At equally myelosuppressive doses in humans, this investigation concluded that epirubicin was less cardiotoxic than doxorubicin (Young, 1984).

Preclinical toxicology testing in rabbits and dogs has also demonstrated epirubicin to have lower cardiotoxicity than doxorubicin (Casazza et al., 1978). Treated intravenously with epirubicin or doxorubicin for 3 consecutive days per week for a total of 6 weeks using three dose levels, the toxic effects were qualitatively similar. Histopathologic findings in normal white rabbits revealed a 25% lower incidence of cardiac lesions in those receiving epirubicin than in those receiving doxorubicin. Histopathologic cardiac lesions were observed in all dogs treated with doxorubicin and absent in all epirubicin-treated dogs (Casazza et al., 1978).

We have observed a reduced potential for the development of cardiac toxicity in dogs treated with epirubicin compared with doxorubicin. Sixty-four dogs with multicentric malignant lymphoma were treated with 180 mg/m² cumulative dose of either epirubicin (n = 32 dogs) or doxorubicin (n = 32 dogs) (30 mg/m² IV every 3 weeks) and evaluated by echocardiography before the first, third, and sixth session of chemotherapy. Six dogs had treatment-related cardiotoxicity (five dogs treated with doxorubicin, one dog treated with epirubicin). Of

the five dogs treated with doxorubicin, abnormalities included reduced echocardiographic left ventricular ejection fraction (four of five), premature ventricular contractions (three of five), left ventricular enlargement (one of five), and histopathologic documented myocardial degeneration (four of five). These five dogs received a cumulative dose of 120 to 300 mg/m² of doxorubicin. In the epirubicin-treated dog, no antemortem clinical signs of cardiotoxicity were noted. Only subtle ultrasonographic evidence of reduced cardiac contractility was noted after receiving a cumulative dose of 240 mg/m². On necropsy, the right ventricular free wall was thin and flaccid and demonstrated histopathologic features consistent with anthracycline toxicity.

CONCLUSION

Epirubicin is similar, in most respects, to its isomeric compound doxorubicin. The plasma distribution, metabolism, and toxicity of epirubicin and doxorubicin are similar in dogs. Epirubicin is as effective as doxorubicin in the induction of clinical remission in canine malignant lymphoma. Conclusive data regarding remission length and survival time in epirubicin-treated compared with doxorubicin-treated dogs with malignant lymphoma are pending, but response appears to be similar. Preclinical toxicology testing and our preliminary clinical trial results indicate a reduced potential for anthracycline-induced cardiotoxicity in dogs treated with epirubicin.

References and Suggested Reading

Arcamone, F., and Penco, S.: Synthesis of new doxorubicin analogs. In Lown, J. W. (ed.): Anthracycline and Anthracenedione-Based Anticancer Agents. New York: Elsevier Science, 1988, p 1.
The pharmacology of the newer synthetic antitumor anthracyclines.

Cammagi, C. M., Comparsi, R., Strocchi, E., et al.: Epirubicin and doxorubicin comparative metabolism and pharmacokinetics: A crossover study. Cancer Chemother. Pharmacol. 21:211, 1988.
The pharmacokinetics and metabolism of doxorubicin and epirubicin are compared in eight cancer patients.

Casazza, A. M., Di Marco, A., Bertazzoli, C., et al.: Antitumor activity, toxicity and pharmacological properties of 4'-epi-Adriamycin. In Siegenthaler, W., and Luthy, R. (eds.): Current Chemotherapy, Proceedings of the 10th International Congress of Chemotherapy. Washington, DC: American Society of Microbiology, 1978, p. 1257.
An investigation of the in vitro and in vivo action of epirubicin in mouse tumor cell lines, normal rabbits, and normal dogs.

Cersosimo, R. J., and Hong, W. K.: Epirubicin: A review of the pharmacology, clinical activity, and adverse effects of an adriamycin analog. J. Clin. Oncol. 4:425, 1986.
A comprehensive review of the antitumor activity of epirubicin in human neoplasms.

Ganzina, F.: 4'-Epi-doxorubicin, a new analogue of doxorubicin: A preliminary overview of preclinical and clinical data. Cancer Treat. Rev. 10:1, 1983.
The pharmacology, antitumor effects, and toxicity of doxorubicin and epirubicin.

Grandi, M., Guiliana, F. C., Verhoef, V., et al.: Screening of anthracycline analogs. In Lown, J. W. (ed.): Anthracycline and Anthracenedione-Based Anticancer Agents. New York: Elsevier Science, 1988, p. 571.

In vitro *and in vivo* methods of screening new anthracycline analogues for antitumor activity and toxicity.

Myers, C. E., Mimnaugh, E. G., Yeh, G. C., et al.: Biochemical mechanisms of tumor cell kill by the anthracyclines. *In* Lown, J. W. (ed.): *Anthracycline and Anthracenedione-Based Anticancer Agents.* New York: Elsevier Science, 1988, p. 527.
The biologic mechanisms of anthracycline cytotoxicity.

Oki, T.: Antitumor anthracycline antibiotics from microbial origins. *In* Lown, J. W. (ed.): *Anthracycline and Anthracenedione-Based Anticancer Agents.* New York: Elsevier Science, 1988, p. 103.
The chemical structure, antitumor activity, and biosynthesis of anthracyclines.

Richardson, R. C., Hahn, K. A., Knapp, D. W., et al.: Hematologic changes associated with epirubicin and doxorubicin during the first 21 days following administration. Proc. Vet. Can. Soc. 8th Annual Conference. Estes Park, CO, 1988, p. 22.
Results of a pilot study.

Young, C. W.: Epirubicin: A therapeutically active doxorubicin analogue with reduced cardiotoxicity. *In* Bonadonna, G. (ed.): *Advances in Anthracycline Chemotherapy: Epirubicin.* Milan: Masson, 1984, p. 183.
Results of a phase II clinical trial in human neoplasms treated with epirubicin.

ADVANCES IN PLATINUM COMPOUND CHEMOTHERAPY

SUSAN A. KRAEGEL
Davis, California

and RODNEY L. PAGE
Raleigh, North Carolina

Platinum complexes, predominately cisplatin (*cis*-diamminedichloroplatinum Platinol, Bristol-Myers Oncology) are among the most active chemical agents available for the treatment of neoplasms in humans. During the past 5 to 10 years, cisplatin has earned a role in veterinary oncology as well. Despite cisplatin's importance, its toxicity profile (nephrotoxicity, neurotoxicity, ototoxicity, and gastrointestinal toxicity) has limited its use. An intensive search for new analogues has led to the development of active platinum compounds with similar efficacy but reduced toxicity compared with cisplatin. Carboplatin (*cis*-diaminocyclobutanedicarboxylatoplatinum Paraplatin, Bristol-Myers Oncology) is the first commercially available drug that fulfills these criteria. This article addresses clinical advances in platinum therapy (see this volume, p. 409, and *CVT X*, pp. 494 and 497, for a complete review of cisplatin pharmacology, administration, and previous clinical experience).

CISPLATIN

Systemic Administration

The current recommendation for cisplatin dose and administration varies from one institution to another. No obviously superior method of infusion has been identified, but all include aggressive saline diuresis to reduce nephrotoxicity. Doses up to 60 to 70 mg/m^2 every 3 weeks for four treatments are well tolerated in most older tumor-bearing dogs.

The cisplatin-based chemotherapy protocol appears to increase survival times after amputation or limb salvage procedures in dogs with *osteosarcoma*. Median survival times range from 9 to 12 months after amputation plus adjuvant cisplatin, versus 4 to 5 months with amputation alone (Kraegel et al., in press). Despite the absence of true, randomized prospective studies to confirm the relative benefit of cisplatin in dogs with osteosarcoma, improvements in median survival of this magnitude suggest that adjuvant cisplatin should be the current treatment of choice. Characterization of predictive indicators related to treatment (i.e., cumulative dose, perioperative chemotherapy timing, and so on) may further increase survival times.

Preliminary studies suggested that cisplatin might be an active agent in canine squamous cell carcinoma, transitional cell carcinoma, and other epithelial tumors. Cisplatin as a single agent has been used to treat transitional cell carcinomas in dogs (Moore et al., 1990). Therapeutic benefit was observed in 6 of 12 evaluable dogs. Three of these six had partial responses (greater than 50% decrease in measured tumor volume). For the other three dogs, tumor progression was not observed during the period of chemotherapy. Azotemia developed in 5 of the 12 dogs, underscoring the need for further development of non-nephrotoxic cisplatin analogues for use in animals with pre-existing renal disease.

Cisplatin can also be incorporated into multimodality treatment regimens. The current use of cisplatin, radiation, and surgery for limb sparing in dogs with osteosarcoma is one example (LaRue et al., 1989). Cisplatin in combination with hyperthermia or radiation is also being vigorously investigated. It is possible that as a result of synergy or potentiation between modalities, tumor responses may be increased without concomitantly increasing toxicities to normal tissues.

Toxicity and Dose Intensity

Dose intensity is defined as the total quantity of a drug administered over a specified time, and increasing dose intensity has been associated with significant improvement of cisplatin anticancer activity in humans (Ozols, 1989). Given the antitumor activity of cisplatin against selected neoplasms of veterinary importance, increasing the dose intensity may improve response rate or response duration or broaden the spectrum of antitumor activity. Whether cisplatin dose intensity can be increased in canine patients depends on whether ways can be found to increase the antitumor efficacy of cisplatin or reduce the toxicity of treatment.

Investigation of methods to reduce toxicity has focused on the principal dose-limiting toxicities. These include gastrointestinal upset (vomiting, diarrhea, anorexia), myelosuppression, and acute or chronic renal disease in dogs.

Although emesis following standard doses of cisplatin is generally acute and self-limiting, the likelihood of vomiting increases at high doses of cisplatin and in low-weight dogs (Ogilvie et al., 1989). Drugs with tranquilizing or antiemetic activity, such as butorphanol (0.2 mg/kg SC before cisplatin infusion and repeated 3 hr later) or chlorpromazine (2 mg/kg SC before cisplatin infusion and repeated 3 hr later), may ameliorate the severity of nausea and vomiting, as may extension of drug infusion time. Myelosuppression is rarely a problem at current doses. The ability to limit myelosuppression with use of stem cell growth factors may become important at higher doses (see this volume, p. 466).

Acute renal disease following cisplatin treatment may necessitate a dose reduction or a treatment delay, thereby reducing significantly the dose intensity. It has been demonstrated that in dogs, like other species, one factor associated with acute renal toxicity is circadian rhythm (Hardie et al., in press). Because of altered drug elimination, cisplatin administration during the middle of the day significantly reduced the acute renal effects of cisplatin compared with early morning administration. Optimal circadian timing of drug infusion to reduce acute toxicity may become even more important in dose-escalation investigations.

Chronic renal disease may develop after multiple courses of cisplatin therapy and is now the most important dose-limiting side effect in dogs. Careful monitoring of renal function before each cisplatin treatment is imperative. Development of renal insufficiency (polyuria/polydipsia without azotemia) usually precedes clinical signs of renal failure and can, in most instances, be managed conservatively for extended periods. Guidelines for dose adjustment based on creatinine clearance are unavailable for dogs, but pre-existing or acquired isosthenuria, proteinuria, or azotemia necessitates dose reduction or discontinuation of treatment. Regional cisplatin infusion, hypertonic (3 to 4%) saline infusion, and non-nephrotoxic analogues have been the most useful strategies for reducing cisplatin-induced nephrotoxicity in humans.

Infusion of cisplatin with hypertonic saline has resulted in almost doubling of the maximally tolerated dose in humans and has eliminated nephrotoxicity as the primary dose-limiting side effect (Ozols, 1989). The dramatic increase in dose intensity with this technique has established a clear dose-response relationship for cisplatin, including the response of "resistant" tumors refractory to lower doses of the drug. Similar studies in dogs are needed.

Regional Administration

One method of increasing the therapeutic index of cisplatin is local dose intensification. Intra-arterial infusion and intracavitary and intralesional administrations of cisplatin have recently been used in dogs with regionally confined neoplasms.

Intra-arterial cisplatin administration yields high local tumor and normal tissue drug concentrations while providing adequate systemic drug levels to control potential metastasis. This technique has been reported for management of primary limb osteosarcomas either before limb-sparing procedures (LaRue et al., 1989) or as primary therapy (Heidner et al., in press). Intra-arterial infusion of cisplatin has also been combined with radiotherapy in the management of two dogs with bladder tumors (McCaw and Lattimer, 1988).

Intracavitary administration of cisplatin has pharmacokinetic advantages relative to systemic therapy for tumors confined to a body cavity (Markman, 1989). Systemic absorption of intraperitoneally delivered cisplatin results in drug delivery to most tissues at levels similar to those attained with intravenous therapy. Intraperitoneal tissues, however, receive higher drug doses as a result of direct diffusion following intraperitoneal injection. Because direct diffusion of cisplatin at high concentra-

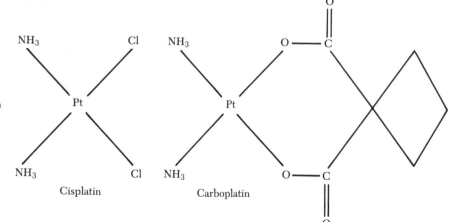

Figure 1. Structures of cisplatin and carboplatin.

tions is limited to the first 1 to 2 mm of exposed cell layers, intracavitary therapy is theoretically most advantageous for patients with microscopic disease or small tumor nodules less than 5 mm. In a limited clinical study, six dogs with malignant pleural or abdominal effusions were treated with 50 mg/m² cisplatin delivered in 0.9% saline following pretreatment intravenous saline diuresis (Moore et al., 1991). Four of the dogs, two with mesotheliomas and two with carcinomas, had long-term palliation of malignant effusions with such therapy.

Intralesional administration of cisplatin provides high, sustained intratumoral drug concentrations and is useful for treatment of nonresectable primary or residual local neoplasms. Collagen, sesame oil, and polylactic acid polymer have been used as matrices to permit sustained release of cisplatin. Preliminary studies in horses and dogs are encouraging (Theon et al., 1990; Withrow et al., 1990). Intralesional treatment combined with radiation therapy provides a convenient method for taking advantage of both direct antitumor activity and radiation-potentiating effects of cisplatin (Theon et al., 1990).

CARBOPLATIN

Carboplatin is a cisplatin analogue in which a 1-cyclobutane dicarboxylate chain is substituted for cisplatin's two chlorine atoms (Fig. 1). In extensive clinical trials in human patients, carboplatin shows decreased nephrotoxicity, neurotoxicity, and emetogenecity compared with cisplatin (Bunn, 1990). The dose-limiting toxicity of carboplatin is bone marrow suppression. Although carboplatin is currently licensed only for palliative therapy in women with refractory ovarian carcinoma, randomized trials comparing the two drugs demonstrate equivalent efficacy against ovarian, testicular, lung, and head and neck malignancies in humans.

Pharmacology

Carboplatin is available as a lyophilized powder with mannitol in 50-mg, 150-mg, and 450-mg vials. It is administered by slow, constant-rate intravenous infusion (15 to 60 min) and can be given without additional fluid diuresis. Unopened vials should be stored at room temperature and protected from light. Reconstituted solutions are stable for only 8 hr at room temperature.

The mechanism of action for carboplatin, like cisplatin, depends on the intracellular formation of highly reactive, positively charged intermediate compounds following aquation of the drug. These active complexes bind to DNA to form intra- and interstrand cross-links and DNA-protein cross-links. Because the aquation of carboplatin to the active intermediate occurs at a much slower rate than the aquation of cisplatin, marked differences occur in the pharmacokinetic disposition and pattern of toxicity of these two drugs. At isoeffective doses, however, both drugs produce equal drug-DNA cross-links and thus equal biologic effects (Schurig et al., 1990). Cross-resistance between the two drugs is common because of their identical cytotoxic intermediate (Ozols, 1989).

Clinical Experience

Phase I and pharmacokinetic studies of older, tumor-bearing dogs have been completed at North Carolina State University. The maximally tolerated dose of multiple courses of carboplatin administered as a 30-min infusion was 300 mg/m² (Fig. 2). Dogs that received 350 mg/m² or had been heavily pretreated with other anticancer drugs developed cumulative toxicity.

The dose-limiting toxicity of carboplatin in dogs was myelosuppression. Both neutropenia and thrombocytopenia occurred with a nadir of 14 days.

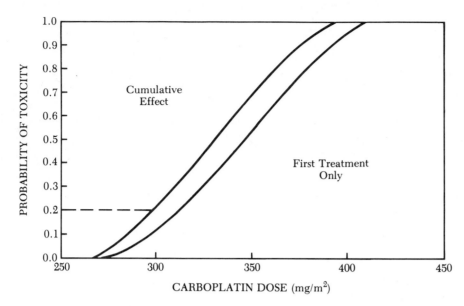

Figure 2. Logistic regression analysis of toxicity as a function of cisplatin dose following the first treatment only or the first and second treatments obtained in a phase I study at North Carolina State University. Toxicity was defined as neutrophil count <2000/μl, platelet count <80,000/μl. The dose associated with 20% probability of toxicity after two treatments is 300 mg/m² and thus represents a safe dose for future use in phase II/III clinical trials.

Anorexia and less frequently emesis occurred several days after treatment but were usually mild. Renal dysfunction, as evidenced by elevations in the blood urea nitrogen or creatinine concentrations, has not been observed. Because carboplatin is rapidly excreted in the urine, however, dose adjustments are necessary in animals with renal dysfunction in order to prevent increased nonrenal toxicities.

Data regarding tumor responses to carboplatin in dogs are limited. At North Carolina State University, 17 dogs with various tumors were treated in a Phase I study. No complete responses were observed. Three dogs had partial responses (one dog each with melanoma, squamous cell carcinoma, and osteosarcoma), and five had stabilization of disease with a median time to progression of 3.5 months. At the University of California at Davis, two of eight dogs with malignant melanoma that received at least two treatments of carboplatin at 300 to 350 mg/m² every 3 weeks had partial remission of 3 and 6 months duration. An additional six dogs with mammary or pulmonary neoplasia treated at least twice showed no measurable responses. Eight dogs received only one treatment as a result of rapid disease progression, including dogs with lymphoma, melanoma, carcinoma, and sarcoma. Hutson and colleagues (1990) reported results from 12 dogs treated with carboplatin at 350 mg/m² every 4 weeks. Two dogs with transitional cell carcinoma of the bladder or urethra had partial responses. Additional data on treatment of dogs with osteosarcoma, transitional cell carcinoma, and squamous cell carcinoma are needed before conclusions on carboplatin's efficacy compared with cisplatin can be reached.

CONCLUSION

Cisplatin chemotherapy is a valuable addition to the management of selected tumors in dogs. With careful management of toxicities and innovative methods of dose intensification, it may be possible to expand the effectiveness of this drug. The new platinum analogue carboplatin is less toxic and easier to administer than cisplatin. Myelosuppression is the dose-limiting toxicity, and gastrointestinal toxicity is mild. Because it is less nephrotoxic than cisplatin, carboplatin can be given to animals with pre-existing renal disease if doses are reduced. The therapeutic spectrum of carboplatin in dogs is not yet known, although substantial overlap with cisplatin is anticipated.

References and Suggested Reading

Bunn, P. A.: Carboplatin: Current status and future directions. *In* Bunn, P. A., Canetta, R., Ozols, R. F., et al. (eds.): *Carboplatin (JM-8).* Philadelphia: W. B. Saunders, 1990, p. 371.
   An overview of phase I, II, and III results for carboplatin therapy in humans.
Hardie, E. M., Page, R. L., Williams, P. L., et al.: The effect of time of administration on cisplatin toxicity and pharmacokinetics in the dog. Am. J. Vet. Res. (in press).
   Evaluation of AM versus PM cisplatin administration in normal dogs.
Heidner, G. L., Page, R. L., McEntee, M. C., et al.: Treatment of canine appendicular osteosarcoma using cobalt-60 radiotherapy and intra-arterial cisplatin. J. Vet. Intern. Med. (in press).
   A prospective study of 12 dogs with osteosarcoma.
Hutson, C. A., Degen, L. A., and Rackear, D. G.: Preliminary results of carboplatin toxicity and efficacy in 12 canines and 4 felines. Proceedings of the Veterinary Cancer Society 10th Annual Conference, Auburn, AL, 1990, p. 87.
   Phase II clinical trial of carboplatin.
Kraegel, S. A., Madewell, B. R., Simonson, E., et al.: Canine osteogenic sarcoma and cisplatin chemotherapy: A case-report study. J.A.V.M.A. (in press).

Data on 16 dogs that received adjuvant cisplatin following amputation, as well as a brief literature review.

LaRue, S. M., Withrow, S. J., Powers, B. E., et al.: Limb-sparing treatment for osteosarcoma in dogs. J.A.V.M.A. 195:1734, 1989.
Clinical study of multimodality limb-sparing treatment in dogs with osteosarcoma.

Markman, M.: Intraperitoneal cisplatin chemotherapy in the management of ovarian carcinoma. Semin. Oncol. 16:79, 1989.
Reviews the initial results of intraperitoneal cisplatin administration in women.

McCaw, D. L., and Lattimer, J. C.: Radiation and cisplatin for treatment of canine urinary bladder carcinoma. Vet. Radiol. 29:264, 1988.
Two case reports on dogs treated with intra-arterial cisplatin combined with radiation.

Moore, A. S., Cardona, A., Shapiro, W., et al.: Cisplatin (cisdiamminedichloroplatinum) for treatment of transitional cell carcinoma of the urinary bladder or urethra. J. Vet. Intern. Med. 4:148, 1990.
A retrospective study of 15 dogs.

Moore, A. S., Kirk, C., and Cardona, A.: Intracavitary cisplatin chemotherapy experience with six dogs. J. Vet. Intern. Med. 5:227, 1991.
Clinical results on intracavitary cisplatin in tumor-bearing dogs.

Ogilvie, G. K., Moore, A. S., and Curtis, C. R.: Evaluation of cisplatin-induced emesis in dogs with malignant neoplasia: 115 cases (1984–1987). J.A.V.M.A. 195:1399, 1989.
A retrospective study of cisplatin-induced emesis.

Ozols, R. F.: Cisplatin dose intensity. Semin. Oncol. 16:22, 1989.
A review of high-dose cisplatin therapy in human clinical trials.

Schurig, J. E., Rose, W. C., Catino, J. J., et al.: The pharmacologic characteristics of carboplatin: Preclinical experience. *In* Bunn, P. A., Canetta, R., Ozols, R. F., et al. (eds.): *Carboplatin (JM-8).* Philadelphia: W.B. Saunders, 1990, p. 3.
Overview of results from preclinical evaluations of carboplatin.

Theon, A. P., Madewell, B. R., Kraegel, S., et al.: Irradiation and intratumoral cisplatin chemotherapy: A pilot study in spontaneous canine tumors. Proceedings of the Veterinary Cancer Society 10th Annual Conference, Auburn, AL, 1990, p. 77.
Results of a clinical trial evaluating the combination of intralesional cisplatin and radiation therapy in 12 dogs.

Theon, A. P., Pascoe, J. R., and Krag, D. N.: Intraoperative cisplatin chemotherapy for the treatment of equine malignancies. Proceedings of the Veterinary Cancer Society 10th Annual Conference, Auburn, AL, 1990, p. 14.
Clinical trial of intralesional cisplatin suspended in sesame oil.

Withrow, S. J., Straw, R. C., Cooper, M., et al.: Local slow release cisplatin therapy after marginal local tumor resection. Proceedings of the Veterinary Cancer Society 10th Annual Conference, Auburn, AL, 1990, insert.
Evaluation of a biodegradable compound containing cisplatin in wounds of normal and osteosarcoma-bearing dogs following surgery.

MITOXANTRONE CHEMOTHERAPY

GREGORY K. OGILVIE

Fort Collins, Colorado

and ANTONY S. MOORE

North Grafton, Massachusetts

Mitoxantrone is a new dihydroxyquinone derivative of anthracene that is related to doxorubicin and daunorubicin (Yap et al., 1981). The drug, which is brilliant blue in color, is available in many countries and is contained in a multidose vial with a long shelf life. Compared with many chemotherapeutic agents, mitoxantrone is relatively nontoxic in tumor-bearing humans, dogs, and cats. An important advantage of mitoxantrone over doxorubicin is a lower likelihood of cardiotoxicity. The only consistent limiting toxic effect of mitoxantrone in humans and cats is myelosuppression in the form of neutropenia, which is generally of short duration and readily reversible. Gastrointestinal toxicity also may be a limiting factor in the cat. This drug has antitumor activity similar to that of doxorubicin for the treatment of a variety of cancers.

Supported in part by US Public Health Service grant PO-1-CA-29582 awarded by the National Cancer Institute, DHHS.

EFFICACY IN THE DOG

In a study involving 129 dogs with histologically confirmed, measurable malignant tumors the response to mitoxantrone was determined (Ogilvie et al., 1991b). Ninety-five dogs had been refractory to one or more previous treatment modalities (surgery, n = 57; chemotherapy other than mitoxantrone, n = 37; radiation, n = 4; whole-body hyperthermia, n = 1). The overall response rate (complete and partial remission) of carcinomas and sarcomas to mitoxantrone therapy was similar to that in a previous report that evaluated the efficacy of doxorubicin (Ogilvie et al., 1989). A partial or complete remission (>50% volume reduction) was obtained in 23% (29/126) of all dogs treated, 20.4% (10/49) of the carcinomas, 34.4% (11/32) of the lymphomas, and 17.7% (8/45) of the sarcomas. Tumors in which there was a partial or complete remission included lymphoma (11/32), squamous cell carcinoma (4/9),

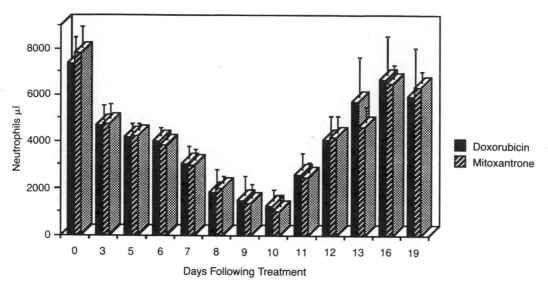

Figure 1. Mean neutrophil counts (± standard deviation) from clinically normal dogs that received mitoxantrone (5 mg/m² IV, n = 7) and doxorubicin (30 mg/m² IV, n = 7). Note that the nadir of both drugs is on day 10 and that mitoxantrone appears to be slightly more myelosuppressive than doxorubicin.

fibrosarcoma (2/9), thyroid carcinoma (1/10), transitional cell carcinoma (1/6), mammary adenocarcinoma (1/6), hepatocellular carcinoma (1/4), renal adenocarcinoma (1/1), chondrosarcoma (1/2), oral malignant melanoma (1/12), cutaneous malignant melanoma (1/1), myxosarcoma (1/1), mesothelioma (1/1), and hemangiopericytoma (1/1). In this study, several dosages and different numbers of treatments per dog were used. In general, the response to chemotherapeutics is directly related to the concentration of the drug multiplied by the time of exposure. The higher response rates to mitoxantrone given at 5 mg/m² IV over 4.5 and <4.5 mg/m² suggest that the responses to therapy may have been higher if all the dogs received 5 mg/m².

Dogs with lymphoma treated with mitoxantrone do not respond as well as to some other drugs. Several reports document a >75% complete remission rate in dogs with lymphoma treated with doxorubicin; however, none of the dogs in these studies had received chemotherapy before the administration of doxorubicin. In one study, mitoxantrone was used as a single agent to treat dogs with lymphoma (Moore et al., 1991). The overall response rate (complete and partial remission) was 43% (complete response, 30%). Forty-four dogs had not received previous chemotherapy, and 13 of these dogs had a complete response for a median of 93 days (range, 49 to 440 days). Forty-four other dogs received mitoxantrone after failing to respond to other chemotherapeutic agents. Thirteen of these dogs had a complete response for a median of 127 days (range, 42 to 792 days). Failure to respond to doxorubicin did not affect response to mitoxantrone, with 9 of 33 dogs achieving complete remission for a median

of 140 days (range, 42 to 792 days). Further studies are needed to determine the therapeutic potential of mitoxantrone for the treatment of lymphoma in the dog.

TOXICOSES IN THE DOG

A study was performed to determine the toxicity of mitoxantrone in 129 older dogs with histologically confirmed, measurable malignant tumors (Ogilvie et al., 1991c). One to ten doses of the drug were administered at 21-day intervals at dosages ranging from 2.5 to 5 mg/m² body surface area IV. In this study, no dogs died of complications resulting from mitoxantrone therapy. Mild depression (18/129 dogs; 34.7% of all toxicoses) and gastrointestinal signs (16/129 dogs; 32.6% of all toxicoses) were the most common adverse effects associated with mitoxantrone therapy. Gastrointestinal side effects were less frequent and less severe than reported with doxorubicin therapy (Ogilvie et al., 1989). As with doxorubicin, vomiting, diarrhea, and clinical signs compatible with colitis may result in part from the cytotoxic effect of the drug on the rapidly dividing cells of the gastrointestinal tract. Dogs did not develop pruritus or anaphylaxis during the administration of the drug, and colitis was infrequently observed; these problems are commonly seen in dogs treated with doxorubicin and are thought to be induced by the release of histamine. The adverse effects associated with the administration of mitoxantrone at a dosage of 5 mg/m² IV were considered significant enough to preclude higher doses. It can be argued, however, that higher doses might be safe and clinically useful in some patients. The drug rarely produced adverse effects on the animals' quality of life.

The dose-limiting toxicoses associated with the administration of mitoxantrone are myelosuppression and thrombocytopenia in humans and also myelosuppression in dogs. The leukopenia in either species generally is neither severe nor life-threatening. To determine the lowest neutrophil count (nadir) resulting from mitoxantrone therapy, mitoxantrone was administered to four normal dogs at a dosage of 5 mg/m² body surface area IV; neutrophil counts were then compared with those of the dogs with cancer. The nadir of neutrophil counts of the normal dogs was seen on day 10 (mean ± SEM: 1159/µl ± 252.86). This is lower than with doxorubicin (Fig. 1). Tumor-bearing dogs did not seem to exhibit the same degree of myelosuppression (mean ± SEM: 6262.8/µl ± 1230.4). Between 2 and 14% of human patients have white blood cell counts of <1000/mm³. This is similar to the observations reported in dogs. Twelve dogs in one study developed clinical signs of sepsis associated with mitoxantrone-induced neutropenia, although none exhibited problems related to thrombocytopenia (Ogilvie et al., 1991c). The neutrophil counts appeared to decrease earlier and to a lesser degree in tumor-bearing dogs than in normal dogs; this may be due to altered pharmacokinetics of mitoxantrone, to a change in the sensitivity of the bone marrow in the older dog with cancer, or to misleading results obtained from the small number of normal dogs. Canine recombinant granulocyte colony–stimulating factor has been shown to reduce the duration and severity of mitoxantrone-induced myelosuppression in the dog (see this volume, p. 399).

One significant advantage that mitoxantrone has over doxorubicin is that the former does not readily produce cardiotoxicity in dogs and monkeys (Henderson et al., 1982). Twenty-four dogs had six to ten treatments of mitoxantrone (5 mg/m² q 21 days IV) without developing clinical evidence of cardiac disease (Ogilvie et al., 1991c). Indeed, none of the 129 dogs reported by our group showed clinical signs of cardiotoxicity. However, the authors recommend close cardiac monitoring until the true potential for cardiotoxicity in dogs is known.

Various risk factors were evaluated to predict toxicosis. As expected, the single most important risk factor examined was the dosage of mitoxantrone. The odds of developing toxicoses increased 5.9-fold for each milligram of mitoxantrone administered. Another clinically important observation was that dogs that develop toxicosis initially are significantly more likely to develop complications to subsequent treatment with mitoxantrone.

FELINE STUDIES

A study has been completed to determine the toxicoses associated with administration of mitoxantrone to 87 cats with histologically confirmed malignant tumors (Ogilvie et al., 1991a). The drug was administered intravenously over 2 minutes at 21-day intervals at dosages ranging from 2.5 to 6.5 mg/m² body surface area. Each cat was evaluated for signs of toxicosis for 3 weeks after each dose was administered or until it developed progressive disease, or until the animal's quality of life diminished to an unacceptable level as determined by the owner or attending veterinarian. Forty-seven cats had been refractory to one or more previous forms of treatment modalities (surgery, n = 35; chemotherapy other than mitoxantrone, n = 12; radiation, n = 2). The most common signs of toxicosis were vomiting, anorexia, diarrhea, depression, sepsis secondary to myelosuppression, and seizures. Two cats died of complications that were attributed to mitoxantrone therapy. No cardiac toxicity was noted. Tumor-bearing cats exhibited some degree of myelosuppression when given mitoxantrone at 6.5 mg/m² (median neutrophil count: 2640; range, 1595 to 6300 cells/µl).

Although the primary purpose of this study reported previously (Ogilvie et al., 1991a) was to determine a clinically useful dosage and to characterize the toxicoses associated with mitoxantrone administration, each cat was monitored for response to therapy (Ogilvie et al., 1991a). Eleven cats with squamous cell carcinoma were treated concurrently with radiation therapy. A partial or complete remission (>50% volume reduction) was obtained in 26.4% (23/87) of all cats treated and in 18.4% (14/76) of cats that received only mitoxantrone. A remission was recorded in 29% (18/62) of the carcinomas, 11.8% (2/17) of the lymphomas, and 37.5% (3/8) of the sarcomas. Tumors in which there was a partial or complete remission include lymphoma (2/17), squamous cell carcinoma (4/32 without concurrent radiation, 9/12 with concurrent radiation), fibrosarcoma (1/6), transitional cell carcinoma (1/1), mammary adenocarcinoma (2/8), nasal carcinoma (1/1), rhabdomyosarcoma (1/1), mast cell tumor (1/1), and apocrine gland adenocarcinoma (1/1). Overall, the response rate was limited. Additional studies are needed to determine the usefulness of mitoxantrone for the treatment of tumors in the cat.

References and Suggested Reading

Henderson, B. M., Dougherty, W. J., James, V. C., et al.: Safety assessment of a new anticancer compound, mitoxantrone, in beagle dogs. Comparison with doxorubicin: clinical observations. Cancer Treat Report 66:1139, 1982.
This study compares the toxicity associated with administration of mitoxantrone and doxorubicin in normal experimental dogs.
Moore A. S., Ogilvie G. K., Ruslander D., et al.: Mitoxantrone for the therapy of canine lymphoma. Proc. 11th Annual Conference, Veterinary Cancer Society, 1991.
This report reviews the response to therapy of a large group of dogs with lymphoma treated with mitoxantrone chemotherapy.
Ogilvie, G. K., Moore, A. S., Obradovich, J. E., et al.: Safety and efficacy

associated with the administration of mitoxantrone to cats with malignant tumors. J.A.V.M.A. Submitted 1991a.
*This prospective study reviews the toxicity and efficacy of mitoxantrone
when used to treat cats with a variety of malignant tumors.*
Ogilvie, G. K., Obradovich, J. E., Elmslie, R. E., et al.: Efficacy of
mitoxantrone against various canine neoplasms. J.A.V.M.A. 198:1618,
1991.
*This prospective study reviews the antitumor activity of mitoxantrone
when used to treat a wide variety of malignant tumors in dogs.*
Ogilvie, G. K., Obradovich, J. E., Elmslie, R. E., et al.: Toxicoses
associated with the administration of mitoxantrone to dogs with malignant tumors. J.A.V.M.A. 198:1613, 1991.
This prospective study documents the clinically significant toxicoses

*associated with the administration of mitoxantrone to dogs with malig-
nant tumors.*
Ogilvie, G. K., Richardson, R. C., Curtis, C. R., et al.: Acute and short-
term toxicoses associated with the administration of doxorubicin to dogs
with malignant tumors. J.A.V.M.A. 195:1580, 1989.
*This prospective study documents the clinically significant toxicoses
associated with the administration of doxorubicin to older, tumor-
bearing dogs.*
Yap, H. Y., Blumenschien, G. R., Schell, F. C., et al.: Dihydroxyanthra-
cenedione: a promising new agent in the treatment of advanced breast
cancer. Ann. Intern. Med. 95:694, 1981.
*This article reviews the biochemical, pharmacologic, and clinical aspects
of mitoxantrone.*

CHEMOTHERAPY: PHARMACOLOGIC AND TOXICOLOGIC CONSIDERATIONS

RODNEY L. PAGE

Raleigh, North Carolina

Despite success in the treatment of lymphopro-liferative tumors in companion animals, the use of chemotherapy has not consistently demonstrated efficacy in the treatment of other tumor types. However, renewed enthusiasm for the role of chemotherapy in the management of neoplasia in animals has been generated from data suggesting improved survival in osteosarcoma and hemangio-sarcoma (Hammer and Couto, 1990; Straw et al., 1990). In addition, identification of factors predictive of poor response or toxicity in chemosensitive neoplasia has helped to define more carefully the indications for drug therapy that ultimately improves results (Matus, 1989). Such progress provides the impetus to further refine the use of chemotherapy in the hope of improved means of tumor control.

If improved control is to be expected, the reasons for treatment failure must be understood. The biologic basis of cytotoxic therapy is the dose-response relationship illustrated in Figure 1, which exists for both tumor and normal tissue. Many factors may affect the clinical manifestation of these relationships. Normal tissue toxicity is governed by patient-related factors such as concurrent disease or poor nutritional status and pharmacologic factors that affect cellular drug delivery. Tumor tissue response is influenced by these same factors in addition to specific tumor-related factors such as inherent che-

mosensitivity, drug resistance, cell kinetic factors, and tumor blood flow.

PHARMACOLOGIC CONSIDERATIONS

Designing dosage regimens to achieve the therapeutic objective of tumor control is the goal of clinical pharmacology. Investigation of appropriate drug prescription and administration, measurement of drug concentrations in various biologic compartments or tissues, and modeling of drug disposition to various tissues may suggest alterations in drug delivery that will ultimately improve the dose-response relationship.

Dose Prescription Base

Unlike most drugs, which act to alter cellular or tissue function, the primary effect of conventional cytotoxic chemotherapeutic agents is cell death. Therefore, some degree of normal tissue toxicity is expected. In view of such a narrow therapeutic index, it is essential that dose prescription be precise.

Unfortunately, no ideal dose prescription base currently exists. Body surface area (BSA) correlates with metabolic rate and may therefore predict tox-

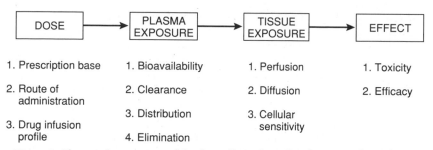

Figure 1. Pharmacologic aspects of the dose-effect relationship for cancer chemotherapy.

icity more accurately than body weight if a drug's action or biotransformation is a function of some metabolic process. A disproportionately greater dose is given to small dogs if dosage is based on BSA, on the assumption that the metabolic rate is increased and thus drug biotransformation and elimination are also increased. However, evidence suggests that, for certain drugs, BSA fails as a uniform prescription base and can result in a relative overdose in small dogs (Ogilvie et al., 1989; Page et al., 1988). In one study, body weight was shown to be a more useful determinant of potential for bone marrow toxicity than BSA for dogs (Page et al., 1988).

The use of BSA as a prescription base for dogs creates several problems. First, the calculation of BSA from body weight suggests that, regardless of conformation, all dogs weighing the same will have the same BSA; thus, a 10-kg dachshund would have the same surface area as a 10-kg whippet. Second, the mathematical derivation of BSA is based on outdated and insufficient data. Third, the metabolic rate may not relate to certain normal tissue end points (e.g., bone marrow function).

Several solutions can be considered. Re-examination of BSA calculation in the dog to include a wide conformational and weight range may reveal a more accurate means of determining BSA. However, a method to directly calculate the surface area of dogs would be preferable. Consideration of each drug's disposition and biotransformation as well as the primary normal tissue target may suggest that its administration should be based on a more appropriate parameter than BSA (e.g., body weight). However, until a better estimate of dose prescription is developed, BSA appears to be a useful criterion for calculating dosage of most chemotherapeutic agents.

Therapeutic Drug Monitoring

It is obvious from Figure 1 that plasma or tissue drug concentrations better reflect the chemotherapeutic end points and thus are associated with fewer potential variables that may confound the dose-response relationship. In many studies, the effect is better correlated with drug concentration in plasma than with the administered dose. Therapeutic drug monitoring involves drug concentration measurements in plasma or other biologic fluids that may help modify the dose-response relationship. Therapeutic drug monitoring is indicated (1) when a dose-effect relationship is not readily measurable, (2) to determine potential causes of therapeutic failure (e.g., interpatient pharmacokinetic variability), and (3) in the presence of hepatic, renal, or other disorders. A thorough understanding of drug pharmacokinetics and the ability to measure drug concentrations are prerequisites to therapeutic drug monitoring.

Such monitoring is only beginning to be used in veterinary oncology to ensure ideal plasma drug concentrations. Plasma drug disposition has been characterized in tumor-bearing dogs for several routine chemotherapeutic agents. It is now possible to study various administration schedules, such as prolonging of infusion periods or circadian timing, that may improve the plasma and tissue drug exposure. Therapeutic drug monitoring may be beyond the scope of individual treatment, but refinement of these clinical pharmacologic end points that correlate to outcome may significantly affect the future of veterinary oncology.

TOXICOLOGIC CONSIDERATIONS

Maximum Tolerated Dose

As previously mentioned, cytotoxic chemotherapy generally exhibits a dose-response relationship with a narrow therapeutic index. Therefore, the highest *tolerable* dose must be administered, since either under- or overdosage may have life-threatening consequences. The maximum tolerated dose (MTD) in older, tumor-bearing dogs or cats can be defined as a dose that can be administered multiple times without dose reduction or treatment delay. However, the MTD is not simply the dose that causes mild or moderate toxic effects; MTD encompasses a broader range of parameters defined by

Table 1. *General Grading of Toxicity Resulting from Chemotherapy in Companion Animals*

Grade	
0	No toxicity
1	Mild toxicity, usually transient, requiring no special treatment and generally not interfering with daily activities
2	Moderate toxicity that may be ameliorated by simple therapeutic maneuvers; usually impairs activities
3	Severe toxicity that requires therapeutic intervention and impairs usual activities; hospitalization may be necessary
4	Life-threatening toxicity requiring hospitalization

the investigator's experience, protocol requirements, and the type of supportive care available. Thus, for any given drug, the MTD may vary. Determination of the MTD is an objective of any phase I study, and such studies should be carefully regulated so that subsequent adjustments can be accurately estimated.

The fundamental considerations of the phase I study are similar in companion animals and in humans, and include the starting dose and dose escalation scheme, a definition of "tolerable" toxicity so that MTD can be defined, and a statistical analysis of data. The concept that tolerable toxicity exists and can be carefully defined is an essential assumption of chemotherapy. Without this understanding, it is impossible to ensure that a drug will have any biologic effects. The MTD concept has evolved in human oncology to consider not only metabolic and hematologic toxicity but also quality-of-life issues. Similar considerations apply to a true MTD for companion animals. Table 1 describes five general levels of toxicity that can be used as guidelines to develop specific criteria for each form of normal tissue toxicity and extrapolated to loosely define quality-of-life issues.

Table 2 suggests criteria for reporting adverse effects of chemotherapy on several body systems. These variables have been developed from phase I studies at the author's hospital but do not represent a consensus of all veterinary oncologists. Similar categories can be established for any system and modified as necessary. The degree of toxicity that is deemed "tolerable" varies with each organ system and clinical situation. Regardless of individual variations, however, a clear description of acceptable and unacceptable toxicity should be established before initiating a phase I study. For example, the MTD of a drug with primary myelosuppressive activity may be defined as that dose associated with moderate toxicity at its peak effect (i.e., <2000 neutrophils/μl or <80,000 platelets/μl in 50% of the patients entered at that dose. A different MTD for the same drug could be defined as the dose associated with severe toxicity in 10% of the patients entered at any one dose. Defining the MTD in several ways using the same organ system may permit a more precise estimate of the therapeutic index for that drug. Criteria for treatment modification or discontinuation must also be established.

Dose Intensity

Dose intensity is defined as the amount of drug administered in a given time (Hryniuk and Levine, 1986). It implies that (1) agents are being used that are active as single agents, (2) the MTD of the drug is administered, and (3) the schedule of drug administration (e.g., frequency, length of infusion, circadian timing) is optimal. Convincing evidence of a dose-response effect in human oncology has accumulated over the past 5 to 10 years. Noteworthy examples include the improvement in response rates after high-dose cisplatin administration in patients with non–small cell lung cancer, ovarian carcinoma, and testicular tumors (Gandara et al., 1989; Ozols, 1989). Pharmacologic techniques have permitted a two-fold escalation in cisplatin dosage and elimination of nephrotoxicity as the limiting side effect. Modification in drug scheduling has

Table 2. *Recommendations for Grading Toxic Effects of Cancer Chemotherapy in Dogs*

System	Normal Range (Grade 0)	Mild Toxicity (Grade 1)	Moderate Toxicity (Grade 2)	Severe Toxicity (Grade 3)	Life-threatening Toxicity (Grade 4)
Hematologic					
Granulocytes (cells/mm^3 × 10^3)	4–10	2–4	1–2*	0.5–1.0	<0.5
Platelets (cell/mm^3 × 10^3)	150–500	80–150	40–80*	10–40	<10
Renal					
Creatinine (mg/dl)	0.1–1.8	1.8–2.5	2.5–3.0*	3.0–4.0	>4.0
Cardiac					
Left ventricular shortening fraction (% ΔD)	28–50	25–28†	23–25*	20–23	<20
Ventricular arrhythmias	None	Occasional	<10/min* unifocal	10–20/min unifocal	>20/min or multifocal

*Assessment of additional clinical data may indicate a more serious grade of toxicity (i.e., hospitalization necessary.)
†*Editor's Note:* Some clinically normal dogs fall within this range of LVSF.

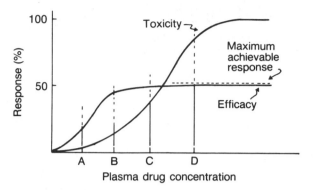

Figure 2. A theoretical concentration-response curve for an antineoplastic agent. The sensitivity of the tumor determines the slope of the curve and the maximum achievable response. Drug concentrations below point A are not associated with significant biologic effect. Increasing the concentration to point B results in maximum tolerated dose as well as maximum achievable response. A further increase in drug concentration will only increase toxicity. (Reprinted with permission from Moore, M. J., and Erlichman, C: Therapeutic drug monitoring in oncology: Problems and potential in antineoplastic therapy. Clin. Pharmacokinet. 13:205, 1987.)

reduced the frequency of severe myelosuppression and neurotoxicity at these high doses.

The greatest potential for improvement in dose intensity in veterinary oncology will initially stem from defining and maximizing the MTD. Additional improvement will likely result from altered infusion schedules. Novel strategies to safely increase doses of chemotherapeutic agents are being vigorously investigated in both human and veterinary oncology (see this volume, p. 466).

CONCLUSION

Figure 2 summarizes the problems associated with optimizimg cancer chemotherapy. Theoretical dose-response curves are shown for both toxicity and efficacy. The maximum tumor response is limited by factors such as inherent chemosensitivity, cell kinetic factors, drug resistance, and tumor blood flow. Toxicity is a function of normal tissue sensitivity and patient tolerance. Drug doses below point

A are associated with minimal biologic effect on either normal or tumor tissue and therefore should not be administered. Increasing the dose from A to B results in moderate increases in toxicity but a greater increase in response (i.e., the MTD). Further increases in dose would not improve response but would increase toxicity. Once the MTD and optimal schedule can be identified so that it is certain that chemotherapy is being administered with the greatest therapeutic potential, more complicated questions, such as how to reduce normal tissue toxicity or increase the maximum achievable tumor response, can be systematically addressed.

References and Suggested Reading

Gandara, D. R., Wold, H., Perez, E. A., et al.: Cisplatin dose intensity in non–small cell lung cancer: Phase II results of a day 1 and day 8 high-dose regimen. J. Natl. Cancer Inst. 81:790, 1989.
Prospective phase II evaluation of 92 human patients treated with a modified cisplatin schedule that supports the potential importance of cisplatin dose intensity.
Hammer, A. S., and Couto, C. G.: Adjuvant chemotherapy for sarcomas and carcinomas. Vet. Clin. North Am. 20:1015, 1990.
A review of the principles of adjuvant therapy and a summary of relevant clinical studies pertaining to adjuvant chemotherapy.
Hryniuk, W., and Levine, M. N.: Analysis of dose intensity for adjuvant chemotherapy trials in stage II breast cancer. J. Clin. Oncol. 4:1162, 1986.
A retrospective survey and re-analysis of chemotherapeutic trials for human breast cancer according to dose intensity.
Matus, R. E.: Chemotherapy of lymphoma and leukemia. In Kirk, R. W. (ed.): Current Veterinary Therapy X. Philadelphia: W. B. Saunders, 1989, p. 482.
A review of diagnosis, treatment, and prognosis of canine and feline lymphoproliferative disorders.
Ogilvie, G. K., Richardson, R. C., Curtis, C. R., et al.: Acute and short-term toxicosis associated with the administration of doxorubicin to dogs with malignant tumors. J.A.V.M.A. 195:1584, 1989.
An analysis of the incidence of and risk factors for toxicosis after doxorubicin therapy.
Ozols, R. F.: Cisplatin dose intensity. Semin. Oncol. 16:22, 1989.
A review of the pharmacologic rationale of high-dose cisplatin and a summary of clinical trials in humans using this technique.
Page, R. L., Macy, D. W., Thrall, D. E., et al.: Unexpected toxicity associated with use of body surface area for dosing melphalan in the dog. Cancer Res. 48:288, 1988.
A comparison of myelosuppression after chemotherapy dosed on a body surface area basis compared with body weight basis.
Straw, R. C., Withrow, S. J., Richter, S. J., et al.: Amputation and cisplatin for treatment of canine osteosarcoma. J. Vet. Intern. Med 5:205, 1991.
A prospective analysis of adjuvant cisplatin after amputation in dogs with appendicular osteosarcoma.

DRUG RESISTANCE IN
CANCER CHEMOTHERAPY

JANE STEWART
and NEIL T. GORMAN
Glasgow, Scotland

Chemotherapy has become a major form of treatment for systemic malignant disease. At the clinical level, resistance to chemotherapeutic drugs can be intrinsic or acquired. Tumor types that rarely respond to chemotherapy are said to be intrinsically resistant, whereas tumors, such as canine lymphosarcoma, that are initially chemosensitive but eventually become refractory to treatment are described as having acquired resistance.

Failure to respond to treatment can be due to cellular resistance or to an inability to deliver a therapeutic dose of the cytotoxic agent to all tumor cells. The latter is termed pharmacologic resistance and will not be discussed in this article. However, it is important to remember that drug distribution may play a decisive role in the clinical outcome. The poor penetration of drugs into the central nervous system (CNS) and testes is well recognized, but even relatively small, solid tumors can have diffusional variations in drug concentration within the mass, which may result in some cells receiving a subcytotoxic dose of drug. These variations could have profound effects on the success of treatment and on the emergence of drug-resistant tumor cells. Neither cellular nor pharmacologic resistance is an all-or-nothing phenomenon. Increasing the amount of drug delivered to a tumor may overcome both cellular resistance mechanisms and intratumor diffusion problems. In patients, dose escalation is seldom possible because of unacceptable host toxicity, and at this stage, treatment failure is inevitable.

CELLULAR RESISTANCE

Cells have a myriad of protection mechanisms against the noxious chemicals (including drugs) that are ubiquitous in the environment. These mechanisms are found in bacteria, plants, parasites, and normal mammalian cells. Therefore drug resistance is a common phenomenon that can result from the improved efficiency of normal protective mechanisms. Unfortunately, the protective mechanisms in *normal* cells that form the basis for the selective cytotoxicity of antitumor drugs are largely unknown.

It is possible to predict that chemotherapeutic drug resistance will involve changes in key aspects of cellular pharmacology, such as permeability, detoxification pathways, and the ability to remove drug-induced lesions in DNA.

Drug resistance appears to arise as a consequence of natural selection. Drug-resistant cells arise spontaneously in a cell population at a rate dependent on the mutation rate within the population. Tumor cells are generally considered to be genetically unstable, and many chemotherapeutic drugs are inherently mutagenic; therefore, the mutation rate may be high within a tumor chronically exposed to antineoplastic drugs. The drugs then act as a selecting agent to allow the preferential survival of drug-resistant subpopulations within the tumor mass. With repeated exposure to the selecting agent, a resistant subpopulation can become the predominant cell within the tumor. Attempts have been made to mathematically model the emergence of drug-resistant cells in tumors. These models predict that as a tumor grows, the likelihood of a drug-resistant clone arising spontaneously is increased. Therefore, to maximize the chances of producing a cure, chemotherapy should be instituted early in the disease. Goldie and Coldman (1984) and Rosenthal (1986) discuss the effects of tumor growth and kinetics on drug sensitivity, and they emphasize that, clinically, early-stage disease is biologically "old" in terms of the number of cell divisions undergone by the time the tumor is detected. This reinforces the importance of starting chemotherapy as quickly as possible after tumor detection.

In tumor cells selected *in vitro*, resistance to a particular drug can be achieved by several distinct mechanisms. Different tumor types that are resistant to the same drug may not employ the same mechanism. Some mechanisms (discussed later) can alter the efficacy of more than one class of drug, and when these mechanisms act simultaneously, the resultant spectrum of drug sensitivity can be extremely complex.

Multidrug Resistance; P-Glycoprotein

P-glycoprotein (P-gp) is a normal cell-surface molecule present in a variety of tissues, including liver,

Table 1. *Antineoplastic Drugs That Are P-gp Substrates and Topoisomerase Poisons*

MDR Drugs	Example	Topoisomerase Poison
Anthracyclines	Adriamycin Daunorubicin Epirubicin	Anthracyclines
Podophyllotoxins	Etoposide (VP-16) Tenoposide (VM-26)	Podophyllotoxin derivatives
Vinca alkaloids	Vinblastine Vincristine	Miscellaneous
Miscellaneous	Actinomycin D Puromycin	Mitoxantrone Actinomycin D

kidney, adrenals, and the gastrointestinal tract of all the species studied so far, including the dog. P-Glycoprotein acts as an energy-dependent export pump for a large range of lipophilic substances, including adriamycin and vincristine, and may represent a cellular waste-disposal system for harmful xenobiotics. Depending on the species, more than one type of P-gp exists.

Tumor cells that overexpress P-gp can maintain a low intracellular concentration of the drugs listed in Table 1 and hence evade the cytotoxic activity of an important range of natural product–based drugs. The *in vitro* pattern of cross-resistance associated with P-gp is called *multi-drug resistance*, or MDR (formerly pleiotropic resistance), but it is important to note that *the cross-resistance does not usually extend to alkylating agents or antimetabolites.*

There is mounting evidence that P-gp may affect tumor sensitivity at the clinical level. Tumors that arise from tissues that would normally express P-gp (e.g., liver and kidney) are invariably intrinsically resistant to MDR drugs. P-Glycoprotein expression has been seen to increase during chemotherapy in a variety of human malignancies. The presence of P-gp in hemopoietic malignancies can correlate with *in vivo* resistance to MDR drugs and is associated with poor clinical performance in some solid tumors.

Some, but not all, MDR drugs can interfere with the function of topoisomerase II. Topoisomerases twist and untwist the DNA helix by making nicks in the DNA strands, which are then immediately religated; this activity is vital for many aspects of DNA function. The formation of drug-enzyme-DNA complexes stabilizes the topoisomerase in its active cleaving form on the DNA strand and can generate lethal DNA double-strand breaks. Unlike most other chemotherapy targets, topoisomerases actually contribute to the cytotoxic effect; therefore, resistance could arise through lowering the topoisomerase concentration or altering its activity. Indeed, adriamycin- and VP-16-resistant cell lines have been isolated with altered topoisomerase II activity. P-Glycoprotein overexpression or alterations in topoisomerase activity can produce similar, but not quite identical, resistance patterns.

Antimetabolites

The antimetabolites inhibit critical biochemical pathways usually involving DNA and RNA synthesis. Methotrexate (MTX), cytosine arabinoside (Ara-C), and the purine analogues (6-mercaptopurine and 6-thioguanine) appear to enter cells by active transport. However, these transport mechanisms are relatively specific such that alterations in MTX transport do not affect the entry of purine analogues or Ara-C into the tumor cell.

Methotrexate resistance has been widely studied and illustrates that multiple mechanisms can interact to produce a drug-resistant phenotype. MTX is a competitive inhibitor of the enzyme dihydrofolate reductase (DHFR), which is important in folate metabolism. In addition to reduced transport into the cell, MTX resistance can be acquired by increasing the DHFR concentration and through variant forms of the enzyme which have reduced affinity for MTX. Multiple copies of the gene encoding DHFR have been found in resistant cells selected *in vitro* and *in vivo*. This gene amplification allows gross overproduction of the DHFR enzyme. Glutamination of MTX within the cell reduces efflux of the drug across the cell membrane. Some resistant cells have decreased polyglutamination of MTX, which means the drug can rapidly exit the cell.

5-Fluorouracil (5-FU) has similar resistance mechanisms to those of MTX in that alterations in the amount and the affinity of its target enzyme, thymidylate synthetase, are found in resistant cells. 5-FU is metabolized to an active form within the cell and inhibition of the enzymes involved in this metabolism (orotate phosphoribosyl transferase, uridine phosphorylase, uridine kinase) can reduce cell sensitivity to 5-FU.

Fortunately, drug resistance to one antimetabolite does not usually result in cross-resistance to other drugs of its class. However, cross-resistance between drugs with very similar mechanisms of action is possible, e.g., between different purine analogues.

Alkylating Agents and Cisplatinum

The alkylating agents such as melphalan, chlorambucil, and cyclophosphamide form covalent attachments to many intracellular molecules, including DNA bases. The presence of a bulky drug adduct in the DNA helix interferes with DNA replication and messenger RNA synthesis.

Drug-resistant cell lines that can rapidly remove these DNA adducts have been identified. DNA repair pathways in mammalian cells are very poorly understood; the best characterized DNA repair protein is O^6-alkylguanine DNA alkyltransferase, which can remove covalently attached alkyl adducts from guanine. Cells deficient in this enzyme are more sensitive to a whole range of alkylating agents.

Excision repair of DNA adducts also occurs. In this system, a DNA adduct is recognized and excised from the DNA strand, and the subsequent gap in the DNA is repaired. Although there may be variations in the ability of cells to recognize different drug adducts, the remainder of this repair pathway is common to all types of DNA-binding drugs. Thus alterations in this repair pathway could result in considerable cross-resistance between different DNA-binding drugs.

Cisplatinum (CDDP) forms both interstrand and intrastrand DNA crosslinks. Comparison between sensitive and resistant tumor cell lines has implicated the ability to repair *intrastrand* cross-links as being an important factor in determining drug tolerance. CDDP is electrophilic and reacts with sulfur-containing nucleophiles, such as metallothionines, which form an intracellular "sink" for CDDP. Increases in metallothionines have been associated with CDDP resistance. Decreased CDDP accumulation has been found in resistant cell lines selected *in vitro*, but the biochemical basis for this is unknown.

Cell lines resistant to alkylating agents are not uncommonly cross-resistant to cisplatinum. As well as sharing DNA repair pathways, these agents also share some detoxification mechanisms. Glutathione S-transferases (GSTs) can convert a variety of electrophilic substrates to less toxic and more easily excreted forms by conjugating the drugs to glutathione. Cyclophosphamide, melphalan, and chlorambucil are all conjugated in this way. Glutathione (GSH) itself, without any enzymatic catalysis, can act as a sink for electrophiles such as CDDP and many of the alkylating drugs. Certain GST isoenzymes have intrinsic peroxidase activity, which may help counteract the reactive oxygen radical intermediates generated by a wide range of drugs, including cisplatinum and the anthracyclines. Elevated levels of GST and GSH have been detected in cells resistant to alkylating agents, CDDP, and adriamycin. Tumor cells isolated from patients following CDDP treatment can have elevated GST and GSH.

GSTs are similar to P-gp in having tissue-specific patterns of expression and therefore may contribute to intrinsic and acquired resistance. Although most drugs are less toxic following conjugation, bleomycin is peculiar in that it is activated by glutathione conjugation.

L-Asparaginase

The bacterial enzyme L-asparaginase depletes serum asparagine. This is of little consequence to most normal cells because they possess sufficient asparagine synthetase to meet their own asparagine requirement. Some leukemic and lymphoma cells cannot synthesize asparagine and are therefore sensitive to this drug. However, resistance arises relatively easily when the cells increase their asparagine synthetase content.

MODULATION OF DRUG RESISTANCE

Now that the biochemical basis for some resistance mechanisms has been elucidated, attention should focus on the potentials of modulating these mechanisms using noncytotoxic drugs.

MDR-resistant cells can become sensitive to MDR drugs if the P-gp pump is blocked by a large variety of substances, including verapamil, quinidine, and cyclosporins. Verapamil and quinidine are currently being used in some human chemotherapy protocols, but as yet, no clear-cut advantage has been shown (Kane, 1989). Verapamil has dose-limiting cardiovascular effects, which makes it difficult to achieve the concentrations that are necessary to modulate P-gp activity (Dalton, 1989).

Cellular glutathione can be depleted by buthionine sulfoxide (BSO), which can increase the *in vitro* sensitivity to a wide range of drugs, including cisplatinum and alkylating agents. However, it is proving difficult *in vivo* to safely lower the intracellular glutathione concentration sufficiently to alter clinical sensitivity.

Chemosensitization is still in its infancy, but more refined modulators, especially of P-gp, can be expected in the future. The development of these agents will be fraught with the same problems as in anti-cancer agent development, in that normal tissue toxicity will undoubtedly be the limiting factor.

CONCLUSION

Many drug-resistance mechanisms have been identified, some of which result in cross-resistance to other agents (Table 2). Most resistance mechanisms for the antimetabolites are unique to the selecting drug. However, adriamycin and vincristine are both affected by overexpression of P-gp. Similarly, the cytotoxicity of both alkylating agents and cisplatinum can be ameliorated by increased DNA repair capacity.

The development of combination chemotherapy has largely been based on empirical methods aimed at reducing normal tissue toxicity. It has been suggested that non–cross-resistant drugs of equal efficacy should be used in alternating cycles to delay the onset of clinical resistance (Goldie and Coldman, 1984). It has been difficult to implement these proposals primarily because it is difficult to find

Table 2. *Cellular Mechanisms of Resistance to Antineoplastic Drugs*

Mechanism	Example
Decreased cell uptake	Methotrexate
Increased cell export	MDR drugs
Increased repair of drug-induced damage	Cisplatinum Alkylators
Reduced drug activation	5-Fluorouracil
Increased drug inactivation	Cytosine arabinoside Alkylators
Quantitative changes in drug targets	Antimetabolites Topoisomerase inhibitors
Alterations in drug targets	Antimetabolites Topoisomerase inhibitors
Bypass in target function	Antimetabolites

drugs with totally different mechanisms of action that have equal efficacy in a given tumor type.

The most common indication for combination chemotherapy in veterinary medicine is in the treatment of canine lymphoma. There are many published treatment protocols for this disease which suggest that once an animal relapses, dose intensification or addition of new drugs into the regimen is required. The choice of new drugs is often limited because, in the case of lymphomas, most first-line protocols use both an MDR drug, such as vincristine, and an alkylating agent, such as cyclophosphamide. Drugs with completely different activities, such as L-asparaginase or methotrexate, can be tried in relapsing dogs. The addition of adriamycin, despite its known cross-resistance with vincristine, can also be effective. This apparent paradox may be related to the antitopoisomerase action of adriamycin. Minor elevations of P-gp in the face of normal topoisomerase activity may be sufficient to cause vincristine resistance but be insufficient to produce adriamycin tolerance. This last point demonstrates that there is still much to learn before it is possible to accurately predict the chemosensitivity of a relapsed tumor.

References

Andrews, P. A., and Howell, S. B.: Cellular pharmacology of cisplatinum: Perspectives on mechanisms of acquired resistance. Cancer Cells 2:35, 1990.
A review of in vitro and in vivo cisplatinum resistance.
Brown, R., and Kaye, S. B.: Drug resistance and the problem of treatment failure. *In* Ponder, B. A. and Waring, M. J. (eds.): *The Science of Cancer Treatment.* Lancaster, U.K.: Kluwer Academic, 1990, p. 55.
Review with a clinical perspective and discussion of chemosensitization.
Carter, R. F., Harris, C. K., Withrow, S. J. et al.: Chemotherapy of canine lymphoma with histopathological correlation: Doxorubicin alone compared to COP as first treatment regimen. J.A.V.M.A. 23:587, 1987.
Results of different first-line treatments plus subsequent use of salvage therapy.
Dalton, W. S., Grogan, T. M., Meltzer, P. S. et al.: Drug resistance in multiple myeloma and non-Hodgkins lymphoma: Detection of P-glycoprotein and potential circumvention by addition of verapamil to chemotherapy. J. Clin. Oncol. 7:415, 1989.
Describes the use of verapamil in clinically drug-resistant patients.
Goldie, J. H., and Coldman, A. J.: The genetic origin of drug resistance in neoplasms: Implications for systemic therapy. Cancer Res. 44:3643, 1984.
Mathematical modeling of tumor growth and drug resistance plus treatment strategies to avoid resistance.
Kane, S. E., and Gottesman, M. M.: Multidrug resistance in the laboratory and clinic. Cancer Cells 1:33, 1989.
Meeting report which gives brief update on modulator studies in humans.
Kartner, N., and Ling, V.: Multidrug resistance in cancer. Scientific American March 1989.
Didactic account of the discovery of P-glycoprotein and its clinical implications.
Rosenthal, R. C.: Drug resistance in cancer chemotherapy. *In* Kirk, R. W. (ed.): *Current Veterinary Therapy IX.* Philadelphia: W. B. Saunders, 1986, pp. 471.
Smith, P. J.: DNA topoisomerase dysfunction: A new goal for antitumour chemotherapy. Bioessays 12:167, 1990.
Review of topoisomerase poisons and putative resistance mechanisms.

PREVENTION AND TREATMENT OF CHEMOTHERAPY COMPLICATIONS

ALAN S. HAMMER
Columbus, Ohio

Some of the concerns veterinarians have regarding chemotherapy relate to the toxicities and complications associated with these antineoplastic agents. Proper intervention, when indicated, is vital and emphasizes the need for both frequent patient monitoring and a well-informed owner to permit timely therapy. Chemotherapy complications to be discussed include hematologic toxicity (most com-

Table 1. *Prevention and Treatment of Myelosuppression*

Dose reduction
Increase interval between treatments
Avoid overlapping myelosuppressive agents
Know when the nadir occurs
Frequent monitoring with CBC
Prophylactic use of antibiotics (e.g., Tribrissen)
Aggressive therapy for febrile, neutropenic patients (e.g.,
    cephalothin and gentamicin)
Myelostimulants
    Lithium
    Colony-stimulating factors (CSFs)
    Complex biologic products

mon), gastrointestinal disturbances, cardiotoxicity, urinary toxicity, pancreatitis, and anaphylactoid reactions. Each toxicity will be discussed in turn regarding preventive methods or treatment of complications as they arise.

HEMATOLOGIC TOXICITY

Myelosuppression is the hallmark toxicity associated with chemotherapy. The high mitotic rate and growth fraction of the bone marrow cells predispose this organ to toxicity from chemotherapeutic agents. Neutropenia is the most common cytopenia and may lead to life-threatening sepsis. The effect of chemotherapy on neutrophils is related to the rapid bone marrow transit time and short circulating half-life. Thrombocytopenia is less commonly observed, and anemia rarely occurs as a direct effect of anticancer drugs.

Several measures may be taken to prevent neutropenia and sepsis (Table 1). Since the degree of myelosuppression is usually dose-related, decreasing the dose of chemotherapy will often improve the patient's hematologic status. Unfortunately, decreasing the dose may also decrease the likelihood of tumor response.

Knowing when the nadir (lowest point) of neutropenia will occur allows the veterinarian to time the chemotherapy treatments so that severe myelosuppression is avoided. Chemotherapy protocols should be designed so that overlapping toxicities are minimized. The nadir of neutropenia associated with most chemotherapeutic agents usually occurs 6 to 10 days following treatment, and the neutrophil count usually returns to normal values within 36 to 72 hours. Frequent monitoring with complete blood counts (CBC) permits intervention with prophylactic antibiotics. Some chemotherapeutic agents cause delayed myelosuppression, which may not be evident for 3 to 4 weeks following treatment. Return to normal hematologic values is also delayed and may take weeks if these agents are used. Table 2

groups the common chemotherapeutic agents by degree of expected myelosuppression.

Neutrophil counts of fewer than 2000 cells/μl predispose the patient to sepsis. Neutrophil counts under 500 cells/μl are almost invariably associated with sepsis. Enteric organisms are usually the source of infection; chemotherapy-induced desquamation of gastrointestinal epithelial cells occurs simultaneously with myelosuppression. Enteric bacteria are absorbed through the damaged mucosal barrier, and the insufficient numbers of neutrophils are not capable of phagocytizing the bacteria; sepsis ensues.

Prophylactic use of antibiotics is recommended with some chemotherapy protocols (e.g., ADIC, VAC, CHOP) (see *CVT X*, pp. 489 and 494) and with neutropenic, afebrile patients. Trimethoprim-sulfadiazine is particularly favored because it is available for oral use, has a broad spectrum of antibacterial activity, and has minimal effect on the anaerobic intestinal flora. Sparing the anaerobic flora decreases the risk of a "super" infection by yeast or Enterobacteriaceae. Trimethoprim-sulfadiazine is also thought to enhance opsonization by neutrophils. Alternative antibiotics to consider in trimethoprim-sulfadiazine–sensitive patients (e.g., Doberman pinschers) include enrofloxacin, amoxicillin–clavulanic acid, and cephalexin. Owners of neutropenic, afebrile animals should be instructed to monitor their pets closely for the next 48 hours, discontinue all anticancer drugs (except corticosteroids), and seek emergency care if fever develops.

Fever in a neutropenic patient constitutes a med-

Table 2. *Classification of Chemotherapeutic Agents by Degree of Myelosuppression*

Delayed myelosuppression (3–4 wk)
    BCNU
    CCNU
    mitomycin C
Severe myelosuppression (7–10 days)
    Doxorubicin
    Cyclophosphamide
    Cytosine arabinoside
    Vinblastine
    Hydroxyurea
Moderate myelosuppression (7–10 days)
    Methotrexate (low dose)
    6-Mercaptopurine
    Vincristine (>0.5 mg/m^2)
    Melphalan
    5-Fluorouracil
    Cisplatin (70 mg/m^2)
    Mitoxantrone
    Actinomycin D
Mild to no myelosuppression
    Bleomycin
    L-Asparaginase
    Corticosteroids
    Vincristine (0.5 mg/m^2)
    Cisplatin (40–50 mg/m^2)

ical emergency. Aggressive management of these presumably septic patients can be rewarding; less than aggressive management usually results in death. The recommended protocol is as follows: complete a thorough physical examination for a septic focus, aseptically place an indwelling intravenous catheter, and start intravenous fluids. Discontinue all antineoplastic drugs except corticosteroids, which should be gradually discontinued because patients on chronic corticosteroid therapy can develop acute hypoadrenocorticism if therapy is abruptly stopped. Blood samples for CBC, electrolytes, glucose, and blood urea nitrogen (BUN) or creatinine are collected; urine samples for analysis and bacterial culture are also obtained. Two to three sets of aseptically collected blood cultures should be obtained for aerobic and anaerobic cultures. These cultures should be collected at 30-minute intervals to maximize the likelihood of a positive culture. After collecting the second set of cultures, therapy with an empirical bactericidal combination of antibiotics is instituted. Gentamicin (2.2 mg/kg IV t.i.d.) and cephalothin (22 mg/kg IV t.i.d.) is an effective broad-spectrum combination. Amikacin (10 mg/kg IV t.i.d.) and ampicillin (22 mg/kg IV t.i.d.) can be substituted.

Once the neutrophil count returns to normal and the patient has recovered (usually within 72 to 96 hours), the antibiotic combination is discontinued, the patient is started on trimethoprim-sulfadiazine (14 to 20 mg/kg PO b.i.d.) for 7 days, and chemotherapy reinstituted. Patients experiencing repeated neutropenic episodes should be kept on trimethoprim-sulfadiazine continuously while undergoing chemotherapy.

An active and exciting area of investigation for the prevention and treatment of hematologic toxicity is the use of various myelostimulants to counteract the side effects of anticancer drugs. Several classes of bone marrow–stimulating agents are being studied, including lithium, recombinant colony-stimulating factors, and complex biologic products.

Lithium was first noted to have myelostimulatory properties when it was observed that psychiatric patients receiving the drug had leukocytosis. Some clinical trials in human cancer patients suggest a beneficial role for lithium; however, lithium does not prevent vinblastine-induced myelosuppression in normal dogs. Lithium therapy in clinical canine cancer patients has failed to demonstrate a consistent beneficial effect. Use of lithium carbonate in cats is not recommended as it is neurotoxic and causes erythroid and myeloid hypoplasia (Dieringer, 1990).

Lithium carbonate is available in 300-mg tablets and is dosed in the dog at 10 mg/kg. It is excreted primarily by the kidneys, and dosage reductions may be necessary in patients with renal disease. Serum lithium concentrations should be monitored closely starting 48 hours after initiating therapy and at 7-day intervals thereafter. Therapeutic serum lithium concentrations are 0.8 to 1.5 mEq/l at the trough.

Colony-stimulating factors (CSFs) and interleukins (ILs) are cytokines—small glycoprotein molecules produced by a variety of normal cells—that work interactively to regulate myeloid and lymphoid cell production and function. Interleukins tend to act on early pluripotent myeloid and lymphoid stem cells, whereas CSFs generally act on committed progenitor cells and their progeny. These growth factors act in combinations at multiple stages of differentiation, and several different factors may act on several cell lineages. Recombinant technology has increased the availability of these factors such that clinical trials are possible. These trials are investigating the use of CSFs and ILs to accelerate granulocyte recovery from chemotherapy-induced neutropenia or bone marrow transplantation and to treat myelodysplastic conditions, congenital cyclic neutropenia, retroviral-induced neutropenia, and severe aplastic anemia. Although CSFs are considered relatively species-specific, several reports indicate some efficacy of recombinant human products in domestic animals. These reports include use of rh-G-CSF in gray Collies with cyclic neutropenia, rh-G-CSF in cattle, and rh-GM-CSF in a dog overdosed with doxorubicin (Ogilvie, 1990). In each report, there was an increase in myelopoiesis, although formation of neutralizing antibodies by days 21 to 28 limited efficacy of this therapy. Recently, the availability of recombinant canine G-CSF (rc-G-CSF) has made possible prolonged studies in dogs. Both dogs and cats developed sustained leukocytosis when injected subcutaneously with this product; neutrophil counts returned to normal values upon discontinuing the injections of rc-G-CSF.

These growth factors are being heralded as the next era in cancer therapy by allowing dose escalation of chemotherapy protocols. However, the potential negative effects of these growth factors as tumor promoters have not been fully evaluated at this time. Also, these agents are not yet commercially available, and it is unlikely that species-specific CSFs will be commercially available for veterinary use. Thus, use of CSFs in veterinary medicine will, for the near future, be limited to rescue of severely myelosuppressed animals with human rG-CSF or in animals undergoing short, single-cycle, intensive chemotherapy or to enhance bone marrow transplantation engraftment.

An alternative to the use of recombinant CSF is the use of complex biologic products to stimulate the release of endogenous CSFs from normal cells. One such product being evaluated is the ribosomal fraction from Serratia marcescens. Serum G-CSF concentrations are elevated as soon as 4 hours after injection (Ogilvie, 1990). Products such as this may represent an alternative to recombinant CSFs for veterinary medicine.

GASTROINTESTINAL TOXICITY

With the advent of aggressive empiric antibiotic therapy and colony-stimulating factors to combat myelosuppression and sepsis, gastrointestinal toxicity is becoming the limiting factor associated with chemotherapy. Gastrointestinal toxicity can be divided into two categories based on when the toxicity occurs in relation to administration of the drug (i.e., acute, within 6 to 12 hours; delayed, 3 to 5 days following administration). Injectable drugs causing acute nausea and vomiting include cisplatin, DTIC, and actinomycin D. Often, this can be alleviated by administering the drug slowly; in the case of actinomycin D, we inject the drug over a 10-minute period. This has almost completely eliminated the immediate nausea seen with this drug. In our hospital, cisplatin and DTIC are administered as slow 8-hour infusions. We feel this diminishes the acute gastrointestinal effects of these two drugs. If persistent vomiting occurs, the use of antiemetics such as metoclopramide (Reglan) 0.1 to 0.3 mg/kg SQ every 4 to 6 hours or prochlorperazine (Compazine) 0.5 mg/kg IM is indicated.

Delayed gastroenterocolitis occurs 3 to 5 days after therapy when desquamation of intestinal crypt cells begins. Drugs particularly associated with these effects include doxorubicin, actinomycin D, and methotrexate. Predicting which patients are likely to suffer gastrointestinal effects following chemotherapy is important so that owners can be forewarned and antiemetics prescribed. We have found that performance status is predictive as to whether a patient will show adverse reactions when treated with actinomycin D. Dogs showing systemic effects from their tumors (poor performance status) are more likely to be ill from actinomycin D therapy than are dogs with good performance status.

Doxorubicin has been shown to be more likely to cause gastrointestinal toxicity in small (less than 20 kg) dogs than in larger dogs (Ogilvie, 1989a). Also, it has been our experience that collies, collie crosses, Old English sheepdogs, and West Highland white terriers are more likely to develop hemorrhagic gastroenteritis following therapy with doxorubicin. Prophylactic treatment with bismuth subsalicylate may ameliorate the clinical signs in these patients. Supportive therapy with fluids and antiemetics should be used if deemed necessary in severely ill animals.

Finally, a prior history of chemotherapy-induced nausea and vomiting indicates that further chemotherapy with that drug at that dose will provoke a similar reaction. This was demonstrated with mi-

toxantrone where a 95-fold increased risk of gastroenteritis was seen in patients who became ill during the previous cycle (Ogilvie, 1989b).

CARDIOTOXICITY

Cardiotoxicity in veterinary oncology practice is primarily associated with the use of doxorubicin in the dog. Doxorubicin-induced cardiotoxicity is classified as acute toxicity (characterized by the development of transient arrhythmias during administration of the drug) or chronic cumulative cardiotoxicity. Chronic doxorubicin cardiotoxicity is characterized by the development of dilated cardiomyopathy (DCM) and is occasionally preceded by electrocardiogram (ECG) abnormalities and arrhythmias. The risk for DCM increases above a cumulative dose of 240 mg/m^2 of doxorubicin; however, individual patients have been reported to develop DCM at lower doses ranging from 100 to 150 mg/m^2 (Hammer, 1990; Loar, 1986). Once DCM develops, the prognosis is poor, as the myocardial lesions are irreversible.

Preventing doxorubicin-induced cardiotoxicity is based primarily on avoiding high peak serum concentrations of doxorubicin as this has been shown to correlate with the development of cardiomyopathy. The following protocol is used at our hospital and has resulted in an acceptable rate of DCM (approximately one case per year out of 30 to 40 dogs treated with doxorubicin). A baseline echocardiogram is obtained, and animals with compromised myocardial function as determined from the fractional shortening are not treated with doxorubicin. Dogs are pretreated with diphenhydramine (Benadryl) (2.2 mg/kg IM) to avoid the anaphylactoid reaction associated with doxorubicin and spontaneous mast cell degranulation; there is some evidence for histamine as a mediator of cardiotoxicity in dogs treated with doxorubicin. Doxorubicin is administered as a slow infusion over 20 to 30 minutes to avoid high peak serum concentrations. The cardiac status of each patient is re-evaluated every three cycles by echocardiography and doxorubicin is discontinued if any significant decline in myocardial function is noted. Finally, most of our protocols are limited to a cumulative dose of doxorubicin of 150 to 180 mg/m^2, which is below the recommended maximum cumulative level of 240 mg/m^2.

Future considerations in preventing cardiotoxicity may include weekly administration of doxorubicin and use of cardioprotectants. One such cardioprotectant, ICRF-187, is close to clinical use. Experimental use of ICRF-187 permitted greater cumulative doses of doxorubicin to be given than that used in control dogs (Herman, 1988).

Other drugs can actually potentiate doxorubicin-

Table 3. Administration of Cisplatin

Phase I
  0.9% NaCl administered for 8 hr at a rate of 1.7 ml/kg/hr
Phase II
  Mannitol (0.5 gm/kg) given IV over 30 min
  Cisplatin diluted in 0.9% NaCl and administered over 8 hr at
    a rate of 1.7 ml/kg/hr
  Administer metoclopramide or prochlorperazine as indicated
    for nausea and vomiting
Phase III
  0.9% NaCl administered for 8 hr at a rate of 1.7 ml/kg/hr

induced cardiotoxicity, and concurrent use with doxorubicin should be avoided. One drug recently demonstrated to have such an effect is verapamil (Bright, 1990).

URINARY TRACT TOXICITY

Two chemotherapy-induced urinary tract complications may arise in small animals: nephrotoxicity and sterile hemorrhagic cystitis.

Several potentially nephrotoxic chemotherapeutic drugs are used in small animals, but only cisplatin (in dogs) and doxorubicin (primarily in cats) are of clinical concern. The limiting toxicity in cats treated with doxorubicin may actually be nephrotoxicity rather than cardiotoxicity (Cotter, 1985). In dogs, doxorubicin may cause nephrotoxicosis in animals with pre-existing renal disease or in animals concurrently receiving other nephrotoxins (e.g., aminoglycosides). Cisplatin is a consistent nephrotoxin in humans and dogs, and proper administration can prevent much of the renal toxicity. The most important feature in administering cisplatin is hydration. Use of the protocol given in Table 3 has resulted in no episodes of acute renal failure at our hospital for the past 6 years.

Sterile hemorrhagic cystitis is a common complication of cyclophosphamide use in dogs; cats rarely develop this complication. This toxicity develops as a result of one of the metabolites of cyclophosphamide, acrolein, which causes mucosal and arteriolar damage. The prevalence of sterile hemorrhagic cystitis in dogs is reported to be 5 to 30% with female dogs at greater risk. The risk of developing sterile hemorrhagic cystitis can be lessened if cyclophosphamide tablets are administered in the morning, the pet allowed to urinate frequently during the day, free access to water provided, and the food salted to encourage water intake. In addition, if prednisone is part of the chemotherapy protocol, it should be given on the same day as the cyclophosphamide for its mild diuretic and anti-inflammatory effects. Furosemide has also been reported to prevent cystitis even at very high oral doses of cyclophosphamide.

Recently, three dogs with peracute hemorrhagic cystitis were reported after intravenous use of cyclophosphamide (Peterson, 1990). Doses ranged from 100 to 250 mg/m². This appears to be an idiosyncratic reaction.

Various sulfhydryl compounds are available to prevent sterile hemorrhagic cystitis. The compounds have been used both intravesically and intravenously; their protectant action does not appear to diminish the antineoplastic activity of the cyclophosphamide. Although these compounds are expensive, their use may permit higher intravenous doses of cyclophosphamide to be administered in dogs and cats.

If sterile hemorrhagic cystitis develops, the offending drug should be discontinued and the urine cultured to detect urinary tract infections. Diuresis should be induced and anti-inflammatory agents such as prednisone administered. Prophylactic antibiotics are recommended to prevent bacterial infection. If the clinical signs continue to worsen despite this approach, 1% formalin in water can be instilled into the bladder under general anesthesia to cauterize the mucosal surface and decrease the hemorrhage.

ANAPHYLACTOID REACTIONS

Several drugs (e.g., doxorubicin, etoposide, L-asparaginase) are capable of inducing acute type I hypersensitivity-like reactions. Doxorubicin-induced anaphylaxis is not a true type I hypersensitivity reaction as mast cell degranulation is induced independently of IgE binding. Etoposide itself may not cause these anaphylactoid reactions, but rather the vehicle, polysorbate 80, has been incriminated (Ogilvie, 1988). Reaction to both doxorubicin and etoposide has been observed on the first administration. L-Asparaginase, as a macromolecule, can induce true type I hypersensitivity reactions, and its use usually requires prior sensitization.

Because these hypersensitivity reactions are life-threatening, they are best prevented. Intravenous etoposide is not recommended for use in dogs and cats. Patients receiving doxorubicin or L-asparaginase should be pretreated with antihistamines (diphenhydramine 2.2 mg/kg IM), and corticosteroid and epinephrine (Adrenalin) should be available should a reaction occur. Antihistamines should be used with caution in cats as severe CNS depression may occur, resulting in apnea.

PANCREATITIS

L-Asparaginase can induce acute pancreatitis in dogs. Its use in dogs with a past history of pancreatitis or of increased serum amylase or lipase concentrations, or in overweight, middle-aged female dogs, is not recommended. Other chemotherapeutic agents are also suspected of occasionally causing pancreatitis (e.g., doxorubicin, DTIC).

IDIOSYNCRATIC TOXICITIES

Species-specific drug toxicities are known, and use of certain drugs in selected species is to be avoided. 5-Fluorouracil results in neurotoxicity in the cat. Neurotoxicosis has also been seen in the dog, but with less frequency. Cisplatin is a documented cause of acute pulmonary toxicity in the cat and should not be used in this species.

SUMMARY

The three important aspects for dealing with chemotherapy complications are knowledge of potential toxicities, patient monitoring for early signs of toxicity, and intervention to prevent or treat complications. Armed with the information discussed earlier, veterinarians can feel confident in monitoring and effectively dealing with chemotherapy complications in their patients.

References and Suggested Reading

Bright, J. M., and Buss, D. D.: Effects of verapamil on chronic doxorubicin-induced cardiotoxicity in dogs. J. Nat'l. Cancer Instit. 82:963, 1990.
Documentation of interaction between doxorubicin and verapamil in causing cardiomyopathy.
Cotter, S. M., Kanki, P. J., and Simon, M.: Renal disease in five tumor-bearing cats treated with adriamycin. J. Am. Anim. Hosp. Assoc. 21:405–409, 1985.
First report of nephrotoxicity of adriamycin in cats.
Dieringer, T. M., Rogers, K. S., Brown, S. A., et al.: Evaluation of lithium carbonate as a bone marrow stimulant in healthy cats. Proc ACVIM, Washington, D.C., 1990, p. 1113 (abstract).
Documents the hematologic and neurologic toxicity of lithium in cats.
Hammer, A. S., Couto, C. G., Getzy, D., et al.: Efficacy and toxicity of VAC chemotherapy in dogs with hemangiosarcoma. J. Vet. Intern. Med. 5:160–166, 1991.
Cardiomyopathy developed in three dogs treated with VAC at doses of 100, 150, and 150 mg/m².
Herman, E. H., Ferrans, V. J., Young, R. S. K., et al.: Effect of pretreatment with IRCF-187 on the total cumulative dose of doxorubicin tolerated by beagle dogs. Cancer Res. 48:6918–6925, 1988.
Documentation of protective effects of IRCF-187 in normal dogs.
Loar, A. S., and Susaneck, S. J.: Doxorubicin-induced cardiotoxicity in five dogs. Semin. Vet. Med. Surg. 1:68–71, 1986.
Series of cases and literature review of adriamycin-induced cardiotoxicity in the dog.
Ogilvie, G. K., Cockburn, C. A., Tranquilli, W. J., et al.: Hypotension and cutaneous administration of etoposide in the dog. Am. J. Vet. Res. 49:1367–1370, 1988.
One of several reports documenting etoposide toxicity in the dog.
Ogilvie, G. K., Richardson, R. C., Curtis, C. R., et al.: Acute and short-term toxicoses associated with the administration of doxorubicin to dogs with malignant tumors. J.A.V.M.A. 195:1584–1587, 1989a.
Evaluation of doxorubicin toxicity in more than 180 dogs.
Ogilvie, G. K., Elmslie, R. E., Obradovich, J. E., et al.: Efficacy and toxicoses associated with mitoxantrone therapy in the dog. Proceedings 9th Annual Vet. Cancer Soc., Raleigh, N.C., 1989b, pp. 3–4 (abstract).
First report of mitoxantrone use in veterinary medicine.
Ogilvie, G. K.: Use of colony-stimulating factors in human and veterinary medicine. Proc ACVIM, Washington, D.C., 1990, pp. 917–920.
Overview of colony-stimulating factors in veterinary medicine, including research results on recombinant canine G-CSF in dogs and cats.
Peterson, J. L., Couto, G. C., Hammer, A. S., and Ayl, R. D.: Acute sterile hemorrhagic cystitis immediately after intravenous cyclophosphamide in three dogs. Proceedings 10th Annual Vet. Cancer Soc., Auburn, AL, 1990, pp 45–46 (abstract)
First report of acute hemorrhagic cystitis in dogs.

LASERS IN VETERINARY ONCOLOGY

ELSA R. BECK
Detroit, Michigan

Although once restricted to the world of science fiction and high technology, lasers today are accessible in such mundane circumstances as grocery store scanners and remote control units for home stereo components. The greatest obstacle to the implementation of laser technology in veterinary medicine has been the cost of equipment. However, rapid expansion of technology has increased the availability of older surplus machinery. Later generation lasers are already available at some teaching hospitals and private referral centers. As this technology has become available, interest regarding laser applications in veterinary oncology has increased. For these reasons, a basic understanding of how lasers work and their possible applications is appropriate for veterinary practitioners.

The term "laser" stands for "*Light Amplification by Stimulated Emission of Radiation.*" A comprehensive explanation of laser design and function is beyond the scope of this review, but lasers function somewhat like a fluorescent light bulb. In both, electricity Stimulates a gas contained within a tube, and Radiation in the form of Light is Emitted. The quantity of light is then Amplified by mirrors inside the laser. Light that leaves the laser chamber can be focused to a very small and precise spot and then coupled to the treatment device.

Lasers are named by the lasing medium, or the substance that produces the light. For example, argon and krypton lasers produce a visible wavelength by means of argon or krypton gas. A Nd:YAG laser produces an infrared wavelength by means of a solid-state crystal of yttrium-aluminum-garnet with impurities of neodymium.

Lasers have various functions in medical technology, based on the different ways in which light can interact with tissue. Within tissue, light energy may be absorbed, reflected, transmitted, or scattered. The interaction that occurs is determined primarily by the wavelength of light. Consequently, the optimum function of a laser is dictated by its wavelength. Slight alterations in wavelength can be achieved by tuning the laser. However, substantial changes must be made by switching the gas contained within the tube or by substituting a liquid or crystal for the gas. In practical terms this means obtaining a different lasing system.

CLINICAL APPLICATIONS

Lasers can be classified according to their clinical application, the lasing medium, or the wavelength produced. For the purposes of this discussion, various types of lasers will be reviewed according to their clinical applications. The most common functions of lasers in veterinary medicine are for surgery, hyperthermia, or photodynamic therapy.

Surgical Lasers

Much of the work regarding the application of lasers in veterinary surgery has not been directly targeted to oncology. Nevertheless, the applications are readily apparent. Lasers can perform a variety of functions, including cutting tissue, coagulating blood, heating to the point of vaporizing, and welding tissue. This allows the surgeon to excise tumors without contaminating the surgical field, without excessive blood loss, and without disseminating tumor cells through lymphatic or vascular channels. Certain lasers allow surgery to be performed through an endoscope; this has obvious appeal when accessibility is limited and general anesthesia is risky. Some laser beams can be focused at a specific depth in the interior of a structure such as the brain. This property may allow surgical ablation without disruption of overlying critical structures.

The benefits of these properties to surgical oncology are obvious. The major lasers employed in general or ophthalmic surgery are the CO_2, Nd:YAG, krypton, and argon lasers.

THE CO_2 LASER

The carbon dioxide laser produces an infrared light (10,600 nm) invisible to the human eye and strongly absorbed by water. This property allows the CO_2 laser to make incisions by vaporizing the cells in its path, but renders it useless in pools of fluid or blood. The power can be adjusted to produce cutting, heating, or tissue welding. These properties make the CO_2 laser an excellent surgical scalpel, especially for microsurgery or superficial ophthalmic procedures.

THE ND:YAG LASER

The Nd:YAG laser produces an infrared wavelength (1064 nm), which penetrates water, hemoglobin, and melanin with minimal absorption. Consequently, tissue coagulation is especially good with this laser. Since the function of the Nd:YAG laser is not negated by pools of fluid or blood, it is ideal for certain intraocular procedures.

THE KRYPTON LASER

This laser produces visible light in a variety of wavelengths, from red to blue (488 to 676 nm). These wavelengths produce good coagulation and can treat tissue despite the presence of blood. Krypton lasers have limited application at this time; they are primarily used in ophthalmology.

THE ARGON LASER

Argon lasers produce visible light in the bluish green wavelengths (488 to 514 nm). These wavelengths are absorbed strongly by hemoglobin and melanin, which limits the penetration depth. However, coagulation is excellent, and the ability to tightly focus the beam allows for very precise dissection during surgery.

SYNOPSIS OF LASERS IN SURGICAL ONCOLOGY

Much remains to be determined regarding the optimal application of lasers in surgical oncology. An advantage of Nd:YAG, krypton, and argon lasers is that their light output can be channeled through fiberoptic cables. This allows surgery to be performed through a flexible endoscope. Only a brief synopsis of their potential roles has been presented here. For more information readers are referred to a review by Klause and Roberts, 1990.

Hyperthermia

Hyperthermia can be an effective adjuvant to other cancer treatments, such as radiation or chemotherapy. Several different techniques are available to induce heating, but each has specific drawbacks. The Nd:YAG laser has been suggested as an alternative because its wavelength is minimally absorbed by water, hemoglobin, or melanin (Panjehpour et al., 1991). This property allows relatively deep penetration. The light can be channeled through fiberoptic cables, allowing heat to be delivered through a flexible endoscope. Clinical experience is quite limited at this time, but the technique does appear feasible.

Photodynamic Therapy

Photodynamic therapy (PDT) is a relatively new treatment modality advocated for a variety of cancers in pet animals (Thoma, 1989). The technique involves the parenteral administration of a photosensitizing compound followed by the activation of that compound by laser-generated light. A series of physical and chemical events is set in motion, and oxygen radicles are generated. Because oxygen radicles are toxic to all cells, the ideal photosensitizing compound would localize exclusively, or at least preferentially, in tumor cells. However, no current photosensitizer has this property.

The agent first employed for PDT was a complex mixture of compounds termed hematoporphyrin derivative, HPD, or Photofrin (Dougherty et al., 1975). This mixture was useful for localization of tumors as well as for treatment, since certain impurities were fluorescent. Purification of this product eliminated the fluorescence but produced the compound dihematoporphyrin ether (DHE, or Photofrin II). Both compounds have been successful in controlling pet tumors (Thoma, 1989). Extensive investigations into alternatives to HPD or DHE have produced several different types of photosensitizers. One new drug, a sulfonated phthalocyanine, has been used in veterinary cancer patients (Roberts et al., 1989). However, none of these drugs have been approved for domestic animals by the FDA.

Two laser systems are used for PDT, gold vapor and argon-pumped dye lasers. The output of either laser can be coupled to a fiberoptic system and then directed to the treatment area. Gold vapor lasers produce light with the appropriate wavelength to activate HPD or DHE. Argon lasers produce a different wavelength that must be converted before it is useful. The high-intensity output of the argon laser is focused and channeled into a dye column. The dye absorbs the energy of the argon light and converts it into the appropriate wavelength. Several dyes are available for this purpose, depending on the wavelength desired. This system is referred to as an argon-pumped dye laser because the light produced by the argon laser is used to power, or pump, the dye laser.

Excellent responses to PDT have been seen in several tumors that respond poorly to traditional treatments. Although protocols have varied, over 200 pets have been treated with PDT. Tumors for which the most information is available to date are squamous cell carcinomas, transitional cell carcinomas, and soft-tissue sarcomas.

SQUAMOUS CELL CARCINOMAS

Squamous cell carcinomas of the head and neck were treated in nine dogs and two cats with PDT using Photofrin II (Beck et al., 1991). All cases were recurrent after at least one surgical removal. Twelve of 14 cases achieved a complete remission after a single PDT treatment. Relapses occurred early, at 2 to 3 months. Eleven of the 14 patients remain in remission, with a median follow-up time of 13 months. These results suggest that local control of many oral squamous cell carcinomas may be possible without disfiguring surgical procedures or other time-consuming forms of therapy.

Cats with cutaneous squamous cell carcinomas of external nonpigmented areas were treated with a sulfonated phthalocyanine (Klein et al., 1989). Approximately 50% of the patients (6 of 13 locations) remained in complete remission at 6 months. Although subsequent observation revealed continued relapses over 12 to 18 months, optimizing treatment parameters or repeated treatments may improve the remission duration (Peavy et al., 1991).

TRANSITIONAL CELL CARCINOMAS

Traditional treatments for tumors of the bladder or urethra in dogs have resulted in poor local control or severe toxicity. However, ten of ten dogs attained a complete remission that persisted from 5 to 14 weeks following a single PDT (Beck et al., 1990a). A second treatment produced a second remission in four of six dogs. One dog has received five treatments over 15 months with no toxicity. Urethral tumors have shown similar responses but require reduced light doses. Although quite preliminary, these results encourage further investigation.

SOFT-TISSUE SARCOMAS

Soft-tissue sarcomas are locally invasive tumors that comprise approximately 15% of all canine malignancies. The most common histologies include fibrosarcomas, hemangiopericytomas, and neurofibrosarcomas. Because they often occur on extremities and infiltrate deeply, these tumors often cannot be completely resected without amputation. Complete remissions have been obtained with PDT of recurrent soft-tissue sarcomas in 10 of 14 dogs (Beck et al., 1990b). Eight of the ten remained free of disease at 12 months. Two other groups have reported variable success, but the numbers of patients were small (Peavy et al., 1991) and multiple treatment protocols were used (Thoma, 1989). In both of these reports, patients were treated after surgical resection without confirming the presence of tumor. In one study, the treatment results from dogs and cats were combined (Thoma, 1989). This may produce misleading results because, in our experience, complete remissions were achieved in ten of 14 dogs, but only three of 11 cats.

TOXICITY

Systemic toxicity from photosensitizing dyes has been minimal and responds to treatment with systemic corticosteroids or antihistamines. Cutaneous photosensitivity appears as facial edema, especially around the muzzle and eyes when the pigmentation is light or the hair coat is thin. Phthalocyanine compounds are less prone to this problem than Photofrin compounds (Klein et al., 1989). Most reactions in dogs occur during the first few days after Photofrin administration, but cats may be photosensitive for weeks. Limiting the exposure to direct sunlight, especially between 10 AM and 4 PM, will prevent photosensitivity in most animals. High-risk patients may need to avoid all sun exposure, even through windows. White cats that fancy sitting on window-sills can present a special challenge. Rapid administration of Photofrin dye may trigger a shocklike reaction, which can be avoided by administering the dye over a 5- to 10-minute period.

Localized treatment reactions, including swelling and discoloration, occur in most patients. Some necrosis of normal tissues adjacent to the tumor can be expected, since current photosensitizers do not localize exclusively in tumor cells. Moreover, what may appear to be "normal" tissue may in fact contain infiltrates of tumor that are not discernible to the naked eye. These reactions can be early indicators that PDT was effective and usually do not require intervention unless occurring around the eyes or nose. Our impression is that PDT is associated with a high rate of post-treatment infections (Beck et al., 1990b). Experimental studies have demonstrated immunosuppression by PDT. Until the importance of this in veterinary patients is defined, antibiotics should be used appropriately. Other complications have occurred which were related to specific treatment situations or sensitive locations. A more complete review is available (Beck et al., 1990b).

SYNOPSIS OF PDT IN VETERINARY ONCOLOGY

The practice of photodynamic therapy involves a complex interaction of light dose, photosensitizer dose, and pharmacokinetics. Transmission characteristics of light in normal and malignant tissues are far from understood. Apparent species differences in response to PDT may relate to altered photosensitizer pharmacokinetics or as yet unidentified factors. In addition, new photosensitizers are constantly being developed and require testing. Tumor location may also exert an unexpected effect, because the tolerance of different normal tissues to treatment is not fully appreciated. Since all these factors are interdependent, seemingly minor alterations can have a profound impact. Nevertheless, promising results have been obtained in tumors that respond poorly to other forms of therapy.

SUMMARY

Application of laser technology in veterinary oncology holds obvious promise. Lasers may facilitate many aspects of the surgical approach to tumors. Nd:YAG laser–induced hyperthermia may be an effective adjuvant to radiation therapy, chemotherapy, or photodynamic therapy. Excellent responses to PDT have been seen in several tumors that respond poorly to traditional forms of treatment. Which particular applications will eventually be accepted into the main stream of cancer therapy remains to be seen. Continued exploration will define the ultimate role of laser technology in a balanced approach to the management of the cancer patient.

References and Suggested Reading

Beck, E. R., Hetzel, F. W., Morris, K. J., et al.: Response of canine transitional cell carcinomas to photodynamic therapy. *In* Proceedings of the 8th Annual Vet. Med. Forum, May 1990a, p. 1121.
  Complete remissions in ten of ten dogs using PDT for bladder tumors.
Beck, E. R., Hetzel, F. W., Morris, K. J., et al.: Systemic toxicities after localized photodynamic therapy. *In* Proceedings of the 8th Annual Vet. Med. Forum, May 1990b, p. 1122.
  Synopsis of toxicities observed in treating 100 patients.
Beck, E., and Hetzel, F. W.: Photodynamic therapy of pet animals with spontaneously occurring head and neck carcinomas. *In* Proceedings of SPIE Meeting, Jan. 1991.
  Complete remissions seen in ten of 11 animals.
Dougherty, T. J., Grindey, G. B., Fiel, R., et al.: Photoradiation therapy II. Cure of animal tumors with hematoporphyrin and light. J. Natl Cancer Inst. 55:115–121, 1975.
  The first report of controlling spontaneous animal tumors with PDT.

Klause, S. E., and Roberts, S. M.: Lasers and veterinary surgery. Comp. Cont. Ed. 12:1565–1576, 1990.
A review of lasers in veterinary surgery.

Klein, M. K., Roberts, W. G., and Berns, M. W.: Photodynamic therapy of cutaneous squamous cell carcinomas of cats using a phthalocyanine photosensitizer. *In* Proceedings of the 9th Annual Conf. Vet. Cancer Soc., Raleigh, N.C., 1989.
Complete remissions at 6 months in six of 13 cats with squamous cell carcinomas.

Panjehpour, M., Overholt, B. F., Klebanow, E. R., et al.: Hyperthermia treatment of spontaneously occurring oral cavity tumors using a computer controlled ND:YAG laser system. *In* Proceedings of SPIE Meeting, Jan. 1991.
Potential of Nd:YAG to produce heat in tumors.

Peavy, G. M., Klein, M. K., Newman, H. C., et al.: Use of chloroaluminum sulfonated phthalocyanine as a photosensitizer in the treatment of malignant tumors in dogs and cats. *In* Proceedings of SPIE Meeting, Jan. 1991.
Results of prolonged observation of patients treated with a phthalocyanine photosensitizer.

Roberts, W. G., Loomis, M., Weldy, S., et al.: Photodynamic therapy with chloroaluminum sulfonated phthalocyanine for the treatment of malignant tumors. *In* Proceedings of the 9th Annual Conf. Vet. Cancer Soc., Raleigh, N.C., 1989.
Early experience with alternative cancer photosensitizers.

Thoma, R. E.: Photodynamic therapy. *In* Withrow, S. J., and MacEwen, E. G. (eds.): *Clinical Veterinary Oncology.* Philadelphia: J. B. Lippincott, 1989, pp. 124–127.
Summary of PDT results in 93 animals.

HYPERTHERMIA: UPDATE AND CURRENT INDICATIONS

DEBORAH M. PRESCOTT
and MARK W. DEWHIRST
Durham, North Carolina

Hyperthermia is defined here as the raising of tissue temperatures to 42 to 50°C for specific periods of time to produce an antitumor effect. The medical use of hyperthermia was documented during the time of the ancient Greeks for treatment of tumors. Fevers were associated with tumor regression in patients during the 1800's. However, it was not until the mid 1900's that several investigators began adopting new techniques from cell biology and radiobiology to study the effects of hyperthermia on both normal and tumorous tissue. From these studies, the biologic rationale for therapeutic hyperthermia was found to be related to cytotoxic effects as well as potentially helpful interactions with radiation and chemotherapy (Gautherie, 1990a).

Although the field of hyperthermia has experienced many significant advancements in the past 5 to 10 years, several basic problems are still being addressed currently. In this article, recent clinical studies, technical advancements, and current limitations are briefly reviewed. The potential use of hyperthermia in veterinary practice is also discussed.

RECENT CLINICAL STUDIES

Hyperthermia Alone

Using spontaneous tumors in pet animals, Dewhirst and colleagues (1982) reported the results of the first phase III randomized trial designed to compare hyperthermia alone, radiation alone, and the two modalities combined. Hyperthermia alone resulted in a significantly lower response rate and shorter response duration than treatment arms containing radiation. The general conclusion reached from this study is that hyperthermia appears to be of little value as a single treatment modality.

Hyperthermia and Radiation

Many phase I and II clinical trials have demonstrated that hyperthermia may significantly enhance the effects of radiation (Overgaard, 1984). In the majority of these studies, the frequency of complete response rates approximately doubled when hyperthermia was used with radiation compared with radiation alone (Table 1). These results have been encouraging; however, very few phase III randomized prospective clinical trials have compared hyperthermia plus radiation with radiation alone. The results of two phase III studies using pet animals are discussed later.

Using various histologic types, Dewhirst and colleagues (1983) demonstrated that the complete response rate differed significantly between radiation alone (32%) and radiation plus hyperthermia (68%). When melanomas were excluded from the analysis, the response duration for hyperthermia plus radia-

Table 1. *Effect of Adjuvant Hyperthermia on Radiation*

Study	No. Patients or No. Tumors	Frequency of Complete Response	
		Radiation Alone	*Radiation + Heat*
Arcangeli et al.	163	38%	74%
U et al.	7	14%	85%
Overgaard	62	34%	67%
Johnson et al.	14	36%	86%
Kim et al.	159	33%	80%
Bide et al.	76	0%	7%
Hiraoka et al.	33	25%	71%
Kochegarov et al.	161	16%	63%
Lindholm et al.	72	29%	39%
Corry et al.	33	0%	62%
Scott et al.	44	64%	86%
Li et al.	124	29%	54%
van der Zee et al.	45	0%	24%
Severson et al.	75	23%	61%

*Reprinted with permission from Overgaard, J.: Rationale and problems in the design of clinical studies. *In* Overgaard, J. (ed): *Hyperthermic Oncology.* Vol 2. London: Taylor & Francis, 1984, pp. 325–338.

tion was significantly improved over that for radiation alone.

In a randomized prospective study using spontaneous canine oral carcinomas, dose-response curves were generated for radiation alone and for radiation plus hyperthermia (Fig. 1). The slope of the dose-response curve was steeper for radiation and hyperthermia than for radiation alone, indicating a decrease in the heterogeneity of tumor response with the combined therapy. Local tumor control after treatment with 40 and 45 Gy alone was 57% and 75%, whereas 100% of the tumors were controlled with 40 and 45 Gy plus hyperthermia (Gillette et al., 1987).

Several prognostic factors that influence the response of tumors to combined hyperthermia and radiation have been identified and summarized (Valdagni et al., 1988). Some major factors that influence

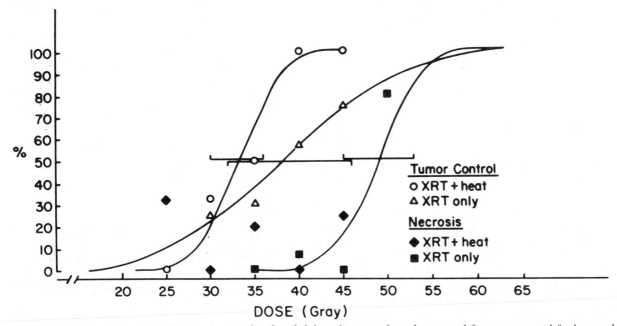

Figure 1. Dose-response curves for tumor control and probability of necrosis for radiation, and for tumor control for heat and radiation. The radiation dose required to control 50% of tumors (TCD_{50}) was 38 Gy for radiation alone and 33 Gy for radiation plus hyperthermia. The dose for 50% probability of late bone necrosis for radiation only was 49 Gy. There was no enhancement of the probability of late bone necrosis with the addition of hyperthermia to radiation. XRT, X-ray therapy. (Reprinted with permission from Gillette, E. L., et al.: Response of canine oral carcinomas to heat and radiation. Int. J. Radiat. Oncol. Biol. Phys. 13:1861, 1987.)

the complete response rates are tumor volume, tumor site for deep-seated tumors, total radiation dose, and minimum tumor temperatures. Maximum tumor temperatures appear to be correlated with complications in normal tissue. Factors that do not appear to influence the complete response rates are tumor histology, tumor site for superficial tumors, and hyperthermia treatment durations greater than 30 min. The optimal total and weekly number of heat treatments, as well as the optimal sequencing of hyperthermia to radiation, is still not known.

Hyperthermia and Chemotherapy

Many chemotherapeutic agents demonstrate significantly increased cell killing at elevated temperatures (Gautherie, 1990a). The amount of thermal enhancement of various drugs depends on the temperature achieved during hyperthermia, the rate at which the temperature is achieved, and the sequencing of drug administration to the hyperthermia treatment. For some drugs, increased thermal sensitization occurs with increasing temperature. For other drugs, there appears to be a threshold with little or no sensitization below 42 to 43°C and a large thermal enhancement above 43°C. Some drugs with no cytotoxic activity at normal temperatures become very cytotoxic at elevated temperatures.

Some common chemotherapeutic agents exhibit thermal enhancement when combined with hyperthermia. *Melphalan* (Alkeran, Burroughs Wellcome) has been used with hyperthermic limb perfusion treatment for malignant melanoma in humans. Thermal sensitization of melphalan was greater at 42°C than at 44°C, and the enhanced toxicity due to this combination was more selective for tumor than normal tissues. The effect of cyclophosphamide (Cytoxan, Bristol) and heat has been investigated in a number of studies with thermal enhancement occurring in a wide temperature range from 41 to 44°C. The greatest thermal enhancement was noted when both modalities were given simultaneously or within 30 to 60 min of each other, provided hyperthermia followed the drug administration. *Cisplatin* (Platinol, Bristol) and hyperthermia are being studied extensively *in vitro* and *in vivo*. Maximum thermal enhancement appears to occur around 42°C, with only a slight increase in enhancement above that temperature. The combination is under investigation for the treatment of metastatic disease. Cisplatin should be administered during the hyperthermia treatment or within an hour afterward. It also appears that resistance to cisplatin may be overcome when it is used at higher temperatures. *Doxorubicin* (Adriamycin, Adria) may be enhanced by hyperthermia. A threshold apparently exists for thermal enhancement of doxorubicin, with no or very little effect observed at temperatures below 42°C, and resistance to doxorubicin appears to develop during hyperthermia treatments longer than 30 to 60 min, depending on the temperature. Furthermore, the thermal enhancement of doxorubicin also decreases as the rate of temperature rise during hyperthermia is prolonged. Further investigation is needed to optimize the combination of hyperthermia and chemotherapy.

TECHNICAL ADVANCEMENTS

Hyperthermia can be categorized into three classes: (1) local hyperthermia, designed to heat small areas; (2) regional hyperthermia, designed to heat whole limbs or body cavities such as the abdomen or pelvis; and (3) systemic (whole body) hyperthermia, designed to heat the whole body. Power needed to heat tissue can be applied externally or internally using microwaves, ultrasound, or radiofrequency currents. The choice of a hyperthermia applicator for a particular patient depends on the tumor location and size. No single hyperthermia device is appropriate for all situations. Readers are referred to recent in-depth reviews of these physical techniques for further information on their advantages and disadvantages (Gautherie, 1990b, 1990c). With the multitude of heating methods available today and the constant development of new equipment by physicists and engineers, adequate training and experience of hyperthermia personnel are imperative. Several hyperthermia workshops are available for individuals wishing to learn these techniques. Information about these workshops can be obtained from the North American Hyperthermia Group, Radiation Research Society, or the American Society of Therapeutic Radiology and Oncology.

Unlike radiotherapy, in individuals receiving hyperthermia, it is impossible to prescribe a specific thermal dose. Hyperthermia treatments are limited in human patients by pain response to increased temperatures in normal tissues and in animal patients, which must be anesthetized, by temperatures monitored in surrounding normal tissues. Therefore, measurement of tissue temperature during hyperthermia is extremely important not only to assess the therapeutic value of a given treatment but also to limit complications in normal tissue.

Thermometry has advanced during the years from a single or a few stationary points measured in a tumor to manually mapped or multipoint measurements (Dewhirst et al., 1990a). Depending on the size of the tumor, from 25 to more than 100 positions can easily be monitored during hyperthermia in animal patients treated at our institution. This increase in the number of points monitored has led to decreased complications of hyperthermia in normal tissue. Methods of predicting or noninvasively measuring the temperature distribution during hyperthermia using heat transfer modeling and nuclear magnetic resonance, respectively, are currently being investigated. Although these techniques may not be used clinically in all patients during hyperthermia, they can be used to answer many questions about thermal dosimetry, tumor blood flow, and selection of an appropriate hyperthermia device.

CURRENT LIMITATIONS

Because the cytotoxic effects of hyperthermia are increased at temperatures greater than 42.5°C, an ideal treatment would be to uniformly heat tumor tissue to above this temperature. However, extensive temperature nonuniformity exists in normal and tumor tissue during local and regional hyperthermia because of tumor blood flow and nonuniform power deposition. This temperature nonuniformity in tumors and surrounding normal tissues during hyperthermia treatments significantly influences tumor response and duration of response as well as complications in normal tissue. The result

is that regions of the tumor near blood vessels remain near body core temperature during the hyperthermia treatment. Methods of increasing tumor temperatures relative to normal tissue temperatures as well as decreasing the heterogeneity of temperatures in both normal and tumor tissues are urgently being sought.

One approach to increasing tumor temperatures and their uniformity has been to combine local hyperthermia with whole-body hyperthermia. During whole-body hyperthermia, the entire body temperature is elevated to approximately 42°C and should result in more uniform tumor temperatures than local or regional hyperthermia techniques. However, temperatures are limited to 42°C or less because of systemic toxicities. By combining whole-body hyperthermia with local hyperthermia, tumor temperature minima have been raised to about 41°C, which is a vast improvement over local hyperthermia alone (Thrall et al., 1990) (Fig. 2). Clinical protocols comparing the efficacy of radiation combined with either local hyperthermia alone or whole-body hyperthermia plus local hyperthermia are currently under way.

Another approach to increasing tumor tempera-

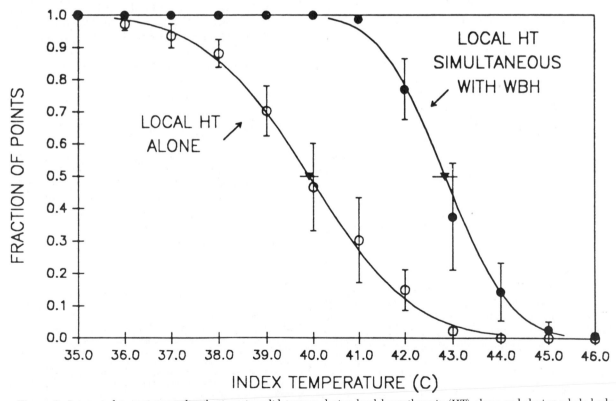

Figure 2. Integrated temperature distributions in solid tumors during local hyperthermia (HT) alone and during whole-body hyperthermia (WBH) and local hyperthermia given simultaneously. Data points are mean values from the five dogs, and error bars are standard error of the mean. Inverted triangles and associated horizontal lines represent the estimated median temperatures and 95% confidence intervals. Simultaneous administration of local and whole-body hyperthermia resulted in higher and more homogeneous temperatures in solid tumors than local hyperthermia alone. (Reprinted with permission from Thrall, D. E., et al.: A comparison of temperatures in canine solid tumours during local and whole-body hyperthermia administered alone and simultaneously. Int. J. Hyperthermia 6:305, 1990.)

tures is to lower tumor blood flow preferentially, thereby decreasing heat loss from the tumor and concurrently increasing temperatures. Vasoactive agents such as hydralazine have been used in both humans and animals to alter tumor temperature distributions during hyperthermia treatment. Because of its prolonged action, the use of orally administered hydralazine in normotensive human patients can lead to side effects such as postural hypotension, nausea, and headaches. Lower doses have been investigated but are ineffective in increasing tumor temperatures (Dewhirst et al., 1990b). Therefore, alternative shorter-acting intravenous vasodilating agents, such as sodium nitroprusside (Nitropress, Abbott), are currently being investigated.

Sodium nitroprusside causes peripheral vasodilation via direct action on vascular smooth muscle. It is administered as an intravenous infusion (0.5 to 10 μg/kg/min) to effect while monitoring arterial blood pressure. When the infusion is stopped, the hypotensive effect dissipates within minutes. Although overdose and prolonged continuous use of this drug can cause cyanide toxicity, sodium nitroprusside infusions during hyperthermia treatments last from 30 to 90 min and should not lead to this problem.

Sodium nitroprusside has been safely administered to tumor-bearing pet dogs during local hyperthermia treatments. Preliminary results show a significant increase in the tumor temperature distribution when sodium nitroprusside is used during hyperthermia. The average tumor temperature increased by approximately 1.5°C, and the minimum tumor temperature increased by approximately 1.0°C. Although there was some temperature increase in normal tissues as well with sodium nitroprusside administration, no toxicities were noted in these initial studies. Further investigations of other vasoactive drugs to manipulate tumor blood flow are currently under way.

Because hyperthermia is more effective against acidic, nutritionally deprived tumor cells, several investigators are trying to manipulate the metabolic status of tumors to enhance thermal cytotoxicity. Administration of glucose to decrease tumor pH, use of lonidamine to interfere with tumor energy metabolism, and depletion of glutathione or polyamines or both are just a few methods now under investigation. Optimization of hyperthermia treatments clinically using the techniques discussed as well as others is likely in future clinical trials.

CURRENT INDICATIONS IN THE VETERINARY COMMUNITY

Hyperthermia has been used in combination with radiation, chemotherapy, and surgery to treat various pet animal tumors. Most recent interest has been in combining hyperthermia with radiation. Although radiotherapy is increasingly available in veterinary medicine and can now be performed at many veterinary schools and some private practices, hyperthermia is offered at only a few of these locations. However, some radiation oncologists at human medical centers are interested in working with veterinarians in the treatment of animal tumors and may be able to offer hyperthermia as well as radiation.

The combination of radiation and hyperthermia can be used to treat various histologic types of tumors including squamous cell carcinoma, fibrosarcoma, melanoma, hemangiopericytoma, liposarcoma, neurofibrosarcoma, leiomyosarcoma, and others. These tumors can be treated in many locations of the body, provided adequate hyperthermia equipment is available. The combination of hyperthermia with radiation appears to enhance control of larger tumor volumes more than smaller volumes; radiation alone can often control small tumor volumes.

Although surgery remains the primary treatment for many cancers in animals, veterinarians must be aware of its limitations. Therefore, when surgery is likely to provide limited local control or will result in severe cosmetic, anatomic, or functional loss, other forms of cancer therapy should be considered. Veterinarians also should consider the use of radiation and hyperthermia to reduce large tumor burdens before surgery.

As the public becomes more aware of the various cancer therapies, their demand for more aggressive treatment for their pets will increase. It is important that veterinarians be aware of new modalities being tested for the treatment of cancer and consider them as alternatives to surgery alone. However, remember that the use of hyperthermia in combination with radiation or chemotherapy is still investigational, and only after these combinations have been tested in appropriate clinical trials should they be attempted in private practices.

References and Suggested Reading

Dewhirst, M. W., Connor, C. G., and Sim, D. A.: Preliminary results of a phase III trial of spontaneous animal tumors to heat and/or radiation: Early normal tissue response and tumor volume influence on initial response. Int. J. Radiat. Oncol. Biol. Phys. 8:1951, 1982.
A prospective study comparing the response of malignant tumors in 77 dogs and cats to hyperthermia and radiation alone with these two modalities combined.
Dewhirst, M. W., Philips, T. L., Samulski, T. V., et al.: RTOG quality assurance guidelines for clinical trials using hyperthermia. Int. J. Radiat. Oncol. Biol. Phys. 18:1249, 1990a.
A summary of the current recommendations for quality assurance for the administration of hyperthermia to patients.
Dewhirst, M. W., Prescott, D. M., Clegg, S., et al.: The use of hydralazine to manipulate tumor temperatures during hyperthermia. Int. J. Hyperthermia 6:971, 1990b.

Results of low-dose hydralazine on tumor temperatures during local hyperthermia in humans and canines.

Dewhirst, M. W., Sim, D. A., Wilson, S., et al.: Correlation between initial and long-term responses of spontaneous pet animal tumors to heat and radiation or radiation alone. Cancer Res. 43:5735, 1983.
A prospective trial comparing response rates for hyperthermia and radiation with those for radiation alone in 130 pet animals.

Gautherie, M.: *Biological Basis of Oncologic Thermotherapy.* Berlin: Springer-Verlag, 1990a.
A review of the biologic and pathophysiologic basis of hyperthermia and its interactions with radiation and chemotherapy.

Gautherie, M.: *Interstitial, Endocavitary and Perfusional Hyperthermia.* Berlin: Springer-Verlag, 1990b.
A review of the technical and clinical state of the art in interstitial hyperthermia and other forms of internal hyperthermia.

Gautherie, M.: *Methods of External Hyperthermic Heating.* Berlin: Springer-Verlag, 1990c.
A review of the electromagnetic and acoustic methods of external hyperthermia.

Gillette, E. L., McChesney, S. L., Dewhirst, M. W., et al.: Response of canine oral carcinomas to heat and radiation. Int. J. Radiat. Oncol. Biol. Phys. 13:1861, 1987.
A prospective study of 38 dogs with oral squamous cell carcinoma using various doses of radiation alone and combined with hyperthermia.

Overgaard, J.: Rationale and problems in the design of clinical studies. In Overgaard, J. (ed.): *Hyperthermic Oncology.* Vol. 2. London: Taylor and Francis, 1984, p. 325.
A review of past clinical results and the need for future clinical trials using hyperthermia in combination with radiation and chemotherapy.

Thrall, D. E., Dewhirst, M. W., Page, R. L., et al.: A comparison of temperatures in canine solid tumours during local and whole-body hyperthermia administered alone and simultaneously. Int. J. Hyperthermia 6:305, 1990.
A comparison of temperature distributions in canine tumors during local and whole-body hyperthermia alone and combined.

Valdagni, R., Liu, F., and Kapp, D. S.: Important prognostic factors influencing outcome of combined radiation and hyperthermia. Int. J. Radiat. Oncol. Biol. Phys. 15:959, 1988.
A review of currently important parameters that may influence the response of tumors to hyperthermia and radiation.

STRATEGIES TO ENHANCE TUMOR RADIORESPONSIVENESS

DONALD E. THRALL

Raleigh, North Carolina

The response of tumors and normal tissues to radiation is characterized by sigmoid dose-response curves (Fig. 1). These curves imply that some minimum dose must be administered before any perceivable response is obtained. Thereafter, as additional dose is applied, the rate of response rises quickly, after which an increased dose provides no additional benefit.

The agent for which dose is expressed on the x axis can be modalities other than radiation. For example, one could depict probability of response versus chemotherapy dose, and the resultant curve would be similar to that in Figure 1. Doses of agents in combination could also be illustrated in this manner. What should be apparent from evaluation of sigmoid dose-response curves is that it is possible, assuming the normal tissue curve is to the right of the tumor curve, to administer a "dose" of some agent or agents sufficient to control a relatively large number of tumors without also producing unacceptable levels of complications in normal tissues. The purpose of this article is to discuss the limitations of radiation as a cancer treatment agent and how improvements in radiation response of tumors can be achieved. The rationale for the use of radiation as a cancer treatment modality is described elsewhere (Thrall, 1982).

LIMITATIONS OF RADIATION THERAPY

Radiation has been in use for treatment of cancer in animals since the early 1900's. Radiation has primarily been used alone, often after other modalities, particularly surgery, have failed to control the tumor. In addition, because animals must be anesthetized or tranquilized for irradiation, the empirical time-dose schemes that have been developed during the years have been composed of a total of 10 to 12 treatments, usually given three times a week on a Monday-Wednesday-Friday schedule. Doses per fraction typically were in the range of 4 to 5 Gy.

When one reviews results of irradiation of animal tumors with these coarse time-dose fractionation schemes, it is apparent that overall long-term control rates could be improved (Thrall and Dewhirst, 1989). Possible reasons for the poor responses thus far obtained include (1) the use of total radiation doses that were too low, (2) the presence of radioresistant tumor cells, (3) the deleterious effect of tumor volume, and (4) the tendency to use single agents, one after another as the preceding one fails, rather than a preplanned strategic combination of multiple agents. Improvement in each of these categories is possible.

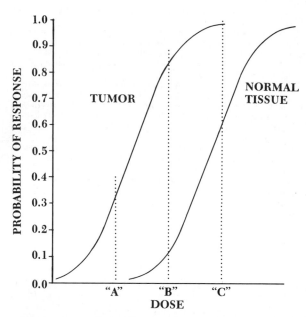

Figure 1. Hypothetical dose-response curves, in which probability of response is plotted as a function of dose, for normal and tumor tissue. Under actual conditions, the slope of the tumor curve is probably not as steep as shown here (see Thrall et al. [1989] for a more complete discussion). The normal tissue curve is to the right of the tumor curve. If this is not the case, no tumor could be cured without unacceptable levels of complications in normal tissue. The agent on the x axis could be radiation, chemotherapy, or a combination of agents. At dose "A," a relatively low number of tumors would be cured, but there would be no serious complications in normal tissue. At dose "B," the tumor response increases dramatically and there is now a small likelihood of complications in normal tissue. At dose "C," tumor response increases only slightly, but there has been a dramatic increase in complications in normal tissue. Assuming that dose "A" represents radiation therapy, one could move to dose "B" by giving radiation in a more effective manner or, for example, by combining radiation with chemotherapy, hyperthermia, or surgery. Careful evaluation of results will be necessary to assure that dose is not increased to the point where normal tissue responses become unacceptable (i.e., dose "C").

The Radiation Dose Issue

Total radiation doses used for treatment of cancer in animals have been coarsely fractionated and low in magnitude compared with those routinely in use for treatment of cancer in humans. One must be cautious in making direct comparisons between treatment of humans and animals, but the poor responses obtained by physicians in treating humans with doses similar to those used in animals, plus the poor results thus far obtained in treatment of cancer in animals, suggest that 40 to 50 Gy, given in 4 to 5 Gy fractions in a three-per-week schedule, is too low. Increasing total radiation dose can be accomplished in several ways.

HIGHER FRACTIONAL DOSES

Higher total doses could be administered without extending overall treatment time by simply admin-

istering higher doses at each treatment. *This method absolutely cannot be recommended.* Evidence from laboratory experimentation and clinical evidence regarding use of large doses per fraction in treatment of cancer in humans support the hypothesis that large doses per fraction result in a disproportionately high incidence of complications in normal tissue. Therefore, an increase in size of dose per fraction does not provide a viable alternative for increasing total dose. In fact, currently used fractional doses of 4 Gy are larger than desired and should be reduced.

INCREASED NUMBER OF FRACTIONS

A larger total dose could be administered by increasing the number of fractions. This idea has not been met with enthusiasm by veterinarians because of the requisite increase in number of anesthetic procedures and demands placed on technical help. However, increasing the number of fractions represents the only viable method by which the total radiation dose can be increased. Modern anesthetic procedures allow anesthesia to be done safely on a daily basis.

Further, increasing the number of fractions should be done by giving more fractions per week rather than by extending overall treatment time, because as treatment time becomes protracted, significant amounts of radiation damage can be offset by proliferation of tumor cells during treatment. However, as mentioned earlier, an increase in the number of fractions without decreasing the fractional dose cannot be recommended because this method carries an increased risk of complications in normal tissue.

It is my opinion that for solid tumors a total dose of 55 to 60 Gy, given in 2.5 to 3.0 Gy daily fractions, over a period of approximately 4 to 5 weeks is a reasonable time-dose scheme to investigate. The total dose is higher than that used in the past, and the fractional dose is lower, thereby reducing the probability of late complications; the total time is reasonable from a patient management standpoint. It may be difficult to administer more aggressive radiation therapy to animals without an undesirably long overall treatment time and also because of the limitations of normal tissue responses. To more completely understand the role of radiation therapy in the management of solid tumors in animals, it will be necessary over the next few years to carefully assess such time-dose schemes as described in this paragraph.

Radioresistant Tumor Cells

INHERENT TUMOR CELL RADIOSENSITIVITY

When the results of a biopsy of a tumor mass become available, there is a tendency to form prognostic assessments based on histologic tumor type. Although histologic type must be known before treatment and such information is valuable in anticipating biologic behavior, in the author's opinion the histologic type of tumor has little significance in terms of predicting response to irradiation.

Although the tendency is to lump certain tumors into radioresistant versus radiosensitive categories based on histologic findings, these categorizations are inaccurate. It has been shown that within groups of tumors of the same histologic type, there is a considerable range of inherent cellular radiosensitivities.

Although methods for assessing inherent cellular radiosensitivity are available, they are not in routine use. Until such methods are in use, the exact role of inherent tumor cell radiosensitivity will remain cloudy. What is important to realize is that accurate prediction of tumor response to treatment should not be based on histopathologic assessment of tumor type.

HYPOXIA

In addition to inherent factors, tumor cell radioresistance is a function of local tissue oxygenation. It has been known for many years that there are regions in solid tumors where tissue oxygenation is reduced, primarily as a result of a mismatch between perfusion and oxygen demand. It is also known that cells that are at reduced oxygen tension are radioresistant. Therefore, a potentially disadvantageous situation exists when some tumor cells are less radiosensitive than normal tissue because of hypoxia. The hypoxia issue has been debated for many years. Some hypoxic cells are probably killed with each radiation fraction, even though the percentage of hypoxic cells killed is less than with oxygenated cells. In addition, hypoxic cells surviving a radiation fraction may become reoxygenated between fractions as a result of revascularization or decreased utilization of oxygen by other lethally irradiated cells. These reoxygenated cells are more likely to be killed by subsequent radiation fractions. Unfortunately, it is still unclear in exactly what situations hypoxia has a significant role in contributing to radiation failures. Some of this uncertainty has resulted from the inability to identify or assess hypoxia in spontaneous solid tumors. Markers of hypoxia that can be detected by immunohistochemical means have been developed, and these have been shown to bind to spontaneous tumors in dogs in a manner consistent with the presence of hypoxia (Cline et al., 1990). Therefore, by careful study of hypoxia in canine tumors, it may be possible to determine if hypoxia plays a part in radiation failures or, alternatively, if specific strategies to kill hypoxic cells can be developed.

The Deleterious Effect of Tumor Volume

A major goal of clinicians treating cancer often is to make the tumor disappear completely. This is gratifying, but one must realize that such a gross response may result from killing only a small fraction of tumor cells present. For example, a tumor is not usually detectable grossly until it reaches approximately 1 cm in diameter. At this time, the tumor contains on the order of 10^9 cells. More typically, tumors are larger when treated and contain between 10^{10} and 10^{11} cells. If one treats a tumor with 10^{11} cells and is successful in killing (by radiation or drugs) or removing (by surgery) 99.9% of the cells (0.1% remaining), the tumor will be undetectable grossly. However, the tumor still contains 10^8 cells ($10^{11} \times 0.1\%$) and will recur. Therefore, the goal of treating solid tumors, whether the treatment is with radiation, surgery, or anticancer agents, should be eradication of all tumor cells, not just the majority.

Use of radiation in higher doses or in conjunction with other modalities is helpful in maximizing tumor cell kill. In addition, concentrated efforts should be made to treat solid tumors when they are as small as possible, because moderate increases in volume can dramatically affect prognosis because of the overall larger number of cells to kill.

Multimodality Cancer Treatment

RADIATION AND CHEMOTHERAPEUTIC AGENTS

There has been little investigation of the combination of radiation and chemotherapeutic agents in animal tumors. There are two possible advantages of such a combination. The first and most commonly cited one is the expectation of some synergistic or supra-additive effect. Although there may be situations in which these interactions are possible, this would be unlikely. An alternative advantage of combining radiation and chemotherapeutic agents would be to increase the "dose" of anticancer therapy administered (see Fig. 1). In this latter situation, and as long as the two agents were not antagonistic, tumor response could be improved without any supra-additive interaction because of the additional cytotoxicity provided by the chemotherapeutic agent.

A major concern in combining radiation and chemotherapeutic agents is enhanced toxicity to normal tissues. Therefore, drug doses may have to be reduced. However, as mentioned earlier, addition of any amount of cytotoxic drug to the conventional dose of radiation may improve tumor response. Both cisplatin and doxorubicin have been used in combination with radiation for treatment of animal tumors. These chemotherapeutic agents are among the more effective against solid tumors and represent logical choices for further investigation.

RADIATION AND HYPERTHERMIA

There is sound biologic rationale for the combination of radiation and hyperthermia (see p. 418; Dewhirst et al., 1989). Briefly, hyperthermia has the potential to (1) kill tumor cells, (2) inhibit the repair of sublethal radiation injury, (3) enhance radiation cytotoxicity, and (4) improve tumor energy status, making tumors more responsive to radiation or chemotherapeutic agents. The full potential of hyperthermia to augment radiation response of solid tumors has been impossible to assess because of the technical limitations in adequately heating most solid tumors. In most instances, heterogeneities of power deposition and of intratumoral blood flow result in extremely nonuniform intratumoral temperatures. These nonuniform intratumoral temperatures make quantification of thermal dose extremely inexact and also make it difficult to assess hyperthermia effects.

Dewhirst and Sim (1984), using radiation and hyperthermia in canine and feline tumors, were the first to show the prognostic importance of minimum intratumoral temperature in predicting response to treatment. A new method for heating solid tumors using the combination of local and whole-body hyperthermia has been assessed in canine tumors (Thrall et al., 1990). This new method, because it increases the temperature of blood circulating through the tumor, results in higher and more uniform intratumoral temperatures (i.e., higher temperature minima) than can be obtained with most local hyperthermia techniques. This heating method in conjunction with radiation has the potential to affect positively the management of soft-tissue tumors in animals and humans.

RADIATION AND SURGERY

In the past, radiation and surgery were often used in the same patient but at different times, when tumors recurred after surgery and were treated with radiation as a salvage procedure. This clearly is not the optimal method of combining the two modalities. Ideally, the most aggressive treatment protocol possible should be administered initially rather than waiting for one modality to fail before instituting another. The more times a tumor is treated and recurs, the more refractory to treatment it becomes.

In a preplanned sense, radiation can be combined with surgery in either a preoperative or postoperative manner (McLeod and Thrall, 1989). Postoperative irradiation has been used most often in animals, and this combination has been shown to have some success in canine nasal cavity tumors, for example (Adams et al., 1987). Unfortunately, the use of preoperative irradiation has not been given as much attention. There are advantages to giving the radiation before surgery, however, particularly in the treatment of soft-tissue tumors: (1) irradiated volume may be smaller when radiation is given before surgery, (2) conservative resections of large tumors may be possible, and (3) metastasis to distant sites may be less likely (McLeod and Thrall, 1989).

There is a need for more complete assessment of the combination of radiation and surgery, with particular attention given to preoperative irradiation. The optimal combination of radiation and surgery requires cooperation between radiation and surgical oncologists and careful preplanning of the treatment strategy. Use of preoperative irradiation has the potential to drastically improve management of tumors such as soft-tissue sarcomas and mast cell tumors.

SUMMARY

Radiation therapy is not optimally applied in veterinary medicine. In this article, methods that may make radiation therapy by itself a more effective treatment were described. In addition, methods for combining radiation with other treatment modalities were discussed, with the hope that these will be assessed in a prospective manner by researchers interested in improving the results of cancer treatment in animals.

References and Suggested Reading

Adams, W. M., Withrow, S. J., Walshaw, R., et al.: Radiotherapy of malignant nasal tumors in 67 dogs. J.A.V.M.A., 191:311, 1987.

Cline, J. M., Thrall, D. E., Page, R. L., et al.: Immunohistochemical detection of a hypoxia marker in spontaneous canine tumors. Br. J. Cancer 62:925, 1990.

Dewhirst, M. W., Page, R. L., and Thrall, D. E.: Hyperthermia. In Withrow, S. J., and MacEwen, E. G. (eds.): Clinical Veterinary Oncology. Philadelphia: J. B. Lippincott, 1989, p. 113.

Dewhirst, M. W., and Sim, D. A.: The utility of thermal dose as a predictor of tumor and normal tissue responses to combined radiation and hyperthermia. Cancer Res. 44(suppl.):4772, 1984.

McLeod, D. A., and Thrall, D. E.: The combination of surgery and radiation in the treatment of cancer—a review. Vet. Surg. 18:1, 1989.

Thrall, D. E.: Radiation therapy in the dog: Principles, indications and complications. Comp. Cont. Ed. Pract. Vet. 4:652, 1982.

Thrall, D. E., and Dewhirst, M. W.: Radiation therapy. In Withrow, S. J., and MacEwen, E. G. (eds.): Clinical Veterinary Oncology. Philadelphia: J. B. Lippincott, 1989, p. 79.

Thrall, D. E., Dewhirst, M. W., Page, R. L., et al.: A comparison of temperatures in canine solid tumours during local and whole-body hyperthermia administered alone and simultaneously. Int. J. Hyperthermia 6:305, 1990.

Thrall, D. R., McLeod, D. A., Bentel, G. C., et al.: A review of treatment planning and dose calculation in veterinary radiation oncology. Vet. Radiol. 30:194, 1989.

CURRENT STRATEGIES
FOR MANAGEMENT OF
METASTATIC DISEASE

E. G. MacEWEN
and E. T. KELLER
Madison, Wisconsin

Metastasis is one of the major causes for mortality in veterinary patients afflicted with cancer. As we learn more about the biology of metastatic disease, we gain greater insight into possible mechanisms for prevention, detection, and therapy of metastasis. Reports regarding the management of tumor metastases are sparse in the veterinary literature, whereas the human literature abounds with clinical trials in regard to metastases.

A basic review of metastatic biology will help guide the clinician in strategic manipulation of metastasis. In general, metastasis occurs as a multistep process involving an ordered sequence of events. This is referred to as the metastatic cascade. Initially, cells detach from the primary tumor and enter the vascular system. These cells are then transported throughout the body, evading host defense mechanisms. They eventually aggregate with platelets and fibrin and arrest within the vascular system. Neoplastic cells then extravasate through the endothelium into the surrounding parenchyma, where they must successfully implant in order to grow. This is considered an inefficient mechanism, since mouse models and human studies demonstrate that when large numbers of tumor cells are within the vascular system, only a small amount (less than 1%) actually form viable metastases. The process of metastasis is selective, and metastases are produced by the nonrandom dissemination and establishment of specialized subpopulations of cells present in the primary tumor. Neoplasms are inherently heterogeneous, and metastatic cells are genetically unstable and rapidly develop resistance to chemotherapy. The successful treatment of metastatic disease will require the development of new strategies with a spectrum of activity that overcomes the existing cellular diversity.

Many neoplasms seen in veterinary medicine are well known for developing metastases. The more common tumors include mammary adenocarcinomas, hemangiosarcomas, osteosarcomas, prostatic adenocarcinomas, and malignant melanomas. Certain organs are also more frequent targets for metastatic disease. The most common sites are lymph node, lung, liver, bone, and brain. This article examines management of metastatic disease of these and other organ systems. Most methods discussed are suggested ideas or based on human studies, since treatment of metastatic disease in veterinary patients has rarely been reported.

Finally, when treating metastatic disease, one must take into account the overall spread of metastases. For example, it would be inappropriate to amputate the leg of a dog with bone metastases if there were multiple other metastases that could not be controlled. Some suggested guidelines and indications for treatment of metastatic disease follow.

SKELETAL METASTASES

Seventeen percent of dogs with malignant tumors and visceral metastasis also have skeletal metastasis. The most common sites for skeletal metastasis are the humerus, femur, and vertebral column. The tumors most frequently associated with skeletal metastasis are mammary, prostate, and thyroid carcinomas, and hemangiosarcomas. Diagnosis of metastatic lesions may be obtained by either radiology or nuclear scintigraphy. Bone scintigraphy allows for early detection of metastases as compared with radiology.

Various surgical regimens may be applicable for control of skeletal metastatic disease. These include limb amputation, tumor curettage combined with internal fixation, segmental resection of bone with a polymethylmethacrylate bone prosthesis, or cryosurgery. Perhaps the most applicable method being performed in veterinary medicine currently is that of the limb salvage procedure. This is used mainly for primary osteosarcomas of the long bones and involves resection of the tumor and replacement of bone with a cortical bone allograft (Thrall, 1990).

Radiation therapy may be used for pain relief from skeletal metastases. The underlying radiosensitivity of the primary tumor will determine if radiation will actually inhibit tumor growth. Currently, we use a total dose of 3000 rads divided into three treatments on days 1, 7, and 21 for primary bone tumors to palliate pain. Effects are usually seen in 1 to 2 weeks and last for several months. This technique may also be suitable for metastatic lesions. Internally administered isotopes are now being evaluated in human medicine for treatment of skeletal metastases. The most promising isotope is samarium-153-EDTMP, a beta emitter, which has a short half-life (46.27 hours) and an avidity for bone involved with cancer.

LYMPH NODE METASTASES

The lymph node is often considered the first barrier to widespread metastatic disease. It is recognized that the draining regional lymph node of a tumor is responsible for both initiation and maintenance of immunity and reactivity to the tumor. In accordance with the important role the lymph node plays, it also often becomes infiltrated with metastatic disease.

If just regional nodes are involved, *en bloc* surgical resection of primary tumor and nodes may be curative. Wide surgical margins should be resected and evaluated histologically for "clean" borders. Surgery can be followed by radiation therapy for any microscopic disease left behind.

Radiation therapy can be used for unresectable lymph node metastasis. Radiation therapy has been described for treatment of seminoma with unresectable metastasis to the iliac lymph nodes in dogs (McDonald, 1988). Cesium-137 teleradiotherapy with a dose of between 17 to 40 Gy in eight to ten fractions, with three fractions weekly, was effective in controlling the metastatic lesions.

Other methods that have been used for treatment of lymph node metastases include transnodal (into the lymph node) injection of chemotherapeutic agents and administration of activated carbon particles with adsorbed anticancer agents. Transnodal injection was used in humans for esophageal carcinoma in which multiple metastatic intrathoracic nodes were impossible to dissect. Humans receiving an intraoperative injection of bleomycin emulsion into the pulmonary hilar nodes demonstrated a decreased recurrence rate of tumor in the nodes compared with controls (Natsuda, 1983). As for the other method, carbon particles with various chemotherapeutic agents adsorbed to them were injected, via gastroscopy, into the gastric walls of patients suffering from gastric carcinoma 2 to 7 days preoperatively. Gastric and regional lymph node resection was performed, and the lymph nodes were analyzed for carbon particle concentration. The authors of this study concluded that this dosage form concentrated the drugs in the regional lymph nodes and hence increased effects of drug on lymph node metastasis and decreased systemic toxicity (Hagiwara, 1985). These are both methods that initially

used dogs as models and certainly could be applicable to lymph node metastases in the dog.

Intravenous cisplatin chemotherapy has been reported to achieve complete remission of digital squamous cell carcinoma metastatic to the popliteal and iliac lymph nodes of a dog (Himsel, 1986). This supports the idea of using intravenous chemotherapy for metastases from primary tumors that have demonstrated sensitivity to chemotherapy.

BRAIN METASTASES

Several exciting innovations in veterinary medicine have been used for treatment of brain tumors and may be applied to metastatic brain lesions also. Radiation therapy using external beam, megavoltage irradiation is used to treat primary tumors. Doses of 4000 to 4800 rads given in 10 to 12 fractions over 22 to 26 days have shown promising results at several veterinary institutions (LeCouteur, 1986). Perhaps radiation therapy would be useful to decrease the effects of multiple small brain metastases.

Immunotherapy has recently been experimentally evaluated for treatment of brain tumors in dogs (Ingram, 1990). Peripheral blood cells are removed ten days prior to surgery for the brain tumor. Lymphocytes are isolated and stimulated with recombinant interleukin-2 (IL-2) *in vitro* (IL-2 stimulates lymphocytes to have increased efficacy of tumor cell killing; these activated lymphocytes are called lymphokine-activated killer cells, or LAK cells). These autologous LAK cells are then transplanted into the tumor bed after surgical removal of the tumor. They may also be injected intracisternally for added effect. Preliminary results are encouraging, with negative CT scans observed for many months after therapy.

Surgical removal of solitary brain metastases can be successfully performed in over 80% of selected human patients. Rigid selection criteria have been suggested for surgery of brain metastatic disease. These include a solitary lesion, limited central neurologic impairment, minimal extra–central nervous system disease, and a long interval from the diagnosis of primary cancer to dissemination in the brain. Recently, humans undergoing excision of brain metastases from malignant melanoma demonstrated minimal morbidity and increased survival (median, 10 months) compared with those treated by radiation therapy or chemotherapy alone (median, 4 months) or those untreated (median, 1 month). These data argue that dogs with individual brain metastases may also benefit from surgical excision. It has been suggested that the combination of surgery and radiation therapy has greater efficacy than surgery alone.

Chemotherapy of brain tumors in humans and dogs is primarily limited to adjuvant therapy. Difficulties encountered include the blood-brain barrier (BBB) and the microenvironment of the brain. These factors are also applicable to metastases. Nitrosoureas are a class of drugs that cross the BBB in sufficient amounts to be partially effective against some brain tumors. Anecdotal reports using carmustine (BCNU) for the treatment of various brain tumors state that this drug successfully decreased clinical signs or tumor size in several veterinary patients. Perhaps the most important chemotherapy for dogs with CNS metastatic disease is symptomatic. Glucocorticoids to decrease brain swelling and phenobarbital to control seizures are probably the most efficacious way to palliate clinical signs for dogs with multiple brain metastases.

PULMONARY METASTASES

Pulmonary metastases are very common for most tumor types. A recent evaluation of pulmonary metastases based on radiographs taken at initial presentation disclosed that dogs with thyroid cell carcinomas and urinary bladder transitional cell carcinomas are particularly prone to the development of early metastatic disease.

Methods to treat pulmonary metastases in veterinary medicine have focused primarily on surgical resection of osteosarcoma metastases. Long-term disease-free survival for approximately 25% of dogs taken to surgery for pulmonary metastasectomy has been reported. Selection criteria included (1) primary tumor under control, (2) fewer than six radiographically visible nodules, (3) no tumor known to be present outside the chest, and (4) tumor diameter doubling time of greater than 40 days. These guidelines could be applied to other metastatic tumors as well. A similar study in humans demonstrated that chemotherapy alone versus surgery was associated with significantly shorter survival times.

Chemotherapy for metastases of tumors other than osteosarcoma may be beneficial. Combination doxorubicin HCl and cyclophosphamide chemotherapy has achieved complete and partial responses in some cats with pulmonary metastases secondary to mammary adenocarcinoma (Jeglum, 1985). For cats with mammary adenocarcinoma with pulmonary metastases that have not yet received chemotherapy (e.g., only surgical resection was performed on the primary tumor), we recommend attempting chemotherapeutic treatment.

Pleural effusion secondary to metastases is a not uncommon presentation of neoplasia. Recently, management of a malignant pleural effusion secondary to metastatic adenocarcinoma of unknown origin was reported in a dog (Shapiro, 1988). Initially, intermittent thoracocentesis and systemic chemotherapy, using a variety of chemotherapeutic agents, including vincristine, doxorubicin, cyclophosphamide, chlorambucil, and cisplatin, palliated clinical signs. Eventually, upon recurrence, chromic phosphate P32 (0.25 mCi/kg) was injected into the pleural space, which maintained the dog free of pleural effusion for 14 weeks. This approach underscores the creativity one must use when attempting to manage metastatic disease.

HEPATIC METASTASES

The liver is very susceptible to metastatic disease because it receives blood supply from both the hepatic artery and the portal vein and therefore has increased exposure to tumor metastases. The most common metastatic tumors identified in the liver are from gastrointestinal tract tumors, hemangiosarcomas, pancreatic tumors, and mammary adenocarcinomas.

The first line of treatment for liver metastasis is surgical resection if possible. Resection of multiple metastases is possible and may either palliate disease or, rarely, increase survival. Unfortunately, by the time liver metastases are detected, they are usually unresectable. Surgical resection of more than four hepatic metastases from colorectal cancer is associated with a very poor prognosis in humans.

Hepatic metastases are considered unresectable if (1) the patient cannot undergo prolonged anesthesia; (2) there are more than four lesions; or (3) there is extensive hepatic replacement by tumor. Unresectable metastases are treated by a variety of methods in humans, which may be applicable to veterinary patients (Levitan and Hughes, 1990). Systemic chemotherapy may be attempted using drugs that are selected based on their efficacy against the primary tumor. Regional chemotherapy can deliver higher doses of drugs to the liver than can be obtained systemically. Both the hepatic artery and the portal vein may be used for access to the liver. In humans it has been reported that liver metastases derive the majority of their blood supply from the hepatic artery, whereas normal liver parenchyma derives the majority from the portal vein. Therefore, it would seem that intra-arterial infusion of drugs would be more effective at delivering drugs directly to the metastases. This unique blood supply also supports the concept of hepatic arterial ligation to destroy tumor blood supply while leaving the blood supply to normal hepatic tissue minimally compromised.

Hepatic irradiation may be helpful for palliative treatment or as a last resort for tumors unresponsive to chemotherapy or surgery. Published randomized prospective clinical trials of this therapeutic modality for treatment of liver metastases are sparse.

METASTASES OF UNKNOWN ORIGIN

We define metastases of unknown origin (MUO) as a metastatic solid tumor for which a primary tumor site cannot be identified after a thorough history, physical examination, basic laboratory testing (including serum chemistry profiles, urinalysis, and complete blood count), noncontrast abdominal and thoracic radiographs, and histopathologic evaluation of biopsy material.

When presented with a patient with MUO, the clinician needs to assess how critical it is to locate the primary tumor. The answer to this query would be based on how management of the primary tumor would aid in patient care. In many instances identity of a primary tumor will have no effect on morbidity and survival. This concept is important, since undertaking a search for a primary tumor may often be expensive and may cause patient discomfort and owner anxiety.

The most important step in patient management is to obtain an accurate histologic diagnosis. Biopsied material should be saved in three portions as follows: formalin for light microscopy, snap frozen for immunohistochemistry, and glutaraldehyde for electron microscopy. As advances in the latter two areas are made in veterinary medicine, these methodologies will have increasing clinical utility. The pathologist and the clinician should work closely together to gain the most information from the biopsy sample. Identification of the tumor type may help direct further diagnostic tests. Also, if a tumor type is identified that is not responsive to current therapies, further search for a primary tumor is generally not warranted.

Specific strategies to identify a primary site include thorough evaluation of the oral cavity, including the nasopharynx and tonsils; thyroid gland; kidney; pancreas; spleen; prostate; and mammary glands for MUO. This can be performed by contrast radiology, endoscopy, computed tomography (CT) scanning, and ultrasonography. Biopsy of any suspicious lesions may be rewarding.

SYSTEMIC THERAPY FOR MICROMETASTATIC DISEASE

Many solid tumors, including osteosarcoma, hemangiosarcoma, and advanced mammary cancer, are now considered systemic or metastatic at the time of diagnosis. A logical consequence of the concept of micrometastatic disease has been the development of combined modality therapy in which local therapy consisting of surgery or radiation therapy is supplemented with adjunctive systemic therapy ("adjuvant therapy"). The rationale for the use of adjuvant therapy is derived from (1) observations that chemotherapy or immunotherapy

Table 1. *Summary of Selected Adjuvant Chemotherapy or Immunotherapy Trials That Demonstrated Prolonged Survival*

Treatment	Tumor
Cisplatin	Osteosarcoma
Cisplatin + doxorubicin	Osteosarcoma
Doxorubicin + cyclophosphamide + vincristine	Hemangiosarcoma
Corynebacterium parvum	Oral melanoma
Liposome MTP-PE	Osteosarcoma

agents have achieved objective reductions in tumor size or have increased the disease-free survival time and (2) studies in experimental animal models indicate that once a primary tumor reaches 1 cm in diameter, the minimum size at which many tumors can be diagnosed by physical examination, it has undergone at least 30 tumor doubling times. The "Goldie-Coldman" hypothesis suggests that the resistance of cells to drugs increases directly with the number of spontaneous mutations and that drug resistance from these mutations is far more likely in advanced versus early neoplasms (Goldie and Coldman, 1986). It therefore makes sense, at least theoretically, to use adjuvant therapy as early as possible in order to eradicate the tumor cells before they have a chance to develop spontaneous drug resistance. Clinical trials in veterinary oncology to evaluate adjuvant therapy have been limited. Table 1 summarizes the most current approaches used today.

NEW APPROACHES TO TREAT METASTASES

The successful approach to the therapy of neoplasms and their metastases may involve the activation of tumoricidal properties of the host's own immune responses (immunotherapy). One area of interest in particular is tumoricidal activation of the host's own macrophages. Severe limitation of many cancer chemotherapies, particularly chemotherapy and radiation, is the lack of selectivity and the resultant toxicity to the patient. Therefore, macrophages must also be able to distinguish between normal and tumorigenic targets so as to avoid nonspecific destruction of normal tissue.

Tumoricidal blood monocytes can discriminate between tumorigenic and nontumorigenic allogeneic cells, even under co-cultivation conditions. Normal cells probably resist macrophage-mediated lysis because macrophages do not bind to normal cells. Activated macrophages and monocytes have been shown to have direct cytotoxic effects on tumor cells or indirect effects through the elaboration of various cytotoxic materials, such as interleukin-1, tumor necrosis factor, proteases, or superoxide radicals.

There are two major pathways to achieve macrophage activation *in vivo*. Macrophages can be activated subsequent to contact with microorganisms or their products, such as endotoxin or cell wall skeleton. Muramyl dipeptide (MDP), a component of the bacterial cell wall, is capable of activating macrophages. A lipophilic MDP derivative, muramyl tripeptide phosphatidylethanolamine (MTP-PE), has also been shown to activate mononuclear macrophages. *In vivo* macrophage activation can also be produced by a family of polypeptides generally referred to as lymphokines. Antigen- and mitogen-stimulated T lymphocytes produce diffusible mediators that interact with target cells bearing appropriate receptors. Macrophage activation is produced by a group of lymphokines termed macrophage-activating factors (MAFs). The best known MAF is gamma-interferon. To activate macrophages, the lymphokines must first bind to surface receptors and then be internalized (Fidler, 1985).

Delivery of activators in synthetic phospholipid vesicles (liposomes) has provided a means of activating macrophages *in situ*. During the last several years, attention has focused on the use of liposomes to deliver drugs to various organ sites *in vivo*. Liposomes can be used to deliver biologic agents to cells of the reticuloendothelial system, resulting in activation of these phagocytic cells to a tumoricidal state.

The distribution of intravenously administered liposomes is determined by their physical size, composition, and charge and the size of the inoculum. In addition, circulating phagocytes are also capable of engulfing liposomes within the vascular compartment. Thus, liposomes are removed from the circulation mainly by fixed or free phagocytic cells, and not by extravasation. Peripheral blood mononuclear cells that have endocytosed liposomes can infiltrate visceral tissues and there differentiate into fixed tissue macrophages and histiocytes.

We have recently completed a prospective double blind clinical trial to evaluate liposome-encapsulated MTP-PE combined with surgical amputation in dogs with osteosarcoma. Twenty-seven dogs were entered into the study. All dogs had histologically documented osteosarcoma and a complete amputation of the primary tumor-bearing limb. Immediately after surgery, dogs were randomized to receive either liposomal MTP-PE or liposomes containing saline (placebo). Infusions (IV) were given twice-weekly for 8 weeks (total of 16 injections). The dose per infusion was 2 mg/m^2 body surface area of MTP-PE (500 mg of phospholipids). Fourteen dogs received liposome MTP-PE, and 13 dogs received liposome saline. The median survival time for the dogs receiving placebo was 77 days. This survival did not differ from that reported with surgery alone.

In contrast, the median survival time for dogs treated with liposome MTP-PE was 222 days ($P < 0.002$). Indeed, four dogs in this group were alive and free of disease 1 year after surgery. Liposomal MTP-PE did not produce toxic effects and was well tolerated (MacEwen, 1989). If a major limitation for treatment of metastasis by macrophage activation is tumor burden, it is probable that in some dogs, the tumor burden (in micrometastases) exceeded the level that can be eliminated by macrophages.

Currently we are conducting a clinical trial combining amputation and chemotherapy (cisplatin) combined with liposomal MTP-PE in dogs with osteosarcoma. The rationale of the combined approach is to use the cytotoxic chemotherapy to reduce the micrometastatic burden in the dog before the initiation of immunotherapy. To date we have 36 dogs entered into this clinical trial. Eleven dogs developed lung metastases during chemotherapy administration and one dog has died of chemotherapy-related toxicity. Twenty-two dogs have completed all phases of treatment, ten received liposomal MTP-PE, and 12 received the liposome placebo. Of the 12 dogs in the placebo group, ten dogs (83%) have died and two dogs are still alive. The median survival time is 10 months. For the ten dogs receiving liposomal MTP-PE, four dogs (40%) died of metastasis. Five of the remaining six liposomal MTP-PE dogs are still alive and free of metastases, and all are alive more than 1 year after surgery. Although preliminary, it appears that liposomal MTP-PE is effective for preventing metastasis when combined with amputation and cisplatin chemotherapy. Liposomal MTP-PE may also be effective in the control of metastasis in other tumors with a high metastatic potential, such as oral melanoma, hemangiosarcoma, and mammary adenocarcinoma.

PLATELETS, COAGULATION, AND METASTASIS

Interaction of tumor cells with host platelets is believed to facilitate metastasis. However, the exact mechanism is unknown. Tumor cells may become shielded within platelet thrombi. This may prevent destruction by the host immune system. Platelets may also enhance tumor cell adhesion to endothelial surfaces via platelet bridges. Tumor cell survival and multiplication may be enhanced owing to the release of platelet mitogenic factors (i.e., platelet-derived growth factor [PDGF]). Finally, platelet- or coagulation protein-derived products may mediate endothelial cell retraction. Tumor cells must initiate endothelial cell retraction before the formation of stable adhesions with the basement membrane. Experimental studies are being conducted to evaluate antiplatelet drugs for their antimetastatic activity. Thromboxane (TXA_2) synthetase inhibitors and prostacyclin (PGI_2) inhibit tumor cell–induced platelet aggregation. PGI_2 has been shown to prevent or reduce the development of lung metastasis in mice injected with B16 melanoma cells (a line of melanoma cells that readily metastasize to the lung). Prevention of platelet protection and arrest of tumor cells may enhance their destruction by the immune system. As an example, the effect of PGI_2 could be abrogated in mice rendered natural killer (NK) cell–deficient (NK cells are cytolytic cells of the immune system).

Detailed understanding of the factors involved in the evolution and control of cellular diversity within malignant tumors is also crucial for the design of more effective protocols for the treatment of metastatic disease. Successful therapy of multiple metastases populated by tumor cells with differing responses to antineoplastic agents will require treatment regimens that are able to circumvent such cellular heterogeneity. In addition, the demonstration that the extent of subpopulation heterogeneity within a neoplastic lesion can influence the rate at which new subpopulations of cells with novel properties are formed raises the disturbing question whether restriction of cellular diversity via therapeutic elimination of susceptible cellular subpopulations might stimulate the rapid formation of new variant and increasingly resistant tumor cells from any surviving subpopulation (Poste, 1985).

References and Suggested Reading

Fidler, I. J.: Macrophages and metastasis—A biological approach to cancer therapy: Presidential address. Cancer Res. 45:4714–4726, 1985.
A review paper on the experimental use of macrophage activation to prevent metastasis.
Goldie, J. H., and Coldman, A. J.: Application of theoretical models to chemotherapy protocol design. Cancer Treat. Rep. 70:127–131, 1986.
A mathematical approach to the problem of acquired drug resistance in cancer.
Hagiwara, A., Ahn, T., Ueda, T., et al.: Anticancer agents adsorbed by activated carbon particles: A new form of dosage enhancing efficacy on lymphnodal metastases. Anticancer Res. 6:1005–1008, 1985.
Clinical trial using intragastric injection of chemotherapeutic agents adsorbed to carbon particles.
Himsel, C. A., Richardson, R. C., and Craig, J. A.: Cisplatin chemotherapy for metastatic squamous cell carcinoma in two dogs. J.A.V.M.A. 189:1575–1578, 1986.
Case report discussing results of chemotherapy.
Ingram, M., Jacques, D. B., Freshwater, D. B., et al.: Adoptive immunotherapy of brain tumors in dogs. Vet. Med. Reports 2:398–402, 1990.
Clinical trial with five dogs using adoptive immunotherapy.
Jeglum, K. A., deGuzman, E., and Young, K.: Chemotherapy of advanced mammary adenocarcinoma in 14 cats. J.A.V.M.A. 187:157–160, 1985.
Clinical trial using cyclophosphamide and doxorubicin HCl.
LeCouteur, R. A., and Turrel, J. M.: Brain tumors in dogs and cats. *In* Kirk, R. W. (ed.): *Current Veterinary Therapy IX.* Philadelphia: W. B. Saunders, 1986, pp. 820–825.
Good general review of clinical diagnosis and management of brain tumors.
Levitan, N., and Hughes, K. S.: Management of non-resectable liver metastases from colorectal cancer. Oncology 4:77–84, 1990.
Review article of various methods for treating hepatic metastases.
MacEwen, E. G., Kurzman, I. D., Rosenthal, R. C., et al.: Therapy for osteosarcoma in dogs with intravenous injection of liposome encapsulated muramyl tripeptide. J. Natl. Cancer Inst. 81:935–938, 1989.
A prospective randomized study comparing surgery with surgery combined with immunotherapy.
McDonald, R. K., Walker, M., Legendere, A. M., et al.: Radiotherapy of metastatic seminoma in the dog. J. Vet. Intern. Med. 2:103–107, 1988.
Describes four dogs treated with cesium-137 teleradiotherapy for metastatic seminoma.
Natsuda, Y., Sugimachi, K., Ueo, H., et al.: Experimental study on transnodal cancer chemotherapy for metastatic lymph nodes. Jap. J. Surg. 13:368–372, 1983.
A description of both technique and several cases using injection of drugs into lymph nodes.
Poste, G.: Tumor cell heterogeneity and the pathogenesis of cancer metastasis. *In* Torisu, M., and Yoshida, T. (eds.): *Basic Mechanisms of Clinical Treatment of Tumor Metastasis.* New York: Academic Press, 1985, pp. 79–100.
A review of the new approaches to treat cancer metastasis.
Shapiro, W., and Turrel, J.: Management of pleural effusion secondary to metastatic adenocarcinoma in a dog. J.A.V.M.A. 192:530–532, 1988.
Single case report describing use of ^{32}P to treat malignant pleural effusion.
Thrall, D. E., Withrow, S. J., Powers, B. E., et al.: Radiotherapy prior to allograft limb sparing in dogs with osteosarcoma: A dose response assay. Int. J. Radiat. Oncol. Biol. Phys. 18:1351–1357, 1990.
Clinical trial using increasing doses of radiation therapy in conjunction with surgical limb salvage.

UNIQUE METABOLIC ALTERATIONS ASSOCIATED WITH CANCER CACHEXIA IN DOGS

GREGORY K. OGILVIE

Fort Collins, Colorado

and DAVID M. VAIL

Madison, Wisconsin

Cancer causes profound alterations in carbohydrate, protein, and lipid metabolism that result in a syndrome known as *cancer cachexia* (Ogilvie, 1989; Ogilvie and Vail, 1990; Vail et al., 1990b). Cancer cachexia, a devastating consequence of malignancy, results in weight loss in the presence of adequate nutritional intake. Unfortunately, cancer cachexia occurs frequently, with an estimated incidence of up to 87% in hospitalized human patients with cancer. Because the incidence of malignant disease is higher in dogs than in humans, there is reason to believe that cancer cachexia is at least as significant a problem in veterinary patients. Human patients affected with cancer cachexia have a decreased quality of life, decreased response to treatment, and a shortened survival time when compared with individuals who have similar neoplastic disease but do not have cachexia. Studies now under way demonstrate that animals and people with suboptimum nutritional intake cannot metabolize drugs adequately. These metabolic alterations are indirectly responsible for increased drug-induced toxicity and a poorer overall response to therapy. The tremendous prognostic significance of cancer cachexia is illustrated by the finding that survival of people affected with some cancers is more accurately predicted when based on the degree of cachexia present than on whether the individual receives treatment.

Alterations in metabolism are most important in the pathogenesis of this complex disorder. We have identified significant alterations in carbohydrate, protein, and lipid metabolism in dogs with cancer, even before clinical evidence of cancer cachexia is apparent (Ogilvie et al., 1988, 1991; Vail et al., 1990c). Many of these findings are identical to what

has been reported in humans with cancer cachexia. The quality of life, response to therapy, and survival time may be improved in animals with cancer by using this knowledge to select appropriate parenteral fluids, diets, and medication for therapy.

CARBOHYDRATE METABOLISM

The profound alterations observed in carbohydrate metabolism in dogs and humans with cancer result in a net energy gain by the tumor and a net energy loss by the host (Ogilvie, 1989; Ogilvie and Vail, 1990; Vail et al., 1990b). Glucose is the preferred substrate for energy production in tumor cells. An understanding of how the tumor uses glucose is essential to minimize metabolic alterations in carbohydrate metabolism in cancer patients.

Instead of completely oxidizing glucose, yielding 36 mol of adenosine triphosphate (ATP) per mole of glucose and forming carbon dioxide and water, as occurs in host cells, glucose enters glycolysis and is incompletely metabolized, yielding only 2 mol of high-energy phosphate bonds in the form of ATP and forming lactate as a metabolite. In order to meet large glucose requirements of the tumor, lactate produced by the tumor is then converted back into glucose by host hepatocytes. An additional energy expenditure of 12 molecules of ATP is incurred by the host for every glucose molecule produced from lactate. The end result is a shift in carbohydrate metabolism by the host from energy-producing oxidative pathways to energy-requiring gluconeogenic pathways. Therefore, the tumor realizes a net energy gain whereas the host has a net energy loss.

Relative insulin resistance has been reported in both humans and dogs with cancer. The insulin resistance may be due to a defect in the insulin

Supported in part by Morris Animal Foundation and by US Public Health Service Grant PO-1-CA-29582 awarded by the National Cancer Institute, DHHS.

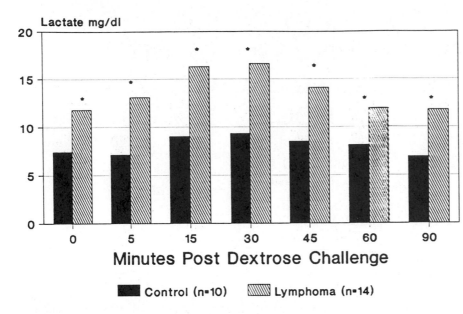

Figure 1. Serum lactate concentrations in dogs with and without lymphoma before and after intravenous administration of 500 mg/kg dextrose. Asterisks (*) indicate values from dogs with lymphoma, which differ significantly ($P<0.001$) from those from control dogs at the same time periods. (Reprinted with permission from Vail, D. M., et al.: Alterations in carbohydrate metabolism in canine lymphoma. J. Vet. Intern. Med. 4:11, 1990.)

receptor (receptor defect) or an abnormality in processing this signal after insulin attaches to the receptor (postreceptor defect). Glucose intolerance thus occurs before other overt signs of cancer cachexia are noted. A review of existing data suggests that dogs with lymphoma may have a postreceptor defect, further implying that dietary therapy may be effective in controlling this problem, as in some patients with type II diabetes.

When dogs with untreated lymphoma but without clinical evidence of cancer cachexia were compared with controls using an intravenous glucose tolerance test, lactate and insulin concentrations were significantly higher at several time intervals before and during the 90-min evaluation period (Figs. 1 and 2)

(Vail et al., 1990c). In the same study, glucose concentrations were determined to be similar to those in controls in response to an intravenous glucose tolerance test. Surprisingly, the increased lactate levels did not normalize after a complete remission was obtained during doxorubicin chemotherapy (Ogilvie et al. [in press], 1991). The dogs had even higher lactate levels when they were reevaluated after they lost their remission and began to show evidence of cachexia. In addition, the hyperinsulinemia did not abate after doxorubicin chemotherapy in dogs with lymphoma. These alterations in carbohydrate metabolism result in part because tumors preferentially metabolize glucose, using anaerobic glycolysis for energy and forming

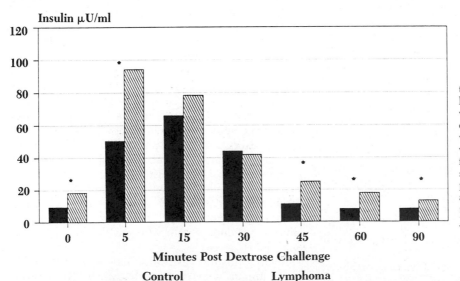

Figure 2. Serum insulin concentrations in dogs with and without lymphoma before and after intravenous administration of 500 mg/kg dextrose. Asterisks (*) indicate values from dogs with lymphoma, which differ significantly ($P<0.001$) from those from control dogs at the same time periods. (Reprinted with permission from Vail, D. M., et al.: Alterations in carbohydrate metabolism in canine lymphoma. J. Vet. Intern. Med. 4:11, 1990.)

lactate as an end product. These results parallel those observed in human patients suffering from cancer cachexia.

The impact of these observations of hyperlactatemia and hyperinsulinemia in dogs with lymphoma is far reaching. Research is under way to determine if these findings should alter the choice of fluids as well as enteral and parenteral feeding products. In one study that we performed, normal dogs were given lactated Ringer's solution and compared with dogs with lymphoma (Vail et al., 1990a). The hyperlactatemia observed in dogs with lymphoma became even more pronounced when lactated Ringer's solution was administered (Fig. 3). Because hyperlactatemia was noted after a simple intravenous glucose tolerance test, fluids that contain dextrose are also likely to cause increased lactate levels. A study is currently under way to determine if lactate-containing fluids will significantly affect quality of life, response to therapy, and survival time in dehydrated, cachectic dogs with cancer.

It can be hypothesized that parenteral and enteral nutrients high in simple carbohydrates as the primary source of calories may result in clinically significant hyperlactatemia and hyperinsulinemia in dogs with cancer. If this increase in the already elevated lactate concentrations lasts for several hours, the patient may be forced into a cachectic state. As mentioned earlier, the host must convert most of this lactate back to glucose, resulting in a net energy gain by the tumor and an energy loss by the host. Therefore, it can be hypothesized that foods that have a minimum of simple carbohydrates may be ideal for dogs with cancer.

PROTEIN METABOLISM

In cancer cachexia, protein degradation exceeds protein synthesis, resulting in a negative nitrogen balance with important clinical implications (Ogilvie, 1989; Ogilvie and Vail, 1990; Vail et al., 1990b). Because all protein is functional, net protein loss in cancer cachexia results in decreased cell-mediated and humoral immunity, gastrointestinal function, and wound healing. Loss of body protein is manifested clinically as atrophy of skeletal muscle and hypoalbuminemia. Amino acids are the primary substrate for gluconeogenesis in cancer cachexia because fatty acids cannot serve as gluconeogenic precursors in these animals. Plasma amino acid profiles in both human patients with cancer and tumor-bearing laboratory animals reveal a pronounced decrease in amino acids that favor gluconeogenic substrates but no decrease in leucine, the only amino acid that cannot serve as a gluconeogenic precursor. We have identified many of the same alterations in amino acid profiles in dogs that have lymphoma and have been previously identified and in people and laboratory animals with cancer. Dogs with lymphoma have significant decreases in threonine, glutamine, glycine, valine, cystine, and arginine. In contrast, isoleucine and phenylalanine levels are significantly increased. These significant alterations do not improve after a remission is obtained. We have also demonstrated that chemotherapy and remission did not significantly improve the amino acid profiles in 16 normal dogs. Correcting some of these abnormalities in amino acid levels may have profound clinical impact. For example,

Figure 3. Blood lactate concentrations in dogs with and without lymphoma before and during intravenous infusion of lactated Ringer's solution (LRS). Asterisks (*) indicate values from dogs with lymphoma, which differ significantly ($P<0.05$) from those from control dogs at the same time periods. Plus sign (+) indicates that values differ significantly ($P<0.05$) from preinfusion baseline values within the same test group. (Reprinted with permission from Vail, D. M., et al.: Exacerbation of hyperlactatemia by infusion of lactated Ringer's solution in dogs with lymphoma. J. Vet. Intern. Med. 4:228, 1990.)

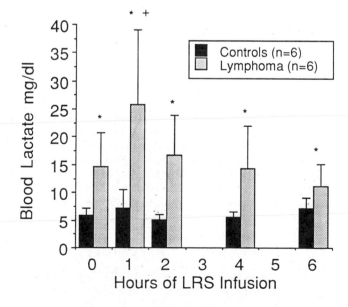

supplementation in arginine-deficient animals with the decreased amino acid has been shown to improve immune function. Therefore, animals with cancer have alterations in protein metabolism that if left uncorrected may result in serious health risks to these patients.

FAT METABOLISM

Most weight loss in cancer cachexia is due to depletion of body fat (Ogilvie, 1989; Ogilvie and Vail, 1990; Vail et al., 1990b). Patients with cancer cachexia have increased fat breakdown that correlates with increased levels of free fatty acids and certain plasma lipoprotein. Knowledge that tumor cells have difficulty utilizing lipids as a fuel may be of value clinically, especially because host tissues can continue to oxidize lipids for energy. Because insulin normally increases triglyceride synthesis in adipose tissue and decreases lipolysis, the insulin resistance identified in humans and dogs with cancer favors the decreased lipid synthesis and increased lipolysis occurring in cancer cachexia. Insulin supplementation in tumor-bearing laboratory animals results in decreased fat loss. We reported that dogs with untreated lymphoma, like humans with the same malignant disease, have significantly higher free fatty acid, total triglyceride, very low-density lipoprotein, and triglyceride serum concentrations when compared with untreated controls. The high-density lipoprotein cholesterol levels were significantly lower than in controls. After treatment with doxorubicin, the dogs with lymphoma also developed significantly elevated total cholesterol levels, as previously noted in humans with cancer.

Specific types of triglycerides and fatty acids have been shown under experimental conditions to minimize cancer cachexia and in some circumstances to have anticancer effects. Medium-chain triglycerides and 3-hydroxybutyrate have been shown to reduce weight loss and tumor size in rodents. The use of diets high in fish oils that are rich in omega-3–type polyunsaturated fatty acids eicosapentaenoic acid (C20:5, omega-3) and docosahexaenoic acid (C22:6, omega-3) have also been shown to be effective for promoting weight gain while having an anticancer effect. Use of diets high in these ingredients may be of value for treating cancer in veterinary patients.

Therefore, animals with cancer have significant alterations in fat metabolism that may have profound implications. The application of this knowledge may be of great benefit when formulating therapeutic protocols for enteral and parenteral therapy.

RESTING ENERGY EXPENDITURE

Increases in basal metabolic rate (BMR) and resting energy expenditure (REE) have been observed in humans and animals with cancer cachexia, and these changes are associated with the earlier mentioned derangements in carbohydrate, protein, and lipid metabolism (Ogilvie, 1989; Ogilvie and Vail, 1990; Vail et al., 1990b). The adaptive decrease in metabolic rate that is observed in healthy humans during fasting states does not occur in humans affected with cancer cachexia. Three phases of cancer cachexia have been identified in tumor-bearing rats using indirect calorimetry: silent or preclinical, hypermetabolic, and hypometabolic. Data that we have acquired reveal that asymptomatic dogs with lymphoma have REEs similar to those of controls but that the REE seems to decrease when these animals enter remission. These dogs may be in the silent or preclinical stage of disease. REE may be an important indicator to monitor response to therapy and to determine the metabolic state of an animal with cancer.

EFFECT OF NUTRITIONAL STATUS ON DRUG METABOLISM

Nutritional status is not usually considered when calculating a dosage of an anticancer drug for a patient. Clinically, it has been observed that well-nourished patients tolerate chemotherapy better than malnourished patients (Anderson, 1988; Krishnaswamy, 1987). Malnourishment, which frequently occurs in cancer patients, has been recognized as a poor prognostic indicator; it correlates with increased drug toxicity. Little is known, however, about the effects of nutritional status on the plasma pharmacokinetics of chemotherapeutic agents. Drugs with narrow margins of safety need to be evaluated in such situations so that more precise individualization of therapy can occur and toxicity predictions based on nutritional status of the patient can be made. Indeed, drug regimens may have to be adjusted in malnourished patients in order to prevent potentially dangerous side effects.

It appears that a normal diet contains xenobiotics that the liver detoxifies and in so doing maintains basal detoxification enzyme activity. The route of delivery of nutritional support appears also to be important, because studies on parenteral versus enteral support give a clear edge to the latter when comparing drug toxicity protection. Research in protein- and calorie-deprived human and laboratory animal models suggest that decreased plasma clearance of a wide array of commonly used chemotherapeutics including doxorubicin, methotrexate, and 5-fluorouracil may account for increased toxicity to patients. Toxicity may result not because of malnourishment *per se* but because of exposure to a higher effective dose of the cytotoxic drug. Nutritional supplementation could potentially reverse depressed drug clearance times.

ENTERAL AND PARENTERAL THERAPY

Nutritional manipulation in human cancer patients, although in its infancy, shows early promise for minimizing the degree of cancer cachexia resulting from metabolic alterations. Detrimental effects, such as increased rate of tumor growth or rate of metastasis, have not been demonstrated after nutritional support of human patients with cancer cachexia. Several investigators have reported that nutrient profiles containing 30 to 50% of nonprotein calories as fat instead of carbohydrate decrease glucose intolerance, fat loss, and tumor growth while increasing host weight, nitrogen, and energy balance. Simply increasing the fat content may decrease the degree of cancer cachexia in dogs with cancer. In essence, cancer-bearing hosts may thrive on nutrient profiles relatively high in certain types of fat and low in carbohydrate. As mentioned earlier, the addition of medium-chain fatty acids and omega-3 fatty acids may be of great value in treating dogs with cancer. This approach is distinct from those that suggest that low-fat diets when fed to species *without* cancer may be vital to *prevent* certain types of cancer. Many commercially prepared dog foods contain large amounts of sugars as the primary source of calories, and these foods may be detrimental to some animals with cancer.

Until more information is available, the following guidelines are suggested:

1. Whenever possible, nourishment should be provided by regular feeding practices. When that is not possible, tube feeding may be necessary. It is hypothesized that enteral products that are fed to debilitated animals through nasogastric, gastrostomy, or jejunostomy tubes should minimize the carbohydrate caloric sources (see this volume, p. 117, and *CVT X*, p. 30, for details concerning enteral feeding methods).

2. Every attempt should be made to increase the appetite of an anorexic animal. Feeding fresh aromatic foods that are warmed to body temperature and using diazepam derivatives or megesterol acetate may be effective for enhancing an animal's appetite.

3. Whenever the gastrointestinal tract cannot be used, parenteral feeding techniques should be employed (see *CVTX*, p. 25, for details concerning parenteral feeding methods).

4. The majority of cancer patients are thought to be hypermetabolic. In addition, many are recovering from surgery, radiation therapy, or chemotherapy. Therefore, many animals with cancer may need a great deal more nutrients than do normal animals. As an example, to calculate the number of calories needed by a dog with cancer, first determine the basal energy requirement (kcal/day) by multiplying 70 times the animal's weight in $kg^{0.75}$ and then multiplying by 2. The protein requirement in dogs without renal disease is approximately 4 to 6 gm/kg/day.

5. Lactate- and glucose-containing parenteral fluids should be avoided in animals that are in critical condition with cancer requiring acute, intensive fluid therapy.

References and Suggested Reading

Anderson, K. E.: Influences of diet and nutrition on clinical pharmacokinetics. Clin. Pharmacokinet. 14:325, 1988.
This review article discusses the mechanisms and clinical consequences of how nutrition can alter drug metabolism and distribution.

Krishnaswamy, K.: Effects of malnutrition on drug metabolism and toxicity in humans. Nutritional Toxicology 2:105, 1987.
This article points out the clinical consequences and drug metabolism in people in various states of malnutrition.

Ogilvie, G. K.: Paraneoplastic syndromes. *In* Withrow, S. J., and MacEwen, E. G. (eds.): *Clinical Veterinary Oncology.* Philadelphia, J. B. Lippincott, 1989, p. 29.
A review of common paraneoplastic syndromes in animals with cancer, with specific emphasis on cancer cachexia.

Ogilvie, G. K., and Vail, D. M.: Nutrition and cancer: Recent developments. *In* Couto, G. M. (ed.): Clinical management of the cancer patient. Vet. Clin. North Am. 20:1, 1990.
This is a comprehensive review of cancer cachexia and potential therapeutic options.

Ogilvie, S. J., Vail, D. M., Wheeler, S. L., et al.: Alterations in fat and protein metabolism in dogs with cancer. Proceedings Veterinary Cancer Society, 1988, p. 31.
A prospective study documenting the unique alterations in fat and protein profiles in dogs with cancer.

Ogilvie, G. K., Vail, D. M., Wheeler, S. J., et al.: Effect of chemotherapy and remission on carbohydrate metabolism in dogs with lymphoma. Cancer Res. (in press).
This prospective study documents that the alterations in carbohydrate seen in dogs with lymphoma do not improve with remission secondary to doxorubicin chemotherapy.

Vail, D. M., Ogilvie, G. K., Fettman, M. J. et al.: Exacerbation of hyperlactatemia by infusion of lactated Ringer's solution in dogs with lymphoma. J. Vet. Intern. Med. 4:228, 1990a.
A prospective study documenting the development of very high lactate levels in dogs with cancer receiving modest doses of lactated Ringer's solution.

Vail, D. A., Ogilvie, G. K., and Wheeler, S. L.: Metabolic alterations in patients with cancer cachexia. Comp. Cont. Ed. Pract. Vet. 12:381, 1990b.
This is a literature review on what is known about cancer cachexia.

Vail, D. M., Ogilvie, G. K., Wheeler, S. L., et al.: Alterations in carbohydrate metabolism in canine lymphoma. J. Vet. Intern. Med. 4:8, 1990c.
This prospective study documents the alterations in carbohydrate metabolism in dogs with lymphoma.

CACHEXIA ASSOCIATED WITH CANCER AND IMMUNODEFICIENCY IN CATS

JAMES R. HARTKE,
JENNIFER L. ROJKO,
and LAWRENCE E. MATHES
Columbus, Ohio

The clinical presentation of cachexia in a well-fed adult cat suggests an underlying chronic disease state. Cachexia is the severe progressive loss of body weight and lean body mass. The cachexic animal is unable or unwilling to correct the severe weight deficit. Common noninfectious causes of cachexia include chronic heart failure, chronic renal failure, hyperthyroidism, diabetes mellitus, and malignancy. Common infectious causes of cachexia include feline leukemia virus (FeLV), feline immunodeficiency virus (FIV), and feline infectious peritonitis (corona) virus.

In any individual cat, cachexia results from a combination of three factors: (1) a variable degree of inappetence, (2) maldigestion or malabsorption, and (3) defects of intermediary metabolism. The net result is a negative energy balance over time, causing a loss of fat stores and, more important, a loss of lean body mass.

ANOREXIA

Anorexia has a large number of causes in cats, ranging from fever to idiopathic appetite depression. The presentation of chronic weight loss with anorexia usually suggests a poor prognosis. Cats are finicky eaters by nature and tend to decrease their food consumption quickly when they are ill. The presence of nausea caused either by the primary disease or by medications administered to treat the disease may create a lasting aversion to specific foods consumed during a period of nausea. This may pose a serious problem in cats accustomed to a particular food. Varying the diet fed to a cat while it is healthy may help the cat accept a greater range of food when it is ill. Central nervous system (CNS) transmitters (serotonin) and plasma mediators (interleukin-1) probably have a role in appetite suppression, but further research is needed to define their contributions (Hellerstein et al., 1989).

MALASSIMILATION

Malassimilation may be a result of maldigestion or malabsorption. The resulting negative nutrient balance will cause a progressive weight loss. Increased food intake may partially compensate for the decreased efficiency of assimilation. Cachectic cats may present with diarrhea as a primary intestinal disorder or secondary to hyperthyroidism, gastrointestinal cancer, or immune suppression. Interestingly, both normal and feline retrovirus-infected cats appear to compensate for periods of decreased energy intake by increasing energy absorption (Hartke, unpublished data, 1990).

INTERMEDIARY METABOLISM

Once nutrients are absorbed, metabolic pathways may not utilize the nutrients to their maximum extent. Nutrients may be "wasted" by futile cycling of metabolism, such as the anaerobic metabolism of glucose to lactate in neoplastic tissue and the regeneration of glucose from lactate in the liver. This cycle wastes four molecules of high energy adenosine triphosphate (ATP) for every molecule of glucose that is converted to lactate and back to glucose. Another common example of nutrient wasting is feline hyperthyroidism where increased food intake (hyperphagia) fails to compensate for the increased metabolic rate and the cat loses weight.

The progression of cachexia in any individual cat is a combination of many different factors. The delicate balance of metabolism is disrupted at different points in each disease process. An understanding of the specific susceptibilities of the cat to cachexia is a benefit in clinical therapy.

This work was supported by grants from the National Institute of Diabetes, Digestive, and Kidney Diseases (RO1DK41066 and RO1DK40640), and the Glen Barber Fund for Amino Acid Research.

438

PATHOGENESIS OF CACHEXIA

The strict carnivorous nature of feline metabolism predisposes the cat to cachexia. Omnivores such as the dog regulate key hepatic enzymes to metabolize meat-based or plant-based diets based on differences in protein and lipid concentrations. The homogeneity of the feline diet during evolution meant these enzymes did not need to be regulated, so in the modern-day cat, deamination enzyme levels are set at a constant rate. The cat also lost many enzymes that convert plant precursors to mammalian nutrients, such as the enzymes to convert linoleic acid to arachidonic acid. The end result is a metabolism that does not adapt well to the stress of neoplasia or disease. Feline idiopathic hepatic lipidosis is a specific example of the peculiarity and the inability of feline metabolism to respond to stress.

Postprandial periods in the cat are characterized by high rates of amino acid deamination and the generation of glucose from abundant amino acids. In fasting states, the low amount of amino acid substrates available limit the rate of deamination and reduce the rate of gluconeogenesis. Blood glucose levels are maintained through glycogen release and, if the fasting occurs for a long enough time period, catabolism of protein stores. Omnivore species regulate the activity level of the deamination enzymes to conserve protein but also eventually resort to protein catabolism to maintain blood glucose. The constitutive nature of deamination enzymes in the feline liver sensitize the cat to reductions in dietary protein or amino acid imbalance (MacDonald et al., 1984b). The cat has also lost the ability to synthesize arginine (through a complex pathway involving citrulline). Arginine deficiency slows urea production, causing the blood ammonia levels to rise. A single meal without arginine results in salivation, dementia, coma, and death in 4 to 6 hours due to a hyperammonemic crisis. Fortunately, arginine is a common constituent of meat-based diets, and as such, a deficiency is rarely observed clinically. Pharmacologic doses of arginine enhance thymic function and induce the secretion of growth hormone and prolactin. Experimentally, arginine promotes wound healing, positive nitrogen balance, and recovery from trauma (Kirk et al., 1990). The inability of the cat to synthesize arginine may cause a relative deficiency in cachexic conditions. Further evaluation is needed before clinical protocols can be suggested. The cat also requires specific amino acids such as taurine to prevent central retinal degeneration and dilated cardiomyopathy. Presumably, these amino acids are in ample supply in a carnivorous diet (MacDonald et al., 1984b).

The cat does not require carbohydrates such as sugars or starches in its diet but will utilize them quite readily as an energy source.

The lipid portion of the feline diet is important as a concentrated source of energy, fat soluble vitamins, and essential fatty acids. Lipids contain 9 kcal/gm compared with 4 kcal/gm for carbohydrates and proteins. The increased caloric density of high-lipid foods means less volume of food needs to be consumed, which may benefit an inappetent cat. Further review of feline nutrient needs and metabolism is available (Hand et al., 1989; Lewis et al., 1987).

Our understanding of intermediary metabolism alterations in cancer cachexia or feline retrovirus-induced (FeLV- or FIV-induced) cachexia is limited. The failure of enteral or parenteral nutrition to prevent or reverse cachexia in these diseases demonstrates that decreased dietary intake or assimilation is not the sole cause of weight loss. Many investigators have suggested an increased metabolic rate or the wasting of absorbed nutrients may contribute to the cachexia. However, the metabolic rate of cachexic animals does not show consistent changes and probably varies with the disease and the stage of weight loss. Wasting of absorbed nutrients such as anaerobic glycolysis with lactate formation in peripheral or neoplastic tissues does occur in specific diseases. Feline retrovirus-infected cats have altered plasma fatty acid profiles with specific decreases in arachidonic acid proportions. These decreases probably are not due to malassimilation alone, as FeLV specifically alters fatty acid metabolism in target lymphocytes *in vitro*, again decreasing arachidonic and also docosahexaenoic acid proportions. Arachidonic acid and docosahexaenoic acid are precursors of prostaglandins, thromboxanes, and leukotrienes, so decreased proportions may alter production of these critical mediators. Cats fed a diet deficient in arachidonic acid have variable degrees of immunosuppression and cachexia (MacDonald et al., 1984a). It may be valuable to evaluate arachidonic acid replacement therapy in cachectic FeLV-infected cats.

CYTOKINE CONTROL MECHANISMS

Cytokines (intercellular mediators produced by the immune system) possess a broad range of effects on cells outside the immune system, such as muscle, adipose tissue, and bone. These endogenous factors that control cachexia are only recently discovered, and their mechanisms of action are not well understood (Beutler and Cerami, 1989). Interleukin-1 (IL-1) is produced by activated macrophages and many other cell types to produce acute phase response proteins. Metabolic effects of IL-1 include anorexia, myalgia, and a negative nitrogen balance (protein catabolism). The parallel discoveries of cachectin, a protein cytokine elevated in cachectic rabbits infected with *Trypanosoma brucei,* and of tumor necrosis factor (TNFα), a cytokine capable of inducing signs of endotoxemia, have begun to elucidate the control mechanisms of cachexia. Recently, through genetic sequencing, cachectin and TNFα have been shown to be the same cytokine. TNFα is normally produced by the fixed macrophage system in response to endotoxins (gram-negative bacteria cell membrane components) and other as yet undefined stimuli. Single-bolus intravenous infusions of cachectin/TNFα produce signs of endotoxemia, such as neutrophil migration and cardiovascular collapse. Cachectin secretion by macrophages appears to be beneficial to the cat in moderate amounts by alerting the immune system to the presence of bacterial invaders. In severe sepsis, the overproduction of cachectin and the resulting endotoxic shock represent the overuse of this beneficial system. Chronic administration of cachectin/TNFα produces cachexia in rats, and TNFα-secreting cells implanted in mice produce cachexia. However, elevated plasma levels of TNFα or IL-1 have not been demonstrated in many cases of cachexia. The absence of plasma elevations of cachectin/TNFα or IL-1 in cachexia may be a result of elevated local production. Cytokines such as TNFα or IL-1 may be produced locally and primarily affect tissues in close association with the fixed macrophage system, such as the Kupffer cells of the liver. In such a case, plasma concentrations of cytokines may not reflect local changes in cytokine control. The hepatic parenchyma may be exposed to increased cytokine concentrations causing changes in metabolism without an increase in plasma concentrations. Endotoxin stimulation of cachectin/TNFα production may occur in immunosuppressed animals through frequent but small breeches of the gastrointestinal tract mucosal barrier. The result would be low-level episodic stimulation of hepatic macrophages. Further understanding of the cytokine control of cachexia may lead to therapeutic measures such as the administration of blocking antibodies to TNFα or IL-1.

Cachexia is an important prognostic factor in many diseases. Correction of cachexia can result in a better response to therapy or a better quality of life in progressive diseases. Treatment of cachexia is especially important in cancer therapy to minimize the side effects of therapeutic protocols.

THERAPY

Correction of cachexia requires minimizing inappetence and malassimilation and controlling the loss of nutrients by an inefficient intermediary metabolism. Treatment of cachexia first involves correction of the underlying disease, if possible, in conjunction with sound supportive therapy.

Appetite may be stimulated by using good nursing practices, such as offering a variety of canned foods, warming the foods to approximately 40°C (100°F) in the microwave to increase the aroma, and offering small amounts frequently. Calorie-dense foods that contain a high percentage of lipids and protein are beneficial since cachectic animals often eat a reduced volume of food. Coaxing the cat to eat from a spoon or flat plate at frequent intervals in a quiet room may also help increase consumption. Cat owners may know of a favorite food or presentation of food that may help to stimulate the appetite. Gentle reassurance, such as petting the cat gently on the back, may increase appetite or encourage the cat to eat (Abood et al., in press; see also CVT X, p. 18). Fish-based diets, which are high in N3 fatty acids, may help to ameliorate the cachexia. Preliminary research shows a decrease in IL-1 secretion and a decrease in the anorexigenic effects of IL-1 in rats fed a fish oil–based diet compared with a corn oil–based diet (Hellerstein et al., 1989).

If the appetite continues to decline, pharmacologic stimulation of appetite may be necessary. Diazepam (Valium, Roche) at a dose of 0.17 to 0.27 mg/kg every 12 to 24 hours IV may stimulate appetite for a few minutes (Helfand, 1990). The effects are short-lived and the volume of food consumed is small. The long-term usage may produce tachyphylaxis as well as the inconvenience of repeated intravenous injections. Oxazepam (Serax, Wyeth-Ayerst) at a dose of 2.0 mg/cat every 12 hours PO provides a less invasive and more easily administered appetite stimulant on a long-term basis, although in many cases it is ineffective. The serotonin antagonist cyproheptadine (Periactin, Merck Sharpe and Dohme) at a dose of 1 mg/cat every 24 hours PO is also reported to increase appetite in healthy cats (see CVT X, p. 23). Caution must be exercised when using benzodiazepines because they may further depress an already listless animal. Also, the consumption of a small amount of food shortly after stimulant administration should not cause the false conclusion that intake levels over a 24-hour period are adequate. The use of appetite-stimulating medications should be used in conjunction with careful measurement of food intake (record volume or weight daily) so that more aggressive measures are not delayed on the assumption that intake levels are adequate (Abood et al., in press). Other long-term stimulants include anabolic steroids such as stanozolol (Winstrol-V, Winthrop) at a dose of 1 mg/cat every 12 hours PO or nandrolone decanoate (Decadurabolin, Organon) at a dose of 2.5 mg/kg every 2 to 3 weeks IM. Clinical prediction of the efficacy of anabolic steroids is difficult because clinically similar cases may show a positive response or no response at all.

Enteral feeding requires more nursing care but offers the strong advantages of frequent feedings, controlled amounts of food, and adequate hydration (see *CVT X*, p. 30). Cats that have lost greater than 10% of their body weight and that cannot be coaxed to eat will benefit from enteral feeding. Enteral feeding on a short-term basis may help return the appetite of the cat through nonspecific gastrointestinal stimulation in some cases. Nasogastric tubes are easily inserted and provide a route for good enteral nutrition for days up to weeks. Longer term enteral nutrition can be provided through a pharyngostomy tube or a gastrostomy tube. The use of enteral feeding in cases where the primary cause of cachexia can be corrected has a high degree of success. Reviews of enteral diets and enteral feeding techniques are available (Donoghue, 1989).

Correction of intermediary metabolism is the most difficult but often most crucial treatment of cachexia. Currently, the best correction of intermcdiary metabolism is the treatment of the inciting disease process. Unfortunately, in many cases this is not possible, and palliative measures are the only therapy available.

Specific nutrient therapy (e.g., restoration of arachidonic acid levels in cachectic, FeLV-infected cats) may prove to have value with further study. Antibodies against feline cachectin/TNFα or IL-1 may provide a method to lower cachectin/TNFα or IL-1 levels, which may reverse the cachexia. Until the mechanisms of cachexia induction are better understood, the best current therapy is correction of the primary disease combined with good supportive care.

References and Suggested Reading

1. Abood, S. K., Mauterer, J. V., McLoughlin, M. A., et al.: Nutritional support of hospitalized patients. *In* Slatter, D. H. (ed.): *Textbook of Small Animal Surgery.* Philadelphia: W. B. Saunders (in press).
2. Beutler, B., and Cerami, A.: The biology of cachectin/TNF—A primary mediator of the host response. Ann. Rev. Immunol. 7:625, 1989.
3. Donoghue, S.: Nutritional support of hospitalized patients. Vet. Clin. North Am. Sm. Anim. Prac. 19(3):475, 1989.
4. Hand, M. S., and Armstrong, P. J.: Nutritional requirements and feeding recommendations. *In* Sherding, R. G. (ed.): *The Cat: Diseases and Clinical Management.* New York: Churchill Livingston, 1989, p. 117.
5. Helfand, S. C.: Supportive care of cats with cancer. Proc 8th ACVIM Forum, Washington D.C., May 1990, p. 405.
6. Hellerstein, M. K., Meydani, S. N., Meydani, M., et al.: Interleukin-1 induced anorexia in the rat. J. Clin. Invest. 84:228, 1989.
7. Kirk, S. J., and Barbui, A.: Role of arginine in trauma, sepsis and immunity. J. Parenter. Enter. Nutr. 14:226, 1990.
8. Lewis, L. D., Morris, M. L., and Hand, M. S.: Anorexia, inanition, and critical care nutrition. *In Small Animal Clinical Nutrition III.* Topeka, KS: Mark Morris Associates, 1987, pp. 5–11.
9. MacDonald, M. L., Anderson, B. C., Rogers, Q. R., et al.: Essential fatty acid requirements of cats: Pathology of essential fatty acid deficiency. Am. J. Vet. Res. 45:1310, 1984a.
10. MacDonald, M. L., Rogers, Q. R., and Morris, J. G.: Nutrition of the domestic cat, a mammalian carnivore. Ann. Rev. Nutr. 4:521, 1984b.

IMMUNOLOGIC ASSESSMENT OF THE SMALL ANIMAL PATIENT

LAUREL J. GERSHWIN
Davis, California

The small animal patient is equipped with an immune system that responds to disease with humoral or cellular defense mechanisms. Failure to respond to infection with a pathogenic agent as well as the occurrence of one or more of the following situations may indicate a defect in the immune system: (1) recurrent infection, particularly with organisms that are not pathogenic in the normal animal, (2) fever of unknown origin, (3) failure to thrive, (4) clinical signs suggestive of an autoimmune or allergic disease, (5) neurologic disease, (6) unusual reactions to medication, and (7) cancer.

DIAGNOSTIC STEPS FOR AN IMMUNOLOGIC WORKUP

The clinical immunology laboratory offers a variety of tests to assist the clinician in detecting suboptimal immune function. However, before specific immunologic tests are requested, it is expected that the initial workup will include: (1) complete history and physical examination, (2) complete blood count (CBC) with total white blood cell count and differential, (3) urinalysis, (4) blood chemistry panel, and (5) organ system–specific tests, such as radiography, as indicated.

Clinical history, including age and breed of the patient, assists in establishing the type of immune defect that is suspected since immune defects can be inherited (primary) or acquired (secondary). Primary immune defects are usually observed early in life, whereas acquired defects occur in animals of all ages. Breed predisposition is seen for several inherited immunodeficiencies, such as IgA deficiency in Sharpei and German shepherd dogs, X-linked severe combined immunodeficiency in Bassett hounds, and canine granulopathy syndrome in Irish setter dogs. Choice of the appropriate immunologic tests to perform can be made most appropriately after consideration of these factors and others. The type of infection, particularly if recurrent, may be important. Patients with T-cell defects will have more severe viral and mycotic disease, while a patient with a phagocytic defect will be most affected by bacterial pathogens.

Immune responses may be exuberant or misdirected as in hypersensitivity and autoimmune disorders. Type 1 hypersensitivity disorders, such as canine allergic inhalant dermatitis, are the result of an exuberant IgE response to an environmental antigen, whereas autoimmune disorders, such as systemic lupus erythematosus, are the result of an immune response to self-antigens. In both cases, a tentative clinical diagnosis can be confirmed by laboratory testing.

Examination of the immune system is best achieved by evaluation of the component parts: (1) humoral immunity (B lymphocytes, immunoglobulins), (2) cellular immunity (T lymphocytes, NK cells), (3) complement, and (4) phagocytic system (polymorphonuclear leukocytes, macrophages). Defects in immune function can occur in each of these components.

EVALUATION OF HUMORAL IMMUNITY

The humoral immune system consists of the B lymphocytes, the plasma cells, and the immunoglobulins or antibodies. Functions of the humoral immune system include: (1) secretion of antibodies specific for the stimulating antigens; (2) defense against bacterial pathogens, particularly encapsulated bacteria, which require opsonization for efficient killing by phagocytes; (3) virus neutralization (IgA is important on mucosal surfaces); (4) detoxification of toxins; and (5) prevention of reinfection by viral and bacterial pathogens. Thus the impairment of these functions may be indicative of a defect in humoral immunity.

Table 1 lists tests that can be used to evaluate B-cell function. Generally, the presence and quantity of each antibody class (IgG, IgM, IgA) is determined as a first step. These assays are described later. The next step in assessing humoral immunity can involve

Table 1. *Tests to Evaluate B-Cell Function*

1. Quantitation of IgG, IgM, and IgA levels by single radial diffusion
2. Quantitation of B-cell numbers in peripheral blood by immunofluorescence
3. Quantitation of immunoglobulin response to specific antigens
4. Identification of bacteria causing recurrent infections: pneumonia, otitis, pyoderma, etc.
5. Enumeration of antibody-producing plasma cells by immunofluorescent staining for cytoplasmic immunoglobulin in biopsy specimens

quantitation of B-cell numbers by immunofluorescence. If normal concentrations of each antibody class are confirmed and B-cell numbers appear adequate, it may be useful to look for a response to a particular antigen, such as tetanus toxoid or leptospira bacterin. In this case the patient's blood should be drawn before and 7 to 10 days after immunization with the vaccine. The laboratory determines the titer using a standard protocol for the particular antigen system. The expected normal result is an increase in titer or seroconversion.

Immunoelectrophoresis

Immunoelectrophoresis (IEP) is a laboratory procedure used to detect the presence of paraproteinemia and some immunoglobulin deficiencies. It is a qualitative procedure, which is performed as a screening test to be followed up by specific antibody class quantitation if a deficiency or a monoclonal gammopathy is suspected.

In performance of the IEP test, a sample of the patient's serum is added to a well on an agarose-covered slide. The slide is placed into an electrophoresis chamber and electrophoretic separation of the serum proteins of the patient is carried out. Immediately after electrophoretic separation, the agar is removed from a trough opposite to the well and antiserum is added. The slide is then incubated overnight to allow diffusion of antigen (serum proteins) and antibodies (present in the antiserum). Arcs of precipitation are seen at the sites where antigen-antibody complexes have formed. By testing the patient's serum with several different antisera (anti-IgG, anti-IgM, anti-IgA), the specific antibody classes can be recognized.

Interpretation of the IEP is performed by comparison of the pattern seen with the patient's serum with that of a normal control serum, which is tested simultaneously. A patient with a monoclonal gammopathy will produce an IEP test that has a thickened area associated with the arc representing the antibody class containing the monoclonal antibody. This so-called "bat wing" appearance is significant and signals the need to perform a quantitative evaluation for that antibody class (see under Single Radial Immunodiffusion).

Another significant observation on the IEP is the absence or near-absence of a particular arc. For example, if the IgA arc is not visible on the patient's IEP profile but is present in the control IEP, the possibility of a selective IgA deficiency in the patient should be further investigated by performing a quantitative assay for IgA. Similarly, IgG and IgM deficiencies can be detected in this way.

Single Radial Immunodiffusion

Concentrations of each antibody class (IgG, IgM, IgA) can be determined from a serum sample by single radial immunodiffusion (SRID). The technique uses an agarose plate that has species-specific heavy chain–specific antiserum incorporated into it. Serum is added to a well, and standards are added to other wells. After 18 to 24 hr of incubation, a ring of precipitate is formed around each well. The diameter of the ring is proportional to the amount of antibody present in the serum sample. The standards are used to establish a line from which unknowns are calculated. The result obtained from SRID is reported in milligrams of antibody of the class tested for per unit volume. In veterinary immunology laboratories at present, there is a lack of standardization for plates and normal values. Therefore, it is best to ask the laboratory for their normal values and to compare your results with these.

EVALUATION OF CELLULAR IMMUNITY

T lymphocytes are important as effector cells in reactions that are classified as cell-mediated immunity. The T-helper subset is also important to humoral immunity in that interactions between T-helper cells and B lymphocytes are required for antibody production to occur. Thus, a defect in T-helper cells (number or function) may be reflected in compromised ability to produce antibodies to a specific antigen. In human AIDS helper T cells are selectively destroyed; the severe repercussions underscore the importance of helper T cells in immune responses.

Additional functions of T lymphocytes include: (1) effector cells against certain viruses, facultative intracellular bacterial pathogens, and fungi, (2) cytotoxic response to tumor cells, (3) initiation of delayed type hypersensitivity, (4) initiation of graft versus host reaction, and (5) rejection of solid tissue grafts.

The function of T cells can be evaluated by a variety of techniques listed in Table 2.

Table 2. *Tests to Evaluate T-Cell Function*

1. Quantitation of stimulation index in response to T cell mitogens: Con A, PHA
2. Peripheral blood lymphocyte count
3. Immunofluorescent quantitation of total T cells and T-cell subsets
4. Development of contact allergy after exposure to 2-4 dinitrochlorobenzene
5. Determination of cell density in paracortical region of stimulated lymph node on biopsy

Lymphocyte Stimulation

Lymphocyte stimulation (blastogenesis, transformation) is an *in vitro* assay performed to evaluate the ability of the patient's lymphocytes to respond to mitogenic stimulation or antigenic stimulation. The mitogens used are plant lectins that stimulate by binding to receptors on the lymphocyte and initiating the process of blastogenesis. Concanavalin A (Con A) and phytohemagglutinin (PHA) stimulate T lymphocytes exclusively, whereas pokeweed mitogen (PWM) stimulates both T and B lymphocytes. These mitogens stimulate all of the T cells, regardless of antigenic specificity. It is possible to evaluate the subset of T cells that respond to a particular antigen by stimulating with that antigen instead of mitogen. In this test the patient's lymphocytes are incubated in wells of a tissue culture dish with mitogen for 3 days; late in incubation tritiated thymidine is added. The cells are harvested, and the amount of incorporated thymidine is determined in a scintillation counter. A stimulation index is calculated based on the counts obtained from the stimulated culture divided by the counts obtained from an unstimulated culture. Cells from a normal control of the same species must be tested alongside those of the patient to be sure the mitogens are functioning as expected.

Macrophage Inhibitory Factor

Macrophage inhibitory factor (MIF) production can be determined in a patient for a specific antigen. Application of this assay is most useful when infection with a viral or fungal agent has been confirmed and there is concern that the T-cell immune response is not effective. Peripheral blood mononuclear cells from the patient are incubated with the antigen in a capillary tube; a control tube lacks antigen. The ability of the macrophages to migrate from the top of the tube is limited by the production of MIF by sensitized T lymphocytes. Thus the tube containing antigen and responsive lymphocytes will show no macrophage migration. If macrophage migration occurs in the tube containing antigen, the lymphocytes are not sensitized to the antigen and there is no T-cell response to that antigen.

Quantitation of T Lymphocytes

T-cell quantitation in peripheral blood is possible using monoclonal antibodies that recognize T-cell determinants. A pan–T-cell antibody will bind to all of the T lymphocytes; an antibody specific for the canine equivalent of CD 4 will bind only to T helper cells; and an antibody that recognizes the CD 8 equivalent will bind to the T suppressor/cytotoxic cell population. Laboratories that are equipped with a fluorescence-activated cell sorter/analyzer use a fluorescein-conjugated antibody to label the cells and then determine the percentage of total lymphocytes that display the marker. Normally T lymphocytes are about 70% of the peripheral blood lymphocytes, and the remaining 30% are B lymphocytes and null cells. Testing with the pan–T-cell antibody will provide a measure of total T cells. The ratio of T4 to T8 cells indicates relative amounts of each subset. Depletion of T helper cells results in a ratio of 1:1 or less.

In Vivo Assessment of Cell-Mediated Immunity

In vitro correlates of cell-mediated immunity can be augmented in cases of suspected T-cell function deficit by a simple *in vivo* test. The chemical hapten 2-4 dinitrochlorobenzene sensitizes for contact allergy when it is applied to the skin in a patch. A typical contact hypersensitivity lesion (indurated, erythematous) will appear within several days if T-cell responses are normal. Failure to elicit a lesion indicates inadequate T-cell responsiveness. Other *in vivo* measurements of T-cell immunity, such as rejection of an allograft of skin, can be performed in cases where additional documentation of T-cell dysfunction is required.

Lymph node biopsy can be a useful adjunct to immunologic evaluation. Aplasia or hypoplasia of the node is indicative of insufficient population of the secondary lymphoid organs by mature T cells. Absence of germinal centers is observed in primary agammaglobulinemia.

EVALUATION OF THE COMPLEMENT SYSTEM

The complement system provides a mechanism by which antibodies and cells of the immune system can kill pathogenic agents. Humoral immunity without complement would be considerably less effective. Because the alternate pathway of complement fixation does not require the presence of specific antibody, complement is an innate defense mechanism as well.

The genetic absence of complement components has been reported in several laboratory animals and in humans. Currently, the only well-documented complement deficiency in small animals is a C3 deficiency in a Brittany spaniel. C3 levels are low in diseases that consume complement, such as immune complex diseases. The unavailability of good assays for each individual complement component has slowed recognition of specific deficiencies. However, most veterinary immunology laboratories can evaluate total hemolytic complement (a measure of effectiveness of the system) and C3 (the pivotal protein in both alternate and classical pathways). Patients with C3 deficiency generally develop highly lethal susceptibility to infections.

The technique of single radial diffusion is used to quantitate C3. It requires that anti-C3 serum (species-specific) be incorporated into the agarose. As in immunoglobulin quantitation, standards must be assayed alongside the samples.

Hemolytic complement 50 (CH_{50}) is a measure of the ability of the patient's serum to serve as a source of complement for lysis of sensitized sheep red blood cells. CH_{50} is the highest dilution of serum that produces 50% lysis of the target cells. To perform the test the patient's fresh serum is diluted and added to sensitized cells. After incubation, the tubes are observed for the presence of hemolysis. Results are reported as CH_{50} units per milliliter of blood. Normal values may vary somewhat between laboratories.

EVALUATION OF PHAGOCYTIC CELL FUNCTION

Evaluation of neutrophil function must include: (1) adequacy of numbers, (2) chemotaxis, (3) phagocytosis, and (4) killing. Defects in one or more of these neutrophil functions will result in decreased effectiveness and consequent failure to combat infection, particularly with extracellular bacterial pathogens.

Neutrophil quantitation is easily accomplished as a part of the CBC. In gray collies in which cyclic neutropenia is an inherited defect, neutrophil numbers should be measured weekly to demonstrate the cyclic nature of the defect. Light and electron microscopy are used to obtain detailed information on cell and organelle morphology.

Measurement of Chemotaxis

Chemotaxis is the movement of neutrophils along a concentration gradient. Chemotactic factors are released from mast cells after immunologic activation; activation of complement creates fragments (C5a) that are chemotactic for neutrophils. The presence of bacteria, such as *Staphylococcus aureus*, is in itself also a chemotactic stimulus for neutrophils. A "lazy leukocyte syndrome" is associated with an increased incidence of infection.

Chemotactic assays are performed to test the ability of a patient's neutrophils to respond to a chemotactic factor. A sample of blood is obtained, and the neutrophils are placed on one side of a Boyden chamber. A micropore membrane separates the neutrophils from a chemotactic factor on the other side. The ability of the cells to move along the concentration gradient is measured after incubation and counting of the number of neutrophils accumulated on the membrane. Percent migration is compared with a normal control.

Measurement of the Ability to Ingest and Kill

Phagocytic index is a measure of the cell's ability to engulf foreign particles. Incubation of the patient's phagocytes with a suspension of bacteria (e.g., *Staphylococcus aureus*) is followed by slide preparation and staining. The numbers of organisms per phagocyte are determined and compared with a normal control. The opsonizing ability of the patient's serum is evaluated by incubation of the patient's cells and bacteria in its own serum (homologous) and incubation of a second aliquot of patient's cells in serum from a normal control prior to slide preparation. Normal phagocytic ability only in the presence of control serum indicates a lack of opsonizing antibody, rather than an innate phagocyte defect. Subnormal ability to phagocytize in both homologous and control serum indicates a defect in the phagocyte's ability to engulf.

Bactericidal assay is performed to evaluate the ability of phagocytes to kill ingested organisms. The patient's leukocytes are washed and incubated with a log phase growing culture of *Staphylococcus aureus*. At time 0 and every 30 min for the next 2 hr, an aliquot of the cell-bacteria mixture is removed, antibiotics are added to kill extracellular organisms, and the neutrophils are ruptured by dilution with distilled water before plating onto blood agar plates. The number of colonies present at each time point is plotted to generate a killing curve. The killing curves for the patient's cells in homologous serum, the patient's cells in control serum, and the control cells in control serum are compared. If there is a defect in killing with the patient's cells that is not correctable by opsonization with normal serum, then a neutrophil defect is present.

Nitroblue tetrazolium test measures the respiratory burst that occurs in neutrophils after phagocytosis. Within the phagocytic vacuole there is production of superoxide anions; this oxidation process is accompanied by the reduction of nitroblue tetrazolium and the consequent formation of a purple cytoplasmic precipitate. The test is performed by incubating the patient's neutrophils with opsonized zymosan particles and measuring dye reduction. Neutrophils defective in the respiratory burst do not reduce the nitroblue tetrazolium.

EVALUATION OF THE IMMUNE SYSTEM FOR DYSPROTEINEMIA

Multiple myeloma involves the formation of malignant clones of plasma cells with the release of immunoglobulin into the serum. The immunoglobulin is monoclonal, identical due to clonal origin of the plasma cells. When the clinician suspects multiple myeloma, the following immunologic tests should be performed: (1) serum electrophoresis, (2) immunoelectrophoresis, and (3) immunoglobulin quantitation by SRD. The serum electrophoresis reveals a monoclonal spike, which can be attributed to a particular antibody class on the IEP. SRD determinations indicate a marked increase in the class containing the monoclonal, while the other classes are often less than normal levels.

An additional test that can be performed is the detection of Bence-Jones protein in the urine. These are homogeneous light chains. The IEP test is performed on concentrated urine using light chain–specific antisera.

Cryoglobulinemia is suspected in the patient that develops loss of circulation in the peripheral tissues, such as those of the feet and ears, when the temperature is less than 37°C. Testing for cryoglobulins requires a sample of serum, which is incubated at 37°C and at 4°C. The formation of a precipitate in the 4°C tube indicates the presence of cryoglobulins.

EVALUATION OF THE IMMUNE SYSTEM FOR AUTOIMMUNITY

The multisystem autoimmune disease, systemic lupus erythematosus (SLE), must often be differentiated from a variety of other diseases, depending on which organ systems are affected. Tests that rely on the detection of antinuclear antibodies are the first choice for narrowing the diagnosis to SLE.

Antinuclear Antibody Test

Diagnosis of the multisystem disorder SLE requires the performance of the antinuclear antibody test (ANA). The presence of a high titer of antinuclear antibodies confirms a clinical diagnosis of SLE. To perform this indirect immunofluorescence test, the patient's serum is diluted serially and added to wells on a slide. These wells contain cells, fixed so that the nuclear antigens are accessible to any antibodies in the serum that are directed toward nuclear antigens. The antibodies bind and are subsequently made visible by the binding of fluorescent conjugated antibody directed against the species antibody. For example, a dog serum sample is tested with antidog IgG, coupled to a fluorescein conjugate. A positive test has bright green fluorescence associated with the nucleus. The fluorescence can occur in one of several patterns. The most common pattern is diffuse homogeneous nuclear staining. This pattern is seen when the antigen is DNA-histones. Other patterns seen less frequently include the rim, or peripheral, pattern and the speckled and nucleolar patterns. Results of the ANA test are reported as positive or negative, and a titer and pattern are reported for those that are positive. A positive ANA test is diagnostic of SLE if the titer is greater than 100. Low titers can be present in aged animals and have no significance relevant to disease. Low titers (1:10 to 1:20) are usually called suspicious, while very high titers are thought to correlate well with the severity of the disease.

LE Cell Test

The LE cell test requires whole blood and can be performed as an adjunct to the diagnosis of SLE. The development of LE cells occurs when neutrophils ingest nuclear material that is opsonized by antinuclear antibodies. Performance of the test requires incubation of the patient's blood after disruption of the cells by vortexing or forcing them through a filter. The neutrophils engulf the opsonized nuclei from the broken cells and become LE cells. These LE cells contain the large homogeneous pink nucleus within the cytoplasm.

Additional tests are performed as indicated by the organ system involved. For example, if there is skin involvement a lesion biopsy can reveal the "lupus band," or if there is kidney dysfunction, a kidney biopsy will reveal the deposition of immune complexes.

Immune Complex Detection in Tissues

Detection of immune complexes is performed by immunofluorescence on kidney, synovium, and skin as indicated by clinical signs. The biopsy is placed in Michel's medium, which contains ammonium sulfate for retention of deposited immune complexes. Upon receipt by the laboratory, the tissue is frozen in liquid nitrogen and sectioned by cryostat. Sections are stained with antispecies-specific heavy-chain sera and with anti-C3, followed by an antiglobulin reagent conjugated with fluorescein. When these tests are positive, deposited immune complexes are visualized as bright green fluorescence in kidney glomeruli, within the walls of small blood vessels in synovium and skin, and along the basal laminae ("lupus band") of the skin.

Immunofluorescence staining of skin biopsy material is an important adjunct to diagnosis of a variety of autoimmune skin diseases. The deposition of immunoglobulin and complement at the dermal-epidermal junction is seen in autoimmune skin diseases other than SLE: bullous pemphigoid, pemphigus erythematous, and discoid lupus. Pemphigus vulgaris is characterized by a reticular "honeycomb" pattern of fluorescence within the epidermis.

Detection of Organ-Specific Autoimmune Disease

Specialized tests for detection of organ-specific autoimmune disease are required for diagnosis of autoimmune blood, muscle, nervous system, skin, and endocrine diseases. For example, autoimmune myasthenia gravis can be detected by staining of biopsy material for the presence of autoantibodies which recognize the motor end-plate of muscle. Autoimmune thyroiditis can be evaluated by immunofluorescence testing of the patient's serum for autoantibodies reactive to thyroid tissue sections. Arthritis can accompany SLE, can be rheumatoid in nature, or can be the result of an immune response to an infectious or unknown cause. Rheumatoid arthritis is associated with the production of rheumatoid factors (IgM antibodies specific for IgG). The presence of RF can be detected in patient's serum using a latex agglutination test.

Autoimmune hemolytic anemia (AIHA) occurs as a distinct disease and as part of the symptom complex of SLE. Detection of autoantibodies specific for erythrocyte antigens is accomplished with the Coombs' test. Coombs'-positive anemia is frequently associated with SLE. To perform this test, the patient's blood is collected in EDTA or ACD anticoagulant and the erythrocytes are washed. Antiglobulin (species specific) is added to the cells, and they are incubated at 37°C (for warm reactive antibodies). If autoantibodies are attached to the patient's erythrocytes, the antiglobulin reagent will cross-link them and cause agglutination.

Autoimmune thrombocytopenia can develop as a primary disorder or in conjunction with SLE or AIHA. If immune-mediated thrombocytopenia is suggested by low platelet counts and clinical signs, a test for autoantibodies reactive with platelets can be performed. The platelet factor 3 test is performed by incubating the patient's serum with platelet-rich plasma from a control animal. If autoantibodies specific for platelets are present, they bind to the

Table 3. *Sampling for Evaluation of Immune Deficiency/Dysfunction*

Test	Sample	Indications
Immunoelectrophoresis	0.5 ml serum	Ab deficiency, myeloma
Single radial diffusion	0.5 ml serum	Ab deficiency, myeloma
B-cell count (IFA)	10 ml blood*	Immunodeficiency
Lymphocyte stimulation	5–10 ml blood* and age-matched control	T-cell dysfunction
T-cell count (IFA)	10 ml blood*	T-cell deficiency
Phagocytic index	10 ml blood* 10 ml clot tube	Neutrophil defect
Bactericidal test	10 ml blood* 10 ml clot tube and age-matched control	Neutrophil defect
NBT test	3 ml blood*	Neutrophil defect
Chemotactic test	3 ml blood*	Neutrophil defect

*Preservative-free heparin

platelets and initiate the release of thromboplastin (platelet factor 3), which results in a fibrin clot.

An alternative test is the performance of direct immunofluorescence on megakaryocytes within a bone marrow biopsy. Platelet-specific autoantibodies bound to the megakaryocytes are stained by the fluorescein-conjugated antiglobulin. The immunofluorescence test is more specific for autoimmune thrombocytopenia than the platelet factor 3 test, but it is also more invasive.

EVALUATION OF HYPERSENSITIVITY DISEASE

Atopic skin disease in the dog is a type 1 hypersensitivity reaction mediated by IgE antibodies. Testing for allergen-specific IgE is performed in two ways: the evaluation of IgE present on mast cells in the skin by intradermal skin testing and the evaluation of circulating IgE using an *in vitro* test. The results of these two tests do not always agree, probably because the half-life of IgE on mast cells is weeks to months and the half-life in serum is about 2.5 days. Intradermal skin testing requires shaving the dog, may be difficult in intractable dogs, and may be tedious. The *in vitro* assays require only a sample of blood, but they are expensive.

For intradermal skin testing the dog must be taken off short-acting steroids and antihistamine drugs for at least 10 days before testing (30 to 60 days may be required for longer-acting corticosteroids). Tranquilization, if necessary, must not be induced with acepromazine, owing to its antihistamine activity. The lateral thorax is clipped, and intradermal injections of allergens common to the geographic area are made. Detailed descriptions of the technique are available elsewhere. Results appear within 20 min of injection, and the size of the wheals are scored from +1 to +4 (the size of the histamine control).

In vitro assays are available from several commercial laboratories and at some clinical immunology laboratories associated with veterinary schools. These assays vary in design but are generally of the enzyme-linked immunosorbent assay (ELISA) or radioallergosorbent test (RAST) format. In these assays the patient's serum is incubated with allergen on a solid phase. After washing off unbound antibody, a conjugated antidog IgE reagent is added and allowed to incubate. The conjugate is an enzyme (ELISA) or a radioisotope (RAST). After the anti-IgE is allowed to bind, the solid phase is again washed and either reacted with substrate (ELISA) for color development or measured for radioactivity bound in a scintillation counter. The amount of color (ELISA) or radioactivity (RAST) is proportional to the amount of IgE bound to the allergen. Correlation between results obtained from the various commercial laboratories is not always good.

SAMPLING

Some of the assays performed by the clinical immunology laboratory require previous notification (lymphocyte stimulation, bactericidal test) and the submission of control material along with the pa-

Table 4. *Sampling for Evaluation of Autoimmunity*

Test	Sample	Indications
Antinuclear antibody	1–3 ml serum	SLE
Rheumatoid factor	1–3 ml serum	Rheumatoid arthritis
LE cell preparation	0.5 ml blood	SLE
Coombs' antiglobulin	1 ml blood (EDTA)	AIHA
Cold agglutinins	1 ml serum*	Cold agglutinin disease
Antiplatelet Ab (IFA) thrombocytopenia	bone marrow	Autoimmune disease
Platelet factor 3 test thrombocytopenia	3 ml plasma (citrated)	Autoimmune disease
Hemolytic complement	1–3 ml serum	Complement deficiency
FA tissue staining	biopsy†	Ig and/or C' deposition
Antithyroglobulin	1 ml serum	Autoimmune thyroiditis
Pemphigus antibody	1 ml serum	Autoimmune skin disease
C1q binding assay	0.5 ml serum	Immune complex disease

*Collect blood and harvest serum at 37°C
†Tissue snap frozen on dry ice or preserved in Michel's medium

tient's sample. Tests that require viable cells require that the blood be carried on ice to the laboratory within several hours. When only serum is required, it should be separated from the clotted blood and sent to the laboratory frozen if significant travel delay is expected. Biopsy samples should be taken at the edge of an active lesion. Tables 3 and 4 list the samples required for tests mentioned in the text.

CONCLUSION

The clinical immunology laboratory performs a variety of tests to assist the clinician in assessing the immune status of the patient. Deficiency or dysfunction, misdirected immune responses (as in autoimmune disease), and exuberant immune responses (as in hypersensitivity disease) can be diagnosed with greater certainty using the laboratory.

An understanding of how each test is performed facilitates appropriate procedures in sample collection and accurate interpretation of the results.

References

Baker, E.: *Small Animal Allergy: A Practical Guide.* Philadelphia: Lea & Febiger, 1990, pp. 61–72.
   An easily understood explanation of how to evaluate IgE responses in small animals.

Barta, O.: *Laboratory Techniques of Veterinary Clinical Immunology.* Springfield, IL: Charles C Thomas, 1984, pp. 43–83, 103–179.
   A manual that explains in detail assays to evaluate immune function in veterinary species.

Bennett, D., and Kerkham, D.: The laboratory identification of serum antinuclear antibodies in the dog. J. Comp. Pathol. 97:523, 1987.
   Description of the ANA test and results obtained with canine serum.

Felsburg, P. J., Glickman, L. T., and Jezyk, P. F.: Selective IgA deficiency in the dog. Clin. Immunol. Immunopath. 36:297, 1985.
   Description of the syndrome.

Lewis, R. M., and Picut, C. A.: *Veterinary Clinical Immunology: From Classroom to Clinic.* Philadelphia: Lea & Febiger, 1989, pp. 230–250.
   An excellent applied text with case histories, diagnostic tests, and treatments.

PRIMARY IMMUNODEFICIENCIES

PETER J. FELSBURG
West Lafayette, Indiana

The immune system is multicellular and composed of two main components—one concerned with nonspecific immune responses and one concerned with specific immune responses. The cells involved in the nonspecific immune response are phagocytic cells, primarily neutrophils and monocytes (macrophages), which are responsible for the engulfment (phagocytosis), digestion, and elimination of foreign substances from the body. The cells of the specific component of the immune system are the lymphocytes. They interact with antigens in a manner that exhibits not only high specificity but also memory to individual antigens. This part of the immune system is divided into two different functional components—the humoral (B cell) and cell-mediated (T cell) immune systems. The primary function of the humoral immune system is the production of antibodies against foreign antigens. The cell-mediated immune system has many functions, including the production of soluble substances called lymphokines, which exert their influence on the cells of the nonspecific component of the immune system, and the destruction of virus-infected

and tumor cells by cytotoxic (killing) mechanisms. Cytokines produced by monocytes and T cells are important in the amplification and down-regulation of the immune system.

Immunodeficiency disease results from abnormalities in one or more of the components of the immune system. *The major clinical manifestation of immunodeficiency is an increased susceptibility to infection. When there is no apparent explanation for recurrent infections in a patient, a primary or acquired immunologic defect should be considered.* The type of infection involved and the clinical signs are influenced by the severity of the defect and which part of the immune system is affected. Some of the more common conditions associated with immunodeficiency diseases are respiratory infections, otitis, dermatitis and pyoderma, diarrhea, growth retardation, adverse reactions to modified-live vaccines, and infection with usually nonpathogenic organisms. Defects in the B-cell system usually predispose an animal to increased susceptibility to bacterial infection. Animals with a defective cell-mediated immunity are more susceptible to fungal, protozoal, and viral infections. Disorders of the phagocytic system are associated with superficial skin infections or systemic infections with pyogenic organisms.

Immunodeficiencies can be classified as either primary (congenital) or secondary (acquired). Primary immunodeficiencies are congenital diseases in which the inherited defect in the immune system predisposes the animal to increased susceptibility to infection. Secondary or acquired immunodeficiencies, on the other hand, are alterations in immunologic function caused by some underlying disease process and increase susceptibility to infection. Animals with acquired immunodeficiencies are born with an intact immune system, but, during or following the underlying disease, their immune system becomes transiently or permanently impaired. Differentiation between a primary or secondary immunodeficiency is important from the standpoint of treatment and prognosis.

PRIMARY IMMUNODEFICIENCIES INVOLVING SPECIFIC COMPONENTS OF THE IMMUNE SYSTEM

There are approximately 30 primary immunodeficiencies that have been documented in humans. The study of primary immunodeficiency diseases in dogs and cats is still in its infancy. The primary immunodeficiency diseases discussed here are congenital or inherited disorders of the specific (lymphocytic) and nonspecific (phagocytic) components of the immune system that have been described in dogs and cats and that are associated with increased susceptibility to infections. Although many of the following diseases have been primarily described in certain breeds, they most likely occur in all breeds of dogs. For example, IgA deficiency, originally described in the beagle and Shar pei, has been observed in many breeds as well as in mixed breed dogs.

X-Linked Severe Combined Immunodeficiency

Severe combined immunodeficiency (SCID) is the most severe of all the primary immunodeficiencies. The term SCID describes a heterogeneous group of disorders that have the common feature of severely deficient humoral and cell-mediated immune responses. Three major types of SCID are observed in man: SCID characterized by a lymphoid stem cell defect in which the patient lacks or possesses few B and T cells; SCID associated with an adenosine deaminase (ADA) deficiency; and SCID with B cells and nonfunctional T cells. The mode of inheritance may be autosomal or X-linked recessive. Since both components of the immune system are deficient, clinical signs occur early in infancy, and affected individuals are susceptible to a wide spectrum of microbial agents, both bacterial and viral. Untreated human patients rarely survive past the first year.

An X-linked form of SCID has been documented in the dog (Felsburg and Jezyk, 1982; Jezyk et al., 1989). These dogs present as early as 3 weeks of age with clinical signs that include pyoderma, otitis, diarrhea, and respiratory infections. These infections, usually of bacterial origin, are unresponsive to antibiotic therapy. A universal finding in affected dogs is a failure to thrive (stunted growth). Affected puppies usually die before 3 to 4 months of age either from overwhelming bacterial infections or from viral infections, primarily distemper. Several affected puppies vaccinated with a modified-live distemper vaccine died 2 to 3 weeks later of distemper induced by the vaccine.

In X-linked SCID, only males are affected whereas females may be carriers of the disease. In the dog, approximately half the males in a litter from a carrier female will be affected and half the females will be potential carriers. It is important to emphasize that carrier females show no clinical or immunologic evidence of any abnormalities.

Laboratory findings include normal numbers of circulating B lymphocytes and normal concentrations of IgM, but low to absent concentrations of serum IgG and IgA, indicating a defect in the differentiation and maturation of IgG and IgA B cells into immunoglobulin-secreting plasma cells. There are low to normal numbers of circulating T cells, but these T cells are nonfunctional as demonstrated by their severely depressed blastogenic response to T-cell mitogens and their inability to support normal B-cell function (see this volume, p. 441).

The typical postmortem findings in X-SCID dogs are a very small thymus characterized by thymic dysplasia and a profound lymphoid hypoplasia. It is difficult to detect any lymph nodes in affected dogs.

The only successful treatment of SCID in man is reconstitution of the patient with lymphoid stem cells by bone marrow transplantation. At present, this is not technically practical in dogs.

Selective IgA Deficiency

Selective IgA deficiency (IgAd) is the most common primary immunodeficiency in man. The prevalence in the "normal" population is approximately 1:600. Affected individuals have absent or markedly reduced levels of serum IgA and, with few exceptions, secretory IgA. Serum IgM and total serum IgG are usually within normal range. IgAd actually represents a heterogeneous group of diseases consisting of three major types: severe IgAd as defined by undetectable IgA as measured by radial immunodiffusion (usually less than 5 to less than 10 mg/dl); partial IgAd as defined by detectable IgA but less than two standard deviations of the mean for age-matched controls; and transient IgAd as defined by undetectable or low IgA with subsequent development of normal IgA concentrations.

Although IgAd is often found among apparently healthy individuals, reduced levels of IgA predispose to a variety of diseases, including recurrent infections, particularly of the upper respiratory tract, autoimmune disease, and atopy. In a large study of pediatric and adult symptomatic IgAd patients, recurrent infections were observed in 55% of the patients, immune-mediated or autoimmune disease in 25% of the patients, and atopy in 20% of the patients. Convulsive episodes of unexplained etiology have also been associated with IgAd.

A perplexing question is why many IgAd individuals show no clinical signs of illness at the time of diagnosis. Recent studies have associated IgG subclass deficiencies with IgAd. It has been suggested that IgAd alone in patients with severe IgAd is sufficient to cause manifestation of clinical disease, whereas in partial IgAd patients, a concomitant IgG subclass deficiency predisposes to disease.

All three forms of IgAd have been documented in the dog (Felsburg et al., 1985; Moroff et al., 1986). Although the initial descriptions were in the beagle and in Shar peis, IgAd has been diagnosed in many different breeds. The clinical presentation in dogs consists of recurrent infections, usually upper respiratory infections, otitis and staphylococcal dermatitis, and atopic dermatitis. As in man, there does not appear to be a difference in the clinical manifestations between dogs with severe IgAd and dogs with partial IgAd. In spite of intranasal vaccination with an effective bivalent vaccine, IgAd dogs develop mild, recurrent upper respiratory infections due primarily to *Bordetella bronchiseptica* and canine parainfluenza virus. The infections associated with IgAd are usually not severe or life-threatening. Several dogs have experienced episodes of convulsion. Recent epidemiologic studies have shown that puppies born of "healthy" IgAd dams are at much higher risk of developing upper respiratory infections than are puppies born of dams with normal concentrations of IgA.

Screening of large populations of clinically normal adult dogs has revealed IgAd in apparently "healthy" adults, just as is seen in man. There appears to be a high incidence of IgAd in Shar peis, which may reflect on their predisposition to upper respiratory infections and atopic disease.

The only abnormal laboratory finding is an absence or a markedly low concentration of IgA when compared with values of age-matched normal dogs. The immunologic defect appears to be in the maturation and differentiation of the IgA B cell.

There is a possibility that some young dogs diagnosed as IgA deficient may have a transient IgA deficiency and will outgrow their tendency for recurrent infections as they become adults.

Transient Hypogammaglobulinemia of Infancy

Transient hypogammaglobulinemia of infancy is a self-limiting immunoglobulin deficiency resulting from an abnormally prolonged delay in the onset of immunoglobulin synthesis by the neonate and young puppy. The puppies show a normal decline in maternal antibody over the first weeks of life, but they fail to synthesize their own immunoglobulins until much later than normal. This disorder is characterized by an increased susceptibility to infection after the disappearance of maternal antibody until the affected puppy's own B-cell system is fully operational.

Affected puppies present with chronic or recurrent bacterial infections of the respiratory tract and skin that start around 2 to 3 months of age, following the disappearance of maternal antibody. Spontaneous recovery occurs as the levels of immunoglobulins become normal, around 5 to 6 months of age (Felsburg et al., manuscript in preparation).

The only significant laboratory finding is a low level of immunoglobulins, compared with those of dogs of comparable age, that occurs after the disappearance of maternal antibody and persists until the puppies are 5 to 7 months of age. It is essential to monitor the immunoglobulin concentrations of puppies diagnosed as immunoglobulin deficient in order to determine whether it is a permanent or transient defect.

PRIMARY IMMUNODEFICIENCIES INVOLVING NONSPECIFIC COMPONENTS OF THE IMMUNE SYSTEM

Canine Cyclic Hematopoiesis

Neutropenia is the most common disorder of the polymorphonuclear phagocytic system in man. Neutropenia results in increased susceptibility to severe bacterial infections and a poor response to antibiotic therapy. Neutropenia can be either acquired or congenital.

A congenital form of neutropenia has been documented in the dog (Lund et al., 1967). Unlike cyclic neutropenia in man, the disease in the dog is characterized by cyclic fluctuations of not only peripheral blood neutrophils but of all cellular blood elements, including platelets. The defect appears to be at the level of the pluripotential stem cell. It was originally reported in gray collies and has been shown to be inherited as an autosomal recessive trait. Cyclic neutropenia generally occurs every 8 to 12 days and lasts 2 to 4 days. Clinical signs are cyclic and are present only during the periods of neutropenia. Affected dogs suffer from severe, recurrent bacterial infections primarily involving the respiratory or gastrointestinal tract. Epistaxis or profuse hemorrhage may be present owing to the associated thrombocytopenia. The infections usually clear when the neutrophils return to normal levels. Affected dogs rarely survive past 3 years of age.

It was originally thought that the recurrent infections occurred because of a lack of sufficient numbers of functional neutrophils during the periods of neutropenia. However, more recent studies have shown that the neutrophils exhibit impaired killing of bacteria because of metabolic abnormalities such as a myeloperoxidase deficiency and a defect in iodination. No other immunologic abnormalities have been documented in these dogs.

The laboratory diagnosis is based on the demonstration of a cyclic neutropenia as well as an abnormal bactericidal assay.

Treatment is primarily supportive antibiotic therapy to control the infections. Other treatments that have been successful are bone marrow transplantation and endotoxin or lithium carbonate therapy (see this volume, p. 409). As mentioned previously, bone marrow transplantation is not practical at this time in veterinary medicine. Although endotoxin or lithium carbonate therapy is effective in controlling the cycling of the neutrophils and platelets, once therapy is discontinued, cycling of the cells and clinical signs reappear. However, chronic therapy with these agents is not suggested owing to their potential toxicity.

Canine Granulocytopathy Syndrome

This disease is a congenital disorder of neutrophil function that is characterized by recurrent life-threatening bacterial infections (Renshaw et al., 1975). These dogs present with a neutrophilia, but, unlike the condition in cyclic neutropenia, these neutrophils are defective in their ability to kill phagocytocized bacteria. The defect is inherited as an autosomal recessive trait.

Clinically, these dogs present at a young age with a history of recurrent episodes of infections with pyogenic bacteria that respond poorly to routine antibiotic therapy. Suppurative skin lesions, pododermatitis, gingivitis, and marked lymphadenopathy are common clinical findings. In advanced states, osteomyelitis may be observed.

Hematologic findings consist of a persistent leukocytosis with a regenerative left shift. Mature neutrophils exhibit prominent nuclear hypersegmentation. These dogs apparently have competent humoral and cell-mediated immune systems. The only functional defect appears to be related to an inability of the neutrophils to kill bacteria as determined by bactericidal assays. This defect is intrinsic to the neutrophil, since serum from these dogs possesses normal opsonizing antibodies for neutrophils from normal dogs.

C3 Deficiency

C3 is a component of the complement system that is important in the opsonization of bacteria. A C3 deficiency has been documented in the dog with an autosomal recessive mode of inheritance (Blum et al., 1985). Dogs that are homozygous for the trait have no detectable C3, whereas dogs that are heterozygous have C3 concentrations that are approximately 50% of normal. Clinical signs are observed only in dogs that are homozygous for the C3 deficiency and are related to an increased susceptibility to bacterial infections, including septicemias, primarily involving gram-negative organisms and clostridia. Signs of renal disease and possibly amyloidosis may be present.

The major immunologic abnormality in these dogs is the absence of serum C3. The renal complications may be due to immune complex disease, and dogs showing symptoms of renal disease may possess rheumatoid factor.

Chédiak-Higashi Syndrome

Chédiak-Higashi syndrome is an autosomal recessive genetic disease of humans and other species, including the Persian cat (Kramer et al., 1977). It is characterized by the presence of abnormally large, eosinophilic granules in neutrophils, basophils, and eosinophils. Enlarged melanin granules are observed in the skin and hair shafts of affected animals.

Affected cats may show an increased susceptibility to infection, particularly to neonatal septicemia and viral respiratory infections. Sudden death due to an increased bleeding tendency may occur. The increased bleeding tendency is thought to be due to abnormal platelet function and can result in major bleeding problems following even minor surgery and hematoma formation following venipuncture. The abnormal melanin granules cause abnormally light coat colors in affected blue smoke Persian cats. Affected cats may also have light-colored irises, reduced fundic pigmentation, photophobia, and an increased incidence of congenital cataracts.

Neutrophils from affected cats exhibit impaired chemotaxis and a defect in intracellular killing of bacteria. Treatment is symptomatic.

Leukocyte Surface Glycoprotein (Mo1) Deficiency

Recently, a combined Mo1 and LFA-1 leukocyte surface glycoprotein deficiency has been described in the dog. Mo1 is a surface glycoprotein found on neutrophils and monocytes that is involved in cell adhesion, chemotaxis, and phagocytosis of complement-opsonized bacteria. LFA-1 (lymphocyte function-associated antigen 1) is expressed on phagocytes and lymphocytes and promotes lymphoid cell adhesion interactions that include lymphocyte proliferation and cytotoxic effector activity. This immunodeficiency is characterized by defective phagocytic function and suppressed cell-mediated immunity.

The clinical presentation in dogs includes deep skin wound infections, pododermatitis, superficial pyoderma, gingivitis, pneumonia, thrombophlebitis, and osteomyelitis. Infection sites usually exhibit a localized cellulitis with impaired pus formation. Poor wound healing is a common feature. The mode of inheritance in the dog appears to be autosomal recessive. In man, both autosomal recessive and X-linked recessive modes of inheritance have been reported.

Laboratory findings include a persistent marked leukocytosis, with most of the cells being mature neutrophils. Neutrophils from affected dogs will show an absence of Mo1 and LFA-1 on their surface as demonstrated by immunofluorescence using monoclonal antibodies to Mo1 and LFA-1. Neutrophil function tests are uniformly abnormal. Lymphocytes from affected dogs will also have a markedly suppressed blastogenic response following mitogenic stimulation.

It has been hypothesized that owing to the clinical and immunologic similarities, canine granulocytopathy syndrome may, in fact, represent a leukocyte adhesion molecule deficiency.

Miscellaneous Neutrophil Immunodeficiencies

A neutrophil bactericidal defect has been reported in eight related Doberman pinschers (Breitschwerdt et al., 1987). These dogs suffered from chronic respiratory infections from birth. The humoral and cell-mediated immune systems appeared to be normal in these dogs. The neutrophil count was normal in these dogs.

A defect in neutrophil oxidative metabolism has been independently described by two groups in a total of 64 related Weimaraner dogs (Couto et al., 1989; Studdert et al., 1984). Clinically, these dogs presented with recurrent febrile episodes, vomiting, diarrhea, pneumonia, pyoderma, lymphadenopathy, and osteomyelitis. Neurologic signs such as ataxia, disorientation, head pressing, and seizures were seen in some of the dogs. The only immuno-

logic abnormality observed in these dogs is reduced neutrophil oxidative metabolism as measured by chemiluminescence.

MANAGEMENT OF ANIMALS WITH IMMUNODEFICIENCY DISEASES

Successful management of patients with immunodeficiency diseases depends on whether the deficiency is primary or secondary and which part or parts of the immune system are affected.

Secondary immunodeficiencies are treated with symptomatic therapy such as antibiotics to control infections while attempts are made to cure or treat the underlying disease process. Once the underlying disease is cured, the immunodeficiency should be resolved.

Primary immunodeficiencies pose a very special problem to the clinician and clinical immunologist. Since these are newly recognized diseases in the dog, our experience in treating them is limited. Nevertheless, we can draw upon the knowledge gained over the past 30 years in treating human primary immunodeficiencies. Antibiotics can be life-saving in the treatment of the infectious episodes of patients with immunodeficiencies.

Humoral immune or B-cell deficiencies with normal T-cell function are the easiest to manage. Aggressive antibiotic therapy should be first used in an attempt to control infections. In cases in which this approach is insufficient, patients may be given gamma globulin preparations to replace the immunoglobulins that they are lacking. In humans, monthly intramuscular injections of gamma globulin preparations at a dosage of 100 mg/kg is sufficient to keep patients symptom-free. If gamma globulin preparations are not available, plasma infusions at a dosage of 20 ml/kg may be employed. The exception to the use of gamma globulin or plasma is selective IgA deficiency. IgA-deficient patients cannot be given preparations that contain IgA, since many will have an anaphylactic reaction to it. In addition, serum IgA probably plays a very minor role in host defense. What really has to be replaced is secretory IgA, and at this time, there is no practical way of passively administering secretory IgA. These patients have to be treated symptomatically.

At this time there is no *practical* way of treating a T-cell deficiency other than by symptomatic therapy. Nonspecific immunostimulators have yet to be shown by well-controlled studies to be of any benefit in treating T-cell deficiencies in the dog. *Do not* use modified-live virus vaccines in animals with a T-cell deficiency or severe combined immunodeficiency. These animals may develop infections from the vaccine itself.

Patients with a neutrophil defect should be treated aggressively with a broad-spectrum *bacte-*

ricidal antibiotic. If the defect is primary or permanent, it is important to initiate therapy with high doses of a bactericidal antibiotic to treat even mild infections.

Most life-threatening infections associated with immunoglobulin deficiencies or neutrophil defects result from delay in diagnosis or treatment. Continuous antibiotic therapy may be required to control infections, depending on the severity of the deficiency.

When the clinician deals with animals with primary immunodeficiencies, perhaps the best reason for understanding why the patient has an increased susceptibility to infection is to be able to advise the client on the prognosis for a cure or successful management of the case. (Some patients may not get better no matter how you or another veterinarian treats them).

References and Suggested Reading

Blum, J. R., Cork, L. C., Morris, J. M., et al.: The clinical manifestations of a genetically determined deficiency in the third component of complement in the dog. Clin. Immunol. Immunopathol. 34:304, 1985.

Breitschwerdt, E. B., Brown, T. T., DeBuysscher, E. V., et al.: Rhinitis, pneumonia, and defective neutrophil function in the Doberman Pinscher. Am. J. Vet. Res. 48:1054, 1987.

Couto, C. G., Krakowka, S., Johnson, G., et al.: In vitro immunologic features of Weimaraner dogs with neutrophil abnormalities and recurrent infections. Vet. Immunol. Immunopathol. 23:103, 1989.

Felsburg, P. J., and Jezyk, P. F.: A canine model for combined immunodeficiency. Clin. Res. 30:347, 1982.

Felsburg, P. J., Glickman, L. T., and Jezyk, P. F.: Selective IgA deficiency in the dog. Clin. Immunol. Immunopathol. 36:297, 1985.

Felsburg, P. J.: Immunodeficiency diseases. *In* Morgan, R. V. (ed.): *Handbook of Small Animal Practice,* New York: Churchill Livingstone, 1988, p. 835.

Giger, U., Boxer, L. A., Simpson, P. J., et al.: Deficiency of leukocyte surface glycoproteins Mo1, LFA-1, and Leu M5 in a dog with recurrent bacterial infections: An animal model. Blood 69:1622, 1987.

Guilford, W. G.: Primary immunodeficiency diseases of dogs and cats. Comp. Sm. Anim. Pract. 9:641, 1987.

Jezyk, P. F., Felsburg, P. J., Haskins, M. E., et al.: X-linked severe combined immunodeficiency in the dog. Clin. Immunol. Immunopathol. 52:173, 1989.

Kramer, J. W., Davis, W. C., and Prieur, D. J.: The Chédiak-Higashi syndrome of cats. Lab. Invest. 36:554, 1977.

Lund, J. E., Padgett, G. A., and Ott, R. L.: Cyclic neutropenia in grey collie dogs. Blood 29:452, 1967.

Moroff, S. D., Hurvitz, A. I., Peterson, M. E., et al.: IgA deficiency in Shar-Pei dogs. Vet. Immunol. Immunopathol. 13:181, 1986.

Renshaw, H. W., Chatburn, C., Bryan, G. M., et al.: Canine granulocytopathy syndrome: Neutrophil dysfunction in a dog with recurrent infections. J.A.V.M.A. 166:443, 1975.

Stiehm, E. R.: *Immunologic Disorders in Infants and Children,* 3rd ed. Philadelphia: W. B. Saunders, 1989.

Studdert, V. P., Phillips, W. A., Studdert, M. J., et. al.: Recurrent and persistent infections in related Weimaraner dogs. Aust. Vet. J. 61:261, 1984.

ACQUIRED IMMUNODEFICIENCY DISEASES

STEVEN KRAKOWKA
Columbus, Ohio

Acquired immunodeficiency disease is a common complicating manifestation of many systemic diseases of diverse causes (Table 1). Clinical expression of this defect varies, but most have as their common denominator enhanced expression of secondary opportunistic or unusual infections. In most cases, the provisional diagnosis of immunologic dysfunction is made by inference once the primary or inciting cause has been identified. For example, failure of passive transport of immunoglobulin is a problem of the neonate; viral infectious diseases are chiefly problems in post-weanling and young adult animals; and cancer is a disease of middle to old age.

While sophisticated laboratory assays are beyond the capabilities of most private practitioners, several presumptive tests are useful in identifying the nature of the dysfunction. Viral antigen assays are especially useful in the evaluation of the feline leukemia virus (FeLV-FIV) complex. Most suppressive diseases are manifested as an absolute lymphopenia easily detected in routine hemograms. Cutaneous skin test responses to mitogens such as PHA or ConA or commonly encountered environmental antigens such as streptokinase-streptodornase (SK-SD) are convenient methods for *in vivo* assessment of cell-mediated immunity. Serum immunoglobulin levels are easily determined by commercially available radial immunodiffusion kits. Successful therapeutic approaches to these diseases revolve around two basic principles: limit or remove the primary cause and institute supportive therapy, including broad-spectrum antimicrobial agents to treat the secondary infections.

Table 1. *An Outline of Recognized General Causes of Secondary Immunodeficiency Diseases in Dogs*

General Etiology	Occurrence	Comments and/or Diagnostic Feature
Failure of passive transport (FPT)	Neonatal animals	Low serum IgG, IgA
Viral infections	Usually young animals	Direct lymphocytolytic or indirect via cytokine disruption
Nutritional disease	Protein-caloric deficiency	Low serum immunoglobulin levels
Metabolic disease	Adults	Secondary infections associated with diabetes, hyperthyroidism, ketosis, etc.
Parasitism	Demodicosis in young animals	*Demodex* spp., pyoderma, circulating immune complexes, soluble suppressive factor(s)
Lymphoreticular neoplasms	Viral in young animals; adult animals	Replacement of lymphoid tissue; disruption of control network
Extra-lymphoid malignant neoplasms	Adult animals	Cachexia plus circulating immune complexes and soluble suppressive factor(s), etc.

SHORT-TERM EFFECTS: CANINE PARVOVIRUS (CPV) AND FELINE PANLEUKOPENIA (FPV)

Parvoviruses are small DNA viruses with a predilection for replication in rapidly proliferating host target cells. Thus, manifestations of infection and, hence, clinical disease are seen primarily in three organ systems: fetal tissues; epithelia, particularly of the gut; and bone marrow cells and associated lymphoid precursor cell population(s) (Kurtzman et al., 1989). Following oronasal infection and local replication in lymphoid tissues, a transient viremia with spread to systemic lymphoid tissues and epithelia occurs (McCartney et al., 1988). The viremia coincides roughly with the onset of leukopenia. Immunosuppression associated with CPV and FPV has been difficult to document, although most studies report decreased lymphocytic responsiveness to mitogens during the course of disease (Phillips and Schultz, 1987). The mechanism for this effect is undoubtedly a direct virolytic effect on replicating lymphocyte populations, although secondary depression of bone marrow (chiefly CFU-GM) contributes to the phenomenon (Kurtzman et al., 1989). Since parvovirus-infected gnotobiotes are clinically asymptomatic, clinical disease characteristic of both CPV and FPV is most likely mediated by secondary factors, chiefly absorbed bacterial endotoxin through the duodenal gut, and is manifested by the effects of endotoxin-stimulated release of tumor necrosis factor and interleukin-1 by macrophages/monocytes (Isogai et al., 1989). Nonetheless, classical immunosuppression is not considered to be a major factor either in expression of disease or in the potentiation of secondary disease syndromes in these species.

FELINE LEUKEMIA COMPLEX OF CATS

There are three currently recognized pathogenic retroviruses of cats: feline leukemia virus (FeLV), feline acquired immunodeficiency disease syndrome (FeLV-FAIDS) (Overbaugh et al., 1988), and feline immunodeficiency virus (FIV, formerly FTLV) (Gardner and Luciw, 1989). All, in their natural expression of disease in cats, are immunosuppressive and are associated with a variety of syndromes, including lymphoreticular neoplasia(s) (FeLV only), wasting, enhanced or unusual manifestations of secondary opportunistic diseases, and immunoregulatory disorders such as immune complex disease (ICD) or Coombs' positive hemolytic disease (Ogilvie et al., 1988). This FeLV-associated suppressive disease is the most common cause of death in this species (Reinacher, 1989). While the pathogenesis of FIV particularly is not yet conclusively established, it is likely that it progresses through a sequence similar to that of FeLV, wherein replication in the local site(s) of infection is followed by a viremia and pantropic infection. Persistently viremic cats are destined to develop one of the clinical syndromes outlined earlier, whereas transiently viremic cats do not.

Mechanisms of suppression are well understood for FeLV (and presumably FeLV-FAIDS). The primary target cell population in cats is the T-helper lymphocyte subset as manifested *in vivo* by delayed allograft skin graft rejections, lymphopenia, thymic atrophy, paracortical (T-cell) lymphoid depletion, and absolute decreases in the circulating CD_4-equivalent (T-helper) cells. *In vitro* changes characteristic of FeLV disease are decreased lymphocyte responsiveness to T-cell mitogens (Con A and PHA) but not B-cell mitogens (protein A and LPS), reduced IgG but not IgM production, and reduced production of interleukin-2 and gamma interferon but not macrophage-origin interleukin-1 (Tomkins et al., 1989). Virus-mediated neutrophil dysfunction in viremic as well as latently infected cats also contributes to the suppressive status of exposed cats (Lafrado et al., 1989). It is important to recognize that these defects are seen in cats (expressing infectious virus) but also many effects can be reproduced by a nonreplicating component of the FeLV envelope, p15E.

Much less is known about the manifestations of

disease induced by a closely related lentivirus, FIV (Pederson et al., 1989). *In vitro*, the virus replicates in feline T-cell lines coinfected with FeLV as well as in interleukin-2–dependent cell lines established from normal cats. Epidemiologic studies associate FIV infection with an AIDS-like syndrome of relentless progression until death. Three phases of infection have been identified: an initial clinical phase of lymphadenopathy, fever, malaise, and leukopenia; an intervening normal clinical phase; and a terminal phase characterized by the appearance of secondary opportunistic infection plus FIV-associated neurologic involvement. Chronic unresponsive stomatitis is present in up to one half of the cats, whereas respiratory disease, dermatitis, and chronic enteritis account for the rest. Although the relationship is unclear, neoplasms of lymphoreticular origin may be associated with terminal stages of FIV.

FELINE INFECTIOUS PERITONITIS (FIP) VIRUS OF CATS

Feline infectious peritonitis is a coronavirus infectious disease of cats. While the majority of infected cats remain asymptomatic, clinically affected animals invariably die of direct viral infection of vital tissues (e.g., brain), systemic disease associated with immune-complex vasculitis, or superimposed opportunistic infection. Unlike the other viral diseases, however, the most common manifestation of disease (the effusive or wet form) appears to be mediated by an induced hyper-reactivity to viral antigen(s). While not delineated in detail, it is tempting to speculate that this hyper-responsiveness is due to FIP-induced dysfunction of the suppressor cell network.

CANINE DISTEMPER VIRUS (CDV) INFECTION OF DOGS

Canine distemper virus (CDV), an enveloped RNA virus of the genus *Morbillivirus* (family Paramyxoviridae) is an important pathogen of canids and their relatives. It is closely related to measles virus, an important human pathogen in which immunosuppression as a part of the disease was first documented by von Pirquet in 1908. In spite of the widespread use of safe and effective modified-live vaccines, CDV remains a serious and frequently fatal pathogen in its own right. Secondary viral, bacterial, and mycotic infections of the respiratory and enteric systems contribute significantly to the overall fatality rates associated with this disease complex (Krakowka et al., 1980; Turnwald et al., 1988).

Following oronasal exposure, virus first replicates in macrophages of local lymphoid tissue and then spreads via a plasma and cell-associated viremia to secondary tissues. As early as 5 days after infection, direct infection of vascular endothelium occurs, which facilitates spread of virus to many extravascular sites, including the brain. Prompt development of circulating virus neutralizing (VN) antibodies correlates with the outcome of the disease process. High VN levels are associated with normal convalescence, intermediate levels with persistent neurologic disease, and low levels with acute onset mortality.

Immunosuppression mediated by CDV is manifested in a number of different ways. The lymphotropic phase of infection results in viremia (in all circulating lymphoid cell leukocytes), nonselective lymphopenia (versus FeLV), hypogammaglobulinemia, and systemic lymphoid necrosis and depletion associated with viral inclusions in syncytial giant cells of mixed (e.g., lymphocyte and macrophage) origin. During this phase of infection, cutaneous allograft rejection times may be delayed and skin test responses to antigens and phytomitogens are suppressed (Krakowka et al., 1980). *In vitro* immunoglobulin production is reduced, yet interleukin-2 production by T lymphocytes is only marginally affected. CDV infection has no effect upon NK-like activity. More important, interleukin-1 production by CDV-infected monocytes is markedly reduced, and prostaglandin E_2 synthesis and release (the major suppressive metabolite of arachidonic acid catabolism) are enhanced (Krakowka et al., 1987). Dogs in nonviremic convalescence exhibit residual immunologic deficits, including delayed *in vivo* response to immunogens, depressed phytomitogen responses, and enhanced nonspecific suppressor cell activity. Thus, for CDV, virus-mediated immunosuppression modulates the outcome of the disease process by regulating the production of protective levels of VN antibody and by facilitating infection by unrelated secondary infectious diseases.

FAILURE OF PASSIVE TRANSFER (FPT) OF MATERNAL IMMUNOGLOBULIN

Failure of passive transport (FPT) is the most common form of acquired immunodeficiency disease and is a major cause of neonatal infections and septicemia, especially of farm animals. Since the neonate depends on maternal-origin IgG through colostrum to combat neonatal pathogens, failure to ingest or absorb colostrum by any mechanism results in immunodeficiency (Lewis and Picut, 1989; Tizard, 1982). For reasons unclear at this time, this phenomenon seems to be less important in companion animals than in farm animals. Nonetheless, if suspected, this form of immunodeficiency is easiest to treat. Intravenous administration of hyperimmune serum plus a supportive regimen of broad-spectrum antimicrobials is frequently successful.

CANCER-ASSOCIATED IMMUNODEFICIENCY

It is well recognized that cancer-bearing animals and humans suffer immunosuppression apart from the general debilitation and cachexia associated with disseminated malignant neoplasms (Pollock and Roth, 1989). For descriptive purposes it is convenient to divide these effects by neoplastic type into lymphoreticular and nonlymphoreticular cancers.

Lymphoreticular neoplasms exert their suppressive effects by replacement of normal lymphocytes with neoplastic lymphocytes, by inappropriate production of immunoregulatory cytokines, or by activation of suppressor cell networks. As a general rule, T-cell origin neoplasms inhibit cell-mediated immune functions whereas B-cell origin neoplasms inhibit B-cell functions. If a virus is involved (for example, FeLV), these effects are additive to direct or indirect viral effects. Immunoglobulin (Ig)-secreting plasma cell myelomas are strongly suppressive, not only by replacement of normal lymphoid tissue by neoplastic cells but also by the downregulating effects of elevated Ig protein secreted by the neoplastic cells.

Nonlymphoid cancers may interfere with normal host immune responses directly by producing suppressive factors and indirectly by overstimulating the host response to tumor antigen, thereby inducing inadvertent activation of down-regulating host immune mechanisms such as the suppressor cell network. Tumors stimulate production of circulating suppressive tumor antigen-antibody immune complexes, acute phase serum reactants, and a number of blocking factors, including prostaglandin E_2, tumor necrosis factor (responsible for host cachexia), a variety of molecules that inhibit protein and DNA synthesis, and inhibitory growth-regulating molecules and hormones, to name a few.

Finally, it is important to recognize that most (if not all) of the drugs used in cancer chemotherapy exert their mode of action chiefly through their toxic antiproliferative effects. Thus, the nonselective nature of these drugs can and does directly affect remaining normal immune responsiveness.

PARASITE-ASSOCIATED IMMUNOSUPPRESSION

Depressed immune responsiveness has been noted in animals with toxoplasmosis, trypanosomi-asis, trichinosis, and demodicosis (Tizard, 1982). For these diseases, our knowledge of the nature of the defects observed has not progressed much beyond the descriptive state. Canine disseminated demodicosis is the most thoroughly understood of these. Lymphocytes from these dogs are poorly responsive to mitogens, and affected dogs demonstrate suppressed responses to skin test antigens. In addition, a plasma-origin suppressive factor inhibits lymphocyte blastogenic responses *in vitro* (most likely parasite antigen-antibody immune complexes). If the skin condition associated with mite infestation is reversed, immune responses return to the normal range.

References and Suggested Reading

Gardner, M. B., and Luciw, P. A.: Animal models of AIDS. FASEB J. 3:2593–2606, 1989.

Isogai, E., Isogai, H., Onuma, M., et al.: Eshcerichia coli associated endotoxemia in dogs with parvovirus infection. Jap. J. Vet. Sci. 51(3):597–606, 1989.

Krakowka, S., Higgins, R. J., and Koestner, A.: Canine distemper virus: Review of structure and functional modulations in lymphoid tissues. Am. J. Vet. Res. 41(2):284–292, 1980.

Krakowka, S., Ringler, S., Lewis, M., et al.: Immunosuppression by canine distemper virus: Modulation of *in vitro* immunoglobulin synthesis, interleukin release, and prostaglandin E_2 production. Vet. Immunol. Immunopathol. 15:181–201, 1987.

Kurtzman, G. J., Platanias, L., Lustig, L., et al.: Feline parvovirus propagates in cat bone marrow cultures and inhibits hematopoietic colony formation *in vitro*. Blood 74(1):71–81, 1989.

Lafrado, L. J., Dezzutti, C. S., Lewis, M. G., et al.: Immunodeficiency in latent feline leukemia virus infections. Vet. Immunol. Immunopathol. 21:39–46, 1989.

Lewis, R. M., and Picut, C. A.: *Veterinary Clinical Immunology: From Classroom to Clinic.* Philadelphia: Lea & Febiger, 1989, pp. 205–209.

McCartney, L., Thompson, H., McCandlish, I. A. P., et al.: Canine parvovirus: Interaction between passive immunity and virulent challenge. Vet. Record 122:573–576, 1988.

Ogilvie, G. K., Tompkins, M. B., and Tompkins, W. A. F.: Clinical and immunologic aspects of FeLV-induced immunosuppression. Vet. Microbiol. 17:287–296, 1988.

Overbaugh, J., Donahue, P. R., Quackenbush, S. L., et al.: Molecular cloning of a feline leukemia virus that induces fatal immunodeficiency disease in cats. Science 239:906–910, 1988.

Pedersen, N. C., Yamamoto, J. K., Ishida, T., et al.: Feline immunodeficiency virus infection. Vet. Immunol. Immunopathol. 21:111–129, 1989.

Phillips, T. R., and Schultz, R. D.: Failure of vaccine or virulent strains of canine parvovirus to induce immunosuppressive effects on the immune system of the dog. Viral Immunol. 1(2):135–144, 1987.

Pollock, R., and Roth, J.: Cancer-induced immunosuppression: Implications for therapy? Semin. Surg. Oncol. 5:414–419, 1989.

Reinacher, M.: Diseases associated with spontaneous feline leukemia virus (FeLV) infection in cats. Vet. Immunol. Immunopathol. 21:85–95, 1989.

Tizard, I.: *An Introduction to Veterinary Immunology.* Philadelphia: W. B. Saunders, 1982, pp. 336–342.

Tompkins, M. B., Ogilvie, G. K., Gast, A. M., et al.: Interleukin-2 suppression in cats naturally infected with feline leukemia virus. J. Biol. Resp. Mod. 8:86–96, 1989.

Turnwald, G. H., Barta, O., Taylor, W., et al.: Cryptosporidiosis associated with immunosuppression attributable to distemper in a pup. J.A.V.M.A. 192:79–81, 1988.

DEVELOPMENT OF VACCINES AGAINST FELINE LEUKEMIA VIRUS

OSWALD JARRETT

Glasgow, Scotland

New techniques in molecular biology offer opportunities to produce effective, safe, and relatively inexpensive vaccines against infectious diseases. Much of the pioneering work in this field has been done with viral diseases since the genomes of viruses are small and therefore relatively easy to manipulate. The reasons for wishing to produce novel vaccines vary according to the type of virus involved. In some cases, the impetus is to produce a vaccine that is more effective than that currently in use. In other cases, these techniques offer the possibility of constructing a vaccine against a virus which is impossible to grow in the laboratory and therefore for which there is no existing vaccine.

In many instances, the viral protein responsible for the induction of a protective immune response has been identified and the gene encoding that protein has been cloned. The goal of the genetic engineer, then, is to use this information to construct vaccines. Several approaches have been considered. Some follow familiar paths such as the modification of viruses for use as live vaccines. The viruses used in most existing modified-live vaccines were obtained more or less by chance or, at best, by selection for growth in unorthodox conditions. More recently, however, wild type viruses have been specifically engineered to inactivate the genes responsible for pathogenicity while retaining those encoding the antigens necessary for induction of immunity. An example of this type of vaccine is that used against Aujesky's disease (pseudorabies) in pigs. In another variant of this approach, recombinant viruses can be made in which a gene encoding the immunogen of the virus of interest is inserted into another virus which acts as a vector to deliver the immunogen into the appropriate host. Viruses shown to be effective as vectors are vaccinia and other poxviruses, adenoviruses, and herpesviruses.

In a second approach, which may be considered as the modern equivalent of an inactivated vaccine, the gene encoding the immunogen can be inserted into bacterial, yeast, insect, or mammalian cells, and the resulting expressed protein can be purified and formulated as a subunit vaccine. This might be the only approach possible for those viruses that cannot be cultivated *in vitro*. A case in point is the vaccine for hepatitis B virus of man. An extension of this approach is to identify the peptide within the immunogenic protein which is the primary antigenic determinant, or epitope, and to use that peptide, together with a much larger carrier molecule, as a vaccine. So far this approach has been used only at the experimental level.

In considering how these techniques might be applied to viruses of small animals, feline leukemia virus (FeLV) is a good example. FeLV has been known as an important pathogen of domestic cats for more than 25 years, but it is only in the past few years that vaccines have been available. This delay is in part a reflection of the fact that the retroviruses, the viral group that includes FeLV, feline immunodeficiency virus and human immunodeficiency virus, have proved to be relatively poorly immunogenic. Therefore, various attempts have been, and are still being, made to overcome this problem.

THE IMMUNE RESPONSE TO FELINE LEUKEMIA VIRUS

In nature, FeLV is often spread by the transmission of virus-containing saliva from a persistently infected carrier cat to a susceptible animal during licking and grooming (Hardy et al., 1973; Jarrett et al., 1973). There are essentially two possible consequences of exposure. First, the virus may spread throughout the body and establish a permanent infection with a characteristic persistent viremia. The immune response to the virus is very limited, and in most cases, no virus neutralizing antibodies are found in the serum. The prognosis for these cats is poor, and about 80% die within 3 years, mainly of FeLV-related diseases.

The second possible outcome is that the cat recovers from the infection, with or without showing signs of a transient viremia, depending on how far the virus spreads before an effective immune response inhibits viral growth. In many cases, the virus is not completely eliminated from the cat and persists for several months as an inapparent, latent infection in the bone marrow or other locus.

The main determinant of which outcome prevails is the age of the cat at exposure; young kittens are very susceptible to becoming viremic while kittens older than 16 weeks are relatively resistant (Hoover et al., 1976). This difference is probably a reflection of the state of maturity of the immune system of the host.

The immunologic mechanism by which the virus is eliminated from the cat is not yet established, but it is generally believed that some form of cell-mediated immunity is involved since not only free virus but also virus-infected cells must be destroyed in the process. While antibody can inactivate viral particles, a cellular response, perhaps involving cytotoxic T lymphocytes, is required to kill infected cells. What is clear, however, is that virus-neutralizing antibodies are important in protecting cats from infection with FeLV. Thus, cats that recover from exposure to the virus often produce virus neutralizing antibodies and are resistant to reinfection (Russell and Jarrett, 1978). Also, passive immunization with antibody is protective: Maternally derived antibody protects kittens from experimental inoculation with high doses of FeLV (Hoover et al., 1977). Further, administration of antibody to older kittens will protect them from challenge if administered up to 6 days after inoculation (Haley et al., 1985). It would seem obvious, therefore, that induction of neutralizing antibodies by vaccination would provide protection from exposure to FeLV in the field. Indeed, this is now the goal of most vaccine developers.

THE IMMUNOGEN REQUIRED FOR FeLV VACCINATION

Virus-neutralizing antibodies are directed against the spike on the surface of the FeLV particle. About 1000 spikes extend from the envelope of the virus particle in a regular array, and each is composed of an aggregate of several copies of two molecules, a glycoprotein, gp70, and a nonglycosylated protein, p15E, which are both encoded by one of the three genes of the virus, the *env* (for envelope) gene. The p15E is embedded in the lipoprotein envelope of the virus, anchoring the gp70, which is thereby exposed on the viral surface. In virus neutralization, binding of antibodies to sites on gp70 prevents the virus from making an infection either by blocking the attachment of the virus to the specific receptors for gp70 on susceptible cells or by disrupting the process by which the virus subsequently enters the cell following attachment.

Evidence for the specificity of the neutralization reaction is that recovered cats make a particularly strong antibody response to gp70, which is corre-lated with resistance to reinfection, and that passive administration of antibodies raised against gp70 protects cats against challenge. Consequently, it seems logical that an effective vaccine against FeLV should contain gp70 in an immunogenic form. As described later, a vaccine incorporating gp70 has recently been shown to be protective.

DESIGN OF FeLV VACCINE TRIALS

In any discussion of FeLV vaccine development, the age-related susceptibility of cats to FeLV must be considered. At present, to show efficacy of a FeLV vaccine, licensing authorities demand that 70% of vaccinated animals be protected against a challenge which will cause a persistent viremia in 80% of nonvaccinated controls. Many consider oronasal challenge to most closely simulate natural transmission of FeLV. However, if this method is to be used without any other modification of the cat's response, the challenge must be given before the kitten is 14 weeks of age, otherwise a very high proportion of the control kittens will naturally recover from exposure and it will be difficult to assess efficacy. Given that usual vaccination practice in kittens is to give two immunizations at 9 and 12 weeks of age, experimental vaccination at these times followed by challenge 2 weeks later should still result in a high proportion of unvaccinated kittens of the same age becoming persistently viremic. However, to enable older animals to be used in trials, ways to circumvent the developing natural resistance of the cat have been found. First, administration of corticosteroid around the time of challenge enhances the effect of the FeLV infection (Lewis et al., 1981). Another method to boost the challenge is to inoculate the virus by the intraperitoneal route (Marciani et al., 1991). Which of these methods most closely resembles the effect of natural exposure remains to be determined.

DEVELOPMENT OF CURRENT FeLV VACCINES

The first reported FeLV vaccine consisted of cells chronically infected with the virus (Jarrett et al., 1975). These workers also found that chemically inactivated cells protected cats from challenge, but the immune response achieved was apparently insufficiently consistent for this type of preparation to be used in a commercial vaccine. The first commercial vaccine (Leukocell) was based on the work of Olsen and his colleagues (Lewis et al., 1981) using the viral components harvested from the same cell line used in the original vaccine trials. They found that when these FL74 cells, a FeLV-producing line of T cells derived from a lymphoma in a cat, were incubated in culture medium deficient in serum (usually necessary for cell growth), viral proteins were released into the culture fluid. This fluid was treated with an inactivating agent to destroy any residual live FeLV, was concentrated and then used as an antigen, together with saponin as an adjuvant, in the vaccine. This vaccine protected approximately 70% of cats against challenge with virulent FeLV.

There has been considerable controversy about the efficacy of this vaccine. While protection against natural challenge in a multicat household containing FeLV-excreting cats was reported (Pollock and Scarlett, 1990), other studies failed to demonstrate significant protection against experimental (Pedersen et al., 1985) or natural (Legendre et al., 1990) infection.

Other conventional vaccines based on inactivated virus have given reasonable levels of protection. Pedersen et al. (1979) used purified virus inactivated with formaldehyde and obtained protection in 70% of vaccinates against a challenge that produced a persistent infection in 90% of unvaccinated kittens. These authors were rather modest in their claims of success since some of their vaccinated kittens showed signs of a transient infection before they recovered. Similar results obtained by others have been the basis of VacSyn/FeLV (Bio-Trends International), Fel-O-Vax (Fort Dodge Laboratories), Fevaxyn FeLV (Solvay Animal Health), and Covenant (Diamond Scientific).

It is clear that these vaccines give some, but not necessarily complete, protection against FeLV infection. There are several obvious reasons for this relatively poor performance. First, the quantity of gp70 antigen in the vaccines may be suboptimal. It has been observed that some vaccines containing relatively small amounts of gp70 may in fact enhance infection rather than protect (Pedersen et al., 1986). Second, the antigen may not be in a particularly immunogenic condition. We found that the concentration of inactivating agent was important in preserving the antigenicity of gp70. A third major determinant of a successful immune response is the efficacy of the adjuvant used in the vaccine. Several manufacturers claim that the efficacy of their vaccine depends on a novel adjuvant formulation.

NEW APPROACHES TO FeLV VACCINATION

Researchers are now attempting to develop "second-generation" vaccines that will protect all vaccinated kittens, and many are approaching this problem using recombinant DNA technology.

The development of a modified-live FeLV vaccine has generally not been considered seriously because of the problem of demonstrating safety. In theory it is perfectly feasible to generate a modified FeLV

that has been so enfeebled that it would replicate for only a short period in a cat and, one hopes, immunize the animal before being eliminated. However, there has been only limited research toward this end.

RECOMBINANT FeLV VACCINES

Much more effort has been expended in developing recombinant viruses into which the *env* gene encoding gp70 has been inserted. At least two viruses have been used as vectors for the FeLV gene, vaccinia virus and feline herpesvirus (FHV). Vaccinia virus has many excellent attributes for use as a vector. For example, the genome of the virus has been extensively characterized, and therefore, the basis for genetic manipulation is well established. It is known that certain vaccinia virus genes are not essential for virus growth and can be replaced by genes of other viruses, which are then expressed when the recombinant virus infects appropriate cells. Also, the virus has a very wide host range, so an efficient vector, once developed, could theoretically be used in vaccines for many viruses in different species. There are several examples of vaccinia recombinants producing excellent protective immune responses in animals. A vaccinia-rabies virus vaccine has produced superior results to a conventional modified-live rabiesvirus vaccine in trials to immunize red foxes in the wild in Belgium. Therefore, it is disappointing that a vaccinia-FeLV vaccine did not produce immunity in cats (Gilbert et al., 1986). The reasons for this failure are not clear. One possibility is that the level of expression of the FeLV *env* gene to produce gp70, which appeared to be reasonable in cell culture, was not sufficient *in vivo* to immunize cats. Another reason may be that the conformation of the gp70 when produced in cells infected with the recombinant virus was in some way different from that in cells infected with FeLV and therefore was not recognized by the feline immune system.

A recombinant FHV-FeLV *env* virus has also been constructed and has been shown to induce good expression of gp70 in cat cells (Cole et al., 1990). The results of immunization trials with this virus are awaited with great interest.

A SUBUNIT FeLV VACCINE

Recently, a subunit FeLV vaccine has been produced and is licensed for use in many European countries (Marciani et al., 1991). The major part of the *env* gene was cloned and expressed in *Escherichia coli*. The resulting protein had a molecular weight of 45,000 rather than the 70,000 of the native gp70 because proteins produced in bacteria are not glycosylated. Doubts have often been expressed about whether or not nonglycosylated viral envelope proteins produced in bacteria would have a secondary or tertiary structure of the native glycoprotein which would be recognized by the immune system of the host. In the case of FeLV, the bacterial protein appears to have the capacity to induce an immune response sufficient to protect the majority of cats against viral challenge. Part of the success of this vaccine may reside in the use of a new adjuvant purified from crude saponin.

FeLV-ISCOM VACCINE

Obviously, adjuvants are extremely important in nonliving vaccines and may be critical in protecting against FeLV infection. The most dramatic example of the importance of antigen presentation has been the demonstration of a very powerful immune response to FeLV induced by a FeLV-ISCOM vaccine (Osterhaus et al., 1989). ISCOMs (immune-stimulating complexes) are cagelike structures, approximately 30 nanometers in diameter, which form when viral envelope glycoproteins, usually obtained from purified virus, are solubilized in an appropriate detergent, a mixture of saponin and lipid is added, and the detergent is then removed (Morein et al., 1984). The array of protein along the edges of the ISCOMs apparently dramatically enhances its immunogenicity. A FeLV-ISCOM vaccine protected cats against FeLV challenge (Osterhaus et al., 1985). In addition, the vaccine induced a dramatic serologic response in pet cats following immunization (Osterhaus et al., 1989), including the production of virus-neutralizing antibodies, which had not been achieved previously with any type of FeLV vaccine. The ISCOM vaccine is now being developed for commercial use. A potential problem with exploitation of this technology is the expense of producing gp70 from purified virus. In future it should be possible to combine the power of the ISCOMs adjuvant system with the relative ease of bacterial expression of antigen to formulate vaccines that will protect all of our cats against FeLV infection.

References and Suggested Reading

Cole, G. E., Stay-Phipps, S., and Nunberg, J. H.: Recombinant feline herpesviruses expressing feline leukemia virus envelope and gag proteins. J. Virol. 64:4930, 1990.

Gilbert, J. H., Pedersen, N. C., and Nunberg, J. H.: Feline leukemia virus envelope protein expression encoded by a recombinant vaccinia virus: Apparent lack of immunogenicity in vaccinated animals. Virus Res. 7:49, 1986.

Hardy, W. D., Jr., Old, L. J., Hess, P. W. et al.: Horizontal transmission of feline leukaemia virus. Nature 244:266, 1973.

Haley, P. J., Hoover, E. A., Quackenbush, S. L. et al.: Influence of antibody infusion on the pathogenesis of experimental feline leukemia virus infection. J. Natl. Cancer Inst. 74:821, 1985.

Hoover, E. A., Olsen, R. G., Hardy, W. D., Jr., et al.: Feline leukemia virus infection: Age-related variation in response of cats to experimental infection. J. Natl. Cancer Inst. 57:365, 1976.

Hoover, E. A., Schaller, J. P., Mathes, L. E., et al.: Evaluation of immunity from dams naturally infected or experimentally vaccinated. Infect. Immunol. 16:54, 1977.

Jarrett, W., Jarrett, O., Mackey, L., et al.: Horizontal transmission of leukemia virus and leukemia in the cat. J. Natl. Cancer Inst. 51:833, 1973.

Jarrett, W., Jarrett, O., Mackey, L., et al.: Vaccination against feline leukemia virus using a cell membrane antigen system. Int. J. Cancer 16:134, 1975.

Legendre, A. M., Mitchener, K. L., and Potgieter, L. N. D.: Efficacy of a feline leukemia virus vaccine in a natural exposure challenge. J. Vet. Intern. Med. 4:92, 1990.

Lewis, M. G., Mathes, L. E., and Olsen, R. G.: Protection against feline leukemia by vaccination with a subunit vaccine. Infect. Immunol. 34:888, 1981.

Marciani, D. J., Kensil, C. R., Beltz, G. A., et al.: Genetically-engineered subunit vaccine against feline leukemia virus: Protective immune response in cats. Vaccine 9:89, 1991.

Morein, B., Sundquist, B., Hoglund, S., et al.: ISCOM, a novel structure for antigenic presentation of membrane proteins from enveloped viruses. Nature 308:457, 1984.

Osterhaus, A., Weijer, K., UytdeHaag, F., et al.: Induction of protective immune response in cats by vaccination with feline leukemia virus ISCOM. J. Immunol. 135:591, 1985.

Osterhaus, A., Weijer, K., UytdeHaag, F., et al.: Serological responses in cats vaccinated with FeLV ISCOM and an inactivated FeLV vaccine. Vaccine 7:137, 1989.

Pedersen, N. C., Johnson, L., and Ott, R. L.: Evaluation of a commercial feline leukemia virus vaccine for immunogenicity and efficacy. Feline Pract. 15:7, 1985.

Pedersen, N. C., Johnson, L., Birch, D., et al.: Possible immunoenhancement of persistent viremia by feline leukemia virus envelope glycoprotein vaccines in challenge-exposure situations where whole inactivated virus vaccines were protective. Vet. Immunol. Immunopathol. 11:123, 1986.

Pedersen, N. C., Theilen, G. H., and Wunner, L. L.: Safety and efficacy studies of live and killed feline leukemia virus vaccines. Am. J. Vet. Res. 40:1120, 1978.

Pedersen, N. C., Theilen, G. H., and Werner, L. L.: Safety and efficacy studies of live and killed feline leukemia virus vaccines. Am. J. Vet. Res. 40:1120, 1979.

Pollock, R. V., and Scarlett, J. M.: Randomized blind trial of a commercial feline leukemia virus vaccine. J.A.V.M.A. 196:611, 1990.

Russell, P. H., and Jarrett, O.: The occurrence of feline leukaemia virus neutralizing antibodies in cats. Int. J. Cancer 22:351, 1978.

IMMUNOREGULATORY CYTOKINES AND THEIR POTENTIAL IN THERAPY

MARY B. TOMPKINS
and WAYNE A. F. TOMPKINS
Raleigh, North Carolina

Cytokines are a group of small-molecular-weight (10,000 to 20,000) proteins or glycoproteins, including interleukins (IL), lymphokines, monokines, interferons (IFN), and certain growth factors that function as regulatory molecules in the immune response and subsequent inflammatory reactions. Cytokines may be produced by lymphocytes, monocytes, endothelial cells, and fibroblasts, usually in response to a stimulus, and generally act in a localized autocrine or paracrine fashion. Some cytokines, most notably IL-1, tumor necrosis factor-α (TNF-α), and IL-6, are able to act also in an endocrine manner. Although many cytokines were initially named on the basis of a single function (e.g., interferon, T-cell growth factor), most are multifunctional, with a wide range of biologic activity and multiple targets. In addition, there is a duplication of function among some cytokines; for example, IL-1 and TNF-α share many of the same functions in the inflammatory response.

Cytokines act by binding to high-affinity cell surface receptors, which then transmit an activation signal intracellularly. Cytokines provide both positive and negative activation signals, proliferation and differentiation signals, and recruitment signals, creating a network that regulates the immune response. The response to receptor binding depends on the cell type, differentiation state, and microenvironment, including the presence or absence of other cytokines. For example, both IL-4 and IFN-γ can independently bind to receptors on macrophages (MPs) and activate them to cytotoxicity, but if MPs are exposed to these two cytokines simultaneously, activation is blocked. Another example is IL-5, which acts as a differentiation/maturation factor for eosinophil precursors in the bone marrow but as a chemotactic and activation factor on mature, circulating eosinophils. In a physiologic setting, these signals produce an ordered sequence of immune response, inflammation, and lesion resolution; in a nonphysiologic setting, they may contribute to immunopathology.

Because of the multiple and often overlapping activities of cytokines, it is difficult to trace the flow of cytokine-receptor signaling and cellular responses through the complex network. A list of cytokines detailing their individual properties does not provide an adequate description of their true function *in vivo*. Therefore, this article does not attempt to document the properties and functions of all the cytokines (for such, readers are referred to several excellent review articles: Arai et al., 1990; Mizel, 1989; O'Garra, 1989a, 1989b) but instead examines cytokine function within the dynamics of the immune response, inflammation, and hematopoiesis.

CYTOKINES AND THE IMMUNE RESPONSE

The immune response is initiated when an antigen is processed by antigen-presenting cells of the monocyte/macrophage lineage. Processing stimulates the production and secretion of IL-1 by these cells; the processed antigen is then presented to T helper (T$_H$) cells. Antigen presentation, in collaboration with the MP-derived IL-1, triggers the T$_H$ cells to synthesize IL-2 and IL-2 receptors. Binding of these high-affinity IL-2 receptors by IL-2 then stimulates the T$_H$ cells to proliferate. Thus an autocrine feedback loop is established to amplify the immune response without needing more antigen (Fig. 1).

Evidence suggests that at least in mice, there are two subsets of T$_H$ cells, T$_H$1 and T$_H$2, each capable of synthesizing distinct cytokines, which then determine what pathway the immune response will follow (cell-mediated, antibody, mucosal, or other). T$_H$1 cells synthesize IL-2, IFN-γ and lymphotoxin (LT) and use IL-2 as an autocrine growth factor. T$_H$2 cells produce IL-4, IL-5, and IL-6 and use IL-4 as an autocrine growth factor. T$_H$2 cells can also respond to IL-2 in a paracrine manner. T$_H$1 cells drive the immune response toward the cell-mediated and delayed-type hypersensitivity (DTH) pathways, whereas T$_H$2 cells mediate antibody responses, mucosal immunity, and immunity to parasites.

461

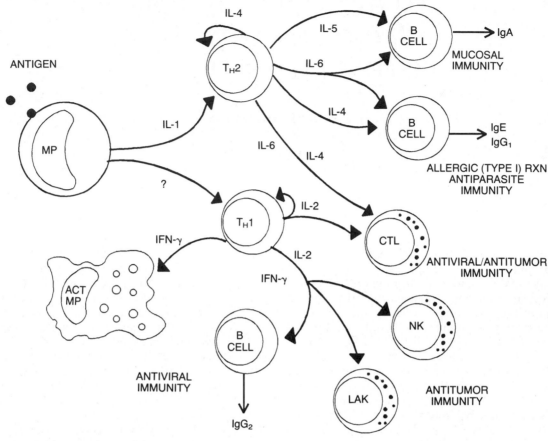

Figure 1. Cytokine regulation of the immune response. ACT MP, activated macrophage; CTL, cytotoxic T lymphocyte; IFN-γ, gamma-interferon; IL-1, interleukin-1; LAK, lymphokine-activated killer cell; MP, macrophage; NK, natural killer cell; RXN, reaction; T_H, T helper cell.

The factors that determine selection of a T_H1 over a T_H2 response are not known, but there is evidence that they require different activation signals. Proliferation of cloned T_H2 cells depends on IL-1, but the activation signal for T_H1 cells is unknown. There is also evidence that these two subsets regulate each other by the cytokines they secrete. T_H2-derived IL-4 can block MP activation by IFN-γ, and IFN-γ can block IL-4–mediated induction of major histocompatibility complex class II molecules (necessary for antigen presentation) on B cells. In addition, IL-10, produced by T_H2 cells, suppresses cytokine production by T_H1 cells (Fiorentino et al., 1989). There is no evidence for the presence of these two separate T_H cell subsets in species other than the mouse. However, DTH responses and antibody responses are often mutually exclusive, suggesting that in other species a mechanism allows for selective production of cytokines that can modulate the T-cell arm or the B-cell arm of the immune response. The factors that determine which pathway will dominate remain a mystery, but factors such as type of antigen, route of administration, and how an antigen is processed are most likely involved.

The B-Cell Response

A number of cytokines secreted by T_H2 cells provide proliferation, differentiation, and activation signals to B cells. In addition to acting as an autocrine growth factor for T_H2 cells, IL-4 is a potent stimulator of B-cell growth and differentiation. IL-4 also enhances the expression of class II molecules on resting B cells, which may enhance the ability of B cells to present antigen to T_H cells and thus initiate an antibody response to that antigen. Finally, IL-4 appears to have an important role in antibody class switch, promoting the production of immunoglobulin E (IgE) and immunoglobulin G_1 (IgG). IL-5, on the other hand, induces B-cell differentiation to immunoglobulin A (IgA)-producing cells and thus the development of the mucosal immune response. IL-5 also appears to enhance the synthesis of IgM and IgG_1. Finally, IL-6 can act on stimulated B cells to enhance antibody synthesis in general.

The T_H1 cytokines IFN-γ and IL-2 also have a role in B-cell regulation and antibody production. IFN-γ is able to inhibit the activity of IL-4. Inhibition of IL-4 activity allows for IFN-γ, in concert with IL-2, to promote the production of immuno-globulin G_{2a} (IgG$_{2a}$), an antibody class generally associated with an effective antiviral immune response.

The T-Cell Response

T cells, like B cells, are regulated by a number of cytokines. The initial activation signal comes from the MP in the form of IL-1 for T_H2 cells. Although the activation signal for T_H1 cells is unknown, resting T cells express high-affinity receptors for IL-6, and it has been suggested that IL-6 may provide the accessory cell signals that are not attributable to IL-1 (O'Garra, 1989). Following the initial signal, T_H1-derived IL-2 and T_H2-derived IL-4 provide the proliferation/differentiation signals to their respective T_H cell subsets. IL-2 and IL-4, in addition to T_H2-derived IL-6, also provide activation signals to terminally differentiated T cells, yielding antigen-specific cytotoxic T lymphocytes (CTL). IL-2, T_H1-derived IFN-γ, and perhaps IL-4 are also capable of inducing and activating natural killer (NK) and lymphokine-activated killer (LAK) cells. T_H1 cells also activate MPs to cytotoxicity via IFN-γ. Activated MPs are critical to host defense against viruses and other intracellular parasites, and they play a part in immunity to tumors.

CYTOKINES IN INFLAMMATION

The development of an inflammatory response depends on recruitment of cells (chemotaxis) and a mechanism for migrating cells to identify the lesion. A number of cytokines provide these signals. An early response to an inflammatory stimulus is the production of IL-1, TNF-α, and IL-6 by MPs, endothelial cells, and fibroblasts. These three cytokines act synergistically to initiate the acute-phase response and the synthesis of acute-phase proteins by the liver. IL-1 is the major endogenous pyrogen, but TNF and possibly IL-6 are also capable of inducing fever.

IL-1 and TNF induce endothelial cells to release a number of chemotactic factors for neutrophils (PMNs) and MPs. IL-8, produced by MPs and endothelial cells, is a family of molecules that act as chemotactic and activation signals for PMNs. A monocyte chemotactic activating factor is also released by endothelial cells stimulated by IL-1. T_H2-derived IL-5 acts as a potent recruitment and activation factor for eosinophils. A number of colony-stimulating factors (CSFs), such as granulocyte-macrophage CSF (GM-CSF), also act on mature cells as chemotactic factors.

An important group of adhesion molecules known as *integrins* provide a means for the migrating inflammatory cell to identify an inflammatory site and remain there. Both IL-1 and TNF-α induce the expression of integrins on vascular endothelial cells. These integrins then function as ligands for circulating PMNs, MPs, and lymphocytes. Similar integrins with recognition sites for endothelial cells are induced by cytokines on activated leukocytes. IL-8, for example, induces the expression of the integrin molecule Mac-1 on the PMN, which then promotes adhesion of PMNs to vascular endothelium.

A final step in inflammation is tissue repair, and cytokines are important in this stage of inflammation as well. IL-1 and TNF-α have major roles in tissue remodeling and wound healing. IL-1 induces the release of neutral proteases from a wide range of connective tissue cells. These proteases then degrade collagen, elastic fibers, and proteoglycan. Both IL-1 and TNF-α activate osteoclasts, leading to bone matrix resorption. These are necessary first steps in tissue remodeling and wound healing. IL-1 and TNF-α also induce fibroblast and mesenchymal cell proliferation and the production of fibroblast growth factors, all of which lead to repair.

CYTOKINES IN HEMATOPOIESIS

In addition to providing signals for inflammation and the immune response, cytokines play a major part in the regulation of hematopoiesis. Binding of IL-1 and TNF-α to receptors on bone marrow stromal cells stimulates the production of IL-6, GM-CSF, and G-CSF. On the other hand, IL-7 and M-CSF are produced constitutively by bone marrow stromal cells. These cytokines then act as differentiation/maturation factors on various bone marrow stem cells.

The most pluripotent of the cytokines is IL-3, which stimulates the maturation of most bone marrow precursors, including early erythroid cells, megakaryocytes, PMNs, MPs, eosinophils, and mast cells. It appears that IL-3 targets the very early stage stem cell and cannot support terminal differentiation. IL-6 appears to enhance the ability of stem cells to respond to IL-3. The major source of IL-3 is the T_H cell, suggesting that this cytokine is an important component of the hematopoiesis that occurs in response to acute inflammation.

Another cytokine that stimulates very early precursor cells is IL-7, which acts on lymphoid cells. The growth of early B-cell precursors (pro-B and pre-B) is supported by IL-7. Interestingly, there is no evidence that IL-7 can induce differentiation of these cells, and mature B cells are not responsive to IL-7. The most immature population of thymocytes also uses IL-7 as a growth factor. In contrast to B cells, mature T cells appear to be able to respond to IL-7.

The differentiation and maturation of later stage precursor cells is supported by GM-CSF, M-CSF, and G-CSF. Eosinophils respond to IL-5, which is a selective differentiation factor for these cells. Both IL-4 and IL-6 can also act synergistically with the CSFs to promote hematopoietic cell differentiation. Interestingly, a number of mature cells continue to express the receptor for their particular maturation factor and thus continue to be regulated by these factors. For example, IL-5 provides a maturation signal to eosinophil precursors in the bone marrow and a powerful chemotactic and activation signal when it binds to the same receptor on mature eosinophils in the circulation. Similarly, GM-CSF is a maturation factor for neutrophil precursors and a chemotactic and activation factor for mature neutrophils. The source of growth factors regulating hematopoiesis usually is the bone marrow stroma, whereas the same factors regulating mature cells are derived from T cells, MPs, and endothelial cells. These cytokines with dual roles (hematopoiesis and activation/chemotaxis) have therapeutic potential, particularly when the state of immunodeficiency is associated with bone marrow suppression.

CYTOKINES IN DISEASE

It should be clear from this discussion that the immune system and inflammatory response are extremely complex and subject to uncountable positive and negative regulatory signals. Disruption of any of these signals leading to over- or underproduction of one or a number of cytokines could easily lead to pathology. For example, high levels of IL-1 may selectively enhance the development of T_H2 cells, leading to the production of IgE, eosinophils, mast cells, and the development of a type I hypersensitivity response (see Fig. 1). On the other hand, selective enhancement of T_H1 cells may lead to a type IV hypersensitivity (DTH) with the activation and recruitment of CTLs and MPs (see Fig. 1). A number of tumors, including cervical cancers, bladder carcinomas, and cardiac myxomas, produce high levels of IL-6, and this cytokine, acting as a polyclonal B-cell stimulator, may be involved in the pathogenesis of autoimmunity associated with these diseases (O'Garra, 1989). IL-6 has also been shown to act as an autocrine growth factor for plasma cell tumors (Whicher and Evans, 1990).

CYTOKINE THERAPY

With the development of recombinant DNA technology, it has become possible to generate large quantities of highly purified cytokines in vitro. This technology, coupled with our increased understanding of the cytokine network, has provided new opportunities for manipulating the immune system in treating disease. Much of the work has been done in mice and humans, but cytokine therapy is rapidly moving into veterinary medicine. With few exceptions, cytokine genes have not been cloned from canine or feline cells. Fortunately, however, many of the cytokines are genetically highly conserved in nature, and the receptor binding sites frequently cross-react among diverse species. A number of recombinant human cytokines have been studied in both dogs and cats.

Because of the pivotal role IL-2 has in the immune response, many immunotherapy studies have focused on this molecule. A number of studies have shown that high doses of recombinant human IL-2 (rHuIL-2), alone or in conjunction with LAK cells, have caused a partial or complete remission of some tumors in humans, including renal cancer, colorectal cancer, melanoma, and non-Hodgkin's lymphomas (Rosenberg et al., 1987). Unfortunately, the effective dose of IL-2 or IL-2 plus LAK cells is near the maximal tolerated dose, and therapy is thus limited by toxic reactions, manifested primarily by an increase in capillary permeability, causing vascular leak syndrome (VLS).

Studies have now demonstrated that canine and feline cells respond well to rHuIL-2. We have demonstrated that infusion of rHuIL-2 into cats induces the proliferation of lymphocytes, when cultured in vitro, into LAK cells. Toxicity was not noted at a dose of 2.5×10^4 units/kg every 12 hr for up to 14 days of treatment. Twice this dose, however, produced lethargy and mild VLS, which resolved with cessation of treatment. Interestingly, these cats also developed a marked and prolonged eosinophilia characterized by selective enhancement of bone marrow eosinophil precursors as well as activation of the circulating eosinophils (Tompkins et al., 1990). Eosinophilia has also been observed in both humans and dogs receiving rHuIL-2. Because IL-2 has no effect on eosinophils and IL-5 is a specific differentiation and activation factor for eosinophils, the observed eosinophilia suggests that treatment with high doses of IL-2 stimulates the production of IL-5.

Both IL-1 and TNF are logical candidates as therapeutic agents because of their cytotoxic activity against tumor cells, their role in targeting leukocytes to inflammatory lesions, and the role of IL-1 in initiating the immune response. Injection of rHuIL-1 into dogs produced within 24 hr a dose-dependent neutrophilia that lasted 5 to 6 days. The neutrophils also appeared to be activated, as measured by increased respiratory burst activity (Neta et al., 1989). Both IL-1 and TNF have the potential for being extremely toxic because of their wide range of activities and target cells, including vascular endothelial cells. Therapy with these two cytokines should thus be carried out with extreme caution.

Because CSFs function as both maturation signals and activation/chemotactic signals for cells of the granulocyte/monocyte lineage, they have good potential as therapeutic agents. A particularly promising clinical role is the protection of myeloid cells from toxicity by cell cycle–active antineoplastic chemicals, thereby allowing for higher or more frequent doses of chemotherapy. A number of studies have documented that when dogs and cats are given rHuCSFs, a neutrophilia develops shortly after the start of treatment and can be maintained up to 3 weeks. Treatment of dogs with genetic cyclic neutropenia with rHuG-CSF was particularly encouraging (Lothrop et al., 1988).

Of all the cytokines, IFN has perhaps commanded the greatest attention as a therapeutic agent. Success of parenteral rHuIFN-α treatment of hairy cell leukemia in humans prompted numerous therapeutic studies, but the response to IFN has for the most part been disappointing and accompanied by toxic signs of fever, nausea, pain, and anorexia. Several studies in feline leukemia virus (FeLV)–infected cats using HuIFN-α have reported some benefit, but the number of treated animals was small. In a more recent study, low doses of natural HuIFN-α given orally prevented or delayed the development of disease associated with experimental infection of cats with the Rickard strain of FeLV (Cummins et al., 1988). Less than 25% of HuIFN-α–treated cats developed clinical signs of disease during the course of the study, whereas 100% of the sham-treated cats developed fatal FeLV-associated disease. Although these results are somewhat surprising, considering the low doses (0.5 to 5.0 units IFN-α) and the route of administration, the responses of the cats are compelling and the oral use of IFN warrants further study.

Unfortunately, there are limitations to the use of heterologous cytokine therapy. Although highly conserved, these cytokines are still interpreted as foreign by the immune system of the patient, and antibodies that inhibit cytokine function and limit the duration of therapy usually develop by 2 weeks of administration. This is illustrated by the decline in neutrophil counts in the cyclic neutropenic dogs during the third week of rHuGM-CSF therapy despite continued treatment (Lothrop et al., 1988). Successful cytokine therapy in dogs and cats requires that the genes for these molecules be identified, cloned, and recombinant products synthesized. This has already been done for the gene for canine G-CSF, which is now being used in several studies with positive results (Obradovitch et al., 1991).

SUMMARY

Although much has been learned about the cytokine network, there are still gaps in our information, and the model discussed here will likely be modified with time. It is possible, however, to seriously consider the clinical application of cytokines as immunotherapeutic agents in canine and feline medicine. However, exploiting the full potential of immunotherapy in veterinary medicine awaits the cloning of the cytokine genes from different species. This work is already in progress in many laboratories.

References and Suggested Reading

Arai, K., Lee, F., Miyajima, A., et al.: Cytokines: Coordinators of immune and inflammatory responses. Annu. Rev. Biochem. 59:783, 1990.
A review of the molecular biology of cytokines and their role in inflammation.
Cummins, J. M., Tompkins, M. B., Olsen, R. G., et al.: Oral use of IFN-α in the cat. J. Biol. Response Mod. 7:513, 1988.
Results of treating 14 FeLV-infected cats with low-dose oral interferon.
Fiorentino, D. F., Bond, M. W., and Mosmann, T. R.: Two types of mouse T helper cell IV. T_{h2} clones secrete a factor that inhibits cytokine production by T_{h1} clones. J. Exp. Med. 170:2081, 1989.
The initial description of a factor (IL-10) secreted by T_H2 cells that inhibits production of cytokines, especially IFN, by T_H1 cells.
Lorthrup, C. D., Warren, D. J., Souza, L. M., et al.: Correction of canine cyclic hematopoiesis with recombinant human granulocyte colony-stimulating factor. Blood 72:1324, 1988.
Results of the use of rHuG-CSF in one normal dog and two dogs with cyclic hematopoiesis.
Mizel, S. B.: The interleukins. FASEB J. 3:2379, 1989.
A review of interleukins 1 through 7, each discussed individually.
Neta, R., Monroy, R., and MacVittie, T. J.: Utility of interleukin-1 therapy of radiation injury as studied in large and small animal models. Biotherapy 1:301, 1989.
A comparison of the effects of IL-1 therapy for radiation injury in mice, monkeys, and dogs.
Obradovich, J. E., Ogilvie, G. K., and Boone, T.: Evaluation of recombinant canine granulocyte colony-stimulating factor as an inducer of granulopoiesis: A pilot study. J. Vet. Intern. Med. 5:75, 1991.
O'Garra, A.: Interleukins and the immune system, Part 1. Lancet 1:943, 1989a.
A discussion of the therapeutic implications of IL-1, IL-2, and IL-6.
O'Garra, A.: Interleukins and the immune system, Part 2. Lancet 1:1003, 1989b.
A brief review of IL-3, IL-4, IL-5, IL-7, and IFN.
Rosenberg, S. A., Lutz, M. T., Mull, M., et al.: A progress report on the treatment of 157 patients with advanced cancer using lymphokine activated killer cells and interleukin-2 alone. N. Engl. J. Med. 316:889, 1987.
A review of the hematologic and therapeutic response of patients with various tumors to either IL-2/LAK treatment or IL-2 alone.
Tompkins, M. B., Novotney, C., Grindem, C. B., et al.: Human recombinant IL-2 induces differentiation and recruitment signals for feline bone marrow eosinophil precursors in vivo. J. Leukoc. Biol. 48:531, 1990.
Hematologic and bone marrow changes in 23 adult cats infused with rHuIL-2.
Whicher, J. T., and Evans, S. W.: Cytokines in disease. Clin. Chem. 36:1269, 1990.
A discussion of cytokines in the immune response and hematopoiesis, different assay methods, and the clinical applications of cytokine measurements.

HEMATOPOIETIC GROWTH FACTORS: CLINICAL USE AND IMPLICATIONS

GREGORY K. OGILVIE

Fort Collins, Colorado

and JOYCE E. OBRADOVICH

Bloomfield Hills, Michigan

Hematopoietic growth factors have made a dramatic entrance in human and veterinary medicine (Elmslie, 1989; Obradovich and Ogilvie [in press]). There is little doubt that these factors will have profound implications for improving animal health for many years to come. At this point, sufficient data are available on the efficacy and safety of erythropoietin and granulocyte colony-stimulating factor (G-CSF) in dogs and cats to review their clinical use in veterinary medicine (see this volume, p. 484, for an excellent discussion on the use of erythropoietin in dogs and cats). Granulocyte-macrophage colony-stimulating factor (GM-CSF) is being used in many clinical trials in human medicine but may have limitations for use in animals. Clinical trials with interleukin 3 (IL-3) and macrophage colony-stimulating factor (M-CSF) have been promising in human medicine; however, IL-3 use in dogs has produced disappointing results. Trials in humans and animals with combinations of these growth factors and with even newer cytokines are too preliminary to review at this time. There is little doubt that the clinical importance of these newer cytokines will be forthcoming in the near future.

GRANULOCYTE COLONY-STIMULATING FACTOR

Natural G-CSF is a glycoprotein produced by bone marrow stromal cells, monocyte/macrophage cells, fibroblasts, and endothelial cells in response to IL-1, IL-3, tumor necrosis factor (TNF), gamma-interferon, and bacteria. Recombinant human and canine G-CSF has been produced in large quantities through recombinant technology using *Escherichia coli* bacteria. Most work done with G-CSF has shown that the cytokine is lineage-specific, acting primarily on committed granulocytic precursors.

The result is an increase in the number and function of neutrophils. Other more recent information has shown that G-CSF *in vitro* may act alone or in combination with other cytokines on early multi-potential progenitors. Like GM-CSF, G-CSF increases neutrophil phagocytosis, superoxide generation, and antibody-dependent cellular cytotoxicity. G-CSF differs from GM-CSF in that it does not inhibit neutrophil migration.

G-CSF causes a dose-dependent increase in neutrophils in dose ranges of 1 to 60 µg/kg/day in humans. The only toxicity noted in the groups given higher doses was mild, transient bone pain.

We have demonstrated a dose-dependent increase in neutrophil and monocyte counts when recombinant *canine* G-CSF (rcG-CSF) was given subcutaneously to normal dogs at dosages ranging from 3 to 25 µg/kg/day (Obradovich et al., 1990a). The only toxicity noted in the dogs was occasional mild irritation at the injection site. Based on clinical studies in humans and our work in dogs, 5 µg/kg/day is currently being used in clinical studies of dogs. A study was recently completed evaluating the changes in neutrophil counts when rcG-CSF was administed at a dose of 5 µg/kg/day. At that dosage, mean neutrophil counts increased significantly to 26,330/µl within 24 hr after the first injection of rcG-CSF (Obradovich et al. [in press]). The neutrophils reached a maximum of 72,125/µl by day 19. The neutrophil counts remained in this range until the cytokine therapy was discontinued. Blood counts returned to normal within 5 days after discontinuing treatment. Prior administration of G-CSF appears to "prime" the bone marrow to subsequent rcG-CSF therapy. Reinitiation of G-CSF treatment resulted in a more rapid, dramatic increase in neutrophil numbers. Our studies have also shown that monocyte numbers increase significantly in response to rcG-CSF. The use of recombinant *human* G-CSF (rhG-CSF) in dogs has been shown to induce significant decreases in neutrophil counts,

Supported in part by the US Public Health Service Grant PO-1-CA-29582 awarded by the National Cancer Institute DHHS.

presumably as a result of formation of antibody to the foreign rhG-CSF (Lorthrup et al., 1988). Our studies suggest that long-term treatment with rcG-CSF does not induce antibody formation in dogs. Therefore, if rhG-CSF is to be used in dogs, it should be used only on a short-term basis.

Work done in our laboratory has shown that rhG-CSF induces a short-term increase in neutrophil numbers in normal cats. After approximately 14 days, the number of neutrophils and their precursors decreased significantly, presumably because rhG-CSF is sufficiently different from a cat's own native G-CSF to induce antibody formation. The use of rcG-CSF in cats does not appear to induce antibody formation in this species (Fig. 1). Recombinant canine G-CSF increases neutrophils in cats to approximately 30,000/μl within 24 hr after initiation of therapy. The neutrophil counts continue to rise, reaching approximately 67,000/μl on day 14 and then remaining within a range of 67,000 to 88,000/μl for 42 days. As in dogs, once the rcG-CSF administration was discontinued, neutrophil counts returned to pretreatment levels within 5 days. Occasional irritation at the injection site was the only toxicity noted.

One of the most promising areas of clinical application of G-CSF is in the prevention and treatment of chemotherapy and radiation-induced cytopenias. Several studies have documented the ability of G-CSF to reduce the duration and severity of myelosuppression associated with single- and multiple-agent chemotherapy in monkeys and humans. We have shown that rcG-CSF was effective for significantly reducing the myelosuppression associated with mitoxantrone chemotherapy in dogs (Fig. 2) (Ogilvie et al. [in press]). The dose-limiting toxicity associated with mitoxantrone therapy in dogs is myelosuppression (see this volume, p. 399, for

additional details). In that study, 10 dogs were given mitoxantrone at a dose of 5 mg/m² body surface area IV. Recombinant canine G-CSF was administered to five of these dogs at a dose of 5 μg/kg/day SC for 20 days starting 24 hr after the chemotherapy was administered. The median neutrophil counts dropped below normal (<3000/μl) for 2 days in the dogs that received rcG-CSF and for 5 days in the dogs that only received mitoxantrone. Four of the five dogs not treated with rcG-CSF and none of the dogs receiving rcG-CSF developed serious neutropenia (<1500/μl). The neutrophil counts were significantly higher in the rcG-CSF–treated dogs at all time points evaluated except before the administration of the cytokine and mitoxantrone and on the sixth day of therapy. Therefore, rcG-CSF appears to be safe and effective for preventing chemotherapy-induced myelosuppression in dogs. It can allow the use of chemotherapy with higher dosages and closer dosing intervals while minimizing toxicity associated with myelosuppression. One area of intense investigation is whether G-CSF and other hematopoietic growth factors enhance or stimulate the growth of tumor cells. To date, most evidence would suggest that this is not a significant problem in most types of cancer.

Investigators have reported that rhG-CSF was effective for reducing the duration and severity of sublethal whole-body irradiation (200 cGy) (Mac-Vittie et al., 1990). The administration of whole-body irradiation (350 cGy) to control dogs resulted in 60% lethality. Treatment with rhG-CSF reduced the lethality of similarly treated dogs to zero. Dogs that did not receive G-CSF required antibiotic therapy for 14 days, whereas those that were treated with rhG-CSF after lethal whole-body irradiation needed only 3 days of antibiotic therapy. Therefore, despite the problems associated with autoantibody

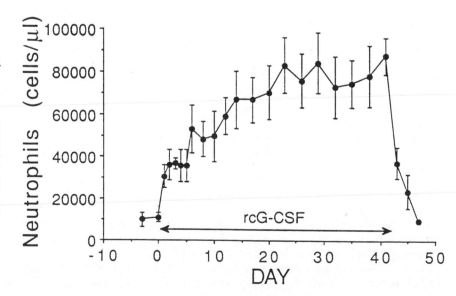

Figure 1. Mean neutrophil counts (± standard deviation) of five normal cats treated with recombinant canine granulocyte colony-stimulating factor (rcG-CSF). Administration of rcG-CSF began on day 0 and ended on day 42 (represented by arrow). Neutrophil counts returned to pretreatment levels within 5 days of discontinuing rcG-CSF. (Reprinted with permission from Obradovich, J. E., et al.: Evaluation of canine recombinant granulocyte colony-stimulating factor in the cat. J. Vet. Intern. Med. [in press].)

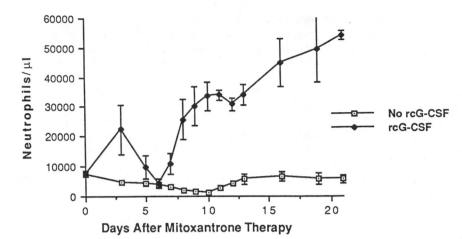

Figure 2. Mean neutrophil counts (± standard deviation) from the two groups of five dogs that received mitoxantrone (5 mg/m² IV) on day 0. Administration of rcG-CSF began on day 1 and continued until day 20 in one of two groups of dogs designated with closed circles. (Reprinted with permission from Ogilvie. G. K., et al.: The use of recombinant canine granulocyte colony-stimulating factor to decrease myelosuppression associated with the administration of mitoxantrone in the dog. J. Vet. Intern. Med. [in press].)

formation, rhG-CSF was effective for short-term use in this setting.

Bone marrow transplantation is becoming an important clinical tool in veterinary medicine for dogs and cats. G-CSF has been shown in monkeys and in humans to be an important therapy for accelerating reconstitution of the neutrophil numbers. The administration of G-CSF can be given to either the donor before or to the recipient after the transplant. Unlike GM-CSF, G-CSF does not stimulate the reconstitution of thrombopoiesis and erythropoiesis. G-CSF may be used in bone marrow transplantation of feline leukemia virus (FeLV)-positive cats to treat bone marrow failure syndromes or the infection itself. Caution has been advised by some because the use of this growth factor may actually accelerate the viral infection.

Clinical trials of rhG-CSF and GM-CSF in gray collies and in people with cyclic neutropenia have been successful in increasing neutrophil counts and decreasing clinical signs associated with prolonged myelosuppression (Lorthrup et al., 1988). Daily treatment is essential to maintain the increased neutrophil counts. Chronic use of rhG-CSF did result in autoantibody formation in the studies investigating cyclic neutropenia in dogs. Both human and canine cyclic neutropenia have been attributed to a regulatory abnormality affecting hematopoiesis at the stem cell level; however, the exact nature of this defect is not yet understood. Other similar diseases such as congenital and idiopathic neutropenia also appear to be responsive to cytokine therapy.

It is not yet clear if G-CSF can be used as a differentiation therapy in the treatment of leukemia in humans, dogs, and cats. *In vitro* studies have shown that the administration of cytokines such as G-CSF inhibit growth or actually induce differentiation of certain types of leukemia. The success of G-CSF differentiation therapies will always depend on the extent to which the growth factor maintains proliferation of leukemic stem cells. It is also possible that G-CSF can be used to accelerate cell entry into S phase for enhanced cell killing by S-phase–specific chemotherapy such as cytosine arabinoside.

As mentioned earlier, G-CSF has been shown to enhance neutrophil function and numbers. Therefore, one important area of application is in the treatment of infectious diseases. G-CSF in combination with appropriate antibiotics has been shown to significantly improve survival over the use of antibiotics alone in cases of overwhelming infection in rodents. One of the many areas of application in dogs and cats is in parvoviral infections due to virus-induced myelosuppression and subsequent bacterial infections.

GRANULOCYTE-MACROPHAGE COLONY-STIMULATING FACTOR

GM-CSF is a glycoprotein that is produced by a number of different tissues in the body including T lymphocytes, monocytes, endothelial cells, and fibroblasts. As its name implies, GM-CSF stimulates the production of granulocytes and macrophages and acts in concert with erythropoietin and IL-3 to stimulate erythroid precursors. This cytokine also acts in concert with IL-3 to regulate thrombopoiesis. This stimulator of multilineage progenitors and committed progenitors also increases the function of mature granulocytes, monocytes, macrophages, and eosinophils. More specifically, the cell-killing activity of neutrophils is enhanced by inhibiting migration of these cells, increasing chemotaxis, adhesion, phagocytosis, and superoxide generation. GM-CSF increases tumoricidal cytotoxicity.

The use of GM-CSF in clinical medicine has the potential for being at least as important and widespread as G-CSF. The only limitation is the availability of a species of GM-CSF that will work in pet animals. We have used rhGM-CSF in dogs with chemotherapy-induced myelosuppression with variable results. One reason why GM-CSF may not have had as profound an impact as G-CSF in dogs is because of variable sequence homology between the recombinant products and the native GM-CSF of dogs. This has been shown in various species. For example, there is only a 57% sequence homology between human and murine GM-CSF and up to 75% homology between human and murine G-CSF. In an attempt to overcome this problem, we have explored the use of nonspecific inducers of hematopoietic growth factors. For example, Imuvert (Cell Technologies), a biologic response modifier composed of ribosomes and other subcomponents of *Serratia marcescens*, is known to induce various cytokines including IL-1, IL-2, and GM-CSF. We have shown that this product induces a transient, profound neutrophilia in dogs and cats. Imuvert decreased the duration and severity of doxorubicin chemotherapy–induced myelosuppression in dogs when compared with controls (Ogilvie et al. [in press]). The mechanism of action of this biologic response modifier in dogs is unknown at the present time; endogenous G-CSF as determined by enzyme-linked immunoassay methodology did not increase in response to administration of Imuvert.

Like G-CSF, GM-CSF has been shown to decrease the duration and severity of chemotherapy- and radiation-induced neutropenia in humans and laboratory animals. Interestingly, after a cesium-137 radiation accident in Brazil, eight patients with bone marrow failure were treated with GM-CSF, and all seven evaluable patients had rapid increases in granulocytes and marrow cellularity. Because GM-CSF affects several cell lines, various disease states can be treated with this growth factor. Diseases linked with leukopenia-associated acquired immunodeficiency syndrome (AIDS), bone marrow failure states such as myelodysplasia, aplastic anemia, as well as chronic and acute bacterial infections have been shown to be substantially improved with GM-CSF therapy. GM-CSF may be more valuable than G-CSF for rapid recovery from bone marrow transplantation. GM-CSF can stimulate some leukemic cells and therefore may be of value for forcing cells into the cell cycle, thus making them more susceptible to cell cycle–specific drugs. Some hypothesize that GM-CSF, like G-CSF, may force leukemic cells to differentiate and die.

INTERLEUKIN-3

IL-3, like GM-CSF, affects multipotential marrow progenitors except that IL-3 appears to have activity at an earlier stage than GM-CSF. People with myelodysplasia and aplastic anemia treated with IL-3 showed dramatic increases in granulocytes, platelets, and red blood cells. Unlike G-CSF and GM-CSF therapy, responses to IL-3 do not occur until the fourth week after the start of treatment. Some investigators have shown that IL-3 can be used to decrease chemotherapy-induced myelosuppression. Sequential administration of IL-3 and GM-CSF has been shown to cause a marked increase in white cells, including myeloid lineages and platelets. The effect was clearly additive.

MACROPHAGE COLONY-STIMULATING FACTOR

M-CSF stimulates the proliferation and differentiation of mononuclear phagocytic progenitors as well as promotes the survival and effector functions of mature monocytes and macrophages. It is produced by endothelial cells, B lymphocytes, fibroblasts, and macrophages. M-CSF production can be increased by other cytokines, including gamma interferon, IL-1, and TNF. M-CSF increases monocyte and macrophage numbers as well as the antitumor activity of these cells. The cytokine causes a release of G-CSF, GM-CSF, IL-1, interferon, and TNF. Several interesting studies have shown beneficial results when M-CSF has been used to decrease myelosuppression associated with chemotherapy and increase cellular recovery in bone marrow transplants. M-CSF retards the growth of human melanoma cells in nude mice and has been shown to cause terminal differentiation of certain types of leukemia cells. M-CSF enhances monocyte/macrophage antimicrobial activity against bacteria, mycobacteria, fungi, and virus in animal models. Although relevant clinical studies thus far are scarce, M-CSF may be of great value in clinical medicine.

References and Suggested Reading

Elmslie, R. E., Dow, S. W., and Ogilvie, G. K.: Interleukins: Their biological properties and therapeutic potential. J. Vet. Intern. Med. 5:283, 1991.
  This article reviews the biology and clinical applications of a wide variety of interleukins, including many of the hematopoietic growth factors.
Lorthrup, C. D., Jr., Warren, D. J., Souza, L. M., et al.: Correction of canine cyclic hematopoiesis with recombinant human granulocyte colony-stimulating factor. Blood 72:1324, 1988.
MacVittie, T. J., Monroy, R. L., Patchen, M. L., et al.: Therapeutic use of recombinant human G-CSF (rhG-CSF) in a canine model of sublethal and lethal whole-body irradiation. Int. J. Radiat. Biol. 57:723, 1990.
  This study demonstrates that the potentially lethal myelosuppression associated with whole-body irradiation can be reduced in severity and duration in dogs.
Obradovich, J. E., and Ogilvie, G. K.: Evaluation of canine recombinant granulocyte colony stimulating factor in the dog. J. Vet. Intern. Med. (in press).
  This article contains a broad review on the background, function, and clinical application of the most common hematopoietic growth factors.

Obradovich, J. E., Ogilvie, G. L., Cooper, M. F., et al.: Effect of increasing dosages of canine recombinant granulocyte colony-stimulating factor on neutrophil counts in normal dogs. Proceedings of the 10th Annual Conference of the Veterinary Cancer Society, Auburn, Alabama, 1990, p. 5.
This abstract reviews the dose-dependent increase in neutrophil counts in dogs treated with rcG-CSF.
Obradovich, J. E., Ogilvie, G. K., Stadler-Morris, S., et al.: Evaluation of canine recombinant granulocyte colony-stimulating factor in the cat. J. Vet. Intern. Med. (in press).
This prospective study documents for the first time that rcG-CSF is safe and effective for expanding the number of neutrophils in normal cats.

Ogilvie, G. K., Elmslie, R. E., and Pearson, F.: The use of a biological extract of *Serratia marcesens* to decrease myelosuppression associated with doxorubicin-induced myelosuppression in the dog. J. Vet. Intern. Med. (in press).
This prospective study demonstrates that a biologic response modifier reduces the duration and severity of doxorubicin-induced myelosuppression in dogs.
Ogilvie, G. K., Obradovich, J.E., Cooper, M. F., et al.: The use of recombinant canine granulocyte colony-stimulating factor to decrease myelosuppression associated with the administration of mitoxantrone in the dog. J. Vet. Intern. Med. (in press).
This prospective study documents that rcG-CSF reduces the duration and severity of mitoxantrone-induced myelosuppression in dogs.

THE FELINE AB BLOOD GROUP SYSTEM AND INCOMPATIBILITY REACTIONS

URS GIGER

Philadelphia, Pennsylvania

Until recently, feline blood groups have received little attention in clinical medicine. It had been common practice to transfuse anemic cats without prior cross matching or blood typing. The risk of encountering significant transfusion reactions was believed to be negligible (Weiser, 1989). Furthermore, in contrast to the case in other species, neonatal isoerythrolysis (NI) had not been considered an important cause of the fading kitten syndrome. Auer and Bell's (1981, 1983, 1986) recent survey in Australia and experimental studies on transfusion incompatibility have, however, revived an interest in feline blood types. This article summarizes our work and the findings of other recent studies on feline blood types in the United States and emphasizes their importance for clinical practice.

FELINE AB BLOOD GROUP SYSTEM

Blood types, also known as blood groups, are antigenic and species-specific genetic markers on the surface of red blood cells. A set of allelic blood type genes make up a blood group system. Although naturally occurring alloantibodies were found in cats at the beginning of this century, the feline blood group system was not discovered until the second half of the century. Today, three blood types have been recognized in the feline AB blood group system: A, the most common blood type; B, a blood type with varied frequency among breeds; and AB, which is extremely rare. There is no type O. They appear to be carbohydrate-containing determinants, but they differ from the human ABO blood group system. No other blood group system has yet been found in cats.

Type A and B are allelic at the same gene locus. The allele for type A is completely dominant over the allele for type B (Giger et al., 1991). Thus, type B cats are homozygous for the B allele (genotype B/B), whereas type A cats can be either homozygous (genotype A/A) or heterozygous (genotype A/B) at that gene locus for the B allele. Breeding of a homozygous type A cat always results in type A offspring even when the type A cat is bred to a type B cat. Matings of two heterozygote type A cats produce offspring with A and B blood types in a phenotypic ratio of 3:1. Offspring of two type B parents will always have type B blood. No AB cats were produced by these matings. However, the appearance of the extremely rare type AB cat could be explained by the presence of a third allele that allows codominant expression of both A and B substance.

FREQUENCY OF BLOOD TYPES

Table 1, updated from our previous surveys (Giger et al., 1989, 1991a, b), shows the frequency

The author's studies were supported by grants from the Robert H. Winn Foundation and the National Institutes of Health (HL02355, RR02512).

Table 1. Blood Type Frequencies in Different Feline Breeds of the United States

Breed (over 6000 cats typed)	Type B Frequency (%)
Siamese, Burmese, Ocicat, Oriental shorthair, Tonkinese	0
DSH/DLH, Maine Coon, Norwegian Forest	≤5
Abyssinian, Himalayan, Japanese Bobtail, Persian, Somali, Sphinx	5–25
British shorthair, Cornish Rex, Devon Rex	25–50

Updated from Giger et al., 1991.

of blood types in over 6,000 cats from the United States. Approximately half of them were domestic short-hair and long-hair (DSH/DLH) cats. Most DSH/DLH cats had blood type A (98.2%), few had blood type B (1.7%), and extremely rarely did we encounter type AB cats (0.1%). The frequency varied significantly between geographic areas of the United States. In the Northeast and Northern Central/Rocky Mountain regions <0.5% were type B cats; in the Southeast and Southwest 1 to 2% and 2 to 3% had type B blood, respectively; and on the West Coast 4 to 6% were blood type B cats. Most type AB cats were found in California. Surveys from other countries conducted since 1950 on 300 to 1800 cats, which presumably were all DSH/DLH cats, also revealed type A as the most common blood type. However, the frequency of types A and B cats did vary geographically, with the proportion of type B cats being 3% in Manchester, England; 10% in Tokyo, Japan; 15% in Paris, France; and 26% in Brisbane, Australia.

Although for some breeds the number of cats studied was small, we can still draw some conclusions regarding the breed's blood type. No type B cats were found among the Siamese or related modern breeds such as the Burmese, Tonkinese, and Oriental short-hair, or American short-hair cats. Nevertheless, we cannot assume that the B allele is entirely absent among these cats. A number of other breeds demonstrated a variably higher proportion of type B cats, with the frequency ranging from 2% to 25% except among the British short-hair, and Cornish and Devon Rex breeds, in which the percentage was about 50%. No geographical variation was observed in purebred cats in the United States. However, certain purebred catteries were found to have nearly exclusively type B cats because of inbreeding practices.

Based on the inheritance pattern of feline A and B blood types, we can estimate the frequency of the B allele in the outbred and purebred cat population. Among the breed populations in which the B allele was found, the frequency is lowest in DSH/DLH cats and highest in the British short-hair.

Moreover, we recently discovered the first pure-bred cats with type AB blood in a family of Birman, British shorthairs, and Scottish fold ear cats.

Since only heterozygous type A kittens (genotype A/B) are at risk for neonatal isoerythrolysis (NI; see section on NI), there is constant selection against heterozygotes; therefore, a stable polymorphic equilibrium cannot be established. This selection, known as heterozygous disadvantage, reduces the frequency of the rarer allele. In populations in which the frequency of the B allele is less than 0.5, in time, natural selection should eliminate the B allele completely. Conversely, in populations in which the B allele is predominant, as in the Devon Rex, the frequency of the A allele should eventually fall to zero. This natural selection process is likely to be further influenced by the breeders' efforts to achieve compatible matings (Giger et al., 1991).

ALLOANTIBODIES

In contrast to dogs, cats have naturally occurring antibodies against the other blood type in their plasma. They are known as allo- or isoantibodies and can easily be identified *in vitro* by hemagglutination or hemolysis reactions. All type B cats have strong hemagglutinins and hemolysins against type A red blood cells. The hemagglutinin and hemolysin titers of anti-A alloantibodies are 1:64 or higher in all cases, reaching 1:2048 in some cats. In contrast, type A cats have weak hemagglutinins and hemolysins with titers typically only 1:2 and reaching 1:32 rarely. Immunologic studies reveal that the hemagglutinins are immunoglobulins of the IgM class, whereas the hemolytic activity is due to IgM and IgG. As expected, the extremely rare type AB cat has no alloantibodies.

Since the feline placenta is of the endotheliochorial type and, therefore, does not allow significant passage of maternal antibodies, newborn kittens do not have any alloantibodies. However, during the first two days of life, maternal alloantibodies of the IgG class and to a lesser extent of the IgM class are transferred to the kitten via colostrum. If the kitten has blood type A and the queen has blood type B, these colostral alloantibodies will bind to and lyse erythrocytes in the newborn, thereby causing NI. No alloantibodies will be detected in the plasma of these kittens, but the Coombs' test may prove positive. If, however, queen and kitten have the same blood type, the kitten's antibody titer may reach a strength similar to that in the queen. Thereafter, over the first few weeks of life, the kitten's alloantibody titer will decline, demonstrating a half-life of approximately 10 days. This process is similar to the disappearance of maternal antibodies against infectious diseases. Particularly in type B cats, a rise in alloantibody titer occurs between 6 and 10 weeks of age, reaching maximal levels at a few months of age, providing evidence for the natural occurrence of these antibodies. While the titer may be further increased by stimulation, no prior transfusion or pregnancy is required for the production of alloantibody. Rather, these alloantibodies are believed to be formed against common food and bacterial antigens very similar to blood type antigens in the intestines.

BLOOD TYPING

To blood-type cats, sera from type A cats with high agglutination titers and any type B cat can be used. The feline blood-typing procedures are simple, and the test results are easy to read. Erythrocytes are separated from the plasma by centrifugation, washed twice, and then resuspended to a 2% to 5% erythrocyte suspension in buffered saline. One drop of erythrocyte suspension is added to two drops of either anti-A or anti-B serum. The mixture is then incubated either at 20°C or 4°C. After 15 to 30 minutes, the presence of agglutination is recorded macroscopically. In the presence of anti-A serum, type A erythrocytes strongly agglutinate, forming one clump; type B erythrocytes, incubated with anti-B serum, form multiple smaller aggregates. Type A and type B cells do not react with the opposite serum, whereas type AB erythrocytes agglutinate with both sera (Auer and Bell, 1981; Giger et al., 1989). Furthermore, lectins can be used instead of anti-sera to type cats.

To confirm these blood-typing test results, one can look for alloantibodies in the plasma (serum) of the cat to be typed. In this test, known as a back-typing test, A and B erythrocytes are incubated with the patient's plasma. Plasma from type B cats will strongly agglutinate type A cells, whereas plasma from type A cats usually shows a weak to moderate agglutination of B cells. This back-typing test is similar to a blood cross-match test when the blood type of the donor is known. That test detects antibodies directed against donor erythrocytes.

These alloantibodies not only are useful diagnostic reagents, but are also responsible for two major incompatibility reactions, which will be discussed later.

NEONATAL ISOERYTHROLYSIS (NI)

NI, or hemolysis of the newborn, results when maternal alloantibodies gain access to the neonate's circulation and cause lysis of the neonate's erythrocytes. Strong maternal anti-A alloantibodies of type B queens are passively transferred via collostrum to the type A neonates and destroy their erythrocytes. Since all type B cats have high allo-antibodies, even primiparous queens can have litters with NI. This differentiates cats from all other species studied, in which a prior sensitization through a previous pregnancy, blood transfusion, or homologous vaccines is generally required to evoke an immune response.

Since 1985, a few case reports of feline NI have been published (Giger, 1991; Hubler et al., 1987). Our recent survey recognized several dozen purebred litters with NI, suggesting that NI is a major cause of the fading kitten syndrome in purebred cats. All of the queens with NI litters had type B blood, with the usual high anti-A titers. All the affected kittens and their sires had type A blood. The type B mothers had to be homozygous (genotype B/B), while the type A fathers were either of the genotype A/A or A/B. If the father is AA, then all of the offspring will be heterozygous (genotype A/B) and at risk for NI. If the father has the genotype A/B, only one half of the offspring will be heterozygotes, with the genotype A/B and at risk for NI. Kittens with the rare AB blood type born to type B queens may also develop NI.

In DSH/DLH cats, in which the frequency of the B allele is very low, less than 1 % of random matings produce litters that are at risk for NI; however, in the Devon Rex and British short-hair breeds, nearly one quarter of all matings are incompatible, thereby producing kittens at risk for NI. Not all at-risk kittens develop overt and fatal clinical signs. Thus, one cannot assume that clinically unaffected kittens have one blood type or the other. Presumably because anti-B titers are typically low, no kittens from type A queens have been found to have NI (Giger, 1991).

Since the endotheliochorial placenta in cats does not allow significant passage of maternal antibodies, type A kittens from type B queens are born healthy and start nursing vigorously. However, as a result of colostrum intake (which contains high titers of maternal alloantibodies of the IgG class), these kittens may develop *clinical signs* within hours or days. In peracute cases, kittens may suddenly die during the first day of life without showing any specific clinical signs. In acute cases, kittens may stop nursing during the first few days of life and fail to thrive. The hallmark clinical finding is dark, brown-red discolored urine caused by severe hemoglobinuria. Breeders and veterinarians are urged to collect urine manually from kittens that fail to thrive, in order to determine the urine color. Affected kittens may develop icterus and anemia and, unless treated during the first week of life, can die. Kittens that survive the acute disease or only exhibit subclinical signs, such as a positive direct Coombs' test, may develop a tail-tip necrosis as part of this syndrome. The severity of clinical signs may depend on the maternal plasma and colostral antibody titer, the amount of colostrum taken in by the kitten, and the ability of the neonate's intestine to absorb maternal antibodies.

Depending on the timepoint of death, the following gross pathologic findings may be encountered: bladder filled with dark, brown-red urine and precipitated hemoglobin; enlarged spleen; jaundice; and rarely tail-tip necrosis. Microscopically, the liver and spleen display extramedullary hematopoiesis and marked erythrophagocytosis. Pyknotic nuclei and eosinophilic droplets in the cortical tubular cells of the kidney and eosinophilic material in the lumen of the cortical medullary tubules are evidence of a chromoproteinuric nephropathy. The systemic effects of immune-mediated hemolysis, disseminated intravascular coagulation, acute renal failure, and anemia are the likely causes of fatal NI (Giger, 1991; Hubler et al., 1987).

NI is best prevented by avoiding incompatible matings between type B queens and type A toms. If an incompatible mating has been performed, NI can still be *prevented* by immediately removing the kitten from the queen after birth and foster nursing it for the first 48 hours. Kittens that were initially allowed to nurse should be removed immediately from their mother at the first recognition of clinical signs, such as pigmenturia, and kept apart from the mother for the first 2 to 3 days of life. Foster nursing can be successfully achieved by feeding a commercial milk replacer and providing other supportive care or by placing the kitten with another queen who has type A blood. Severely anemic kittens may require a transfusion of washed type B blood during the first 3 days of life or a transfusion of type A blood thereafter, which may be administered intramedullary.

TRANSFUSION REACTIONS

Based on the blood types of donor and recipient, transfusions can be either matched or mismatched. The characteristics of feline transfusions with type A and type B blood are shown in Table 2. AB matched transfusions in cats have a long survival rate with an erythrocyte half-life ranging from 29 to 39 days (Giger and Bucheler, 1991). They are well tolerated in both type A and type B cats and can

be highly effective in clinical practice. The absence of any reactions following AB-matched transfusions suggests a lack of any other clinically important feline blood group aside from the AB blood group system.

First and subsequent AB-mismatched transfusions, however, cause acute hemolytic incompatibility reactions in cats. Because of the natural occurrence of alloantibodies, erythrocytes are immediately destroyed (within minutes or days). This reaction is in contrast to the delayed transfusion reactions seen in dogs, where erythrocytes are removed only after an immune response develops, usually 1 to 2 weeks following the first transfusion (although immediately after the second transfusion).

Although type A cats have generally low anti-B alloantibodies, the mean half-life of transfused type B erythrocytes is only 2 days. The recipient's IgM and IgG alloantibodies bind the transfused erythrocytes. This leads to the activation of a small amount of complement and slight intravascular hemolysis. Minor clinical signs characterized by discomfort, listlessness, tachycardia, and tachypnea may be observed during the first few minutes after the transfusion has been started. However, most of the erythrocytes are steadily removed from circulation owing to IgG-mediated extravascular hemolysis. Thus, type B blood transfused into type A cats may not cause obvious, serious clinical signs, but because of the short erythrocyte survival, these transfusions are clinically ineffective.

In contrast, clinical cases of acute hemolytic transfusion reactions in type B cats receiving type A blood have been documented (Giger and Akol, 1990) in Abyssinian, Persian, and DSH (Wilkerson et al., 1991) cats and have been studied experimentally (Auer and Bell, 1983, 1986; Giger and Bucheler, 1991). In type B cats, transfused type A erythrocytes are destroyed within minutes or hours. The large amount of IgM anti-A alloantibodies in type B cats causes rapid and marked IgM binding to transfused erythrocytes, which results in severe complement binding and activation. This leads to massive intravascular hemolysis and serious clinical signs. One milliliter of type A blood can cause clinical signs. Cats become restless, vocalize, and attempt to get free from restraints. Then they exhibit lateral recumbency, become depressed, and

Table 2. Feline Transfusions

| Transfusion Types | Blood Types | | Cross Match | | Recipient | | |
	Recipient	Donor	Major	Minor	Alloantibody Titer (mean)	Erythrocyte Half-Life	Clinical Reactions
Matched	A	A		Compatible	1:16	32.8 ± 3.1 d	None
	B	B		Compatible	1:128	34.4 ± 2.8 d	None
Mismatched	A	B	microagglut	4+ macroagglut	1:16	2.1 ± 0.2 d	Mild
	B	A	macroagglut	microagglut	1:128	1:3 ± 2.3 h	Severe

urinate, vomit, or salivate. Transient apnea or hypopnea, bradycardia, cardiac arrhythmia, and hypotension can be observed. This first phase of the transfusion reaction lasts 1 to 3 minutes and may cause death or can be followed by compensatory tachycardia and tachypnea. Abnormal cranial nerve signs and an increased bleeding tendency may also be noted. Animals usually recover from this second phase within hours. Signs of hemolysis include massive transient hemoglobinemia and hemoglobinuria and later, mild icterus and bilirubinuria. Renal failure due to hemolysis has not been observed. Since a type B cat that is transfused for the first time with type A blood may experience a life-threatening incompatibility reaction after receiving only one milliliter of blood, mismatched transfusions should be avoided by *typing all donors and recipients* or performing major and minor cross-match tests. This testing is particularly important in purebred cats.

It would be best to transfuse the anemic cat who has the rare AB blood type with blood from a type AB cat, but blood from cats with type A can also be used safely, since type AB cats lack naturally occurring alloantibodies.

RECOMMENDATIONS

Based on our recent survey of feline blood types in outbred and purebred cats, as well as studies of the efficacy, safety, and danger of transfusions in cats and recognition of neonatal isoerythrolysis reactions as a major cause of the fading kitten syndrome, the following recommendations are offered:

To avoid transfusion reactions:

1. All feline blood donors should be typed. Feline blood typing is readily available through our laboratory and many veterinary teaching hospitals or commercial laboratories.

Most blood donors will have type A blood; type B donors are available at the University of Pennsylvania and other institutions. Although type B blood is rarely required, a healthy type B cat should be located near each veterinary clinic for emergency transfusions.

2. Prior to their first transfusion, cats should be blood typed to provide a safe, matched transfusion. If time constraints make blood typing impossible, both a major and a minor cross-match test should be performed on both the typed blood donor and the recipient. Cross-match tests may be considered even after blood typing to determine blood incompatibilities that fall outside the AB system.

3. The practice of administering small amounts of blood to check for compatibility should be discontinued, since even this may induce serious transfusion reactions.

To prevent neonatal isoerythrolysis:

1. Blood typing is indicated before breeding purebred cats to assure blood compatibility of the males and avoid NI. In particular, type B queens should be bred to type B males. NI can occur in the first or subsequent litter of a queen and may affect one, several, or all kittens in the litter.

2. In breeds with low (less than 5%) type B frequency, cats with type B blood should not be used for breeding, to avoid further problems in that breed.

3. Type A kittens born to type B queens and therefore at risk for developing NI can be protected by removing them from the queen at birth and foster nursing them for the first 2 days of life with a milk replacer or with another type A queen. Another (though less safe option) is to allow the kittens to nurse until the first clinical signs (pigmenturia, fading) are observed and then to separate them from the queen for 2 days.

References and Suggested Reading

Auer, L., and Bell, K.: The AB blood group system of cats. Anim. Blood Group Biochem. Genet. 12:287, 1981.
   A study on the frequency of blood type A, B, and AB in domestic cats from Australia.
Auer, L., and Bell, K.: Transfusion reactions due to AB blood group incompatibility. Res. Vet. Sci. 35:145, 1983.
   Experimental study on the clinical features of feline transfusion reactions.
Auer, L., and Bell, K.: Feline blood transfusion reactions. In Kirk, R. W. (ed.): *Current Veterinary Therapy IX*. Philadelphia: W. B. Saunders, 1986, p. 515.
   A review of clinical signs and management of feline transfusion reactions.
Giger, U., Kilrain, C. G., Filippich, L. J., et al.: Frequencies of feline blood groups in the United States. J.A.V.M.A. 195:1230, 1989.
   A survey on the blood type frequency in domestic cats in the USA.
Giger, U., Bucheler, J., and Patterson, D. F.: Frequency and inheritance of A and B blood types in feline breeds of the United States. J. Hered. 82:15, 1991a.
   Study on the inheritance of A and B blood types and a survey of purebred cats.
Giger, U., and Akol, K. G.: Acute hemolytic transfusion reaction in an Abyssinian cat with blood type B. J. Vet. Intern. Med. 4:315, 1990.
   A clinical transfusion reaction in a purebred cat is described.
Giger, U., and Bucheler, J.: Transfusion of type A and B blood in cats. J.A.V.M.A. 198:411, 1991.
   An experimental study on the survival of transfused type A and B erythrocytes in cats.
Giger, U., Griot Wenk, M., Bucheler, J., et al.: Geographical variation of the feline blood type frequencies in the United States. Feline Pract. 19(6):5, 1991b.
   A survey on the geographical distribution of blood types in the USA.
Giger, U.: Feline neonatal isoerythrolysis: A major cause of the fading kitten syndrome. Proc. Am. Coll. Vet. Med. 1991, p. 347.
   A review on neonatal hemolysis in newborn kittens.
Hubler, M., Kaelin, S., Hagen, A., et al.: Feline neonatal isoerythrolysis in two litters. J. Sm. Anim. Pract. 28:833, 1987.
   A description of clinical and pathologic findings of feline neonatal isoerythrolysis.
Weiser, M. G.: Erythrocytes and associated disorders. In Ettinger, S. J. (ed.): *Textbook of Veterinary Medicine*, 3rd ed. Philadelphia: W. B. Saunders, 1989, p. 2145.
   A discussion on transfusion of cats.
Wilkerson, M. J., Wardrop, K. J., Giger, U., et al.: Two cat colonies with A and B blood types and a clinical transfusion reaction. Feline Practice 19:22, 1991.
   A transfusion reaction in a DSH cat.

PRACTICAL GUIDELINES FOR TRANSFUSION THERAPY

MICHAEL S. STONE
Ontario, Canada

and SUSAN M. COTTER
North Grafton, Massachusetts

SEROLOGY

Dog erythrocyte antigen (DEA) groups are shown in Table 1, and the most clinically important antigens, DEA 1.1 or DEA 1.2, are present in approximately 60% of the canine population. Dogs with either DEA 1.1 or 1.2 antigen are referred to as group A positive and dogs with neither are group A negative. Clinically significant, naturally occurring antibodies against group A antigens do not occur but can develop after exposure to A positive blood (Table 2). Antibodies against DEA 1.1 or 1.2 render a dog susceptible to future reaction if given A positive blood. All blood donors should be typed for DEA 1.1 and 1.2 and be group A negative. Testing for DEA 7 is not routinely done, but this antigen may also elicit an antibody response in dogs lacking that antigen. The other antigens are either weakly reactive, very prevalent, or rare, so that donor and recipient are likely to match for some of these antigens. Because typing is not done for all known (or unknown) antigens, dogs that have received previous transfusions should be cross matched before subsequent transfusions. Only a major crossmatch (testing donor red cells against recipient plasma) is necessary, since donor plasma would not have antibodies unless the donor has been previously transfused (see this volume, p. 470).

COMPONENT THERAPY

In many veterinary practices fresh whole blood is collected from an available donor and administered for all situations requiring transfusion therapy. Component therapy supplies only what the patient needs, thus avoiding fluid overload and minimizing exposure to foreign proteins or citrate. Local blood banks may separate components for veterinarians, or components may be ordered from commercial suppliers (Animal Blood Bank, Vacaville, CA). Fresh-frozen plasma may be kept for patients with deficiencies of clotting factors. Blood component preparation, storage, and administration have been reviewed (Authement, 1987).

Whole blood or packed red blood cells (PRBC) may be administered immediately or stored in CPD-A$_1$ for at least 21 days. Fresh-frozen plasma (FFP) maintains adequate levels of labile clotting factors for up to 1 year. Frozen plasma, stored longer than 1 year, has low levels of factors V, VIII, and von Willebrand factor (vWF) but adequate levels of vitamin K–dependent factors. Cryoprecipitate, produced from fresh-frozen plasma, contains high concentrations of factors VIII, vWF, fibrinogen, and fibronectin and may be stored up to 1 year. Platelet rich plasma must be used within 24 hours of collection. Dog blood is drawn into human "unit" bags holding 450 ml blood and 50 ml of anticoagulant and stored as approximately 225 ml "units" of PRBC, 225 ml "units" of plasma, or 80 ml "units" of cryoprecipitate. For cats, the unit is often defined as 50 ml since this is the maximum amount safely drawn from a 10- to 12-lb. cat.

INDICATIONS FOR COMPONENT THERAPY

Acute Blood Loss

Acute blood loss may not alter the hematocrit for several hours, despite the loss of significant red cell mass. The hematocrit will decrease once the intravascular fluid volume is replenished from extravascular fluid equilibration or exogenous fluid admin-

Table 1. Dog Erythrocyte Antigen Groups

Blood Group	Prevalence (%)
DEA 1.1	40
DEA 1.2	20
DEA 3	5
DEA 4	98
DEA 5	25
DEA 6	98
DEA 7	45
DEA 8	40

Table 2. *Possible Interactions with Group A Negative and Positive Blood Transfusions*

Recipient Blood Group	Antibodies Against DEA 1.1 or 1.2	Donor Blood Group	Reaction to Transfusion?
A +	Not possible	A −	No
A +	Not possible	A +	No
A −	No	A −	No
A −	No	A +	No
A −	Yes (sensitized by prior transfusion with A + blood)	A −	No
A −	Yes	A +	Yes

istration. The initial therapy for acute blood loss is volume restoration with crystalloid or colloid fluids or hypertonic saline. The best replacement fluid is controversial, with both crystalloids and colloids having proponents, while some advocate a combination of the two. Most animals do not require red cell replacement in acute blood loss until 25 to 30% of the blood volume is lost. Whole blood may be used, but in most cases, PRBC along with crystalloid fluids are preferred. Plasma and interstitial proteins equilibrate rapidly, and approximately half of the albumin lost is replaced within 24 hours from the extravascular space. Because 2,3-diphosphoglycerate (DPG) levels may fall in blood stored longer than 2 weeks, there is a theoretical advantage to the administration of relatively fresh red cells in the severely anemic patient (Ou, 1975). Red cells should be administered to keep the hematocrit above 15%. For dogs greater than 10 kg, most transfusions are given in unit volumes, and the hematocrit is raised into the safe range. One unit/20 kg of PRBC or whole blood should be administered and the response monitored. Clotting factor depletion may occur after massive transfusion with PRBC and require replacement either by fresh-frozen plasma or fresh whole blood. This is generally not a problem until a patient has received a transfusion equivalent of one blood volume.

Anemia

HEMOLYTIC ANEMIA

Many patients with a hematocrit of 10% are stable as long as they are confined to a cage. The rapidity of the decrease of the hematocrit is an important determinant of how well the animal tolerates the anemia since a rapid drop does not allow time for compensation for hypoxia. The decision to transfuse depends as much on clinical judgment as it does on the hematocrit. Dyspnea may be a sign of hypoxia from anemia, but pulmonary thromboembolism is common in dogs with hemolytic anemia and should

be considered in the dyspneic patient with a hematocrit greater than 15% (Klein, 1989; see also this volume, p. 104). The concept that patients with hemolytic anemia should not be transfused because "fuel will be added to the fire" is not necessarily true. The animal must be supported until drug therapy can control hemolysis. PRBCs are the component of choice since plasma is not required. Typing and cross-matching may be difficult or impossible if the dog is strongly Coombs' positive or if autoagglutination is present. Ongoing destruction of red cells makes prediction of the post-transfusion hematocrit difficult. Serial measurements of the hematocrit are necessary.

IRON DEFICIENCY ANEMIA

Unless the anemia is life-threatening, iron deficiency should be treated with iron, not blood. More severe anemia may initially respond to transfusion but later recur unless supplemental iron is added to the diet and the cause removed. Blood is a rich source of iron; each ml of whole blood contains approximately 1 mg of iron, but even so, 50 to 300 mg/day ferrous sulfate should be added to the diet for several months (Mahaffey, 1986). The overuse of blood donors may lead to iron deficiency, and supplemental iron should be supplied to their diet.

NONREGENERATIVE ANEMIA

Since the rate of decline of the hematocrit determines the tolerance to anemia, the hematocrit may drop very low before transfusion is needed. PRBCs are the components of choice, but whole blood may be used if PRBCs are unavailable. As a guideline, 10 ml/kg of PRBC or 20 ml/kg of whole blood can be expected to increase the hematocrit 10%. A more accurate estimate of the volume for transfusion may be calculated from Table 3. Normal blood volume is 85 to 90 ml/kg for dogs and 65 to 75 ml/kg for cats. The half-life of transfused allogenic red cells is about 35 days in the dog and cat. Unexpected

Table 3. *Example of Estimating Volumes for Transfusion**

30 kg dog with Hct = 10%; desired Hct = 18%; donor blood with Hct = 50%.
1. Total blood volume = (90 ml/kg) (30 kg) = 2700 ml
2. Existing red cell mass = (2700 ml) (10%) = 270 ml
3. Desired red cell mass = (2700 ml) (18%) = 490 ml
4. Required PRBC volume = 490 ml − 270 ml = 220 ml
5. Required whole blood volume = (220 ml)/(50%) = 440 ml

*Modified from O'Rourke, L. G.: Practical blood transfusions. In Kirk, R. W. (ed.): Current Veterinary Therapy VIII. Philadelphia: W. B. Saunders, 1983, p. 410.

decreases in the hematocrit may represent occult hemolysis or bleeding.

Coagulopathies

THROMBOCYTOPENIA

Platelet counts greater than 30,000/μl are rarely associated with clinical bleeding. Recently released platelets function better than older ones, and patients with accelerated platelet destruction may maintain normal coagulation function with platelet counts as low as 10,000/μl. Platelet transfusions from fresh whole blood or platelet rich plasma (PRP) may be considered, but the half-life of platelets in the presence of accelerated destruction is often in the range of minutes, not days. One unit/20 kg of PRP or fresh whole blood may be administered and the platelet count repeated in 1 hour. If elevation of the platelet count is not observed, further platelet transfusions are unlikely to be of benefit. If the platelet count has increased, repeated transfusions are given as needed to control bleeding. In most cases, platelet transfusions are of little benefit because of accelerated platelet destruction, inadequate dosing, or the development of alloantibodies. PRBC are used to support the patient until the thrombocytopenia resolves.

VITAMIN K ANTAGONISTS

After the administration of vitamin K, 8 to 12 hours are necessary for the regeneration of sufficient clotting factors to correct hemostasis. In the asymptomatic or mildly affected patient, vitamin K administration with careful observation should be adequate. If there is profuse bleeding, the administration of plasma will immediately correct the coagulopathy. Either FFP or frozen plasma is appropriate since the vitamin K–dependent factors are stable with storage. Ten to 20 ml/kg (1 unit/10–20 kg) is administered and prothrombin time (PT) or partial thromboplastin time (PTT) repeated 1 hour later. Clinical bleeding is unlikely unless the PT or PTT is greater than 1.5 times normal. If the hematocrit is less than 15% or if the animal is hypoxic, red cell support may also be necessary.

DISSEMINATED INTRAVASCULAR COAGULATION

Therapy must be individualized for each patient with disseminated intravascular coagulation. If an underlying cause is found (e.g., bleeding splenic neoplasm), this must be corrected or removed before control can be obtained. Support can be given to the actively bleeding patient by administration of FFP. Approximately 1 unit/20 kg is administered, and coagulation tests are repeated 1 hour later. Repeated administration may be necessary. The PT or PTT must be prolonged approximately 1.5 times normal for active bleeding to occur, and it is therefore not necessary to normalize the laboratory values to control active bleeding. The use of heparin is controversial. It is contraindicated in the actively bleeding patient without concurrent replacement of clotting factors. Prophylactic heparin therapy may be administered to the patient without clinical signs of hemorrhage but at risk for the development of disseminated intravascular coagulation (DIC) (e.g., heat stroke).

HEMOPHILIA AND VON WILLEBRAND'S DISEASE

Hemophiliac patients require only intermittent transfusion therapy. Cryoprecipitate is the preferred therapy for hemophilia A or von Willebrand's disease, but FFP can be used if cryoprecipitate is not available. The preferred therapy for hemophilia B is frozen plasma or FFP. One unit/20 kg of cryoprecipitate, FFP, or frozen plasma should be administered and clinical response and PTT (or activated clotting time if PTT is not available) measured 1 hour post-transfusion. Transfusions are repeated until bleeding stops, which usually occurs when the PTT decreases to below 1.5 times normal. Red cells are indicated if bleeding is severe and either PRBC plus FFP or fresh whole blood may be administered to provide both red cells and clotting factors.

Hypoproteinemia

The benefit of plasma transfusion to the hypoproteinemic patient is limited. Intravascular albumin is in equilibrium with albumin in the interstitial space, and calculation of the total body deficit must take this into account. Only 40% of body albumin is in the intravascular space while 60% resides in the interstitial space (Table 4). The half-life of albumin is very short with protein-losing diseases, and hyperalimentation is probably of more benefit than transfusion. Plasma may be beneficial to patients with acute reversible decreased production or loss of albumin such as occurs with severe liver disease or inflammatory bowel disease. Colloidal alternatives such as dextrans or hetastarch may be useful in the short-term management of peripheral edema or ascites, but their half-lives are also relatively short.

***Table 4.** Albumin Deficit in a Hypoalbuminemic 30-kg Dog with Serum Albumin 1.8 gm/dl*

1. Total blood volume (30 kg) (90 ml/kg) = 2700 ml
2. Total plasma volume (2700 ml) (60%) = 1620 ml
3. Total plasma albumin (16.20 dl) (1.8 gm/dl) = 29 gm
4. Normal plasma albumin (16.2 dl) (3 gm/dl) = 48.6 gm
5. Plasma deficit of albumin (48.6) − (29) = 19.6 gm
6. If only 40% of body albumin is in the plasma, total body deficit (19.6 gm)/(40%) = 49 gm
7. Amount of albumin in one unit FFP: 250 ml = 2.5 dl. (2.5 dl) (3 gm/dl) = 7.5 gm
8. Number units necessary (49 gm)/(7.5 gm/unit) = 6.5 units

SIDE EFFECTS OF TRANSFUSIONS

Acute hemolysis is probably the most feared reaction to transfusion but is fortunately also one of the rarest. Intravascular destruction of red blood cells causes hemoglobinemia and hemoglobinuria and releases thromboplastic substances which may cause DIC. The potential for acute renal failure also exists. Signs of an acute hemolytic reaction include fever, tachycardia, weakness, tremors, vomiting, and collapse. If signs occur, the transfusion should be stopped and a blood sample drawn from the recipient into EDTA and also spun in a capillary tube to check for hemoglobinemia. Any remaining donor blood in the bag should be saved for further testing for incompatibility or for bacteriologic evaluation by Gram's stain and culture. The major aims of treatment are to maintain blood pressure and renal blood flow and prevent DIC. Crystalloid fluid therapy is begun at two to three times maintenance and continued for at least 6 hours. Prophylactic furosemide should be administered and urine output monitored.

Apparent hemolytic reactions can occur when blood is inadvertently hemolyzed prior to transfusion. Causes include freezing or overheating of blood beyond 50°C, mixing with hypo-osmotic solutions such as 5% dextrose in water, pushing blood or clots through small needles, and contamination with hemolytic bacteria. Since acute hemolytic reactions from immunologic causes are rare in animals, these causes must be considered if such a reaction occurs.

Delayed hemolysis is suspected when an unexplained decrease in the hematocrit occurs 2 days to 2 weeks after the transfusion. This occurs most frequently in previously transfused dogs that developed an antibody titer too low to be detected on crossmatch. Hemoglobinemia and hemoglobinuria are absent as are signs of acute hemolysis. Treatment is unnecessary but concern should be given to careful matching of future transfusions.

The development of fever during transfusion could indicate bacterial contamination of blood; however, this is rarely the case. If blood is contaminated, the reaction is usually immediate and severe and resembles the acute hemolytic reaction. Management includes the immediate cessation of the transfusion, intravenous antibiotics, and treatment for shock. Most febrile reactions are related to leukocyte antigens, generally mild, and more commonly seen in cats. Despite the fever, the patient usually is clinically improved after the transfusion. In this situation, it is often advantageous to monitor without treatment for 24 hours since nonspecific transfusion-induced fevers often spontaneously resolve within that time. Some fevers may be caused by the animal's underlying disease (e.g., FeLV-related infection) and become evident after a moribund or hypothermic cat is transfused.

Allergic reactions are rare but occasionally occur in dogs and are manifested by urticaria and angioneurotic edema. If an allergic reaction occurs, the transfusion is stopped and intravenous antihistamines such as diphenhydramine are given. If the reaction subsides, the transfusion is slowly given. These reactions are rarely severe enough to require epinephrine and corticosteroids.

Circulatory overload is most likely to occur when large volumes of blood are given to cats, small dogs, or patients with underlying cardiac insufficiency. If overload is suspected, the transfusion is stopped and furosemide and oxygen are administered. Anemic animals susceptible to circulatory overload should always be given slow infusions of PRBC, not whole blood.

Citrate toxicity may occur during rapid administration of plasma or whole blood and is caused by an acute decrease in the ionized serum calcium. Animals with portosystemic shunts, severe liver disease, or hypothermia will metabolize citrate slowly and are more prone to toxicity. Signs include muscle tremors, facial twitches, and seizures. Diagnosis cannot be made by measuring serum calcium since only the ionized fraction is decreased. In most cases symptoms resolve if the transfusion is stopped for 5 minutes and restarted at a slower rate. If signs do not resolve quickly, injectable calcium gluconate may be used.

Ammonia levels rise with prolonged storage of PRBC and whole blood. Although the ammonia is of minimal consequence to most patients, encephalopathy could be precipitated in animals with portosystemic shunts or severe liver disease. If necessary, treatment would be the same as that for hepatic encephalopathy.

References and Suggested Reading

Authement, J. M., Wolfsheimer, K. J., and Catchings, S.: Canine blood component therapy: Product preparation, storage, and administration. J. Am. Anim. Hosp. Assoc. 23:483, 1987.

Cotter, S. M.: Clinical transfusion medicine. *In* Cotter, S. M. (ed.): *Comparative Transfusion Medicine.* Orlando: Academic Press (in press).

Klein, M. K., Dow, S. W., and Rosychuk, R. A. W.: Pulmonary thromboembolism associated with immune-mediated hemolytic anemia in dogs: Ten cases (1982–1987). J.A.V.M.A. 195:246, 1989.

Mahaffey, E. A.: Disorders of iron metabolism. In Kirk, R. M. (ed.): Current Veterinary Therapy IX. Philadelphia: W. B. Saunders, 1986, p. 521.

Ou, D., Mahaffey, E., and Smith, J. E.: Effect of storage on oxygen dissociation of canine blood. J.A.V.M.A. 167:56, 1975.

APLASTIC ANEMIA

DOUGLAS J. WEISS

St. Paul, Minnesota

Aplastic anemia (also termed aplastic pancytopenia and myeloaplasia) includes a group of disorders characterized by pancytopenia and generalized bone marrow suppression without underlying disease. Excluded from this are pancytopenias associated with myelophthisic disorders, such as leukemia and myelofibrosis, myelodysplastic disorders in which the marrow is usually normocellular or hypercellular, and pure red cell aplasia in which only red blood cell production is suppressed.

NORMAL HEMATOPOIESIS

Hematopoiesis is regulated by hematopoietic growth factors, biologic response modifiers, and marrow stromal cells which form a supportive microenvironment (Groopman et al., 1989). The microenvironment appears to affect the earliest stem cells in the marrow by directing stem-cell renewal but may inhibit stem-cell differentiation and entry into the cell cycle. These effects are mediated either by cell-to-cell contact or by as yet unidentified cytokines. Hematopoietic growth factors are glycoprotein cytokines that regulate differentiation and proliferation of the more differentiated progenitor cells. These factors exert their effects at different stages of cell differentiation. Interleukin-1, interleukin-4, and interleukin-6 appear to act at the stem-cell stage. The major function of IL-1 is likely indirect through induction of expression of genes for IL-6, granulocyte-monocyte colony-stimulating factor (GM-CSF), and granulocyte colony-stimulating factor (G-CSF). Interleukin-3 (IL-3) and GM-CSF act primarily at the multipotential progenitor cell stage (see this volume, p. 466). G-CSF, M-CSF, erythropoietin, and Meg-CSF/thrombopoietin act on lineage-specific progenitor cells committed to granulocyte, monocyte, erythroid, and megakaryocyte production, respectively. Other molecules, including interferon, tumor necrosis factor, transforming growth factor, and prostaglandins, can influence hematopoiesis either directly or indirectly but are not considered primary hematopoietic growth factors.

PATHOGENESIS

Studies involving naturally occurring and induced models of aplastic anemia suggest that multiple rather than singular mechanisms are involved in the pathogenesis of aplastic anemia. Mechanisms that could lead to suppression of hematopoiesis and subsequent pancytopenia include: (1) toxic destruction of stem cells, (2) proliferation of stem cells with decreased self-renewal capacity or decreased proliferation or differentiation capacity, (3) immune-mediated destruction of stem cells, (4) altered marrow microenvironment, (5) lack of hematopoietic growth factors, and (6) presence of inhibitors of hematopoiesis. The latter three mechanisms have not been documented as causes of aplastic anemia. Direct destruction of stem cells caused by exposure to drugs or chemicals, such as hydroxyurea, trimethoprim/sulfadiazine, and quinidine, result in acute marrow failure and pancytopenia. Clinical signs related to leukopenia and thrombocytopenia usually develop within 2 weeks of initial treatment (Weiss and Klausner, 1990). Discontinuation of the agent often results in recovery within 2 weeks, and stem-cell numbers return to normal. Other drugs and chemicals, such as busulfan and cyclophosphamide, produce dose-dependent acute aplasia, but recovery is associated with a persistent decrease in stem-cell numbers. Recent studies suggest that the chronic depletion of stem cells is the result of damage to the marrow microenvironment. Repair of defects in the microenvironment is limited and slow, and recovery may take weeks or months. Persistent depletion of stem cells after remission of idiopathic aplastic anemia in humans suggests that stromal damage was involved in the pathogenesis.

The role of immune-mediated suppression in

naturally occurring aplastic anemia is controversial. Several studies report supression of *in vitro* colony formation by lymphocytes from human patients with idiopathic aplastic anemia or altered subsets of T and B lymphocytes. Others have reported defective monocyte maturation. The interpretation of these findings is limited by lack of understanding of the effects of lymphoid cells on normal hematopoiesis. Immune-mediated suppression of hematopoiesis has not been studied in dogs or cats.

ETIOLOGY

Aplastic anemia may be idiopathic or induced by irradiation, drugs, chemicals, or infectious agents (Table 1). The aplasia may be acute or chronic. Acute aplastic anemia is characterized by severe granulocytopenia and thrombocytopenia with mild to nonexistent anemia. Chronic aplastic anemia develops over a prolonged period and is characterized by severe anemia and variable degrees of leukopenia and thrombocytopenia.

Drug-Induced Aplasia

ESTROGEN INTOXICATION

Dog bone marrow is highly susceptible to estrogen-induced supression (Shelly, 1988; Weiss and Armstrong, 1984). Estrogens derived from endogenous as well as exogenous sources have been incriminated. Experimental injection of a single large dose of natural or synthetic estrogens produces a predictable hematologic response in blood and bone marrow. Thrombocytopenia, leukocytosis, and mild but progressive anemia develop in the first 3 weeks after injection. During this period the bone marrow has normal cellularity owing to myeloid hyperplasia, but erythropoiesis and thrombocytopoiesis are depressed. Pancytopenia and marrow hypoplasia/aplasia develop 3 to 4 weeks after injection. Dogs begin to recover by 30 days after injection. However, some clinical cases develop severe chronic aplasia, particularly when multiple doses are administered (Weiss and Klausner, 1990). The potential reversibility of the chronic phase is uncertain since many dogs have been euthanatized shortly after diagnosis. At least four reported cases, which were given prolonged supportive treatment, recovered several months after initial diagnosis. One case, treated with multiple transfusions of platelet-rich plasma, began to recover 10 weeks after estradiol cyclopentyl propionate (ECP) administration (Weiss and Klausner, 1990).

NONSTEROIDAL ANTI-INFLAMMATORY DRUGS

Nonsteroidal anti-inflammatory drugs have been incriminated as causes of aplastic anemia. At least ten cases of phenylbutazone-associated and one case of meclofenamic acid (arquel)-associated blood dyscrasia have been reported. Phenylbutazone-associated granulocytopenias and aplastic anemia occur sporadically, often after long-term treatment, and are not dose dependent. Most affected dogs died or were euthanatized when symptomatic treatment failed to resolve the condition.

CHEMOTHERAPEUTIC DRUGS

Suppression of hematopoiesis is the most common toxicity associated with administration of chemotherapeutic drugs (Couto, 1986). Drugs with high myelosuppressive potential include cyclophosphamide, cytosine arabinoside, doxorubicin, vinblastine, and hydroxyurea. The high mitotic rate of bone marrow precursor cells predisposes them to destruction. Since stem cells do not have a high mitotic rate, they are usually spared. Therefore, hematologic recovery usually occurs after discontinuation of the drug. The associated hypoplasia/aplasia is of the acute type and is characterized by leukopenia and thrombocytopenia. Neutropenia usually develops within 5 to 7 days after drug administration, and thrombocytopenia develops in 7 to 10 days. Neutrophil counts return to normal in 36 to 72 hours after discontinuing the drug. Animals with less than 200 segmented neutrophils/μl are highly susceptible to bacterial sepsis. Thrombocytopenia associated with administration of chemotherapeutic drugs is usually not severe enough to cause spontaneous hemorrhage.

TRIMETHOPRIM-SULFADIAZINE

Six cases of a sulfadiazine-induced allergy have been reported in Doberman pinschers. Clinical signs included polyarthritis, lymphadenopathy, polymyositis, glomerulonephritis, retinitis, anemia, leukopenia, and thrombocytopenia. Clinical signs resolved after discontinuing treatment. One case of trimethoprim-sulfadiazine–associated acute aplastic anemia in a non-Doberman breed has been reported (Weiss and Klausner, 1990). The hematologic dyscrasia resolved when the drug was discontinued.

OTHER DRUGS

Other drugs causally associated with aplastic anemia in the dog or cat include quinidine, griseofulvin, and thiacetarsamide (Table 1). The animals re-

Table 1. *Reported Causes of Aplastic Anemia in the Dog and Cat*

Cause	Dog	Cat	Type of Aplasia	Number of Reported Cases	Outcome
Idiopathic	X	X	Chronic	One	Irreversible
Drug-associated					
Estrogen	X		Acute/chronic	Many	Reversible/irreversible
Chemotherapy	X	X	Acute	Many	Reversible
Phenylbutazone	X		Acute	Many	Most irreversible
Meclofenamic acid	X		Acute	One	Irreversible
Trimethoprim/sulfadiazine	X		Acute	Eight	Reversible
Quinidine	X		Acute	One	Reversible
Thiacetarsamide	X		Acute	One	Reversible
Griseofulvin		X	Acute	One	Reversible
Infectious					
Ehrlichia	X		Acute/chronic	Many	Reversible/irreversible
Parvovirus	X	X	Acute	Many	Reversible
Feline leukemia virus		X	Chronic	Many	Irreversible

covered promptly after discontinuation of the drug (Shelly, 1988; Weiss and Klausner, 1990). Chloramphenicol, when given in therapeutic doses, may cause mild bone marrow suppression in both dogs and cats, but the severe aplastic anemia reported in human patients has not been documented.

Infectious Agents

Infectious causes of aplastic anemia include ehrlichiosis, parvovirus, and feline leukemia virus infections (Shelly, 1988; Weiss and Armstrong, 1984). Feline leukemia virus produces selective suppression of erythropoiesis (nonregenerative anemia), suppression of all hemic cells (aplastic anemia), hemolytic anemia, or proliferative disorders, including myelodysplasia and leukemia. The marrow dyscrasia is frequently accompanied by macrocytosis in the blood.

Peripheral blood cytopenias occur in both the acute and chronic forms of ehrlichiosis. In the acute form, bone marrow is hypercellular, suggesting that the cytopenias are the result of cell destruction in the peripheral blood. In the chronic form, the marrow is hypocellular, consistent with a diagnosis of aplastic anemia. In the acute form, treatment with tetracycline usually results in rapid hematologic recovery, but in the chronic form, recovery is less predictable and protracted.

Parvovirus infection, in both dogs and cats induces acute aplastic anemia. Examination of bone marrow aspirates revealed hypocellularity and degenerative changes in all hematopoietic cell lines. Hematologic recovery is usually rapid if the animal survives the acute stages of the disease.

Idiopathic Aplastic Anemia

Only one case of idiopathic aplastic anemia has been reported in dogs. This paucity of reported cases suggests that the incidence of idiopathic aplastic anemia is low in the dog when compared with humans, where 40 to 90% of aplastic anemia cases are idiopathic.

DIAGNOSIS

Minimum clinical evaluation of a patient with suspected aplastic anemia includes a complete history with questions pertaining to exposure to drugs, chemicals, and infectious agents, complete blood count, blood smear evaluation, and bone marrow aspiration and core biopsy. A diagnosis of aplastic anemia cannot be made without evaluation of bone marrow (see this volume, p. 488). Bone marrow aspiration smears permit identification of individual cells, while core biopsy sections are essential for evaluating marrow cellularity and architecture. Without a core biopsy, differentiation of hypocellular aspirates from poor sampling technique is difficult. Cellularity in the core biopsy is assessed by estimating the relative percentage of the marrow space occupied by hemic cells. In aplastic anemia, hemic tissue occupies less than 25% of the marrow space, with the remainder replaced by adipose tissue. Frequently, only small islands of hemic cells remain and consist mainly of lymphocytes and plasma cells. In acute toxic aplastic anemia, rapid destruction of hemic cells may result in multifocal areas of necrosis in the tissue section.

In acute aplastic anemia, particular attention should be given to drug or chemical exposure 2 to 3 weeks before clinical signs develop. The patient with acute aplastic anemia presents with signs referable to neutropenia and thrombocytopenia. Anemia is usually mild but may be progressive over time. Drug toxicities, acute ehrlichiosis, and parvovirus infection should be considered as possible causes. Ehrlichiosis can be evaluated through examination of blood smears for organisms or by determining antibody titers. Capillary blood, obtained by an ear prick, is the best specimen for identification of the organism. Generally, discontinuation of the drug or successful treatment of the infection results in prompt hematologic recovery.

In the chronic form of aplastic anemia, animals usually present with signs referable to severe anemia. Although variable degrees of leukopenia and thrombocytopenia accompany the anemia, enough residual granulopoiesis and thrombopoiesis remain to prevent infection and hemorrhage and permit development of anemia over weeks or months.

TREATMENT

Supportive Care

Treatment of aplastic anemia depends on whether the aplasia is of the acute or chronic type and on the severity of the cytopenias in the blood. Because many drugs and chemicals can induce aplastic anemia, all drug therapy given before diagnosis should be discontinued if possible, and the animal's environment should be inspected for potential toxins. Additionally, drugs that adversely affect neutrophil or platelet function should be avoided.

Severe leukopenia (i.e., segmented neutrophils < 200/μl) is associated with markedly increased susceptibility to bacterial infection. Administration of a broad-spectrum antibiotic is essential to control infection. The first antibiotic is usually effective for 5 to 7 days in controlling fever and infection. Administration of a second antibiotic controls infection for up to 5 days while subsequent antibiotics may control infection for only a day or two. Choice of antibiotic should be based on bacterial culture and sensitivity whenever possible. In the absence of culture and sensitivity results, broad-spectrum antibiotics, such as cephalosporins, or a combination of antibiotics should be used. A combination of gentamycin (1 mg/lb IV t.i.d.) and cephalothin (20 mg/lb IV t.i.d.) or gentamycin and ticarcillin (20 mg/lb IM q.i.d.) has been recommended to treat neutropenic animals that are febrile (Couto, 1986).

Glucocorticoids have been recommended to attenuate hemorrhage associated with thrombocytopenia. Glucocorticoids suppress neutrophil function, however, and may therefore increase susceptibility to infection.

Whole Blood and Blood Components

Aplastic anemia is frequently a chronic condition that may require multiple transfusions. To prevent alloimmunization and subsequent transfusion reactions, all donors should be DEA 1.1, 1.2, and 7 negative, and crossmatches should be done before each transfusion (see this volume pp. 470 and 475). Since multiple transfusions are often necessary, blood typing of the recipient is preferred. Blood-typing kits for dogs are available commercially (Stormont Labs, Inc., Woodland, CA). Blood component therapy to treat specific cytopenias is preferable to whole blood transfusion. Animals with chronic aplastic anemia are frequently severely anemic, with packed cell volumes less than 10%. Administration of washed RBC helps to minimize leukocyte, platelet, and plasma sensitizations. In acute aplastic anemia, severe leukopenia or thrombocytopenia may require attention. Administration of platelet-rich-plasma, sufficient to increase platelet counts to between 25,000 and 75,000/μl should maintain platelet counts above 5000/μl for 3 to 5 days. Alloimmunization to platelets occurs over time, and subsequent transfusions may be ineffective in increasing platelet counts.

The benefit of granulocyte transfusion remains controversial in human medicine and has been used infrequently in veterinary medicine (Quie, 1987). Early and intensive antibiotic therapy is of critical importance in treating and preventing sepsis associated with neutropenia. However, if the invading organisms are resistant to antibiotics, or if neutropenia persists for more than 10 days, granulocyte transfusions would likely be beneficial. Granulocytes can be collected by filtration leukapheresis, gravity leukapheresis, continuous-flow leukapheresis, or intermittent-flow leukapheresis. A minimum of four daily granulocyte transfusions should be given. Granulocytes contain a variety of neutrophil-specific and nonspecific antigens, including RBC antigens and major histocompatibility antigens. Alloimmunization can be minimized by RBC and leukocyte crossmatching. Leukocyte-specific antigens can be evaluated by leukoagglutination or by immunofluorescence.

Immunosuppression

Immunosuppressive therapy has not been extensively evaluated in dogs or cats, nor has an immune basis for aplastic anemia been established. In human medicine, immunosuppressive therapy has been effective for treatment of idiopathic aplastic anemia. Treatment with either antithymocyte globulin or high-dose methylprednisolone resulted in sustained improvement in 45 to 70% of human patients (Doney et al., 1987). Methylprednisolone was given at 20 mg/kg/day intravenously on days 1 through 4; 10 mg/kg/day intravenously on days 5 through 8; 2 mg/kg/day on days 9 to 16, and 1.5 mg/kg/day PO on days 17 through 24. From days 25 to 38, a fixed dose of 4 mg was given daily PO. Methylprednisolone, when given intravenously, was infused over a 4-hour period. Another report suggested that administration of 1 gm of methylprednisolone IV per day for 3 days may be effective. In human patients, antithymocyte globulin was administered at a dose of 15 mg IgG/kg body weight/day intravenously for 10 days. The dose was administered over 6 to 12 hours. Cyclosporine has also been reported to induce remission in some human patients. It has been administered orally at 6 mg/kg b.i.d. Veterinary studies are lacking.

Bone Marrow Stimulation

Nonspecific bone marrow stimulants include anabolic steroids, cobalt, growth hormone, lithium, and plasma infusions. Despite widespread use of anabolic steroids, controlled studies of their use in human aplastic anemia indicate that they are not an effective therapy. However, remission of one canine case of aplastic anemia after treatment with oxymetholone (2 mg/kg PO divided b.i.d.) was reported. No controlled studies have been done to indicate therapeutic efficacy of growth hormone, cobalt, lithium, or plasma infusions.

Recently, recombinant hematopoietic growth factors have become available for research applications and clinical trials in dogs. Granulocyte-macrophage colony-stimulating factor has been used to treat severe aplastic anemia in human patients. In separate studies, 10 of 10 and 6 of 8 human patients had transient improvement in neutrophil and monocyte counts and had increased bone marrow cellularity without increases in numbers of colony-forming units (Ogilvie and Obradovich, 1990) (see this volume, p. 466). Studies to date suggest that GM-CSF reduces the need for transfusion in aplastic anemia by stimulating existing residual hematopoiesis but does not ameliorate the underlying defect in hematopoiesis. Combination therapy, using two or more hematopoietic growth factors and growth factors that act at the stem-cell level (i.e., interleukins 1 and 6), is being investigated at present.

GM-CSF has been administered to healthy dogs by continuous intravenous infusion for 14 days (Ogilvie and Obradovich, 1990). The infusion was well tolerated, and neutrophil counts increased to three to six times preinfusion numbers. Neutrophil counts returned to pretreatment numbers 3 to 7 days after discontinuation of infusion.

Bone Marrow Transplantation

The dog has been used as a model for bone marrow transplantation for many years; therefore, techniques are well established (Storb et al., 1984). Bone marrow transplantation for aplastic anemia is limited by a lack of compatible donors. Dogs have at least two polymorphic histocompatibility systems in addition to the DLA system. Rejection of bone marrow transplants appears to be mediated by non–T lymphocytes. Treatment with procarbazine and antilymphocyte serum or with cyclosporine before total body irradiation resulted in sustained engraftment in most normal dogs. The rejection rate is increased by prior blood transfusion. Despite improved engraftment, graft versus host disease, and other associated diseases, such as neurologic disease and malignancy, are significant side effects. Studies in humans with aplastic anemia suggest that transplantation is superior to immunosuppressive therapy only when HLA-identical related donors are available (see this volume, p. 493).

PROGNOSIS

Predicting the outcome of aplastic anemia and its response to specific treatments depends on the cause and whether it is acute or chronic. Generally, acute aplastic anemias are reversible after elimination of initiating agents, such as drugs, toxins, or infectious agents, provided adequate supportive care is given. Nonsteroidal anti-inflammatory drugs are an exception. With present approaches to treatment of phenylbutazone-associated aplastic anemia, most affected dogs do not recover.

Chronic aplastic anemia is less amenable to treatment. With supportive care, recovery weeks to months after initial diagnosis has been reported (Weiss and Klausner, 1990). In the future, more extensive use of blood component therapy, recombinant hematopoietic growth factors, and bone marrow transplantation should further increase survival time and remission rates.

References

Couto, C. G.: Toxicity of anticancer chemotherapy. *In* Campfield, W. W. (ed.): *Kal Kan Symposium for the Treatment of Small Animal Diseases.* Vermon, CA.: Kal Kan Pet Foods, 1986, p. 37.
  A review of the toxic side effects associated with administration of anticancer chemotherapy.
Doney, K., Storb, R., Buckner, C. D., et al.: Treatment of aplastic anemia with antithymocyte globulin, high-dose corticosteroids, and androgens. Exp. Hematol. 15:239, 1987.
  A review of the treatment of human aplastic anemia with antithymocyte globulin and high-dose methylprednisolone.
Groopman, J. E., Molina, J. M., and Scadden, D. T.: Hematopoietic growth factors: Biology and applications. N. Engl. J. Med. 321:1449, 1989.
  A review of recombinant growth factors and their clinical application.
Ogilvie, G. K., and Obradovich, J.: Use of colony-stimulating factors in human and veterinary medicine. Proceedings of the 8th Am. College of Vet. Internal Med. Forum. Washington, D.C., 1990, p. 917.
  An introduction to the clinical use of recombinant hematopoietic growth factors in veterinary medicine.
Quie, P. G.: The white cell: Use of granulocyte transfusion. Rev. Infect. Dis. 9:189, 1987.
  A review of the usefulness of granulocyte transfusions in human patients.
Shelly, S. M.: Causes of canine pancytopenia. Compend. Cont. Ed. 10:9, 1988.
  A review of the causes of pancytopenia in dogs.

Storb, R., Thomas, E. D., Buckner, C. D., et al.: Marrow transplantation for aplastic anemia. Semin. Hematol. 21:27, 1984.
A review of bone marrow transplantation in dogs, mice, and humans.
Weiss, D. J., and Armstrong, P. J.: Nonregenerative anemias in the dog. Compend. Cont. Ed. 6:452, 1984.
A review of the primary and secondary causes of bone marrow suppression in the dog.

Weiss, D. J., and Klausner, J. S.: Drug-associated aplastic anemia in dogs: Eight cases (1984–1988). J.A.V.M.A. 196:472, 1990.
A retrospective study of eight dogs with aplastic anemia which may have been caused by therapeutic drugs.

APPLICATION OF RECOMBINANT HUMAN ERYTHROPOIETIN IN DOGS AND CATS

LARRY D. COWGILL

Davis, California

REGULATION AND DISORDERS OF ERYTHROPOIETIN

Erythropoietin is the principal regulatory hormone for red blood cell (RBC) production by the bone marrow. It is produced in the renal cortex by peritubular endothelial cells, and in some species (but not dogs) the liver also contributes to a minor degree. Regulation of erythropoietin is coupled inversely to the availability of oxygen to the kidneys. Reduced oxygen supply secondary to anemia, hypoxia, or interference with oxygen transfer from hemoglobin activates erythropoietin messenger RNA (mRNA) production and elaboration of functional erythropoietin within hours of the stimulus. Increased oxygen availability due to polycythemia or hyperoxia down-regulates erythropoietin secretion and reduces RBC production by a classic stimulus-effector feedback control system. Erythropoietin interacts with high-affinity receptors on target cells in the bone marrow to promote an increase in RBC mass. It most effectively stimulates committed erythroid progenitor cells (colony-forming units—erythrocyte [CFU-E]), which are activated to differentiate and develop into mature RBCs. Erythropoietin also promotes hemoglobin synthesis and accelerates the egress and release of newly formed RBCs and reticulocytes into the circulation.

Pathologic conditions related to disordered regulation of erythropoietin may be categorized into secondary polycythemia subsequent to excessive production of erythropoietin or anemia coincident with its diminished production. Secondary polycythemias are relatively uncommon and are characterized by an increase in RBC number, hematocrit, hemoglobin, and absolute RBC mass. Secondary polycythemia is recognized as a physiologic response to hypoxemia in animals living at high altitudes, in patients with congenital cardiovascular disorders (e.g., tetralogy of Fallot) with right-to-left shunting of blood away from the lungs, and in patients with diffuse pulmonary diseases that prevent adequate hemoglobin saturation. In most circumstances, these conditions can be diagnosed on the basis of history and physical findings, demonstration of abnormally low arterial oxygen saturation, and elevated serum or urinary erythropoietin concentrations.

Secondary polycythemia can also result from pathologic stimulation of erythropoietin by various neoplastic, cystic, infiltrative, or space-occupying diseases of the kidneys. The cause of the excessive erythropoietin production is not entirely defined but likely is due to unregulated secretion from the lesion *per se* or from intrinsic renal production subsequent to interference with oxygen delivery to regional renal parenchyma. These disorders can be distinguished from physiologic causes of polycythemia by the adequacy of arterial oxygen saturation and demonstration of discrete renal lesions through radiographic or ultrasonic imaging. An elevated erythropoietin concentration is the distinguishing feature of all forms of secondary polycythemia.

Erythropoietin deficiency with hypoproliferative anemia is the most clinically significant and common disorder of erythropoietin metabolism. Progressive destruction of renal parenchyma causes diminished erythropoietin secretory capacity, and the association between progressive renal failure and the development of anemia is well recognized in companion animals. Although a generally inverse correlation between hematocrit reading and serum creatinine level exists in dogs and cats, considerable variation is apparent owing to differences in the stage and causes of renal failure and clinical variations among patients. In individual patients, however, the progression of anemia with progressive deterioration of renal function is a predictable and inevitable consequence of the uremic syndrome. Reticulocyte counts are dependably low, and bone marrow cytology reveals an increased myeloid:erythroid ratio that is characteristic of erythropoietin deficiency and erythroid hypoplasia. Measurements of serum erythropoietin concentrations in dogs with naturally occurring and experimental forms of renal failure reveal low to normal serum erythropoietin concentrations and support the tenet of absolute or *relative* erythropoietin deficiency (King et al. [in press]; Petrites-Murphy et al., 1989).

The contributions of anemia to the clinical consequences of end-stage renal disease (ESRD) have been poorly characterized in companion animals and are generally combined conceptually into the multisystemic syndrome of uremia. However, in recent studies of both dogs and cats with ESRD, when the anemia was corrected independently of changes in azotemia, significant improvements in the inappetence, weakness, fatigue, lethargy, cold intolerance, social apathy, and clinical well being that characterize the uremic syndrome in these species were documented (Cowgill et al., 1990). Erythropoietin deficiency and anemia can no longer be considered inevitable features of ESRD that are conveniently tolerated and therapeutically abandoned; their resolution yields clinical benefits that dramatically influence the spectrum of renal failure.

TREATMENT OF ERYTHROPOIETIN DEFICIENCY

Until recently there was no specific or consistently effective therapy for erythropoietin deficiency except intermittent blood transfusion. The development and availability of recombinant human erythropoietin (r-HuEPO, EPOGEN [epoetin alfa], AMGEN Inc., Thousand Oaks, CA) has revolutionized the ability to treat this inevitable consequence of progressive renal failure. Recombinant human erythropoietin is a therapeutic dividend of molecular biology in which the human genome is probed to isolate specific segments of DNA responsible for the coding of erythropoietin. This genetic information is then expressed in cultured mammalian cells that "manufacture" the replica hormone. The mature recombinant protein contains 165 amino acids and has a molecular weight of approximately 34,000 daltons. Recombinant human erythropoietin has the same primary structure as human urinary erythropoietin and is a faithful molecular and biologic reproduction of the natural hormone (Egrie et al.,

1986). EPOGEN consists of r-HuEPO (2000, 3000, 4000, or 10,000 units/ml) in 0.25% human serum albumin USP, buffered by 20 mM sodium citrate and 100 mM sodium chloride at pH 6.8.

In clinical trials in human patients maintained on chronic hemodialysis, r-HuEPO reversed the anemia and transfusion dependency in virtually every patient. It normalized the hematocrit, hemoglobin concentration, and RBC count in a dose-dependent manner after intravenous or subcutaneous doses between 50 and 300 units/kg three times weekly (Eschbach, 1990; Eschbach et al., 1987). Concomitantly with the hematologic changes, human patients reported improvements in their sense of wellbeing, appetite, strength, exercise capacity, sleep habits, hair growth, and sexual performance (Delano, 1989).

The erythropoietin molecule maintains a high degree of homology among mammalian species, and preliminary trials with r-HuEPO in dogs and cats with naturally occurring renal failure demonstrated erythropoietic and clinical effects comparable to those described in human patients (Cowgill et al., 1990). It effectively reversed the decline in hematocrit associated with chronic renal failure and promoted an approximate 1 vol%/day increase in hematocrit during the first month of therapy. RBC count, hematocrit, and hemoglobin concentrations were normalized within 3 to 4 weeks of initiating therapy in most patients (Figs. 1 and 2). The hypoplastic bone marrow converted to an active erythroid proliferative state. Recombinant human erythropoietin had no effects on white blood cells or platelet counts or on the leukocyte distribution in either canine or feline patients, consistent with its specificity for CFU-E precursors. Concomitantly with resolution of anemia by r-HuEPO, there were incontrovertible improvements in clinical well

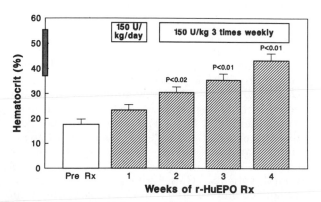

Figure 1. Change in hematocrit before and during treatment with r-HuEPO for 4 weeks in uremic dogs. Each bar represents the mean ± SE hematocrit in six dogs. Statistically significant differences are compared with the pretreatment value, and the shaded area on the vertical axis depicts the reference range. The r-HuEPO was administered subcutaneously at 150 units/kg/day for 7 days, then at 150 units/kg three times a week.

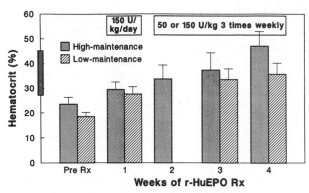

Figure 2. Change in hematocrit before and during treatment with r-HuEPO for 4 weeks in uremic cats. Bars represent the mean ± SE hematocrit in three cats (high maintenance) or four cats (low maintenance) before and during treatment with r-HuEPO for 4 weeks. The shaded area on the vertical axis depicts the reference range. The r-HuEPO was administered SC at 150 units/kg/day for 7 days, then at 150 units/kg (high maintenance) or 50 units/kg (low maintenance) three times a week.

being, appetite, activity level, playfulness, weight gain (typically 10 to 12%), and physical strength. Decreased sleep requirements, increased affection, and return of old behaviors were noted also.

Despite its consistent erythroid stimulation and benefits in clinical well being, r-HuEPO therapy predisposes to both theoretic and predictable adverse effects. In human patients, the most consistent and notable *adverse events* are (1) systemic hypertension, (2) iron deficiency, (3) hyperkalemia, (4) seizures, and (5) interference with hemodialysis efficiency (Eschbach, 1990). Systemic hypertension may develop in normotensive patients or become exacerbated in previously hypertensive patients in association with r-HuEPO therapy in humans.

Its heterology for dogs and cats and current formulation in human serum albumin could promote both local and systemic *allergic reactions*. Cellulitis, fever, arthralgia, and mucocutaneous ulcerations have been rarely recognized coincident with r-HuEPO therapy. An allergic basis for these reactions could not be demonstrated by intradermal skin testing, but all manifestations resolved within days of discontinuing r-HuEPO therapy. In preliminary trials, anti–r-HuEPO antibodies were detected in both dogs and cats after variable courses of treatment with EPOGEN. The formation of antibody correlated with development of profound anemia, arrest of erythropoiesis, and transfusion dependency and was detectable in 20 to 50% of treated patients. These adverse events must be recognized and factored into risk-versus-benefit decisions confronting r-HuEPO therapy. When the anemia is profound and associated with overt clinical signs, the risks of treatment with EPOGEN are generally warranted and the results beneficial. In patients with mild anemia, a more cautious therapeutic approach is in order.

The role of r-HuEPO in other types of anemia remains speculative and untested. In most hypoproliferative anemias uncomplicated by ESRD, high concentrations of endogenous erythropoietin are documented (Wardrop et al., 1986), and the efficacy of further bone marrow stimulation must be questioned. Potential applications of r-HuEPO include autotransfusion before elective surgery and as an adjunct to chemotherapy using myelosuppressive pharmaceuticals.

Treatment Guidelines for Dogs and Cats

EPOGEN is not currently licensed for use in companion animals, nor does the manufacturer endorse its administration to dogs or cats. No express therapeutic indications for r-HuEPO have been advocated, but its use as replacement therapy in the anemia of ESRD seems implicit. Specific guidelines for EPOGEN therapy in dogs and cats with renal failure or other conditions will not be forthcoming until greater clinical experience and controlled clinical trials in patients with naturally occurring disease have been completed. However, the following recommendations are extrapolated from available recommendations for human patients and preliminary experiences in dogs and cats.

Recombinant human erythropoietin is logically indicated for erythropoietin replacement in uremic dogs and cats demonstrating hypoproliferative anemia and its attendant consequences of weakness, fatigue, inappetence, social apathy, cold intolerance, or altered behavior. Hematocrits below 30% for dogs and 25% for cats are consistent with the development of these signs and represent general starting points for therapy. Treatment should be withheld from patients with systemic hypertension or iron deficiency until these conditions have been corrected. Because more than 60% of patients with renal disease have systemic hypertension and perhaps 20 to 40% of uremic patients have low serum iron concentrations (personal observation), it is important that both blood pressure and serum iron be measured before r-HuEPO therapy.

In both dogs and cats, r-HuEPO therapy is initiated at 100 units/kg body weight SC three times weekly. This dosage is maintained for the first 12 weeks of therapy or until the target hematocrit of 37 to 45% for dogs or 30 to 40% for cats is achieved. Once the lower range of the target hematocrit is reached, the dosage interval is decreased to twice weekly to prevent overshooting the target range. If further modification is required to prevent polycythemia, the dosage interval is changed to once per week. If anemia redevelops with twice-weekly administration, a thrice-weekly dosage schedule is reinstituted. If adequate control cannot be achieved within these dosage intervals, the dose may be increased by 25 to 50 units/kg, but, in general, the dosage interval should not exceed thrice weekly or be less than once weekly. The maintenance dosage to sustain the hematocrit within the target range must be established individually for each patient by judicious adjustment of the dosage or interval of administration, as well as adequate surveillance of the patient's responses. Dosages of 75 to 100 units/kg two to three times weekly generally are sufficient. Once-weekly administration may be inadequate to maintain an effective response.

Failing an adequate response, the patient should be evaluated for iron deficiency, external blood loss, hemolytic disease, or concurrent infectious, inflammatory, or neoplastic diseases that could blunt or prevent erythropoiesis. The dosage or interval of administration should not be adjusted more frequently than every 3 weeks because of the prolonged lag time for changes in hematocrit after dosage modifications. More rapid adjustments result in large fluctuations in the hematocrit and the tendency to therapeutically "chase" the excursions. Treatment should be temporarily withheld if the hematocrit exceeds normal limits until it is reestablished within the target range.

The profound erythropoiesis promoted by r-HuEPO administration significantly influences iron homeostasis. The rapid demands for iron can deplete body iron stores and promote iron depletion. Consequently, most patients require *iron supplementation* to prevent this complication and to foster the therapeutic response. Serum iron concentrations, total iron binding capacity, and transferrin saturation should be normalized before initiating r-HuEPO therapy by administration of ferrous sulfate, 100 to 300 mg/day PO for dogs and 50 to 100 mg/day PO for cats. Maintenance iron therapy with multivitamin preparations that contain ferrous sulfate should be provided until a stable hematocrit is achieved.

The erythropoietic potency of r-HuEPO and the need for lifelong therapy necessitate regular evaluation of patients to ensure maximal therapeutic efficacy and recognition of untoward effects of treatment. The hematocrit should be monitored at weekly intervals until it is established within the target range and an appropriate dosage regimen has been determined to maintain a stable hematocrit in this range for at least 4 weeks. Thereafter, a complete blood cell count should be performed at monthly or bimonthly intervals to ensure adequacy of the erythropoietic response and to monitor for adverse effects.

Serum iron, total iron-binding capacity, and the erythrocytic indices (mean corpuscular volume, mean corpuscular hemoglobin, mean corpuscular hemoglobin concentration) should be monitored 3 to 4 weeks after starting r-HuEPO therapy and regularly for the duration of treatment. Systemic blood pressure should be determined by direct or indirect methods at least monthly during the initiation phase of therapy and monthly or bimonthly thereafter. Development or exacerbation of systemic hypertension refractory to antihypertensive therapy warrants temporary or permanent discontinuation of r-HuEPO treatments. Pain, inflammation, or discoloration at injection sites should be evaluated regularly to ascertain sensitivities to the drug.

The development of refractory anemia in the presence of adequate doses of r-HuEPO and normal iron metabolism is a potentially serious consequence of r-HuEPO therapy. A bone marrow aspirate demonstrating erythrocytic hypoplasia suggests depvelopment of anti–r-HuEPO antibodies and contraindicates its further administration. The myeloid:erythroid ratio is a sensitive monitor of this untoward event, and increases in the myeloid:erythroid ratio may precede notable decreases in hematocrit. Ratios greater than 6 with adequate r-HuEPO administration predict antibody formation and dictate discontinuation of r-HuEPO.

References and Suggested Reading

Cowgill, L. D., Feldman, B., Levy, J. et al.: Efficacy of recombinant human erythropoietin (r-HuEPO) for anemia in dogs and cats with renal failure. J. Vet. Intern. Med. 4:126, 1990.
Abstract of preliminary trial of r-HuEPO administration to dogs and cats with ESRD.

Delano, B. G.: Improvements in quality of life following treatment with r-HuEPO in anemic hemodialysis patients. Am. J. Kidney Dis. 14 (suppl. 1):14, 1989.
Quantitative analysis of quality of life assessment in hemodialysis patients with anemia subsequent to treatment with r-HuEPO.

Egrie, J. C., Strickland, T. W., Lane, J., et al.: Characterization and biological effects of recombinant human erythropoietin. Immunobiology 172:213, 1986.
This article describes the molecular and immunologic characterization of r-HuEPO and compares its structure and function with purified human erythropoietin.

Eschbach, J. W.: Erythropoietin therapy for the anemia of chronic renal failure. Kidney Int. 22:1, 1990.
Review of the physiology, pharmacokinetics, hematologic effects, clinical use, and adverse effects of r-HuEPO in human patients.

Eschbach, J. W., Egrie, J. C., Downing, M. R., et al.: Correction of the anemia of end-stage renal disease with recombinant human erythropoietin: Results of a combined phase I and II clinical trial. N. Engl. J. Med. 316:73, 1987.
Elaboration of the results of the initial phase I and II clinical trials or r-HuEPO administration to human patients with ESRD.

King, L. G., Giger, U., Diserens, D., et al.: Anemia of chronic renal failure in dogs. J. Vet. Intern. Med. (in press).
Clinical and hematologic evaluation (including serum erythropoietin) of dogs with naturally occurring renal failure.

Petrites-Murphy, M. B., Pierce, K. R., Lowry, S. R., et al.: Role of parathyroid hormone in the anemia of chronic terminal renal dysfunction in dogs. Am. J. Vet. Res. 50:1898, 1989.
Comparison of erythropoietin concentration and erythropoietic potential in control dogs and dogs with experimentally induced renal insufficiency.

Wardrop, K. J., Kramer, J. W., Abkowitz, J. L., et al.: Quantitative studies of erythropoiesis in the clinically normal, phlebotomized, and feline leukemia virus-infected cat. Am. J. Vet. Res. 47:2274, 1986.
Experimental evaluation including measurements of serum erythropoietin, ferrokinetic analysis, and proliferative responsiveness of erythroid progenitors in normal and phlebotomized cats and FeLV-afflicted cats naturally infected with anemia.

BONE MARROW BIOPSY: INDICATIONS AND TECHNIQUES

DEBORAH A. O'KEEFE

Urbana, Illinois

The purpose of this article is threefold: to describe bone marrow biopsy techniques, to briefly describe how a clinical pathologist evaluates a bone marrow sample, and to discuss the indications for bone marrow biopsy. The term *bone marrow biopsy* here includes both needle aspiration and core biopsy. When distinction between the two is necessary, the specific term is used.

BONE MARROW BIOPSY TECHNIQUES

Bone marrow samples can be obtained by needle aspiration or core biopsy. Needle aspirates provide marrow smears for cytologic evaluation, whereas core biopsy samples allow histologic examination. Diseases that affect the marrow architecture or are focal in distribution are more readily evaluated with core biopsies. Diseases in which cell morphology is critical are best examined cytologically. Table 1 outlines which procedures are generally most helpful in specific diseases. Optimal evaluation of the bone marrow, however, is achieved when both a marrow smear and a biopsy sample are obtained at the same time. A complete blood count (CBC), including a peripheral blood smear, should be submitted with the marrow sample so that the marrow results can be correlated with the peripheral blood picture.

BIOPSY NEEDLES

Figure 1 illustrates the more common needles available for aspiration and core biopsy. All of these needles can be used for marrow aspiration, whereas core biopsies are performed with a Jamshidi's biopsy

Table 1. *Most Reliable Biopsy Technique for Specific Diseases*

Aspiration	Core Biopsy
Leukemias	Myelofibrosis
Dysplasias	Metastatic neoplasia
Maturation defects	Lymphoma
	Infectious granuloma
	Megakaryocyte number

needle. Both types of needles are available in stainless steel, which can be autoclaved and reused. The needles with plastic parts (Fig. 1B, C) were designed for single use in human medicine; however, they can be gas sterilized and reused several times before becoming dull.

BIOPSY SITES

The most common sites include the iliac crest and the femoral neck. I prefer the iliac crest for medium to large dogs and the femoral neck for cats and small dogs. Bone marrow can also be easily obtained from the proximal humeral metaphysis. The ribs and sternebrae contain active bone marrow; however, these sites should be avoided because of the risk of slipping off the bone and entering the thoracic cavity.

ANESTHESIA AND PATIENT PREPARATION

Table 2 summarizes the necessary supplies. Because bone marrow samples clot very quickly, it is important to have all supplies readily at hand. Coating the lumen of the biopsy needle and syringe with a small amount of 2% ethylenediaminetetraacetic acid (EDTA) may also help prevent clotted samples. Both aspiration and core biopsies can usually be done in docile animals using only a local anesthetic. Other chemical restraint may be necessary in cats or excitable dogs. The animal is usually placed in lateral recumbency, although iliac crest aspiration can be done in sternal recumbency. The biopsy site is clipped and scrubbed with antiseptic solution. The skin, subcutis, and periosteum are infiltrated with 1 to 2 ml of 2% lidocaine. A small stab incision is then made in the anesthetized skin.

Aspiration Biopsy

ILIAC CREST

The needle is placed into the wing of the ileum at approximately a 45° angle to its long axis and is

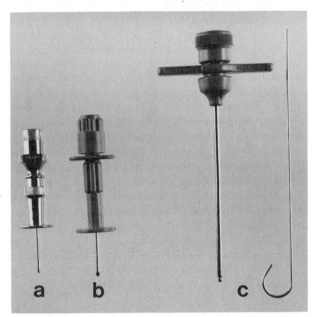

Figure 1. Bone marrow aspiration and core biopsy needles. A, Stainless steel University of Illinois sternal needle (15 and 18 gauge, Baxter V. Mueller, McGaw Park, IL). B, Jamshidi's disposable University of Illinois sternal/iliac aspiration needle (15 and 18 gauge, Baxter Healthcare, Valencia, CA). C, Jamshidi's disposable bone marrow biopsy/aspiration needle (11 and 13 gauge, Baxter Healthcare, Valencia, CA).

rotated in an alternating clockwise-counterclockwise motion under moderate pressure until it is well seated in the marrow cavity. The stylet is then removed, and a 12- to 20-ml syringe is securely attached to the needle. Negative pressure is applied by rapidly pulling back on the syringe plunger. Repeated applications of negative pressure are often necessary to obtain a sample. A reaction to pain usually signifies that the needle is in the marrow cavity. Negative pressure is released as soon as a few drops of marrow are obtained in the syringe. Continued pressure results in dilution of the marrow sample with peripheral blood. Once a sample has been obtained, the needle is removed from the bone, and smears are quickly made as described later. Bone marrow occasionally is not obtained on the first aspiration. If this occurs, the needle should be repositioned in the marrow cavity. First, it

Table 2. *Supplies for Needle and Core Bone Marrow Biopsies*

2% lidocaine
Sterile biopsy needle
Sterile gloves
Scalpel blade
12–20 ml syringe
Clean glass slides
2% ethylenediaminetetraacetic acid (optional)
10% formalin (core biopsy)

should be advanced deeper; if no marrow is obtained, the needle should be slowly withdrawn, keeping gentle suction on the syringe. If marrow still cannot be obtained, a core biopsy sample should be taken.

FEMUR

The aspiration needle is placed into the marrow cavity through the trochanteric fossa in a manner similar to that used when placing an intramedullary pin. A right-handed person uses the left hand to stabilize the animal's left leg. The left thumb is placed on the femur parallel to its long axis, thus aiding in determining the location of the marrow cavity. The needle is then guided along the medial aspect of the greater trochanter until it is in contact with the trochanteric fossa. Seating of the needle and marrow aspiration are done in a similar manner to that described earlier, making sure to keep the needle parallel to the long axis of the femur.

SAMPLE HANDLING

The contents of the syringe and needle are quickly expelled onto glass slides that are held at a 45° angle, allowing blood to run off and leaving the marrow spicules on the slide. Clean slides are placed over the spicules, the marrow is allowed to spread slightly, and the slides are gently pulled apart to make smears. Six to eight smears can usually be made. One smear should be stained with new methylene blue or Diff-Quik to ensure that an adequate sample has been obtained. The remaining slides should be sent unstained to a hematopathologist for evaluation.

Core Biopsy

Core biopsy samples are taken with a Jamshidi's biopsy needle (see Fig. 1). When evaluating hematologic abnormalities, specimens are usually taken from the ileum. The iliac crest can be sampled in the same site as described earlier, or the needle can be seated in the flat portion of the ileum, perpendicular to the wing. The needle is advanced into cortical bone with an alternating clockwise-counterclockwise motion. Once the needle is seated, the stylet is removed and the needle is advanced 1 to 2 cm farther into cancellous bone, thus driving a core of tissue into the needle. To detach the core from surrounding bone, the needle is rocked back and forth and rotated in both directions. The needle is then removed by applying upward pressure while rotating it back and forth.

The core is pushed out of the needle by introducing the probe into the needle's tapered cutting end. Impression smears for cytologic examination can be made by gently rolling the core on a glass slide. The core is then placed in either 10% formalin or Zenker's solution for fixation.

Core biopsy specimens can also be used to evaluate lytic bone lesions. Radiographs and palpation are used to determine the areas to be sampled. Material should be taken from both the center and periphery of the lesion. Radiographs can be made to ensure that appropriate areas were sampled.

BONE MARROW EVALUATION

The interpretation of bone marrow cytologic and histopathologic findings requires a great deal of expertise and should be done by those trained in veterinary hematopathology. Clinicians should provide the pathologist with as much clinical and laboratory information as possible. A CBC and peripheral blood smear taken at the same time as the marrow sample are essential. The bone marrow elements evaluated by the pathologist are briefly described next.

CELLULARITY

Bone marrow spicules must be present for accurate assessment of overall bone marrow cellularity. Hemodilution falsely decreases the perceived cellularity. Cellularity is decreased with hypoproliferative disorders and is increased when peripheral utilization or destruction is occurring. Neoplastic infiltration also can cause hypercellularity.

MYELOID:ERYTHROID RATIO

A comparison is made between the numbers of myeloid and erythroid cells, and the ratio is determined to be normal, high, or low. A high ratio is noted with both myeloid hyperplasia and erythroid hypoplasia. Conversely, a low ratio is reported with myeloid hypoplasia and erythroid hyperplasia. The CBC results help differentiate which cell line is abnormally represented.

MATURATION AND MORPHOLOGY OF ERYTHROID AND MYELOID SERIES

Maturation should progress in an orderly fashion from blast to mature granulocyte or red blood cell. A left shift in the peripheral blood should be reflected by an increased percentage of young cells in the marrow. The term *ineffective myelopoiesis* or *erythropoiesis* is used to describe marrow hyperplasia that is not accompanied by an appropriate response in the peripheral blood. This is often accompanied by what is termed *maturation arrest*; maturation is orderly through a particular stage and then declines, causing a paucity of cell types beyond that stage. Ineffective hematopoiesis can occur with myeloproliferative disease or with immune-mediated disease when the antibodies are directed at the marrow precursor cells. It also occurs when the bone marrow is recovering from a previous hypoproliferative state.

Dysmyelopoiesis and dyserythropoiesis are characterized by asynchronous maturation accompanied by nuclear and cytoplasmic morphologic abnormalities. These changes are due to abnormal RNA and DNA synthesis, which can be caused by vitamin deficiencies (folate and vitamin B$_{12}$), chemotherapeutic drugs, or myeloproliferative disease.

THROMBOPOIESIS

Megakaryocytes are not distributed evenly throughout a marrow smear, making quantitation of their number difficult. Although estimates can be made from a marrow smear, megakaryocyte number is best evaluated by core biopsy.

NEOPLASTIC CELLS

When large numbers of neoplastic cells are present, they can be easily recognized on a marrow smear. However, neoplastic infiltrates are often present in small, focal accumulations that are more readily identified on core biopsy specimens.

IRON STORES

Iron is normally stored in bone marrow macrophages. Adequacy of iron stores can be estimated by a careful examination of these cells.

MISCELLANEOUS ABNORMALITIES

Other abnormalities include increased numbers of plasma cells or mast cells and the presence of infectious agents such as *Histoplasma*, *Ehrlichia*, and *Leishmania*.

INTERPRETATION

The bone marrow sample is interpreted in light of the clinical and hematologic data. When given sufficient information, a pathologist can make an assessment of what disease processes would be consistent with the marrow findings.

INDICATIONS FOR BONE MARROW BIOPSY

Table 3 lists indications for bone marrow biopsy along with commonly associated diseases. These indications are discussed in greater detail in the following paragraphs.

Cytopenias

Cytopenias can be caused by decreased production, increased peripheral destruction or utilization, and increased loss. Bone marrow biopsy can help differentiate problems in production from increased consumption and can often determine the underlying cause. An accurate diagnosis is essential in determining prognosis and therapy.

PANCYTOPENIA

Decreased marrow production is usually present when two or more cell lines are depressed. Mye-

lophthisis, the replacement of normal marrow elements by abnormal cells, and marrow hypoplasia or aplasia are common causes of pancytopenia. Myelophthisis is often caused by lymphoid or myeloid leukemia. It is important to remember that leukemia begins in the bone marrow, and marrow infiltration can be present before atypical cells appear in the peripheral blood. Leukemia can usually be diagnosed by marrow aspirate, although determining the involved cell type may require special cytochemical stains (Facklam and Kociba, 1985).

Myelodysplasia, a form of dysmyelopoiesis that sometimes precedes myeloid leukemia, can also be diagnosed by a marrow aspirate. It is characterized by an increase in myeloblasts with or without dysplastic changes, an increased myeloid:erythroid ratio, and erythroid hypoplasia, usually with megaloblastic changes.

If an aspirate is hypocellular, a core biopsy is indicated to look for marrow aplasia or myelofibrosis. Myelofibrosis is the replacement of bone marrow by fibrous tissue, and it can occur secondary to neoplastic or inflammatory bone marrow disorders. If aplasia is present, the animal should be evaluated for an underlying etiology (e.g., ehrlichiosis, hyperestrogenism, feline leukemia virus).

Table 3. Indications for Bone Marrow Aspiration/Biopsy

Listed under each indication are commonly associated diseases.
Pancytopenia (aplastic anemia)
  Myelophthisis
  Ehrlichiosis
  Hyperestrogenism
  Myelodysplasia
  Marrow necrosis
  Idiopathic
Nonregenerative anemia
  Folate or B_{12} deficiency
  Pure red blood cell aplasia
  Immune-mediated
  Feline leukemia virus (FeLV)
  Myelophthisis
Thrombocytopenia
  Immune-mediated
  Myelophthisis
  Ehrlichiosis
  Hyperestrogenism
Neutropenia
  Myelophthisis
  Viral (FeLV, feline immunodeficiency virus)
  Immune-mediated drug reaction
Atypical cells in peripheral blood
  Lymphoproliferative neoplasia
  Myeloproliferative neoplasia
Monoclonal gammopathies
  Multiple myeloma
  Lymphoma
  Ehrlichiosis
  Systemic mycosis (uncommon)
Neoplasia
  Nonhematologic bony metastases
  Clinical staging of lymphoma and mast cell tumors

ANEMIA

Marrow examination is helpful in evaluating nonregenerative anemia when extramarrow causes (iron deficiency, chronic inflammatory disease, renal disease) have been ruled out. A regenerative anemia usually indicates that red blood cell production is adequate, making examination of the bone marrow unnecessary.

THROMBOCYTOPENIA

There is no method comparable to the reticulocyte count for evaluating platelet production; accordingly a bone marrow biopsy is indicated in all cases of persistent thrombocytopenia when evidence for increased platelet loss (severe hemorrhage, vasculitis, disseminated intravascular coagulation) is not present. Immune-mediated thrombocytopenia is most often associated with megakaryocyte hyperplasia, whereas megakaryocyte hypoplasia is encountered with the other common causes of thrombocytopenia (myelophthisis, ehrlichiosis, hyperestrogenism). Immune-mediated thrombocytopenia is occasionally due to destruction of megakaryocytes, leading to megakaryocyte hypoplasia. This is often accompanied by abnormalities in megakaryocyte morphology.

NEUTROPENIA

Neutrophil production also cannot be satisfactorily evaluated on a peripheral blood smear, so marrow examination is indicated in cases of persistent neutropenia. Myeloid hypoplasia occurs with many conditions that cause neutropenia, including myelophthisis, viral diseases, and drug reactions. Myeloid hyperplasia could be encountered with immune destruction or increased peripheral utilization of neutrophils.

Atypical Cells in Peripheral Blood

Atypical cells are most often associated with some form of leukemia. Circulating malignant lymphocytes can also be found with lymphoma. A bone marrow biopsy specimen confirms the presence of abnormal cells in the marrow cavity and indicates how severely the normal marrow precursors are depleted. It is important to differentiate lymphoid neoplasms from myeloproliferative disorders because the prognosis and therapy of each condition are different. It can be difficult to classify the neoplastic cells based on cellular morphology alone. Special cytochemical stains can be used to help establish the correct diagnosis (Facklam and Kociba, 1985).

Monoclonal Gammopathies

Multiple myeloma is the most common cause of a monoclonal gammopathy, although it can also be encountered with lymphoma, erhlichiosis, and systemic mycoses. A bone marrow aspirate can be helpful in establishing the correct diagnosis. If lytic bone lesions are present, the aspirate should be taken from these areas. Bone marrow normally has approximately 1 to 2% plasma cells. Plasma cells exceeding 20% of the marrow, particularly if present in clusters or sheets, would be consistent with multiple myeloma. In most cases, the morphology of the plasma cells is relatively normal, although large cells with nucleoli or double nuclei may be seen. Marrow plasma cells can also be increased with any disease that causes prolonged antigenic stimulation, so the marrow aspirate must be considered in light of the entire clinical picture. If systemic mycosis is a consideration, careful evaluation of the marrow smear for intracellular fungal organisms is important. *Histoplasma capsulatum* can often be identified in the bone marrow, even in the absence of lytic bone lesions.

Neoplasia

NONHEMATOLOGIC BONY METASTASES

Nonhematologic neoplasms, particularly carcinomas, can metastasize to the bone marrow, producing painful osteolytic lesions or cytopenias. Because of the focal nature of these neoplasms, neoplastic infiltrates are detected more readily by core biopsy. If bone lysis is present, the biopsy sample should be taken from an affected area.

CLINICAL STAGING OF LYMPHOMA AND MAST CELL TUMORS

Bone marrow evaluation is often used in the clinical staging of lymphoma and mast cell tumors. Although needle aspiration is the method most commonly used, core biopsy is more sensitive for detecting lymphomatous infiltrates (Raskin and Krehbiel, 1989). Small numbers of mast cells are normally present in bone marrow samples; however, more than 10 mast cells per 1000 nucleated cells should be considered abnormal (O'Keefe et al., 1987).

References and Suggested Reading

Facklam, N. R., and Kociba, G. J.: Cytochemical characterization of leukemic cells from 20 dogs. Vet. Pathol. 22:363, 1985.
A description of the cytochemical staining characteristics of canine leukemic cells.
Harvey, J. W.: Canine bone marrow: Normal hematopoiesis, biopsy techniques, and cell identification and evaluation. Comp. Cont. Ed. Pract. Vet. 6:909, 1984.
A review of normal hematopoiesis, bone marrow biopsy techniques, and cytologic evaluation, with illustrative photomicrographs.
Jacobs, R. M., and Valli, V. E. O.: Bone marrow biopsies: Principles and perspectives of interpretation. Semin. Vet. Med. Surg. 3:176, 1988.
A review of indications for and interpretation of bone marrow biopsy.
O'Keefe, D. A., Couto, C. G., Burke-Schwartz, C., et al.: Systemic mastocytosis in 16 dogs. J. Vet. Intern. Med. 1:75, 1987.
A retrospective study of the clinicopathologic findings in dogs with systemic mastocytosis.
Raskin, R. E., and Krehbiel, J. D.: Prevalence of leukemic blood and bone marrow in dogs with multicentric lymphoma. J.A.V.M.A. 194:1427, 1989.
A prospective study evaluating the sensitivity of peripheral blood smear, bone marrow aspirate, and core biopsy in the diagnosis of marrow involvement with lymphoma.
Valli, V. E. O.: Techniques in veterinary cytopathology. Semin. Vet. Med. Surg. 3:85, 1988.
A review of various cytopathologic techniques including bone marrow biopsy, fine-needle aspiration, Tru-Cut biopsy, and fluid analysis.

BONE MARROW TRANSPLANTATION: UPDATE AND CURRENT CONSIDERATIONS

PETER W. GASPER,
RONNA FULTON,
and MARY ANNA THRALL
Fort Collins, Colorado

Bone marrow transplantation therapy (BMT) is a powerful therapy that offers a potential cure for many malignant and nonmalignant disorders. BMT differs from solid organ transplantation in two major ways. First, in BMT, one simply infuses cells intravenously and the marrow "organ" assembles itself with pluripotent stem cells, seeding the recipient with a lifelong source of donor origin lymphohematopoietic cells. Second, because marrow transplant recipients acquire a new immune system of donor origin, marrow grafts can mount immune reactions against normal recipient tissues—a condition termed *graft-versus-host disease*. This article addresses the current status of BMT in veterinary medicine. It focuses primarily on the results of the first 90 allogeneic marrow transplants performed on cats at the Colorado State University Marrow Transplant Laboratory, and it presents BMT as possible therapy for feline retrovirus infections to illustrate the potential of BMT for treatment of veterinary patients. A background and description of BMT methodologies can be found elsewhere (Gasper, 1989).

CURRENT STATUS

The application of BMT to treat humans has grown exponentially since its clinical introduction more than two decades ago. In 1990, more than 4000 allogeneic BMTs were estimated to have been completed in humans, in contrast to 169 in 1977. Fifty-seven publications in 1970 described BMT studies. There were 174 such publications in 1980 and at least 1109 in 1990. Although some animals have received BMT to treat their specific diseases, most BMTs in animals continue to be performed to obtain information to treat humans more effectively. As progress continues in our understanding of small animal hematology, oncology, and immunology, we anticipate that more BMTs will be performed for the benefit of veterinary patients.

The use of BMT in veterinary medicine is stimulated by the progress in humans and is impeded by the complexity and related expense of management of patients after BMT. Marrow transplant therapy is currently the preferred treatment for certain leukemias and aplastic anemias in humans, and we anticipate that clients may seek similar treatments for their pets. The actual transplant procedure is simple and relatively inexpensive. However, the management of immune-suppressed BMT recipients after transplantation and before hematologic and immunologic reconstitution or during graft-versus-host disease can be difficult and expensive. The current average cost for performing an allogeneic BMT in humans is $150,000. An analysis of the cost-effectiveness of BMT versus conventional chemotherapy for the treatment of nonlymphocytic leukemias in humans revealed that the costs per year of life saved were less for patients who underwent BMT because of their better rate of disease-free survival (Welch and Larson, 1989). No veterinary practices are currently performing BMTs as a routine service for client-owned animals, so comparable costs for the procedure are not available. A number of practitioners have attempted BMTs, generally as a last resort for severely ill dogs or cats.*

The largest number of BMTs for dogs and cats have been performed in studies designed to develop new techniques and new therapies for certain in-

---

*Dr. Robert C. Rosenthal (Veterinary Specialists of Rochester, 2816 Monroe Ave., Rochester, NY 14618; telephone [716] 271–7700) may accept certain dogs (preferably dogs up to 10 years old, weighing less that 45 kg, and in first complete remission) for autologous BMTs. The Colorado State University Marrow Transplant Laboratory (Department of Pathology, College of Veterinary Medicine and Biomedical Sciences, Fort Collins, CO 80523; telephone [303] 491–7593) may accept certain cats with lymphohematopoietic neoplasias, aplastic anemias, and feline retroviruses (see criteria later) for allogeneic BMTs.

Table 1. *Cats Receiving Allogeneic Marrow Transplants*

No. Cats	Reason for Transplantation
15	Normal controls
	Inherited metabolic diseases therapy
25	Mucopolysaccharidosis VI–affected
7	Chédiak-Higashi syndrome–affected
6	G_{M1} Gangliosidosis–affected
1	Alpha Mannosidosis–affected
1	Mucopolysaccharidosis I–affected
	Feline retrovirus therapy
33	Feline leukemia virus–infected
2	Feline immunodeficiency virus–infected

herited and acquired diseases for which there are human analogues. Examples of past and present studies include BMT therapy for cyclic neutropenia, pyruvate kinase deficiency, mucopolysaccharidosis VII, and mucopolysaccharidosis I in dogs. BMT therapy has been performed for Chédiak-Higashi syndrome, mucopolysaccharidosis VI, mucopolysaccharidosis I, alpha mannosidosis, GM_1 gangliosidosis, and retrovirus infections in cats. In addition to the stated objectives of BMT studies, insight is gained into the basic science of each condition, and techniques that are learned can be applied to performing BMTs for client-owned animals. Marrow transplants in animals will lead the way for some exciting new therapies, such as gene therapy (Lehn, 1990), fetal liver transplantation, use of non–histocompatibility-matched marrow donors (Kaminski, 1989), and intrauterine BMT therapy.

MARROW TRANSPLANTS IN CATS

Cats appear to be uniquely suited for marrow transplantation. They keep themselves clean, thus decreasing the incidence of secondary infections while they are immunosuppressed, and they seem to conserve energy by expending just the amount needed for a particular activity in accordance with their state of health. Less is known about the feline histocompatibility system than about these systems in humans and dogs. Although one can identify the usual components of the histocompatibility complex in cats, results from performing 90 feline allogeneic BMTs suggest that cats have a lower incidence of graft-versus-host disease (19% versus 45% in dogs and people), and they are more likely to accept nonsibling marrow grafts than other outbred mammals (Kaminski, 1989).

The Colorado State University Marrow Transplant Team has performed more than 90 allogeneic bone marrow transplants in cats during the past 7 years, with our two objectives being to develop new therapies for inherited metabolic diseases and to treat retrovirus infections. Table 1 lists the number of cats receiving BMT for each condition treated. The overall rate of successful BMT (stable donor-origin lymphohematopoietic engraftment) is 79%. This figure compares well with the success rate in dogs and humans, which is between 60 and 80% depending on the studies evaluated. The longest-living BMT recipients are 6½ years post-transplantation. Table 2 lists the evolution of protocol used for the 90 transplants. Our present preferred regimen is pretransplant enrofloxacin (Batril, Haver Mobay; 2.5 mg/kg PO once daily) for gastrointestinal decontamination (from day −6 through day +14 or onset of fever), total-body irradiation (TBI) (10.00 Gy divided into six 1.67-Gy fractions delivered twice, 6 hr apart on days −2, −1 and 0 via a 6-meV linear accelerator), and cyclosporin (15 mg/kg a day on days −1, 0 and +1 and then from the day of engraftment until day +100). The marrow is harvested from the donor and administered to the recipient cat on day 0 (following TBI) and again on day +5 (Gasper, 1989). We house the cats conventionally, provide food and water *ad libitum*, evaluate them at least twice a day, and provide nutritional support, fluids, and antibiotics as needed.

Cats have a high incidence of bone marrow disorders (aplastic anemias, immunodeficiencies, and myeloproliferative and lymphoproliferative neoplasms). As promising a therapy as BMT is for these fatal diseases, further investigations are needed to make this therapy available to more practices or regional veterinary hospitals. The linear accelerator at Colorado State University is the only one of its kind at a veterinary hospital. Chemotherapeutic ablation of marrow would eliminate the need for a radiation source to perform pretransplant conditioning. We are currently evaluating a combination of cyclophosphamide (Cytoxan, Mead Johnson) and busulfan (Myleran, Burroughs Wellcome) as a possible alternative to TBI for myeloablation. Ninety-five percent of human BMT recipients develop an infection (usually bacterial), with an overall mortality of 20 to 40%. The advancements in molecular

Table 2. *Evolution of Allogeneic Marrow Transplant Methods*

Method	No. Cats
Pretransplant antibiotics	
Polymixin B and neomycin	42
Enrofloxin	48
Pretransplant conditioning	
7.0 Gy single fraction	1
12.0 Gy (5 × 2.4 Gy)	4
6.5 Gy (3 × 2.2 Gy)	4
10.0 Gy (5 × 2.0 Gy)	46
10.0 Gy (6 × 1.7 Gy)	33
12.0 Gy (6 × 2.0 Gy)	2

Neomycin 40 mg/kg PO once a day; polymixin B 10,000 units/kg PO once a day.

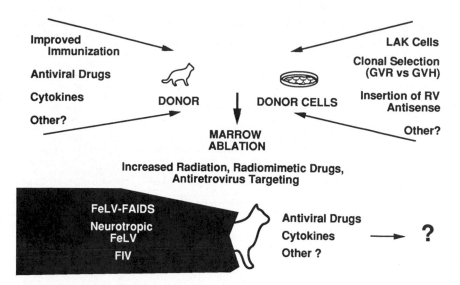

Figure 1. Possible future studies to treat cats infected with retroviruses by BMT. This figure illustrates the three sites where therapy can be implemented: to the donor, to the donor cells, and to the retrovirus-infected recipient cat. FAIDS, feline acquired immune deficiency syndrome; FeLV, feline leukemia virus; FIV, feline immunodeficiency virus; GVH, graft versus host; GVR, graft versus retrovirus; LAK, lymphocyte-activated killer cells; RV, retrovirus.

biology that have made large quantities of hematopoeitic growth factors available may soon provide us with means to accelerate engraftment, thereby preventing life-threatening leukopenias and thrombocytopenias, and to enhance cats' immune responses once they develop a post-transplant infection (see this volume, p. 466).

MARROW TRANSPLANTATION FOR FELINE RETROVIRUS INFECTIONS

Allogeneic BMT offers a fresh approach for treating persistent retrovirus infections. The strategy is to eliminate provirus-bearing lymphohematopoietic cells and to reconstitute with retrovirus-free marrow. The challenge is to protect the newly infused virus-naive progenitor cells from becoming infected during the critical period of hematologic engraftment. We have performed allogeneic BMTs in 33 feline leukemia virus (FeLV)-infected cats and in 2 feline immunodeficiency virus (FIV)-infected cats. In all cats, we have observed a decrease in detectable retrovirus after TBI. In studies using donors immunized with a custom vaccine (formalin-inactivated FeLV of the same strain with which the recipient cats were infected), two of four cats remained FeLV-positive, one became latently infected, and we could not detect FeLV in one cat's tissues when it died of a pulmonary embolus at day +64. In further studies using similarly immunized donors and treating six of nine transplanted cats with 3′-azido-3′deoxythymidine ([AZT] zidovudine) 15 mg/kg PO t.i.d. × 90 days), four of nine cats remained FeLV-positive, four of nine cats became latently infected, and one cat had no detectable FeLV in its marrow and was FeLV-negative by indirect immunofluorescent assay; however, FeLV

provirus could be recovered from some of its tissues by polymerase chain reaction (PCR).

Similar allogeneic BMTs have now been performed on humans infected with HIV. Notably, no HIV could be detected by PCR in one patient who was treated with BMT and AZT and who died at day +47 after a relapse of his lymphoma (Holland et al., 1989). BMT for retrovirus infections is currently in a research and development phase in which there have been a few successes but the patients have not survived long term. Figure 1 illustrates the various possible future studies that could be performed to perfect this aggressive but potentially curative approach to retrovirus therapy.

The criteria we are now using to select ideal feline patients are: age less than 5 years; full sibling available for marrow donation; anemia, leukopenia, or leukemia present; no other apparent organ involvement (such as liver or kidney failure); platelet count not less than 20,000/μl; no previous blood transfusions; patient still ambulatory and eating; FeLV and FIV status determined; and referring veterinarian willing and able to collaborate and provide follow-up data.

SUMMARY

BMT offers a potential cure for many feline and canine conditions that have until now been considered fatal. It is a simple procedure that requires state-of-the-art patient management. BMT is currently not a practical therapy for veterinary patients; however, we may be near the end of considering BMT solely an experimental procedure.

References and Suggested Reading

Barker, J. E.: Marrow transplantation in the treatment of murine hereditary diseases. Bone Marrow Transplant. 3:501, 1988.

A review of BMT in Mus musculus *with hereditary anomalies in order to analyze the curative potential of BMT therapy.*

Ferrara, J. L. M., and Deeg, H. J.: Mechanisms of disease: Graft-versus-host disease. N. Engl. J. Med. 324:667, 1991.

A review of the definition and cause, clinicopathologic spectrum, immunopathophysiology, and prophylactic and therapeutic interventions associated with graft-versus-host disease in humans.

Gasper, P. W.: Bone marrow transplantation. *In* Kirk, R. W. (ed.): *Current Veterinary Therapy* X. Philadelphia: W. B. Saunders, 1989, p. 515.

An overview and description of BMT methodologies.

Holland, K. H., Saral, R., and Rossi, J. J.: Allogeneic bone marrow transplantation, zidovudine and human immunodeficiency virus type I (HIV-I) infection: Studies in a patient with non-Hodgkin lymphoma. Ann. Intern. Med. 111:97, 1989.

Kaminski, E. R.: How important is histocompatibility in bone marrow transplantation? Bone Marrow Transplant. 4:439, 1989.

A retrospective study on the importance of the major histocompatibility complex and of minor histocompatibility systems in allogeneic BMT in humans.

Lehn, P. M.: Gene therapy using bone marrow transplantation: A 1990 update. Bone Marrow Transplant. 5:287, 1990.

A review of the improvements made in retroviral technology for gene transfer using BMT and of the problems still associated with such technology.

Sullivan, K. M.: Current status of bone marrow transplantation. Transplant. Proc. 21 (suppl. 1):41, 1989.

A review of the indications, techniques, and results associated with 3000 allogeneic, autologous, and syngeneic transplants performed for various life-threatening hematologic disorders, discussed in the context of the clinical care of the marrow graft recipient.

Welch, H. G., and Larson, E. B.: Cost effectiveness of bone marrow transplantation in acute nonlymphocytic leukemia. N. Engl. J. Med. 321:807, 1989.

An evaluation of the resources used in the care of adult human patients with acute nonlymphocytic leukemia to compare the cost-effectiveness of BMT and conventional chemotherapy.

Witherspoon, R. P., Fisher, L. D., Schoch, G., et al.: Secondary cancers after bone marrow transplantation for leukemia or aplastic anemia. N. Engl. J. Med. 321:785, 1989.

Results of a study of patients who received allogeneic, syngeneic, or autologous marrow transplants for leukemia (n = 1926) or aplastic anemia (n = 320) to determine the incidence of secondary cancers after transplantation.

Section
7

DERMATOLOGIC DISEASES

WILLIAM H. MILLER, Jr.
Consulting Editor

THE EFFECT OF GLUCOCORTICOID THERAPY ON DIAGNOSTIC PROCEDURES IN DERMATOLOGY

JAMES O. NOXON

Ames, Iowa

Glucocorticoids (GCs) are among the most commonly used medications in canine and feline dermatology. One important ramification of GC therapy is the effect of these drugs on commonly used diagnostic procedures. Many patients have received GCs as empirical or symptomatic therapy before the clinician sees the patient for the first time or before the owner will consent to diagnostic testing. In other cases, the clinician may prescribe GCs for one problem and then desire to perform diagnostic tests for an unrelated problem that develops later. Therefore, it is important to review the current knowledge of the effects of these drugs on the diagnostic procedures commonly used in dermatology cases.

DERMATOLOGIC/PHYSICAL EXAMINATION

Glucocorticoids may reduce the inflammation associated with dermatologic disease, regardless of the underlying etiology. Through their anti-inflammatory properties, glucocorticoids will often reduce pruritus, resulting in clinical improvement of the patient. Patients may then have clinical signs discordant with their clinical history and underlying disease. The decreased severity of inflammation and pruritus may mislead the clinician into believing the disease is truly GC responsive, when the improvement is temporary and incomplete.

Examples of this potential deception include the dog with scabies that shows dramatic clinical improvement when given GCs; and the pruritic dog with staphylococcal infection that becomes less pruritic while receiving GCs but in which the pyoderma persists. The astute clinician should not allow symptomatic and often incomplete improvement of the patient due to GC therapy to influence the natural progression of diagnostic tests.

HEMATOLOGY

The effects of GCs on the hemogram have been well described. Glucocorticoid therapy will result in leukocytosis, lymphopenia, eosinopenia, and monocytosis. Eosinopenia is the most consistently reported abnormality. This "stress leukogram" may follow one dose of a short-acting GC; however, it is more consistently seen in patients receiving inappropriate (daily) short-acting GC therapy and in patients receiving repeated injections of long-acting GCs. Lymphopenia may persist for up to 1 month following oral treatment with prednisone. These findings are, to a degree, dose dependent and vary with the formulation of GC used and the duration of therapy.

BIOCHEMISTRIES

Biochemical tests are used in dermatology as screening tests for internal disease that has dermatologic manifestations. Administration of GCs will affect various biochemical parameters. These effects vary with the dose, formulation, duration, and frequency of GC administration.

The most consistent biochemical alteration following GC therapy is elevation of serum alkaline phosphatase (ALP) enzyme levels. Both endogenous and exogenous GCs are known to induce production of a specific ALP isoenzyme. This may create some diagnostic confusion since elevated serum levels of ALP are often used as an indicator of spontaneous hyperadrenocorticism, a disease in which up to 90% of canine patients present with elevated ALP levels.

Daily or alternate-day administration of prednisone or prednisolone, short-acting GCs, may result in dramatic and prolonged ALP serum levels. One dose of methylprednisolone acetate has been shown to result in elevated serum ALP levels for up to 32 weeks. Also, administration of otic medications containing triamcinolone or dexamethasone to dogs has been shown to result in mild to moderate increases in serum alkaline phosphatase, alanine aminotransferase, and gamma-glutamyltransferase concentrations (Meyer et al., 1990) The solution containing dexamethasone caused greater increase than the

498

solution containing triamcinolone. Serum bile acid and lipoprotein-X concentrations were not affected by these otic preparations. This effect of GC therapy on serum concentrations of ALP complicates the clinical case in which spontaneous hyperadrenocorticism is suspected and the patient has been receiving GCs for pruritus or other dermatologic signs.

Glucocorticoids can result in elevated serum levels of glucose in dogs and cats, although this elevation occurs inconsistently. Glucocorticoid therapy may also lead to elevated concentrations of alanine aminotransferase, cholesterol, and triglycerides. However, these biochemical parameters were shown to be inconsistently affected in several clinical studies, and in some studies, no alterations in serum concentrations were seen. Clinicians should be aware that GC therapy *may* result in elevations of these parameters. Elevated serum levels of these substances should be interpreted with caution in dogs with a history or prior GC administration. Whenever possible, GCs should be withheld prior to biochemical testing.

URINALYSIS

Urinalysis is not a diagnostic test often indicated in the evaluation of a patient with dermatologic disease. However, a urinalysis may be part of a complete workup on a patient with suspected autoimmune disease, endocrine imbalance, or internal disease with cutaneous manifestations.

Glucocorticoids may interfere with urinary concentrating mechanisms, resulting in lowered urinary specific gravity. A complete history should alert the clinician to this possible cause of hyposthenuria. Long-term GC therapy has also been reported to be associated with urinary tract infections. One study (Ihrke et al., 1985) revealed urinary tract infections in 39% of dogs receiving alternate-day GC therapy for 6 to 60 months. The majority of these patients had little evidence of urinary tract infection on the routine urine sediment analysis. These findings suggest that GC therapy may mask urinary tract infection by reducing the inflammatory reaction in the urine.

THYROID FUNCTION TESTS

The effects of parenteral administration of GCs on thyroid function in the dog have been well documented. Glucocorticoids may suppress thyroid hormone concentrations by several mechanisms, including altered thyroid hormone secretion and protein binding, decreased thyrotropin secretion, and altered peripheral metabolism of thyroid hormones. A single dose of prednisolone may result in decreased T_4 concentrations for 24 to 48 hours after

administration. A single dose of dexamethasone or prednisolone will also decrease resting T_3 concentrations and increase reverse T_3 concentrations in dogs.

Glucocorticoids suppress basal concentrations of T_4 and T_3 and will blunt the release of T_4 and T_3 following TSH stimulation. Resting T_4 and T_3 concentrations were shown to be decreased during prednisone treatment (2.2 mg/kg, IM, every other day; Kemppainen et al., 1983) or prednisolone therapy (1.0 mg/kg, PO, b.i.d.; Torres, 1989). Thyroxine and T_3 responses to thyrotropin (TSH) administration are also suppressed; however, T_4 and T_3 concentrations still increase significantly above baseline levels following either TSH or thyrotropin-releasing hormone administration. These effects of glucocorticoids are similar to findings in dogs with spontaneous hyperadrenocorticism.

A single dose (10 mg) of prednisone will decrease circulating total T_4 concentrations for 24 hours in euthyroid cats, but significant abnormalities are not detected 1 or 2 weeks following a single injection of methylprednisolone acetate.

Thyroid evaluation using measurements of total T_4 levels should be delayed for 2 weeks, and preferably 4 weeks, following short-term daily or alternate-day therapy with short-acting glucocorticoids. However, thyroid function may be accurately evaluated in those patients by measuring total T_4 concentrations before and after TSH administration.

ADRENAL FUNCTION TESTS

Adrenal function tests are performed in dermatology cases to identify animals with spontaneous or iatrogenic hyperadrenocorticism. The most frequently used adrenal function tests include the adrenocorticotropin (ACTH) stimulation test, the low-dose dexamethasone suppression test, the high-dose dexamethasone suppression test, and the measurement of plasma ACTH concentrations.

Adrenal suppression has been shown to occur in normal dogs following oral, parenteral, otic, ophthalmic, or topical administration of GCs. The duration and severity of the suppression varies with the formulation, the duration of administration, and the route of administration. Short-acting GCs, given orally or intramuscularly at doses typical of those used in dermatologic cases, will result in adrenocortical suppression, lasting for up to 2 weeks after therapy is discontinued (Chastain and Graham, 1979). Table 1 illustrates the adrenal suppressive effects of a single injection of various GC preparations in the dog.

Repeated injections of GCs, especially long-acting formulations, will cause prolonged suppression of basal cortisol concentrations and adrenal response to ACTH stimulation. These effects may persist for

Table 1. *Effects of a Single Injection of Glucocorticoids on Adrenal Gland Function in Dogs*

Drug	Dose	Route	Duration of Suppression
Triamcinolone acetonide	0.22 mg/kg	IM	≤ 4 wk
Prednisone	2.2 mg/kg	IM	< 24 h
Prednisolone	2.2 mg/kg	IM	1 wk
Dexamethasone 21-isonicotinate suspension	0.1 mg/kg	IM	10 d
Dexamethasone 21-isonicotinate suspension	1.0 mg/kg	IM	4 wk
Dexamethasone or dexamethasone sodium phosphate	0.01 mg/kg	IV	< 24 h
Dexamethasone	0.1 mg/kg	IV	32 h
Dexamethasone sodium phosphate	0.1 mg/kg	IV	< 24 h
Methylprednisolone acetate	2.5 mg/kg	IM	≤ 5 wks
Dexamethasone alcohol	1 mg/kg	IM	24–48 h

Modified with permission from: Romatowski, J.: Iatrogenic adrenocortical insufficiency in dogs. J.A.V.M.A. 196:1144–1146, 1990.

several months following administration of long-acting GCs, such as methylprednisolone acetate and betamethasone.

The precise effects of GC therapy on the adrenal function tests in dogs with spontaneous hyperadrenocorticism are unclear. Theoretically, high-dose GC therapy in a patient with pituitary-dependent hyperadrenocorticism could override pituitary resistance to negative feedback mechanisms and result in artificially lowered plasma cortisol and ACTH concentrations. In those cases, both the ACTH stimulation test and dexamethasone suppression tests could be affected. However, this does not seem to be a major source of error or confusion in clinical cases. Short-term therapy or long-term alternate-day glucocorticoid therapy with short-acting GCs should not affect the interpretation of test results in patients with hyperadrenocorticism. Whenever possible, GCs should be withheld for 2 to 4 weeks prior to testing.

Differentiation of iatrogenic from spontaneous hyperadrenocorticism in the patient that is receiving GCs may be a diagnostic dilemma. The ACTH stimulation test is recommended for screening in these patients, since animals receiving GCs in doses high enough to create clinical changes generally will have suppressed serum basal and post-ACTH cortisol concentrations.

Synthetic GCs may interfere with cortisol measurement by cross-reacting with cortisol in some assays, resulting in artificially high cortisol levels. The degree of cross reactivity varies with the diagnostic kit and procedure. Serum or plasma levels of orally administered prednisone should be sufficiently cleared by the body within 48 hours to allow for accurate testing in most cases.

SEX HORMONE DETERMINATIONS

Determinations of plasma levels of testosterone, progesterone, and estrogen are occasionally indicated in suspected cases of hormonal imbalance. Glucocorticoids may affect plasma levels of these hormones as a result of a negative feedback on the pituitary, resulting in decreased release of gonadotropic hormones. They may also directly inhibit testicular and ovarian function. Male dogs with spontaneous hyperadrenocorticism have depressed plasma testosterone concentrations that significantly increase following successful treatment of the Cushing's disease. Administration of GCs may result in decreased circulating levels of testosterone in male dogs and suppression of estrus in the bitch. The degree and duration of specific sex hormone interference following GC therapy are unclear and probably vary with the dose, formulation, and duration of GC therapy.

INTRADERMAL SKIN TESTING

Intradermal skin testing is indicated to confirm a diagnosis and identify causative allergens in patients with inhalant allergies (atopy) and flea allergy dermatitis. There is general agreement among veterinarians who perform these tests on a regular basis that GCs reduce the reactivity of the skin to intradermal challenge with allergens. These impressions were reflected in a recent survey of veterinarians, who recommended different periods of GC withdrawal, depending on the formulations used, prior to skin testing (Table 2). These opinions are based on clinical observations and experiences associated with skin testing.

Actual clinical data resulting from controlled studies in this area are sparse in the veterinary litera-

Table 2. *Opinions Regarding Adequate Withdrawal Times for Various Glucocorticoid Treatment Regimens Prior to Intradermal Skin Testing*

Drug	Regimen	Adequate Withdrawal Time (wk*)
Prednisolone	2 wk, PO	2.6 ± 1.6
Prednisolone	2 mo, PO	4.1 ± 5.6
Prednisolone	≥ 6 mo, PO	5.5 ± 4.8
Triamcinolone acetonide	1–2 injections	5.3 ± 4.3
Methylprednisolone acetate	1 injection	6.5 ± 4.2
Methylprednisolone acetate	≥ 3 injections	9.0 ± 6.2

Reprinted with permission from: DeBoer, D. J.: Survey of intradermal skin testing practices in North America. J.A.V.M.A. 195:1357–1363, 1989.
*Expressed as mean ± SD

ture. One injection of betamethasone or methyl-prednisolone acetate was shown to interfere with wheal diameter posthistamine injection in two dogs, each for at least 30 days (Baker, 1971). One injection of prednisone (2.2 mg/kg, IM) or one injection of triamcinolone (0.22 mg/kg, IM) caused wheals, following intradermal injection of histamine phosphate, to be significantly smaller on post-treatment day 6, but not on day 13 or 30 (Kemppainen et al., 1982). Therefore, one injection of a short-acting GC may suppress skin reactivity to intradermal histamine for up to 2 weeks, and one injection of a long-acting glucocorticoid may suppress skin reactivity for 30 days. These findings are consistent with the opinions expressed in Table 2 regarding GC withdrawal prior to skin testing in dogs.

Application of glucocorticoids in topical, ophthalmic, and otic formulations clearly results in adrenal suppression for periods up to 2 to 8 weeks, depending on the formulation. If the preparation is sufficiently potent to cause adrenal suppression for these time periods, it would seem likely that it could also be capable of suppressing skin reactions in patients undergoing intradermal testing for atopy. Topical application of GCs at the site of intradermal testing will suppress wheal size following antigen challenge in atopic human patients. Controlled studies have not been reported in this area in veterinary medicine.

In conclusion, intradermal skin tests are considered to be suppressed by glucocorticoid therapy. Recommendations for steroid withdrawal vary with the formulation, route of administration, and duration of GC therapy. I am in agreement with the average withdrawal times listed in Table 2. Otic, ophthalmic, and topical GCs should be discontinued for 2 to 8 weeks before intradermal testing. Negative responses to skin testing in patients with clinical features strongly suggestive of atopy may require longer withdrawal in those cases.

IN VITRO ALLERGY TESTING

Both enzyme-linked immunosorbent assay (ELISA) and radioallergosorbent assay (RAST) tests are commercially available for the diagnosis of allergic disease of the dog. In addition, an ELISA test is available for cats. Recommendations regarding withdrawal of GCs prior to testing vary with the laboratory performing the test. One laboratory (ELISA test) recommends cessation of GC therapy in a similar manner as in preparation for intradermal skin testing: 2 weeks if alternate-day short-acting GCs are involved, up to several months if repeated injections of long-acting GCs have been administered, and at least 2 weeks for otic, ophthalmic, and topically applied GCs.

Other laboratories claim no GC interference with their testing methods and results. Data from studies performed on canine allergy patients are not readily available to support these claims. Nonpublished data from clinical trials suggest that GCs do have suppressive effects on the findings of in vitro tests (Griffin, personal communication, 1990). Until controlled studies in dogs and cats are available, I recommend withdrawal of GCs prior to in vitro allergy testing in the same manner as for intradermal skin testing.

SKIN BIOPSY

Skin biopsy is useful in dermatologic disease to rule out specific etiologies of skin disease, to clarify the pathologic process involved in the dermatosis, and to identify specific causes of pathologic changes. The effects of endogenous GCs on the skin are well described, and examination of the skin in hyperadrenocortical patients may show the following histologic changes: hyperkeratosis; hair follicles predominantly in telogen, epidermal, and follicular atrophy; thin dermis; thickened dermis; sebaceous atrophy; dystrophic mineralization; and other histologic changes (Scott, 1982). The excessive use of GCs in dogs will result in similar histologic alterations. In one study, prednisone (0.55 mg/kg PO every 24 hours) for 4 weeks resulted in no gross changes in the skin of dogs, but epidermal atrophy, hyperkeratosis, follicular hyperkeratosis, and atrophy of the adnexal glands was observed histologically (Chastain and Graham, 1979). Subcutaneously administered GCs may induce cutaneous atrophy, alopecia, or calcinosis cutis at the site of injection. Topical glucocorticoids may also result in epidermal and dermal atrophy, alopecia, and pigmentary changes. In addition, the anti-inflammatory properties of GCs may decrease the inflammation associated with some pathologic processes, masking the primary disease process and making accurate diagnosis difficult.

Previous administration of topical, parenteral, or oral GCs will not likely deter skin biopsy in those cases where this procedure is indicated. However, clinicians should alert the pathologist of previous GC therapy so that accurate interpretation of the histologic changes can be made.

DIRECT IMMUNOFLUORESCENCE TESTING

Direct immunofluorescence tests (DIT) are used to detect the presence of immunoglobulin or complement in the skin of patients suspected of having autoimmune or immune-mediated dermatoses. One study of 20 canine patients with clinical and histologic evidence of autoimmune skin disease demonstrated fewer positive DIT tests in skin from patients previously receiving GCs (Griffin and Rosenkrantz, 1987). No conclusions could be drawn regarding the time required for return to positive reactivity. Until conclusive evidence about the effects and duration of DIT interference by exogenous GCs is available, it seems prudent to recommend GC withdrawal in a similar manner to skin testing.

I am not aware of any data regarding the effects of GC therapy on immunoperoxidase staining of skin for immunoglobulin.

SEROLOGY

Various serologic procedures are indicated in selected dermatologic conditions. Serologic tests that detect serum antibody levels should not be influenced to a major extent by GC therapy, since GCs exert their immunomodulating effects primarily by interfering with cellular reactions (inhibiting chemotaxis, paralyzing receptors, etc.). The degree to which there is decreased antibody production as a result of GC therapy is not clear, but it appears to be small.

Antinuclear antibody titers used to support the diagnosis of selected immune-mediated diseases are reported to be relatively resistant to interference from previous GC administration. The exact amount and duration of GC therapy that is tolerated before the test is influenced is unknown.

SUMMARY

Glucocorticoid therapy can significantly affect the diagnostic tests and procedures commonly used in dermatology cases. Specific recommendations regarding withdrawal of GCs are often unclear, since the degree and duration of test interference are affected by many factors. General recommendations are to postpone diagnostic tests for 2 to 4 weeks following short-term (2 weeks or less) administration of short-acting GCs. Whenever possible, diagnostic testing should be delayed for 1 to 2 months after a single injection of a long-acting GC. Repeated injections of long-acting glucocorticoids may preclude accurate testing for longer periods of time.

References and Suggested Reading

Baker, K. P.: Intradermal tests as an aid to the diagnosis of skin disease in dogs. J. Sm. Anim. Pract. 12:445, 1971.
This paper describes intradermal skin testing in normal and allergic dogs.

Chastain, C. B., and Graham, C. L.: Adrenocortical suppression in dogs on daily and alternate-day prednisone administration. Am. J. Vet. Res. 40:936, 1979.
This study evaluated adrenal function, hepatic, and extrahepatic effects of three regimens of prednisone therapy in dogs.

DeBoer, D. J.: Survey of intradermal skin testing practices in North America. J.A.V.M.A. 195:1357, 1989.
Results of a survey of opinions concerning various aspects of intradermal skin testing in dogs and cats.

Griffin, C. E., and Rosenkrantz, W. S.: Direct immunofluorescent testing: A comparison of two laboratories in the diagnosis of canine immune-mediated skin disease. Semin. Vet. Med. Surg. 2:202, 1987.
A prospective comparison of immunofluorescent testing results on paired samples sent to two different laboratories and the effects of prior glucocorticoid therapy on the results.

Griffin, C. E.: Personal communication, 1990.

Ihrke, P. J., Norton, A. L., Ling, G. V., et al.: Urinary tract infection with long-term corticosteroid administration in dogs with chronic skin diseases. J.A.V.M.A. 186:43, 1985.
A study demonstrating increased urinary tract infections in dogs receiving glucocorticoid therapy.

Kemppainen, R. J., Lorenz, M. D., and Thompson, F. N.: Adrenocortical suppression in the dog given a single intramuscular dose of prednisone or triamcinolone acetonide. Am. J. Vet. Res. 42:204, 1982.
Evaluation of several parameters, including skin response to intradermal histamine injection, following injection of glucocorticoids.

Kemppainen, R. J., Thompson, F. N., Lorenz, M. D., et al.: Effects of prednisone on thyroid and gonadal endocrine function in dogs. J. Endocrinol. 96:293, 1983.
A study evaluating the effects of intramuscular administration of prednisone on thyroid function tests and gonadal function tests in dogs.

Meyer, D. J., Moriello, K. A., Feder, B. M., et al.: Effect of otic medications containing glucocorticoids on liver function test results in healthy dogs. J.A.V.M.A. 196:743, 1990.
A study demonstrating the effects of otically administered dexamethasone and triamcinolone on various liver function tests.

Romatowski, J.: Iatrogenic adrenocortical insufficiency in dogs. J.A.V.M.A. 196:1144, 1990.
A review of the effects of various glucocorticoid preparations and formulations on adrenal function in dogs.

Scott, D. W.: Histopathologic findings in endocrine skin disorders of the dog. J. Am. Anim. Hosp. Assoc. 18:173, 1982.
A review of histopathologic features of skin changes associated with various endocrine disorders.

Torres, S.: Effect of prednisolone on thyroid function in dogs. Proc. Ann. Members' Meetings AAVD & ACVD 5:11, 1989.
A study evaluating thyroid function tests on dogs following prednisolone administration.

THE VALUE OF IMMUNOFLUORESCENCE TESTING

KATHLEEN M. KALAHER

Baltimore, Maryland

Immunofluorescence testing is a valuable adjunct to the clinical and histopathologic evaluation of patients with suspected immune-mediated or autoimmune dermatoses. In order to maximize the value of immunodiagnostics, the practitioner must be familiar with both the technical aspects of these studies and the limitations of these tests.

DIRECT IMMUNOFLUORESCENCE TESTING

Direct immunofluorescence testing (DIT) refers to the examination of tissues for various immunoreactants (immunoglobulin, complement). Tissue for DIT is submitted in the form of punch or excisional biopsies. Formalin-fixed specimens cannot be used for DIT. Tissue may be sent immediately (within several hours of biopsy) to the laboratory in saline-soaked gauze, quick frozen (using isopentane or liquid nitrogen), or placed in a special transport medium (Michel's fixative). The use of Michel's fixative is ideal for the general practitioner since it allows for postal shipment at ambient temperatures. Specimens can be reliably preserved for 7 to 14 days. To ensure adequate tissue preservation, it is generally recommended that specimens be no larger than 3 mm. If 6-mm punch biopsies are taken, they may be split with a blade prior to submission. The laboratory should be consulted if appropriate sample size is not specified. Vials containing Michel's fixative are usually available from the laboratory performing the testing. Specimens for histopathology must be submitted separately in formalin.

The laboratory procedure itself involves the preparation of frozen sections of tissue which are then incubated with fluorescein-labeled species-specific antisera. If immunoreactants are present in the tissue, the fluorescein-conjugated antiglobulin will bind to them and fluorescence will be observed when the sections are examined under a fluorescent microscope. Positive DIT may be seen as fluorescence in the intercellular spaces of the epidermis, at the basement membrane zone (BMZ), or within blood vessel walls.

The immune-mediated and autoimmune dermatoses are characterized by specific patterns of fluorescence. In the pemphigus complex, immunoreactant deposition occurs within the intercellular spaces of the epidermis. Positive BMZ fluorescence is seen in cases of discoid and systemic lupus erythematosus, bullous pemphigoid, and linear IgA dermatosis. Pemphigus erythematosus is characterized by both intercellular and BMZ immunofluorescence. Immunoreactant deposition occurs in blood vessel walls in cases of vasculitis. The correct interpretation of DIT findings, however, requires an awareness of existent pitfalls which may result in false-positive and false-negative results.

Immunoreactant deposition can occur in diseases other than those mentioned above. Intercellular immunofluorescence has been reported in dogs with staphylococcal folliculitis and mycosis fungoides (Scott et al., 1987a). Patchy, focal deposition of immunoreactants in the intercellular spaces may be seen in any condition in which the epidermis is edematous (Muller et al., 1989). BMZ immunofluorescence has been described in cases of staphylococcal folliculitis, dermatophytosis, drug eruption, and the Vogt-Koyanagi-Harada-like syndrome (Scott et al., 1987a).

Positive DIT has also been seen in clinically normal dogs and cats. IgM deposition has been demonstrated at the BMZ of tissue from the normal canine and feline nasal planum and the normal canine footpad. Granular deposition of IgM at the dermoepidermal junction was documented in 11 of 15 (73%) dogs with normal noses (Scott et al., 1983a), in five of 11 (45%) dogs with normal footpads (Scott et al., 1983b), and in three of 28 (11%) cats with normal noses (Kalaher et al., 1990). DIT of normal feline footpad epithelium was consistently negative in one study (Kalaher et al., 1990) as was DIT of the normal canine lip (Scott et al., 1983a). Since immune-mediated and autoimmune dermatoses often affect the nasal planum and footpads and biopsies from these sites are often submitted for DIT, the demonstration of immunoglobulin at the BMZ, notably IgM, must be interpreted with caution.

Conversely, negative DIT does not rule out the presence of immune-mediated or autoimmune disease. The use of glucocorticoids or other immunosuppressive drugs can lead to false-negative results. It is recommended that these drugs (both systemic and topical) be discontinued for at least several weeks prior to biopsy if possible. Improper lesion selection and handling is another major cause of false-negative results. In pemphigus erythematosus, pemphigus foliaceous, and bullous pemphigoid early intact vesicles/pustules, and perilesional skin should be biopsied. Old lesions, excoriated lesions, erosions, and ulcers should be avoided. In cases of pemphigus vulgaris and bullous pemphigoid, which often present as ulcerative dermatoses, tissue should be submitted from the edge of fresh lesions. If discoid or systemic lupus erythematosus is suspected, older nonulcerated lesions are preferred. If DIT is performed in cases of vasculitis, tissues must be biopsied within 4 hours of lesion formation (Muller et al., 1989). The submission of multiple specimens will decrease the incidence of false-negative results.

Since there are numerous procedural pitfalls inherent in the performance of DIT, specimens should be sent to a reliable laboratory with a proven record in veterinary immunopathology. It is imperative that species-specific antiglobulin be used. It is also important to test for various immunoreactants as only a single immunoglobulin class or only complement may be deposited in tissues. Griffin and Rosenkrantz (1987) compared the results of DIT from two different laboratories to determine the frequency and accuracy of positive DIT in canine patients with immune-mediated skin disease. Of 23 cases diagnosed on the basis of history, clinical findings, histopathology, and response to therapy, 13 (57%) were positive on DIT. Of these 13 cases, six were positive from one laboratory only. In six cases both laboratories reported positive DIT, although the immunoreactants (five cases) or pattern (two cases) varied. Identical results were reported in only one case.

The use of DIT as a routine diagnostic test in all cases of suspected autoimmune or immune-mediated disease is controversial. Werner et al. (1983/1984) conducted a retrospective survey of 230 canine cases in which DIT was requested. Based on clinical findings and either supportive immunohistologic criteria or therapeutic response, only 84 of these dogs were ultimately diagnosed with autoimmune skin disease. The value of DIT versus histopathology in establishing the diagnosis was also assessed. Histopathology was diagnostic in 69% of the cases. DIT was positive in 52% of the dogs.

Only 33% of the cases had both histologic and immunopathologic evidence of autoimmune disease. Given these findings, it may be prudent to use DIT as a confirmatory rather than a screening procedure, especially in those cases where the index of suspicion is not high. Tissue may be held in Michel's fixative pending histopathology results, or (if the same institution is used for both studies) both specimens may be submitted with a request that DIT be performed only if a morphologic diagnosis of autoimmune disease is established. If the workup is limited by financial constraints, histopathology should take precedence over DIT.

Recently, immunoperoxidase methods for the detection of tissue immunoreactants have been described. Although these procedures can be performed on formalin-fixed specimens and use light rather than fluorescent microscopy, the advantages are outweighed by the fact that false-positive results are frequently encountered. At present, DIT remains the test of choice.

INDIRECT IMMUNOFLUORESCENCE TESTING

Indirect immunofluorescence testing (IIT) refers to the examination of serum for the presence of circulating autoantibodies. Although IIT is used in the evaluation of human patients with vesicobullous disorders, it is usually negative in cases of canine and feline pemphigus and canine pemphigoid. For this reason, IIT is not currently recommended for the diagnosis of autoimmune dermatoses.

References and Suggested Reading

Griffin, C. E., and Rosenkrantz, W. S.: Direct immunofluorescent testing: A comparison of two laboratories in the diagnosis of canine immune-mediated skin disease. Semin. Vet. Med. Surg. (Sm. Anim.) 2:202, 1987.
  A comparison of the frequency and accuracy of DIT from two different laboratories.
Kalaher, K. M., Scott, D. W., and Smith, C. A.: Direct immunofluorescence testing of normal feline nasal planum and footpad. Cornell Vet. 80:105, 1990.
  The results of DIT of nasal and footpad epithelium in 28 normal cats.
Muller, G. H., Kirk, R. W., and Scott, D. W.: *Small Animal Dermatology*, 4th ed. Philadelphia: W. B. Saunders, 1989, p. 441.
  A discussion of direct and indirect immunofluorescence testing.
Scott, D. W., Walton, D. K., Lewis, R. M., et al.: Pitfalls in immunofluorescence testing in dermatology. II. Pemphigus-like antibodies in the cat, and direct immunofluorescence testing of normal dog nose and lip. Cornell Vet. 73:275, 1983a.
  The results of IIT in 75 cats and DIT of nasal and lip epithelium from 15 normal dogs.
Scott, D. W., Walton, D. K., Manning, T. O., et al.: Pitfalls in immunofluorescence testing in canine dermatology. Cornell Vet. 73:131, 1983b.
  The results of IIT in 100 dogs and DIT of footpad epithelium from 11 normal dogs.
Scott, D. W., Walton, D. K., Slater, M. R., et al.: Immune-mediated dermatoses in domestic animals: Ten years after—Part I. Compend. Cont. Ed. Pract. Vet. 9:423, 1987a.

A detailed study of cases of pemphigus and pemphigoid, including results of DIT.

Scott, D. W., Walton, D. K., Slater, M. R., et al.: Immune-mediated dermatoses in domestic animals: Ten years after—Part II. Compend. Cont. Ed. Pract. Vet. 9:539, 1987b.
A detailed study of cases of lupus erythematosus, vasculitis, and linear IgA dermatosis, including DIT findings.

Werner, L. L., Brown, K. A., and Halliwell, R. E. W.: Diagnosis of autoimmune skin disease in the dog: Correlation between histopathologic, direct immunofluorescent and clinical findings. Vet. Immunol. Immunopathol. 5:47, 1983/1984.
A study of the reliability of histopathology and DIT as diagnostic aids in canine autoimmune dermatoses.

IMMUNOTHERAPY IN CANINE ATOPY

DONNA WALTON ANGARANO
and JOHN M. MacDONALD
Auburn, Alabama

THEORY AND INDICATIONS

Hyposensitization (immunotherapy) is the art of administering allergen extract to allergic patients in an attempt to decrease their clinical response to exposure of natural allergens. The concept of immunotherapy was initiated by Pasteur, Jenner, and others in their early work with vaccinations. The application to allergy was first used in 1911 by two English physicians, Noon and Freeman, who attempted to immunize hay-fever sufferers with injections of grass-pollen extract.

Our understanding of immunology and allergic diseases has led to progress in immunotherapy, although the exact method by which hyposensitization works remains controversial. A variety of immunologic changes have been demonstrated during hyposensitization.

The most consistent immunologic change reported in patients undergoing immunotherapy is an initial increase in serum IgE followed by a subsequent decrease. This observation has been used to support several theories for the possible mechanism of hyposensitization, which include the following: (1) development of blocking antibodies, (2) the induction of suppressor T cells, (3) the formation of anti-idiotype antibodies, and (4) altered susceptibility of mediator-secreting cells.

Additional immunologic changes observed during hyposensitization include:

1. An increase in the level of allergen-specific IgG, in particular IgG_4, which is implicated as a short-term sensitizing antibody;
2. A decrease in the amount of histamine that is released upon addition of allergen to basophils in a leukocyte suspension;
3. A reduction in the ability of peripheral blood lymphocytes to transform *in vitro* in response to allergen (Halliwell and Gorman, 1989).

In general, there has been a poor correlation of these immunologic observations with clinical response to hyposensitization.

While the role of IgE and immediate reactions in allergic inhalant dermatitis (atopy) has been clearly demonstrated, evidence suggests that late-phase allergic reactions may also be involved (Kaliner, 1984). These late-phase inflammatory responses occur 4 to 8 hours after the initial mast cell–dependent allergic reaction. Additional studies are needed to assess both the mechanism by which atopy occurs, as well as the mode of action for its treatment.

Hyposensitization has been used in the treatment of canine atopy since the late 1960's with numerous reports of success. Most accepted therapeutic regimens have an empirical origin with minimal scientific basis. A common practice is the limitation of antigens for hyposensitization to ten or less. The rationale for this suggestion is that additional antigens either increase the likelihood of severe side effects or that dilution of specific antigen may result in a decreased rate of success. Thus, in patients that show allergic reactions to large numbers of antigens, the veterinarian and owner must select a limited number of antigens based on importance. Response to this approach may have limited benefit. As a result, the owner and veterinarian are frequently frustrated and continue to rely heavily on chemical suppression as a means of maintaining the animal's comfort.

HYPOSENSITIZATION PROCEDURES

At the Auburn University College of Veterinary Medicine, intradermal allergy testing and hyposensitization are accomplished using aqueous antigens (Greer Laboratories, Inc., Lenoir, NC). Therapeutic antigens are diluted for allergy testing every 4 weeks. Intradermal allergy testing is performed with 61 antigens (Table 1) according to standard allergy testing procedures. (The reader is referred to other articles for information regarding intradermal allergy testing.) The recommendation of hyposensitization is based on test credibility and historical correlation. Antigens showing reactions of 2, 3, or 4 + (range = 0 − 4) are included in the mixture. The hyposensitization formula varies depending on (1) exposure to the antigen, (2) seasonality of the antigen, (3) the number of total antigens in the solution, and (4) the intradermal reaction score. The amount of each antigen added to a 10-ml vial is variable, but usually not less than 0.25 ml. The majority of antigens used are 20,000 PNU (protein nitrogen units) per ml concentration or the maximum if less than that.

The maintenance solution is used to produce two other solutions representing 1:10 and 1:100 dilution, respectively. A standard 5-ml vial containing 4.5 ml of phenolized saline is purchased for this procedure. Color-coded caps are recommended to avoid wrong selection during dilution and therapy.

Table 1. *Antigens Used by the Authors for Intradermal Allergy Testing*

Grasses	Trees/Shrubs	Trees/Shrubs
Bahia	Ash	Maple
Bermuda	Beech, American	Eastern oak mix
Meadow fescue	Birch	Virginia live oak
Johnson	Box elder	Pecan
Kentucky blue	Red cedar	Pine mix
Orchard	Eastern cottonwood	Sweet gum
Perennial rye	Elm	Sycamore, Eastern
Red top	Hackberry	Black walnut
Sweet vernal	Hickory	Black willow
Timothy		

Weeds	Molds	Miscellaneous
Baccharis	*Alternaria*	Flea
Cocklebur	*Aspergillus*	House dust
Dock-Sorrel mix	*Curvularia specifera*	Cockroach,
Dog fennel	*Fusarium*	American
English plantain	*Helminthosporium*	Cotton linters
Golden rod	*sativum*	Epidermal mix
Lamb's-quarter	*Hormodendrum*	(horse, cat, dog,
Marsh elder	*hordei*	goat, cow)
Pigweed, rough	*Mucor plumbeus*	Feather mix
Ragweed	*Penicillium mix*	Kapok
Sagebrush	*Pullaria pullalans*	Nylon
	Rhizopus arrhizus	Pyrethrum
		Sheep's wool
		Silk
		Tobacco

Table 2. *Hyposensitization Schedule for Aqueous Allergenic Extracts*

Day	1:100 Dilution Vial 1 (Blue)	1:10 Dilution Vial 2 (Yellow)	Maintenance Solution Vial 3 (Red)
0	0.2 ml		
2	0.4		
4	0.6		
6	0.8		
8	1.0		
10		0.2 ml	
12		0.4	
14		0.6	
16		0.8	
18		1.0	
20			0.2 ml
22			0.4
24			0 6
26			0.8
28			1.0
38			1.0
48			1.0
68			1.0
88			1.0
108			1.0

The owner is instructed in proper administration of subcutaneous injections. Either 1.0- or 1.25-ml syringes are dispensed with instructions to discard after each injection. The hyposensitization solution should be refrigerated. Animals should be observed for 30 to 60 minutes after each injection for any sign of reaction. A recent report suggests that feeding at or near the time of administration may increase the likelihood of anaphylactic reactions (Reedy and Miller, 1989), although this has not been an observation of the authors.

An induction phase is begun with the most dilute solution (1:100). Injections are given every other day with the volume gradually increasing to a maximum of 1.0 ml. The next most concentrated (1:10) dilution is then used in a comparable manner (Table 2). Administration of maintenance solution follows in a similar method until 1.0 ml volume is attained on day 28. Following day 28, the interval of treatment is extended to 10 days, then 20 days.

If 20 or fewer antigens are desired for hyposensitization, they are mixed in appropriate amounts in the 10-ml vial. If more than 20 antigens are selected, they are divided into two groups and two solutions are prepared, each with the respective dilutions. The major reasons for dividing antigens into two solutions are first, too many different antigens in one vial may result in such a low concentration of each antigen that it may not be effective. Second, increasing the number of antigens mixed together may increase the likelihood of cross-reactions of the antigens. The antigens are generally divided into seasonal and nonseasonal categories when preparing a multivial formulation. The solutions are labeled for proper identification (e.g., A and B). During the induction phase, both solutions are administered concurrently. Once the maintenance phase is reached, the two solutions are given at different times (for instance, an injection from Vial A may be given on days 10, 30, and 50 while solution from Vial B is given on days 20, 40, and 60). No more than two solutions are used in any particular patient.

Maintenance therapy is usually 1.0 ml (approximately 20,000 PNU) administered SQ every 20 days. The schedule may be modified depending on the animal's response to therapy. Some animals do well with 10,000 to 15,000 PNU given every 20 days. Others do best if given 10,000 PNU every 10 days. Close client communication and patient re-evaluation is necessary to modify the treatment schedule for optimal effect. Schedule modification may also be required, depending on the time of year and presence of other pruritogenic factors, such as fleas. Owners frequently discontinue hyposensitization either because it does not appear to be working or because the animal no longer demonstrates a problem. Most owners come to realize the value of immunotherapy when the signs return or worsen. Maintenance therapy is generally continued for as long as the animal continues to be exposed to its allergens. On rare occasions, an animal will appear to become desensitized and hyposensitization is discontinued.

SUCCESS OF HYPOSENSITIZATION

A review of 78 patients beginning hyposensitization therapy during an 8-month period was conducted. The patients' response to therapy was based on owners' assessments. All patients included in this review were dogs. There were eight mixed-breed dogs in addition to 34 other breeds. The most common breeds were golden retriever (7), Labrador retriever (7), cocker spaniel (5), Shar pei (3), West Highland white terrier (3), Shih tzu (3), English bulldog (3), miniature schnauzer (3), and dachshund (3). Included in this study were dogs ranging in age from 7 months to 12 years. The average age at the time of intradermal allergy testing and initiation of hyposensitization was 4.8 years. Many animals were tested and began hyposensitization at a young age. It is not uncommon to have initial improvement with subsequent relapses in these cases. It may be necessary to repeat the intradermal allergy test and modify the immunotherapy to include additional antigens. Owners are informed of this possibility at the time of the initial allergy test. The majority of owners of intensely allergic young dogs are willing to participate in such a diagnostic and therapeutic plan simply to avoid excessive glucocorticoid therapy.

The number of allergens used in hyposensitization ranged from 1 to 50 (Table 3). Thirty-two (41%) of these patients were hyposensitized for ten or fewer antigens. The remaining 36 patients (59%) were hyposensitized with more than ten antigens, which is above that recommended in most veterinary dermatology textbooks.

Success with hyposensitization may be difficult to determine. The placebo effect observed in humans receiving hyposensitization therapy has been reported as high as 65%. Multiple pruritic diseases in dogs receiving hyposensitization therapy often obscure the true benefit derived. Most patients on immunotherapy also receive other treatment such as antibiotics, antihistamines, shampoo therapy, parasiticidal treatment, and essential fatty acid supplements. The variability of allergen load and individual pruritic threshold influences the extent of control. Most atopic dogs in the southeastern United States require supplemental medical therapy to the immunotherapy, particularly spring through fall. A minority of animals may be controlled exclusively with hyposensitization.

Response to hyposensitization therapy usually requires 45 to 90 days, but optimal response may require as long as 1 year. Glucocorticoid therapy (alternate-day prednisolone/prednisone) may be administered during immunotherapy, although it should be restricted to a minimum. Alternative nonsteroidal medication is often combined with glucocorticoid treatment. Reduction of prednisone dosage is attempted during hyposensitization therapy.

Success is measured in most instances by patient comfort and requirement for glucocorticoid therapy and a decrease in the relapse rate of bacterial pyoderma. In most cases, either previous medical therapy by itself was insufficient to control the dog's symptoms, or side effects from medical therapy (glucocorticoids) restricted its use.

Flea allergy is frequently a major complication in the atopic dog. Similar to other studies, 62 (79%) of the dogs in this study were also flea allergic. Flea exposure is an additional problem during hyposensitization of coexistent atopy/flea allergy dogs. Hyposensitization for inhalant allergens only is used initially in combination with parasiticidal treatment for flea control. In those cases with both inhalant allergy and flea allergy, additional medical therapy may be needed during the height of the flea season.

Table 3 shows response with immunotherapy in dogs that are atopic and flea allergic compared with those that have only inhalant allergy. Although immunotherapy was directed only toward inhalant allergens, 81% of the flea allergic, atopic dogs showed response to hyposensitization, while only 75% of non–flea allergic, atopic dogs showed improvement. It is likely that response in flea allergic, atopic dogs is also related to flea control. This

Table 3. *Response* of Dogs with Atopy to Hyposensitization Therapy with Inhalant Allergens*

No. of antigens	Atopic Dogs		Atopic and Flea Allergic Dogs	
	No. evaluated	No. improved (%)	No. evaluated	No. improved (%)
≤ 10	6	5 (83)	26	18 (69)
11–15	6	3 (50)	16	15 (94)
16–20	2	2 (100)	13	12 (92)
21–40 (1 vial)	0		2	2 (100)
21–40 (2 vials)	1	1 (100)	3	3 (100)
41–50 (2 vials)	1	1 (100)	2	0 (0)
Overall success	16	12 (75)	62	50 (81)

*Based on owner assessment

supports the concept of summation of effect in that a reduction in any of the pruritigenic factors may result in overall improvement.

As can be seen in Table 3, 72% of dogs that were hyposensitized to ten antigens or less showed improvement. This compares well with previously published response to hyposensitization (DeBoer, 1989 and Willemse et al., 1984). In dogs receiving immunotherapy to 11 to 20 antigens, 86% showed response, and of the nine dogs that were hyposensitized for greater than 21 antigens, seven (78%) showed improvement. This later success rate is especially significant because immunotherapy is twice as expensive in patients receiving multiple vials of antigen. The dogs in this category (greater than 21 antigens) that responded to immunotherapy were being hyposensitized for 21 and 34 antigens (one vial) and 26, 31, 32, 40, and 49 antigens (two vials). The two dogs in which large, multiantigen hyposensitization was not continued were receiving 41 and 43 antigens split into two vials.

A concern regarding multiantigen hyposensitization is the frequency of undesired reactions. An increase in pruritus immediately following immunotherapy may be observed but usually subsides in time. Some cases are severe enough to warrant concurrent administration of antihistamines or glucocorticoids. More severe reactions are uncommon. In this review, four dogs (5%) showed significant adverse reactions to immunotherapy. Of these, only one was severe enough to warrant discontinuation of immunotherapy. The first case involved a 2-year-old Shar pei receiving immunotherapy with 19 antigens. The dog developed edema and irritation at the injection site. This was corrected by a further dilution of the immunotherapy. The second reaction was in a 12-year-old Pekinese being hyposensitized with ten antigens. The dog experienced a seizure on one occasion following antigen therapy. A cause-effect relationship was not determined. This did not recur with subsequent injections. The third case occurred in a 10-year-old schipperke whose immunotherapy contained six antigens. The dog developed a mild anaphylactic reaction, with tachycardia, pale mucous membranes, and depression. It responded to conventional therapy. The dosage of immunotherapy was reduced and administered following antihistamine therapy with no recurrence. The most severe reaction was observed in a 2-year-old English bulldog being hyposensitized with four antigens. The dog showed a severe anaphylactic reaction but did respond when taken to the local veterinarian and given conventional therapy. Immunotherapy was discontinued. Based on these results, there does not appear to be a relationship between the number or amount of allergen used and adverse reactions.

Immunotherapy is a cost-effective method for treating canine atopy. From the 78 cases in this study, it would appear that immunotherapy with large, multiantigen solutions produces a clinical response, although numerous variables exist which make exact comparisons difficult.

References and Suggested Reading

Creticos, P. S., and Norman, P. S.: Immunotherapy with allergens. J.A.M.A. 258:2874, 1987.
A review of the use of immunotherapy in man.

DeBoer, D. J.: Survey of intradermal skin testing practices in North America. J.A.V.M.A. 195:1357, 1989.
Results of a mail-out survey to veterinarians regarding intradermal allergy testing methods and response.

Halliwell, R. E. W., and Gorman, N. T.: *Veterinary Clinical Immunology*. Philadelphia: W. B. Saunders Company, 1989, p. 232.
A textbook chapter with current information regarding proposed mechanisms and methods of allergy testing and immunotherapy.

Kaliner, M.: Hypotheses on the contribution of late-phase allergic responses to the understanding and treatment of allergic diseases. J. Allergy Clin. Immunol. 73:311, 1984.
An editorial regarding the importance of late-phase allergic reactions in allergic disease.

Reedy, L. M., and Miller, W. H.: *Allergic Skin Diseases of Dogs and Cats.* Philadelphia: W. B. Saunders, 1989, p. 111.
A textbook chapter with a practical description of methods of and response to immunotherapy.

Willemse, A., Van den Brom, W. E., and Rijnberk, A.: Effect of hyposensitization on atopic dermatitis in dogs. J.A.V.M.A. 184:1277, 1984.
Results of a double-blind study in dogs using treatment with a placebo or with alum-precipitated allergen solutions.

FELINE ATOPY

DIDIER N. CARLOTTI

Carbon-Blanc, France

Allergic inhalant dermatitis (atopy) is thought to exist in the cat. Although reaginic antibodies have not been identified and inherited predisposition has not been demonstrated in this species, other features of the disease are typical of canine atopy (Halliwell and Gorman, 1990). The amazing tolerance of the cat to the side effects of massive corticosteroid and megestrol acetate therapy may explain why immunologic studies have not been performed until recently.

ETIOLOGY AND PATHOGENESIS

During the sensitization phase, aeroallergens are inhaled and induce the production of reaginic antibodies. It is likely that these allergens are the same in all species. They may be seasonal, i.e., pollens, or nonseasonal, such as house dust mites (see later section, Diagnosis). To date, there are no published reports on the identification and purification of feline IgE. However, a study has demonstrated that hypersensitivity to *Otodectes cynotis* was mediated by a heat-labile, mercaptoethanol-sensitive antibody whose physicochemical characteristics were compatible with its designation as a reaginic antibody (Powell et al., 1980). A recent study on passive cutaneous anaphylaxis (PCA) testing in cats showed a 40% rate of transferability for the allergens tested (Bevier, 1990). The positive reactions could be eliminated when the donor's serum was heat treated at 36°C for 4 hours. These results support the presence of IgE or an IgE-like antibody in the cat. One laboratory in the United States claims to have purified feline IgE via genetic engineering and hybridoma technology.

When the cat is re-exposed to sensitizing aeroallergens, the allergens combine with reaginic antibodies, which have been fixed on inflammatory cells (mainly mast cells and possibly basophils). These cells degranulate and release many mediators of inflammation and pruritus. In dogs, proteolytic enzymes, histamines, and leukotrienes are thought to be important, and this probably also is true for the cat.

Central to the understanding of atopic disease in the cat and its successful management is the concept of a pruritic threshold. Each animal will tolerate some level of pruritic stimulation without clinical itching. This pruritic threshold varies from animal to animal and can be altered by the health status of the cat or by medications. If the allergic but as of yet nonpruritic cat is given additional pruritic stimulation, either of an allergic or nonallergic basis, itching will result. If a cat has only one allergic condition, i.e., atopy or flea allergy, it will not itch until the pollen or flea load reaches some critical level. If the cat is multiply sensitive, i.e., atopic and also flea allergic, it will itch sooner or more intensely when the pollens appear because its other allergens have lowered its pruritic threshold.

CLINICAL SIGNS

No breed or sex predilections have been demonstrated in the cat. One author reported that five of 16 atopic cats had affected relatives and that 75% of these cats developed their initial clinical signs between 6 months and 2 years of age (Scott et al., 1986). Others have been unable to demonstrate familial tendency or age predilection (Carlotti and Prost, 1988; MacDougal, 1986; Reedy, 1982).

The clinical features of feline atopy are highly variable, but pruritus is always present and often is the chief complaint. However, the pruritus may not be seen by the owner as some cats are night lickers and scratchers or even hide to lick and scratch themselves during the day. The pruritus can be seasonal (summer or winter) or nonseasonal.

The pruritus in atopic cats can be localized or generalized, and the cat may or may not have any primary skin lesions. Many atopic cats will start to scratch at apparently normal skin and may create visible lesions. The pruritus often is focused on the head (particularly the face), in the ears (with an erythematous otitis externa), or on the neck, but it may be generalized. Some atopic cats do not scratch but rather lick their skin. During the licking, the hairs are broken off, giving the cat the appearance of one with "psychogenic" alopecia. The alopecia is most commonly seen on the thighs, abdomen, flanks, and tail. In some cases, the cat eventually will excoriate the skin in the hairless areas.

Skin lesions that can be seen in atopic cats include crusted papules (miliary dermatitis), indolent ulcers, eosinophilic plaques, and linear granulomas. These lesions appear spontaneously, and then the cat responds to them by licking or scratching.

Respiratory signs may be seen in feline atopy

(Halliwell and Gorman, 1990). Chronic cough (suggestive of allergic bronchitis), respiratory difficulty accompanied by an expiratory wheeze (compatible with asthma), and rhinoconjunctivitis are the main respiratory features of atopic disease in the cat. In ten atopic cats, the author had five owners report that their cat sneezed as well as itched (Carlotti and Prost, 1988).

DIAGNOSIS

As always, a complete history and a thorough, exhaustive clinical examination are the first steps to lead to the tentative diagnosis of atopic disease. Confirmation of the disease can be obtained by ruling out the other differential diagnoses and by allergy testing.

The differential diagnoses include other hypersensitivities (flea allergy dermatitis, food allergy, intestinal parasite hypersensitivity, drug eruption, contact dermatitis), ectoparasitism (notoedric mange, cheyletiellosis, otoacariasis, demodicosis), dermatophyte infection, bacterial folliculitis (rare), true psychogenic alopecia (self-induced), true endocrine alopecias (e.g., Cushing's disease), telogen effluvium, and idiopathic symmetric alopecia. Response to flea control, elimination diet, coproscopy, response to drug elimination and contact avoidance, multiple skin scrapings, microscopic examination of cerumen, Wood's light examination, microscopic examination of hair, fungal culture, endocrine tests, "behavioral" therapy trials, and biopsy will be useful in many instances. One of the most difficult challenges is to differentiate symmetric alopecia (endocrine, telogen effluvium, idiopathic) from self-induced alopecia. In the latter, hair is not epilated easily, appears broken under the microscope, and regrows when an Elizabethan collar is put on the cat for 1 month.

In Aquitaine, France, the most common cause of pruritus in the cat is flea allergy dermatitis. I think that skin testing cats with a flea extract leads to numerous false-negative reactions, at least with the HAL extract (HAL Laboratories, Haarlem, Holland), although this procedure is highly reliable in the dog. Therefore, if a cat is thought to have an allergic skin disease, exhaustive flea control is first prescribed. If there is little or no response to this treatment, an elimination diet to confirm or exclude the diagnosis of food allergy is instituted. If after at least 3 weeks of dietary elimination there is no response, the owner is told that the atopy is the logical diagnosis even if a partial response to flea control is seen. There is no reason why flea allergy and atopy could not occur simultaneously. Allergy tests are indicated. In the United States, and recently in Europe, one laboratory offers serologic allergy testing for the cat, but the reliability of this test is unknown. Intradermal testing works well in the cat and, at present, is the preferred method of allergy testing in cats.

The length of time that anti-inflammatory agents can interfere with intradermal testing in cats largely is unknown. On an empirical basis, I would recommend waiting 6 weeks after an injection of a long-acting glucocorticoid, 3 weeks after an oral or topical glucocorticoid, 1 week after an oral antihistamine, and probably several months after megestrol acetate therapy.

Allergens must be selected carefully and should be similar to those used in testing dogs. A recent study indicates that, for the majority of allergens, the allergen concentrations used to skin-test dogs are also appropriate for the cat (Bevier, 1990). General anesthesia is often necessary to skin-test cats. Although ketamine (5 mg/kg IV or 10 mg/kg IM) has been recommended, I prefer to use the combination glycopyrrolate (Robinul V) 0.01 mg/kg IV or IM, and tiletamine-zolazepam (Zoletil) 5 mg/kg IV or 10 mg/kg IM because no hyperexcitation is seen.

About 0.05 ml of each extract is injected intradermally as well as the two controls (histamine and diluent). The injections can be difficult because cat skin is very thin and resistant. The author uses the same syringes on different patients without problems. However, if viral diseases (FeLV, FIV) are common in the practice area, new needles should be used for each cat.

In the cat, interpretation of the skin test is much more difficult than in the dog since the positive reactions in the cat are small, flat, diffuse wheals. Erythema is also minimal so that palpation will be useful to recognize an increase in the thickness of the skin (Halliwell and Gorman, 1990). I read the tests in an obliquely directed light, and observe the area continuously during 20 minutes to avoid missing any transient wheal. Delayed reactions may be seen (up to 48 hours), but their significance is unknown (Halliwell and Gorman, 1990; Muller et al., 1989).

The reactions can be scored by measuring the wheals at their largest size. Positive reactions are indicated by those wheals that have a diameter equal to or greater than the mean diameters of the histamine and negative controls. A positive reaction means only that the cat has reaginic antibodies against inhaled allergens. Correlation with the history must be good. For instance, seasonal pruritus can be correlated with positive reactions to pollens alone or to pollens and nonseasonal allergens, but not to nonseasonal allergens only. Nonseasonal pruritus cannot be explained by positive reactions to pollens only, at least at the earliest stage of the disease.

False-positive and false-negative reactions may occur. One study has demonstrated that false-positive reactions are rare in normal cats. The percentage of normal cats reacting to various extracts varied from 0 to 30, with irritating allergens (e.g., house dust, feathers) showing the highest reactivity. In the same study, young cats and dark cats showed more reactions (Bevier, 1990). One should remember that irritant, contaminated, poorly injected allergens can lead to false-positive reactions. On the other hand, true positive reactions demonstrate that the patient has fixed antibodies, which may or may not be clinically important. All reactions must be evaluated in light of the history.

False-negative reactions are mainly due to previous anti-inflammatory therapy. Other causes include poor technique (too few allergens, subcutaneous injections, air injections), poor allergens (e.g., mixed extracts, outdated, insufficient concentration), and probably other factors not well understood. On an empirical basis, I think that skin testing with pollens should be done at the end of the pollination period to avoid false-negative reactions. Good training and expertise are needed to perform and interpret skin tests in the cat, and the clinician must do testing on a regular basis to maintain the appropriate level of expertise.

Published results on skin tests in cats are variable (Carlotti and Prost, 1988; MacDougal, 1986; Reedy, 1982; Scott et al., 1986). Nevertheless, multiple sensitization is almost always demonstrated, and "house dust" or "house-dust mite" extracts often give positive reactions. I have had 100% reactivity to the house-dust mite *Dermatophagoides farinae* in ten cats. The variation in reaction to different allergens can be due to the practice area, the cat's environment, the allergenic extracts, and the scoring method.

THERAPY

Therapy is required in feline atopy since spontaneous desensitization does not seem to occur. Avoidance of the offending allergen would be the ideal therapy, but unfortunately, this is very difficult in atopy. Some nonseasonal allergens can be removed from the animal's environment (e.g., wool, kapok, feathers). As polysensitization is common, the removal of one allergen, when it is possible, may push the patient below its allergic threshold and thus reduce itching. Such a therapeutic opportunity should not be neglected.

Medical therapy is very useful in feline atopy. Glucocorticoids are widely used in the cat with good results, at least at the beginning of the treatment. Long-acting corticosteroid injections are effective (e.g., methylprednisolone acetate, 20 mg/cat IM). This can be an acceptable form of therapy in the cat if only three to four injections are required per year. Triamcinolone acetonide (5 mg/cat SQ) can be used similarly. After a few years, response to repeated injection can decrease and side effects may occur, so another form of therapy should be investigated. Oral glucocorticosteroids are preferable in the cat for long-term usage. Short-acting compounds such as prednisone, prednisolone, or methylprednisolone may be administered at the dose of 1 to 2 mg/kg/day for 5 to 7 days, and then the same dose should be given on an alternate-day basis. Cats that are active during the night should receive the medication in the evening, while those cats that are more active during the day should be medicated every-other morning. Long-term therapy can be achieved with such a method, while minimizing side effects. The amount of drug administered is adjusted according to the needs of the patient.

Response to this therapy also can decrease progressively, and sometimes side effects occur (most often after a few months or years of therapy, but sometimes much sooner). In such cases, intermediate-acting oral glucocorticoids (e.g., triamcinolone, 0.5 to 1 mg/kg/day) or long-acting oral glucocorticoids (e.g., dexamethasone or betamethasone, 0.1 mg/kg/day) should be tried. However, alternate-day therapy is not possible with these compounds.

Generally speaking, my first therapeutic approach for seasonal atopic pruritus in a cat would be glucocorticoids. However, other forms of medical therapy can be used. Megestrol acetate has been widely used in feline dermatology because of its strong anti-inflammatory effects. However, long-term therapy is required, and side effects such as polyphagia with obesity, polyuria-polydipsia with or without diabetes mellitus, mammary hypertrophy, and even mammary carcinoma may occur. Because of these intolerable side effects, I *strongly* recommend that this drug not be used in cats.

Nonsteroidal anti-inflammatory medications are routinely used in the management of chronic canine pruritus (see this volume, p. 563). Far less information is available in the cat. A recent study (Miller and Scott, 1990) has shown that chlorpheniramine maleate (2 mg every 12 hours) can successfully control the pruritus in approximately 70% of allergic cats. In Europe, products containing both chlorpheniramine and hydroxyzine are licensed for use in dogs and cats. This drug has a strong sedative effect, and its safety and efficacy in the cat has not been evaluated. Cats, in general, can be very sensitive to antihistamines, so new drugs must be investigated carefully. To my knowledge, H_2 blockers have not been evaluated in the cat.

Hyposensitization (immunotherapy) is indicated when avoidance of the offending allergens is impossible and when medical therapy has decreasing effectiveness or increasing side effects. The owner of the cat must be seriously motivated, and the cat should be healthy and not too old. In the cat, only four studies on the effectiveness of hyposensitization

Table 1. *Hyposensitization Schedules with Alum-Precipitated Allergens*

HAL Extracts		
Week No.	*Injection No.*	*Dose in ml (SQ)*
1	1	0.02
2	2	0.05
3	3	0.1
5	4	0.2
7	5	0.4
9	6	0.8
12	7	1
15	8	1
19	9	1
23	10	1
27	11	1

are available (Carlotti and Prost, 1988; MacDougal, 1986; Reedy, 1982; Scott et al., 1986). Aqueous allergens which require frequent injections (a potential problem in some aggressive cats) have been used on a weekly basis in two studies with good results in 3 of 3 (100%) cases (Scott et al., 1986), and 9 of 13 (69%) cats (MacDougal, 1986). Alum-precipitated allergens, which are "intermediate" as far as number of injections and time required for hyposensitization are concerned, were used in two studies with good results in 11 of 15 (73%) cats (Reedy, 1982) and 4 of 6 (67%) cats (Carlotti and Prost, 1988). The schedule I use is given in Table 1. In all these studies, a good result meant at least a 75% improvement in the clinical signs or a very large reduction in the cat's glucocorticoid requirement. I have successfully hyposensitized more than 20 cats and am aware of many other unpublished cases successfully managed by hyposensitization.

As in dogs, immunotherapy in cats probably will be required life-long. Adverse reactions have not been reported in the cat. Steroid therapy can be used during hyposensitization but should be at the lowest oral dosage possible (i.e., on an alternate-day basis).

CONCLUSION

Further studies are needed to increase our knowledge of the pathogenesis of feline atopy and to evaluate therapeutic possibilities on a larger basis, particularly hyposensitization. However, at present, clinical aspects of this disease are well known, diagnosis by skin testing seems to be quite reliable, and medical or immunologic therapy is possible.

References and Suggested Reading

Bevier, D. E. The reaction of feline skin to the intradermal injection of allergenic extracts. Passive cutaneous anaphylaxis using serum from skin test positive cats. *In* Von Tscharner, C. and Halliwell, R. E. W. (eds.): *Recent Advances in Veterinary Dermatology*, vol. 1. London: Baillière Tindall, 1990, pp. 126–136.
Two excellent fundamental studies.
Carlotti, D. N., and Prost, C.: L'atopie féline. Point Vét. 20:777, 1988.
A review and report of ten cases of feline atopy.
Halliwell, R. E. W., and Gorman, N. T.: *Veterinary Clinical Immunology*. Philadelphia: W. B. Saunders, 1990, p. 248.
A complete handbook of veterinary immunology, including a chapter about atopic diseases.
MacDougal, B. J.: Allergy testing and hyposensitization for three common feline dermatoses. Mod. Vet. Pract. 81:629, 1986.
A well-documented report.
Miller, W. H. Jr., and Scott, D. W.: Efficacy of chlorpheniramine maleate for management of pruritus in cats. J.A.V.M.A. 197:67, 1990.
A new therapeutic approach of the pruritic cat.
Muller, G. H., Kirk, R. W., and Scott, D. W.: *Small Animal Dermatology*, 4th ed. Philadelphia: W. B. Saunders, 1989, p. 450.
The classical and exhaustive handbook.
Powell, M. B., Weisbroth, S. H., Roth, L., et al.: Reaginic hypersensitivity in *Otodectes cynotis* infection of cats and mode of mite feeding. Am. J. Vet. Res. 41:877, 1980.
A strong suggestion of the existence of a reaginic antibody in the cat.
Reedy, L. M.: Results of allergy testing and hyposensitization in selected feline skin diseases. J. Am. Anim. Hosp. Assoc. 18:618, 1982.
The first clinical study of atopic disease in the cat; well documented.
Reedy, L. M., and Miller, W. H. Jr.: *Allergic Skin Diseases of Dogs and Cats*. Philadelphia: W. B. Saunders, 1989, pp. 46, 131.
A very useful and practical handbook.
Scott, D. W., Walton, D. K., and Slater, M. R.: Miliary dermatitis: A feline cutaneous reaction pattern. Proc. 2nd Ann. Kal Kan Seminar, Eastern States Vet. Conf., Orlando: 1986, p. 11.
An interesting review, including reports of cases of atopy.

FOOD HYPERSENSITIVITY

STEPHEN D. WHITE

Fort Collins, Colorado

Adverse reactions to foods have been well documented in small animals. The terms "food allergy" and "food hypersensitivity" have been used interchangeably in the human and veterinary medical literature to describe symptoms induced by food ingestion in which there are demonstrable or highly suspected immunologic reactions. Food intolerance and occasionally food sensitivity have been used where immunologic etiology is unlikely or has not been established. Although the etiology of abnormal reactions to ingested foods has not always been well established in small animals, common usage dictates the use of the terms food hypersensitivity or food allergy. I prefer the former as being more accurate in describing an abnormal response of the immune system.

ETIOLOGY

The exact pathomechanisms of food hypersensitivity have not been delineated in dogs and cats. Reactions to food that could be termed immediate (hypersensitivity type I: occurring within minutes to hours after ingestion) and delayed (type IV: occurring within hours to days of ingestion) have been noted in the dog and cat.

Food contaminants such as pathogenic bacteria or other toxins, food additives such as tartrazines, and vasoactive amines such as tyramine in cheese have all been implicated or suspected as mimicking food hypersensitivity in humans. While their importance in small animals is unknown, I know of one dog that was documented as having an allergic reaction to the additive gum carrageenan (Harvey, R. G., personal communication, 1990).

SIGNALMENT, HISTORY, AND CLINICAL SIGNS

No age, breed, or sex predilections have been noted in dogs or cats with food hypersensitivity. Age of onset is variable, with most animals having been fed the offending diet for at least 2 years. Owners seldom relate the onset of clinical signs with any recent change in diet.

Clinical signs are variable. Pruritus is the most common sign, although nonpruritic dogs are reported rarely. The pruritus is often distributed similar to that of inhalant allergies; i.e., feet, ears, face, and axilla. Cutaneous lesions noted in dogs include papules, erythema, epidermal collarettes, pododermatitis, seborrhea sicca, and otitis externa. In cats with food hypersensitivity, generalized pruritus, miliary dermatitis, facial and head pruritus, pruritic angioedema-urticaria, eosinophilic plaque, eosinophilic ulcers, and erythema have been reported.

Gastrointestinal signs (vomiting, diarrhea) have also been noted. In cats, food hypersensitivity has been manifested as lymphocytic-plasmacytic colitis, although there is little evidence to support dietary allergy as a cause of lymphocytic-plasmacytic enteritis in dogs. Neurologic signs (epileptiform seizures, malaise) and respiratory distress (asthma-like syndromes) have been reported rarely. Multiple organ involvement is uncommon.

LABORATORY DATA

There is no consistent laboratory finding in small animals with food hypersensitivity. Peripheral eosinophilia may or may not be present. Histopathology is nondiagnostic, usually characterized by a perivascular dermatitis with neutrophils or mononuclear cells predominating and variable secondary suppurative changes. Tissue eosinophilia is uncommon but has been reported.

DIAGNOSIS

Intradermal skin testing has usually been unrewarding in humans and small animals, possibly owing to changes in composition of the allergen with digestion or to improper dilution of the test allergen. Serologic diagnostics using the radioallergosorbent test (RAST) or the enzyme-linked immunosorbent assay (ELISA) for reaginic antibodies have been used in human beings and correlate with history and provocative exposure tests in perhaps over 50% of the cases reported. However, the data from two recent studies, one using RAST (White and Mason, 1990) and one using the ELISA test (Jeffers et al., 1991) are far less promising. The RAST study showed all healthy dogs (n = 5) and 75% of pruritic dogs without food hypersensitivity (n = 4) as having positive test reactions to various

513

foods. In addition, dogs with food hypersensitivities (n = 7) often tested positive to foods that they were able to be fed without eliciting clinical signs. Similar results were documented in the ELISA study, which showed no predictive value for that test.

Preliminary findings in France have shown some value in the basophil degranulation test as a diagnostic aid in canine food hypersensitivity (Prelaud, 1990).

The most commonly employed means of diagnosis is the restricted (hypoallergenic) test diet. The animal is fed a diet with a very limited number of foodstuffs, preferably ingredients to which the animal has had little or no previous exposure. I usually use a diet limited to (noninstant) rice and lamb in a 1:1 mix for dogs, and a lamb-based baby food (strained lamb baby food, Gerber, Freemont, MN) for cats, simply because most small animals in my practice area are not exposed to lamb on a routine basis. However, test diets must be individualized on the basis of a careful dietary history. Hypoallergenic diets should be free of colorings, preservatives, and flavorings. Palatable medications, such as certain heartworm preventatives, should be stopped (another type of heartworm preventative should be given for the duration of the diet), as well as all vitamin and mineral supplements. Commercially prepared pet foods, including prescription diets, diets containing no preservatives, or diets marketed as "natural" are *not* adequate test diets. Presumably, all these products contain too many foodstuffs or manufacturers process those foodstuffs in varying ways so they cannot be considered true restricted test diets. I (and other investigators) have diagnosed pets with food hypersensitivity whose clinical signs have recurred when their diets have been switched from the home-prepared test diet to the aforementioned prescription or "natural" foods.

Occasionally, an animal may be presented to the clinician with such intense pruritus that the administration of oral corticosteroids is indicated while the diet is in progress. Such administration should be limited to prednisone (or prednisolone or methylprednisolone) and will obviously obscure any positive response to the diet. I generally give a corticosteroid (0.5 to 1.0 mg/kg PO every 24 hours) for 10 days, then stop. In such cases, the diet should be continued for a minimum of 2 weeks beyond the discontinuation of the medication in order to properly evaluate response to diet. The same rules for time of administration apply to antibiotics given to animals with secondary pyoderma.

Clinical improvement has been reported to occur within periods varying from 24 hours to a full 3 weeks. Thus the recommended duration of diet also varys from 3 days to 8 weeks. I have found 3 to 4 weeks to be a reasonable length of time in which to expect some improvement. Improvement is best defined as a reduction of pruritus (or other clinical signs if pruritus is absent). If only partial improvement is noted, the diet may not have been given long enough for full effectiveness. Alternatively, the restricted diet's content should be re-evaluated and possibly changed (i.e., potatoes substituted for rice) or other concurrent hypersensitivities (to fleas or inhalant allergens) evaluated.

MANAGEMENT

Once improvement is noted, several alternatives are open to the clinician. Ideally, the animal should be challenged with its original diet in order to substantiate the diagnosis. The literature usually recommends adding individual foodstuffs to the restricted diet at 5- to 10-day intervals until a balanced diet is achieved or the offending allergen(s) is discovered. Unfortunately, I have found that many owners are unwilling to exacerbate a clinically improved animal or separate out various components of foods to determine potential allergens. They may be more interested in achieving a balanced (and if feeding lamb, less expensive) diet as soon as possible. Once maximum improvement is noted on the test diet, I usually change the animal's diet to either a lamb-based (Prescription Diet d/d [canned], Hill's Pet Products, Topeka, KS) or egg-based (Prescription Diet d/d [dry], Hill's Pet Products, Topeka, KS) prescription diet, or one of several commercial diets without commercial additives (Cornucopia Natural Pet Foods, Huntington, NY; Nutro Max, Nutro Products, Inc., City of Industry, CA). If the new diet is not tolerated, most animals show a recurrence of clinical signs within 72 hours, although a few pets may take longer. If the animal will not tolerate a commercial diet, a home-prepared diet must be used. Such diets should consist of a protein and starch source supplemented with vitamins, minerals, and, for cats, sufficient taurine (approximately 60 to 100 mg of taurine/cat/day). The previous recommendation of supplementation with 0.5 teaspoon of clam juice per day is *not* adequate taurine supplementation.

Reports of suspected or proven dietary allergens are numerous in the literature, and such allergens include beef, pork, chicken, cow's milk, horsemeat, eggs, wheat, oats, fish, whale meat, soy, fungal contaminants in drinking water, and others. I have diagnosed fish as an offending allergen in 50% of cats with food hypersensitivity. The vast array of foodstuffs used in commercial pet foods, as well as variable processing methods, probably accounts for the large numbers of allergens reported.

References and Suggested Reading

Carlotti, D. N., Remy, I., and Prost, C.: Food allergy in dogs and cats. A review and report of 43 cases. Vet. Dermatol. 1:55, 1990.

Jeffers, J. G., Shanley, K. J., and Meyer, E. K.: Diagnostic testing for canine food hypersensitivity. J.A.V.M.A. 198:245, 1991.

Pion, P. D., Power, H. T., Rogers, Q. R., et al.: Taurine for cats (letter). J.A.V.M.A. 194:1005, 1989.

Prelaud, P.: The basophil degranulation test in the diagnosis of canine allergic skin disease. *Advances in Veterinary Dermatology*, vol. 1. London: Baillière Tindall, 1990, pp. 117–125.

Rosser, E. J.: Food allergy in the dog: A prospective study of 51 dogs. Proceedings American Academy of Veterinary Dermatology and American College of Veterinary Dermatology, 1990.

White, S. D.: Food hypersensitivity in 30 dogs. J.A.V.M.A. 188:695, 1986.

White, S. D., and Sequoia, D.: Food hypersensitivity in cats: 14 cases (1982–1987). J.A.V.M.A. 194:692, 1989.

White, S. D., and Mason, I. S.: Proceedings of the Dietary Allergy Workshop. In *Advances in Veterinary Dermatology*, vol 1. London: Baillière Tindall, 1990, pp. 404–406.

FOLLICULAR DISORDERS OF THE DOBERMAN PINSCHER

WILLIAM H. MILLER, JR.

Ithaca, New York

Disorders of the hair follicle are common in all dogs. When a Doberman pinscher develops a skin disease, it often has a follicular orientation. Careful examination of the history and patient often will allow the clinician to formulate an appropriate list of differential diagnoses but will not identify the specific cause of the problem. Diagnostic testing must be done. The purpose of this article is to describe the causes of generalized follicular disease in the Doberman pinscher so that the diagnostic effort can be well focused.

THE FOLLICULOPATHY

Follicular pathology can be a result of inflammation (folliculitis) or follicular inactivity. With follicular inactivity, the hairs eventually fall out, leaving exposed, noninflamed skin. Follicular inactivity usually is induced by severe stress (i.e., telogen effluvium) or an endocrine disorder such that many of the hair follicles are affected at the same time. Accordingly, the hair loss seen involves large areas of the body.

Folliculitis, regardless of the cause, also will result in hair loss, but because not all hair follicles are equally affected, the hair loss will be patchy. In short-coated dogs with a widespread folliculitis, the dog's coat will look moth-eaten with multifocal, small areas of alopecia. In suppurative folliculitis, one will see erythema and scale in the hairless areas, and possibly papules or pustules. Once the cause of the folliculitis is eliminated and the inflammation subsides, the skin will heal and the hair will regrow. Although uncommon in dogs, the hair at the first regrowth may be lighter in color, even white.

The following discussion describes the follicular disorders to which the Doberman pinscher appears to be predisposed. Since a secondary bacterial folliculitis often is superimposed on a disorder of follicular inactivity, both patterns of follicular disease may be seen in the same patient.

BACTERIAL FOLLICULITIS

The most common follicular disorder of the Doberman pinscher, or, for that matter, any breed of dog, is a bacterial folliculitis. Depending on the cause, the lesions may be fairly localized or widespread. In the localized category, the Doberman pinscher is predisposed to develop muzzle folliculitis and acral lick dermatitis (see this volume, p. 552). Although the reason why some dogs develop muzzle folliculitis (canine acne) is unknown, friction with subsequent hair impaction may play an important part in the disease. Minimization of chin friction by the elimination of chew toys, rough playing, and so forth can help in the treatment of the disorder. Widespread bacterial folliculitis in the Doberman pinscher can be secondary to some underlying sterile follicular disorder, described subsequently. (For current information on the treatment of bacterial disease in the dog, see this volume, p. 539.)

GENERALIZED DEMODICOSIS

The *Demodex canis* mite typically has a commensal relationship with its host but occasionally becomes a true parasite and causes demodicosis. The reason(s) why certain dogs develop disease is uncertain, but genetic susceptibility plays a central role. Textbooks on veterinary dermatology list the Doberman pinscher as a breed prone to generalized demodicosis, and the results of a retrospective study I conducted confirm those observations. In that study, the odds ratio for generalized demodicosis in the Doberman pinscher was 5:2, which shows a strong breed susceptibility. These data should reinforce the need to neuter dogs with generalized demodicosis.

Although one can see classic lesions of folliculitis in Doberman pinschers with generalized demodicosis, these dogs usually have large areas of hair loss, erythema, seborrhea, and bacterial pyoderma. If one follows the basic tenet of dermatology, scrape everything, the diagnosis should be straightforward.

Not all dogs, especially puppies, with generalized demodicosis will need intense miticidal therapy. Assisted self-cure can occur. Once a dog reaches 12 to 18 months of age, its demodicosis will require treatment. Today, the topical application of an amitraz solution (Mitaban, UpJohn) is the most widely used method of treatment. In the United States, this product is licensed for use at 250 ppm, once every 14 days. There are a variety of conflicting reports on the efficacy of this protocol. Without needlessly prolonging this discussion, one can safely say that not all dogs can be cured with semi-monthly dips of a 250 ppm solution. If the owners of these incurable dogs are happy with the thought of maintenance therapy, lifelong dipping should keep the mite under control.

For the dog owner who wants to exhaust all modes of treatment so that his dog can be cured and not just controlled, other options are available. *None however are licensed for use in dogs.* Full disclaimers by informed owners who understand and accept the risks are mandatory before usage. Most widely used is the amitraz solution, but with more frequent application, and often at greater concentrations. Typically, the 250 ppm solution will be applied once weekly for 4 weeks. If a positive response is seen, the protocol is followed until the mites are eradicated and then continued for an additional 30 days. Mite eradication must be determined by the examination of multiple skin scrapings and not just by visually inspecting the dog's skin. If the weekly application of the 250 ppm solution fails to eliminate the mites, the concentration can be increased to 500 ppm or even 1000 ppm. At these concentrations, therapy becomes expensive and chances of intoxication are increased. I have never used the 1000 ppm solution, but I have not seen any intoxication at the 500 ppm level. If these measures do not work, the dog probably cannot be cured with amitraz.

The thought of an oral or parenteral method of treatment for generalized demodicosis always has been appealing but, to date, has not been achieved. Parenteral weekly administration of ivermectin at 400 µg/kg failed to cure three of four dogs to which it was given. Further refinement of the protocol might improve the efficacy, but since large doses of this product are known to occasionally cause serious, even fatal, adverse reactions, little work has been done.

Recently the author has participated in a study on the efficacy of oral milbemycin (Interceptor, Ciba-Geigy) in the treatment of generalized demodicosis. The drug is given daily for a minimum of 90 days at a dose of 0.5 to 1.0 mg/kg. In its licensed application, heartworm and hookworm prevention, the drug is given at the 0.5 mg/kg level, once monthly. Accordingly, the dosage used to treat demodicosis is 90 to 180 times the recommended dose. At this writing, 23 dogs have entered the study, and no adverse reactions have been seen in any dog. Ten dogs have finished their treatment. Two dogs could not be made mite free, and negative skin scrapings were achieved in eight dogs. Three of these eight dogs had a relapse after the drug was discontinued. The other five dogs remain clinically normal with the shortest follow-up time being 6 months. These data give an apparent cure rate of 50%, but the final figure will not be available until all dogs have completed their treatment and have been untreated for 1 year.

If the milbemycin is too cost prohibitive or proves to be ineffective and amitraz will not cure the dog, the old-fashioned method of treatment with topical organophosphates can be used. The reader is referred to older literature for a complete description of the protocol. Although highly effective, the organophosphates are messy and toxic, and most owners will not complete a course of treatment. If nothing presently available will cure the dog, the owner should be encouraged to adopt the control method of treatment with the amitraz. This should keep the dog relatively normal while new modes of therapy are developed. Again, the dog with generalized demodicosis, regardless of how good it looks, should never be used for breeding. All dogs with generalized demodicosis, especially those who are being kept "normal" by artificial means, should be neutered.

PEMPHIGUS FOLIACEUS

Pemphigus foliaceus is a rare autoimmune skin disease that has been documented in many breeds of dogs. Many cases have been recognized in Doberman pinschers. This may indicate a genetic susceptibility or simply be a chance occurrence due to the popularity of the breed. Most Doberman pinschers with pemphigus foliaceus have a pronounced papulocrustus disorder of the face, ears, feet, and footpads. Pustular lesions often are seen in conjunction with the crusty lesions. Since the other disorders described in this article do not have such a striking clinical presentation, they usually can be dismissed fairly quickly. However, some Doberman pinschers do not have the classic lesions of pemphigus foliaceus, but rather just have widespread pustular or follicular lesions. If intact pustules are present, cytologic evaluation of their content, to search for the presence of numerous acanthocytes, should suggest the diagnosis of pemphigus. Skin biopsies should be done to confirm that diagnosis.

HYPOTHYROIDISM

Hypothyroidism is the most common endocrine disorder of the dog and the Doberman pinscher is known to be prone to develop this disease. Although there are a myriad of signs of hypothyroidism, an affected Doberman pinscher usually will present with a recurrent bacterial folliculitis without an endocrine-type of hair loss, an endocrine-type of hair loss with or without a secondary bacterial folliculitis, or multiple areas of acral lick dermatitis. Since hypothyroidism is common in this breed, one can never be sure if the hypothyroidism is the cause of the problem or just a coincidental, but significant, finding. The animal's response to therapy will answer that question. (For a current discussion on the diagnosis and treatment of hypothyroidism, see this volume, p. 330.)

COLOR DILUTION ALOPECIA

Color dilution alopecia, more commonly known as color mutant alopecia, is a disorder that causes tardive, permanent hair loss in dogs with a dilute coat color. Blue, a dilution of black, or fawn, a dilution of brown, are the two commonly recognized dilute coat colors. Although the disorder has been recognized in a variety of breeds, it appears to be most common in the Doberman pinscher. In a retrospective and prospective study of color dilution alopecia in Doberman pinschers, the author found that approximately 90% of adult blue or fawn Doberman pinschers examined at the New York State College of Veterinary Medicine had color dilution alopecia. There was a tendency for darkly diluted dogs, those with a steel-blue or dark fawn coat, to be normal or to develop their hair loss during their third to fifth year of life.

Since color dilution alopecia is linked to the dilute coat color, a genetic trait, the hair loss typically starts early in life, between 6 and 12 months of age in most dogs. Lesions are first noted over the dorsum. Although the pathogenesis of the disorder is unknown, the hair loss first seems to be due to fracture of the hair shafts at or below the skin surface. This microtrauma induces a sterile folliculitis, which often is compounded by secondary bacterial invasion. Early on, treatment with antibiotics or antibacterial shampoos will resolve the lesions and some hair regrowth will be noted. This improvement will be short-lived. New and more widespread lesions will be seen, and the hair loss will become permanent. This degenerative process will continue at a variable rate until all the dilute hairs are lost, leaving a bald-and-tan dog. The tan hairs at the points are not diluted, so they will remain intact.

The tentative diagnosis of color dilution alopecia usually is straightforward. The dog has a diluted coat color and develops hair loss and folliculitis early in life. Skin scrapings, fungal cultures, and cytology should be performed to exclude other differentials. Microscopic examination of plucked hairs is very useful. Nondiluted dogs have small pigment granules evenly distributed along the hair shaft. Diluted dogs, whether they have color dilution alopecia or not, have large pigment granules (macromelanosomes) with an uneven distribution. In dogs with color dilution alopecia, the macromelanosomes are very large and can distort the hair shafts. If hair examination shows these large macromelanosomes, the diagnosis of color dilution alopecia is almost a certainty. Skin biopsies will absolutely confirm the diagnosis.

Coat color dilution is due to the influence of recessive alleles at the D, or dilution, locus. Coat color dilution occurs in most species of animals, but color dilution alopecia is seen only in dogs. There are many diluted dogs that do not lose hair, so there must be something special about dogs that do. The author has postulated that dogs with color dilution alopecia have a lethal allele at the D locus, which ultimately destroys the hair follicle. If this is true, that gene would appear to be widespread in the Doberman pinscher such that it would be difficult, if not impossible, to eliminate it. Certainly, dogs with color dilution alopecia should not be used for breeding. Once the hair loss starts, there is nothing that can be done to prevent it. Antibiotics or antibacterial shampoos should eliminate any secondary infections and may slow the rate of progression, but the hair loss will continue. With good common sense measures, avoidance of long exposure to sun, cold, and dry heat, and periodic bathing, the dog can lead a very normal life.

FOLLICULAR DYSPLASIA

With the high incidence of hypothyroidism and color dilution alopecia in Doberman pinschers, truncal hair loss is a common complaint. Some black or red dogs will present for a persistent dorsal hair loss. These dogs will start to lose hair in their flank areas as young adults, typically between 1 and 2 years of age, and the hair loss will progress ever so slowly to involve the dorsum and flank region from the midthorax to the rump. Bacterial infections may or may not occur. These dogs are euthyroid or fail to respond to adequate thyroid supplementation, do not have hyperadrenocorticism, and do not respond to neutering or sex hormone supplementation. Skin biopsies show histologic changes of follicular dysplasia and color dilution alopecia.

Although the pathogenesis of this disorder is uncertain, it appears that problems in pigment transfer, as are seen in color dilution alopecia, are present in these dogs. It may be that these dogs are carrying the lethal recessive allele at the D locus and that somehow it is being expressed in a regionalized fashion.

Through a retrospective review of case material from 1975 through 1987, the author could identify only three dogs with this disorder. Since then, ten dogs have been recognized. This dramatic increase in frequency could simply reflect an awareness of the condition on my part or a true increase in frequency. I favor the latter explanation. If the disorder is associated with a recessive coat color gene or some other gene, its frequency should increase unless some restrictive breeding program is instituted.

Any Doberman pinscher with a persistent dorsal hair loss should have skin biopsies taken early in the course of the evaluation. If the changes of follicular dysplasia are seen, the hair loss will be permanent. Pedigree analysis, with special attention to the coat color of the relatives, may shed some light on the etiology of this disorder.

VITILIGO

Vitiligo is an uncommon, acquired depigmentary process to which the Doberman pinscher appears predisposed. Affected dogs lose the pigment in their skin (leukoderma) and hair (leukotrichia) as young adults. Usually the skin of the nose, lips, and buccal mucosa is affected, and patchy areas of color change are seen over the body and limbs. In this classical presentation, the tentative diagnosis of vitiligo is straightforward and can be confirmed by skin biopsy. Occasionally, one will examine a Doberman pinscher for discrete, scattered truncal leukotrichia. Without a skin biopsy, it is impossible to tell if this pigment loss is the first sign of vitiligo or could be the result of previous follicular inflammation. If the dog has vitiligo, the depigmentation will progress for 6 to 12 months. Once the pigment loss stops, the dog usually will maintain that degree of depigmentation for the remainder of its life. Affected dogs should not be used for breeding.

CONCLUSION

The Doberman pinscher can develop a wide variety of follicular disorders, the most common of which is bacterial folliculitis. If the dog's clinical disease is treated on an empiric basis with antibiotics and does not improve or the condition recurs, the follicular disorders described herein should be considered.

References and Suggested Reading

Miller, W. H., Jr.: Color dilution alopecia in Doberman pinschers with blue or fawn coat colors: A study on the incidence and histopathology of this disorder. Vet. Dermatol. 1:113, 1990.
  A study on the incidence of color dilution alopecia in 57 dogs.
Miller, W. H., Jr.: Follicular dysplasia in adult black and red Doberman pinschers. Vet. Dermatol. 1:181, 1990.
  A study of the disorder in six dogs.
Miller, W. H., Jr.: Canine demodicosis. Compend. Cont. Ed. 2:334, 1980.
  A review of the causes, clinical features, and methods of treatment of generalized demodicosis.
Muller, G. H., Kirk, R. W., and Scott, D. W.: *Small Animal Dermatology*, 4th ed. Philadelphia: W. B. Saunders, 1989.

SKIN DISORDERS OF THE SHAR PEI

CRAIG E. GRIFFIN
and WAYNE S. ROSENKRANTZ
Garden Grove, California

The Chinese Shar pei breed has become very popular in the past 15 years. The recognition of frequent and numerous skin diseases paralleled the breed's rise in popularity (Table 1). The Shar pei is reported to be predisposed to atopy, demodicosis, folliculitis, body-fold dermatitis, hypothyroidism, and seborrhea (Muller et al., 1989). The Chinese Shar pei has been shown to have the highest relative risk factor for generalized demodicosis, atopic disease, and hypothyroidism (Miller et al., 1990). Normally rare disorders such as IgA deficiency and cutaneous mucinosis have also been found frequently in the Chinese Shar pei. Other clinical observations suggest that the Shar pei may manifest some cutaneous problems differently from other breeds. Regardless of these problems, the breed is growing in popularity. For these reasons it is important for the clinician to be familiar with dermatologic disorders of the Chinese Shar pei.

Table 1. *Incidence of Dermatologic Disease in Shar Peis Presented with Skin Disease to Two Veterinary Clinics*

Disease	N = 119* % affected	N = 58† % affected
Bacterial folliculitis		
secondary	48.7	48.3
idiopathic	9.2	25.9
Atopy	66.4	
Food allergy	15.1§	44.8‡
Flea allergy	20.2	
Demodex	14.2	8.6
Hypothyroidism	3.4	1.7
Mucinosis	12.6	10.3
IgA deficiency	NE	8.6
Idiopathic seborrhea	4.2	5.2
Pemphigus foliaceus	1.7	0
Possibly immune mediated	0	3.4
Miscellaneous contagious diseases	1.7	3.4

*Unpublished review by Rosenkrantz and Griffin.
†Miller, W. H., Wellington, J. R., and Scott, D. W.: Dermatologic disorders of the Chinese Shar-Pei: A retrospective analysis of 58 cases (1981 to 1989). J.A.V.M.A. (in press).
‡All three allergic diseases grouped.
§Restricted diets maintained for 3 weeks.
N, total number of cases with skin disease in specific review; NE, cases not examined for this disease.

ALLERGIC DISEASES

In one study, 67.2% of Shar peis with skin disease were felt to have some type of allergic dermatitis, and in 44.8%, the allergy was associated with folliculitis. The relative risk factor for atopy was higher than that for any other breed (Miller et al., 1990). Our study found allergic dermatitis in 71.4% of the Shar peis. Atopy was the most common disease in 66.4%. Food allergy was present in 15.1% of the Shar peis and the only allergic disease in 4.7%. Food allergy was present as an intercurrent condition in 16.5% of the atopic dogs. Flea allergy is considered the most common allergic skin disease but was diagnosed in 20.2% of the Shar peis seen at our clinic and was the only diagnosis in less than 1%. The same clinic finds flea allergy in 60% of all atopic dogs, but only 29% of atopic Shar peis had a concurrent immediate flea allergy.

The diagnosis of allergic dermatitis may be tentatively made by the history and physical examination findings. Pruritus with no rash or with erythematous papules is classically seen. Nonseasonal pruritus is common, and therefore the major differential is usually sarcoptic mange. Greater than 25% of the allergic dogs have at least two or three types of allergy. For the most effective management it is important to try and identify which allergies are present.

Atopic Disease

Atopic disease is the most common skin disease in the Shar pei and usually presents with pruritus. Affected dogs may have no lesions or erythematous macules and patches. The majority present with folliculitis. The face, paws, flexor elbows, axilla, and flankfold are most commonly affected. Otitis externa is common and, in many Shar peis, is often complicated by the presence of stenotic ear canals. Interdigital swelling and erythema or hyperpigmentation is common. Chronic cases often develop hyperpigmented, lichenified plaques in the flankfolds and axilla.

519

The age of onset is different from what is normally reported for atopic disease. Thirty-seven percent of atopic Shar peis develop disease by 6 months, 82.3% by 1 year of age.

The tendency to spontaneously outgrow clinical atopic disease is described by many breeders. The incidence of this is not reported by breeders or in the literature. In one placebo controlled study on hyposensitization of atopic dogs, 21% of the placebo adjuvant treated group did improve by greater than 50% (Willemse et al., 1984). The effect of the adjuvant is unknown, but this study indicates that at the most, 21% of atopic dogs may improve on their own.

Atopic disease is best identified by intradermal testing with aqueous allergens (Halliwell and Gorman, 1989; Reedy and Miller, 1989). *In vitro* tests may be used but are not the optimum approach owing to false-positive results (Griffin, 1989). Other pruritic diseases must be ruled out prior to performing *in vitro* allergy tests. Favorable results are achievable with hyposensitization based on *in vitro* test results. Therefore this testing and treatment is preferred to lifelong glucocorticoid therapy.

Food Allergy

Food allergy frequently may not be differentiated clinically from atopic disease. If the pruritus is seasonal, food allergy will not be the only disease present. The presence of primary lesions that are not pyoderma makes food allergy more suspect in allergic cases. Food allergy is best identified by feeding a restricted diet followed by provocative exposure (see this volume, p. 513). The diet used should have completely different ingredients from the previous dog food. Homecooked diets are preferred. The belief that food allergy is common in the Shar pei has prompted many breeders to recommend lamb- and rice-based diets to new owners. Lamb and rice may be allergenic, so in these cases, a different diet such as potatoes and beans, fish, or tofu may be used. The majority of food allergic Shar peis have another allergic disease and therefore may show only partial improvement with the new diet. It is important for clients to grade pruritus. A food allergy case not only improves with the new diet but becomes more pruritic when exposed to the original diet. Provocative exposure is necessary to confirm food allergy. In cases where clients will not homecook a diet, or once a food allergy has been confirmed, limited-ingredient commercial diets may be used.

The feeding of limited-ingredient, unbalanced homecooked diets in young growing puppies is a concern to many owners. In these cases, vitamins, minerals, and essential fatty acids must be added.

Here fish is preferred to vegetable proteins, or the diet test can be delayed. In other cases, Nature's Recipe Puppy Performance may be used. If the puppy previously ate a lamb diet, Protocal 4R and Science Dry DD may be tried. Again any trial with a commercial diet is not 100% effective in ruling out a food allergy.

Flea Allergy

The one allergic disease that the Shar pei is not unusually prone to is flea allergy dermatitis. Most cases occur in conjunction with atopic disease. Flea allergy will typically manifest with primary lesions consisting of macules and papules. The lesions and pruritus are most prominent in the dorsal lumbar and sacral regions though other areas may be affected.

If fleas are not controlled and flea allergy is present, these cases tend to respond poorly to nonsteroidal allergy treatments. The best diagnostic test for flea allergy is the intradermal test with aqueous flea antigen. We prefer flea antigen (Greer) at 1:1000 W/V. *In vitro* tests have very poor correlation with clinical disease and intradermal tests. If intradermal testing cannot be done, then a clinical diagnosis is preferred to *in vitro* tests. The clinical diagnosis is made by finding evidence of fleas, an erythematous papular rash, and pruritus in the dorsal lumbar and sacral regions.

Since most allergic Shar peis have multiple types of allergy, the treatment usually involves a plan consisting of multiple therapies. Antibiotics for the folliculitis, bathing programs, and supplements containing gamma linolenic acid and eicosapentaenoic acid (DVM Derm Caps) are the most common initial treatments. If fleas are present, environmental and topical flea control measures are essential. A trial with several different antihistamines is often the next step (see this volume, p. 563). In greater than 60% of the cases, these initial treatments will be ineffective and intradermal testing and hyposensitization or a hypoallergenic diet is then recommended. Following hyposensitization and dietary modification, 20 to 30% of the allergic Shar peis may require oral alternate-day glucocorticoids for long-term control. Clients should be counseled about probable relapses that may require adjustments in the therapeutic plan.

FOLLICULITIS

Folliculitis is the most common presenting dermatologic abnormality of the Chinese Shar pei. Folliculitis is inflammation of the hair follicle, not a specific diagnosis. Infection with *Staphylococcus intermedius* is the most common cause. Demodex is the next most common cause of folliculitis and dermatophytosis the next. Rare cases of noninfectious folliculitis are described in other breeds.

Folliculitis clinically presents with multiple circular alopecic areas typically ½ to 1 cm in diameter. They may coalesce, producing larger serpiginous, circinate, or archiform patches of alopecia. Classically the lesions start with erythematous papules or pustules that may raise the involved hairs above the normal surrounding haircoat. The lesions may crust, the hairs fall out, and the inflammation subsides. Shar peis with folliculitis often present with few erythematous papules, and the skin lesions look noninflammatory. Instead, scaling and hyperpigmentation are the most common lesions in the alopecic areas. The multiple areas of alopecia give an appearance that is referred to as "moth-eaten." Once the clinical diagnosis is suspected, the etiology of folliculitis must be determined.

Bacterial Folliculitis

Bacterial folliculitis is the most common folliculitis seen in Shar peis, comprising 74% of the dogs in one study (Miller et al., 1990) and 58% in our study. If pustules or papules are present, the diagnosis can be made by cytologic examination of the fluid expressed from them. Culture and sensitivity may be performed; however, staphylococcal isolation does not document disease. Many cases present without any papules or pustules. In these cases a tentative diagnosis is made by ruling out the major differentials by skin scrapings and fungal cultures. The diagnosis is confirmed with a complete response to antibiotic therapy.

Treatment for bacterial folliculitis requires systemic antibiotics appropriate for *S. intermedius* and topical therapy. Since active inflammatory lesions may not be visible, treatment must continue until obvious regrowth of hair is occurring, with no new areas of alopecia occurring for at least 1 week. A minimum of 3 weeks is usually required. Topical antimicrobial shampoos should be used at least weekly.

Bacterial folliculitis is almost always secondary to another disease. Allergic dermatitis is most common, and recurrences of bacterial folliculitis will continue until the allergic dermatitis is controlled. The other major differentials for chronic recurrent bacterial folliculitis are demodicosis, hypothyroidism, idiopathic mucinosis, and IgA deficiency syndrome.

Demodicosis

Demodectic folliculitis is a common disease in the Shar pei, with a frequency of 8.6 to 14.2%. In Miller's study, the Shar pei had the highest relative risk factor of any breed for generalized demodex. When it is not complicated with secondary pyoderma, demodectic folliculitis is usually not grossly inflammatory. In some cases, there are erythematous macules or scales. The index of suspicion for demodectic folliculitis should be increased when follicular casts or comedones are present.

The diagnosis of demodicosis is confirmed by finding the mites on skin scrapings. In other breeds with demodicosis, finding the mites is relatively easy and routine. In the Shar pei, a negative skin scraping does not conclusively rule out the diagnosis. We have seen cases that required skin biopsies to find the demodectic mites. Even after confirming the diagnosis, further skin scrapings were negative.

Treatment of generalized demodicosis in young dogs can vary from just shampoos and systemic antibiotics for secondary pyoderma to amitraz (Mitaban) therapy. Many young dogs with generalized demodicosis will spontaneously cure. According to many breeders, this seems to be especially common in the Shar pei. In support of this, we have yet to see a Shar pei that has not self-cured or been cured with amitraz therapy. In contrast to an 80% response to amitraz in other breeds, the Shar pei approaches 100%. Unfortunately, this has led some breeders to believe that generalized demodicosis in the Shar pei is not serious enough to warrant removing affected individuals from a breeding program. This should be discouraged. All dogs that require amitraz therapy should be altered or their owners strongly counseled against breeding them.

IDIOPATHIC MUCINOSIS

Idiopathic mucinosis has been identified primarily in the Shar pei (Dillberger and Altman, 1986; Rosenkrantz et al., 1987). Normal Shar peis have more dermal mucin than any other breed examined. This may relate to the genetic selection for the wrinkled, thickened skin desired by breeders.

In mammals, mucin is a component of the dermal ground substance and is composed of a variety of mucopolysaccharides, most notably hyaluronic acid. The substances function in dermal structure, support, nutrition, and mineral balance. The primary source of mucin production is thought to be the dermal fibroblast; however, small amounts may be produced by epidermal keratinocytes.

Idiopathic mucinosis may present in two clinical forms. The most common is a thickened, edematous condition, most notably involving the extremities and ventral cervical and thoracic regions. These same cases can also have intradermal vesicles present. Pruritus is not a common feature. The second form seen are cases with intradermal vesicles only. Either form may present with concurrent folliculitis and alopecia. Age at onset is variable, but most cases generally present at 4 months to 1 year of age. Although hypothyroidism has been associated with mucinosis, all the cases seen by us (15) and those in Miller's study (3) were considered or tested to be euthyroid. No sex predilection has been determined.

The diagnosis is made on history, physical examination, intradermal prick test, and skin biopsies. The intradermal prick test is performed by pricking the edematous area with the bevel of a hypodermic needle. Positive tests exude a thick, clear, sticky fluid from the puncture site. Skin biopsies can be stained for mucin with a variety of stains, but generally the mucin is so marked, it can be seen on routine hematoxylin-eosin stain.

Most cases outgrow the disease by the time they are 2 to 5 years of age. In cases where treatment is deemed desirable, immunosuppressive doses of systemic glucocorticoids may be beneficial. Prednisone (2.2 mg/kg) should be divided and given twice daily for 3 days; then once daily for 3 days; and then slowly tapered and discontinued after 1 month. For years, many breeders have complained that glucocorticoids caused decreased skin thickness and wrinkling (deflation) of their Shar peis. The glucocorticoids most likely affect the mucin production from the dermal fibroblasts. Cases that resolve on their own probably do so because of maturation and changes in dermal mucopolysaccharide composition.

IgA DEFICIENCY

Selective IgA deficiency is the most common immunodeficiency of man and has been reported in German shepherds, beagles, and Chinese Shar peis (Moroff et al., 1986; see also this volume, p. 528).

The most common signs are respiratory infections and skin disease. In the Shar pei, 30 of 39 normal dogs (76.9%) had deficient IgA levels (Moroff et al., 1986). Serum IgA levels were measured in seven dogs in which skin disease was the primary presenting problem (Miller et al., 1990), and all seven dogs were IgA deficient (less then 15 mg/dl). Four of these dogs had allergic skin disease with recurrent

folliculitis, one had a polyarthropathy, and two had a recurrent nonpruritic folliculitis. One case was also hypothyroid.

The significance of IgA deficiency is not known. Based on one report, Shar peis have a very high incidence of IgA deficiency as compared with other breeds. This may reflect what is normal for the Shar pei breed. In the one study that evaluated skin disease, 100% had deficient levels but only five (71%) had signs typical of IgA deficiency in humans. IgA deficiency may be a primary underlying problem in Shar peis with chronic skin disease. It may also be normal for this breed or secondary to the skin disease. Additional research is needed to evaluate this finding.

References and Suggested Reading

Dillberger, J. E., and Altman, N. H.: Focal mucinosis in dogs: 7 cases and review of cutaneous mucinosis of man and animals. Vet. Pathol. 23:132, 1986.
A review of disorders that have abnormal mucin deposition associated with them.
Griffin, C. E.: RAST and ELISA testing in canine atopy. *In* Kirk, R. W. (ed.): *Current Veterinary Therapy X.* Philadelphia: W. B. Saunders, 1989, p. 592.
A review of in vitro testing, including problems with these tests in making the diagnosis of atopy.
Halliwell, R. E., and Gorman, N. T. (eds.): *Veterinary Clinical Immunology.* Philadelphia: W. B. Saunders, 1989, pp. 232–247.
A chapter with in-depth discussion of skin history and hyposensitization.
Miller, W. H., Wellington, J. R., and Scott, D. W.: Dermatologic disorders of the Chinese Shar-Pei: A retrospective analysis of 58 cases (1981 to 1989) J.A.V.M.A. (in press).
A survey of Shar peis presented to a university and the dermatologic diagnoses made.
Moroff, S. D., Hurvitz, A. I., Peterson, M. E., et al.: IgA deficiency in Shar Pei dogs. Vet. Immunol. Immunopathol. 13:181, 1986.
First report describing low levels of IgA and signs associated with this in the Shar pei.
Muller, G. H., Kirk, R. W., and Scott, D. W.: *Small Animal Dermatology,* 4th ed. Philadelphia: W. B. Saunders, 1989.
Breed predisposition to dermatologic diseases are listed.
Reedy, L. M., and Miller, W. H., Jr.: *Allergic Skin Diseases of Dogs and Cats.* Philadelphia: W. B. Saunders, 1989, pp. 81–109.
Provides a complete discussion of allergy testing.
Rosenkrantz, W. S., Griffin, C. E., Walder, E. J., et al.: Idiopathic cutaneous mucinosis in a dog. Comp. Anim. Pract. 1:39, 1987.
A case report comparing mucin deposition in an abnormal Shar pei to normal Shar peis.
Willemse, A., van den Brom, W. E., and Rijnberk, A.: Effect of hyposensitization on atopic dermatitis in dogs. J.A.V.M.A. 184:1277, 1984.
A double-blind placebo controlled study that showed hyposensitization is efficacious.

TREATMENT OF SEBORRHEA IN THE AMERICAN COCKER SPANIEL

KENNETH W. KWOCHKA

Columbus, Ohio

One of the most difficult and frustrating skin diseases to manage is primary seborrhea of American cocker spaniels. The term "seborrhea" is reserved for the primary scaling disorder seen in this breed. This dermatosis appears to have a hereditary basis with certain lines of purebred cocker spaniels having a higher incidence. Seborrhea usually develops within the first 1 to 3 years of life and may stay mild or progress to a severe, uncontrollable dermatitis, sometimes resulting in a decision for euthanasia.

CLINICAL FEATURES

Seborrheic cocker spaniels have varying degrees of generalized dry, waxy, or greasy scale formation. There are usually regions of the body with more severe greasy scale, including the lips, periocular skin, ventral neck, axillae, perineum, tail, and interdigital skin. In the acute stages of the disease, these areas are alopecic, erythematous, and pruritic and have secondary pyoderma. As the condition becomes chronic, the affected sites become extremely hyperpigmented and lichenified. Some seborrheic dogs will also develop multifocal, erythematous plaques on the ventrum which are covered by thick, yellow scales and crusts (hyperkeratotic seborrheic plaques). It is common to see comedones, follicular casts, and secondary pyoderma. Most of these dogs also have a ceruminous otitis externa.

DIAGNOSIS

These clinical signs may also be seen secondary to other dermatoses. The practitioner has a difficult task to determine if primary seborrhea is present or if the signs are simply secondary to another treatable disease. Important differentials include demodicosis, scabies, cheyletiellosis, pyoderma, dermatophytosis, hypothyroidism, hyperadrenocorticism, pemphigus foliaceus, mycosis fungoides, atopy, food allergy, flea allergy, and vitamin A–responsive der-

matosis. In my practice the most important differentials are demodicosis, pyoderma, dermatophytosis, hypothyroidism, and allergy. It is also possible for more than one dermatosis to be present. I have several patients with primary seborrhea and allergic disease and primary seborrhea and hypothyroidism.

If the owner is interested in establishing a definitive diagnosis, the medical evaluation should include skin scrapings, fungal and bacterial cultures, allergy testing, hypoallergenic food trial, complete blood count (CBC), serum biochemical profile, baseline T_4 value, and skin biopsy. A definitive diagnosis of seborrhea is achieved if the results of the tests are normal or negative and the biopsy findings are suggestive of a keratinization defect. Histologic findings are characterized by orthokeratotic and parakeratotic hyperkeratosis, follicular hyperkeratosis, and dyskeratosis. The follicular abnormalities are generally more severe than changes in the surface epidermis. A superficial perivascular dermatitis with a mixed-cell infiltrate is also seen.

A more complete description of the diagnostic approach to seborrhea, including a valuable diagnostic flow chart, has been published (Kunkle, 1983).

PATHOPHYSIOLOGY

In order to establish effective treatment programs for seborrhea, much information is needed about the pathophysiology of the dermatosis. Some work has been done in cocker spaniels with primary seborrhea. The basal cell labeling indices are three to four times greater for the seborrheic epidermis, hair follicle infundibulum, and sebaceous glands, indicating that these structures are hyperproliferative (Kwochka and Rademakers, 1989). The cell renewal time for the viable epidermis is decreased from 22 to 8 days. This accelerated cell renewal results in overproduction of corneocytes and visible scale.

There is evidence that the cell proliferation abnormalities are a result of a primary epidermal cell defect. The cells remain hyperproliferative when grown in pure cell culture without dermal components (Kwochka et al., 1987). Additionally, the seborrheic epidermis remains hyperproliferative 6 weeks after being grafted onto the dermis of normal dogs (Kwochka and Smeak, 1990). Finally, both *in vivo* and *in vitro*, the total cell cycle time of the basal epidermal keratinocyte is significantly shortened in seborrheic versus normal dogs (Kwochka, unpublished data, 1990).

Cutaneous lipids and fatty acid production have also been evaluated in seborrheic dogs. A recent study reported elevated cutaneous levels of arachidonic acid in seborrheic dogs (14 of 21 dogs studied were cocker spaniels) and suggested that this might be partially responsible for epidermal hyperproliferation and inflammation (Campbell, 1990).

TREATMENT AND MANAGEMENT

Although there have been some important recent advances in our understanding of the pathophysiology and treatment of seborrhea in cocker spaniels, this is still considered a controllable and not a curable disease. However, because of these advances, our ability to more adequately control the dermatosis has improved. Several drugs or groups of drugs should be considered in the management of seborrhea. These include topical keratolytic and keratoplastic agents, fatty acids, antibiotics, topical and systemic glucocorticoids, and retinoids.

Antiseborrheic Shampoos

Topical therapy is a very important part of any program to manage seborrhea. In mild cases, topical therapy may be all that is required to control the dermatosis. Since seborrhea is usually generalized, shampoo formulations containing keratolytic and keratoplastic agents are the best alternatives for topical therapy. Degreasing agents are usually also indicated since most cocker spaniels have greasy scale.

Bathing is instituted two to three times per week until the scale, greasiness, and odor are controlled. This is followed by a maintenance program of bathing as infrequently as possible. Unfortunately, in a greasy, malodorous cocker spaniel, this may still necessitate bathing fairly often. Most of the products used to help control scale require a 10- to 15-minute contact time for adequate activity. Owners should be encouraged to actually use a watch to time the bath, not start timing until the dog is completely lathered, and continue a gentle lathering during the entire time.

Some of these cocker spaniels will have such a thick accumulation of scale and greasy exudate that bathing first with a mild detergent (Palmolive Liquid, Colgate-Palmolive; Ivory Liquid, Procter & Gamble) will allow this material to be removed before use of the more expensive antiseborrheic shampoos. Topical ceruminolytic agents such as dioctyl sodium sulfosuccinate (Clear-x Ear Cleansing Solution, DVM) are helpful when applied, 15 minutes before bathing, to focal areas of severe greasy scale such as the neck, axillae, and ventral plaques.

Antiseborrheic agents incorporated into veterinary shampoos are keratolytic, keratoplastic, or both. A keratolytic agent causes cellular damage of corneocytes, resulting in ballooning of the cells and subsequent cell shedding. Thus, the stratum corneum is softened and removed, resulting in better control of scale formation. A keratoplastic agent results in "normalization" of epidermal cell kinetics and keratinization, usually by cytostatic effects on the basal cell layer. Common antiseborrheic agents include sulfur, salicylic acid, benzoyl peroxide, coal tar, and selenium sulfide. A more complete description of the mechanisms of action and use of these agents has been published (Kwochka, 1988).

Sulfur and salicylic acid have synergistic keratolytic and keratoplastic activity and are incorporated in veterinary shampoos in approximately equal concentrations (SebaLyt, DVM; Sebolux, Allerderm/Virbac). SebaLyt also contains the antiseptic agent triclosan, which makes this product helpful when a secondary pyoderma is present. Sulfur and salicylic acid are not good degreasing agents. These shampoos may be effective in mild cases of seborrhea with minimal greasiness.

Since most seborrheic cocker spaniels have moderate to severe greasy scale formation, a keratolytic or keratoplastic agent with good degreasing activity, such as benzoyl peroxide or coal tar, is desired. Benzoyl peroxide (OxyDex, DVM; Pyoben, Allerderm/Virbac) is a good keratolytic, superior antimicrobial, and excellent degreasing agent, which is very useful in severe cases of greasy seborrhea, especially with a secondary bacterial component. Follicular flushing activity helps remove keratinous material, glandular secretions, and bacteria from plugged hair follicles. Even greater antiseborrheic activity is achieved when sulfur is added to a benzoyl peroxide shampoo formulation (Sulf-OxyDex, DVM). Benzoyl peroxide is very drying owing to its degreasing activity. This is beneficial in the typical greasy seborrheic cocker spaniel. However, a small number of these dogs may become excessively dry with chronic use of benzoyl peroxide shampoos.

Coal tar shampoos are also used for their keratoplastic and degreasing activity. However, care should be exercised when tar shampoos are used since they may be irritating, malodorous, staining, and photosensitizing, especially at the higher concentrations. Because of their potential as irritants,

I prefer to use a tar shampoo only if a sulfur-salicylic acid or benzoyl peroxide shampoo has proven to be ineffective.

Many veterinary tar shampoos are available. Most also contain sulfur and salicylic acid for enhanced keratolytic and keratoplastic activity. The primary difference between these products is the concentration of coal tar and the refinement process used. Because of the potential for irritation, it is best to start with a low concentration 2% solubilized coal tar extract shampoo (Clear Tar, Veterinary Prescription). If this is not effective, then a 3% juniper tar product with sulfur and salicylic acid is tried (LyTar, DVM). Finally, a 4% tar product (Allerseb-T, Allerderm/Virbac) may be necessary, but only for severe, recalcitrant cases of oily seborrhea. When using these higher concentrations, owners should be advised to lather the shampoo gently, rinse it off very well, watch for the development of excessive drying, and observe for signs of irritation such as "hivelike" lesions with pruritus.

Selenium sulfide is also keratolytic, keratoplastic, and degreasing. The veterinary formulations have limited usefulness because they tend to be staining, drying, and irritating, especially to mucous membranes and the scrotum. Selenium sulfide is considered in cocker spaniels with severe oily seborrhea that is nonresponsive to sulfur, salicylic acid, benzoyl peroxide, or coal tar. The human product (Selsun Blue, Abbott) should be used since it is less irritating, contains the same concentration of selenium, and is in a pleasant-scented detergent vehicle.

In general, it is best to start with a sulfur-salicylic acid shampoo for 2 to 3 weeks. If there is no response, the next choice is a benzoyl peroxide-sulfur shampoo, and finally a coal tar product. In cases that appear to be getting too dry on therapy, the benzoyl peroxide or tar product should be alternated with a sulfur-salicylic acid or hypoallergenic-moisturizing (HyLyt*efa, DVM; Allergroom, Allerderm/Virbac) shampoo, and an emollient rinse (HyLyt*efa Bath Oil Coat Conditioner, DVM; Humilac, Allerderm/Virbac) should be considered after each bath. For severe, greasy seborrhea complicated by pyoderma, alternating a benzoyl peroxide and coal tar product at each bathing is useful. It may be possible to switch from degreasing to nondegreasing shampoos after initial control of the seborrhea. Some seborrheic cocker spaniels will have dry scale on the dorsal aspect of the trunk but be greasy on other parts of the body. In such cases it is valuable to use two different shampoos at the same time, a less drying shampoo on top and a good degreasing agent on other parts of the body. Many cocker spaniels will be much easier to bathe and will have their scale controlled better if the haircoat is clipped and kept short.

Fatty Acids

Clinical signs in seborrheic cocker spaniels mimic what is seen in experimental essential fatty acid deficiency. Some dogs seem to benefit from an increased level of fatty acids in the diet. This may be due to an increased requirement at the skin level, especially the epidermis, in these dogs or to favorable modification of arachidonic acid metabolism. Such modification may result in the production of eicosanoids (prostaglandins, leukotrienes, thromboxanes) with anti-inflammatory activity and thus lead to better control of associated inflammation and pruritus and maintenance of normal epidermal integrity.

At the same time that the topical therapy program is started, dietary modifications are made. Dogs that are on dry, semimoist, or home-cooked diets are switched to a high-quality commercial canned food if the owners are agreeable to such a change. Even this modification may not be enough of a change since the actual polyunsaturated fatty acid content of most foods is not well known. There may be variability from batch to batch in the type and quality of fat added, in storage, and in chemical processing.

A polyunsaturated fatty acid supplement is added with or without a change in diet. Corn, sunflower, or safflower oil will increase dietary polyunsaturates. The current recommendation (based on good results in a recent study) is to supplement with 1.5 ml/kg, every 24 hours, PO, of sunflower oil (Campbell, 1990). A commercial fatty acid supplement (DVM Derm Caps, DVM) containing omega-6 and omega-3 fatty acids may also be used. In all cases of dietary modification and supplementation, changes should be given a minimum of 8 to 12 weeks before a determination of efficacy is made. Caloric intake may need to be reduced with high-level fatty acid supplementation, and caution should be exercised in dogs predisposed to pancreatitis.

Topical application of fatty acids (HyLyt*efa Bath Oil Coat Conditioner, DVM) sprayed onto the skin and haircoat daily for 8 to 12 weeks may also be helpful. However, few clients are willing to spray an oil preparation on an already greasy dog.

Antibiotics

The abnormalities in epidermal cell kinetics and keratinization associated with seborrhea result in altered epidermal barrier function. In many cocker spaniels this results in increased colonization and infection of the skin with coagulase-positive staphylococci. Bacterial infection is a major cause of the pruritus and inflammation associated with seborrhea. Some of the circular scaly lesions along the ventrum of seborrheic cocker spaniels are pyoderma lesions, and not hyperkeratotic seborrheic plaques. A 3- to 4-week course of antibiotics based on culture and susceptibility results along with an antibacterial shampoo (SulfOxyDex, DVM; OxyDex, DVM; Pyoben, Allerderm/Virbac) is warranted. Periodic antibiotics may be necessary until epidermal barrier function is normalized.

Seborrheic cocker spaniels may also develop secondary colonization of the skin surface with *Malassezia canis*. These are usually identified by cytologic examination of surface material collected from the ventral neck and between the toes by vigorously rubbing a wet swab over the skin surface. Slides are stained with new methylene blue or Diff-Quick (American Scientific Products) and examined with oil immersion objectives for large numbers of budding yeasts. Like staphylococci, *Malassezia canis* does not represent a primary problem but a secondary infection that may further contribute to the inflammation and pruritus associated with the seborrhea. *Malassezia canis* may be controlled with selenium sulfide or benzoyl peroxide shampoos given three times a week for a month. Ketoconazole shampoo (Nizoral Shampoo, Janssen) is now available in the United States but is expensive. Severe cases will benefit from a 4-week course of systemic ketoconazole (Nizoral, Janssen) at 10 mg/kg, every 24 hours, PO. Again, periodic treatment may be necessary if the primary seborrhea cannot be controlled and the yeast becomes a chronic recurrent problem.

Otic Preparations

One of the most frustrating conditions associated with seborrhea in cocker spaniels is ceruminous otitis externa. The ear canal is lined with sebaceous and ceruminous glands. In seborrhea the glands are hyperplastic, the barrier function of the epithelium is compromised, and the canals become greasy, inflamed, pruritic, and secondarily infected with bacteria and yeast. Ear canals may become stenotic and calcified, making medical management of the otitis virtually impossible.

During the initial examination, swabs should be used to collect exudate for cytologic examination to determine if infectious agents are present. A short course of prednisone or prednisolone at 1.0 mg/kg, every 24 hours, PO, for 7 to 10 days, is often helpful to bring the inflammation, stenosis, edema, and pruritus under control to allow easier examination and topical treatment of the canals. A ceruminolytic agent (Clear-x Ear Cleansing Solution, DVM; Pan-Otic, Adams/Norden) is necessary to adequately remove the greasy exudate from the canals. This should be used daily until the otitis is controlled. Since most seborrheic ears are initially inflamed and infected, a combination product containing an

antibiotic and a steroid (Cortisporin Otic Solution, Burroughs Wellcome; Gentocin Otic, Schering), or an antibiotic, steroid, and antifungal agent (Tresaderm, Merck) is usually employed. Aqueous preparations are chosen over creams or ointments since these ears are usually moist and greasy and are only further moistened and occluded if such formulations are used.

The ears should be re-evaluated every 2 to 3 weeks until the canals are fairly normal and cytologic evaluation shows that bacteria and yeast organisms are gone. In many cases, long-term control is achieved by use of a ceruminolytic agent periodically as needed. This is easiest to do at the time of bathing. In order to keep the canal as clean and dry as possible, a cleaning and drying agent (Epi-Otic, Allerderm/Virbac; Otic Domeboro, Dome; Oti Clens, Beecham; Panodry, Solvay) is used after the bath. In severe cases where inflammation, edema, pruritus, and a copious exudate continue to be a problem but infection has been eliminated, periodic use of a steroid otic preparation (Synotic, Syntex) is indicated as needed. Many cocker spaniels can be maintained using this fluocinolone acetonide-dimethyl sulfoxide solution once or twice a week. A topical steroid may also help control the ventral, seborrheic hyperkeratotic plaques on the body which do not respond to shampoos and antibiotics.

Many seborrheic cocker spaniels can be adequately controlled with the treatments described earlier. However, those that are most severely affected may remain scaly, greasy, inflamed, pruritic, and malodorous with multiple hyperkeratotic plaques. The two alternatives in these cases are to try systemic steroids or one of the retinoids.

Systemic Glucocorticoids

Systemic glucocorticoids at low doses may be helpful because of their ability to inhibit epidermal cell renewal, suppress sebaceous gland function, and inhibit arachidonic acid release. Prednisone or prednisolone, used at 0.5 to 1.0 mg/kg, every 48 hours, PO, may control the dermatosis with minimal side effects. However, these dogs should be monitored every 6 months for potential development of any severe side effects (iatrogenic hyperadrenocorticism, infections, diabetes mellitus, gastric ulceration, pancreatitis) since lifetime therapy will most likely be needed.

Retinoids

The term "retinoids" refers to the entire group of naturally occurring and synthetic vitamin A derivatives. Vitamin A compounds have profound effects on regulation of cell proliferation and differentiation, especially of keratinizing epithelia. Thus, they are helpful in the treatment of primary scaling disorders, including seborrhea of cocker spaniels.

A small subset of seborrheic cocker spaniels have a vitamin A–responsive dermatosis that responds to vitamin A alcohol (retinol) given at 625 to 800 IU/kg, every 24 hours, PO (Scott, 1986). Clinically, these dogs have marked follicular plugging and hyperkeratotic plaques with surface "frondlike" plugs of keratinous material from the follicles. These lesions are present on the ventral and lateral thorax and abdomen. The histologic abnormalities are very distinct and dramatic with marked orthokeratotic hyperkeratosis and severe dilation of hair follicles. Response to medication is seen within 4 weeks, with complete remission by 10 weeks. Treatment is needed for life, but retinol at this dose appears to be well tolerated in dogs without side effects. It is important to stress that this syndrome is very distinct and represents only a small portion of cocker spaniels with seborrhea. However, it is logical to try a course of retinol in those dogs with ventral hyperkeratotic plaques which do not respond well to topical therapy and antibiotics. Retinol is inexpensive in comparison to the synthetic retinoids.

Two synthetic retinoids have been used in seborrheic cocker spaniels. Isotretinoin (Accutane, Roche) has shown minimal efficacy. Recently, etretinate (Tegison, Roche) was evaluated in 15 cocker spaniels with primary seborrhea (Power and Ihrke, 1990). Dogs were treated for 4 months at a dosage of 0.75 to 1.0 mg/kg, every 24 hours, PO. All 15 dogs showed a good to excellent response with a decrease in scale, a softening and thinning of seborrheic plaques, reduced odor, and decreased pruritus. Most dogs showed some response within the first 2 months and continual improvement over the next 2 months. Some severely affected dogs were treated for 6 months. Unfortunately, etretinate did not improve the ceruminous otitis externa. Clinical signs returned on discontinuation of therapy, but response was again seen with readministration of the drug. Some dogs have been maintained over several months on alternate-day therapy.

The synthetic retinoids appear to be better tolerated in companion animals than in humans. However, animals on etretinate therapy should be monitored for dry skin, conjunctivitis, keratoconjunctivitis sicca, arthralgias, myalgias, hyperactivity, vomiting, diarrhea, and elevations in cholesterol, triglycerides, and liver enzymes. When observed, these have been mild and completely reversible. The synthetic retinoids are highly teratogenic and *should not be used in breeding animals*. With etretinate there may be a prolonged period of time after discontinuation of therapy before breeding can

be safely undertaken. Clients must also be warned about the potential risk from accidental human ingestion. With chronic usage, the possibility of skeletal changes must be considered. Radiographs should be taken every 6 months and evaluated for cortical hyperostosis, demineralization of long bones, and periosteal calcification. Most of these changes are asymptomatic. They have been created experimentally in dogs, but only with chronic administration of very high doses.

In spite of this early success in treating seborrheic cocker spaniels with etretinate, this retinoid is usually reserved for severe cases which do not respond to other forms of therapy. Price of the drug is a limiting factor, with treatment of the typical cocker spaniel costing approximately $1.50 per day. With time, this cost will be significantly decreased as new analogs are produced for human use and current human products are licensed for use in dogs.

References and Suggested Reading

Campbell, K. L.: Effects of oral sunflower oil on serum and cutaneous fatty acids in seborrheic dogs. *In Sixth Proceedings*, Annual Membership Meeting, Am. Acad. Vet. Dermatol. Am. Coll. Vet. Dermatol., 1990, p. 44.
Results of treatment with sunflower oil in 21 dogs with seborrhea.
Kunkle, G. A.: Managing canine seborrhea. *In* Kirk, R. W. (ed.): *Current Veterinary Therapy VIII*. Philadelphia: W. B. Saunders, 1983, p. 518.
A review of the clinical signs, differential diagnosis, diagnostic approach, and treatment of seborrhea with special attention to the Doberman pinscher, Irish setter, and cocker spaniel.
Kwochka, K. W.: Rational shampoo therapy in veterinary dermatology. *In* Campfield, W. W. (ed): *Proceedings of The 11th Annual Kal Kan Symposium for the Treatment of Small Animal Diseases*. Vernon, CA: Kal Kan Foods, 1988, p. 87.
A review of all aspects of shampoo therapy in veterinary dermatology, including general principles, mechanisms of action of active ingredients, specific products, and indications for use.
Kwochka, K. W., and Rademakers, A. M.: Cell proliferation kinetics of epidermis, hair follicles, and sebaceous glands of cocker spaniels with idiopathic seborrhea. Am. J. Vet. Res. 50:1918, 1989.
Results of a study comparing cutaneous cell proliferation rates between normal and seborrheic cocker spaniels.
Kwochka, K. W., Rademakers, A. M., Schultz, K. T., et al.: Development and characterization of an *in vitro* cell culture system for the canine epidermis. *In Third Proceedings*, Annual Membership Meeting, Am. Acad. Vet. Dermatol. Am. Coll. Vet. Dermatol., 1987, p. 9.
Results of epidermal cell growth characteristics for normal and seborrheic canine keratinocytes grown in a cell culture system.
Kwochka, K. W., and Smeak, D. D.: The cellular defect in idiopathic seborrhoea of cocker spaniels. *In* Von Tscharner, C., and Halliwell, R. E. W. (eds.): *Advances in Veterinary Dermatology*, Vol. 1. London: Bailliere Tindall, 1990, p. 265.
Histologic and epidermal cell kinetic results of epidermal-dermal recombinant grafting in normal beagles and seborrheic cocker spaniels.
Power, H. T., and Ihrke, P. J.: Synthetic retinoids in veterinary dermatology. Vet. Clin. North Am. Sm. Anim. Pract. 20:1525, 1990.
A review of vitamin A metabolism, pharmacokinetics, clinical use, and toxicity, including results of treatment of seborrheic cocker spaniels with etretinate.
Scott, D. W.: Vitamin A-responsive dermatosis in the cocker spaniel. J. Am. Anim. Hosp. Assoc. 22:125, 1986.
Results of treatment with vitamin A alcohol (retinol) in five cocker spaniels with a seborrheic syndrome.

IgA DEFICIENCY AND
SKIN DISORDERS

KAREN L. CAMPBELL
Urbana, Illinois

and PETER J. FELSBURG
West Lafayette, Indiana

FUNCTIONS OF IgA

The mucosal surfaces are in direct contact with the external environment and are, therefore, a major site of antigenic exposure. The external secretions that bathe these surfaces form a unique immunologic mechanism involved in host defense—the mucosal immune system. The organ systems involved in the mucosal immune systems include the gastrointestinal tract, respiratory tract, urogenital tract, salivary glands, lacrimal glands, mammary glands, and the skin.

There are both immune and nonimmune defense mechanisms functioning to prevent infection at the mucosal surfaces. The nonimmunologic host protective mechanisms of the mucosal organs are related to the physical properties of the individual organs. For example, the skin acts as a physical barrier to invading microorganisms. The skin also has a dense and stable resident bacterial flora whose composition is regulated by a number of factors such as desquamation, desiccation, and a relatively low pH that is due, in part, to the presence of fatty acids in the sebum. If any of these environmental factors is altered, the composition of the skin flora is disturbed, its protective properties reduced, and colonization of pathogens may occur. The resident flora of the gastrointestinal tract is essential not only for the control of potential pathogens but also for digestion. If the natural flora of the intestine is altered (e.g., antibiotic therapy), dietary disturbances result, and the overgrowth of potential pathogens may occur. The flushing action of saliva and intestinal motility are also important physical features in preventing bacterial colonization. The mucociliary tree of the upper respiratory tract is an important physical factor in regulating colonization of the respiratory tract with potential pathogens. The flushing action of the urogenital system and mammary glands is important in limiting bacterial growth in these organs.

The primary immune effector molecule of the mucosal immune system is a special form of IgA called secretory IgA (SIgA).

IgA found in the serum is primarily a monomer or a single IgA molecule. IgA found in secretions consists of a dimer of IgA, two IgA molecules bound together, surrounded by another molecule referred to as secretory component or secretory piece. The secretory component is thought to increase the stability of SIgA, making it less susceptible to digestion by the various proteolytic enzymes found in the various secretions of the organs comprising the mucosal immune system. SIgA is produced by plasma cells residing in the mucosa of the mucosal organs. In the skin, IgA is found in the apocrine sweat glands, suggesting that it functions as a cutaneous secretory immunoglobulin (Garthwaite, 1983).

Since SIgA is found in the secretions covering the mucosal surfaces, it provides the first line of defense against infectious disease agents, primarily toxins, bacteria, and viruses. SIgA is capable of neutralizing toxins before they bind to their cellular receptors. The antibacterial activity of SIgA relates to its ability to bind antigenic determinants on the bacteria, thereby inhibiting adherence and colonization of the bacteria. SIgA binds to viruses to prevent adherence. If the virus cannot adhere to the epithelial surface, infection is prevented. SIgA has also been shown to inhibit absorption of macromolecular antigens such as potential allergens. In summary, the interaction of SIgA with the various nonimmunologic defense mechanisms is important in preventing infection of the mucosal organs.

A deficiency of IgA results in the failure to mount a local immune response to viruses and bacteria and predisposes the individual to infections. IgA-deficient individuals also have an increased absorption of antigens, predisposing them to the potential development of allergies and other immune-mediated diseases.

CLINICAL SIGNS ASSOCIATED WITH IgA DEFICIENCY

IgA deficiency (IgAd) is the most common primary immunodeficiency in man. The prevalence of

IgAd is approximately 1:700 in western populations. IgAd in man and the dog actually represents a heterogeneous group of diseases consisting of three major clinical syndromes: severe IgAd defined by an undetectable IgA level measured by radial immunodiffusion (usually less than 5 to less than 10 mg/dl); partial IgAd, defined by a detectable IgA level but less than two standard deviations of the mean for age-matched individuals; and transient IgAd, defined by undetectable or low IgA levels with subsequent development of normal IgA concentrations.

Although IgAd is often found among apparently healthy people and dogs, reduced levels of IgA predispose to a variety of diseases, including recurrent infections, particularly upper respiratory infections, atopy, and autoimmune disease. In man, approximately 50% of the symptomatic IgAd patients present with recurrent infections, 25% with autoimmune disease, and 20% with atopy. Approximately 7% of IgAd people have recurrent or chronic skin infections. The onset of clinical signs associated with IgA deficiency is often early childhood. Up to 60% of atopic IgA-deficient children have a history of nonspecific dermatitis or eczema. The incidence of IgA deficiency in humans with atopy is 6 to 8%, which is much higher than the incidence in the general population (0.2%). IgA-deficient humans also have an increased incidence of rheumatoid arthritis, systemic lupus erythematosus, autoimmune thyroiditis, dermatomyositis, autoimmune hemolytic anemia, Sjörgen's syndrome, and chronic active heptatis. Thirty-five per cent of IgA-deficient humans are positive for rheumatoid factor, and 7% have a positive antinuclear antibody titer.

The limited number of reports in man, and our work in the dog, suggests that individuals with parital IgAd or transient IgAd have the same clinical problems with respiratory and skin infections, atopy, and autoimmune disease as do individuals with severe IgAd (see this volume, p. 448).

A perplexing question that remains to be answered is why many IgAd individuals show no clinical signs of illness at the time of diagnosis. Low serum IgA levels have been reported in clinically normal German shepherd and Shar pei dogs. Recent studies have suggested that IgAd alone in patients with severe IgAd is sufficient to cause manifestation of clinical disease, whereas in partially IgAd individuals, a concomitant IgG subclass deficiency is required to predispose to clinical disease. Humans with IgA deficiency frequently have increased levels of IgM-secreting plasma cells in the lamina propia of their intestines and increased levels of IgM in gastrointestinal secretions.

Although upper respiratory infections are the predominant infections observed in human IgAd patients, chronic or recurrent skin infections appear to be the predominant infection in the dog.

A large commercial beagle colony with a 30% incidence of IgAd in the breeding dogs has a high incidence of recurrent *Bordetella bronchiseptica* upper respiratory tract infections, canine parainfluenza virus upper respiratory tract infections, and parvovirus enteritis, despite an intensive preventive vaccination program. Two per cent of the adult dogs in the colony have chronic/recurrent dermatitis, and 1% have chronic/recurrent otitis externa. Puppies from dams with low serum IgA levels have an increased incidence of coughing, sneezing, and nasal discharge (25.3% affected with signs of upper respiratory tract infections), conjunctivitis (13.4% affected), diarrhea (1.7% affected), otitis externa (1.4% affected), and dermatitis (0.6% affected) in the first 18 weeks of life. Within this kennel, puppies born to healthy IgAd dams had a 3.5 times increased relative risk of developing upper respiratory tract infections compared with puppies born of dams with normal serum IgA concentrations. Puppies born to dams with low levels of IgA receive little IgA in colostrum, and the lack of IgA predisposes them to infections early in life. Puppies sired by dogs with low IgA levels show an increased incidence of infections after 10 weeks of age, suggesting that genetic factors are also involved (Felsburg et al., 1985; Glickman et al., 1988; Shofer et al., 1990).

Seven of ten dogs with chronic/recurrent dermatitis in the above colony were tested and found to be deficient in serum IgA concentrations. Five of these ten beagle dogs were also positive for rheumatoid factor. Two Shar pei dogs with IgAd and chronic sinopulmonary disease have been reported. One of these Shar pei dogs also had an atopic-like dermatitis. It was hypothesized that the high incidence of atopy and food allergy in Shar pei dogs may be associated with the high incidence of IgA deficiency in the breed.

Forty dogs were identified as being deficient in IgA based on serum immunoglobulin quantitation at the University of Illinois from 1986 to 1990. Affected breeds included the cocker spaniel (8), Shar pei (5), Doberman pinscher (4), German shepherd (4), miniature schnauzer (3), miniature dachshund (3), Akita (2), Yorkshire terrier (1), Welsh corgi (1), Newfoundland (1), West Highland white terrier (1), Keeshond (1), Irish setter (1), Irish wolfhound (1), Wheaten terrier (1), Old English sheepdog (1), and mixed breed dogs (2). Each of the 40 dogs had been brought to the Veterinary Medical Teaching Hospital for evaluation of chronic skin diseases. Diagnoses made for these animals included chronic/recurrent staphylococcal pyoderma (12), atopy with secondary staphylococcal pyoderma (14), atopy and food allergy with secondary staphylococcal pyoderma (1), food allergy with secondary staphylococcal pyoderma (2), demodicosis with secondary staphylococcal pyoderma (3), bullous pemphigoid (1), chronic/recurrent otitis externa (8), chronic staphylococcal pyoderma and chronic bronchitis (1), chronic staphylococcal pyoderma and chronic *Escherichia coli* urinary tract infection (1) and hypothyroidism (7). No age or sex predilection was apparent.

Over a 2-year period, six partially IgAd dogs in our breeding colony of IgAd dogs developed a nonspecific dermatitis. Three of the six dogs' skin tested positive to several environmental allergens, suggesting these dogs developed an atopic dermatitis. The strong association of IgAd with atopic dermatitis in the dog is more marked than that in man, probably owing to the fact that atopy in man is primarily manifested by respiratory signs and in the dog by dermatologic signs.

In a recent study of a large population of dogs with a history of recurrent or chronic skin infections, we found 70% of the dogs to be IgA deficient. We have also recently associated IgAd with a systemic, necrotizing vasculitis in the dog.

IMMUNOPATHOGENESIS OF IgA DEFICIENCY

Although various clinical immunologic abnormalities have been well documented in IgAd, the basic underlying immunologic defect in IgAd still remains to be determined.

The defect may be intrinsic to the IgA B lymphocytes or regulatory T lymphocytes, since normal production of IgA is highly T-cell dependent. Although IgAd individuals appear to have normal numbers of IgA B cells, 89% of these IgA B cells also express IgM on their surface, similar to that of newborns. Normal adult IgA B cells express IgA only on their surface. This suggests the presence of an "immature IgA B cell" which has been arrested at an early stage of its maturation.

The clinical manifestations of selective IgAd are heterogeneous, suggesting there may be several subgroups with differing immunologic responsiveness. Indeed, studies of humans with IgAd have demonstrated a heterogeneity of immunologic defects, including B-cell defects. Functional studies using various *in vitro* techniques have reported defects intrinsic to the IgA B cell, defective helper T-cell function, excessive IgA-specific suppressor T-cell activity, anti-IgA antibodies, and a combination of B- and T-cell defects. Probably the most current hypothesis is that IgAd is a manifestation of a regulatory T-cell defect that affects only the IgA B cell.

Dogs with IgAd have normal numbers of peripheral B and T lymphocytes, normal *in vitro* lymphocyte blastogenic responses to mitogenic stimulation, and normal primary and secondary IgM and IgG humoral responses following immunization. In several IgAd dogs, a defect in the maturation and terminal differentiation of IgA B cells into IgA-secreting plasma cells has been identified. Following *in vitro* polyclonal activation with pokeweed mitogen, the peripheral blood lymphocytes from these dogs generate normal numbers of IgG- and IgM-secreting plasma cells; however, few, if any, IgA-secreting plasma cells are found.

Increased levels of IgG are frequently present in the serum of humans and dogs with IgA deficiency. This may be due to increased penetration of antigens that are restricted to mucosal surfaces in normal individuals. The elevated levels of IgG could also be a result of an underlying immunologic regulatory defect.

The association of IgAd with autoimmune disease and atopic disease may be due to increased absorption of foreign antigens across the mucosal surface that cross-react with self-antigens or that stimulate IgE production, resulting in the production of autoantibodies or atopy, respectively.

Severe neutrophilic chemotactic defects have been found in 10 of 12 humans with selective IgAd. Hypotheses for the relationship between the chemotactic defects and the IgAd include a common abnormality affecting microtubules or microfilaments or exaggerated T suppressor cell activity affecting both immunoglobulin production and neutrophil chemotactic function. Defects in neutrophil chemotaxis predispose individuals to cutaneous infections. Neutrophil chemotactic defects have been reported in dogs with recurrent staphylococcal pyoderma; however, the serum immunoglobulin levels in these dogs were not reported.

Familial aggregation in humans and dogs suggests a genetic basis for IgAd. Hypothesized patterns of inheritance in humans include autosomal recessive, autosomal dominant with low penetrance, multifactorial, and polygenic. There is a weak association of human leukocyte antigens A, B, C, and DR with IgAd; this association is usually in individuals with coexisting autoimmune disease, diabetes mellitus, or epilepsy. In humans, there is a higher association of IgAd relating mother to child than father to child. The increased transfer from mother to child may be a result of transplacental transfer of maternal anti-IgA antibodies.

The mode of inheritance of IgAd in dogs has not been reported. A familial aggregation is apparent. Four of five littermates of two IgA-deficient beagles were also IgA deficient. A breeding of two IgAd dogs produced four IgAd puppies in a litter of five. The mode of inheritance remains to be resolved.

DIAGNOSIS

Levels of serum IgA are low in all puppies. By 3 to 4 months of age, serum IgA levels have increased to levels where normal and IgAd individuals can be identified. Unlike IgM and IgG, serum IgA concentrations do not reach normal adult levels until 12 to 18 months of age. *It is imperative to evaluate a young, potentially IgAd dog with values for age-matched normal dogs.* Dogs diagnosed as IgAd before 1 year of age may, in fact, have a transient IgAd. This is an important consideration from the standpoint of a long-term prognosis. We have recently shown that 90% of dogs diagnosed as IgAd at 1 year of age or greater remain IgAd on follow-up testing 1 year later; however, approximately 20% of dogs diagnosed as IgAd prior to 1 year of age will revert to normal IgA levels between 12 to 18 months of age (transient IgAd). Dogs with transient IgAd may be predisposed to the development of allergies owing to their increased exposure to foreign antigens early in life.

The diagnosis of an IgAd in man and dogs is based upon the quantitation of serum IgA. The reason for this is that although the clinically relevant IgA that is deficient is SIgA, there is only one documented case where a diagnosis of IgAd was made based upon serum, and the patient had normal levels of SIgA. It is far easier to quantitate serum IgA than it is SIgA.

The most commonly used method of quantitating serum IgA is single radial immunodiffusion (SRID). Values obtained by SRID are highly reproducible within a laboratory. Each individual laboratory should generate its own normal values for various age groups of dogs, especially younger dogs. The normal reference range from different laboratories may vary owing to difference in buffer systems and other methodologic techniques. It should be stressed that the immunologic diagnostic criteria for the various categories of IgAd are based upon SRID values.

Recent trends favor the use of enzyme-linked immunosorbent assay (ELISA) and radioimmunoassays. These techniques are easier to perform and more sensitive than SRID. Most depend on binding of the anti–class-specific antibody to a solid ligand; the antibody reacts with immunoglobulins in the test serum. The interaction is identified by the subsequent addition of either enzyme-linked or radiolabeled anti–class-specific antibody. Normal reference ranges for canine sera using these methods must be established for various age groups.

In humans, there are no differences in normal IgA levels between the sexes, but there are differences between races. Breed differences may be present in dogs since clinically healthy adult German shepherd and Shar pei dogs have lower serum IgA levels than Irish setter and mongrel dogs.

In humans, individual immunoglobulin concentrations are considered characteristic for the person (low longitudinal variation). Over a 6-month period, weekly quantitations varied within ± 17% (2 SD)

of their mean. Greater biologic variability has been found in dogs. Beagle dogs with two quantitations taken at a 2-year interval showed a regression toward the population mean. The mean IgA concentrations of low IgA dogs increased from 17 mg/dl to 23 mg/dl; the mean of medium IgA dogs stayed constant at 70 mg/dl; and the mean of high IgA dogs decreased from 163 mg/dl to 140 mg/dl. Despite these variations, an adult dog with low IgA on one test is likely to remain IgA deficient.

MANAGEMENT OF DOGS WITH IgA DEFICIENCY

Treatment of patients with IgAd has been limited to the symptomatic treatment of the various infections, allergies, or autoimmune diseases. No specific immunotherapy exists for the treatment of the IgAd itself.

The staphylococcal pyoderma frequently found in IgAd dogs responds to conventional antibiotic therapy; however, the pyoderma frequently recurs within days to weeks of discontinuation of the antibiotic. Likewise, the otitis externa of IgAd dogs improves during conventional therapy with otic preparations and then recurs following discontinuation of the treatment.

Three dogs diagnosed with concurrent IgAd and dietary hypersensitivity at the University of Illinois showed improvement of their dermatitis (decrease in itching) following placement on a restricted diet of home-cooked lamb and rice. Eight of 14 dogs diagnosed with concurrent IgAd and atopy had a favorable response (decrease in itching) to immunotherapy using allergens selected based on intradermal skin test reactivity. Follow-up immunoglobulin quantitation has not been done for any of these cases. The allergic diseases of IgAd humans are reported as being harder to control than those of people with normal IgA levels.

There have been few reports on the usage of immunomodulating agents in the therapy of individuals with IgAd. Immunomodulating agents with the potential to enhance antibody production include levamisole, bacille Calmette-Guérin vaccine, Staphylococcal phage lysate (SPL; Delmont Laboratories, Swarthmore, PA), *Propionibacterium acnes* vaccine (Immunoregulin; Immunovet, Tampa, FL), and soluble mediators such as interleukins and interferons. Recent placebo-controlled studies have demonstrated the efficacy of SPL and *P. acnes* vaccines in the treatment of recurrent staphylococcal pyodermas in dogs. These reports did not include any reference to the immunoglobulin concentrations in the affected dogs. Six dogs with IgAd and chronic/recurrent staphylococcal pyoderma were treated at the University of Illinois with SPL (0.5 ml/dog SQ every Monday and Thursday) for a minimum of 10 weeks. The mean serum IgA levels in these dogs increased from 13.8 mg/dl (pretreatment) to 41.8 mg/dl (post-treatment). Four of the six dogs had a beneficial clinical response (regression of the pyoderma with decreased frequency of recurrence while off antibiotic therapy). Additional placebo-controlled, blind studies will be needed to document the efficacy of SPL and other immunomodulating agents in the management of skin diseases associated with IgAd in the dog.

References and Suggested Reading

Ammann, A. J., and Hong, R.: Selective IgA deficiency: Presentation of 30 cases and review of the literature. Medicine 50:223, 1971.
A review of immunologic findings and clinical symptoms associated with IgA deficiency in humans.
Becker, A. M., Janik, T. A., Smith, E. K., et al.: *Propionibacterium acnes* immunotherapy in chronic recurrent canine pyoderma. J. Vet. Int. Med. 3:26, 1989.
A randomized, double-blind, placebo-controlled study of P. acnes as an adjuvant to antibiotic therapy in 15 dogs (13 controls).
DeBoer, D. J., Moriello, K. A., Thomas, C. B., et al.: Evaluation of a commercial staphylococcal bacterin for management of idiopathic recurrent superficial pyoderma in dogs. Am. J. Vet. Res. 51:636, 1990.
A double-blind, placebo-controlled study of a commercial staphylococcal bacteria as an adjuvant to antibiotic therapy in 13 dogs (8 controls).
Felsburg, P. J., Glickman, L. T., and Jezyk, P. F.: Selective IgA deficiency in the dog. Clin. Immunol. Immunopathol. 36:297, 1985.
This study documented selective IgA deficiency in two dogs and screened littermates, offspring, and other breeding stock in a large beagle colony for immunoglobulin levels and incidence of clinical disease.
Garthwaite, G., Lloyd, D. H., and Thomsett, L. R.: Location of immunoglobulins and complement (C$_3$) at the surface and within the skin of dogs. J. Comp. Pathol. 93:185, 1983.
Results of immunofluorescence studies of skin biopsies and immunoelectrophoresis of eluted proteins from the skin of dogs are reported.
Glickman, L. T., Shofer, F. S., Payton, A. J., et al.: Survey of serum IgA, IgG, and IgM concentrations in a large beagle population in which IgA deficiency had been identified. Am. J. Vet. Res. 49:1240, 1988.
Results of immunoglobulin quantitations of 829 adult beagles in a colony with IgA deficiency are compared with those of 100 adult beagles in a control kennel with analysis of covariance for age, sex, and kennel.
Halliwell, R. E. W., and Gorman, N. T. (eds.): *Veterinary Clinical Immunology.* Philadelphia: W. B. Saunders, 1989, pp. 19, 55, 449, 504.
A review of immunology. Relevant chapters include "The immunoglobulins, structure, genetics, and function"; "Immunoglobulin quantitation and clinical interpretation"; "Diseases associated with immunodeficiency"; and "Anti-inflammatory drugs, immunosuppressive agents, and immunomodulators."
Moroff, S. D., Hurvitz, A. I., Peterson, M. E., et al.: IgA deficiency in Shar pei dogs. Vet. Immunol. Immunopathol. 13:181, 1986.
Describes the clinical history and immunologic evaluation of two Shar pei puppies with chronic infections and a population of 39 normal adult Shar pei dogs from two colonies.
Shofer, F. S., Glickman, L. T., and Payton, A. J.: Influence of parental serum immunoglobulins on morbidity and mortality of beagles and their offspring. Am. J. Vet. Res. 51:239, 1990.
A review of the incidence of disease in 5,796 beagle puppies from 856 litters whelped over a 4-month period in a beagle colony with correlations to the IgA levels in the dams and sires.
Whitbread, T. J., Batt, R. M., and Garthwaite, G.: Relative deficiency of serum IgA in the German Shepherd dog: A breed abnormality. Res. Vet. Sci. 37:350, 1984.
Compares serum immunoglobulin concentrations in 13 clinically healthy adult German shepherd dogs to those in 14 Irish setter and 13 mixed breed dogs.

ZINC-RELATED CUTANEOUS DISORDERS OF DOGS

TON WILLEMSE
Utrecht, The Netherlands

A genetic defect in the intestinal utilization of zinc has been shown in malamutes and bull terriers. In the latter, an autosomal recessive mode of inheritance has been found. Symptoms usually appear at a few months of age, and multiple dogs from the same litter are often affected (Jezyk et al., 1986; Muller et al., 1989; Mundell, 1988). Although the nature of the inheritance has not been established in Siberian huskies, zinc-related dermatosis has been presumed to be inherited in this breed also. Thoday (1989) believes that zinc-dependent skin disorders in malamutes and Siberian huskies were more common in the late 1970's and early 1980's but have disappeared almost entirely at the present time. In contrast, the disorder in bull terriers now has a much higher incidence.

High-cereal, high-soy, and corn-based diets containing increased amounts of phytates, as well as high-calcium diets, may cause decreased zinc absorption because of their binding of intestinal zinc. Excesses of other trace elements (e.g., iron, copper, cadmium, and chromium) reduce absorption by competing with zinc for absorption sites. A relative zinc deficiency may occur in dogs on nonstandardized dog foods and in fast-growing puppies of large breeds, such as Great Danes, German shepherds, and Labrador retrievers (Bremner, 1983; Muller et al., 1989).

CLINICAL FEATURES

Two clinical syndromes may be differentiated on the basis of the type of lesion.

The first group of dogs exhibits hyperkeratotic plaques with soft-feeling surface keratin at one or more sites, such as around the eyes, lips, inner sides of the ears, vulva, anus, and prepuce and on the elbows and footpads. The coat is dull and dry. These manifestations are more common in Siberian huskies, malamutes, and rapidly growing dogs and are usually noted before puberty, although they may occur first in adult dogs.

In the second group of dogs, the onset is usually at 1 to 2 months of age. Early erythema rapidly progresses to a suppurative dermatitis with crusts, scales, and alopecia. These lesions are mainly observed on the head, elbows, and footpads and around joints and are more common in bull terriers. A dull coat with a puppylike texture, seborrhea, depression, and growth retardation are common (Sanecki et al., 1981). Intestinal disturbances are rare, but lowered serum zinc concentrations are common. Acrodermatitis enteropathica in humans has similar clinical features. In humans, an inborn error of zinc metabolism has been shown, together with diminished 24-hr urinary zinc excretion and a prompt response to oral supplementation of zinc sulfate (Fine and Moschella, 1985). Because bull terriers do not fulfill these criteria (Muller et al., 1989; Mundell, 1988), the name *acrodermatitis enteropathica* should not be used for their zinc-related disease.

RELIABILITY OF DIAGNOSTIC TESTS

A preliminary diagnosis of a zinc-related cutaneous disorder in dogs is made on the basis of the history, physical examination, and histopathology of skin biopsy specimens, which reveal a hyperplastic superficial perivascular dermatitis with marked diffuse and follicular parakeratotic hyperkeratosis.

Otherwise, zinc deficiency currently is difficult to diagnose (Birnstingl et al., 1956; Patrick and Dervish, 1970). Response to therapy and relapse with withdrawal probably are the only truly acceptable evidence of zinc deficiency. Plasma and hair zinc levels are extremely difficult to interpret under conditions of mild zinc deficiency without concurrent malnutrition. Plasma and hair zinc concentrations have only a corroborative value in the diagnosis (Van den Broek and Stafford, 1988), whereas leukocyte zinc concentrations were similar in both normal and diseased animals. However, as we understand more of the pathophysiology of zinc, it is likely that more sophisticated measurements of subcellular components will allow the subdivision of zinc deficiency into that due to negative balance and that due to the absence of receptor sites, binding proteins, or transport systems (Mundell, 1988).

Zinc excretion studies performed in our institute with orally administered radiolabeled ^{65}Zn showed that some Siberian huskies with clinical features of zinc-related dermatosis had diminished intestinal absorption of zinc (65% compared with normal Siberian huskies). In addition, after intravenous administration of ^{69m}Zn, a biphasic excretion pattern was observed in normal dogs, whereas in Siberian huskies with the disease, a monophasic excretion was seen. The significance of this observation has not been elucidated so far.

In a similar study of two bull terriers with presumed acrodermatitis enteropathica, we found that intestinal zinc absorption was comparable to that of the control dogs. These findings have been confirmed in a study by Mundell (1988).

CLINICAL MANAGEMENT

Rapidly growing dogs respond promptly to oral treatment with zinc sulfate (10 mg/kg/day). Other dietary imbalances should be corrected. In other dogs with a suspected zinc-related dermatosis, the response to oral zinc is unpredictable. In some dogs, treatment with zinc sulfate or zinc methionine (Zinpro, Norden; 2 mg/kg PO of elemental zinc daily divided every 12 hr) is effective, whereas in others no beneficial effect is noted. In the latter group, weekly administration of zinc sulfate* (10 to 15 mg/kg IV, diluted 1:1 with saline) for at least 4 weeks may be effective. In the majority of dogs treated in this way, maintenance therapy with an interval between 1 and 6 months is required. Concurrent seborrhea should be treated separately.

In bull terriers with zinc-related dermatosis, supplementation of zinc in any form has been shown to be of no value. Almost all of these dogs die before 2 years of age as the result of a severe bronchopneumonia and immunologic incompetence, and not even a temporary beneficial effect has been observed.

Breeding should be discouraged in affected malamutes, Siberian huskies, and bull terriers because of the hereditary nature of the disease. Related siblings and parents of affected bull terriers should also not be used for breeding, because two thirds may be carriers.

References and Suggested Reading

Birnstingl, M., Stone, B., and Richards, V.: Excretion of radioactive zinc in bile, pancreatic, and duodenal secretions of the dog. Am. J. Physiol. 186:377, 1956.
   A study of intestinal zinc excretion in dogs.

Editor's Note: The zinc sulfate used by Dr. Willemse contains 50 mg of zinc sulfate per milliliter, which is equivalent to approximately 0.2 mg elemental zinc per milliliter. The injection should be given very slowly. Panting for 1 to 2 min has been the only observed side effect.

Bremner, I.: The role of metallothionine in the metabolism of copper and zinc. Ann. Rep. Stud. Anim. Nutr. All. Sci. 39:13, 1983.
    A review of carrier substances in zinc and copper metabolism.
Fine, J. D., and Moschella, S. L.: Diseases of nutrition and metabolism. *In* Moschella, S. L., and Hurley, H. J. (eds.): *Dermatology.* Philadelphia: W. B. Saunders, 1985, p. 1422.
    A review of the etiology, pathology, clinical manifestations, and treatment of acrodermatitis enteropathica in humans.
Jezyk, P. F., Haskins, M. E., MacKay-Smith, W. E., et al.: Lethal acrodermatitis in bull terriers. J.A.V.M.A. 8:833, 1986.
    The first report about lethal acrodermatitis in dogs.
Muller, G. H., Kirk, R. W., and Scott, D. W.: *Small Animal Dermatology III.* Philadelphia: W. B. Saunders, 1989, p. 801.
    A review of zinc-responsive dermatosis in dogs.
Mundell, A. C.: Mineral analysis in bull terriers with lethal acrodermatitis. Proc. Am. Acad. Vet. Dermatol. Washington, DC, 1988, p. 22.

Results of kidney and liver mineral analysis and zinc absorption tests in bull terriers with presumed acrodermatitis enteropathica.
Patrick, J., and Dervish, C.: Leukocyte zinc in the assessment of zinc status. Crit. Rev. Clin. Lab. Sci. 20:95, 1970.
    A review of the value of leukocyte zinc determination in zinc deficiency.
Sanecki, R. K., Corbin, J. E., and Forbes, R. M.: Tissue changes in dogs fed a zinc-deficient ration. Am. J. Vet. Res. 43:1642, 1981.
    A report on poor wound healing and growth retardation in zinc-deficient dogs.
Thoday, K. L.: Diet-related zinc-responsive skin disease in dogs: A dying dermatosis? J. Small Anim. Pract. 30:213, 1989.
    A critical review of the incidence of diet-related zinc-dependent cutaneous disease in dogs.
Van den Broek, A. H. M., and Stafford, W. L.: Diagnostic value of zinc concentrations in serum, leukocytes and hair of dogs with zinc-responsive dermatosis. Res. Vet. Sci. 44:41, 1988.
    A study of diagnostic tests for canine zinc-responsive dermatosis.

SEBACEOUS ADENITIS

EDMUND J. ROSSER, Jr.

East Lansing, Michigan

Sebaceous adenitis is an inflammatory disease process directed against the sebaceous glands of the skin. It is most commonly recognized in standard poodles, Akitas, Samoyeds, and Vizslas (Griffin, 1988; Muller et al., 1989; Rosser, in press; Rosser et al., 1987; Rosser and Sams, 1991). In the United States, an increased incidence of this condition is noted in standard poodles. This observation has led to test breeding studies to attempt to determine the mode of inheritance of the disease in standard poodles. The etiology and pathogenesis of sebaceous adenitis are currently unknown. Speculations on the pathophysiology include the following: (1) the sebaceous gland destruction is a developmental and genetically inherited defect; (2) the sebaceous gland destruction is an immune-mediated or autoimmune disease directed against a component of sebaceous glands; (3) the initial defect is a keratinization abnormality with subsequent obstruction of the sebaceous duct resulting in sebaceous adenitis; and (4) the sebaceous adenitis and keratinization abnormality are the result of an abnormality in lipid metabolism affecting keratinization and the production of sebum (Rosser et al., 1987; Scott, 1986).

CLINICAL FEATURES

Sebaceous adenitis occurs primarily in young adult and middle-aged dogs, with no apparent sex predisposition. The disease can present in one of two forms, with differences in the clinical presentation and histologic changes observed in each type.

The first form occurs in long-coated breeds of dogs, the standard poodle being the most closely studied (Rosser et al., 1987). Similar findings have been observed in the Akita and Samoyed, but these breeds should be more closely examined. Sebaceous adenitis in standard poodles was first reported only in black and apricot colors but has now been recognized in all color variants. The first signs noted are a symmetric and partial alopecia with excess scaling and dull, brittle hairs. Lesions are most often observed along the dorsal midline. Affected areas may include the dorsal planum of the nose, top of the head, dorsal neck and trunk, tail, and pinnae. In the early stages of the disease, patients are usually nonpruritic, and there is no complaint of an offensive odor. In some instances, the disease never progresses beyond this stage. In instances in which the disease does progress, tightly adherent silver-white scales develop around hair shafts (follicular casts), often forming small tufts of matted hair. At this stage, a dog is predisposed to the development of a secondary bacterial folliculitis and subsequent pruritus and malodor. Additionally, the clinical course may have a cyclic nature with periods of spontaneous improvement or worsening independently of treatment. Some of the dogs may have concurrent idiopathic epilepsy (Powers, H., personal communication, 1990). The condition in Akitas tends to be the more severe form of the disease with a chronic secondary bacterial folliculitis. These dogs may show signs of systemic illness.

The second form of sebaceous adenitis occurs in short-coated breeds of dogs, with Vizslas seemingly predisposed. The first signs noted are a moth-eaten to diffuse alopecia with mild scaling that may affect the trunk, head, and ears. This form is usually nonpruritic, and the development of a secondary bacterial folliculitis is rare.

A case of a granulomatous sebaceous adenitis has been described in a cat (Scott, 1989). The cat presented with a nonpruritic skin disease with multiple annular alopecic and hyperkeratotic lesions involving the trunk, neck, and head. Results of tests to demonstrate a bacterial or fungal etiology were negative. Various treatments attempted were ineffective, and the dermatosis remained stable while being evaluated for 1½ years.

DIAGNOSIS

The breed affected, the historic development of the problem, and the physical findings are what lead a clinician to suspect sebaceous adenitis. The diagnosis is confirmed by the histopathologic examination of several skin biopsy samples representative of the different degrees of severity noted on physical examination. Sites selected for biopsy should include clinically normal skin, mildly affected areas, and severely affected areas. The most common histologic finding is a nodular granulomatous to pyogranulomatous inflammatory reaction at the level of the sebaceous glands. Results of special stains and cultures to examine for evidence of bacterial or fungal agents are usually negative. The exception is noted when a secondary bacterial folliculitis has developed, often due to *Staphylococcus intermedius*. In long-coated breeds, a moderate to marked orthokeratotic hyperkeratosis and keratinous follicular cast formation are noted. In short-coated breeds, the hyperkeratotic changes are mild or absent. The advanced stages of the disease are marked by a complete loss of the sebaceous glands, which are replaced by fibrotic tissue. On rare occasions, the entire hair follicle and adnexal structures may be destroyed. In cats with sebaceous adenitis, the histopathologic examination of skin biopsy specimens reveals a pyogranulomatous perifolliculitis with loss of the sebaceous glands (Scott, 1989).

TREATMENT AND MANAGEMENT

Long-term management of sebaceous adenitis can be a frustrating experience for owners and veterinarians because the response to therapy varies depending on the severity of the disease at the time of diagnosis as well as the lack of a consistent response to any single treatment regimen. This problem has led to several treatment recommendations and much confusion about which treatments should be tried. For this reason, I recommend a systematic approach to the treatment of sebaceous adenitis in dogs.

The goal of therapy should be to remove the excess scales, improve the luster of the haircoat, and regrow hair whenever possible (in standard poodles, the hair regrowth is usually straight rather than curled). When response to treatment is observed, some level of maintenance therapy is usually required to control the disease. In severe or chronic cases, when the sebaceous glands have been completely lost, the prognosis for accomplishing these goals is guarded to poor. In mildly affected dogs, regular use of antiseborrheic shampoos, conditioners, emollients, and essential fatty acid dietary supplements may be effective. If the response is inadequate, then two other treatments may be considered. The first is the use of a 50 to 75% mixture of propylene glycol and water applied once daily as a spray to the affected areas (Griffin, 1988). The propylene glycol acts a hygroscopic lipid solvent that penetrates the horny layer and increases water content. The second is the use of essential fatty acids orally at high doses (Marshall and Williams, 1990; Powers, H., personal communication, 1990). One protocol uses the following empiric dosing regimen: essential fatty acid dietary supplement (Derm Caps ES, Dermatologics for Veterinary Medicine; one capsule PO every 12 hr) and evening primrose oil (EPO, Efamol, 500 mg PO every 12 hr). Occasionally observed side effects include vomiting, diarrhea, and flatulence. These treatments may also be tried for moderate or severely affected patients. When these treatments have been ineffective, two other treatment protocols may be considered. The first treatment (Stewart et al., 1991) is the use of the retinoid isotretinoin (Accutane, Roche), 1 mg/kg PO every 12 hr for 1 month (see *CVT X*, p. 553). If improvement is noted, the dosage should be reduced to 1 mg/kg PO every 24 hr for another month. If improvement continues, the long-term goal is to control the disease with either 1 mg/kg PO every 48 hr or 0.5 mg/kg PO every 24 hr. The second treatment (Carothers et al., 1991) is the use of cyclosporine (Sandimmune, Sandoz), 5 mg/kg PO every 12 hr (see *CVT X*, p. 570).

This condition appears to be relatively refractory to the beneficial effects of either anti-inflammatory or immunosuppressive doses of corticosteroids. In cases in which a secondary bacterial folliculitis is present, the treatment should include the use of an appropriate systemic antibiotic along with a keratolytic, antibacterial, and follicular flushing shampoo (Sulf Oxydex, Dermatologics for Veterinary Medicine). Of the predisposed breeds discussed, the Akita appears to the most refractory to successful treatment (Powers, H., personal communication, 1990).

References and Suggested Reading

Carothers, M. A., Kwochka, K. W., and Rojko, J. L.: Cyclosporine responsive granulomatous sebaceous adenitis in a dog (abstract). Proc. Am. Acad. Vet. Dermatol. Am. Coll. Vet. Dermatol. Annual Meeting, 1991.

Griffin, C. E.: Common dermatoses of the Akita, Shar Pei and chow chow. Am. Acad. Vet. Dermatol. Annual Meeting, Washington D.C., 1988, p. 31.

Marshall, C., and Williams, J.: Re-establishment of hair growth, skin pliability and apparent resistance to bacterial infection after dosing fish oil in a dog with sebaceous adenitis. In von Tscharner, C., and Halliwell, R. E. W. (eds): Advances in Veterinary Dermatology, vol 1. London: Baillière Tindall, 1990, p. 446.

Muller, G. H., Kirk, R. W., and Scott, D. W.: Small Animal Dermatology, 4th ed. Philadelphia: W. B. Saunders, 1989.

Rosser, E. J.: Sebaceous adenitis. In Griffin, C. E., MacDonald, J. M., and Kwochka, K. W. (eds.): Current Veterinary Dermatology. St. Louis: C. V. Mosby (in press).

Rosser, E. J., and Sams, A. W.: Scaling dermatoses. In Allen, D. G. (ed.): Small Animal Medicine. Philadelphia: J. B. Lippincott, 1991, p. 679.

Rosser, E. J., Dunstan, R. W., Breen, P. T., et al.: Sebaceous adenitis with hyperkeratosis in the standard poodle: A discussion of 10 cases. J. Am. Anim. Hosp. Assoc. 23:341, 1987.

Scott, D. W.: Granulomatous sebaceous adenitis in dogs. J. Am. Anim. Hosp. Assoc. 22:631, 1986.

Scott, D. W.: Adenite sebacee pyogranulomateuse sterile chez un chat. Point. Vet. 21:107, 1989.

Stewart, L. J., White, S. D., and Carpenter, J. L.: Isotretinoin in the treatment of sebaceous adenitis in two Vizslas. J. Am. Anim. Hosp. Assoc. 27:65, 1991.

STERILE PYOGRANULOMATOUS AND GRANULOMATOUS DISORDERS OF DOGS AND CATS

RADA PANIĆ

Ithaca, New York

Most granulomatous or pyogranulomatous skin lesions appear clinically as nodules. The skin lesions may be solitary or multiple, localized or generalized, and appear as papules, nodules, or plaques. The lesions may be alopecic or haired and may or may not be ulcerated. Lesions can be firm to fluctuant in consistency and vary in size from a few millimeters to several centimeters in diameter. Clinically, it can be difficult to differentiate these lesions from certain tumors. Numerous infectious and noninfectious agents have been implicated in the induction of granulomatous inflammation. Diagnostic procedures to define the etiologic agent should include bacterial and fungal cultures and skin biopsies in all cases. Noninfectious causes include endogenous foreign bodies (hair, sebum, keratin, calcium, urates) and exogenous substances (e.g., plant material, sutures, silica, beryllium, embedded insect mouth parts). These materials may be visible in skin biopsy specimens. Idiopathic sterile granulomas for which no inciting factors could be found have been described in dogs and cats and are discussed subsequently.

CUTANEOUS HISTIOCYTOSIS

Cutaneous histiocytosis is a rare disorder in which cytologically normal histiocytes proliferate. The dis-order is characterized by the presence of variable numbers of dermal to subcutaneous nodules or plaques. Large lesions may be alopecic, ulcerated, and occasionally umbilicated. Affected sites have included the face, neck, and the trunk. In addition, the nasal mucosa may be involved, resulting in respiratory stridor. Histopathologic examination of skin biopsy specimens reveals nodular to diffuse dermal or subcutaneous infiltrates of morphologically normal histiocytes. Cultures, special stains, and electron microscopy do not reveal an etiologic agent.

Lesions typically wax and wane with no specific treatment. The response to prednisolone administered at 2.2 to 4.4 mg/kg/day is variable. In some dogs, no change in the lesions is seen with glucocorticoid therapy, whereas a remission can be achieved in others. Surgical excision frequently results in recurrence at excision sites or at new locations. The chronic and recurrent nature of the disease warrants a guarded prognosis.

SYSTEMIC AND MALIGNANT HISTIOCYTOSIS

Systemic and malignant histiocytosis are rare disorders that have been described most frequently in related Bernese Mountain Dogs. Dogs of other breeds can also be affected. In both disorders, dogs show systemic signs of illness, most commonly anorexia, weight loss, and lethargy. Peripheral lymphadenopathy is often present.

In systemic histiocytosis, the skin lesions are striking and include numerous papules, nodules, plaques, and ulcers. In some areas, the skin can be crusted and hypotrichotic. Skin biopsy samples reveal a superficial to deep perivascular as well as a nodular to diffuse accumulation of predominantly histiocytes with small numbers of interspersed neutrophils, eosinophils, lymphocytes, and plasma cells. On electron microscopy, these histiocytes appear normal. The course of the disease is variable, ranging from rapid progression with a fatal outcome to a prolonged period of remission and exacerbation. In advanced cases, histiocytes infiltrate the lungs, liver, spleen, bone marrow, and lymph nodes, at which point euthanasia becomes a humane consideration. Treatment with standard immunosuppressive chemotherapeutics and systemic glucocorticoids has generally not been effective. It has been speculated that the disease responds favorably to immunoregulatory therapy with bovine thymosin (Moore, 1984); however, this was not well established.

In malignant histiocytosis, systemic signs predominate; skin lesions, typically firm dermal to subcutaneous nodules, are uncommon. Typical histopathologic findings in skin include nodular to diffuse infiltrates of large pleomorphic mononuclear cells and multinucleated histiocytic giant cells in the deep dermis and subcutis. The histiocytes are cytologically atypical, with large and frequently multiple nucleoli. A high mitotic index with bizarre mitotic figures is often seen. There appears to be no effective treatment at present.

STERILE PYOGRANULOMA/GRANULOMA SYNDROME

Canine sterile pyogranuloma/granuloma syndrome is an uncommon disorder. There seems to be no age predilection; however, male dogs are overrepresented. Breeds predisposed to this disorder are the collie, boxer, Great Dane, Weimaraner, and golden retriever (Panić et al., in press). Typical skin lesions include papules, nodules, and plaques, found most commonly on the head (periocular region, muzzle, bridge of nose) and feet. Bacterial and fungal cultures are consistently negative. Pedal lesions, as a result of their anatomic location and susceptibility to trauma, tend to become secondarily infected with bacteria, resulting in ulceration and formation of exudative draining tracts. These dogs are systemically healthy.

Typical histopathologic findings include nodular to diffuse granulomatous to pyogranulomatous dermatitis. The inflammatory cell infiltrate closely follows or tracks hair follicles, forming vertically oriented, oblong granulomas, without invading the follicular epithelium. Histiocytes, plasma cells, lymphocytes, and occasional multinucleated histiocytic giant cells are the predominant cell types in granulomatous lesions, with neutrophils being abundant in pyogranulomatous lesions.

Response to immunosuppressive doses of glucocorticoids is generally very good. Prednisone is used at 2.2 to 4.4 mg/kg/day initially until remission is achieved, usually within 7 to 14 days. The amount is then gradually tapered to the lowest possible alternate-day dose. Prolonged courses of therapy are typically necessary to maintain a remission, but some dogs do not require long-term treatment. Surgical excision of solitary lesions is curative in most dogs.

An idiopathic sterile granulomatous/pyogranulomatous dermatitis has been reported in four cats (Scott et al., 1990). Based on the clinicopathologic findings, two distinct groups were defined. The first two cats, both females, had bilateral, pruritic, preauricular, orange-yellow plaques. Skin biopsy specimens showed diffuse granulomatous dermatitis with pleomorphic histiocytes, purpura, and erythrophagocytosis. The other two cats, both males, had multiple erythematous to violaceous pruritic papules, nodules, and plaques on the head, pinnae, feet, and perineum. The histopathologic findings in these cats showed a perifollicular pyogranulomatous dermatitis. Special stains as well as bacterial and fungal cultures did not reveal an etiologic agent. In three cats in which follow-up information was available, the lesions underwent spontaneous resolution in 3 to 9 months. Anti-inflammatory doses of glucocorticoids were of no benefit, and no recurrences were seen in these cats. Conroy (1983) reported a sterile perifollicular granulomatous to pyogranulomatous syndrome in cats, characterized by nodules and plaques on the head and extremities. This condition, unlike that reported by Scott and colleagues, was responsive to glucocorticoids but frequently recurred.

STERILE PANNICULITIS

Panniculitis is characterized by inflammation of the subcutaneous adipose tissue. It is an uncommon disorder in both dogs and cats. The disease has been associated with infectious agents (bacteria, actinomycetes, mycobacteria, fungi), immune-mediated disorders (systemic lupus erythematosus, drug eruption), nutritional imbalances, metabolic disorders, and other factors. Bacterial and fungal cultures are indicated in all cases to rule out infectious causes. The presence of foreign bodies may be disclosed with polarized light microscopy. Idiopathic sterile panniculitis, however, appears to be the most common form.

In a recent retrospective study of sterile panniculitis, no age, breed, or sex predilection could be established (Scott and Anderson, 1988). However, previously it was generally considered that dachshunds were a breed at risk. The typical skin lesions were subcutaneous firm to fluctuant nodules of variable size. Lesions were most commonly solitary and occurred on the ventrolateral thorax, neck, and abdomen, as well as at other sites. Although most dogs and cats have solitary lesions, multiple lesions can be seen. Approximately one third of the lesions ulcerate, resulting in fistula formations that discharge yellowish-brown to bloody oily material. Systemic signs (pyrexia, anorexia, lethargy) are occasionally noted.

Histologically, the panniculitis can be characterized as lobular, septal, or diffuse. However, such anatomic classification appears to be of minimal diagnostic and prognostic significance in dogs and cats. The inflammatory cell infiltrates form pyogranulomas and granulomas with various degrees of suppuration, necrosis, and fibrosis. Fibrinoid vascular thrombosis within adipose tissue may be seen.

Surgical excision of solitary lesions is usually curative, with no recurrence. Multiple lesions have been successfully treated with oral prednisone (2.2 mg/kg body weight every 24 hr) for an average period of 3 to 8 weeks until remission is achieved. Cats require higher doses—namely, up to 4.4 mg/kg every 24 hr. Alternate-day steroid therapy for prolonged periods is required in recurrent cases.

GRANULOMATOUS SEBACEOUS ADENITIS

Granulomatous sebaceous adenitis is a rare, idiopathic granulomatous disorder of the sebaceous glands of dogs and cats. In dogs, no sex predilection exists; however, the disease occurs most commonly in young adult dogs, especially the Vizsla, Akita, Samoyed, and standard poodle (see this volume, p. 534).

Biopsy specimens reveal pronounced surface hyperkeratosis and a nodular granulomatous to pyogranulomatous inflammatory infiltration at the level of the sebaceous glands in early lesions. The complete absence of sebaceous glands is typical in advanced cases, when perifollicular fibrosis and follicular atrophy are common findings. Early cases may respond to systemic glucocorticoids (prednisone, 2.2 mg/kg PO every 24 hr). Antiseborrheic shampoos, emollient rinses, or humectants (total body spraying with 75% propylene glycol in water) may be beneficial for symptomatic relief. In general, the prognosis for recovery is poor. Experience with retinoids at the New York State College of Veterinary Medicine has not been rewarding. Two dogs

have been treated with isotretinoin (1 mg/kg every 12 hr), and two dogs have been treated with etretinate (0.75 mg/kg every 24 hr). None of these dogs improved with treatment. The reason for the failure in these dogs could be the advanced stage of their disease when the treatment was initiated. The results of treating long-haired dogs with retinoids have not been as rewarding as those reported in short-haired breeds. In none of the dogs were sebaceous glands visible histologically.

STERILE SARCOIDAL GRANULOMATOUS SKIN DISEASE

A sterile sarcoidal granulomatous skin disorder has been reported in three dogs (Scott and Noxon, 1990). These dogs had skin lesions consisting of multiple firm erythematous papules, plaques, and nodules on the pinnae, head, and trunk. Most lesions were covered by a mild surface scale and did not appear to be pruritic. Some were alopecic and remained unchanged during a follow-up period of 1½ years. Systemic signs were not present in two dogs; however, the third animal had a dilated cardiomyopathy. Because cardiac biopsies were not performed, it was not possible to confirm sarcoidal granulomatous disease of the heart.

Skin biopsy specimens were characterized by multiple tightly packed or diffuse sarcoidal (epithelioid) granulomas in the deep dermis and subcutis. The granulomas varied in shape and were surrounded by small numbers of lymphocytes and occasional multinucleated histiocytic giant cells. Sarcoidal granulomas by definition lack prominent peripheral lymphocytic and fibroblastic inflammatory components. Results of skin scrapings, tissue bacterial and fungal cultures, hemograms, and serum chemistry panels were negative or unremarkable. Results of special stains and polarized light examination of tissue were also negative.

Two dogs were treated with prednisone (2.2 mg/kg PO every 24 hr), and the lesions resolved within 10 days. The disease spontaneously regressed in the third dog after 1 year.

CONCLUSION

Sterile granulomatous and pyogranulomatous disorders of the skin are uncommon in dogs and cats. The importance of their recognition is their differentiation from neoplastic and infectious disorders. A systematic diagnostic approach, including skin biopsies for histopathology as well as bacterial and fungal culture, should be undertaken in all cases. Fine-needle aspiration of lesions and cytologic evaluation yield useful information. The definitive diagnosis should, however, be based on interpolation of histopathologic findings, bacterial and fungal culture results, and the presence or absence of foreign material.

References and Suggested Reading

Conroy, J. D.: An overview of immune-mediated diseases in the dog and cat, Part II. Other diseases based on immunologic mechanisms. Am. J. Dermatopathol. 5:595, 1983.
  A review of immune-mediated diseases of dogs and cats.
Moore, P. F.: Systemic histiocytosis of Bernese mountain dogs. Vet. Pathol. 21:554, 1984.
  A description of clinical signs, pathologic findings, and preliminary therapy of a histiocytic proliferative disorder in six Bernese Mountain dogs.
Panić, R., Scott, D. W., and Miller, W. H.: Canine sterile pyogranuloma/granuloma syndrome: A retrospective analysis of 29 cases. J. Am. Anim. Hosp. Assoc. (in press).
  A retrospective study of clinical signs, histopathologic findings, and therapy of canine cutaneous pyogranuloma/granuloma syndrome.
Rosser, E. J., Dunstan, R. W., Breen, P. T., et al.: Sebaceous adenitis

with hyperkeratosis in the standard poodle: A discussion of 10 cases. J. Am. Anim. Hosp. Assoc. 23:341, 1987.
  The hyperkeratotic skin lesions, histopathologic findings, and treatment modalities in ten standard poodles with sebaceous adenitis.
Scott, D. W.: Granulomatous sebaceous adenitis in dogs. J. Am. Anim. Hosp. Assoc. 22:631, 1986.
  Granulomatous sebaceous adenitis in three adult male dogs, including histopathologic features and response to therapy.
Scott, D. W., and Anderson, W.: Panniculitis in dogs and cats: A retrospective analysis of 78 cases. J. Am. Anim. Hosp. Assoc. 24:551, 1988.
  A retrospective study of 78 cases of panniculitis in dogs and cats with descriptions of skin lesions, etiology, histopathologic features, and response to therapy.
Scott, D. W., and Noxon, J. O.: A sterile sarcoidal granulomatous skin disease of dogs. Canine Pract. 15:11, 1990.
  A description of dermal lesions, histopathologic findings, and therapeutic response in three dogs with a sterile sarcoidal granulomatous skin disorder.
Scott, D. W., Buerger, R. G., and Miller, W. H.: Idiopathic sterile granulomatous and pyogranulomatous dermatitis in cats. Vet. Dermatol. 1:129, 1990.
  A description of four cats with idiopathic sterile granulomatous and pyogranulomatous dermatitis, including skin lesions, histopathologic findings, and response to therapy.

THERAPY FOR CANINE PYODERMA

DAVID H. LLOYD
London, England

Pyoderma is a syndrome of skin infection with pyogenic microorganisms, most commonly bacteria. Normal skin is resistant to bacterial infection, and pyoderma arises only after some event or events degrade this resistance. The location, extent, and severity of the pyoderma depend on the nature of the event. As a result, pyoderma can appear in many different clinical forms, often with little or no obvious sign of pus. Diagnosis and effective therapy depend on recognition of both the nature of the pyoderma and the factors that underlie it. This article concentrates on the measures required to eliminate bacterial infection and re-establish effective skin resistance to reinfection. The bacteria involved and their roles as both residents and pathogens thus must be understood.

ROLE OF THE NORMAL MICROFLORA

The skin surface in animals and humans is colonized by bacteria that are well adapted to the microenvironment of the superficial stratum corneum and the hair follicles. A close relationship exists between the different members of the flora,

enabling them to efficiently utilize the nutrient supply provided by the skin secretions and to fully occupy the available sites. Invading organisms thus find it difficult to gain a foothold and establish infection. In this way, the normal flora contributes to skin immunity, and this factor has been used in humans and, experimentally, in pigs to control staphylococcal disease (Allaker and Noble, 1992). Hence, factors that upset the equilibrium of the skin surface ecosystem may predispose to infection by pathogens. Such factors include not only pathologic processes that impair skin function but also inappropriate use of antimicrobial and other medications that eliminate the normal flora or adversely affect their habitat.

PATHOGENIC BACTERIA

Canine pyoderma normally involves infection with pathogenic staphylococci. Three species are recognized. *Staphylococcus intermedius*, formerly known as *S. aureus* biotypes E and F, is now known to be responsible for more than 90% of cases. The remainder of cases may involve *S. aureus* or, on rare occasions, *S. hyicus*. The first two species are coagulase positive, but some strains of *S. hyicus* are not and may thus be classified along with the other coagulase-negative staphylococci and remain unrecognized. The latter are generally considered to be nonpathogenic but are sometimes identified in cases of pyoderma in which the well-established pathogenic strains are not found. It is, of course, important to identify the pathogen in order to correctly assess antibiotic sensitivity; this information may also be useful in identifying the source of the infecting strain. It should be remembered that more than one species or strain of pathogenic *Staphylococcus* may sometimes be isolated from lesions in a single animal, and these isolates may differ in antibiotic sensitivity. Tests on a single isolate thus are not always reliable. Antibiotic resistance plasmids are also readily transferred both among and between the pathogenic and nonpathogenic species. Sudden changes in resistance may occur in bacteria from dogs that are in contact with animals or humans carrying resistant strains of these organisms.

Little is known of the ecology of *S. aureus* and *S. hyicus* from dogs. However, *S. intermedius* is present in the upper respiratory tract, on the buccal mucosa, on the anal mucosa, and in the perineal regions of most dogs. It can also be found at other sites on the coat and at the skin surface, particularly on the ventral abdomen. However, its presence on the skin at these sites is sporadic, and it seems likely that the skin surface is constantly seeded with *S. intermedius* from the oronasal region and perineum as dogs groom themselves and interact with others. Long-term establishment of the pathogenic staphylococci at such sites may depend initially on the presence of an unusually favorable environment caused by disruption of the normal skin surface microenvironment, either directly or as a result of pathologic changes within the skin. Mason and Lloyd (1986) have postulated that such changes might explain, at least in part, the development of pyoderma in cases of allergic skin disease in dogs. Once infection is established, the production of virulence factors may be sufficient to enable a vicious cycle of skin damage and bacterial proliferation to be instituted. *S. intermedius* produces various virulence factors (Allaker et al., 1991), but their significance in the pathogenesis of canine pyoderma is still poorly understood; the existence of virulent, epidemic strains of pathogenic staphylococci in dogs has not yet been documented, although it is well recognized in humans.

Various other bacteria including gram-negative organisms such as *Pseudomonas*, *Proteus*, and *Escherichia coli* can often be isolated from pyoderma, particularly from moist lesions and in traumatized and debilitated skin. However, these bacteria are usually secondary invaders that follow infection by the pathogenic staphylococci. More rarely, deep granulomatous lesions, involving actinomycetes, mycobacteria, and *Actinobacillus*, and cellulitis, associated with anaerobic infections ("gas gangrene") including *Clostridium* and *Bacteroides*, are encountered.

DIAGNOSTIC APPROACH

Readers are referred to other texts (Muller et al., 1989; White and Ihrke, 1987) for detailed descriptions of the different forms of canine pyoderma. These are generally classified according to the depth and severity of the disease (Table 1). This classification is useful because it unites forms of the syndrome with a similar prognosis and therapeutic approach. However, it is important to appreciate that merely classifying the form of pyoderma does not necessarily constitute a diagnosis. Identification of the underlying cause is usually necessary so that both this and the infection can be treated or controlled.

Definition of underlying causes is sometimes straightforward, as in skinfold pyoderma, but in other cases can be difficult or impossible. In the latter situation, the disease has to be described as idiopathic. A wide variety of investigative techniques may be necessary, and it is beyond the scope of this article to consider them in detail. In principle, any deficiency of nonspecific or specific immunity and any factor that damages the skin or alters the surface microenvironment may be responsible. No reliable routine tests of immune function are available for dogs. Hematologic examination can give general information on a dog's ability to mount a response to infection. Neutrophilia will be noted in most cases, and the lymphocyte count should be greater than 1000/ml. Serum electrophoresis should reveal a rise in beta and gamma globulins. More complex assays of canine neutrophil function and T-cell activity are not routinely available at present.

Evaluation of the pyoderma itself can be done rapidly in most cases by preparation of smears of pus from the lesions. Pus can be obtained on swabs or by aspiration, or impression smears may be made

***Table 1.** Classification of Canine Pyoderma*

Surface pyodermas
    Acute moist dermatitis (pyotraumatic dermatitis, "hot spots")
    Skinfold pyoderma (intertrigo)
Superficial pyoderma
    Impetigo ("puppy pyoderma")
    Superficial folliculitis
    Dermatophilosis
Deep pyoderma
    Muzzle folliculitis and furunculosis ("canine acne")
    Localized deep pyodermas (nasal, pedal, pressure point)
    Generalized deep pyoderma
    Bacterial granulomas

directly from the lesions. When possible, aseptic methods should be used. In this way, sterile lesions, as occur in pemphigus, will be recognized and the significance of any bacteria present can be more easily assessed. Staining with hematologic stains such as Diff-Quik (Harleco) or Giemsa's is sufficient in most cases. Any cocci found probably are staphylococci, whereas rods are likely to be secondary invaders. An absence of phagocytosed cocci may point toward some form of immunodeficiency.

Isolation of the causative organisms is useful to confirm involvement of staphylococci and to enable antibiotic sensitivity tests. If possible, intact lesions should be swabbed aseptically and cultured without delay or sent to the laboratory in transport medium. Failure to isolate pathogenic staphylococci may indicate poor sampling or processing of the swab, and the procedure should be repeated. Staphylococci from animals that have had little previous antibiotic therapy are likely to be sensitive to a wide range of antibiotics, and sensitivity testing may not be warranted. However, in deep pyodermas and when prolonged therapy is needed, sensitivity testing is always advisable. If the involvement of uncommon pathogens, such as *Dermatophilus* or mycobacteria, is suspected, the laboratory must be alerted because special isolation techniques are required.

When there is doubt about the underlying problem, biopsy sampling will almost always shed valuable light on the problem, particularly in deep pyodermas. Specimens from representative primary lesions should be submitted to an experienced veterinary histopathologist with a special interest in dermatology. Bacteriologic cultures and impression smears can also be made from biopsy specimens.

TREATMENT AND CONTROL OF PYODERMA

Therapeutic Strategy

Effective treatment of pyoderma requires control of the infecting pathogen and correction of the factors that predisposed the skin to disease. However, antibacterial therapy alone can be successful when the underlying problem is transient. It is important to remember that pathogenic staphylococci are probably resident in the anal or oronasal regions and that even prolonged and vigorous therapy may not completely eliminate them even if the pyoderma is cured.

Surface pyodermas (see Table 1) are moist lesions that generally involve various organisms that are relatively easily removed from the skin surface by the use of antibacterial shampoos and washes. In acute moist dermatitis, the causal factor is usually marked pruritus leading to self-trauma, often associated with flea allergy. Short-term treatment with

oral corticosteroids (prednisolone or prednisone, 1 mg/kg/day for up to 1 week) coupled with gentle cleansing and clipping of the adjacent coat is usually sufficient. However, "hot spots" may conceal deep pyoderma, and if evidence of this is found, systemic antibiotic therapy is required and corticosteroids are contraindicated. When moist dermatitis lesions are thickened and papules or pustules are present in adjacent areas of skin, deep pyoderma should be suspected. Biopsy examination is necessary in cases that do not show a rapid response. In the skinfold pyodermas, regular treatment with benzoyl peroxide shampoo or gel or with ethyl lactate shampoo may provide control, but surgery or weight loss in obese animals is the definitive treatment.

Impetigo differs from the other forms of superficial pyoderma in not having a follicular pattern of infection. The subcorneal pustules are readily accessible to topical therapy, and when it occurs in puppies, the condition can be controlled with antibacterial shampoos, such as benzoyl peroxide and ethyl lactate, used every second or third day for 4 weeks. When impetigo is seen in adults, systemic antibiotic treatment may be required. Superficial folliculitis can also be controlled by the regular use of antibacterial shampoos using the regimen described earlier (Ascher et al., 1990), and this may be necessary if the underlying causes cannot be identified or eliminated. Once the condition is controlled, the frequency of shampooing can often be reduced. However, systemic antibiotic therapy is more effective and should be used in the first instance. Treatment should be continued for at least 2 weeks after lesions have disappeared. Dermatophilosis also tends to localize in the hair follicles, but the organism is protected by the crusts that form at the surface. Treatment with tetracyclines for 7 days stops the infection, but the crusts remain infective and are a potential hazard to other animals and to humans. Daily antibacterial washes are advisable, and crusts should be removed and destroyed as they loosen from the skin.

Deep pyodermas involve the hair follicles and dermal tissue. Cellulitis may also occur. Muzzle folliculitis and furunculosis can be quite mild, and treatment may not be required. Benzoyl peroxide shampoo used daily or 5% benzoyl peroxide gel used once or twice daily often gives control. Treatment subsequently may be reduced to every 2 to 3 days. More severe infections should be treated the same as the other deep pyodermas. These are serious diseases that always require a systemic antibiotic. Therapy should continue for at least 7 to 10 days after lesions are healed. Topical therapy with shampoos, soaks, and whirlpool baths helps to cleanse and detoxify the skin and may reduce pain and pruritus. Care should be taken to avoid further damage to the affected skin.

When chronic granulomatous lesions are encountered, possible infection with mycobacteria, actinomycetes (*Nocardia* and *Actinomyces*), and *Actinobacillus* should be considered. In cases of cellulitis, anaerobic infection including clostridia, *Bacteroides*, peptostreptococci, and enterobacteria may occur. Treatment of these conditions is beyond the scope of this article, and readers should refer to a more detailed text (Muller et al., 1989).

Despite careful diagnostic analysis and vigorous treatment, a proportion of cases of both superficial and deep pyoderma fail to respond fully or recur repeatedly. Immunotherapy with staphylococcal vaccines or immunostimulants is effective in some cases, but continual antibiotic therapy is occasionally necessary.

Systemic Antibiotic Therapy

Systemic antibiotic therapy normally eliminates skin infection in pyoderma if properly applied (Table 2). Ideally, choose a narrow-spectrum bactericidal agent that is known to be effective against the bacterial pathogen, usually *S. intermedius*. Bactericides do not depend on host resistance to eliminate the infection, and narrow-spectrum agents are less likely to affect the normal microflora adversely. This ideal often cannot be achieved, and in practice, the use of broad-spectrum and bacteriostatic agents seldom causes problems. However, relatively high doses are needed to establish effective levels within the avascular epidermis and to penetrate swollen, debilitated, or granulomatous lesions. If possible, doses should be based on actual body weights. Treatment for an adequate duration is also critical, and elimination of infection from deep pyoderma may require therapy lasting for periods of 3 months or more.

Selection of the particular antibiotic to be used depends on the nature of the infection and previous treatment history. In most cases, staphylococci are the primary pathogen. These organisms tend to be beta-lactamase producers and are thus resistant to penicillin G and amoxicillin. Tetracycline resistance is also common. These antibiotics should not be used unless indicated by sensitivity tests. Resistance to erythromycin, lincomycin, and clindamycin (10 to 25%) and to trimethoprim-sulfonamide (about 9%) is less frequent. Resistance to chloramphenicol, cephalosporins, synthetic penicillins such as oxacillin, and methicillin and to the amoxicillin/clavulanic acid combination is rare. In relatively mild superficial infections in dogs with little previous exposure to antibiotic therapy, bacterial isolation and sensitivity testing may not be warranted. Empirically based treatment with any of the previously listed antibiotics, except the tetracyclines and beta-lactamase–sensitive penicillins, may be effective. However, vomiting commonly occurs with erythromycin, and there is increasing evidence of drug side effects with trimethoprim-potentiated sulfonamides. In some countries, the use of chloramphenicol is reserved for severe infections. It has also been proposed that the cephalosporins should be reserved for life-threatening disease because of evidence of emerging resistance (White and Ihrke, 1987). Resistance to gentamicin and similar aminoglycosides (amikacin, tobramycin) is rare, but these drugs may be toxic and require parenteral administration and careful monitoring. They should only be used when no less-toxic alternative is available. Enrofloxacin, a recently developed quinolone carboxylic acid derivative, is a broad-spectrum, bactericidal antibiotic that has shown promise in initial studies in canine pyoderma reported by Paradis and colleagues (1990). However, the investigators emphasize that therapy must continue for at least 1 week after clinical cure.

Topical Therapy

Topical therapy is an important component of the treatment of most pyodermas. It should aim to remove scales, crusts, and exudate from the skin surface; to promote drainage of deeper lesions; to unblock hair follicles; and to reduce the bacterial populations to normal levels. It may also play a part in reducing pain and pruritus. It is often necessary to clip part or all of the coat to gain adequate access to the skin, and sedation may be necessary to achieve this. Cosmetic considerations should not be allowed to override the need for clipping, which also helps to convince the owner of the seriousness of the problem. Cleaning the skin and coat also has social benefits and tends to improve morale in both the dog and its owner. Treatments that occlude the surface (e.g., ointments), that are excessively drying, that change skin pH, or that draw the dog's

Table 2. *Antibiotic Doses Used in Canine Pyoderma*

Antibiotic	Dose (mg/kg)	Dosage Interval (hr)	Route
Oxacillin (C)	22	8	PO
Amoxicillin/Clavulanic acid (C)	12.5–25	12	PO
Enrofloxacin (C)	2.5	12	PO
Cephalexin and Cephadroxil (C)	22	12	PO
Gentamicin (C)	1	8	SC
Trimethoprim-sulfonamide (C)	30	12	PO
Erythromycin (S)	15	8	PO
Lincomycin (S)	22	12	PO
Chloramphenicol (S)	50	8	PO, IV

C, bactericidal; IV, intravenous; PO, orally; S, bacteriostatic; SC, subcutaneous.

attention to the affected area should be avoided. It is important to remember that damage to the skin may make it fragile, and overzealous cleaning may lead to disruption of hair follicles with subsequent alopecia and scarring.

Shampoos are the most acceptable and readily applied mode of therapy in the majority of pyodermas. Benzoyl peroxide shampoo has antimicrobial, follicle-flushing, and degreasing properties, which are very important. However, it is moderately irritating and should not be used on open wounds. At concentrations of 3% or less, it is well tolerated by most dogs. It does cause irritant reactions in some animals, particularly if it is applied too vigorously. These reactions can be recognized by the appearance of erythema and increased pruritus within 2 hr of use. Apparently allergic reactions can also occur after about 24 hr, but this event is quite uncommon. Benzoyl peroxide is normally used initially at 2- to 3-day intervals. When control has been established, it can be used weekly to monthly as a prophylactic measure for recurrent pyodermas. When used more frequently, benzoyl peroxide can be associated with excessive drying of skin. In such cases, moisturizers can be employed, but selection of a less-drying shampoo is preferable. Ethyl lactate shampoo (Etiderm, Allerderm), a new product, is nonirritating and nondrying and is useful in superficial and surface pyodermas. More powerful antibacterial and emollient actions can be obtained with shampoos containing chlorhexidine, such as ChlorhexaDerm (Dermatologics for Veterinary Medicine).

Soaks or whirlpool baths are valuable, particularly for severe exudative pyodermas. In such cases, crusting and matting of the coat tend to restrict access to the skin and it is necessary to soak and soften the affected areas first. The coat should be clipped around these areas, and lesions not previously apparent may be revealed. These dogs should be immersed up to the neck for 15 min or more in water containing antibacterial agents such as chlorhexidine (Nolvasan, Fort Dodge) or povidone-iodine (Betadine, Purdue Frederick). Soaks or preferably whirlpool baths should be repeated once or twice daily until healing of the skin surface and control of the pyoderma have been achieved. Shampooing may then be used on a regular basis, if necessary, to inhibit recurrence of the pyoderma.

Creams, gels, and ointments are seldom used in the treatment of pyoderma. They tend to attract dogs' attention to the treated site and are licked off quite readily. Ointments, which occlude the skin surface, are generally contraindicated. Benzoyl peroxide 5% gel (Oxydex Gel, Dermatologics for Veterinary Medicine; Pyoben Gel, Allerderm) is an exception. It is quite effective in the management of canine acne and skinfold pyodermas. It can also be used to control localized papular dermatitis in relatively alopecic areas, and in some cases its use may enable intervals between shampooing to be extended.

Immunomodulatory Therapy

Staphylococcal bacterins have long been used on an anecdotal basis to treat chronic pyodermas. They generally are used only for cases that are not responsive to other forms of therapy. Staphoid-AB (Jensal) is a cell wall antigen and toxin product. Staphage Lysate (Delmont) is made from human S. aureus lysed by bacteriophage. Controlled studies have confirmed that Staphage Lysate is beneficial. Ihrke (1986) concluded that about 20% of dogs with antibiotic-responsive, recurrent, pruritic pyoderma would respond to subcutaneous administration of 1 ml of Staphage Lysate weekly. In Britain, autogenous bacterins are also used quite commonly. These are prepared from staphylococci isolated from the affected animals, normally S. intermedius, and contain killed bacterial cells. In theory, better immunity should be generated by autogenous bacterins, but no comparisons have been made. The preparation and administration protocols vary considerably, but the vaccines are generally given weekly for a period of several weeks and then at 6-month intervals. Good control is obtained initially in some dogs but often is maintained for only a year or so. Both local and systemic adverse reactions have been observed after treatment with staphylococcal bacterins. Owners should be warned of this possibility, and following injection, dogs should be kept under observation for at least half an hour.

Levamisole has also been used in pyoderma when immunodeficiency is suspected. It has immunostimulatory effects and may restore phagocytic activity and T-cell function. However, it appears to be effective over only a narrow dose range that is not well defined, and inappropriate dosage may cause immunosuppression rather than immunostimulation. White and Ihrke (1987) use 2.2 mg/kg PO three times weekly. Various side effects, including neurologic signs, vomiting, and diarrhea, have been reported but are uncommon.

References and Suggested Reading

Allaker, R. P., and Noble, W. C.: Microbial interactions on the skin. In Noble, W. C. (ed.): The Skin Microflora in Health and Disease. Cambridge: Cambridge University Press, 1992.
A review of bacterial interaction at the skin surface in animals and humans.
Allaker, R. P., Lamport, A. I., Lloyd, D. H., et al.: Production of virulence factors by Staphylococcus intermedius isolates from cases of canine pyoderma and healthy carriers. Micr. Ecol. Hlth. Dis. 4:169, 1991.
Comparison of virulence factors from strains of S. intermedius derived from dogs with pyoderma and normal dogs.
Ascher, F., Maynard, L., Laurent, J., et al.: Controlled trial of ethyl

lactate and benzoyl peroxide shampoos in the management of canine surface pyoderma and superficial pyoderma. *In* von Tscharner, C., Halliwell, R. E. W. (eds.): Advances in Veterinary Dermatology. Vol. I. London: Baillière Tindall, 1990, p. 375.
Comparison of the two shampoos showing equivalent efficacy.

Devriese, L. A., and De Pelsmaecker, K.: The anal region as a main carrier site of *Staphylococcus intermedius* and *Streptococcus canis* in dogs. Vet. Rec. 121:302, 1987.
A study of the locations of these organisms and indications of their populations at different sites.

Ihrke, P. J.: Antibacterial therapy in dermatology. *In* Kirk, R. W. (ed.): *Current Veterinary Therapy IX.* Philadelphia: W. B. Saunders, 1986, p. 566.
A review of antibacterial treatment methods in pyoderma.

Kwochka, K., and Kowalski, J. J.: Prophylactic efficacy of four antibacterial shampoos against *Staphylococcus intermedius* in dogs. Am. J. Vet. Res. 52:115, 1990.
An evaluation of long-term use of antibacterial shampoos.

Mason, I. S., and Lloyd, D. H.: The role of allergy in the development of canine pyoderma. J. Small Anim. Pract. 30:216, 1986.
Research leading to a hypothesis of the way in which skin allergic reactions may predispose to pyoderma.

Medleau, L., Long, R. E., Brown, J., et al.: Frequency and antimicrobial susceptibility of *Staphylococcus* species isolated from canine pyodermas. Am. J. Vet. Res. 47:229, 1986.
An examination of the antibiotic sensitivity patterns of the different staphylococcal species isolated in canine pyoderma.

Muller, G. H., Kirk, R. W., and Scott, D. W.: *Small Animal Dermatology.* Vol. IV. Philadelphia: W. B. Saunders, 1989.
The definitive small animal text with detailed descriptions of the different forms of pyoderma.

Paradis, M., Lemay, S., Scott, D. W., et al.: Efficacy of enrofloxacin in the treatment of bacterial pyoderma. Vet. Dermatol. 1:123, 1990.
Excellent responses to treatment were observed in 28 of 30 dogs with pyoderma.

White, S. D., and Ihrke, P. J.: Pyoderma. *In* Nesbitt, G. H. (ed.): *Contemporary Issues in Small Animal Practice.* Vol. VIII. Dermatology. New York: Churchill Livingstone, 1987, p. 95.
Chapter devoted to clinical aspects of pyoderma in dogs and cats.

MALASSEZIA DERMATITIS AND OTITIS

KENNETH V. MASON

Springwood, Queensland, Australia

Malassezia pachydermatis (also known as *Pityrosporum pachydermatis* and *Pityrosporum canis*) is a lipophilic nonmycelial yeast with a characteristic slightly elongated oval shape, a thick wall, and unipolar budding. It is commonly found on normal and abnormal canine skin and within the ear canal, anal sacs, vagina, and rectum. There is an increase in the number of organisms in some cases of otitis and dermatitis. The role of *Malassezia* as a disease-producing organism has been unclear and controversial. It is becoming increasingly clear that this commensal organism can become a significant secondary invader or pathogen, in the presence of the appropriate surface microclimate and if the host's defense mechanism fails or is overwhelmed. Surface microclimatic factors leading to *Malassezia* proliferation are wax or sebum production, accumulation of moisture, disruption of the epidermal barrier function, and exacerbation of allergic and bacterial skin diseases. Staphylococci have been demonstrated *in vitro* to enhance the yeast's growth, as has an oily film over dextrose agar. These two factors may also be important *in vivo*. The host's defense response, which is normally responsible for recovery from acute infection or the prevention of disease by normal fungal flora, is associated with the development or presence of T-cell–mediated hypersensitivity to the fungus.

It is now clear that *Malassezia*, like staphylococci, is an opportunistic pathogen; in my opinion, both together have a significant role in seborrheic (oily and scaly) dermatitis as well as otitis. *Malassezia*-associated dermatitis should not be thought of as uncommon but should be considered in any scaly, erythematous, or oily pruritic dermatitis in which other diagnoses and treatments have failed to resolve the condition.

CLINICAL DISEASE

Mycotic otitis associated with *Malassezia* may take three common clinical forms, all of which may have the following clinical signs: head hanging and shaking, ear scratching, excessive aural discharge, pain on palpation of the ear, and an offensive odor. On otoscopic examination, one may see a generalized erythema and fine scaling or waxy covering of the external pinna and external meatus. Another common finding, usually associated with more chronic disease, is an external meatus full of thick yellow wax or a flaky black wax. The latter is often misdiagnosed as ear mites. The third form is a yellow purulent discharge associated with erythema and ulceration, principally of the external meatus but possibly spilling over onto the pinna. This latter form is a mixed infection of *Staphylococcus intermedius*, sometimes streptococci, and *Malassezia*.

When presented with an otitis, especially a *Malassezia* mycotic otitis, performing a complete dermatologic examination and obtaining a history are important. The first two forms of mycotic otitis are often associated with allergic (atopy or food allergy, flea allergy) dermatitis or superficial staphylococci pyoderma or *Malassezia* dermatitis. Unless the underlying dermatitis is addressed, the otitis will respond only temporarily to treatment. Waxy otitis may also be seen with hypothyroidism. The conformation of the ear canal and opening may also predispose a dog to recurrent infections. The finding of hairy, narrowed canals in flopped-down ears that are typical of some water sporting breeds (e.g., cocker spaniels, Springer spaniels) and poodles may be a sufficient explanation for recurrent mycotic otitis. Surgical intervention to open the canal should thus be considered. In erect-eared dogs like the German shepherd, mycotic otitis is often associated with allergic skin disease and other seborrheic skin diseases.

Superficial *Malassezia* dermatitis can occur as a regional disease or a generalized disorder. As mycotic otitis externa is associated with a moist and oily environment, similar considerations can lead to *Malassezia* cheilitis and pododermatitis. Poodles, Silky terriers, Australian terriers, Maltese terriers, and Shetland sheepdogs seem predisposed to the regional forms of the disease. The presenting complaint can be face rubbing, either as a mild but persistent habit, or a frenzied fit of nose and lip scratching with the front paws. The skin may look mildly erythematous and scaly, with associated secondary alopecia and excoriation from self-inflicted trauma. The dermatitis can be overlooked because the skin is obscured by long hair. Some animals that exhibit the frenzied scratching are misdiagnosed as having fitting behavior of central nervous system origin and are treated with anticonvulsants. The pododermatitis is more easily recognized as foot licking. One or more paws may be erythematous between the pads, and the dorsal surface may show alopecia and scale (yellow or slate gray).

Generalized *Malassezia* dermatitis is usually associated with intense pruritus, although some cases may be less pruritic. Poodles, Maltese terriers, Chihuahuas, and Shetland sheepdogs seem predisposed. I have identified the disease mainly in small breeds of dogs such as dachshunds, most terrier breeds including the West Highland white terrier, and schnauzers, and in only a few large breeds, two cases in German shepherds. There was no age or sex predilection. As with *Malassezia* otitis, there are three clinical forms of superficial *Malassezia* dermatitis.

Affected animals may exhibit patches of erythema and scale that coalesce and appear serpiginous or may show a generalized exfoliative erythroderma. The third presentation is seen as hyperpigmented,

lichenified areas of alopecia that may have obvious gray to white scale. Gray to white scaly plaques may be found as the main feature or in association with the erythematous and hyperpigmented lesion already described. The degree of wax or oily seborrhea varies, as does the associated offensive odor.

DIAGNOSIS

The most useful and readily available tool for the diagnosis of *Malassezia* dermatitis or otitis is cytologic study. I use a cotton swab vigorously rubbed onto affected skin or wiped onto the discharge in the ear then pressed and rolled onto a glass slide. Tape strips pressed onto glass slides are also valuable, as is a superficial scrape with a blunt spatula or scalpel blade. All material is heat fixed and stained in Diff-Quik or new methylene blue and examined under high power or oil immersion. Biopsy for histopathology of affected skin is also useful, but the correct interpretation depends on the dermatopathologic knowledge of the service to which the sample is sent. Until recently, the finding of *Malassezia* organisms in skin biopsy specimens was considered to be insignificant. Such an interpretation may still persist in some pathology services. Routine cultures of skin surfaces more often than not fail to isolate the organism. If the laboratory is alerted to look for *Malassezia*, an oil-covered dextrose agar can be used with better results. *Malassezia* may occasionally grow on dermatophyte medium. Overall, culture is not a reliable method to identify the presence of *Malassezia* in a dermatitis or otitis. The demonstration of *Malassezia* does not confirm that the organism is the cause of the skin disease, because these yeasts are often present on diseased skin. I believe that if *Malassezia* is easily demonstrated by cytologic study, numerous colonies of the yeast probably are present. High numbers of either *S. intermedius*, *Malassezia*, or both when present probably contribute significantly to the disease process present.

Because the clinical signs of *Malassezia* dermatitis are a pruritic, erythematous, scaly, hyperpigmented and lichenified dermatitis and otitis, the differential diagnosis can be extensive. Even more perplexing is a situation in which the *Malassezia* dermatitis is associated with or triggered by most of the potential differential diagnoses. The prime differential diagnoses and associated predisposing diseases are atopy, flea allergy, food allergy, superficial pyoderma, and all etiologic factors considered in an oily seborrhea and waxy, scaly seborrhea complex.

The only way to resolve the issue of whether a commensal organism has become pathogenic and has a contributory role in the dermatitis present is to remove that organism. When *Malassezia* is demonstrated cytologically and the dermatitis fails to resolve with removal of other identified factors, then trial therapy with ketoconazole at 10 mg/kg b.i.d. for 2 weeks would be a suitable action to investigate the yeast's role in the dermatitis. An alternative and more tentative approach would be to select a severely affected area and treat it twice per day for 2 weeks with a miconazole cream. An improvement in the treated area in comparison with a nontreated spot would encourage a further treatment trial with ketoconazole.

TREATMENT

Several treatments have been recommended for *Malassezia* otitis. Vinegar and water and other mild acidic solutions have been recommended. I do not find these preparations to be very effective. Nystatin is a topical antifungal drug found in many otic preparations. *In vitro* tests demonstrate that nystatin is not as effective as drugs of the ketoconazole and miconazole group. In my experience, nystatin otic preparations need to be used for 10 to 14 days in cases of *Malassezia* otitis. Miconazole-containing otic preparations are more effective. The combination of antibiotics and corticosteroids does speed resolution of clinical signs. Effective resolution of predisposing causes (e.g., atopy and flea allergy or ear conformational defects) helps ensure that recurrences of the otitis are minimal.

The treatment of *Malassezia* dermatitis is effectively accomplished with 30 days of ketoconazole therapy (10 mg/kg b.i.d.). Vomiting and vague signs of malaise are occasionally encountered and can often be overcome by giving food with the tablets. Rarely, liver damage is known to be associated with ketoconazole use in humans.

Local treatment with a miconazole cream can be valuable in pododermatitis and cheilitis, as well as in the most severely affected areas in cases of generalized dermatitis. Selenium sulfide shampoo baths are recommended to remove scale on which the yeasts are surviving. These baths have also been demonstrated to have a direct effect on the organism. I recommend 10-minute selenium sulfide soaks twice per week for the first 2 weeks, then once per week thereafter until the dermatitis is resolved. It is a good idea to continue using a selenium sulfide or chlorhexidine shampoo for regular bathing.

Some cases of generalized mycotic dermatitis have benefited from povidone-iodine rinses after a selenium sulfide or chlorhexidine shampoo. In animals unable to tolerate ketoconazole, a combination of the previously described topical treatments may be effective. Griseofulvin is not effective against *Malassezia*. Ketoconazole, unlike griseofulvin, is secreted via the sebaceous glands onto the epidermal surface, thus explaining why ketoconazole is effective against such a surface-dwelling organism. Secondary predisposing causes must be addressed, because this type of mycotic dermatitis frequently recurs.

CONCLUSION

Since *Pityrosporum* was first described by Rivolta in 1873 and Malassez in 1874 suggested its role in dandruff, several studies have demonstrated that this yeast fulfills Koch's postulate as the cause of seborrheic dermatitis in humans. Despite this proof, seborrheic dermatitis continued until recently to be considered a hyperproliferative disorder of the epidermis (Shuster, 1988). The veterinary profession must now decide what role, if any, *Malassezia* has in seborrheic dermatitis of dogs.

References and Suggested Reading

Dufait, R.: *Pityrosporum canis* as the cause of canine chronic dermatitis. Vet. Med. Small Anim. Clin. 78:1055, 1983.
Mason, K. V., and Evans, A. G.: Dermatitis associated with *Malassezia pachydermatis* in eleven dogs. J. Am. Anim. Hosp. Assoc. 37:13, 1991.
Scott, D. W., and Miller, W. H.: Epidermal dysplasia and *Malassezia pachydermatis* infection in West Highland white terriers. Vet. Dermatol. 1:25, 1989.
Shuster, S.: Introduction: A history of seborrhoeic dermatitis and dandruff in fungal disease. *In* Shuster, S., and Blatchford, N. (eds.): *International Congress and Symposium Series. No. 132*. London: Royal Society of Medicine Service, 1988, p. 3.

FELINE DERMATOPHYTOSIS

LINDA MEDLEAU
Athens, Georgia

and KAREN A. MORIELLO
Madison, Wisconsin

Dermatophytosis is the most common fungal disease of cats. Elimination of dermatophyte infections requires identifying infected cats, treating them with appropriate antifungal drugs, and instituting measures to prevent reinfection.

ETIOLOGY

Infection occurs when a dermatophyte penetrates the stratum corneum and invades anagen hair follicles. Fungal hyphae invade the ostium of a hair follicle, proliferate on the surface of the hair, and migrate downward to the hair bulb. The dermatophyte produces keratinolytic enzymes that allow penetration of the hair cuticle and growth within the hair shaft until the keratogenous zone is reached. At this point, the dermatophyte either establishes equilibrium between its downward growth and hair growth or it is expelled.

Although *Microsporum gypseum* and *Trichophyton mentagrophytes* occasionally cause dermatophyte infections in cats, *Microsporum canis* is most commonly isolated. *M. canis* may live on the hair and skin of cats with or without eliciting an inflammatory reaction. Infected cats that have no lesions are commonly referred to as asymptomatic carriers.

CLINICAL SIGNS

Many cats are asymptomatic carriers of *M. canis*, and infection may not be noticed until dermatophytosis develops in a human or animal contact. Careful inspection of suspect carriers may reveal patchy areas of partial alopecia, scaling, or broken hairs.

Dermatophytosis is classically considered nonpruritic, but cats may be moderately to even intensely pruritic. Localized dermatophytosis is less common than generalized dermatophytosis in cats. Cats, especially kittens, may have what appears to be a localized infection. However, if lesional hairs and normal-appearing hairs elsewhere on the body are cultured separately, *M. canis* is usually isolated from both sites, indicating that the infection is really generalized (Moriello, 1990).

In kittens, lesions are often first seen on the face, ears, or forelegs. Patchy or circumscribed areas of alopecia that may be scaly, crusty, and erythematous are common. Hairs at the margin of lesions are frequently broken and frayed.

In adult cats, dermatophytosis typically presents as patchy areas of alopecia that may be focal, multifocal, or generalized. Secondary scaling, crusting, or erythema may be present. Less commonly, dermatophytosis appears as a diffuse folliculitis or as miliary dermatitis. Other uncommon manifestations of dermatophytosis include recurrent feline chin acne, chronic blepharitis (due to infection of the periocular hairs and cornea), kerion reactions, and pseudomycetomas.

In dermatophyte pseudomycetomas, the dermatophyte infection involves the deep dermal and subcutaneous tissues. All reported cases of dermatophyte pseudomycetomas in cats have been caused by subcutaneous infection with *M. canis* (Medleau, 1990). To date, all infected cats have been Persians. Clinically, cats present with firm nodules that may ulcerate and drain. The dorsum of the trunk or base of the tail usually is affected. Some cats have a history of superficial dermatophyte infection before development of pseudomycetomas. Affected cats may also be asymptomatic carriers of *M. canis*.

DIAGNOSIS

Diagnostic aids commonly used include ultraviolet Wood's light examination, direct microscopic examination of scales and hairs for fungal elements, histopathologic examination of skin biopsy samples, and fungal culture. Of these, the Wood's light examination is the easiest screening test for dermatophytosis.

The Wood's light is an ultraviolet light filtered through a cobalt or nickel glass filter. The light must be allowed to warm up for 5 to 10 min before it is used. The cat is then placed in a dark room, and its haircoat is examined with the Wood's light. When exposed to the Wood's light, hairs invaded by fluorescing strains of *M. canis* glow yellow green. However, approximately 50% of *M. canis* isolates do not fluoresce, and *M. gypseum* and *T. mentagrophytes* never fluoresce. Also, some topical medications such as iodine destroy fluorescence. Thus, the lack of fluorescence does not rule out dermatophyte infection.

False-positive fluorescence may occur if topical ointments or solutions have been applied to the haircoat. Thus, positive fluorescence is not necessarily diagnostic of dermatophytosis. The Wood's light is best used as an aid in choosing hairs for fungal culture.

The fungal culture is the most reliable method for confirming dermatophyte infection. Dermatophyte test medium (DTM) is the most commonly used fungal culture medium. DTM is available commercially in glass screw-cap containers (Fungassay, Pitman Moore) or in dual-compartment plates with DTM on one side and plain Sabouraud's dextrose agar on the other (Sab-Duets, Bacti-Labs). DTM contains the pH indicator phenol red, chlortetracycline, and gentamicin to inhibit bacterial growth, and cycloheximide, which inhibits some saprophytic fungi. When cultured on DTM, dermatophytes prefer to utilize protein, which causes the medium to turn red. The color change occurs simultaneously with the appearance of colony growth. Color change and colony growth usually occur within 3 to 7 days of culture inoculation but may take up to 21 days. Dermatophyte colonies are white, cream, or buff in color. Saprophytic fungi may also grow on DTM cultures. Saprophytes prefer to utilize carbohydrates, so that as the colony appears, the medium remains yellow. After all carbohydrates are utilized, saprophytes may then use protein. However, colony growth will be well established before the color change occurs, indicating that the fungus is not a dermatophyte. Consequently, DTM cultures should be examined daily in order to determine if any color change occurs with colony growth or afterward. Also, darkly colored colonies are saprophytes regardless of when color change occurs.

For culture, hairs that fluoresce with Wood's light should be selected and plucked with forceps. If no fluorescence is noted, hairs within and adjacent to lesions should be cultured. However, if noninfected hairs are plucked, fungal culture results will be falsely negative.

The best way to collect hairs for culture when no fluorescence is seen is to use the toothbrush technique, because this technique minimizes the chances of false-negative cultures and maximizes identification of carriers. A new toothbrush in the original cellophane packaging is sterile for fungi. If any suspect lesions are present, they should be thoroughly combed with the toothbrush; otherwise, the cat's entire body should be combed. Afterward, the toothbrush should contain hairs. If it does not, the combing was not aggressive enough. The col-

lected hairs are then cultured on DTM. *M. canis* colonies will usually grow within 7 to 10 days. Cultures from asymptomatic cats may take as long as 14 to 21 days to grow if a low number of infective spores was obtained. Positive identification of the fungus should be made by examining slide preparations of the culture colony. The sticky surface of acetate tape is touched to the surface of the culture colony. The tape is then pressed, sticky side down, on a slide with a drop of lactophenol cotton blue stain and examined under the microscope. Gross and microscopic descriptions of dermatophyte colonies can be found in most veterinary microbiology books.

A diagnosis of dermatophyte pseudomycetoma is best made by histopathologic examination of skin biopsy specimens and by fungal culture of the lesions. Histologically, the lesions are characterized by a pyogranulomatous to granulomatous panniculitis. Granulomas are usually composed of an amorphous eosinophilic material (Splendori-Hoeppli reaction) in which irregularly shaped aggregates of distorted septate hyphae and thick-walled fungal cells are embedded. The inflammatory response is usually characterized by the presence of neutrophils, macrophages, epithelioid cells, and multinucleated giant cells. Fibroplasia may surround the granulomas. Fungal elements are often not detected in the hair shafts or epidermis of the overlying skin. Fungal cultures of dermatophyte pseudomycetomas have so far yielded *M. canis* in all cats.

Because asymptomatic infection of hairs in cats with pseudomycetomas is possible, the haircoat should be examined carefully for stubbled or broken-off hairs. A Wood's light examination as well as fungal culture of suspect hairs should be performed. Hairs should be collected for fungal culture using the toothbrush technique.

TREATMENT

Localized Dermatophytosis

Because cats with only a few clinical lesions may also have infected hairs elsewhere on the body, culturing the entire haircoat using the toothbrush technique should be done to rule out the possibility of generalized infection (Moriello, 1990). When localized dermatophytosis is diagnosed, the affected areas should be clipped and the lesions treated twice daily with a topical antifungal product. The antifungal product is also applied to the skin and hairs surrounding the lesion in order to prevent the fungal infection from spreading outward. Treatment is continued 2 weeks after apparent clinical cure and negative fungal culture results. Antifungal products that may be used in treating localized lesions are listed in Table 1. Several newer topical products

Table 1. Topical Antifungals for Localized Dermatophytosis

Generic Name	Trade Name
Chlorhexidine ointment	Nolvasan (Fort Dodge)
Povidone-iodine ointment	Betadine (Purdue Frederick)
Thiabendazole	Tresaderm (MSD Agvet)
Miconazole cream or solution	Micatin (Advanced Care)
	Conofite (Pitman-Moore)
	Monistat (Ortho)
Haloprogin cream or solution	Halotex (Westwood)
Econazole cream	Spectrazole (Ortho)
Clotrimazole	Lotrimin (Schering)
	Mycelex (Miles)

for human dermatophytosis have not yet been evaluated in cats. These products include ketoconazole cream (Nizoral, Janssen), sulconazole nitrate cream and solution (Exelderm, Westwood), oxiconazole nitrate cream (Oxistat, Glaxo), and naftifine hydrochloride cream (Naftin, Herbert). Several imidazole antifungal drugs are undergoing clinical tests in humans but are not yet available for topical use. These drugs include tioconazole, bifonazole, and isoconazole. Tioconazole has fungicidal activity and may lead to more rapid clearing of infection than the other imidazoles. Terconazole, a triazole antifungal agent, is also in an investigational phase and is not yet available in the United States. It may be more active against dermatophytes than are the imidazoles. Regardless of the topical product used, cats with refractory or recurring lesions should be treated for generalized dermatophytosis.

Generalized Dermatophytosis

Standard therapy for generalized dermatophytosis involves long-term treatment with both topical and systemic antifungal products. Affected cats with medium or long haircoats should be clipped with a number 10 cutting blade in order to remove infected hairs. The cat's entire body should be treated with an antifungal solution once or twice a week until fungal cultures are negative (4 to 16 weeks of treatment or longer). Antifungal products for topical treatment of generalized dermatophytosis include lime sulfur solution (LymDyp, Dermatologics for Veterinary Medicine), chlorhexidine solution (Nolvasan, Fort Dodge), povidone-iodine solution (Betadine, Purdue Frederick), Captan (Orthrocide Garden Fungicide), sodium hypochlorite (e.g., Clorox), and enilconazole (Imaverol, Janssen) (Table 2). Enilconazole, an imidazole, is available in Europe and Canada but is not yet approved for use in the United States.

Before topical application, the individual performing the treatment should remove any jewelry and don protective clothing and rubber gloves. The antifungal solution is applied to the cat's body with a sponge until the haircoat and skin are completely saturated. The entire body is treated, including the face, but contact with the eyes should be avoided. The solution is not rinsed off but is allowed to dry on the cat.

Griseofulvin is the drug of choice for systemic treatment, but it must be used in conjunction with topical antifungal therapy. Griseofulvin *must* be administered every day and is poorly absorbed unless given with a high-fat meal. The particle size of griseofulvin affects absorption, and microsize or ultramicrosize forms should be used. The dosage of microsized griseofulvin is 50 mg/kg PO every 24 hr. Microsize griseofulvin is available as tablets (Fulvicin U/F, Schering) and pediatric suspension (Grifulvin V, Ortho Pharmaceutical). Because the tablets are difficult to administer to small kittens, the pediatric suspension, which contains 125 mg of griseofulvin per 5 ml, may be preferable instead. Ultramicrosize griseofulvin is available as tablets (Gris-PEG, Herbert), and its dosage is 30 mg/kg PO every 24 hr. If no response is seen after 2 weeks of therapy, the dose of griseofulvin should be doubled. Treatment is continued until follow-up fungal cultures are negative (minimum, 4 weeks treatment).

Griseofulvin is teratogenic and is contraindicated in pregnant animals. Gastrointestinal side effects (nausea, vomiting, diarrhea) may occur. These side effects may be alleviated by dividing the total daily dosage into two or three doses. Idiosyncratic reactions in cats have also been reported and include anemia, leukopenia, depression, ataxia, and pruritus (Helton et al., 1986).

Ketoconazole (Nizoral, Janssen) is also effective in the treatment of dermatophyte infections. In humans, ketoconazole probably reaches the skin surface via eccrine sweat gland secretions (Clissold, 1987). Measurable concentrations of ketoconazole remain in the skin for as long as 10 days after cessation of treatment, suggesting that ketoconazole binds to skin proteins (Clissold, 1987). Results of a study of rats and guinea pigs led the investigators to propose that in animals, ketoconazole reaches the skin surface via sebum (Clissold, 1987). In another study, ketoconazole cleared dermatophyte infections in guinea pigs beginning at the base of the hairs (Adamson's fringe) (Odds et al., 1980). Thus, ketoconazole is distributed not only to the skin surface but also to hairs, where it prevents fungal invasion of the hair shaft.

In one study, ketoconazole alone (without clipping or topical therapy) was found effective in the treatment of generalized dermatophytosis in cats (Medleau and Chalmers, 1990). Cats were treated with ketoconazole, 10 mg/kg PO every 12 to 24 hr with food, until they were clinically resolved and follow-up fungal cultures were negative. Duration

Table 2. *Topical Antifungals for Treating Generalized Dermatophytosis*

Generic Name	Trade Name	Dilution	Side Effects
Lime sulfur solution	LymDyp (Dermatologics for Veterinary Medicine)	25 ml/L water	Stains fabrics and white haircoats, tarnishes jewelry
Chlorhexidine solution	Nolvasan (Fort Dodge)	25 ml/L water	Local irritation, corneal ulcers
Povidone-iodine solution	Betadine (Purdue Frederick)	42 ml/L water	Irritating to cats, stains white haircoats
Captan 50% powder	Orthrocide Garden Fungicide	1.5 teaspoons/L water	Contact sensitizer in humans, possible carcinogen
Sodium hypochlorite	Clorox	100 ml/L water	Discolors haircoats

of therapy ranged from 2 to 10 weeks (median duration, 6 weeks). Because ketoconazole is not approved for use in animals, its use should be reserved for those cats that cannot tolerate or are resistant to griseofulvin. *It is imperative to obtain client waivers when using any of the nonapproved medications discussed here.*

Side effects of ketoconazole in cats include depression, anorexia, weight loss, vomiting, diarrhea, high serum liver enzyme (alanine aminotransferase [ALT]) levels, and jaundice (Greene, 1990). If side effects occur, ketoconazole therapy should be halted, the cat's serum ALT level should be measured, and supportive care (i.e., fluid therapy) should be initiated if needed. Therapy with ketoconazole is reinstituted at a lower dose, given on an alternate-day basis, or both after the serum ALT level returns to normal and the side effects abate. Because mummified fetuses and stillbirths have been found in ketoconazole-treated bitches, ketoconazole is contraindicated for use in pregnant animals.

Itraconazole (Janssen), a new investigational triazole antifungal compound, has shown promise as a systemic antifungal agent. It shares its basic principles of activity with ketoconazole and is also administered orally but appears to have fewer side effects in humans. Itraconazole is currently being investigated in the treatment of dermatophyte infections in cats (Medleau, unpublished data, 1991). To date, seven cats (four long-haired and three short-haired) have been successfully treated with itraconazole for generalized dermatophytosis. Haircoats were not clipped, and topical therapy was not used. Cats were given itraconazole, 10 mg/kg PO every 24 hr with food. Duration of itraconazole treatment ranged from 4 to 20 weeks in these cats. Itraconazole is also being evaluated for treatment of widespread dermatophytosis in a Persian cat cattery. If found effective, treatment with itraconazole may become a therapeutic option for cattery owners who do not want to clip their cats. Unfortunately, treatment results of this study are not yet available.

Itraconazole side effects may occur in cats and appear to be dose related. Side effects may include anorexia, depression, vomiting, weight loss, elevated serum ALT level, jaundice, and hepatotoxic-

ity. If side effects occur, itraconazole therapy is halted, the cat's serum ALT level is measured, and supportive care (i.e., fluid therapy) is initiated if needed. Itraconazole therapy is reinstituted at a lower dose, given on an alternate-day basis, or both once the serum ALT level returns to normal and the side effects have abated.

In dermatophyte pseudomycetomas, surgical excision of the lesions does not result in cure because lesions tend to recur at the surgical site. Because so few cats have been studied, the medical treatment of choice is not yet known. Two cats have been treated with griseofulvin. In one cat, lesions resolved after treatment for 2 months with griseofulvin, 30 mg/kg PO every 24 hr (Bourdin et al., 1975). Another cat did not improve when treated with griseofulvin, 65 mg/kg daily for 2 months. This cat also failed to respond to treatment with ketoconazole, 37 mg/kg daily (Miller and Goldschmidt, 1986).

Two cats are currently being treated with itraconazole. One cat remains clinically controlled but not cured after 18 months of therapy with itraconazole, 25 mg/day (Mundell, unpublished data, 1990). Because this cat's serum ALT level increased after 5 months of therapy, a higher dose of itraconazole has not been used for fear that clinical side effects might occur. In the other cat, clinical cure appears to have been achieved after 10 months of therapy with itraconazole (Medleau, unpublished data, 1991). The dosage in this cat has varied from 10 mg/kg every 24 hr (lesions initially improved, then worsened) to 20 mg/kg every 24 hr (lesions improved, but side effects developed) to 20 mg/kg every 48 hr (apparent resolution of lesions and numerous repeat negative fungal cultures).

Cattery Situations

In a multiple-cat household or cattery situation, the veterinarian and owner need to know which cats are infected with *M. canis* so that these cats can be separated from the noninfected ones. In order to identify asymptomatic carriers, all cats should be cultured using the toothbrush technique.

When a large number of cats are infected, three

therapeutic options exist. The first option involves treating the cats with only topical therapy. Culture-positive cats should be separated from culture-negative cats to prevent further spread of the infection. Culture-positive cats are clipped, and all cats are treated topically with an antifungal product (see Table 2) once or twice weekly. All cats (including previously culture-negative cats) should be recultured for dermatophytes every 2 to 4 weeks using the toothbrush technique. Treatment is continued until all cats are culture negative, plus an additional month for insurance. Clients that choose this regimen should be warned that it may be necessary to start systemic therapy at a later date because topical therapy alone is not always effective. The second option is to treat all cats aggressively in the cattery or household with clipping, topical therapy, and systemic therapy. Because of the systemic therapy (griseofulvin or ketoconazole), the cats cannot be bred during treatment. Also, cats should not be shown, sold, or loaned for breeding, nor should new cats be added to the colony for the duration of treatment. Culture-positive cats should be separated from culture-negative cats to prevent further spread of the infection. All cats should be cultured for dermatophytes every 2 to 4 weeks using the toothbrush technique. Treatment is continued until all cats are culture-negative, plus an additional month for insurance. Depending on the number of cats, the cost of this treatment program can be very high. The third option is to treat only infected kittens. This option is pursued if a cattery owner is only interested in producing kittens that are not infected and cannot or will not treat the entire cattery. Breeding and pregnant queens are isolated from the remainder of the cattery. The queens should be clipped and then treated topically every 5 days with chlorhexidine shampoo or dip. After queening, therapy with oral griseofulvin is initiated in the queen. When weaned, the kittens should be isolated from the rest of the colony and cultured for dermatophytosis. Culture-positive kittens should be treated topically with chlorhexidine shampoos and orally with griseofulvin. Those that culture negative should be prophylactically treated topically with chlorhexidine shampoo every 5 days until they are sold.

Preventive Measures

Because fungal spores remain viable on shed hairs for as long as 18 months, cat hairs must be removed from the environment to prevent reinfection. Carpeted areas and furniture should be vacuumed at least once weekly, with the vacuum bag discarded after each use. Cattery owners should thoroughly vacuum the rooms where cats are kept, including heating ducts, ceiling, ventilation ducts, and transportation vehicles. Hard surfaces such as floors, countertops, litter boxes, and cages must be disinfected at least once a week with sodium hypochlorite diluted 1:10 in water. Cages should be cleaned once daily with a 1:4 dilution of chlorhexidine solution. Brushes, bedding, combs, and toys should be disinfected or destroyed.

To prevent *M. canis* from being introduced into a cattery, newly acquired cats, cats that have been at cat shows, or cats that were on breeding loan should be cultured for *M. canis* and kept isolated from the other cats in the colony until culture results are known. Pending culture results, isolated cats should be treated with topical antifungal shampoos or dips every 5 days. To prevent infection at cat shows, cats should be handled as little as possible and groomed using only the handler's grooming equipment in an area free of other cats.

References and Suggested Reading

Bourdin, M., Destombes, P., Parodi, A. L., et al.: Premiere observation d'un mycetome a Microsporum canis chez un chat. Rec. Med. Vet. 151:475, 1975.
Clinical signs, diagnosis, and treatment of dermatophyte pseudomycetoma in a cat.

Clissold, S. P.: Pharmacokinetic properties. *In* Jones, H. E. (ed.): *Ketoconazole Today: A Review of Clinical Experience.* Manchester: ADIS Press, 1987, p. 22.
Pharmacokinetic properties of ketoconazole in laboratory animals and humans.

Greene, C. E.: Antifungal therapy. *In* Greene, C. E. (ed.): *Infectious Diseases of the Dog and Cat.* Philadelphia: W. B. Saunders, 1990, p. 649.
A review of antifungal drugs, their uses, and their side effects.

Helton, K. A., Nesbitt, G. H., and Caciola, P. L.: Griseofulvin toxicity in cats: Literature review and report of seven cases. J. Am. Anim. Hosp. Assoc. 22:453, 1986.
A review of griseofulvin side effects in cats.

Medleau, L.: Recently described feline dermatoses. Vet. Clin. North Am. Small Anim. Pract. 20:1615, 1990.
Includes a review of the cause, clinical signs, diagnosis, and treatment of feline dermatophyte pseudomycetomas.

Medleau, L., and Chalmers, S. A.: Ketoconazole for treatment of dermatophytosis in cats. J.A.V.M.A. (in press).
Ketoconazole was successfully used to treat dermatophytosis in cats.

Miller, W. H., and Goldschmidt, M. H.: Mycetomas in the cat caused by a dermatophyte: A case report. J. Am. Anim. Hosp. Assoc. 22:255, 1986.
A case report and review of dermatophyte pseudomycetomas in cats.

Moriello, K. A.: Management of dermatophyte infections in catteries and multiple cat households. Vet. Clin. North Am. Small Anim. Pract. 20:1457, 1990.
A review of the etiology, diagnosis, and treatment of dermatophytosis in cats.

Odds, F. C., Milne, L. J. R., Gentles, J. C., et al.: The activity *in vitro* and *in vivo* of a new imidazole antifungal, ketoconazole. J. Antimicrob. Chemother. 6:97, 1980.
Mechanism of action of ketoconazole.

PSYCHOGENIC DERMATOSES

KEVIN SHANLEY
and KAREN OVERALL
Philadelphia, Pennsylvania

Psychogenic dermatoses that may have tandem behavioral and dermatologic causality include numerous diseases (Table 1) with a tremendous variation in suspected etiologies. It is frequently difficult to distinguish the role of pruritus versus the role of behavioral abnormalities.

By definition, psychogenic dermatoses present with both behavioral and dermatologic components; therefore, it is inappropriate to address only one of these aspects. In general, the first step in approaching these cases is to take thorough behavioral and medical histories and perform a complete physical examination. Multiple deep skin scrapings, fungal culture, bacterial culture and sensitivity testing, and other laboratory tests should be done when deemed appropriate. After all dermatologic causes are ruled out and secondary problems such as bacterial infection are resolved, the behavioral diseases should be pursued.

Even when medical causes have been ruled out or treated, it can still be difficult to isolate the behavioral diagnosis. Psychogenic dermatoses with underlying behavioral etiologies consist of three classes: (1) those that respond to behavioral therapy only, (2) those that respond to behavioral therapy plus pharmacologic intervention, and (3) those that do not respond to behavioral therapy at all and may not respond to traditional pharmacologic therapy. This latter category represents those conditions that may be obsessive-compulsive types of disorders. Most of the refractory cases probably fall within this category.

PATHOPHYSIOLOGY

The pathophysiology of pruritus is unclear. Pruritus is best understood as a primary sensory modality. Current research proposes the following sequence of events for pruritus:

$$stimulus \rightarrow mediator \rightarrow receptor \rightarrow$$
$$peripheral\ pathway \rightarrow$$
$$central\ processing \rightarrow$$
$$central\ interpretation \rightarrow response$$

Various types of itching that may have significant roles in psychogenic dermatoses include spontaneous itch, epicritic itch, protopathic itch, conversion itch, and pathologic itch (Shanley, 1988). We suggest that a local stimulus or trauma may induce a well-localized itch that persists briefly after the stimulus or trauma is removed (spontaneous itch). Additionally, a normal cutaneous sensory experience, such as touch, may be perceived as pruritus (conversion itch). These may lead to an intense skin response occurring with pathologic changes that provokes severe scratching (pathologic itch). Endorphins may be released, causing an "endorphin high," which results in positive feedback that stimulates additional scratching and continues the cycle.

The gate control theory of pruritus states that cells of the substantia gelatinosa of the dorsal horn of the spinal cord act as a swinging gate to dampen or accentuate afferent nerve patterns from large and small nerve fibers before they stimulate central transmission cells in the dorsal horn. These transmission cells activate nerve fibers to cause stimulation of an action system that is responsible for pruritus perception and response of the individual. Central factors such as anxiety, previous experiences, boredom, or other competing cutaneous sensations may act as a check-and-balance system on the substantia gelatinosa cells to reduce or amplify the sensation of pruritus.

Table 1. Psychogenic Dermatoses

	Canine	Feline
Acral lick dermatitis	X	—
Psychogenic alopecia	X	X
Psychogenic dermatitis	X	X
Trichotillomania	—	X
Flank sucking	X	—
Tail chasing, sucking, or mutilation	X	X
Limb biting	X	X

ACRAL LICK DERMATITIS

Acral lick dermatitis (ALD) remains one of the most frustrating and challenging problems in veterinary dermatology. Numerous underlying causes and therapies have been suggested. Most veterinarians and veterinary dermatologists have a routine approach to ALD, yet we all have numerous failures of a wide variety of therapeutics. Most cases of ALD do not have primary psychogenic abnormalities as the underlying etiology.

In general, a diagnosis of ALD can be made within a few seconds after looking at the lesion. These patients present with one or more areas of firm, raised, ulcerative plaques frequently located on the dorsal aspect of the carpus, metacarpus, tarsus, or metatarsus. Extensive ulceration appears to be associated with severe licking, whereas chronicity correlates directly with thickness, firmness, and degree of elevation of the plaque. In a period from March, 1989, through September, 1990, 98 biopsy specimens submitted to the Surgical Pathology Laboratory at the Veterinary School of the University of Pennsylvania were diagnosed as ALD. When known, the location of these biopsy samples was equally divided between front (39) and rear (38) legs. When compared with the total in-hospital pool of 44,960 cases seen during this same time period, Doberman pinschers ($P \leq 0.001$) and Labrador retrievers ($P \leq 0.007$) were significantly over-represented. Akitas, Dalmations, English setters, Maltese, peke-a-poo, Shar pei, standard schnauzer, and Weimaraners had relative risks of at least 2; however the sample pool was too small to be statistically significant. Additional studies of these breeds may identify other breeds at risk for developing ALD. No sex predilections could be identified.

Because the majority of cases of ALD that present to the Veterinary Hospital of the University of Pennsylvania (VHUP) are advanced, a high percentage have significant perforating folliculitis. Therefore, skin scrapings, fungal culture, and bacterial culture and sensitivity testing are important initial diagnostics. Obtaining biopsy specimens for culture and histopathologic study is often pursued. If results of the fungal culture and skin scrapings are negative, appropriate antibiotics are administered for a period of 6 to 16 weeks or occasionally longer. Another rule of thumb in treating the bacterial component of ALD is to treat for 3 to 4 weeks after resolution of the infection. Many severe ALD lesions respond dramatically or completely resolve with antibiotic therapy alone. *Staphylococcus intermedius* is the most frequently identified pathogen. Gram-negative bacteria may be present as a secondary pathogen. As with most deep skin infections, the ideal antibiotic is one to which both organisms are susceptible; if this is not the case, treatment for the *S. intermedius* often results in elimination of the gram-negative organism as well, because it is dependent on the *S. intermedius* to thrive. Cephalexin (Keflex, Lilly; 22 mg/kg PO every 12 hr) usually has excellent efficacy. Erythromycin (9 to 13 mg/kg PO every 8 hr) is another reliable choice if the sensitivity results concur, because it is inexpensive and may have other anti-inflammatory effects in addition to its antibacterial actions. The trimethoprim-sulfa antibiotics often have poor efficacy in deep pyodermas, particularly ALD.

It is important to pursue other diagnostic methods after initiating antibiotic therapy. The history, signalment, and physical examination findings may provide important clues that suggest an underlying etiology. If the age at onset of the skin disease is less than 5 years, allergic inhalant dermatitis and food allergy should be considered and intradermal allergy testing and an elimination diet trial should be performed. Hypothyroidism may be the underlying cause and is more common in middle-aged to older animals. Hyperadrenocorticism is an uncommon cause of ALD. Obtaining biopsy specimens for dermatohistopathologic study is helpful to confirm a diagnosis of ALD and to quantitate the degree of infection and scar tissue formation present. It may also identify *Demodex canis*, dermatophytes, or foreign bodies or may suggest an underlying allergic component. Radiographs help identify neoplasia, serious trauma, radiopaque foreign bodies, and degenerative changes. The most common radiographic changes are periosteal reaction deep to the ALD and surrounding soft-tissue swelling. Nerve conduction studies and biopsy of nerve are rarely helpful. Conduction velocities may be abnormal, but according to the cases handled by one of us (K.S.), this change has always been bilateral, even though the ALD is unilateral. In some cases, sensory nerve dysfunction has been implicated in dogs with ALD (Van Nes, 1986); in these animals, affected limbs and nonlicked limbs show no difference in amplitudes of sensory evoked potentials. It is possible that such a dysfunction is associated with behavioral attributes, including decreased sensitivity to an injury, which might promote chewing.

The lack of any "clues" to suggest a specific underlying disease should not eliminate that disease from the differential diagnosis. That is, ALD may be the only sign to indicate a specific cause such as atopy, food allergy, flea allergy, or hypothyroidism.

Once all dermatologic causes have been ruled out, patients who remain affected are addressed as having an underlying behavior abnormality. Therapy is directed at treatment for an obsessive-compulsive or self-mutilation disorder. Antihistamines such as hydroxyzine or chlorpheniramine, narcotic antagonists such as naltrexone, or tricyclic antidepressants (TCAs) such as doxepin or amitriptyline are used (see later).

SELF-MUTILATION

It is frequently difficult to distinguish between primary self-mutilation and self-mutilation that is secondary to an obsessive-compulsive type of disorder. In the latter case, self-mutilation may be just one of a constellation of symptoms in a poorly understood complex.

Many people and some animals with mutilatory lesions may have decreased sensitivity to pain (Brown et al., 1987; Dodman et al., 1988). It has been postulated that this may be mediated by endorphin (opiate) receptor sites. If so, such patients should have increases in the number, affinity, or activity of endorphin receptor sites. For some of these patients, the increase in endorphin levels may be noted in blood but not in the cerebrospinal fluid. Should this be the case, morphine, an exogenous narcotic, should stimulate endorphin receptors, producing an exaggerated response. This technique can be used diagnostically, but caution is urged because the diagnosis could be confused by an endorphin-induced histamine-evoked pruritus. It is important to obtain a definitive diagnosis before resorting to progestins and corticosteroids, which can mask physiologic complications or contributory factors and may cause other behavioral problems.

The conditions that may respond to behavioral modification alone include attention-seeking behavior and boredom. The role of boredom has been vastly over-rated as an underlying cause of self-mutilatory conditions including ALD. Boredom as a diagnosis is frequently an artifact of incomplete medical and behavioral histories. It is critical to distinguish boredom from confinement. Confined dogs may be maintained on inappropriate substrates or exposed to irritants. These inappropriate management practices may predispose dogs to conversion itch and pathologic itch. To attribute such conditions to an impoverished sensory environment, implicit in the diagnosis of boredom, is simplistic and wrong. If boredom is truly thought to be the diagnosis, enrichment of the sensory environment should ameliorate the situation. This may include giving the animal more space to explore, additional toys, toys that "play back" (e.g., squeak toys), or canine or feline companions. If these do not help, the animal was not bored.

Attention-seeking behavior occurs when an animal exhibits a behavior, including limb chewing or tail chasing, in order to get a response from the owner. It is important to remember that for animals who get very little attention from their owners, negative attention is better than no attention. Animals can learn this behavior and may start to exhibit it whenever their owner is present but ignoring them. The nature of the condition becomes apparent when the behavior resolves when the owner learns not to react. For the animal's sake, it is critical also to give attention and praise when it is calm.

Self-mutilation is infrequent in dogs experiencing separation anxiety; when it occurs, it is secondary. Dogs with separation anxiety cannot be left alone by their owners without panicking and becoming destructive. It is important to distinguish random damage from that done by an animal that, in the process of seeking stimulation, unrolls and shreds a roll of toilet paper. Toilet paper and the contents of trash baskets may play back. These behaviors may occur when the owner is home and not paying attention to the animal and are easily distinguished from the severe destruction that occurs in separation anxiety. In the process of destroying the area in which they are confined, dogs with separation anxiety sometimes damage themselves. These lesions may then become secondary foci for self-mutilation. Such conditions are best treated with a combination of behavior modification (Voith and Borchelt, 1982) and antianxiety medication. As a sole therapy, behavior modification that teaches a dog not to react to the absence of its owners seldom works. Amitriptyline HCl (Elavil, Stuart; canine dose, 1 to 2 mg/kg PO every 12 hr; feline dose, 5 to 10 mg PO per *cat* every 12 to 24 hr) is the drug of choice in these conditions because TCAs do not interfere with the ability to learn and so can be used with behavioral modification programs. Benzodiazepines interfere with the ability to learn and therefore should not be used in these situations.

OBSESSIVE-COMPULSIVE DISORDERS

Behavior modification has almost no role in treating self-mutilation that is part of an obsessive-compulsive disorder. When all medical causes are ruled out, all secondary infections are treated, and traditional behavioral and pharmacologic therapy are unsuccessful, the mutilation may be due to an obsessive-compulsive disorder. In those cases seen at the Behavior Clinic at VHUP, the behavior is ritualistic, stereotypic, and may or may not involve mutilation. A newer TCA, clomipramine HCl (Anafranil; Ciba-Geigy), has been inordinately successful in treating obsessive-compulsive disorders in humans, including trichotillomania. Studies are ongoing at VHUP to establish dose levels and identify side effects in dogs and cats. This drug alleviates obsessive-compulsive effects separately from antidepressant effects (Ananth, 1986; Goldberger and Rappaport, 1991). This suggests that efficacy with this drug is diagnostic of an obsessive-compulsive disorder. The investigators postulate that many canine psychogenic dermatoses that have no detectable underlying medical or dermatologic etiology may be obsessive-compulsive disorders. Treatment of most human obsessive-compulsive disorders is continual, and drug withdrawal results in relapse. The same is probably true of dogs. Owners give animals with ALD attention during both self-mutilating and quiescent periods. It is unlikely that these severe cases are manifestations of attention-seeking behavior; many ALD and self-mutilation conditions probably have an obsessive-compulsive component. This would certainly account for the high recidivism rate of these syndromes. It is important to emphasize that owners are often successful in inhibiting a dog from chewing while they are present; this does not mean that the dog no longer has the urge to chew. Again, this is often true in obsessive-compulsive disorders.

FELINE PSYCHOGENIC ALOPECIA AND DERMATITIS

Feline psychogenic alopecia is an uncommon disease that presents as traumatic (stubble) alopecia that usually is bilaterally symmetric. Flea allergy, food allergy, and allergic inhalant dermatitis are the most common causes of traumatic alopecia in cats and must be ruled out before considering a diagnosis of feline psychogenic alopecia. The dermatitis form, neurodermatitis, is characterized by excoriations that manifest as hemorrhagic crusting and are present in addition to the alopecia. This is a poorly characterized entity in cats and is most frequently reported in high-strung breeds of cats (Siamese, Burmese, and Abyssinian) of various ages and sexual status. Although a supportive history is frequently lacking, these lesions are induced by overzealous self-grooming. These cats are often referred to as "closet lickers" because they often perform their excessive grooming when their owners are absent. The most important diagnostic clue is broken distal ends of hairs in the affected areas, confirming self-induced traumatic alopecia. The differential diagnosis for this type of alopecia includes any pruritic skin disease such as flea allergy dermatitis, food allergy, allergic inhalant dermatitis, dermatophytosis, otodectic mange, cheyletiellosis, notoedric or demodectic mange, allergic reaction to intestinal parasites, or other ectoparasite or immunologic disorders, as well as psychogenic alopecia. Feline endocrine alopecia is extremely rare and should present with complete alopecia rather than traumatic alopecia, with the majority of remaining hairs in telogen rather than anagen. Historic findings may help suggest a psychogenic problem, although all causes of pruritic skin disease should be ruled out before a diagnosis of psychogenic alopecia or dermatitis can be confirmed. There is no single confirmatory test to diagnose psychogenic skin disease.

The pattern of traumatic alopecia or dermatitis is variable, but affected sites often have well-delineated borders. Most animals referred to us with a tentative diagnosis of psychogenic alopecia or dermatitis are actually diagnosed as having an underlying pruritic dermatologic abnormality. Flea allergy dermatitis is the most common reason for misdiagnosis of psychogenic dermatitis.

Once a diagnosis of psychogenic alopecia and dermatitis has been made, treatment is based on eliminating the underlying cause if possible. Usually this is not possible, and various therapeutics such as chlorpheniramine (Chlor-Trimeton, Schering; 0.4 to 0.7 mg/kg PO) and amitriptyline HCl may help. In the future, clomipramine HCl may be helpful.

THERAPY

Numerous therapies for psychogenic dermatoses have been uniformly unsuccessful in our experience. These include physical restraint, surgery, amphetamines, topical therapy, and tranquilizers. The use of Elizabethan collars, bandages, and other physical restraint devices to prevent animals from traumatizing themselves usually has very limited success. The key to successful treatment of ALD, self-mutilation, and obsessive-compulsive disorders is to extinguish the desire for focusing on an area and thus eliminate the self-trauma. Physical restraint devices probably only increase the desire to attend to an area and the frustration in not being able to satisfy that desire. However, in the most severe cases, when permanent physical damage will occur if self-trauma continues, these devices may provide needed temporary restraint. Elizabethan collars are most effective in these situations. Bandaging with the application of bitter-tasting chemicals rarely provides adequate protection for more than a few hours. Also, patients may fixate on traumatizing new areas just proximal or distal to the bandaged area, creating a new lesion and complicating the initial problem.

Topical use of corticosteroids, anti-inflammatory drugs, or antibacterial agents is usually unsuccessful in treating ALD. Of the patients with ALD seen by the Dermatology Service at VHUP, less than 10% respond to flunixin meglumine (Banamine, Schering) and flucinolone acetonide-dimethyl sulfoxide (Synotic, Diamond) combination therapy. It is possible that this product will help early cases of ALD, but is clearly insufficient for severe, chronic cases. Topical use of mupiricin (Bactoderm, Beecham) has had limited success in those cases with significant bacterial complications. Topical 5% benzoyl peroxide gel (OxyDex, Dermatologics for Veterinary Medicine; Pyoben, Allerderm) has also been helpful in a small percentage of cases with significant infection, when exudate and crusting are present. Other antibacterial agents have not been successful. Application of topical agents may also increase an animal's attention to the affected area, thus causing negative results.

Surgical removal of the offending limb may be necessary in cases of extreme mutilation when there is no hope of reconstruction or healing. Surgical ablation is unsuccessful as a treatment, because the dog further mutilates more proximate regions of the limb.

Tranquilizers cannot treat psychogenic dermatoses and may confound accurate diagnosis, because tranquilized animals do not exhibit a typical behavioral response to either the condition or any stimuli.

Amphetamines are frequently misused to treat dogs in which practitioners attribute psychogenic dermatoses to boredom and overactivity. Truly overactive dogs are rare and should manifest continuous, noninterruptable, noncircadian activity.

Progestins are among the most inappropriately and overprescribed medications for psychogenic dermatoses. Their mode of action is probably attributable to their effects on specific hypothalamic nuclei and their prolonged glucocorticoid-like effects (Romatowski, 1989). Megestrol acetate (Ovaban, Schering; Megace, Bristol-Myers; canine dose, 2 to 4 mg/kg PO every 24 hr; feline dose, 2.5 to 5.0 mg PO per *cat* every 48 hr for 7 to 14 days, then 2.5 to 5.0 mg PO per *cat* every 7 to 14 days) and medroxyprogesterone acetate (Depo-Provera, Upjohn; canine dose, 20 mg/kg SC, repeat in 4 to 6 months if needed; feline dose, 50 to 100 mg SC per *cat,* repeat in 4 to 6 months if needed) may decrease pruritus at the risk of gynecomastia, mammary neoplasia, alterations of the pituitary-adrenal axis, polyuria, polydypsia, alterations in carbohydrate metabolism including diabetogenesis, and bone marrow suppression. They further predispose the animal to frequent urination, with occasional incontinence and decrease in bladder tone, and so can be a factor in elimination problems in felines. They can render any aggressive animal more unpredictable. Finally, progestins can cause profound cutaneous changes including alopecia and cutaneous atrophy. All of these effects are more pronounced in cats than in dogs. It is difficult to conceive of a rational role for these drugs in the treatment of psychogenic dermatoses. However, if these drugs are used, they should be administered at the lowest possible efficacious dose and always with frequent laboratory monitoring.

Corticosteroids

It is important to remember that previous medical therapy may either exacerbate the condition or mask both dermatologic and behavioral symptoms. Corticosteroids and progestins are notorious in this respect and appear to be used so uncritically that a discussion of their rational and irrational use is germane. Behavioral problems commonly attributed to these drugs include increased drinking and attendant urination, alterations in bladder tone and possible incontinence, and unpredictable mood swings. Both dogs and cats maintained on steroid therapy can develop inappropriate substrate preferences for urination after first soiling the areas accidentally. Dogs that are aggressive may become more reactive, unpredictable, and dangerous when on steroids. Because these drugs are appetite stimulants, it is critical that they be used with the utmost caution in dogs having food-related aggression.

Narcotic Antagonists

Narcotic antagonists may be useful for animals with aberrant endorphin metabolism or receptors and have been successfully used to treat some tail chasing or mutilation (Dodman et al., 1988). Naloxone blocks central endorphin receptors, affording relief from the described stereotypic symptoms. Its main role may be as a diagnostic agent: if the response is not blocked, the etiology of the lesion is not at the level of aberrant endorphin metabolism. Drawbacks include administration route (pure naloxone is available only in injectable form (dogs, 11 to 22 μg/kg IM, IV, SC as needed) and the need to administer the drug continually or full relapse results. The oral form, a mixed narcotic agonist/antagonist, is available as Talwin (Winthrop; 50 mg pentazocine plus 0.5 mg naloxone PO every 12 hr). Naltrexone HCl (Trexan, DuPont), a pure opioid antagonist, has been used at a dosage of 25 to 50 mg/day PO in cats and 2.2 mg/kg PO every 12 to 24 hr in dogs.

Hydroxyzine Hydrochloride

Hydroxyzine hydrochloride (Atarax, Roerig; 2.2 mg/kg PO every 8 hr) is classified as a piperazine H_1 antihistamine. Its duration of action in humans is 6 to 24 hr, and it has a central depressant activity that may account for its prominent antipruritic action (Garrison, 1990). It is available as oral tablets, an oral liquid, or an injectable medication. Antipruritic efficacy occurs in 20 to 50% of patients. Side effects include sedation and are uncommon. Regarding antihistamines and TCAs, a general rule of thumb we suggest is initially to use trade name products until a response is seen, then switch to a less expensive generic equivalent; it is important to make sure the same degree of response is observed with the generic.

Tricyclic Antidepressants

TCAs have a role in psychogenic dermatoses that have a component of anxiety—that is, the animal exhibits the symptoms primarily when left alone. They may also be useful for animals with healing lesions because the animal is less anxious about the lesion and so may not lick as much. The antihistaminic effects of most antidepressants were known long before the discovery of their antidepressant effects. TCAs cross the blood-brain barrier and appear to inhibit serotonin reuptake. Amitriptyline HCl is very safe in dogs and cats and has a half-life of 6 to 8 hr in dogs, taking about 3 to 4 days to reach a steady-state level. In humans, the peak serum concentration of TCAs after an oral dose is 2 to 8 hr, and the elimination half-life is approximately 24 hr. After absorption, the TCAs bind to plasma proteins, are lipophilic, and become widely distributed. They are metabolized by hepatic microsomal enzymes and eliminated exclusively via the liver. Uncommon withdrawal side effects (diarrhea, restlessness, anxiety piloerection, and hot and cold flushes) may occur 48 hr after abrupt cessation. No major long-term side effects have been reported. Because TCAs are protein bound and soluble in lipids, steady-state levels may be reached later in obese animals. When used at the Behavior Clinic at VHUP, these drugs are dosed as discussed later for the first 7 to 10 days; if no noticeable calming effect is observed after that time, the dose is doubled. At high doses, rare instances of paradoxical excitement have been seen. This effect resolves on drug withdrawal. If there is no effect 10 days after the dose is doubled, amitriptyline will not work and should be stopped. For management of behavioral conditions, maintenance is an option. Most patients are kept on the drug for 1 to 2 months or for 3 to 4 weeks after all behavioral symptoms have resolved. At that point, the drug can either be stopped abruptly or reduced over a period of 3 weeks; a few dogs have relapsed on abrupt withdrawal, and reinstitution of the drug at slightly higher levels causes symptoms to abate. TCAs are contraindicated in animals with extant cardiac disease including pronounced arrhythmias. Side effects of all TCAs include a dry mouth and occasional increased water consumption in dogs, possibly necessitating more frequent urination. These drugs are used extensively at the Behavior Clinic at VHUP, and very few clients note this effect. Occasional arrhythmias and tachycardias occur at high doses; these resolve on drug withdrawal. Reduced doses are urged for animals with ongoing renal or hepatic disease. If lethargy ensues, stop the drug immediately.

Amitriptyline HCl has been useful in early and very mild psychogenic dermatoses and in those cases that have an allergic component. Caution is urged for dogs that may have concurrent thyroid abnormalities. Hypothyroidism can present with both dermatologic and behavioral components. The latter may include fearfulness, uneasiness in new circumstances, and uneven responses in familiar situations. Although amitriptyline can relieve these signs, TCAs have been associated with sick euthyroid syndrome in humans.

Doxepin HCl (Sinequan, Roerig; Adapin, Fisons; canine dose, 3 to 5 mg/kg PO every 12 hr; maximum dose is 150 mg every 12 hr) is a TCA with potent antihistaminic (H_1), anticholinergic, and alpha$_1$-adrenergic blocking properties. In humans, doxepin, amitriptyline, and trimipramine are the most effective TCAs for the treatment of primary dermatologic problems such as urticaria and pruritus in patients without concomitant psychologic abnormalities. The doses of these drugs for their antipruritic effects are lower than required for their antidepressant effects. Also, the response to therapy is quicker (2 to 4 weeks) when treating pruritic disorders compared with treating depressant disorders (4 to 6 weeks). Doxepin HCl is 800 times more potent an H_1 receptor antagonist than diphenhydramine HCl (Benadryl) and 67 times more potent than hydroxyzine HCl. It also has more significant anticholinergic effects than hydroxyzine or diphenhydramine. It is six times more potent than cimetidine as an H_2 antihistamine (Gupta et al., 1987).

In humans, doxepin and other TCAs have the potential for cardiotoxicity, primarily ventricular arrhythmias, because of their anticholinergic and quinidine-like effect on the heart. Doxepin is relatively less cardiotoxic than the others. In general, TCAs should not be used with monoamine oxidase inhibitors, clonidine, anticonvulsants (especially phenytoin), oral anticoagulants, steroid hormones, antihistamines, or aspirin (Gupta et al., 1987). Other side effects include hyperexcitability, lethargy, vomiting, and diarrhea. Doxepin in particular is contraindicated in animals with glaucoma or urinary retention.

SUMMARY

Psychogenic dermatoses are a poorly understood group of diseases. Current thinking suggests that most patients with ALD and feline traumatic alopecia have common primary dermatologic diseases as underlying causes. The most severe, chronic cases of these diseases, as well as most cases of obsessive-compulsive or self-mutilation disorders, probably have underlying psychological abnormalities. New therapeutic agents with both antihistaminic and antidepressant actions may help many patients with true psychogenic disorders. It will continue to be difficult to separate chewing, licking, and sucking due to pruritus from that due to psychogenic factors.

References and Suggested Reading

Ananth, J.: Clomipramine: An antiobsessive drug. Can. J. Psychiatry 31:253, 1986.
Brown, S. A., Crowell-Davis, S., Malcolm, T., et al.: Naloxone-responsive compulsive tail chasing in a dog. J.A.V.M.A. 190:884, 1987.

Dodman, N. H., Shuster, L., White, S. D., et al.: Use of narcotic antagonists to modify stereotypic self-licking, self-chewing and scratching behavior in dogs. J.A.V.M.A. 193:815, 1988.

Garrison, J. C.: Histamine, bradykinin, 5-hydroxytryptamine and their antagonists. *In* Goodman, L. S., Gilman, A., Rall, T. W., et al. (eds.): *Goodman and Gilman's the Pharmacological Basis of Therapeutics*, 8th ed. New York: Pergamon Press, 1990, pp. 575–599.

Goldberger, E., and Rappaport, J. L.: Canine acral lick dermatitis: Response to the antiobsessional drug clomipramine. J. Am. Anim. Hosp. Assoc. 27:179, 1991.

Gupta, M. A., Gupta, A. K., and Ellis, C. N.: Antidepressant drugs in dermatology. Arch. Dermatol. 123:647, 1987.

Romatowski, J.: Use of megestrol acetate in cats. J.A.V.M.A. 194:700, 1989.

Shanley, K. J.: Pathophysiology of pruritus. Vet. Clin. North Am. Small Anim. Pract. 18:971, 1988.

Van Nes, J. J.: Electrophysiological evidence of sensory nerve dysfunction in 10 dogs with acral lick dermatitis. J. Am. Anim. Hosp. Assoc. 22:157, 1986.

Voith, V. L., and Borchelt, P. L.: Introduction to animal behavior therapy. Vet. Clin. North Am. Small Anim. Pract. 12:565, 1982.

TREATMENT OF *SARCOPTES* AND *CHEYLETIELLA* INFESTATIONS

KAREN A. MORIELLO

Madison, Wisconsin

During the past several years, I have noted a significant increase in the number of cases of scabies and cheyletiellosis diagnosed at the Veterinary Medical Teaching Hospital (VMTH), School of Veterinary Medicine, University of Wisconsin. The most interesting finding with this resurgence is the difficulty encountered in treating these mite infestations and the surprising need for environmental treatment, especially for cheyletiellosis.

SCABIES

Scabies is caused by the mite *Sarcoptes scabiei* var. *canis*. The entire life cycle is completed on the host within 21 days. Mites live in the superficial noncornified layers of the epidermis, where they burrow, breed, and lay eggs. Clinical signs are the result of hypersensitivity reactions to mites and the mechanical irritation produced by burrowing. Transmission occurs most commonly from direct contact. Fomite transmission and environmental contamination may be under-recognized sources of contagion because of the difficulty encountered in eliminating the infestation, in some cases until environmental treatment is instituted. The disease is most common in young dogs, dogs that have been recently kenneled, and small dogs that frequent professional grooming establishments.

The hallmark of this disease is an intense pruritus that is incompletely responsive to corticosteroids. Classic scabies begins ventrally on the abdomen, inner leg region, and thorax. As the mites burrow, a papular eruption develops. The pruritus results in various degrees of self-trauma, and with time, excoriations, alopecia, and crusting of elbows, ear margins, and hocks develops. If left untreated, the lesions may become generalized. Fever, lymphadenopathy, weight loss, secondary pyodermas, and even death may occur. Scabies incognito is a manifestation of this parasitic disease that occurs in well-groomed pets. These dogs present with intense pruritus but have few dermatologic abnormalities. Rarely are skin scrapings positive.

In a busy practice situation, there are two methods of diagnosis—skin scrapings and response to specific therapy (see later). Skin scrapings are most likely to be positive from areas with new lesions and little evidence of self-inflicted trauma.

Treatment Recommendations

Previously efficacious chemicals (e.g., malathion, phosmet) have lately become increasingly less reliable for the treatment of scabies. Regardless of the treatment prescribed, no therapy is 100% effective, and this fact should be emphasized to clients. I

Editor's Note: Extralabel use of ivermectin as described in this article is not approved by the Food and Drug Administration for use in the United States.

prefer to use amitraz, lime sulfur, or ivermectin. The choice of product depends on the circumstances and, of course, the client. All dogs in the house should be treated. I do not recommend the routine treatment of cats because only four cases of *Sarcoptes* infestations have been reported in cats (Hawkins et al., 1987). If necessary, secondary medical problems should be treated before parasiticidal therapy. Clipping of long or matted haircoats is recommended. A cleansing bath in a mild hypoallergenic shampoo will facilitate treatment. A warm lime sulfur dip (LymDyp, Dermatologics for Veterinary Medicine; 4 oz/gal) every 5 to 7 days for 8 weeks is the treatment of choice for puppies less than 12 weeks of age, pregnant or nursing bitches, or other debilitated animals. In addition to being miticidal, lime sulfur is mildly antipruritic. For older puppies and adult dogs, amitraz (Mitaban, UpJohn) dip every 2 weeks for three treatments is effective and more readily accepted by clients. If clients with puppies refuse to use lime sulfur, I suggest amitraz at half the manufacturer's recommended dilution until the puppies are older than 12 weeks. Ivermectin is highly effective in the treatment of scabies. It can be administered orally or by injection, and there is some evidence to suggest that injection may be more effective (Barragry, 1987). The most commonly used product is the bovine injectable (Ivomec, Merck), which is a 1% solution (10,000 μg/ml).* This can be precisely diluted in propylene glycol for accurate doses in small dogs. I use 200 μg/kg three times at 2-week intervals. This drug should not be used in "herding breeds" of dogs, and the reader is directed to an excellent review of the drug (Paradis, 1989). Although not recommended, I have administered ivermectin in puppies less than 6 weeks of age and to pregnant bitches without adverse effects.

Organophosphates, carbamates, pyrethrins, pyrethroids, and citrus-derived flea control products are not recommended for treatment of canine scabies. In particular, I avoid the use of phosmet (Paramite, Vet-Kem) because of numerous treatment failures (diagnosed on the basis of positive skin scrapings) even when the product was used as recommended. Apparently there are geographic differences in organophosphate efficacy, because these products are reported to be still effective in Australia (Shaw, S., Murdoch University, W. Australia, personal communication, 1987). As mentioned earlier, no product is 100% efficacious, and I have observed two cases of amitraz failure and know of one ivermectin failure (Schultz, K., University of Wisconsin, School of Veterinary Medicine, personal communication, 1989).

Environmental Treatment

Textbooks of veterinary dermatology rarely recommend environmental treatment because the mite is considered very susceptible to desiccation. Research on scabies mite "host-seeking" behavior and survival has shown that dislodged mites are sources of infestation. Scabies mites use host odor and thermal stimuli to find their hosts (Arlian et al., 1984b). Canine scabies mites can survive off the host and be infective for 3 days in warm, dry temperatures and up to 18 to 21 days in cool, moist environments (Arlian et al., 1984a). I have encountered numerous cases in which scabies infestation could not be eliminated until environmental treatment was instituted. Therefore, I routinely recommend routine cleaning of the environment and treatment of the premises with a premises flea spray (Siphotrol Plus II House Treatment, Vet-Kem).

CHEYLETIELLOSIS

Cheyletiellosis is caused by an infestation of a mite, *Cheyletiella*. Like *Sarcoptes*, this mite spends its entire life (3 weeks) on the host (dogs, cats, or rabbits) under ideal situations. The mites live and burrow in the cornified epidermis of the skin. In contrast to scabies, the mites lay their eggs on the host's haircoat, and this difference becomes an important consideration in transmission and elimination of the infestation. Clinical signs are most likely the result of hypersensitivity to the mite and mechanical irritation. Like *Sarcoptes*, *Cheyletiella* is highly contagious, and infestation is the result of contact with an infested animal. Because eggs are attached to hairs that can be shed into the environment and serve as sources of reinfestation, I strongly believe that the environment is also a potential source of infestation. The disease is most common in young animals, in multipet households, in pet store kittens and puppies, and in animals kenneled or professionally groomed.

The hallmark of this disease is excessive scaling and pruritus. The pruritus usually is mild to moderate in severity, and rarely clients complain about their pets scratching all night long. The disease has a predominantly dorsal distribution; however, generalized infestations can occur. A papular, crusted eruption may be present or just excessive scaling. Cats may present with miliary dermatitis. In all target species, asymptomatic carriers are common. Although "cheyletiellosis" incognito is not commonly observed, I have seen it in both dogs and

---

*The 1% solution can be diluted very easily for accurate dosing. One milliliter (10,000 μg/ml) mixed with 9 ml of propylene glycol results in a dilution of 1000 μg/ml or 100 μg/0.1 ml. This diluted solution should be kept at room temperature, in a tightly closed container, and protected from light.

cats. This disease, like scabies, is a zoonosis, and owners may be affected.

Skin scrapings, acetate tape preparations, and flea combings can be used to diagnose infestations. In my experience, skin scrapings and acetate tape preparations are the *least* reliable diagnostic aids. I prefer to collect hairs and scale with a flea comb and inspect the debris with a hand-held magnifying lens or dissecting microscope. Hairs should be carefully examined for the presence of eggs glued to their shafts.

Treatment Recommendations

It is commonly believed that this disease is easy to treat and that many owners eliminate infestations on their pets by using flea shampoos or sprays. My experience, especially during the past several years, has been strikingly different. Flea shampoos, flea sprays, and powders have *not* been effective as sole therapeutic agents. Additionally, successful treatment has required therapy for *6 to 8 weeks, as opposed to previous recommendations of 3 weeks.* *All* animals in the household should be treated at the same time. Clipping of the haircoat of all medium- and long-haired animals will greatly increase efficacy of treatment and decrease contagion. Animals should be bathed in a mild hypoallergenic shampoo to remove excess scale and crusts. All animals should be treated for a minimum of 6 to 8 weeks. Pregnant or lactating animals, kittens and puppies, or debilitated animals should be dipped weekly in warm lime sulfur (4 oz/gal) or a pyrethrin dip diluted according to label instructions. Amitraz dips every 2 weeks for three to four treatments are also effective. Amitraz can be toxic to cats and rabbits, and its use is best avoided in these species. When this therapy fails or client compliance is poor, I recommend ivermectin, 300 µg/kg SC repeated three times at 2-week intervals. In addition, twice-weekly applications of a pyrethrin-based flea spray are necessary to kill migrating or newly hatched mites.

Environmental Treatment

In the past, aggressive environmental treatment has not been recommended; however, I have found instances when it was difficult to eliminate infestations from homes without treating the environment. In one instance, the owner was bitten by mites every time she sat on a cloth couch in her home. The owner vacuumed the couch, and I found live mites and numerous hairs with eggs attached in the debris. In three other cases (all cats), topical lime sulfur dips appeared to be ineffective. After determining that client compliance was good and that untreated animals were not the source of reinfestation, I instructed the owner to institute environmental treatment. This finally eliminated the infestation. I currently recommend that owners use an environmental flea control product every 2 weeks during the treatment period. It appears that veterinarians may have underestimated the longevity of these mites in the environment.

CONCLUSION

Sarcoptes and *Cheyletiella* infestations have become increasingly more difficult to treat. Current recommendations for successful elimination of infestations include treatment of all animals in the household, clipping of the haircoat of medium- and long-haired animals, extended topical therapy (6 to 8 weeks) or extended ivermectin therapy (6 to 8 weeks), and treatment of the environment.

References and Suggested Reading

Arlian, L. G., Runyan, R. A., Achar, S., et al.: Survival and infestivity of *Sarcoptes scabiei* var. *canis* and var. *hominis*. J. Am. Acad. Dermatol. 11:210, 1984a.

Arlian, L. G., Runyan, R. A., Sorlie, B. S., et al.: Host-seeking behavior of *Sarcoptes scabiei*. J. Am. Acad. Dermatol. 11:594, 1984b.

Barragry, T. M.: A review of the pharmacology and clinical uses of ivermectin. Can. Vet. J. 28:512, 1987.

Hawkins, J. A., McDonald, R. K., and Woody, B. J.: *Sarcoptes scabiei* infestation in a cat. J.A.V.M.A. 190:1572, 1987.

Paradis, M.: Ivermectin in small animal dermatology. *In* Kirk, R. W. (ed.): *Current Veterinary Therapy X*. Philadelphia: W. B. Saunders, 1989, p. 560.

NECROLYTIC MIGRATORY ERYTHEMA IN DOGS: A CUTANEOUS MARKER FOR GASTROINTESTINAL DISEASE

WILLIAM H. MILLER, Jr.
Ithaca, New York

The term *necrolytic migratory erythema* (NME) was coined in 1973 to describe the skin rash in a person with a pancreatic carcinoma. Today in human dermatology, NME is considered a paraneoplastic dermatosis that is a distinctive cutaneous marker for a glucagon-secreting pancreatic tumor (glucagonoma). Patients with NME have various medical complaints, which include diabetes mellitus (85%), anemia (61%), hypoalbuminemia (81%), and hypoaminoacidemia (97%). Approximately 90% of patients with a glucagonoma will develop NME, but the eruption can occasionally be recognized in association with other serious gastrointestinal disorders, especially hepatic cirrhosis.

In 1986, Walton first introduced NME to veterinary medicine. That initial work suggested that the skin eruption was in some way related to diabetes mellitus. Today, it is known that NME in dogs is a distinctive cutaneous marker for a serious gastrointestinal disorder. In contrast to the findings in humans, NME in dogs usually is associated with hepatic cirrhosis because glucagonomas are rare.

CLINICAL FEATURES

At the time of this writing, NME has been reported in 18 dogs, but I am aware of another 20 cases. From the published data, NME occurs in old dogs (mean age, 10.25 years) with no apparent breed or gender predisposition. Most of these animals were healthy throughout their lives and showed few, if any, constitutional signs of illness before the skin eruption was noticed. At presentation, 7 dogs were normoglycemic, whereas 11 had clinical or laboratory evidence of glucose intolerance or overt diabetes mellitus. In the hyperglycemic dogs, seven developed the diabetes mellitus after the skin disease, three had both problems recognized simultaneously, and one was a confirmed diabetic for 6 months before the NME occurred. Five of the seven normoglycemic dogs became hyperglycemic during the course of their disease, giving an overall frequency of 88.9% of diabetes mellitus in dogs with NME.

Specific laboratory data were available for 16 of the 18 reported cases. A mild to severe nonregenerative anemia was seen in 12 of 15 (80%) dogs. Biochemical abnormalities were observed in all 16 dogs and were as follows: elevated alkaline phosphatase (16/16), elevated alanine transaminase (15/16), hyperglycemia (11/16), and hypoalbuminemia (9/16). Eleven dogs had their liver function evaluated by a sulfobromophthalein retention test or by the pre- and postprandial measurement of bile acids, and chronic liver disease was documented in nine (81.8%). One distracting finding was a low-titer positive antinuclear antibody (ANA) test result in three of eight dogs tested.

The skin lesions of NME are dramatic but not unique for that disorder. They typically are discrete to coalescent crusted erosions on an erythematous base. Intact superficial vesicles or bullae can occasionally be seen. Older lesions, especially those in areas of trauma (i.e., footpads, pressure points), are very hyperkeratotic and crusted. Lesions can occur anywhere, but frequent sites of involvement are the feet and footpads (18/18), face (14/18), external genitalia (13/18), distal extremities (12/18), skin on the ventrum (9/18), pressure points (7/18), and pinnae (7/18).

Although striking, the clinical lesions of NME are not pathognomonic for that disorder and can be seen in drug eruption, pemphigus foliaceus, lupus erythematosus, zinc-responsive dermatosis, and generic dog food dermatosis. One dermatologist treating human patients has gone so far as to recommend that one consider NME "when nothing else makes sense" (Hanifin, 1980).

DIAGNOSIS

As in many other skin conditions, the diagnosis of NME is made by skin biopsy findings. The unique features of this eruption are a diffuse parakeratotic hyperkeratosis and high-level epidermal edema. With advancing age or trauma, the high-level epidermal edema can be lost, so it is imperative that multiple biopsy samples be taken. Even then, it may be impossible to make the definite diagnosis of NME.

NME and the other differential diagnoses have an "autoimmune" clinical appearance, so most dogs undergo biopsy early in the course of their disease. Depending on the clinician and the client's finances, routine hematologic and biochemical data may or may not be collected before the biopsies are performed. If at all possible, these laboratory data should be gathered before, or at least simultaneously with, the biopsy samples. With their liver disease, these dogs may be an anesthetic risk. More importantly, it may be impossible to diagnose NME without this supporting laboratory work. If the high-level epidermal edema is absent, a pathologist is likely to give a differential diagnosis of a nutritional or an autoimmune disease. Nutritional supplements are of little benefit in these dogs but should not harm them. Immunosuppressive doses of glucocorticoids are another matter. Although the lesions of NME do improve with glucocorticoid therapy, approximately 89% of these dogs have a glucose intolerance, and a disastrous diabetic condition can be created with the glucocorticoid therapy. None of the differential diagnoses for NME, including systemic lupus erythematosus, have the laboratory features of this disease. The combination of the biopsy results, even if they are not specific, with the laboratory results should make the diagnosis of NME secure.

In the 18 reported cases, pancreatic glucagonomas were found only in two dogs. I have also documented a glucagonoma in one dog. In only one of these dogs was the tumor suggested by ultrasonographic examination of the abdomen. However, this procedure is a valuable diagnostic tool because the size and shape of the liver can be evaluated. The liver is typically small, with a nodular appearance that corresponds to the nodular hyperplasia seen microscopically.

To complete the evaluation of a dog with NME, an exploratory celiotomy should be performed. If a pancreatic tumor is identified, it should be removed. In most cases, even my one case of a glucagonoma, no tumor is visible and liver biopsy samples should be taken. In humans, glucagon levels and amino acid profiles are routinely determined. Although dogs typically have elevated glucagon levels (Miller et al., 1989) and hypoaminoacidemia (Gross et al., 1990), these tests are not widely available for dogs and appear to be of limited diagnostic or therapeutic value.

TREATMENT AND PROGNOSIS

As mentioned previously, corticosteroids resolve the skin lesions of NME but do nothing for the underlying cause and can induce a diabetic crisis. Other forms of therapy, although not harmful, are of little or no value. In humans, amino acid hyperalimentation or the use of somatostatin improves the skin rash. Although both of these therapies are used in veterinary medicine, they are expensive and of unproven value in NME. More importantly, they could only be considered palliative measures because they do not address the underlying problem.

In dogs, the development of NME is a poor prognostic sign. In one study (Miller et al., 1989), the mean survival time from diagnosis was 1.6 months. Unless the dog has a pancreatic tumor that can be removed or a safe and effective method to treat canine cirrhosis is developed, these dogs should be considered untreatable and should be euthanized when constitutional signs of the liver disease develop or if the skin lesions become unbearable.

References and Suggested Reading

Gross, T. L., and O'Brien, T. D.: Superficial necrolytic dermatitis (diabetic dermatopathy) in two dogs with glucagon-producing pancreatic endocrine tumors. Proc. Am. Coll. Vet. Dermatol./Am. Acad. Vet. Dermatol. p. 59, 1989.
A formal presentation on 2 dogs with reference to 10 other dogs without a pancreatic tumor.
Gross, T. L., O'Brien, T. D., Davies, A. P., et al.: Glucagon-producing pancreatic endocrine tumors in two dogs with superficial necrolytic dermatitis. J.A.V.M.A. 197:1619, 1990.
A complete report on the two previous cases.
Hanifin, J. M.: Glucagonoma syndrome. *In* Demis, D. J. (ed.).: Clinical Dermatology. Philadelphia: Harper & Row, 1980:1, Unit 4-12A, pp. 1–4.
A review of the disorder in human beings.
Miller, W. H., Jr., Scott, D. W., Buerger, R. G., et al.: Necrolytic migratory erythema in dogs: A hepatocutaneous syndrome. J. Am. Anim. Hosp. Assoc. 1989.
A study on the clinical, laboratory and histologic findings in 11 dogs with NME.
Turnwald, G. H., Foil, C. S., Wolfsheimer, K. J., et al.: Failure to document hyperglucagonemia in a dog with diabetic dermatopathy resembling necrolytic migratory erythema. J. Am. Anim. Hosp. Assoc. 25:363, 1989.
A report on one case.
Walton, D. K., Center, S. A., Scott, D. W., et al.: Ulcerative dermatosis associated with diabetes mellitus in the dog: A report of four cases. J. Am. Anim. Hosp. Assoc. 22:79, 1986.
A study on four diabetic dogs with NME.

NONSTEROIDAL THERAPY FOR CANINE AND FELINE PRURITUS

MANON PARADIS
St. Hyacinthe, Québec

and DANNY W. SCOTT
Ithaca, New York

Pruritus is a frequent reason for consultation in dermatology. The ideal treatment for canine and feline pruritus is the identification and removal of the cause, which usually is detectable with a complete history, physical examination, and various diagnostic tests. In addition, a therapeutic trial is often needed to definitively rule out bacterial pyoderma or ectoparasitism. Atopy, flea-bite hypersensitivity, and idiopathic pruritus (dermatoses wherein the historical, clinical, and therapeutic features are suggestive of allergy but diagnostic testing is negative or not performed) are the major pruritic skin diseases in the dog and cat. Long-term medical management is often indicated and justified in these cases.

Traditionally, medical management of these diseases has been accomplished with systemic glucocorticoids. Although glucocorticoids are highly effective in the management of many hypersensitivity disorders in pets, the potential side effects of these drugs (especially in the dog) stimulate constant investigations for alternative drugs or methods that will allow the clinician to stop or reduce the dose of glucocorticoids.

Many mediators and modulators of pruritus have been studied, including histamine, proteases (proteolytic enzymes, kallikrein), peptides (bradykinin, substance P), serotonin, prostaglandins, leukotrienes, and opioid peptides. However, the mediator(s) or modulator(s) of prime importance in the vast array of pruritic dermatoses is unclear in most instances. Recent clinical studies have suggested that histamine and leukotrienes are particularly important in dogs with cutaneous hypersensitivity disorders and that histamine plays a central role in cats with allergic pruritus.

NONSTEROIDAL THERAPY FOR CANINE PRURITUS

Clinical interest in the nonsteroidal management of canine pruritus—especially with the use of antihistamines and omega-3 and omega-6 fatty acid products—has recently surged. As a result, information gathered from clinical trials is replacing anecdotal data found in the older veterinary literature.

Antihistamines

For many years, antihistamines were considered ineffective in dogs because histamine was not thought to be a major mediator of pruritus. Recent studies have shown that antihistamines can be very effective in some patients and should be considered for use in patients with chronic pruritus of undetermined etiology, in patients with short- or long-term pruritus that do not tolerate glucocorticoids well, and in patients in which the use of glucocorticoids is undesirable or contraindicated.

The antihistamines most commonly used are H_1 blockers. These drugs exert their antipruritic action by inhibiting the effects of histamine at H_1 receptors and by exerting some local anesthetic actions and central nervous system sedative effects. There are seven classes of antihistamines with variable sedation as a side effect. Classical antihistamines are liposoluble and easily cross the blood-brain barrier. The sedative effect of most classical antihistamines is caused by the blockage of central histaminergic receptors and may play an important role in the control of pruritus. The new generation of nonsedating antihistamines (e.g., astemizole) is not as liposoluble and do not readily cross the blood-brain barrier, thus producing fewer central nervous system side effects.

Recent clinical studies have evaluated the antipruritic potential of several antihistamines in dogs (Table 1). In one study (Scott and Buerger, 1988), the H_1-blocking antihistamines hydroxyzine, diphenhydramine, and chlorpheniramine produced moderate to excellent control of pruritus in 24.5%, 22.3%, and 17.8%, respectively, of 45 dogs with allergic skin disease. The most commonly reported side effect was drowsiness, varying from 15.6% for hydroxyzine and diphenhydramine to 26.7% for

563

Table 1. *H_1-Antagonist Antihistamine Use in Dogs*

Drug Class	Drug Name	Oral Dosage		% of Dogs with Good to Excellent Control of Pruritus
Ethanolamine	Diphenhydramine	1.0–2.0 mg/kg	q 8–12 h	22.3
	Clemastine	0.5–1.5 mg	q 12 h	30
Piperazine	Hydroxyzine	2.2 mg/kg	q 8 h	24.5
Alkylamine	Chlorpheniramine	2.0–12.0 mg	q 8 h	17.8
Phenothiazine	Trimeprazine	0.5–2.0 mg/kg	q 12 h	3.3
Miscellaneous				
Nonsedative	Astemizole	2.5–10 mg	q 24 h	3.3
Tricyclic antidepressants with	Doxepin	10–30 mg	q 8 h	0
potent antihistamine effects	Amitriptyline	1.0–2.0 mg/kg	q 12 h	28

chlorpheniramine. Another clinical study (Paradis et al., 1991) evaluated the antipruritic potential of several other antihistamines and the ability of one antihistamine to reduce required glucocorticoid dose in pruritic dogs. Thirty allergic dogs were treated in a double-blind, placebo-controlled trial using a series of six drugs with potential antipruritic action: astemizole (nonsedating H_1-blocking antihistamine), doxepin (tricyclic antidepressant with potent antihistaminic activity), clemastine and trimeprazine (two conventional H_1-blocking antihistamines), trimeprazine plus prednisone (Vanectyl-P [Rogar/STB] in Canada, and Temaril-P [Smith Kline Beckman] in the United States), and prednisone. The combination product was included in the study because of anecdotal reports that indicated that the addition of the antihistamine allowed a reduction in the daily glucocorticoid requirement. In an attempt to assess the benefits of the combination product, prednisone and trimeprazine were also investigated individually, at doses equivalent to those found in the combination product. The average dose of prednisone administered alone or combined with trimeprazine was 0.2 mg/kg (every 12 hr). As expected, glucocorticoid-containing products were the most effective in controlling pruritus. The trimeprazine-prednisone combination product controlled pruritus in 76.7% of dogs, and prednisone alone was satisfactory in 56.7%; however, trimeprazine alone was effective in only 3.3%. Although trimeprazine was ineffective when used alone, it decreased the alternate-day glucocorticoid requirement by an average of 30% in nine of 12 allergic dogs. These findings suggest that there is a synergistic effect between antihistamines and glucocorticoids. Clemastine offered satisfactory control of pruritus in 30% of dogs, by far the best reported performance by an antihistamine alone. This control was achieved in all dogs without visible side effects. Astemizole was effective in only 3.3% of dogs. None of the 30 dogs showed improvement with doxepin, in spite of its potent antihistaminic effect. Recently, amitriptyline, another tricyclic antidepressant with potent antihistaminic activity, successfully controlled pruritus in 32.2% of 31 allergic dogs (Miller et al., 1991). Side effects were rarely seen.

Anecdotal reports have suggested that the combination of an H_1- and an H_2-blocking agent was superior to either agent alone. However, cimetidine, an H_2-blocking antihistamine, was found to be ineffective—whether administered alone or in combination with an H_1-blocking antihistamine, diphenhydramine—in the management of canine pruritus (Miller, 1989).

Fatty Acids

Essential fatty acids and other fatty acids found in fish oil or evening primrose oil have been described as useful for the treatment of a variety of cutaneous and noncutaneous disorders. Recently, preparations containing omega-3 fatty acids (also referred to as cold-water fish–oils) and omega-6 fatty acids have been clinically evaluated for their use as antipruritic drugs by many researchers. Of the several omega-3 fatty acids investigated, eicosapentaenoic acid has been shown to be structurally similar to arachidonic acid and competes for the utilization of the lipoxygenase and cyclo-oxygenase enzyme pathways, which results in the formation of eicosanoids with markedly reduced inflammatory properties. DVM DermCaps (Dermatologics for Veterinary Medicine, Inc.) has been used by many investigators for the treatment of allergic pruritus. In one study (Miller et al., 1989), 18.3% of 93 allergic dogs showed an excellent response, while another 17.2% experienced a substantial reduction in, but not the elimination of, pruritus. A second study (Scott and Buerger, 1988) reported an excellent response in 11.1% of 45 allergic dogs and a moderate response in another 11.1%. A third study (Pukay, 1987) reported a decrease in pruritus of more than 50% in eight out of 20 dogs. In a fourth study (Paradis et al., 1991), pruritus was satisfactorily controlled in 26.7% of 30 allergic dogs.

Because of anecdotal reports from veterinary practitioners that DermCaps were "often" more effective in controlling canine pruritus when given at twice the manufacturer's recommended dosage, 20 allergic dogs known to be unresponsive to the manufacturer's recommended dosage of DermCaps received the latter at twice the manufacturer's recommended dosage (Scott and Miller, 1990). Not a single dog experienced a reduction in its level of pruritus. It is conceivable, nonetheless, that further increases in the dosage of DermCaps could be more effective in some dogs. In human medicine, the dosage of some of the DermCaps constituents used for the treatment of various dermatoses (e.g., psoriasis, acne, atopic dermatitis) approximate 35 to 200 mg/kg of eicosapentaenoic acid and 25 to 160 mg/kg of docosahexaenoic acid per day. In contrast, the dosages used in dogs with manufacturer's recommended and double dosages of DermCaps approximate 1.6 to 3.2 mg/kg of eicosapentaenoic acid and 1.1 to 2.2 mg/kg of docosahexaenoic acid per day. Approximating the dosages used in humans would make DermCaps prohibitively expensive in the dog.

In the United Kingdom (Lloyd, 1989), a fatty-acid product containing evening primrose oil (omega-6) improved the coat quality and decreased the amount of seborrheic changes in ten atopic dogs, but there was no change in the level of pruritus. The addition of eicosapentaenoic acid to evening primrose oil had no apparent synergistic effect. In more recent work with an evening primrose oil/eicosapentaenoic acid supplement that contains vitamins and minerals (EfaVet, EfamolVet, Woodbridge Meadows), the same author reported results to be excellent in 18% and good in 76% of 33 atopic dogs. Improvement included a decrease in both seborrheic signs and pruritus.

Although the success rates vary, all the above studies clearly show that fatty-acid supplements containing omega-3 and omega-6 fatty acids (eicosapentaenoic acid and evening primrose oil) can be beneficial in the treatment of allergic pruritus in dogs. These supplements may also allow the clinician to use lower doses of glucocorticoids. One product containing omega-3 and omega-6 fatty acids (DermCaps) has been reported to allow a 50% reduction in the required alternate-day dosage of glucocorticoids in some allergic dogs (Miller, 1989).

Combination of Antihistamines and Fatty Acids

Since it is known that various antipruritic drugs exert their action at different points in the inflammatory process, it is logical to believe that, by using two or more drugs with differing antipruritic actions, we might observe a synergistic effect. Recently, a synergistic effect was demonstrated in 23 pruritic dogs known to be unresponsive to chlorpheniramine and DermCaps when either drug was used alone (Scott and Miller, 1990). Pruritus was satisfactorily controlled in 34.8% of the dogs when they received chlorpheniramine in combination with DermCaps. In a similar study (Paradis et al., 1991), a synergistic effect was demonstrated with the combination of clemastine and DermCaps in three of 30 dogs with allergic pruritus.

Miscellaneous Nonsteroidal Agents

A large number of other nonsteroidal anti-inflammatory drugs exist, and more are being developed. For most of these agents, little information about their clinical pharmacology in small animals is available.

Clinical trials with vitamin E and zinc methionine (Miller, 1989), and aspirin and erythromycin (Scott and Buerger, 1988) indicated that these drugs were of minimal to no benefit in the management of canine allergic pruritus. Other drugs, such as gold salts or cytotoxic immunosuppressants (e.g., cyclophosphamide, azathioprine), potentially could have some antipruritic action because of their respective modes of action. However, because of their potential toxicities and more complicated surveillance protocols, these agents will not be routinely used in allergic patients.

Nonsteroidal Therapy for Feline Pruritus

The nonsteroidal management of feline pruritus has received considerably less attention than its canine counterpart. This is probably because of the relatively lower incidence of side effects that cats develop with the prolonged use of glucocorticoids and the difficulties encountered in giving many cats oral medication over a prolonged period of time. Chlorpheniramine was administered orally (2 mg, every 12 hr) to 26 cats with pruritic skin disease (Miller and Scott, 1990). In 19 cats (73.1%), pruritus was completely eliminated; one cat had 50% reduction in pruritus; and six cats had no response to treatment. Serious or long-lasting clinical side effects were not observed in any cats. Two cats had transient drowsiness for the first few days of treatment, and two cats developed an aversion to the bitter taste of the medication. The low incidence of side effects suggest that this drug is safe for use in cats, but safety needs to be defined by toxicologic studies. Clinical observations on a small number of cats indicated that the lack of efficacy and side effects seen with the use of diphenhydramine (hyperexcitability), hydroxyzine (polydipsia) and amitriptyline (hypersalivation and vomiting) may preclude the use of these drugs in cats (Miller and Scott, 1990). Caution should be exercised in the selection of other drug protocols in this species. A clinical trial using a product containing omega-3 and omega-6 fatty acids (DVM DermCaps) in 28 allergic cats indicates a 46.4% good to excellent clinical response (Miller et al., 1991). Side effects have not been observed.

SUMMARY

Glucocorticoids are highly effective in managing pruritus in dogs and cats, but because of the serious potential side effects, alternatives are constantly being sought. It is becoming increasingly clear that various H_1-blocking antihistamines, fatty acids, or combinations thereof can be of great benefit in controlling pruritus in allergic dogs and cats. It is also clear that the clinician has no way to predict which antihistamine, fatty-acid supplement, or combination will be successful in any given patient. Frequently, a series of antipruritic agents must be tried to determine which is most effective, least toxic, and so on. Currently, most dosages are extrapolated from human data. Because of multiple ongoing trials in small animals, more accurate information on optimal dosages of various drugs should be available in the near future. Nevertheless, for dogs or cats with chronic pruritus that do not tolerate glucocorticoids or in which glucocorticoids are contraindicated, it is worthwhile to offer clients the choice of trying fatty-acid supplements or various antihistamines, with the hope of finding a nonsteroidal alternative that controls pruritus in their pets or, at least, reduces the amount of glucocorticoid required.

References and Supplemental Reading

Lloyd, D., and Thomsett, L. R.: Essential fatty acid supplementation in the treatment of canine atopy: A preliminary study. Vet. Dermatol. 1:41, 1989.
A prospective study on ten atopic dogs treated with EFA.

Miller, W. H. Jr.: Nonsteroidal anti-inflammatory agents in the management of canine and feline pruritus. *In* Kirk, R. W. (ed.): *Current Veterinary Therapy X.* Philadelphia: W. B. Saunders, 1989, p. 566.
An overview of antipruritic agents useful in dogs and cats.

Miller, W. H. Jr.: Fatty acid supplements as anti-inflammatory agents. *In* Kirk, R. W. (ed.): *Current Veterinary Therapy X.* Philadelphia: W. B. Saunders, 1989, p. 563.
A discussion of the potential role of fatty-acid supplements in companion animals.

Miller, W. H. Jr., Griffin, G. E., Scott, D. W., et al.: Clinical trial of DVM DermCaps in the treatment of allergic disease in dogs: A nonblinded study. J. Am. Anim. Hosp. Assoc. 25:163, 1989.
A prospective study on 93 allergic dogs treated with DermCaps.

Miller, H. W., and Scott, D. W.: Efficacy of chlorpheniramine maleate for management of pruritus in cats. J.A.V.M.A. 197:67–70, 1990.
A prospective study on 26 allergic cats treated with chlorpheniramine.

Miller, W. H. Jr., Scott, D. W., and Wellington, J. R.: Nonsteroidal management of canine pruritus with amitriptyline. Cornell Vet. (in press).

Miller, W. H. Jr., Scott, D. W., and Wellington, J. R.: Efficacy of DVM DermCaps Liquid™ in the management of allergic and inflammatory dermatoses of the cat. J. Am. Anim. Hosp. Assn. (in press).

Paradis, M., Lemay, S., and Scott, D. W.: The efficacy of clemastine (Tavist®), a fatty acid supplement (DermCaps®), and the combination of both products in the management of canine pruritus. Vet. Dermatol. J. (in press).
A prospective study on 30 dogs in which the antipruritic efficacy of clemastine (Tavist®), DermCaps, or the combination of both products was investigated.

Paradis, M., Scott, D. W., and Giroux, D.: Further investigations on the use of nonsteroidal anti-inflammatory drugs in the management of canine pruritus. J. Am. Anim. Hosp. Assoc. 27:44, 1991.
A prospective study of 30 dogs in which the antipruritic efficacy of clemastine, astemizole, doxepine, trimeprazine, trimeprazine plus prednisone, and prednisone was investigated.

Pukay, B. P.: A clinical evaluation of the efficacy of omega-3 fatty acid in the treatment of pruritus in canine atopy. Can. Acad. Vet. Dermatol. Bull. 4:4, Fall 1987.
A prospective study on 20 allergic dogs treated with DermCaps.

Scott, D. W., and Buerger, R. G.: Nonsteroidal anti-inflammatory agents in the management of canine pruritus. J. Am. Anim. Hosp. Assoc. 24:423, 1988.
A prospective study on 45 dogs in which the antipruritic efficacy of chlorpheniramine, hydroxyzine, diphenhydramine, DermCaps, aspirin, and erythromycin was investigated.

Scott, D. W., and Miller, W. H. Jr.: Nonsteroidal management of canine pruritus: Chlorpheniramine and a fatty acid supplement (DVM DermCaps) in combination, and the fatty acid supplement at twice the manufacturer's recommended dosage. Cornell Vet. 80:381, 1990.
A prospective study on 43 allergic dogs treated with DermCaps and chlorpheniramine in combination (23) or DermCaps at twice the manufacturer's recommended dosage (20).

GASTROINTESTINAL DISORDERS

DAVID C. TWEDT

Consulting Editor

FELINE GINGIVITIS, STOMATITIS, AND PHARYNGITIS

ALICE M. WOLF

College Station, Texas

Inflammation, proliferation, or ulceration of the oral/pharyngeal mucosa occurs as a primary disease or secondary to a systemic disorder. Local causes include chemical or physical irritation, foreign bodies, trauma, neoplasia, periodontal disease, lymphocytic-plasmacytic gingivitis/stomatitis, and eosinophilic granuloma complex. Systemic causes for oral lesions include metabolic diseases (e.g., uremia, diabetes mellitus), infectious diseases (e.g., herpesvirus, calicivirus, feline leukemia virus, feline immunodeficiency virus, systemic mycoses), immune-mediated diseases, toxins (e.g., thallium), and immunologic (e.g., neutropenia) or nutritional deficiencies.

PATIENT EVALUATION

Clinical Signs

Clinical signs of inflammatory, proliferative, or ulcerative oropharyngeal diseases may be absent initially or if the lesions are mild. Chronic or severe lesions may cause partial or complete anorexia, changes in food preference (e.g., soft versus dry foods), dysphagia, ptyalism, halitosis, pain on opening the mouth, and rubbing or pawing at the face or mouth. Weight loss, lethargy, and other systemic signs may occur if the disorder is chronic or systemic in origin.

History and Physical Examination

The clinician should elicit a thorough history and perform a complete physical examination to detect systemic problems and carefully inspect the tissues of the oral cavity and oropharynx, noting the size, symmetry, location, and relationship of lesions to other structures (e.g., teeth, tongue). It may be helpful to observe the cat attempting to eat to determine if dysphagia is associated with the oral disorder. Sedation or anesthesia is usually required to examine the oral cavity because of the cat's temperament or because of pain associated with

examination of this area. Associated cranial and cervical structures should be evaluated for involvement (e.g., regional lymph nodes, bony structures, and cranial nerves).

Diagnostic Evaluation

Laboratory studies are indicated if a cause for the oral lesions is not apparent from the history and physical examination. The diagnostic database should include a complete blood count, biochemistry profile, urinalysis, and tests for feline leukemia virus antigen and feline immunodeficiency virus antibody. These tests will help to determine if a systemic disorder is causing or is associated with the oral disease. Other laboratory studies can be performed as directed by findings on these initial tests. Radiography of the oral cavity or pharynx should be performed with the cat under anesthesia. Radiography is indicated for cats with severe periodontitis, dysphagia, or pain of unknown cause or if swelling or distortion of the bone or soft tissues is present. Further local investigation in the oral cavity can be performed during the same anesthetic procedure and may include exfoliative cytology, biopsy, or bacteriologic or mycologic culture.

LOCAL DISORDERS

Chemical or Physical Irritation

Cats are usually fastidious eaters and generally avoid purposefully ingesting foreign substances. Chewing on decorative houseplants such as dieffenbachia, poinsettia, and Christmas trees is a common cause of oral irritation. Irritating chemicals may be picked up on the fur or feet and ingested by the cat because of its grooming habits. Cleansing and disinfecting agents, pesticides, and fertilizers may be ingested in this manner. Chemical irritants often produce large lingual ulcers and ulceration of other oral tissues and the esophagus. Systemic signs of illness, including lethargy and fever, may be present in some of these cats. Modified-live herpesvirus and calicivirus vaccines may cause local oral ulceration if they are deposited on the skin and ingested. Physical irritation can occur secondary to physical

568

trauma from a number of causes and also occurs on buccal membranes in contact with heavily tartared teeth. Treatment of physical and chemical irritation includes removal of the source of irritation, local treatment or tissue débridement, and fluid and nutritional support until the oral tissues heal.

Oral Foreign Bodies and Traumatic Lesions

The most common feline oral foreign bodies are string, thread, and needles. Strings and thread are usually found beneath the tongue and may become imbedded in the lingual frenulum. Lingual, oral, and pharyngeal ulceration can result from the "sawing" action of these materials. Needles may become imbedded in the tongue, cheek, or oropharynx. Bone fragments and plant awns and other plant materials may also become lodged in the oral cavity. Bone fragments can become wedged between premolars or molars across the hard palate, causing pressure necrosis of soft tissue and bone in this area. Plant awns penetrate oral soft tissues or imbed in the gingival sulci around teeth or in the tonsillar fossa. Grass blades may lodge dorsal to the soft palate, the dangling end causing pharyngeal irritation and gagging. Treatment consists of removal of the foreign body and local or supportive treatment as mentioned earlier.

Severe oral trauma can result from the "high-rise syndrome" (falling from the balcony, window, and so forth) and vehicular trauma. The most common injuries include mandibular and maxillary fractures and avulsion of the lower lip from the mandibular symphysis. Electrical cord injury damages any part of the oral cavity but especially the hard palate, gingiva, and the commissures of the lips. Initially, electrical burns appear as gray discoloration of the tissue, but extensive tissue and bone damage may have occurred that is not immediately obvious. One must also monitor for late-developing signs of electrical shock injury (e.g., cardiac arrhythmias, pulmonary edema, and seizures). The owner should be warned that extensive tissue or bone sloughs may require future reconstructive surgery.

Neoplasia

Gingival or lingual squamous cell carcinoma is the most common feline oral tumor (Cotter, 1981). These lesions are usually erosive and may invade underlying bone. Fibrosarcomas, tonsillar or pharyngeal lymphosarcomas, ameloblastomas, adamantinoma, melanomas, giant cell tumors, and other miscellaneous carcinomas and sarcomas have also been reported (Cotter, 1981; Stover, 1987). Diagnostic evaluation for neoplasia includes deep biopsy and radiography of the lesion. Although most of these tumors are locally invasive and slow to metastasize, if neoplasia is confirmed, thoracic radiography and biopsy of the local lymph nodes are indicated before aggressive surgery, radiation, or chemotherapy is performed. Successful treatment of oral neoplasia requires early recognition and prompt treatment. Surgical resection may be curative for some tumors of the mandible and maxilla. Successful radiation and cryotherapy have also been reported for some squamous cell carcinomas; lymphosarcoma may respond to chemotherapy. Solid-tissue sarcomas respond poorly to radiation and chemotherapy, and successful treatment is unlikely unless complete surgical removal is possible.

Periodontal Disease

Periodontitis associated with dental disease is a common feline problem. Treatment consists of thorough dental scaling, root planing, and gingival resection (Sams and Harvey, 1989). Loose and fractured teeth should be removed. Subgingival tooth root erosion ("neck lesions") causes extreme dental sensitivity and pain (Sams and Harvey, 1989). Teeth with root erosion should be removed or restored with amalgam or glass ionomer (Eisner, 1989). A broad-spectrum antibiotic with efficacy against anaerobes should be administered just before a dental procedure and should be continued for 3 to 5 days following a procedure.

Recurrence of gingivitis associated with dental disease may be retarded by feeding a dry food diet and encouraging home dental care. Many cats will tolerate daily tooth brushing using a childs' toothbrush with the bristles cut down or with gauze wrapped around a finger. Abrasive veterinary dental pastes or powders are available in flavors acceptable to cats. Oral flushing with germicidal solutions has been recommended by some clinicians; however, most cats vigorously resist this procedure.

Lymphocytic-Plasmacytic Gingivitis and Stomatitis

Lymphocytic-plasmacytic gingivitis and stomatitis (LPGS) is one of the most common feline oral soft-tissue diseases. The etiology of LPGS is unknown, but it is suspected to have an immunologic basis because of the character of the cellular infiltrate. Calicivirus has been isolated from some affected cats (Knowles et al., 1989).

Lymphocytic-plasmacytic gingivitis and stomatitis most commonly affect young to middle-aged cats, but a cat of any age may be affected. There is no particular breed predilection for LPGS. Abyssinian and Somali cats have a high incidence of a similar but milder type of gingivitis called "red gum" by cat breeders. The gingival lesions in these breeds can appear by 6 months of age and remain mild or progress in severity.

Lymphocytic-plasmacytic gingivitis and stomatitis cause proliferative, friable, and painful proliferation of the gingiva. The buccal gingiva near the cheek teeth is most severely involved; the lingual gingiva and that around the canines and incisors is infrequently affected. Subgingival tooth root erosion commonly accompanies the gingival lesions in this disease (Sams and Harvey, 1989). LPGS may also affect the palatine arches, the lesions ranging from small erythemic papules to severe mucosal proliferation (Johnessee and Hurvitz, 1983). Complete blood counts are usually normal; serum biochemistry profiles may reveal increased serum globulin concentrations (Johnessee and Hurvitz, 1983). Feline leukemia virus antigen and feline immunodeficiency virus antibody tests are usually negative. Biopsies or deep scrapings examined by exfoliative cytology will reveal mucosal hyperplasia with large numbers of lymphocytes and plasma cells. Neutrophils and macrophages are also present in variable numbers.

No treatment has been uniformly successful in resolving LPGS. The owner should be warned at the time of diagnosis that response to therapy is often poor and relapses are common (Sams and Harvey, 1989). Dental prophylaxis, including restoration or removal of teeth with subgingival root erosion, should be performed in all affected cats. Parenteral antibiotic therapy with a broad-spectrum agent (e.g., amoxicillin [Amoxi-Tabs, Beecham] 22 mg/kg PO every 12 hr) or one with a good anaerobic spectrum (e.g., metronidazole [Flagyl, Searle] 50 mg/kg PO every 24 hr) may provide some improvement, most likely because of a reduction in secondary bacterial infection. Immunosuppressive drugs, including corticosteroids (e.g., prednisone) 2 to 4 mg/kg PO every 24 hr, megestrol acetate (Ovaban, Schering; 5 mg PO every 7 days), azathioprine (Imuran, Burroughs Wellcome; 2.2 mg/kg PO every 24 to 48 hr), and aurothioglucose (Solganol, Schering; test dose of 1 mg IM, then 0.5 to 1.0 mg IM weekly until remission), then reduce frequency, have been used with variable degrees of success. Each of these drugs can be associated with significant side effects, and therapy must be closely monitored. Resection of proliferative gingiva using electrocautery with a ball tip used at low power is beneficial in some patients. Full mouth extraction of all cheek teeth has been successfully used as a salvage procedure in cats that fail to respond to medical therapy.

Eosinophilic Granuloma Complex

Eosinophilic ulcers, plaques, and granulomas can occur in the oral cavity. Eosinophilic ulcers are most frequently found on the upper lip opposite the lower canine teeth. They are usually deforming and red-brown and may have a yellowish center. Eosinophilic plaques and granulomas occur less frequently and may occur anywhere in the oral cavity. Peripheral eosinophilia is present in some cats with oral eosinophilic granuloma complex. Other laboratory abnormalities have not been reported.

Although biopsy of any ulcerative oral lesion is recommended, eosinophilic ulcers on the lips are usually diagnosed by their classical clinical appearance. Biopsy should be used to confirm the diagnosis of the other eosinophilic lesions and to exclude more serious disorders such as neoplasia.

Eosinophilic granuloma complex is usually responsive to high-dose corticosteroid therapy (e.g., methylprednisolone acetate [Depo-Medrol, Upjohn] 20 mg IM every 2 weeks for three treatments). Recently, some corticosteroid-resistant lesions responded to therapy with trimethoprim-sulfadiazine (Tribrissen, Burroughs Wellcome; 30 mg/kg PO every 12 hr) or to nonspecific immunomodulators such as mixed bacterial vaccine or levamisole (Levasole, Pitman-Moore; 5 mg/kg PO three times a week) (Rosenkrantz, 1989). Initial therapy should be aggressive because eosinophilic granuloma complex lesions become more resistant to treatment after relapse.

SYSTEMIC DISORDERS

Infectious Diseases

RETROVIRUS INFECTIONS

Gingivitis and stomatitis are the most common physical findings associated with feline immunodeficiency virus infection (Yamamoto et al., 1989). Clinical signs often include fever, malaise, anorexia, weight loss, or lymphadenopathy. Oral lesions in feline immunodeficiency–positive cats may be proliferative but are more often ulcerative and necrotic. These lesions are probably not a direct viral effect but rather secondary to the viral immunosuppressive effects, allowing proliferation and invasion of oral flora. Similar lesions are seen in cats with feline leukemia virus infection (Knowles et al., 1989). Treatment is symptomatic and supportive.

OTHER VIRAL INFECTIONS

Lingual or hard-palate ulceration commonly occurs during acute, symptomatic infection with feline herpesvirus and calicivirus. Associated signs include fever, lethargy, and oculonasal discharge. As previously mentioned, feline calicivirus may be associated with lymphocytic-plasmacytic stomatitis and gingivitis. Feline parvovirus (panleukopenia) has caused necrotic gingivitis, ulcerative stomatitis, and palatine ulcerations in a few cats (Sams and Harvey, 1989). Treatment is symptomatic and supportive.

MYCOTIC STOMATITIS

Candida albicans is a rare cause of stomatitis in the cat (Harvey, 1989). Granulomatous oral lesions have been observed in some cats with *Cryptococcus* and *Histoplasma* infection. Diagnosis is made by exfoliative cytology, biopsy, or culture of the lesions. Local therapy with nystatin solution may be beneficial for cats with oral candidiasis. Systemic antifungal treatment is required for the deep mycotic diseases.

BACTERIAL STOMATITIS

Primary feline bacterial stomatitis is a controversial diagnosis. Secondary bacterial infection is likely following any oral tissue damage or immunosuppression. An apparent clinical response of oral lesions to antibiotic therapy does not confirm the diagnosis of bacterial stomatitis, and a thorough diagnostic evaluation should be performed to search for underlying primary diseases.

Metabolic Diseases

Stomatitis associated with renal failure is caused by ammonia produced by bacterial action on urea excreted in saliva. The effects of ammonial irritation may be more severe in dehydrated patients with dry oral mucous membranes (Harvey, 1989). Local treatment of the lesions is ineffective in uremic patients, and therapy must be directed at reversing the renal insufficiency. Diabetic cats have reduced resistance to infection and may have problems with severe periodontitis and dental disease. Treatment consists of control of the diabetic condition and local therapy for dental disease and periodontitis.

Immune-Mediated Diseases

Pemphigus and systemic lupus erythematosus may rarely cause oral ulceration (Stover, 1987). Other signs of skin involvement are present in most cats. The mucocutaneous junctions are most frequently involved, although these diseases may affect any cutaneous surface. The lesions arise as vesicles or bullae, but the thin feline epidermis ruptures easily, producing ulcers or crusts. Malaise, fever, and anorexia are often present. Systemic lupus erythematosus is a polysystemic disease, and other abnormalities, including blood dyscrasias, polyarthritis, myositis, neuritis, or glomerulonephritis, may be present in these patients.

Routine hematologic and biochemical parameters are often normal in cats with pemphigus. Cats with systemic lupus erythematosus may have a variety of laboratory abnormalities, depending on the extent and severity of organ system involvement. Immune-mediated skin disease can be confirmed with histopathologic examination and direct immunofluorescent antibody testing of skin biopsy specimens. Antinuclear antibodies may be present in some cats with pemphigus and should be present in high titer in cats with systemic lupus erythematosus. Unfortunately, the antinuclear antibodies test is often unreliable in cats, and false-negative or false-positive results are common.

Immune-mediated diseases are treated initially with corticosteroids. Those failing to respond to this therapy may be given other immunosuppressive drugs, including azathioprine; cyclophosphamide (Cytoxan, Mead Johnson; 1 mg/kg PO every 24 hr, for 4 consecutive days each week); and aurothioglucose; these drugs may be used as single agents or as combination therapy.

Toxic Disorders

Oral ulceration may accompany other signs of drug eruption or toxic epidermal necrolysis. Thallium toxicosis causes severe oral and cutaneous ulceration. Other heavy metal intoxications occasionally cause oral lesions (Harvey, 1989). Diagnosis is usually based on a history of exposure to drugs or toxins and an appropriate time interval between exposure and development of the oral lesions. Treatment consists of removal of the toxic agent (e.g., bathing, emesis), specific treatment for intoxication, and supportive care.

Nutritional Disorders

Oral lesions can result from defective epithelial development secondary to vitamin deficiency (Lyon, 1988). These disorders are very rare because most cats are fed nutritionally balanced, commercially prepared diets. Diagnosis is made on the basis of dietary history. Treatment consists of correction of the dietary deficiency.

References and Suggested Reading

Cotter, S. M.: Oral pharyngeal neoplasms in the cats. J. Am. Anim. Hosp. Assoc. 17:917, 1981.
  Review of the incidence and approach to treatment of oral neoplasms in the cat.

Eisner, E. R.: Chronic subgingival tooth erosion in cats. Vet. Med. 84:378, 1989.
Excellent description of this problem, with a thorough, illustrated discussion of therapy.

Harvey, C. E.: Oral, dental, pharyngeal, and salivary gland disorders. *In* Ettinger, S. J. (ed.): *Textbook of Veterinary Internal Medicine*, 3rd ed. Philadelphia: W. B. Saunders, 1989, p. 1226.
Overview of some disorders causing oral lesions in the cat.

Johnessee, J. S., and Hurvitz, A. J.: Feline plasma cell gingivitis-pharyngitis. J. Am. Anim. Hosp. Assoc. 19:179, 1983.
The most definitive description of this condition in the cat.

Knowles, J. O., Gaskell, R. M., Gaskell, C. J., et al.: Prevalence of feline calicivirus, feline leukaemia virus and antibodies to FIV in cats with chronic stomatitis. Vet. Rec. 124:336, 1989.
Comparative study of the prevalence of these infectious diseases in cats with gingivitis in the U.K. and U.S.

Lyon, K. F.: Approach to feline oral disease. J. Vet. Dent. 5(3):11, 1988.
Review of the differential diagnosis for oral lesions in the cat.

Rosenkrantz, W.: Eosinophilic granuloma complex (confusion). Vet. Focus 1:29, 1989.
Excellent review of the diagnosis and management of feline eosinophilic granuloma complex.

Sams, D. L., and Harvey, C. E.: Oral and dental diseases. *In* Sherding, R. G. (ed.): *The Cat: Diseases and Clinical Management.* New York: Churchill Livingstone, 1989, p. 879.
Thorough discussion of dental disease and an overview of other oral lesions in the cat.

Stover, S. C.: A differential for oral ulcers in cats. Feline Health Topics (Cornell Feline Health Center) 2:1, 1987.
Review of disorders causing oral ulceration in the cat.

Yamamoto, J. K., Hansen, H., Ho, E. W., et al.: Epidemiologic and clinical aspects of feline immunodeficiency virus infection in cats from the continental United States and Canada and possible mode of transmission. J.A.V.M.A. 194:213, 1989.
Oral lesions were the most common clinical finding in a survey of 310 FIV-infected cats.

DYSPHAGIA AND SWALLOWING DISORDERS

M. D. WILLARD

College Station, Texas

There are three major causes of canine and feline dysphagia: (1) anatomic abnormalities of the oral cavity or pharynx, (2) pain associated with apprehension, mastication, or swallowing, and (3) neuromuscular dysfunction of cranial or pharyngeal muscles (Table 1). Dysphagia *per se* may be identified if either the client or veterinarian sees repeated efforts or inability to swallow, obvious difficulty or discomfort during swallowing, or aspiration and gagging when swallowing (especially liquids). These signs may be intermittent, necessitating repeated observations to recognize the problem. Some dysphagic animals may be anorexic (especially if swallowing is painful), making their problem harder to detect and define. Drooling, being "head-shy," regurgitation, coughing (due to aspiration), gagging, or weight loss may also be associated with disorders causing dysphagia. Many affected patients evidence multiple signs simultaneously.

DIAGNOSTIC APPROACH

The first step is to use the history to determine if rabies is likely (i.e., consider the locale and the pet's vaccination status), whether the dysphagia began acutely or gradually (i.e., is trauma or a foreign object likely?), if the dysphagia is stable or progressive, and whether the patient swallows solids better than liquids (suggestive of pharyngeal dysfunction). If rabies seems possible, precautions should immediately be initiated to lessen human exposure (i.e., do not handle the animal unless absolutely necessary, use gloves when working with the patient, properly disinfect the environment, contact public health officials).

Physical examination is used next to define the problem more clearly and look for causes. Observe the animal's eating, because it may offer clues. Search for pain, crepitus, masses/swellings, muscle atrophy or nerve deficits in the head and neck, halitosis, cervical esophageal dilatation, and evidence of aspiration disease (e.g., drooling and pulmonary crackles). Check the eyes for displacement (i.e., exophthalmos, strabismus) or inflammation suggesting a retrobulbar mass or inflammation.

Oral examination is the most important part of the physical examination and, if possible, should be performed while the patient is conscious. Do not hesitate to use chemical restraint if a patient will not allow an adequate oral examination (see this volume, p. 27); however, first perform a complete blood count (CBC), serum chemistry profile, and urinalysis and be prepared to perform adjunct diagnostic procedures (e.g., static image radiographs, biopsies) during anesthesia. A laryngoscope is indis-

Table 1. *Major Causes of Dysphagia in Dogs and Cats*

Anatomic disease
  Tumor (squamous cell carcinoma, fibrosarcoma, melanoma)
  Eosinophilic granuloma
  Lymphadenopathy (especially retropharyngeal)
  Fracture (mandible, maxilla, hyoid)
  Sialocele
  Cleft palate/short soft palate
  Loss of anterior tongue (uremic)/abnormal frenulum
  Laryngeal/pharyngeal trauma

Pain
  Stomatitis/glossitis
  Foreign object (penetrating, linear)
  Fracture
  Temporomandibular joint disease
  Tooth problems
  Retrobulbar abscess/soft-tissue abscess

Neuromuscular
  Rabies
  Masseter myositis
  Oral dysphagia (cranial nerves V, VII, XII)
  Pharyngeal dysphagia (cranial nerves VII, IX, X)
  Cricopharyngeal dysfunction

pensable in searching for anatomic defects, oral swellings, masses, inflammation, foreign objects, and fractures. Note deviation from the normally bilateral symmetry of the patient's head and neck, to detect submucosal swelling. Masses and swellings that do not disrupt the mucosa may be difficult to appreciate, especially those on the midline (e.g., dorsal to the larynx). Foreign objects may penetrate the mucosa without obvious signs of local trauma, especially in the posterior pharynx. Feeling this area with your fingertips may allow detection of a mass or foreign object that is not grossly obvious. Finally, check to see if the teeth are loose.

Absence of a normal structure suggests a congenital defect, trauma, scarring, or necrosis (e.g., uremia causing lingual necrosis, masseter myositis causing cranial muscular loss, infection causing tissue or bone necrosis). Patients with chronic infections should be screened (i.e., CBC, serum chemistry profile, urinalysis) for systemic disease (e.g., hyperadrenocorticism) that allowed the infection to occur and persist. If rabies seems likely, then immunofluorescence of biopsy specimens from tactile hair roots may be considered in addition to confinement and observation (contact the local health department).

If a mass, swelling, or inflamed area is found, biopsy should be performed. One cannot reliably distinguish neoplastic from non-neoplastic lesions visually, nor prognosticate based on a lesion's size or appearance. Fine-needle aspiration is recommended initially, especially of deeper lesions (e.g., enlarged lymph nodes). Lymphadenopathy of retropharyngeal nodes or masses dorsal to the larynx

may be difficult to appreciate grossly (i.e., one only feels the normal surrounding structures, which are pushed out and made more prominent) and hard to approach, except by fine-needle aspiration biopsy. Radiography plus ultra-sonographic imaging of this area (Fig. 1) is informative and aids in obtaining representative needle biopsy specimens. Fine-needle aspiration may also reveal a retropharyngeal mass as a zygomatic gland sialocele.

If a fine-needle aspirate biopsy cannot be done or is nondiagnostic, an incisional or excisional biopsy is needed. When performing incisional biopsies in the oral cavity, one must remember that the ulceration, necrosis, and inflammation caused by the normal oral flora in the superficial mucosa will obscure the diagnosis. Therefore, the incision must be extended deeply enough to provide artifact-free tissue. Such biopsies often cause substantial hemorrhage; cautery (e.g., silver nitrate) can control bleeding unless major vessels (e.g., palatine artery) are severed. Excisional biopsies should be well planned (i.e., evaluate regional lymph nodes and surrounding osseous tissues for evidence of neoplastic metastasis) lest the surgery be inadequate and a second procedure be necessary.

Static radiographs are often performed while a patient is anesthetized for the oral examination. They are useful in that they may alter the prognosis or treatment of oral neoplasms and they may detect occult neoplastic bone involvement, fractures, tooth root abscesses, soft-tissue abscesses, temporomandibular arthropathies, deeply embedded radiopaque foreign objects, or enlarged lymph nodes (see Fig. 1). Adequate radiographic evaluation of the head almost always necessitates careful and exacting dorsoventral, lateral, open mouth, or oblique views; these require anesthesia. The hyoid apparatus should be included in cases of dysphagia.

NEUROMUSCULAR DISEASE

Dysphagic patients that do not have detectable anatomic lesions or oral pain should be examined for neuromuscular dysfunction. Neuromuscular disorders are often subdivided into three major categories to facilitate their understanding, diagnosis, and treatment. Swallowing may be simplistically divided into oral (also called prehensile), pharyngeal, and cricopharyngeal phases. The oral phase includes placing food in the mouth and chewing it. Lower motor neuron dysfunction due to masseter myositis or deficits of cranial nerves (especially V, VII, or XII), may prevent the patient from placing or keeping food in its mouth when chewing or attempting to swallow. Cranial nerve deficits responsible for such problems are usually obvious from physical and neurologic examinations. Neurogenic oral dysphagia is typically associated with

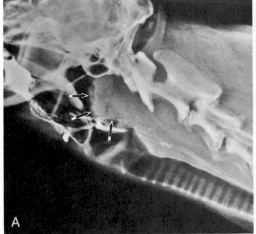

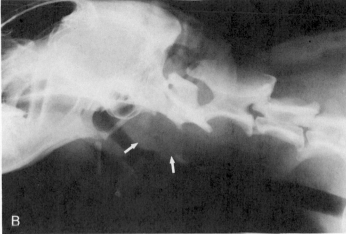

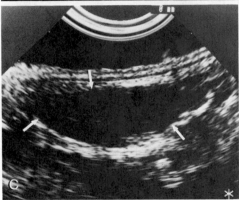

Figure 1. *A*, Lateral barium contrast radiograph of a dog's head and neck that demonstrates ventral displacement of the larynx by an obvious, large squamous cell carcinoma in the posterior pharynx (arrows). *B*, Lateral radiograph of a dog's head and neck, demonstrating ventral displacement of the larynx by a soft-tissue mass (arrows) that is not well demarcated. Compare this radiograph with *A*, in which the mass is much more obvious. Ultrasonography-assisted fine-needle aspiration demonstrated this circumscribed mass to be a lymph node. *C*, Ultrasonographic image of the mass seen in *B*. It is an enlarged lymph node (arrows) that is dorsal to the larynx and ventral to the cervical vertebrae. The ultrasound unit was used to facilitate fine-needle aspiration of the node, which was found to be reactive.

normal or flaccid jaw tone and is often due to bilateral cranial nerve defects or a central lesion (e.g., trauma, hydrocephalus).

It is important to distinguish neurologic disorders causing oral disorders from myositis of the masseter and temporalis muscles. Acute myositis may cause so much pain that a patient refuses to open its mouth. The temporal and masseter muscles typically are swollen and painful. Chronic myositis causing marked fibrosis and atrophy of the muscles of mastication prevents eating because the patient cannot open its mouth, even when anesthetized. Systemic signs of myopathy usually are not present in dogs with masseter myositis. If uncertain, one may check for antibodies to 2M muscle fibers because they are principally found in masseter myositis but not polymyositis (Shelton and Cardinet, 1989). Although uncommon, tetanus may also cause spasticity of the muscles of mastication; however, these patients usually have signs of generalized muscle spasticity.

Patients with oral dysphagia due to idiopathic cranial nerve deficits usually must be managed by conservative dietary therapy. Many affected animals modify their eating behavior and compensate for the problem. Making food into small balls and "throwing" them into the back of the pet's mouth

may work in other cases. Most affected animals will be able to drink if provided with a deep bowl or bucket that allows them to insert their mouth and suck up the water. Atrophic/masseter myositis usually responds well to high-dose corticosteroid therapy (e.g., prednisolone 2.2 mg/kg/day), especially when combined with azathioprine. However, do not reduce the dose too quickly lest the disease return and be harder to bring under control.

The pharyngeal phase involves forming a food bolus at the base of the tongue and pushing it back to and through the cricopharyngeal sphincter. Dysfunctions of this phase of swallowing typically cause repeated attempts to swallow, difficulty swallowing (as manifested by repeatedly flexing or stretching the neck), regurgitation during or after swallowing (regurgitation can occur immediately or hours later if food has been impacted in the pharynx), aspiration, or gagging. The signs associated with pharyngeal dysphagia may mimic those of cricopharyngeal dysfunction/achalasia, especially if regurgitation occurs immediately after swallowing. Many affected patients have more difficulty handling liquids than solids, probably because the liquids are easier to aspirate.

If pharyngeal dysphagia is suspected, contrast radiographs are needed to detect and distinguish it

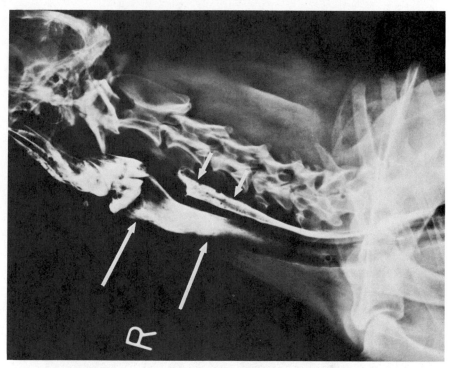

Figure 2. A lateral contrast radiograph of a dog with apparent neurogenic pharyngeal dysfunction. There is retention of barium in the pharynx. More importantly, note the barium in the trachea (long arrows) due to aspiration plus the retention of barium in the esophagus (short arrows) due to concurrent esophageal dysfunction.

from cricopharyngeal dysfunction. Static image radiographs are usually inadequate as fluoroscopy or cinefluorography is needed to delineate pathology of the swallowing process. Barium sulfate paste is a good choice for such procedures, but some patients may have to be evaluated with liquid preparations. Iodine contrast agents are not recommended.

It is also important to check for concurrent esophageal weakness in patients with pharyngeal dysfunction (Fig. 2). Proximal esophageal dilatation or food retention may confuse the diagnostician, and its presence has prognostic implications, especially if cricopharyngeal myotomy is considered. If possible, patients with esophageal weakness should have the competence of their cricopharyngeus muscle evaluated fluoroscopically to see if there is spontaneous leakage of esophageal contents back into the oropharynx (Fig. 3). Such incompetence suggests a more guarded prognosis, because aspiration tends to be more frequent and severe.

One should look for underlying causes of acquired pharyngeal dysfunction, especially myopathies, neuromuscular junction disorders, and neuropathies. Myasthenia gravis has been recognized to affect principally the esophagus or pharyngeal muscles in some dogs. As in cases of generalized myasthenia gravis, these patients have measurable circulating antibodies against acetylcholine receptors (Shelton et al., 1990). Antinuclear antibodies and serum T_3 and T_4 concentrations should also be evaluated because systemic lupus erythematosus and hypothyroidism may produce myoneuropathies.

Electromyography and biopsy of pharyngeal muscles may be helpful. Care must be taken not to inadvertently transect the cricopharyngeus muscle during a biopsy procedure.

If an underlying cause is found, it should be treated. Localized esophageal dysfunction and megaesophagus resolve in some hypothyroid patients following supplementation with thyroxine. Acetylcholinesterase inhibitors (e.g., pyridostigmine [Mestinon, Roche]) may be tried in patients with idiopathic localized myasthenia gravis, but care must be taken to avoid toxicity from overdose. Cricopharyngeal myotomy is of dubious value in pharyngeal dysfunction and is seemingly contraindicated in patients with abnormal retention of food or barium in the proximal esophagus. In these latter patients, such surgery often produces severe aspiration (Watrous and Suter, 1983).

If an underlying cause of pharyngeal dysfunction cannot be found, symptomatic dietary management may be tried. Pharyngeal dysfunction is typically found as an acquired disorder in older animals. However, it occasionally occurs in young dogs, which may seemingly "grow out" of it, much like some cases of congenital megaesophagus. If aspiration is severe, a pharyngostomy or gastrostomy tube may be placed. An alternative is to create a permanent cervical esophageal fistula through which clients can intermittently pass a tube to feed and water the animal.

The cricopharyngeal phase involves coordinated relaxation of the cricopharyngeus muscle, allowing food boluses to pass into the esophagus, where

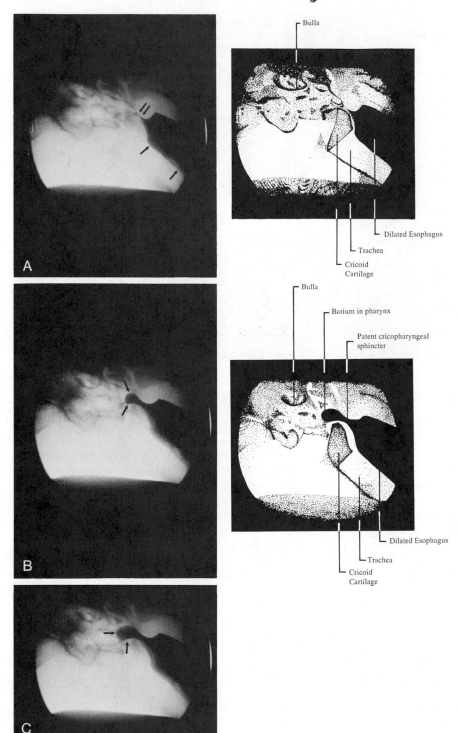

Figure 3. Three consecutive fluoroscopic images of the cricopharyngeal region of a dog with regurgitation and aspiration. Note that the image is reversed (i.e., the barium is a dark black shadow). *A* and *B* include labeled drawings corresponding to the fluoroscopic images. *A*, The proximal esophagus is dilated with barium liquid (single arrows), and the cricopharyngeal region is denoted by a narrowed area (double arrows). *B*, The cricopharyngeal area is opening and allowing barium in the esophagus to leak back into the pharynx (arrows). *C*, More barium is entering the pharynx through the incompetent cricopharyngeal sphincter (arrows). This dog had severe aspiration disease. (Reprinted with permission from Allen, D. [ed.]: *Small Animal Medicine.* Philadelphia: J.B. Lippincott, 1991, p. 492.)

primary esophageal waves carry them to the stomach. Cricopharyngeal disease usually consists of failure of the cricopharyngeus muscle to relax or failure to coordinate this relaxation with the pharyngeal phase. Principally diagnosed in young dogs, cricopharyngeal dysfunction occasionally occurs as an acquired disorder of older animals. Cricopharyn-

geal dysfunction classically produces regurgitation that occurs immediately after swallowing, although rare patients become anorexic, ostensibly because of discomfort when attempting to swallow or when regurgitating. Aspiration is less common than in pharyngeal dysfunction, but emaciation may occur as a result of diminished caloric intake.

Dynamic contrast radiography is needed for definitive diagnosis of cricopharyngeal dysfunction. One needs to be certain of the diagnosis because cricopharyngeal myotomy, although curative of this disorder, may kill animals with pharyngeal dysfunction. Postoperatively, the prognosis is favorable if there is no cicatrix formation.

References and Suggested Reading

Shelton, G. D., and Cardinet, G. H. III: Canine masticatory muscle disorders. *In* Kirk, R. W. (ed.): *Current Veterinary Therapy X.* Philadelphia: W. B. Saunders, 1989, pp. 816–819.
A discussion of the diagnosis and treatment of masticatory myositis, including the use of serologic study.
Shelton, G. D., Willard, M. D., Cardinet, G. H. III, et al.: Acquired myasthenia gravis: Selective involvement of esophageal, pharyngeal, and facial muscles. J. Vet. Intern Med. 4:281, 1990.
This article describes the syndrome of localized myasthenia causing regurgitation in dogs.
Suter, P. F., and Watrous, B. J.: Oropharyngeal dysphagias in the dog: A cinefluorographic analysis of experimentally induced and spontaneously occurring swallowing disorders. Vet. Radiol. 21:24, 1980.
One of the initial and classic descriptions of neurologic dysphagia in dogs, involving nine dogs with spontaneous disease.
Watrous, B. J.: Clinical presentation and diagnosis of dysphagia. Vet. Clin. North Am. 13:437, 1983.
An excellent synopsis of neurologic dysphagia in dogs.
Watrous, B. J., and Suter, P. F.: Oropharyngeal dysphagias in the dog: A cinefluorographic analysis of experimentally induced and spontaneously occurring swallowing disorders. Vet. Radiol. 24:11, 1983.
Twelve cases of spontaneous neurologic dysphagia in dogs are discussed, plus six cases of experimentally induced defects.
Willard, M. D., Burns, J., Jennings, D., et al.: Progressive oropharyngeal dysfunction in a dog. J.A.V.M.A. 183:1009, 1983.
A report of a dog with spontaneous neurologic dysphagia that responded to corticosteroids.

MANAGEMENT OF ESOPHAGEAL FOREIGN BODIES

BRENT D. JONES
Columbia, Missouri

Despite the distensibility of the normal esophagus, partial or complete luminal obstruction caused by the presence of foreign bodies is a common problem in dogs. Foreign body obstruction is reported to be six times more common in dogs than in cats (Ryan and Greene, 1975). Indiscriminate eating habits and inadequate mastication may contribute to the higher incidence of esophageal foreign bodies in dogs than in cats. Cats are usually more fastidious eaters than dogs but can still acquire foreign bodies because of their hunting or playing behaviors. Common types of esophageal foreign bodies are steak, chicken, and pork chop bones; wood; string; and fishhooks, needles, and other metal objects. In my experience, bones are the most commonly encountered foreign body, followed by fishhooks. The extent of foreign body-induced esophageal injury in dogs and cats is largely determined by the duration of the obstruction as well as by the size, contour, and type of object.

Anatomically, the esophagus has several narrow areas where swallowed foreign bodies tend to lodge. These are the cranial esophageal sphincter; the thoracic inlet, where adjacent soft tissues impede esophageal dilation; the heart base, where the aorta moves the esophagus to the right; and the region of the distal esophageal hiatus. Except for impeded fishhooks, most foreign bodies are found near the distal esophageal hiatus. A significant number also lodge in the cervical esophageal region.

CLINICAL SIGNS

Clinical signs are related to either partial or complete obstruction of the esophagus or to inflammation associated with the presence of the foreign body. Acute signs include regurgitation, painful dysphagia, ptyalism, persistent gulping, and anorexia. Chronic signs include depression, weight loss, and signs of complications that include severe esophagitis, mucosal lacerations, esophageal stricture, diverticula, perforated esophagus, pleuritis, mediastinitis, and pyothorax. Liquids and semisolids may bypass partial obstructions, and regurgitation may only be evident after eating solid foods. Respiratory distress secondary to airway impingement may occur if the ingested object is very large. Clinical signs of dyspnea and wheezing predominate in these patients. Significant airway obstruction can result in the formation of pulmonary edema. Results of the physical examination are usually supportive of the clinical findings; however, physical examination should include careful observation of the base of the tongue for the presence of linear foreign objects that may extend into the esophagus.

DIAGNOSIS

Most esophageal foreign bodies are found in animals 2 to 3 years old or younger. Diagnosis is often aided by the history of foreign body ingestion. A definitive diagnosis is determined by clinical findings, radiographic evaluation, or esophagoscopy. Radiographic examination should include the entire length of the esophagus. Radiopaque foreign objects are readily visualized on survey radiographs, but positive contrast agents are needed to outline and localize radiolucent objects. If a foreign body is obstructing the esophagus, air is frequently visualized cranial to the foreign body. If gas is visualized radiographically in the adjacent mediastinal or pleural space, perforation of the esophagus should be considered. If an esophageal perforation is suspected, the use of barium sulfate as a contrast agent is contraindicated. By providing direct visualization, *esophagoscopy* is the best method of diagnosing esophageal foreign bodies. Esophagoscopy is superior to radiography in recognizing inflammation, punctures, and lacerations, and it allows assessment of the extent of esophageal injury.

TREATMENT

Because the incidence of complications increases with the duration of the disease process, the management of esophageal foreign bodies must be considered an *emergency*. Esophageal foreign bodies may be removed by esophagoscopy or surgery. Esophagoscopy is less traumatic than esophagotomy, and most patients undergoing esophagoscopy for foreign body removal are released within a few hours after the procedure. In my experience, most (85 to 90%) esophageal foreign bodies can be removed by esophagoscopy, although embedded fishhooks are by far the most difficult to remove. Therefore, surgery should only be considered if esophagoscopy has failed or is unavailable.

In cases of suspected esophageal foreign body, I initially pass a flexible endoscope into the esophagus to visualize the foreign body and to inspect the mucosa for any damage (Fig. 1). If the foreign body is small, it can frequently be removed by passing flexible four-prong grasping forceps through the endoscope, clasping the foreign body, and pulling it and the endoscope retrograde (Fig. 2) out of the esophagus. If the foreign body is too large for the flexible grasping forceps, rigid grasping forceps may be passed alongside of a flexible endoscope (Fig. 3). Once grasped, the foreign body and the endoscope can be pulled retrograde through the mouth (Fig. 4). The foreign body frequently becomes dislodged from the forceps as it passes through the cranial esophageal sphincter. At this point, the foreign body can be easily retracted using large surgical forceps

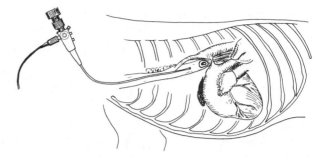

Figure 1. The use of a flexible endoscope to visualize a bone foreign body lodged at the base of the heart. (Reprinted with permission from Roudebush, P., et al.: Medical aspects of esophageal disease. *In* Jones, B. D. [ed.]: *Canine and Feline Gastroenterology.* Philadelphia: W. B. Saunders, 1986, p. 69.)

with a more secure grip, but these forceps are too short to be used in the more distal esophagus. If flexible endoscopes are unavailable, rigid endoscopes work well (Figs. 5 through 7).

If the foreign body cannot be removed in a retrograde manner, the second procedure of choice is to advance it into the stomach. Once in the stomach, the foreign body may pass into the intestine, where it may be later excreted in the feces. Most bone foreign bodies are digested by the acid in the stomach and then are eliminated in the feces in 7 to 10 days. A series of abdominal radiographs should be taken to confirm that the foreign body has left the stomach and to make sure that it does not cause an obstruction distally in the intestine. If the foreign body is too large to pass into the intestine, it may be removed by gastrostomy, which

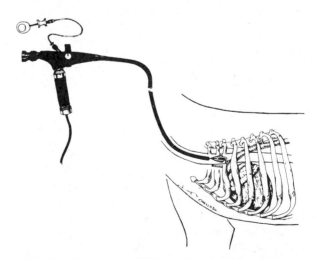

Figure 2. The use of a flexible endoscope with a four-prong grasping forceps being passed through the operating channel. The grasping forceps are holding the bone foreign body. Small foreign bodies can then be removed by pulling the endoscope and grasping forceps retrograde through the mouth. (Reprinted with permission from Roudebush, P., et al.: Medical aspects of esophageal disease. *In* Jones, B. D. [ed.]: *Canine and Feline Gastroenterology.* Philadelphia: W. B. Saunders, 1986, p. 69.)

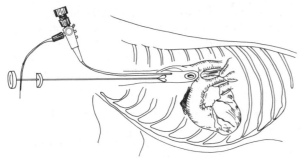

Figure 3. Rigid grasping forceps are passed alongside the flexible endoscope to clasp the bone foreign body. The foreign body can easily be held as one visually observes the grasping forceps and foreign body through the endoscope. (Reprinted with permission from Roudebush, P., et al.: Medical aspects of esophageal disease. *In* Jones, B. D. [ed.]: *Canine and Feline Gastroenterology.* Philadelphia: W. B. Saunders, 1986, p. 70.)

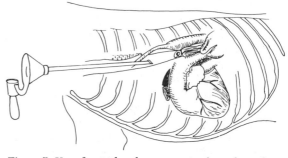

Figure 5. Use of a rigid endoscope to visualize a bone foreign body lodged at the base of the heart. A human sigmoidoscope can sometimes be used as a rigid endoscope. (Reprinted with permission from Roudebush, P., et al.: Medical aspects of esophageal disease. *In* Jones, B. D. [ed.]: *Canine and Feline Gastroenterology.* Philadelphia: W. B. Saunders, 1986, p. 70.)

is an easier procedure with far less morbidity and mortality than esophagotomy. Use care when advancing a foreign body into the stomach, because the distal esophageal deviation at the gastroesophageal junction causes resistance to the passage of the foreign body into the stomach. All manipulations of foreign bodies with the endoscopic equipment must be carefully performed in order to minimize further esophageal trauma.

In cases in which an embedded fish hook could not be removed by esophagoscopy (approximately 75 to 80%), I have used a combination of surgery and endoscopy. The surgeon can cut off the point of the hook as it emerges through the esophageal wall, and the remaining part of the fishhook can then be removed from the esophageal lumen via esophagoscopy. By using this method, the surgeon can avoid making an incision into the poorly healing esophagus.

After the foreign body has been removed (either retrograde or anterograde), the esophageal damage should be assessed. The esophageal mucosa should be visually examined by passing an endoscope

through the entire length of the esophagus. The degree of mucosal disease present usually is directly proportional to the duration of the foreign body in the esophagus. Erythema and mild ulceration at the site of entrapment are common. Pay special attention to any evidence of tears, lacerations, or perforations of the esophageal wall. Survey thoracic radiographs should be taken after removing all esophageal foreign bodies, because a pneumothorax or a pneumomediastinum may be present if the esophagus was perforated.

In my experience, mild tears, lacerations, and ulcerations will heal with the symptomatic treatment described for esophagitis (Jones et al., 1989). Larger esophageal lacerations and perforations may need to be treated with pharyngotomy tubes, chest drainage, and supportive management (Ryan and Greene, 1975). The use of pharyngotomy or gastrostomy tubes allows enteral alimentation of an animal while resting the esophagus. Disadvantages of the use of a pharyngotomy tube include continued irritation of the esophagus from the physical presence of the tube and the possibility of reflux of gastric contents into the esophagus due to interference of gastroesophageal sphincter closure (Lantz

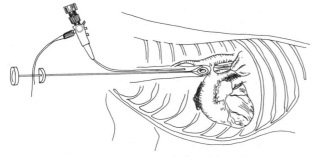

Figure 4. The grasping forceps and flexible endoscope in place. These two instruments are then pulled retrograde to extract the foreign body from the esophagus. (Reprinted with permission from Roudebush, P., et al.: Medical aspects of esophageal disease. *In* Jones, B. D. [ed.]: *Canine and Feline Gastroenterology.* Philadelphia: W. B. Saunders, 1986, p. 70.)

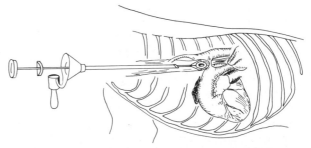

Figure 6. Grasping forceps passing through the rigid endoscope to clasp the bone esophageal foreign body. (Reprinted with permission from Roudebush, P., et al.: Medical aspects of esophageal disease. *In* Jones, B. D. [ed.]: *Canine and Feline Gastroenterology.* Philadelphia: W. B. Saunders, 1986, p. 70.)

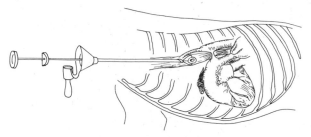

Figure 7. Grasping forceps and rigid endoscope being pulled retrograde to remove the bone foreign body. Note that the foreign body is pulled snug against the rigid endoscope to facilitate removal as the endoscope dilates the esophagus while being pulled retrograde. (Reprinted with permission from Roudebush, P., et al.: Medical aspects of esophageal disease. *In* Jones, B. D. [ed.]: *Canine and Feline Gastroenterology.* Philadelphia: W. B. Saunders, 1986, p. 71.)

et al., 1983). Large esophageal rents and signs of mediastinitis or other thoracic cavity involvement demand surgical exploration and repair.

PROGNOSIS

Approximately one third of the animals with esophageal foreign bodies will develop complica-

tions (Strombeck and Guilford, 1990). Most complications are relatively minor and include esophagitis and mucosal lacerations. Serious complications such as esophageal perforation, mediastinitis, and pleuritis are rare. It is my opinion that the incidence of complications is greatest when foreign objects become lodged between the heart and diaphragm. This observation may, however, just be a reflection of the increased frequency of foreign bodies found in this area. Stricture, diverticulum formation, and local deficits in motility may occur several weeks after successful removal of a foreign body.

References and Suggested Reading

Jones, B. D., Jergens, A. E., and Guilford, W. G.: Diseases of the esophagus. *In* Ettinger, S. J. (ed.): *Textbook of Veterinary Internal Medicine.* Philadelphia: W. B. Saunders, 1989, p. 1255.
Lantz, G. C., et al.: Pharyngostomy tube induced esophagitis in the dog: An experimental study. J. Am. Anim. Hosp. Assoc. 19:207, 1983.
Ryan, W. W., and Greene, R. W.: The conservative management of esophageal foreign bodies and their complications: A review of 66 cases in dogs and cats. J. Am. Anim. Hosp. Assoc. 11:243, 1975.
Strombeck, D. R., and Guilford, W. G.: Diseases of swallowing. *In* Strombeck D. R. (ed.): *Small Animal Gastroenterology.* Davis, CA: Stonegate, 1990, p. 140.

MEGAESOPHAGUS SECONDARY TO ACQUIRED MYASTHENIA GRAVIS

G. DIANE SHELTON
La Jolla, California

Acquired myasthenia gravis (MG) is an autoimmune disorder of neuromuscular transmission resulting from the actions of autoantibodies against nicotinic acetylcholine receptors (AChRs) at neuromuscular junctions (see this volume, p. 154). Although megaesophagus associated with generalized canine acquired MG has been well documented, a focal form has recently been recognized. In this form, megaesophagus and regurgitation in the absence of detectable generalized weakness are the principal clinical signs. Some dogs with this focal form of MG may concurrently have weakness involving the pharyngeal and laryngeal muscles, resulting in dysphagia and dyspnea or weakness of the facial muscles and a decreased palpebral reflex.

In two different studies of dogs with idiopathic megaesophagus, 18 of 48 dogs (37%; Lennon, V. A., personal communication, 1989) and 40 of 152 dogs (26%; Shelton, 1990) were found to have elevated serum antibody titers to AChRs, diagnostic of acquired MG. In the study of 152 dogs, numerous breeds of dogs had esophageal dilatation associated with antibodies to AChR; however, golden retrievers (7 of 20, 35%) and German shepherd dogs (8 of 25, 32%) were the breeds most often affected. These same breeds were also highly represented in studies of generalized canine acquired MG (Shelton, 1989; Shelton et al., 1988). Age of onset of idiopathic megaesophagus as compared with focal MG is shown in Figure 1. Although dogs with acquired idiopathic megaesophagus tend to have later onset, those with focal MG had a bimodal age of onset as in generalized MG, with a younger group of dogs showing clinical signs at 2 to 4 years of age and an older group at 9 to 13 years of age. The prevalence of increased serum antibody titers was not significantly different among sex groupings. The clinical course after diagnosis was available for 35 of 40 cases of focal MG. Six dogs died of aspiration pneumonia or choking, and 12 were euthanatized with no treatment attempted because of the poor prognosis that was given. For the remaining 17 dogs (48%), clinical improvement or remission of clinical signs was reported, in all cases associated with decreased titers of antibody to AChRs. Radiographic resolution of the megaesophagus was reported in six dogs in complete clinical remission.

CLINICAL SIGNS

Clinical signs are expressed in an adult animal without a previous history of regurgitation or dysphagia. Clinical signs referable to esophageal or pharyngeal weakness include regurgitation, increased drooling or salivation, and repeated attempts at swallowing with extension or twisting of the head and neck. Clinical signs may often be attributable only to the respiratory system and include purulent nasal discharge, moist cough, and dyspnea due to a resultant aspiration pneumonia. It is important to differentiate vomiting from regurgitation, because a differential diagnosis of vomiting would lead a clinician down the wrong diagnostic pathway.

DIAGNOSIS

Swallowing disorders can be frustrating problems, and the underlying cause of the dysfunction very often is not determined. If a structural abnormality cannot be identified, a search must be made for a functional abnormality. Functional abnormalities are the result of either primary or secondary neuromuscular disorders with a loss of motor function. Because the muscles involved in the swallowing process are predominantly striated, any disorder that can produce limb muscle weakness can theoretically result in dysphagia or megaesophagus. In some cases, however, a diagnosis can be made and treatment of the underlying problem can resolve clinical signs. MG is one such disorder.

Clinical evaluation of dysphagia and megaesophagus must be approached in a systematic manner. A complete physical and neurologic examination should be performed, with particular emphasis on muscle groups innervated by cranial nerves. A complete blood count, serum chemistry profile,

AGE DISTRIBUTION
DOGS WITH MEGAESOPHAGUS

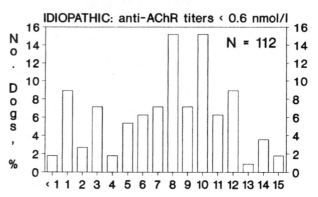

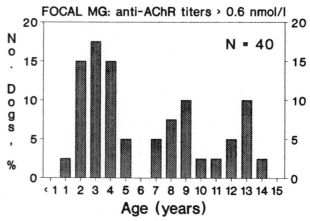

Figure 1. Dogs with acquired megaesophagus and focal myasthenia gravis (MG) have a bimodal age of onset of clinical signs very similar to that in generalized canine MG. Although younger dogs are affected with idiopathic megaesophagus of other causes (serum acetylcholine receptor [AChR] antibody titers <0.6 nmol/L), a later age of onset seems to predominate. (Reprinted with permission from Shelton, G. D., et al.: Acquired myasthenia gravis: Selective involvement of esophageal, pharyngeal, and facial muscles. J. Vet. Intern. Med. 4:283, 1990.)

electrolyte measurements, creatine kinase determination, and evaluation of thyroid and adrenal gland function are indicated in all cases to rule out an underlying metabolic disorder. The diagnostic assay for focal MG, as in acquired generalized MG, is demonstration of circulating antibodies against canine AChR by immunoprecipitation radioimmunoassay. Because MG may be the underlying problem in a large proportion of cases of acquired megaesophagus, a serum AChR antibody titer should be performed as part of the minimum database in all cases.

An edrophonium chloride (Tensilon; Roche) challenge test can be performed to provide a presumptive diagnosis if a decreased or absent palpebral reflex is present. Following the intravenous administration of 0.1 to 0.2 mg/kg of the short-acting anticholinesterase drug, an increase in strength of the blink reflex may be noted. Further, if fluoroscopy is available, evaluation of the passage of an isotonic water-soluble contrast agent or a small volume of a dilute barium solution from the oral cavity to the stomach before and after edrophonium may give some indication of whether anticholinesterase drugs may be of benefit in improving pharyngeal or esophageal function.

Radiographic contrast studies using barium should be performed with caution, especially if esophageal dilatation is readily visualized on survey radiographs, and they should be done only if fluoroscopic and cineradiographic capabilities are available. It is not worth the risk of barium aspiration pneumonia just for additional confirmation of the presence of a megaesophagus. Although the prognosis for resolution of clinical signs is favorable for MG in the absence of barium aspiration pneumonia, the prognosis for recovery from barium aspiration pneumonia often is poor.

TREATMENT

Alteration of feeding procedures is an important initial step in the therapy of dogs with megaesophagus and regurgitation secondary to MG. A high-calorie semiliquid gruel should be fed from an elevated position with the dog held in a standing position for 10 min after a meal. If anticholinesterase drugs are part of the treatment regimen, they should be given 1 hr before feeding. If significant regurgitation is still a problem after this procedure, placement of a percutaneous gastrostomy tube should facilitate maintenance of nutrional support and drug delivery (Bright and Burrows, 1988).

Although anticholinesterase drugs are the cornerstone of therapy for generalized MG, their value in focal MG is yet to be determined. Although no physiologic studies are yet available, the esophagus may not be as responsive clinically to this therapy as limb muscles, and the chance of overdose due to inadequate monitoring of clinical signs is increased. If oral dosing is impossible as a result of severe regurgitation and aspiration, injectable neostigmine (Prostigmin, Roche) at a dosage of 0.04 mg/kg IM every 6 hr is given until the animal is able to handle oral medication or can be medicated through a gastrostomy tube. Once the animal can handle oral medication, pyridostigmine bromide syrup or tablets (Mestinon; Roche) at a dosage of 0.5 to 1.0 mg/kg every 8 to 12 hr may be initiated. The low end of the dosage range is suggested for cases of focal MG, because clinical responses may be difficult to evaluate and drug overdose may be misinterpreted as progressing muscular weakness. In some cases, pyridostigmine has lessened clinical signs of regurgitation. If aspiration pneumonia is present, treatment for it should also be initiated.

In the absence of aspiration pneumonia, immunosuppressive doses of corticosteroids may be useful. Care must be taken when using corticosteroids in combination with anticholinesterase drugs, because muscle weakness may be enhanced. Whether or not corticosteroids are actually of benefit is also open to question, because many dogs go into spontaneous remissions in the absence of any drug treatment (G. D. Shelton, 1990).

Other drugs, including cholinergics and anticholinergics that act on smooth muscle, have not been shown to improve esophageal function in canine megaesophagus. Calcium channel antagonists have been evaluated in dogs with megaesophagus, and there is no reliable evidence that they are of any value (Strombeck, 1990). Care must be taken when giving drugs such as aminoglycoside antibiotics, antiarrhythmic agents, phenothiazines, or methoxyflurane to myasthenic patients. Caution must also be used when giving magnesium, either parenterally or in cathartics, to these patients. These drugs have been shown to reduce the safety margin of neuromuscular transmission and can potentiate neuromuscular weakness.

After diagnosis, the serum AChR antibody titer should be rechecked at 4 to 6-week intervals to determine the course of the disorder and to make adjustments in therapy. Treatment should be continued until the serum antibody titer is within the normal range. Some dogs progress to the generalized form of MG; however, if they are going to do so, it is usually within the first few weeks after onset of clinical signs. Dogs with only focal MG may represent a milder form of the disease. A large percentage of the dogs will have spontaneous remissions in which the serum antibody titer returns to the normal range and the megaesophagus may no longer be radiographically apparent. The time course from onset of clinical signs until remission can vary from days to months. During clinical remissions, all medication can be discontinued. However, owners should be advised that the disease may recur.

In some dogs, serum AChR antibody titers remain elevated and clinical signs persist. A search should be made in this group of dogs for evidence of other concurrent autoimmune or neoplastic disorders, and appropriate treatment should be initiated. In particular, thyroid function should be evaluated and a careful search made for cranial mediastinal mass.

PROGNOSIS

In the absence of aspiration pneumonia, the prognosis for full recovery of function in cases of MG with only megaesophagus can be favorable. If pharyngeal paralysis is concurrently present, the prognosis becomes guarded because of difficulties in management. The key to a successful outcome in cases of focal MG with only megaesophagus is prevention of aspiration pneumonia through careful management of feeding and very restricted use of barium.

References and Suggested Reading

Bright, R. M., and Burrows, C. F.: Percutaneous endoscopic tube gastrostomy in dogs. Am. J. Vet. Res. 49:629, 1988.
  Placement of gastrostomy tubes for myasthenic dogs that cannot tolerate oral feeding or medication.
Shelton, G. D.: Disorders of neuromuscular transmission. Semin. Vet. Med. Surg. (Small Anim.) 4:126; 1989.
  General overview of disorders affecting neuromuscular transmission, with emphasis on MG.
Shelton, G. D., Cardinet, G. H. III, and Lindstrom, J.: Canine and human myasthenia gravis autoantibodies recognize similar regions on the acetylcholine receptor. Neurology 38:1417, 1988.
  Clinical characteristics of 35 dogs with generalized MG.
Shelton, G. D., Willard, M. D., Cardinet, G. H. III, et al.: Acquired myasthenia gravis: Selective involvement of esophageal, pharyngeal, and facial muscles. J. Vet. Intern. Med. 4:281, 1990.
  Study of 152 dogs with idiopathic megaesophagus, with the diagnosis of MG in 40 of the dogs.
Strombeck, D. R.: Diseases of swallowing. In Strombeck, D. R., and Guilford, W. G.(eds.): Small Animal Gastroenterology. Davis: Stonegate, 1990, p. 140.
  In-depth information on the physiology, pharmacology, and management of swallowing disorders.

ACUTE VOMITING: A DIAGNOSTIC APPROACH AND SYMPTOMATIC MANAGEMENT

MICHAEL S. LEIB

Blacksburg, Virginia

Vomiting is common in dogs and cats. Occasional vomiting may be considered normal (especially in cats); more frequent vomiting is associated with gastrointestinal (GI) disorders or metabolic diseases. Because vomiting is a clinical sign of many disorders, an accurate and efficient diagnosis can most easily be reached by following a logical diagnostic plan. To reduce the number of potential diagnoses and available diagnostic tests, it is helpful to classify vomiting dogs and cats as having acute or chronic disease. The duration of clinical signs for acute vomiting is usually less than 5 days. Some acutely vomiting dogs and cats have life-threatening diseases and need in-depth diagnostic evaluation and vigorous therapy, while many others have self-limiting disorders and need only minimal diagnostic testing and simple supportive therapy. Chronically vomiting animals require thorough diagnostic evaluation that often includes endoscopic examination. When differentiating acute and chronic cases, it is important to remember that chronic vomiting starts acutely. Failure to identify a cause of acute vomiting when clinical signs persist indicates the animal should be reclassified as chronically vomiting and a different diagnostic plan followed. This chapter will review the author's approach to the diagnosis of dogs and cats that acutely vomit. Further informa-tion concerning individual diseases or fluid therapy can be found within this volume.

PATHOPHYSIOLOGY

Vomiting is a centrally mediated reflex controlled by the vomiting center in the medulla (dorsal lateral reticular formation). Input can reach the vomiting center by four pathways (Davis, 1980): (1) Efferent impulses from receptors in the pharynx, stomach, duodenum, jejunum, liver, gall bladder, and other abdominal organs travel to the vomiting center via vagal and sympathetic pathways. These receptors are stimulated by distention, irritation, hyperosmolarity, and certain chemicals; (2) Circulating substances may stimulate the vomiting center via the chemoreceptor trigger zone (CRTZ). The CRTZ is located on the floor of the fourth ventricle and is not protected by the blood-brain barrier. Free nerve endings are in direct contact with cerebral spinal fluid (Willard, 1984). Stimulation of the CRTZ results in dopamine release and subsequent stimulation of the vomiting center. CRTZ stimulation can occur with substances such as digoxin, apomorphine, cancer chemotherapeutics (cisplatin), and uremic toxins; (3) Input from the semicircular canals is responsible for vomiting associated with motion sickness and rarely otitis media; (4) The vomiting center may be stimulated by input from the cerebral cortex or limbic system, probably of minor importance in small animals.

Regardless of the stimulus, the vomiting center initiates the complex act of vomiting. Nausea is the initial event and results in salivation, depression, anxiety, and frequent swallowing efforts. Nausea is an imprecisely defined, unpleasant sensation believed to be caused by mild activation of the same pathways that mediate vomiting. Retching precedes the expulsion of gastric and duodenal contents and is associated with deep inspiration, elevation of the soft palate, closure of the glottis, inhibition of esophageal and proximal gastric motility, and relaxation of the caudal esophageal sphincter. Expulsion occurs as the duodenum, antrum and pylorus, abdominal musculature, and diaphragm vigorously contract, forcing gastric and duodenal contents into the pharynx and triggering a gag reflex that expels ingesta from the mouth. The respiratory center is inhibited to prevent aspiration.

Occasional vomiting results in few pathophysiologic consequences to the animal but may be unpleasant and inconvenient for owners. Profuse and protracted vomiting can lead to dehydration, loss of electrolytes (chloride and sodium, and to a lesser degree hydrogen, potassium, and bicarbonate) and acid-base derangement. Mildly vomiting dogs and cats usually maintain normal acid-base status, but severe vomiting can lead to metabolic acidosis. Animals vomiting because of an obstructed pylorus can develop metabolic alkalosis, as vomitus is limited to gastric contents and duodenal bicarbonate is retained. Vomiting can also result in aspiration pneumonia.

DIAGNOSTIC PLAN

The most critical step during initial evaluation of small animals that present for acute vomiting is to differentiate between true vomiting and regurgitation. Expulsion of swallowed food is often described by owners as vomiting when regurgitation of retained esophageal contents may actually be occurring. Regurgitation requires an alternate diagnostic plan. In most cases, a thorough detailed history will allow accurate problem identification.

Vomiting is associated with salivation, retching, and violent abdominal contractions. Expulsion of yellow material suggests bile-stained duodenal contents and vomiting. Regurgitation is a passive process that occurs when esophageal disorders result in retention of food within the esophagus. As the esophagus distends, increased intrathoracic pressure or gravity causes the retained material to move along the path of least resistance, often into the pharynx, where initiation of a gag reflex occurs and results in expulsion from the mouth.

Table 1. *Some Causes of Acute Vomiting*

Self-Limiting	Potentially Life-Threatening
Acute gastritis	Acute gastritis
dietary indiscretion	Gastric-duodenal foreign body
drugs	Gastric-duodenal ulcer
chemicals	Intussusception
foreign material	*Giardia*
bacteria	Canine distemper
Ascaris	Feline panleukopenia
Giardia	Infectious canine hepatitis
Motion sickness	Canine parvovirus
Otitis media	Canine coronavirus
	Leptospirosis
	Salmon poisoning
	Hemorrhagic gastroenteritis
	Acute gastric dilatation-volvulus
	Acute pancreatitis
	Acute renal failure
	Acute hepatic failure
	Hypoadrenocorticism
	Peritonitis
	Pyometra
	Septicemia
	Central nervous system edema

After acute vomiting has been identified, the next important step is to determine if the animal has either a self-limiting or possible life-threatening problem. This crucial assessment is based on a thorough history, careful physical examination, clinical experience and judgment, and understanding of the differential diagnosis of acute vomiting (Table 1) (Thayer, 1981; Twedt, 1983). Animals with a self-limiting problem require minimal diagnostic testing (Table 2) and symptomatic treatment and often cease vomiting within 12 to 24 hr of initial presentation. Life-threatening cases of acute vomiting require an in-depth diagnostic evaluation (Table 2), vigorous symptomatic management, and often specific therapy directed at the underlying cause. Continuation or progression of clinical signs in animals thought to have a self-limiting problem, especially after appropriate symptomatic therapy, suggests the possibility of a life-threatening disorder.

Dogs and cats with self-limiting acute vomiting have a history of infrequent vomiting of food, mucus, bile, or foreign material and ingestion of table scraps or other forms of dietary indiscretion. Ques-

Table 2. *Minimum Database for Acute Vomiting*

Self-Limiting	Potentially Life-Threatening
Packed cell volume	Complete blood count
Total solids	Biochemical profile
Zinc sulfate fecal flotation	Urinalysis
Digital rectal examination	Digital rectal examination
	Zinc sulfate fecal flotation
	Amylase/lipase
	Survey abdominal
	radiographs

tioning may uncover the administration of drugs (aspirin, ibuprofen, erythromycin) or exposure to chemicals (herbicides, fertilizers, cleaning agents) that may be the cause of acute vomiting, which often resolves with removal of the offending agent and symptomatic therapy. The presence of mild diarrhea may indicate dietary indiscretion or gastrointestinal parasites such as *Ascaris* (puppies or kittens) or *Giardia* as the cause of the acute vomiting.

Physical examination is often normal; however, mild depression and signs of mild to moderate dehydration (e.g., slightly dry mucous membranes, slight loss of skin turgor, slightly prolonged capillary refill time, mild enophthalmus) may be seen. Abdominal palpation is often normal, although evidence of mild abdominal pain may be found. A digital rectal examination should be performed to evaluate fecal consistency.

A minimum database for animals with self-limiting vomiting should include determination of packed cell volume (PCV) and total solids, zinc sulfate fecal flotation, and digital rectal examination (see Table 2). The PCV and total solids help assess hydration and will also provide a baseline reference if clinical signs persist or progress. A digital rectal examination allows immediate collection of feces for flotation and establishes the presence or absence of diarrhea. If diarrhea is present, it can intensify dehydration and more aggressive fluid therapy may be required. Zinc sulfate fecal flotation is often necessary to identify *Giardia* cysts (Kirkpatrick, 1987).

Animals thought to have a life-threatening cause of acute vomiting have a history of profuse or persistent vomiting that may be increasing in frequency. These animals may vomit blood (hematemesis) or "coffee grounds" (partially digested blood) (see this volume, p. 572). Vaccination status may be incomplete, supporting the possibility of an infectious cause of acute vomiting, especially in the puppy or kitten. Owners may report moderate to severe abdominal pain, depression, or diarrhea. In addition, reclassification to life-threatening status may be indicated if an animal initially assessed as having self-limiting acute vomiting continues to vomit despite appropriate symptomatic therapy.

Physical examination in animals with potentially life-threatening causes of acute vomiting may reveal moderate to severe dehydration. Abdominal palpation often demonstrates moderate to severe pain and may identify such abnormalities as thickened small intestinal walls, distended loops of bowel, an intestinal foreign body, or an abdominal mass. The presence of metabolic diseases that can cause vomiting may be suggested by pyrexia, lymphadenopathy, icterus, respiratory crackles, and similar symptoms.

The initial minimum database for an animal with potentially life-threatening, acute vomiting includes a complete blood count, biochemical profile, urinalysis, zinc sulfate fecal flotation, serum amylase and lipase, and survey abdominal radiographs (see Table 2). Complete laboratory evaluation will help to eliminate infectious or metabolic causes of acute vomiting (acute renal failure, acute hepatic failure, hypoadrenocorticism, and acute pancreatitis) and allow assessment of fluid, electrolyte, and acid-base derangements secondary to vomiting. Multiple fecal examinations may identify parasites such as *Giardia* or *Ascaris*. Survey abdominal radiographs will help rule out radiodense foreign bodies, small intestinal obstructions, or linear foreign bodies (Felts et al., 1984). In some instances, initial evaluation indicates the necessity for additional diagnostic studies such as determination of acid-base status, upper GI endoscopy, upper GI barium series, abdominal ultrasound, ACTH-response testing, or surgical exploration of the abdomen.

THERAPY: SELF-LIMITING VOMITING

If an underlying cause for self-limiting acute vomiting can be identified, it should be corrected or removed. Many dogs and cats with self-limiting acute vomiting can be successfully managed by withholding food and water and correcting dehydration, if present. Animals should be given nothing per os (NPO) until vomiting ceases for 12 to 24 hr, after which small amounts of water or ice cubes should be offered frequently. If vomiting does not occur, small volumes of a bland diet can be offered every 2 to 4 hr. During the next 2 to 3 days, food quantity should be gradually increased and the frequency of meals gradually decreased until daily caloric maintenance requirements can be supplied. The animal's original diet should be slowly introduced. Table scraps, snacks, and other treats should be avoided.

Maintaining the animal NPO allows the inflamed gastrointestinal mucosa to rest and reduces gastric secretions. Gastric acid can back-diffuse across damaged mucosa, preventing healing of eroded or ulcerated tissue and causing further damage. Dietary proteins in the stomach and gastric distention are potent stimuli for the release of gastric acid. Withholding of food followed by frequent feeding of small meals low in protein helps to minimize gastric acid secretion and additional mucosal injury. The initial diet should be soft in consistency, low in fat, and high in carbohydrates (especially rice, which is highly digestible). Fats are the most complex nutrient to be digested and absorbed. Poorly assimilated fat can lead to diarrhea by stimulating secretion, inhibiting absorption, and altering gastrointestinal motility. Low-fat diets promote efficient assimilation of nutrients and minimize the potential for developing fatty acid–induced diarrhea. Homemade diets of chicken or lean hamburger and rice

Table 3. *Potassium Supplementation**
for Vomiting Dogs and Cats

Serum Potassium	mEq KCl/L Maintenance Fluids
<2.0	80
2.0–2.5	60
2.5–3.0	40
3.0–3.5	20

*Rate not to exceed 0.5 mEq/kg per hour.

or gastrointestinal diets such as Hill's Prescription Diet i/d are recommended.

Animals with minimal dehydration can receive subcutaneous or short-term intravenous fluid therapy with isotonic, polyionic fluids. If vomiting and diarrhea continue and cause progressive dehydration despite subcutaneous fluid therapy, intravenous fluids are indicated and a more aggressive diagnostic approach for a potentially life-threatening disorder should be pursued.

THERAPY: LIFE-THREATENING VOMITING

If a precipitating cause for life-threatening acute vomiting can be identified, specific treatment and fluid therapy should be administered. A fluid therapy plan must correct dehydration, provide for daily maintenance requirements, and replace ongoing losses. Most animals that are moderately or severely dehydrated (8 to 12%) require intravenous fluid administration. Estimated deficits secondary to dehydration should be replaced during the first 24 hr of hospitalization. Maintenance fluid requirements are approximately 60 ml/kg per day. Continued losses due to vomiting and diarrhea should be estimated and immediately replaced.

Replacement fluids such as lactated Ringer's solution are suitable for most vomiting dogs and cats. Maintenance fluids should be supplemented with potassium chloride based on the recommendations in Table 3 (Twedt and Grauer, 1982). Even if serum potassium is normal, 20 mEq/L of potassium chloride should be added, as a body potassium deficiency is probably occurring. Potassium should not be administered at a rate greater than 0.5 mEq/kg/hr, as it is cardiotoxic. Animals should be frequently monitored during the administration of fluid therapy and the rate adjusted accordingly. Parameters such as body weight, mucous membrane moisture, capillary refill time, eye position, skin turgor, thoracic auscultation, extremity temperature, PCV, total solids, and central venous pressure should be frequently evaluated to assess hydration status. After rehydration, body weight should remain relatively constant.

ANTIEMETICS

Antiemetics should be used judiciously in vomiting patients. Persistent vomiting associated with appropriate NPO therapy is often a sign of deterioration or progression of the underlying disease. Continued vomiting is a sign that more aggressive diagnostic testing and therapy may be needed. Masking this important monitoring parameter with antiemetics may provide a false impression that diagnostic testing and therapy are adequate and thus restrict additional diagnostic testing or administration of more aggressive therapy. The author uses antiemetics in the following situations: (1) continued vomiting interferes with the patient's requirements for rest, (2) continued vomiting makes maintenance of fluid, electrolyte, and acid-base status difficult, and (3) the owners of an self-limiting outpatient case cannot cope with continued vomiting at home and do not wish to have the animal hospitalized. It is important to be confident of the underlying diagnosis before antiemetics are used on an outpatient basis.

Metoclopramide has both central and peripheral antiemetic affects. As a dopamine antagonist, it blocks the CRTZ and prevents emesis associated with chemotherapy. Peripherally, metoclopramide increases tone of the caudal esophageal sphincter, and it increases gastric antral contractions while relaxing the pylorus and duodenum. These peripheral actions inhibit the vomiting reflex. Metoclopramide can be given at 0.2 to 0.4 mg/kg IM or SC every 8 hr or in some cases 1 to 2 mg/kg every 24 hr by continuous intravenous infusion. Metoclopramide is contraindicated if gastrointestinal obstruction is suspected. Although metoclopramide has been frequently recommended in preventing emesis associated with chemotherapy, a recent report showed that pretreatment did not significantly reduce the incidence of vomiting (Ogilvie et al., 1989). Further study of preventive protocols is necessary to develop adequate antiemetic prophylaxis for chemotherapy-induced emesis in dogs and cats.

Phenothiazines block both the CRTZ and the emetic center but may not effectively reduce efferent impulses due to severe gastrointestinal irritation. Due to their alpha-adrenergic blocking activity, they can produce vasodilation and should not be used in dehydrated animals. They can also cause mild depression, making patient monitoring more difficult. Phenothiazines should not be used in epileptic animals, as they may lower seizure threshold. Recommended drugs and dosages include chlorpromazine 0.5 mg/kg IM or SC every 6 to 8 hr and prochlorperazine 0.1 to 0.5 mg/kg IM or SC every 6 to 8 hr. Some preparations (e.g., Compazine, Smith Kline Beckman) come in suppository form and can be conveniently administered to outpatients. Antihistamines block input from the vestibular system and help prevent vomiting due to motion sickness. Diphenhydramine 2 to 4 mg/kg every 8 hr PO and dimenhydrate 25 to 50 mg every 8 hr PO can be given to produce sedation and prevent motion sickness.

Other dopamine antagonists may be able to block CRTZ-stimulated vomiting when the previously described antiemetics do not (Willard, 1984). Haloperidol is a butyrophenone that can prevent vomiting for up to 4 days in dogs at a dose of 100 μg/kg. Pimozide, a long-acting diphenylbutylpiperidine, may protect dogs from drug-induced emesis for up to 6 days when given at 100 μg/kg. Clinical experience in veterinary medicine with these dopamine antagonists is minimal, and caution should be used if they are instituted in cases of refractory vomiting believed to be initiated by the CRTZ. Further clinical experience with these drugs is necessary to identify potential side effects in dogs and cats.

SUMMARY

Vomiting is the expulsion of gastric and duodenal contents and results from a centrally mediated reflex. Vomiting is a clinical sign of many gastrointestinal disorders and metabolic diseases. Profuse and persistent vomiting can lead to dehydration, hypokalemia, hypochloremia, and metabolic acidosis. Most cases of acute vomiting can be classified as self-limiting or life-threatening based on history and physical examination. Animals with self-limiting vomiting can be managed by maintaining an NPO status and administering subcutaneous fluid therapy. Life-threatening cases of acute vomiting often require in-depth diagnostic evaluation and vigorous intravenous fluid therapy. Antiemetics can reduce the frequency of vomiting but should be used cautiously so they do not mask the signs of progression of the underlying cause of vomiting.

References and Suggested Reading

Davis, L. E.: Pharmacologic control of vomiting. J.A.V.M.A. 176:241, 1980.
A review of the vomiting reflex and antiemetic drug therapy.
Felts, J. F., Fox, P. R., and Burk, R. L.: Thread and sewing needles as gastrointestinal foreign bodies in the cat: A review of 64 cases. J.A.V.M.A. 184:56, 1984.
A study of the history, clinical signs, and radiographic and surgical findings in 64 cases of linear foreign body.
Kirkpatrick, C. E.: Giardiasis. Vet. Clin. North. Am. Small Anim. Pract. 17:1377, 1987.
A review of the life cycle, clinical signs, and treatment of Giardia.
Ogilvie, G. K., Moore, A. S., and Curtis, C. R.: Evaluation of cisplatin-induced emesis in dogs with malignant neoplasia: 115 cases (1984–1987). J.A.V.M.A. 195:1399, 1989.
A retrospective review of factors that may influence the incidence of vomiting in dogs treated with chemotherapy.
Thayer, G. W.: Vomiting: A clinical approach. Comp. Cont. Ed. Pract. Vet. 3:49, 1981.
A review of the diagnosis and therapy of acute and chronic vomiting in small animals.
Twedt, D. C., and Grauer, G. F.: Fluid therapy for gastrointestinal, pancreatic, and hepatic disorders. Vet. Clin. North. Am. Small Anim. Pract. 12:463, 1982.
A thorough review of fluid therapy for many gastrointestinal disorders.
Twedt, D. C.: Differential diagnosis and therapy of vomiting. Vet. Clin. North Am. Small Anim. Pract. 13:503, 1983.
A complete review of the diagnosis and therapy of acute and chronic vomiting in small animals.
Willard, M. D.: Some new approaches to the treatment of vomiting. J.A.V.M.A. 184:590, 1984.
A review of drugs not commonly used in veterinary medicine that may be useful as antiemetics.

ADVERSE REACTIONS TO FOOD

W. GRANT GUILFORD
Palmerston North, New Zealand

Adverse reactions to food are frequently observed in dogs and cats. They are composed of a variety of subclassifications (Table 1). Most adverse reactions to food result from ingestion of the inciting agent, followed by interaction of the agent with a cellular or noncellular biologic amplification system that leads to inflammation and the generation of clinical signs. The amplification system varies considerably with the inciting agent but may include mast cells, phagocytes, the autonomic nervous system, the antigen-specific immune system, the arachidonic acid cascade, the complement cascade, and the kinin system. At times, sufficient toxic material is present in food to produce clinical signs without need for amplification.

CLINICAL SIGNS AND DIAGNOSIS OF ADVERSE REACTIONS TO FOOD

Adverse reactions to food (food sensitivities) are suspected when an association is noted between the ingestion of a certain foodstuff and the appearance of a particular clinical sign or group of signs. The clinical signs are usually dermatologic or gastrointestinal (Table 2). Diagnosis is confirmed by reso-

Table 1. Major Subclassifications of Adverse
Reactions to Food*

Adverse reaction (sensitivity) to food—general terms applied to
   a clinically abnormal response attributed to an ingested food
   or food additive.
Food allergy (hypersensitivity)—an adverse reaction to food
   with a proven immunologic basis.
Food intolerance—a general term describing an adverse
   reaction to food that does not have an immunologic basis.
Food idiosyncrasy—a quantitatively abnormal response to a
   food or food additive that resembles a hypersensitivity
   response but does not involve immune mechanisms.
Pharmacologic reactions to food—an adverse reaction to food
   as a result of a naturally derived or added chemical that
   produces a druglike or pharmacologic effect in the host.
Metabolic reactions to food—an adverse reaction to food due to
   an effect of a substance upon the metabolism of the host, or
   as a result of defective metabolism of a nutrient by the host.
Food poisoning—an adverse reaction to food caused by the
   direct action of a toxin.

*The terms and definitions are those recommended by the American
Academy of Allergy and Immunology.

lution of clinical signs after the elimination of the
suspected food, followed by recrudescence of the
signs when the patient is subsequently challenged
with the incriminated foodstuff. A protocol for an
elimination-challenge trial is presented in Table 3.
The success of elimination-challenge trials depends
on good client cooperation. Patients undergoing
food challenges must be closely observed. Short
periods of avoidance of the food to which an animal
is sensitive may markedly exacerbate adverse signs
when the food is reintroduced ("unmasking").

To reiterate, elimination-challenge trials confirm
or rule out food sensitivities. Definitive differentiation of food allergy or intolerance necessitates immunologic investigations. The latter are often omit-
ted because the management of most patients will
not be altered whether the clinical signs result from
food allergy or from food intolerance.

FOOD ALLERGY

The term food allergy has been overused in the
veterinary literature, obscuring the true incidence
of the condition. The cause of food allergy is unknown. Most evidence points to a failure of the
immunologic mechanisms that mediate oral tolerance or to a breakdown of the mucosal permeability
barrier. In cases of a breakdown of the mucosal
permeability barrier, food allergies may be precipitated by viral or chronic inflammatory disorders of
the bowel. The pathogenesis of the disorder can
involve type I, III, or IV hypersensitivity.

Chemistry of Food Antigens

Food allergens are almost exclusively proteins.
There is little evidence that food additives act as
allergens. Additives are, however, thought to be an
important cause of food intolerances. Foods suggested to be prevalent causes of food allergy in dogs
and cats include milk, beef, soy, tuna, wheat, eggs,
chicken, and corn. On most occasions, the protein
to which an animal is allergic will be the one that
is present in greatest quantity in its usual diet.
Cross-reactivity is particularly common with sea-
foods and legumes.

Clinical Features

The history usually reveals adverse reactions that
are uniform in clinical manifestation and that consistently occur on exposure to a food. On rare
occasions, a suspected food may fail to consistently
lead to the expected clinical signs. One reason for
such inconsistency is an altered method of preparation of the food. The clinical signs are nonseasonal
(in contrast to many inhalation allergies) and often
occur suddenly after months of consuming the diet
containing the inciting foodstuff (in contrast to most
food intolerances). A wide age range of dogs and
cats can be affected, including animals less than 1
year of age.

Table 2. Proven or Suspected Clinical Signs or
Disorders Associated with Food Sensitivity

Dermatologic
   Excessive grooming
   Eosinophilic dermatitis
   Hyperesthesia
   Miliary dermatitis
   Otitis externa
   Papules and erythema
   Pododermatitis
   Pruritus (head and neck; face, feet, ears; generalized)
   Seborrhea
   Urticaria or angioedema

Gastrointestinal
   Abdominal pain
   Colitis
   Diarrhea
   Vomiting
   Eosinophilic gastroenteritis
   Gluten-sensitive enteropathy
   Oral and pharyngeal pruritus

Respiratory
   Asthma?
   Bronchitis?
   Nonseptic pneumonitis?
   Rhinitis?

Miscellaneous
   Anal pruritus?
   Anaphylaxis
   Glomerulonephritis?
   Hyperactivity?
   Malaise?
   Polyarthritis?
   Vasculitis?

? Reported in humans but as yet not in dogs and cats.

Table 3. *Suggested Protocol for Elimination-Challenge Trials for the Diagnosis of Adverse Reactions to Food**

Elimination trial

1. Place the patient on a controlled diet of a single protein source and a single carbohydrate source until signs resolve, e.g., lamb and boiled white rice, or cottage cheese and rice, or tofu and rice.
2. After 2 symptom-free weeks, add to the controlled diet a small quantity of the incriminated food (100 gm) or food additive for the first 3 days of the week (or for less time if clinical signs occur rapidly). The dose of the food additive used is the calculated average daily dietary intake of the additive.
3. Observe for clinical signs during the 3-day challenge period and the 4 days thereafter during which the patient is returned to the controlled diet without the incriminated agent.
4. If no evidence of clinical abnormality occurs, repeat the procedure using another food or additive every week, until a dietary component is identified that appears to cause clinical signs.
5. If a prolonged trial becomes necessary, supplement the diet with appropriate quantities of vitamins and minerals.

Challenge trial

6. After a suspected food or food additive has been identified, immediately remove it from the diet, and observe for evidence of resolution of signs.
7. Wait a minimum of 1–2 weeks from the last ingestion of the suspected agent and until the patient is symptom free, and then, under close observation, challenge the patient with the suspected food or additive to ensure that similar signs are manifested on the second exposure.

*Modified with permission from Strombeck, D. R., and Guilford, W. G.: *Small Animal Gastroenterology*, 2nd ed. Davis, CA: Stonegate Publishing, 1990, p. 344.

Food allergy may potentially result in any of the clinical signs of food sensitivity listed in Table 2, but dermatologic and gastrointestinal manifestations appear to predominate. Gastrointestinal signs need not be present to attribute a dermatologic abnormality to a food allergy.

Diagnosis of Food Allergy

The diagnosis of food allergy requires that an adverse reaction to a food first be confirmed by elimination-challenge trials (Table 3). Second, the adverse reaction to the food must be proved to have an immune-mediated basis. Tests used for this purpose include skin tests, radioallergosorbent test, enzyme-linked immunosorbent assay, assays of cell-mediated immune reactions and mast-cell degranulation, endoscopic intragastric challenge tests, and gastrointestinal biopsy (see this volume, p. 441). All of these procedures have significant limitations.

Intradermal skin testing detects antigen-specific IgE in the skin. Food allergies with symptoms restricted to the gastrointestinal tract or those predominantly caused by non–IgE-mediated processes

are rarely diagnosed by skin tests. The specificity of skin testing for foods has also been questioned, with some studies yielding a high incidence of false-positive results. These observations suggest that skin testing cannot be relied on to confirm food allergy or to predict which foods the patient should avoid, particularly if the predominant manifestation of the allergy is gastrointestinal.

The concentration of antigen-specific IgE in the serum can be measured by radioallergosorbent test or enzyme-linked immunosorbent assay. In humans and dogs, poor correlations between these tests and oral challenge, skin, and intragastric tests have usually been observed. This poor correlation is to be expected because an elevated serum level of antigen-specific IgE indicates only that the patient has the *potential* to manifest a reaginic response to the food antigen. A multitude of other factors determines whether the elevated level of IgE actually will produce clinical signs. Radioallergosorbent test and enzyme-linked immunosorbent assay should be regarded as screening tests for only one form of food allergy—that mediated by IgE released in sufficient quantities to enter the systemic circulation in measurable amounts. Tests to measure canine and feline reaginic antibody levels are commercially available (Bio-Medical Services, Austin, TX).

Endoscopic intragastric testing can be used to evaluate the acute response of the gastrointestinal mucosa to food antigens. Extracts of foods (0.5 ml; 1000 PNU; Greer Labs, Lenoir, N.C.) are dripped onto an area of gastric mucosa and the mucosal response is observed. In food-sensitive dogs, welts develop within minutes at the site of antigen application. The diagnostic accuracy of this technique is as yet unknown.

Gastrointestinal biopsy is rarely helpful in the confirmation of food allergy because many of the acute-phase changes, such as edema, are transient, and there are no pathognomonic histologic features that differentiate food hypersensitivity from other causes of chronic intestinal inflammation. Eosinophilic infiltration is compatible with, but not diagnostic of, food allergy.

Treatment of Food Allergy

Treatment of food allergy depends on elimination of the allergen from the diet for a minimum of 6 months, whereafter oral tolerance to the foodstuff is sometimes regained. Because most true food allergies are caused by dietary proteins, successful control of the clinical signs of animals with allergies to specific foods can often be achieved by changing to a high-quality commercial brand of pet food that does not contain the protein to which the patient is allergic. This will rarely be successful, however, in animals with food *intolerance* rather than food allergy (see later). Similarly, in patients predisposed to acquiring multiple allergies, such as atopic animals or those with chronic gastrointestinal inflammatory disorders, different commercial foods are likely to offer only transient benefit. To reduce the likelihood of clinical relapses caused by acquired hypersensitivities, predisposed animals should be placed on a "hypoallergenic" diet or, alternatively, on a rotation diet.

So-called hypoallergenic or oligoantigenic diets vary greatly in their hypoallergenicity. The least allergenic of the hypoallergenic diets available for use in dogs and cats are elemental diets. Enteral diets composed of protein hydrolysates are less antigenic than intact proteins. Homemade diets composed of single protein and carbohydrate sources may also be considered less antigenic than commercial diets containing a variety of different protein sources. Commercial hypoallergenic pet foods are the most convenient but least effective of the hypoallergenic diets because most contain intact proteins from a number of different sources and a variety of food additives.

Elemental diets such as Vivonex (Norwich Eaton, Norwich, NY) are useful for short-term use in dogs with multiple allergies. Most dogs will readily drink Vivonex. Its major drawback is expense. Enteral diets containing protein hydrolysates (e.g., Criticare HN, Mead Johnson) or purified proteins (e.g., Pulmocare, Ross Labs) are potential alternatives to Vivonex. These products need supplemental calcium and phosphorus and, for use in cats, additional protein (15 to 30 gm of casein powder per can) and taurine (250 mg per can).

Homemade hypoallergenic diets are beneficial for animals with allergies to one or more proteins or intolerances to food additives. They should be composed of a single, high-quality protein source, a gluten-free carbohydrate source such as rice (rice also contains some protein), and a vitamin and mineral supplement (avoid those labeled "palatable" or "chewable"). The use of a single protein source lowers the antigenicity of the diet. The protein should be provided in minimal quantity (approximately 2 gm/kg and 3.5 gm/kg for adult dogs and cats, respectively, unless concomitant protein-losing enteropathy is suspected). Most animal proteins are suitable for inclusion in hypoallergenic diets. The choice of protein should be based on the results of the patient's elimination-challenge trial and on practical constraints such as cost. Contrary to popular belief, there is nothing inherently "hypoallergenic" about lamb. Dogs and cats can readily acquire allergies to sheep meats if such meats form a regular part of their diet. It is important to note that because both homemade and commercial hypoallergenic diets contain intact proteins, it is not uncommon for animals with gastrointestinal inflammatory disorders to rapidly acquire sensitivities to the proteins in these diets.

Rotation diets can be used to delay or prevent the acquisition of new dietary allergies in predisposed patients. The protein sources in the diet are changed every few days on a rotating basis. It is thought that the brief period of oral exposure to each protein is insufficient to incite a clinically significant hypersensitivity response. Moreover, if acquired allergies do develop, they are easily diagnosed. The optimal duration of ingestion of each protein and the minimum interval between reingestion have not been determined.

Anti-inflammatory drug therapy can be used if the food allergen(s) cannot be eliminated from the diet. Diphenhydramine (2.0 to 4.0 mg/kg PO) or prednisone (0.5 mg/kg PO) administered before meals may temper signs of the allergy. Hyposensitization therapy has no proven benefit in food hypersensitivity. Symptomatic therapy with antiseborrheic shampoos, antibiotics, and moisturizing rinses, or with fluids and electrolytes, and motility modifiers may assist in control of dermatologic and gastrointestinal signs, respectively.

FOOD INTOLERANCES

Nonimmunologic adverse reactions to foods are collectively termed food intolerances. The majority of food sensitivities in humans are thought to be food intolerances. A similar situation may exist in dogs and cats, partly explaining the frequent failure of skin and radioallergosorbent tests to correctly identify animals suffering from food sensitivity and the poor efficacy of antihistamines and corticosteroids in its treatment. Food intolerances result in the same range of clinical signs as food allergy, but the signs may occur on the first exposure to the food, and for some categories of intolerance, large quantities of food may have to be ingested before signs develop.

Food Idiosyncrasy

A wide variety of food additives have been noted to produce adverse reactions to food in susceptible people and may also affect dogs and cats in an idiosyncratic manner. These reactions closely mimic food allergies, but with the exception of certain contact urticarias, most appear to be mediated by nonimmunologic mechanisms such as direct initiation of the arachidonic acid cascade. Identification of offending additives requires the use of elimination-challenge diets. No in vitro tests are available. A partial list of incriminated food additives commonly included in pet foods is given in Table 4. Treatment is by avoidance of the additive.

Table 4. *Partial List of Potentially Adverse Additives Commonly Added to Pet Foods and Treats*

Additive	Clinical Signs in Humans or Animals
Artificial colorings	Asthmatic attacks,* urticaria*
Butylhydroxyanisole (BHA)	Urticaria*
Carrageenan	Colitis,† urticaria*
Metabisulfite	Asthmatic attacks,* hypotension*
Monosodium glutamate	Headache,* chest pain*
Propylene glycol	Heinz body anemias‡
Sodium nitrite	Urticaria,* diarrhea*† Methemoglobinemia*
Sulfur dioxide	Asthmatic attacks,* hypotension*
Sorbic acid	Urticaria,* angioneurotic edema*
Spices	Urticaria*
Vegetable gums	Urticaria*

*Reported in humans
†Reported in laboratory animals
‡Reported in cats

Pharmacologic Reactions to Food

A variety of foods contain vasoactive amines and other pharmacologically active substances capable of inducing a wide range of signs. Histamine is a vasoactive amine present in high amounts in yeast and poorly preserved tuna and mackerel. In humans, ingestion of spoiled tuna can lead to diarrhea, nausea, urticaria, or bronchospasm. Histamine potentially could cause similar adverse reactions in cats. Psychoactive agents and stimulants are contained in some foods. Theobromine, for instance, is the major toxicant in chocolate.

Metabolic Adverse Reactions to Food

Lactase deficiency is a common metabolic defect in dogs and cats that results in diarrhea, bloating, and abdominal discomfort following ingestion of moderate amounts of lactose. Collectively, inborn errors of metabolism are important causes of metabolic adverse reactions to food in humans and also occur in animals, for example, urea cycle enzyme deficiencies (see this volume, p. 18). Treatment involves minimizing the intake of the poorly tolerated food.

Food Toxicity

Food poisoning is a frequent cause of gastrointestinal disease in small animals. Poisoning can result from foodstuffs that are inadequately prepared, spoiled, or contaminated by microorganisms or their toxins. Many foods contain natural toxicants. For example, ingestion of onions by dogs can cause Heinz body anemia probably caused by N-propyl disulfide; undercooked red kidney beans contain lectins that can cause intense epithelial inflammation, diarrhea, and abdominal pain; excessive quantities of preserved meats containing nitrates and nitrites can lead to methemoglobinemia and diarrhea; high levels of oxalates and anthraquinone glycosides contained in spinach and beets can lead to a corrosive gastroenteritis; and large quantities of spices can cause abdominal discomfort.

Gluten-Sensitive Enteropathy

Gluten-sensitive enteropathy has been described in Irish setter dogs and is characterized by poor weight gain, mild chronic intermittent diarrhea, partial villus atrophy, and brush-border enzyme defects that are particularly severe in the proximal small intestine. The cause of the gluten sensitivity is unknown. The disease may affect dogs other than Irish setters, perhaps accounting for some cases incorrectly labeled as idiopathic lymphocytic-plasmacytic enteritis. Diagnosis is made by intestinal biopsy and elimination-challenge trials with gluten-containing cereals. Treatment is by elimination of wheat, barley, rye, buckwheat, and oats from the diet. Gluten-free diets such as d/d (Hill's Pet Products) are available. Avoidance of gluten-containing diets during rearing may prevent the disease.

References and Suggested Reading

American Academy of Allergy and Immunology Committee on Adverse Reactions to Foods. National Institute of Allergy and Infectious Diseases: *Adverse Reactions to Foods.* NIH Publ. No. 84–2442, July 1984. *A review of adverse reaction to foods with emphasis on correct terminology.*

August, J. R.: Dietary hypersensitivity in dogs: Cutaneous manifestations, diagnosis, and management. Comp. Cont. Ed. Pract. Vet. 7:469, 1985. *Review of cutaneous manifestations of food sensitivity.*

Batt, R. M., and Hall, E. J.: Chronic enteropathies in the dog. J. Small Anim. Pract. 30:3, 1989. *Review of chronic enteropathies, including gluten enteropathy.*

Brostoff, J., and Challacombe, S. J.: *Food Allergy and Intolerance.* London: Bailliere Tindall, 1987. *A textbook with detailed coverage of every aspect of adverse reactions to foods.*

Kniker, W. T.: Immunologically mediated reactions to food: State of the art. Ann. Allergy 59:60, 1987. *A review of food allergy in humans.*

Strombeck, D. R., and Guilford, W. G.: *Small Animal Gastroenterology,* 2nd ed. Davis, CA: Stonegate Publishing, 1990, p. 344. *A review of adverse reactions to foods in dogs and cats.*

White, S. D.: Food hypersensitivity in 30 dogs. J.A.V.M.A. 188:695, 1986. *Description of the clinical manifestations of food sensitivities in dogs.*

DIETARY FIBER IN THE MANAGEMENT OF GASTROINTESTINAL DISEASE

DONNA S. DIMSKI

Baton Rouge, Louisiana

Dietary fiber has recently been shown to influence many functions of the gastrointestinal tract in laboratory animals, humans, and companion animals. Fiber has become popular for the treatment of many disorders in humans, although much controversy exists over its therapeutic effects. The purposes of this paper are to define *dietary fiber* and to review current recommendations for its use in gastrointestinal diseases of dogs and cats.

DEFINITION AND COMPOSITION OF FIBER

Fiber is the polysaccharide and lignin portion of the plant cell wall that is resistant to animal digestive enzymes. Dietary fiber can be classified by structure, by source, or by its physical, chemical, and physiologic properties. These properties are important in choosing an appropriate fiber source for the treatment of gastrointestinal disease. However, many natural sources contain both soluble and insoluble fiber, with variable physiologic properties.

Soluble Fiber

Soluble fiber has great water-holding capacity, forms viscous solutions in water, and is easily degraded by the gastrointestinal microflora. The sources of soluble fiber in foods include pectin, some hemicelluloses, and vegetable gums. Foods high in soluble fiber include the parenchymatous portions of fruits and vegetables, oats, oat bran, barley, citrus fruits, legumes (such as beans and lentils), and psyllium husk.

Insoluble Fiber

In contrast to soluble fiber, insoluble fiber has minimal water-holding capacity and does not form solutions. Insoluble fiber is not degraded completely by gastrointestinal microflora. The extent to which the fiber is degraded depends on the fiber type and source. Insoluble fibers are primarily found in cereal grains and seed coats. Celluloses, some hemicelluloses, and lignin are the major types of insoluble fiber. Vegetables, wheat, wheat bran, and other cereal grains are the most common sources of insoluble fiber in diets.

EFFECTS OF FIBER ON GASTROINTESTINAL FUNCTION

Fiber alters gastrointestinal function in many ways, depending on the fiber type and source. Although most studies on the physiologic effects of fiber have been performed in humans, much of the data can likely be extrapolated to small animals. The effects of dietary fiber are summarized in Table 1.

Satiety

Satiety, the feeling of fullness, is difficult to assess in animals. However, studies in humans show that diets high in soluble or insoluble fiber may increase ingestion time and stimulate centrally mediated satiety signals that occur with chewing and gastric distention (Krotkiewski, 1985). In one study, humans given high-fiber foods became full at approximately half the caloric intake of low-fiber, high-energy density foods (Duncan et al., 1983). This property of dietary fiber is used extensively in the formulation of weight-reduction diets for companion animals.

Table 1. *Physical, Chemical, and Physiologic Properties of Dietary Fiber*

Property	Soluble Fiber	Insoluble Fiber
Water-holding	Maximal	Less than soluble
Viscosity	Maximal	Less than soluble
Fermentation	Maximal	Less than soluble
Gastric emptying	Slowed	Not predictable
Intestinal transit time	Slowed	More rapid
Feces weight	Little effect	Increased

592

Gastric Emptying

Soluble fiber, with increased jelling properties, has been shown to slow gastric emptying time in humans. In contrast, insoluble fiber has a less predictable effect; tests in humans have reported more rapid to delayed gastric emptying, depending on the fiber source, amount given, and method of measurement of gastric emptying (Pilch, 1987).

Digestion and Absorption in Small Intestine

The ingestion of dietary fiber can influence intestinal motility, nutrient absorption, and mucosal morphology. Gastrointestinal transit time, a measurement of intestinal motility, accelerates significantly with the addition of insoluble fiber (cellulose) to the diet of humans and dogs (Burrows et al., 1982). The effects on transit time and myoelectrical activity in the small intestine vary with fiber type, making generalizations about the action of fiber on motility difficult.

Fiber can also inhibit absorption of nutrients from the small intestine, presumably by altering intestinal transit time, interfering with mucosal surface-nutrient contact, or increasing the thickness and viscosity of the unstirred water layer at the mucosal surface (Pilch, 1987). Fiber may also decrease the activity of some brush-border enzymes required for nutrient digestion and absorption (Stock-Damge et al., 1983). Therefore, digestion and absorption of sugars, fats, amino acids, and minerals may be decreased. Although dietary fiber may impair mineral absorption to a degree, it is unlikely that clinical effects of decreased mineral absorption would be seen in healthy adult dogs and cats.

Fiber alters the morphology and epithelial cell turnover rate of the villi of the small intestine (Pilch, 1987). Although the effects of soluble and insoluble fiber on cell turnover rate in laboratory animals have been studied, the results are variable. The effects on health of changes in villi morphology and cell turnover rate are not known.

Colonic Function and Fecal Characteristics

Insoluble fiber alters canine colonic myoelectrical activity, which is a stimulus for colonic motility (Burrows and Merritt, 1983). In addition, increased fiber in the colon promotes increased bacterial growth and fermentation of fiber, with the production of energy, gas, and short-chain fatty acids. The short-chain fatty acids acidify colonic contents and may serve as an energy source for colonocytes (Strombeck and Guilford, 1990).

Since dietary fiber is fermented to variable degrees, the impact on fecal bulking depends on fiber type. Insoluble fiber adds bulk to the feces, increasing fecal wet weight (Burrows et al., 1982). Soluble fiber is more completely fermented but adds to fecal bacterial content.

Pancreatic Function

Dietary fiber modifies the secretion of pancreatic digestive enzymes, contributing to a change in nutrient absorption. Studies in dogs have demonstrated that the addition of bran to the diet resulted in an increase in total pancreatic juice output and a decrease in pancreatic lipase production (Stock-Damge et al., 1983).

Bile Acid Metabolism

Dietary fiber will absorb bile acids within the gastrointestinal tract, which increases fecal bile acid output and decreases the amount of bile acids returned to the liver via enterohepatic circulation (Pilch, 1987). Soluble fiber and lignin increase fecal bile acid output to a greater degree than most insoluble fibers. This binding effect increases the synthesis of more primary bile acids, although the type of bile acids produced is modified (Pilch, 1987).

USES OF FIBER IN GASTROINTESTINAL DISEASE

Dietary fiber has received increased attention in both human and veterinary medicine for its uses in gastrointestinal diseases. Various sources of dietary fiber are available for small animals, ranging from specially formulated high-fiber diets to over-the-counter fiber supplements (Table 2). Although few controlled studies have been performed in small animals, many gastroenterologists believe that dietary fiber therapy may be beneficial in the treatment of some cases of diarrhea and constipation in small animals. Further research in this field may be beneficial in outlining the uses of the specific fiber types in gastrointestinal diseases of small animals.

Diarrhea

Diarrhea is a sign of underlying intestinal dysfunction and not a diagnosis. Diarrhea can result whenever there is an alteration in the normal motility or fluid movement within the gastrointestinal tract. Addition of fiber to the diet has achieved some success in treating diarrhea in both human and veterinary patients.

Fiber in the gastrointestinal tract can be of benefit

Table 2. *Sources of Dietary Fiber for the Treatment of Gastrointestinal Diseases*

Fiber Source	Fiber Type	Recommended Dose
High-fiber diets		
Prescription Diet r/d (Hill's Pet Products, Topeka, KS)	Insoluble	To meet energy requirements
Prescription Diet w/d (Hill's Pet Products, Topeka, KS)	Insoluble	To meet energy requirements
Fiber Formula (Stewart Nutritional Products, South Bend, IN)	Insoluble	To meet energy requirements
Fit-N-Trim (Ralston Purina Co., St. Louis, MO)	Insoluble	To meet energy requirements
Fiber food supplements		
Coarse wheat bran	Insoluble	1–2 tbsp daily with food
Canned pumpkin	Insoluble	1–4 tbsp daily with food
Bran cereals	Insoluble	3–5 tbsp daily with food
Oat bran	Soluble	1–2 tbsp daily with food
Fiber medical supplement		
Psyllium hydrocolloid (Metamucil, Searle Consumer Products, Chicago, IL; Vetasyl, Veterinary Prescription, Harbor City, CA)	Soluble and insoluble	1–2 tsp daily with food

in treating diarrhea for several reasons. In the colon, abnormal motility can be normalized by increased insoluble fiber (Willard, 1988). The water-holding properties of fiber contribute to a reduction in free fecal water, which may reduce diarrhea. The viscosity of soluble fiber causes an increase in intestinal transit time, allowing for greater water absorption. The organic binding properties of fiber may be useful in secretory or osmotic diarrhea by neutralizing toxins within the gastrointestinal lumen. Finally, the alteration of intestinal microflora may reduce the number of pathogenic bacteria in cases of primary bacterial diarrhea or secondary bacterial overgrowth. These effects must be contrasted to the negative effects of dietary fiber on nutrient digestion and absorption.

SMALL BOWEL DIARRHEA

Soluble fiber has been used as an adjunct therapy for small bowel diarrhea, such as in kaolin-pectin suspensions (Kaopectate, Upjohn). However, no controlled studies have proved their usefulness in treating diarrhea other than increasing the jelling properties of the feces. Since small bowel diarrhea may be complicated by maldigestion and malabsorption, the addition of fiber may impair nutrient assimilation. Therefore, the addition of soluble or insoluble dietary fiber to diets used in the management of small bowel diarrhea is not routinely recommended (Strombeck and Guilford, 1990).

LARGE BOWEL DIARRHEA

Dietary fiber therapy shows more promise in the treatment of large bowel diarrhea in small animals.

In one study, seven of eight dogs with idiopathic large bowel diarrhea resembling human irritable bowel syndrome had marked improvement in clinical signs when treated with a bland diet supplemented with psyllium (Leib, 1990). Some dogs and cats may respond to specially formulated high-fiber diets or bran supplementation of the normal diet (see this volume, p. 604).

Insoluble or soluble fiber may be useful as primary or adjunctive therapy in inflammatory colitis in dogs and cats (Willard, 1988). The addition of a dietary fiber source such as psyllium to a hypoallergenic diet may be an appropriate therapy for small animals with inflammatory colitis, since elimination diets are also used (Willard, 1988). Although fiber supplementation may be useful in dogs when combined with other therapies, some cats will respond to fiber supplementation alone (Willard, 1988). Regardless of the dietary choice, the high-fiber diet trial should be evaluated for at least 6 weeks.

Constipation

Constipation occurs when feces are retained in the colon for too long, allowing excess absorption of water from the feces. Therapy for constipation may include enemas, laxatives, and the addition of fiber to the diet. Of these therapies, the addition of fiber to the diet is recommended for long-term prophylaxis of repeated bouts of constipation. Insoluble fiber is primarily used in the prevention of recurrent constipation, either in a specially formulated diet or as a supplement. Psyllium may also be used as a dietary supplement. Canned pumpkin is a surprisingly palatable source of insoluble fiber for both dogs and cats. Provision of dietary fiber to a dehydrated, constipated patient could cause fecal impaction, so monitoring of patients receiving fiber supplementation is advised (Willard, 1988) (see this volume, p. 619).

References and Suggested Reading

Burrows, C. F., Kronfeld, D. S., Banta, C. A., et al.: Effects of fiber on digestibility and transit time in dogs. J. Nutr. 112:1726, 1982.
A study of the effects of cellulose on intestinal transit in dogs.

Burrows, C. F., and Merritt, A. M.: Influence of alpha-cellulose on myoelectric activity of the proximal canine colon. Am. J. Physiol. 245:G301, 1983.
A study of the effects of cellulose on colonic motility in dogs.

Duncan, K. H., Bacon, J. A., and Weinsier, R. L.: The effects of high and low energy density diets on satiety, energy intake and eating time of obese and nonobese subjects. Am. J. Clin. Nutr. 37:763, 1983.
A study of the effects of dietary fiber on satiety in humans.

Krotkiewski, M.: Uses of fibres in different weight reduction programs.

In Bjoerntorp, P., Vahouny, G. V., and Kritchevsky, D. (eds.): *Current Topics in Nutrition and Disease*, Vol. 14: *Dietary Fiber and Obesity*. New York: Alan R. Liss, 1985, p. 85.
A review of the uses of dietary fiber in managing human obesity.

Leib, M. S.: Fiber-responsive large bowel diarrhea. In ACVIM Proceedings, 1990, p. 817.
A study of the effects of psyllium supplementation in eight dogs with idiopathic large bowel diarrhea.

Pilch, S. M. (ed.): *Physiological Effects and Health Consequences of Dietary Fiber*. Washington: Federal Drug Administration, Center for Food Safety and Applied Nutrition, 1987, p. 28.
A comprehensive review of all studies of the effects of dietary fiber in humans.

Stock-Damge, C., Bouchet, P., Dentinger, A., et al.: Effect of dietary fiber supplementation on the secretory function of the exocrine pancreas in the dog. Am. J. Clin. Nutr. 38:843, 1983.
A study of the effect of fiber on intestinal and pancreatic function in dogs.

Strombeck, D. R., and Guilford, W. G.: *Small Animal Gastroenterology*. Davis, CA: Stonegate Publishing, 1990, p. 690.
A review of the physiologic effects of fiber on gastrointestinal function in small animals.

Willard, M. D.: Dietary therapy in large intestinal diseases. In ACVIM Proceedings, 1988, p. 713.
A review of the uses of high fiber and hypoallergenic diets in the management of large bowel diarrhea in dogs and cats.

GASTROINTESTINAL NEOPLASIA IN DOGS AND CATS

C. GUILLERMO COUTO

Columbus, Ohio

Gastrointestinal (GI) neoplasms account for approximately 2% of all canine and feline neoplasms, with malignant neoplasms being more common than benign ones; over two thirds of GI neoplasms in dogs and cats are malignant (Priester, 1980). Therefore, patients with confirmed or suspected GI neoplasms should be approached more aggressively than patients with tumors in other organ systems. In both dogs and cats, intestinal tumors are more common than gastric neoplasms; histologically, most neoplasms are adenocarcinomas, although lymphomas are quite common in both species.

Most dogs and cats with GI neoplasia are middle-aged or older (7 to 10 years old), and there is a definite sex predisposition in dogs with adenocarcinoma and lymphoma (most dogs with these tumor types are males). There is no apparent sex predisposition in cats with GI neoplasia, but Siamese cats appear to be at higher risk for the development of adenocarcinomas of the intestine.

The information presented in this article is mainly derived from two previous publications (Birchard et al., 1986; Couto et al., 1989). Given the fact that nonlymphoid neoplasms possess different clinicopathologic features, they will be discussed separately from lymphomas.

CLINICAL APPROACH TO DOGS AND CATS WITH GASTROINTESTINAL NEOPLASIA

Most dogs and cats with GI neoplasia are examined for vomiting, diarrhea, blood in the stool or vomitus, tenesmus, abdominal effusion, lethargy, weight loss, hypoproteinemia, anemia, or edema. Microcytic, hypochromic anemia is commonly seen in dogs with GI neoplasms, particularly in patients with leiomyomas and leiomyosarcomas of the intestine. In most cases the clinical signs are chronic, although in some dogs with gastric or duodenal carcinomas, the signs may be acute and may mimic GI obstruction caused by a foreign body. Occasionally, an episode of acute abdominal pain after a protracted course of GI disturbances prompts the owner to seek veterinary attention. In these cases, tumor-related GI perforation, obstruction, or intussusception should be considered likely differential diagnoses.

Physical abnormalities in dogs and cats with GI neoplasia are mainly nonspecific and include pallor, emaciation or cachexia, edema, palpable abdominal masses, abdominal effusion, hepatomegaly or splenomegaly, and evidence of diarrhea. Careful abdominal and rectal palpation are of utmost importance in detecting intra-abdominal neoplasms or enlarged lymph nodes.

Clinical evaluation of patients with suspected or confirmed GI neoplasms should also include examination of serum biochemical and hematologic parameters, urinalysis, abdominal and thoracic radiography, and, when possible, endoscopy and abdominal ultrasonography.

A cytologic or histopathologic diagnosis should be obtained before instituting chemotherapy or radiotherapy, particularly if a lymphoid neoplasm is suspected and these modalities will be the primary treatment. Lymphoid neoplasms of the GI tract are best treated with chemotherapy; in the case of solitary GI lymphomas, adjuvant chemotherapy is recommended following surgical resection. In my opinion most nonlymphoid gastrointestinal malignancies are surgical diseases (i.e., chemotherapy and radiotherapy are of little or no benefit).

GASTRIC ADENOCARCINOMAS

Gastric adenocarcinomas are rare in dogs and exceedingly rare in cats. In a series of 350 canine and 40 feline cases of GI neoplasia, gastric carcinomas/adenocarcinomas were diagnosed in 61 (17%) dogs, while no such tumors were seen in cats (Priester, 1980). Gastric carcinomas comprise 47 to 76% of all gastric malignancies in dogs and are therefore the most common gastric neoplasm. Mature male dogs are at high risk for developing gastric carcinomas, but there is no apparent breed predilection for this tumor type.

Clinical signs include protracted vomiting of food or of gastrointestinal contents (with or without blood), anorexia, weight loss, melena, and lethargy. Vomiting is the most common client complaint. Although the stomach is not easily palpated when empty, large gastric masses can occasionally be detected on abdominal palpation. Small intra-abdominal masses may represent lymphadenopathy secondary to metastatic disease.

Survey abdominal radiographs may reveal thickening of the gastric wall, absence of a normal rugal fold pattern, or intra-abdominal masses in the gastric region. Positive-contrast radiographs using oral barium sulfate may outline an intraluminal mass and reveal thickening of the gastric wall, loss or derangement of rugal folds, ulcers, filling defects, or delayed gastric emptying. Similar changes may be evident on gastroscopic examination. Ultrasonographic evaluation of the abdominal cavity may

Table 1. *World Health Organization Staging Form for Canine and Feline Nonlymphoid Gastrointestinal Neoplasms*

T:	**Primary Tumor**
T0	No evidence of tumor
T1	Tumor not invading serosa
T2	Tumor invading serosa
T3	Tumor invading neighboring structures
N:	**Regional Lymph Nodes (RLN)**
N0	No evidence of RLN involvement
N1	RLN involved
N2	Distant LN involved
M:	**Distant Metastases**
M0	No evidence of distant metastases
M1	Distant metastases detected—specify site _____

No stage grouping is at present recommended.

reveal additional masses not previously detected on physical examination, lymphadenopathy, mild abdominal effusion, or liver metastases.

The diagnosis can be confirmed by means of a biopsy, procured either by endoscopy or during an exploratory laparotomy. Over one half of gastric adenocarcinomas occur in the pyloric region; the greater curvature of the stomach is the second most common site. Exploratory laparotomy is usually indicated when therapy is contemplated because partial, subtotal, or total gastrectomy is the main therapeutic approach for patients with gastric carcinomas. Moreover, visualization of the abdominal organs provides ample information for staging of the neoplasm. For this purpose, the local lymph nodes should be carefully palpated and excised if the surgeon believes them to be abnormal. Regional lymph node metastases are common, occurring in as many as 75% of cases, while liver metastases are present in 20 to 30% of patients. Thoracic radiographs should also be included as part of the initial evaluation because up to 30% of dogs with gastric carcinoma can have visible metastatic lung lesions on initial presentation. A staging form for gastrointestinal neoplasms is presented in Table 1.

Hematologic and serum biochemical changes in dogs with gastric carcinoma are nonspecific. Normocytic-normochromic or microcytic-hypochromic anemia can occur as a consequence of "anemia of chronic disease" or chronic blood loss (iron-deficiency anemia), respectively, but are very uncommon. Neutrophilic leukocytosis secondary to tumor necrosis or to nonspecific chemotactic stimuli from the neoplastic tissue can also occur. Biochemical abnormalities vary and are usually related to the metastatic sites rather than to the primary tumor.

Surgical excision of the primary mass is the main approach to therapy. If the tumor is small and limited to the gastric wall, prolonged survival after wide surgical excision is not uncommon. The prognosis is poor when there is invasion of the serosa or of neighboring structures or metastases to the lymph nodes or other distant organs.

Table 2. Combination Chemotherapy Protocols for Dogs and Cats with Gastrointestinal Adenocarcinoma

Protocol	Dosage
*CF protocol (dogs)**	
5-Fluorouracil†	150 mg/m², IV, once/wk
Cyclophosphamide‡	50 mg/m², PO, q.o.d.
CMF protocol (dogs)	
As above +	2.5 mg/m², PO, 2 or 3 times/wk
Methotrexate§	
FAC protocol (dogs)	
Doxorubicin‖	30 mg/m², IV, on day 1 of the cycle
Cyclophosphamide	100 mg/m², IV, on day 1 of the cycle
5-Fluorouracil	150 mg/m², IV, on days 8 and 15 of the cycle
	Cycles consist of 21 days
AC protocol (cats)	
Doxorubicin	20–25 mg/m², IV, on day 1
Cyclophosphamide	200–300 mg/m², PO, day 13 *or* 14
	Cycles consist of 21 or 28 days (depending on side effects)
VAC protocol (cats)	
Vincristine¶	0.5–0.6 mg/m², IV, days 8 and 15 (and 21)
Doxorubicin	20–25 mg/m², IV, on day 1
Cyclophosphamide	200–300 mg/m², PO, day 13 *or* 14
	Cycles consist of 21 or 28 days (depending on side effects)
MA protocol (cats)	
Mitoxantrone**	3–3.5 mg/m², IV, day 1
Cyclophosphamide	200–300 mg/m², PO, day 13 *or* 14
	Cycles consist of 21 days

*Treat for 5 consecutive weeks, discontinue 1 week, and repeat. Number of cycles varies, but chlorambucil (Leukeran, Burroughs Wellcome Co.) should be substituted for cyclophosphamide if more than three cycles are used (it decreases prevalence of cyclophosphamide-induced hemorrhagic cystitis).
†5-FU, Roche Laboratories
‡Cytoxan, Mead Johnson Pharmaceutical Div.
§Methotrexate, Lederle Laboratories
‖Adriamycin, Adria Laboratories Inc.
¶Oncovin, Eli Lilly and Co.
**Novantrone, Lederle

Intraoperative radiotherapy can be used successfully in patients with neoplasms localized to the gastric wall. Combination chemotherapy, including 5-fluorouracil derivatives and mitomycin C, has improved the 5-year survival rate in humans with gastric carcinomas, although it has been of little or no benefit in dogs with this disease. I have used several drug combinations in dogs with gastric adenocarcinoma with discouraging results (i.e., no partial or complete responses documented) (Table 2). Chemotherapy for cats with intestinal adenocarcinomas has not been beneficial in our clinic.

NONLYMPHOID INTESTINAL NEOPLASMS

We retrospectively evaluated the clinical features, pathologic findings, and survival after surgery (without adjuvant chemotherapy) in 32 dogs and 14 cats with nonlymphoid intestinal neoplasia (Birchard et al., 1986). Tumors of the duodenum, jejunum, ileum, and colon were included (gastric and rectal neoplasms were excluded from this study). Tumor types in dogs included adenocarcinomas (53%), leiomyosarcomas (19%), fibrosarcomas (13%), leiomyomas (9%), undifferentiated sarcoma (3%), and benign polyp (3%); all the tumors in cats were adenocarcinomas. The anatomic location of the tumors is presented in Table 3.

The mean ages at presentation were 9.2 years for dogs (range: 1 to 14 years) and 8.7 years for cats (range: 2 to 17 years). Although no breed of dogs was overrepresented in the study, Siamese cats comprised 10 of 14 affected cats (71%), compared with a hospital population of Siamese cats of 7.8%. The male:female ratio was 1.9 for dogs and 0.55 for cats.

Weight loss was the most common presenting sign in both dogs (37.5%) and cats (93%). Fifty-eight percent of the dogs with weight loss had tumors of the jejunum, while cats with weight loss had tumors equally distributed among jejunum, ileum, and colon. Vomiting was the second most common presenting sign in dogs (28.1%). The majority of these dogs (78%) had tumors of the duodenum and jejunum. Anorexia was the second most common sign in cats (50%). The tumors in anorexic cats were equally distributed among jejunum, ileum, and colon.

Six of eight dogs (75%) with diarrhea and five of six dogs (83%) with tenesmus had colonic neoplasia. Four cats (28.6%) were presented for evaluation of diarrhea; two had ileal tumors and two had colonic tumors. One cat was presented for tenesmus and also had an ileal tumor.

During physical examination, an abdominal mass was palpable in 56% of the dogs and in 57% of the cats. The majority of the dogs had duodenal or jejunal tumors, while 50% of cats with a palpable abdominal mass had ileal tumors. Other physical examination findings in dogs were less common and included abdominal pain (12.5%) and emaciation (9.4%); dehydration was also common in cats (28%).

Plain abdominal radiography revealed an abdominal mass in 43% of the dogs and in 14% of the cats.

*Table 3. Location of Nonlymphoid Intestinal Neoplasms in 32 Dogs and 14 Cats**

Location	Dog			Cat
	Carcinomas	Sarcomas	Benign	Carcinomas
Duodenum	3	2	0	0
Jejunum	2	8	3	5
Ileum	3	1	0	5
Colon	9	0	1	4

*Reprinted with permission from Birchard, S., Couto, C. G., and Johnson, S.: Non-lymphoid intestinal neoplasia in dogs and cats. J. Am. Anim. Hosp. Assoc. 22:533, 1986.

An intestinal obstructive pattern was evident in 10% of the dogs and in 7% of the cats. Positive-contrast upper gastrointestinal studies were performed on seven dogs and eight cats; intestinal filling defects were evident in four of the dogs (57%) and three of the cats (37.5%), while an intestinal obstructive pattern was detected in six cats (75%). No evidence of metastatic pulmonary disease was detected in 30 dogs evaluated by means of plain thoracic radiography; radiographic changes compatible with lung metastases were detected in two of the 14 cats evaluated (14%). The metastatic pattern of these tumors is summarized in Table 4.

Hematologic abnormalities were nonspecific. Anemia was detected in 40% of the dogs and almost 70% of the cats from which complete blood cell counts were available for evaluation. The anemia was microcytic-hypochromic in three of the eight anemic dogs and normocytic-normochromic in the remaining five dogs and in all the cats. Leukocytosis with neutrophilia and regenerative left shift was observed in approximately 40% of the patients, while monocytosis was detected in 25% of the dogs and 15% of the cats evaluated. Serum biochemical abnormalities were also nonspecific. Investigation of the feline leukemia virus status of ten cats was accomplished by peripheral blood immunofluorescence or enzyme-linked immunosorbent assay, and all ten were found to be negative; because the test was not available at that time, the feline immunodeficiency virus status of these cats was not evaluated.

Six dogs, including those with benign tumors, were eliminated from the survival data, since they were lost to follow-up. For 12 untreated dogs, the mean survival time was 12 days (range 1 day to 2 months); eight of these dogs were euthanized. Twelve dogs had intestinal resection and anastomosis, with a mean survival time of 114 days. Dogs with sarcomas appeared to live longer postoperatively (mean = 182 days) than dogs with carcinomas (mean = 55 days), and dogs with no metastatic

Table 4. *Location of Metastases in 17 Dogs and 14 Cats with Intestinal Carcinoma**

Location	Dog	Cat
	Number (%)	*Number (%)*
Mesenteric lymph nodes	9 (53%)	5 (36%)
Liver	3 (18%)	1 (7%)
Mesentery	2 (12%)	0
Lung	0	2 (14%)
Spleen	1 (6%)	0
Kidney	1 (6%)	0
Vertebrae	1 (6%)	0
Peritoneum carcinomatosis	2 (12%)	4 (29%)

*Reprinted with permission from Birchard, S., Couto, C. G., and Johnson, S.: Non-lymphoid intestinal neoplasia in dogs and cats. J. Am. Anim. Hosp. Assoc. 22:533, 1986.

Table 5. *Chemotherapy Protocols for Dogs with Gastrointestinal Sarcomas*

ADIC protocol	
Doxorubicin	30 mg/m², IV, on day 1
Dacarbazine*	1 gm/m², IV drip (over 8 hr in 5% dextrose), on day 1
	Repeat cycle every 21 days
VAC protocol	
Vincristine	0.75 mg/m², IV, on days 8 and 15
Doxorubicin	30 mg/m², IV, on day 1
Cyclophosphamide	100–200 mg/m², IV, day 1
	Cycle is repeated every 21 days

*DTIC Dohme, Miles, Inc.

disease appeared to live longer postoperatively (mean = 135 days) than dogs with metastatic disease (mean = 79 days), although none of these data were statistically significant.

The mean survival for seven untreated cats was 3 days (range 1 to 6 days); six of these cats were euthanized. Seven cats had intestinal resection and anastomosis with a mean postoperative survival time of 7 days (range 1 to 13 days).

Diagnosis of neoplasms of the small intestine generally requires an exploratory laparotomy because these tumors are not usually accessible via endoscopy. Exploratory surgery also provides ample visualization of the primary tumor and of possible metastatic sites, allowing for surgical resection of the mass(es), if indicated. Staging is usually achieved by direct visualization of the abdominal organs as well as by evaluation of thoracic radiographs for the presence of metastatic lesions (see Table 1).

In my experience, postoperative adjuvant chemotherapy appears to be of little or no benefit in dogs and cats with intestinal adenocarcinoma. The drugs and dosages are the same as those used for gastric adenocarcinomas (see Table 2). 5-Fluorouracil is contraindicated in cats because of severe, potentially fatal neurotoxicity.

Several chemotherapy protocols have been used in our clinic for dogs and cats with GI adenocarcinomas, either following surgical resection or as primary treatment (see Table 2). Although beneficial responses were documented, they were anecdotal. Overall, no clinical benefit was seen in dogs or cats with GI carcinomas treated with chemotherapy. Also, a limited number of dogs with GI leiomyosarcomas and fibrosarcomas received ADIC chemotherapy (Table 5) in conjunction with surgery; responses were rare and of brief duration. Side effects with some of these protocols (i.e., VAC, FAC, ADIC) are common (Couto, 1990).

Radiation therapy has been used to treat rectal adenocarcinomas with encouraging results. Intraoperative radiation is used to deliver 20 to 25 Gy in a single dose to the affected area. This procedure can be followed by external-beam irradiation of the rectal area (20 to 24 Gy in 5 to 6 fractions). Side effects include transient, self-limiting proctitis and, in some cases, permanent rectal strictures secondary to tumor death and subsequent fibrosis.

LYMPHOMA

The GI tract is the most common site of extranodal lymphoma in cats and dogs. Most GI lymphomas in both species arise from the "gut-associated lymphoid tissue" and are therefore primarily of B-lymphocyte origin. Gastrointestinal lymphoma in cats and dogs will be discussed separately.

Feline Gastrointestinal Lymphoma

The prevalence of the GI form of lymphoma in cats varies in different parts of the world. In most studies, alimentary lymphomas represent the most common anatomic form, comprising approximately 20% of all GI malignancies and 15 to 40% of all lymphomas. In contrast to cats with multicentric and mediastinal lymphoma, most cats with alimentary lymphoma (70 to 80%) proved negative for feline leukemia virus on enzyme-linked immunosorbent assay or indirect immunofluorescence test. This is not surprising, since feline leukemia virus usually affects T lymphocytes, causing either their proliferation (e.g., lymphoma) or atrophy (e.g., thymic atrophy); as discussed above, GI lymphomas are primarily B-lymphocyte neoplasms.

Lymphocytic-plasmacytic gastroenteritis may constitute a prelymphomatous disorder in some dogs and cats (Couto et al., 1989; Davenport et al., 1987). Three of nine cats with lymphocytic-plasmacytic gastroenteritis diagnosed during a 1-year period subsequently developed GI lymphoma 9 to 18 months after the initial diagnosis. The initial clinical signs resolved in all nine of the cats following dietary manipulation (hypoallergenic diets) but recurred in the three cats with lymphoma. In this report, the initial diagnosis of lymphocytic-plasmacytic gastroenteritis was established by means of full-thickness gastrointestinal biopsies in all cats, thus ruling out biopsy artifact (see later). Two cats with lymphocytic-plasmacytic gastroenteritis evaluated in our clinic also developed gastric lymphoma several months after the initial diagnosis; in these two cats, the initial diagnosis was obtained by means of endoscopic biopsies.

Clinically, cats with GI lymphoma are examined for protracted and vague clinical signs, which usually progress to anorexia, vomiting, or diarrhea. Physical examination may reveal intra-abdominal masses, abdominal effusion, thickened bowel loops, or emaciation. Anemia is uncommon because the red cell aplasia seen in cats with feline leukemia virus–positive lymphoma is usually the result of a direct viral effect on the bone marrow cells, and most cats with GI lymphoma are feline leukemia virus negative.

Two main forms of presentation, solitary and diffuse (multifocal), are commonly seen. In the former, a single tumor mass is present in the GI tract; the mesenteric lymph nodes may or may not be affected. Cats with diffuse (multifocal) GI lymphoma show involvement of several segments of the alimentary tract, and the mesenteric lymph nodes are commonly affected. Some reports suggest a high frequency of renal involvement in cats with GI lymphoma.

Hematologic and serum biochemical abnormalities in cats with GI lymphoma are highly variable and nonspecific. Anemia, neutrophilic leukocytosis, lymphocytosis, and hypoproteinemia are some of the changes detected in these patients.

Radiographic changes are nonspecific, although abdominal masses or a GI obstructive pattern may be seen. Positive-contrast radiographs are of foremost importance in assessing the extent of GI involvement and in formulating a diagnostic and therapeutic plan. Solitary masses can be surgically excised, resulting in effective tumor debulking prior to chemotherapy. If diffuse GI involvement is evident on radiographic examination and if palpable intra-abdominal masses are present, a fine-needle aspiration of one of these masses usually yields sufficient material to obtain a cytologic diagnosis. Intestinal biopsies in cats with diffuse GI lymphoma should be performed with caution, since dehiscence of the suture line may occur.

Endoscopic biopsies can be obtained in cats with gastric, upper small intestinal, or colonic masses. In these instances, it is important to obtain not only mucosal but also submucosal tissue, since early GI lymphomas usually affect only the latter, without causing significant histologic changes in the mucosa.

Detailed studies of therapeutic responses in cats with GI lymphoma are scarce. In most cases, cats with several anatomic forms of lymphoma were evaluated, and the survival and remission times for the entire group were given. Cotter (1983), however, reported seven cats with GI lymphoma treated with chemotherapy. Three of these cats had solitary lymphomatous masses that were surgically excised prior to chemotherapy. Remission was induced in six of seven cats (86%), and the median duration of remission was 4.5 months (range 3 to 13+ months).

Cats with solitary GI lymphoma appear to have a better prognosis than cats with diffuse intestinal involvement. Surgical excision of solitary masses alone can result in survival times in excess of 2 to 3 months. Because diffuse GI lymphoma usually results in severe metabolic derangement (e.g., anemia, hypoproteinemia, cachexia, dehydration), these patients are often presented in poor physical condition and may thus be poor candidates for treatment.

Three cats with localized gastric lymphoma treated in our clinic with cyclophosphamide, vincristine, cytosine arabinoside, and prednisone (COAP) followed by LMP chemotherapy (see Table 6) had survival times in excess of 1 year. Thus, this anatomic form appears to have a better prognosis than other GI lymphomas.

Multiple-agent chemotherapy is recommended for cats with GI lymphoma. We currently use the COAP protocol (Table 6) with encouraging results in cats with solitary GI lymphoma; results of treatment in cats with diffuse GI involvement are discouraging. Adjuvant chemotherapy is also indicated following surgical excision of a solitary lymphomatous mass; in these instances, either the COAP or LMP protocol may be used, although subjectively, remission and survival times are longer when using the former. In every patient, treatment of the neoplasm has to be coupled with nutritional and metabolic support. Moreover, because the GI mucosal barrier is usually affected, sepsis caused by enteric organisms is not unusual.

Canine Gastrointestinal Lymphoma

Gastrointestinal lymphomas are believed to be less common in dogs than in cats, representing between 5 to 7% of all GI neoplasms and approximately 7% of all lymphomas.

Twenty dogs with GI lymphoma were diagnosed at the Veterinary Teaching Hospital of The Ohio State University between January 1970 and June 1984 (Couto et al., 1989). Based on strict criteria, 15 neoplasms were classified as primary GI lymphoma, while five dogs had multicentric lymphoma with secondary GI involvement. Age at presentation ranged from 17 months to 13 years (mean = 6.7 years). Five of the affected dogs (25%) were of mixed breeding. Breeds in which there were more than one affected dog included Scottish terrier (n = 3), poodle (n = 3), Basset hound (n = 2), boxer (n = 2), and German shepherd (n = 2). Breeds with one affected dog each included golden retriever, Doberman pinscher, and soft-coated wheaten terrier. Eighteen dogs (90%) were males (13 intact, five castrated), and two (10%) were females (both Basset hounds), compared with a hospital population of 48.8% males and 51.2% females; thus, male dogs were overrepresented. The body weight in the affected dogs ranged from 4 to 35 kg (mean = 18 kg).

Clinical signs included depression (90%), vomiting (85%), anorexia (70%), diarrhea (65%), weight loss (50%), icterus (5%), and tenesmus (5%). Vomiting and diarrhea usually occurred together; how-

Table 6. *Chemotherapy Protocols for Cats and Dogs with Gastrointestinal Lymphoma*

COAP protocol*	
Cyclophosphamide	50 mg/m² BSA, PO, 4 days/wk or every other day for 8 wk
Vincristine	0.5 mg/m² BSA, IV, once/wk, for 8 wk
Cytosine arabinoside†	100 mg/m² BSA, IV or SQ, divided b.i.d., for 4 days
Prednisone	40–50 mg/m² BSA, PO, s.i.d. for a wk; then 20–25 mg/m² BSA, PO, every other day for 7 wk
CHOP protocol (21-day cycle)	
Cyclophosphamide	100–150 mg/m² BSA, IV, day 1
Doxorubicin	30 mg/m² BSA, IV, day 1
Vincristine	0.75 mg/m² BSA, IV, days 8, 15
Prednisone	40–50 mg/m² BSA, PO, s.i.d. days 1–7; then 20–25 mg/m² BSA, PO, q.o.d., days 8–21
Sulfadiazine-trimethoprim (Tribrissen), at a dose of 13 mg/kg, PO, b.i.d. is recommended to decrease the prevalence of septic episodes secondary to neutropenia	
LMP protocol (used for maintenance after COAP or CHOP)	
Chlorambucil‡	20 mg/m² BSA, PO, every other week
Prednisone	20–25 mg/m² BSA, PO, every other day
Methotrexate§	2.5–5 mg/m² BSA, PO, twice a week

*In cats, cytosine arabinoside is used for only 2 days, and the remaining 3 drugs (cyclophosphamide, vincristine, prednisone) for 6 wk rather than 8 wk.
†Cytosar-U, Upjohn
‡Leukeran, Burroughs Wellcome
§Methotrexate, Lederle

ever, vomiting alone was noted in five dogs (25%) and diarrhea alone in one (5%). Vomiting was reported in 11 of 12 dogs (92%) with gastric involvement and in seven of 14 dogs (50%) with intestinal involvement. The vomitus or feces contained visible blood in nine dogs (45%).

The duration of clinical signs ranged from 3 days to 13 weeks (mean = 6.1 weeks), and the signs in most dogs gradually increased in frequency and severity, responding poorly to symptomatic treatment. Acute exacerbation of clinical signs in two dogs was caused by acute peritonitis resulting from perforation of tumor-associated gastric ulcers.

Physical examination was abnormal in 17 dogs (85%). Abnormalities included poor body condition (40%), presence of a midabdominal or cranial abdominal mass (25%), abdominal pain (20%), pyrexia (20%), and hepatomegaly (10%). Enlarged tonsils, splenomegaly, and diffusely thickened bowel were each noted once (5%).

Hematologic findings were abnormal in 17 dogs (85%). Six dogs (30%) were anemic (packed cell volume range, 19 to 34%; mean = 27.2%; reference range, 37 to 52%). With only one exception, all anemic dogs were also hypoproteinemic. Hypoproteinemia and anemia were seen mostly in dogs with diffuse GI lymphoma. The anemia was normochromic-normocytic in four dogs and microcytic-hypochromic in two additional dogs. Morphologic red blood cell abnormalities included target cells (25%), fragments (20%), and mild to moderate anisocytosis and polychromasia (20%).

Eight of the 20 dogs were treated. Five dogs treated with glucocorticosteroids alone or in combination with azathioprine or vincristine responded only briefly or not at all, and all but one died or were euthanized within 3 to 14 weeks of diagnosis. Multiple agent chemotherapy with cyclophosphamide, vincristine, L-asparaginase (Elspar, Merck, Sharpe & Dohme), and prednisone (CLOP protocol) was used in one dog and COAP protocol in two dogs. One of these had an objective response to therapy but was euthanized 5 weeks later because of thrombosis of the iliac arteries. One dog was lost to follow-up, and one dog with colorectal lymphoma had a survival time in excess of 5 years. Four of the dogs not treated with chemotherapy died, three of them from postoperative bowel dehiscence. One dog was lost to follow-up, and the other seven dogs were euthanized at the time of diagnosis.

Histopathologically, all the lymphomas appeared to originate in the submucosa, with six arising in the stomach (40%), seven in the small intestine (47%), and two in the large intestine (13%). Most lesions involved diffuse infiltrates of noncleaved cells in the submucosa and lamina propria. While lymphocytic-plasmacytic inflammation occurred in conjunction with tumors of both gastric and intestinal origin, it was found more frequently in association with tumors involving the intestine. Specifically, marked to severe lymphocytic-plasmacytic inflammation was present adjacent to, or occasionally distant from, the neoplastic foci in eight of 15 dogs (53%) with primary GI lymphoma and in one of five dogs (20%) with multicentric lymphoma. The junctional region between neoplastic and non-neoplastic tissue was not sharply demarcated, and often an inflamed mucosa overlaid a submucosal lymphomatous focus.

The high prevalence of extensive mucosal lymphocytic-plasmacytic inflammation suggests either that lymphocytic-plasmacytic gastroenteritis represents a prelymphomatous change in the GI tract or, alternatively, that some plasma-cell–rich areas within a heterogeneous lymphomatous infiltration may resemble lesions of lymphocytic-plasmacytic gastroenteritis. A syndrome of immunoproliferative disease of the small intestine characterized by lymphocytic-plasmacytic gastroenteritis has been described in three Basenji dogs that subsequently developed GI lymphoma (Breitschwerdt et al., 1982). The problem is highlighted by recent reports that indicate that immunohistochemical stains are the only reliable method for differentiating benign (pseudolymphomatous) GI lymphoplasmacytic infiltrations from GI lymphomas in human patients (Kahn and Mir, 1984). In some of these dogs the occurrence of neoplastic and lymphocytic-plasmacytic infiltrates in adjacent areas in the same dog supports the fact that the diagnosis of lymphoma depends on the site selected and the depth of the biopsy (i.e., exploratory laparotomies had higher diagnostic yield than endoscopic biopsies).

In addition to the information presented earlier, it is my clinical impression that dogs with GI lymphoma have shorter survival times than dogs with other anatomic forms of the disease (approximately 6 to 8 months versus 10 to 18 months) and that diffuse small intestinal lymphomas bear a worse prognosis than localized lymphomas. In our clinic we routinely use a doxorubicin-containing protocol (CHOP, see Table 6) for dogs with diffuse GI lymphoma; although we have documented some prolonged remissions, they are mostly anecdotal.

A form of GI lymphoma with a more benign biologic behavior is that of lymphomatous lesions confined to the colon and rectum. We have treated four such dogs in our clinic using COAP and LMP chemotherapy, obtaining remission in all dogs and survival times ranging from approximately 2 to 5 years. In one dog, chemotherapy was discontinued after the patient had remained in remission for 2 years, at which time the tumor recurred. Remission was reinduced with COAP chemotherapy, and the patient remained tumor-free for 3 additional years. When he died of unrelated causes, no tumor could be found at necropsy.

References and Suggested Reading

Birchard, S., Couto, C. G., and Johnson, S.: Non-lymphoid intestinal neoplasia in dogs and cats. J. Am. Anim. Hosp. Assoc. 22:533, 1986.

Breitschwerdt, E. B., Waltman, C., Hagstad, H. V., et al.: Clinical and epidemiologic characterization of a diarrheal syndrome in Basenji dogs. J.A.V.M.A. 180:914, 1982.

Cotter, S. M.: Treatment of lymphoma and leukemia with cyclophosphamide, vincristine, and prednisone: II. Treatment of cats. J. Am. Anim. Hosp. Assoc. 19:166, 1983.

Couto, C. G.: Complications of anticancer chemotherapy. Vet. Clin. North Am. 20:1037, 1990.

Couto, C. G., Rutgers, C., Sherding, R. G., et al.: Gastrointestinal lymphoma in 20 dogs: A retrospective study. J. Vet. Intern. Med. 3:73, 1989.

Davenport, D. J., Leib, M. S., and Roth, L.: Progression of lymphocytic-plasmacytic enteritis to gastrointestinal lymphosarcoma in three cats. Proc. Vet. Cancer. Soc. 7th Annual Conf. Madison, WI, 1987 (addendum).

Kahn, L. B., and Mir, R.: Lymphoid proliferations of the gastrointestinal tract. In Levin, B., and Riddell, R. H. (eds.): Frontiers in Gastrointestinal Cancer. New York: Elsevier, 1984, p. 19.

Owen, L. N. (ed.): TNM Classification of Tumors in Domestic Animals. Geneva: World Health Organization, 1980.

Priester, W. A.: The occurrence of tumors in domestic animals. Natl. Cancer Inst. Monograph 54, 1980.

CLOSTRIDIUM PERFRINGENS–
ASSOCIATED ENTEROTOXICOSIS
IN DOGS

DAVID C. TWEDT

Fort Collins, Colorado

Clostridium perfringens is an enteric, anaerobic, gram-positive rod bacterium associated with disease in humans and animals. In animals, it has most often been associated with the effects of the systemic, lethal toxins it produces. *C. perfringens* type A causes gastrointestinal distress as the result of an enterotoxin that locally affects the intestinal epithelium. Enterotoxin-producing *C. perfringens* type A is known to be one of the most common causes of food poisoning in humans and recently has been identified as a cause of gastrointestinal disease in dogs. This organism has been linked to nosocomial and acquired acute and chronic diarrhea in dogs.

C. perfringens is normally found in a vegetative form in dogs. The enterotoxin, a component of the spore coat released during the sporulation process, causes fluid accumulation in the intestines. The enterotoxin also causes intestinal damage by binding and inserting itself into the brush-border membrane of the intestinal epithelium. This results in bleb formation within the cell membrane and altered permeability to ions, amino acids and nucleotides. Membrane holes subsequently enlarge, proteins are lost, and macromolecular synthesis is inhibited. This direct damage to the intestinal epithelium causes secretion of fluid and sodium chloride into the lumen, inhibition of glucose transport, sloughing of epithelial cells, and weakening of peristalsis.

The stimulus for sporulation and enterotoxin production is unknown. The organism tends to colonize and sporulate in the alkaline environment of the distal small intestine and upper colon. It is not known whether specific enterotoxin-producing strains behave as true infectious agents in producing disease or if an alteration of the enteric environment allows the organism to increase beyond its normally small population. Nutrient changes, bacterial ecologic alteration, or intestinal epithelial damage may be responsible for initiation of disease.

The isolation of *C. perfringens* following fecal culture in humans with enterotoxicosis does not necessarily correlate with clinical disease. The presence of enteric disease correlates better with high spore counts in the feces, and more specifically with presence of the enterotoxin in the feces. Fecal *C. perfringens* enterotoxin, detected by a reverse passive agglutination test, is considered to have excellent specificity and sensitivity for the disease, as fecal enterotoxin is rarely found in asymptomatic patients.

CLINICAL FINDINGS

The following clinical information is based on experience at Colorado State University.

C. perfringens enterotoxicosis occurs in dogs of all ages and breeds and occasionally in cats. The infection may result from either an acquired nosocomial (hospital-acquired) or as a naturally occurring disease. Nosocomial disease is characterized by signs appearing during or shortly following hospitalization. The gastrointestinal signs associated with *C. perfringens* can be either acute or chronic. Chronic signs may have persisted for weeks to years in some dogs, with intermittent episodes as frequently as once every several weeks. Acute signs generally resolve within 5 to 7 days.

Most dogs with *C. perfringens* exhibit signs of large-bowel diarrhea. Fecal mucus and fresh blood, scant stools, tenesmus, and increased frequency of bowel movements are characteristic. Occasionally, dogs will have small-bowel diarrhea characterized by large volumes of a watery stool. Vomiting may occur and in a few cases sometimes is the only gastrointestinal sign observed. Flatulence, abdominal discomfort, and failure to gain weight were observed in one dog with high levels of *C. perfringens* enterotoxin in the feces. Fever or evidence of systemic involvement is uncommon. Enterotoxin has also been identified in the stools of some dogs with acute hemorrhagic gastroenteritis (HGE) syndrome, parvovirus enteritis, giardiasis, and inflammatory bowel disease. Dietary change, stress, or concurrent disease appear to be predisposing in some dogs.

DIAGNOSIS

The diagnosis of *C. perfringens* enterotoxicosis should be considered in dogs exhibiting either acute or chronic gastrointestinal signs. An animal with chronic intermittent signs should be examined during a clinical episode because there is usually no evidence of clostridial enterotoxin or spores during asymptomatic periods. Results of a complete blood count and serum biochemical tests are usually unremarkable. The definitive diagnosis is identification of *C. perfringens* enterotoxin in the feces. The assay of fecal material is relatively simple, involving a reverse passive latex agglutination test (PET-RPLA Kit, Oxoid USA, Columbia, MO). The assay was developed for use in humans but is also accurate in dogs and cats, as the enterotoxin produced by all strains of *C. perfringens* appears to be antigenically similar. A few veterinary diagnostic laboratories and many human diagnostic laboratories can perform the assay on a small (pea size) sample of stool. Because *C. perfringens* is a normal intestinal flora, positive fecal culture does not always correlate with clinical disease, but only suggests a possible etiology.

The presence of *C. perfringens* enterotoxin correlates well with fecal spore counts of > 10^6 organisms per gram of feces in humans. *C. perfringens* spores are rarely present (< 10^3 organisms per gram) in the feces of healthy dogs or dogs with diarrhea due to other causes. Fecal spores of other enteric bacteria may also on occasion be identified in low numbers in normal dogs. Fecal cytology to identify spores is a quick and simple screening test, as identification of numerous spores in dogs with clinical disease tends to correlate well with spore cultures and fecal toxin assay. A very thin smear of feces is placed on a microscope slide, air-dried or heat-fixed, stained, and examined under microscopic high-power oil immersion for spores. Most cytology stains, such as Diff-Quik or Wright's stain, are adequate. The spores are quite easy to identify, as they are larger than most bacteria and have a "safety pin" appearance. Only the remains of the vegetative cell (a dense body usually located at one end of the spore) and the spore wall will stain (Fig. 1). Spore counts of 2 to 3 or greater per each high-power oil immersion field is considered abnormal (generally > 10^6 organisms per gram of feces) and suggests *C. perfringens* enterotoxemia as an etiology.

Additional diagnostics may be required for definitive diagnosis, as some cases of *C. perfringens* enterotoxicosis develop in conjunction with other conditions. Endoscopy and colonic biopsy should be considered in workups of chronic gastrointestinal disease to exclude concurrent enteric disorders. In cases of enterotoxicosis the colon may appear hemorrhagic, hyperemic, or ulcerated and mucosal biopsies may show a catarrhal or suppurative colitis. Colon biopsies taken during an asymptomatic period are generally normal.

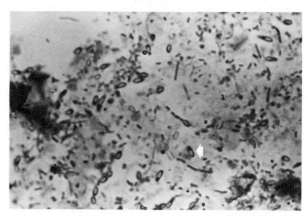

Figure 1. A Diff-Quik–stained fecal smear on high-power oil immersion showing numerous *Clostridium perfringens* spores (arrow) found in a dog positive for *Clostridium perfringens* enterotoxin.

TREATMENT

Acute *C. perfringens* gastrointestinal disease is often self-limiting. If *C. perfringens* enterotoxigenic gastroenteritis is documented, the treatment regimen should include oral antibiotics directed against *C. perfringens*. Recommended antimicrobial agents include ampicillin, amoxicillin, or metronidazole given for 7 days. Metronidazole is given at a rate of 5 to 7.5 mg/kg PO every 8 to 12 hr. Most animals will respond quickly to antibiotic therapy, and signs resolve in approximately 3 to 5 days. Occasionally, a second course of therapy may be required.

Animals exhibiting chronic intermittent signs are more difficult to treat. They frequently respond to short-term antibiotic therapy but relapse following discontinuation of treatment. Most cases with chronic intermittent signs require long-term antibiotic therapy. It appears that enteric antibiotic concentrations need not be high and that submicrobial inhibitory concentrations of antibiotics may actually function by altering the enteric microflora and preventing sporulation rather than by reducing enteric *C. perfringens* counts. Effective antibiotics include ampicillin, tetracycline, metronidazole, and tylosin. Doses of ampicillin, tetracycline, and metronidazole can often be tapered to once a day or every other day or whatever frequency of administration prevents clinical signs from reoccuring. Recent antibiotic sensitivity testing for *C. perfringens* obtained from affected dogs at Colorado State University has identified an occasional strain of the organism as being resistant to ampicillin, tetracycline, and metronidazole but none as yet that are resistant to tylosin.

Tylosin is an enteric antibiotic that has been advocated for years in the treatment of chronic diarrhea in dogs and cats. Tylosin causes minimal bacterial antibiotic resistance, does not significantly alter enteric microflora, and has no systemic toxic side effects. The previous commercial source of oral tylosin is no longer available; tylosin tartrate (Tylan Soluble, Elanco) is currently recommended. Each teaspoon supplies approximately 2.27 gm of tylosin, and the suggested dose is 10 to 20 mg/kg PO every 12 hr mixed with food. An approximate dose range is 1/16 teaspoon in dogs under 25 lb, 1/8 teaspoon for dogs around 50 lb, and ¼ teaspoon in larger dogs, given twice a day mixed with food. Dispensing such small quantities of tylosin is difficult, especially in small animals, but Tylan Soluble can be expanded with dextrose for ease of administration. Mixing 290 gm of dextrose powder with 28.6 gm of Tylan Soluble will yield approximately 300 mg of tylosin per teaspoon.

Some dogs respond to dietary modification alone. A few dogs with clinical signs of chronic intermittent large-bowel disease seem to improve when placed on high-fiber diets. It is postulated that fiber either decreases colonic pH and thus inhibits sporulation or that it alters the bacterial microflora environment, preventing *C. perfringens* proliferation and enterotoxin production.

The prognosis for dogs with acute *C. perfringens* enterotoxicosis is good. Animals with chronic intermittent signs generally require long-term or possibly lifelong therapy. If the animal has a concurrent disease, that must also be specifically treated.

PREVENTION

Infection is associated with environmental contamination. Because the organism is shed in the spore form, it is quite resistant to environmental degradation, making nosocomial infections prevalent. Careful decontamination of the environment with disinfectants effective against bacterial spores is required.

References and Suggested Reading

Harmon, S. M., and Kautter, D. A.: Evaluation of a reverse latex agglutination test kit for *Clostridium perfringens* enterotoxin. J. Food Proc. 49:523, 1986.
An evaluation of the toxin assay in determining Clostridium perfringens *enterotoxin.*
Kirth, S. A., Prescott, J. F., Welch, M. K., et al.: Nosocomial diarrhea associated with enterotoxigenic *Clostridium perfringens* infection in dogs. J.A.V.M.A. 195:331, 1989.
A clinical description of a nosocomial outbreak of Clostridium perfringens *in a veterinary teaching hospital.*
Mattson, A., Twedt, D. C., and Jones, R. L.: Community-acquired canine enteritis associated with enterotoxigenic *Clostridium perfringens* infection. J. Am. Animal Hosp. Assoc. (in press).
Clinical findings of 26 cases associated with Clostridium perfringens *enterotoxin.*
McClane, B. A., Hanna, P. C., and Wnek, A. P.: *Clostridium perfringens* enterotoxin. Microbial Pathogenesis 4:317, 1988.
A description of the pathogenesis of Clostridium *and toxin production.*
Twedt, D. C., Jones, R. L., Collins, J. K., et al.: *Clostridium perfringens* enterotoxin associated with diarrhea in dogs. ACVIM Scientific Proceedings, 1989, p. 1046.
An abstract of clinical findings in dogs with Clostridium perfringens.

IRRITABLE BOWEL SYNDROME

TODD R. TAMS
West Los Angeles, California

The irritable bowel syndrome (IBS) is a chronic disorder characterized by variable signs of gastrointestinal dysfunction or distress in the absence of underlying structural causes for the symptoms. It has also been termed spastic colon, nervous colon, spastic colitis, and mucous colitis. IBS has been well recognized in man for many years and is classified as a *functional* bowel disorder. The term *functional disorder* indicates disordered or abnormal physiologic function in the absence of pathologic lesions. IBS in humans is characterized by intermittent disturbances of intestinal function with unpredictable periods of exacerbation and remission. Sometimes bouts occur in response to nonspecific emotional stresses or other psychologic factors. Clinical experience, based on detailed patient evaluation (including negative enteroscopies and colonoscopies) and no evidence of organic disease in a number of patients with compatible signs, strongly suggests that a similar syndrome occurs in small animals, especially in dogs.

Functional bowel disorders are the most common reason for a human patient to be referred to a gastroenterologist and may affect 8 to 17% of the general population (Greenbaum et al., 1987). By definition, a patient is not diagnosed as having IBS unless recognizable organic diseases (inflammatory, infectious, parasitic, anatomic, or neoplastic) are convincingly excluded. Thorough diagnostic testing is therefore necessary before a diagnosis of IBS can be made. This article will review current recommendations regarding diagnostic evaluation of patients with suspected IBS and will describe a suggested strategy for management of IBS in dogs.

CLINICAL PRESENTATION

Humans

The most common clinical signs experienced by humans with IBS include abdominal pain, altered stools (either diarrhea or constipation, or both), excessive flatulence, urgency, and passage of mucus in the stools. Intermittent abdominal pain is sometimes the predominant symptom. The disorder is chronic, and the symptoms may vary (e.g., diarrhea and constipation sometimes alternate). The prognosis in terms of life expectancy is good. Patients with IBS often report that stress is a major factor in precipitating symptoms. Although psychiatric disorders, including anxiety and depression, were previously thought to play an important role in the syndrome, investigators who have successfully identified objective, physiologic abnormalities in IBS patients are now finding few psychiatric deviations from normal (Kellow and Phillips, 1987). This suggests that as diagnostic methods for IBS become more sophisticated and the pathophysiology is more clearly elucidated, less emphasis will be placed on psychiatric aberrations as a common cause of IBS in humans.

Animals

The clinical presentation in dogs with IBS most often involves signs of a large bowel disorder. Intermittent passage of small amounts of mucoid stool, with or without dyschezia, and increased frequency of defecation are commonly observed. Hematochezia may occur but is infrequent. There are occasional episodes of urgency to defecate, perhaps because of a sensation of incomplete evacuation. Stools may be soft but formed or watery. Unlike the situation in humans, in my experience, constipation does not commonly occur in dogs with IBS.

Often, other signs occur, with or without diarrhea, that heighten the clinician's suspicions that IBS may be present. Intermittent bloating, nausea, vomiting, and abdominal pain may also be present. There may be evidence of significant distress (e.g., reluctance to move, groaning, pacing) associated with cramping. It is emphasized that IBS is a chronic disorder characterized by an intermittent or cyclic pattern of symptoms. The clinician should evaluate the history carefully, with particular interest in determining what, if any, stressful or disruptive events occur in close association with clinical signs. Stressful factors may include being left alone for a longer period of time than the animal is accustomed to, household conflict between humans, or other environmental stimuli, such as work details for police or other performance dogs. Pecking order problems with other dogs in the immediate environment may also be a factor. While some dogs with IBS are timid and reserved or, alternatively, hyperactive, many other dogs seem to be well adjusted, and stressful factors cannot be reliably implicated as a cause. In these situations, distinct periodic aberrations in normal motility patterns (involving either small or large bowel or both) may be involved, and stress may play no role at all. Alternatively, perhaps overresponsive, "doting" owners may themselves represent a significant "stress" factor.

There is no known sex or breed predilection for IBS. I have examined a number of both large breed dogs (police, guard, seeing eye) and small to medium-size dogs in which clinical signs were consistent with IBS and in which detailed diagnostic evaluations failed to provide any positive diagnostic information for the presence of organic disease. Veterinarians are cautioned that dogs that have an acute but short-term bout of diarrhea associated with the first day or two in a boarding facility or a stressful visit to a veterinary hospital waiting room should not be automatically assumed to have IBS. These animals generally do not have any history of pre-existing gastrointestinal symptomatology, and the acute diarrhea is most likely mediated by the autonomic and enteric nervous systems (Strombeck and Guilford, 1990). The diarrhea generally resolves quickly and uneventfully in these patients. It is strongly suggested that a diagnosis of IBS be limited to patients that have undergone detailed diagnostic evaluation, lest the term be used too loosely to describe conditions with a provable cause for which the clinician has failed to investigate thoroughly.

PATHOPHYSIOLOGY

The pathophysiology of IBS has not been clearly defined. A number of explanations, including disturbed intestinal motility, dietary intolerances, disturbances in neural or neurochemical regulation, and psychologic factors, have been proposed. The most likely cause of clinical signs is deranged bowel motility. Although in many IBS patients signs of large bowel dysfunction predominate or at least are prominent in the overall symptomatology, it has been shown that abnormalities in motility in *both* the small and large bowel can occur in human IBS patients (Kellow and Phillips, 1987).

Interdigestive migrating motor complexes ("housekeeper contractions"), peristaltic waves that occur during unfed states, clear nondigestible material and bacteria from the bowel. Studies performed to characterize myoelectrical activity of the intestine have identified three different patterns: no motility (phase I), propulsive activity that is similar to peristaltic waves associated with feeding (phase II), and maximum propulsive activity of housekeeper contractions (phase III) (Strombeck and Guilford, 1990). A study at the Mayo Clinic evaluated 16 human patients with IBS and 16 age-matched controls (Kellow and Phillips, 1987). Periodicities of the interdigestive migrating motor complexes were found to be shorter in IBS patients. Diurnal cycles were much shorter in patients with diarrhea than in controls. Ileal propulsive waves and clusters of increased jejunal pressure activity were found to be more common in IBS patients. A correlation of certain motor patterns with exacerbation of clinical signs was made in some of the patients. Cramping abdominal pain was usually noted when ileal motility was propulsive (termed prolonged propagated contractions) and in some instances in conjunction with jejunal bursts. These findings implicate the distal small intestine as the site of origin of symptoms in some patients with IBS. The phenomenon of prolonged propagated contractions has also been identified in dogs, and these contractions are characteristic of peristaltic wave activity. Although detailed motility studies have not been performed in dogs with IBS, it seems reasonable to speculate that similar motility aberrations occur in both human and canine patients.

DIAGNOSIS

The diagnosis of IBS is complicated by the fact that similar clinical signs can be caused by a number of gastrointestinal disorders (i.e., functional disorders may resemble the presentation of organic disorders) potentially involving any area of the gastrointestinal tract. Since there are no histologic changes identifiable in patients with IBS, no hematologic or biochemical abnormalities, and no pathogens to identify on culture or serology, IBS is truly a *diagnosis of exclusion*.

The clinician can only be confident of a diagnosis of IBS once all other conditions have been excluded. In my experience, abnormal gastric motility, inflammatory bowel disease, and chronic idiopathic colitis are the most commonly encountered disorders that must be differentiated from IBS. As the treatment course and prognosis for these disorders can vary considerably, it is strongly recommended that patients with chronic signs be thoroughly evaluated so that the best possible therapeutic regimen can be instituted.

Since most IBS patients are presented with a history of chronic, intermittent signs *without* physical deterioration, the clinician generally has the opportunity to be selective in choosing diagnostic tests. A detailed history is extremely important as positive clues may be elucidated (e.g., characteristic cycles of clinical signs; symptoms appearing primarily in conjunction with stressful events; or intermittent bloating with attendant abdominal pain, suggesting motility aberrations). It is important that the clinician take the time necessary to gain the client's trust. Often, owners of dogs with IBS arrive prepared to give a detailed history, and any sign of indifference can be particularly damaging to the veterinarian-client relationship. Physical examination is often unrevealing. Occasionally there is evidence of abdominal pain or rectal sensitivity. Dietary intolerances and occult parasitism (especially *Giardia* and *Trichuris* infections) should be ruled out by appropriate tests and therapeutic trials.

If clinical signs are poorly responsive to initial treatments, the clinician should undertake a more detailed investigation, including a complete blood count, biochemical profile, and fecal cytology. (Increased numbers of neutrophilic leukocytes suggest inflammatory small or large bowel disease or invasive bacterial enteritis.) Since chronic *Clostridium perfringens* enterotoxemia can cause chronic signs very similar to those of IBS, tests (fecal cytology with identification of spores, fecal culture, and toxin analysis) should be done to evaluate for this pathogen (see this volume, p. 602). Abnormal cobalamin and folate assays may suggest intestinal bacterial overgrowth. Contrast radiographic studies (food mixed with barium or radiopaque markers) should be considered if a gastric motility disorder is suspected (stomach should be empty by 8 to 10 hours after a meal). Contrast studies are generally done if the patient is primarily experiencing signs referable to a gastric or gastroesophageal problem. If small and large intestinal signs predominate, I generally prefer to do gastroscopy, enteroscopy (both duodenum and ileum), and colonoscopy as the next step after blood and fecal analyses are completed. The diagnostic yield is considerably greater with endoscopy than with survey and contrast radiography.

In most IBS patients, there are no significant gross abnormalities. Occasionally, mild mucosal hyperemia, increased intraluminal mucus, increased tone and hypermotility, and spasm activity are observed. Since inflammatory diseases of the small and large intestine more commonly cause symptomatology similar to that of IBS than any other GI disorder, histologic examination of the intestine is extremely important. Intestinal biopsies are normal in IBS patients. It is emphasized that multiple (six to ten) biopsy samples should be obtained from the colon, representing various sites in the ascending, transverse, and descending colon, because idiopathic colitis is characterized in some patients by patchy rather than diffuse inflammatory cell infiltrates. The cecum should be examined as well. If only a small number of histologically normal tissue samples are examined, inflammatory disease cannot be definitively excluded.

TREATMENT

Management of IBS poses a significant challenge to both primary care veterinarians and specialists. Because symptoms and timing of episodes are so variable, response to treatment is sometimes unpredictable, and the disorder is incurable, clients can easily become frustrated with their inability to effect better control over their pets' condition. One of the most important initial steps for the veterinarian to undertake is to secure the client's confidence. Credibility is best established by thoroughly excluding organic causes and then spending time educating the client about the nature of IBS. Reassurance that no serious disease exists and that life expectancy should not be altered with IBS should be conveyed.

Next, a therapeutic strategy for control of symptoms is formulated and tailored to the predominant clinical signs of the patient. General categories of primary symptomatology include diarrhea (most common), abdominal pain, and vomiting, or a combination of these signs. Treatment generally includes either individually or in combination, dietary modification and use of fiber supplementation, antidiarrheal drugs, anticholinergics, and tranquilizers. Most patients can be managed successfully with dietary adjustments and *intermittent* pharmacotherapy.

The most commonly recommended treatment for humans with IBS in recent years has been dietary fiber supplementation (see this volume, p. 592). Potentially beneficial effects of fiber include alteration of abnormal intestinal myoelectrical activity and normalization of gut transit times. Recent well-controlled human studies, however, have failed to prove that fiber supplements are of any greater benefit than placebo in improving symptoms (Cook et al., 1990; Lucey et al., 1987). In studies that support fiber efficacy, the symptoms that most often improve include constipation and abdominal pain. Fiber supplementation has been used in canine IBS patients with variable results. In my experience, only a small number of IBS patients with chronic diarrhea experience complete resolution of clinical signs on a long-term basis when fiber supplementation is the sole therapy used. Patients whose symptom pattern includes acute, intermittent (days to weeks) flare-ups of large bowel diarrhea sometimes have fewer episodes, but clinical signs rarely abate completely. Still, it makes sense to initiate dietary trials for IBS because even a partial response may be quite beneficial. Highly digestible diets (e.g., Iams Eukanuba; Prescription Diets, i/d, d/d,

Hill's Pet Products) divided into two to three meals a day, alone or with fiber supplementation (1 to 6 teaspoons of unprocessed bran or a psyllium product, such as Metamucil or Fiberall), are recommended. Commercial high-fiber diets (e.g., Hill's w/d, r/d) can also be used. The owner is encouraged to maintain careful records regarding compliance with fiber consumption and clinical response (i.e., frequency and duration of any episodes, degree of alteration of symptoms, and so forth).

Pharmacotherapy for diarrhea-predominant IBS includes use of motility-modifying drugs such as loperamide (Imodium, Janssen) at 0.1 to 0.2 mg/kg every 8 hr, PO, or diphenoxylate (Lomotil, Searle) at 0.05 to 0.1 mg/kg every 8 to 12 hr, PO. Loperamide is a potent antidiarrheal drug that decreases intestinal secretions, enhances absorption, stimulates rhythmic segmentation contractions, and increases anal sphincter tone. There is often significant improvement in stool consistency and abatement of pain and urgency following loperamide therapy. Although loperamide can be used safely on a long-term basis, several days to 1 to 2 weeks of therapy is often sufficient to normalize stools. After the first several days of therapy, it may be possible to decrease administration to once or twice daily.

Patients with abdominal pain (cramping, bloating, assuming an arched-back stance, reluctance to move, loud abdominal gurgling sounds) or those with signs of general distress, such as pacing, are treated with combination antispasmodic-tranquilizer preparations. Chlordiazepoxide (a centrally acting sedative) and clidinium bromide (an anticholinergic agent) are combined in the capsule preparation Librax (Roche). Chlordiazepoxide is a benzodiazepine with peripheral smooth-muscle relaxant properties as well as central nervous system (CNS) effects. This combination seems to be especially effective in relieving the discomfort that may be associated with increased colonic motor function. The dose of Librax (chlordiazepoxide 5 mg and clidinium 2.5 mg) is 0.1 to 0.25 mg/kg clidinium every 8 to 12 hr, PO. The drug is generally used on a short-term basis (1 day to 2 weeks), and clients are instructed to administer it at the first sign of cramping or abdominal pain. Occasionally, long-term use is necessary (one to two doses a day). As some IBS patients are affected by unpredictable flare-ups of abdominal distress, a supply of this drug should be kept at home for immediate use. Other drugs that combine anticholinergic and CNS-depressant activity include isopropamide and prochlorperazine (Darbazine) and hyoscyamine plus phenobarbital (Donnatal, Rorer). Occasionally, anticholinergic drugs without an added tranquilizer provide effective relief. These include hyoscyamine (Levsin, Schwarz Pharma) 0.003 to 0.006 mg/kg every 8 to 12 hr, PO, dicyclomine (Bentyl, Merrell Dow) 0.15 mg/kg every 8 to 12 hr, PO, and propantheline (Pro-Banthine, Searle) 0.25 mg/kg every 8 to 12 hr, PO. My preference is to use chlordiazepoxide/clidinium initially for antispasmodic effect. If the desired response is not achieved, other preparations are tried, since their effectiveness may vary among individuals.

Certain IBS patients occasionally experience such severe distress that abdominal discomfort is accompanied by groaning, relentless pacing, nausea, and sometimes vomiting. Oral medications are either ineffective for providing prompt relief or inappropriate (vomiting patient). Injectable (preferred) or suppository medications should be administered promptly in these situations. When these signs are first recognized, the patient is best treated and monitored in a hospital setting so that response to treatment can be carefully evaluated. The drug most commonly used in our hospital is chlorpromazine (Thorazine, Smith Kline Beckman), a potent broad-spectrum antiemetic with tranquilizer effect (0.2 to 0.5 mg/kg every 6 to 24 hr, SC or IM). If there is a good response, future episodes can be treated by the client (preloaded syringes are provided for home use) at the onset of signs. Alternatively, a suppository such as prochlorperazine (Compazine, Smith Kline Beckman) can also be used. Once nausea and vomiting are under control, clidinium bromide and chlordiazepoxide are instituted.

Combination therapy may be necessary in some cases. For example, a patient with signs predominantly characterized by diarrhea and abdominal pain may respond better to loperamide and clidinium/chlordiazepoxide used concurrently. Despite any objective reason for its use, sulfasalazine (Azulfidine, Pharmacia) (22 to 30 mg/kg every 8 hr, PO), an anti-inflammatory drug useful in the treatment of colitis, sometimes provides symptomatic relief, especially when used in combination with loperamide or clidinium, for IBS patients with significant

dyschezia and increased evacuation of small volumes of loose, mucoid stool. This relief has been observed in patients in which multiple colon biopsies and careful evaluation for pathogenic intestinal organisms have proved negative. Likewise H_2 receptor blockers such as famotidine (Pepcid, Merck, Sharp & Dohme) at dosages of 0.5 to 1 mg/kg every 24 hr, PO, used in combination with clidinium or isopropamide, may provide better control of IBS-related nausea or vomiting than either drug alone.

Finally, the patient's environment should be evaluated in an effort to identify stress (i.e., antagonistic) factors, if any exist. These should be altered or alleviated whenever possible. Veterinary clinicians are reminded that being available for communication and providing support for clients whose pets are affected by the variable and unpredictable symptoms of IBS are extremely important in the overall management scheme. Some patients will be subject to intermittent lifelong disturbances of gastrointestinal function, while in others, as occurs in some humans, IBS symptoms completely abate at some point, with only rare short-term recurrences.

References and Suggested Reading

Cook, I. J., Irvine, E. J., Campbell, D., et al.: Effect of dietary fiber on symptoms and rectosigmoid motility in patients with irritable bowel syndrome. Gastroenterology 98:66, 1990.

Greenbaum, D. S., Mayle, J. E., Lawrence, M. D., et al.: Effects of despiramine on irritable bowel syndrome compared with atropine and placebo. Dig. Dis. Sci. 32:257, 1987.

Kellow, J. E., and Phillips, S. F.: Altered small bowel motility in irritable bowel syndrome is correlated with symptoms. Gastroenterology 92:1885, 1987.

Lucey, M. R., Clark, M. L., Lowndes, J. O., et al.: Is bran efficacious in irritable bowel syndrome? A double blind placebo controlled cross-over study. Gut 28:221, 1987.

Strombeck, D. R., and Guilford, W. G.: Motility disorders of the bowel. In Strombeck, D. R., and Guilford, W. G., (eds.): Small Animal Gastroenterology. Davis, CA: Stonegate Publishing, 1990, p. 442.

INTESTINAL HISTOPLASMOSIS

ROBERT G. SHERDING
and SUSAN E. JOHNSON
Columbus, Ohio

The cause of histoplasmosis, *Histoplasma capsulatum*, is a dimorphic soilborne fungus found in many temperate and subtropical regions of the world. In North America, the disease is most prevalent in the river valley regions of the central United States, especially in areas bordering the Mississippi River and its tributaries. At ambient temperature, soil enriched by decomposing nitrogenous matter (e.g., feces of birds or bats) provides an ideal growth medium for the mycelial phase of *Histoplasma*. The principal route of infection is by inhalation of airborne spores and mycelial fragments in windblown soil; however, intestinal infection from ingestion may also occur. At body temperature (37°C), *Histoplasma* organisms transform into a yeast phase that causes intracellular infection of macrophages.

Histoplasmosis primarily invades the lungs and cells of the mononuclear phagocyte system, but widespread hemolymphatic dissemination to virtually any tissue or organ system can occur. Animals less than 5 years of age are most often affected. Inapparent infections without evidence of clinical disease are common. In the dog, intestinal histoplasmosis is the most common disseminated or extrapulmonary form of the disease, while in cats intestinal involvement is relatively rare. Intestinal involvement may result from extrapulmonary dissemination or primary infection by ingestion.

CLINICAL MANIFESTATIONS

Intestinal histoplasmosis is a chronic debilitating disease that may affect the colon, small intestine, or a combination of both. Lesions are characterized by extensive granulomatous inflammation of the bowel wall, often with associated mesenteric and visceral lymphadenopathy. Intractable diarrhea and progressive weight loss are the most consistent clinical signs. The colon is most frequently affected, resulting in severe, bloody-mucoid large bowel diarrhea and tenesmus. Small bowel involvement is characterized by malabsorption syndrome with voluminous watery feces and sometimes protein-losing enteropathy. Intestinal lesions often cause thickening and ulceration of the bowel, which may result in intestinal blood loss from melena or hematochezia. Other signs may include fever, pallor, inappetence, vomiting, and lethargy. Abdominal palpation may reveal diffuse thickening of the colon or small intestine, focal tumor-like (granulomatous) thickenings in the intestinal tract or mesentery, mesenteric lymphadenopathy, or abdominal effusions. When the rectum is involved, mucosal proliferations may be detected by digital palpation of the rectum.

Additional manifestations may involve other sites of dissemination such as the liver (hepatomegaly, icterus, ascites), spleen (splenomegaly), peritoneum (omental masses, mesenteric adhesions, nodular or granular serosal surfaces), bone marrow (anemia), peripheral lymph nodes (lymphadenopathy), eyes (exudative anterior uveitis, multifocal granulomatous chorioretinitis, optic neuritis), central nervous system (ataxia, seizures), skin (fistulous tracts that drain pus or subcutaneous nodules), bone (lameness associated with proliferative or lytic bony lesions), or oral cavity (ulcers).

DIAGNOSIS

Intestinal histoplasmosis should be suspected in young animals (less than 5 years of age) with chronic intractable diarrhea that live in endemic areas. Definitive diagnosis requires identification of *Histoplasma* organisms in cytology, biopsy, or culture specimens.

Exfoliative cytology and fine-needle aspiration are generally the most practical and high-yield methods for definitive diagnosis of histoplasmosis. For animals with intestinal involvement, cytologic specimens may include smears of rectal mucosal scrapings, impression smears of endoscopic biopsies, and fine-needle aspirates of abdominal lymph nodes or intestinal masses. Endoscopic examinations of the colon and duodenum, especially colonoscopy, should be considered for the collection of diagnostic cytology or biopsy specimens. Histoplasmosis lesions appear endoscopically as areas of irregular mucosal thickening and proliferation that produce a corrugated or cobblestone appearance, with or without mucosal hemorrhage and ulceration.

In addition, *Histoplasma* organisms are also frequently found in bone marrow aspirates and buffy-coat smears of peripheral blood from dogs with disseminated histoplasmosis. Other sources of cytologic specimens with potential diagnostic benefit depend on the sites of involvement and may include effusions, peripheral lymph node aspirates, liver or spleen aspirates, skin lesion impression smears, oculocentesis, and respiratory cytologies (bronchoscopic alveolar lavage, transtracheal washing, fine-needle lung aspirate). Wright's, Giemsa's, or Diff-Quik stain (American Scientific Products, McGaw Park, IL) is ideal for identification of *Histoplasma* in cytology preparations. The organisms are found most often intracellularly within the cytoplasm of macrophages as round to oval bodies, 2 to 4 μm in size, surrounded by a characteristic clear halo, or "pseudocapsule," that results from shrinkage during staining.

Biopsies of the intestinal tract or other affected tissues reveal granulomatous inflammation, but organisms are usually sparse and difficult to see with hematoxylin-eosin stain. Detection of organisms in biopsies may be facilitated by use of special fungal stains such as periodic acid-Schiff, Grocott-Gomori methenamine-silver nitrate, or Gridley.

Any of the specimens mentioned earlier for cytologic or biopsy identification of *Histoplasma capsulatum* can also be used to culture the fungi in Sabouraud's medium; however, the organism is difficult to isolate in culture and requires 10 to 14 days for growth.

Serologic tests that detect anti-*Histoplasma* antibodies are not sufficiently reliable for definitive diagnosis; thus, every effort should be made to confirm infections through identification of the *Histoplasma* organisms. Nevertheless, a complement fixation titer of 1:16 or greater or a positive agar-gel immunodiffusion (precipitin) test is considered strongly suggestive of histoplasmosis. Unfortunately, these tests often yield false-negative results in animals with intestinal histoplasmosis. In addition, other mycotic infections (e.g., blastomycosis) may cross react on serodiagnostic tests for histoplasmosis, and anticomplementary sera may make complement fixation unusable in some animals.

The results of ancillary laboratory and radiographic evaluations in animals with intestinal histoplasmosis are variable. The hemogram may reveal normochromic-normocytic nonregenerative anemia, neutrophilic leukocytosis or neutropenia with left shift, monocytosis, and thrombocytopenia. The anemia may be attributed to a number of mechanisms, including the effects of chronic inflammation, dissemination of *Histoplasma* into the bone marrow, intestinal blood loss, and hemolysis. Thrombocytopenia is usually mild and subclinical; however, platelet counts of less than 50,000/μl are occasionally seen in association with macroplatelets in the circulation and increased megakaryocytes in the bone marrow, suggesting platelet consumption or destruction. *Histoplasma* organisms may be seen within circulating monocytes or neutrophils on routine blood smears, especially if 1000 cells are examined in differential cell counts or if buffy-coat smears are examined.

Hypoalbuminemia, with or without concomitant hyperglobulinemia, is a common serum chemistry abnormality and may be pronounced in dogs with severe protein-losing enteropathy. Serum liver enzymes may be increased in animals with hepatic dissemination. Diffuse involvement of the small intestine is likely to cause malabsorption, which can be evaluated by a xylose absorption test, fecal fat determination, or serum assays for folate and cobalamin. Results of these tests, however, are inconsistent in affected animals and not specific for histoplasmosis.

Contrast barium radiography of the upper gastrointestinal tract or colon may demonstrate irregularity of the intestinal mucosa and thickening of the bowel wall. These are nonspecific findings indicative of a diffuse infiltrative lesion. Other radiographic findings, depending on sites of dissemination, may include hepatosplenomegaly, abdominal or thoracic effusions, and lytic-proliferative bone lesions.

TREATMENT

Disseminated histoplasmosis involving the intestinal tract is generally progressive without treatment. Effective treatment regimens have included (1) an azole derivative, such as either ketoconazole (Nizoral, Janssen) or itraconazole (Janssen), as single drugs, (2) amphotericin B (Fungizone, Squibb) as a single drug, or (3) dual therapy using a combination of amphotericin B and ketoconazole. Regardless of regimen, the unpredictable response to treatment in the disseminated form of the disease should dictate a guarded prognosis.

The oral azoles, such as ketoconazole and itraconazole, are currently the first-choice antifungal drugs for single-agent treatment of histoplasmosis if the disease is not fulminating or life-threatening. The newer generation azole, itraconazole, appears to be particularly promising and should be commercially available in the near future. Preliminary results have suggested that itraconazole may be more effective than ketoconazole because it has better absorption, greater potency, quicker onset of action, longer duration of action, and less toxicity.

The major disadvantages of amphotericin B are that it must be given intravenously and it is frequently nephrotoxic. Nevertheless, amphotericin B can be combined with ketoconazole or itraconazole for the initial treatment of advanced or rapidly progressing infections because of its more rapid onset of antifungal activity and because clinical experience suggests combination antifungal therapy may be more effective than either drug alone.

Ketoconazole

The advantages of ketoconazole (Nizoral, Janssen), a synthetic imidazole, as a first-choice drug for treatment of histoplasmosis are the convenience of oral administration and the absence of nephrotoxicity. Ketoconazole inhibits the biosynthesis of ergosterol in the fungal cell membrane. Since the onset of this fungistatic effect may be delayed for 1 to 2 weeks after therapy is initiated, the clinical response to ketoconazole may be slow. Ketoconazole depends on hepatobiliary metabolism and excretion, and it is distributed widely except in the central nervous system, eye, and testes.

The usual oral dosage of ketoconazole for induction therapy in both dogs and cats has ranged from 10 to 30 mg/kg/day (in divided doses b.i.d. or t.i.d.). Dogs are usually initiated at the higher end of this range (20 to 30 mg/kg/day). Since cats are generally more susceptible to the side effects of ketoconazole, they are started at the lower end of this dosage range (10 to 20 mg/kg/day, or a total dose of 50 mg once daily); however, if tolerance is still a problem in a cat, another option is to administer a dosage of 20 mg/kg on alternate days. Acidity is required for optimal absorption of ketoconazole; thus, concurrent use of antacids or drugs such as H_2 blockers that inhibit gastric acid secretion should be avoided. There is conflicting evidence as to whether the drug is absorbed better in fasted or fed animals; however, since nausea and vomiting seem to be less of a problem if the daily dosage is divided and given with food, we recommend this approach.

Once remission is achieved, ketoconazole is continued at a maintenance dosage of at least 10 mg/kg/day for an additional 3 to 4 months. The total duration of therapy is usually at least 4 to 6 months. Since ketoconazole is a fungistatic drug, the duration of therapy is variable, and relapses have occurred up to 1 year after therapy was discontinued. If recrudescence occurs, a full course of ketoconazole is reinstituted for at least another 6 to 8 months.

For initial treatment of advanced or rapidly progressing disseminated infections, combination use of amphotericin B (see later) with ketoconazole for the first few weeks provides quicker antifungal action and may increase the remission rate. If there is central nervous system or ocular involvement, the initial daily dosage of ketoconazole may need to be 40 mg/kg to reach effective tissue concentrations, although this dosage will increase the risk of side effects.

The most common immediate side effects of ketoconazole are anorexia, vomiting, and diarrhea. Longer term side effects may include hepatotoxicity (hepatomegaly, elevated serum liver enzymes, icterus), weight loss, and haircoat changes (lightening of color, alopecia). Because of hepatic effects it is advisable to monitor serum liver enzymes monthly during treatment. The liver, GI, and haircoat reactions are usually reversible with reduction in dosage. Anorexia and vomiting can usually be minimized by dividing the daily doses and administering them with food.

Ketoconazole inhibits adrenal and testicular steroidogenesis. In dogs but not cats, ketoconazole diminishes serum testosterone and cortisol while increasing serum progesterone. Ketoconazole is also embryotoxic and teratogenic and thus should not be used in pregnant animals (see this volume, p. 349).

Itraconazole and Other Newer Azoles

Itraconazole is a newer generation azole derivative that should soon be available commercially as an oral antifungal drug. Itraconazole has successfully treated disseminated histoplasmosis in both dogs and cats at dosages of 5 mg/kg, once or twice daily. Although itraconazole may cause anorexia and hepatotoxicity, it has less liver and GI side effects than ketoconazole, especially in cats, and it does not appear to inhibit adrenal and testicular steroidogenesis. In experiments, dogs have received daily dosages of 40 mg/kg for 3 months without toxicity. An occasional side effect that has been noted in treated animals is vasculitis, which produces ulcerative skin lesions and limb edema. This adverse reaction appears to be dose dependent and reversible. As with ketoconazole, consideration should be given to combining amphotericin B with itraconazole as initial therapy in animals with rapidly progressive, life-threatening histoplasmosis.

In the future it is likely that fluconazole and other azoles currently in development or under investigation may be found to be effective for treatment of intestinal or disseminated histoplasmosis. Although documented reports of successful use of these agents in animals are lacking, these drugs generally have improved potency and a broader spectrum of antifungal activity with less toxicity. The major advantage of fluconazole over other azoles is its much better penetration of the central nervous system in fungal meningitis.

Amphotericin B

Amphotericin B (Fungizone, Squibb) is a polyene antibiotic for intravenous use that has both fungicidal and fungistatic actions. It binds to ergosterol of fungal cell membranes, thereby causing cell membrane damage and leakage of cell contents. Amphotericin B distributes well into most tissues except for the central nervous system and eye. It is metabolized locally in the tissues; thus, its elimination is not impaired if nephrotoxicity occurs.

Amphotericin B is supplied as a powder in a 50-mg vial. The powder is first reconstituted with 10 ml of sterile water that does not contain any preservatives. Since amphotericin B forms a precipitate in acidic or electrolyte solutions, only a 5% solution of dextrose in water should be used for the final dilution. The drug is also light sensitive and thus should be protected from prolonged exposure to direct light. The reconstituted product has stable potency for 1 day at room temperature and 7 days at refrigerator temperature (4°C).

In dogs, amphotericin B is administered intravenously at a dosage of 0.5 mg/kg on alternate days for 3 days a week, such as a Monday-Wednesday-Friday schedule. Because of greater sensitivity to the toxic effects of the drug in cats, a lower dosage of 0.15 to 0.25 mg/kg is used. There are two basic methods of administration: rapid and slow intravenous infusion techniques. In the rapid infusion technique, the dosage of amphotericin B is diluted in 20 to 60 ml of 5% dextrose solution and given as an intravenous injection over 3 to 5 minutes. In the slow infusion technique, the dosage is diluted in 250 to 500 ml of 5% dextrose solution and given as a constant-rate intravenous infusion over a period of 4 to 6 hours or more. The slower and more diluted drip method of delivery is preferred since this may reduce the nephrotoxicity of amphotericin B, although this is unproved.

When used in combination with ketoconazole to induce remission, amphotericin B is given for the first 3 to 4 weeks until the total cumulative dose reaches 4 to 6 mg/kg, at which time ketoconazole is continued alone for maintenance. If amphotericin B is used as a single drug, treatment should be continued for 6 to 12 weeks until a minimum total cumulative dose of 9 to 12 mg/kg is achieved or until at least 1 month beyond clinical remission. In advanced life-threatening fungal disease, either a high-dose protocol of 1.0 mg/kg every other day or an accelerated protocol of 0.5 mg/kg daily can be used. Both of these methods increase the risk of nephrotoxicity, although less so with the high-dose, alternate-day protocol.

The major side effect of amphotericin B is nephrotoxicity. Other side effects in dogs and cats include transient fever of 24 to 36 hours' duration after the first dose, anorexia, nausea/vomiting, thrombophlebitis (local irritant effect), and perivascular irritation if extravasated. Nephrotoxicity is due to a combination of reduced renal blood flow (arteriolar vasoconstriction) and direct renal tubular injury. Thus, urinalysis should be performed and renal function (serum creatinine, blood urea nitrogen) should be evaluated before initiating amphotericin B therapy, and the animal should be monitored frequently during treatment. Although there is considerable individual variation in susceptibility to nephrotoxicity, most animals treated with amphotericin B show some degree of renal dysfunction. In general, the earliest evidence of a renal effect is decreased urine specific gravity; this is followed by abnormal numbers of renal cells and casts in the urine sediment. Eventually, azotemia may develop.

If blood urea nitrogen exceeds 50 mg/dl or serum creatinine exceeds 2.5 mg/dl during therapy, treatment should be suspended until blood urea nitrogen/creatinine return to normal. Azotemia in most cases is reversible when the drug is discontinued.

Renoprotective measures aimed at enhancing renal blood flow and glomerular filtration rate have been recommended to reduce nephrotoxicity, although efficacy has not been well documented. First, hydration of the patient before treatment is an important consideration for preventing nephrotoxicity. Second, the dilution of amphotericin in 5% dextrose solution and administration by the slow intravenous infusion method over a period of 4 to 6 hours or more seem to lower the risk of nephrotoxicity. In addition, one or more of the following proposed renal-sparing treatments may be given with each amphotericin treatment: (1) concurrent administration of mannitol (0.5 to 1.0 gm/kg, IV); (2) saline loading to promote a sodium diuresis (0.9% sodium chloride solution, 50 ml/kg, IV, given over a period of 1 to 3 hours before amphotericin therapy is initiated, or it may be given concurrently using a different vein to avoid amphotericin precipitation); (3) furosemide (Lasix, 2 mg/kg, IV); or (4) aminophylline.

References and Suggested Reading

Clinkenbeard, K. D., Cowell, R. L., and Tyler, R. D.: Disseminated histoplasmosis in dogs: 12 cases (1981–1986). J.A.V.M.A. 193:1443, 1988.

Clinkenbeard, K. D., Wolf, A. M., Cowell, R. L., et al.: Canine disseminated histoplasmosis. Comp. Cont. Ed. Pract. Vet. 11:1347, 1989.

Cole, C. R., Farrell, R. L., Chamberlain, D. M., et al.: Histoplasmosis in animals. J.A.V.M.A. 122:471, 1953.

Dillon, A. R., Teer, P. A., Powers, R. D., et al.: Canine abdominal histoplasmosis: A report of four cases. J. Am. Anim. Hosp. Assoc. 18:498, 1982.

Ford, R. B.: Canine histoplasmosis. Comp. Cont. Ed. Pract. Vet. 2:637, 1980.

Grant, S. M., and Clissold, S. P.: Itraconazole. A review of its pharmacodynamic and pharmacokinetic properties, and therapeutic use in superficial and systemic mycoses. Drugs 37:310, 1989.

Graybill, J. R., and Craven, P. C.: Antifungal agents used in systemic mycoses: Activity and therapeutic use. Drugs 25:41, 1983.

Greene, C. E.: Antifungal chemotherapy. In Green, C. E. (ed.): Infectious Diseases of the Dog and Cat. Philadelphia: W. B. Saunders, 1990, pp. 649–658.

Mahaffey, E., et al.: Disseminated histoplasmosis in three cats. J. Am. Anim. Hosp. Assoc. 13:46, 1977.

Medleau, L.: Imidazoles and triazoles. In Kirk, R. W. (ed.): Current Veterinary Therapy X. Philadelphia: W. B. Saunders, 1989, p. 577.

Mitchell, M., and Stark, D. R.: Disseminated canine histoplasmosis: A clinical survey of 24 cases in Texas. Can. Vet. J. 21:95, 1980.

Moriello, K. A.: Ketoconazole: Clinical pharmacology and therapeutic recommendations. J.A.V.M.A. 188:303, 1986.

Noxon, J. O.: Systemic antifungal chemotherapy. In Kirk, R. W. (ed.): Current Veterinary Therapy X. Philadelphia: W. B. Saunders, 1989, p. 1101.

Patnaik, A. K., et al.: Canine histoplasmosis: A report of two cases. J. Am. Anim. Hosp. Assoc. 10:493, 1974.

Pyle, R. L.: Clinical pharmacology of amphotericin B. J.A.V.M.A. 179:83, 1981.

Robinson, V. B., and McVickar, D. L.: Pathology of spontaneous histoplasmosis. A study of twenty-one cases. Am. J. Vet. Res. 13:214, 1952.

Stark, D. R.: Primary gastrointestinal histoplasmosis in a cat. J. Am. Anim. Hosp. Assoc. 18:154, 1982.

Stickle, J. E., and Hribernik, T. N.: Clinicopathological observations in disseminated histoplasmosis in dogs. J. Am. Anim. Hosp. Assoc. 14:105, 1978.

Willard, M. D.: Treatment of fungal and endocrine disorders with imidazole derivatives. In Kirk, R. W. (ed.): Current Veterinary Therapy X. Philadelphia: W. B. Saunders, 1989, p. 82.

Wolf, A. M., and Belden, M. N.: Feline histoplasmosis: A literature review and retrospective review of 20 new cases. J. Am. Anim. Hosp. Assoc. 20:995, 1984.

Wolf, A. M., and Troy, G. C.: Deep mycotic diseases. In Ettinger, S. J. (ed.): Textbook of Veterinary Internal Medicine. Philadelphia: W. B. Saunders, 1989, pp. 341–372.

DISEASES OF THE RECTUM AND ANUS

KEITH P. RICHTER

Rancho Santa Fe, California

Anorectal diseases are not uncommon in small animals. The purpose of this article is to review the management of selected disorders of the rectum and anus.

NORMAL ANATOMY AND FUNCTION

The rectum represents the terminal portion of the colon, beginning at the pelvic inlet, with an indistinct boundary between the colon and rectum. The rectal wall is similar to the colon, although rectal mucosa contains more mucous cells than colonic mucosa. At the caudal aspect of the rectum, the smooth muscle (muscularis layers) forms the internal anal sphincter. Striated muscle surrounds the internal anal sphincter and forms the external anal sphincter. Dorsally, the external sphincter blends with the rectococcygeal muscle, which attaches to the coccygeal vertebrae, and thus provides an attachment of the rectum to the vertebrae.

The external anal sphincter is innervated by branches of the pudendal nerve, originating from the sacral spinal cord segments. Bilateral transection of the pudendal nerve or sacral cord lesions result in fecal incontinence, whereas unilateral transection does not result in incontinence. The internal anal sphincter is innervated by branches of the pelvic nerve, carrying afferent impulses to the sacral spinal cord. The efferent motor fibers are carried in the pudendal, hypogastric, and pelvic nerves and are autonomic in nature. Parasympathetic fibers in the pelvic nerve are motor to the rectum and colon and inhibitory to the internal anal sphincter. Sympathetic fibers in the hypogastric nerve are inhibitory to the rectum and motor to the internal anal sphincter. The normal anal sphincter maintains a zone of high pressure in the anal canal during fecal storage. The high-pressure zone decreases when the rectum is distended (the rectosphincteric reflex) and during defecation. The rectosphincteric reflex results in relaxation of the internal anal sphincter. Voluntary cortical control can inhibit the act of defecation by conscious contraction of the external anal sphincter.

Motor activity in the colon is similar to that in the small bowel, consisting of propulsive movements (peristalsis) and segmental contractions acting to delay transit. The colon possesses another type of electrical activity characterized by prolonged bursts originating in the middle of the colon and progressing in the aboral direction. This activity is responsible for rapid discharge of colonic contents during defecation. The main stimulus for motility in the large intestine is distention by intraluminal contents, causing stimulation of segmental contractions, thus limiting transit of intraluminal contents. Distention will also stimulate the mass propulsive activity, thus allowing evacuation of the colon. This explains the paradoxical beneficial effect of bulk agents with both diarrhea and constipation. With diarrhea, adding bulk to stimulate segmental contractions slows transit and allows more complete absorption. With constipation, increasing bulk will stimulate the mass propulsive activity necessary for fecal evacuation. These concepts are important to understanding proper therapeutic interventions with motility-modifying drugs.

ANORECTAL DISORDERS

Constipation/Obstipation

CLINICAL FINDINGS

Constipation can be defined as absent, infrequent, or difficult defecation, whereas obstipation results from prolonged constipation in which feces

Table 1. *Causes of Constipation in Dogs and Cats*

Obstruction
  Extraluminal
    Perirectal/perianal tumors
    Prostatomegaly
    Prostatic cyst/abscess
    Pelvic bone fractures
    Perineal hernia
    Pseudocoprostasis
  Intraluminal
    Rectal/anal stricture
      Neoplasia
      Trauma
    Rectal/anal neoplasia
    Intraluminal foreign object
    Congenital imperforate anus
Abnormal motility
  Inflammatory bowel diseases
  Lumbosacral spinal cord lesions
  Peripheral neuropathies
  Electrolyte abnormalities
  Drugs
  Idiopathic
Pain during defecation
  Proctitis
  Anal sacculitis
  Anal neoplasia
  Perianal fistula
  Pelvic trauma

become progressively harder and drier until the act of defecation becomes impossible. Clinical signs of constipation are variable. Some animals will display frequent or painful attempts to defecate with little or no fecal passage. When the condition is prolonged, there is often lethargy, anorexia, and occasionally vomiting. With certain anorectal diseases, the animal may cry in pain during the act of defecation (dyschezia). Tenesmus (straining while defecating) should not be confused with constipation, since tenesmus is commonly seen with many inflammatory diseases of the colon that result in diarrhea without constipation. When there is fecal impaction or a rectal stricture, small amounts of thin feces may be passed, giving the false impression of diarrhea. Causes of constipation are listed in Table 1.

Physical examination findings depend on the cause of constipation. Careful attention must be paid to abdominal palpation, feeling for mass or inflammatory lesions near the rectum. Occasionally, it may be difficult to distinguish a hard mass of fecal material from a mass within or outside the bowel. A digital rectal examination should also be performed, palpating for perianal masses, rectal masses, anal gland disorders, size of prostate, pelvic bone conformation, and so forth. A careful neurologic examination should assess lumbosacral nerve function. Laboratory work should be obtained to rule out metabolic problems that can cause peripheral neuropathies or electrolyte imbalances that result in constipation. A complete blood count

serum chemistry profile, urinalysis, and thyroid function tests should be obtained. Abdominal radiographs and ultrasonography (if available) should be obtained to confirm the presence of constipation and to look for mass lesions, abnormalities of the prostate, and vertebral lesions. If no other cause of constipation is identified, colonoscopy should be performed. It may be difficult to adequately evacuate fecal material from the colon to enable a complete examination. Oral lavage solutions (GoLYTELY, Braintree Laboratories) are contraindicated in colonic obstruction, and enemas may be damaging or painful. If an adequate preparation of the rectum and distal colon is possible, it can be examined for the presence of a stricture, mass, inflammatory disease, or other intraluminal abnormality.

TREATMENT

The treatment of constipation depends on the severity of the problem and the underlying cause. If the underlying cause can be corrected, management of constipation will more likely be successful. Animals with complete obstipation must have the feces manually removed. This can be accomplished with carefully administered warm water enemas in the awake state in a few animals, but it usually requires general anesthesia. Enemas and sponge forceps are used to evacuate the colon in these patients. Care must be taken to avoid colonic perforation since in some cases the wall is thin. Once the colon is completely evacuated, further management is usually necessary. Supportive care may also be necessary in severe cases, including volume expansion and correction of electrolyte abnormalities. This discussion will pertain to conditions that have no underlying cause that can be identified or treated.

When constipation is mild, simple dietary changes are often effective. These include adding fiber or other bulk agents to the diet. This can be accomplished by using high-fiber diets (Prescription Diets r/d or w/d, Hill's Pet Products) or by adding fiber or other bulk laxatives to the diet. These agents act to increase the water content of the feces and therefore increase fecal volume. Since this results in colonic distention, it will stimulate mass propulsive activity necessary for fecal evacuation. Insoluble fiber may be given in the form of wheat or oat bran, in psyllium-containing products, or as indigestible cellulose products. Examples of these products include Siblin (Parke-Davis), Metamucil (Searle Consumer Products), Konsyl (Lafayette Pharmacal), or generic equivalents. The dosage of wheat bran is approximately 1 tablespoon per 5 to 10 kg of body weight per meal. The dosage of psyllium- or cellulose-containing products is ap-

Table 2. *Causes of Fecal Incontinence in Dogs and Cats*

Neurogenic
  Spinal cord lesions
  Pudendal nerve damage
    Iatrogenic (surgery)
    Peripheral neuropathies
    Trauma
    Fight wound
  Idiopathic
Urgency
  Idiopathic inflammatory bowel disease/proctocolitis
  Bacterial proctocolitis
  Other inflammatory diseases
  Neoplasia
Anal Sphincter Trauma/Damage
  Neoplasia
  Iatrogenic (surgery)
  Fight wound
  Perianal fistula
Miscellaneous
  Behavior problem
  Overflow incontinence (obstipation, stricture, etc.)

proximately 1 teaspoon per 5 to 10 kg of body weight per meal.

In more severe cases, additional laxative therapy may be necessary. Emollient laxatives, such as docusate sodium (Colace, Mead Johnson Pharmaceuticals), are often effective when combined with bulk laxatives (50 to 200 mg every 8 hr). In refractory cases, loose feces or diarrhea can be induced with the osmotic cathartic lactulose (Duphalac, Reid-Rowell; Chronulac, Merrell Dow). This drug is a nonabsorbed disaccharide that osmotically draws water into the lumen of the bowel. In addition, it is fermented by colonic bacteria to acid end-products. The lowered colonic pH also acts to stimulate colonic motility. The dosage should be titrated to achieve loose, but not liquid, feces. A typical starting dosage is 1 ml/kg every 8 to 12 hr. Finally, the occasional use of suppositories may be helpful in stimulating the act of defecation. Glycerin pediatric suppositories or bisacodyl suppositories (an irritant that stimulates the defecation reflex) may be useful for this purpose.

Details of management of idiopathic megacolon are contained elsewhere (see this volume, p. 619).

Fecal Incontinence

ETIOLOGY

Fecal incontinence can be defined as the inability to retain feces until defecation is desired. It can be caused by a variety of conditions related to abnormal rectal and anal function (Table 2). The earlier section "Normal Anatomy and Function" will be helpful in understanding the mechanism of incontinence for the various problems listed in Table 2.

DIAGNOSTIC EVALUATION

A careful history and physical examination helps the clinician understand possible mechanisms of fecal incontinence in an individual patient. If possible, the client should attempt to distinguish abnormal urgency to defecate (which may be associated with inflammatory colorectal diseases) from uncontrollable dribbling of feces not associated with the act or posture of defecation (which may be associated with neurogenic causes or anal sphincter damage). The client should also be questioned about urination. Simultaneous fecal and urinary incontinence is highly suggestive of a neurogenic cause. In addition, the history may suggest the possible presence of systemic diseases, trauma, previous surgical procedures, and progression of the problem.

Physical examination should carefully evaluate the neurologic status of the patient. Attention should be directed to sacral spinal cord function by evaluating anal tone and the perineal (anal) reflex. In addition, a careful digital rectal examination should be performed to evaluate anal tone and to determine the presence of possible anal lesions and disorders. Laboratory evaluation should screen for causes of peripheral neuropathies (such as endocrinopathies) and other changes that may be associated with any of the disorders listed in Table 2. If a neurologic cause is suspected, special studies such as plain radiography, myelography, epidurography, cerebrospinal fluid analysis, and electrophysiologic testing of anal sphincter function should be considered. Rectoanal manometry may also be helpful in selected cases. If abnormal urgency to defecate is associated with fecal incontinence, proctoscopy or colonoscopy and mucosal biopsy may be helpful to obtain a definitive diagnosis.

TREATMENT

If a primary cause of incontinence is identified (see Table 2), the treatment is usually aimed at the underlying cause. In many cases, incontinence will resolve when the primary disease resolves. In many cases, however, the primary disease cannot be successfully treated (especially many neurogenic disorders and anal sphincter damage). In these cases, symptomatic treatment may be helpful.

Dietary therapy is often helpful in cases of fecal incontinence. To reduce the frequency of defecation and fecal volume, a low-residue, highly digestible diet is helpful. Some commercial diets are helpful (Prescription Diet i/d, Hill's Pet Products), but homemade diets are more effective. Cottage cheese or tofu and rice is a highly digestible diet for this purpose. Additional medical management should include drugs that decrease colonic transit rate.

This is best accomplished by narcotic motility-modifying drugs, such as loperamide (Imodium, Janssen) and diphenoxylate (Lomotil, Searle). These drugs act to increase rhythmic segmental contractions of the colon and thus help slow passage of feces. In addition, these drugs help to re-establish normal colonic secretion and absorption. Their combined effects will also reduce fecal volume. These drugs may also increase anal sphincter tone. Loperamide should be given at a dosage of 0.1 to 0.2 mg/kg every 8 to 12 hr. Diphenoxylate should be given at a dosage of 0.1 to 0.2 mg/kg every 8 hr.

The author has also had success in a limited number of patients with abnormal anal sphincter function using the alpha-adrenergic agonist phenylpropanolamine. This drug is much more effective in cases of urinary incontinence caused by primary urethral sphincter incompetence. Although most animals with fecal incontinence do not improve with administration of phenylpropanolamine, some animals will benefit. The dosage is 1.5 to 2.0 mg/kg every 8 to 12 hr. Side effects are minimal.

Additional treatment measures can include surgical palliation. A modified fascial sling procedure has been described in dogs. A strip of fascia lata is sutured to the muscles at the base of the tail and then brought over the base of the tail and sutured to itself (Leeds and Renegar, 1981). In addition, a polyester-impregnated silicone elastomer sling implanted in the perianal region, forming a band surrounding the anus, has also been used successfully in the dog (Dean et al., 1988). The sling was well tolerated and successfully achieved complete fecal continence in five of six dogs that underwent bilateral pudendal neurectomy. The material is relatively inexpensive, readily available, and requires a minimal amount of equipment and surgical expertise to implant. Various surgical procedures have also been described for use in humans (Guilford, 1990). Finally, regular enema administration to evacuate feces from the colon may be helpful to prevent inadvertent leakage of feces from the colon.

Proctitis

ETIOLOGY

Proctitis (inflammation of the rectum) can develop in conjunction with colitis or as an isolated entity. When proctitis occurs without concurrent colitis, there is usually no known underlying etiology. As with idiopathic inflammatory bowel disease of the large intestine, lymphocytic-plasmacytic infiltration is the most common histologic finding. Most of the evidence available suggests that immunologic factors play a major role in lymphocytic-plasmacytic inflammatory bowel disease of the large intestine. The presence of these inflammatory cells may represent a nonspecific immune response of the large intestine to a variety of antigens, including bacterial and dietary or those contained within the mucosal epithelium. If antigenic stimulation persists, the immune response continues, resulting in continued inflammation and, eventually, fibrosis. Additional evidence for immune-mediated causes is positive response to hypoallergenic diets and to immune-modulating drugs. Despite these observations, there is no direct evidence for an immune-mediated etiology, and a multifactorial etiology and pathogenesis involving bacterial, dietary, and intestinal antigens has been proposed (Richter, 1989).

CLINICAL FINDINGS

The most common signs exhibited by dogs with proctitis are tenesmus and pain during the act of defecation. Dogs may take several minutes to complete a bowel movement. Often, signs are mistaken for constipation when the fecal consistency and appearance are often normal. Occasionally, there will be fresh blood on the surface of well-formed feces, usually in the beginning of the bowel movement. When there is concurrent involvement of the colon, other signs of large bowel diarrhea will accompany those mentioned earlier.

Physical examination findings may be normal, or abnormalities may be detected during digital rectal examination. There is often irregularity of the rectal mucosa and thickened tissue with a "cobblestone" texture just inside the mucocutaneous junction. The formation of small coalescing polyps also gives the impression of marked irregular mucosa. Finally, pain and bleeding may occur during the examination.

Proctoscopy and anoscopy usually reveal thickened irregular mucosa with a cobblestone-like or granular appearance beginning at the mucocutaneous junction and extending in a cranial direction for a variable distance into the rectum. There are often superficial ulcers and erosions, with marked hyperemia and friable tissue that bleeds easily following introduction of the scope. Polyp formation can occur as a sequela to chronic inflammation and may appear as a solitary mass or as small multiple coalescing polyps, giving the surface a nodular appearance.

TREATMENT

Dietary management is often helpful in managing chronic proctitis. Since dietary antigens are the cause of the inflammatory response in some patients, a hypoallergenic diet designed to use a single protein and carbohydrate source that is highly digestible is indicated to minimize such antigens. In addition, a low-residue diet may be helpful in some animals to minimize the pain during the act of defecation. Cottage cheese and rice is an appropriate diet in most cases. Commercial diets, such as Prescription Diet dry d/d (Hill's Pet Products), are also effective. Occasionally, stool softeners are helpful, including bulk agents (bran, psyllium- or cellulose-containing products), docusate sodium, or lactulose. The reader is referred to the earlier section on constipation for details on the use of these agents.

Anti-inflammatory drugs are also helpful in managing chronic proctitis. Local administration is often effective and reduces the likelihood of systemic side effects. Corticosteroids can be given locally by rectal infusion. Steroid absorption from the rectum and colon is about half that after ingestion. The effects of a true retention enema are difficult to achieve in animals because of a lack of cooperation; nonetheless, local infusion is often very effective. Several rectal infusion products are available, including hydrocortisone acetate foam (Cortifoam, Reed & Carnrick), hydrocortisone acetate mixed with an anesthetic foam containing pramoxine (Proctofoam-HC, Reed & Carnrick), hydrocortisone retention enema (Cortenema, Reid-Rowell Laboratories), and hydrocortisone acetate suppositories (Cort-Dome, Miles Pharmaceuticals; Corticaine, Glaxo). Of these products, the author prefers Proctofoam-HC. Steroid-containing lotions and creams (Cort-Dome, Miles Pharmaceuticals; Corticaine, Glaxo; Cortaid, Upjohn) and other soothing lotions (Balneol, Reid-Rowell Laboratories) are also helpful when applied to the anus and surrounding skin for decreasing anal irritation and inflammation.

Systemic anti-inflammatory drugs may also be helpful, especially when there is concurrent involvement of the colon. The initial drug of choice is sulfasalazine (Azulfidine, Pharmacia), given at a dosage of 20 to 30 mg/kg every 8 hr. This drug is a combination of the sulfa drug sulfapyridine and the antileukotriene and antiprostaglandin 5-aminosalicylate. The 5-aminosalicylate portion is the active moiety in the colon, where it is active locally and binds to colonic connective tissue. The most common side effect of sulfasalazine therapy is keratoconjunctivitis sicca, attributed to the sulfa moiety.

Since the only purpose of the sulfa moiety is to act as a delivery system of the active drug to the colon, it would be desirable to eliminate the sulfa portion without decreasing the concentration of 5-aminosalicylic acid reaching the colon. Therefore, new products have been developed to allow delivery of the active drug to the colon without the sulfa moiety. The most effective of the newer agents for treating proctitis may be mesalamine (Rowasa, Reid-Rowell), a 5-aminosalicylic acid–containing enema. In this formulation, there is no sulfa moiety that could potentially cause systemic side effects. Rectal administration allows delivery of a high concentration of the active drug. I have found the drug to be effective and well tolerated in a dog with severe chronic proctitis. Other formulations containing 5-aminosalicylic acid have been developed to allow delivery to the large intestine after oral administration. I have successfully used Asacol (Norwich Eaton) in a dog with severe proctitis. This drug is a pH-sensitive polymer-coated 5-aminosalicylic acid. The polymer coating allows delivery of the active drug to the large intestine. Other drugs with future promise include olsalazine (Dipentum, Pharmacia) and Pentasa. Additional systemic drugs that may be effective for proctitis include metronidazole (Flagyl, Searle) and prednisone.

Rectal and Anal Tumors

INCIDENCE

Neoplasms of the large intestine represent 36 to 60% of all canine and 10 to 15% of feline alimentary tract neoplasia. The most common tumor of the rectum in the dog is the benign adenomatous polyp (Holt and Lucke, 1985). Other common tumors of the rectum of the dog include rectal carcinoma, carcinoma *in situ* within an adenomatous polyp, lymphosarcoma, leiomyosarcoma, anaplastic sarcoma, extramedullary plasmacytoma, mast cell tumor, and leiomyoma (Richter, 1989). Lymphosarcoma is the most common rectal tumor in the cat (Richter, 1989). Adenocarcinomas can be variable in appearance and behavior. They can (1) infiltrate the rectal wall, creating a fibrotic stricture, (2) cause ulceration of the mucosa, (3) proliferate within the lumen of the rectum and subsequently ulcerate, or (4) infiltrate the submucosa without causing an obstruction. All types are usually slowly progressive and do not cause symptoms until they result in a severe stricture, ulceration and frank hemorrhage, or metastasis. Most animals are more than 8 years of age; there may be an increased incidence in males; and West Highland white terriers, collies, and German shepherds may have a higher incidence than other breeds (Holt and Lucke, 1985). Survival following successful surgical removal is approximately 1 year (White and Gorman, 1987).

In addition to tumors of the colon and rectum, tumors of the pararectal tissues, including the anal sac, apocrine glands of the anal sac, and connective tissue of the rectal wall and pelvis, occur in the dog and cat. The most common tumor of the pararectal tissue is the perianal apocrine adenoma in the male dog (White and Gorman, 1987). Other pararectal tumors include perianal gland adenocarcinoma, apocrine gland carcinoma of the anal sac, and tumors derived from the skin and connective tissue around the anus. In addition, prostatic adenocarcinomas can infiltrate the pararectal and perineal areas. Apocrine gland carcinomas of the anal sac are almost exclusively seen in female dogs and are frequently associated with hypercalcemia.

CLINICAL FINDINGS

Clinical signs vary with the type and location of the neoplasm and are essentially the same as those of inflammatory and obstructive processes (see this volume, p. 595). Often the signs are slowly progressive. Most animals are in good physical condition until late in the course of disease, when there is severe mucosal ulceration, obstruction, or metastasis (White and Gorman, 1987). Adenocarcinomas usually metastasize to local lymph nodes, liver, and occasionally the lungs. Metastasis to adjacent blood vessels and lymphatics can occur, resulting in circulatory obstruction and subsequent inguinal and hind-leg edema. Many animals are asymptomatic and present with perineal swelling or a visible anal or protruding rectal mass.

Lymphosarcoma can diffusely infiltrate the colonic and rectal mucosa, remaining confined to this area of the bowel or involving other regions of the intestine and the liver. Clinical signs depend on the extent of involvement, including large bowel signs only or a mixture of large and small bowel signs. Lymphosarcoma can also appear as a discrete mass infiltrating the rectal wall. This can result in ulceration or obstruction.

Diagnostic findings in cases of anorectal neoplasia depend on the nature of the tumor. Palpation of the lesion by digital rectal or transperineal approach is often valuable in detecting rectal and pararectal tumors. Fecal examination and laboratory tests generally do not contribute to the diagnosis with the exception of the finding of hypercalcemia in cases of apocrine gland carcinoma of the anal sac. Survey abdominal radiographs may show a large intraluminal mass if it is contrasted with gas in the rectum. Fecal impaction may be seen if the lesion is causing an obstruction. Sublumbar lymph node enlargement may also be seen radiographically or ultrasonographically if metastasis has occurred. Demonstration of rectal neoplasia is best accomplished with proctoscopy and subsequent biopsy. The limitations of biopsies performed in this manner are that lesions not involving the mucosa may be missed, since only superficial samples are obtained. Biopsy instruments capable of taking deeper samples carry an increased risk of perforation. Barium enema radiography may be helpful in selected cases if proctoscopy is not available. Anal and pararectal lesions are usually easily biopsied directly with percutaneous biopsy instruments, such as a skin biopsy punch or a core-biopsy needle.

TREATMENT

The initial treatment of most rectal and pararectal tumors is surgical removal. The location and extent of the lesion determine which surgical approach is used. In general, rectal surgery carries more risk and potential complications than in other areas of the bowel. Superficial anal and perineal tumors are removed by complete surgical excision. Care must be taken to avoid transection of both pudendal nerves to avoid the development of fecal incontinence (unilateral transection does not result in fecal incontinence). For rectal tumors, local excision may be achieved in many cases by everting the rectum and performing a full-thickness mucosal or submucosal resection and simple interrupted closure. For tumors more cranial in location that cannot be exposed by simple eversion, more complicated surgical procedures will be necessary for resection. In my practice, the use of an end-to-end transanal stapling device intended for use in human beings was used successfully in three dogs with rectal tumors 10 to 12 cm from the anus. Other surgical techniques include the abdominoanal pull-through resection and the anal pull-out resection. These techniques have been described in detail (White and Gorman, 1987).

Certain neoplasms, such as lymphosarcoma and mast cell tumors may be amenable to chemotherapy. I have successfully treated two cases of undifferentiated carcinoma of the perianal area with cisplatin. Adjuvant chemotherapy may have a role following surgical removal of anorectal carcinomas to control metastasis and improve survival times. Prospective clinical trials are needed to substantiate the use of adjuvant chemotherapy in this setting. Adenocarcinomas have also been treated successfully with single high-dose radiation (Turrel and Theon, 1986). In this study, there was a complete response in six of seven dogs with rectal carcinomas, with a 67% 1-year survival rate and mean survival time of 11.3 months.

The prognosis for benign or localized slow-growing malignant tumors or carcinoma *in situ* is good if surgical removal is successful. Poorly differentiated or advanced malignant tumors have a poor prognosis because local recurrence or metastasis usually occurs.

References and Suggested Reading

Dean, P. W., O'Brien, D. P., Turk, M. A. M., et al.: Silicone elastomer sling for fecal incontinence in dogs. Vet. Surg. 17:304, 1988.
   A description of a successful surgical procedure to treat fecal incontinence in dogs.
Guilford, W. G.: Fecal incontinence in dogs and cats. Comp. Cont. Ed. Pract. Vet. 12:313, 1990.
   A review article on fecal incontinence.
Holt, P. E., and Lucke, V. M.: Rectal neoplasia in the dog: A clinicopathological review of 31 cases. Vet. Rec. 116:400, 1985.

A detailed retrospective review of 31 cases of rectal neoplasia in the dog.

Leeds, E. B., and Renegar, W. R.: A modified fascial sling for the treatment of fecal incontinence—Surgical technique. J. Am. Anim. Hosp. Assoc. 17:663, 1981.
A description of a surgical technique used successfully to correct fecal incontinence in a dog.

Richter, K. P.: Diseases of the large bowel. *In* Ettinger, S. J. (ed.): *Textbook of Veterinary Internal Medicine*, 2nd ed. Philadelphia: W. B. Saunders, 1989, p. 1397.
A detailed review of diseases of the large intestine.

Rosin, E., Walshaw, R., Mehlhaff, C., et al.: Subtotal colectomy for treatment of chronic constipation associated with idiopathic megacolon in cats: 38 cases (1979–1985). J.A.V.M.A. 193:850, 1988.
Retrospective review of 38 cats that underwent subtotal colectomy.

Sherding, R. G.: Management of constipation and dyschezia. Comp. Cont. Ed. Pract. Vet. 12:677, 1990.
A review article on constipation and dyschezia.

Turrel, J. M., and Theon, A. P.: Single high-dose irradiation for selected canine rectal carcinomas. Vet. Rad. 27:141, 1986.
A description of the successful treatment of dogs with rectal carcinomas using single high-dose irradiation.

White, R. A. S., and Gorman, N. T.: The clinical diagnosis and management of rectal and pararectal tumours in the dog. J. Small Anim. Pract. 28:87, 1987.
A detailed retrospective review of 42 dogs with rectal and pararectal tumors.

CHRONIC FELINE CONSTIPATION/OBSTIPATION

ROBERT C. DeNOVO, Jr.,
and RONALD M. BRIGHT

Knoxville, Tennessee

Constipation is a common clinical sign of many diseases in the cat. In general, constipation is characterized by tenesmus, infrequent or absent defecation, and retention of hard feces in the colon and rectum. Episodes of mild constipation are easily treated with laxatives, enemas, and dietary changes and usually cause no long-term problems. Obstipation is a much more serious condition of chronic intractable constipation in which fecal impaction becomes so severe that defecation cannot occur.

Megacolon is a disorder in which the colon becomes markedly dilated and flaccid, a condition that is usually irreversible. Acquired megacolon can occur secondary to any disorder that prevents normal defecation for prolonged periods of time, most notably mechanical obstruction or neurologic defects caused by distal spinal lesions. In the cat, megacolon most frequently occurs in the absence of an identifiable lesion and is known as idiopathic megacolon, one of the most common causes of chronic constipation and obstipation. Idiopathic megacolon is thought to be caused by primary colonic neuromuscular degeneration resulting in an irreversibly dilated and hypomotile colon. As such, medical management of idiopathic megacolon is frustrating and unrewarding; however, subtotal colectomy is proving to be a successful treatment.

PATHOPHYSIOLOGY

The colon has three major functions: absorption of electrolytes and water from fecal material, storage and delivery of feces, and maintenance of an abundant growth of microbes that contribute to the digestive process. The movements of the colon produce slow flow and adequate mixing to facilitate these functions. The primary activity in the proximal colon of the cat is retrograde peristalsis, intermittent contractions that move colonic contents into the proximal colon and cecum. These contractions churn and mix colonic contents, optimizing active absorption of electrolytes and subsequent passive diffusion of water into the mucosal cells. Entry of new matter from the ileum causes strong contractions of the proximal colon and cecum so that some contents are pushed distally. Distention of the distal transverse and descending colon stimulates phasic contractions of circular and longitudinal muscles to form a peristaltic wave. These tonic constrictions slowly move colonic contents distally. Intermittent strong contractions known as mass peristalsis move large amounts of colonic content distally, which empties the distal colon and facilitates defecation.

Any disorder that prolongs fecal transit time allows continued absorption of water, producing a drier and harder fecal mass that contributes to the development of constipation. Fecal concretions can damage the colonic mucosa, causing inflammation and increased colonic secretions. These secretions are usually insufficient to soften the fecal mass. Subsequently, intermittent episodes of watery diarrhea occur despite the constipation as liquid passes around the fecal mass. Fluid, electrolyte, and protein loss can be significant and cause rapid deterioration of condition. Recurrent constipation and obstipation disrupt the coordinated movements of the colon. Prolonged colonic emptying and chronic distention cause degeneration of colonic smooth muscle, resulting in a dilated and flaccid colon.

CAUSES OF CONSTIPATION

Constipation is a symptom of a variety of diseases and a differential diagnosis is required. Primary causes and conditions that predispose to constipation include dietary and environmental factors, mechanical obstruction, metabolic and neuromuscular diseases, anorectal pain, and the effects of some drugs.

Ingestion of foreign material, especially hair swallowed during grooming, can contribute to the formation of a hard fecal mass. Occasionally, obstipation occurs following ingestion of birds or rodents. Diets low in fiber content have been implicated but not proved as a cause of constipation in the cat.

A number of environmental and behavioral factors are known to inhibit defecation in cats. Changes in housing or daily routine (e.g., hospitalization or boarding) or the addition of a new cat to the environment may change elimination habits. Also, the stimulus to defecate is inhibited by conditions causing painful defecation or an inability to posture to defecate. This occurs most frequently in cats with pelvic or rear limb fractures or those with dislocated hips. Less commonly, inflammatory anorectal diseases may decrease the frequency of defecation and predispose to constipation.

Mechanical obstruction of defecation from intraluminal and extraluminal lesions is a common cause of constipation in the cat and usually occurs with a narrowed pelvic canal from a healed pelvic fracture. Occasionally, stenotic neoplastic or inflammatory lesions in the colon, rectum, or anus impede passage of feces. Obese, sedentary cats tend to become constipated more frequently than active, lean cats. Excessive intrapelvic fat may interfere with normal passage of feces.

Several neuromuscular diseases should be considered when evaluating the chronically constipated cat. Diseases affecting the lumbosacral spinal cord can cause constipation by interfering with colonic innervation; however, such circumstances are uncommon in the cat. Sacral spinal deformity in Manx cats can result in both constipation and fecal incontinence. Constipation is also a consistent symptom of feline dysautonomia (Key-Gaskell) syndrome, a progressive and fatal polyneuropathy of the autonomic nervous system generally seen in young adult cats.

Idiopathic megacolon is an acquired disorder primarily affecting adult male cats. Although the cause is uncertain, it is thought to result from a degenerative neuromuscular disease of the colon that eventually causes severe colonic distention, loss of motility, and intractable obstipation. Idiopathic megacolon may be caused by a functional abnormality of the rectum resulting in outlet obstruction and subsequent constipation and dilation of the colon. This circumstance might be similar to congenital aganglionic megacolon or Hirschsprung's disease in humans. Hirschsprung's disease is caused by a segmental lack of intramural ganglion cells in the enteric, nonadrenergic, noncholinergic nervous system. The smooth muscle of the aganglionic segment is persistently contracted, causing dilation of the proximal colon. Although aganglionosis of the distal colon or rectum has not been documented in cats affected with idiopathic megacolon, additional functional and morphologic studies are needed.

Dehydration and electrolyte imbalances, most notably hypokalemia, predispose to constipation by causing excessive absorption of water from the feces and diminished smooth muscle function. This is particularly true for cats that have been anorectic and debilitated for a long period. Drug-induced constipation occurs infrequently but should be considered when anticholinergics, opiates, antihistamines, diuretics, phosphate binders, or barium sulfate are used.

HISTORY AND CLINICAL SIGNS

Constipated cats are usually presented for absence of defecation. Tenesmus and frequent attempts to defecate with passage of scant or no feces are typically observed. Small amounts of diarrheal liquid, sometimes containing blood or mucus, may be passed. Systemic signs vary depending on severity, duration, and the presence of underlying disease. Anorexia, vomiting, lethargy, and weight loss are common in obstipated cats. Idiopathic megacolon tends to affect adult males more frequently and is characterized by recurrent episodes of obstipation and poor response to treatment with laxatives, fecal softeners, enemas, and high-fiber diets. Physical examination findings are usually nonspecific except for the presence of an obviously distended and firm colon. Cats with simple constipation are usually normal on physical examination.

Chronically obstipated cats are typically dehydrated, debilitated, and weak, often with a distended and painful abdomen. Cats with constipation due to dysautonomia may have other signs of autonomic nervous system failure, such as regurgitation due to megaesophagus, urinary and fecal incontinence, bradycardia, mydriasis, decreased lacrimation, and prolapse of the nictitating membrane.

DIAGNOSIS

Diagnosis is straightforward and is based on history and clinical evaluation. The primary diagnostic goal is to determine an underlying cause for the constipation/obstipation. Physical examination should include a digital rectal exam and a complete neurologic evaluation. Abdominal radiographs help determine the severity of constipation and may identify predisposing causes such as foreign material in the feces, abdominal masses, and pelvic or spinal lesions. Generalized and extreme colonic dilation without obstructing lesions usually indicates irreversible idiopathic megacolon. Endoscopy will help to identify intraluminal tumors, inflammatory lesions, and strictures. If endoscopy is unavailable, barium enema radiographs are indicated after removal of feces when an intraluminal obstruction or colonic stricture is suspected. A complete blood count, biochemical profile, and urinalysis is needed for all chronically constipated or obstipated cats to detect underlying systemic disease and direct supportive therapy.

TREATMENT

The therapeutic plan is determined by severity of disease, which ranges from simple constipation with no systemic illness to severe obstipation accompanied by debility, dehydration, and megacolon. Fluid, electrolyte, and metabolic abnormalities must be corrected initially to help restore normal intestinal motility and secretions. Methods of removal of fecal impaction depend on the severity and underlying causes of constipation, which must be corrected. Long-term management with laxatives and dietary fiber prevents reoccurrence (see this volume, p. 592). Subtotal colectomy should be considered for cats with chronic obstipation and megacolon unresponsive to medical management.

Removing the Fecal Impaction

Simple constipation is easily treated with the use of enemas or suppository laxatives to soften and lubricate the feces and stimulate defecation. Initially, 5 ml/kg body weight of a warm-water or isotonic saline enema is slowly infused; a well-lubricated rubber feeding tube attached to a large syringe facilitates a gentle and controlled infusion. Enemas given too rapidly are quickly expelled without adequate time to soften the fecal mass; rapid colonic distention also stimulates vomiting. The addition of 5 to 10 ml of an emollient laxative such as docusate sodium (Colace, Mead Johnson Pharmaceuticals) or docusate calcium (Surfak, Hoechst-Roussel) or a mild soap such as povidone iodine soap (1 ml per 10 ml of enema) will help soften dry feces and stimulate colonic secretions. Rectal infusion of lubricants is helpful if large fecal concretions are present. Sterile lubricant jelly mixed with equal parts of warm water is particularly effective; mineral oil can be used as an alternative. Suppositories can be given by the owner as needed to treat mild constipation. Bisacodyl (Dulcolax, Boehringer Ingelheim) and docusate suppositories are more effective than glycerine preparations; if the response to one or two pediatric suppositories given 6 hr apart is inadequate, enemas must be given.

Several precautions must be observed when choosing enema solutions for cats. Soaps containing hexachlorophene will cause neurotoxicity if absorbed. Sodium phosphate enemas are contraindicated in cats because they can cause life-threatening hypernatremia, hyperosmolality, hyperphosphatemia, and hypocalcemia (see this volume, p. 376). Additionally, since docusate promotes mucosal absorption of mineral oil, these two agents should not be mixed.

Relief of obstruction in the severely obstipated cat often requires manual removal of the fecal mass in combination with liberal colonic irrigation. After fluid and electrolyte balance have been restored, the cat should be anesthetized using an endotracheal tube to prevent aspiration should colonic manipulation induce vomiting. Warm saline enemas should be infused into the colon and the fecal mass gently compressed by abdominal palpation. As the mass loosens, it can be gently milked into the rectum and removed digitally or with the use of sponge forceps. Patience and caution are essential as the colonic wall in obstipated patients is susceptible to trauma and perforation. In some instances it is advisable to remove the impaction with repeated enemas and manual extraction over a period of several days providing the patient can tolerate repeated procedures. Infrequently, colotomy is necessary when more conservative efforts have failed to remove the impaction or foreign bodies.

Laxatives

Most laxatives work by promoting some of the mechanisms involved in the pathogenesis of diarrhea, specifically decreased water and electrolyte absorption, increased electrolyte and fluid secretion, increased intraluminal osmolarity, and stimulation of motility. Laxatives are classified as (1) lubricant, (2) emollient, (3) osmotic, (4) stimulant, and (5) bulk-forming (Table 1).

LUBRICANTS

Mineral oil and petrolatum products are the major lubricant laxatives and can be given orally or rectally. Lubricants allow easier passage of coated feces and soften the fecal mass by decreasing colonic reabsorption of fecal water. Lubricants are the pri-

Table 1. Selected Laxative Treatments for Constipation/Obstipation in Cats

Laxative Treatment*	Commercial Product (Manufacturer)	Route	Suggested Daily Dosage
Lubricant Laxatives†			
Mineral oil‡	(Many)	Oral	10–25 ml (flavored
		Rectal (enema)	1–2 ml/kg
White petrolatum	Laxatone (Evsco)	Oral	1–5 ml
Sterile lubricant jelly	(Many)	Rectal (enema)	5–10 ml mixed with warm water
Emollient Laxatives‡			
Docusate sodium	Colace (Mead Johnson Pharmaceuticals)	Oral	1 50-mg capsule
		Rectal (suppository)	1 pediatric suppository q 6 hr; discontinue if no response following second dose
		Rectal (enema)	10–30 ml alone or added to warm water enema
Docusate calcium	Surfak (Hoechst-Roussel)	Oral	1–2 50-mg tabs
		Rectal (enema)	10–30 ml alone or added to warm water enema
Osmotic Laxatives			
Lactose	Milk		Add to diet to effect
Lactulose	Duphalac Syrup (Reid-Rowell)	Oral	0.5 ml/kg q 8 hr initially; adjust dosage as needed to produce soft stool
	Cephulac (Merrell Dow)	Oral	As above
Glycerin	(Many)	Rectal (suppository)	1–2 pediatric suppositories
Polyethylene glycol-electrolyte solutions§	Colyte (Reed & Carnrick)	Oral (stomach tube)	25 ml/kg; repeat in 2–4 hr
	GoLYTELY (Braintree Laboratories)	Oral (stomach tube)	As above
Stimulant Laxatives			
Bisacodyl	Dulcolax (Boehringer Ingelheim Pharmaceuticals)	Oral	1 5-mg tab
		Rectal (suppository)	1–3 pediatric suppositories
	Fleet Bisacodyl Enema (C.B. Fleet)	Rectal (enema)	1 ml/kg
Castor oil§	Emulsoil (Paddock Laboratories)	Oral	5–10 ml
Bulk-Forming Laxatives			
Psyllium	Metamucil (Procter & Gamble)	Oral	1–2 tsp. mixed with moist food
Canned pumpkin	Pie filling	Oral	1–2 tsp. mixed with moist food

*Cat should be hydrated prior to use of laxatives and enemas. Provide fresh drinking water, clean litter pan, and quiet environment. Enema fluid dosage = 5–10 ml/kg warm water or saline.

†Treat between meals with long-term use to avoid malabsorption of fat-soluble vitamins.

‡Do not give mineral oil concurrently with emollients.

§Primarily used to prepare bowel for endoscopy/radiology; contraindicated if animal is obstructed/obstipated.

mary ingredients in many commercial veterinary laxatives and are most useful as hairball treatment or as an aid to relieve minor constipation. Because mineral oil is tasteless and can easily be aspirated, its use is preferably limited to rectal administration. Mineral oil and docusates should not be used concurrently. Mineral oil interferes with the emollient effects of docusates and docusates enhance mucosal absorption of mineral oil, potentially causing lymphatic foreign-body reaction. Chronic use of oral lubricant laxatives can reduce absorption of fat-soluble vitamins; treatment between meals will reduce this effect.

EMOLLIENTS

Emollient laxatives are surfactants that facilitate the mixture of water and fat-soluble material to soften the fecal mass. They also stimulate secretion of fluid into the bowel. These mild laxatives are available in oral and enema preparations and are recommended for the treatment of constipation with hard, dry feces. Patients should be adequately hydrated prior to the use of emollients because they increase intestinal fluid loss. Oral preparations may require 24 to 72 hr to take effect. Because emollients may promote intestinal absorption of other agents, these products should not be given concurrently with other oral drugs.

OSMOTICS

Osmotic retention of water in the bowel maintains fecal hydration and subsequently stimulates intestinal motility by increasing intraluminal pressure. Unabsorbed carbohydrates such as lactose (milk) or lactulose (Cephulac, Merrell Dow; Duphalac, Reid-Rowell) are effective osmotic laxatives especially useful for long-term management of recurrent constipation in cats. Milk has a mild laxative effect in some cats if consumed in amounts sufficient to exceed the digestive capacity of intestinal lactase. Lactulose is a more effective alternative. In addition to its osmotic effects, lactulose is metabolized by colonic bacteria to lactic acid and other organic ions that lower colonic pH, which subsequently increases colonic peristalsis. Lactulose consistently produces a soft stool when given at a dose of 0.5 ml/kg body weight every 8 to 12 hr. Flatulence and watery diarrhea will occur in some cats but is easily corrected by decreasing the dosage until a soft stool is produced. This drug is an especially effective adjunct to dietary management for the treatment of recurrent constipation in cats. It is readily consumed when mixed with food and long-term use is without adverse effect.

Many over-the-counter drugs have magnesium hydroxide (Phillips' Milk of Magnesia, Glenbrook Laboratories) as an osmotic agent. Poor patient acceptance limits their practical use. Additionally, magnesium products are contraindicated for use in renal failure. Oral polyethylene glycol-electrolyte solutions (Colyte, Reed & Carnrick; GoLYTELY, Braintree Laboratories) are effective osmotic cathartics for bowel preparation for endoscopy. They are not intended for use as laxatives and are specifically contraindicated if bowel obstruction is suspected.

STIMULANTS

Several types of stimulant laxatives are available that increase the propulsive contractions of the colon. Bisacodyl stimulates the nerve plexus of the colon, causing contractions of the entire colon and decreasing water absorption in the small and large intestine. Short-term use of this drug is well-tolerated in the cat and is a useful adjunct to enemas for the treatment of mild to moderate constipation. Castor oil, another stimulant laxative, is metabolized to ricinoleic acid, which stimulates intestinal fluid secretion and motility and decreases intestinal glucose absorption. Poor patient acceptance tends to limit this effective laxative to in-hospital use. In general, stimulant laxatives should be avoided in the presence of severe obstipation or obstructive lesions.

BULK FORMERS

Dietary modification with high-fiber diets is the mainstay of long-term control of constipation. Fiber therapy is more physiologic, better tolerated, and more effective than long-term use of other laxatives. Adding fiber to the diet increases fecal bulk, softens stool consistency, and decreases intestinal transit time. Insoluble fiber from wheat bran, cereal grains, and vegetables increases fecal bulk most effectively because the cellulose fraction of these fibers is poorly digested. Increased fecal bulk also stimulates the defecation reflex due in part to the effect of mechanical distention in the proximal colon. Bacterial fermentation of fiber releases fatty acids that act as secretagogues, further stimulating colonic motility and secretions. Fecal water retention is enhanced by rapid intestinal transit and by undigested fiber particles that absorb water. Fiber-rich diets are commercially available (Prescription Diet Feline w/d and r/d, Hill's Pet Products). These calorie-restricted diets are most useful in preventing the recurrence of constipation. If these foods are refused, fiber can be added by mixing coarse bran, canned pumpkin, or a commercial psyllium product (Metamucil, Procter & Gamble) to canned cat food.

Surgical Palliation

For cats unresponsive to medical therapy, subtotal colectomy should be considered. Approximately 95% of the colon is removed with or without the ileocolic valve (ICV). The authors prefer to preserve the ICV when possible.

Bowel preparation in the form of oral antibiotics and multiple enemas is not necessary. Perioperative administration of a second-generation cephalosporin (cefmetazole [Zefazone, Upjohn] or cefoxitin [Mefoxin, Merck Sharp & Dohme]) is given starting 20 to 30 min before surgery. Mefoxin is given intravenously and intramuscularly, concurrently, at a dosage rate for each route of 30 mg/kg. Zefazone is given intravenously only at a dose of 20 mg/kg. An additional dose is given intravenously 1.5 hr later.

A ventral midline caudal abdominal incision is used to exteriorize the small and large bowel. The

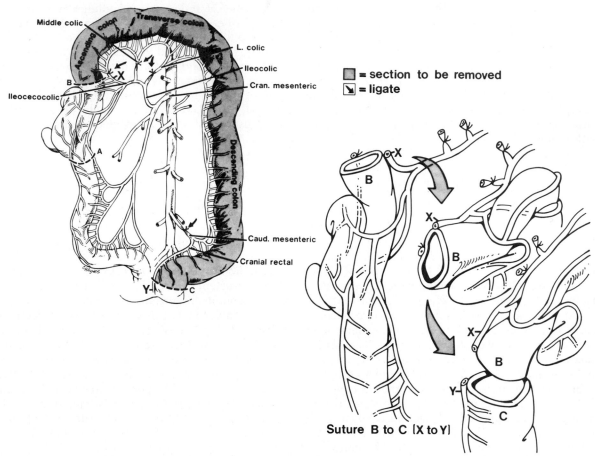

Figure 1. Colocolostomy with preservation of the ileocolic valve (ICV). The shaded area between B and C is removed when the ICV is left intact. Appropriate blood vessels are ligated *(small arrows)*. The mesenteric sides of the two bowel segments are aligned (X and Y) before the anastomosis.

middle and left colic and the caudal mesenteric vessels are double ligated (Fig. 1).

When the ICV valve is preserved, the entire colon is resected except for a 1- to 2-cm segment of the ascending colon and a similar length of colon just cranial to the pubis. If the ICV is removed, most of the ileum should be retained for anastomosis to the distal colonic segment. The ileocecocolic vessels must also be ligated (Fig. 2).

A colocolostomy (see Fig. 1, adjoining B to C) will reestablish bowel continuity with ICV preservation. When the ICV is removed, an ileocolostomy (see Fig. 2, adjoining A to C) is performed. Nonabsorbable or synthetic absorbable suture (3 or 4-0 size) is used in a simple interrupted appositional pattern. Lumen disparity can be corrected several ways, but the authors prefer partial closure of the larger colonic segment using the same suture pattern (Fig. 3). Gentle and accurate placement of all sutures is mandatory. Straight Doyen's noncrushing intestinal clamps are used to help appose the two bowel segments during the placement of sutures. The sutures are not pulled excessively tight. A piece

of omentum is tacked to the bowel above and below the anastomotic site.

The surgeon should not be tempted to resect only the portion of the colon that appears to be pathologic. Partial or segmented colectomies have resulted in recurrences of constipation.

For 5 to 7 postoperative days, tenesmus may be observed. A liquid-to-semisolid stool will eventually form over a period of 5 to 14 days. Most cats will increase frequency of defecation. Incontinence is not usually a problem.

Food intake is strongly encouraged within 24 to 36 hr of surgery. The authors recommend giving the cat any type of food necessary to encourage eating. After the cat gains a good appetite, the owner is instructed to experiment with various brands and types of food until satisfactory stool consistency is attained.

Within 2 or 3 weeks, most cats return to normal activity and regain any weight loss associated with the constipation/obstipation problem. The convalescent period appears to be shorter in cats when the ICV is retained. In addition, these cats will be less

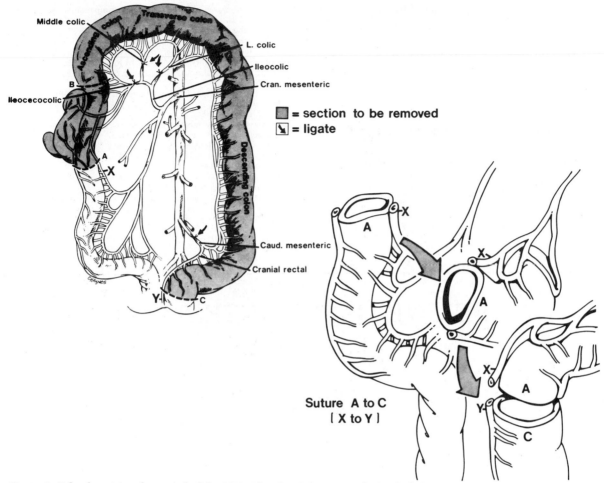

Figure 2. Colocolostomy with removal of the ICV. After the ICV is removed, the shaded area between A and C is resected and an additional set of blood vessels is ligated (ileocecocolic artery and vein). The ileum is anastomosed to the colonic segment.

Figure 3. Lumen disparity corrected by oversewing the larger bowel segment using the same suture pattern as for the anastomosis (simple interrupted appositional).

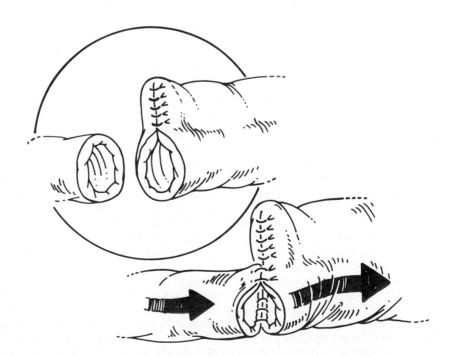

likely to have steatorrhea caused by bacterial overgrowth syndrome. On rare occasions fresh blood may be seen in the stool, but this is probably related to irritation from the nonabsorbable suture used in the anastomosis. Using a synthetic, absorbable suture may eliminate this problem.

References and Suggested Reading

Bright, R. M., Burrows, C. F., Goring, R., et al.: Subtotal colectomy for treatment of acquired megacolon in the dog and cat. J.A.V.M.A. 188:1412, 1986.
A retrospective study reviewing the history, clinical signs, pathologic changes, and long-term results of subtotal colectomy for treatment of acquired megacolon in four cats and a dog.
Burrows, C. E.: Constipation. *In* Kirk, R. W. (ed.): *Current Veterinary Therapy IX.* Philadelphia: W. B. Saunders, 1986, p. 904.
A review of causes and treatments for constipation in the cat and dog.
Burrows, C. E.: Evaluation of a colonic lavage solution to prepare the colon of the dog for colonoscopy. J.A.V.M.A. 195:1719, 1989.
Discussion of the efficacy and safety of an orally administered colonic lavage solution as a means of colon preparation for endoscopy in dogs.
Christensen, J.: Motility of the colon. *In* Johnson, L. R. (ed.): *Physiology of the Gastrointestinal Tract.* 2nd ed. New York: Raven Press, 1987, p. 665.
A review of comparative colonic anatomy, patterns of contraction and flow in the colon, effects of drugs on colonic contractions, and disordered colonic motility.
Edwards, C. A.: The mechanisms of action of dietary fiber in promoting colonic propulsion. Scand. J. Gastroenterol. 22:97, 1987.
Jenkins, D. J. A., Jenkins, A. L., Wolever, T. M. S. et al.: Fiber and starchy foods: Gut function and implications in disease. Am. J. Gastroenterol. 81:920, 1986.
A review of the effects of dietary fibers on gastrointestinal function in the healthy and diseased gut.
Sherding, R. G.: Diseases of the intestines. *In* Sherding, R. G. (ed.): *The Cat: Diseases and Clinical Management.* New York: Churchill Livingstone, 1989, p. 955.
A review of pathophysiology, diagnosis, and clinical management of feline intestinal disorders.

FELINE GASTROINTESTINAL PARASITES

CRAIG R. REINEMEYER
Knoxville, Tennessee

Most domestic cats probably experience some type of gastrointestinal parasitism during their lifetime. Parasitism is highly prevalent in young kittens because certain routes of transmission are unique to neonatal animals and because acquired immunity may not yet be effective. In mature cats, however, infection most commonly results from predation of intermediate hosts. The transmission of parasites to feline and intermediate hosts is markedly reduced by the domestic cat's habitual burial of feces.

Gastrointestinal parasitism in cats is usually diagnosed by demonstration of parasitic organisms or their reproductive products in feces. The most common diagnostic procedure is fecal flotation, a concentration technique that is adequately described in other sources (Georgi and Georgi, 1990; Sloss and Kemp, 1978). A fecal smear is an acceptable substitute when only a small sample is available. A few feline parasitisms are diagnosed more readily by techniques other than flotation, and those exceptions will be noted. For identification of parasites and parasitic products in feces, readers should consult standard textbooks and diagnostic manuals containing photomicrographs of parasitologic specimens (Georgi and Georgi, 1990; Sloss and Kemp, 1978; Williams and Zajac, 1980).

Many gastrointestinal parasitisms of cats are not accompanied by obvious clinical signs, and the benefits of treatment may be equivocal. Nevertheless, some feline parasites represent important zoonotic threats, and control is desirable from a public health standpoint.

The common gastrointestinal parasites of cats may be classified in three major taxonomic groups: nematodes, cestodes, and protozoa.

NEMATODE PARASITES OF CATS

Ascarids or Roundworms

Toxocara cati is the most prevalent feline ascarid, and patent infections are common in cats of all ages. The major route of transmission for mature cats is by ingestion of paratenic hosts; ingestion of embryonated eggs is a potential, yet minor, source. Kittens can be infected by the lactogenic route, in which arrested *Toxocara* larvae in the tissues of pregnant queens are stimulated by the hormones of pregnancy and lactation and migrate to the mammary glands. Larvae are subsequently ingested by nursing kittens. *T. cati* causes visceral larva migrans in humans, but less commonly than *T. canis*.

Toxascaris leonina is less prevalent than *Toxocara*

Table 1. *Anthelmintics Effective against Gastrointestinal Nematodes of Cats*

Approved for Cats		
Drug	**Spectrum**	**Regimen**
Dichlorvos (Task Tabs, Fermenta)	A, H	11 mg/kg, PO
Disophenol (D.N.P., Mobay)	H	10 mg/kg, SC
Febantel + Praziquantel (Vercom, Mobay)	A, H	10 mg/kg, q 24 hr 3 days, PO
Piperazine (Sergeants, ConAgra)	A	55 mg/kg, PO
Not Approved for Cats		
Fenbendazole (Panacur, Hoechst)	A, H	50 mg/kg, q 24 hr 3 days, PO
	M	50 mg/kg, q 24 hr 10–21 days, PO
Pyrantel pamoate (Nemex, Pfizer)	A, H	20 mg/kg, PO
Thiabendazole (Equizole, MSD Agvet)	S	125 mg, q 24 hr 3 days, PO

A = ascarids; H = hookworms; M = Miscellaneous nematodes; S = *Strongyloides.*

in domestic cats but is common in captive felines in zoos. Ingestion of embryonated eggs or paratenic hosts (birds and small mammals) is the only route of infection. *T. leonina* occurs in canids as well as felids but does not migrate systemically and has no zoonotic potential.

CLINICAL SIGNS AND DIAGNOSIS

Infected cats are often asymptomatic, but kittens may exhibit poor growth, diarrhea, rough haircoat, and abdominal enlargement. Patent ascarid infections are diagnosed by demonstration of ova with fecal flotation or by observation of adult and juvenile worms in vomitus or feces.

TREATMENT

Approved, single-treatment anthelmintics for ascarids include piperazine (Sergeants, ConAgra) and dichlorvos (Task Tabs, Fermenta). Piperazine is very safe, but caution should be used in administering organophosphates to young or debilitated kittens. A combination of febantel and praziquantel (Vercom, Mobay) kills ascarids when given for 3 consecutive days. Unapproved, yet safe, anthelmintics include pyrantel pamoate (Nemex, Pfizer) given once (Reinemeyer and DeNovo, 1990), and fenbendazole (Panacur, Hoechst) for 3 days (Roberson and Burke, 1980). See Table 1 for dosages and regimens. Since none of these products is known to be effective against systemic larvae, it may be advisable to

repeat treatment in 2 to 3 weeks, when larvae that were migrating at the time of the first treatment have reached the gut.

PREVENTION

Feces containing ascarid ova should be disposed of daily, and predation must be curtailed if reinfection is to be avoided. Patent *Toxocara* infections of kittens could be prevented by repeated treatments, e.g., at 2, 4, 6, and 8 weeks of age. This rigorous program is not warranted, however, because of the limited public health significance of *T. cati.* Regimens to remove *Toxocara* larvae from the tissues of pregnant queens have not been evaluated, but they seem similarly unnecessary.

Hookworms

Ancylostoma tubaeforme, the most common hookworm of cats, is more prevalent in the southern United States. Cats are infected by ingestion of infective larvae or paratenic hosts. *A. braziliense* is a less pathogenic hookworm of cats and dogs transmitted by the same routes; larvae of *A. braziliense* also can penetrate intact skin and may cause human cutaneous larva migrans. *A. tubaeforme* larvae apparently are incapable of percutaneous infection.

CLINICAL SIGNS AND DIAGNOSIS

A. tubaeforme is an avid blood sucker and causes anemia, melena, and poor growth in young kittens. Signs of *A. braziliense* infection usually consist of mild anemia or hypoproteinemia. Clinical signs in adult cats are less severe. The typical strongylate ova are demonstrated by fecal flotation.

TREATMENT

Although unapproved for cats, pyrantel pamoate (Nemex, Pfizer) combines the rapid action and high margin of safety needed for clinical hookworm disease (see Table 1). Of the approved drugs, disophenol (D.N.P., Mobay) kills worms too slowly to be of immediate benefit to an anemic kitten, and dichlorvos (Task Tabs, Fermenta) is contraindicated in debilitated animals. Similarly, febantel plus praziquantel (Vercom, Mobay) (approved) and fenbendazole (Panacur, Hoechst) (unapproved) require 3 days for optimal efficacy. Severely anemic kittens may require supportive therapy. A fecal sample should be checked 2 to 3 weeks after treatment to

Table 2. *Miscellaneous Gastrointestinal Nematodes of Cats*

Nematode	Site	Transmission	Signs	Diagnosis
Capillaria putorii	Small intestine	Ingestion of ova	None	Flotation
Ollulanus tricuspis	Stomach	Ingestion of larvae	Vomiting	Larvae or adults in vomitus
Physaloptera spp.	Stomach	Arthropod IH	Vomiting	Flotation; adults in vomitus
Strongyloides tumefasciens	Colon	Larvae ingested or percutaneously	Diarrhea	Baermann test for larvae
Trichuris campanula	Cecum, colon	Ingestion of ova	None?	Flotation

detect new adults arising from larvae that were migrating during the initial treatment.

PREVENTION

Daily disposal of feces will prevent the accumulation of infective larvae in the environment. Predation should be restricted.

Miscellaneous Nematodes

Cats are the definitive hosts of numerous other gastrointestinal nematodes that occur less commonly than ascarids and hookworms. These nematodes, along with their major biologic, pathogenic, and diagnostic features, are listed in Table 2; proposed therapies are presented in Table 1. For more complete details, readers are referred to Georgi and Georgi (1990) and Malone et al. (1977).

CESTODE PARASITES OF CATS

All cestode infections of cats are transmitted by ingestion of intermediate hosts. The usual intermediate host is a flea in the case of *Dipylidium caninum;* rodents and other small mammals are intermediate hosts of *Taenia* spp. and *Echinococcus multilocularis*. Small mammals, reptiles, and birds are the intermediate hosts of *Mesocestoides* and *Spirometra* spp. *Dipylidium* and *Taenia* spp. are the most common cestodes of domestic cats in North America.

CLINICAL SIGNS AND DIAGNOSIS

Although various gastrointestinal, pulmonary and even central nervous system syndromes have been attributed to tapeworms, most cestode infections are virtually innocuous. Larval stages of *Echinococcus* and *Mesocestoides* may cause severe disease in intermediate hosts but are harmless to cats.

Cestode infections are diagnosed by observation of proglottids, either on the feces or in the environment or attached to the host. Although cestode eggs are recovered occasionally by fecal flotation, this technique is inconsistent because eggs may not be released within the host. Specific identification of the cestode infection is desirable so that potential intermediate hosts can be recognized. This is easiest when eggs are recovered by flotation, but crushing fresh, gravid proglottids between two microscope slides releases eggs for microscopic examination and specific identification. The typical, operculate eggs of *Spirometra* are best demonstrated by fecal sedimentation, but some may be recovered by flotation. Eggs of *Dipylidium, Mesocestoides,* and *Spirometra* are distinctive, whereas *Taenia* and *Echinococcus* spp. produce identical ova.

TREATMENT

Therapeutic decisions are based as much on the aesthetic concerns of the client as on perceived or actual health threats. Numerous products are effective against cestodes of cats (Table 3). Praziquantel (Droncit, Mobay) and epsiprantel (Cestex, SmithKline Beecham) have excellent activity against *Taenia* and *Dipylidium* with a single treatment; febantel plus praziquantel (Vercom, Mobay) and fenbendazole (Panacur; Hoechst-Roussel) (unapproved) perform similarly when given for 3 days. Vomiting is observed occasionally after cestocidal

Table 3. *Anthelmintics Effective against Gastrointestinal Cestodes of Cats*

Drug	Spectrum	Regimen
Bunamidine (Scolaban, Coopers)	T, ± D	25–50 mg/kg PO
Epsiprantel (Cestex, SmithKline Beecham)	T,D	2.75 mg/kg, PO
Febantel + Praziquantel (Vercom, Mobay)	T,D	10 mg/kg, q 24 hr 3 days, PO
Fenbendazole (Panacur, Hoechst)	T	50 mg/kg, q 24 hr 3 days, PO
Praziquantel (Droncit, Mobay)	T,D,E, M,S	3–7 mg/kg, PO, SC 10 mg/kg, q 24 hr, PO, SC; repeat as necessary

D = *Dipylidium;* E = *Echinococcus multilocularis;* M = *Mesocestoides;* S = *Spirometra;* T = *Taenia* spp.
± indicates marginal efficacy.

treatment. In comparison, an older cestocide, bunamidine (Scolaban, Coopers) demonstrates slightly reduced efficacy against *Taenia* and *Dipylidium*. This product requires fasting before administration and subsequent vomiting is common. *Echinococcus* in cats is probably most susceptible to praziquantel (Droncit, Mobay). An elevated dosage (10 mg/kg) of praziquantel may be necessary to kill *Mesocestoides* and *Spirometra* in cats; complete removal may require repeat doses for several days (see Table 3). Most modern cestocides cause dissolution of tapeworms, so a visible mass of worms does not pass after treatment. The reappearance of proglottids shortly after treatment may indicate anthelmintic failure, but reinfection is another possibility because *Dipylidium* and *Mesocestoides* have prepatent periods as short as 2 weeks (Georgi and Georgi, 1990).

A comprehensive flea control program is required to avoid reinfection with *D. caninum*. Similarly, access to vertebrate intermediate hosts must be denied to prevent infections with *Taenia*, *Mesocestoides*, *Echinococcus*, and *Spirometra*.

PROTOZOAN PARASITES OF CATS

Unlike the parasites discussed earlier, protozoa are one-celled animals that can multiply asexually. Most protozoan parasites of cats are opportunists; infection is common, but clinical signs appear mainly in kittens or adults with deficient immunologic mechanisms. Protozoal infections with a typically temporary course of disease can become chronic in immunocompromised hosts. Drugs used in antiprotozoal therapy often merely suppress parasitic reproduction, and the infection ultimately is eliminated by host defense mechanisms. No antiprotozoal drugs are approved for this use in cats. Environmental sanitation is critical for the prevention of infection because some protozoa are infective as soon as they leave the host.

Coccidia

Isospora felis and *I. rivolta* are the most frequently diagnosed gastrointestinal protozoans of cats and kittens and are acquired by ingestion of sporulated oocysts or rodent intermediate hosts.

CLINICAL SIGNS AND DIAGNOSIS

Most coccidial infections are asymptomatic, but some animals exhibit diarrhea and hematochezia. Despite the concurrent passage of oocysts, severe diarrheas are more likely to be caused by other enteric pathogens (Kirkpatrick and Dubey, 1987).

Table 4. *Compounds Effective against Gastrointestinal Protozoa of Cats*

Drug	Spectrum	Regimen
Furazolidone (Furoxone, Norwich Eaton)	*Giardia*	4 mg/kg, q 12 hr 7–10 days, PO
Metronidazole (Flagyl, Searle)	*Giardia*	10 mg/kg, q 12 hr 5 days, PO
Sulfadimethoxine (Albon, Roche; Bactrovet, Pitman Moore)	*Isospora*	55 mg/kg, q 24 hr day 1, PO, followed by 27.5 mg/kg, q 24 hr days 2–10
Trimethoprim + Sulfadiazine (Tribrissen, Coopers)	*Isospora*	30 mg/kg, q 24 hr 10 days, PO

The usual method of diagnosis is demonstration of unsporulated or sporulated oocysts by fecal flotation.

TREATMENT

Sulfadimethoxine (Albon, Roche; Bactrovet, Pitman Moore) and trimethoprim plus sulfadiazine (Tribrissen, Coopers) decrease asexual multiplication and reduce oocyst production (Table 4). Symptomatic improvement, however, may be due to the activity of these drugs against bacterial enteritis. Treatment of mature cats with an asymptomatic coccidial infection is unnecessary unless they are a source of contamination for susceptible kittens. The complete elimination of a coccidial infection usually requires an immunocompetent host.

PREVENTION

Sanitation and frequent disposal of feces reduce the number of oocysts in the environment. Cleaning cages and litter pans with strong sodium hydroxide solutions is reportedly effective (Kirkpatrick and Dubey, 1987). Predation should be discouraged.

Miscellaneous Coccidia

Cats are the definitive hosts of other protozoans with numerous similarities to *Isospora*. Some of these are transmitted only by ingestion of an intermediate host (*Besnoitia*, *Hammondia*, *Sarcocystis*), whereas others are acquired only by ingestion of oocysts (*Cryptosporidium*). *Toxoplasma* infects cats by either route; *Toxoplasma* infection is also congenital.

CLINICAL SIGNS AND DIAGNOSIS

Of these genera, only *Cryptosporidium* causes severe diarrhea. *Toxoplasma* causes systemic disease in cats, but the enteric phase is essentially harmless. *Toxoplasma, Besnoitia,* and *Hammondia* all produce oocysts of 10 to 12 μ that cannot be differentiated microscopically. Fecal flotation recovers these oocysts and the sporocysts of *Sarcocystis. Cryptosporidium* has oocysts of 4 to 6 μ that are demonstrated by sucrose centrifugation or by a variety of staining procedures.

TREATMENT

The intestinal phases of sarcocystosis and cryptosporidiosis are not susceptible to drugs. Similarly, oocyst shedding by *Toxoplasma* and its relatives cannot be terminated by simple chemotherapy.

PREVENTION

Cats should be confined indoors to avoid contact with sporulated oocysts in the environment. Predation of birds and mammals must be eliminated, and only commercial cat foods should be provided to prevent ingestion of tissues from potential intermediate hosts. *Cryptosporidium* and *Toxoplasma* are zoonotic, and feces containing their oocysts should be disposed of promptly.

Other Protozoan Parasites

Feline giardiasis is more common than suspected, especially in kittens. *Giardia* is transmitted directly by ingestion of the organism. Cats develop immunity to giardiasis, but relapses or reinfection may occur.

CLINICAL SIGNS AND DIAGNOSIS

Giardiasis is characterized by small bowel diarrhea with pale, foul-smelling, steatorrheic stools. If the diarrhea becomes chronic, weight loss or poor growth may result. Giardiasis frequently goes undetected because of the use of improper diagnostic techniques and failure to recognize the organism. Trophozoite and cyst forms occur in feces, but the former is seen only infrequently. Cysts in feces are best demonstrated by a centrifugation/flotation technique using zinc sulfate or saturated sucrose. Oocysts are shed inconsistently, and three samples taken on alternate days should be examined to rule out infection (Kirkpatrick, 1987). Cysts and trophozoites stain with iodine, and this can be used to differentiate *Giardia* from similar protozoa.

TREATMENT

Kirkpatrick (1987) recommends furazolidone (Furoxone, Norwich Eaton) over metronidazole (Flagyl, Searle) for cats because palatability and acceptance are better (Table 4). Regardless of the clinical response, fecal flotation should be repeated at the end of a treatment regimen to detect persistent shedding. If retreatment is required, elevated dosages or lengthened regimens may provide better results.

PREVENTION

Rigid environmental sanitation provides the best prevention. Feces should be removed daily, and the premises kept as dry as possible. Applications of o-benzyl-p-chlorophenol (Lysol, Lehn and Fink) or dilute chlorine bleach may reduce the infection potential of the environment (Kirkpatrick, 1987). *Giardia* is a zoonotic agent, and kennel/cattery workers should be instructed in appropriate hygienic procedures to minimize accidental exposure to organisms while cleaning cages and litter pans.

References and Suggested Reading

Georgi, J. R., and Georgi, M. E.: *Parasitology for Veterinarians*, 5th ed. Philadelphia: W. B. Saunders, 1990.
    A textbook presenting fairly complete information on the biology, diagnosis, and management of parasitic infections of cats and other domestic animals.
Kirkpatrick, C. E.: Giardiasis. Vet. Clin. North Am., Small Anim. Pract. 17:1377, 1987.
    A review of the biology and clinical management of Giardia *infections in small animals.*
Kirkpatrick, C. E., and Dubey, J. P.: Enteric coccidial infections. Vet. Clin. North Am. Small Anim. Pract. 17:1405, 1987.
    A review of the biology, pathogenesis, and management of infections with Isospora *and other coccidia of the gastrointestinal tract.*
Malone, J. B., Butterfield, A. B., Williams, J. C., et al.: *Strongyloides tumefasciens* in cats. J.A.V.M.A. 171:278, 1977.
    A case history of S. tumefasciens *infection in a cat, describing clinical signs, diagnosis, and therapy.*
Reinemeyer, C. R., and DeNovo, R. C.: Evaluation of the efficacy and safety of two formulations of pyrantel pamoate in cats. Am. J. Vet. Res. 51:932, 1990.
    A report of the efficacy and safety of pyrantel pamoate against ascarid and hookworm infections in cats and kittens.
Roberson, E. L., and Burke, T. M.: Evaluation of granulated fenbendazole (22.2%) against induced and naturally occurring helminth infections in cats. Am. J. Vet. Res. 41:1499, 1980.
    A report of the efficacy of fenbendazole against ascarid, hookworm, and cestode infections of cats.
Sloss, M. W., and Kemp, R. L.: *Veterinary Clinical Parasitology*, 5th ed. Ames, IA: Iowa State University Press, 1978.
    A manual of diagnostic techniques and photomicrographs of common parasites of domestic animals.
Williams, J. F., and Zajac, A. M.: *Diagnosis of Gastrointestinal Parasitism in Dogs and Cats*. St. Louis: Ralston Purina Company, 1980.
    A manual of diagnostic techniques and photographs and photomicrographs of gastrointestinal parasites of dogs and cats.

ACUTE PANCREATITIS

DAVID A. WILLIAMS

Manhattan, Kansas

The major function of the acinar cells of the exocrine pancreas is to secrete a fluid rich in digestive enzymes that degrade proteins, lipids, and polysaccharides (Table 1). This protein-rich secretion is diluted and carried along the duct system by the profuse, watery, bicarbonate-rich secretion of the centroacinar and duct cells and is discharged into the duodenal lumen. Pancreatic secretion related to feeding occurs as a response to cephalic stimulation (e.g., the anticipation and smell of food) as well as to gastric and intestinal stimulation due to the presence of food in the stomach and small intestine. Secretin and cholecystokinin, released into the blood from the proximal small intestine when acid and partly-digested food are emptied from the stomach into the duodenum, stimulate the secretion of bicarbonate-rich and enzyme-rich components of pancreatic juice, respectively.

Several mechanisms discourage autodigestion of the pancreas by the enzymes it secretes. First, proteolytic and phospholipolytic enzymes are synthesized, stored, and secreted by the pancreas in the form of catalytically inactive zymogens (Table 1). These zymogens are activated by enzymatic cleavage of a small *activation peptide* from the amino terminal of the polypeptide chain (Fig. 1). Enzymes from several sources, including some lysosomal proteases, are capable of activating pancreatic zymogens, but activation of zymogens does not ordinarily occur until they are secreted into the small intestine. The enzyme enteropeptidase, synthesized by the enterocytes lining the duodenal mucosa, is particularly effective at cleaving the activation peptides from trypsinogens to form trypsins. Active trypsins subsequently cleave the activation peptides from other digestive zymogens (Fig. 2).

Second, as synthesis of digestive enzymes begins, they are segregated, along with potentially damaging lysosomal enzymes, into the lumen of the rough endoplasmic reticulum. This is part of the cisternal space of the acinar cell, a compartment separate from the cell cytosol that contains other enzymes with the potential to activate the zymogens. Segregation is due to the presence of a transient peptide extension on the amino terminal of the enzymes as they are translated from mRNA on the ribosomes. This extension, the *signal sequence* or *signal peptide*, routes the protein being synthesized into the cisternal space. The signal peptide is subsequently removed by the action of a *signal peptidase* located on the inside surface of the lumen of the rough endoplasmic reticulum. Segregation of enzymes in the cisternal space continues as they are processed through the Golgi apparatus, where lysosomal enzymes are selectively routed to lysosome. The digestive enzymes are incorporated into *condensing vacuoles* and ultimately into *zymogen granules* for storage prior to secretion (Fig. 3).

Finally, the acinar cells contain a specific trypsin inhibitor that is synthesized, segregated, stored, and secreted along the digestive enzymes. This low-molecular-weight *pancreatic secretory trypsin inhibitor (PSTI)* is distinct from the much larger

Table 1. *Major Secretory Proteins of the Canine Exocrine Pancreas**

Enzymes secreted as inactive zymogens
  Trypsinogens: trypsins
  Chymotrypsinogens: chymotrypsins
  Proelastases: elastases
  Procarboxypeptidases: carboxypeptidases
  Prophospholipase A_2: phospholipase A_2

Coenzyme
  Procolipase: colipase

Enzymes
  Alpha-amylase
  Lipase

Inhibitor
  Pancreatic secretory trypsin inhibitor

*Modified from Williams, D. A.: Exocrine pancreatic disease. In Ettinger, S. J. (ed.): Textbook of Veterinary Internal Medicine, 3rd ed. Philadelphia: W. B. Saunders, 1989, p. 1529.

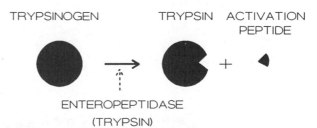

Figure 1. Diagrammatic representation of zymogen activation (activation of trypsinogen to trypsin by enteropeptidase with liberation of a small activation peptide fragment). (Modified with permission from Williams, D. A.: Exocrine pancreatic disease. In Ettinger, S.J. [ed.]: *Textbook of Veterinary Internal Medicine*, 3rd ed. Philadelphia: W. B. Saunders, 1989, p. 1530.)

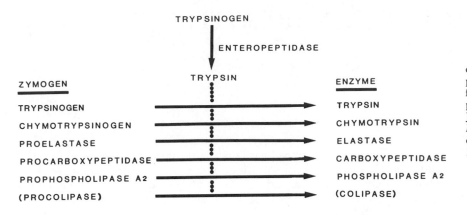

Figure 2. Activation of pancreatic proteases and phospholipase. (Reprinted with permission from Williams, D. A.: Exocrine pancreatic disease. *In* Ettinger, S. J. [ed.]: *Textbook of Veterinary Internal Medicine,* 3rd ed. Philadelphia: W. B. Saunders, 1989, p. 1530.)

plasma protease inhibitors (Table 2). It is believed that PSTI immediately inhibits any trypsin activity produced should there be activation of trace amounts of trypsinogen within the acinar cell or duct system and therefore blocks further intrapancreatic activation of the digestive enzymes (Fig. 4).

It is normal for trace amounts of zymogens of pancreatic proteases as well as active amylase, lipase, and other enzymes to be present in the blood. These enzymes and their zymogens leak directly from the pancreas into the blood stream, from which they are cleared by glomerular filtration, with subsequent variable degradation by renal tubular epithelial cells.

PATHOLOGY AND PATHOPHYSIOLOGY

When examined during exploratory laparotomy or necropsy, the acutely inflamed pancreas is often edematous, swollen, and soft, and there may be adhesions to adjacent organs. Severely affected areas of the pancreas may be liquefied and form sterile pseudocysts, while secondary infection with enteric organisms may produce pancreatic abscesses. Hemorrhage may be present in the omentum and the pancreas, and there are often chalky areas of abdominal fat necrosis. The peritoneal cavity may contain a small amount of blood-stained fluid with fat droplets. In some cases, the pancreas

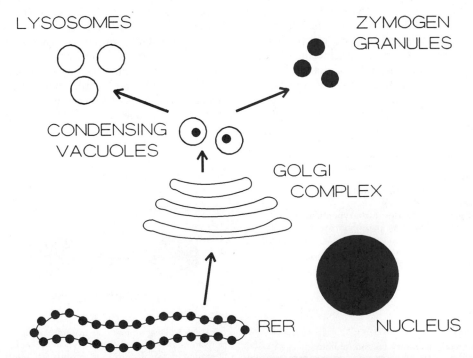

Figure 3. Normal intracellular routing of digestive and lysosomal enzymes to separate compartments within the pancreatic acinar cell. RER, rough endoplasmic reticulum. (Modified with permission from Williams, D. A.: Exocrine pancreatic disease. *In* Ettinger, S. J. [ed.]: *Textbook of Veterinary Internal Medicine,* 3rd ed. Philadelphia: W. B. Saunders, 1989, p. 1531).

Table 2. *The Role of Enzymes in the Pathophysiology of Pancreatitis**

Enzyme	Pathophysiologic Action
Trypsin	Activation of other proteases
	Coagulation and fibrinolysis
	(disseminated intravascular coagulation)
Phospholipase A₂	Hydrolysis of cell membrane phospholipids
	Pulmonary surfactant degradation
	Demyelination
	(cell necrosis and liberation of toxic substances such as myocardial depressant factor); (respiratory distress); (neurological signs: pancreatic encephalopathy)
Elastase	Degradation of elastin in blood vessel walls (hemorrhage, edema, respiratory distress)
Chymotrypsin	Activation of xanthine oxidase and subsequent generation of oxygen-derived free radicals (membrane damage)
Kallikrein	Kinin generation from kininogens
Kinins	Vasodilation, pancreatic edema (hypotension, shock)
Complement	Cell membrane damage, aggregation of leukocytes (local inflammation)
Lipase	Fat hydrolysis (local fat necrosis, hypocalcemia)

*Reprinted with permission from Williams, D. A.: Exocrine pancreatic disease. *In* Ettinger, S. J. (ed.): *Textbook of Veterinary Internal Medicine*, 3rd ed. Philadelphia: W. B. Saunders, 1989, p. 1533.

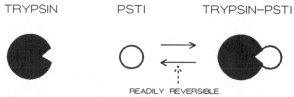

READILY REVERSIBLE

Figure 4. Pancreatic secretory trypsin inhibitor (PSTI) is a low-molecular-weight (6000), trypsin-specific inhibitor protein present in pancreatic zymogen granules and pancreatic juice. It prevents intrapancreatic cascade activation of pancreatic enzymes following spontaneous autoactivation of trace amounts of trypsin within the pancreas. A transient inhibitor only, it is eventually digested in the duodenum by the trypsin that it temporarily inhibits. (Modified with permission from Williams, D. A.: Exocrine pancreatic disease. *In* Ettinger, S. J. [ed.]: *Textbook of Veterinary Internal Medicine,* 3rd ed. Philadelphia: W. B. Saunders, 1989, p. 1530.)

may appear deceptively normal on gross examination, but histologically there may be extensive multifocal infiltration by neutrophils and varying degrees of hemorrhage, necrosis, edema, and vessel thrombosis. Irreversible destruction of pancreatic tissue in patients with chronic pancreatitis may reduce the gland to a few distorted lobules.

It is generally believed that pancreatitis develops upon activation of digestive enzymes within the gland with resultant pancreatic autodigestion. Current evidence suggests that the site of initiation of enzyme activation is often intracellular rather than in the intercellular space or duct system as previously assumed. Several experimental models have shown that abnormal fusion of lysosome and zymogen granules occurs prior to the development of overt pancreatitis, probably due to failure of normal intracellular transport, storage, or exocytosis of zymogen granule contents (Fig. 5). Lysosomal proteases then activate trypsinogen because PSTI (see above) is ineffective at the acidic pH level present in lysosome.

After intracellular and intraductal activation of trypsinogens to trypsins takes place, further activation of all enzymes, particularly elastase and phospholipase, will amplify pancreatic damage. Activation of progressively larger amounts of protease and phospholipase within the gland is associated with transformation of mild pancreatic inflammation to severe hemorrhagic or necrotic pancreatitis with

multisystem involvement and consumption of plasma protease inhibitors (Fig. 6) (Table 2).

Plasma protease inhibitors are vital in protecting against the otherwise fatal effects of proteolytic enzymes in the vascular space. Alpha-macroglobulins (Fig. 7) are particularly important in this regard. Intravascular pancreatic enzymes are tolerated without adverse effects provided that free alpha-macroglobulins are available to bind the active proteases. However, once alpha-macroglobulins are no longer available, acute disseminated intravascular coagulation, shock, and death occur within minutes as the free proteases activate the kinin, coagulation,

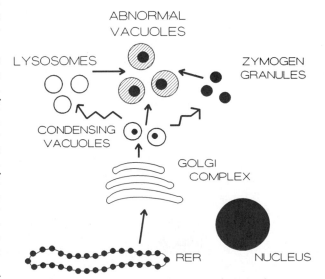

Figure 5. Abnormal intracellular routing of digestive and lysosomal enzymes within acinar cells results in mixing of zymogens and lysosomal proteases in abnormal intracellular vacuoles. Subsequent activation of zymogens by lysosomal proteases at the acidic pH level in these vacuoles may result in pancreatitis. RER, rough endoplasmic reticulum. (Modified with permission from Williams, D. A.: Exocrine pancreatic disease. *In* Ettinger, S. J. [ed.]: *Textbook of Veterinary Internal Medicine*, 3rd ed. Philadelphia: W. B. Saunders, 1989, p. 1531.)

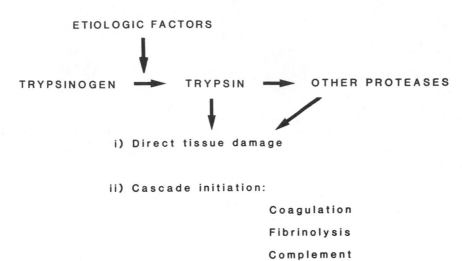

ETIOLOGIC FACTORS

TRYPSINOGEN → TRYPSIN → OTHER PROTEASES

i) Direct tissue damage

ii) Cascade initiation:

              Coagulation

              Fibrinolysis

              Complement

              Kallikrein–kinin

Figure 6. Local and systemic effects of trypsin in pancreatitis. (Reprinted with permission from Williams, D. A.: Exocrine pancreatic disease. *In* Ettinger, S. J. [ed.]: *Textbook of Veterinary Internal Medicine,* 3rd ed. Philadelphia: W. B. Saunders, 1989, p. 1533.)

fibrinolytic, and complement cascade systems (see Fig. 6 and Table 2).

Binding of proteases by alpha-macroglobulin results in a change in conformation (see Fig. 7), which allows the complex to be recognized and rapidly cleared from the plasma by the reticuloendothelial system. This removal is important because alpha-macroglobulin–bound proteases retain catalytic activity, particularly against low-molecular-weight substrates; normal functioning of the reticuloendothelial system is an important factor determining survival in experimental pancreatitis.

Eighty percent of plasma alpha-protease inhibitor (Fig. 8) is still available to bind proteases when alpha-macroglobulins are saturated with trypsin, but the alpha-protease inhibitor is not lifesaving. While pancreatic proteases bound to alpha-protease inhibitor are effectively inhibited, the binding is reversible (Fig. 8). Alpha-protease inhibitor probably functions largely as a transient inhibitor and an intermediary in the transport of protease to alpha-macroglobulins, particularly in the extravascular spaces into which the large alpha-macroglobulin and molecules cannot permeate.

ETIOLOGY

The cause of spontaneous canine and feline pancreatitis is usually unknown, but the following

TRYPSIN   α–M   TRYPSIN–α–M

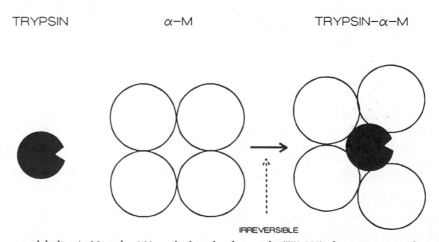

IRREVERSIBLE

Figure 7. Alpha-macroglobulins (α-M_1 and α-M_2) are high-molecular-weight (750,000) plasma proteins. They are highly effective "lifesaving" inhibitors when large amounts of almost any proteolytic enzyme, including pancreatic digestive proteases, are released into the vascular space. The complexes of enzyme and inhibitor are rapidly cleared by the reticuloendothelial system. Dogs with experimental pancreatitis die within minutes when these inhibitors are no longer available to bind with enzymes released into the vascular space. (Modified with permission from Williams, D. A.: Exocrine pancreatic disease. *In* Ettinger, S. J. [ed.]: *Textbook of Veterinary Internal Medicine,* 3rd ed. Philadelphia: W. B. Saunders, 1989, p. 1530.)

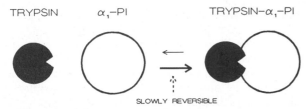

TRYPSIN α_1–PI TRYPSIN–α_1–PI

SLOWLY REVERSIBLE

Figure 8. Alpha$_1$-protease inhibitor (α_1-antitrypsin, α_1-PI) is an albumin-sized (molecular weight: 55,000) protein present in plasma and intercellular fluid. It probably functions primarily as an inhibitor of neutrophil elastase and other proteolytic enzymes released during inflammation, thus localizing the inflammatory response. It may act as a minor temporary inhibitor of proteases released into the intercellular fluid and blood during acute pancreatitis but is not lifesaving. (Modified with permission from Williams, D. A.: Exocrine pancreatic disease. *In* Ettinger, S. J. [ed.]: *Textbook of Veterinary Internal Medicine*, 3rd ed. Philadelphia: W. B. Saunders, 1989, p. 1530.)

should be considered as potential inciting factors or exacerbating influences.

HYPERTRIGLYCERIDEMIA. Hypertriglyceridemia, often grossly apparent, is common in dogs with acute pancreatitis, and may also develop secondary to pancreatitis as a result of abdominal fat necrosis. It may also be a cause of the disease, however, since toxic concentrations of fatty acids may be generated by the action of lipase on abnormally high concentrations of triglycerides in pancreatic capillaries. Some familial hyperlipoproteinemias of human beings are associated with frequent episodes of pancreatitis that respond to control of serum triglyceride levels. There is anecdotal evidence that pancreatitis in dogs may develop after a fatty meal and may be particularly prevalent in miniature schnauzers with idiopathic hyperlipoproteinemia.

DRUGS. A number of drugs have the potential to induce pancreatitis. Suspect drugs used in veterinary medicine include thiazide diuretics, furosemide, azathioprine, L-asparaginase, sulfonamides, and tetracycline. It is controversial whether or not corticosteroids induce pancreatitis, although they have the potential to exacerbate the severity of disease by inhibiting the function of the reticuloendothelial system.

INFECTION. Viral and parasitic infections may be associated with pancreatitis, although this is usually recognized as part of a more generalized disease. Bacterial infection may increase the severity of pancreatitis and lead to complications.

DUCT OBSTRUCTION. Experimental obstruction of the pancreatic ducts produces inflammation when the pancreas is subsequently stimulated. While rare, partial or complete obstruction of the pancreatic ducts may occur with compression, spasm, or edema of the duct or duodenal wall secondary to neoplasia, parasite migration, trauma, or surgical interference. Congenital anomalies of the duct system may also predispose to pancreatitis.

DUODENAL REFLUX. Enteropeptidase, activated pancreatic enzymes, bacteria, and bile present in the duodenal juice may all contribute to development of pancreatitis. Under normal circumstances, such reflux is unlikely to occur because the duct opening is surrounded by a specialized, compact, smooth mucosa over the duodenal papilla and is equipped with an independent sphincter muscle. This antireflux mechanism may sometimes fail in the face of abnormally high duodenal pressure, however, such as may occur with vomiting.

ISCHEMIA AND TRAUMA. Experimental and clinical reports have implicated ischemia in the pathogenesis of acute pancreatitis; it presumably disrupts acinar cell function. Pancreatic ischemia may develop during shock and secondary to hypotension during general anesthesia. Surgical manipulation, automobile accidents, and falls are potential causes of pancreatic trauma and ischemia, but reports of pancreatitis following such insults are rare, and injury to the pancreas is probably mild or unrecognized in most cases of abdominal trauma. Pancreatitis is a rare complication of pancreatic biopsy with wedge or needle techniques and is also uncommon following resection of pancreatic neoplasms.

MISCELLANEOUS. Hypercalcemia, uremia, and toxins such as cholinesterase inhibitors, cholinergic agonists, and scorpion venom may induce pancreatitis, probably secondary to hyperstimulation of secretion. Pancreatitis and gastrointestinal hemorrhage have been reported in association with intervertebral disk disease in dogs, although it is not known if this arises as a direct consequence of spinal cord trauma, corticosteroid therapy, or a combination of these factors.

DIAGNOSIS

History and Clinical Signs

Animals with acute pancreatitis are usually presented because of depression, anorexia, vomiting, and in some cases diarrhea. Severe acute disease may be associated with shock and collapse, while other cases may have a history of less dramatic signs extending over several weeks. Signs of pain may be elicited on abdominal palpation but it must be noted that some animals with severe pancreatitis do not react. An anterior abdominal mass is palpable in some cases. Many affected animals are mildly to moderately dehydrated and febrile. Uncommon systemic complications of pancreatitis that may be apparent on physical examination include jaundice, dyspnea, cardiac arrhythmias, and signs of impaired hemostasis.

Radiographic and Ultrasonographic Signs

History and clinical signs associated with pancreatitis are nonspecific and common to numerous gastrointestinal and metabolic disorders. Abdominal radiographs may provide evidence for one of these alternative diagnoses or support a tentative diagnosis of pancreatitis. Radiographic signs that may be seen with pancreatitis include increased density, granularity and diminished contrast in the right cranial abdomen, displacement of the stomach to the left, and widening of the angle between the pyloric antrum and the proximal duodenum due to the presence of a mass medial to the descending duodenum. A static gas pattern and corrugated walls may be seen in the duodenum and transverse colon owing to impaired motility, and there may be gastric distention due to gastric outlet obstruction. Unfortunately, the most common radiographic finding in acute pancreatitis is a somewhat subjective loss of visceral detail ("ground glass appearance") in the cranial abdomen.

Ultrasonography may reveal nonhomogeneous masses and loss of echodensity and is particularly valuable for localizing pancreatic masses. Cytologic and bacteriologic evaluation of needle aspiration from such masses facilitates differentiation between pseudocysts and abscesses.

Laboratory Aids to Diagnosis

Leukocytosis is common in acute pancreatitis. The hematocrit may be increased as a result of dehydration, although in some cases unexplained anemia is observed. Prerenal azotemia is frequently present, but there may sometimes be acute renal failure arising secondary to pathophysiologic sequelae of pancreatitis itself. Liver enzyme activities are often increased, reflecting hepatocellular injury as a result of either hepatic ischemia or exposure of the liver to high concentrations of toxic products in portal blood. In some cases, the enzyme changes suggest an obstructive hepatopathy (marked elevation of serum alkaline phosphatase) with hyperbilirubinemia, indicating intrahepatic or extrahepatic obstruction to bile flow.

Hyperglycemia is common as a result of hyperglucagonemia and stress-related increases in the concentrations of catecholamines and cortisol, though some animals are diabetic during and following recovery owing to destruction of islet cells. Mild hypocalcemia is often present, but only very rarely are there signs of tetany due to severe hypocalcemia. Hypercholesterolemia and hypertriglyceridemia are common, and hyperlipemia may be grossly apparent.

Assays of pancreatic enzymes and zymogens in serum provide more specific tests for pancreatitis. Numerous assay methods exist, including conventional catalytic assays and newer, highly specific immunoassays (Fig. 9). It is imperative that an appropriate method for each species be utilized, as immunoassays are generally only applicable to the species for which they were developed. Clinical and experimental observations have involved primarily amylase and lipase, but recently phospholipase A_2 and serum trypsin-like immunoreactivity (TLI) have been investigated.

Experimental studies in general indicate parallel changes in results of different enzyme determinations during the course of canine pancreatitis, except that serum TLI tends to increase earlier and decrease sooner during the course of the disease than do other enzymes, reflecting its shorter half-life. Serum TLI is pancreas-specific in origin, whereas amylase, lipase, and phospholipase activities originate from pancreatic and extrapancreatic sources. In dogs with spontaneous disease, however, there may be elevations of one enzyme accompanied by minimal increases in another; persistently normal activities are seen in some cases. It is probable that by the time some clinical cases are investigated, the inflamed pancreas is depleted of stored enzymes, synthesis of new enzymes is disrupted, and therefore release into the blood stream is no longer increased. Similar reasoning may explain the lack of correlation between the magnitude of the increases in enzyme activities and the clinically perceived severity of disease and eventual outcome.

Increased concentrations of circulating pancreatic enzymes may also arise secondary to reduced clearance from the plasma as happens in severe renal failure. Because azotemia is common in acute pancreatitis, it is sometimes difficult to determine whether increased levels of pancreatic enzymes are due to pancreatic inflammation or renal disease. Increases greater than two to three times above the upper limit of normal are unlikely to result from

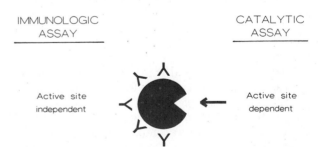

Figure 9. Immunoassays (such as that used to assay trypsin-like immunoreactivity) measure the concentration of antigenic determinants on the surface of enzyme molecules and therefore usually detect both zymogens and active enzymes. In contrast, catalytic assays (such as those commonly used to assay amylase and lipase) measure substrate degrading activity of the enzyme and therefore do not detect inactive zymogen. (Modified with permission from Williams, D. A.: Exocrine pancreatic disease. *In* Ettinger, S. J. [ed.]: *Textbook of Veterinary Internal Medicine*, 3rd ed. Philadelphia: W. B. Saunders, 1989, p. 1536.)

renal dysfunction alone, however, and serum pancreatic enzyme levels are normal in the majority of animals with even severe chronic renal dysfunction.

Amylase, lipase, and phospholipase originate from both pancreatic and extrapancreatic sources, and serum activities may increase in dogs with hepatic, renal, or neoplastic disease in the absence of pancreatitis. Lipase and phospholipase activities have been reported to have more reliability as markers for pancreatitis than does amylase. However, dexamethasone administration has been shown to increase canine serum lipase activity up to fivefold without histologic evidence of pancreatitis, although parallel increases in amylase activity do not occur. Moderate elevations of serum lipase in dogs receiving dexamethasone should therefore not be taken as strong evidence for pancreatitis unless amylase is also increased. Assay of lipase and TLI in serum collected soon after presentation is most likely to reliably identify affected dogs.

The presence of trypsin complexed with plasma alpha$_1$-protease inhibitor (see Fig. 8) or of trypsinogen activation peptides (TAP; see Fig. 1) in serum or urine is a specific marker for pancreatitis because in the absence of pancreatitis only trypsinogen is present in the plasma. Furthermore, there is clinical evidence that the concentration of these markers correlates with the severity and clinical course of the disease. At present, technical complexities limit the usefulness of species-specific trypsin alpha$_1$-protease inhibitor complex assay, but assays for TAP, which are similar in different species and more readily measured, may prove to be of practical value.

Reports of acute pancreatitis in cats are few, but elevations of serum amylase and lipase are less than in dogs, as are normal activities of these enzymes. An experimental study demonstrated that while serum lipase increased significantly in cats following induction of pancreatitis, amylase activity never increased above normal but rather decreased significantly during the course of the disease.

As there is no widely available ideal test or combination of tests for the diagnosis of acute pancreatitis, in the absence of direct examination of pancreatic tissue the diagnosis can only be tentative. Nonetheless, careful evaluation of the entire clinical picture can provide a high degree of confidence in the presumptive diagnosis. If gross or histopathologic confirmation of the diagnosis is required or the possibility of other abdominal disease is to be eliminated, it is important that attention be given to stabilization of fluid, plasma protein, and electrolyte status prior to general anesthesia and surgical exploration of the abdomen.

TREATMENT

The basis for therapy of acute pancreatitis is maintenance of fluid and electrolyte balance while the pancreas is "rested" by withholding food and thereby allowed to recover from the inflammatory episode. Sufficient balanced-electrolyte solution should be given intravenously to replace fluid deficits and provide maintenance requirements while all oral intake is suspended for 3 or 4 days. Potential etiologic factors (see earlier) should be identified and rectified if possible. In particular, if drug-induced pancreatitis is suspected, the incriminated agent should be withdrawn and replaced by an unrelated alternative drug if necessary.

Mild cases of pancreatitis are self-limiting and spontaneously improve after 1 or 2 days. Other patients require aggressive fluid therapy over several days to treat severe dehydration and ongoing fluid electrolyte loss due to vomiting and diarrhea. Hypokalemia is common during such therapy and intravenous fluids should be supplemented as needed with potassium chloride. Acid-base abnormalities should be corrected as indicated by evaluation of laboratory test results. Parenteral antibiotics are commonly given during this supportive period, particularly when toxic changes are evident in the hemogram or when the patient is febrile. Trimethoprim-sulfadiazine may be considered, as it penetrates well into the canine pancreas and is effective against many common pathogens isolated from human patients with pancreatitis.

If abdominal pain is severe, analgesic therapy (such as meperidine hydrochloride 2 to 5 mg/kg SC every 6 hr) should be given to provide relief (see this volume, p. 82). Hyperglycemia is often mild and transient, but if frank diabetes mellitus is present, treatment with insulin is indicated. Respiratory distress, neurologic problems, cardiac abnormalities, bleeding disorders, and acute renal failure are all poor prognostic signs. Attempts should be made to manage these complications with appropriate supportive measures, but recovery is unlikely unless the underlying pancreatitis resolves.

Some affected animals do not improve or continue to deteriorate in spite of supportive care. In severe pancreatitis there is marked consumption of plasma protease inhibitors as activated pancreatic proteases are cleared from the circulation. Saturation of available alpha-macroglobulins is followed within minutes by acute disseminated intravascular coagulation, hypotensive shock, and death (see Fig. 6). Transfusion of plasma or whole blood to replace alpha-macroglobulins may be lifesaving in these circumstances and has the additional benefit of maintaining plasma albumin concentrations. The oncotic properties of albumin not only help maintain blood volume and prevent pancreatic ischemia but also limit pancreatic edema formation. Low-molecular-weight dextrans have also been used to expand plasma volume, but they may aggravate bleeding tendencies, contain no protease inhibitor, and provide no major advantages over plasma administration.

The use of corticosteroids in pancreatitis has been recommended because they stabilize lysosomal membranes, reduce inflammation, and alleviate shock, but they have not been shown to be of value in acute experimental studies. Corticosteroids should be given only on a short-term basis to animals in shock associated with fulminating pancreatitis and then in concert with fluids and plasma as described earlier. Long-term administration is contraindicated because corticosteroids may impair removal of alpha-macroglobulin–bound proteases from the plasma by the reticuloendothelial system, with resultant complications due to systemic effects of circulating uninhibited proteolytic enzymes.

Peritoneal dialysis to remove toxic material from the peritoneal cavity is beneficial experimentally and may be of value in some clinical cases that are not progressing well. When acute pancreatitis is confirmed during exploratory laparotomy, removal of as much free fluid as possible by abdominal lavage is advisable. In some cases, pancreatitis may be localized to one lobe of the gland, and surgical resection of the affected area may be followed by complete recovery. Surgical intervention is generally inadvisable unless either specific foci of necrosis or infection are to be resected or drained or biliary tract obstruction is to be relieved in patients that are not responding favorably to conservative therapy.

Indirect approaches to inhibition of pancreatic secretion that have been employed in addition to the withholding of food include nasogastric suctioning of gastric secretions and inhibition of gastric secretion by use of antacids or cimetidine. None of these methods has been consistently shown to be effective, and their use is not recommended. Attempts to rest the pancreas by use of direct inhibitors of secretion such as atropine, acetazolamide, glucagon, calcitonin, and somatostatin or its analogues have also not been proved effective. Pancreatic gamma irradiation is an effective but impractical method that reduces pancreatic secretion and lessens the severity of experimental pancreatitis. Administration of a variety of naturally occurring and synthetic enzyme inhibitors with selective actions against individual pancreatic digestive enzymes has shown promise in experimental studies, as has the administration of free radical scavengers, but the value of these and other experimental approaches remains to be demonstrated in clinical trials.

As soon as there has been no vomiting for 1 or 2 days, small amounts of water should be offered, and if there is no recurrence of clinical signs, food may be gradually reintroduced. The diet should have a high carbohydrate content (rice, pasta, potatoes) because protein and fat are more potent stimulants of pancreatic secretion and are more likely to promote a relapse. If there is continued improvement, gradual introduction of a low-fat maintenance diet should be attempted. Another period of food deprivation should be initiated if signs of pancreatitis recur.

In many patients, a single episode of pancreatitis occurs and the only long-term therapy necessary is to avoid feeding meals with an excessively high fat content. In other patients repeated bouts of pancreatitis occur, and it may be beneficial to feed a moderately or severely fat-restricted diet permanently, although some animals will still experience recurrent disease.

Oral pancreatic enzyme supplements decrease the pain that accompanies chronic pancreatitis in human beings, probably by feedback inhibition of endogenous pancreatic enzyme secretion. It is not known if they are of similar value in dogs or cats, but in individuals with chronic or recurrent signs attributed to pancreatitis a trial period of enzyme therapy is warranted.

PROGNOSIS

Pancreatitis is an unpredictable disease of widely varying severity, and it is difficult to give a prognosis even when a diagnosis is definitively established. Life-threatening signs accompanying acute fulminating pancreatitis are usually followed by death in spite of supportive measures, but some dogs recover fully following an isolated severe episode. In other cases, relatively mild or moderate chronic or recurrent pancreatitis persists despite all therapy, and the patient either dies in an acute severe exacerbation of the disease or is euthanatized because of failure to recover and the expense of long-term supportive care. Most patients with uncomplicated pancreatitis probably recover spontaneously after a single episode and do well if high-fat diets are avoided.

References and Suggested Reading

Bradley, E. L.: Antibiotics in acute pancreatitis: Current status and future directions. Am. J. Surg. 158:472, 1989.
A review of what is known about antibiotic therapy in acute pancreatitis.
Cuschieri, A., Cumming, J. R. G., Meehan, S. E. et al.: Treatment of acute pancreatitis with fresh frozen plasma. Br. J. Surg. 70:710, 1983.
Clinical study evaluating the value of plasma in therapy of pancreatitis in human patients.
Edwards, D. F., Bauer, M. S., Walker, M. A., et al.: Pancreatic masses in seven dogs following acute pancreatitis. J. Am. Anim. Hosp. Assoc. 26:189, 1990.
A retrospective study of pancreatitis cases in which pancreatic masses were documented and in which six or seven dogs died.
Gudgeon, A. M., Heath, D. I., Hurley, P., et al.: Trypsinogen activation peptide assay in the early prediction of severity of acute pancreatitis. Lancet 335:4, 1990.
Trypsinogen activation peptides in urine reflect abnormal intrapancreatic enzyme activation, and their concentration predicts severity of disease in human patients.
Lasson, A.: Acute pancreatitis in man: A clinical and biochemical study of pathophysiology and treatment. Scand J Gastroenterol 99(suppl):1, 1984.
A detailed review of the pathophysiology of human pancreatitis with emphasis on the role of plasma protease inhibitors.
McMahon, M. J., Bowen, M., Mayer, A. D., Cooper, E. H.: Relation of

alpha$_2$-macroglobulin and other antiproteases to the clinical features of acute pancreatitis. Am. J. Surg. 147:164, 1984.
  A clinical study in human patients documenting consumption of alpha$_2$-macroglobulin in severely affected individuals.

Poston, G. J., and Williamson, R. C. N.: Surgical management of acute pancreatitis. Br. J. Surg. 77:5, 1990.
  A review of the limitations of and indications for surgical intervention in acute pancreatitis, one of the conclusions of which is that fluid replacement is the only treatment of proven value.

Salisbury, S. K., Lantz, G. C., Nelson, R. W., et al.: Pancreatic abscess in dogs: Six cases (1978–1986). J. A. V. M. A. 193:1104, 1988.
  Three of six dogs with sterile pancreatic masses recovered after surgical debridement and abdominal drainage.

Simpson, K. W., Batt, R. M., McLean, L., et al.: Circulating concentra-

tions of trypsin-like immunoreactivity and activities of lipase and amylase after pancreatic duct ligation in dogs. Am. J. Vet. Res. 50:629, 1989.
  Serum TLI tended to peak earlier and to decrease more rapidly than lipase and amylase in this experimental model of mild pancreatitis.

Steer, M. L., and Meldolesi, J.: The cell biology of experimental pancreatitis. N. Engl. J. Med. 316:144, 1987.
  A review of recent advances in understanding the subcellular pathophysiology of pancreatitis.

Williams, D. A.: Exocrine pancreatic disease. In Ettinger, S. J. (ed.): *Textbook of Veterinary Internal Medicine*. Philadelphia: W. B. Saunders, 1989, p. 1528.
  A detailed review of canine and feline pancreatitis with an extensive bibliography.

HEPATIC ENCEPHALOPATHY

ROBERT M. HARDY

St. Paul, Minnesota

Hepatic encephalopathy (HE) is a clinical syndrome characterized by abnormal mental status, an altered state of consciousness, and impaired neurologic function in a patient with advanced liver disease or severe portosystemic shunting (Fraser and Arieff, 1975). Other terms used to describe this syndrome are *hepatic coma* and *portosystemic encephalopathy*.

CLINICAL FINDINGS

HE is recognized most often in dogs or cats with congenital anomalies of the portal vascular system; however, it may be found in acute fulminant hepatic failure or in association with chronic progressive hepatic disorders that lead to end-stage liver failure (cirrhosis).

Signs associated with HE in dogs and cats can be grouped into two general categories. The first group includes signs associated with liver failure; they are nonspecific and are often encountered in non-neurologic and nonhepatic diseases. These include anorexia, depression, weight loss, lethargy, polydipsia, polyuria, nausea, hypersalivation, vomiting, and diarrhea. Rare pica and polyphagia may be noted as well. The second group of signs are those that typically relate to the central nervous system (CNS) but are induced by HE. Such signs include bizarre behavioral changes or dementia characterized by hysteria, unpredictable bouts of aggression, staggering, pacing, compulsive circling, ataxia, head pressing, amaurotic (cortical) blindness, intermittent deafness, tremors, seizures, and ultimately coma. The severity of clinical signs depends on the acuteness with which the liver disease has developed, the extent of functional injury that is present,

and the degree of portosystemic shunting that exists. The slower the onset of failure, the less dramatic the signs. Animals with stable liver disease may develop an episode of HE in association with some precipitating event. In my experience, the most commonly identified precipitating factors in animals are the ingestion of high-protein meals, gastrointestinal (GI) bleeding, and azotemia. HE also often follows administration of anesthetics or sedative drugs. Other potential precipitating factors are hypokalemia, hyponatremia, analgesic medications, infections, hypoxia, hypoglycemia, metabolic or respiratory alkalosis, and constipation.

Animals with HE associated with acute severe viral or toxic hepatitis often have a fatal outcome, regardless of the nature of therapeutic intervention. In contrast, animals with HE associated with chronic progressive hepatic disease and extensive portosystemic shunting (cirrhosis) have intermittent signs interspersed with relatively long periods of normal behavior. Because the coma that accompanies fulminant hepatic failure is associated with reversible pathologic changes (edema) and the coma of chronic hepatic failure is often rapidly and completely reversible, it is assumed that neither clinical syndrome results from permanent morphologic abnormalities of the brain. Thus, HE should be approached as a potentially reversible metabolic abnormality of cerebral metabolism that is induced by biochemical alterations associated with hepatic failure.

PATHOGENESIS

The pathogenesis of HE is incompletely understood. It is likely that multiple factors are capable of inducing the syndrome that is recognized clinically as HE. It is accepted that a healthy liver is necessary for normal brain function and that alterations in normal liver function lead to abnormal cerebral function. The fundamental hypothesis regarding the pathogenesis of HE incorporates two basic concepts. First, HE results when a diseased liver fails to remove toxic products of gut metabolism from portal blood. Second, HE may also develop because of failure of the diseased liver to synthesize factors other than glucose that are necessary for normal brain function (Jones et al., 1989). Factors considered most important in the production of HE are (1) cerebral toxin accumulation (ammonia, mercaptans, short-chain fatty acids [SCFA], and gamma-aminobutyric acid [GABA] agonists); (2) alterations in plasma amino acids, which on reaching the CNS impair normal cerebral function; and (3) increased cerebral sensitivity.

Cerebral Toxins

AMMONIA

Ammonia is considered one of the key cerebral toxins in HE. Blood ammonia arises primarily from the colon and from renal tubular synthesis from glutamine. Colonic ammonia production results from the conversion of intraluminal urea to ammonia by urease-producing bacteria. Ammonia diffuses readily out of the colon and enters the portal vein. A normal liver extracts from 81 to 87% of portal vein ammonia and converts it again to urea in the Krebs-Henseleit urea cycle. The remaining 16% of gastrointestinally derived ammonia is left to enter the systemic circulation (Aldrete, 1975). The liver is the sole site of urea synthesis in the body and the major organ of ammonia detoxification. Elevations in blood ammonia concentrations occur in liver failure when insufficient numbers of functional hepatocytes remain to convert the normal daily load of ammonia to urea or when acquired or congenital portal vein shunting leads to diversion of portal vein ammonia directly into the systemic circulation, bypassing hepatic metabolism.

METHIONINE/MERCAPTANS

Metabolic by-products of oral methionine are capable of inducing encephalopathy in dogs with hepatic failure (Merino et al., 1975). Methionine is degraded by gut flora to a group of by-products collectively called *mercaptans* (methanethiol, ethanethiol, dimethyl sulfide). The toxicity of methionine is a result of its metabolism by GI bacteria to mercaptans, because intravenous methionine has no effect on patients in liver failure. Signs of methionine toxicity can be reversed by prior treatment with oral antibiotics that suppress GI flora (Breen, 1972). Doses of 25 gm of oral methionine will induce encephalopathy in dogs with portocaval shunts (Merino et al., 1975).

SHORT-CHAIN FATTY ACIDS (SCFA)

SCFA (5-6-8-carbon; butyric, octanoic, valeric acids) have also been implicated in the production of HE in animals and humans, although evidence of their role in encephalopathy is more circumstantial than that of ammonia or mercaptans (Breen and Schenker, 1972, Schenker et al., 1974, Zieve, 1981). They arise primarily from dietary medium-chain triglycerides but may also be synthesized from carbohydrates and amino acids by intestinal bacteria. SCFA are known to act synergistically with ammonia and mercaptans, and their effects are augmented by increased concentrations of aromatic amino acids in blood (Zieve, 1981).

ALTERATIONS IN CIRCULATING AMINO ACIDS— BRANCHED CHAIN VS. AROMATIC AMINO ACID IMBALANCE

Alterations in the concentrations of circulating amino acids are consistently identified in patients with liver failure and considered to have a role in the genesis of HE. The normal ratio between the concentration of circulating branched-chain amino acids (BCAA) (leucine, isoleucine, valine) and the aromatic amino acids (AAA) (phenylalanine, tyrosine, and tryptophan) is 3.03:1.0. This ratio is disrupted in hepatic failure. In hepatic failure, the serum BCAA:AAA ratio is 1.5:1 or less (Fanelli et al., 1986). BCAA are utilized by the brain for synthesis of the normal excitatory neurotransmitters norepinephrine and dopamine. They compete with AAA for entry into the brain. When the BCAA:AAA ratio decreases, the potential for increased entry of AAA into the CNS is enhanced. When large quantities of AAA gain entry into the CNS, they are utilized in the synthesis of both weak neurotransmitters and inhibitory neurotransmitters.

In liver failure, accelerated uptake of BCAA by muscle tissue occurs, decreasing serum concentrations of BCAA. The liver is the primary site of AAA metabolism by the body, and in liver failure, decreased removal of AAA occurs. The increase in circulating AAA favors their entry into the brain and is hypothesized to result in increased synthesis of false and inhibitory neurotransmitters, leading to depressed neurologic function (Jensen, 1986). Unfortunately, evidence now casts doubt on the importance of false or weak neurotransmitters in the production of HE (Zieve, 1981). It appears that altered BCAA:AAA ratios correlate better with the severity of portosystemic shunting and the degree of liver failure than with the presence or absence of HE (Eriksson and Conn, 1989).

GAMMA-AMINOBUTYRIC ACID

The newest research into the pathogenesis of HE suggests that a disruption in the fine balance between normal excitatory and inhibitory neurotransmitter substances within the brain is tilted toward inhibition (Jones et al., 1984). The most important inhibitory mediators in the CNS are GABA and glycine. The GABA receptor is complexed with separate binding sites for both benzodiazepines and barbiturates, which mediate the centrally active hypnotic and sedative effects of these drugs. An increase in receptor density of affinity may explain the heightened sensitivity of patients in hepatic failure to small amounts of these compounds (Jones et al., 1984). GABA is produced endogenously in the brain, but compounds with GABA-like activity are also present in portal blood and are produced by GI bacteria (*Escherichia coli* and *Bacteroides fragilis*) (Jones et al., 1984). Hemorrhage into the GI tract is also associated with increased absorption of substances with GABA-like activity from the bowel (Jones et al., 1984). The liver is the main site of clearance of these substances with GABA-like activity from portal blood, and in liver failure, concentrations of GABA increase in plasma. Uncontrolled clinical trials in humans suggest that dramatic reversal of HE may occur following the use of an experimental benzodiazepine antagonist, flumazenil (Ferenci et al., 1989). This class of compounds may offer unique alternatives to therapy of HE in the future if further studies validate their effectiveness.

SYNERGISM THEORY—INCREASED CEREBRAL SENSITIVITY

Because no single theory has been able to explain all cases of HE, several of the previously mentioned factors are proposed to work synergistically to induce coma. This has been shown to be true for ammonia, SCFA, methionine, and methanethiol (Merino et al., 1975; Zieve et al., 1974). Coma can be precipitated in susceptible individuals by drugs and other factors (infection, sedatives, electrolyte imbalances, hypoxia) that are well tolerated by normal individuals (Breen and Schenker, 1972). Certainly, the increased sensitivity that patients with liver failure have to barbiturates and benzodiazepines may now be explained by the new information about the GABA receptor complex (Basile and Gammal, 1988; Jones et al., 1989). Clinicians

must be cautious when using any drug in animals with liver failure, because precipitation of encephalopathy is a real possibility, and it may not be recognized that the coma was iatrogenically induced.

DIAGNOSIS

HE is a clinical syndrome. It is diagnosed by a combination of historical information, physical examination findings, and laboratory data supporting that significant liver disease is present in a patient in which no other cause for encephalopathy can be identified. In many cases, the diagnosis is one of exclusion, and therapeutic response is the best support for the diagnosis. Clinicians must maintain a high index of suspicion for HE in cases of unexplained coma or bizarre neurologic behavior in patients with no prior history of liver disease. Routine screening biochemical profiles are usually abnormal in these animals; however, in young dogs or cats with congenital portosystemic shunts or urea cycle enzyme deficiencies, function tests (bromosulfophthalein, ammonia tolerance, fasting and postprandial bile acid assay) may be necessary to appreciate the severity of liver failure.

The laboratory test most often used to support a diagnosis of HE is the blood ammonia concentration. The disadvantages of this test are its relatively limited clinical availability, the unreliability of samples that are not run within 30 min of collection, and the finding that some patients with HE have normal blood ammonia concentrations. Fasting arterial ammonia concentrations have been the most reliable in human patients for documenting HE (Jensen, 1986). Results of other routine screening or function tests for liver disease may be abnormal but do not clearly define whether the identified liver abnormality is the cause of CNS signs in a particular patient. If other metabolic and organic diseases that can cause encephalopathy are ruled out, then HE is probable.

THERAPY

The goal of therapy in patients with HE is to control the pathophysiologic mechanisms responsible for inducing the encephalopathy while the liver attempts to regenerate or maintain sufficient function to support life. This is accomplished by (1) early recognition and correction of precipitating causes of the encephalopathy, (2) reducing the entry, production, and absorption of gastrointestinal "toxins," (3) and providing supportive and symptomatic care.

Important precipitating causes of HE were discussed previously. Clinicians should avoid the use of sedatives, anesthetics, and analgesics unless absolutely indicated. Infectious complications should be looked for and treated aggressively. Hypoxia and other causes of acid-base abnormalities (metabolic and respiratory alkalosis) should be corrected if present. Electrolyte abnormalities such as hypokalemia or hyponatremia must be corrected. Finally, hypoglycemia, renal failure, GI bleeding, and constipation should be controlled or eliminated.

Reducing the entry, production, and absorption of GI toxins is accomplished by elimination or reduction of protein intake, suppression or elimination of urease-producing intestinal bacteria, and catharsis. For animals exhibiting signs of encephalopathy, all oral intake of food should cease until CNS signs abate. This is particularly important for protein. Cessation of food intake eliminates dietary sources of ammonia, toxic amines, AAA, and SCFA, which induce encephalopathy. Next, complete catharsis of the colon should be done. Emptying the colon rapidly decreases numbers of colonic bacteria and removes potentially toxic by-products of bacterial metabolism. Although warm water enemas are most often used, a more effective method combines substances that impair ammonia production or absorption in the enema solution. Using a 10% povidone-iodine solution as the enema fluid or adding liquid neomycin sulfate (22 mg/kg) to the enema fluid results in more efficient, rapid suppression of colonic bacteria, which generate the majority of the blood ammonia. Enemas should be repeated until no fecal material is evident in the evacuated fluid.

Another drug that is highly effective in lowering blood ammonia concentrations when added to enema fluid is lactulose (1-4-beta-galactosidofructose [Cephulac, Merrell Dow]). When lactulose reaches the colon, intestinal bacteria hydrolyze it to lactic, acetic, and formic acids, which dramatically lower colon pH. The large quantities of unabsorbed solutes produced after lactulose metabolism also induce an osmotic diarrhea (Fingl, 1980). Blood ammonia concentrations are lowered through several unique attributes of lactulose. By-products of lactulose fermentation produce what is termed *ionic trapping* of ammonia within the colon. In an acid environment, ammonia (NH_3) accepts a proton to form ammonium (NH_4^+). Ammonium is much less diffusible than ammonia. Thus, ammonium ions remain within the colon and are excreted rather than absorbed. This effect occurs at a colon pH of 6.2 or less and is most noticeable if the colon pH is 5.0 or less (Vince and Burridge, 1980). Lactulose also inhibits ammonia generation by colonic bacteria through a process known as *catabolite repression* (Vince and Burridge, 1980). By providing a carbohydrate source to intestinal bacteria, less proteolysis, peptide degradation, and deamination of bacterial proteins occur. Significantly less ammonia

thus is generated by colonic bacteria than they would produce under other circumstances, and this effect is independent of the pH effect. Improvement is noted in 80 to 90% of human patients using lactulose enemas, whereas warm water enemas benefit only 20% (Uribe et al., 1987). Lactulose is diluted with warm water (30% lactulose, 70% water) and given as a retention enema. Approximately 20 to 30 ml/kg is infused and retained in the colon for 20 to 30 min before evacuation. The pH of the evacuated fluid is measured, and if greater than 6.0, another lactulose enema should be administered. Improvement in neurologic status can occur within 2 hr.

As soon as patients are able to tolerate oral liquids, attempts should be made to decrease urease-containing bacteria within the gut by using nonabsorbable intestinal antibiotics. The antibiotic used most commonly for this purpose is neomycin sulfate, although kanamycin, vancomycin, and paromomycin may be used interchangeably. The recommended dosage of neomycin sulfate in dogs and cats is 20 mg/kg every 6 to 8 hr. Other beneficial effects of the use of oral antibiotics are to decrease bacterial deamination of amino acid and reduce the production of AAA, circulating false neurotransmitters, mercaptans, and SCFA by gut bacteria (Breen and Schenker 1972; Fischer et al., 1974; Schenker et al., 1974). In human patients, chronic use of neomycin is associated with rare complications, including ototoxicity and nephrotoxicity, severe diarrhea, and intestinal malabsorption. A number of other systemically absorbed antibiotics may be used as alternatives to aminoglycosides in animals with hepatic failure. One that has received a great deal of interest is metronidazole (Flagyl, Searle). Metronidazole is active against many urease-positive, gram-negative anaerobes that are potent generators of ammonia in the intestinal tract (Morgan et al., 1982). Most clinical studies have indicated that metronidazole is equal in effectiveness to neomycin in controlling blood ammonia concentrations (Morgan et al., 1982). The recommended dosage is 20 mg/kg every 8 hr. Neurotoxicity following metronidazole use has been reported in dogs, and this adverse reaction may be more likely to develop in animals in hepatic failure. This is because the half-life of this drug can increase by as much as threefold in the presence of decreased hepatic clearance (Loft et al., 1987). In humans, therapeutic blood levels may be achieved through once-daily or every-other-day administration. Neurotoxic manifestations of metronidazole toxicity may be confused with signs of HE (Loft et al., 1987). Many animals also respond to other antibiotics, such as ampicillin, that are effective against intestinal anaerobes. Animals improve clinically while receiving antibiotics but develop signs of illness when antibiotics are stopped. This phenomenon likely corresponds to the effects the drug has on GI flora, an effect that stops soon after it is discontinued.

Oral lactulose may be used as an alternative to or in conjunction with intestinal antibiotics in the management of hepatic coma. Most surveys indicate that either latulose or neomycin alone provides clinical improvement in 80% of humans with chronic encephalopathy (Atterbury et al., 1978). Additional patients will benefit from the combination of neomycin and lactulose because the drugs are sometimes synergistic. Neomycin inhibits bacterial degradation of lactulose in less than a third of patients (Orlandi et al., 1981). Lactulose is degraded by lactulosophilic bacteria, of which *Bacteroides* predominates. *Bacteroides* is fairly resistant to the effects of neomycin. To determine whether effective latulose degradation is occurring in animals receiving both drugs, measure stool pH after 7 to 14 days of combined therapy. If the stool pH is less than 6, lactulose is being metabolized and neomycin is not impairing its effectiveness. If stool pH remains around 7, lactulose will be ineffective and should be discontinued. Lactulose is dosed so that a decrease in fecal pH is produced, but diarrhea is avoided. Cats usually require 2.5 to 5.0 ml every 8 hr, and dogs require 2.5 to 25.0 ml every 8 hr. If watery diarrhea develops, the dose should be reduced.

Alternative methods of controlling HE may be tried but are not likely to be as effective as lactulose and neomycin. Attempts may be made to repopulate the colon with lactose-fermenting, non–urease-containing bacteria such as lactobacilli. Unfortunately, supplementing the diet with lactobacillus-containing drugs or yogurt in quantities sufficient to maintain desirable flora in adequate numbers has not met with clinical success.

Specifically formulated intravenous solutions containing primarily BCAA as the nitrogen source have been marketed for use in the therapy of acute hepatic encephalopathy (Hepatamine, American McGaw). These solutions are designed to help normalize plasma amino acid patterns by decreasing muscle catabolism. Decreasing muscle breakdown reduces the concentration of circulating AAA. Experimental work in encephalopathic dogs indicated that use of these preparations resulted in marked improvement in neurologic status (Fruend et al., 1979). However, the majority of the published results in humans with chronic encephalopathy does not support that it provides significant benefit over other well-balanced amino acid solutions (Michel et al., 1985). Clinicians must be extremely cautious when using inexpensive intravenous protein hydrolysates in animals in hepatic coma. Such solutions have extremely high ammonia concentrations, 1500 to 1900 μgm/dl, and may rapidly worsen the clinical status of the patient (Strombeck et al., 1975). Stored blood may also be dangerous in this regard.

Another drug that may be considered for use in encephalopathic dogs or cats that fail to respond to traditional therapy is L-dopa (Larodopa, Roche). L-dopa is a precursor to norepinephrine and dopamine, and when given orally, it raises cerebral dopamine concentrations (Szcerban and Rozya, 1979). Evidence now suggests that the beneficial effects of L-dopa result from increased renal ammonia elimination and not from improved cerebral neurotransmitter concentrations (Jensen, 1986). It has been used with some success in acute hepatic coma. Human patients usually respond by regaining full consciousness in 6 to 12 hr. Unfortunately, responses may be transient even though therapy is continued. The recommended dosages, based on those used in humans, would be an initial dose of 6.8 mg/kg followed by 1.4 mg/kg every 6 hr. No information regarding the safety or efficacy of L-dopa in animals is available.

Additional supportive measures may be necessary in the management of animals with HE. Parenteral fluid therapy is often required for several days in patients with hepatic failure, and the fluid chosen can be an important therapeutic decision. Animals with chronic liver failure are often hypokalemic, alkalotic, and prone to sodium retention (Twedt, 1985). The ideal fluid should be supplemented with potassium; it should also be low in sodium and nonalkalizing. Sodium bicarbonate is given only if metabolic acidosis develops and is severe (pH < 7.1). Fluids containing lactate may be ineffective as alkalizing agents because the liver is the site of conversion of lactate to bicarbonate and glucose. Either half-strength saline (0.45%) or half-strength saline plus 2.5% dextrose is a good choice for fluid needs in an animal with liver failure. These fluids should be supplemented with approximately 20 mEq/L of potassium chloride. Glucose supplementation is beneficial in preventing hypoglycemia and in decreasing peripheral catabolic processes; it may also directly decrease brain ammonia concentrations.

FULMINANT HEPATIC FAILURE

Fulminant hepatic failure is a syndrome associated with acute, massive necrosis of parenchymal cells and sudden severe impairment of hepatic function. It is uncommon in small animals but deserves special mention because the approach to therapy differs from that of more chronic, less aggressive forms of liver failure. Before beginning intensive supportive therapy, attempts should be made to determine whether an acute process is present and not the end stages of chronic progressive hepatic disease. Although the prognosis for survival is generally guarded to poor initially, these animals have the potential for complete recovery if they survive the first few days of acute illness. Patients with chronic progressive liver failure with end-stage clinical signs will not survive their illness, and heroic efforts are unwarranted.

Patients that die in fulminant hepatic failure do so because of cerebral edema, hemorrhage and sepsis, not because of the loss of hepatic parenchyma (Corall and Williams, 1986; Hetzel, 1985; Payne, 1986). Cerebral edema may develop rapidly in patients with HE, particularly those with acute fulminant hepatic failure. CNS signs are due to the combined effects of HE and edema on the brain. The edema is primarily of vasogenic origin (Corall and Williams, 1986). Permeability of the blood-brain barrier is altered, allowing circulating toxins and plasma proteins to egress from intracranial capillaries into the extracellular space. In the presence of hypoalbuminemia, this process is accelerated. Determining whether the CNS signs present in a patient with HE are due to liver failure or cerebral edema is difficult (Ede and Williams, 1986). The diagnostic test of choice in humans is computed tomography. Cerebrospinal fluid pressure is constantly measured with a manometer. Papilledema is a rare finding. Changes in pupillary light response in one or both pupils are a reliable indication of increased intracranial pressure (Ede and Williams, 1986). Increases in muscle tone of the arms and legs, hyperventilation, and decerebrate posture all can be seen (Ede and Williams, 1986). Any rapid deterioration in the state of consciousness suggests that cerebral edema is developing. In general, if a patient's neurologic status continues to deteriorate despite aggressive management of HE, it is wise to treat for cerebral edema for 12 to 24 hr rather than do nothing.

Therapy of cerebral edema in fulminant hepatic failure involves the use of mannitol and furosemide. Furosemide is synergistic with mannitol in dogs (Ede and Williams, 1986). Steroids are ineffective in this form of edema (Payne, 1986). A 20% solution of mannitol is given at a dose of 1 gm/kg IV over 30 min and is repeated every 4 hr if the patient does not improve neurologically. Furosemide is given simultaneously at 1 to 2 mg/kg IV every 8 hr for two to three doses. If hypoproteinemia is present, plasma transfusions are indicated to increase plasma oncotic pressure.

Hypoglycemia may be severe in fulminant hepatic failure. Blood glucose concentrations must be closely monitored and, if low, treated aggressively. Intravenous glucose may have to be given as 10 to 20% solutions in order to maintain normal blood glucose concentrations.

Sepsis is the cause of death of 10 to 15% of humans with fulminant hepatic failure. It is extremely important that great care be taken to prevent sepsis during catheter placement and to rapidly control any infections that develop. Broad-spectrum antibiotics (ampicillin plus aminoglycosides, cephalosporins, quinolones) should routinely be administered.

Hemorrhage occurs early and often in fulminant hepatic failure. Bleeding from any location in the body may be evident. Hemorrhage is usually secondary to decreases in prothrombin-dependent clotting factors. Increasing the gastric pH to > 4 with intravenous cimetidine (Tagamet, Smith Kline Beckman; 5 mg/kg every 4 to 6 hr) or ranitidine (Zantac, Glaxo; 2 mg/kg every 8 hr) significantly reduces GI bleeding (Hetzel, 1985). Fresh whole blood is needed to control acute bleeding in these situations. The use of injectable vitamin K_1 (1.0 to 2.5 mg/kg SC every 24 hr) is indicated because it may be rapidly incorporated into prothrombin by newly regenerating hepatocytes.

Renal failure occurs in as many as 40% of patients with fulminant hepatic failure and is termed *hepatorenal syndrome*. When it is present, the prognosis is usually very poor. Hepatorenal syndrome appears to result from intense renal vasoconstriction, which may cause acute tubular nephrosis. Therapeutic measures are often ineffective in reversing this problem. Prerenal components must be reversed rapidly. Hemodialysis is often necessary to support patients with this syndrome (Corall and Williams, 1986).

Glucocorticoids do not appear to offer significant benefit to patients with fulminant hepatic failure, particularly if it is viral in origin. Experimental work in toxic hepatic failure now suggests that methylprednisolone may improve survival (Miuk et al., 1986). Because steroids may aggravate GI bleeding tendencies and impair the host defense mechanisms against infection, they should be used with caution.

References and Suggested Reading

Aldrete, J. S.: Quantification of the capacity of the liver to remove ammonia from the circulation of dogs with portacaval transposition. Surg. Gynecol. Obstet. 141:399, 1975.
Experimental study to determine the ability of a dog's liver to remove ammonia from portal blood.
Atterbury, C. E., Maddrey, W. C., and Conn, H. O.: Neomycin-sorbitol and lactulose in the treatment of acute portal systemic encephalopathy. Dig. Dis. Sci. 23:398, 1978.
Human clinical trial comparing efficacy of neomycin, sorbitol, and lactulose in HE therapy.
Basile, A., and Gammal, S.: Evidence for the involvement of the benzodiazepine receptor complex in hepatic encephalopathy: Implications for treatment with benzodiazepine receptor antagonists. Clin. Neuropharmacol. 11:410, 1988.
Experimental study of CNS receptors important in HE and the possibility of using benzodiazepine antagonists.
Breen, K. J., and Schenker, S.: Hepatic coma: Present concepts of pathogenesis and therapy. *In* Popper, H., and Schaffner, F. (eds.): *Progress in Liver Disease IV.* New York: Grune & Stratton, 1972.
Excellent review article on hepatic encephalopathy.
Corall, I., and Williams, R.: Management of liver failure. Br. J. Anaesth. 58:234, 1986.
Good review of therapy of fulminant hepatic failure.
Ede, R. J., and Williams, R.: Hepatic encephalopathy and cerebral edema. Semin. Liver Dis. 6:107, 1986.

Discussion of the pathogenesis of cerebral edema in fulminant hepatic failure.

Eriksson, L. S., and Conn, H. O.: Branched-chain amino acids in the management of hepatic encephalopathy: An analysis of variants. Hepatology 10:228, 1989.
Questions the pathogenesis of HE in terms of BCAA:AAA imbalances.

Fanelli, F. R., Cangiano, C., Capocaccio, L., et al.: Use of branched chain amino acids for treating hepatic encephalopathy: Clinical experiences. Gut 27:111, 1986.
Therapeutic trial in humans supporting value of BCAA in therapy of HE.

Ferenci, P., Grimm, G., Meryn, S., et al.: Successful long-term treatment of portal-systemic encephalopathy by the benzodiazepine antagonist flumazenil. Gastroenterology 96:240, 1989.
One of first uncontrolled observations to support the value of benzodiazepine antagonists in therapy of chronic HE.

Fingl, E.: Laxatives and cathartics. In Goodman, A., and Gillman, L. S. (eds.): The Pharmacological Basis of Therapeutics, 6th ed. New York: MacMillan, 1980, p. 1009.
Pharmacology of lactulose.

Fischer, J. E., Deane, J., Dodsworth, J., et al.: An alternative mechanism for beneficial effects of intestinal sterilization in hepatic encephalopathy. Surg. Forum 25:369, 1974.

Fraser, C. L., and Arieff, A. I.: Hepatic encephalopathy. N. Engl. J. Med. 313:865, 1975.
Good review article on the pathogenesis of HE.

Fruend, H., Yoshimura, N., and Fischer, J.: Chronic hepatic encephalopathy. Long-term therapy with a branched-chain amino acid enriched diet. J.A.M.A. 24:347, 1979.
Clinical trial in humans supporting the value of BCAA-enriched diets for therapy of HE.

Hetzel, D. G.: Fulminant hepatic failure. Anaesth. Intensive Care 13:272, 1985.
Review of hepatic failuure.

Jensen, D. M.: Portal systemic encephalopathy and hepatic coma. Med. Clin. North Am. 70:1081, 1986.
Good review article of the etiopathogenesis of HE.

Jones, E. A., Schaffner, D. F., Ferenci, L., et al.: The neurobiology of hepatic encephalopathy. Hepatology 4:1235, 1984.
Discussion of new information on GABA receptors in the CNS.

Jones, E., Skolnick, P., Gammal, S., et al.: NIH conference: The gamma-aminobutyric acid-a (GABA) receptor complex and hepatic encephalopathy: Some recent advances. Ann. Intern. Med. 110:532, 1989.
Discusses the interaction between GABA, barbiturates, and benzodiazepines on CNS receptor sites.

Loft, S., Sonne, J., and Dossing, M.: Metronidazole pharmacokinetics in patients with hepatic encephalopathy. Scand. J. Gastroenterol. 22:117, 1987.
Documents the prolonged half-life of metronidazole in humans with HE.

Merino, G. E., Jetzer, T., Dorzaki, W. F. D., et al.: Methionine induced hepatic coma in dogs. Am. J. Surg. 130:41, 1975.
Experimental study of effects of methionine on CNS function in dogs with HE.

Michel, H., Bories, P., Aubin, J. P., et al.: Treatment of acute hepatic encephalopathy in cirrhotics with a branched chain amino acid enriched vs a conventional amino acid mixture: A controlled study of 70 patients. Liver 5:282, 1985.

Clinical trial in humans with HE refuting the benefit of BCAA-enriched diets over conventional methods.

Miuk, G. Y., Sherman, T. A., Shaffer, E. A., et al.: A comparative study of the effects of insulin/glucagon infusions, parenteral amino acids and high dose corticosteroids on survival in a rabbit model of fulminant hepatitis. Hepatology 6:73, 1986.
Experimental study in rabbits supporting the role of prednisolone in acute therapy of hepatic failure.

Morgan, M. H., Read, A. E., and Speller, D. C. E.: Treatment of hepatic encephalopathy with metronidazole. Gut 23:1, 1982.
Compares metronidazole with other antibiotics in HE of humans.

Orlandi, F., Freddara, U., Candelaresi, M. T., et al.: Comparison between neomycin and lactulose in 173 patients with hepatic encephalopathy: A randomized clinical study. Dig. Dis. Sci. 26:498, 1981.
Clinical trial in humans supporting the benefit of combined neomycin and lactulose in chronic HE.

Payne, J. A.: Fulminant hepatic failure. Med. Clin. North Am. 70:1067, 1986.
Good discussion of pathogenesis and therapy.

Schafer, D. F.: Hepatic coma: Studies on the target organ. Gastroenterology 93:1131, 1987.
Review of pathogenesis.

Schenker, S., Breen, K. J., and Hoyumpa, A. M.: Hepatic encephalopathy: Current status. Gastroenterology 66:121, 1974.
Excellent review article on the pathogenesis of HE.

Strombeck, D. R., Weiser, M. G., and Kaneko, J. J.: Hyperammonemia and hepatic encephalopathy in the dog. J.A.V.M.A. 166:1105, 1975.
Clinical study of blood ammonia alterations in hepatic failure in dogs.

Szcerban, J., and Rozya, J.: Treatment of acute and chronic portal encephalopathy with the precursors of dopamine. Acta Med. Pol. 20:249, 1979.
Clinical application of L-dopa in the treatment of HE.

Twedt, D. C.: Cirrhosis: A consequence of chronic liver disease. Vet. Clin. North Am. 15:151, 1985.
Reviews therapeutic principles for dogs with chronic liver failure.

Uribe, M., Campollo, O., Vargas, F., et al.: Acidifying emenas (lactitol and lactulose) vs. non-acidifying enemas (tap water) to treat acute aportal systemic encephalopathy: A double-blind, randomized clinical trial. Hepatology 7:639, 1987.
Documents the benefit of lactulose or lactitol over warm water enemas in spontaneous liver failure in humans.

Vince, A. J., and Burridge, S. M.: Ammonia production by intestinal bacteria: The effects of lactose, lactulose and glucose. J. Med. Microbiol. 13:177, 1980.
Experimental study on mechanisms by which lactulose lowers blood ammonia.

Weber, F. L., Fresare, K. M., and Lally, B. R.: Effects of lactulose and neomycin on urea metabolism in cirrhotic subjects. Gastroenterology 82:213, 1982.
Study documenting the benefit of lactulose and neomycin in humans with spontaneous chronic liver failure.

Zieve, L., Doizaki, W. M., and Zieve, F. J.: Synergism between mercaptans and ammonia or fatty acids in the production of coma: A possible role for mercaptans in the pathogenesis of hepatic coma. J. Lab. Clin. Med. 83:16, 1974.
Proposed synergism theory of HE.

Zieve, L.: The mechanism of hepatic coma. Hepatology 1:360, 1981.
Good review article on the pathogenesis of HE.

Section
9

CARDIOPULMONARY DISEASES

BRUCE W. KEENE

Consulting Editor

CAUSES AND PREVALENCE OF CARDIOVASCULAR DISEASE

JAMES W. BUCHANAN
Philadelphia, Pennsylvania

The types and prevalence of heart disease in dogs in the Philadelphia area were characterized 30 years ago in a survey of 5000 dogs at the University of Pennsylvania (Detweiler and Patterson, 1965). Eleven per cent of the dogs had reliable signs of heart disease, and another 9% had possible heart disease. Congenital heart disease (CHD) was recognized in 0.56% of the dogs (1% if referral cases were included). In recent years, the overall prevalence of heart disease appears to be similar, but comparable epidemiologic data for acquired abnormalities in the United States are not available. A clinical review in Italy found heart disease in 11% of 7148 dogs (Fioretti and Delli Carri, 1988).

CHD may have increased in overall frequency compared with 30 years ago. At the University of Pennsylvania during 1987 to 1989, CHD was diagnosed in 150 of 22,283 dogs (0.67%). The nationwide Veterinary Medical Data Base (VMDB) at Purdue University during the same period recorded CHD in 1320 of 154,233 dogs (0.85%). However, the same source in 1964 to 1971 reported CHD in only 642 of 138,921 dogs (0.46%) (Mulvihill and Priester, 1973). The increased rate of diagnoses may be due to increased prevalence of CHD, but it is more likely that improved diagnostic methods and more trained cardiologists nationwide account for the increased rate of recorded CHD. It should be recognized also that prevalence rates are influenced by denominator differences in hospital populations such as heartworm incidence, breed predispositions, and breed popularity in different areas and countries; thus crude (unadjusted) prevalence rates should be viewed with caution.

The specific causes of some diseases have been identified in recent years, and it is apparent that genetic factors have a role in some "acquired" abnormalities as well as most congenital abnormalities. Because of space limitations here and thorough reviews in other textbooks, only the most common abnormalities and those with breed predispositions or recently reported relevant information will be reviewed here.

CANINE CONGENITAL HEART DISEASE

Breed predispositions for certain forms of CHD were suggested in the pioneering epidemiologic studies by Detweiler and Patterson. Specific predispositions and heritability were subsequently confirmed by examination of related animals, breeding experiments, and genetic analyses (Patterson, 1968). Nearly all breeding experiments yielded positive results and supported the hypothesis that common congenital cardiac abnormalities in dogs are usually inherited as polygenic threshold traits (Patterson, 1989).

Although many of the breed predispositions observed 25 to 30 years ago still exist, there have been several additions and changes, and some anomalies now occur more frequently and predominantly in breeds that apparently were not previously predisposed. The best example is the occurrence of subvalvular aortic stenosis (SAS) in golden retriever and Rottweiler dogs in recent years. Other investigators also have noted increased frequency of SAS in these breeds, but published data have not included reference population information, so breed-specific relative risks could not be assessed. Other breed-associated abnormalities also have been mentioned by various investigators, but population data usually have not been given. Such reports are helpful in identifying familial disease patterns and alerting others to new diseases in certain breeds but have not permitted estimation of relative risk.

In order to determine current breed risks more accurately, CHD diagnoses in 1320 dogs registered in the VMDB in 1987 to 1989 were evaluated. Results for the most common diseases are summarized in Tables 1 through 6.

Patent ductus arteriosus (PDA) is still the most common form of CHD nationwide (Table 1). In a total of 418 dogs, it occurred in 61 different breeds. Females outnumbered males by 3:1. The odds ratios (OR) in breeds represented by 5 or more affected animals indicate increased risk in several breeds in addition to those previously identified (Ackerman et al., 1978; Patterson, 1968). Although the disease is still common in toy and miniature poodles, the estimated relative risks in Maltese, Pomeranians, Shetland sheepdogs, English springer spaniels, keeshonden, and bichons frises are greater (Table 2).

Supported by the Bernard and Muriel Freeman Heart Research Fund.

Table 1. *Comparative Frequencies of Congenital Heart Disease in Dogs*

	% of All Canine CHD Cases		
	UP-1 Series (n=276)	UP-2 Series (n=150)	VMDB Series (n=1320)
Patent ductus arteriosus	25.3	24.7	31.7
Pulmonic stenosis	17.6	11.3	18.3
Aortic stenosis	12.3	34.6	22.1
Persistent right aortic arch	7.1	3.3	4.5
Ventricular septal defect	6.2	7.3	6.6
Atrial septal defect	3.7	3.0	0.7
Tetralogy of Fallot	3.4	4.0	2.7
Tricuspid dysplasia	—	7.3	2.4
Other defects	23.4	4.5	10.9
	100.0	100.0	100.0

UP-1: University of Pennsylvania, 1958–1965 (Patterson, 1968).
UP-2: University of Pennsylvania, 1987–1989.
VMDB: Veterinary Medical Data Base at Purdue University, 1987–1989.
—, Frequency less than 3.4%; included in other defects.

Inheritance of PDA and ductus diverticulum occurred as a polygenic threshold trait in a mixed poodle strain of dogs developed by Patterson and colleagues (1971). Failure of ductus closure in this strain had a morphologic basis and was due to graded hypoplasia of ductus-specific smooth muscle and elastic wall substitution in areas that should have been muscular (Buchanan, 1978). Similar abnormalities were found in serial section histologic studies of PDAs in Pomeranian, keeshond, collie, and cocker spaniel dogs, indicating that the pathogenesis of PDA in most dogs is probably the same as in the strain of dogs with hereditary PDA.

Aortic stenosis is the most common CHD observed at this institution but was second in fre-

quency nationwide (see Table 1). There was no significant gender predilection. The data include all forms of left ventricular outflow tract (LVOT) obstruction, because it is often difficult to determine the level of obstruction without angiocardiography or necropsy. In confirmed cases, nearly all dogs with LVOT obstruction have fibrous or fibromuscular SAS. However, studies now suggest that hyperdynamic functional LVOT obstruction in golden retrievers may be more common than indicated by previous studies (Jones, 1989) (see this volume, p. 760). Newfoundlands still have the greatest risk for SAS, but golden retrievers were observed more frequently because of their greater breed popularity (Table 3). Hereditary transmission and pathology in Newfoundlands was demonstrated several years ago (Pyle et al., 1976). German shepherds represent a large proportion of clinical cases because of their breed popularity, but they have only a mildly increased relative risk as a breed. Screening clinics to detect SAS in high-risk breeds have been recommended, but the results are difficult to interpret. A recent survey of 83 asymptomatic golden retrievers at an auscultation clinic revealed that 60% of the dogs had grade I–II/VI systolic murmurs "typical of subaortic stenosis" (O'Grady et al., 1989). Doppler echocardiography to measure blood flow velocity is used to confirm the diagnosis of LVOT obstruction, but there is disagreement about the definition and significance of mildly increased flow velocities. Peak LVOT flow velocities less than 1.5 m/sec are normal, and most cardiologists regard velocities greater than 2.5 m/sec as indicative of organic or functional obstruction.

Pulmonic stenosis is the third most frequent CHD (see Table 1). Nationwide it was most common by far in English bulldogs, but that breed was not represented among 17 dogs with pulmonic stenosis in our series of 150 dogs with all forms of CHD. It occurred with equal frequency in males and females of all breeds except English bulldogs, of which 24 of 30 (80%) were males (Table 4). Studies indicate

Table 2. *Patent Ductus Arteriosus—Estimated Relative Risks (Odds Ratios) by Breed (n=418)**

Breed ≥ 5 Cases	No.	Odds Ratio	95% Confidence Limits	P
Maltese	15	9.6	5.5–16.5	<.0001
Pomeranian	18	7.0	4.2–11.5	<.0001
Shetland sheepdog	35	5.3	3.7–7.6	<.0001
English springer spaniel	29	4.9	3.3–7.2	<.0001
Keeshond	6	4.8	1.9–11.1	.002
Bichon frise	5	4.1	1.5–10.5	.008
Toy poodle	20	3.5	2.1–5.5	<.0001
Miniature poodle	30	3.1	2.1–4.6	<.0001
Yorkshire terrier	14	2.9	1.6–5.1	<.001
Chihuahua	6	2.1	0.8–4.9	NS
Collie	14	2.0	1.1–3.4	.022
Standard poodle	10	1.8	0.9–3.5	NS
Cocker spaniel	26	1.4	0.9–2.1	NS
German shepherd	27	1.3	0.8–1.9	NS

*Data from Veterinary Medical Data Base (VMDB) at Purdue University, 1987–1989.
NS, not significant.

Table 3. *Aortic Stenosis—Estimated Relative Risks (Odds Ratios) by Breed (n=292)**

Breed ≥ 5 Cases	No.	Odds Ratio	95% Confidence Limits	P
Newfoundland	41	40.5	28.4–57.5	<.0001
Golden retriever	78	7.2	5.5–9.4	<.0001
Rottweiler	29	7.1	4.8–10.7	<.0001
Boxer	16	5.4	3.2–9.2	<.0001
Samoyed	7	2.8	1.2–6.1	.016
Bulldog	6	2.7	1.1–6.4	.026
Great Dane	6	2.4	1.0–5.7	.041
German shepherd	32	2.3	1.5–3.3	<.0001

*Data from Veterinary Medical Data Base (VMDB) at Purdue University, 1987–1989.

Table 4. Pulmonic Stenosis—Estimated Relative Risks (Odds Ratios) by Breed (n = 298)*

Breed ≥ 5 Cases	No.	Odds Ratio	95% Confidence Limits	P
English bulldog	30	19.2	12.8–28.7	<.0001
Mastiff	5	11.6	4.2–29.4	<.0001
Samoyed	11	5.4	2.8–10.1	<.0001
Miniature schnauzer	14	3.5	2.0–6.2	<.0001
West Highland white terrier	5	3.3	1.2–8.3	.020
Chow chow	5	2.2	0.8–5.5	NS
Cocker spaniel	18	1.7	1.0–2.8	.026

*Data from Veterinary Medical Data Base (VMDB) at Purdue University, 1987–1989.
NS, not significant.

that an important cause of pulmonic stenosis in this breed is external compression of the pulmonic valve by an anomalous left coronary artery (Buchanan, 1990). The left main coronary artery arises from a single right coronary artery and encircles and compresses the right ventricular outflow tract adjacent to the base of the pulmonic valve, producing a banding effect.

Valvular pulmonic stenosis was reported in four male Boykin spaniels in Georgia (Jacobs et al., 1990). This breed is a common hunting dog in the Southeast but is not reflected significantly in national data. However, two Boykin spaniels with pulmonic stenosis were recorded in the VMDB, including one from Georgia and one from Alabama. We have studied one female Boykin spaniel (from Virginia) with pulmonic stenosis, indicating that both sexes may have the disease. Valvular pathology described by Jacobs and colleagues and angiocardiography in our case indicate that thickened, dysplastic valves are the cause of the stenosis. A similar form of pulmonic stenosis in beagles was shown to be hereditary (Patterson et al., 1981).

Ventricular septal defects have been recognized in various breeds. Among 87 VMDB entries, only English bulldogs were substantially over-represented (n = 9, OR 15.2). Other breeds with three dogs each include Newfoundland (OR 8.3), chow chow (OR 4.7), Brittany spaniel (OR 4.2), and Samoyed (OR 4.0). Significant sex differences were not observed.

Tricuspid dysplasia has increased in frequency in recent years and currently shares fourth place with ventricular septal defect at our institution (see Table 1). It occurred predominantly in Labrador retrievers in our clinic as well as nationwide. VMDB entries on 32 dogs in 1987 to 1989 included nine Labrador retrievers (OR 5.7), seven German shepherds (OR 5.1), and 3 boxers (OR 9.6). A significant predominance of males (21 of 32 dogs) was noted.

Persistent right aortic arch and related vascular abnormalities were recorded in 60 dogs in the VMDB. German shepherds continue to show moderately increased incidence (n = 8, OR 3.2), but Great Danes had a higher risk estimate (n = 5, OR 11.9). Cocker spaniels were mildly over-represented (n = 5, OR 2.2). Various other breeds were represented with one to three animals, but no Irish setters were recorded.

Tetralogy of Fallot is a relatively uncommon abnormality, and individual breed totals were insufficient for meaningful statistics. Significant sex differences were not observed. The total of 41 dogs with tetralogy of Fallot included 3 golden retrievers and 2 each of the wirehaired fox terrier, Labrador retriever, Siberian husky, and toy poodle breeds. Various other breeds including the keeshond and English bulldog had one affected animal each. These and other breed predispositions suggested or confirmed by others are indicated by asterisks in Table 5.

Portacaval shunts are the second most common congenital cardiovascular malformation in dogs, and they were found with a frequency equal to that of aortic stenosis. The vascular communications allow portal venous blood to bypass the liver and enter the central venous system, with resultant neurologic signs due to elevated ammonia levels. Analysis of 1987 to 1989 VMDB entries for 298 dogs with portacaval shunts revealed an approximately equal sex distribution and several breed predispositions especially for Yorkshire terriers (Table 6). Portacaval shunts are excluded from Tables 1 and 5 because they are noncardiac abnormalities.

FELINE CONGENITAL HEART DISEASE

CHD appears to occur less commonly in cats than in dogs. Combined data on 287 cats with CHD indicated an overall prevalence of approximately 0.2% (Harpster and Zook, 1987). The types and frequencies of various anomalies also were different. Mitral and tricuspid valve malformations were most common (17%), followed by ventricular septal defect (15%), endocardial fibroelastosis (11%), PDA (11%), vascular anomalies (8%), aortic stenosis (6%), tetralogy of Fallot (6%), atrial septal defect (4%), common atrioventricular (AV) canal (4%), and pulmonic stenosis (3%). Male predominance was reported for AV valve malformation (5:1), aortic stenosis (3:1), endocardial fibroelastosis (9:5), and tricuspid dysplasia (6:1).

VALVE AND ENDOCARDIAL DISEASE

Chronic Valvular Disease

Chronic mitral valvular disease (CVD or endocardiosis) is the most common acquired cardiac abnor-

Table 5. Breed Predilections in Dogs with Congenital Heart Disease*

Airedale terrier	Pulmonic stenosis (PS)-2
Beagle	PS†
Bichon frise	Patent ductus arteriosus (PDA)-2
Boxer	Aortic stenosis (AS)-3
Boykin spaniel	PS†
Bull terrier	Mitral dysplasia (MD)†
Chihuahua	PS†, PDA†
Cocker spaniel	PDA-1, PS-1
Collie	PDA-1
Doberman pinscher	Atrial septal defect (ASD)†
English bulldog	PS-3, ventricular septal defect (VSD)-3, AS-1, tetralogy of Fallot (TF)†
English springer spaniel	PDA-2
German shepherd	Tricuspid dysplasia (TD)-3, AS-1, persistent right aortic arch (PRAA)-2, MD†, PDA†
German short-hair pointer	AS†
Golden retriever	AS-3, TD†
Great Dane	AS-1, PRAA-3, MD†, TD†
Irish setter	PRAA†
Keeshond	PDA-2, TF†
Kerry blue terrier	PDA-3
Labrador retriever	TD-3
Maltese	PDA-3
Mastiff	PS-3
Miniature schnauzer	PS-2
Newfoundland	AS-3
Pomeranian	PDA-3
Poodles	PDA-2
Rottweiler	AS-3
Samoyed	PS-3, AS-1, ASD†
Scottish terrier	PS-2
Shetland sheepdog	PDA-3
West Highland white terrier	PS-3
Weimaraner	TD†, peritoneopericardial hernia†
Yorkshire terrier	PDA-1

*Data from Veterinary Medical Data Base (VMDB) at Purdue University, 1987–1989: 1320 dogs with CHD out of 154,233 dogs. Numbers 1–3 identify predisposed breeds represented by four or more affected dogs in which relative risk for the indicated abnormality was significantly elevated in this series ($P < .05$ to $P < .0001$).

-1: mildly increased risk (Odds ratio 1.5–2.9 times all other dogs).
-2: moderate risk (Odds ratio 3–4.9 times others).
-3: marked risk (Odds ratio >5 times others).
†Breed-associated diseases not confirmed in this study but suggested or confirmed by others.
Sex predominance: PDA (females 3:1), PS in English bulldogs (males 4:1), mitral and tricuspid dysplasia (males 2:1).

mality in dogs. It is a myxomatous degenerative process and affects more than one third of dogs over 10 years of age. When the disease is moderate to severe or a chorda tendinea ruptures, mitral regurgitation occurs and can lead to left heart enlargement and congestive heart failure. Tricuspid valve involvement in the same animals is also frequent but usually less severe. CVD occurs with relatively greater frequency in small dogs, especially the poodle, miniature schnauzer, Chihuahua, cocker spaniel, fox terrier, and Boston terrier breeds (Buchanan, 1977). The disease is slightly more common and more severe in males. An exceptional occurrence of CVD has been noted in Cavalier King Charles spaniel (CKCS) dogs in Great Britain, along with a moderately increased risk in Chihuahuas, miniature poodles, male miniature pinschers, and male whippets (Thrusfield et al., 1985). Stethoscopic examination of 431 CKCSs at dog shows in Great Britain revealed mitral regurgitation murmurs in 31% of all dogs and 59% of those 4 years of age and older (Darke, 1987). Examination of 225 CKCSs at a show in Baltimore, Maryland, in 1990 revealed grades I–V/VI systolic left apical murmurs in 23% of all dogs and 54% of those 4 years and older (Beardow and Buchanan, submitted, 1991).

The clinical course of CVD usually extends over several years, but an abrupt onset of congestive heart failure may occur if major chordae tendineae rupture and mitral regurgitation suddenly becomes severe. Secondary partial or perforating rupture of the left atrium also may occur, and some dogs develop acquired atrial septal defects or hemopericardium. These complications have been observed mainly in male miniature poodles, cocker spaniels, and dachshunds (Sadanaga et al., 1990).

Comparative pathologic studies have confirmed the similarity of CVD in dogs and mitral valve prolapse in humans (Kogure, 1980). The cause of CVD is still unknown, but genetic factors involving collagen degeneration and glycosaminoglycan accumulation are suspected because of the nonrandom breed predispositions and histologic appearance of affected valves. Experimental studies of high-carbohydrate diet and treadmill exercise in 24 dogs older than 3 years showed increased edema of heart valves and decreased uptake of radiolabled sulfate and proline (Schole et al., 1982). The investigators suggested that alterations in adrenal hormones and growth hormone–dependent anabolic factors associated with exercise contribute to the pathogenesis of CVD. Acquired valvular disease in cats is rare.

Bacterial Endocarditis

Bacterial endocarditis is a relatively rare condition. Lombard and Buergelt (1983) found echocar-

Table 6. Portacaval Shunts—Estimated Relative Risks (Odds Ratios) by Breed (n = 298)*

Breed ≥ 5 Cases	No.	Odds Ratio	95% Confidence Limits	P
Yorkshire terrier	56	19.9	14.6–26.9	<.0001
Pug	11	10.0	5.2–18.8	<.0001
Miniature schnauzer	32	6.9	4.7–10.1	<.0001
Maltese	12	5.4	2.9–9.9	<.0001
Pekingese	7	3.7	1.6–8.1	.004
Shih tzu	11	3.4	1.8–6.4	<.001
Standard schnauzer	5	3.7	1.3–9.2	.014
Lhasa apso	8	2.4	1.1–5.0	.022

*Data from Veterinary Medical Data Base (VMDB) at Purdue University, 1987–1989.

diographic signs of endocarditis in 10 of 345 dogs (3%) in a cardiology clinic. However, in the absence of an echogenic thrombus or aortic regurgitation, a clinical diagnosis of endocarditis is difficult to confirm, and most epidemiologic data are based on necropsy studies. The overall prevalence at necropsy varies 100-fold, from 0.06 to 6.6%, and is probably influenced more by the diligence and interest of the investigator than by true differences in the prevalence at various institutions. In dogs, the high-pressure valves (aortic and mitral) are most often affected, and the most common organisms isolated are *Staphylococcus aureus*, *Streptococcus*, and *Escherichia coli* (Calvert et al., 1985) (see this volume, p. 752). Others have suggested that pre-existing heart disease predisposes dogs to the development of endocarditis, but that has not been my experience.* In practical terms, the major etiologic factors are the virulence of the organism and the presence of chronic infection elsewhere in the body. Prostate infections were most frequent in 40 dogs with endocarditis at this institution (Anderson and Dubielzig, 1984). In an association reported between joint disease and bacterial endocarditis, both infective and noninfective arthritis were found in 12 dogs with endocarditis (Bennett and Taylor, 1988). The cause-and-effect relationship was not certain, although the investigators presumed embolic disease was the cause of the infective arthritis. They hypothesized that immune-mediated disease was the cause of arthritis in noninfected joints.

Endocardial Fibroelastosis

Endocardial thickening with mild fibrosis and increased elastic fibers may occur in response to chronic dilatation and diastolic pressure overload. The degree of secondary thickening in this circumstance is not clinically significant, and signs are related to the underlying valvular or myocardial disorder. More severe primary endocardial fibroelastosis with clinical signs indistinguishable from those of dilated cardiomyopathy was reported in four young dogs by Lombard and Buergelt (1984). Although the cause was unknown, the age of the dogs suggests that it was a congenital abnormality. In a hereditary form of fibroelastosis in Burmese cats, the endocardium progressed from normal histology at birth to symptomatic fibroelastosis by 2 months of age (Zook et al., 1981). Dilated lymphatics were the first change noted, followed by increased fibrous tissue and elastic fibers.

Editor's Note: In my practice, there appears to be an inordinately high incidence of bacterial endocarditis in dogs with congenital SAS.

Endomyocardial Fibrosis

Endomyocardial fibrosis occurs more commonly in cats than dogs and causes restrictive "cardiomyopathy" when the subendocardial myocardium is significantly involved and restrictive scar formation develops. Although this condition is distinguishable from congenital anomalous mitral valve complex (also common in cats) at necropsy, the two entities may have similar clinical and echocardiographic features. The cause of the restrictive scarring is unknown, but the process may be the healed result of active endomyocarditis. This phenomenon has been observed in several young (1- to 3-year-old) cats at this and other institutions. Excessive left ventricular false tendons (moderator bands) also are commonly found in cats, but their significance is uncertain (Liu, 1987).

MYOCARDIAL DISEASE

Myocardial diseases of various types have been recognized with increased frequency in recent years. In 1958 to 1960, the prevalence of myocardial disease in 5000 dogs was 0.45%, based mainly on the detection of arrhythmias in electrocardiograms. In a 1988 study of 7148 dogs, 1.1% were found to have dilated cardiomyopathy (Fioretti and Delli Carri, 1988). The increased frequency is due in part to improved diagnostic capability with the advent of echocardiography, but also it reflects an increased incidence of diseases such as cardiomyopathy in Doberman pinscher and boxer dogs. Indirect evidence for the increased prevalence of myocardial disease is the fact that most cardiomyopathies are associated with arrhythmias and congestive heart failure, and these complications would not have been recognized in the years before the advent of echocardiography.

In addition to improved diagnostic methods, the prevalence of myocardial disease varies with geographic factors (e.g., Chagas' disease in southern border states), the nature of the study (clinical or pathologic), and criteria selected. Necropsy studies generally reveal a higher prevalence of myocardial disease than do clinical investigations. As an example, a histopathologic study of the myocardium in 50 apparently healthy cats found only 15 cats (30%) without lesions (Nobel et al., 1974).

The types and pathology of most myocardial diseases in all species of animals have been reviewed by Van Vleet and Ferrans (1986). Clinical aspects of myocardial diseases in small animals, including types, prevalence, and causes, have been described well in various textbooks (Fox, 1989; Keene, 1989; Thomas, 1987b), and updates are included elsewhere in this volume.

Feline Cardiomyopathy

The major change regarding the prevalence of myocardial disease has been the reduced frequency of dilated cardiomyopathy (DCM) in cats following the discovery of plasma taurine deficiency as the principal cause of this condition and subsequent taurine supplementation in commercial cat foods (Pion et al., 1989). In one study, diagnoses of feline DCM decreased from 61 of 221 echocardiograms (28%) in 1986 to 12 of 207 (6%) in 1989, whereas the occurrence of hypertrophic cardiomyopathy did not change (Skiles et al., 1990). DCM is seldom seen in our clinic now, and most cats with cardiomyopathy have primary hypertrophic or restrictive forms or thyrotoxicosis.

Canine Cardiomyopathy

Various types of myocardial disease that were not present or not recognized 30 years ago are now seen commonly in dogs. Large breeds of dogs, especially males, were and still are predisposed to dilated (congestive) cardiomyopathy, but a particular susceptibility has now been recognized in Doberman pinscher dogs. Of 68 dogs with DCM at the University of Georgia, 39 (57%) were Dobermans (Calvert, 1986). The cause is uncertain, but myocardial L-carnitine deficiency was detected in 13 of 18 affected Doberman pinschers despite normal plasma carnitine levels in most of the dogs (Keene et al., 1989). Taurine deficiency does not appear to have a role in the etiology of DCM in dogs, based on the finding of normal plasma taurine levels in affected animals (Kramer and Fox, 1989).

Other breed-associated cardiomyopathies include DCM in Old English sheepdogs (Thomas, 1987a), familial cardiomyopathy in English cocker spaniels (Gooding et al., 1986), Duchenne's X-linked muscular dystrophy cardiomyopathy in male golden retriever dogs (Valentine et al., 1989), and arrhythmogenic cardiomyopathy in boxer dogs (Harpster, 1983). Hypertrophic cardiomyopathy is quite rare in dogs, but a hereditary form has been reported in pointer dogs (Sisson, 1990; Thomas, 1987b). The frequency of parvovirus myocarditis has diminished greatly since the advent of vaccination programs, and no cases have been recognized in our clinic in recent years. Occasional dogs with arrhythmias are seropositive for *Borrelia burgdorferi*, but the significance of titers in our region is uncertain, and it is difficult to substantiate a clinical diagnosis of Lyme disease myocarditis (Henes, 1989; Keene, 1989). Chagasic myocarditis due to *Trypanosoma cruzi* still appears to be limited to occasional dogs in southern border states (Barr et al., 1989)

Breed-Associated Arrhythmias

Most forms of cardiomyopathy have nonspecific ventricular or atrial arrhythmias, but certain breeds have characteristic arrhythmias that may occur with or without significant cardiomegaly or signs of congestive heart failure. Most notable in this regard is *sick sinus syndrome* (SSS). The original report characterizing the disorder in female miniature schnauzers (Hamlin et al., 1972) has been supported by recent tabulations. Fifteen dogs with SSS at this institution in 1987 to 1989 included 10 miniature schnauzers (6 females), whereas the breed constitutes only 1.6% of our clinic population (OR 129). Analysis of VMDB breed risk data on 318 dogs with SSS during the same period confirmed increased risk of SSS in miniature schnauzers (OR 6.9) as well as in Pomeranians (OR 3.5), boxers (OR 2.6), and cocker spaniels (OR 1.7). Most of the miniature schnauzers were females (34/44), and 32 of 34 (96%) had been neutered. Sex differences were not significant in other breeds.

Boxer dogs have a sufficiently high incidence of ventricular tachyarrhythmias and fainting or sudden death to deserve the special designation of arrhythmogenic *boxer cardiomyopathy* (Harpster, 1983). Although this often occurs in the absence of cardiomegaly and congestive heart failure, other investigators have observed the latter complications more frequently and suggest that there may be variations in the nature of boxer cardiomyopathy in different parts of the country (Keene, 1989). Biochemical analyses and therapeutic trials indicate that myocardial L-carnitine deficiency had a central role in the pathogenesis of dilated cardiomyopathy in a family of boxer dogs (Keene et al., 1991).

Persistent atrial standstill (silent atrium), characterized by thin-walled, dilated atria and absence of P waves, was observed in six young dogs (1 to 3 years old) with ascites at this institution 10 to 12 years ago, but none have been diagnosed here since then. Four of the dogs were English springer spaniels. Similar findings have been reported by others and are reviewed elsewhere (see this volume, p. 786).

Ventricular ectopy with paroxysmal ventricular tachycardia, flutter, and fibrillation has been recognized as a familiial arrhythmia causing sudden death in a family of German shepherds (see this volume, p. 749). Other presumably breed-associated arrhythmias reported years ago include AV conduction block in pugs with hereditary stenosis of the bundle of His (James et al., 1975) and sudden death in Doberman pinschers (James and Drake, 1968).

PERICARDIAL DISEASE

Several types of primary and secondary pericardial diseases occur and have been reviewed in previous volumes. An update is also given elsewhere in this volume.

From a prevalence standpoint, changes have occurred in recent years. The most common disorder, pericardial effusion, now occurs almost exclusively in large breeds of nonbrachycephalic dogs of either sex. It is usually secondary to primary or metastatic hemangiosarcoma or mesothelioma rather than chemodectomas, as in previous years. Occasional dogs with idiopathic benign pericardial effusion, pericarditis, congestive heart failure, or ruptured left atrium are also recognized. The frequency of diagnosis of pericardial effusion has increased with the advent of echocardiography, but it is also likely that the incidence of pericardial effusion has increased, particularly in certain breeds. In a series of 92 dogs with pericardial disease in 1987 to 1989, we observed an increased risk of pericardial effusion in golden retrievers (n = 22, OR 7.4), German shepherds (n = 14, OR 2.3), Laborador retrievers (n = 8, OR 2.2), German short-hair pointers (n = 4, OR 9.5), and Akitas (n = 3, OR 6.5). Brachycephalic breeds were uncommon and were represented by only three boxer dogs (OR 1.5), one bulldog, and one Boston terrier.

Pericardial disease (mainly effusion) in 66 of 2852 feline necropsies (2.3%) has been reviewed by Rush and colleagues (1990). In most instances, it was associated with other illnesses including feline infectious peritonitis, cardiomyopathy, renal failure, systemic infection, coagulopathies, or neoplasia (lymphosarcoma or metastatic carcinoma). Hemangiosarcoma and benign idiopathic pericardial effusion were not observed.

VASCULAR DISEASE

Pulmonary vascular disease is most often due to *Dirofilaria immitis* infection, which has been reviewed in previous editions of this book. The disease occurs in cats much less frequently than in dogs. In endemic areas, 11 necropsy surveys showed average heartworm infection rates of 1.9% in cats and 34.6% in dogs (Kume, as cited by Rawlings, 1990). Pulmonary thromboembolism also occurs in other diseases but was suspected clinically in only 2 of 47 dogs with emboli at necropsy (LaRue and Murtaugh, 1990). The most commonly associated diseases were cardiac (15), neoplasia (14), and disseminated intravascular coagulopathy (10). Another necropsy survey of vascular thrombosis in 59 dogs excluded those conditions (Van Winkle et al., 1989). Pulmonary thromboemboli were found in 27 of 59 dogs, and the most commonly associated conditions were renal disease (11 of 27) and hyperadrenocorticism or steroid therapy (11 of 27). Portal vein thrombi (12 of 59) were mainly associated with

steroid therapy (4 of 12) and pancreatic necrosis (4 of 12).

Primary systemic vascular disease is uncommon, but atherosclerosis and aortic or coronary thrombosis are occasionally recognized, particularly in dogs with hypothyroidism and elevated cholesterol levels (Liu et al., 1986). Primary renal disease was found in 7 of 23 dogs with systemic arterial thrombi (Van Winkle et al., 1989). Congenital or acquired peripheral arteriovenous fistulas also occur, usually in limbs and secondary to trauma (Suter, 1989). Spontaneous, asymptomatic coronary artery vasculitis of unknown etiology has been recognized in up to 34% of young laboratory beagles histopathologically (Hartman, 1987; Spencer and Greaves, 1987). Systemic vasculitis causing a canine pain syndrome also has been noted in young laboratory beagles (Scott-Moncrieff et al., 1990)

Secondary aortic thromboembolism in cats may occur with any of the forms of cardiomyopathy and represents the most frequent vascular abnormality encountered in small animal medicine. Although aspirin is often given in the hope of avoiding this complication, no controlled studies have been reported to confirm that such therapy is effective, and we continue to receive patients that have aortic embolism and have been on recommended doses of prophylactic aspirin therapy. The prevalence is highest in emergency clinics because most animals are presented as emergencies with sudden onset of posterior paralysis.

HYPERTENSION

Hypertension in small animals appears to be more common than studies indicated 30 years ago. Conservative criteria for the diagnosis of hypertension are blood pressures above 180 mm Hg systolic or 100 mm Hg diastolic in untrained dogs or 170/90 in trained animals. Surveys revealed pressures above these levels in 1 to 2% of dogs (Spangler et al., 1977). About one third of dogs with hypertension have chronic renal disease, and one third have hyperadrenocorticism (Littman, 1991b). The presenting complaint is often a sudden onset of blindness due to retinal hemorrhage and other ocular changes (Dimski and Hawkins, 1988; Littman, 1991; Littman et al., 1988). Spontaneous essential hypertension also has been recognized, and two colonies of dogs with the disorder have been established (Bovee et al., 1989; Tippett et al., 1986). Hypertension also has been recognized in cats in association with chronic renal disease or hyperthyroidism (Kobayashi et al., 1990; Littman, 1991a; Morgan, 1986). Sudden onset of blindness was reported in a total of 35 cats with hypertension, and most of them had laboratory or necropsy evidence of chronic renal disease (Littman, 1991a; Morgan, 1986).

References and Suggested Reading

Ackerman, N., Burk, R., Hahn, A. W., et al.: Patent ductus arteriosus in the dog: A retrospective study of radiographic, epidemiologic and clinical findings. Am. J. Vet. Res. 39:1805, 1978.

Anderson, C. A., and Dubielzig, R. R.: Vegetative endocarditis in dogs. J. Am. Anim. Hosp. Assoc. 20:149, 1984.

Barr, S. C., Simpson, R. M., Schmidt, S. P., et al.: Chronic dilatative myocarditis caused by *Trypanosoma cruzi* in two dogs. J.A.V.M.A. 195:1237, 1989.

Bennett, D., and Taylor, D. J.: Bacterial endocarditis and inflammatory joint disease in the dog. J. Small Anim. Pract. 29:347, 1988.

Bovee, K. C., Littman, M. P., Crabtree, B. J., et al.: Essential hypertension in a dog. J.A.V.M.A. 195:81, 1989.

Buchanan, J. W.: Chronic valvular disease (endocardiosis) in dogs. Adv. Vet. Sci. Comp. Med. 21:75, 1977.

Buchanan, J. W.: Morphology of the ductus arteriosus in fetal and neonatal dogs genetically predisposed to patent ductus arteriosus. *In* Rosenquist, G. C., and Bergsma, D. (eds.): *Morphogenesis and Malformation of the Cardiovascular System.* New York: Alan R. Liss, Birth Defects: Original Article Series 14:349, 1978.

Buchanan, J. W.: Pulmonic stenosis caused by single coronary artery in dogs: Four cases (1965–1984). J.A.V.M.A. 196:115, 1990.

Calvert, C. A.: Dilated congestive cardiomyopathy in Doberman pinschers. Comp. Cont. Ed. Pract. Vet. 8:417, 1986.

Calvert, C. A., Greene, C. E., and Hardie, E. M.: Cardiovascular infections in dogs: Epizootiology, clinical manifestations, and prognosis. J.A.V.M.A. 187:612, 1985.

Darke, P. G. G.: Valvular incompetence in Cavalier King Charles spaniels. Vet. Rec. 120:365, 1987.

Detweiler, D. K., and Patterson, D. F.: Prevalence and types of cardiovascular disease in dogs. Ann. N. Y. Acad. Sci. 127:481, 1965.

Dimski, D. S., and Hawkins, E. C.: Canine systemic hypertension. Comp. Cont. Ed. Pract. Vet. 10:1152, 1988.

Fioretti, M., and Delli Carri, E.: Epidemiological survey of dilatative cardiomyopathy in dogs. Veterinaria 2:81, 1988.

Fox, P. R.: Myocardial diseases. *In* Ettinger, S. J., (ed.): *Textbook of Veterinary Internal Medicine.* Philadelphia: W. B. Saunders, 1989, pp. 1097–1131.

Gooding, J. P., Robinson, W. F., and Mews, G. C.: Echocardiographic characterization of dilatation cardiomyopathy in the English cocker spaniel. Am. J. Vet. Res. 47:1978, 1986.

Hamlin, R. L., Smetzer, D. L., and Bresnock, E. M.: Sinoatrial syncope in miniature schnauzers. J.A.V.M.A. 161:1022, 1972.

Harpster, N. K.: Boxer cardiomyopathy. *In* Kirk, R. W. (ed.): *Current Veterinary Therapy VIII: Small Animal Practice.* Philadelphia: W. B. Saunders, 1983, p. 329.

Harpster, N. K., and Zook, B. C.: The cardiovascular system. *In* Holzworth, J. (ed.): *Disease of the Cat: Medicine and Surgery.* Philadelphia: W. B. Saunders, 1987, pp. 820–933.

Hartman, H. A.: Idiopathic extramural coronary arteritis in beagle and mongrel dogs. Vet. Pathol. 24:537, 1987.

Henes, M. G.: Myocardial dysfunction associated with Lyme disease. Vet. Med. 84:982, 1989.

Jacobs, G., Mahaffey, M., and Rawlings, C. A.: Valvular pulmonic stenosis in four Boykin spaniels. J. Am. Anim. Hosp. Assoc. 26:247, 1990.

James, T. N., and Drake, E. A.: Sudden death in Doberman pinschers. Ann. Intern. Med. 68:821, 1968.

James, T. N., Robertson, B. T., Waldo, A. L., et al.: Hereditary stenosis of the His bundle in pug dogs. Circulation 52:1152, 1975.

Jones, C. L.: Inheritable left ventricular outflow obstruction in the golden retriever. ACVIM Scientific Proceedings, 1989, pp. 851–853.

Keene, B. W.: Canine cardiomyopathy. *In* Kirk, R. W. (ed.): *Current Veterinary Therapy X: Small Animal Practice.* Philadelphia: W. B. Saunders, 1989, p. 241.

Keene, B. W., Kittleson, M. D., Rush, J. E., et al.: Myocardial carnitine deficiency associated with dilated cardiomyopathy in Doberman pinschers. J. Vet. Intern. Med. 3:126, 1989.

Keene, B. W., Panciera, D. P., Atkins, C. E., et al.: Myocardial L-carnitine deficiency in a family of dogs with dilated cardiomyopathy. J.A.V.M.A. 198:647, 1991.

Kobayashi, D. L., Peterson, M.E., Graves, T. K., et al.: Hypertension in cats with chronic renal failure or hyperthyroidism. J. Vet. Intern. Med. 4:58, 1990.

Kogure, K.: Pathology of chronic mitral valvular disease in the dog. Jpn. J. Vet. Sci. 42:323, 1980.

Kramer, G. A., and Fox, P. R.: Plasma taurine concentrations in dogs with acquired heart disease. J. Vet. Intern. Med. 3:126, 1989.

LaRue, M. J., and Murtaugh, R. J.: Pulmonary thromboembolism in dogs: 47 cases (1986–1987). J.A.V.M.A. 197:1368, 1990.

Littman, M. P.: Spontaneous systemic hypertension in 24 cats. J. Vet. Intern. Med. 1991a (in press).

Littman, M. P., Spontaneous systemic hypertension in dogs. BSAVA Congress 1991b, p. 119.

Littman, M. P., Robertson, J. L., and Bovee, K. C.: Spontaneous systemic hypertension in dogs: Five cases (1981–1983). J.A.V.M.A. 193:486, 1988.

Liu, S. K.: Left ventricular false tendons associated with cardiac malfunction in 101 cats. Lab. Invest. 56:44A, 1987.

Liu, S. K., Tilley, L. P., Tappe, J. P., et al.: Clinical and pathologic findings in dogs with atherosclerosis: 21 cases (1970–1983). J.A.V.M.A. 189:227, 1986.

Lombard, C. W., and Buergelt, C. D.: Vegetative bacterial endocarditis in dogs: Echocardiographic diagnosis and clinical signs. J. Small Anim. Pract. 24:325, 1983.

Lombard, C. W., and Buergelt, C. D.: Endocardial fibroelastosis in four dogs. J. Am. Anim. Hosp. Assoc. 20:271, 1984.

Moise, N. S.: Sudden cardiac death in related German shepherds. ACVIM Scientific Proceedings, 1990, p. 855.

Morgan, R. V.: Systemic hypertension in four cats: Ocular and medical findings. J. Am. Anim. Hosp. Assoc. 22:615, 1986.

Mulvihill, J. J., and Priester, W. A.: Congenital heart disease in dogs: Epidemiologic similarities to man. Teratology 7:73, 1973.

Nobel, T. A., Newmann, F., and Klopfer, U.: Histopathology of the myocardium in 50 apparently healthy cats. Lab. Anim. 8:119, 1974.

O'Grady, M. R., Holmberg, D. L., Miller, C. W., et al.: Canine congenital aortic stenosis: A review of the literature and commentary. Can. Vet. J. 30:811, 1989.

Patterson, D. F.: Epidemiologic and genetic studies of congenital heart disease in the dog. Circ. Res. 23:171, 1968.

Patterson, D. F.: Hereditary congenital heart defects in dogs. J. Small Anim. Pract. 30:153, 1989.

Patterson, D. F., Haskins, M. E., and Schnarr, W. R.: Hereditary dysplasia of the pulmonary valve in beagle dogs. Am. J. Cardiol. 47:631, 1981.

Patterson, D. F., Pyle, R. L., Buchanan, J. W., et al.: Hereditary patent ductus arteriosus and its sequelae in the dog. Circ. Res. 29:1, 1971.

Pion, P. D., Kittleson, M. D., and Rogers, Q. R.: Cardiomyopathy in the cat and its relation to taurine deficiency. *In* Kirk, R. W. (ed.): *Current Veterinary Therapy X: Small Animal Practice.* Philadelphia: W. B. Saunders, 1989, pp. 251–262.

Pyle, R. L., Patterson, D. F., and Chacko, S.: The genetics and pathology of discrete subaortic stenosis in the Newfoundland dog. Am. Heart J. 92:324, 1976.

Rawlings, C. A.: Pulmonary arteriography and hemodynamics during feline heartworm disease. J. Vet. Intern. Med. 4:285, 1990.

Rush, J. E., Keene, B. W., and Fox, P. R.: Pericardial disease in the cat: A retrospective evaluation of 66 cases. J. Am. Anim. Hosp. Assoc. 26:39, 1990.

Sadanaga, K. K., MacDonald, M. J., and Buchanan, J. W.: Echocardiography and surgery in a dog with left atrial rupture and hemopericardium. J. Vet. Intern. Med. 4:216, 1990.

Schole, J., Sallman, H. P., Brass, W., et al.: Experimentelle Untersuchungen zum Bindegewebesstoffwechsel des Hundes bei unterschiedlichen Haltungs- und Futterungsbedingungen, unter besonderer Berucksichtigung der Endokardiose. Zentralbl. Veterinarmed. [A] 29:253, 1982.

Scott-Moncrieff, J. C., Snyder, P. W., Glickman, L. T., et al.: Systemic vasculitis (canine pain syndrome) in young laboratory beagles. J. Vet. Intern. Med. 4:112, 1990.

Sisson, D. D.: Heritability of idiopathic myocardial hypertrophy and dynamic subaortic stenosis in pointer dogs. J. Vet. Intern. Med. 4:118, 1990.

Skiles, M. L., Pion, P. D., Hird, D. W., et al.: Epidemiologic evaluation of taurine deficiency and dilated cardiomyopathy in cats. J. Vet. Intern. Med. 4:117, 1990.

Spangler, W. L., Gribble, D. H., and Weiser, M. G.: Canine hypertension: A review. J.A.V.M.A. 170:995, 1977.

Spencer, A., and Greaves, P.: Periarteritis in a beagle colony. J. Comp. Pathol. 97:121, 1987.

Suter, P. F.: Peripheral vascular disease. *In* Ettinger, S. J. (ed.): *Textbook of Veterinary Internal Medicine.* Philadelphia: W. B. Saunders, 1989, p. 1189.

Thomas, R. E.: Canine idiopathic congestive cardiomyopathy: Breed incidence from a series of 17 cases. Vet. Rec. 121:423, 1987a.

Thomas, W. P.: Myocardial diseases of the dog. *In* Bonagura, J. D. (ed.): *Cardiology.* New York: Churchill Livingstone, 1987b, p. 117.

Thrusfield, M. V., Aitken, C. G. G., and Darke, P. G. G.: Observations on breed and sex in relation to canine heart valve incompetence. J. Small Anim. Pract. 26:709, 1985.

Tippett, F., Padgett, G., Eyster, G. E., et al.: Primary hypertension in a colony of dogs. Hypertension 4:170, 1986.

Valentine, B. A., Cummings, J. F., and Cooper, B. J.: Development of Duchenne-type cardiomyopathy: Morphologic studies in a canine model. Am. J. Pathol. 135:671, 1989.

Van Vleet, J. F., and Ferrans, V. J.: Myocardial diseases of animals. Am. J. Pathol. 124:98, 1986.

Van Winkle, T., MacDonald, M., and Hendricks, J.: Thrombosis of the portal vein, pulmonary arteries, and aorta in the dog (abstract). Proc. Am. Coll. Vet. Pathol. 40th Annual Meeting, 1989.

Zook, B. C., Paasch, L. H., Chandra, R. S., et al.: The comparative pathology of primary endocardial fibroelastosis in Burmese cats. Virchows Arch. [A] 390:211, 1981.

ANESTHESIA IN PATIENTS WITH CARDIOPULMONARY DISEASE

PETER W. HELLYER

Raleigh, North Carolina

CARDIOVASCULAR DISORDERS

Anesthetic Principles

Animals with cardiovascular disorders often need anesthesia. These patients have invoked various degrees of compensatory mechanisms, related to the severity of their disease, to maintain cardiovascular homeostasis. Virtually all anesthetics and anesthetic adjuvants either depress cardiovascular function directly or modify reflex cardiovascular regulatory mechanisms. Thus, patients with cardiovascular disease, whether compensated or decompensated, are susceptible to acute destabilization as result of anesthesia (Barker et al., 1987). The severity, etiology, and functional classification of the cardiovascular disorder should be assessed before administration of any anesthetic drug. An anesthetic plan should be formulated in which adequate degrees of anxiety relief and analgesia are provided while invoking only minimal alterations in cardiovascular homeostasis. Although routine anesthetic techniques are well tolerated by healthy animals, these techniques may destabilize patients with cardiovascular disease.

PREMEDICATION

Preanesthetic medications that reduce anxiety or minimize pain are used before the induction of general anesthesia or in combination with local or regional anesthetic techniques. Pain and anxiety can alter autonomic tone and may adversely affect patients with limited cardiovascular reserves (Seeler et al., 1988). Preanesthetic medications that are routinely administered to patients with cardiovascular disease include the benzodiazepines and opioids (narcotics) (Table 1). Doses are titrated according to the severity of cardiovascular disease and the behavioral characteristics of the animal. Generally, relatively calm animals are administered a benzodiazepine intravenously just before anesthetic induction to relieve anxiety and reduce the required dose of induction drug. Opioids are commonly administered intramuscularly 20 to 30 min before intravenous catheter placement. Respiratory depression must be monitored after intramuscular narcotic administration and oxygen delivered by face mask if hypoventilation becomes significant.

Table 1. Anesthetic Drugs and Adjuvants

Drug	Trade Name	Dose/Route
Anticholinergics		
Atropine sulfate		0.02–0.04 mg/kg IV or IM
Glycopyrrolate	Robinul – V (Robins)	0.01–0.02 mg/kg IV or IM
Benzodiazepines		
Diazepam		0.2–0.4 mg/kg IV
Midazolam	Versed (Roche)	0.2–0.4 mg/kg IV or IM
Narcotics		
Morphine sulfate		0.4–1.0 mg/kg IM
Oxymorphone	Numorphan (DuPont Pharmaceuticals)	0.05–0.2 mg/kg IV or IM
Fentanyl		1–3 µg/kg IV
Sufentanil citrate	Sufenta (Janssen)	1–5 µg/kg IV
Induction drugs		
Thiopental sodium		8–12 mg/kg IV
Ketamine		1–5 mg/kg IV
Etomidate	Amidate (Abbott)	0.5–2.0 mg/kg IV

Preanesthetic medications that should be *avoided* include the alpha-2 agonists (xylazine and detomidine), acepromazine, Telazol, and high doses (>5 mg/kg IM) of ketamine (cats). All these drugs produce profound cardiovascular changes that may be poorly tolerated in animals with limited cardiovascular reserves. Anticholinergics, atropine, and glycopyrrolate should only be used as needed in patients with bradycardia or atrioventricular block. Anticholinergics alter autonomic balance and may induce sinus tachycardia and tachyarrhythmias.

INDUCTION

Injectable anesthetic drugs used to induce general anesthesia should be administered in as low a dose as possible in order to minimize deleterious cardiovascular side effects (see Table 1). Preanesthetic medication leading to a calm, pain-free patient will minimize struggling and excitement when low doses of induction drugs are used. Animals that will tolerate a face mask are preoxygenated with 100% oxygen for 3 to 5 min before induction. The thiobarbiturates, thiamylal sodium and thiopental sodium, induce marked cardiovascular and respiratory depression when used in anesthetic doses. Cardiopulmonary depression is minimized when thiobarbiturates are administered as a slow bolus in doses less than 8 mg/kg IV. Patients with severe cardiovascular disease generally do not tolerate even low doses of thiobarbiturates. An alternative to the thiobarbiturates is etomidate, an ultra–short-acting hypnotic that induces general anesthesia with minimal to no cardiovascular depression. Similarly, narcotics (oxymorphone, fentanyl, sufentanil) in combination with a benzodiazepine are suitable induction drugs in severely compromised patients. Mask induction with halothane or isoflurane is not recommended because of the marked cardiovascular depression associated with induction doses of the inhalant anesthetics.

ANESTHETIC MAINTENANCE

Maintenance of general anesthesia is most readily accomplished with inhalation anesthetics. Halothane and isoflurane can be used for maintenance in patients with cardiovascular disease. Methoxyflurane anesthesia, characterized by slow induction, slow recovery, and dose-dependent cardiovascular and respiratory depression, is a poor choice for patients with cardiovascular disease. Halothane and isoflurane should be titrated to effect. Nitrous oxide combined with oxygen (50% N_2O/50% O_2) may be used to reduce the dose of halothane and isoflurane necessary for anesthesia. Although nitrous oxide is a myocardial depressant, it generally causes less cardiovascular depression than halothane or isoflurane. Nitrous oxide should be discontinued in the presence of deteriorating cardiovascular performance or hypoxemia. Intravenous narcotics (oxymorphone, fentanyl, sufentanil) are recommended for use intraoperatively to provide analgesia and reduce the dose of inhalant. Ventilation should be supported with intermittent positive-pressure ventilation (IPPV) performed either manually or using a mechanical ventilator. Hypoventilation and respiratory acidosis occur commonly when large doses of intraoperative narcotics are used in combination with inhalation anesthesia. Respiratory acidosis, particularly in the presence of a pre-existing metabolic acidosis, is poorly tolerated in patients with compromised cardiopulmonary function.

MONITORING

Patients with cardiovascular disease should be closely monitored throughout the entire anesthetic period. The minimum amount of monitoring consists of close observation of the subjective signs of cardiopulmonary function (heart rate, pulse quality, color and capillary refill time of mucous membranes, color of tissues, and the presence or absence of hemorrhage at surgical sites) and an electrocardiogram (ECG). Pulse oximetry, arterial blood pressure (indirect or direct), and central venous pressure (CVP) monitoring may be essential in decompensated patients. Assessment of fluid volume (serial determinations of packed cell volume [PCV], total protein [TP], and CVP) and renal function (blood urea nitrogen, urine production) should be performed frequently in patients with large fluid losses and fluid shifts. Urine production should be measured in patients to be anesthetized for prolonged periods and should be maintained greater than 1 ml/kg/hr.

Close observation and monitoring of patients must be continued well into the postoperative period. Patients that tolerated the anesthetic period may decompensate during recovery for various reasons, including hypothermia, hypoventilation resulting in hypoxemia and hypercarbia, hypotension, the effects of unrelieved anxiety and pain, ongoing fluid shifts, and residual anesthetic effects. If supportive measures were instituted during the operative period (e.g., intravenous fluids, dobutamine or dopamine, oxygen), they may be needed in the postoperative period until the patient is stabilized. Appropriate techniques in critical care during the recovery period often yield a successful outcome.

HYPERTROPHIC CARDIOMYOPATHY

The primary goal during the anesthetic period for patients with hypertrophic cardiomyopathy (HCM) is to maintain hemodynamic stability. Asymmetric septal hypertrophy may result in dynamic subaortic obstruction to left ventricular outflow (Fox, 1989), and increases in sympathetic tone and myocardial contractility further contribute to subaortic obstruction. Consequently, an anesthetic care plan that avoids increases in sympathetic tone should be formulated. Equally important is attention to ventricular filling. Diastolic compliance (distensibility) is reduced and ventricular relaxation is prolonged in HCM. Decreases in left ventricular diastolic compliance are compensated by maintaining adequate (or high) left ventricular filling pressures and maintaining normal sinus rhythm (Reich et al., 1990). Tachycardia or hypotension may cause ischemia and increase ventricular stiffness. Cardiac medications, particularly propranolol or diltiazem, are maintained up until the anesthetic period. Premedication is essential in order to avoid anxiety and stress with associated increases in myocardial contractility or ventricular stiffness. Cats, particularly older and debilitated patients, respond favorably to premedication with oxymorphone and midazolam. I prefer to avoid the use of ketamine in cats with HCM, although low doses (<5 mg/kg IM) may not necessarily be detrimental. Diazepam or midazolam, administered intramuscularly concurrently with ketamine, may blunt ketamine-induced increases in sympathetic tone. Adequate doses of anesthetic drugs should be administered to ensure smooth induction, free from struggling or excitement. Supplemental doses of anesthetic should be administered if necessary to prevent coughing and gagging at the time of endotracheal intubation. Light planes of general anesthesia, with associated increases in sympathetic tone, are to be avoided. Anesthesia is maintained with either halothane or isoflurane. Halothane may be a better choice, however, because it decreases myocardial contractility more and causes less vasodilation (less decrease in preload, less decrease in coronary perfusion pressure) than isoflurane. Intraoperative narcotics (oxymorphone, fentanyl) are often indicated to maintain an adequate plane of anesthesia without excessive depression of the myocardium. Maintaining adequate blood volume necessitates the judicious use of intravenous crystalloid fluids (3 to 5 ml/kg/hr) during the anesthetic period. Arterial hypotension may be treated by decreasing the dose of inhalant, increasing the rate of intravenous fluid administration, and administering an alpha-adrenergic agonist (phenylephrine 10 to 100 μg/kg IV). Beta agonists are relatively contraindicated because they increase myocardial contractility and may increase left ventricular outflow obstruction. Tachycardia and tachyarrhythmias increase myocardial oxygen consumption and increase the chance of myocardial ischemia and lung edema. Arrhythmias should be treated with either lidocaine or a short-acting beta-blocker

(esmolol [Brevibloc, DuPont Pharmaceuticals] initially 50 to 200 μg/kg/min IV followed by a continuous IV infusion, 50 to 200 μg/kg/min, if necessary). Sinus tachycardia may be slowed by deepening the plane of anesthesia or administering narcotics. Postoperative control of pain and anxiety is essential to avoid potentially deleterious increases in sympathetic tone and cardiac work (see this volume, p. 82).

DILATED CARDIOMYOPATHY

The hemodynamic features of dilated cardiomyopathy (DCM) are characterized by decreased myocardial contractility, high ventricular filling pressures, and an inverse relationship between peripheral vascular resistance and cardiac output (Fox, 1989). The goals of anesthesia are to (1) minimize decreases in myocardial contractility, (2) avoid increases in systemic vascular resistance, (3) avoid extremes of heart rate (bradycardia, tachycardia), and (4) maintain adequate filling volume without overloading the heart. Inotropic support may be necessary to offset the decreases in contractility induced by anesthetic drugs. Dobutamine (1 to 10 μg/kg/min IV) or dopamine (1 to 5 μg/kg/min) are the inotropes of choice. Excessive doses of dopamine (>10 μg/kg/min) increase systemic vascular resistance, which may further decrease cardiac output. Anesthetic induction drugs and doses should be chosen to minimize depression of contractility. Patients should be adequately premedicated (oxymorphone, morphine) to avoid struggling and to minimize the dose of the induction drug. Ketamine may be used as a premedication in cats; however, the dose should be low (≤5 μg/kg IM) to prevent tachycardia and increases in systemic vascular resistance. Induction in severely compromised patients may be accomplished with intravenous diazepam (or midazolam) followed by oxymorphone or sufentanil. Bradycardia is common after sufentanil induction, and patients should be pretreated with an anticholinergic unless tachycardia is already present. Etomidate or low doses of thiobarbiturates may also be used for induction after adequate premedication. Isoflurane is preferred over halothane for anesthesia maintenance, because it causes less depression of cardiac contractility for a given depth of anesthesia. Supplemental doses of intravenous narcotics (oxymorphone, fentanyl, buprenorphine sufentanil) should be administered in order to avoid excessive concentrations of isoflurane (preferably <1.5%). Patients with severe DCM may not tolerate the cardiac depressant properties of either inhalant agent and may need to be maintained with a balanced technique (i.e., diazepam, fentanyl, or sufentanil, and N_2O/O_2). Local and regional techniques are a reasonable alternative for lower abdominal and limb procedures. Epidural anesthesia may cause peripheral vasodilation, hypotension, and decreases in venous return (preload); consequently, intravenous fluid therapy needs to be adjusted to maintain vascular volume and preload.

MITRAL VALVE INSUFFICIENCY

Most patients with early compensated mitral valve insufficiency tolerate general anesthesia without problems. The primary hemodynamic goals are to avoid significant decreases in heart rate and increases in systemic vascular resistance (afterload), which increase regurgitant fraction. Decreased heart rates may reduce cardiac output and should be treated with intravenous anticholinergics. Vascular volume is maintained by intravenous fluids administered at reduced rates (3 to 5 ml/kg/hr). CVP should be monitored to assess right-sided filling pressures in dogs with severe mitral insufficiency and signs of congestive heart failure. Moderate decreases in systemic vascular resistance (afterload) increase cardiac output and are generally beneficial. Anesthetic drugs (acepromazine, droperidol) or techniques (lidocaine epidural) that can cause significant and prolonged vasodilation and hypotension should be used with caution. Excessive vasodilation and hypotension may decrease venous return and reduce cardiac output and coronary perfusion, further compromising cardiac function. Drugs that cause vasoconstriction (ketamine, Telazol, nitrous oxide) should be avoided, because they may increase afterload with subsequent increases in regurgitant flow and decreases in forward blood flow. The extent to which dogs with mitral insufficiency can tolerate decreases in myocardial contractility depends on the stage of heart disease. Dogs with early mitral insufficiency and normal myocardial contractility tolerate the depressant effects of inhalant anesthetics fairly well. In contrast, dogs with advanced mitral insufficiency, depressed myocardial contractility, and signs of congestive heart failure may destabilize during inhalant anesthesia. These dogs can be maintained on low doses of isoflurane with supplemental doses of narcotics (oxymorphone, fentanyl) if needed. Inotropic support, with dopamine or dobutamine (preferably), may be necessary to maintain cardiac output and treat hypotension.

PERICARDIAL DISEASE

The hemodynamic consequences of pericardial disease depend on the degree to which ventricular diastolic filling is impaired. Pericardial tamponade and constrictive pericarditis are characterized by a decreased end-diastolic volume, reduced stroke volume, and decreased arterial blood pressure (Lake, 1983). Compensatory mechanisms invoked to improve cardiac output include increases in blood volume and venous pressure, heart rate, and myocardial contractility. Consequently, the goals of the anesthetic care plan are to maintain or expand vascular volume, prevent decreases in heart rate, and avoid depression of contractility. Pericardiocentesis under a local block (lidocaine 2%) should be performed on patients with tamponade *before* induction of anesthesia (see this volume, p. 725). After pericardiocentesis, patients with stable cardiovascular function may be induced using a standard protocol of a premedication and a thiobarbiturate. Patients with tamponade that cannot be relieved before anesthesia may not tolerate the venodilation often induced by thiobarbiturates. CVP monitoring is helpful to titrate the rate of intravenous fluid administration necessary to maintain adequate filling pressures (generally 5 to 20 ml/kg/hr). Heart rate is maintained by the judicious use of anticholinergics. IPPV with high peak inspiratory pressure is often poorly tolerated by patients with unrelieved tamponade or constrictive pericarditis. The adverse effects of IPPV are diminished after pericardiocentesis or on opening the thorax. Pericardectomy of an adhered pericardial sac is often associated with significant hemorrhage and arrhythmogenesis. Antiarrhythmic therapy with a continuous infusion of lidocaine (50 to 80 μg/kg/min) may be necessary to control arrhythmias. Whole blood or packed cells should be available if hemorrhage during pericardiectomy is extensive.

HEARTWORM DISEASE

Heartworm-infected dogs and cats may be asymptomatic or display clinical signs of right heart failure, low cardiac output, and pulmonary thromboembolism. Asymptomatic patients generally tolerate thiobarbiturates well and respond favorably to routine general anesthesia. These patients should be monitored closely for arrhythmias and hypotension. Dehydration, excessive vasodilation (acepromazine), or hemorrhage will be poorly tolerated if high right ventricular filling pressures are required to maintain cardiac output. Patients with advanced heartworm disease are prone to hypoxemia and may have pulmonary vasoconstriction that is oxygen responsive. Thus, they should be supplemented with oxygen in the induction and recovery periods and given 100% oxygen during the procedure. Fluid management is more difficult in patients with advanced heartworm disease. Excessive fluid administration may overload an already compromised right heart, whereas hypovolemia may result in inadequate filling pressures. It is better to err on the side of volume, as hypotension is more life-threatening than ascites. CVP monitoring provides a useful guide for intravenous fluid administration. Patients with advanced heartworm disease generally have low cardiac output and do not tolerate decreases in contractility or heart rate. Anticholinergics should be administered if needed to maintain heart rate. Patients may tolerate low doses of thiobarbiturates (<8 mg/kg IV) after premedication (oxymorphone plus diazepam intravenously). Etomidate is a useful alternative, because it causes less cardiovascular depression than the thiobarbiturates. Premedication reduces the dose and cost of an etomidate induction. Isoflurane is the preferred inhalant, although low doses of halothane may be tolerated. Intraoperative narcotics should be used to minimize the dose of inhalant. The safety of ketamine as an induction drug is uncertain and depends on the relative effects of increased sympathetic stimulation on the heart and vasculature: ketamine-induced increases in heart rate and contractility may beneficially increase cardiac output, whereas ketamine-induced increases in systemic vascular resistance may decrease cardiac output. Consequently, if ketamine is to be used, it should be administered with caution and in low doses. Myocardial dysfunction may require inotropic support with dopamine or dobutamine to maintain cardiac output and arterial blood pressure. High doses of dopamine (>10 μg/kg/min) increase systemic vascular resistance and may be detrimental. Ideally, these patients should be monitored with ECG, direct arterial blood pressure measurement, CVP assessment, and intermittent blood gas determinations.

RESPIRATORY DISORDERS

Anesthetic Considerations

Virtually all anesthetic drugs produce some degree of respiratory depression, which may precipitate a respiratory emergency in patients with pre-existing respiratory disorders. Profound hypoventilation causes hypoxemia (Pa_{O_2} < 80 mm of Hg) and respiratory acidosis (elevated Pa_{CO_2}). Hypoxemia may decrease oxygen delivery, causing tissue hypoxia, cardiovascular instability, and eventual cardiovascular collapse. Ensuring a patent airway and adequate gas exchange are essential during the entire anesthetic period. Supplementation with 100% oxygen (by face mask, nasal cannula, endotracheal tube) is always indicated in patients with compromised ventilation. Procedures requiring restraint are often best performed under general anesthesia after endotracheal intubation with assisted or controlled ventilation. Local anesthetic techniques in sedated animals may be useful for short procedures; however, these patients must be monitored closely for hypoxemia. The choice of anesthetic drugs is dictated by a patient's degree of respiratory compromise as well as the status of the cardiovascular system. Drugs with profound and prolonged cardiopulmonary effects, such as xylazine, detomidine, Telazol, and pentobarbitol, should be avoided. Dose requirements of anesthetic drugs are often significantly reduced in patients with respiratory compromise. Minimum effective doses of anesthetic drugs should be used to avoid excessive cardiopulmonary depression. Ideally, recoveries should be rapid, with no residual anesthetic-induced respiratory depression and the patient free of pain and anxiety. Animals that are anxious or in pain may become excited and struggle, worsening pre-existing respiratory compromise. An animal in pain, particularly after thoracotomy, may be reluctant to expand its chest, further compromising ventilation. Consequently, judicious use of analgesics (narcotics) and tranquilizers is often indicated in the postoperative period in patients with compromised ventilation (see this volume, p. 82). The advantages of postoperative tranquilizers and analgesics generally outweigh the disadvantages, provided that patients are monitored and oxygen is supplemented as needed.

Upper Airway Disease

Patients presenting with partial airway obstruction are at greatest risk during the induction and recovery periods. Anxious or excitable animals (particularly brachycephalic breeds) often become profoundly dyspneic when struggling during restraint. Premedication with acepromazine or oxymorphone is indicated to decrease the amount of struggling and respiratory distress. Induction of anesthesia should be routine, provided that the patient is not hypoxemic and the cardiovascular system is normal. Preoxygenation for 3 to 5 min before induction is indicated if the patient will tolerate a face mask. Thiobarbiturates are generally satisfactory and allow rapid intubation and securing of a patent airway. Ketamine (5.5 mg/kg IV) and diazepam (0.28 mg/kg IV), combined in the same syringe, provide for slower induction with less respiratory depression than the thiobarbiturates. Ketamine-diazepam inductions are useful to visualize the larynx for suspected laryngeal paralysis. Anesthesia may be maintained with either halothane or isoflurane, depending on a patient's cardiovascular status. Ventilation should be supported with IPPV either manually or mechanically. Anti-inflammatory doses of corticosteroids are administered to reduce upper airway swelling after laryngeal surgery. Patients that have partial upper airway obstruction or that have undergone airway surgery must be monitored closely during the recovery period. The endotracheal tube should be left in place as long as possible. Brachycephalic dogs, particularly if they have received narcotics, often tolerate the endotracheal tube until they are ready to stand. Patients should have a patent intravenous catheter during recovery. A face mask, for delivery of oxygen and tranquilizers (acepromazine, diazepam), should also be at hand during recovery. Patients with severe upper airway disease should be monitored continuously until they are fully awake and able to walk back to their cage. Clinicians should be prepared to reanesthetize the patient, intubate the trachea, and maintain anesthesia until laryngeal swelling subsides or perform a tracheostomy if necessary.

PLEURAL CAVITY DISEASE

Patients with pleural cavity disease (pneumothorax, pleural effusions, diaphragmatic hernia, flail chest) are at risk of hypoventilation, hypoxemia, respiratory acidosis, and cardiopulmonary collapse. Compromised patients may be recumbent, dyspneic, or anxious and reluctant to be restrained. Oxygen should be supplemented with a loose-fitting face mask. Aspiration of fluid or air from the pleural cavity should be accomplished before induction of anesthesia. Patients requiring continuous pleural suction (tension pneumothorax) should have a chest tube placed under local anesthesia (lidocaine 2%). Intravenous oxymorphone provides additional analgesia during chest tube placement. Induction of anesthesia should occur after preoxygenation, stabilization, and aspiration of the pleural cavity. Severely compromised patients may be intubated after intravenous diazepam and oxymorphone. Thiobarbiturates (<8 mg/kg) are useful for a quick induction

to obtain a patent airway. Intravenous ketamine is a less satisfactory induction drug, because intubation and securing a patent airway are slower. IPPV with 100% oxygen should begin immediately on intubation, before beginning gas anesthesia. The choice of inhalant anesthesia depends on a patient's physical status, with isoflurane being preferred for severely compromised patients. Hypoxemia during recovery is a frequent complication and may result from hypoventilation, ventilation-to-perfusion ratio inequalities, and intrapulmonary shunting. Oxygen should be supplemented in an oxygen cage or by a nasal cannula during the recovery period. Adequate doses of opioids (oxymorphone, morphine) should be administered to both dogs and cats to control postoperative pain.

References and Suggested Reading

Barker, S. J., Gamel, D. M., and Tremper, K. K.: Cardiovascular effects of anesthesia and operation. Crit. Care Clin. 3:251, 1987.
  A review of the effects of anesthetic drugs and surgery on the normal and diseased cardiovascular system.
Fox, P. R.: Myocardial diseases. In Ettinger, S. J. (ed.): Textbook of Veterinary Internal Medicine. Philadelphia: W. B. Saunders, 1989, p. 1097.
  A review of the etiology, physiology, and pathology of canine and feline cardiomyopathy.
Lake, C. L.: Anesthesia and pericardial disease. Anesth. Analg. 62:431, 1983.
  A review of the diagnosis, pathophysiology, and anesthetic management of pericardial disease.
Reich, D. L., Brooks, J. L., and Kaplan, J. A.: Uncommon cardiac diseases. In Katz, J., Benumof, J. L., and Kadis, L. B. (eds.): Anesthesia and Uncommon Diseases. Philadelphia: W. B. Saunders, 1990, p. 333.
  A review of the pathophysiology and anesthetic management of uncommon cardiovascular diseases.
Seeler, D. C., Dodman, N. H., Norman, W., et al.: Recommended techniques in small animal anaesthesia: IV anaesthesia and cardiac disease. Br. Vet. J. 144:108, 1988.
  A review of the pathophysiology of common cardiac disorders and the anesthetic management of patients.

CURRENT USES AND HAZARDS OF BRONCHODILATOR THERAPY

BRENDAN C. MCKIERNAN
Urbana, Illinois

Bronchodilators have been used since the early part of this century in veterinary medicine. Their use has been based mostly on extrapolations of the therapeutic actions and effective ranges in human medicine.

In 1953, the *Veterinary Drug Encyclopedia and*

Therapeutic Index listed methylxanthines as therapeutic agents (either alone or in combination) for relief of "difficult breathing" and for cardiac asthma (Stephenson and Mittelstaedt, 1953). In 1964, Jackson and Secord recommended the use of either ephedrine, aminophylline, or atropine for the treatment of bronchospasm in dogs. In addition, Jones and colleagues (1977) suggested that methylxanthines or ephedrine could be used in the treatment of pulmonary edema, "broken wind" in horses, and "bronchial asthma" in cats.

Despite continued widespread clinical use, many concerns still remain about dosage, efficacy, and toxicity of these drugs. It is only in the last decade that research has begun to critically evaluate these drugs in animals.

As of this writing, there are no bronchodilators specifically approved for use in veterinary medicine. Given the expense involved in research and development to obtain formal approval for a new drug, it is unlikely that any bronchodilator will be approved for use in small animals.

This does not mean, however, that these drugs should be avoided in the clinical setting. A number of recent studies have documented the pharmacokinetics, pharmacodynamics, efficacy, and toxicity of many of the bronchodilators used in small animals. It is the goal of this article, based on some of these studies, selected review articles, and the author's experience, to provide the clinician with an objective means of prescribing bronchodilators in small animals.

CONTROL OF BRONCHOMOTOR TONE

Changes in bronchomotor tone that lead to bronchoconstriction are the logical basis for bronchodilator therapy. Considerable advancements in understanding the factors that influence mammalian bronchomotor tone have been made in the past decade. Recent reviews of the mechanisms involved in the control of airway smooth muscle have been published (Barnes, 1991). Briefly, there are three systems that influence airway caliber in most species: the parasympathetic, the sympathetic, and the recently recognized nonadrenergic, noncholinergic (NANC) systems.

The parasympathetic system, thought to be the dominant airway constrictor in animals, is mediated by acetylcholine release from cholinergic nerves. Adrenergic receptors on postganglionic parasympathetic nerves may help modulate and regulate the constrictor response in this system.

The degree of sympathetic innervation of mammalian airways varies considerably. Adrenergic receptors (both alpha and beta) clearly exist on a variety of target cells within the respiratory tract. Alpha-receptors, although not demonstrable in resting canine airways, may be unmasked following nonspecific irritant (e.g., histamine) inhalation and lead to a marked bronchoconstrictor response (Barnes, 1991). Beta-receptors mediate the sympathetic relaxation of airway smooth muscle, with $beta_1$-receptors being activated following sympa-

thetic nerve stimulation and $beta_2$-receptors responding to exogenously administered beta-agonists. Norepinephrine and epinephrine, released from adrenergic nerves and the adrenal medulla, respectively, are the mediators of the sympathetic system.

The complexity of neural control of mammalian airways increased with the relatively recent discovery of the NANC system, which exerts control through nonadrenergic, noncholinergic mechanisms. It is generally believed that the neurotransmitters involved in the NANC system are neuropeptides such as vasoactive intestinal peptide (VIP). VIP is an extremely potent bronchodilator in human bronchial smooth muscle, much more potent than isoproterenol. Both inhibitory (relaxant) and excitatory (constrictive) NANC nerves have been demonstrated in different species. An inhibitory response (bronchodilation) has been shown in cats following appropriate NANC stimulation. Research involving the NANC system will undoubtedly continue and provide better understanding of airway control.

Three classes of bronchodilators have been identified: (1) the anticholinergics (e.g., atropine), (2) the beta- (specifically beta-2) adrenergic agonists (e.g., terbutaline), and (3) the methylxanthines (e.g., theophylline). Most of the bronchodilator research in veterinary medicine has involved theophylline.

INDICATIONS FOR BRONCHODILATOR USE

The classic indication for the use of bronchodilators in human medicine is in the treatment of reversible airway disease (e.g., asthma). Methylxanthines (theophylline and caffeine) have also been used in the treatment of neonatal apnea, chronic respiratory failure (as a positive inotrope to the diaphragm), and chronic pulmonary disease (i.e., cor pulmonale).

Reversibility of airway disease has been based on the significant improvement in pulmonary function tests (PFTs) noted in humans following bronchodilator therapy. Airway narrowing results in changes in many PFTs, including increases in lung resistance and expiratory time and decreases in maximal expiratory flow rates and maximal forced expiratory volume at 1 sec (FEV_1). The availability and routine use of these tests has allowed for the relatively easy determination of bronchodilator efficacy. Unfortunately, these PFTs are neither available nor applicable to clinical veterinary medicine primarily because of the need for patient cooperation and maximal voluntary effort. Only recently (mostly on a research basis) have any of the PFTs been used in veterinary medicine to evaluate the efficacy of bronchodilators.

Measurement of pulmonary function (lung resistance and dynamic compliance) is being utilized at the University of Illinois for the determination of reversible airway disease in cats, but use of these and other measurements of pulmonary function (e.g., arterial blood gases, tidal breathing flow-volume loop analysis, lung perfusion scans) is not widespread in veterinary medicine.

Lacking PFT results, the clinical indications for bronchodilator therapy remain somewhat subjective. Evaluation of changes in the pattern of breathing (e.g., increased expiratory time), radiographic or physical evidence of air trapping (e.g., a flattened diaphragm, wheezing, or forced expiratory effort), and chronic coughing can be used as clinical indicators of the need for a therapeutic bronchodilator trial. No other drugs should be given during this trial period, as it is difficult to interpret the response to multiple drug therapies when faced with either a beneficial or potentially toxic effect.

METHYLXANTHINES

The N-methyl–substituted xanthines, (i.e., theophylline, theobromine, and caffeine) constitute a family of closely related chemical compounds. All are natural alkaloids found in various plants worldwide and in foods such as tea, coffee, and cocoa. Caffeine was recommended for use in dogs and cats over 75 years ago for a variety of conditions including relief of spinal paralysis, acute heart weakness, and incipient lung edema. The first articles suggesting the usefulness of theophylline in treating human asthma were published in the early 1920's, although it was not until the mid-1930's that routine use of theophylline for this purpose began.

Theophylline is one of the major drugs for the treatment of asthma and other chronic obstructive pulmonary diseases in man. During the past 10 to 20 years, active theophylline research in human medicine has led to renewed interest and new research into the use of theophylline in veterinary medicine.

Theophylline

Theophylline is a "parent" or active compound. Aminophylline (the ethylenediamine salt of theophylline) is a soluble complex used for intravenous injections. The amount of the parent compound, theophylline, determines the activity of its formulations. Recommendations for theophylline dosage must be based on theophylline content and not salt content (Table 1). To prevent confusion on this point, most drug labels now include a statement of actual theophylline content of the product. In this

Table 1. *Common Salts of Theophylline Used in Small Animal Medicine*

Trade name	Aminophylline	Choledyl SA
Theophylline salt	Ethylenediamine	Oxtriphylline
Manufacturer	Various	Parke-Davis
Theophylline equivalency	78%	64%
Route of administration	PO, IV*	PO
Animal for which kinetic data are available	Dog, cat	Dog

*Aminophylline should not be given by IM injection due to its basic pH level.

article, all doses will be based on theophylline content unless otherwise specified.

MECHANISM OF ACTION

A number of mechanisms have been proposed to explain the actions of theophylline on the respiratory system. Increased levels of intracellular cyclic adenosine monophosphate (cAMP) are associated with bronchial smooth muscle relaxation, probably through secondary activation of protein kinases that leads to eventual cross-bridging between myosin and actin and muscle contraction. Phosphodiesterase (PDE) is the enzyme that catalyzes the breakdown of cAMP to inactive 5'AMP and is inhibited by theophylline. Inhibition of PDE with subsequent increase in the intracellular levels of cAMP was presented in the early 1970's as the explanation for the relaxant (bronchodilatory) effects of theophylline. Although one of the classic PDE inhibitors, it has since been noted that this effect occurs at plasma theophylline concentrations well above those associated with PFT improvement in man.

Other mechanisms of action suggested to explain the therapeutic effects of theophylline include adenosine antagonism (through competition for receptor sites), catecholamine release (from the adrenal gland), prostaglandin antagonism, and alteration of intracellular calcium. It is now apparent that theophylline's many therapeutic (and probably toxic) effects may be attributed to one or more of these mechanisms of action.

PHARMACOLOGY

Methylxanthines are metabolized in the liver by the mitochondrial P-450 enzyme systems. Metabolism involves either N-demethylation or 8-hydroxylation. Of the major metabolites, only 3-methylxanthine has been shown to be active, but due to a very short plasma half-life it is not considered to be a clinically active metabolite in man. All metabolites are excreted in the urine. Although 7% to 15% of a human theophylline dose is excreted unchanged in the urine, decreased renal function does not usually warrant dosage adjustments. Theophylline metabolites have not been quantified in veterinary medicine, although in the late 1890's theophylline metabolites in the dog were found to be similar to those reported in man.

The beneficial effects of theophylline on the respiratory system include bronchodilation (via smooth muscle relaxation), enhanced mucociliary clearance, stimulation of the respiratory center, increased sensitivity to Pa_{CO_2}, increased diaphragmatic contractility, and stabilization of mast cells. Various mechanisms of action are probably responsible for these different effects. Diaphragmatic contractility appears to be modulated through intracellular changes in calcium (as it can be blocked with the calcium channel blocker verapamil). The mechanism of action for bronchodilitation is probably multifactorial and includes calcium changes, adenosine antagonism, catecholamine release, and (probably as a secondary messenger) increases in intracellular cAMP. That many of the respiratory effects are not primarily caused by an increase in cAMP is based on the observation that PDE inhibition occurs at theophylline concentrations considerably above the human therapeutic range. Adenosine, an important inflammatory mediator, is one of many substances that can bind to the cell membrane of mast cells and lead to degranulation. This latter effect can be blocked by methylxanthines and is the basis for references to theophylline as an antianaphylactic drug.

The effects of various drugs and disease states on theophylline metabolism are well documented in human medicine. As a result, plasma theophylline concentrations may change significantly (potentially becoming either toxic or ineffective) following the use of certain drugs or due to various disease states (Table 2). It is not known whether theophylline metabolism is similarly affected in dogs and cats.

PHARMACOKINETICS IN DOGS AND CATS. Despite many years of methylxanthine use in dogs and cats, it was not until the early 1980's that the pharmacokinetics of theophylline were determined. Initial studies demonstrated a definite difference between the dose requirements in these two species. Based on the accepted plasma therapeutic range in human medicine of between 5 to 20 μg/ml, these studies reported immediate-release theophylline dose requirements varying from b.i.d. for the cat to q.i.d. for dogs (Table 3). Realizing that owner compliance with these recommendations might be poor, additional studies using some of the sustained-release (SR) theophylline preparations were undertaken. Some were determined suitable for once- (cat) or twice- (dog) daily administration while maintaining relatively flat plasma theophylline concentrations within the human therapeutic range (Dye et al.,

Table 2. *Significant Effects of Various Drugs, Diseases, and Other Factors on Theophylline Metabolism and Plasma Concentration in Humans**

Factor	Effect on Theophylline	
	Drug Clearance	Concentration
Drugs		
Enzyme inhibitors— Erythromycin†, troleandomycin†, cimetidine† chloramphenicol‡	Decrease	Increase
Enzyme inducers— Phenobarbital§, phenytoin†	Increase	Decrease
Disease States		
Liver disease†,‖	Decrease	Increase
Cor pulmonale†	Decrease	Increase
Acute pulmonary edema†	Decrease	Increase
Febrile viral respiratory tract infections†	Decrease	Increase
Miscellaneous		
Geriatrics	Decrease	Increase

*Adapted from Hendles, L., and Weinberger, M.: Theophylline: A "state of the art" review. Pharmacotherapy 3:2, 1983.

†Effect may be and require a dosage adjustment.

‡Ed. note: Although not included in the study adapted here, chloramphenicol is a potent hepatic microsomal enzyme inhibitor and should logically be included in this group.

§Effect not large, and may not require dosage adjustment.

‖Includes cirrhosis, acute hepatitis, and cholestasis.

1989; Koritz et al., 1986) (Table 3). It must be stressed that these recommendations are product specific; the results *cannot* be extrapolated to other SR products. Two products not listed in Table 3 (Theo-24, Searle; Theo-Dur *Sprinkle*, Key Pharmaceuticals) have also been evaluated in the dog but were found unsuitable due to poor or erratic bioavailability.

An increased incidence of nocturnal symptoms has been noticed in people with asthma due to circadian bronchomotor tone fluctuations (possibly mediated by decreases in circulating catecholamines and their inhibition of cholinergic-mediated bronchomotor tone). It is unknown whether feline airways demonstrate a similar circadian rhythm. Based on work by Dye et al. (1990), it appears that the kinetics of once-daily SR theophylline administration in the cat favors evening rather than morning dosing.

EFFICACY

The determination of theophylline efficacy in humans involves the use of pulmonary function testing. Since most PFTs depend upon patient cooperation and maximal effort, they have not been

Table 3. *Theophylline Dosages in the Dog and Cat**

Product	Dose (mg/kg by species)		Frequency	Time to Peak Concentration
	As Salt	As Theophylline		
Injectable theophylline products†				
Aminophylline	11 D	8.5 D	q 6 hr	Immediate
	5 C	4 C	q 8–12 hr	Immediate
Immediate-release oral theophylline products				
Aminophylline	11 D	8.5 D	q 6 hr	1.5 hr
	5 C	4 C	q 8–12 hr	1.5 hr
Sustained-Release oral theophylline products				
Theo-Dur *Tablets* (Key Pharmaceuticals)	NA	20 D	q 12 hr	4.7 hr
	NA	25 C	q 24 hr (in PM)‡	12 hr
	NA	25 C	q 24 hr (in AM)	8 hr
Slo-bid Gyrocaps (Rorer Pharmaceuticals)	NA	20–25 D	q 12 hr	4.0 hr
	NA	25 C	q 24 hr (in PM)‡	12 hr
	NA	25 C	q 24 hr (in AM)	8 hr
Choledyl-SA Tablets (Parke-Davis)	39–47 D	25–30 D	q 12 hr	3.9 hr

*These dosages are based on pharmacokinetic parameters and are predicted to result in steady-state plasma theophylline concentrations of 5 to 20 μg/ml. Dose recommendations are product-specific and should not be extrapolated to other products or formulations. Time to peak may be used to measure plasma theophylline concentrations when checking for therapeutic or potential toxic plasma concentrations. Plasma samples obtained from EDTA (ethylenediaminetetracetic acid) blood should be separated and kept frozen until submitted for analysis.
†Should only be given intravenously and slowly; intramuscular injection is contraindicated.
‡Evening dosing time is recommended for once-daily sustained-release products in cats.
C, cat; D, dog; NA, not applicable.

widely utilized in veterinary medicine. Nevertheless, efficacy of theophylline has been determined for some animal species and for some of the drug's effects.

EFFICACY IN COMPANION ANIMALS. Although bronchodilation (decrease in airway resistance) has been documented in the heavey pony at theophylline concentrations of 10 to 15 μg/ml, similar data has not been published for the dog and cat. A preliminary study in dogs indicated some theophylline protection against histamine-induced bronchoconstriction. Protection against antigen-induced bronchoconstriction has been documented in the dog using aerosolized dyphylline. Experimentally, an increase in mucociliary clearance, protection against diaphragmatic fatigue, and a 25% increase in diaphragmatic contractility have been shown to occur at plasma theophylline concentrations near 15 μg/ml in the dog, well within the plasma theophylline concentrations that the dosages in Table 1 are predicted to achieve. Clearly, more research is needed to document minimum effective and toxic theophylline concentrations, thereby better defining the role of theophylline in veterinary medicine.

CARDIOVASCULAR EFFECTS. The cardiovascular effects of theophylline have been extensively studied, yet many questions still exist. Theophylline is reported to be a positive inotrope and chronotrope in humans and animals. Increases in heart rate, stroke volume, cardiac output, right and left ventricular ejection fraction (primarily in chronic pulmonary disease states), force of ventricular papillary muscle contraction, rate of ventricular automaticity, and conduction velocity have been reported. On the other hand, theophylline decreases systemic vascular resistance, right and left end-diastolic pressures, and pulmonary capillary wedge and artery pressure. In humans, an important adverse cardiac effect of theophylline is its arrhythmogenic action. cAMP accumulations and release of catecholamines are the proposed mechanisms of action for most of these cardiac effects. In the heart, theophylline's adenosine antagonism is primarily (but not universally) reported to cause coronary vasoconstriction.

CENTRAL NERVOUS SYSTEM EFFECTS. Methylxanthine stimulation of the central nervous system (CNS) is common knowledge today. The resultant stimulation may manifest itself in humans as muscle tremors, irritability, hyperactivity, arousal, and insomnia. The antagonism of adenosine (a CNS depressant and vasodilator) is the probable mechanism of action. These CNS effects may occur within the therapeutic (bronchodilating) range in man. Caffeine is a recognized stimulant, but its CNS arousal effects are also useful as medical therapy for neonatal apnea (based on the ability of methylxanthines to decrease central chemoreceptor threshold to CO_2 and increase respiratory center output). Use of methylxanthines in the management of brachycephalic dogs with sleep-disordered breathing problems (hypersomnolence, apnea, and oxygen desaturation) may be a veterinary corollary to the use of methylxanthines in human infants.

MISCELLANEOUS EFFECTS. Many other effects of theophylline have been reported. For the most part they are of less clinical significance but may be apparent as toxic effects in cases of theophylline overdose. These effects include gastrointestinal, renal, skeletal muscle, metabolic, thermogenic, and anti-inflammatory effects.

TOXICITY

Methylxanthine toxicity is essentially an extension of the mechanisms of action. Signs of toxicity frequently occur in humans when plasma theophylline concentrations exceed 20 μg/ml, although minor (and usually transient) toxic effects may occur below this level. In humans, theophylline toxicities may be described as transient, minor, or major. Nausea, abdominal cramps, insomnia, and headaches are transient theophylline side effects and may be seen within the therapeutic range. Although there has been some concern regarding possible effects on immune system response in humans, there have been no studies to substantiate this concern in veterinary medicine.

Tolerance to methylxanthines is rapidly acquired. Minor signs of toxicity include persistent nausea, vomiting, mild CNS stimulation (manifested as excitability, irritability, and agitation), muscular tremors, and sinus tachycardia. In general, these effects are reported with plasma theophylline concentrations of 20 to 35 μg/ml. The major side effects of theophylline, which may be life-threatening, most often occur at plasma concentrations above 35 μg/ml and include seizures and ventricular arrhythmias in humans.

Theophylline toxicity in veterinary medicine has only recently been evaluated, mostly with acute administration (e.g., intravenous or oral) of large theophylline doses in laboratory animals or in anesthetized animals where the combined effects of anesthesia and theophylline administration may be hard to separate. There are species differences in susceptibility to theophylline toxicity, as well as differences due to the route of administration (e.g., intravenous versus oral) and the duration of therapy (e.g., acute versus chronic). In awake dogs, Munsiff et al. (1988) found that acute oral toxicity occurs at much higher plasma theophylline concentrations than in humans and that no serious toxicity was observed despite theophylline concentrations near 100 μg/ml.

The most commonly reported clinical side effects of theophylline in the dog relate to the CNS and gastrointestinal systems. Hyperexcitability, vomiting, and diarrhea have been reported, although the author knows of no measurements of actual plasma theophylline concentrations for evaluating possible toxicity. The toxicities and corresponding plasma theophylline concentrations reported by Munsiff et al. are summarized in Table 4. Others have reported cardiac arrhythmias in the dog following intravenous

Table 4. Theophylline Toxicity and Plasma Theophylline Concentrations in Six Healthy, Awake Pointer Dogs*

Route of Administration	Toxicity	Mean Plasma Theophylline Concentration
Oral	Cardiac†	68.0 μg/ml
	Central nervous system‡	
	Restlessness	37.3 μg/ml
	Excitability	50.1 μg/ml
	Vomiting	59.6 μg/ml
Intravenous	Cardiac†	19.8 μg/ml
	Central nervous system‡	
	Restlessness	11.9 μg/ml
	Excitability	22.9 μg/ml
	Vomiting	not observed

*Adapted from Munsiff, I. J. et al. Determination of the acute oral toxicity of theophylline in conscious dogs. J. Vet. Pharmacol. Ther. 11:381, 1988.
†Cardiac toxicity was defined as sinus tachycardia (heart rate 180 beats/min). No ventricular arrhythmias were noted in these clinically normal dogs.
‡The central nervous system signs observed included excitement and restlessness. No seizures were noted in any dog.

aminophylline administration, but these studies often utilized extremely large doses of theophylline (e.g., 140 mg/kg) in dogs under various gas anesthetics, making interpretation and application to the awake animal difficult.

MEASURING PLASMA THEOPHYLLINE CONCENTRATIONS. Determination of plasma theophylline concentrations in cats and dogs with possible theophylline toxicity is necessary to establish any specific correlation between reported signs and the dosages given. Most hospitals routinely determine human plasma theophylline concentrations and can usually rapidly analyze a sample. Proper sample timing is important to accurately measure peak plasma concentration. Table 3 includes a listing of the times blood samples should be drawn postdose based on the type of product administered.

BETA-ADRENERGIC AGONISTS

RATIONALE FOR USE

Both beta₁- and beta₂-receptors have been discovered in lung tissue from many different animal species. Beta-agonists, unlike anticholinergic agents, act to reverse bronchoconstriction regardless of the source of the stimulus (Barnes, 1991). Due to the potential side effects associated with the use of nonselective beta-agonists (i.e., those having both beta₁ and beta₂ actions), it is preferable to utilize beta₂-specific agonists (e.g., terbutaline, albuterol) in the treatment of bronchoconstriction. Even the beta-2–specific agonists may be associated with toxicity when given in large doses.

Table 5. *Doses of Beta-agonists and Anticholinergic Agents Recommended or Evaluated for the Treatment of Bronchospasm in Dogs and Cats**

Product	Indication†	Dose (mg/kg by species)	Route
Beta-agonists			
Epinephrine	E	20 µg/kg (C) q 30 min	IM,IV,SC
Ephedrine	E	2–5 mg total (C)	PO
	M	1–2 mg/kg q 8–12 hr (D)	PO
Isoproterenol	E	0.44 mg/kg q 6–12 hr (C)	PO
Terbutaline	M	1.25 mg total q 12 hr (C)	PO
	M	0.625 mg total q 12 hr (C)	PO
	M	1.25–5 mg total q 8–12 hr (D)	PO
Albuterol	M	50 mg/kg q 8 hr (D)	PO
Anticholinergics			
Atropine	E	0.02–0.04 mg/kg (C)	IV,IM,SC
Glycopyrrolate	E	0.01–0.02 mg/kg p.r.n. (C)	IV,IM,SC

C, cat; D, dog; IM, intramuscular; IV, intravenous; SC, subcutaneous.
*Data compiled from Boothe (1990), McKiernan et al. (1991), and Padrid et al. (1990).
†Indications are for emergency (E) relief of respiratory distress or for maintenance (M) therapy in chronic obstructive pulmonary diseases.

PHARMACOLOGY AND MECHANISM OF ACTION

Beta agonists bind to receptors on the surface of cells and stimulate the enzyme adenylate cyclase to increase production of cAMP. Increased levels of intracellular cAMP lead to bronchial smooth muscle relaxation similar to the action described for theophylline. In addition to bronchodilation, beta-agonists are also reported to decrease mediator release from mast cells (thereby helping to control inflammation by limiting the release of mediators), increase ciliary beat frequency, modify parasympathetic tone, and play a role in the modulation of mucosal edema by decreasing microvascular leakage. (Barnes, 1991; Boothe, 1990)

BETA-AGONISTS IN DOGS AND CATS. A number of selective beta-2 agonists (e.g., terbutaline, albuterol, metaproterenol) have been recommended for use in dogs and cats, although pharmacokinetic studies of beta agonists in companion animals have not been published (Boothe, 1990; Prueter and Sherding, 1985). An albuterol dose of 50 mg/kg t.i.d. in dogs with chronic bronchial disease was effective in a study by Padrid et al. (1990). Preliminary data suggest that oral terbutaline at a dose of 0.15 mg/kg (approximately 0.625 mg total) b.i.d. may be used in cats (McKiernan et al., 1991). Currently recommended dosages of beta-agonists in dogs and cats are summarized in Table 5.

Epinephrine is the drug of choice for the treatment of status asthmaticus in humans. Epinephrine, ephedrine, and isoproterenol have been recommended for the emergency relief of respiratory distress in cats (Boothe, 1990). Epinephrine and ephedrine stimulate alpha receptors and may result in vasoconstriction and hypertension. Isoproterenol has also been recommended in companion animals but lacks the specificity needed to avoid stimulation of beta-1 receptors (and the problems of hypoten-

sion and tachycardia). Aerosolized beta agonists are readily available in human medicine, but due to difficulty in administration are rarely used in routine veterinary practice.

EFFICACY IN DOGS AND CATS. Preliminary work at the University of Illinois has shown terbutaline efficacy in some (but not all) cats with chronic bronchial disease (Fig. 1). Clinical, radiographic, and tidal breathing flow-volume loop improvement was noted in most cases following a 2-week therapeutic trial with albuterol in 12 dogs with chronic bronchial disease (Padrid et al., 1990). Transient signs of toxicity (nervousness, muscle tremors) were reported in some of these dogs at the start of albuterol therapy.

Signs of beta-agonist toxicity usually relate to

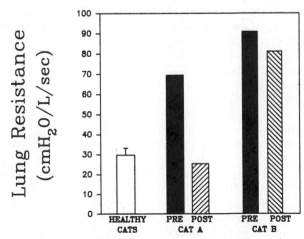

Figure 1. Immediate effect of intravenous terbutaline (0.01 mg/kg) on lung resistance (R_L) measured in two cats presented with signs of chronic bronchial disease compared to the mean lung resistance obtained in eight healthy cats. Note that although apparently similar in presentation, only cat "A" demonstrated a favorable response to acute bronchodilator therapy.

beta-1 stimulation and most notably include hypotension and tachycardia. Stimulation of peripheral $beta_2$-receptors may also result in signs of toxicity. Experimentally, the combined use of theophylline and beta agonists has been associated with toxic changes (e.g., focal myocardial necrosis secondary to hypoxic vasoconstriction) (Hendles and Weinberger, 1983). Although combined beta-agonist and methylxanthine therapy has been suggested in severe or refractory cases, clinicians should be aware of this potential toxicity.

ANTICHOLINERGIC AGENTS

A small amount of resting bronchomotor tone is reported to exist in many animals, including cats. Following lung irritant or stretch receptor stimulation, afferent cholinergic impulses reach the brain and result in stimulation of the parasympathetic nervous system. Efferent impulses travel via the vagus nerves and lead to subsequent bronchoconstriction. Atropine readily blocks this reflex arc response (as well as resting tone) by actively competing against acetylcholine for receptor sites on the effector cells (i.e., the bronchial smooth muscle).

CLINICAL USE AND RECOMMENDATIONS

Anticholinergics provide little protection against agents that exert their effect through the local release of mediators (Barnes, 1991). Beta-blockade–induced bronchoconstriction (seen occasionally in cats treated with propanolol) is a specific indication for the use of anticholinergic agents in veterinary medicine. Recommended canine and feline dosages of anticholinergic agents are summarized in Table 5.

EFFICACY AND TOXICITY

Although effective in blocking all types of muscarinic receptors, atropine's lack of specificity may result in adverse side effects that limit its chronic use in the treatment of bronchoconstriction. The unwanted side effects of atropine include drying of respiratory tract secretions, interference with normal mucociliary clearance mechanisms, tachycardia, meiosis, and possible alterations in gastrointestinal and urinary tract function. Atropine and glycopyrrolate can be used in conjunction with beta agonists during the initial management of the acutely dyspneic cat (Boothe, 1990).

IPRATROPIUM. An aerosol-administered, synthetic anticholinergic, ipratropium bromide has been used in human medicine for a number of years. Due to its poor absorption from the respiratory tract, ipratropium use has generally not been associated with the adverse effects noted with atropine use (Boothe, 1990). Although the efficacy of ipratropium has been documented experimentally in the dog, the lack of clinical experience to date and the difficulty of using an aerosolized drug limits its use in clinical veterinary practice.

SUMMARY

Successful bronchodilation should in theory, provide relief of respiratory distress and improve ventilation perfusion ratios in the lung. Unfortunately little scientific information on the pharmacokinetics and pharmacodynamics of these drugs is available for veterinary species. The determination of plasma concentrations (e.g. theophylline) in cases where ineffective clinical results and/or toxicity are suspected will greatly improve our understanding of these drugs in clinical practice. Continued research in the area of kinetics and dynamics will help future clinicians in making rational therapeutic choices when selecting a bronchodilator for their patients.

References and Suggested Reading

Barnes, P. J.: Neural control of airway smooth muscle. *In* Crystal, R. G., West, J. B. et al. (eds.): *The Lung.* New York: Raven Press, 1991, p. 903.
Provides a current, in-depth review of the mechanisms of airway neural control by one of the experts in the field

Boothe, D. M.: Feline respiratory pharmacology. Sheba Symposium Proceedings, Orlando, FL, 1990, p. 27.
Comprehensive review of the pharmacology for feline respiratory diseases.

Dye, J. A., McKiernan, B. C., Jones, S. D., et al.: Sustained-release theophylline pharmacokinetics in the cat. J. Vet. Pharmacol. Ther. 12:133, 1989.
Provides pharmacologic background for the use of sustained-release theophylline formulations in the cat as well as a review of earlier theophylline kinetics in this species.

Dye, J. A., McKiernan, B. C., Neff-Davis, C. A., et al.: Chronopharmacokinetics of theophylline in the cat. J. Vet. Pharmacol. Ther. 13:278, 1990.
Explains the rational for once-daily dosing of sustained-release theophylline formulations in the cat, with a short review of other drugs that demonstrate circadian fluctuations.

Hendles, L., and Weinberger, M.: Theophylline: A "state of the art" review. Pharmacotherapy. 3:2, 1983.
Comprehensive review of the pharmacology of theophylline in human medicine.

Jackson, W. F.: Dyspnea. *In* Kirk, R. W. (ed.): Current Veterinary Therapy. Philadelphia: W. B. Saunders, 1964, p. 55.
An early discussion of dyspnea in the dog and cat and its treatment.

Jones, L. M., Booth, N. H., and McDonald, L. E. (eds.): *Veterinary Pharmacology and Therapeutics,* 4th ed. Ames, IA: Iowa State Press, 1977, p. 413.
Discussion of the pharmacokinetics and clinical use of methylxanthines.

Koritz, G. D., McKiernan, B. C., Neff-Davis, C. A., et al.: Bioavailability of four slow-release theophylline formulations in the beagle dog. J. Vet. Pharmacol Therap 9:293, 1986.
Description of the pharmacokinetics of four sustained-release theophylline formulations in the dog.

McKiernan, B. C., Dye, J. A., Powell, M., et al.: Terbutaline pharmacokinetis in cats. (Abstract.) J. Vet. Intern. Med. 5:122, 1991.

Munsiff, I. J., McKiernan, B. C., Neff-Davis, C. A., et al.: Determination of the acute oral toxicity of theophylline in conscious dogs. J. Vet. Pharmacol. Ther. 11:381, 1988.
Provides specifics on the toxicity observed following the administration of variable doses of sustained-release theophylline formulations to awake, healthy dogs.
Padrid, P. A., Hornof, W. J., Kurpershoek, C. J., et al.: Canine chronic bronchitis. J. Vet. Intern. Med. 4:172, 1990.
Reviews the clinical and pathologic findings in a series of 18 bronchitic dogs and details their response to short-term oral albuterol therapy.

Prueter, J. C., and Sherding, R. G.: Canine chronic bronchitis. Vet. Clin. North Am. 15:1085, 1985.
Provides a review of canine bronchitis, including etiology, clinical presentation, pathology, diagnosis, and treatment.
Secord, D. C.: Pulmonary emphysema. *In* Kirk, R. W. (ed.): Current Veterinary Therapy. Philadelphia: W. B. Saunders, 1964, p. 293.
Rationale for using ephedrine and aminophylline in chronic bronchitis.
Stephenson, H. C., and Mittelstaedt, S. G. (eds.): *Veterinary Drug Encyclopedia and Therapeutic Index.* New York: Drug Publications, 1953, pp. 83, 86, 96.

CURRENT USES AND HAZARDS OF DIURETIC THERAPY

PHILIP R. FOX

New York, New York

Diuretics are the foundation of congestive heart failure (CHF) therapy. Their importance in small-animal practice is underscored by statistics showing that manufacturer sales of veterinary-labeled diuretics totaled $2.9 million to $3.6 million annually from 1984 through 1989. Furosemide accounted for 73 to 93% of these sales.

The routine use of diuretics reflects several realities. First, they have a relatively low and predictable toxicity when administered appropriately. Second, loop diuretics rapidly and reliably reduce venous pressures (preload), making them effective agents for treating moderate and severe CHF. Third, these agents are easily affordable.

Pharmacologic mechanisms of action vary among diuretic classes, but all have the common action of inhibiting renal ion transport. They promote negative sodium balance by limiting sodium reabsorption from renal tubular fluid into systemic circulation.

Diuresis and natriuresis depend upon several factors including drug potency relative to inhibition of electrolyte reabsorption, site of drug action in the nephron, and factors related to heart failure that may counter diuretic actions (e.g., excess aldosterone, antidiuretic hormone, circulating blood volume).

Successful application of diuretics requires a basic understanding of their pharmacology, systemic and hemodynamic effects, and potential for adverse drug interactions, as well as a prompt and accurate diagnosis, knowledge of underlying disease pathophysiology, complete patient database, and clearly defined and monitored therapeutic end points.

RENAL ALTERATIONS IN HEART FAILURE

The kidney plays a central role in modulating neurohumoral responses to heart failure. Compensatory mechanisms are initially beneficial by maintaining cardiac performance. For example, salt and water retention initially restores effective circulating blood volume, increases cardiac filling (preload), and sustains cardiac output. Compensatory mechanisms eventually become ineffective, produce excessive physiologic responses, and contribute to cardiac decompensation (congestive heart failure).

SODIUM RETENTION. Several mechanisms promote sodium reabsorption in heart failure. As cardiac output falls, renal prostaglandins and concentrations of circulating catecholamines and angiotensin II are increased. These effects maintain glomerular filtration rate by increasing the filtration fraction (the ratio of glomerular filtration rate to renal blood flow). However, the amount of sodium reabsorbed from the proximal tubule is also increased and is further enhanced by blood flow redistribution from cortical to juxtamedullary nephrons, which demonstrate more efficient sodium reabsorption capability.

By these mechanisms, urine volume is reduced and water and solutes are conserved at a time when increased thirst (stimulated by angiotensin II) may be promoting water intake. The circulatory system and failing heart are thus presented with an increased fluid volume for distribution as ascites, effusions, or edema according to prevailing hydrostatic and oncotic forces.

ACTIVATION OF THE RENIN-ANGIOTENSION-AL-DOSTERONE SYSTEM. Renin is released by renal juxtaglomerular cells when stimulated by changes in afferent arteriole transmural pressure, sodium delivery, or sympathetic activity. The proteolytic enzyme renin converts an alpha globulin in the liver to angiotensin I, which is transformed in the lungs by a converting enzyme into angiotensin II, a potent vasoconstrictor that increases systemic vascular resistance and afterload.

In addition, the concentration of circulating plasma aldosterone may be increased. Factors include enhanced adrenal synthesis and release stimulated by angiotensin II and decreased aldosterone metabolism related to hepatic congestion and reduced splanchnic blood flow. Aldosterone enhances renal sodium reabsorption with accompanying expansion of extracellular and intravascular fluid volumes.

WATER RETENTION. Increased total body sodium promotes water retention in heart failure. Contributing factors include elevated plasma antidiuretic hormone (ADH) levels, which reduce renal free-water clearance; increased circulating angiotensin II, which stimulates thirst; resetting of atrial pressure receptors, which blunts the normal diuretic response to left atrial distention mediated by atrial natriuretic factor; and renal sodium retention.

Azotemia. Prerenal azotemia is common in decompensated heart failure patients. This is especially true in cats, which often display anorexia and vomiting with CHF. Elevated blood urea nitrogen (BUN) results principally from reduced glomerular filtration rate and from lesser factors such as augmented passive urea reabsorption in the distal nephron and a catabolic state associated with chronic heart failure. Serum creatinine may be initially preserved in mildly decompensated animals. Severe heart failure may markedly reduce renal blood flow and glomerular filtration rate, elevating serum creatinine.

Mild to moderate prerenal azotemia in feline CHF is not a poor prognostic sign and should be anticipated. In dogs, prerenal azotemia is usually mild and transitory. Severe azotemia is often a poor prognostic sign, especially if atrial fibrillation, hyponatremia, and advanced right-sided heart failure are present.

POTASSIUM HOMEOSTASIS. Several mechanisms may contribute to hypokalemia in animals with heart failure. Distal tubular exchange of sodium for potassium and hydrogen may be associated with enhanced aldosterone secretion and also promotes sodium and potassium exchange with resulting kaliuresis. Anorexia is a common cause of hypokalemia in decompensated animals, and affected cats are frequently mildly hypokalemic (3.1 to 3.5 mEq/ml). This may be exacerbated by pre-existing chronic polyuric renal disease, nutritional influences, or overzealous diuretic therapy. Thiazide or loop diuretic therapy inhibits sodium reabsorption proximal to aldosterone's site of action. Dogs, on the other hand, are usually unaffected unless prolonged anorexia and concurrent high-dose diuretic therapy have been present.

DIURETIC MECHANISMS AND SITES OF ACTION

Basic knowledge of renal physiology and diuretic pharmacology is useful when planning and modifying therapy. The clinician should be familiar with diuretic drug mechanisms as they relate to renal physiology, sites of drug activity, drug potencies, onset of action, duration of expected effects, and untoward complications. Therapeutic end points should be clear and monitored.

PROXIMAL TUBULE. Approximately two thirds of filtered sodium is isotonically reabsorbed here. Several factors govern the absolute quantity of solute and water reabsorption; the most significant are the volume of glomerular filtrate and the net effect of Starling's forces on transtubular ion and water transport. While active solute reabsorption occurs, it is less important.

Proximal tubular sodium exchange depends upon a basolateral cell membrane sodium pump (Na^+, K^+-ATPase) and carbonic anhydrase. The latter generates intracellular hydrogen protons that exchange with sodium on the luminal side of the tubule. Brush-border membrane carbonic anhydrase converts luminal carbonic acid to carbon dioxide and water intracellularly, increasing net bicarbonate reabsorption. A specific apical cell membrane sodium-proton exchanger modulates net luminal bicarbonate and sodium absorption.

For a diuretic to significantly inhibit proximal tubular sodium reabsorption, it must act either on the basolateral sodium pump, sodium-proton exchanger, or carbonic anhydrase. At normal *in vivo* concentrations, diuretics do not directly block either of the first two mechanisms. Agents that act in the proximal tubule exert their effect on carbonic anhydrase.

HENLE'S LOOP. Approximately one third of the glomerular filtrate arrives at the descending limb of Henle's loop. No active solute reabsorption occurs here. Water is reabsorbed from the highly permeable tubular epithelium through an increasingly hyperosmotic medullary interstitium. Medullary interstitial hypertonicity is maintained by the thick ascending limb of Henle's loop, which is impermeable to water. Here, an electroneutral process occurs in which a sodium-potassium (Na^+/K^+) cotransport system is coupled to active uptake of two chloride ions bringing sodium, potassium, and two chloride ions into the cell. The energy process is dependent upon a sodium gradient created by Na^+,K^+-ATPase in the basolateral cell membrane. This cotransporter creates an electrochemical gradient for chloride to enter the blood. Most potassium that enters the cell via the electroneutral carrier is recycled back into luminal urine across the apical cell membrane. Movement of chloride from cell to blood and recycling of potassium from cell to tubule contributes to a transepithelial positive potential that drives sodium out of the luminal thick ascending limb through paracellular spaces. Passive reabsorption of calcium and magnesium occur here as well. This $Na^+/K^+/2Cl$ cotransport system is the receptor for loop diuretics.

DISTAL TUBULE. This segment is largely ADH-insensitive and impermeable to water, allowing formation of dilute urine. Sodium, chloride, and other ions are absorbed here. An electroneutral sodium chloride cotransporter in apical cell membranes mediates their reabsorption. Very high furosemide concentrations and lower concentrations of thiazides and metolazone inhibit this coupled sodium chloride transport entry step in the distal tubule membrane.

COLLECTING DUCT. This duct is divided into cortical and medullary segments; ADH augments the water permeability of both segments, but only the former is sensitive to effects of aldosterone. Aldosterone binds to a cytoplasmic receptor protein, which increases apical membrane sodium permeability. Increased intracellular sodium is pumped out into the blood by basolateral cell membrane Na^+,K^+-ATPase. A luminal negative potential is thereby created that favors potassium and chloride secretion back into the lumen. Antialdosterone drugs like spironolactone competitively inhibit aldosterone from binding to its receptor. This limits apical cell membrane permeability to sodium, reduces the negative luminal potential, and decreases active sodium transport from cell to blood by Na^+,K^+-ATPase

DIURETIC THERAPY

The goal of heart failure therapy is to prolong and improve the quality of life. Clinical signs relate primarily to impaired cardiac output, abnormal regional blood flow, and circulatory congestion. Judicious diuretic administration is an essential component of heart failure therapy.

Diuretics are used to reduce congestion by lowering cardiac preload (although some studies indicate that they also increase stroke volume from the failing left ventricle by reducing peripheral vascular resistance and afterload). Pulmonary edema due to elevated left-heart filling pressures in dogs can occur with volume overload (e.g., mitral regurgitation, left-to-right shunts) or myocardial failure. In cats,

lung edema most commonly results from reduced left ventricular diastolic compliance (e.g., left ventricular hypertrophic diseases). Right-sided heart failure usually causes pericardial, pleural, or abdominal effusions and occasionally peripheral edema. This may be associated with elevated right-heart filling pressures from volume overload (e.g., tricuspid regurgitation), pulmonary hypertensive disorders, or left-heart diseases. Furosemide is the diuretic most commonly used to reduce cardiac filling pressures. Dietary sodium restriction and venodilator drugs represent two additional methods to control preload.

DIURETIC AGENTS

Four classes of diuretics are generally available. They include carbonic anhydrase inhibitors, loop diuretics, thiazides, and potassium-sparing agents. Comparative diuretic effects on urinary electrolytes are contrasted in Table 1. Diuretic actions, dosages, and adverse effects are listed in Table 2.

Carbonic Anhydrase Inhibitors

PHARMACOLOGY AND MECHANISMS

Represented by acetazolamide, this class is among the weakest of the diuretic drugs. Promoting less than 5% fractional sodium excretion, it is relegated to non–heart failure conditions where negative sodium balance is unimportant (e.g., glaucoma therapy). The primary diuretic effect is due to inhibition of sodium bicarbonate absorption in the proximal tubule. The increased distal sodium bicarbonate delivery exceeds absorption capabilities there and results in increased urinary excretion of bicarbonate. Potassium wasting may follow because bicarbonate acts as a nonreabsorbable anion.

CLINICAL USE

Carbonic anhydrase inhibitors are rarely employed in heart failure therapy. Acute administration induces increased urinary excretion of bicarbonate and urinary alkalinization; the latter effect could theoretically enhance excretion of certain weak acids such as aspirin during overdose.

Loop Diuretics

PHARMACOLOGY AND MECHANISMS

Loop or "high-ceiling" agents are the most potent of the listed diuretic categories and can induce

Table 1. *Effects of Diuretics on Urinary Electrolyte Excretion*

Agent	FE_{Na}	Na^+	K^+	Cl^-	HCO_3^-	Ca^{++}	Mg^{++}
Weak Diuretics							
Carbonic anhydrase inhibitors (acetazolamide)	<5	+	+	0	+ +	+	↓
Potassium-sparing (spironolactone, amiloride)	<5	+	↓, ↓ ↓	(+)	+	0	↓
Moderately Potent Diuretics							
(Thiazides and related compounds)	8–10	+ +	+	+ +	(+)	↓	+
Potent Diuretics							
Loop diuretics (furosemide, bumetanide, ethacrynic acid)	20–25	+ + +	+	+ + +	0	+ +	+

(+), +, + +, + + +, Degree of potency from minimum to maximum; ↓, Reduction of urinary excretion; Fe_{Na}, Fractional excretion of sodium (%).

natriuresis approximating 20 to 25% of filtered sodium. They are weak acids extensively bound to plasma proteins and reach their tubular site of action by active secretion in the proximal tubule. Of the available loop diuretic drugs—ethacrynic acid, bumetanide, and furosemide—only furosemide is administered routinely in veterinary therapy.

All three agents inhibit chloride and sodium reabsorption in the thick ascending Henle's loop by actively blocking sodium-potassium-chloride cotransport. They increase and may redistribute renal blood flow from juxtamedullary to outer cortical regions. Unlike thiazides, they do not induce compensatory reduction of glomerular filtration rate (GFR) by glomerulotubular feedback mechanisms, and loop diuretics promote natriuresis even with decreased GFR and renal blood flow.

In addition to their intrarenal properties, loop diuretics exert important extrarenal effects. Although controversial, there is evidence that intravenous furosemide may acutely increase venous capacitance, presumably due to release of vasodilatory prostaglandins. This action may occur even before natriuresis.

Table 2. *Diuretics: Action and Dosage*

Diuretic	Trade Name (Manufacturer)	Site; Mechanism of Action	Effect on Blood Electrolytes, Acid-Base	Available Forms	Dosage
Thiazides		Distal tubule; inhibit NaCl transport	↓ Na^+, ↓ Cl^- ↑ HCO_3, ↑ Ca^{++}; mild metabolic alkalosis		
Chlorothiazide	Diuril (Merck Sharp & Dohme)			250- and 500-mg tabs	20–40 mg/kg b.i.d.
Hydrochloro-thiazide	HydroDIURIL (Merck Sharp & Dohme)			25- and 50-mg tabs	2–4 mg/kg b.i.d.
Loop Diuretics		Thick ascending limb, Henle's loop; inhibit Na/K/Cl cotransporter	↓ K^+, ↓ Cl^-, ↓ Na^+ ↑ HCO_3; hypochloremic metabolic acidosis		
Furosemide	Lasix (Hoechst-Roussel)			12.5- and 50-mg tabs; 50-mg/ml injection	Dog: 1–4 mg/kg s.i.d.–t.i.d. Cat: 0.9–1.8 mg/kg s.i.d.–b.i.d.
Bumetanide	Bumex (Roche Laboratories)			0.1-, 1-, and 2-mg tabs	
Potassium-Sparing Diuretics		Collecting duct	↑ K^+; metabolic acidosis		
Spironolactone	Aldactone (Searle)	Aldosterone antagonist		25-mg tabs	2 mg/kg/day
Triamterene	Dyrenium (Smith Kline & French)	Inhibits apical membrane Na^+ conductance		100-mg capsules	2–4 mg/kg/day
Amiloride	Midamor (Merck Sharp & Dohme)	Impairs Na^+ entry in distal nephron; spares K^+			

Onset of action is rapid. Intravenous administration of furosemide and bumetanide promotes diuresis within minutes, peaking within 30 min and returning to baseline within 2 or 3 hr.

Oral administration, however, may result in variable absorption, and natriuresis with orally administered furosemide and bumetanide may be attenuated in CHF. Causes include delayed intestinal absorption and reduced drug delivery to tubular receptor sites. Optimally, onset of action after oral administration is between 30 to 60 min, peaking at 30 to 120 min and returning to baseline in 2 to 3 hr.

Bioavailability differences have been documented between Lasix (Hoechst-Roussel) and some generic furosemide preparations. Lasix has been shown to be significantly superior to several generic furosemide preparations in establishing maximal furosemide plasma levels and in bioavailability. Inequivalence between formulations and product may reduce the effectiveness of diuretic therapy, and this concern bears consideration in the treatment of moderate to severe heart failure.

Saluretic and diuretic effects of intramuscularly administered furosemide have been experimentally evaluated in normal cats and dogs. In cats, 10 mg/kg caused apathy for 5 hr and reduced appetite for 24 hr postinjection. Normal dogs, however, tolerated this dose with no adverse effects. Compared to the dog, cats responded to intramuscular furosemide with stronger and more rapid saluresis and diuresis.

Bumetanide has pharmacokinetic and pharmacodynamic properties similar to furosemide in man. However, it is absorbed more quickly, has greater bioavailability (80% versus 40% with furosemide), and has greater potency (40:1). Elimination half-lives are approximately 1 to 2 hr, but that of bumetanide is a little shorter due to more rapid clearance. Bumetanide does not possess greater efficacy than furosemide and has not been extensively evaluated in spontaneous animal heart failure models.

CLINICAL USE

Furosemide's rapid onset of action, high potency, and ability to induce diuresis when renal blood flow is reduced make it the agent of choice to treat moderate and severe CHF. Intravenous administration induces natriuresis quickly, decreases extracellular volume, and may increase venous capacitance; this rapidly reduces cardiac preload and pulmonary congestion. In appropriately selected patients with CHF, maintenance furosemide therapy, especially when combined with a low-salt diet, will reduce congestion with minimal reduction in cardiac output. However, increased morbidity may result from overzealous diuresis with both acute and chronic administration. Dosage is variable and must be modified according to prevailing physiologic conditions and concurrent drug therapies.

The standard canine dosage varies from 1 to 4 mg/kg s.i.d. to t.i.d. PO, IV, IM, or SC. Dose selection and administration route depend upon onset and severity of congestive signs. For small-breed dogs in sinus rhythm with chronic acquired atrioventricular valvular insufficiency (myxomatous degeneration), with an otherwise uncomplicated first onset of mild to moderate pulmonary edema, an average oral starting dose is 2 mg/kg s.i.d. to b.i.d. When coupled with cage rest and dietary sodium restriction, clinical signs often resolve within 24 to 48 hr. Maintenance therapy employs the lowest effective dose, typically 2 mg/kg s.i.d. to b.i.d. initially. Drug resistance and chronic progressive cardiac disease may require doubling these doses, with t.i.d. administration in some cases.

For moderate to severe pulmonary edema in the dog, furosemide may be administered intravenously to promote rapid diuresis. It may be initially dosed at 2 to 3 mg/kg b.i.d. or s.i.d. IV to promote clinical resolution of dyspnea. Dogs with renal failure may require a higher initial dose to deliver sufficient furosemide to the distal nephron. Dogs with refractory ascites often respond much better to parenteral furosemide than to equivalent doses of an oral preparation. This may be related to malabsorption of the oral agent in dogs with intestinal congestion.

Some canine patients, and Doberman pinschers as a breed, may be very sensitive to diuretic-induced preload reduction in the setting of severe myocardial failure. The furosemide dose may need to be reduced 25 to 50% in these settings.

Cats are more sensitive than dogs to the diuretic effects of furosemide. With parenteral administration, overdiuresis can quickly occur. Because anorexia has often been present for 24 to 48 hr preceding patient examination, mild to moderate dehydration and hypokalemia may already be present. Following furosemide administration, further dehydration, hypovolemia, and hypotension may occur unless these side effects are recognized and monitored. Therefore, furosemide dosage for cats is less than that for dogs.

For acute pulmonary edema in cats, furosemide is dosed at 0.9 to 1.8 mg/kg s.i.d. to b.i.d. parenterally; intravenous injection is the preferred route if stress can be avoided. Practically speaking, this amounts to about 5 to 10 mg in a large cat and 2.5 to 5 mg for a small cat, once to twice daily, often combined with venodilator therapy (e.g., 2% transdermal nitroglycerin ointment). Dosage is reduced as soon as significant improvement is noted.

Maintenance furosemide therapy in the cat also utilizes the lowest effective dose. This is typically one quarter to one half of a 12.5-mg tablet given every other day to twice daily. The average oral maintenance dose after resoluton of pulmonary edema in the cat is 6.25 mg daily. With exacerbations of heart failure, chronic, refractory effusions, or diuretic resistance during long-term maintenance therapy, oral furosemide may need to be increased to 1.5 to 4.5 mg/kg s.i.d. to t.i.d.

Functional renal insufficiency must be avoided when angiotensin-converting enzyme (ACE) inhibitors (e.g., captopril, enalapril, or lisinopril) are administered concurrently with diuretics and sodium-restricted diets. In low-output states, angiotensin II–mediated vasoconstriction becomes an important factor in maintaining systemic blood pressure, renal perfusion pressure (by intrarenal vasoconstriction), and GFR. ACE inhibition coupled with dietary salt restriction and diuretic-induced natriuresis and diuresis must therefore be closely evaluated in these situations. Should drug-induced azotemia occur (without edema), resolution may be facilitated by fluid therapy, replenishing total body sodium (decreasing or eliminating dietary sodium restriction), and diuretic dose reduction.

Noncardiac indications for furosemide include symptomatic hypercalcemia, nephrotic syndrome, and hypertension. Furosemide may also be used to treat cirrhosis with ascites refractory to spironolactone and dietary salt restriction and to avert oliguria in acute renal failure after intravascular volume expansion.

Thiazides and Related Agents

PHARMACOLOGY AND MECHANISMS

These drugs induce a fractional sodium excretion of approximately 10% and are categorized as moderately potent diuretics. Their usefulness is limited because large quantities of solute are already reabsorbed in the nephron at sites proximal to a thiazide's distal site of action. The thiazides are pharmacologically similar and have equivalent maximal diuretic efficacy but differ in potency and elimination half-life. The more lipid-soluble agents have greater volumes of distribution, lower renal clearance, and longer duration of action. They are highly plasma-protein bound, are mainly secreted in the proximal renal tubule, and act by inhibiting distal tubular sodium chloride reabsorption. These agents reduce urinary calcium excretion but promote potassium and magnesium wasting. They may become relatively ineffective in advanced renal failure due to decreased glomerular filtration.

In addition to the renal effects described above, thiazides have antihypertensive activity. This is not related solely to their ability to reduce intravascular fluid volume; it is also associated with reduction of systemic vascular resistance.

Three related drugs used in human medicine have not been well evaluated in veterinary therapy. Chlorthalidone displays a longer half-life than do the thiazides. Metolazone is more potent than thiazide agents and maintains natriuresis in advanced renal failure with greatly reduced GFR. Indapamide is very lipid soluble, has a longer duration of action, and has antihypertensive activity at doses that are minimally diuretic.

CLINICAL USE

Thiazides have been historically employed for chronic maintenance therapy of mild to moderate heart failure, although low-dose furosemide is equally efficacious. However, thiazide monotherapy is not advocated for management of acute pulmonary edema or severe right-sided heart failure. Treatment of the rapidly progressive and potentially lethal edema state with slower-acting and less-potent thiazide agents puts some patients at risk. Moreover, thiazides may not be efficacious with the severely reduced glomerular filtration that accompanies renal failure, while furosemide's activity is relatively uneffected by renal insufficiency. Absorption of oral thiazide agents in heart failure is not well studied in animals.

Dosages for oral chlorothiazide as monotherapy in the dog and cat are 20 to 40 mg/kg b.i.d.; onset of action is within 1 hr, peak effect occurs at about 4 hr, and duration may extend 6 to 12 hr. Hydrochlorothiazide dosage is 2 to 4 mg/kg b.i.d.; onset of action occurs within 2 hr and peak effect is in 4 hr with a 12-hr duration of effect. It has been successfully used in cats as an adjunct (5 to 10 mg s.i.d. to b.i.d.) to furosemide for refractory right-sided heart failure.

Extracardiac use of thiazides occurs in antihypertensive therapy, nephrotic syndrome and cirrhosis with ascites (second-choice agents), and nephrogenic diabetes insipidus.

Potassium-Sparing Diuretics

PHARMACOLOGY AND MECHANISMS

These drugs induce a fractional sodium excretion of less than 5% and are weak diuretics. This is because their physiologic actions are limited to a late portion of the nephron reached by a relatively small fraction of sodium. Drugs of this category inhibit sodium reabsorption and reduce potassium and hydrogen ion secretion by one of two different mechanisms of action: aldosterone antagonists (spironolactone) and direct inhibitors of sodium transport (amiloride, triamterene).

Aldosterone antagonists (e.g., spironolactone) competitively bind to cytoplasmic receptor protein in aldosterone-responsive cells of the distal tubule and early collecting duct. They block potassium-sodium exchange, thereby conserving potassium while promoting sodium excretion. Thus, they have little effect when aldosterone concentrations are low but are more effective with hyperaldosteronism, especially in combination with another diuretic. They do not affect free water production or reabsorption because their site of action is distal to free water formation or generation of medullary interstitial tonicity.

Spironolactone is protein bound. It induces hepatic cytochrome P-450 and may alter hepatic microsomal metabolism of other drugs. Canrenone, a metabolite of spironolactone, and the related agent canrenoate potassium are also commercially available.

Amiloride and triamterene block the sodium entry channel. They prevent sodium transport from the distal tubule lumen into tubular cells regardless of circulating aldosterone concentrations. This reduces the quantity of sodium available for sodium-potassium pumps, decreasing potassium secretion and promoting its conservation. Reduced sodium reabsorption also makes the luminal potential less negative and limits potassium and hydrogen secretion.

CLINICAL USE

As monotherapy agents, potassium-sparing diuretics are not useful for management of routine heart failure because they induce only mild natriuresis and diuresis. Their diuretic effect is enhanced as adjuncts in combined therapy with furosemide or thiazides, especially to attenuate potassium loss.

The aldosterone antagonist spironolactone may be effective in conditions associated with high aldosterone concentrations, such as some cases of CHF or ascites due to cirrhosis. Spironolactone in dogs is orally dosed at 2 to 4 mg/kg/day. It has a gradual onset of action. Peak effect occurs 2 to 3 days after therapy is initiated and lasts 2 to 3 days after treatment is discontinued. In cats, a combination spironolactone-thiazide product (Aldactazide, Searle) is dosed at 2.2 to 4.4 mg/kg b.i.d. PO.

Triamterene dosage in dogs is 2 to 4 mg/kg/day orally. Onset begins within 2 hr, peak activity occurs at 6 to 8 hr, and duration of effect extends 12 to 16 hr. Absorption in animals with heart failure has not been closely evaluated.

Potassium-sparing diuretics are generally contraindicated with hyperkalemia. Therefore, their use with oral potassium supplements, feline thromboembolic disease, or renal insufficiency should be limited. Concomitant effects with ACE inhibitors have not been well studied in animals with heart failure, and because of the potential for excess potassium retention, this combination is not generally recommended.

Combination Diuretic Therapy

Refractory edema or effusion may occasionally require addition of a second diuretic agent. Combination diuretic drug therapy induces a potentiated effect due to varied mechanisms of action and different sites of activity in the nephron. Thiazides can be successfully used as an adjunct to furosemide for this purpose. Potassium-sparing drugs can be added to furosemide to increase diuresis and decrease renal potassium wasting. Alterations in electrolyte and acid-base homeostasis can be encountered during combination diuretic therapy, so caution must be exercised.

COMPLICATIONS OF DIURETIC THERAPY

While acute mortality from diuretic misuse is rare, morbidity is common. Inappropriate diuretic administration may create systemic, hemodynamic, electrolyte, or acid-base derangements and render concomitant drug therapy ineffective or harmful.

Cardiac Function and Hemodynamics

Overdiuresis and resultant circulatory impairment is a frequent complication of diuretic therapy, especially with loop diuretics. Severe intravascular volume contraction may follow when the dosage is excessively high, especially when initial doses are unaltered after congestion resolves. Stroke volume and cardiac output depend on adequate cardiac filling pressures. Thus, cardiac performance can deteriorate and cause systemic hypotension, reflex sinus tachycardia, poor tissue perfusion, and organ impairment (e.g., muscle weakness, renal insufficiency). Additional factors that can exacerbate this problem include dehydration associated with anorexia, vomiting, diarrhea, heart failure, azotemia, water restriction, or drug toxicity. Furosemide-treated animals should be closely monitored by measuring heart rate, blood pressure, urine output, femoral arterial pulse pressure, general mentation and strength, radiographic changes, renal function tests, and electrolytes.

Reducing cardiac filling pressures with diuretics will benefit patients whose cardiac performance operates on the relatively flat portion of the ventricular function curve (Fig. 1, curve A). These may

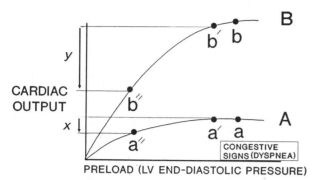

Figure 1. Effects of diuretic-induced preload reduction on cardiac function (cardiac output). Diuretics will lower preload and ventricular filling pressures. In patients with elevated ventricular filling pressures and whose cardiac performance operates at the flat portion of the ventricular function curve (*curve A*), judicious diuretic administration reduces pulmonary edema without severe impairment of cardiac output (a–a'). However, cardiac output may fall (*x*) when diuresis and preload reduction are excessive, especially when filling pressures are only moderately elevated (a'–a''). When diuretics are administered to animals requiring maximal preload (*curve B*) and whose cardiac performance operates on the ascending limb of the ventricular function curve (b'–b''), precipitous decline in cardiac output (*y*) may result. LV, left ventricular.

include animals with chronic volume overload from mitral regurgitation or myocardial failure. However, patients whose cardiac performance operates on the ascending limb of the curve may experience precipitous decline in cardiac output if filling pressures are too severely reduced. Examples include normal animals with pulmonary disease, cats with hypertrophic cardiomyopathy and impaired ventricular compliance, and dogs with left ventricular hypertrophy from aortic stenosis, constrictive pericardial or myocardial disorders, cardiac tamponade, and chronic, severe hypertension (Fig. 1, curve B).

Diuretic Effects on Other Systemic Diseases

Volume depletion from excessive diuresis may develop with thiazide and loop diuretics, particularly in animals fed salt restricted diets. This can exacerbate pre-existing renal insufficiency and alter excretion of drugs dependent upon renal elimination (e.g., digoxin).

Diuretics administered to patients with primary pulmonary diseases (whose clinical signs may be misdiagnosed as CHF) may cause dehydration, dry airway secretions or make them more tenacious, and inhibit mucociliary clearance mechanisms. A therapeutic principle for treatment of pneumonia bronchitis is maintenance of systemic hydration and airway moisture to decrease the viscosity and tenacity of airway secretions.

Furosemide potentiates the nephrotoxicity of the aminoglycoside antibiotics, and these combinations should be avoided.

Electrolyte Disturbances and Acid-Base Alterations

Because diuretics affect renal potassium transport, hypokalemia is always a potential side effect of their use. Additional factors may contribute to potassium wasting. For example, chronic renal disease is associated with hypokalemia in a large number of cats. Compensatory aldosterone secretion may result from diuretic-induced hypovolemia, especially in animals fed sodium-restricted diets. Aldosterone stimulates renal sodium conservation through exchange with potassium.

In cats, mild hypokalemia due to anorexia is often present at the time of examination. Because signs of mild to moderate potassium depletion are subtle and often overlooked, hypokalemia may be worsened by diuretic therapy. It is therefore prudent to monitor serum potassium concentrations in cats and either administer supplemental potassium as soon as hypokalemia is detected or attempt to prevent hypokalemia by sprinkling potassium chloride salt on their food (⅛ teaspoon).

In dogs, diuretic-induced hypokalemia is uncommon unless prolonged anorexia has been present. Potassium supplementation is usually unnecessary, especially if appetite resumes once heart failure is controlled.

Hyperkalemia is a potential complication of potassium-sparing diuretics. It is most likely to occur with conditions predisposing to hyperkalemic states, such as severe acute renal insufficiency, or in animals taking ACE inhibitors or large doses of oral potassium supplements.

Hyponatremia is occasionally encountered, particularly in decompensated heart failure. Predisposing causes include diuretic-induced inhibition of free water clearance; inappropriately high vasopressin levels related to decreased cardiac output and renin-angiotensin activity; excessive thirst; and reduced intracellular potassium concentrations with replacement by sodium. Mild hyponatremia may respond to fluid restriction and moderate dietary salt reduction. Severe hyponatremia, however, is a poor prognostic sign. Judicious therapy with loop diuretics, positive inotropic agents, intravenous 0.9% sodium chloride administration (controversial, as total body sodium may be increased), and possibly ACE inhibitors have been advocated in this setting. Future development of drugs that block vasopressin may be useful in these seriously ill patients.

Acid-base disturbances may occur with diuretic therapy. Persistent chloride depletion with loop diuretics can induce hypochloremic metabolic alkalosis, especially in salt-restricted, potassium-depleted animals. Because multiple systemic, metabolic, and respiratory derangements can be present in heart failure patients, mixed acid-base abnormalities are common.

References and Suggested Reading

Brater, D. C.: Disposition and response to bumetanide and furosemide. Am. J. Cardiol. 57:20A, 1986.

Feig, P.: Cellular mechanism of action of loop diuretics: Implications for drug effectiveness and adverse effects. Am. J. Cardiol. 57:14A, 1986.

Fox, P. R.: Feline myocardial disease. In Fox, P. R. (ed.): Canine and Feline Cardiology. New York: Churchill Livingstone, 1988, p. 435.

Fox, P. R., and Papich, M. G.: Complications of cardiopulmonary drug therapy. In Kirk, R. W. (ed.): Current Veterinary Therapy X. Philadelphia: W. B. Saunders, 1989, p. 308.

Klatt, P., Muschaweck, R., Bossaller, W., et al.: Method of collecting urine and comparative investigation of quantities excreted by cats and dogs after administration of furosemide. Am. J. Vet. Res. 36:919, 1975.

Meyer, B. H., Muller, F. O., Swart, K. J., et al.: Comparative bioavailability of four formulations of furosemide. S. Afr. J. 68:645, 1985.

Packer, M., Lee, W. H., Medina, N., et al.: Functional renal insufficiency during long-term therapy with captopril and enalapril in severe chronic heart failure. Ann. Intern. Med. 106:346, 1987.

Smith, T. W., Braunwald, E., and Kelly, R. A.: The management of heart failure. In Braunwald, E. (ed.): Heart Disease. 3rd ed. Philadelphia: W. B. Saunders, 1988, p. 485.

Wilson, J. R., Reicheck, N., Dunkman, W. B., et al.: Effect of diuresis on the performance of the failing left ventricle in man. Am. J. Med. 70:234, 1981.

CURRENT USES AND HAZARDS
OF BETA-BLOCKERS

WENDY A. WARE

Ames, Iowa

ADRENERGIC RECEPTORS

The sympathetic nervous system influences many physiologic and metabolic events through the actions of the catecholamines norepinephrine and epinephrine. Adrenergic receptors are distributed widely throughout various body tissues and are located at presynaptic (prejunctional) and postsynaptic (postjunctional) sites. These receptors have been classified into alpha-1, alpha-2, beta-1, and beta-2 subtypes. Presynaptic adrenoceptors are mostly the alpha-2 and beta-2 subtypes. Stimulation of alpha-2 receptors causes inhibition of norepinephrine release from the nerve terminal; thus, intrasynaptic norepinephrine inhibits its own release as part of a negative feedback mechanism. In contrast, presynaptic beta-2 stimulation increases endogenous norepinephrine release from the nerve ending, whereas blockade of these receptors inhibits norepinephrine release. Postsynaptic alpha-1 receptors are located mainly in vascular smooth muscle and mediate vasoconstriction, although other alpha-1 receptors mediate increased contractility in cardiac muscle. Some postsynaptic alpha-2 receptors mediate vasoconstriction; these are thought to be primarily responsive to circulating catecholamines because they are located outside the nerve synapse. Beta-1 receptors are mainly located within the myocardium and mediate increases in heart rate, contractility, atrioventricular (AV) conduction velocity, and automaticity in specialized fibers. The majority of postsynaptic beta-2 receptors are located in vascular and bronchial smooth muscle; they mediate vasodilation and bronchodilation, respectively. Other peripheral beta-2 receptors mediate the release of renin and insulin. Beta-2 receptors are also found in the myocardium, in extrasynaptic locations; they mediate increased contractility.

Adrenergic receptors are not static. Multiple factors dynamically regulate their concentration and alter tissue sensitivity to catecholamines. For example, the number of beta-1 receptors in the myocardium of humans with chronic heart failure, a condition associated with increased sympathetic activation, decreases as a result of a reversible conformational change in the receptor. This down-regulation of available receptors results in diminished myocardial sensitivity to the effects of catecholamines. Conversely, after chronic exposure to beta-receptor blocking drugs (antagonists), the number

Table 1. Pharmacodynamic Properties of Various Beta-Blockers

Drug	Beta-Blocking Potency Ratio (Propranolol = 1)	Relative Beta-1 Selectivity	Intrinsic Sympathomimetic Activity
Acebutolol	0.3	+	+
Atenolol	1.0	+ +	0
Betaxolol	—	+	0
Bevantolol	0.3	+ +	0
Bisoprolol	10.0	+ +	0
Bucindolol*	0.1	0	+ ?
Carteolol	10.0	0	+
Celiprolol†	0.4	+	+ ?
Esmolol	0.02	+ +	0
Labetalol*	0.3	0	+ ?
Metoprolol	1.0	+ +	0
Nadolol	1.0	0	0
Oxprenolol	0.5–1.0	0	+
Penbutolol	1.0	0	+
Pindolol	6.0	0	+ +
Propranolol	1.0	0	0
Sotalol‡	0.3	0	0
Timolol	6.0	0	0

*Has additional alpha-1 blocking activity and direct vasodilatory actions.
†Also has possible alpha-2 blocking effects at high doses.
‡Also has class III antiarrhythmic activity.

of beta-receptors increases (up-regulation). Other factors can also influence the number of receptors. Hyperthyroidism has been associated with an increase, and hypothyroidism with a decrease, in beta-receptor binding sites. Reduced numbers of beta-receptors are also associated with advancing age.

BETA RECEPTOR ANTAGONISTS

Drugs classified as beta-adrenergic receptor antagonists competitively inhibit catecholamine binding to beta-receptors so that a greater concentration of agonist is required to stimulate a given level of response. The clinical effects of beta-blocking drugs are directly related to the prevailing level of sympathetic activation as well as plasma drug concentration. The most pronounced effects occur in the presence of increased sympathetic tone. Many drugs that block the stimulation of beta receptors have been and continue to be developed. Some of these drugs are considered nonselective because they have antagonist effects at both beta-1 and beta-2 receptor sites. Others possess various degrees of selectivity for one receptor subtype. Still others may also have some intrinsic sympathomimetic activity (ISA), alpha-blocking ability, or membrane-stabilizing effects (Table 1). The potency of a beta-blocker refers to the amount of drug necessary to inhibit an adrenergic agonist's effects. The relative potency of the various beta-blockers is usually established with respect to propranolol (Table 2).

Drug potency influences the dose required for effective beta blockade but otherwise has little impact on the choice of agent for clinical use. However, differences in the pharmacokinetic properties of the various beta-blockers may influence how well an individual patient tolerates a particular drug.

Some beta-blockers (e.g., propranolol) have a quinidine-like (membrane-stabilizing) effect on cardiac tissues unrelated to their beta-blocking effects. However, this effect is seen only at high drug concentrations, not with usual therapeutic doses. Most beta-blockers are available as racemic mixtures of the L- and D-stereoisomers, with the L-isomer having the majority of beta-blocking activity. The only D-isomer thought to have potential clinical value is D-sotalol, which has class III antiarrhythmic properties.

Selectivity of Beta Blockade

Nonselective beta-blockers have effects on both beta-1 (predominantly cardiac) and beta-2 (predominantly vascular and bronchial smooth muscle) receptor subtypes. Selective beta-1 receptor blocking agents primarily affect cardiac beta-1 receptors, with relatively little antagonism of bronchial and vascular beta-2 receptors, especially at low doses. This is clinically advantageous in animals with asthma or obstructive lung disease, in which beta-2 blockade could trigger bronchospasm. Selective beta-1 agents should also be preferable in patients prone to hypoglycemia or with peripheral vascular disease or thrombosis. Receptor subtype selectivity is only relative; at higher doses, these agents also antagonize beta-2 receptors.

Intrinsic Sympathomimetic Activity

A few beta-blocking drugs also have partial agonist or ISA (e.g., pindolol). They block catecholamine access to the receptor sites while simultaneously causing mild receptor stimulation. These drugs may help protect against cardiac failure, severe bradycardia, bronchospasm, depression of AV conduction, and marked increases in peripheral vascular resistance. It appears that the partial agonist effect is most noticeable when sympathetic tone is low; during times of sympathetic stimulation (e.g., exercise), the beta-blocking effects predominate (Frishman, 1988). Although they generally are effective antiarrhythmic agents in human patients, exacerbation of ventricular arrhythmias has occurred with pindolol. It is unknown if such drugs offer a clinical advantage in the treatment of cardiac disease in animals.

Table 2. Pharmacokinetic Parameters of Various Beta-Blockers*

Drug	Main Route of Elimination†	Lipophilicity	Oral Bioavailability	Effective Plasma Concentration (Human)	Elimination Half-Life (hr)‡	Active Metabolites
Acebutolol	B	Moderate	Moderate	0.2–2.0 μg/ml	3–4§	Yes
Atenolol	RE	Low	Good	0.2–5.0 μg/ml	6–9 (3.2 D‖)	No
Betaxolol	B	Low	Good		14–22	
Bevantolol	HM	Moderate	Good	0.1–3.0 μg/ml	2–4	No
Carteolol	RE	Low	Good	40–160 ng/ml	5–6	Yes
Celiprolol	B	Low	Poor		5	Yes
Esmolol	BE	Low	—	0.2–1.0 μg/ml	9–10 min	No
Labetalol	HM	Low	Poor	0.7–3.0 μg/ml	3–4	No
Metoprolol	HM	Moderate	Moderate	50–100 ng/ml	3–4 (1.3 C, 1.6 D‖)	No
Nadolol	RE	Low	Poor	50–100 ng/ml	14–24 (3.6 D‖)	No
Oxprenolol	HM	Moderate	Moderate	80–100 ng/ml	2–3	No
Penbutolol	RE	High	Good		27	No
Pindolol	B	Moderate	Good	5–15 ng/ml	3–4	No
Propranolol	HM	High	Poor (variable)	50–100 ng/ml	3–4 (0.5 C, 0.6–1.5 D‖)	Yes
Sotalol	RE	Low	Good	0.5–4.0 μg/ml	9–10	No
Timolol	RE	Low	Good	5–10 ng/ml	4–5 (0.8 D‖)	No

*Most values from human literature (see Frishman, 1988); information from dog and cat studies as noted.
†HM, hepatic metabolism; RE, renal excretion; B, both important; BE, blood esterases.
‡D, dog; C, cat.
§Has active metabolite with half-life of 8 to 13 hr in humans.
‖See Muir and Sams, 1984.

Alpha-Adrenergic Blocking Activity

Several beta-blockers (e.g., labetalol) also have alpha-adrenergic blocking ability. These drugs reduce peripheral vascular resistance, although less so than phentolamine. Applications in human patients have included hypertension and hypertensive emergencies, arrhythmias, angina pectoris, and dilated cardiomyopathy.

Pharmacokinetic Characteristics

The various beta-blocking drugs may differ markedly with regard to their pharmacokinetic properties, although their therapeutic effects are similar (see Table 2). Some beta-blockers, such as propranolol and metoprolol, are eliminated mainly by hepatic metabolism. These drugs tend to be lipid soluble. They rapidly cross biologic membranes and are well absorbed by the small intestine. Lipophilic beta-blockers have large volumes of distribution and low renal clearances. However, their rapid hepatic metabolism (first-pass effect) often produces relatively short plasma half-lives and variable bioavailability. The oral dose of such drugs depends largely on the magnitude of the first-pass effect. Lipophilic agents like propranolol, timolol, and metoprolol can reduce their own clearance and that of other drugs (e.g., lidocaine) that are largely dependent on liver blood flow, by reducing cardiac output. Other causes of reduced liver blood flow, such as dehydration, congestive heart failure, shock, anesthesia, and hepatic cirrhosis, or a reduction in hepatic mass and function can decrease their clearance as well.

Higher serum concentrations of propranolol have been documented in elderly humans (Frishman, 1988).

Some beta-blockers, like nadolol, are more water soluble, are not extensively reabsorbed in the renal tubules, and are largely eliminated unchanged by the kidneys. These generally have longer half-lives and more consistent bioavailability. Patients with renal disease or otherwise-reduced glomerular filtration rate have slower elimination of these drugs and may experience elevated plasma concentrations. Active metabolites, often eliminated by the kidneys, result from beta-blockers like metoprolol and propranolol. Timolol is metabolized into inactive metabolites and may be beneficial in animals with renal disease (Muir and Sams, 1984).

Esmolol, an ultra–short-acting beta-1 selective agent, is unique in that it is metabolized by blood esterases (Turlapaty et al., 1987). With a half-life of less than 10 min, it is most effectively given by constant intravenous infusion in acute care situations. Because of its short half-life, it has found use as a "trial agent" to assess the acute effects of beta-blockade in a specific clinical situation. Drugs with longer half-lives generally require less frequent dosing, although some drugs with shorter half-lives (hours) can be given once or twice a day. Sustained-release preparations (e.g., of propranolol) can produce a smoother daily plasma concentration curve and fewer side effects, at least in human patients (Frishman, 1988).

Drug interactions between beta-blockers and other medications may be clinically important. Table 3 outlines some possible interactions. Table 4 lists some available beta-blockers.

Table 3. Interactions Between Beta-Blockers and Other Drugs

Drug	Possible Effects
Aluminum hydroxide gel	Reduces beta-blocker absorption and therapeutic effects
Calcium entry blockers	Potentiate bradycardia, atrioventricular block, myocardial depression, and hypotension
Cimetidine	Prolongs half-life of propranolol
Digoxin	Potentiates bradycardia
Epinephrine	Hypertension; bradycardia
Indomethacin	Inhibition of antihypertensive response to beta blockade
Lidocaine	Propranolol increases blood levels of lidocaine
Phenobarbital	Hepatic enzyme induction may decrease propranolol and metoprolol blood levels
Phenothiazines	Potentiates hypotensive effects
Phenylpropanolamine	Severe hypertensive reaction
Phenytoin	Additive cardiac depressant effects
Quinidine	Additive cardiac depressant effects
Theophylline	Nonselective agents antagonize bronchodilating effect and may reduce clearance

CLINICAL USES OF BETA-BLOCKERS

Uses in Cardiovascular Disease

Beta-blocking drugs are used in the treatment of many cardiac as well as several noncardiac disorders. The effects of beta-blocker therapy depend largely on the contribution of sympathetic tone to the disease process. Because sudden antagonism of sympathetic activation may be deleterious in certain diseases, beta-blocker therapy is begun with a low dose; this is slowly increased to effect over several dosage intervals. The risk of adverse reactions is minimized by carefully individualizing each patient's dosage and monitoring the effects of therapy.

CARDIAC ARRHYTHMIAS

The clinically important antiarrhythmic effects of beta-blocking drugs arise from their inhibition of adrenergic effects on cardiac pacemaker action potentials. Beta-blockers slow the spontaneous rate of discharge of sinus and ectopic pacemaker cells by decreasing the slope of phase 4 depolarization and therefore are useful for controlling arrhythmias caused by enhanced automaticity. Conditions associated with enhanced automaticity include digitalis toxicity, hyperthyroidism, pheochromocytoma, and myocardial infarction. It appears that at equivalent levels of beta blockade, all beta-blockers are comparably effective in reducing automaticity. Certain beta-blockers may have additional antiarrhythmic effects as well: D-sotalol prolongs action potential

duration (class III antiarrhythmic effect) and delays depolarization. Propranolol also has quinidine-like (class I antiarrhythmic) effects on cardiac tissues; however, these are only manifested at very high or toxic doses and are not believed to be important in most clinical situations.

Supraventricular arrhythmias, such as frequent atrial premature beats and supraventricular tachycardia, are often responsive to beta blockade. Propranolol has traditionally been considered the second drug of choice for these arrhythmias, after digitalis. However, beta-blockers may be more advantageous in certain situations, especially in animals in which digitalis glycosides are not indicated or not well tolerated. Intravenous administration provides rapid onset of action with some beta-blockers. More experience has been acquired with propranolol, but this drug may have significant cardiodepressant effects in animals with heart failure and is a nonselective beta-blocker. Esmolol has been useful in humans because of its rapid onset of action, beta-1 selectivity, short duration of action, and lesser cardiodepressive effects compared with propranolol.

Supraventricular tachycardias caused by re-entry through the AV node or an accessory pathway, as well as atrial flutter, may be responsive to beta-blockers. Because beta blockade slows AV conduction and prolongs the refractory period of re-entrant pathways, the circuit motion may be extinguished, abolishing the arrhythmia. Alternatively, a slowing in the ventricular response rate may occur. Repetition of a previously unsuccessful vagal maneuver may, after beta blockade, terminate an acute arrhythmia.

Atrial fibrillation in small animals usually occurs in the presence of severe underlying cardiac disease, and as such, return to sustained sinus rhythm is uncommon. Beta-blockers, like propranolol and atenolol, are generally ineffective in converting atrial fibrillation to sinus rhythm, but they slow the ventricular response rate by increasing AV nodal refractoriness. In cases in which underlying myocardial contractility is poor (e.g., dilated cardiomyopathy) and the patient is dependent on high sympathetic tone and heart rate to maintain cardiac output, care must be taken that further depression of myocardial function or bradycardia does not occur. A beta-blocker often is administered in conjunction with a positive inotropic agent, like digoxin, in these situations.

Ventricular arrhythmias that result from excess sympathetic stimulation are lessened in severity or abolished with beta-blocker therapy. Generally the initial treatment of ventricular arrhythmias in dogs consists of class I antiarrhythmic agents such as lidocaine, quinidine, or procainamide; however, the addition of a beta-blocker to this background therapy is sometimes effective when the initial drug was

Table 4. Commercially Available Beta-Blockers

Drug	Trade Name (Manufacturer)	Forms Available	Suggested Dosage*
Acebutolol	Sectral (Wyeth-Ayerst)	200, 400 mg caps	—
Atenolol	Tenormin (ICI Pharma)	50, 100 mg tabs; 5 mg/10 ml injection	12.5–50 mg once or twice a day, dogs
Betaxolol	Kerlone (Searle)	10, 20 mg tabs	—
Carteolol	Cartrol (Abbott)	2.5, 5 mg tabs	—
Esmolol	Brevibloc (DuPont Pharmaceuticals)	10, 250 mg/ml injection	500 μg/kg slow IV load, 50–200 μg/kg/min infusion
Labetalol	Normodyne (Schering) and Trandate (Allen & Hansburys)	100, 200, 300 mg tabs; 5 mg/ml injection	—
Metoprolol	Lopressor (Geigy)	50, 100 mg tabs; 1 mg/ml injection	5–50 mg t.i.d., dogs
Nadolol	Corgard (Princeton)	40, 80, 120, 160 tabs	5–40 mg b.i.d.–t.i.d., dogs
Penbutolol	Levatol (Reed & Carnrick)	20 mg tabs	—
Pindolol	Visken (Sandoz)	5, 10 mg tabs	1–3 mg t.i.d., dogs
Propranolol	Inderal (Wyeth-Ayerst, others) (Roxane)	10, 20, 40, 80, 90 mg tabs.; 1 mg/ml injection 4, 8, 80 mg/ml oral solution	5–40 mg t.i.d., dogs; 2.5–5 mg b.i.d.–t.i.d., cats
	Inderal LA (Wyeth-Ayerst)	80, 120, 160 mg caps	—
Timolol	Blocadren (Merck Sharp & Dohme)	10, 20 mg tabs	0.5–5 mg t.i.d., dogs

*The dosage for all beta-blockers is dependent on a patient's level of sympathetic activation as well as the underlying disease process; therefore, the initial dose of any beta-blocker should be low. Careful individual dosage titration should follow.

not. In cats, a beta-blocker (most commonly propranolol) is often the drug of first choice for ventricular tachyarrhythmias. Arrhythmias secondary to myocardial ischemia may respond well to beta blockade, and this may be important in animals with hypertrophic cardiomyopathy, other diseases causing myocardial hypertrophy, and myocardial infarction. If sympathetic stimulation underlies recurrent ventricular arrhythmias, beta-blocker therapy should be effective. In human patients, beta-blockers also have been shown to prevent exercise-induced ventricular tachycardia (Frishman, 1988). By decreasing sympathetic stimulation of the heart, beta-blockers may also reduce the potential for reentrant ventricular arrhythmias and sudden death. It has been shown that beta blockade increases the ventricular fibrillation threshold in ischemic myocardium (Frishman, 1988). The beneficial effects of beta-blockers on human survivors of acute myocardial infarction include reductions in mortality (including sudden and nonsudden cardiac deaths) and incidence of fatal reinfarctions.

CARDIOMYOPATHY

HYPERTROPHIC CARDIOMYOPATHY. Propranolol has long been a mainstay of therapy for cats with hypertrophic cardiomyopathy, although its use may be eclipsed by the calcium blocker diltiazem. Beta-blockers have been useful in reducing dyspnea and syncopal attacks, and the increased left heart filling pressures and reduced ventricular compliance exacerbated by sympathetic stimulation may be ameliorated by beta blockade. By lowering heart rate and myocardial oxygen demand, beta-blockers can reduce ischemia and control arrhythmias. Effects on myocardial diastolic function are unresolved. Beta-blockers also reduce the severity of ventricular outflow gradient in hypertrophic obstructive cardiomyopathy. The beta-1-blocker esmolol has been successful for this purpose in cats given 500 μg/kg IV over 1 min followed by an infusion of 100 μg/kg/min (Bonagura et al., 1991).

DILATED CARDIOMYOPATHY. Mounting evidence from cases of human dilated cardiomyopathy suggests that beta-blockers, when tolerated by a patient, have a favorable effect on disease progression and possibly mortality rate. Adverse effects of excessive adrenergic stimulation in chronic heart failure include myocardial catecholamine depletion, direct toxic effects on the myocardium, down-regulation of beta-receptors, increased vascular resistance, further stimulation of renin release, increased production of angiotensin II and aldosterone, and increased release of vasopressin. Worsening of congestive heart failure, low output signs, and increased likelihood of ventricular arrhythmias result. In human clinical trials using various beta-blockers, improved cardiac function and clinical status have been noted in many patients (Frishman, 1988; Waagstein et al., 1989). Drugs with ISA have not shown clinical benefit in patients in heart failure; they appear to inhibit up-regulation of beta-receptors. Selective beta-1-blocking drugs, such as metoprolol or atenolol, may be preferred over nonselective drugs like propranolol; however, studies using nonselective beta-blocking drugs with vasodilatory properties (bucindolol, labetalol) have also had favorable results (Gilbert et al., 1990; Leung et al., 1990). Clinical studies of animals with dilated cardiomyopathy are needed before specific therapeutic recommendations can be made regarding beta blockade.

HYPERTENSION

Beta-blockers have often been effective in veterinary as well as human patients for the control of hypertension. Hypertensive cats have been reported to respond well to propranolol (2.5 mg PO every 12 hr) and a low-sodium diet, either initially or when added to a diet and diuretic regimen that failed to control blood pressure (Morgan, 1986). In dogs, propranolol has been variably effective in controlling clinical hypertension when used with a low-salt diet and diuretic; in some cases, the substitution or addition of an angiotensin-converting enzyme inhibitor was more effective (Littman et al., 1988). The mechanism by which beta-blockers reduce blood pressure is controversial; it is likely that differences in the underlying cause of hypertension are influential. Postulated mechanisms include reduced cardiac output secondary to slowed heart rate and reduced contractility, a central nervous system effect, reduced renin release (nonselective beta-blockers), enhancement of baroreceptor sensitivity, and blockade of prejunctional beta-receptors (which mediate norepinephrine release). Peripheral vascular resistance is not directly reduced by nonselective beta-blockers; rather, blockade of postsynaptic (vasodilatory) beta-2 receptors would leave alpha-1 (vasoconstrictor) receptors unopposed. There are theoretic advantages to using beta-1 selective agents or those with alpha antagonist (labetalol) activity or ISA (pindolol) for hypertension, although beta-1 selectivity tends to diminish at the higher drug doses that may be needed in hypertension. In a study of human patients (van den Meiracker et al., 1989), no difference in antihypertensive effect was found between propranolol, pindolol, atenolol, and acebutolol; interference with vasoconstriction through blockade of central or peripheral prejunctional beta-receptors was thought to explain the antihypertensive effects.

OTHER CARDIAC APPLICATIONS

MYOCARDIAL INFARCTION. Myocardial infarction occurs sporadically in dogs (see this volume, p. 791), and beta-blockers may provide appropriate therapy. The reduced heart rate and contractility caused by beta-blockers results in lowered myocardial oxygen demand and longer diastolic filling time. As noted earlier, beta-blockers reduce mortality associated with myocardial infarction in humans. This is attributed to the antiarrhythmic as well as the anti-ischemic effects of these drugs. Propranolol, timolol, metoprolol, and atenolol have been used, although other beta-blockers would also be expected to have beneficial effects.

OBSTRUCTIVE HEART DISEASE. In certain diseases, increased sympathetic activity occurring with exercise, stress, or excitement leads to tachycardia, dynamic muscular outflow obstruction, reduction of cardiac output, and myocardial ischemia. In children with tetralogy of Fallot, beta-blockers have decreased severe hypoxic and cyanotic spells (Frishman, 1988). Myocardial hypertrophy in the right ventricular outflow tract can cause additional systolic outflow obstruction in this anomaly; reduced heart rate and contractility caused by beta blockade should lessen this obstruction and improve pulmonary blood flow. Animals with secondary dynamic outflow obstruction such as congenital subaortic stenosis and possibly isolated pulmonic stenosis may also benefit from the anti-ischemic, negative inotropic and chronotropic, and antiarrhythmic effects of beta blockade during times of sympathetic stimulation.

Uses in Noncardiac Diseases

THYROTOXICOSIS

Controversy surrounds the mechanisms of apparent sympathetic excess in hyperthyroidism. Nonetheless, beta-blocking drugs can suppress many sympathomimetic effects of excess thyroid hormone. Severe manifestations of hyperthyroidism, including tachycardia, fever, and disorientation, may be rapidly alleviated with beta blockade. However, beta-blockers are not a substitute for specific antithyroid therapy, because they do not reduce thyroid hormone secretion and cannot fully eliminate the signs and physiologic effects of thyrotoxicosis (see this volume, p. 338).

PHEOCHROMOCYTOMA

Beta-blockers have been used to control tachycardia and arrhythmias in patients with pheochromocytoma, but they must be used in conjunction with alpha-blockers to avoid severe hypertensive reactions.

OPEN-ANGLE GLAUCOMA

Topical application of beta-blockers has been effective in lowering intraocular pressure in humans, although the efficacy of this therapy is questionable in animals. Systemic levels of topically applied beta-blockers are minimal, but some adverse effects could occur in susceptible patients.

TOXICITIES

CAFFEINE, THEOBROMINE (CHOCOLATE), AND THEOPHYLLINE TOXICITY. Caffeine, theobromine (chocolate), and theophylline toxicity may be associated with tachycardia and arrhythmias. Beta-blocker therapy, in conjunction with other supportive measures, may be helpful in controlling heart rate and arrhythmias (see *CVT IX*, p. 191). Metoprolol may be preferred over propranolol because the latter has been shown to reduce theophylline clearance in humans. For either drug, an initial dose of 0.1 mg/kg (given IV at a rate of no more than 1 mg/2 min) up to 0.3 mg/kg t.i.d. and continued as needed has been used. Esmolol has been used for treating caffeine toxicity in humans. Beta-blockers may also help control tachyarrhythmias secondary to amphetamine ingestion.

CARDIAC GLYCOSIDES. Beta-blockers may have a role in the therapy of digoxin/digitoxin overdose or accidental ingestion by blocking the effects of digitalis-induced enhancement of central sympathetic tone and norepinephrine release from postganglionic sympathetic nerves. Propranolol has been used in conjunction with phenytoin, potassium supplementation, and atropine. Beta-blockers also have been used in the treatment of animals poisoned by digitalis-like substances. Examples include toxic plants such as oleander and foxglove, the rodenticide red squill (see *CVT X*, p. 116), and toad (*Bufo*) poisoning (see *CVT VIII*, p. 160).

COCAINE. Tachycardia, hypertension, and myocardial ischemia develop after ingestion or absorption of cocaine. Treatment of the hyperadrenergic state induced by accidental or excessive therapeutic cocaine exposure with esmolol has been suggested for human patients. The use of a beta-1 selective agent, in contrast to a nonselective agent, should alleviate further coronary arterial and peripheral vasospasm secondary to unopposed alpha receptor stimulation. Esmolol should allow gradual reduction of heart rate while severe hypertension and bronchospasm are avoided. As the cocaine effects dissipate over an hour or so, esmolol infusion can be discontinued with no prolonged beta-blocking effects. Diazepam, oxygen, and other supportive measures may be indicated as well. Use of the nonselective beta-blocker propranolol has been shown to increase coronary vasoconstriction and is not advised (Lange et al., 1990).

PORTAL HYPERTENSION

Propranolol has been effective in reducing the incidence of gastrointestinal bleeding secondary to portal hypertension in humans. The nonselective blocker propranolol has been more effective for this than beta-1 selective drugs. It is thought that splanchnic vasoconstriction secondary to beta-2 receptor blockade may lead to reduced portal pressure.

ADVERSE EFFECTS OF BETA-BLOCKERS

Adverse effects caused by beta antagonists usually result from the excessive blockade of beta-adrenergic receptors; clinical features are similar for all agents and are independent of the dose used. Some animals are unable to tolerate even small doses of beta-blockers, and the importance of careful dosage titration from an initial low level cannot be overemphasized. Because the sympathetic nervous system is involved in the regulation of many physiologic processes, the adverse effects of beta blockade impact on many body systems. Adverse reactions are thought to be more common in older animals with heart failure or azotemia (Muir and Sams, 1984). Precipitation of congestive heart failure, bradyarrhythmias, depression, hypotension, bronchospasm, and hypoglycemia have resulted from high doses. Overdose of a beta-blocker can be treated by infusion of a beta agonist such as dobutamine (3 to 5 μg/kg/min IV) or isoproterenol (0.01 to 0.09 μg/kg/min). If catecholamines are not effective in treating overdose, in humans, intravenous glucagon has been used. Bradyarrhythmias can be treated with atropine (0.01 to 0.02 mg/kg IM or IV) or glycopyrrolate (0.005 to 0.01 mg/kg IM or IV). Serum glucose levels should be monitored and dextrose given if needed.

Discontinuation of beta-blocker therapy should be accomplished gradually during a period of several days. A withdrawal syndrome has been described in human beings after abrupt cessation of chronic beta-blocker therapy. This condition is more likely to develop in patients with little myocardial oxygen reserve (e.g., ischemic heart disease). Worsening of angina, persistent tachycardia or arrhythmias, and even acute myocardial infarction and death have occurred (Frishman, 1988). Up-regulation of beta-receptors, allowing excessive response to catecholamines once beta blockade is removed, is a likely mechanism. Other postulated mechanisms for this withdrawal reaction include increased platelet aggregability, elevation in thyroid hormone activity, and an increase in circulating catecholamines.

Adverse Effects of Beta Blockade on the Heart

MYOCARDIAL FAILURE

Beta-blockers cause little negative inotropic effect in normal animals. However, when severe underlying myocardial disease or acute heart failure is present, the animal may depend on the effects of high sympathetic tone to maintain cardiac output. The negative inotropic and chronotropic effects of beta-blockers can precipitate or worsen clinical signs of heart failure in these cases. Nonselective beta-blockers might cause further detriment by contributing to increased vascular resistance. Theoretically, a beta-blocker with ISA would be less likely to precipitate heart failure, and one with alpha-blocking effects might offset increased vascular resistance from beta-2 blockade. In general, animals with myocardial failure in which a beta-blocker is indicated are treated first with a positive inotropic agent; in cases in which persistent, rapid tachyarrhythmias appear to be further compromising cardiac output, initial cautious use of a beta-blocker may be of benefit. Intravenous esmolol may be better tolerated than propranolol because it has less myocardial depressant effect and is able to be quickly titrated using a constant rate infusion.

ATRIOVENTRICULAR CONDUCTION DELAY

Animals with partial or complete AV conduction disturbances may experience serious bradyarrhythmias after beta blockade. A drug with ISA may minimize this; however, AV conduction disturbance remains a contraindication to beta-blocker use. Beta-blockers enhance the depression of AV conduction produced by digitalis, class I antiarrhythmic drugs, and calcium entry blockers. The simultaneous use of a beta-blocker and calcium entry blocker must be undertaken with great caution and can lead to marked decreases in heart rate as well as myocardial contractility.

SINUS NODE DYSFUNCTION

The resting heart rate in normal individuals is slowed by beta-blocker treatment, although to a lesser degree with those drugs having ISA. In animals with sick sinus syndrome, all beta-blockers are contraindicated unless an artificial pacemaker has been implanted. Even in normal animals, sinus arrest or sinoatrial block can result from large doses of beta-blockers.

Noncardiac Adverse Effects of Beta Blockade

BRONCHIAL DISEASE

Blockade of bronchial beta-2 receptors may precipitate bronchospasm, especially in patients with underlying asthma or chronic bronchitis. Chronic reactive airway disease is a relative contraindication for nonselective beta-blocker therapy. Drugs with beta-1 selectivity, ISA, or alpha-receptor blocking ability are less likely to stimulate bronchospasm in human asthma sufferers. However, this protection is relative because high doses of beta-1 selective blockers may also cause some degree of beta-2 receptor blockade.

PERIPHERAL VASCULAR DISEASE

Nonselective beta-blockers in particular may further compromise reperfusion of ischemic tissues after arterial thromboemolism in cats with cardiomyopathy. Therapy with a beta-blocker is best delayed until return of limb perfusion, if possible. In human medicine, Raynaud's phenomenon and worsening of intermittent claudication in patients with peripheral vascular disease have been reported with beta-blocker therapy (especially with nonselective agents).

HYPOGLYCEMIA

Although studies of normal humans have shown that propranolol does not change resting glucose levels, it does blunt the hyperglycemic response to exercise. Severe hypoglycemia has occurred in some humans after beta blockade; some were insulin-dependent diabetic patients, but others were not diabetic. Beta-blockers, especially nonselective agents, blunt isoproterenol-stimulated increases in plasma glucose, insulin, and lactate; they also reduce the tachycardia resulting from hypoglycemia-induced sympathetic activation and may interfere with the compensatory response to hypoglycemia. Selective beta-1 drugs or those with ISA may only minimally affect insulin-induced hypoglycemia and its hemodynamic consequences.

CENTRAL NERVOUS SYSTEM EFFECTS

In humans, the central nervous system side effects of insomnia, dreams, hallucinations, and depression have occasionally occurred with beta-blocker therapy. Their incidence is highest with the more lipophilic drugs, which achieve greater concentration in brain tissues. The possible occurrence and incidence of these side effects in animals is not known.

OTHER SIDE EFFECTS

Gastrointestinal signs have occasionally occurred with various beta-blockers; these have included diarrhea, nausea, gastric pain, constipation, and flatulence. Rarely, thrombocytopenia and agranulocytosis have been reported in humans using propranolol.

References and Suggested Reading

Bonagura, J. D., Stepien, R. L., and Lehmkuhl, L. B.: Acute effects of esmolol on left ventricular outflow obstruction in cats with hypertrophic cardiomyopathy (abstract). Proceedings of the American College of Veterinary Internal Medicine. Washington, DC, 1991, Vol. 5, p. 123.
Esmolol decreases subaortic obstruction as measured by Doppler echocardiography.

Frishman, W. H.: β-Adrenergic blockers. Med. Clin. North Am. 72:37, 1988.
An overview of beta-blocking drugs and their indications and side effects in human medicine.

Gilbert, E. M., Anderson, J. L., Deitchman, D., et al.: Long-term β-blocker vasodilator therapy improves cardiac function in idiopathic dilated cardiomyopathy: A double blind, randomized study of bucindolol versus placebo. Am. J. Med. 88:223, 1990.

Lange, R. A., Cigarroa, R. G., Flores, E. D., et al.: Potentiation of cocaine-induced vasoconstriction by beta-adrenergic blockade. Ann. Intern. Med. 112:897, 1990.
Clinical study of the effects of propranolol on coronary vasoconstriction in humans after low-dose cocaine.

Leung, W. H., Lau, C. P., Wong, C. K., et al.: Improvement in exercise performance and hemodynamics by labetalol in patients with idiopathic dilated cardiomyopathy. Am. Heart J. 119:884, 1990.

Littman, M. P., Robertson, J. L., and Bovee, K. C.: Spontaneous systemic hypertension in dogs: Five cases (1981–1983). J.A.V.M.A. 193:486, 1988.
Clinical findings and therapeutic response in dogs with hypertension.

Morgan, R. V.: Systemic hypertension in four cats: Ocular and medical findings. J. Am. Anim. Hosp. Assoc. 22:615, 1986.
Clinical findings and results of therapy in four original, plus seven subsequent, cases of spontaneous hypertension in cats.

Muir, W. W., and Sams, R.: Clinical pharmacodynamics and pharmacokinetics of β-adrenoceptor blocking drugs in veterinary medicine. Comp. Cont. Ed. Pract. Vet. 6:156, 1984.

Turlapaty, P., Laddu, A., Murthy, V. S., et al: Esmolol: A titratable short-acting intravenous beta blocker for acute critical care settings. Am. Heart J. 114:866, 1987.
A review of human and animal studies of the effects and uses of esmolol.

van den Meiracker, A. H., Man in 't Veld, A. J., Boomsma, F., et al.: Hemodynamic and β-adrenergic receptor adaptations during long-term β-adrenoceptor blockade. Circulation 80:903, 1989.
A comparison of the effects of four beta-blockers on systemic and renal hemodynamics, hormones, fluid volume, and lymphocyte beta-receptor density in hypertensive humans.

Waagstein, F., Caidahl, K., Wallentin, I., et al.: Long-term β-blockade in dilated cardiomyopathy. Circulation 80:551, 1989.
Study of metoprolol in humans with dilated cardiomyopathy; useful reference list.

CURRENT USES AND HAZARDS OF CALCIUM CHANNEL BLOCKING AGENTS

PAUL DAVID PION
Davis, California

The term *calcium antagonist* was first used to describe two potential coronary vasodilators, prenylamine and verapamil. These drugs do not, as the term suggests, antagonize the intracellular actions of calcium but instead block the entry of calcium into cells. Thus, the preferred terms today are *calcium channel blocker, calcium entry blocker,* or *slow channel blocker.* Worldwide there are at least 29 different agents in clinical use classified as calcium channel blocking agents. Three of these, verapamil (Calan, Searle; Isoptin, Knoll), diltiazem (Cardizem, Marion), and nifedipine (Procardia, Pfizer), have been used extensively in the United States. Because there are no reports in the veterinary literature describing clinical use of nifedipine and only a small number describing the use of verapamil or diltiazem, clinical use of these drugs is based primarily upon data derived *in vitro* in experimental dogs and cats and from clinical experience in humans.

BASIC PHARMACOLOGY

Interference with calcium movement across excitable membranes is the primary pharmacologic basis for the therapeutic and toxic effects of calcium channel blockers. Being a charged ionic species, calcium (Ca^{2+}) does not freely diffuse across cell membranes. Instead, it moves via transmembrane calcium channels.

Calcium channels must be in an open configuration for calcium to enter the cell. Stimuli capable of signaling for calcium channels to open include membrane potential (voltage-operated calcium channels), hormones or neurotransmitters present on the outside of cells (receptor-operated calcium channels), intracellular second messengers such as inositol triphosphate (second messenger–operated calcium channels), and physical membrane perturbations (stretch-operated calcium channels). Several types of calcium channels have been described.

Table 1. *Relative Sensitivity of Vascular and Myocardial Tissues to Calcium Channel Blocking Agents**

Compound	Relative Activity (Vascular:Myocardial)
Verapamil	1:1
Diltiazem	7:1
Nifedipine	14:1

*Reprinted with permission from Struyker-Boudier, H. A. J., et al.: The pharmacology of calcium antagonists: A review. J. Cardiovasc. Pharmacol. 15(suppl 4):S1–S10, 1990.

Detailed description of these subclasses of calcium channels is not necessary for the purpose of this chapter. It is important to note that not all calcium channels are sensitive to the effects of the calcium channel blockers in clinical use. Therefore not all cellular events mediated by calcium are affected by calcium channel blocker administration. Furthermore, not all calcium channel blocker–sensitive tissues are equally responsive to the calcium channel blocking agents in clinical use.

Effects on Vasculature

All calcium channel blockers dilate arterioles to varying degrees. Nifedipine and other dihydropyridines are the most potent vasodilators. Table 1 lists the relative vascular:myocardial potency of the calcium channel blocking agents.

Net vascular tone is the sum of the basal tension maintained by local autoregulatory mechanisms (myogenic tone), which is then modulated by neurohumoral control mechanisms mediated by the autonomic nervous system (e.g., norepinephrine), local vasoactive substances (e.g., histamine, bradykinin), and products of endothelial cells (e.g., endothelium-derived relaxant factor and endothelin). Both the myogenic vascular tone and neurohumoral modulation are calcium-dependent events (Fig. 1) that can be modified by administration of calcium channel blockers.

The systemic resistance vessels and to some extent the large arteries respond to calcium channel blockers in a dose-dependent manner. The venous capacitance vessels and pulmonary vasculature are much less sensitive to the vasodilatory effects of calcium channel blocking agents. This class of drugs is thus much more clinically useful for modulating systemic arterial blood pressure than venous or pulmonary blood pressures.

Effects on the Heart

The actions of calcium channel blockers on the heart may be divided into effects on myocardial contractility, the sinoatrial (SA) node, the atrioventricular (AV) node, coronary vascular tone, cardiac metabolism following ischemia, and possibly cardiac hypertrophy.

The events underlying contraction of cardiac and skeletal muscle differ from those in vascular smooth muscle (see Fig. 1). Entry of extracellular calcium through transarcolemmal (cardiac muscle cell membrane) calcium channels is required for contraction of cardiac muscle. This differs from skeletal muscle, in which contraction can continue in the absence of extracellular calcium. It is believed that the amount of calcium entering through calcium channels is a determinant of the magnitude of calcium released from the sarcoplasmic reticulum and the maximum intracytoplasmic calcium concentration during the plateau of the cardiac action potential in individual myocytes, thereby affecting the strength of the resultant cardiac contraction.

Administration of calcium channel blocking agents decreases the amount and rate of calcium entering the cardiac myocyte during the plateau of the action potential and thus decreases the strength of contraction. The magnitude of the negative inotropic effects is determined by a complex interaction between the direct effects on the cardiac muscle, the sensitivity of the vasculature (vasodilatory effect) to the agent administered, and cardiovascular reflex

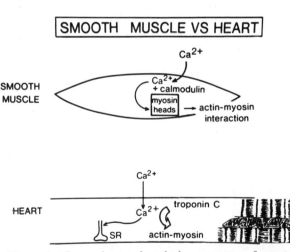

Figure 1. The mechanism by which contraction of arterial smooth muscle is mediated by increased intracellular calcium concentration differs from that in cardiac muscle. In smooth muscle, intracellular calcium ions (Ca^{2+}) bind to calmodulin (a cytoplasmic calcium-binding protein). This calcium-calmodulin complex activates enzymes that phosphorylate myosin, which then promotes myosin-actin interactions and contraction. In cardiac and skeletal muscle, calcium binding to the regulatory protein troponin sets off a cascade of events culminating in cross-bridging of myosin head groups and actin. Repeated binding and release of myosin head groups to actin molecules as the myofilaments slide past one another are translated into gross shortening of the myocyte, and the muscle contracts. SR, sarcoplasmic reticulum. (Modified with permission from Opie, L. H., et al.: *Drugs for the Heart*, 2nd ed. Philadelphia, W. B. Saunders, 1987, p. 37)

Table 2. *Expected Cardiovascular Effects of Calcium Channel Blockers in Healthy Animals*

Parameter	Verapamil	Diltiazem	Nifedipine
Chronotropic (heart rate)	0 or −	0 or =	0
Dromotropic (AV conduction)*	=	=	0
Inotropic (strength)	−	0 or −	0†
Peripheral resistance	−	−	=
Coronary resistance	−	−	=

*This effect is rate dependent and is more pronounced at higher heart rates.

†Nifedipine does have potent negative inotropic effects on isolated cardiac muscle, but baroreceptor reflex–mediated cardiac neural stimulation usually overcomes the direct negative inotropic effects with a net result of no change or a mild positive inotropic effect.

0, no change; −, mild to moderate decrease; =, moderate to marked decrease.

mechanisms. Agents like nifedipine are potent vasodilators and cause a marked decrease in arterial blood pressure. In response to increased baroreceptor discharge, a rise in sympathetic activity and in the strength and rate of cardiac contraction is seen. Thus, an initial positive rather than negative inotropic response is observed. In contrast, following the administration of diltiazem both vasodilation and the baroreceptor-induced cardiac stimulation are of smaller magnitude but sufficient to approximately cancel the direct negative inotropic effects of the drug. After the administration of verapamil, a net negative inotropic response is usually observed. These effects on cardiac inotropy are a major source of concern regarding the adverse effects of calcium channel blocker therapy, especially when used in patients with myocardial failure or in conjunction with other potentially negative inotropic agents such as the beta-adrenergic blocking agents (e.g., propranolol).

The depolarizing currents of the SA node and the upper and middle AV nodal regions are primarily carried by calcium. Verapamil and diltiazem, but not nifedipine, inhibit these currents, reducing the rate of SA node discharge and slowing conduction through the AV node. These agents also prolong the refractory period of nodal tissues. Clinically, effects on the AV node (AV conduction) are more pronounced than those on the SA node (sinus rate). The effects of verapamil and diltiazem on AV nodal conduction are dose dependent and more pronounced at higher heart rates. These actions are useful in the management of supraventricular tachyarrhythmias.

The calcium channel blockers, especially nifedipine, dilate small and large coronary vessels (Table 2). This action, coupled with systemic vasodilatation (afterload reduction) and the ability of calcium channel blockers to partially protect against ischemia-induced acute calcium overload, may be beneficial in cases of cardiac arrest, during cardiac surgical

procedures, and in circulatory failure or during cardiopulmonary resuscitation.

Studies in hypertensive animals treated with calcium channel blockers have demonstrated a reduction in cardiac hypertrophy beyond that expected for the degree of afterload reduction alone. Along with clinical improvement in human and feline patients with hypertrophic cardiomyopathy treated with calcium channel blockers, the data suggest a possible role for these drugs in modulating cardiac hypertrophy.

Effects on Other Systems

Calcium channel blockers have also been used to treat a wide range of noncardiovascular, pathophysiologic conditions because intracellular calcium concentration and calcium currents affect function in most tissues. Further discussion of indications outside the cardiovascular system is beyond the scope of this chapter, but side effects on noncardiovascular systems should be considered when treating cardiovascular disorders with this class of drugs and vice versa.

SPECIFIC INDICATIONS

Supraventricular tachyarrhythmias represent the principal indication for calcium channel blockers in dogs. Re-entrant circuits (see *CVT # X*, p. 271), many involving the AV node, are believed to underlie many paroxysmal supraventricular tachyarrhythmias. Verapamil and diltiazem can terminate many of these arrhythmias in dogs as indicated by several case reports. In one series of cases, intravenous verapamil acutely terminated supraventricular tachyarrhythmias in 12 of 14 (86%) dogs (Kittleson et al., 1988). Although not reported, the efficacy of beta-adrenergic blocking agents is probably not as high. The effects of chronic oral administration of verapamil for therapy of recurrent supraventricular tachyarrhythmias have not been reported in the veterinary literature. While not studied in a controlled manner, diltiazem is emerging as the preferred calcium channel blocker for chronic oral treatment of paroxysmal supraventricular tachyarrhythmias in dogs because it is thought to be equally effective to and safer than verapamil. There are no published reports on the use of verapamil or diltiazem for termination of supraventricular tachyarrhythmias in cats, though both drugs have been clinically effective.

Atrial fibrillation or flutter is most commonly identified in dogs with primary myocardial disease (dilated cardiomyopathy) or advanced mitral regurgitation secondary to chronic progressive degeneration of the mitral apparatus. A less common presentation is atrial fibrillation in dogs without identifiable cardiac disease or significant atrial enlargement.

Controlling the ventricular rate is the usual end point of drug therapy for atrial fibrillation in patients with significant atrial enlargement. By slowing conduction through and prolonging the refractory period of the AV node, verapamil and diltiazem may effectively control the ventricular rate response in dogs with atrial fibrillation.

Conversion of atrial fibrillation and prolonged maintenance of sinus rhythm has been achieved in dogs without congestive heart failure (CHF) or significant atrial enlargement or disease following both verapamil and diltiazem therapy. Intravenous verapamil and oral diltiazem are alternatives to quinidine therapy for this purpose (see *CVT X*, p. 271). In cases of recurrent paroxysmal atrial fibrillation, diltiazem may maintain normal sinus rhythm. The relative efficacy and risks of these therapies have not been adequately assessed in veterinary patients, but diltiazem would appear to have a more advantageous profile (see this volume, p. 676).

Calcium channel blockers are potentially effective in cases of *ventricular ectopy* that are resistant to antiarrhythmic drugs such as procainamide or quinidine, but they should be considered a drug of last choice and extreme care should be taken to avoid excessive hypotension.

Hypertension is poorly defined in veterinary clinical practice. All of the three calcium channel blockers described earlier are effective hypotensive agents in human patients with hypertension. Experience in dogs and cats is minimal.

Evidence documenting the beneficial effects of calcium channel blockers in cases of *hypertrophic cardiomyopathy* in humans and cats is accumulating. The mechanisms responsible are not well defined and the long-term benefits are as yet unknown (see this volume, p. 766).

CLINICAL APPLICATION

As with most drugs, the bioavailability, metabolism, and elimination of calcium channel blockers vary according to the individual. Therefore, the following treatment generalizations should prove more useful than tables of pharmacokinetic values.

VERAPAMIL. In dogs, the half-life for elimination of verapamil ranges between 1 and 5 hr (mean = 2.5 hr). Lengthening of the P-R interval is correlated with serum concentration. A large first-pass effect exists owing to hepatic extraction, so the oral dose is approximately ten times those of the intravenous dose. The half-life and pharmacodynamics in cats are reported to be similar to those in dogs and humans (Pion et al., 1986).

An oral dose of 0.5 to 1.0 mg/kg every 8 hr is recommended for control of atrial fibrillation, atrial flutter, or asymptomatic supraventricular tachyarrhythmia. Beginning with the lower dose is advisable, especially in patients with underlying cardiac disease. Because of lack of evidence documenting differences in efficacy in veterinary patients and the more pronounced negative inotropic effects of verapamil, the author prefers diltiazem in patients with underlying cardiac disease. When treating symptomatic supraventricular tachyarrhythmias intravenously, verapamil should be administered conservatively. Slow (over 10 to 30 min) injection of 0.05 mg/kg is used while monitoring the electrocardiogram. Two to four additional injections of 0.025 mg/kg may be administered cautiously at 5-min intervals to a maximum cumulative dose of 0.15 mg/kg or until the desired effect is achieved (up to 0.2 mg/kg may be required, but the risk of toxicity is increased). Pretreating patients with intravenous calcium salts may decrease the incidence of hypotension associated with intravenous verapamil administration (Barnett and Touchon, 1990), but this approach is not typical.

In cats with symptomatic supraventricular tachyarrhythmias, slow injection of 0.025 mg/kg repeated up to eight times at 3- to 5-min intervals is recommended. Chronic oral therapy in cats and small dogs (0.5 to 1.0 mg/kg PO every 8 hr) is inconvenient owing to the size of available tablets. The deleterious (and sometimes fatal) effects of administering excessive doses of verapamil were illustrated in two early reports in which the commercially available dosage form was administered to small dogs (Hamlin, 1986) and cats (Pion et al., 1986). Most pharmacists, if asked, will formulate smaller-sized capsules. Again, experience is limited, so these recommendations should be taken as guidelines.

Adverse reactions observed after administering verapamil to dogs and cats include first-degree heart block, second-degree heart block, complete heart block, AV dissociation with an accelerated idioventricular rhythm, hypotension, collapse, and sudden death. Administration of calcium chloride, sympathomimetic drugs, or amrinone has been reported to be efficacious in reversing these excessive negative inotropic and vasodilatory responses. Atropine is also recommended to increase sinus rate and AV conduction.

DILTIAZEM. Diltiazem is rapidly becoming the most popular drug of this class among veterinary cardiologists. Theoretically, it is an ideal calcium channel blocker for use in veterinary patients because, when administered at recommended dosage levels, it has effective antiarrhythmic properties with minimal depression of inotropy.

First-pass effect through the liver is not as great as that with verapamil, and half-life in dogs is reported to be similar to verapamil. Diltiazem is available only in oral form (in the United States), so verapamil remains the calcium channel blocker of choice for acute termination of symptomatic supraventricular tachyarrhythmias.

Dosage recommendations for treatment of supraventricular tachyarrhythmias are 0.5 to 1 (up to 1.5) mg/kg PO every 8 hr in dogs and cats and also 7.5 mg PO t.i.d. in cats for treatment of hypertrophic cardiomyopathy. Potential adverse effects and therapy are similar to those for verapamil.

DRUG INTERACTIONS

Both verapamil and diltiazem are reported to have significant drug interactions in humans. They are significant hepatic microsomal enzyme inhibitors and thus affect clearance of drugs such as propranolol, theophylline, and quinidine (Husum et al., 1990). Both are metabolized in the liver, and thus serum concentrations may rise when administered with other hepatic microsomal enzyme inhibitors such as cimetidine.

Verapamil and diltiazem may increase serum levels of digoxin in human patients with heart disease. These alterations in digoxin kinetics are thought to be due to reduction in renal and extrarenal clearance of digoxin. Many authors have advised assessment of serum digoxin concentrations 4 to 7 days after prescribing either of these agents to animals receiving digoxin.

Caution should be used when prescribing calcium channel blockers in conjunction with other negative inotropic (e.g., beta-adrenergic blockers), dromotropic (e.g., propranolol, digoxin) or vasodilating agents. Measurement of serum verapamil concentrations is thought to be of limited diagnostic value (Husum et al., 1990).

CONCLUSION

The future for calcium channel blocker therapy in dogs and cats appears promising. However, as with most drugs used in veterinary medicine, recommendations for use are based largely on data in normal animals, reports on small numbers of veterinary patients, extrapolation from literature describing treatment of human patients, and clinical impression. Veterinary researchers are only beginning to understand the appropriate uses, along with the hazards, of these drugs. In clinical therapy, careful monitoring for signs of efficacy and toxicity is essential. As with all drugs, there is no single effective dose, but only a dose range. Titrating the dose in individual patients is always superior to simply prescribing the recommended dose.

References and Suggested Reading

Allert, J. A., and Adams, H. R.: New perspectives in cardiovascular medicine: The calcium channel blocking drugs. J.A.V.M.A. 190:573, 1987.
A minireview of the pharmacology of calcium entry blockers.
Barnett, J. C., and Touchon, R. C.: Short-term control of supraventricular tachycardia with verapamil infusion and calcium pretreatment. Chest 97:1106, 1990.
A prospective study of the effects of pretreating human patients with intravenous calcium prior to intravenous administration of verapamil.
Hamlin, R. L.: Clinical and experimental studies with verapamil in the dog. Proceedings of the Fifth Biennial Symposium on Veterinary Pharmacology and Therapeutics, 1986, p. 89.
A report describing early adverse clinical experience in which high doses of verapamil were administered to dogs, it includes the effects of administering a high oral dose (4 mg/kg) to experimental dogs and explanation of the adverse clinical responses.
Hunt, B. A., Bottorff, M. B., Herring, V. L., et al.: Effects of calcium channel blockers on the pharmacokinetics of propranolol stereoisomers. Clin. Pharmacol. Ther. 47:548, 1990.
A study evaluating the effects of verapamil and diltiazem administration on the disposition and metabolism of propranolol in healthy humans.
Husum, D., Johnsen, A., and Jensen, G.: Requirements for drug monitoring of verapamil: Experience from an unselected group of patients with cardiovascular disease. Pharmacol. Toxicol. 66:163, 1990.
A prospective study evaluating the diagnostic value of routine serum verapamil concentration in human patients receiving verapamil orally.
Kittleson, M. D., Keene, B., Pion, P., et al.: Verapamil administration for acute termination of supraventricular tachycardia in dogs. J.A.V.M.A. 193:1525, 1988.
A prospective clinical study evaluating the efficacy and safety of intravenous verapamil administration in dogs with spontaneous supraventricular arrhythmias.
Lewis, R. V., and McDevitt, D. G.: Factors affecting the clinical response to treatment with digoxin and two calcium antagonists in patients with atrial fibrillation. Br. J. Clin. Pharmacol. 25:603, 1988.
A double-blind, crossover study comparing digoxin and calcium channel blocker (verapamil or diltiazem) therapy on exercise tolerance and post-exercise heart rate in human patients with atrial fibrillation.
Opie, L. H., and Singh, B. N.: Calcium channel antagonists (slow channel blockers). In Opie, L. H. (ed.): Drugs for the Heart, 2nd ed. Philadelphia, W. B. Saunders. 1987, p. 34.
An excellent chapter on the basic and clinical pharmacology of calcium channel blockers in humans.
Pion, P. D., Babish, J., Schwark, W., et al.: Pharmacokinetics and electrocardiographic study of verapamil in the cat. Proceedings of the Fifth Biennial Symposium on Veterinary Pharmacology and Therapeutics, 1986, p. 89.
An experimental study evaluating the pharmacokinetics and pharmacodynamics of intravenous, acute oral, and chronic oral administration of verapamil in normal cats.
Struyker-Boudier, H. A. J., Smits, J. F. M., and DeMey J. G. R.: The pharmacology of calcium antagonists: A review. J. Cardiovasc. Pharmacol. 15 (suppl 4):S1–S10, 1990.
The keynote article in a symposium on the vascular effects of calcium channel blockers—an excellent review of the basic pharmacology of this class of drugs.

CURRENT USES AND HAZARDS
OF THE DIGITALIS GLYCOSIDES

PATTI S. SNYDER

Madison, Wisconsin

and CLARKE E. ATKINS

Raleigh, North Carolina

The cardiac glycosides have been used amid controversy for over two centuries and are still widely prescribed for the management of human and veterinary cardiac disorders. The terms digitalis, digitalis glycoside, and cardiac glycoside are often used interchangeably and refer to their source: the plants *Digitalis lanata* (digoxin) and *Digitalis purpurea* (digitoxin). The compounds are closely related chemically and share identical mechanisms of pharmacologic action despite widely differing pharmacokinetic profiles. This discussion centers on the most commonly used digitalis glycosides, digoxin and digitoxin.

MECHANISM OF ACTION

Digitalis exerts important inotropic and neurotropic effects. The major positive *inotropic* action of digitalis results from inhibition of sodium-potassium–activated adenosine triphosphatase (Na-K ATPase). Inhibition of Na-K ATPase leads to a transient increase in intracellular sodium ions (Na^+). A sodium-calcium exchange mechanism present in the cell membrane mediates the interchange of Na^+ with extracellular calcium ions (Ca^{++}), leading to increased intracellular Ca^{++} and increased myocardial contractility. Recent evidence suggests that digitalis also increases diaphragmatic contractility by similar mechanisms.

Evidence is accumulating that many veterinary and human heart failure patients experience activation of the sympathetic nervous system and renin-angiotensin-aldosterone axis. This activation often precedes, rather than results from, congestive heart failure (CHF). The extent of this neurohumoral excitation is inversely correlated with prognosis. Digitalis may exert a variety of beneficial effects in heart failure; mechanisms of action include enhancing receptor discharge rate, decreasing sympathetic nerve activity, and sensitizing cardiac and arterial baroreceptors. These *neurotropic* effects appear to be independent of any inotropic action of the drug and have been shown to decrease heart rate, improve muscle blood flow and cardiac output, and reduce pulmonary venous pressures in human patients with chronic CHF.

The therapeutic *electrophysiologic* effects of digitalis are primarily mediated by the autonomic nervous system. By increasing vagal activity, conduction is slowed and the refractory period is lengthened in the atrioventricular (AV) junctional tissues. This action accounts for the efficacy of digitalis in the management of atrial fibrillation and other supraventricular tachyarrhythmias, as well as for the AV block sometimes observed in toxicity. Parasympatholytic agents (e.g., atropine) and increased sympathetic activity can reduce the negative chronotropic effects of digitalis, and this is commonly observed during exercise or deterioration of heart failure. In addition to its vagally mediated effects, digitalis may enhance oscillatory afterpotentials (triggered activity), potentially causing or worsening ventricular arrhythmias.

INDICATIONS

In both human and veterinary medicine, the indications for cardiac glycoside therapy include systolic myocardial dysfunction and supraventricular tachyarrhythmias, especially when the two occur simultaneously. Systolic myocardial dysfunction is the hallmark of dilated cardiomyopathy and may complicate the course of valvular, congenital, nutritional, endocrine, ischemic, septic, and toxic heart diseases. Digitalis may be indicated in the therapy for heart failure associated with any of these conditions, and recent studies suggest that digitalis may produce a stronger inotropic response than beta-adrenergic agonists in septic human patients.

Controversy remains regarding the use of digitalis in dogs that have CHF due to primary atrioventricular valvular insufficiency but without echocardiographic evidence of myocardial failure. Because global ventricular performance appears to be normal in most cases, some authors have argued that there is no indication for inotropic support in patients

689

Table 1. Available Digitalis Formulations

	Bioavailability
Digoxin (Cardoxin, Evsco; Lanoxin, Coopers)	
Tablet: 0.125, 0.25, 0.5 mg	50–80%
Elixir: 0.05, 0.15 mg/ml	60–80%
Capsule: 0.05, 0.1, 0.2 mg	80–100%
Injectable: 0.1, 0.25 mg/ml	100%
Digitoxin (Foxalin, Standex; Crystodigin, Lilly)	
Tablet: 0.05, 0.1, 0.15, 0.2 mg	80–100%

with sinus rhythm. Others believe that many animals eventually develop myocardial failure and that digitalization is indicated because echocardiographic assessment of ventricular function in the setting of mitral regurgitation is inaccurate. Others advocate digitalization only in the late stages of CHF. Current evidence suggests that digitalization early in CHF may reduce neurohumoral activation and restore baroreceptor sensitivity, benefits that accrue independently of inotropic support. Unfortunately, there have been few clinical trials evaluating the efficacy of digitalis in naturally occurring chronic valvular insufficiency, as well as in other conditions such as dirofilariasis, and until such studies are performed in veterinary medicine, this controversy will continue.

The digitalis glycosides are indicated in the management of many (particularly chronic) supraventricular tachyarrhythmias, especially atrial fibrillation, and notably when these rhythm disturbances occur in the setting of heart failure. Many times, however, a beta-blocker or calcium channel antagonist must be used concurrently to control the ventricular rate response to atrial fibrillation adequately (see this volume, p. 745).

PHARMACOKINETIC PROPERTIES

The therapeutic index of the digitalis glycosides is relatively narrow. Appreciation for the pharmacokinetic properties and the appropriate use of serum digitalis levels in making therapeutic decisions can help prevent digitalis toxicity. Although there is a positive correlation between elevated serum digoxin concentrations and clinical signs of toxicity, overlap between therapeutic and toxic serum concentrations exists. Interpretation of these values should therefore be made in light of the patient's history, physical findings, and ECG.

Absorption of digoxin after oral administration varies from 50 to 100% depending on the formulation; the capsule and alcohol-based elixir are more readily absorbed than the tablet (Table 1). Although the elixir is reported to be unpalatable to cats, the authors have not found this to be universally true. Because administration of digoxin with food may result in up to a 50% reduction in serum concentra-

tions, it is best given between meals. In general, parenteral digoxin should be avoided except when rapid digitalization is indicated (i.e., in sepsis, to control supraventricular tachyarrhythmias, or prior to dobutamine infusion in patients with atrial fibrillation) or when digoxin cannot be given orally. Since erratic absorption and intense pain often follow subcutaneous or intramuscular injection of digoxin, neither of these routes is recommended. There is a potential for vasoconstriction when cardiac glycosides are given intravenously, and therefore when indicated for intravenous use they should be administered by slow infusion over at least 15 minutes (0.01 to 0.02 mg/kg IV in two to four doses divided over 4 hr). There are no parenteral formulations of digitoxin. The oral absorption of most digitoxin preparations is 90 to 99% and this is also affected by concurrent feeding.

Despite the large distributive volume of digoxin, dosing should be based on lean body weight, because it is minimally distributed to adipose tissue. Digitoxin is more extensively protein bound, has a smaller volume of distribution, and is more lipid soluble than digoxin, and its dosage need not be adjusted for obesity.

Both drugs are metabolized to some extent by the liver, but digoxin is eliminated via the kidneys and digitoxin via the liver. The reported half-life for digoxin in the dog is about 20 to 30 hr; the half-life for digitoxin in the dog is approximately 6 to 14 hr. Since digoxin is excreted primarily by glomerular filtration and tubular secretion, dosage reduction is required for patients with impaired renal function. Many aging patients may have prolonged digoxin half-life because of subclinical renal dysfunction. Unlike the observations made in humans, poor correlation has been noted between the degree of azotemia and digoxin clearance in dogs, making precise adjustments difficult. Tilley and Scialli (1979) suggested a 50% reduction in digoxin dosage for every 50 mg/dl increase in the serum urea nitrogen. If available and practical, digitoxin is preferred in animals with renal failure because of its primary hepatic excretion. Miyazawa and colleagues (1990) recently described alterations in some of the pharmacokinetic properties of digitoxin in dogs with experimentally induced cholestasis, although extensive hepatocellular injury has previously been shown not to affect the disposition of digitoxin. It may be prudent to evaluate hepatic function in animals before prescribing digitoxin if there is biochemical or clinical evidence of cholestatic liver disease.

The use of loading doses of digoxin to rapidly achieve therapeutic serum concentrations generally is not recommended because of the increased potential for toxicity. Although many practitioners prefer to administer digoxin on the basis of body surface area (0.22 mg/m² b.i.d.), dogs weighing less

Table 2. *Conditions Probably Associated with Increased Risk of Digoxin Intoxication*

Concomitant drug therapy
  Quinidine
  Verapamil
  Furosemide/aspirin/sodium restriction (cats)
  Spironolactone
Metabolic derangements
  Hypokalemia
  Hypomagnesemia
  Hypercalcemia
  Acute hypoxia
  Hypothyroidism
  Obesity
  Myocardial infarction
  Renal insufficiency

than 22 kg usually receive an approximate oral maintenance dose of digoxin of 0.01 mg/kg b.i.d. These dosages are based on lean body weight (assuming a normal 15% body fat), and appropriate adjustments should be made for obesity or cachexia. In the cat, the pharmacokinetic properties of digoxin are more variable, as evidenced by reported elimination half-lives ranging from 10 to 79 hr. The authors recommend an oral digoxin dose at 0.01 mg/kg every 48 hr PO for the cat. This dose should be reduced by one third if the cat is receiving concomitant furosemide, aspirin, and sodium restriction.

Digitoxin is administered to dogs at an oral dose of 0.033 mg/kg b.i.d.–t.i.d. Since the elimination half-life of digitoxin in the cat is in excess of 100 hr, it should not be used in this species. Because of more convenient milligram tablet sizes, increased availability to the practitioner, and the need for less frequent administration, digoxin is the preferred glycoside in most veterinary practices.

Disorders of clinical importance, and drug interactions that have been shown to alter the pharmacokinetic properties of, or sensitivity to, digoxin and predispose to toxicity, are presented in Table 2. In dogs and cats, heart failure has not been shown to alter the pharmacokinetic properties of digoxin. However, since cardiac patients commonly lose weight during the course of their illness, it may be necessary to decrease the doses of digoxin. Careful assessment of the animal's clinical and renal status is important when digoxin is used in patients with renal failure.

Since adjustments in digoxin dosages may be necessary for a multitude of reasons (Table 2), evaluation of serum digoxin concentrations helps to ensure adequate digitalization after achieving steady state (three to five half-lives; 3 to 10 days) and is strongly recommended. Most hospitals for humans and many referral veterinary hospitals and laboratories have access to commercially available radioimmunoassays for digoxin. Dogs receiving digoxin twice daily and cats receiving digoxin every 48 hours should have serum concentrations measured 8 hr after administration of digoxin; serum levels of 0.8 to 2 ng/ml are considered to be within the therapeutic range. Therapeutic digitoxin concentrations are reported to be 15 to 35 ng/ml (6 to 8 hr after digitoxin administration).

EFFICACY

Kittleson (1971) reported an improvement in cardiac performance (as determined by M-mode echocardiography and venous PO_2) in 40% of cardiomyopathic dogs given digoxin. Responding dogs lived significantly longer than nonresponders. However, a later study by the same investigator failed to corroborate this finding (only one of 12 additional dogs responded); when both studies were combined, an overall improvement was achieved in 23% of dogs. On the basis of M-mode echocardiographic determinants in cats with myocardial failure, Atkins and colleagues showed echocardiographic improvement in four of six cats within 10 days of initiating digoxin therapy.*

Only a few inconclusive studies have evaluated the efficacy of digitalis glycosides in dogs with mitral regurgitation. In an early study by Hamlin and colleagues (1971), improvement after glycoside therapy was seen in six dogs with mitral insufficiency and heart failure as judged by the investigators, referring veterinarians, and owners. Three of these six dogs also had concurrent atrial fibrillation, which may have influenced their positive response.

Although digitalis compounds are weak-positive inotropic agents in comparison with the sympathomimetic agents and bipyridine compounds, digitalis is inexpensive, tachyphylaxis does not develop, dosing is oral, and the drug is thus well suited for chronic administration. The recently elucidated neurotropic effects of digitalis make it attractive for the management of chronic CHF. In addition, digoxin may prove useful in the treatment of circulatory failure due to septic shock. Results of a recent human study showed an improvement of 75% in left ventricular stroke work index, a measure of myocardial function, in septic patients treated with intravenous digoxin, compared with 13% improvement when similar patients were given dopamine.

HAZARDS

Digitalis intoxication is a dangerous and all too common complication of glycoside therapy in both

---

*Editors' Note: However, the overall sensitivity of echocardiography as a suitable method by which to evaluate digoxin therapy has not been determined.

human and veterinary patients. Although the incidence of digitalis intoxication has declined as digoxin assays have become more readily available, serious and life-threatening complications still occur. Studies, based on either clinical signs or serum drug concentrations, suggest that up to 25% of canine patients receiving cardiac glycosides are toxic.

The most commonly recognized signs of digitalis toxicity (anorexia, vomiting, diarrhea, depression, and cardiac arrhythmias) are believed to be neurally mediated. Anorexia, nausea, and vomiting are produced centrally by chemoreceptors in the area postrema of the medulla oblongata. Since gastrointestinal signs do not necessarily precede the arrhythmias, there may be no warning signs of impending cardiac toxicity.

Rhythm disturbances reported with digitalis intoxication include a variety of brady- and tachyarrhythmias and result from the indirect effects of digitalis on the autonomic nervous system as well as direct actions on the myocardial cell. Since the diseased myocardium appears to be particularly sensitive to the toxic effects of digitalis, the likelihood and severity of cardiac arrhythmias may be related to both the degree of intoxication and the severity of the underlying cardiac disease. Ventricular arrhythmias may be exacerbated, may be unaffected, or may improve in patients receiving digoxin. Ventricular arrhythmias (especially bigeminy) observed after digitalization should be attributed to intoxication until proved otherwise. Digitalis is not recommended in patients with Wolff-Parkinson-White syndrome who are prone to either atrial fibrillation or flutter, since the drug can promote conduction through the accessory pathway and lead to ventricular fibrillation.

Drug interactions are an important contributing factor to the high incidence of digitalis intoxication. Recognition of drug interactions can be challenging, because the adverse effects must first be recognized and an association made with concomitant drug therapies. Several compounds reduce oral digoxin absorption, producing potentially subtherapeutic serum concentrations. These include kaolin-pectin, metoclopramide, neomycin, antacids, and dietary bran. If digitalization is accomplished while the animal is receiving one of these compounds, toxicity may result if the concurrent therapy is discontinued. In approximately 10% of human patients there is substantial intestinal conversion of digoxin to cardioinactive products by enteric bacteria, thereby requiring high doses to attain therapeutic efficacy. These patients may be predisposed to toxicity if there is an abrupt alteration in gut flora, as may occur with oral antibiotic therapy.

Since digoxin is minimally metabolized in veterinary patients and is not highly protein bound, drugs that induce hepatic metabolism or inhibit protein binding have little consequence on digoxin pharmacokinetics or serum concentrations.

Table 3. Drugs Used in Management of Digitalis-associated Arrhythmias

Lidocaine
  Dog: 2–4 mg/kg IV bolus, followed by 20–80 µg/kg/min IV infusion
  Cat: 0.25–0.5 mg/kg *slow* IV bolus
Phenytoin
  Dog: 2–10 mg/kg *slow* IV bolus
      35 mg/kg PO q 8 hr
Procainamide
  Dog: 5–10 mg/kg IV, up to 20 mg/kg in 30 min
      20–50 µg/kg/min IV infusion
  Cat: 3–6 mg/kg IV
      63 mg PO q 8 hr
Atropine
  Dog or cat: 0.02–0.04 mg/kg SC, IM, IV

In humans, hydralazine and nitroprusside have been reported to increase the excretion of digoxin, while captopril, verapamil, and spironolactone decrease its excretion. The pharmacokinetic interaction of quinidine with digoxin is well recognized in both human and veterinary medicine. Since quinidine decreases the clearance of digoxin, a 50% reduction in the digoxin dose (or substitution of digitoxin) is recommended if quinidine must be used concomitantly. Cats receiving digoxin in conjunction with furosemide, aspirin, and a sodium-restricted diet have also been shown to have reduced digoxin clearance and are predisposed to digoxin toxicity, necessitating appropriate adjustments in digoxin dosage.

If digitalis intoxication is suspected, the serum digoxin concentration should be measured and the drug temporarily discontinued until the result is known and/or the clinical signs of toxicity abate. An electrocardiogram should be evaluated for the presence of arrhythmias and conduction disturbances. Life-threatening or symptomatic ventricular arrhythmias believed to be associated with digitalis intoxication should be controlled with lidocaine, phenytoin, or procainamide (Table 3). If the patient becomes symptomatic for digitalis-induced bradyarrhythmias, atropine may be helpful.

Since hypokalemia has been shown to exacerbate digitalis intoxication (by increasing digitalis binding to Na-K ATPase and by reducing the renal clearance of digoxin) and decrease the efficacy of antiarrhythmic agents, serum electrolyte concentrations should be measured and corrections made if abnormalities are present. Recurrence of digitalis intoxication is prevented by dosage adjustment and/or correction of inciting causes of toxicity (e.g., hypokalemia, renal insufficiency, and discontinuation or dosage reduction of drugs that interact with digitalis). If a recent massive overdose of the cardiac glycosides has occurred, activated charcoal or the steroid-binding resin cholestyramine may be administered to decrease intestinal absorption of the drug.

Table 4. *Guide to Successful Use of Digoxin*

1. Choose digoxin dosage carefully with considerations for obesity, age, renal function, electrolyte disturbances, and concomitant drug therapies. Begin conservatively with alterations in dose based on response to therapy and measurement of serum digoxin concentrations.
2. Educate client as to common clinical signs of digoxin intoxication.
3. After attaining steady state (approximately 7–14 days of therapy), measure serum digoxin concentration approximately 8 hr after dosing.
4. Be cognizant of changes in patient's renal status and body weight, and of addition of other therapeutic agents to treatment regimen.

Although costly, digoxin antibodies (Fab fragments) are available to treat life-threatening toxicities. These compounds complex to digoxin and digitoxin molecules and hasten their elimination. Each vial of Fab fragments (40 mg) binds 6 mg of digoxin or digitoxin at a cost of $150 per vial.

THERAPEUTIC END POINTS

Determination of the ideal digitalis dosage depends on the reasons for the initiation of digitalis therapy in the individual animal. Patients with supraventricular tachyarrhythmias are considered adequately digitalized when their arrhythmia is abolished, or in the case of atrial fibrillation, when their ventricular response rate is reduced to within the normal heart rate range (dogs, under 160 beats/min; cats, under 200 beats/min). If this cannot be achieved at therapeutic serum digoxin concentrations (a common situation), or if further reductions in rate are desired, additional antiarrhythmic therapy may be indicated (see *CVT X,* p. 271). Assessment of digitalis as an effective inotropic and neurotropic agent is more difficult. Subjective improvements in attitude, activity, appetite, and dyspnea indicate that adequate digitalization has probably been achieved, but other concurrently administered therapeutic agents (diuretics, vasodilators) complicate the issue. M-mode and two-dimensional echocardiographic examinations or radionuclide ventriculography provide useful, but relatively insensitive, noninvasive serial evaluations of ventricular function. Invasive hemodynamic measurements are generally impractical, but can be made.

In summary, digitalis therapy is initiated only after careful consideration of the indications in a particular patient (Table 4). The owner should be aware of the potential hazards and signs of digitalis intoxication. Routine follow-up examinations are recommended to evaluate the patient's cardiac status, monitor serum digoxin concentrations, and assess the efficacy of and ongoing need for therapy.

References and Suggested Reading

Atkins, C. E., Snyder, P. S., and Keene, B. W.: Effect of aspirin, furosemide, and commercial low salt diet on digoxin pharmacokinetic properties in clinically normal cats. J.A.V.M.A. 193:1264, 1988.
A prospective study of the effects of concurrent drug therapy on digoxin pharmacokinetics.
Atkins, C. E., Snyder, P. S., Keene, B. W., et al.: Efficacy of digoxin for treatment of cats with dilated cardiomyopathy. J.A.V.M.A. 196:1463, 1990.
A discussion of the efficacy of digoxin in six cats with myocardial failure.
DeRick, A., Belpaire, F. M., Bogaert, M. G., et al.: Plasma concentrations of digoxin and digitoxin during digitalization of healthy dogs and dogs with cardiac failure. Am. J. Vet. Res. 39:811, 1978.
A discussion of digoxin pharmacokinetics in the dog.
Ferguson, D. W., Berg, W. J., Sanders, J. S., et al.: Sympathoinhibitory responses to digitalis glycosides in heart failure patients. Circulation 80:65, 1989.
A discussion of newly described mechanisms of vasodilation in patients receiving digitalis.
Hamlin, R. L., Dutta, S., and Smith, C. R.: Effects of digoxin and digitoxin on ventricular function in normal dogs and dogs with heart failure. Am. J. Vet. Res. 32:1391, 1971.
A presentation of both objective and subjective data regarding the efficacy of digitalis in heart failure.
Hoffman, B. F.: The pharmacology of cardiac glycosides. *In* Rosen, M. R., and Hoffman, B. F. (eds.): *Cardiac Therapy.* Boston: Martinus Nijhoff, 1983, p. 387.
A good summary article regarding the use of digitalis in human medicine.
Kittleson, M. D.: Management of heart failure: Concepts, therapeutic strategies, and drug pharmacology. *In* Fox, P. R. (ed.): *Canine and Feline Cardiology.* New York: Churchill Livingstone, 1988, p. 171.
Includes a discussion of pharmacokinetics of, indications for, and efficacy of cardiac glycosides.
Miyazawa, Y., Sato, T., Kobayashi, K., et al.: Influence of induced cholestasis on pharmacokinetics of digoxin and digitoxin in dogs. Am. J. Vet. Res. 51:605, 1990.
Recent developments in the pharmacokinetics of digitalis glycosides in the dog.
Nasraway, S. A., Rackow, E. C., Astiz, M. E., et al.: Inotropic response to digoxin and dopamine in patients with severe sepsis, cardiac failure and systemic hypoperfusion. Chest 95:612, 1989.
A comparison of digoxin and dopamine as inotropic agents in the setting of sepsis.
Rawlings, C. A.: The patient with congestive heart failure. *In* Rawlings, C. A. (ed.): *Heartworm Disease in Dogs and Cats.* Philadelphia: W. B. Saunders, 1986, p. 116.
A discussion of the use of digitalis in dogs with heartworm disease–induced heart failure.
Smith, T. W.: Digitalis: Mechanism of action and clinical use. N. Engl. J. Med. 318:358, 1988.
An excellent review article with an extensive reference list.
Tilley, L. P., and Scialli, V. T.: *Digitalis: Clinical Indications and Practical Usage.* Research Triangle Park, NC: Burroughs Wellcome, 1979, p. 1.
A discussion of the indications for digoxin in comparison animals.

CURRENT USES AND HAZARDS OF VENTRICULAR ANTIARRHYTHMIC THERAPY

ROBERT L. HAMLIN
Columbus, Ohio

Veterinarians are quite able to identify irregularities in the heartbeat, but know much less about their significance (i.e., Are they innocuous or potentially lethal?) or their mechanism (i.e., Are they caused by re-entry, afterpotentials, or increased automaticity?). Their counterparts in human medicine are not much further advanced. One essential difference between treatment of arrhythmias by physicians and veterinarians is that physicians utilize drugs approved for that purpose by the FDA, whereas veterinarians often utilize the very same drugs without FDA approval because neither safety nor efficacy has been proved for the target species. Thus, veterinarians must address a critical issue: can they select appropriate cases for therapy and appropriate drugs for patients? The purpose of ventricular antiarrhythmic therapy is to prevent hemodynamic compromise (i.e., syncope due to a rapid, sustained ventricular tachycardia) or sudden death from the arrhythmia degenerating into ventricular fibrillation.

Selection of appropriate antiarrhythmic therapy from the many available drugs can be difficult. Ideally, one should: (1) identify the arrhythmia, (2) determine the severity of the arrhythmia (i.e., the need for therapy), (3) establish a putative mechanism, (4) select the antiarrhythmic that exerts its effect primarily on that mechanism, (5) administer the antiarrhythmic at the most efficacious dose and frequency, and (6) determine the patient's clinical response to the antiarrhythmic. Unfortunately, theory is much further advanced than practice, and it is often difficult or impossible to follow the ordered sequence to achieve a satisfactory outcome; in fact, the outcome has often been termed a "misadventure" (Goldstein et al., 1984).

Identifying the Arrhythmia

When it may be observed electrocardiographically, identification is seldom a problem, although with conventional electrocardiography the so-called "wide-QRS" supraventricular tachycardia (Fig. 1A) or atrial fibrillation with right bundle branch block (Fig. 1B) may resemble a ventricular tachycardia (Fig. 1C). Most arrhythmias are episodic; that is, they consist of single premature depolarizations or short paroxysms of ventricular tachycardia that are unlikely to be identified during casual monitoring for 15 sec every 7 days or so. If there are over 10,000 premature beats (out of a total of 150,000 heartbeats) per day and if the premature beats are distributed evenly throughout the day, more than one premature beat would occur among 15 sinus beats. If the heart rate was 100 beats per minute and the recording was for 15 sec, then there would be approximately 25 beats and at least one ventricular premature depolarization should be identified during routine monitoring. However, if there are only 1000 premature beats per day, distributed evenly throughout the day, it is unlikely that a premature beat would be identified in 15 sec of monitoring. On the other hand, if by chance a single brief paroxysm of ventricular tachycardia is noted during the 15-sec recording, a grossly overinflated idea of arrhythmia frequency may result. To circumvent this problem, the electrocardiogram (ECG) may either be monitored for 24 or 48 consecutive hours (i.e., Holter's monitoring), or the arrhythmia provoked by exercise, electrophysiologic testing (i.e., searching for repetitive ventricular responses), or pharmacologic means (e.g., digitalis, epinephrine, vasopressin).

Determination of Severity

It would be convenient if the number of premature depolarizations per minute or the heart rate during ectopic paroxysms (Fig. 2A and B), or the degree of pleomorphism (Fig. 2C), or the presence of premature depolarizations on the T-wave of the preceding beat (Fig. 2D) correlated well with the likelihood that an arrhythmia would result in either syncope or sudden death. Unfortunately there are no data in animals supporting any of these claims. There is no evidence that a paroxysm of rapid, pleomorphic ventricular tachycardia is a better predictor of sudden death than is a single ventricular

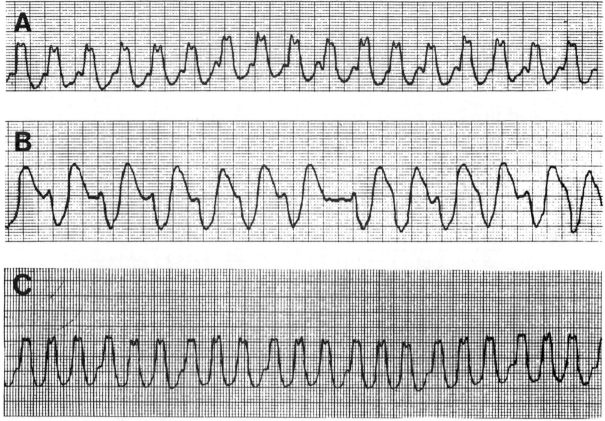

Figure 1. *A*, Lead II ECG (50 mm/sec paper speed) showing "wide-QRS" supraventricular tachycardia appearing like a ventricular tachycardia originating from the right ventricle (because the QRS complexes are positive in lead II). *B*, Lead II ECG (50 mm/sec paper speed) showing atrial fibrillation with right bundle branch block appearing like a ventricular tachycardia originating from the left ventricle (because the QRS complexes are negative in lead II). *C*, Lead II ECG (50 mm/sec paper speed) showing ventricular tachycardia originating from the right ventricle (because the QRS complexes are positive in lead II).

premature depolarization occurring relatively long after the preceding normal beat (Fig. 2*E*).

The reasons for interest—except for intellectual pursuit—in the nature of the arrhythmia are for prognosis and to determine if therapy is required. The latter reason would be less formidable if not for the fact that *the very agents used to terminate arrhythmias may exaggerate them and even lead to sudden death.* Thus, we need to know whether a ventricular arrhythmia is responsible for syncope or, of greater importance, may lead to sudden death. It is thought that rapid, pleomorphic ventricular tachycardias are at one end (the serious end) of the spectrum and occasional ventricular premature depolarizations are at the other end (the trivial end). Two algorithms for determining severity of arrhythmia in humans have been proposed and are in use; however, the search continues for more sensitive and specific methods to identify which arrhythmias require treatment. Currently, most physicians agree that arrhythmia leading to ventricular fibrillation or sustained ventricular tachycardia in a patient with known heart disease must be treated.

Identification of the Arrhythmic Mechanism

Arrhythmias may result from: (1) increased automaticity (i.e., increased slope of phase 4 of the action potential of those tissues that normally possess rhythmicity), (2) oscillatory afterpotentials (i.e., spontaneous fluctuations in the membrane potential triggered by the previous depolarization (also called delayed afterdepolarizations), and (3) re-entry (i.e., an impulse entering a slowly conducting region of the myocardium and "echoing" back to re-excite the normal region).

Although the origin of arrhythmia may be one mechanism (e.g., increased automaticity), maintenance of the arrhythmia may be by another (e.g., triggered activity, re-entry). Thus, a single ventricular premature depolarization may degenerate into a re-entrant tachycardia or a tachycardia sustained by triggered activity. The theoretical value in understanding the putative mechanisms of arrhythmias is that a more rational selection of antiarrhythmic agents may be made. Unfortunately, identifying the mechanism of arrhythmia is often difficult or nearly impossible by routine electrocardiography. Observ-

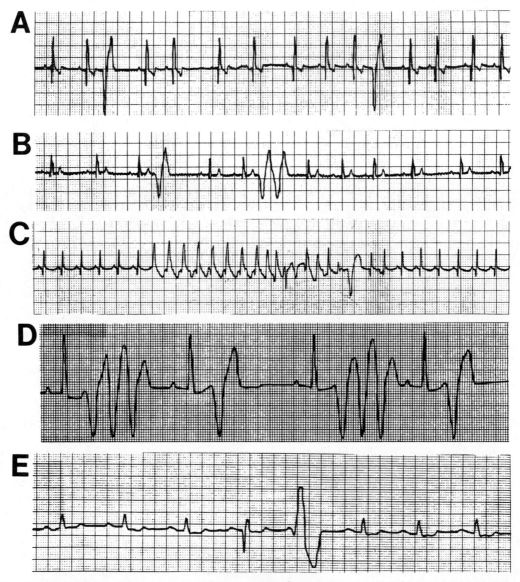

Figure 2. *A*, Lead II ECG (25 mm/sec paper speed) showing isolated ventricular premature depolarizations originating from the left ventricle (because the QRS complexes for the premature depolarization are negative). *B*, Lead II ECG (25 mm/sec paper speed) showing a paroxysm (burst) of ventricular premature depolarizations originating from the left ventricle (because the QRS complexes for the premature depolarizations are negative in lead II). *C*, Lead II ECG (25 mm/sec paper speed) showing pleomorphic (i.e., QRS complexes for premature depolarizations of varying contour in lead II) ventricular premature beats occurring singly and in bursts. *D*, Lead II ECG (50 mm/sec paper speed) showing ventricular premature depolarizations occurring in bursts, with the QRS complex of one premature depolarization occurring on the T-wave of the beat preceding. *E*, Lead II ECG (50 mm/sec paper speed) showing ventricular premature depolarization occurring from the right ventricle (i.e., QRS complex for premature depolarization is positive) and relatively long after the preceding normal T-wave.

Table 1. Ventricular Antiarrhythmics Commonly
Used in Dogs*

Drug	Dosage/Route	Remarks
Lidocaine	2–6 mg/kg 50–75 μg/kg/min infusion	Emergency drug of choice; therapeutic plasma concentrations 1.5–6 μg/ml
Tocainide	10–20 mg/kg t.i.d. oral	"Oral lidocaine"
Mexiletine	4–8 mg/kg t.i.d. oral	Similar to lidocaine
Phenytoin	30 mg/kg t.i.d. oral 10 mg/kg slow IV	Primarily for digitalis toxicity, sometimes effective in combinations for refractory arrhythmias; rapid intravenous injection may cause cardiorespiratory arrest
Procainamide	5–15 mg/kg IV 25–40 μg/kg/min infusion 10–20 mg/kg t.i.d. oral	Therapeutic plasma concentrations 4–10 μg/ml, may extend to 20 μg/ml; use sustained release (SR) prep for t.i.d. oral dosing
Quinidine	5–15 mg/kg t.i.d. oral 5–15 mg/kg t.i.d. IM	Sustained release prep recommended for t.i.d. dosing; intravenous injection may cause hypotension; digoxin interaction predisposes to toxicity; therapeutic plasma concentration 2–7 μg/ml
Propranolol	0.25–1 mg/kg t.i.d. oral 0.1–0.3 mg/kg IV	Beta-blocker, gradually titrate dosage; beware of low-output signs
Esmolol	0.5 mg/kg slow IV load 50–200 μg/kg/min infusion	Ultra-short–acting intravenous beta-blockade

*Drugs used to treat life-threatening ventricular arrhythmias (sustained ventricular tachycardia or complex ventricular arrhythmias in hemodynamically compromised patients) are often chosen sequentially based on response to therapy. Before instituting specific ventricular antiarrhythmic therapy, the patient's hydration, electrolyte, and ventilatory status is evaluated as quickly and thoroughly as possible. Appropriate supportive care is critical to success. Lidocaine is usually the drug of first choice in emergency situations, followed by intravenous procainamide if lidocaine proves ineffective. Lack of response should prompt electrocardiographic confirmation of the diagnosis and detailed evaluation of electrolyte (especially sodium, potassium, and magnesium) and ventilatory (blood gas) status. Additional supportive care (e.g., supplemental oxygen) and specific antiarrhythmic therapy (e.g., test-dose beta-blockade with esmolol) should be attempted to terminate the arrhythmia. DC cardioversion of sustained ventricular tachycardia is performed under narcotic sedation in cases that are refractory to pharmacotherapy.

ing a single ventricular premature depolarization or even a paroxysmal ventricular tachycardia during casual electrocardiography may provide little insight into its mechanism or mechanisms. Even more elaborate electrophysiologic testing may not identify the precise mechanism. Fortunately, the inability to identify the mechanisms of arrhythmia need not obstruct treatment.

Selection of Treatment

Once the decision is made to treat an arrhythmia, selection of an antiarrhythmic regimen is based predominantly on the focus of origin (e.g., supraventricular or ventricular) of the arrhythmia, the pharmacology (e.g., membrane stabilizing, calcium channel blocker) of the antiarrhythmic, and auxilliary features such as the underlying disease and electrolyte balance (Table 1). Agents of choice for treating ventricular arrhythmias are lidocaine (a class IB antiarrhythmic), used predominantly for life-threatening, sustained ventricular tachycardia; procainamide or quinidine (class IA antiarrhythmics), used for arrhythmias that are less likely to degenerate suddenly to ventricular fibrillation; and propranolol and other (class II) beta-blockers, often used concomitantly with class IA drugs. There is a plethora of other antiarrhythmics, some of which are pharmacologically similar (e.g., disopyramide [IA], tocainide, mexiletine [IB]) to those already mentioned and some of which exert their action by dissimilar routes (e.g., flecainide, encainide [class IC], amiodarone [class IV]). If serum potassium is normal, most ventricular arrhythmias may be terminated—at least for the short term—by these agents.

Administration

Almost all ventricular arrhythmias can be terminated within 5 min by intravenous lidocaine if the serum potassium is normal. After the arrhythmia is terminated by boluses of lidocaine, the patient may be given a continuous infusion of lidocaine or switched to quinidine or procainamide. If lidocaine infusion is sustained, there is no information about how long the infusion should be continued before switching to oral quinidine or procainamide. There is also no information about whether, if the animal is switched to quinidine or procainamide, the desired end point should be abolition of the ectopic activity or merely suppression to reduced frequency. In any case, the animal should be monitored electrocardiographically and clinically at frequent intervals.

Precisely how an antiarrhythmic is used depends upon experience of the veterinarian, how closely (e.g., seen four times a day or once every week) and by what means (e.g., physical exam, electrocardiography) the animal is followed, time constraints on the veterinarian, and financial constraints imposed by the owner. As mentioned earlier, most cardiologists prefer treating rapid, ventricular tachycardias with lidocaine or procainamide given intravenously in the hospital. If, on the other hand, there is no other urgent reason (e.g., trauma, severe metabolic derangement) for hospitalizing the ani-

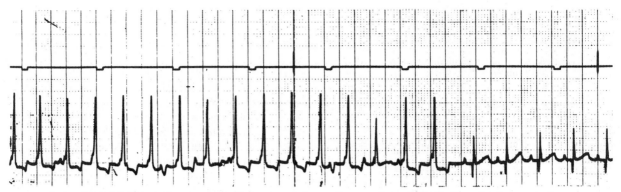

Figure 3. Lead II ECG (25 mm/sec paper speed) showing abolition of ventricular tachycardia (run of right ventricular premature depolarizations) by lidocaine infusion.

mal, there is no evidence that dogs with these tachycardias do any worse if treated at home with quinidine or procainamide given orally. In fact, when at home the dog may manifest reduced sympathoadrenal discharge and be *less likely* to die suddenly from ventricular tachycardia degenerating into ventricular fibrillation. The difference in cost to the client may also be formidable!

Determination of Clinical Response

If it were known how long a given patient would live untreated and if the antiarrhythmic regimen prolonged or shortened life, then the regimen could

be assessed as either effective or dangerous. Unfortunately, we do not know the natural course of most arrhythmias left untreated and so cannot answer questions about danger or efficacy. The author knows of no data supporting the contention that ventricular antiarrhythmic therapy prolongs an animal's life even a single day.

But do antiarrhythmics improve the quality of life by decreasing frequency or duration of syncope? Again, there is anecdotal evidence suggesting symptomatic improvement but no hard data supporting that contention. There are numerous reports demonstrating either apparent abolition (Fig. 3) or suppression (Fig. 4) of ventricular arrhythmia, and there are obvious instances in which arrhythmia is

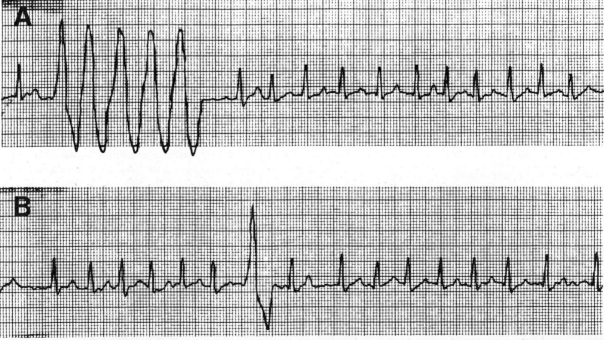

Figure 4. *A*, Lead II ECG (25 mm/sec paper speed) showing decrease in frequency of ventricular premature depolarizations *(B)* as a result of favorable response to oral quinidine.

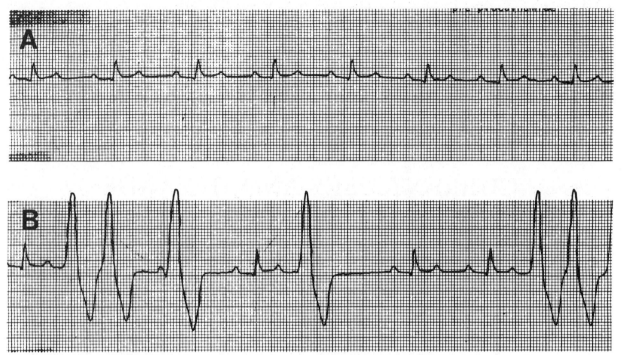

Figure 5. A, Lead II ECG (50 mm/sec paper speed) showing apparent worsening of arrhythmia (B) indicated by more frequent ventricular premature depolarizations after dog received oral procainamide.

apparently worsened (Fig. 5). An important caveat is in the word "apparent" because the contentions are generally based on casual, intermittent monitoring for rather brief periods. It has been reported, that 60% of human patients with ventricular arrhythmias monitored for 2 hr before and after placebo administration have indication of antiarrhythmic effect of the placebo. When monitored for 48 hr, however, the placebo effect disappears. This points to the need for long-term monitoring and to the danger of claiming antiarrhythmic efficacy based on monitoring for short periods. Another caveat: just because an arrhythmia is suppressed or abolished or becomes worse does not mean that the patient feels better and lives longer or feels worse and dies sooner.

Conclusion

The client has a right to know whether or not a pet's life will be altered by use of an antiarrhythmic. As of now, such information does not exist. The consensus among veterinary cardiologists seems to be:

Ventricular arrhythmias are best identified by monitoring a lead II ECG taken at either 25 or 50 mm/sec paper speed for an interval of 15 sec to 1 min.

Mechanisms of ventricular arrhythmias do not con-

tribute substantially to decisions to treat and what agents to use.

Ventricular premature depolarizations are usually treated if the patient is syncopal, if they occur in paroxysms, if there are more than 15 per min, and if the dog is thought to be at high risk for sudden death (i.e., Doberman pinschers, traumatized large-breed dogs).

Lidocaine is used for rapid ventricular tachycardia or paroxysmal tachycardia; class IA antiarrhythmics with or without a beta-blocker are used for less life-threatening arrhythmias or after conversion with lidocaine.

Results of antiarrhythmic therapy are seldom documented. Change in symptoms (e.g., syncope) or frequency of premature depolarizations are used occasionally.

For additional considerations regarding therapy, see CVT X, p. 278.

References and Suggested Reading

Goldstein, R. E., Tibbits, P. A., and Oetgen, W. J.: Proarrhythmic effects of antiarrhythmic drugs. In Greenberg, H. M., Kulbertus, H. E., Moss, A. J. and Schwartz, P. J. (eds.): Clinical Aspects of Life-Threatening Arrhythmias. Ann. N.Y. Acad. Sci., 427:94, 1984.
Hoffman, B. F., and Rosen, M. R.: Cellular mechanisms for cardiac arrhythmias. Circ. Res. 49:1, 1981.
Lown, B., and Graboys, T. B.: Evaluation and management of the patient with ventricular arrhythmia. Cardiac Impulse 6:1–5, 1985.

McGovern, B.: Hypokalemia and cardiac arrhythmias: Editorial views. Anesthesiology 63:127, 1985.

Muir, W. W., and Bonagura, J. D.: Aprindine for treatment of ventricular arrhythmias. Am. J. Vet. Res. 43:1815, 1982.

Opie, L. H.: Drugs and the heart. IV. Antiarrhythmic agents. Lancet 1:861, 1980.

Singh, B. N., and Hauswirth, O.: Comparative mechanisms of action of antiarrhythmic drugs. Am. Heart J. 87:367, 1974.

Tilley, L. P.: *Essentials of Canine and Feline Electrocardiography.* Philadelphia: Lea & Febiger, 1985, pp. 125–247.

Torres, V., Flowers, D., and Somberg, J. C.: The arrhythmogenicity of antiarrhythmic agents. Am. Heart J. 109:1090, 1985.

Vaughan-Williams, E. M.: Classification of antiarrhythmic drugs. Pharmacol. Ther. 1:115, 1975.

Vlay, S. C.: How the university cardiologist treats ventricular premature beats: A nationwide survey of 65 university medical centers. Am. Heart J. 110:904, 1985.

Winkle, R. A.: Antiarrhythmic drug effect mimicked by spontaneous variability of ventricular ectopy. Circulation 57:1116, 1978.

CURRENT USES AND HAZARDS OF VASODILATOR THERAPY IN HEART FAILURE

LAURA A. DeLELLIS

Bloomfield Hills, Michigan

and MARK D. KITTLESON

Davis, California

Vasodilator therapy, once considered a specialized therapeutic concept, is now common in veterinary and human medicine. Clinicians today know more about the role and response of peripheral circulation in heart failure and have become familiar with the associated drugs.

Vasodilators are classified based on their primary site of action (Table 1). Venodilators dilate systemic veins and so initially reduce venous return to the heart, decreasing intracardiac blood volume and diastolic intracardiac pressures. Consequently, they are used to treat edema that develops in heart failure. Venodilators include the nitrates—nitroglycerin and isosorbide dinitrate.

Arteriolar dilators dilate systemic arterioles and so decrease resistance to forward (systemic arterial) blood flow. Hydralazine is the best example. Agents with both systemic arteriolar and venous dilating action are known as mixed or balanced vasodilators and include sodium nitroprusside, prazosin, and angiotensin-converting enzyme (ACE) inhibitors. Vasodilators are also classified according to their mechanism of action (Table 1).

While vasodilators often improve therapeutic results, their use includes the potential for adverse effects. These drugs are often used in critically ill canine and feline patients or those with multiple problems that may be receiving several medications

Table 1. Vasodilator Drugs Commonly Used in Veterinary Medicine

Vasodilator	Type (mechanism)	Route	Dose in Dogs	Dose in Cats
Hydralazine	Arteriolar ($\uparrow$ PGI$_2$ [?])	PO	1–3 mg/kg q 12 hr	2.5–10 mg q 12 hr
Prazosin	Combination (alpha$_1$-blocker)	PO	0.5–2 mg/dog q 8 hr–q 12 hr	
Nitroglycerin	Venous (cGMP formation)	Cutaneous	One-fourth inch per 5 kg q 6 hr–q 8 hr	One-fourth inch q 6 hr–q 8 hr
Nitroprusside	Combination (cGMP formation)	IV	1–15 µG/kg/min	
Captopril	Combination (ACE inhibitor)	PO	0.5–2 mg/kg q 8 hr	3–6 mg q 8 hr
Enalapril	Combination (ACE inhibitor)	PO	0.5 mg/kg q 12 hr–q 24 hr	0.25 mg/kg q 12–24 hr

ACE, angiotensin-converting enzyme; cGMP, cyclic guanosine monophosphate; PGI$_2$, prostaglandin I$_2$.

at one time. These patients, in general, are at greater risk from adverse effects. Avoiding adverse events and using a vasodilator wisely require understanding of the mechanism of action, dosage, side effects, drug interactions, and patient risks involved. Clinicians must be able to differentiate a life-threatening adverse event from a relatively benign complication and understand how to manage serious complications of drug therapy. An accurate diagnosis is required prior to initiation of therapy; otherwise, more frequent complications are likely. Thoracic radiographs, an electrocardiogram, and an echocardiogram are frequently required to establish a correct diagnosis.

HEART FAILURE AND VASODILATORS

Heart failure is a pathophysiological condition in which abnormal systolic or diastolic cardiac function is responsible for failure of the heart to maintain normal ventricular filling pressures or to deliver blood at a rate required for tissue metabolism. Heart failure is represented clinically as congestion and edema (so-called backward or congestive heart failure [CHF]) or poor tissue perfusion (so-called forward or low-cardiac-output failure).

The heart's primary function is to pump a normal quantity of blood through the vascular beds. Cardiac output is influenced by systolic and diastolic func-tions of the heart. Systolic function is determined by preload, afterload, contractility, heart rate and rhythm, and the size of the ventricles. The amount of blood pumped to the body (the effective cardiac output) is also affected by the presence of shunts or regurgitant valves in the system (Fig. 1). These factors can be adjusted to compensate for the failing cardiovascular system and frequently for impaired cardiac function in the face of disease. It is not unusual for compensatory mechanisms like cardiac hypertrophy to maintain cardiovascular function for years in the face of mild to moderate heart disease. Once disease becomes severe, however, these compensatory mechanisms can be overwhelmed and actually contribute to the signs of heart failure. Ventricular diastolic function is an important determinant of ventricular filling. Abnormal diastolic function is common in heart disease and results in elevations of diastolic pressure and eventually edema.

Arteriolar dilators are used to alter afterload. They act to decrease systemic vascular resistance and consequently reduce systemic arterial blood pressure, systolic intraventricular pressure and tension, and afterload. Afterload is systolic wall stress, the force that the ventricular muscle must overcome to shorten and move blood into the aorta. A primary determinant of systolic wall stress is the systolic intraventricular pressure that must be generated (see Fig. 1). A reduction in afterload facilitates

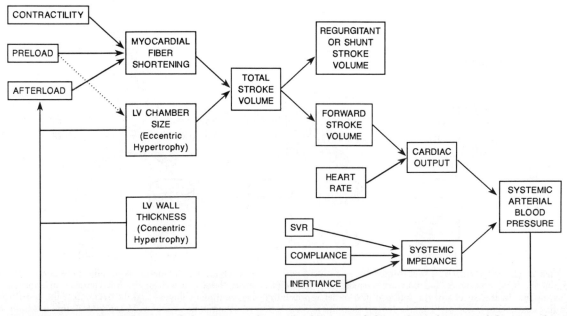

Figure 1. The factors that influence and determine cardiovascular function and their relationships. LV, left ventricular; SVR, systemic vascular resistance.

myocardial shortening, resulting in a greater expulsion of blood. In mitral and aortic valvular regurgitation or in left-to-right shunts, the amount of abnormal blood flow and the amount of blood flow into the aorta relate directly to the resistance to flow through the two orifices. In mitral regurgitation, this relationship is represented by the resistances to flow through the mitral valve orifice and aorta. A decrease in resistance to flow through the systemic arteriolar bed increases ventricular ejection into the aorta and decreases mitral regurgitation. (Fig. 2) Arteriolar dilators can also decrease shunting in a left-to-right shunt. Venodilators affect preload, also a determinant of ventricular systolic function. Their primary beneficial effect, however, occurs in diastole. By pooling blood peripherally, venodilators decrease diastolic intraventricular pressures and reduce edema formation.

The cardiovascular system performs three basic hemodynamic functions: (1) maintaining systemic arterial blood pressure, (2) maintaining cardiac output, and (3) maintaining a normal, low venous pressure. The major priority among these three functions is to maintain systemic blood pressure to ensure perfusion and oxygen delivery to the essential organs (heart, brain, kidney). Arterial pressure is determined by cardiac output and peripheral vascular resistance (primarily by the radius of the systemic arteriolar vascular bed; see Fig. 2). Following a decrease in cardiac output, compensatory mechanisms (increased sympathetic tone, increased formation of angiotensin II) lead to peripheral vasoconstriction to maintain normal blood pressure. Normal blood pressure, however, is approximately 40 to 50 mm Hg greater than is absolutely required for perfusion. The baroreceptors are set to maintain a mean systemic arterial blood pressure of 100 to 110 mm Hg, whereas clinical signs of hypotension are not observed until blood pressure decreases below a level of about 60 mm Hg. The body will not utilize this reserve; however, clinicians, through the use of arteriolar dilators, can take advantage of it.

Monitoring Therapy

The usual therapeutic end points of vasodilator therapy for patients in heart failure are reduction in edema (reduced pulmonary capillary pressure and venous pressures) for venodilators and improved tissue perfusion (elevation of cardiac output) for arteriolar dilators. When valvular regurgitation or left-to-right shunting is present, arteriolar dilators reduce the degree of edema and improve forward flow. While it may not be feasible to measure these parameters directly, close monitoring of clinical signs and radiographic examination of

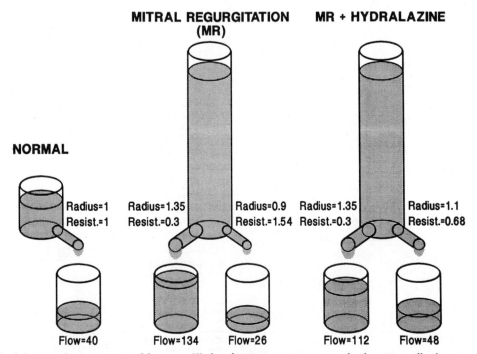

Figure 2. The left ventricle is represented by a can filled with water emptying into a bucket. Normally there is only one spigot or outlet for flow. Resistance and flow are normal. In mitral regurgitation, there is a leak in the left ventricle in addition to the normal outlet. In this situation, the radius of the outlet representing the regurgitant flow is slightly larger than the normal outlet. Note that resistance, however, is markedly less than the normal outlet, resulting in greater flow. When hydralazine is administered, the radius of the normal outlet increases, resulting in a decrease in resistance. Flow increases through the normal outlet as a result, and flow through the regurgitant outlet decreases. Resistance (Resist.) = 1/radius⁴.

the lungs are realistic. Therapeutic response is seen as a decrease in cough, return of normal respiratory rate and effort, improved capillary refill time and color (sometimes hyperemic), improved distal extremity perfusion and temperature, improved attitude and possibly exercise tolerance, resolution of ascites, and radiographic resolution of pulmonary edema or pleural effusion. Blood lactate concentration and venous oxygen tension should become normal following arteriolar dilator therapy if they were initially abnormal. Mean or systolic systemic arterial blood pressure is usually reduced by 10 to 40 mm Hg after the administration of an arteriolar dilator. Mean systemic arterial blood pressure should generally be maintained at approximately 70 mm Hg or above. Although this benefit is unproven in animals, vasodilator therapy has the potential to increase longevity in patients with heart failure.

Adverse Effects

The primary adverse effect of vasodilator therapy is hypotension. This usually occurs as an isolated event following administration of the first doses of drug or during titration of the dose and may warrant only a decrease in the dose rather than discontinuation of the drug. The additive effects of a diuretic and a vasodilator can be a factor in producing hypotension. This most often occurs in the dog; however, in the authors' clinical experience, it is unlikely unless the patient is clinically dehydrated and severely volume depleted. Patients that become anorexic (from medication, azotemia, or the primary disease) while on diuretic therapy can rapidly dehydrate. Owners should be warned of this complication. If a patient is eating and drinking normally, it is difficult to produce clinically significant dehydration and volume depletion with chronic diuretic therapy.

It is important to recognize systemic arterial hypotension. If it is misinterpreted as incomplete response to medication or progression of the disease, further doses could result in added complications. Acute onset of weakness and lethargy following drug administration is the most common clinical sign of hypotension.

Webster's dictionary defines hypotension as an abnormally low blood pressure, difficult to specify in precise terms or numbers, whereas the medical literature defines it as any systemic arterial blood pressure less than normal. Clinically significant hypotension, however, represents more than a mild to moderate decrease in blood pressure. For this discussion, hypotension is defined as systemic arterial blood pressure low enough to cause clinical signs. To produce clinical signs, systemic arterial blood pressure must decrease to a point that blood will not flow through particular vascular beds. When

mean systemic arterial blood pressure decreases to less than approximately 50 to 60 mm Hg, flow becomes compromised. Normal mean arterial blood pressure is 100 to 110 mm Hg. Therefore, there is a blood pressure reserve of about 50 mm Hg. Arteriolar dilators take advantage of this reserve and in patients with heart failure cause mild to moderate decreases in blood pressure as a therapeutic effect. Often, mean systemic arterial blood pressure decreases to 70 to 80 mm Hg following vasodilator therapy. This is an expected and therapeutic effect that causes no obvious clinical signs of hypotension. On the contrary, clinical signs are generally improved because of the increase in systemic blood flow brought about by the decrease in afterload.

Specific Vasodilators

ANGIOTENSIN-CONVERTING ENZYME INHIBITORS

The effects of ACE inhibitors are a consequence of decreased concentration of circulating angiotensin II. Angiotensin II has several important effects: (1) it is a potent vasopressor, (2) it stimulates the release of aldosterone from the adrenal gland, (3) it stimulates vasopressin (ADH) release from the posterior pituitary gland, (4) it facilitates the central and peripheral effects of the sympathetic nervous system, and (5) it preserves glomerular filtration when renal blood flow is decreased. ACE inhibitors have several effects in patients with heart failure. Arteriolar and venous dilation occur owing to the decreased concentration of angiotensin II; therefore, ACE inhibitors are classified as vasodilators. Moreover, ACE inhibitors also decrease plasma aldosterone concentration, and this may be their most important role in some patients. When the stimulus for aldosterone secretion is lessened, Na^+ and water excretion are enhanced and the degree of edema decreases.

ACE inhibitors act as arteriolar dilators. In the majority of canine patients, however, the effect is relatively mild compared with the effects of a drug like hydralazine. This explains the reduced number of hypotensive events observed with ACE inhibitors. This probably also explains why the effect of ACE inhibitors on pulmonary edema and cardiac output in dogs with mitral regurgitation is usually not as profound as with hydralazine. This gradual onset of action makes other vasodilators or combinations (e.g., hydralazine-nitrate or sodium nitroprusside) preferable to ACE inhibitors in life-threatening congestive heart failure. The reduction in aldosterone and ADH release promotes Na^+ and water loss, thereby reducing edema. In human patients, exercise tolerance has been shown to improve over a period of several weeks. In dogs and cats, mild to profound improvement in clinical signs has been observed in the majority of patients over several weeks.

The risks of interfering with angiotensin II formation lie in its important role in preserving systemic blood pressure and glomerular filtration rate (GFR) as renal artery perfusion pressure and renal blood flow decrease. Blocking the action on peripheral arterioles can result in hypotension and cerebral hypoperfusion. Dizziness is seen in 15% of humans taking ACE inhibitors. There are no data on hypotension following ACE inhibitor administration in veterinary medicine.

Angiotensin II preserves glomerular filtration rate in low flow states by constricting the efferent glomerular arteriole. This increases the glomerular capillary pressure needed to maintain overall filtration. Thus, GFR is preserved despite the decrease in flow, and normal serum urea nitrogen (SUN) and serum creatinine concentrations are maintained. The filtration fraction (ratio of GFR to renal plasma flow) may suddenly decrease following ACE inhibition, causing a decrease in GFR and an increase in SUN and serum creatinine. This is reported in up to 35% of human patients receiving ACE inhibitors.

The risk of acutely decreasing glomerular filtration in patients dependent on angiotensin II to maintain GFR is also present in veterinary practice. When angiotensin II concentration is decreased in these patients, GFR decreases and acute azotemia results. The azotemia is generally mild but in some cases can be severe. It can be prevented in some patients by reducing the dose of the concurrent diuretic and can be treated by intravenous fluids (administered carefully) or by discontinuing the ACE-inhibitor.

Recommended guidelines for ACE inhibitor therapy include (1) identify high-risk patients (those with renal insufficiency, proteinuria, other renal diseases) prior to therapy, (2) ensure that the patient is not clinically dehydrated and provide adequate fluid intake throughout therapy, (3) evaluate renal function periodically (e.g., every 2 weeks for the first month after commencing therapy, monthly for the following 2 to 3 months and then every 2 to 6 months as indicated), (4) immediately evaluate the patient's renal function if acute depression or vomiting develops, (5) decrease or discontinue the drug if renal insufficiency or other side effects develop, and (6) consider titrating the dose gradually over 2 to 3 weeks, especially in patients with hyponatremia because this is a marker of renin-angiotensin system activation.

The clinical benefits of ACE inhibitors in heart failure are reasonably evident in human studies. They have been shown to lessen symptoms and prolong life. A combination of hydralazine and isosorbide dinitrate has also been shown to prolong

survival time in humans. It should be noted, however, that vasodilator therapy is still palliative and that even in humans the duration of survival in advanced heart failure is relatively short despite intervention with ACE inhibitors.

There are three ACE inhibitors available: captopril, enalapril, and lisinopril. Generally they have similar, long-term effects, although short-term effects may vary. Lisinopril is the longest acting and is advocated for once-daily use in humans. Its use in veterinary medicine has not been evaluated. (For a complete review of the mechanisms surrounding the actions of ACE inhibitors, see *CVT IX*, p. 334.)

Captopril

Captopril (Capoten, Squibb) has a half-life in dogs of about 2.8 hr. Captopril is almost exclusively eliminated by the kidneys. Biliary excretion is negligible. In patients with altered renal function, a decrease in dose interval or dose is recommended. Captopril is 40% protein bound.

Recommended dosage is 0.5 to 2.0 mg/kg every 8 hr PO. Doses of 3.0 mg/kg every 8 hr have been associated with glomerular lesions and renal failure in experimental dogs and clinical canine patients. In a study performed by one of the authors, the onset of activity of captopril was within 1 hr following the first dose. Drug effect lasted less than 4 hr. A dose of 1 mg/kg produced slightly greater effects than a dose of 0.5 mg/kg. A dose of 2 mg/kg produced no additional benefit.

In this same study, the primary effect of captopril in the dog following its first dose was arteriolar dilation. Little change in pulmonary capillary pressure was noted; consequently, captopril is not a good emergency drug in dogs with severe pulmonary edema. Edema reduction appears to take more than 48 hr to develop, after which profound reductions in pulmonary capillary pressure can be noted.

Side effects include first-dose hypotension, anorexia, vomiting, diarrhea, and azotemia. Captopril's side effects are like those of other ACE inhibitors (i.e., hypotension and inability to maintain GFR in the face of decreased renal artery perfusion, resulting in azotemia). Urine protein concentration, SUN, and electrolytes should be monitored.

Enalapril

Studies examining enalapril's effectiveness in dogs with heart failure are currently in progress. Enalapril (Vasotec, Merck Sharp & Dohme) should have hemodynamic and clinical benefits similar to those of captopril because its actions are very similar. The pharmacokinetics of enalapril, however, are quite different from those of captopril. Enalapril has a longer duration of effect (12 to 14 hr in dogs), a slower onset of effect (4 to 6 hr in dogs) due to required hydrolysis of the pro-drug enalapril in the liver to the active form, enalaprilat, and lacks an active sulfhydryl (SH) group in its structure. The latter is thought to lessen or eliminate the risk of immune-based side effects in man. Enalapril is excreted by the kidney and the dose should be reduced in renal insufficiency. Although some studies suggest oral absorption is not affected by food in the gastrointestinal tract, the manufacturer suggests it be administered on an empty stomach. Recommended dose in dogs is 0.5 to 1.0 mg/kg every 12 to 24 hr. The initial dose in cats appears to be 0.25 mg/kg orally once or twice daily.

In healthy dogs administered doses up to 15 mg/kg/day over 1 year, drug-induced renal lesions were not seen. At 30 mg/kg/day, increasing degrees of renal damage observed were shown to be a direct nephrotoxic response of enalapril on proximal tubular epithelium. This damage was permanent only when potentiated by marked hypotension. Acute renal failure that is reversible with fluid therapy has been observed in a number of dogs following treatment with enalapril.

Side effects include anorexia, vomiting, and diarrhea. These side effects in dogs appear to be less frequent with enalapril than with captopril. Hypotension can also be observed. Extreme care should be taken when administering enalapril to patients that are dehydrated or hyponatremic.

HYDRALAZINE

Hydralazine (Apresoline, CIBA; Alazine, Major) is an arteriolar dilator whose precise mechanism of action is unknown. It probably induces an increase in local prostacyclin concentration.

Apresoline is rapidly absorbed after oral administration. Onset of action in the dog is within 30 to 60 min, peak effect occurs between 3 and 5 hr, and duration of effect is 11 to 13 hr. It is metabolized in the liver by acetylation and undergoes first-pass effect. Uremia may affect biotransformation, so the dose should be decreased in renal insufficiency. Generic hydralazine is not recommended by the authors.

Presumably because of varied bioavailability of hydralazine per individual, hydralazine must be titrated to an effective end point in each dog. The initial dose is 0.5 to 1 mg/kg every 12 hr, which can be titrated up to 3 mg/kg every 12 hr in the dog. The dose in cats is 2.5 mg to 10 mg every 12 hr. The dose can be titrated quite rapidly in the dog if blood pressure can be monitored. When monitoring blood pressure, the clinician is generally looking for a 20 to 40 mm Hg decrease in either mean or systolic (Doppler) systemic arterial blood pressure. In this situation, a dose of approximately 1 mg/kg is administered following measurement of baseline blood pressure. One hour later, blood pressure is measured again. If no decrease is identified, another 1 mg/kg dose is administered. Because the drug

effect lasts 12 hr, the cumulative dose is now 2 mg/kg. Blood pressure is measured again in 1 hr, and if no response is identified another 1 mg/kg dose is administered. The cumulative dose is now 3 mg/kg. The effective cumulative dose is administered every 12 hr. If blood pressure cannot be monitored, titration is performed more slowly and clinical and radiographic signs are monitored. Baseline assessments of mucous membrane color, capillary refill time, murmur intensity, heart rate, cardiac size on radiographs, and severity of pulmonary edema are made. A dose of 1 mg/kg is administered every 12 hr and repeat assessments are made in 12 to 48 hr. If no response is identified, the dose is increased to 2 mg/kg and then to 3 mg/kg if no response is seen at the previous dose.

Mucous membrane color, capillary refill time, and arterial pulse pressure will become noticeably improved in about 50% to 60% of dogs. In most dogs with mitral regurgitation, the severity of the pulmonary edema will lessen within 24 hr. In many of these dogs the size of the left ventricle will decrease. In some dogs, obvious improvement will not be sufficient to identify with certainty. In these cases, the titration may continue with the realization that some dogs will be mildly overdosed and clinical signs of hypotension may become evident. Owners should be warned to watch for signs of hypotension and notify the clinician if they are identified. In most situations, the dog can be observed until the drug effect wears off (11 to 13 hr later), at which time the drug dose should be reduced. If a dog becomes severely or persistently weak and lethargic following hydralazine administration, it should be reevaluated. In the rare event that signs of shock become evident, fluids and vasopressors may be administered.

In emergency situations such as severe mitral regurgitation due to a ruptured chorda tendineae, hydralazine in combination with furosemide can be very effective therapy for pulmonary edema. In this situation, the authors prefer to start the titration dose at about 2 mg/kg PO. An intravenous preparation is available, but as onset of action is within 30 minutes following oral administration, the authors have not identified a true need for this route of administration.

When hydralazine is used as the only agent in patients with hypertension and normal cardiac function, it induces a reflex increase in sympathetic nervous system tone. The increased sympathetic drive increases myocardial contractility and heart rate. Consequently, cardiac output increases dramatically, offsetting the effect of the arteriolar dilation. The net result is no change in systemic arterial blood pressure. When a beta-adrenergic–receptor blocker is added to the therapeutic regimen, the reflex effect is blocked and systemic arterial blood pressure decreases. Although hydralazine is not commonly used to treat hypertension in veterinary medicine, this same response would be expected in a misdiagnosed patient administered hydralazine when that animal is not in heart failure. In patients with heart failure, the sympathetic nervous system is already activated, but the heart's ability to respond to sympathetic activity is blunted. Therefore, when hydralazine is administered to patients with heart failure, reflex tachycardia may not develop and systemic arterial blood pressure routinely decreases.

Hydralazine is a very potent arteriolar dilator. In dogs it is able to decrease systemic vascular resistance to about 50% of baseline compared with captopril, which can only decrease systemic vascular resistance by about 25%. Hydralazine's potency can be both beneficial and detrimental. Its potency is of benefit because it results in moderate to profound improvement in the majority of patients in which it is indicated. Its potency can be detrimental if it results in hypotension.

In patients with mitral or aortic valvular regurgitation or in cases of left-to-right shunting, hydralazine decreases the amount of regurgitation or shunting. Subsequently, forward flow into the systemic arterial system increases while left ventricular volume overload and diastolic pressure decrease. The net result is improvement in those clinical signs pertaining to edema or poor perfusion. The mechanism of reduction in regurgitation is explained in Figure 2. In dogs with mitral regurgitation, the response to hydralazine is generally profound and rapid. Following the administration of an appropriate dose, pulmonary edema generally clears, the size of the left ventricle on radiographs often decreases, and peripheral perfusion markedly improves in many instances, resulting in bright pink mucous membranes and a capillary refill time of less than 0.5 sec.

In patients with dilated cardiomyopathy, hydralazine increases cardiac output but, as opposed to cases of pure mitral regurgitation, often has little effect on the degree of edema. In the authors' experience, dogs with dilated cardiomyopathy improve very little following hydralazine administration. The primary clinical abnormalities in these dogs are pulmonary edema, ascites, and exercise intolerance. Therefore, agents that reduce the degree of edema (e.g., ACE inhibitors) are usually more effective.

Resistance to cerebral, coronary, renal, and splanchnic flow decreases more than does that to skeletal muscle and skin perfusion. Thus, an increase in cardiac output does not necessarily improve exercise tolerance. Hydralazine may be preferred, however, when renal blood flow is decreased in patients with severe heart failure. This can result in poor delivery of furosemide to Henle's loop and is one mechanism by which a patient may become refractory to furosemide administration. Hydralazine increases renal blood flow and may restore the effectiveness of furosemide.

Common side effects include first-dose hypotension, anorexia, vomiting, and diarrhea. Anorexia or vomiting occurs in approximately 20% to 30% of patients and may be intractable, forcing discontinuation of the drug. If hypotension occurs, it is generally manifested as weakness and lethargy and rarely is life-threatening. Severe and even lethal hypotension may develop when two vasodilators are administered concomitantly.

Systemic lupus erythematosus syndrome, drug fever, and peripheral neuropathy have been reported in some people given hydralazine. Reflex sympathetic tachycardia is not as common in heart failure patients as in patients with systemic hypertension but may require the addition of beta-blocking drugs or digoxin to control. Rebound increases in renin release and Na^+ and water retention may occur. This is generally not a clinical problem in patients receiving furosemide.

Hydralazine is used in only about 5% of human patients with heart failure. It is the authors' impression that hydralazine may be similarly unpopular in veterinary medicine as well, probably because of adverse effects of the drug. Nevertheless, hydralazine is an effective and well-tolerated drug in many patients and may be superior to other vasodilators in many cases of CHF. Certainly, intractable anorexia and vomiting in a patient warrant discontinuing the drug in that patient. Similarly, hypotension during drug titration is of concern to the clients and the clinician; however, the clinician must be aware that hypotension in this situation is reversible and generally without sequelae.

PRAZOSIN

Prazosin (Minipress, Pfizer) is a balanced vasodilator that acts primarily by selectively blocking postsynaptic alpha$_1$-adrenergic receptors and may also inhibit phosphodiesterase in vascular smooth muscle. It is effective in reducing filling pressures and increasing cardiac output in humans. It causes less reflex tachycardia and activation of the renin-angiotensin-aldosterone system than does hydralazine. Elimination and metabolism are primarily hepatic, and no adjustment is made for renal insufficiency. Prazosin is effective in reducing mean arterial blood pressure in some dogs with renal hypertension. Development of tachyphylaxis (loss of effectiveness following the first doses) has been observed in humans and some experimental animals. In human studies, it is ineffective in prolonging life when compared with placebo. It may cause marked first-dose hypotension, anorexia, vomiting, diarrhea, and syncope.

Prazosin is available in 1-, 2-, and 5-mg capsules only, and owing to the difficulty in dosing, other vasodilators are more commonly used in veterinary medicine. The starting dose in dogs less than 15 kg is 1 mg every 8 hr and in dogs greater than 15 kg is 2 mg every 8 hr. The dosage is then titrated to an effective end point.

NITRATES AND NITROPRUSSIDE

Nitrates and nitroprusside form nitric oxide (NO), which stimulates guanylate cyclase to produce cyclic guanosine monophosphate (GMP). Cyclic GMP accelerates calcium loss from the vascular smooth muscle cell, which results in vasodilation. Sulfhydryl (SH) groups are necessary for stimulation of guanylate cyclase, and tolerance develops if SH groups are depleted. Methionine administration restores sulfhydryl groups and nitrate effectiveness in humans.

Nitrates are metabolized in the liver by nitrate reductase to two active major metabolites, 1,2- and 1,3-dinitroglycerols. Although less active than their parent compounds, they have longer half-lives and are present in substantial plasma concentrations. Consequently, they may be responsible for some of the pharmacologic effect.

Nitroprusside

Nitroprusside (Nipride, Roche Laboratories; Nitropress, Abbott) is a very potent arteriolar and venous dilator. Nitroprusside is administered intravenously and results in rapid reduction in systemic vascular resistance and systemic arterial blood pressure (onset 1 to 2 min). It reduces both systemic and pulmonary vascular resistance (thus increasing cardiac output) and decreases ventricular filling pressures (thereby reducing pulmonary capillary wedge pressure). Nitroprusside is useful in the short-term management of severe, acute, life-threatening heart failure or severe systemic hypertension. It is especially useful in canine patients with severe heart failure due to dilated cardiomyopathy, where it can be administered in combination with dobutamine. It is also useful in severe heart failure due to mitral or aortic regurgitation.

Initial infusion rates in dogs are 1 to 5 μg/kg/min. The dose is titrated to effect, increasing by increments of no more than 3 to 5 μg/kg/min every 5 to 10 min. Arterial blood pressure must be monitored, preferably by invasive means. The most common side effect is hypotension, which can develop very suddenly but is reversed within 1 to 10 minutes of stopping the infusion. Nitroprusside should be gradually discontinued following prolonged administration because abrupt withdrawal can cause a rebound increase in systemic vascular resistance and ventric-ular filling pressures. These occur 10 to 30 min after stopping therapy and can be avoided by starting oral vasodilator therapy prior to discontinuation of the infusion.

Nitroprusside is metabolized to cyanide. Prolonged administration of high doses can result in toxicity. Cyanide accumulation can result in lactic acidosis, altered behavior, convulsions, and death. Plasma concentration of thiocyanate should be measured in dogs with renal insufficiency and when high doses are administered for more than 2 days. A plasma concentration above 10 mg/dl is considered toxic; a concentration greater than 20 mg/dl is generally lethal. Other side effects in humans include nausea, vomiting, anorexia, flushing, and headache.

Isosorbide Dinitrate

Isosorbide dinitrate (Isordil, Wyeth-Ayerst; Isonate, Major; Sorbitrate, ICI Pharma) is a nitrate absorbed after oral administration. Venodilation predominates; thus, it helps with venous congestion but is not very effective at increasing cardiac output. In humans, vasodilation peaks in 1 hr with a duration of effect of 4 to 6 hr. Isosorbide is eliminated by the kidney. Tachycardias usually do not occur in patients with CHF and elevated venous pressures. There is little information concerning use of this drug in veterinary medicine.

Nitroglycerin

Nitroglycerin (Nitro-Bid, Marion; Nitrol, Adria; Nitrong, Wharton; Nitrostat, Parke-Davis) is primarily a venodilator with little effect on the arterial vessels when administered transcutaneously. It may decrease ventricular filling pressures and relieve signs of edema. When nitroglycerin (Nitro-Bid IV, Marion; Nitrostat IV, Parke-Davis; Nitroglycerin, Quad; and Tridil, DuPont Pharmaceuticals) is administered intravenously, however, it acts as both a potent arteriolar dilator and venodilator. Onset of action after intravenous administration is similar to nitroprusside. The initial recommended administration rate in humans is 5 μg/min (not μg/kg/min). This dose is increased in increments of 10 to 20 μg/min until an effect is identified. There is no fixed optimum dose. Effective doses in small animals have not been identified and so must be extrapolated from the human literature. Side effects in humans include headache, weakness, dizziness, and increased intraocular pressure.

Topical nitroglycerin is available as an ointment or patch for cutaneous application. It is applied to a hairless area. Peak effect in humans occurs within 1 hr. Duration of effect is 4 to 6 hr.

The recommended dose for nitroglycerin cream

in dogs and cats is ¼ to 2 inches applied cutaneously every 6 to 8 hr. One inch of ointment contains about 15 mg nitroglycerin. Controlled studies of efficacy in veterinary medicine are lacking.

We have compared the effects of nitroglycerin ointment with those of petroleum jelly in four dogs equipped with a Swan-Ganz and an arterial catheter. Ointments were applied to a large, shaved area on the lateral thorax. Studies were performed in a blinded fashion. All dogs had pulmonary edema and elevated pulmonary capillary wedge pressure secondary to dilated cardiomyopathy. Cardiac output, pulmonary capillary wedge pressure, systemic arterial blood pressure, and clinical signs were monitored periodically for 24 hr. The dose used was up to four times the recommended dose. There was no change in any measured parameter or clinical signs. It may be that cutaneous absorption from this area on the body in dogs is different from that in humans or that the drug was placed in a less than optimal area. However, this limited information indicates a need for more studies of topical nitrates in animals.

References and Suggested Reading

Amsterdam, E. A. (ed.).: *Cardiology Drug Facts*. St. Louis: J. B. Lippincott, 1989.

Atlas, S. A., Case, D. B., Yu, Z. Y., et al.: Hormonal and metabolic effects of angiotensin-converting enzyme inhibitors: Possible differences between enalapril and captopril. Am. J. Med. 77:13–17, 1984.

Cohn, J. N., Archibald, D. G., Ziesche, S., et al.: Effect of vasodilator therapy on mortality in chronic congestive heart failure. N. Engl. J. Med. 314:1547, 1986.

CONSENSUS Trial Study Group. Effects of enalapril on mortality in severe congestive heart failure. N. Engl. J. Med. 316:1429, 1987.

Creager, M. A., Massie, B. M., Faxon, D. P., et al.: Acute and long-term effects of enalapril on the cardiovascular response to exercise and exercise tolerance in patients with congestive heart failure. J. Am. Coll. Cardiol. 6:163–70, 1985.

Hollenberg, N. K.: Control of renal perfusion and function in congestive heart failure. Am. J. Cardiol. 62:72E–75E, 1988.

Kittleson, M. D.: Cardiovascular physiology and pathophysiology. *In* Slatter, D. H. (ed.): *Textbook of Small Animal Surgery*. Philadelphia: W. B. Saunders, 1985, pp. 1039–1050.

Kittleson, M. D., Eyster, G. E., Olivier, N. B., et al.: Oral hydralazine therapy for chronic mitral regurgitation in the dog. J.A.V.M.A. 182:1205, 1983.

Kittleson, M., and Hamlin, R.: Hydralazine pharmacodynamics in the dog. Am. J. Vet. Res. 44:1501, 1983.

Knowlen, G. G., and Kittleson, M. D.: Captopril therapy in dogs with heart failure. *In* Kirk, R. W. (ed.): *Current Veterinary Therapy IX*. Philadelphia: W. B. Saunders, 1986, pp. 334–339.

Knowlen, G. G., Kittleson, M. D., Nachreiner, R. F., et al.: The relationship of plasma aldosterone concentration to the clinical status in a group of dogs with heart failure. J.A.V.M.A. 183:991, 1983.

Levine, T. B., Francis, G. S., Goldsmith, S. R., et al.: Activity of the sympathetic nervous system and renin-angiotensin system assessed by plasma hormone levels and their relationship to hemodynamic abnormalities in congestive heart failure. Am. J. Cardiol. 49:1659–66, 1983.

MacDonald, J. S., Bagdon, W. J., Peter, C. P., et al.: Renal effects of enalapril in dogs. Kidney International 31 (suppl 20):S148–S153, 1987.

Opie, L.: *Drugs for the Heart*. 2nd ed. Philadelphia, W. B. Saunders, 1987.

Packer, M.: Converting-enzyme inhibition in the management of severe chronic congestive heart failure: Physiologic concepts. J. Cardiovasc. Pharmacol. 10 (Suppl 7):S83–S87, 1987.

Packer, M., Lee, W. H., Yushak, M., et al.: Comparison of captopril and enalapril in patients with severe chronic heart failure. N. Engl. J. Med. 315:847–53, 1986.

Pfeffer, J. M., Pfeffer, M. A., and Braunwald, E.: Hemodynamic benefits and prolonged survival with long-term captopril therapy in rats with myocardial infarction and heart failure. Circulation 75:I-149, 1987.

Plante, G. E., Chainey, A., Sirois, P., et al.: Angiotensin converting enzyme inhibition and autoregulation of glomerular filtration. Journal of Hypertension 6:(suppl 3):S69–S73, 1988.

Riegger, G. A., Liebau, G., Holzschuh, M., et al.: Role of the renin-angiotensin system in the development of congestive heart failure in the dog as assessed by chronic converting-enzyme blockade. Am. J. Cardiol. 53:614–618, 1984.

Singhoi, S. M., Peterson, A. E., Ross, J. J., et al.: Pharmacokinetics of captopril in dogs and monkeys. J. Pharm. Sci. 70:1108–1112, 1981.

Sweet, C. S., Ludden, C. T., Frederick, C. M., et al.: Comparative hemodynamic effects of MK-422, a converting enzyme inhibitor, and a renin inhibitor in dogs with acute left ventricular failure. J. Cardiovasc. Pharmacol. 6:1067–1075, 1984.

UPDATE: TRANSVENOUS CARDIAC PACING

PETER G. G. DARKE
Edinburgh, Scotland

Cardiac pacing has become the definitive treatment for symptomatic bradyarrhythmias in small animals (see *CVT X*, p. 286). Epicardial pacing leads are usually employed in veterinary medicine, although these have long been superseded by transvenous endocardial leads for the majority of human patients. The author has employed endocardial leads in over 30 small animals.

INDICATIONS

The most common indications for cardiac pacing in dogs include advanced second-degree or complete atrioventricular (AV) block and various forms of "sick sinus syndrome." The latter comprise dysrhythmias such as sinus arrest, sinus bradycardia, and sinus bradycardia-tachycardia. Bradycardias tend to cause cardiac output failure, with exercise intolerance, weakness, or collapse. They may also contribute to congestive cardiac failure.

Most of these bradydysrhythmias are idiopathic. However, the possibility of metabolic, endocrine, or neurologic disturbances must be considered, especially in sinus bradycardias. The myocardium should also be assessed for signs of progressive disease (e.g., infection, neoplasia, idiopathic cardiomyopathy), that may be relative contraindications for cardiac pacing.

PACING LEADS

Temporary pacing has often been advocated as immediate therapy for bradydysrhythmias; however, as described later, the permanent transvenous pacing electrode can also be used to gain heart rate control and stabilize the patient prior to induction of general anesthesia. In situations where sustained temporary pacing is required, a temporary transvenous pacing catheter should be advanced into the right ventricle with the patient under sedation and local anesthetic. For temporary pacing, a bipolar lead is usually placed transvenously in the right ventricle. Either a unipolar or bipolar lead can be employed for permanent pacing. Advantages of bipolar leads include reduced likelihood of electrical interference with pacing (especially from peripheral muscle potentials) or muscle twitching around the pacing generator. However, these leads tend to be larger, less compliant, and more expensive than unipolar leads.

Epicardial leads are placed by transthoracic or transabdominal surgery (Fox et al., 1986). The electrode at the tip of the lead is screwed or sutured into place. The site of placement is certain and attachment is initially secure. However, epicardial leads can pull free, there is a serious risk of cardiac arrest during anesthesia for many animals with bradycardia (especially if they are dependent on an escape rhythm and are not temporarily paced by a transvenous method), and invasive surgery can cause complications. Risks of cardiac arrest are minimized by employing temporary transvenous pacing prior to surgery, but the patient requires very close observation to avoid disturbance to a temporary lead and it may be argued that if a lead is to be placed, even noninvasively, a permanent lead is preferable. Permanent transvenous pacing is much less invasive, cheaper, and more rapidly accomplished, and it can even be achieved without general anesthesia.

Lead displacement is the greatest potential disadvantage of permanent transvenous pacing. The simple electrodes usually employed in humans have been reported to be easily displaced in dogs. However, the effectiveness of "tined" leads (which have small plastic hooks near the tip) has been demonstrated. The tines engage in the endocardial trabeculae during lead placement. Displacement occurred within 48 hours of installation in two dogs, but the leads were easily replaced at this stage, after which they remained stable. Late displacement (at 1 year) occurred in one dog. The author's experience with other, plain-ended or "finned" leads was disappointing (Darke et al., 1989).

DUAL-CHAMBERED PACING

Whether epicardial or endocardial leads are employed, two-chambered pacing can be considered. With dual-chambered systems, one lead is attached to the right ventricle and the other to the right atrium. This enables ventricular beats to be synchronized with atrial contractions, providing so-called physiologic pacing. Either a VAT or a DDD pacemaker can be used (for codes, see *CVT X*, p. 286). The VAT type senses atrial P waves and triggers the ventricles in synchrony; this is most useful in advanced AV block with normal atrial function (Fig. 1). The DDD functions similarly to a VAT type, but it can also trigger the atria if there is sinus arrest.

The author has employed both types in dogs, with the DDD used for dogs with sick sinus syndrome and complete AV block. In a vigorously active dog, a sophisticated two-chambered system may permit better exercise tolerance than a simple ventricular (VVI) system. Two-chambered pacing is readily achieved transvenously. The second (atrial) lead is maneuvered to the right auricular appendage with the aid of fluoroscopy, and an endocardial electrocardiogram (ECG) is checked to ensure that P-wave voltage is sufficient to trigger the system. However, even specialized atrial, tined, "J" leads have a tendency to displacement in humans, and the risk may be similar in dogs. Attempts to use a purely atrial system (AAI) in dogs with sick sinus syndrome have been frustrated by the induction of AV block or atrial fibrillation.

PACEMAKER PROGRAMMING

Many pacing generators in current human use are multiprogrammable: sensitivity to inhibition, output voltage, and rate can be adjusted after installation. More sophisticated generators can control other parameters. Programming is of particular value in small animals, for which the heart rate from conventional human generators (usually set at 70 beats/min) is usually inadequate to sustain exercise. Observations suggest that pacing at 100 to 110 beats/min is required for dogs and at least 120 beats/min for cats. However, low heart rates and low

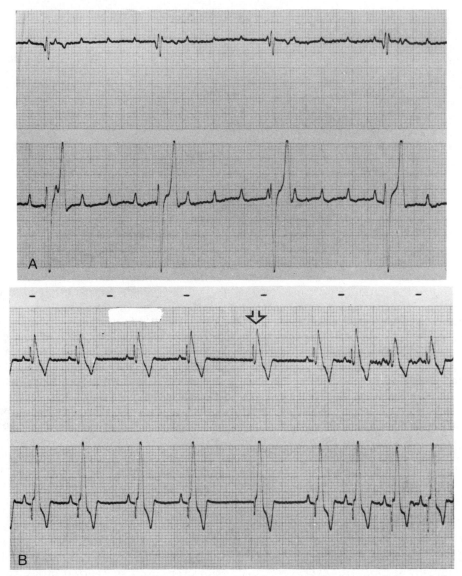

Figure 1. ECGs (Leads I and II, 1 cm/mV and 25 mm/sec) recorded from a Labrador retriever before and after dual-chambered pacing (with a VAT generator). *A* shows complete atrioventricular block, with escape QRS complexes independent of P waves. *B* shows atrioventricular synchrony. P waves are usually sensed, and these trigger the right ventricle via the generator to give QRS complexes. One ventricular beat is generated by the pacemaker without a P wave *(arrow)*; the pacemaker is programmed to pace the ventricles independently if no P wave is sensed during a prolonged pause.

current settings ensure maximum life from the lithium batteries. Battery life ranges from 5 to 15 years according to type of pacemaker, pacing mode, and programmed output.

Activity-induced, rate-responsive pacing is useful in sustaining the heart rate for exercise while conserving battery life and optimizing hemodynamic function in dogs (Cobb et al., 1990). Rather than employing an atrial sensing lead to increase the ventricular rate during excitement or exercise, these generators are sensitive to movement. The author has successfully programmed a resting rate of 60 beats/min and an activity-responsive rate of 125 beats/min in a dog. However, few generators of this type are yet available for recycling and purchase of new units would be very expensive.

COMPLICATIONS OF PACING

Although transvenous cardiac pacing has become the routine treatment for symptomatic bradycardias in the author's clinic (Darke et al., 1989) and mean survival times have been better than reported by other techniques (Bonagura et al., 1983), there have been disappointments. In early installations before the adoption of a Dacron pouch for the generator, seromas developed in most dogs. In two cases a sinus developed that led to intractable secondary infection. Infection (at surgical sites or at the endocardium) is a dangerous complication of pacing that the author has not yet encountered. Lead displacement has been the minor complication. Malignant dysrhythmias, particularly tachycardias, may be anticipated in pacing, but these have not yet been seen. However, electrical or lead failure with dual-chambered systems is suspected in two dogs that died suddenly. Muscle twitching over the generator can be a minor irritation, apparently more annoying to owners than to dogs. Movement of the generator or reprogramming pacer output can cure this.

One dog in this series died with ventricular fibrillation at induction of general anesthesia. However, the most common cause of death or euthanasia, apart from unrelated causes, has been progressive dilated cardiomyopathy (in five animals) or mitral regurgitation, the latter in two aging dogs. These dogs had all benefitted from pacing for months or years, but finally succumbed to unresponsive congestive cardiac failure.

PROCEDURE FOR TRANSVENOUS PACING

Medical Assessment

Each animal should receive a thorough assessment before being involved in the expense and potential complications of pacing. A full physical examination, complete blood count, and biochemical screen should be employed to exclude any neurologic, metabolic, or endocrine disturbance that might nullify the expense and effort of pacing. For example, dogs with brain tumors, hypothyroidism, hypoxia, or hypoadrenocorticism are unsuitable candidates for pacing to treat bradycardias.

A thorough cardiac investigation is essential. Many animals with symptomatic bradycardias have cardiac murmurs. In most cases, Doppler investigation indicates that these are physiologic murmurs caused by increased stroke volume. In some cases, atrioventricular valve regurgitation may be exacerbated by pacing. Radiography demonstrates mild volume overload in most animals that require pacing. However, pacing may also help to resolve congestive cardiac failure. Electrocardiography is essential to define precisely the bradyarrhythmia, and when in doubt, 24-hr (Holter) ECG monitoring can determine the presence of transient arrhythmias. Alternatively, a simple device such as the "Chiltern Box" can be used to record an ECG at the time of collapse or seizure (Brownlie, 1987).

Intermittent arrhythmias can be observed in the cat. Frequently cats with AV conduction disease may not manifest an arrhythmia during a routine ECG examination. Repetitive or Holter ECG monitoring may be required to document high-grade, second-degree, or complete AV block.

Echocardiography is of particular value. Any evidence of myocardial disease, particularly dilated cardiomyopathy, weakens the prognosis. However, despite the expense and effort, pacing may still benefit the animal for a while, giving the owner time to accept the animal's limited future.

Preparation

Various items of equipment are either essential or desirable for efficient transvenous pacing. A suitable generator (the author uses shelf-life–expired packs or pacemakers recycled after brief human use, resterilized with ethylene oxide), a new, tined ventricular pacing lead, a Dacron pouch for the generator (Parsonnet Pulse Generator Pouch; Bard Cardiosurgery Division (BARD), Billerica, MA), a temporary external pacemaker and leads, a vascular surgical pack, and ECG monitoring are essential.* Radiographic fluoroscopy is desirable for optimal lead placement. Electric defibrillator and resuscitation equipment should be available. A pacemaker programmer is also desirable but may be too expensive for purchase in view of the wide variety of available generators. Generators can be preprogrammed to likely settings. Assessment and further programming is carried out after 1 to 2 weeks, if necessary, with the cooperation of medical cardiologists or company representatives, as pacing threshold may change during this time.

The animal is prepared for surgery by a thorough clip of the entire length of the left (or right) side of the neck from the crest to the ventral midline, followed by antiseptic preparation and local analgesia over the ipsilateral jugular vein. Good sedation is essential. The author employs an opioid (buprenorphine, Buprenex, Norwich Eaton, at 0.01 mg/kg), with a low dose of acetylpromazine (0.03 mg/kg) intravenously. Broad-spectrum antibiotic cover is also given.

Lead Placement

The animal is restrained manually. After a skin incision, the jugular vein is penetrated and the permanent pacing lead is guided to the apex of the right ventricle by fluoroscopy. Positive engagement in the trabeculae is ensured by gentle traction on the lead. Temporary pacing is started. Previously sterilized wires are used to connect a temporary pacemaker with the permanent pacing lead. At-

---

Editor's Note: While a pulse generator pouch is useful and may prevent pacemaker migration, uncovered implants can be positioned under subcutaneous muscle if required.

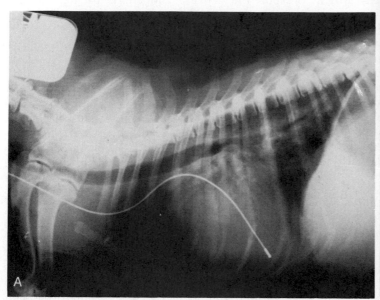
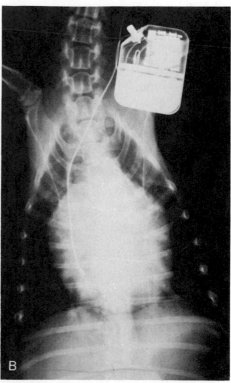

Figure 2. Lateral (A) and dorsoventral (B) thoracic radiographs from a West Highland White terrier with a transvenous endocardial pacing wire in place. Note the loop of lead in the cranial vena cava to prevent dislodgement of the lead by tension from the neck. The lead-tip electrode is at the apex of the right ventricle. (Reprinted with permission from Darke, P. G., McAreavey, D., and Been M.: Transvenous cardiac pacing in 19 dogs and one cat. J. Small Anim. Pract. 30:494, 1989.)

tached to these wires are an alligator clip at one end and a male plug at the other. One alligator clip is connected to the proximal end of the permanent pacing lead and the other clip is attached to the patient's skin. The male ends of the wires are connected to the temporary pacer. This creates a temporary unipolar system that can control the heart rate and stabilize hemodynamics prior to induction of general anesthesia. The patient is paced at a sufficient rate to stabilize blood pressure (100 to 150 beats/min) and improve tissue perfusion. The threshold (the lowest setting at which capture is consistently maintained) is checked with the temporary pacemaker. The author accepts a placement that requires a current less than 0.5 mA (usually about 0.2 mA).

The proximal end of the lead is secured at the point of entry into the jugular vein. A small loop of lead is deliberately left in the cranial vena cava (Fig. 2) to allow for movement that might exert traction on the electrode.

Generator Placement

General anesthesia is induced with thiopentone, and the animal is intubated and transferred to gaseous anesthesia. A system was placed in one dog entirely under sedation and local analgesia. Close attention is paid to the cardiac rhythm during anesthetic induction. When adequately anesthetized, a subcutaneous pocket is created near the top of the dog's neck for the generator. The permanent pacing lead is then tunnelled through to this site and attached to the generator, which is then covered by the Dacron pouch. The generator is inserted into the surgical pocket with surplus lead coiled beneath it. Wounds are closed routinely, the neck is bandaged to prevent trauma by the patient, and antibiotic cover is administered for at least a week. The animal is sedated for several days to reduce the risk of lead displacement. Sutures are removed routinely at 10 days.

Postoperative Care

Initial checking and programming are carried out in approximately 1 week. Thereafter, pacemaker checks should be made at least every 3 to 6 months. Electronic indicators give prolonged advance warning of failure of lithium batteries, and the pacing threshold is also assessed. A rising threshold that requires an increase in pacemaker output can result from fibrosis at the electrode tip or from lead displacement, although this has not proved to be a problem. Radiography is employed to indicate signs of lead displacement or congestive cardiac failure. Echocardiography is desirable to check myocardial function.

Clients are advised to restrain the animal for a few weeks, but then to allow normal activity if cardiac disease permits. A shoulder harness or halter is preferred to a neck collar. Any episodes of weakness or collapse should indicate urgent recall to assess the pacer, check for development of other arrhythmias, and rule out myocardial failure. Clients can be trained to assess the heart rate by palpating the apex beat. Reversion to bradycardia may indicate pacemaker system failure. Exercise intolerance can sometimes be relieved by reprogramming, particularly by increasing the heart rate, but this will reduce battery life. Trauma to the generator or jugular vein must be avoided, and the use of antibiotic cover is advised for routine surgical procedures or with infections to prevent bacterial endocarditis.

Transvenous pacing is relatively simple, effective, and minimally invasive. The reduction in surgical and anesthetic risks offered by this technique should ensure that it becomes the technique of choice for symptomatic bradyarrhythmias.

References and Suggested Reading

Bonagura, J. D., Helphrey, M. L., Muir, W. W.: Complications associated with permanent pacemaker implantation in the dog. J.A.V.M.A. 182:149, 1983.
A review of cardiac pacing in dogs, with clinical experiences and complications.
Brownlie, S. E.: Evaluation for veterinary use of the Chiltern Box: A device for home electrocardiographic monitoring. Vet. Rec. 120:85, 1987.
A description of a simple device for use by a client in recording 15 minutes of ECG at the time of weakness or collapse.
Cobb, M. A., Nolan, J., Brownlie, S. E., et al.: Use of a programmable, activity-sensing, rate-regulating pacemaker in a dog. J. Small Anim. Pract. 31:398, 1990.
Use of a modern multiprogrammable pacemaker to improve exercise tolerance in a dog.
Darke, P. G. G., Been, M., Marks, A.: Use of a programmable, 'physiological' pacemaker in a dog with total atrioventricular block. J. Small Anim. Pract. 26:295, 1985.
A description of dual-chambered transvenous pacing in a dog.
Darke, P. G. G., McAreavey, D., Been, M.: Transvenous cardiac pacing in 19 dogs and one cat. J. Small Anim. Pract. 30:491, 1989.
A description of the authors' technique and experiences in transvenous pacing in small animals.
Fox, P. R., Matthiesen, D. T., Purse, D., et al.: Ventral abdominal transdiaphragmatic approach for implantation of cardiac pacemakers in the dog. J.A.V.M.A. 189:1303, 1986.
A description of epicardial pacing via the abdomen in dogs.
Sisson, D.: Bradyarrhythmias and cardiac pacing. *In* Kirk, R. W. (ed.): *Current Veterinary Therapy X.* Philadelphia: W. B. Saunders, 1989, p. 286.
A review of the diagnosis and management of bradycardias in small animals.

EMERGENCY THERAPY AND MONITORING OF HEART FAILURE

JOHN E. RUSH
North Grafton, Massachusetts

Emergencies of the cardiovascular system can be both challenging and rewarding. Animals with congestive heart failure (CHF) are often acutely and severely ill, with marked dyspnea, weakness, or collapse owing to poor cardiac performance. Rapid identification of heart failure and prompt initiation of appropriate therapy is essential for effective treatment. Many new cardiovascular medications are highly effective and some have the potential to improve the quality and prolong the patient's life. Because many cardiac drugs have a narrow therapeutic index, inappropriate or inadequate therapy can cause death. A specific diagnosis is needed to initiate the most appropriate therapy; however, in the emergency room it may be difficult to establish a definitive diagnosis before initiating therapy for heart failure. In the interim between admission and diagnosis, the following monitoring techniques and therapeutic strategies can be used to stabilize patients.

MONITORING THE CARDIAC PATIENT

Optimal management of animals with severe heart failure is achieved with 24-hour monitoring and nursing care. Continuous care allows treatment to be tailored to meet the changing needs of the patient. Some of the monitoring techniques described in this article may be unavailable to many practices, but it is stressed that some of the most valuable information can be gained by repeated physical examination and attentive nursing care. Recording simple parameters such as respiratory rate, pulse rate and quality, body temperature, mucous membrane color, and capillary refill time every 2 to 4 hours allows trends in patient condition to be discovered, and subsequent therapeutic adjustments made. Body weight should be measured daily to evaluate fluid gain or loss.

Electrocardiographic Monitoring

Electrocardiographic monitoring can be accomplished by recording the electrocardiogram (ECG) intermittently or by continuous ECG display using an oscilloscope. Intermittent ECG monitoring is usually accomplished by obtaining a lead II rhythm strip for 2 minutes at 4- or 6-hour intervals throughout the day, but this method is less desirable because it may fail to identify significant ECG trends and may miss intermittent arrhythmias. Continuous ECG monitoring is performed by transmitting the patient's ECG to an oscilloscope. The hair is clipped in three areas, usually on both sides of the chest, for placement of adhesive ECG electrode pads to the skin. These electrodes are connected by lead wires to either a telemetry pack or a cable to the main ECG terminal. A continuous ECG display is visualized on the oscilloscope. Central monitoring terminals may permit simultaneous display of multiple ECGs and also allow for real-time "hard copy" recordings.

Continuous ECG monitoring is generally indicated for animals with recurrent ventricular or supraventricular arrhythmias to determine the efficacy of drug therapy. In this fashion, arrhythmia trends can be monitored, drug dosages adjusted, or additional drug therapy initiated. Continuous ECG monitoring permits identification of significant trends in heart rate. This is particularly useful for animals receiving dopamine or dobutamine infusions, those with bradycardia, and those in which cardiac pacing is required. In animals at risk for cardiopulmonary arrest, ECG monitoring may reveal bradycardia or changes in cardiac rhythm that may signal an impending cardiopulmonary emergency.

Thoracic Radiographs

Thoracic radiographs should be obtained as soon as possible in every patient with suspected heart failure. Some animals are so dyspneic that oxygen therapy, furosemide, and/or thoracocentesis must be performed to permit safe patient positioning for radiography. Baseline thoracic radiographs are required to confirm the diagnosis of heart failure, and to allow therapeutic response, or lack of response, to be tracked on follow-up radiographs. When treatment of heart failure is effective, resolution or partial resolution of pulmonary edema or pleural effusion can be detected within 2 or 3 days. Thoracic radiographs are also useful to further evaluate the heart and pleural cavity after drainage of pleural or pericardial effusions.

Clinical Pathology

Laboratory parameters commonly followed in cardiovascular patients include packed cell volume and total serum protein, serum electrolyte (sodium, potassium, and chloride levels), and serum creatinine levels. Packed cell volume and total protein are usually followed daily and, in combination with skin turgor and body weight, serve as a measure of hydration status. Excessive diuresis leads to substantial elevation of these parameters, and this finding should dictate a reduction in the diuretic dose, especially if heart failure is controlled.

Serum electrolyte levels are commonly checked every other day to follow hydration status and water balance (sodium) and to monitor the serum potassium level. Hypokalemia is a common cause of deterioration in anorectic, critically ill animals. High doses of furosemide can lead to renal potassium loss. Hypokalemia also predisposes patients to cardiac arrhythmias and can render common antiarrhythmic agents (including lidocaine and procainamide) ineffective. In addition, hypokalemia predisposes the patient to digitalis intoxication. When serum potassium is low, potassium supplementation can be achieved by adding potassium chloride to intravenous fluids or, in less critically ill patients, by giving oral potassium supplements. Potassium loss can be minimized by using potassium-sparing diuretics (see this volume, p. 668) or angiotensin-converting enzyme (ACE) inhibitors (see this volume, p. 700).

Animals with cardiovascular disease may become azotemic owing to diminished cardiac output or to excessive diuresis and resultant decreased renal perfusion. Renal function is usually estimated daily using an Azostix (Miles, Inc., Elkart, IN), and serum creatinine levels are usually measured every second or third day.

Central Venous Pressure

Central venous pressure (CVP) monitoring is usually accomplished using a long, jugular venous catheter that is advanced to the cranial vena cava near the entrance of the right atrium (see *CVT VIII*, p. 11). This catheter is attached to a manometer, and CVP is recorded serially. Measurement of CVP is useful to evaluate filling pressures of the right side of the heart and to help assess hydration status in cardiac patients receiving intravenous fluids and diuretics. Unfortunately, CVP is of very limited value in most patients with pulmonary edema due to left heart failure (see pulmonary arterial catheterization below). Monitoring trends in serial measurements of CVP, usually every 4 hours, often proves more useful than monitoring one isolated value. Animals with heart failure may have mild initial elevations of CVP, yet be in need of fluid infusions to administer drugs or to improve renal function. When CVP continues to rise as these fluids are administered, the volume of fluids infused must be reduced. Elevations in excess of 5 cm of water over the baseline are cause for concern and should dictate a reduction in the rate of fluid administration.

Arterial Blood Pressure Monitoring

Serial evaluation of arterial blood pressure can be especially useful in the management of animals with severe heart failure and low cardiac output. In hypotensive patients with severe myocardial failure, blood pressure usually increases after initiation of an appropriately dosed dobutamine or dopamine infusion. Similarly, arterial blood pressure monitoring may be useful to detect hypotension after initiation of vasodilator therapy (see this volume, p. 700). Both direct and indirect blood pressure monitoring techniques can be employed (see this volume, p. 834, and *CVT IX*, p. 360). Direct blood pressure monitoring is usually accomplished by placing an over-the-needle catheter directly into the dorsal tibial artery and monitoring blood pressure through a fluid-filled, domed transducer. Direct blood pressure monitoring is associated with more complications, including catheter-related sepsis, arterial thrombosis, and catheter disconnection leading to blood loss. Owing to difficulties associated with arterial blood pressure monitoring and increased patient discomfort with this technique, indirect blood pressure monitoring techniques are used more frequently in many practices. Both Doppler and oscillometric techniques can provide reliable results. We find the oscillometric technique (DINAMAP, Critikon, Inc., Tampa, FL) to be most useful in large dogs and in animals with heart rates less than 200 beats/min. In cats and in animals with heart rates greater than 200 beats/min, we find the Doppler technique (Ultrasonic Doppler Flow Detector, Parks Medical Electronics, Inc.) to be more accurate and easier to use.

Echocardiographic Monitoring

Serial echocardiograms can be performed during the course of hospitalization. However, with the exception of certain specific disease processes, we have not found serial echocardiographic monitoring to be nearly as useful as other monitoring techniques. Pericardial effusion is a notable exception in which recurrence or resolution of pericardial effusion and cardiac tamponade can be most effectively identified by serial echocardiograms. The echocardiogram is usually not sensitive enough to reliably detect changes in myocardial function that attend drug therapy, and in fact with many therapies (e.g., diuretics, vasodilators) routine echo measurements of myocardial function are unchanged. Introduction of Doppler echocardiographic indices of ventricular function (e.g., aortic acceleration) may prove more useful for quantifying drug effects. Currently, the end result of improved cardiovascular function is best documented by other means such as thoracic radiography, hemodynamic monitoring, electrocardiography, and patient evaluation.

Blood Gas Determinations

Evaluation of arterial and venous blood gases is often useful. Arterial blood gas samples are usually obtained by direct puncture of the femoral artery. When Pa_{O_2} decreases to less than 60 or 65 mm Hg, administration of supplemental oxygen is indicated. In animals in which Pa_{CO_2} is elevated or when Pa_{O_2} remains below 50 mm Hg after oxygen therapy, mechanical ventilation is needed. (see this volume, p. 98). Following effective treatment of heart failure, supplemental oxygen therapy is usually discontinued when Pa_{O_2} rises above 75 or 80 mm Hg without oxygen.

Venous blood gas determinations can also be useful. We utilize venous blood gases in two settings: (1) in animals with CHF and suspected low cardiac output and (2) in animals recovering from cardiopulmonary arrest. Although a central venous sample obtained from the pulmonary artery is preferred, venous blood gases are often obtained from a free-flowing *jugular* venous sample. In addition to evaluation of blood pH in the postarrest situation, Pv_{O_2} may be useful in determining whether tissues are receiving adequate blood flow. When Pv_{O_2} falls below 30 mm Hg (and when Pa_{O_2} is greater than 65 mm Hg), it is reasonable to assume that blood flow to the peripheral tissues is diminished and that these tissues are extracting more oxygen than normal. In these settings, additional therapy (either infused inotropic drugs or a vasodilator) is usually indicated to attempt to improve oxygen delivery to peripheral tissues.

Pulmonary Arterial Catheterization

Pulmonary arterial catheterization can also be used to monitor response to drug therapy in animals with acute severe heart failure. A specialized balloon-tipped, Swan-Ganz catheter is inserted into the jugular vein and passed into the pulmonary artery. The Swan-Ganz catheter has a distal port, a small balloon just proximal to the distal port, and a proximal port. When the catheter is properly positioned, the proximal port lies in the right atrium so that central venous pressure can be monitored. The distal port, in the pulmonary artery, measures both pulmonary arterial pressure and (when the balloon is inflated and arterial flow occluded), pulmonary capillary wedge pressure (PCWP). PCWP measurements, which estimate left atrial pressure, are made by inflating the small balloon just proximal to the end hole of the catheter. PCWP is increased in animals with elevated left ventricular diastolic pressures and left-sided heart failure and is a sensitive indicator of improvement in cardiovascular function. In animals with severe pulmonary edema, PCWP consistently decreases after initiation of effective drug therapy with diuretics, dobutamine, and certain vasodilators. The drop in PCWP usually precedes clinical and radiographic evidence of improvement. Catheters equipped with a temperature sensor can be used to monitor cardiac output by thermodilution if a cardiac output computer is available. Owing to the expense and intensive nursing care associated with placement of Swan-Ganz catheters, this technique is infrequently used in veterinary patients, and is probably underutilized in the management of critically ill veterinary patients.

TECHNIQUES FOR CARDIOVASCULAR EMERGENCIES

Oxygen Therapy

Oxygen is commonly employed in the initial management of acute, severe heart failure. One hundred per cent oxygen can be administered for short periods, usually 1 to 12 hours. Sustained administration of 100% oxygen can lead to pulmonary toxicity, so 40 to 50% is commonly administered when oxygen therapy must be continued for longer periods. Some animals tolerate oxygen administered through a cone or face mask, but others resist greatly, and the resultant stress is detrimental. Oxygen cages are useful in relieving some of the stress associated with oxygen administration. The oxygen cage must be adjusted to maintain a normal temperature (20° to 22°C, 68° to 72°F) and appropriate humidity (45 to 55%) while delivering 40% oxygen.

Oxygen can also be administered through nasal oxygen catheters in dogs of medium to large breed. Viscous lidocaine is applied to the end of the catheter, usually a no. 5 to 8 French red rubber feeding tube, and the catheter is advanced up the ventral nasal meatus to the level of the fourth premolar (carnassial tooth). The tube is sutured to the skin at the edge of the nostril and again on the top of the head. The catheter is attached to an oxygen source, and an Elizabethan collar is placed on the dog to prevent it from removing the catheter. Oxygen administered through a nasal catheter should be humidified (Bubble Humidifier, Becton Dickinson and Co., Lincoln Park, NJ). The oxygen flow rate is adjusted to between 50 to 100 ml/kg/min to achieve inspired oxygen concentrations of 40 to 50% (Fitzpatrick and Crowe, 1986).

Thoracocentesis

Thoracocentesis can be a life-saving procedure and is indicated in animals with pleural effusion of any cause. Pleural effusion most often follows biventricular heart failure, and should be suspected in animals with short, rapid respirations; muffled heart or ventrally muffled lung sounds; and dull percussion of the chest cavity. Animals with cardiogenic pleural effusion usually have jugular venous distention and hepatomegaly, while concurrent ascites is more common in dogs than in cats. In severely dyspneic animals suspected of having pleural effusion, thoracocentesis can be performed before radiographic confirmation of pleural effusion; a negative tap rarely results in patient deterioration. Thoracentesis, which is usually performed at the seventh or eighth intercostal space (see *CVT XIII*, p. 225) should almost always be carried out as both a therapeutic and a diagnostic procedure. Whenever thoracentesis is performed, as much pleural effusion as possible should be removed. This promotes expansion of collapsed or partially atelectatic lung lobes, increases lung volume, and improves respiratory effort quickly. Some cats with marked dyspnea may resist thoracentesis, and mild sedation with ketamine and valium may be useful to help calm them during the procedure.

Abdominocentesis

There are advantages and disadvantages to removing ascitic fluid in animals with CHF. In animals with voluminous ascites, respiratory compromise results from fluid compressing the diaphragm. Abdominocentesis to remove some of the fluid can improve respiratory character and patient comfort. Unfortunately, this fluid contains protein, and its removal contributes to protein loss and cardiac cachexia. When it is possible to mobilize ascites with rest, drug therapy, and sodium restriction, these therapies are preferred. Acute cardiovascular collapse has occasionally been reported after removal of large volumes of ascitic fluid, especially in animals with no other fluid accumulation or edema; this is another reason to remove only enough fluid to improve respiratory character and patient comfort.

Pericardiocentesis

Pericardiocentesis is another procedure that can be life saving. It can be performed with the patient in sternal or lateral recumbency, generally at the right hemithorax, and with simultaneous ECG monitoring (see this volume, p. 725). Ultrasonography is often useful to help direct catheter placement during pericardiocentesis. In animals with cardiac tamponade, no other therapy or drug provides the immediate relief afforded by this technique.

Cardiac Pacing

Temporary transvenous cardiac pacing is useful in animals with primary bradycardia and resultant heart failure. When bradycardia or relative bradycardia (rate <70 in the dog or <90 in the cat) accompanies heart failure, cardiac pacing will probably result in symptomatic improvement. Placement of temporary transvenous pacemakers is described elsewhere (see this volume, p. 708).

DRUGS COMMONLY USED FOR ACUTE HEART FAILURE

More complete discussions of the general usage and hazards of drugs commonly used in the therapy of heart failure appear elsewhere in this volume. The following brief discussion and Table 1 provide guidelines for emergency therapy only.

Furosemide

Furosemide (Lasix, Hoechst-Roussel) is the diuretic of choice in the emergency management of heart failure. It is potent, and intravenous administration in most instances results in a rapid diuresis. The dosage is highly variable and dependent on the response desired. In animals with acute severe heart failure, high doses of furosemide (up to 4 mg/kg every 2 hr) may be indicated to relieve life-threatening pulmonary edema. Furosemide can be administered intravenously, intramuscularly, subcutaneously, or orally, but the intravenous route is preferred for acute, severe heart failure.

Table 1. Drugs Used for Emergency Therapy of Acute Heart Failure

Furosemide (Lasix, Hoechst-Roussell): IV, IM, or PO
  Dog: 1 mg/kg b.i.d. for mild heart failure up to 4 mg/kg
      t.i.d. for severe heart failure; 4 mg/kg q 2 hr for severe
      pulmonary edema
  Cat: 1 mg/kg every other day up to 2 mg/kg b.i.d. for severe
      heart failure; 4 mg/kg q 2 hr for severe pulmonary
      edema
Captopril (Capoten, E. R. Squibb and Sons): 0.5 to 2 mg/kg
  PO t.i.d., dog and cat
Enalapril (Vasotec, Merck, Sharp & Dohme): 0.5 mg/kg PO
  s.i.d. to b.i.d., dog and cat
Nitroglycerin ointment: ¼ to 1 in. transcutaneously q 4–6 hr,
                           dog
                         ⅛ to ¼ in. transcutaneously q 4–6 hr,
                           cat
Transdermal nitroglycerin patches
  Dog: ¼ to 1 patch q 24 hr (2.5-mg patch 0.1 mg/hr)
  Cat: ¼ patch q 24 hr (2.5-mg patch 0.1 mg/hr)
Sodium nitroprusside (Nipride, Hoffman-La Roche)
  Dog: 1–10 µg/kg/min continuous rate infusion IV
Morphine
  Dog: 0.05 mg/kg IM or SQ to 1 mg/kg q 6 hr
  Cat: 0.05 to 0.1 mg/kg IM or SQ q 6 hr
Dobutamine
  Dog: 2.5–10 µg/kg/min continuous rate infusion IV
  Cat: 0.5–2 µg/kg/min continuous rate infusion IV
Dopamine (Intropin, American Critical Care)
  Dog and cat: 3–10 µg/kg/min continuous rate infusion IV
Acepromazine
  Cat: 0.05–0.1 mg/kg SQ

Angiotensin-Converting Enzyme (ACE) Inhibitors

Captopril (Capoten, E.R. Squibb and Sons) and enalapril (Vasotec, Merck, Sharp & Dohme) are ACE inhibitors used to treat chronic CHF. ACE inhibitors act as balanced vasodilators by abating the vasoconstrictive effects of angiotensin II on arteries and veins in addition to reducing the retention of sodium and water by secondarily inhibiting aldosterone release. These drugs have a fairly rapid onset of action (less than 4 hr) and can be useful in the combined drug therapy for acute, severe CHF; however, other drugs may be superior for life-threatening lung edema caused by cardiomyopathy or valvular disease (see later).

Side effects of ACE inhibitors include hypotension and deterioration of renal function, both of which can be successfully relieved when the dose of diuretic is reduced and intravenous fluids are administered. Anorexia, depression, and gastrointestinal disturbances (vomiting, diarrhea or both) occur more commonly with captopril. Low initial doses with gradual upward dose titration are recommended to minimize hypotension.

Nitroglycerin

Nitroglycerin, the prototypic venodilator, causes direct relaxation of venous smooth muscle and increases systemic venous capacitance. The resultant reduction in preload is potentially useful in animals with acute cardiogenic pulmonary edema, although studies of efficacy are lacking. Because nitroglycerin paste (2% = 15 mg/inch) is readily absorbed transcutaneously, nonpermeable gloves should be worn during application, and adhesive tape labeled "nitrol" is placed on the outer surface of the ear to alert anyone working with the dog to avoid contact with the site of application. Newer, self-adhesive transdermal delivery systems (Nitro-Dur, 2.5 mg (0.1 mg/hr) and 5 mg (0.2 mg/hr) patches, Key Pharmaceuticals) provide sustained nitroglycerin release for 24 hr. Prolonged daily use of nitroglycerin may be limited by the development of tolerance, and in the author's practice the drug is usually used for 2 to 4 days and then discontinued.

Sodium Nitroprusside

Sodium nitroprusside (Nipride, Hoffman-La Roche), a balanced vasodilator, acts directly on arterial and venous vascular smooth muscle. It is an excellent drug for immediately reducing wedge pressure and decreasing left ventricular afterload. Intravenous administration of sodium nitroprusside by continuous infusion is required, because the drug has a rapid onset and short duration of action. In canine patients with severe heart failure or lung edema refractory to furosemide or other vasodilators, nitroprusside may be effective. Use of sodium nitroprusside is limited because it is a potent hypotensive agent and should be used only when close monitoring of the arterial blood pressure, the ECG, and the patient is possible. The drug is susceptible to degradation in light, and the prepared solution must be wrapped in the foil provided (read directions carefully). Initial doses are 1 to 2 μg/kg/min; heart rate and blood pressure must be monitored.

Hydralazine

The direct-acting arteriolar dilatator hydralazine (Apresoline, CIBA) can be used to decrease mitral regurgitant fraction in dogs with severe left-sided CHF. Details are provided elsewhere (see this volume, p. 700).

Morphine

Morphine (0.1 mg/kg IM, IV) is commonly used in anxious, dyspneic dogs with CHF. The sedative effects of morphine may relieve some of the anxiety associated with hospitalization and dyspnea. Morphine may change the respiratory character from rapid, less effective ventilations to somewhat deeper ventilations. This is not always the case, however, because some animals pant after administration of morphine and at times ventilation is depressed. Morphine may also be useful as a mild venodilator to facilitate movement of blood from the lungs to the capacitance veins. Morphine is frequently used in dogs that are anxious and dogs in which the stress of hospitalization leads to barking, pawing at the cage, and excitability.

Dobutamine

Dobutamine (Dobutrex, Eli Lilly and Co.) is usually the sympathomimetic drug of choice in the management of acute severe myocardial failure (dilated cardiomyopathy). Dobutamine, a beta$_1$ agonist with mild alpha$_1$ and beta$_2$ stimulatory properties, increases cardiac contractility and cardiac output. The changes in the peripheral vasculature are minimal at low doses, and undesirable side effects (increased heart rate and arrhythmia formation) are less commonly observed than with other catecholamines. Dobutamine has a short half-life and must be given by continuous intravenous infusion, preferably administered through an infusion pump where the rate can be closely controlled. Continuous ECG monitoring is desirable. Increases in heart rate and the onset of new arrhythmias are usually treated by discontinuation of the dobutamine infusion for 10 to 20 min followed by reinitiation at a lower dose. Side effects include tachyarrhythmias, vomition, nervousness, and seizures (cats).

Dopamine

Dopamine (Intropin, American Critical Care, Dopastat, Parke-Davis) is less expensive than dobutamine and may be used for a variety of reasons in critically ill animals. Like dobutamine, dopamine has a short half-life and must be given by continuous rate infusion. Low doses of dopamine (1 to 3 μg/kg/min) stimulate dopaminergic receptors in renal, mesenteric, coronary, and cerebrovascular beds, causing vasodilation. These lower doses may improve renal blood flow and are used in patients with acute oliguric renal failure. Intermediate infusion rates (3 to 10 μg/kg/min) result in increased cardiac output with little change in peripheral resistance and minimal change in heart rate. At midrange doses, dopamine may be used as a substitute for dobutamine in the management of animals with severe heart failure. High infusion rates (10 to 20 μg/kg/min) stimulate both alpha- and beta-adrenergic receptors and cause increases in heart rate, inotropic state, and blood pressure. Higher doses, which can be arrhythmogenic, are generally used to increase cardiac output and support blood pressure in patients with acute cardiovascular depression. These higher doses are usually given during cardiopulmonary resuscitation efforts and in animals with anesthesia-related cardiovascular depression.

Digoxin

Digoxin is infrequently required for its positive inotropic effects in the management of acute heart failure. When digoxin is given in the emergency setting, it is usually for its antiarrhythmic actions. Animals with rapid ventricular response to atrial fibrillation and those with heart failure and supraventricular tachycardia are candidates for intravenous digitalization. The latter is often used in dogs with atrial fibrillation who require dobutamine or dopamine infusions, because these drugs may facilitate impulse conduction through the atrioventricular (AV) node, increasing the rate of ventricular response to atrial fibrillation. In animals with atrial fibrillation and less severe forms of heart failure, routine oral digitalization is adequate.

Fluid Therapy

Optimal cardiac performance in patients with heart failure requires optimal preload (CVP approximately 10 cm H_2O; PCWP approximately 15 mm Hg). Some authors suggest that it is counterproductive and inappropriate to administer both intravenous fluids and diuretics to a patient with heart failure. In spite of this rational argument, even edematous patients have daily fluid requirements, and many cats and some dogs with both heart failure and azotemia appear to benefit from concurrent administration of furosemide and intravenous fluids. Other patients require drugs (lidocaine, dobutamine, dopamine) that must be administered by continuous infusion. The fluid rate is usually calculated to administer 50 to 75% of the maintenance fluid requirement. Potassium chloride is usually added to prevent or treat hypokalemia. Lactated Ringer's solution can be administered, but 5% dextrose solution or 0.45% saline and 2½% dextrose provides less of a sodium load to the heart failure patient. Whenever intravenous fluids are administered to critically ill patients in CHF, a central venous or pulmonary arterial pressure monitoring line is placed and monitored frequently or continuously to maintain target pressures.

MANAGEMENT OF THE PATIENT WITH ACUTE PULMONARY EDEMA

Cardiogenic pulmonary edema commonly results from chronic mitral valve insufficiency in the dog, dilated cardiomyopathy in the dog, hypertrophic cardiomyopathy in the cat, and certain congenital heart diseases including patent ductus arteriosus, ventricular septal defect, and congenital mitral valve dysplasia in both species. Animals with acute cardiogenic pulmonary edema usually receive supplemental oxygen immediately. In addition to oxygen therapy, dietary sodium restriction, cage rest, and stress reduction are necessary. Diuretics and vasodilators are the backbone of initial therapy.

Furosemide is the diuretic of choice for the management of acute pulmonary edema. In animals with acute severe pulmonary edema, high doses of furosemide (up to 4 mg/kg every 2 hr) may be required to induce a diuresis. After a diuresis is initiated and the dog is symptomatically improved, the dose is markedly reduced, usually to 2 to 4 mg/kg every 12 hr in the dog. To treat acute severe heart failure, intravenous furosemide is preferred initially. High doses of furosemide are less well tolerated by cats and certain breeds of dogs, including Doberman pinschers (see this volume, p. 668). After initial stabilization, many cats can be maintained on 1 to 2 mg/kg every 12 to 24 hr or less frequently.

Nitroglycerin is often used empirically in animals with severe pulmonary edema. Nitroglycerin paste can be applied to the inner surface of the pinna of the ear or over a clipped square of skin (¼ to 1 inch every 6 hr in dogs, ⅛ to ¼ inch every 6 hr in cats). Nitroglycerin is typically used for only 2 or 3 days, until life-threatening edema has resolved, otherwise drug tolerance may develop. Nitroglycerin in sustained-release 2.5- or 5-mg patches can also be used.

ACE inhibitors and arterial dilators such as hydralazine are also useful in the management of severe pulmonary edema. Some clinicians have suggested that dogs receiving captopril may fail to show significant hemodynamic improvement when therapy is first initiated, but others have argued that higher doses of captopril are required to obtain early hemodynamic changes. Studies are currently under way to evaluate the efficacy of enalapril in the management of acute severe heart failure. The initial dose of captopril in the dog is usually 0.5 mg/kg every 8 hr with upward dose titration to 2 mg/kg every 8 hr based on clinical response. Enalapril is started at 0.5 mg/kg every 24 hr and may be increased to 0.5 mg/kg every 12 hr. Most cardiologists prescribe an ACE inhibitor for severe CHF due to dilated cardiomyopathy, but many prefer hydralazine when the cause of severe lung edema is mitral regurgitation (see this volume, p. 700).

Morphine can be used to calm animals that are anxious because of hypoxia or the stress of hospitalization. The initial dose in dogs is 0.05 to 0.1 mg/kg, usually given IM up to four times a day. Morphine is rarely needed to control anxiety in cats with heart failure, but when it is used, low doses (0.05 to 0.1 mg/kg every 6 hr) are administered. Acepromazine (0.05 to 0.1 mg/kg SC) may be substituted for morphine in cats.

In animals with very severe pulmonary edema who do not respond initially to furosemide, nitroglycerin, and an ACE inhibitor or hydralazine, sodium nitroprusside may be useful. The initial dose of 1 μg/kg/min is titrated up as the arterial blood pressure, ECG, CVP, and in some cases PCWP are serially monitored. A drop in PCWP and CVP and a small drop in arterial blood pressure are indicators of successful therapy. Hypotension is a common side effect at high dosages, necessitating serial blood pressure measurement. The effective dose in dogs is usually 2 to 10 μg/kg/min.

MANAGEMENT OF THE PATIENT WITH CARDIOGENIC PLEURAL EFFUSION

Pleural effusion rarely develops from isolated right-sided heart failure (pulmonic stenosis, tricuspid dysplasia, tricuspid valve endocardiosis), or more commonly from biventricular heart failure or superimposition of atrial fibrillation on a right-sided cardiac lesion. Dogs with dilated cardiomyopathy, pericardial disease, or chronic valvular insufficiency due to endocardiosis and cats with congenital heart disease or any form of cardiomyopathy, may develop biventricular heart failure. When pleural effusion is thought to contribute significantly to dyspnea, bilateral thoracocentesis is indicated. In animals with tense ascites and respiratory compromise, abdominocentesis is performed and fluid that is sufficient to relieve dyspnea is removed.

In addition to fluid centesis, sodium restriction, exercise and stress reduction, and oxygen therapy, furosemide is indicated. More conservative doses of furosemide (2 to 4 mg/kg every 12 hr) can often be used in these animals, although those with concurrent pulmonary edema may require the same high doses described for acute pulmonary edema. ACE inhibitors are also useful, but nitroglycerin seems less effective in this setting.

MANAGEMENT OF ANIMALS WITH CONGESTIVE HEART FAILURE AND EVIDENCE OF DECREASED CARDIAC OUTPUT

Animals with signs of congestion and diminished cardiac output (cardiogenic shock) are the most difficult to treat. In addition to fluid accumulations, these animals have cold extremities, a subnormal body temperature, mucous membrane pallor, slow capillary refill time, azotemia, weakness, and decreased blood pressure (mean <70 mm Hg and/or systolic <95 mm Hg). Venous blood gas determinations (free-flowing jugular venous samples) are useful in the evaluation of oxygen delivery to peripheral tissues. When Pa_{O_2} is 65 mm Hg and Pv_{O_2} falls below 30 mm Hg, cardiac output and peripheral perfusion are assumed to be compromised.

Physical warming is accomplished using either a circulating hot water blanket or hot water bottles. Thoracocentesis is done if required. Strict exercise restriction is enforced. Oxygen therapy is delivered and diuretics, and often nitroglycerin are given to decrease edema. Vasodilators should not be administered until cardiac output has been increased (generally in 1 to 4 hr) with dobutamine or dopamine. Once blood pressure has increased, nitroprusside, hydralazine, or an ACE inhibitor can be administered judiciously if required to treat CHF.

Dobutamine is administered especially to patients with dilated cardiomyopathy. The infusion rate is adjusted upward from 2.5 μg/kg/min until signs of improved cardiac function (increased blood pressure, warmer limbs, improved mucous membrane color and capillary refill time [CRT], and higher body temperature) are noted. When blood pressure monitoring is available, the dosage of dobutamine is adjusted to maintain the mean arterial pressure in excess of 70 mm Hg and the systolic pressure above 95 mm Hg in the dog. Serial evaluations of venous blood gases should result in elevation of Pv_{O_2} above 35 mm Hg. Doses of dobutamine in excess of 10 μg/kg/min are rarely required. Increases in heart rate greater than 20% above baseline, heart rates above 190 beats/min, or arrhythmia formation dictate dose reduction. Patients with atrial fibrillation or supraventricular tachycardia depend on functional AV block to maintain a reasonable ventricular rate, and may experience enhanced AV nodal conduction during dobutamine or dopamine infusion. These patients should be intravenously digitalized before or coincident with initiation of sympathomimetic drugs. Dobutamine infusions are usually continued for 1 to 3 days and then tapered as other medications (vasodilators or digoxin) are initiated. Some data suggest that patients may experience a sustained beneficial effect for weeks after dobutamine infusion. Cats with dilated cardiomyopathy commonly experience seizures, vomition, and (in some cases) cardiac arrest when dobutamine is administered in the typical range of 5 to 10 μg/kg/min. In cats, dobutamine is administered at 0.5 to 2 μg/kg/min.

Once edema or effusions are relieved and perfusion and arterial pressure have been stabilized, attention can be directed toward titrating the dosage of other drugs, initiating digitalization (if this has not yet been started), and choosing an orally administered vasodilator (usually an ACE inhibitor).

References and Suggested Reading

Bonagura, J. D.: Fluid and electrolyte management of the cardiac patient. Vet. Clin. North Am. 12:501, 1982.

Fitzpatrick, R. K., and Crowe, D. T.: Nasal oxygen administration in dogs and cats: Experimental and clinical investigations. J. Am. Anim. Hosp. Assoc. 22:293, 1986.

Fox, P. R.: Critical care cardiology. Vet. Clin. North Am. 19:1095, 1989.

Harpster, N.: Pulmonary edema. In Kirk, R. W. (ed.): Current Veterinary Therapy X. Philadelphia: W. B. Saunders, 1989, pp. 385–392.

Johnson, R. A., and Fifer, M. A.: Heart failure. In Eagle, K. A., Haber, E., DeSanctis, R. W., and Austen, W. G. (eds.): The Practice of Cardiology. Boston: Little, Brown & Co., 1989, pp. 65–133.

Keene, B. W., and Rush, J. E.: Therapy of heart failure. In Ettinger, S. J. (ed.): Textbook of Veterinary Internal Medicine. Philadelphia: WB Saunders, 1989, pp. 939–975.

Muir, W., and Bonagura, J.: Cardiovascular emergencies. In Sherding, R. G. (ed.): Medical Emergencies. New York: Churchill Livingstone, 1985, pp. 37–93.

Schertel, E. R., and Muir, M. W.: Shock: Pathophysiology, monitoring, and therapy. In Kirk, R. W. (ed.): Current Veterinary Therapy X. Philadelphia: W. B. Saunders, 1989, pp. 316–330.

Ware, W. A., and Bonagura, J. D.: Pulmonary edema. In Fox, P. R. (ed.): Canine and Feline Cardiology. New York: Churchill Livingstone, 1988, pp. 205–217.

HEARTWORM CAVAL SYNDROME

CLARKE E. ATKINS

Raleigh, North Carolina

A severe variant of heartworm disease, variably termed dirofilarial hemoglobinuria, liver failure syndrome, acute hepatic syndrome, venae cavae syndrome, venae cavae embolism, postcaval syndrome, or caval syndrome, is characterized by high mortality, heavy and atypically located worm burden, hemoglobinemia and hemoglobinuria, anemia, and hepatic and renal dysfunction. The incidence of caval syndrome (CS), which can account for up to 20% of cases of heartworm infection (HWI) in highly endemic areas, varies with the overall prevalence of dirofilariasis, as well as the diligence with which prophylactic measures are applied.

PATHOGENESIS

Caval syndrome is associated with heavy infestation of *Dirofilaria immitis* and is typically seen in the spring and early summer. Although primarily a disease of dogs, there is a recent report of feline CS (Takehashi et al., 1988). In the dog, CS is characterized by a worm burden of greater than 60 worms (>200 in some cases), with 55 to 84% residing in the cranial and caudal venae cavae and the right atrium (Fig. 1). The exact reason that some heartworm-infected dogs develop this syndrome while others do not is unclear but probably involves factors beyond the absolute or even relative (worms/ kg body weight) worm burden (Atkins et al., 1988). The mean age of onset is 5 years (range of 1.5 to 10 years), which is similar to the mean age of diagnosis for heartworm disease (HWD). Most studies have

shown a marked sex predilection with 75 to 90% of cases involving male dogs.

Current evidence suggests that CS results from the retrograde migration of adult heartworms to the cavae and right atrium. The syndrome develops in dogs with severe pulmonary hypertension. The worm mass interferes with the tricuspid valve apparatus and causes tricuspid insufficiency with re-

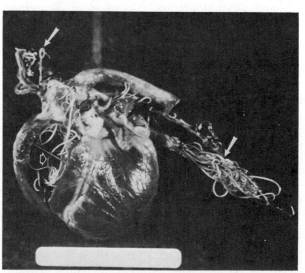

Figure 1. The heart of a dog with caval syndrome (CS). Note the large number of worms in the cavae (*solid white arrows*) and small number in the right ventricle (*open arrow*). (Reprinted with permission from Atkins, C. E.: Semin. Vet. Med. Surg. (Small Anim.) 2:64, 1988.)

sultant systolic murmur, jugular pulsations, elevated central venous pressure, and diminished cardiac output (Fig. 2). In addition to the dramatic fall in cardiac output, this constellation of events precipitates hemolytic anemia secondary to red blood cell (RBC) trauma caused by passage through a sieve of heartworms partially occluding the venae cavae, as well as by transit through fibrin strands in capillaries if disseminated intravascular coagulation (DIC) has developed. The effect of this trauma is magnified by increased RBC fragility that results from changes in serum-free and esterified cholesterol concentrations and lecithin acyltransferase activity. Hemoglobinemia, hemoglobinuria, and hepatic and renal dysfunction are observed in many dogs. Intravascular hemolysis, metabolic acidosis, and diminished hepatic function with impaired removal of circulating procoagulants contribute to the development of DIC. If untreated, death typically ensues within 24 to 72 hr due to cardiogenic shock complicated by anemia, metabolic acidosis, and DIC.

DIAGNOSIS

Clinical Presentation

Owner complaints and physical findings include sudden onset of anorexia, depression, weakness, and possibly cough, accompanied in most dogs by dyspnea and hemoglobinuria. Hemoglobinuria is almost universally noted in acute CS and has been considered pathognomonic by some (although it is not). Physical examination also reveals variable body temperature, mucous membrane pallor, prolonged capillary refill time, weak pulses, jugular distention and pulsation, hepatosplenomegaly, and dyspnea. Thoracic auscultation may disclose adventitious lung sounds, a systolic heart murmur of tricuspid insufficiency (87% of cases), loud, split second heart sound (S2) (67%), and cardiac gallops (20%) (Ogburn et al., 1977). Other reported findings include ascites (29%), jaundice (19%), and hemoptysis (6%).

Laboratory Abnormalities

The clinicopathologic features of CS have been described (Atwell and Farmer, 1982; Ishihara et al., 1978). Hemoglobinemia and microfilaremia are present in 85% of dogs suffering from CS. Moderate regenerative anemia (mean packed cell volume [PCV], 28%), characterized by the presence of reticulocytes, nucleated RBC, and increased mean corpuscular volume (MCV) is seen in the majority of cases. Leukocytosis with neutrophilia, eosinophilia, and left shift has been described. Affected dogs with DIC typically exhibit coagulopathy characterized by thrombocytopenia and hypofibrinogenemia, prolonged one-stage prothrombin time, partial thromboplastin time, activated clotting time, and high fibrin degradation product concentrations.

Serum chemistry analysis has revealed increased activities of aspartate amino transferase (AST), alanine amino transferase (ALT), and alkaline phosphatase. Increased blood urea nitrogen (BUN) is typically associated with a normal serum creatinine concentration. Total and direct serum bilirubin concentrations are usually moderately high and sulfobromophthalein (BSP) retention is prolonged. Urinalysis reveals high bilirubin and protein in 50% of cases. Urine hemoglobin concentrations range from 5 to 700 mg/dl, and small numbers of intact RBCs are frequently observed on examination of urine sediment.

Other Studies

Central venous pressure (CVP) is high in 80 to 90% of cases, with a mean value of approximately 10 cm H_2O. Electrocardiographic abnormalities may include sinus tachycardia, atrial and ventricular premature complexes, and evidence of right ventricular enlargement. Thoracic radiography reveals signs of (in descending order of frequency) severe HWD with right-sided cardiomegaly, main pulmonary arterial enlargement, increased pulmonary vascularity, and pulmonary arterial tortuosity.

Massive worm inhabitation of the right atrium with movement into the right ventricle during diastole is evident echocardiographically and is considered pathognomonic for caval syndrome in the appropriate clinical setting. The right ventricular lumen is enlarged and the left diminished in size, suggesting pulmonary hypertension accompanied by reduced left ventricular loading (Fig. 3). Paradoxical septal motion, caused by high right ventricular volume and pressure, is commonly observed.

TREATMENT

Preoperative Medical Therapy

Caval syndrome is complex, characterized by hemolytic anemia, biochemical aberrations, diminished cardiac output, diminished tissue perfusion, hepatic and renal dysfunction, the potential for pulmonary embolization, hypoalbuminemia, hemoglobinemia and hemoglobinuria, metabolic acidosis, and in some cases DIC. It follows that treatment also is complex and requires careful monitoring. Prognosis is poor unless the cause of the crisis—the right atrial and caval heartworms—is removed. Even with extirpation of the obstructive mass, mortality ranges from 14 to 42% or higher and subsequent adulticide therapy is still necessary (discussed later).

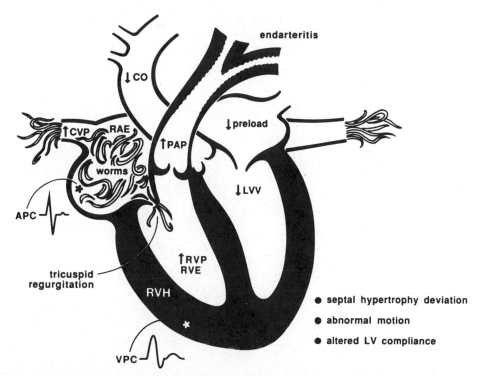

Figure 2. Schematic representation of the sequence of events leading to the development of cardiac dysfunction in caval syndrome. Caval syndrome complicates chronic heartworm disease when retrograde worm migration from the pulmonary arteries occurs, with the majority of worms relocating in the venae cavae and right atrium. Resultant tricuspid regurgitation, superimposed on pulmonary hypertension, results in congestive and low-output failure. Right ventricular inflow obstruction and cardiac arrhythmias probably contribute minimally in most instances. Septal deviation and abnormal motion may contribute to diminished left ventricular (LV) preload and cardiac output (CO). APC, atrial premature complexes; CVP, central venous pressure; LVV, left ventricular volume; PAP, pulmonary artery pressure; RAE, right atrial enlargement; RVE, right ventricular enlargement; RVH, right ventricular hypertrophy; RVP, right ventricular pressure; VPC, ventricular premature complexes. (Reprinted with permission from Atkins, C. E.: Pathophysiology of heartworm caval syndrome: Recent advances. *In* Otto, G. F. (ed.): *Proceedings of the Heartworm Symposium '89.* Washington, D.C.: American Heartworm Society, 1989, p. 27.)

It is desirable to establish the degree of involvement of various organ systems. The database should include thoracic radiographs, PCV, total serum protein, activated clotting time, AST, BUN, serum alkaline phosphatase, CBC, urinalysis, and CVP for determining the severity of cardiac dysfunction and monitoring fluid therapy. Ideally, prothrombin time, partial thromboplastin time, fibrin degradation products, platelet count, and arterial (or venous) blood gases should be evaluated as well. While this information is important, substantial delays in worm removal while awaiting laboratory results are inadvisable.

Fluid therapy is needed to improve cardiac output and tissue perfusion (especially to liver and kidney), prevent or help to reverse DIC, prevent hemoglobin nephropathy, and help correct metabolic acidosis caused by diminished tissue perfusion. Overexuberant fluid therapy, however, may worsen or precipitate signs of congestive heart failure. Ideally, a left jugular catheter is placed and fluid therapy instituted with 5% dextrose in water or 2.5% dextrose in water with 0.45% saline solution intravenously. The catheter should not enter the cranial vena cava because it will interfere with worm embolectomy. A cephalic catheter may be substituted for the less convenient jugular catheter, but this does not allow monitoring of CVP. The infusion rate for intravenous fluids is dependent on the condition of the animal. A useful guideline is to infuse crystalloids as rapidly as possible (up to one cardiovascular volume during the first hour) without raising the CVP, or without raising it above 10 cm H_2O if it was normal or near normal at the outset. Initial therapy should be aggressive (40 to 80 ml/kg/hr for the first hr) if shock is accompanied by a normal CVP (<5 cm H_2O) and should be reduced to approximately 1 to 2 ml/kg/hr if CVP is 10 to 20 cm H_2O. Whole blood transfusion is not indicated in most cases because anemia is typically not severe, and transfused coagulation factors may worsen DIC. Sodium bicarbonate is not indicated unless metabolic acidosis is severe (pH 7.15 to 7.20). Broad-spectrum antibiotics and aspirin (5 mg/kg/day) should be administered. Because cardiac contractility is generally not impaired, positive inotropic drugs are not employed. Except in rare instances—when cardiac arrhythmias are contributing signifi-

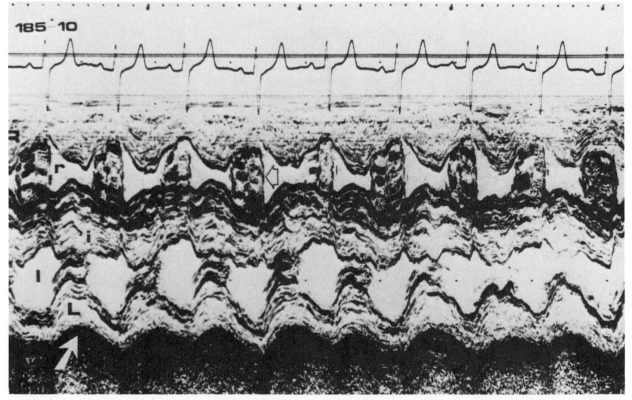

Figure 3. An M-mode echocardiogram from a dog with recent-onset CS demonstrating thickening of the right ventricular (R) and intraventricular (i) septal walls, right ventricular dilatation (r), and a small left ventricle (L). The echogenic mass *(open arrow)* in the right ventricle represents heartworms in the atrium and atrioventricular valve area, which "fall" into the ventricle only during diastole. Paradoxical septal motion is also evident. The left ventricular posterior wall is labeled L, and the pericardium is denoted by a *solid white arrow*. (Reprinted with permission from Atkins, C. E.: Semin. Vet. Med. Surg. (Small Anim.) 2:64, 1988.)

cantly to the animal's hemodynamic compromise or appear to be life-threatening—specific antiarrhythmic therapy is unnecessary.

Treatment for heartworm-associated DIC has been described (Calvert and Rawlings, 1986). Cage rest and supportive care are adequate in most cases. Platelet count should be monitored closely, and if platelets fall below 50,000/mm³ aspirin should be discontinued. Some authors recommend treatment with vincristine at this point, but this is controversial. Heparin may be administered (at 200 units/kg, every 8 hr SC) for chronic or low-grade DIC; the authors recommend 500 units/kg every 8 hr SC for acute DIC and 200 units/kg every 8 hr SC for end-stage DIC. The prognosis for acute or end-stage DIC is dismal.

Surgical and Adulticide Therapy

The technique for surgical removal of caval and atrial heartworms was developed by Jackson (Jackson et al., 1977). This procedure should be undertaken as *early in the course of therapy* as is practical. Sedation is often unnecessary, and the procedure can be accomplished with local anesthesia. The dog is restrained in left lateral recumbency after surgical clipping and preparation. The right jugular vein is isolated distally in the caudal cervical jugular furrow. A ligature is placed loosely around the cranial aspect of the vein until it is incised, after which the ligature is tied. A 20- to 40-cm alligator forceps (preferably of small diameter), a sterile basket catheter (such as is used for endoscopy), or a human urethral stone loop catheter is guided gently down the vein while being held loosely between the thumb and forefinger. The jugular vein can be temporarily occluded with umbilical tape. With the use of forceps, if difficulty is encountered in its passage, gentle manipulation of the dog by assistants to further extend the neck will assist in passage past the thoracic inlet, while medial direction of the forceps may be necessary at the base of the heart. Once the forceps have been placed, the jaws are opened, the forceps are advanced slightly, the jaws are closed, and the worms are removed. One to four worms usually are removed with each pass. This process is repeated until five to six successive attempts are unsuccessful. An attempt should be made to remove 35 to 50 worms. Following worm removal, the jugular vein is ligated distally and subcutaneous and skin sutures are placed routinely.

A drop in CVP after worm removal is expected and is associated with a reduction in the intensity of the cardiac murmur and jugular pulsation, rapid clearing of hemoglobinemia and hemoglobinuria, and eventual normalization of serum enzymes. Improvement in cardiac function is immediate and continues over the following 24 hours. Clinical findings of hypothermia, ascites, and CVP >20 cm H_2O carry a poor prognosis. It is important to realize that removal of worms does nothing to reduce right ventricular afterload (increased pulmonary vascular resistance associated with endarteritis), and hence fluid therapy must be monitored carefully before and after surgery to avoid precipitation of right heart failure. Substantial improvement in anemia should not be expected for 2 to 4 weeks.

Adulticide therapy (sodium caparsolate at 2.2 mg/kg every 12 hr IV for 4 doses) is instituted approximately 2 weeks after stabilization and worm removal. The development of flexible alligator forceps should permit the removal of worms from the pulmonary arteries and may preempt drug therapy in these high-risk cases. Careful scrutiny of BUN and liver enzyme concentrations should precede treatment. Aspirin therapy and strict exercise restriction are continued for 3 to 4 weeks after adulticide therapy to minimize embolic complications. Microfilaricides are usually needed and are administered 6 weeks after completion of therapy.

References and Suggested Reading

Atkins, C. E.: Caval syndrome in the dog. Semin. Vet. Med. Surg. 2:64, 1987.
A comprehensive review of caval syndrome.

Atkins, C. E.: Pathophysiology of heartworm caval syndrome: Recent advances. In Otto, G. F. (ed.): *Proceedings of the Heartworm Symposium '89.* Washington, D.C.: American Heartworm Society, 1989, p. 27.
A review of recent advances in the understanding of risk factors, natural history, precipitating factors, and pathophysiology of caval syndrome.

Atkins, C. E., Keene, B. W., and McGuirk, S. M.: Investigation of caval syndrome in dogs experimentally infected with Dirofilarial immitis. J. Vet. Intern. Med. 2:36, 1988a.
A study of the epidemiology, risk factors, and precipitating factors of an experimental model of caval syndrome.

Atkins, C. E., Keene, B. W., and McGuirk, S. M.: Pathophysiology of cardiac dysfunction in an experimental model of heartworm caval syndrome in the dog: An echocardiographic study. Am. J. Vet. Res. 49:403, 1988b.
A study of the cardiovascular, functional, anatomic, and electrical abnormalities associated with caval syndrome and postulation of the pathophysiological mechanisms involved in this syndrome.

Atwell, R. B., and Farmer, T. S.: Clinical pathology of the "caval syndrome" in canine dirofilariasis in Northern Australia. J. Small Anim. Pract. 23:675, 1982.
A description of hematologic, biochemical, and urinary abnormalities associated with caval syndrome.

Calvert, C. A., and Rawlings, C. A.: Therapy of canine heartworm disease. In Kirk, R. W. (ed.): *Current Veterinary Therapy IX.* Philadelphia: W. B. Saunders, 1986, p. 406.
An excellent overview of all aspects of heartworm disease.

Ishihara, K., Kitagwa, H., Ojima, M., et al.: Clinicopathological studies on canine dirofilarial hemoglobinuria. Jpn. J. Vet. Sci. 40:525, 1978.
A description of hematologic, biochemical, and urinary abnormalities associated with caval syndrome.

Jackson, R. F., Seymour, W. G., Growney, P. J., et al.: Surgical treatment of the CS of canine heart worm disease. J.A.V.M.A. 171:1065, 1977.
Original illustrated description of worm removal in caval syndrome via jugular venotomy.

Ogburn, P. N., Jackson, R. F., Seymour, G., et al.: Electrocardiographic and phonocardiographic alterations in canine heart worm disease. Proceedings of the Heartworm Symposium '77. Bonner Springs, KS: Veterinary Medical Publishing, 1977, p. 67.
Description of electrocardiographic and phonocardiographic abnormalities in heartworm disease of varying severity.

Takehashi, N., Matsui, A., Sasai, H., et al.: Feline caval syndrome: A case report. J. Am. Anim. Hosp. Assoc. 24:645, 1988.
A case report of successful management of feline caval syndrome.

PERICARDIAL DISEASE

MATTHEW W. MILLER
and THERESA W. FOSSUM
College Station, Texas

Diseases of the pericardium represent a fairly small percentage of acquired cardiovascular diseases in dogs and cats; however, they are an important cause of right heart failure in both species. Pericardial disease is one of the more commonly misdiagnosed or overlooked types of cardiovascular disease in dogs. Pericardial diseases are much less common in cats; thus, canine pericardial disease will be emphasized in this chapter. For information regarding feline pericardial disease, the reader is referred to a recent review (Rush et al., 1990) and this volume, p. 647.

Pericardial disease is usually not considered as a differential diagnosis unless there is evidence of right heart failure caused by cardiac tamponade; however, pericardial disease may be present in animals that do not exhibit clinical signs. Cardiac tamponade is the unchecked rise of intrapericardial pressure causing alterations in cardiac filling and reductions in cardiac output. The majority of symptomatic patients with pericardial disease have cardiac tamponade and thus exhibit signs compatible with right heart failure.

PATHOPHYSIOLOGY

An understanding of the pathophysiology of pericardial disease is essential to fully appreciate the diversity of clinical presentation, diagnosis, and therapy of patients with pericardial disease. Pericardial disease causes *diastolic* cardiac dysfunction, with minimal, if any, alterations in systolic function. Elevated intrapericardial pressure inhibits diastolic cardiac filling, causing a reduction in preload for a given venous filling pressure. This reduction in preload results in decreased cardiac output, assuming heart rate, cardiac contractility, and vascular resistance are unchanged.

The body responds to decreased cardiac output by increasing sympathetic tone and activating the renin-angiotensin-aldosterone system (RAAS). Increased sympathetic tone causes elevations in heart rate and augmentation of cardiac contractility. Activation of the RAAS causes renal retention of sodium and water and increased peripheral vascular resistance. The increase in plasma volume elevates venous filling pressures, thereby augmenting preload. The combination of increased preload, elevated heart rate, and augmented cardiac contractility initially restores cardiac output to near normal levels.

Although cardiac output may increase secondary to the aforementioned responses, the increased preload causes elevated venous filling pressures manifested as signs of congestion. Although the elevation of intrapericardial pressure is the same on both sides of the heart, the thin-walled right heart is more sensitive to this elevation and signs of right-sided or biventricular congestive heart failure (e.g., jugular venous distention, ascites, hepatomegaly, pleural effusion) predominate.

ETIOLOGY

Reported causes of pericardial disease are listed as follows; in small animal patients, only a few of these are commonly encountered. General statements regarding etiology can be made based on signalment: (1) young animals most commonly have congenital defects or infectious disease, (2) middle-aged, large-breed dogs most frequently have idiopathic hemorrhagic pericardial effusion, and (3) dogs older than 6 or 7 years of age (especially German shepherds, golden retrievers, Labrador retrievers, boxers, and bulldogs) typically have cardiac neoplasia. It must be stressed that these are general statements and exceptions do occur.

Peritoneopericardial diaphragmatic hernia (PPDH) is by far the most commonly encountered congenital pericardial malformation. The Weimeraner dog is predisposed and cats are often affected. PPDH may be undetected for years and is commonly an incidental finding at necropsy or during the course of evaluation for unrelated problems. Gastrointestinal (e.g., anorexia, vomiting) and cardiopulmonary (e.g., dyspnea, coughing) signs are the most common abnormalities noted in patients with PPDH. These patients occasionally have other concurrent defects, including sternal malformations, umbilical hernias, and ventricular septal defects.

Not all patients with pericardial disease have an obvious effusion or a space-occupying lesion. Constrictive pericardial disease is caused by thickening of the pericardium and resultant constriction of the heart (Thomas et al., 1984a). Although some echocardiographic findings suggest the presence of constrictive pericardial disease (abnormal septal motion, thickened pericardium, large right atrium, flattened left ventricular free wall, minimal or absent effusion), cardiac catheterization is frequently required to establish a definitive diagnosis (Voelkel et al., 1978). Recently, computed tomography scans and magnetic resonance imaging have been used to evaluate pericardium thickness and aid diagnosis of constrictive pericardial disease. Constrictive pericardial disease represents a small percentage of pericardial abnormalities in veterinary patients.

DIAGNOSIS

Physical Examination

Animals with pericardial disease are typically presented with abdominal distention secondary to free abdominal fluid. Jugular venous distention is invariably present, although commonly overlooked. In some cases, the jugular venous distention may be subtle; therefore, clipping the jugular furrow and evaluating the patient for hepatojugular reflux may be beneficial. Hepatojugular reflux is invoked by applying gentle pressure to the liver or cranial abdomen for approximately 10 to 15 sec while simultaneously evaluating the jugular vein. Compressing the liver or cranial abdomen increases venous return to the right side of the heart; if the jugular veins distend or pulsate while the pressure is being applied, it suggests right heart dysfunction and further cardiac evaluation is warranted. Although this provocative test is not specific for pericardial disease, it is very useful for detecting subtle right heart dysfunction.

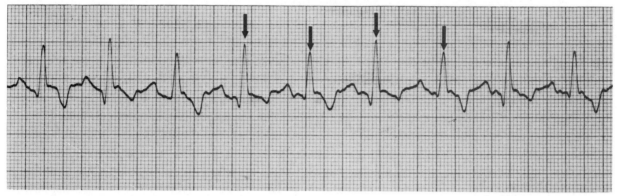

Figure 1. Lead II electrocardiogram obtained from a dog with pericardial effusion. Note the small complex size and the alternation in R wave amplitude *(arrows)*. Lead II, 50 mm/sec, 20 mm = 1 mV.

The heart rate and femoral pulse quality varies depending on the severity of hemodynamic compromise. In cases of pericardial disease with cardiac tamponade, the heart rate is elevated and femoral pulse quality diminished. Auscultatory abnormalities are dependent on the nature and severity of the disease. Although pericardial friction rubs are commonly mentioned in reference to pericardial disease, in the authors' experience they are infrequently recognized in small animals. Large volumes of pericardial or pleural fluid will commonly cause muffled heart and lung sounds. Cardiac murmurs are the exception rather than the rule, unless concurrent valvular heart disease is present. The presence of a third heart sound (gallop rhythm) may be detected in patients with dilated cardiomyopathy or may represent a pericardial knock in constrictive disease. The latter is produced by the rapid cessation of cardiac filling once the elastic limit of the pericardium is reached.

Radiography

Thoracic radiography typically demonstrates a markedly enlarged, globoid cardiac silhouette. It is common to find pulmonary underperfusion in patients with significant reductions in cardiac output. Pleural effusion may or may not be present. In cases of PPDH, variable radiographic densities suggesting the presence of abdominal contents (air-filled, fluid dense, or fat) within the pericardial sac and sternal abnormalities may be noted; a persistent pleural fold is evident ventral to the caudal vena cava. The size of the cardiac silhouette seldom correlates with the severity of clinical signs.

Electrocardiography

Although there is no pathognomonic electrocardiographic finding for pericardial disease, electro-cardiographic abnormalities that should alert the clinician to the possibility of pericardial disease include diminished complex size, electrical alternans, and ST segment elevation (Fig. 1); however, the absence of any or all of these findings does not negate the possibility of pericardial effusion. The degree of reduction in complex size depends on several factors, including the nature and volume of effusion present. Other conditions including pleural effusion, hypovolemia, and obesity can also result in diminished complex size. Electrical alternans may be present in cases of large-volume pericardial effusion and should alert the clinician to the possibility of this condition. Clinicians should avoid confusing alterations in complex size associated with respiration with true electrical alternans. Sinus tachycardia is the most frequently recognized arrhythmia, but supraventricular tachycardia, paroxysmal atrial tachycardia, and ventricular premature contractions are occasionally noted depending on the underlying etiology.

Echocardiography

Echocardiography is the most sensitive and specific noninvasive test available for diagnosing pericardial effusion (Thomas et al., 1984b); it can detect as little as 15 to 20 ml of pericardial effusion. Echocardiographic evaluation will establish the diagnosis and also rule out concurrent disease such as dilated cardiomyopathy, valvular heart disease, and severe congenital disease.

In animals with pericardial effusion, an echo-free space is evident between the myocardium and pericardium (Fig. 2). When imaging from the right hemithorax, the right ventricular free wall (RVFW) commonly appears hyperechoic due to the dramatic difference in echogenicity between the pericardial effusion and epimyocardium. This finding should not be interpreted as an abnormality of the RVFW. Pleural effusion, dramatic left atrial enlargement, and a markedly dilated coronary sinus or persistent left cranial vena cava can sometimes be misinterpreted as pericardial effusion.

Whenever possible, it is best to perform echocardiographic evaluations prior to the removal of pericardial fluid. Small amounts of air introduced during pericardiocentesis may interfere with visualization of cardiac structures, whereas pericardial fluid improves the ability to detect cardiac mass lesions. Special care should be taken to thoroughly examine the right atrium, right auricle, parietal pericardium, and aortic base when a cardiac or heart base mass is suspected (Fig. 3).

Pericardial and Abdominal Fluid Analysis

Since most patients with pericardial disease are presented for abdominal distention, obtaining abdominal fluid for evaluation is frequently indicated. The ascites caused by pericardial effusion is a modified transudate and typically has a total protein of greater than 2.5 to 3.0 gm/dl and low cellularity. An abdominal fluid protein of less than 2 gm/dl is unusual in pericardial disease, unless the animal is markedly hypoproteinemic. Some patients with chronic right heart failure may become hypoproteinemic due to excessive fluid retention by the

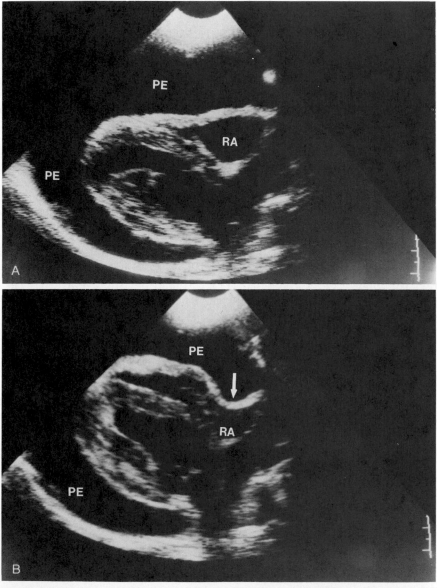

Figure 2. Right parasternal long-axis echocardiogram obtained from a dog with idiopathic, hemorrhagic pericardial effusion. *A,* This systolic image demonstrates the marked pericardial effusion (PE) surrounding the heart. RA, right atrium. *B,* The diastolic frame again documents the presence of pericardial effusion but also reveals diastolic collapse of the right atrium *(arrow)*. This collapse, in addition to being echocardiographic evidence of cardiac tamponade, interferes with diastolic filling and causes reductions in preload and cardiac output.

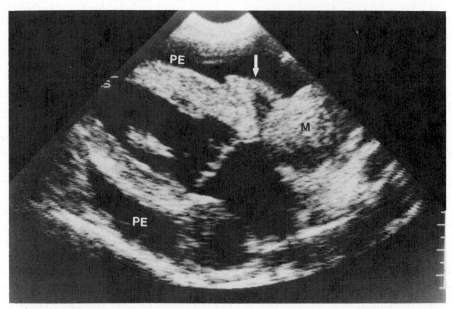

Figure 3. Right parasternal long-axis echocardiogram obtained from a dog with pericardial effusion secondary to a right atrial hemangiosarcoma. Note the PE and mass (M) lesion located within the right atrium. The right auricular appendage can be seen adjacent to the mass lesion *(arrow)*.

kidneys, protein loss in the ascites, concurrent liver dysfunction, or acquired intestinal lymphangiectasia (IL) caused by abdominal venous hypertension. Acquired IL also may affect absorption of orally administered medications in these patients.

Pericardial fluid is routinely submitted for cytologic evaluation and culture (aerobic and anaerobic). Intrapericardial pressure can be measured using a central venous pressure manometer. In most cases of tamponade, the fluid level is >10 cm H_2O and declines to <6 once sufficient fluid has been withdrawn. Gross examination of pericardial fluid is of little diagnostic benefit, as the vast majority of fluid samples have a "port wine" appearance, regardless of etiology. Laboratory and cytologic evaluation can identify chylous, mycotic, or suppurative pericardial effusions but are unreliable for differentiation of idiopathic and neoplastic effusions (Sisson et al.,

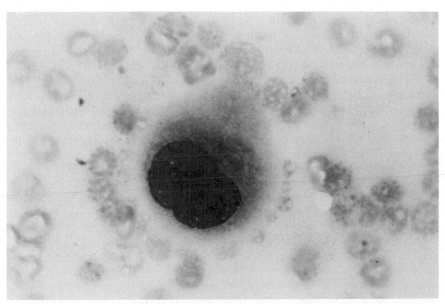

Figure 4. Cytologic specimen of pericardial effusate from a dog with idiopathic pericardial effusion and cardiac tamponade. Note the binucleate, reactive mesothelial cell with the fringed periphery. The cytologic interpretation suggested neoplasia; however, there was no evidence of neoplasia at surgery or on pericardial biopsy. ×100.

1984). Care must be exercised when evaluating cytologic reports on pericardial fluid because mesothelial cells lining the pericardium can become reactive and may exfoliate in the effusion; these reactive cells are easily confused with neoplastic cells (especially mesothelioma) (Fig. 4). Tumors commonly found within the pericardium (e.g., hemangiosarcoma and chemodectoma) seldom exfoliate into the effusion, resulting in frequent false-negative cytologic evaluations.

THERAPY

Medical

Because systolic function is usually normal, positive inotropic support is seldom indicated in patients with pericardial disease. Although many of the clinical signs detected in these patients are due to elevated venous pressures, attempts to significantly lower venous pressures with medical therapy (i.e., diuretics) should be avoided. Cardiac preload is dependent on these elevated venous filling pressures and aggressive diuresis will reduce cardiac preload and can significantly reduce cardiac output, causing hypotension or syncope. Vasodilators often cause significant hypotension, especially when used in combination with diuretics.

Therapy of patients with pericardial effusion is directed at acutely reducing intrapericardial pressure; physical drainage of the pericardial space is the therapeutic measure of choice. Treatment modalities include pericardiocentesis or surgical drainage via subtotal pericardiectomy. The treatment modality selected should be based on the severity of clinical signs, results of diagnostic evaluation, and historic response to therapy. If the animal requires immediate pericardial drainage due to severe cardiac dysfunction, pericardiocentesis should be performed for initial patient stabilization.

Pericardiocentesis is a fairly simple and safe procedure when performed correctly with appropriate precautions. Sedation or general anesthesia is seldom required; the procedure can usually be performed with a local anesthetic. Pericardiocentesis is performed in the authors' hospital with the patient in sternal or left lateral recumbency with constant electrocardiographic monitoring. The authors' prefer to perform pericardiocentesis from the right hemithorax using a 12- to 16-gauge, 4- to 6-inch, over-the-needle catheter (Surflo, The Burrows Co., Wheeling, IL) in medium and large dogs and an 18- to 20-gauge, 1.5- to 3-inch, over-the-needle catheter in small dogs and cats. Two or three extra side holes should be cut in the catheter and the catheter attached to a three-way stopcock and extension tubing to allow drainage of the pleural and pericardial spaces. The cardiac notch between the

lung lobes is larger on the right, and because the majority of the coronary arteries are on the left side, lung puncture and coronary artery laceration is less common when the procedure is performed from the right side. Although the exact site of puncture should be determined from the thoracic radiograph, generally the fifth or sixth intercostal space is used.

A local anesthetic block is performed and a large area of the thorax clipped and aseptically prepared. It is important to block the pleura at the site of insertion, as penetration of the pleura seems to result in significant patient discomfort. A small stab incision is made through the skin to facilitate insertion of the large-bore catheter. Constant negative pressure is applied while the catheter is slowly advanced into the pleural space, and some pleural fluid may be aspirated. As the pericardium is encountered, a subtle scratching sensation will be noticed. At this point, further advancement of the catheter should be performed cautiously to avoid accidental epicardial contact or perforation of the thin right ventricle. If the epicardium is contacted, the clinician will note a jumping motion in the catheter or feel a prominent tapping sensation, either of which should prompt withdrawal of the catheter. Moreover, ventricular premature complexes will be noted on the electrocardiogram and will usually be positive in lead II. This arrhythmia usually disappears once the catheter is withdrawn; however, lidocaine should be available if the arrhythmia persists. It should be emphasized that if the needle is directed too dorsad, the atrium can be punctured, yet no arrhythmia noted.

Once the pericardium is entered, the catheter is advanced over the needle and the needle withdrawn. Most pericardial effusates are "port wine" in color and are difficult to differentiate from venous blood obtained by inadvertent cardiac penetration. Unless the effusion is due to acute hemorrhage, pericardial effusates do not clot (unless agitated or mixed with air) and generally have a much lower packed cell volume than peripheral blood. The initial sample is submitted for cytologic evaluation and culture. The pericardium should be drained as completely as possible; this may be facilitated by altering the position of the patient during the procedure. When the pericardium has been completely evacuated, the catheter is removed. If significant pleural effusion is present, the same catheter may be used to evacuate the pleural space.

In cases of idiopathic pericardial effusion, pericardiocentesis followed by steroid administration (prednisone 1 mg/kg/day for 2 to 3 weeks, then tapered) may be curative. The authors usually place animals on ampicillin immediately following pericardiocentesis and do not institute steroid therapy unless results of microbial culture are negative. Approximately 50% of dogs with idiopathic pericardial effusion respond to one or two pericardial taps and steroid therapy and do not have recurrence of the effusion within 1 year. If an animal requires a third pericardial tap, a subtotal pericardiectomy is indicated. Long-term follow-ups of dogs treated conservatively have not been published.

Surgical

Pericardiectomy is indicated when pericardiocentesis has not significantly palliated clinical signs associated with pericardial effusion, when multiple attempts at pericardiocentesis have failed to resolve the effusion, or when neoplastic or infectious processes involving the pericardium are suspected.

Pericardiectomy may be performed through either a left or right, fourth- or fifth-space intercostal thoracotomy or through a median sternotomy; there are advantages and disadvantages associated with both approaches. An intercostal thoracotomy may be rapidly opened and closed; however exposure of the pericardium on the cardiac surface opposite the approach is limited, making removal of much of the pericardium difficult. Median sternotomies, on the other hand, while affording access to the entire pericardium, generally require increased operative time and, if closure of the sternum is inadequate, may be associated with increased postoperative pain. However, if several sternebrae are left intact so that the sternum will not shift following surgery, postoperative pain does not appear to be greater than with an intercostal thoracotomy. Because of superior pericardial exposure, median sternotomy is the authors' preferred approach, unless a heart base tumor is suspected from echocardiography. For tumors arising from the right atrial appendage, a right, fourth intercostal thoracotomy is preferred.

When performing a pericardiectomy, as much of the pericardium should be removed as possible. If only a small window is made in the pericardium, adhesion of the remaining pericardium to the epicardium may occur, resulting in recurrence of the effusion and associated clinical signs. Removal of the pericardium around the base of the heart is facilitated by dissecting the phrenic nerves from the pericardium. If the phrenic nerves are incorporated in a granulomatous reaction, the pericardium can only be removed from the apex of the heart to the level of the nerves (Eyster and Probst, 1985).

Complications associated with pericardiectomy include hemorrhage, pleural effusion, arrhythmias associated with manipulation of the heart, and recurrence of the pericardial effusion. Hemorrhage can generally be controlled with electrocautery. Pleural effusion may be managed postoperatively by tube thoracostomy. Thoracic radiographs and echocardiography should be performed postoperatively to monitor the development of pleural or pericardial effusion.

The prognosis following pericardiectomy depends on the underlying disease. Idiopathic, hemorrhagic pericardial effusions have excellent prognosis following pericardiectomy if the underlying etiology is controlled or corrected. In dogs with neoplastic disease, pericardiectomy may be a palliative procedure as many tumors have either metastasized (e.g., hemangiosarcoma) or are too expansive to be removed (e.g., chemodectoma, mesothelioma) at the time a diagnosis is established.

References and Suggested Reading

Eyster, G. E., and Probst, M.: Basic cardiac procedures. *In* Slatter, D. H. (ed.): *Textbook of Small Animal Surgery.* Philadelphia: W. B. Saunders, 1985, p. 1125.

Rush, J. E., Keene, B. W., and Fox, P. R.: Pericardial disease in the cat: A retrospective evaluation of 66 cases. J. Am. Anim. Hosp. Assoc. 26:39, 1990.

Sisson, D., Thomas, W. P., Ruehl, W. W., et al.: Diagnostic value of pericardial fluid analysis in the dog. J.A.V.M.A. 184:51, 1984.

Thomas, W. P.: Pericardial disease. *In* Ettinger, S. J. (ed.): *Textbook of Veterinary Internal Medicine.* 3rd ed. Philadelphia: W. B. Saunders, 1989, pp. 1080–1097.

Thomas, W. P., Reed, J. R., Bauer, T. G., et al.: Constrictive pericardial disease in the dog. J.A.V.M.A. 184:546, 1984a.

Thomas, W. P., Sisson, D., Bauer, T. G., et al.: Detection of cardiac masses in dogs by two-dimensional echocardiography. Vet. Radiol. 25:65, 1984b.

Voelkel, A. G., Pietro, D. A., Folland, E. D., et al.: Echocardiographic features of constrictive pericarditis. Circulation 58:871, 1978.

FELINE ARRHYTHMIAS: DIAGNOSIS AND MANAGEMENT

NEIL K. HARPSTER

Boston, Massachusetts

Cardiac arrhythmias are a well recognized and reported finding in cats with underlying cardiac disease and have also been identified as a consequence of certain noncardiac influences (Tilley, 1977). However, the frequency of serious arrhythmias as well as their effect on the morbidity and mortality of cats with significant cardiac disease seems much less than that seen in humans and dogs. One reason for this is unquestionably the fast resting heart rate of the domestic cat, which inhibits the discharge of many spontaneous-firing ectopic foci. Another likely reason is the smaller heart that is less supportive of re-entry fibrillatory mechanisms.

Many of the arrhythmias recognized in the cat on auscultation and as part of a basic cardiac evaluation are relatively benign and do not require specific therapy. They will often diminish in frequency or disappear when effective treatment is instituted for the pre-existing cardiac disease. Nevertheless, when malignant arrhythmias are present and interfere with the establishment of cardiac stability or persist beyond the period of acute manifestations, specific therapy to control these arrhythmias seems indicated.

EFFECT OF ARRHYTHMIAS ON CARDIAC PERFORMANCE

The clinical importance of any arrhythmia depends upon a number of variables: the specific nature of the arrhythmia, the presence or absence of underlying heart disease, activity level and emotional makeup of the patient, and sometimes the presence of concomitant disease processes.

Simply stated, arrhythmias exert a negative influence on cardiac performance by: (1) causing an effective heart rate that is either faster or slower than the optimal rate for a given level of activity, (2) impairing cardiac filling, or (3) altering the method of ventricular activation and subsequent

Table 1. Incidence of Cardiac Arrhythmias in 500 Consecutive Cats

Rhythm/Arrhythmias	Hypertrophic Cardiomyopathy (n = 118)	Intermediate Cardiomyopathy (n = 81)	Dilated Cardiomyopathy (n = 65)	Systemic Thromboembolism (n = 18)	Congenital Heart Disease (n = 34)	Hyperthyroidism (n = 51)
Normal sinus rhythm	82 (69.5)	60 (74.1)	40 (61.5)	10 (55.6)	20 (58.8)	22 (43.1)
Sinus tachycardia	26 (22.0)	9 (11.1)	20 (30.8)	7 (38.9)	10 (29.4)	27 (52.9)
Sinus bradycardia	7 (5.9)	8 (9.9)	2 (3.1)	—	4 (11.8)	1 (2.0)
Sinus node abnormalities, other	1 (0.8)	2 (2.5)	1 (1.5)	—	1 (2.9)	—
Atrioventricular conduction abnormalities	—	2 (2.5)	1 (1.5)	—	—	—
Supraventricular premature beats	2 (1.7)	6 (7.4)	5 (7.7)	1 (5.6)	—	4 (7.8)
Paroxysmal supraventricular tachycardia	—	3 (3.7)	1 (1.5)	1 (5.6)	1 (2.9)	5 (9.8)
Atrial fibrillation	3 (2.5)	3 (3.7)	2 (2.1)	1 (5.6)	—	1 (2.0)
Pre-excitation syndrome	3 (2.5)	—	3 (4.6)	—	2 (5.9)	—
Ventricular premature beats	8 (6.8)	20 (24.7)	9 (13.8)	8 (44.4)	—	9 (17.6)
Paroxysmal ventricular tachycardia	1 (0.8)	2 (2.5)	3 (4.6)	2 (11.1)	—	—
Atrioventricular dissociation	—	1 (1.2)	1 (1.5)	—	—	1 (2.0)

Parenthetical figures in headings (clinical diagnoses) indicate the total number in each group; parenthetical figures within table represent percentage within each individual group. Data from Angell Memorial Animal Hospital.

ventricular ejection. For each species (and perhaps each heart) there is an optimal heart rate. Cardiac output (CO) is the product of heart rate and ventricular stroke volume; thus, inappropriate heart rates are one mechanism by which arrhythmias reduce cardiac output. Cardiac filling consists of a rapid, "passive" phase and an additional atrial contribution or "atrial kick"; these are often altered with cardiac arrhythmias. Ventricular stroke volume also can be reduced by abnormal cardiac electrical activity because the activation process dictates the subsequent mechanical activity.

A number of examples demonstrate the impact of arrhythmias on cardiac performance. Heart rates that are excessively slow, as with atrioventricular block or sinus node dysfunction, limit cardiac output during activity, may cause syncope, and can prevent sufficient cardiac compensation in patients with heart failure. Tachyarrhythmias may encroach on the period of rapid ventricular filling and lead to a decrease in CO. Sustained tachycardia also increases oxygen demand, reduces coronary perfusion time, and can lead to a loss of myocardial contractility—the potentially reversible cardiomyopathy of tachycardia. Irregularity of cardiac contraction, as encountered with premature atrial and ventricular beats, limits cardiac filling time and may cause asynchronous activation of the ventricles. Furthermore, ventricular and junctional rhythms lead to atrioventricular (AV) dissociation, and the atrial contribution to ventricular filling becomes haphazard and often useless. Atrial fibrillation similarly causes a loss of atrial contribution to filling because the atria no long contract; this loss is amplified by the severe tachycardia and irregular ventricular filling that attends atrial fibrillation in cats.

How do these effects on cardiac performance relate to the clinical setting? When significant increases or decreases in the effective heart rate are brief (i.e., less than 3 to 5 sec), clinical consequences are unlikely even during vigorous activity. However, when these heart rates are extreme, or last for relatively longer periods of time, cardiovascular syncopal episodes (i.e., Stokes-Adams syndrome) can be anticipated. With more severe or prolonged compromises in CO, deterioration of a ventricular arrhythmia to ventricular fibrillation and sudden death is possible. Prolonged reduction in CO as a consequence of arrhythmia usually reduces exercise tolerance in the short-term setting, and congestive heart failure (CHF) can develop when these abnormal circumstances persist.

Incidence of Arrhythmias

The frequency of cardiac arrhythmias found in a group of 500 cats at Angell Memorial Animal Hospital, Boston, MA, is presented in Table 1. These cases were collected over a 4-year period (July 1985 through June 1989) from cats presented for cardiac evaluation. All cats were examined clinically by thoracic radiography and with multiple lead electrocardiograms (ECGs). In most cats, both two-dimensional (2-D) and M-mode echocardiographic studies (ECHOs) were also recorded, although nonselective angiocardiographic studies were carried out in place of cardiac ultrasound in some cats and as an addi-

with Presumed Cardiopulmonary Disease

Mitral Insufficiency, Unknown Cause (n = 75)	Myocardial Disease, Other (n = 22)	Pleural Effusion, Noncardiac (n = 20)	Primary Pulmonary Disease (n = 11)	No Diagnosis (n = 12)	Systemic Hypertension (n = 6)	Pericardial Disease (n = 11)	Congestive Heart Failure Present (n = 103)
59 (78.7)	14 (63.6)	17 (85.0)	7 (63.6)	8 (66.7)	5 (83.3)	8 (72.7)	67 (65.0)
11 (14.7)	3 (13.6)	3 (15.0)	3 (27.3)	3 (25.0)	1 (16.7)	3 (27.3)	32 (31.1)
5 (6.7)	4 (18.2)	—	1 (9.1)	1 (8.3)	—	—	4 (3.9)
—	1 (4.5)	—	—	—	—	—	2 (1.9)
—	2 (9.1)	—	—	—	—	—	—
—	4 (18.2)	—	1 (9.1)	—	1 (16.7)	—	4 (3.9)
—	—	—	—	—	—	—	5 (4.9)
—	1 (1.5)	—	—	—	—	—	—
—	1 (4.5)	—	—	—	—	—	1 (1.0)
4 (5.3)	11 (50.0)	1 (5.0)	—	—	—	—	20 (19.4)
1 (1.3)	7 (31.8)	—	—	—	—	—	1 (1.0)

tional procedure in others. Postmortem examinations were performed when possible to confirm or broaden the clinical diagnosis.

Several headings in Table 1 need further clarification. All cats in the category "mitral insufficiency, unknown cause" had holosystolic murmurs of mitral valve incompetence (usually both left and right apex). However, many of these cats were aged and had other serious, noncardiac conditions, including renal insufficiency, anemia, hypoproteinemia, or neoplastic processes, or were young with totally normal cardiac studies. Echocardiographic studies demonstrated either changes consistent with a volume-overloaded left ventricle (i.e., left ventricular end-diastolic dimensions ranging from 1.5 to 1.8 cm with a fractional shortening of 55% or greater) accompanied by a normal-sized left atrium or a totally normal echocardiographic study. In addition, normal thyroxine (T_4) levels were required for all cats 7 years of age or older for inclusion in this category. The category "myocardial disease, other" consisted of cats with either known causes of myocardial disease (i.e., bacterial endocarditis, toxoplasmosis, traumatic myocarditis) or more commonly those with either bradyarrhythmias or tachyarrhythmias in the absence of definable abnormalities on thoracic radiography or echocardiography. The majority of cats in this group were young (range: 8 months to 14 years; mean: 5 years; median: 4 years). In the category "pericardial disease" the most common scenario was pericardial effusion as a consequence to either hypertrophic cardiomyopathy or hyperthyroidism and subsequent CHF. However, in four cats neither a primary cardiac condition nor a multisystem disorder could be identified to explain the pericardial effusion, and pericardial disease was felt to be the primary disorder. Lastly, cats fulfilling the criteria for the category "no diagnosis" were presented for some presumed cardiorespiratory problem and may or may not have had mild cardiac enlargement on survey thoracic radiographs. However, further cardiac studies were within normal limits, and heart disease was not considered significant or responsible for the clinical signs.

Overview of Rate and Rhythm Disturbances

Control of heart rate and rhythm in all warm-blooded animals is in large part the responsibility of the autonomic nervous system (ANS). The final product is largely determined by the mix of sympathetic (excitatory) and parasympathetic (inhibitory) input, which permits precise control of cardiac rate. In the normal cat, heart rhythm as controlled by discharge of the sinoatrial (SA) node is termed *normal sinus rhythm*. This is usually a regular rhythm, characterized on an ECG tracing by regularly occurring P waves with a fixed relationship to subsequent QRS-T complexes, occurring at a rate of 150 to 219/min. When the resting rate is 220/min or greater and the same P-QRS-T relationship exists, the term *sinus tachycardia* is used; *sinus bradycardia* describes the opposite extreme in which the heart rate is less than 150/min.

The incidence of sinus tachycardia differs in the various forms of heart disease (see Table 1). The high incidence of sinus tachycardia in the hyperthyroid group is expected, as thyroid hormones have both a direct stimulant effect on the heart and an exciting effect on the sympathetic nervous system (Bond, 1986). Other categories in which the frequency of sinus tachycardia exceeds 30% include severe cardiovascular stress states: "systemic thromboembolism," "CHF present," and "dilated cardiomyopathy." In the latter category, 70% of the cats were in biventricular heart failure with pleural effusion. Cats in the "congenital heart disease" category were considerably younger than those in the other categories (mean age: 10.4 months; median age: 6 months), making the previously defined criteria for sinus tachycardia of questionable validity.

Significant bradyarrhythmias occur far less frequently than tachyarrhythmias; of these latter arrhythmias, ventricular outnumber supraventricular by nearly 2:1. The high frequency of ventricular arrhythmias in the category "systemic thromboembolism" is not unexpected, as various contributing factors were present, including myocardial fibrosis, CHF, or thromboembolism to the myocardium. Acute myocardial strain or hypoxia probably account for many of the ventricular arrhythmias in the "CHF present" category, as the frequency of these tended to diminish significantly following stabilization of heart failure. The higher incidence of ventricular arrhythmia in the intermediate form of cardiomyopathy than with other forms of cardiomyopathy is more difficult to explain. More extensive myocardial fibrosis, inflammation, or other degenerative changes are strong considerations.

BRADYARRHYTHMIAS

By definition, bradyarrhythmia in the cat indicates a ventricular rate of less than 150/min. This may be the result of abnormal function of the sinoatrial node or interference with impulse conduction through the AV nodal region. Significant cardiac dysfunction is likely at rates of 100/min or less in the cat. Factors responsible for the development of bradyarrhythmias are outlined in Table 2.

Abnormalities of Impulse Generation (Sinoatrial Node Dysfunction)

Abnormalities in sinus node function include a slowing of the discharge rate (i.e., bradycardia) or

Table 2. *Factors Contributing to Cardiac Arrhythmia*

Arrhythmia	Spontaneous Causes	Drugs Responsible
Sinus node dysfunction	Organic heart disease Increased vagal tone Hyperkalemia Hypoxemia Acidosis Hypothermia	Digitalis Beta-adrenergic blockers Calcium channel blockers Quinidine Edrophonium Anesthetic agents
Atrioventricular conduction abnormalities	Organic heart disease Increased vagal tone Hyperkalemia Hypokalemia Endocarditis Amyloidosis	Digitalis Beta-adrenergic blockers Calcium channel blockers Procainamide Morphine derivatives Anesthetic agents
Supraventricular tachyarrhythmias	Organic heart disease (atrial enlargement with stretch, ischemia, focal necrosis/fibrosis) Hyperthyroidism Fever Neoplasia Shock, postshock Blunt chest trauma Hypertension (systemic) Hypothermia	Atropine sulfate Glycopyrrolate Sympathomimetic amines (epinephrine, dopamine, dobutamine, isoproterenol) Thyroid drugs Ketamine hydrochloride
Ventricular tachyarrhythmias	Organic heart disease Hyperthyroidism Shock, postshock Infection Fever Blunt chest trauma Neoplasia	Atropine sulfate Glycopyrrolate Sympathomimetic amines (epinephrine, dopamine, dobutamine, isoproterenol) Digitalis Thyroid drugs Aminophyllin Doxorubicin Anesthetic agents

complete failure of the sinus node to discharge (i.e., sinus arrest or sinus pause). Less commonly, functional abnormalities of the sinus node are the result of organic lesions within or surrounding the sinus node (i.e., sinoatrial block). Electrocardiographically, sinus arrest is characterized by a pause that is greater than the normal P-P interval, whereas in sinoatrial block the pause should be twice the P-P interval (i.e., 2 P-P) or some other multiple of this interval. The normal physiologic response to prolonged sinus arrest or sinoatrial block is the spontaneous firing of a subsidiary pacemaker in either the AV nodal region (i.e., junctional escape beat) or the ventricular conduction tissue (i.e., ventricular

escape beat). In some instances, early discharge of subsidiary pacemaker tissue interferes with the ability to differentiate between sinus arrest and sinoatrial block.

Abnormalities of sinus node function are infrequently identified in the cat. The most common cause of apparent sinus arrest (sinoventricular rhythm with absence of P waves) is hyperkalemia and possibly the associated hypocalcemia and metabolic acidosis that occurs with urethral obstruction of 24-hr duration or longer (Schaer, 1977). Treatment with sodium bicarbonate, calcium gluconate, and intravenous fluids following relief of the obstruction should be curative within 12 hr (Harpster, 1987). Sinus bradycardia is most commonly observed following anesthesia or the use of beta-adrenergic blocking agents for the management of hypertrophic cardiomyopathy or cardiac arrhythmias, or as a result of organic heart disease.

When high vagal tone influences are responsible for abnormalities in sinus node function, the administration of parasympatholytic agents such as atropine sulfate (0.044 mg/kg IV or IM) should be beneficial in the short-term setting (Fig. 1). In the cat in which a cause for the vagotonia cannot be identified or corrected, the use of orally administered parasympatholytic agents should be tried (i.e., propantheline bromide—1.5 to 3.0 mg/kg t.i.d. to q.i.d. or isopropamide [Darbid, Smith Kline & French] 2.5 to 5.0 mg/kg b.i.d. to t.i.d.). However, when clinical signs persist despite medical therapy and particularly when organic heart disease is responsible for the sinus node dysfunction, only permanent pacemaker implantation is likely to be curative.

Abnormalities in Atrioventricular Conduction

Conduction abnormalities include impedance to conduction in the AV node proper, the bundle of His, and the right and left bundle branches. Isolated abnormalities of conduction in the right or left bundle branch/fascicular system, and the fascicular block pattern seen most commonly in cats with hypertrophic cardiomyopathy cause a widening of the QRS complex or changes in the morphology of the QRS complex that are characteristic for each individual bundle/fascicular branch block. The presence of a bundle branch block implies at least a localized myocardial lesion and in many instances a more generalized myocardial disorder exists. However, the bundle branch block serves only as a marker, since clinical signs are absent and specific treatment is not warranted for these abnormalities. The reader is encouraged to consult standard textbooks of veterinary electrocardiography to review the characteristic changes in the QRS pattern that

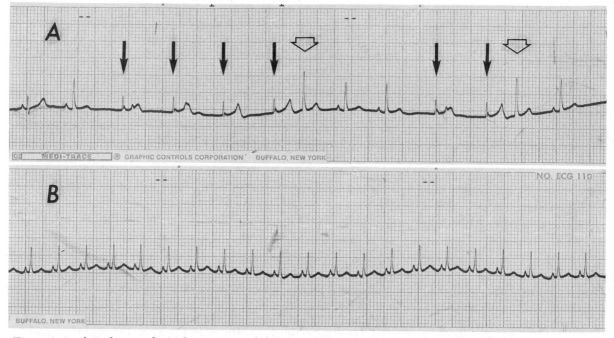

Figure 1. Lead II electrocardiographic strip recorded from an 18-month-old, male (N), domestic short-hair cat with allergic bronchitis. An electrocardiogram (ECG) was taken to further evaluate the slow resting heart rate. On the initial tracing (A), the sinus rate ranges from 85 to 95/min. A secondary pacemaker, probably from a high intraventricular septal focus, captures intermittent control of the heart rate at a rate of 100/min *(arrows)*. The higher-amplitude QRS complexes closely coupled to the intraventricular escape beats *(arrowheads)* are most likely of sinus origin but differ from the other sinus beats because of partial refractoriness of intraventricular conduction pathways. At 90 sec following administration of atropine sulfate (0.2 mg) intravenously (B), sinus node function is enhanced and captures control at 180/min, suggesting that vagal nerve influence may be partially responsible for the slow resting heart rate. (1 mV = 10 mm; 25 mm/sec)

attend these conduction abnormalities (Edwards, 1987; Tilley, 1985).

When alterations develop that affect conduction in the AV node proper, the bundle of His, or the proximal bundle branches bilaterally, more significant abnormalities in conduction can evolve. The mildest of these is termed first-degree AV block and is characterized by prolongation of the P-R interval to or beyond 0.11 sec while the QRS-T complexes should remain normal. As with the isolated bundle branch blocks, first-degree AV block is strictly an electrocardiographic phenomenon; the cat remains asymptomatic relative to the abnormality and treatment is not required unless an underlying cause is detected. Periodic ECG monitoring is warranted to identify progression to more severe AV conduction abnormalities.

Transition to more severe alterations in AV conduction is characterized by the presence of dropped beats, (i.e., the occurrence of P waves without the consistent accompaniment of QRS and T complexes). Mobitz type I second-degree AV block (Wenckebach phenomenon) is recognized by a progressive prolongation of the P-R interval until a P wave is blocked. The pattern seen electrocardiographically is an inconstant repetition pattern with every third to seventh P wave blocked. Mobitz type I second-degree AV block is most commonly an

effect of extracardiac influences rather than intrinsic organic heart disease. Increased vagal tone can be responsible, as well as a variety of pharmacologic agents that either enhance vagal tone, directly depress AV conduction tissue, or both (see Table 2). Organic heart disease is more commonly the cause of Mobitz type II second-degree AV block, which frequently progresses to more advanced forms of second-degree and to third-degree AV block. Mobitz type II AV block is characterized by an occasional blocked P wave, usually every fourth or fifth (i.e., 4:3 or 5:4 AV conduction ratio). The P-R interval of conducted beats may be normal or prolonged but is fixed, unlike the variation seen in Mobitz type I AV block. Advanced second-degree AV block is distinguished by a higher degree of block, usually with a fixed ratio of P wave to QRS-T complexes (i.e., 2:1, 3:1, 4:1). The P-R interval of conducted beats should be constant and is usually prolonged (Fig. 2). With third-degree AV block there is complete dissociation of the P waves and the QRS-T complexes. The P waves occur at the intrinsic rate of the SA node, while the QRS-T complexes occur much slower at the inherent rate of the secondary pacemaker tissue (AV junctional or ventricular in origin). The P-R interval is totally inconstant; QRS complexes tend to be wide and bizarre, their configuration determined by the site of origin of the

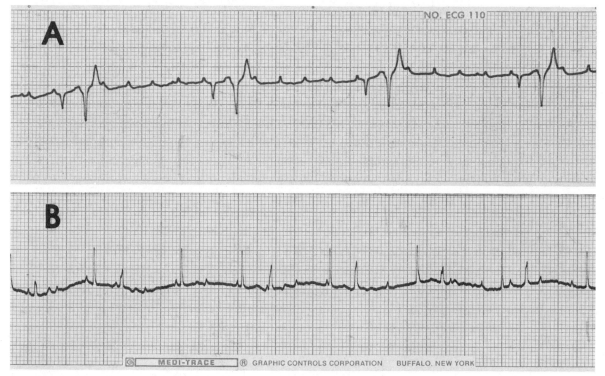

Figure 2. Lead II electrocardiographic recordings taken from a 12-year-old, male (N), Himalayan cat. In the initial tracing (*A*), the basic rhythm is sinus tachycardia at 230/min. However, only every sixth beat is conducted; this is advanced second-degree atrioventricular (AV) block. Note that the P-R interval of conducted beats is constant (0.09 sec). The widened QRS complex that follows the conducted beat is a ventricular premature or ectopic beat and is the result of a re-entry mechanism in the ventricles. This coupling pattern, called ventricular bigeminy, is commonly seen with AV conduction abnormalities. In the lower tracing taken 8 months later (*B*), the conformation of the QRS complexes is totally different; they are narrow, suggesting a supraventricular origin. Now, however, there is no fixed relationship between the P waves and the QRS complexes, implying progression to third-degree AV block. The secondary pacemaker is most likely originating in either an AV junctional or high intraventricular septal focus, and the bigeminal pattern persists as in *A* (i.e., now an AV junctional bigeminal rhythm). This cat had no clinical signs despite a functional heart rate of 68 to 75/min. (1 mV = 10 mm; 25 mm/sec)

secondary pacemaker tissue. The ventricular rate in *cats* should be under 120/min when the secondary pacemaker arises from an AV junctional focus and under 70/min from a secondary pacemaker at the ventricular level.

Specific management of Mobitz type I AV block is optional, as the conduction abnormality alone is not symptomatic. A thorough search is required to identify extracardiac influences that may be responsible and these factors corrected when possible. When therapy administered for other conditions appears responsible for the disturbance, drug dosages should be reduced or alternative agents substituted.

When Mobitz type II AV block is found, a complete investigation should be initiated to see if a specific cardiac cause can be established and corrected. If this proves fruitless and the cat's clinical signs appear unrelated to the conduction abnormality, a periodic re-evaluation program should be instituted. Progression to more severe forms of AV block frequently occurs. In cats, intermittent, high-grade, second-degree or third-degree AV block is

not uncommon. Periods of block may precipitate syncope at home; however, following presentation to the veterinarian, only normal sinus rhythm or sinus tachycardia may be recorded. Intermittent conduction disturbances like these require diligence and a high level of suspicion to diagnose, and identification may require sequential ECGs or Holter ECG monitoring.

Unfortunately, the more advanced forms of AV block are almost invariably the result of organic heart disease and are largely unresponsive to medical therapy. If there are relevant clinical signs (i.e., lethargy, weakness, syncopal episodes), progressive cardiac enlargement by thoracic radiography or echocardiography, or CHF, then only permanent pacemaker implantation is likely to provide a long-term benefit (see this volume, p. 708).

Supraventricular Tachyarrhythmias

The term supraventricular tachyarrhythmia implies early discharge from a focus (or foci) in the

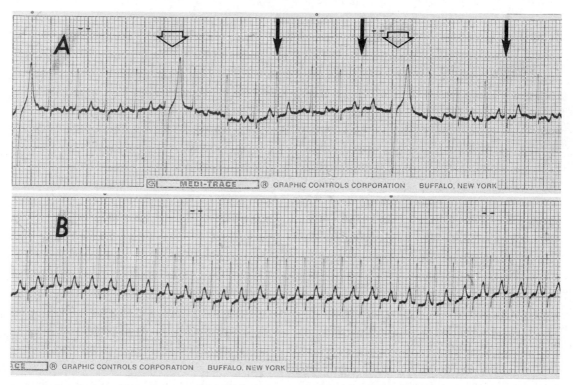

Figure 3. Lead II electrocardiographic strips recorded from a 16-year-old, female (S), domestic long-hair cat with hyperthyroidism. In *A*, the basic rhythm is normal sinus at approximately 200/min, but this is interrupted frequently by both singly occurring supraventricular premature beats *(arrows)* and ventricular premature beats *(arrowheads)*. During ECG recording there were intermittent bursts of supraventricular tachycardia at 300/min as seen in *B*. (1 mV = 10 mm; 25 mm/sec)

atrial or AV junctional tissue for a single or a series of beats. The mildest of these, *supraventricular premature (ectopic) beats,* are characterized electrocardiographically by the early inscription of a QRS complex with a configuration identical or similar to that of the normal QRS complex that follows sinus node discharge. Identifiable P waves may or may not precede supraventricular premature beats. Exceedingly early discharge from an atrial focus frequently results in obliteration of the atrial depolarization wave by the antecedent T wave. Premature beats originating in the AV junctional tissue frequently result in simultaneous depolarization of the atria and ventricles, causing simultaneous inscription of the P wave and QRS complex and obscuring the P wave. When P waves are recognizable, they tend to be positive (i.e., upward deflection in lead II) when the ectopic focus arises in the upper or middle portions of the atria, whereas the P waves are negative (i.e., downward deflection) when the ectopic focus is in the lower atrial regions or within the confines of the AV junctional tissue.

Supraventricular premature beats are usually a consequence of atrial myocardial disease, particularly atrial enlargement and stretch and focal areas of necrosis that are seen with cardiomyopathies, advanced stages of hyperthyroidism, and certain congenital anomalies. Other potential associations

include neoplastic processes (i.e., lymphoma, metastatic pulmonary neoplasms), severe infections (i.e., endocarditis, septicemia), pericarditis, and blunt chest trauma. The administration of parasympatholytic drugs (i.e., atropine, glycopyrrolate) and the sympathomimetic amines (i.e., epinephrine, dopamine, isoproterenol, etc.) may also be responsible (see Table 2). Specific treatment of isolated supraventricular premature beats is not warranted. A thorough workup should be undertaken to identify the nature of the underlying disease process. Treatment of the cardiac or extracardiac condition responsible for the premature beats may be helpful in reducing their frequency.

A series of consecutive supraventricular premature beats constitutes a *supraventricular tachycardia*. When intermittent (i.e., starting and stopping abruptly), it is commonly referred to as *paroxysmal supraventricular tachycardia* (PSVT). Similar to supraventricular premature complexes, PSVT may be accompanied by positively deflected P waves (i.e., paroxysmal atrial tachycardia) or by negatively deflected P waves (i.e., paroxysmal AV junctional or re-entrant tachycardia). However, P waves are rarely seen except following a vagal maneuver (Fig. 3).

Etiologic considerations for PSVT are similar to those for supraventricular premature beats, but the

Table 3. Therapeutic Options in Supraventricular Tachyarrhythmias

Arrhythmia	Hypertrophic Cardiomyopathy	Hyperthyroidism	Intermediate or Dilated Cardiomyopathy
Paroxysmal supraventricular tachycardia*	Diltiazem 7.5 to 15 mg t.i.d. *or* Propranolol 2.5 to 5.0 mg t.i.d. Verapamil 0.05 mg/kg IV over 15 min, repeat to 0.2 mg/kg IV	Methimazole 5.0 mg b.i.d. to t.i.d. *and* Propranolol 2.5 to 5.0 mg t.i.d. *or* Diltiazem 7.5 to 15 mg t.i.d.	Digoxin 0.031 mg q 48 hr *and/or* Propranolol 1.25 to 2.5 mg b.i.d. to t.i.d.
Atrial flutter	Diltiazem 7.5 to 15 mg t.i.d. *or* Propranolol 2.5 to 5.0 mg b.i.d.	Same	Digoxin 0.031 mg q 48 hr alone, *or* in combination with Diltiazem 7.5 to 15 mg t.i.d. *or* Propranolol 1.25 to 2.5 mg b.i.d. to t.i.d.
Atrial fibrillation*	Propranolol 2.5 to 5.0 mg b.i.d. *or* Diltiazem 7.5 to 15 mg t.i.d.	Same	Digoxin 0.031 mg q 48 hr alone, *or* in combination with Diltiazem 7.5 to 15 mg t.i.d. *or* Propranolol 1.25 to 2.5 mg b.i.d. to t.i.d.

*For the acute termination of accelerated paroxysmal supraventricular tachycardia and atrial fibrillation, a vagal maneuver should be tried initially. The response to a vagal maneuver may be enhanced by a single intravenous injection of digoxin (0.03 to 0.06 mg).

similarity ends there. Paroxysmal supraventricular tachycardia is not a benign arrhythmia. It is commonly associated with atrial and associated ventricular heart rates of 280 to 400/min. Intermittent heart rates in this range can result in syncopal episodes, while prolonged tachycardia can lead to weakness, CHF, and sudden death. The initial treatment of choice is a vagal maneuver (i.e., carotid sinus massage, eyeball pressure) to terminate the tachycardia. If this fails, either verapamil or adenosine can be effective therapy. A thorough evaluation should then be initiated to determine a specific cause or the nature of the underlying heart disease; evaluation should include thoracic radiographs, complete laboratory testing (including T_4 level), and an echocardiogram. When active CHF is present, aggressive management of CHF alone (i.e., thoracentesis, intravenous furosemide, oxygen therapy) may be extremely beneficial. Beyond this, specific therapy is based on the nature of the underlying heart disease (Table 3).

Atrial flutter is extremely rare in the cat, whereas atrial fibrillation is recognized more commonly than PSVT. Atrial fibrillation, from an electrophysiologic standpoint, is the result of continuous, chaotic depolarization of the atria, with impulses arriving frequently and irregularly at the AV node. Conduction to the ventricles occurs whenever the AV nodal region is in a nonrefractory state. Electrocardiographically, it is characterized by an absence of P waves, which are replaced by either an isoelectric baseline or fine, irregularly occurring fibrillation (f) waves and a totally irregular ventricular response (i.e., marked variation in R-R intervals, but with QRS duration usually normal or only mildly prolonged) (Fig. 4).

Etiologic implications for atrial fibrillation in the cat are similar to those for the other supraventricular tachyarrhythmias (see Table 2). In general, atrial fibrillation suggests a more chronic, advanced form of heart disease, usually cardiomyopathy, and a poorer long-term prognosis. Management is directed first at control of the normally present heart failure, then specific treatment is instituted based on the underlying form of heart disease (see Table 3). The author suggests a therapeutic goal of maintenance of the ventricular rate at 150/min or less for cats with hypertrophic cardiomyopathy and other causes of left ventricular hypertrophy and between 180 and 220/min when other forms of heart disease are present. Thromboembolism is a common and life-threatening complication of acquired heart disease in the cat; whenever the echocardiographic left atrial to aortic ratio exceeds 1.25:1, the use of antithrombogenic agents (i.e., aspirin 1.25 grains every 48 hr or 2.50 grains twice weekly) should be routine.

Ventricular Pre-Excitation Syndrome

Ventricular activation earlier than would be expected from conduction over normal AV pathways is termed *ventricular pre-excitation*. The accelerated AV conduction occurs via an accessory pathway that partially or completely bypasses the AV node.

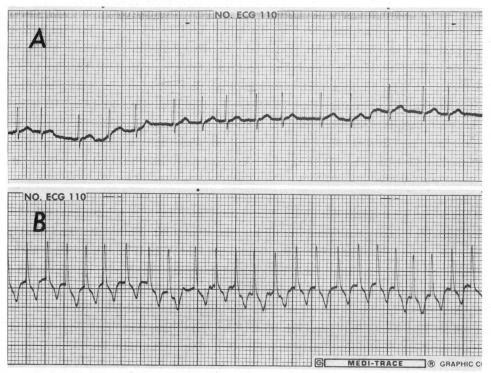

Figure 4. Examples of feline electrocardiograms demonstrating atrial fibrillation. In *A*, taken from a 10-year-old, male (N), domestic long-hair cat with intermediate (i.e., restrictive) feline cardiomyopathy, note the totally irregular ventricular rhythm and the absence of P waves. This cat was receiving digoxin at the time this tracing was taken, which explains the normal heart rate of 180/min. Similar ECG findings are seen in *B*, but the ventricular rate is accelerated to 270/min. This recording was taken from a 6-year-old, male (N), domestic short-hair cat with hypertrophic cardiomyopathy; treatment had not been started at the time of this tracing. (1.0 mV = 10 mm; 25 mm/sec)

Ventricular pre-excitation syndrome (VPS) is the occurrence of a tachyarrhythmia as a result of this defect and has been reported in both the dog and the cat (Flecknell et al., 1979; Hill and Tilley, 1985; Ogburn, 1977).

The electrocardiographic features of ventricular pre-excitation include a short P-R interval (usually with a prolongation of the QRS duration) and a delta wave (Fig. 5). The delta wave refers to the initial deflection of the QRS complex, which is slowed and deformed, indicating early activation of part of the ventricle by the accessory pathway. These characteristic ECG findings are diagnostic of the classic Wolff-Parkinson-White type of ventricular pre-excitation. Sometimes the only electrocardiographic abnormality is a short P-R interval, the QRS interval being normal and the delta wave absent. This is the pattern expected with the atriofascicular tract accessory pathway, often referred to as the Lown-Ganong-Levine syndrome (Lown et al., 1952).

These various manifestations of VPS have in common a tendency for the development of a tachycardia as a result of the two separate AV pathways linking together and establishing a circulus movement between the atria and the ventricles. The resulting tachycardia may be paroxysmal or sus-tained, and while the QRS complexes may be narrow suggesting a supraventricular origin, more commonly they have a bizarre conformation with widening of the QRS.

Only rarely will cats develop syncopal episodes or acute CHF as a sequelae to VPS. The disorder is usually recognized when cats are being evaluated for some other cardiac or pulmonary condition, and the resting ECG provides the diagnosis. However, when a cat is presented with syncopal-like episodes and the ECG supports a diagnosis of VPS, a thorough workup and treatment is required. This could include a period of ECG monitoring if an appropriate system is available, although most Holter monitoring systems are too bulky for normal-sized cats. It has been reported that the majority of cats with VPS also have hypertrophic cardiomyopathy (Hill and Tilley, 1985), but this has not been a strong association in the author's experience.

A general approach to the medical management of VPS is presented in Figure 6. In theory, there are certain therapeutic agents with a significant effect on inhibiting conduction in the AV node, while other agents have a greater effect on inhibition of conduction in the accessory pathway. Only encainide and amiodarone have a significant effect on both pathways in human patients. Treatment should

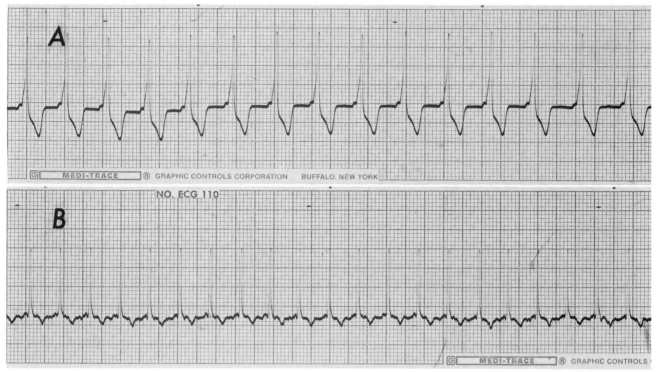

Figure 5. Electrocardiographic recordings from two cats exhibiting several different patterns seen with ventricular pre-excitation. The classic Wolff-Parkinson-White (WPW) pattern is seen in *A*, also called Kent's bundle syndrome and the AV connection. Note the short P-R interval, wide QRS interval, and the delta wave (i.e., the initial slur seen in the upstroke of the QRS complex). This tracing was taken from an 18-month-old, male (N), domestic short-hair cat with an intermediate form of cardiomyopathy. This cat had several acute episodes of weakness associated with a tachycardia (ventricular rate to 340/min). The narrow QRS interval associated with the Lown-Ganong-Levine form of ventricular pre-excitation is presented in *B*. This form has also been called the James fibers syndrome and the atriofascicular tract variety. Notice the short P-R interval, normal QRS interval, and absence of a delta wave. This tracing was recorded from a 3-year-old, male (N), Siamese cat with dilatative cardiomyopathy. Both leads are base-apex. (1.0 mV = 10 mm; 25 mm/sec)

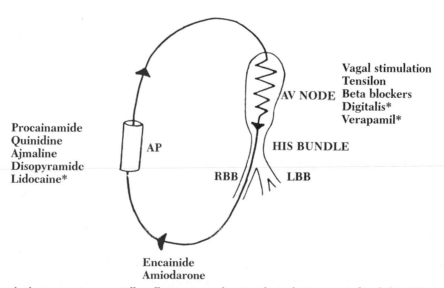

Figure 6. Antiarrhythmic agents potentially effective in prolonging the refractory periods of the AV conduction pathways responsible for recurrent tachyarrhythmias in the pre-excitation syndrome. Drugs on the left exert their major effect on the accessory pathway (AP), while those on the right have a predominant influence on the AV node. Encainide and amiodarone prolong the refractory periods of both pathways. An *asterisk* indicates agents that can increase the ventricular response during atrial fibrillation by increasing the number of pre-excited QRS complexes. RBB, right bundle branch; LBB, left bundle branch.

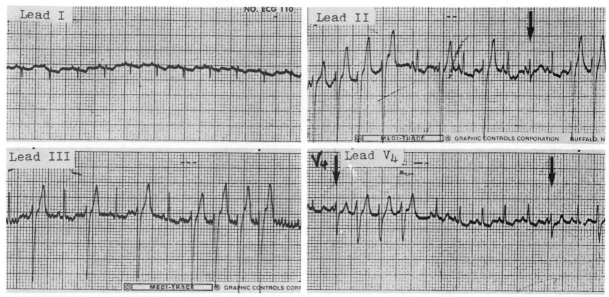

Figure 7. Four-lead electrocardiogram recorded from a 4-year-old, male (N), domestic short-hair cat with an intermediate form of cardiomyopathy. The basic rhythm as seen in lead I is normal sinus at 175/min. The remaining leads show electrocardiographic evidence of ventricular irritability on the basis of frequent ventricular premature beats, fusion beats *(arrows)*, and short runs of paroxysmal ventricular tachycardia (to 270/min). The base-line interference in lead III is an artifact. This cat had a recent thromboembolic episode (i.e., saddle embolus). It is assumed that coronary thromboembolism was in part responsible for these arrhythmias. (1.0 mV = 10 mm; 25 mm/sec)

be considered in the cat with VPS and proved tachycardia as well as in the cat with a history of syncopal episodes that have typical ECG findings of VPS. In the management of a cat with both hypertrophic cardiomyopathy and VPS, propranolol or other beta-adrenergic–blocking agents (at 2.5 to 5.0 mg t.i.d.) would seem a reasonable starting point. If syncopal episodes of tachycardia persist despite adequate control of the sinus node rate (i.e., 150/min or less), then the addition of procainamide (62.5 mg t.i.d.) or quinidine sulfate (31 to 62 mg t.i.d.) should be considered. When dilated cardiomyopathy and VPS coexist, digoxin is preferable to propranolol (though there are potential concerns if the cat should develop atrial fibrillation) because of potentially greater benefit to overall myocardial performance.

Ventricular Tachyarrhythmias

Ventricular tachyarrhythmia is characterized by the occurrence of single or repetitive ventricular premature complexes (VPCs). Isolated ventricular premature complexes appear to be the most benign of ventricular arrhythmias in cats, particularly when they occur infrequently and are of the same configuration (i.e., uniform, unifocal). A potentially more serious circumstance exists when VPCs occur frequently and are of varying configuration (i.e., multiform or multifocal). The occurrence of two consecutive ventricular premature beats is termed a *pair*,

three is termed a *run*, and four or more is called *paroxysmal ventricular tachycardia* (PVT). Even though ventricular arrhythmias occurred 50% more frequently than all other arrhythmias combined (see Table 1), the majority of these were of the infrequent, singly occurring, benign variety.

Electrocardiographically, ventricular arrhythmias are distinguished by widened, bizarre QRS complexes that differ significantly from those QRS complexes that result from sinus node discharge. Although P waves may be seen interspersed among the VPCs, there should be no fixed relationship between them. With PVT, the ventricular rate should be 150/min or greater in the cat, unless antiarrhythmic therapy is being administered (Fig. 7). When the PVT rate is 100 to 150/min, it is not considered a tachycardia and has been termed an enhanced ventricular rhythm or idioventricular tachycardia (Tilley, 1985). This latter ECG pattern could easily be confused with *atrioventricular dissociation* in which the atria and ventricles are discharging independently of one another but at nearly the same rates. Atrioventricular dissociation is not an arrhythmia per se but a descriptive term caused by a mismatch between the sinus node discharge rate, the rate of firing of a secondary pacemaker focus (i.e., from an AV junctional or ventricular position), and the intrinsic rate of conduction via the AV node. With AV dissociation, the sinus node is responsible for depolarizing the atria, while the secondary pacemaker is independently depolarizing the ventricles. Even though the relationship be-

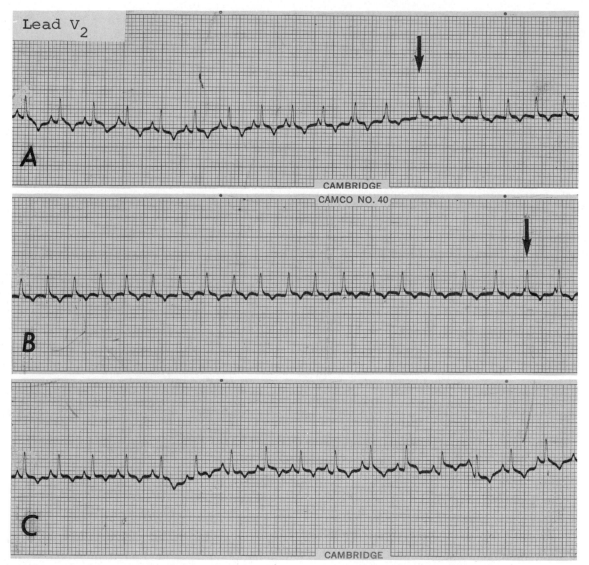

Figure 8. Continuous lead V_2 electrocardiographic recording taken from a 10-year-old, female (S), domestic long-hair cat with systemic hypertension. In *A*, note that the P-R interval gradually shortens until the P wave completely disappears *(arrow)*. This is accompanied by a constancy of the QRS conformation, but there is a gradual acceleration of the ventricular rate from 175 to 200/ min. The P waves remain obscured until the last two complexes in *B (arrow)*, when they begin to emerge. Note that the reappearance of the P waves is again associated with a change in the ventricular rate. This electrocardiographic abnormality is called accelerated idioventricular rhythm or AV dissociation; it is the result of two independent and unassociated pacemakers that occur at nearly equal rates, one controlling the rate of the atria (usually the sinus node) and the other the rate of the ventricles (usually arising in the lower portions of AV node or proximal interventricular septum). When the rates differ slightly, as in *A* and *B*, the term accrochage has been used. In *C*, the rates of the two pacemakers have apparently become equal and constant, as the P-R interval remains at 0.09 sec. This pattern of a constant rate relationship between two separate pacemakers has been termed synchrony. These ECG abnormalities have been reported secondary to digitalis administration and myocardial disease. (1.0 mV = 10 mm; 25 mm/sec)

tween the P waves and the QRS-T complexes appears fixed during a short tracing, the two are occurring independently of one another (Fig. 8).

Ventricular arrhythmias can be the result of a variety of cardiac and extracardiac conditions and influences (see Table 2) but are far more commonly detected in cats with significant heart disease. This is clearly demonstrated in Table 1 by the low incidence of ventricular arrhythmias in cats with

congenital heart disease, primary pleural or pulmonary disease, and those without defined heart disease (no diagnosis) as compared with the combined group of cats with cardiomyopathy (i.e., hypertrophic, intermediate, and dilatative) in which the incidence was 20.5% (54/264).

Treatment of singly occurring ventricular premature beats and probably even coupled ventricular premature beats is not warranted provided there are no related clinical signs. (The ideal approach for coupled ventricular premature beats is a 12- or 24-hr period of ECG monitoring to evaluate for potentially more serious arrhythmias). Runs of ventricular premature beats and episodes of PVT should be treated aggressively, as the potential for compromised cardiac function and sudden death is a concern. Malignant ventricular arrhythmias can be successfully treated with either lidocaine (0.5 to 1.0 mg/kg bolus over 5 min followed by an infusion at 10 to 20 mcg/kg/min [beware of neuroexcitability]) or procainamide (1.0 to 2.0 mg/kg bolus followed by an infusion at 10 to 20 mcg/kg/min). Alternatively, the author has used intramuscular procainamide (7.5 to 15 mg/kg) with good success in some cats. Another method is slow intravenous injection of propranolol (0.25 to 0.50 mg over 3 to 5 min) followed by full oral doses (2.5 to 5.0 mg t.i.d.). For chronic management of serious ventricular arrhythmias, the author has used procainamide (10 to 20 mg/kg t.i.d.), quinidine sulfate (10 to 20 mg/kg t.i.d.), and propranolol (2.5 to 10.0 mg t.i.d.). In several cats, procainamide and propranolol have been used in combination with some improvement over the effect of either drug used alone. Some of the newer antiarrhythmic agents have been tried in a few cats, but the sample size is too small to arrive at any conclusions.

A few words of caution should be voiced concerning the aggressive management of ventricular arrhythmias in cats. Electrocardiographic monitors should be used in patients that are receiving intravenous infusions. Intravenous boluses and infusions of lidocaine can result in neurotoxicity (i.e., depression, seizure) and pacemaker depression. The treatment of choice for this complication is diazepam (0.25 to 0.5 mg/kg IV). Similar reactions can occur with intravenous administration of procainamide but much less frequently. Intravenous administration of propranolol can cause marked hypotension; this drug should be given slowly with ECG monitoring, and only to effect. Finally, the chronic oral administration of quinidine sulfate can result in gastrointestinal signs, particularly a reduced appetite and diarrhea. These intolerance problems may require reducing the dosage or even stopping the quinidine.

References and Suggested Reading

Bond, B. R.: Hyperthyroid heart disease in cats. *In* Kirk, R. W. (ed.): *Current Veterinary Therapy IV*. Philadelphia: W. B. Saunders, 1986, pp. 399–402.

Chung, K. V., Walsh, T. J., and Messre, E.: Wolff-Parkinson-White Syndrome. Am. Heart J. 69:116, 1965.

Edwards, N. J.: *Bolton's Handbook of Canine and Feline Electrocardiography*. 2nd ed. Philadelphia: W. B. Saunders, 1987.

Flecknell, P. A., Gruffydd-Jones, E. L. C., Brown, C. M., et al.: A case of suspected ventricular pre-excitation in the cat. J. Small Anim. Pract., 2:57, 1979.

Gallagher, J. J., Sealy, W. C., Anderson, R. W., et al.: Cryosurgical ablation of accessory atrioventricular connections: A method for correction of the pre-excitation syndrome. Circulation 55:471, 1977.

Harpster, N. K.: The cardiovascular system. *In* Holzworth, J. (ed.): *Diseases of the Cat*, Vol. 1. Philadelphia: W. B. Saunders, 1987, p. 909.

Hill, B. L., and Tilley, L. P.: Ventricular pre-excitation in seven dogs and nine cats. J.A.V.M.A. 187:1026, 1985.

Katz, L. N., and Shaffer, A. B.: The effect of cardiac arrhythmias on the performance of the heart. *In* Dreifus, L. S., and Likoff, W. (eds.): *Mechanisms and Therapy of Cardiac Arrhythmias*. New York: Grune & Stratton, 1966, pp. 1–20.

Lown, B., Ganong, W. F., and Levine, S. A.: The syndrome of short P-R interval, normal QRS complex and paroxysmal rapid heart action. Circulation 5:693, 1952.

Ogburn, P. N.: Ventricular pre-excitation (Wolff-Parkinson-White syndrome) in a cat. J. Am. Anim. Hosp. Assoc. 13:171, 1977.

Prystowsky, E. N., Miles, W. M., Heger, J. J., et al.: Pre-excitation syndrome: Mechanisms and management. Med. Clin. North Am., 68:831, 1984.

Schaer, M.: Hyperkalemia in cats with urethral obstruction. Electrocardiographic abnormalities and treatment. Vet. Clin. North Am. 7:407, 1977.

Sealy, W. C., Gallagher, J. J., and Wallace, A. C.: The surgical treatment of Wolff-Parkinson-White syndrome: Evolution of improved methods for identification and interruption of the Kent bundle. Am. Thorac. Surg., 22:443, 1976.

Tilley, L. P.: Feline cardiac arrhythmias. Vet. Clin. North Am. 7:273, 1977.

Tilley, L. P.: *Essentials of Canine and Feline Electrocardiography*. 2nd ed. Philadelphia: Lea & Febiger, 1985.

THERAPY OF SUPRAVENTRICULAR TACHYCARDIA AND ATRIAL FIBRILLATION

ROBERT L. HAMLIN
Columbus, Ohio

Heart rate is an extremely important parameter of cardiovascular function, and when it exceeds requirements for meeting the metabolic demands of the body, serious consequences may result (Berne and Levy, 1967). In particular, elevation of heart rate increases demand of the myocardium for oxygen and coronary blood flow that carries it, decreases time for coronary blood flow, and decreases time for ventricular filling to an extent that end-diastolic volume is inadequate to permit a forceful contraction. Heart rate may be elevated when the ventricles are driven too rapidly as a result of waves of depolarization entering them through the atrioventricular (AV) transmission system from supraventricular foci (i.e., foci "above" the ventricles).

Supraventricular tachycardias may originate from the sinoatrial (SA) node, from the specialized conductile pathways (internodal tracts) that extend from the SA node to the AV node, or from the tissue around the AV node (i.e., junctional tissue), but usually not from the AV node proper. Supraventricular tachycardias develop most commonly in dogs and cats with extremely large left atria as caused by mitral regurgitation (in small dogs), dilated cardiomyopathy (in large dogs), or hypertrophic cardiomyopathy (in cats). They occur less often in patients with patent ductus arteriosus, tricuspid and mitral valve dysplasia, ventricular septal defect, or aortic stenosis—congenital heart defects in which the atria may enlarge. Supraventricular tachycardias seem to require stretch of atrial myocardial fibers for their occurrence (Boyden et al., 1982). They occur uncommonly with only right atrial enlargement. Thyrotoxicosis (in cats), atrial myocardial fibrosis, and neoplasia have been incriminated in their origin. Junctional tachycardias occur rather frequently as a result of digitalis intoxication.

The clinical and electrocardiographic features of various supraventricular tachycardias have been described elsewhere (see *CVT X*, p. 271). The purpose of this article is to review the most recent experience in the therapy of supraventricular tachyarrhythmias and atrial fibrillation.

RECOGNITION

Supraventricular tachycardias may be recognized best by electrocardiography and must be considered in any dog or cat with an extremely rapid heart rate (Fig. 1). Atrial fibrillation is also recognized best by electrocardiography (Fig. 2) and should be suspected in dogs or cats that (1) are known to have long-standing heart disease, (2) have rapid and irregularly irregular heart rates, and (3) have many fewer femoral pulsations than heartbeats (i.e., pulse deficit) (Bohn et al., 1971; Bolton and Ettinger, 1971; Bonagura and Ware, 1986; Johnson, 1985). Supraventricular tachycardias may occur as short bursts (i.e., paroxysms) or may be sustained (i.e., the beginning or end of the tachycardia is not observed). They are recognized electrocardiographically by (1) a rapid heart rate, (2) QRS complexes and ST-T segments that are (usually) normal or nearly normal for the particular dog or cat, and (3) P waves that are either absent or immediately preceding or following the QRS complex (in junctional tachycardias) or bizarre in contour (in atrial tachycardias) (see *CVT X*, p. 271, for details of these rhythm disturbances).

Supraventricular tachycardias may occasionally generate wide QRS complexes with ST-T complexes that appear nearly identical with those that occur with ventricular tachycardia. The P waves may be buried within the ST-T complex and be virtually invisible. This is termed a *wide QRS supraventricular tachycardia*. The pattern occurs because the AV conduction system is bombarded so quickly by the rapidly discharging supraventricular pacemaker that the impulses are conducted with bundle branch block. It may be virtually impossible to differentiate wide QRS supraventricular tachycardia from ventricular tachycardia by conventional electrocardiography unless P waves are identified within the ST-T-complex.

TREATMENT

Treatment of supraventricular tachycardias is focused on terminating the rapidly discharging supra-

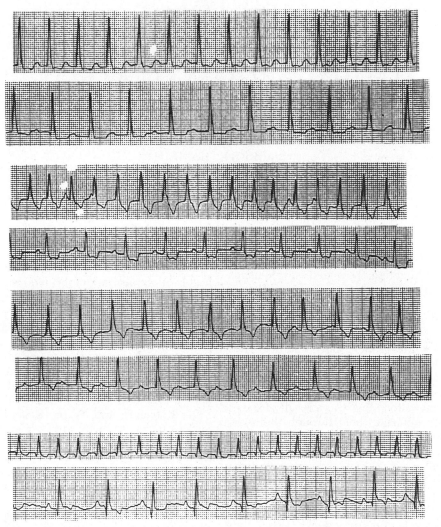

Figure 1. Electrocardiograms (ECGs) from four dogs (*A through D*) with supraventricular tachycardias. In each ECG, records were taken before (*top*) and after diltiazem (*bottom*). Notice the dramatic deceleration in heart rate after therapy.

ventricular pacemaker or decreasing the likelihood of sustaining a circus path; if that is impossible, slowing the ventricular response is the goal. It may be difficult in some circumstances to distinguish a persistent sinus tachycardia from a regularly discharging or conducing ectopic atrial tachycardia. Similarly, atrial flutter can be conduced regularly into the ventricle, and re-entrant supraventricular tachycardia is often quite regular. Atrial fibrillation, conversely, is a straightforward diagnosis because the ventricular rate response is irregular. Generally speaking, sinus tachycardia is treated by first controlling the underlying cardiac disorder. Before heroic efforts are made to terminate supraventricular tachycardia, the pet should be monitored at home to make certain that the tachycardia is not analogous to "white coat" hypertension in humans—hypertension resulting only from interaction with the physician in the office or hospital. If the tachycardia is sinus in origin and is caused by pain or

excitement, when these causes are eliminated, the tachycardia should abate.

Stimulation of the trigeminal-vagal reflex by applying pressure to almost any point on the head—in particular to the eyeballs—may increase vagal efferent traffic sufficiently to abolish the tachycardia (Besbasi, 1989). Emetics such as apomorphine may also abolish the tachycardia via increment in vagal efferent traffic. To avoid injury to the globe, applied pressure should not exceed 50 mm Hg (practice pushing in a blood pressure cuff). A vagal maneuver may not be sufficient to abolish a regular supraventricular tachycardia (especially when the rhythm is unrelated to AV nodal re-entry); however, it may be diagnostically helpful by causing transient AV conduction delay, which can unmask underlying atrial flutter or tachycardia.

Some supraventricular tachycardias appear to develop in conjunction with sympathetic activity or anxiety. Beta-blocking drugs like propranolol (0.5

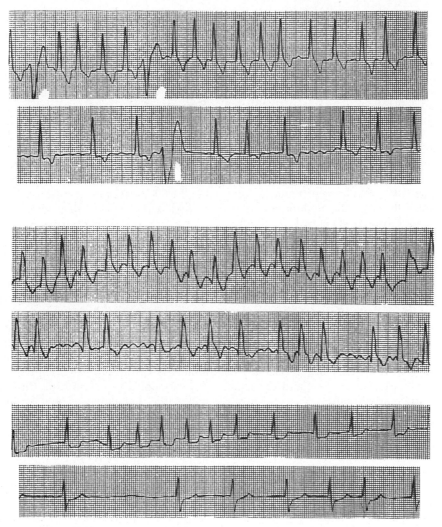

Figure 2. ECGs from three dogs (*A through C*) with atrial fibrillation. In each ECG, records were taken before (*top*) and after (*bottom*) treatment with diltiazem. As in Figure 1, notice the dramatic deceleration in heart rate after therapy.

to 1.0 mg/kg PO b.i.d. to t.i.d.) and atenolol (1 mg/ kg PO once daily) may be beneficial in these cases. Even tranquilizing drugs like diazepam (0.5 mg/kg PO t.i.d. for dogs, b.i.d. for cats) may achieve clinical benefit. If beta-adrenergic blockers are used, the veterinarian must be cautious of the potential for an acute asthmatic episode provoked by blocking the bronchodilator, beta-2 receptors or for worsening of heart failure as a result of negative inotropism of beta-blockers. An ultra–short-acting beta blocker—esmolol (100 to 200 μg/kg/min IV)— may be given (Platia et al., 1989). With esmolol, the beta-blocking activity stops almost immediately after the intravenous infusion is discontinued, so the veterinarian can determine if the beta-blocker terminates the tachycardia or if it provokes asthma or worsens heart failure.

For more resistant and often more rapid and serious tachycardias, more aggressive action is needed. Digitalis glycosides (of which digoxin [0.005

mg/kg PO b.i.d. dogs or cats] is the compound used most commonly) or calcium channel blockers (of which diltiazem [0.5 to 1.5 mg/kg PO b.i.d. to t.i.d. for dogs or cats] is the best), alone or in combination with each other or with a beta-blocker, will terminate most supraventricular tachycardias or will slow the rapid ventricular response with atrial fibrillation (Liu et al., 1984; Salerno et al., 1989) (see Figs. 1 and 2). Increases in AV nodal refractoriness can also be achieved with the newly released drug adenosine (Adenocard).

For dogs with documented nonsinus tachycardia and neither clinical symptoms nor signs of heart failure, my preference is to use diltiazem as monotherapy. In almost all instances, diltiazem slows the ventricular response or terminates the supraventricular tachycardia. If the tachycardia accompanies heart failure, I usually give the recommended oral daily dose of digitalis on day 1 and every day thereafter, and on day 2 begin diltiazem and titrating the dose incrementally. Although diltiazem may slightly decrease myocardial contractility, it also decreases left ventricular afterload and should result in little or no substantial decrease in left ventricular performance (Kulick et al., 1987).

I believe that many dogs with supraventricular tachycardias and most dogs with atrial fibrillation due to dilated cardiomyopathy manifest down-regulation of beta receptors (Waagstein et al., 1975). Therefore, I often give small doses of beta-blockers (1) to promote up-regulation of beta receptors, (2) to further slow the heart rate, (3) to counter the tendency of digitalis to provoke ventricular ectopy, and (4) to attempt to decrease the amount of digitalis or diltiazem or both required to control the rhythm. The value of this therapy is speculative.

My experience has been that small dogs with minimal cardiomegaly often have very rapid supraventricular tachycardias that terminate easily with diltiazem and can be maintained in sinus rhythm with minimal doses of beta-blockers. Large dogs with dilated cardiomyopathy or small dogs with severe mitral regurgitation and pendulous left atrial enlargement most often have atrial fibrillation that requires tritherapy with digitalis and diltiazem (and sometimes a beta-blocker) to achieve and to sustain a satisfactory ventricular response.

WHAT IS THE DESIRED HEART RATE?

When supraventricular tachycardias are abolished, the heart rate does not have to be adjusted further because it usually achieves a value determined by existing autonomic activity or metabolic demands. However, when treating atrial fibrillation, unless treatment causes conversion to a sinus rhythm, therapy must be sustained in order to keep the ventricular rate from accelerating. Before the availability of diltiazem and propranolol, when only digitalis—which exerts its cardiac slowing via a vagal route—was used, determining a final rate was no problem because nontoxic doses of digitalis would only cause slowing to a modest degree. However, by double or even triple drug therapy* (i.e., digitalis, diltiazem, propranolol), we are able to decrease the ventricular rate to any degree we desire—some that may be too low to sustain cardiac output. In particular, the question arises about how high heart rate should be in patients with atrial fibrillation because they lack the atrial contribution to ventricular filling. Because the atrial "kick" is

absent, some argue that heart rate must be more rapid to account for the reduction in left ventricular end-diastolic volume resulting from lack of the atrial contraction (Atwood et al., 1988). On the other hand, enlarged hearts may be more efficient at slower heart rates (Barany, 1967; Guth et al., 1987; Harrison et al., 1984); and because many dogs and cats with atrial fibrillation have significant cardiomegaly, it may be that the target heart rate should be even lower than for a heart of normal size. Our counterparts in human cardiology treating people with atrial fibrillation seek heart rates in the range of 60 to 90 beats per minute because patients seem to feel better when their rates are in that range. There are no data supporting that range as permitting maximal cardiac output and regional distribution of cardiac output or minimal left atrial pressure and pulmonary congestion, nor do we have data on optimal heart rates for dogs or cats. This shortcoming is compounded by the fact that heart rate measured in the hospital is usually significantly higher than at home. Thus I instruct the owners on how to take heart rate by auscultation of the thorax with an inexpensive ($6) stethoscope when the animal is resting quietly. They count the numbers of beats per 15 sec, multiply the number by four, and write that down as the resting heart rate. In my opinion, a target range should be between 70 and 110 beats per minute for dogs and 80 to 140 beats per minute for cats. If the pet appears active at rates as low as 60 or as high as 120 for dogs or 160 for cats, I am not concerned.

My clinical impression is that prognosis is more favorable in dogs with dilated cardiomyopathy and in atrial fibrillation in which heart rate can be kept in the acceptable range. Prognosis appears still more favorable if the deceleration in heart rate can be achieved with either monotherapy or various combinations of digitalis/diltiazem/propranolol.

References and Suggested Reading

Atwood, J., Myers, J., and Sullivan, M.: Maximal exercise testing and gas exchange in patients with chronic atrial fibrillation. J. Am. Coll. Cardiol. 11:508, 1988.

Barany, M.: ATPase activity of myosin correlated with the speed of muscle shortening. J. Gen. Physiol. 50:197, 1967.

Berne, R., and Levy, M.: Cardiovascular Physiology. St. Louis: C.V. Mosby, 1967.

Besbasi, F.: Studies on Sinus Node Function in the Dog. Ph.D. Dissertation, The Ohio State University, Columbus, OH, 1989.

Bigger, J., and Goldreyer, B.: The mechanism of supraventricular tachycardia. Circulation 42:673, 1970.

Bohn, F., Patterson, D., and Pyle, L.: Atrial fibrillation in dogs. Br. Vet. J. 127:485, 1971.

Bolton, G., and Ettinger, S.: Paroxysmal atrial fibrillation in the dog. J.A.V.M.A. 158:64, 1971.

Bonagura, J., and Ware, W.: Atrial fibrillation in the dog: Clinical findings in 81 cases. J. Am. Anim. Hosp. Assoc. 22:111, 1986.

Boyden, P., Tilley, L., and Pham, T.: Effects of left atrial enlargement on atrial transmembrane potentials and structure in dogs with mitral valve fibrosis. Am. J. Cardiol. 49:1896, 1982.

Guth, G., Heusch, G., Seitelberger, R., et al.: Elimination of induced

---

Editors' Note: The combined use of digoxin, diltiazem, and a beta-blocker should be approached cautiously, because each drug depresses AV nodal conduction and the beta-blockers and calcium channel blockers can depress myocardial contractility. Most dogs tolerate digoxin plus additional agents well if the drug is initiated at a low dose and titrated to an effective dose based on resting heart rate response.

regional myocardial dysfunction by a bradycardic agent in dogs with chronic coronary stenosis. Circulation 75:661, 1987.

Harrison, T., Ashman, R., and Larson, R.: Congestive heart failure: The relation between the thickness of the cardiac muscle fiber and the optimum rate of the heart. Arch. Intern. Med. 49:151, 1934.

Hoffman, B., and Rosen, M.: Cellular mechanisms for cardiac arrhythmias. Circ. Res. 49:1, 1981.

Johnson, J.: Conversion of atrial fibrillation in two dogs using verapamil and supportive therapy. J. Am. Anim. Hosp. Assoc. 21:429, 1985.

Kulick, D., McIntosh, N., Campese, V., et al.: Central and renal hemodynamic effects and hormonal response to diltiazem in severe congestive heart failure. Am. J. Cardiol. 59:1138, 1987.

Liu, S., Peterson, M., and Fox, P.: Hypertrophic cardiomyopathy and hyperthyroidism in the cat. J.A.V.M.A. 185:52, 1984.

Maragno, I., Santostasi, G., Gaion, R., et al.: Low- and medium-dose diltiazem in chronic atrial fibrillation: Comparison with digoxin and correlation with drug plasma levels. Am. Heart J. 116:385, 1988.

Platia, E., Michelson, E., Porterield, J., et al.: Esmolol versus verapamil in the acute treatment of atrial fibrillation or atrial flutter. Am. J. Cardiol. 63:925, 1989.

Salerno, D., Dias, V., Kleiger, R., et al.: Efficacy and safety of intravenous diltiazem for treatment of atrial fibrillation and atrial flutter. Am. J. Cardiol. 63:1046, 1989.

Waagstein, F., Hjalmarson, A., Varnauskas, E., et al.: Effect of chronic β-adrenergic blockade in congestive heart failure. Br. Heart J. 37:1022, 1975.

Wit, A., and Cranefield, P.: Reentrant excitation as a cause of cardiac arrhythmias. Am. J. Physiol. 235:H1, 1978.

INHERITED SUDDEN CARDIAC DEATH IN GERMAN SHEPHERDS

N. SYDNEY MOISE
and ROBERT F. GILMOUR, Jr.
Ithaca, New York

Ventricular arrhythmias (ectopy) are among the most common cardiac arrhythmias seen in dogs and cats. Ventricular ectopy includes premature ventricular complexes, ventricular bigeminal or trigeminal rhythms, ventricular couplets or runs, and ventricular tachycardia. Animals with ventricular ectopy frequently have some structural abnormality of the heart (e.g., dilated cardiomyopathy, mitral insufficiency, congenital heart disease) or systemic abnormality affecting the heart (e.g., acidosis, hypoxia, septicemia). The incidence of ventricular ectopy in dogs without identifiable structural cardiac disease is only 0.17%, with a 0% incidence of ventricular tachycardia (Patterson et al., 1961). The purpose of this chapter is to describe German shepherds that have inherited ventricular ectopy and sudden cardiac death without any identifiable structural lesions.

CLINICAL PRESENTATION

Affected dogs are usually detected during routine examination for other purposes (e.g., vaccinations, deworming, neutering). Most are between 4 and 12 months of age. The arrhythmias are diagnosed by electrocardiography after auscultation reveals an irregular rhythm. Other than the irregular rhythm and associated pulse deficits, physical examination is normal, as are blood chemistries, electrolytes, thoracic radiographs, and echocardiograms (Fig. 1). Dogs are not syncopal, have no exercise intolerance,

and appear robust, energetic, and healthy (Fig. 2). Male and female dogs are affected with equal frequency. Owners may report that siblings have died of unknown causes. Death is most common between 4 and 8 months of age and frequently occurs during sleep or during rest following exercise. A prodrome to the sudden death is absent. Breeding studies confirm that this disorder is inherited, although the means of inheritance has not yet been determined.

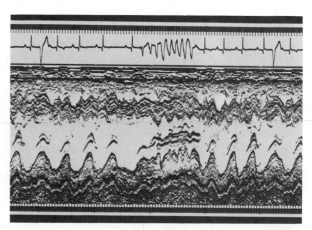

Figure 1. M-mode echocardiogram and simultaneous electrocardiogram recorded from a German shepherd with rapid, nonsustained ventricular tachycardia. The echocardiogram was normal. The dog died during sleep at 1 year of age. Routine postmortem examination could not identify the cause of death. (Paper speed 50 mm/sec.)

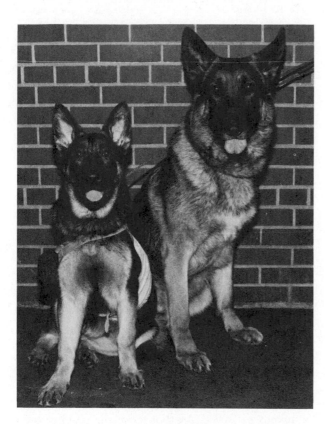

Figure 2. Five-month-old German shepherd with sire. The dog is wearing a Holter monitor harnessed to its body. This dog appeared healthy and active, but died while sleeping in its pen 2 hr after this photograph was taken and the monitor removed.

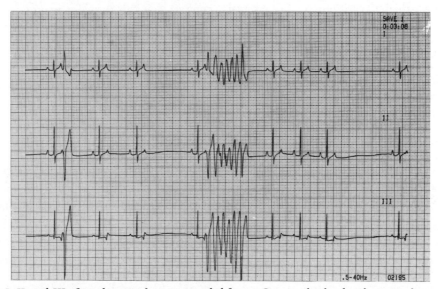

Figure 3. Leads I, II, and III of an electrocardiogram recorded from a German shepherd with ventricular arrhythmias. Four of this dog's siblings died during sleep between 16 and 18 weeks of age. This dog was examined because the referring veterinarian auscultated an arrhythmia. (Paper speed 25 mm/sec; 1 cm = 1 mV.)

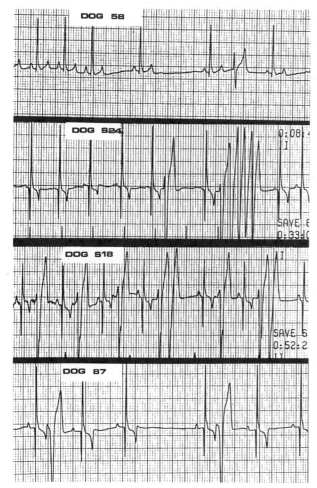

Figure 4. Lead II electrocardiogram recorded from four related German shepherds with ventricular ectopy. These electrocardiograms show the spectrum of ventricular ectopy, including single premature ventricular complexes (dogs 58 and 87), ventricular bigeminy and couplets (dog S18), and nonsustained ventricular tachycardia (dog S24).

of dying. Sustained ventricular tachycardia (greater than 30 complexes) is not characteristic. Because dogs are not syncopal yet die suddenly, ventricular fibrillation is the presumed fatal arrhythmia.

TREATMENT

Approximately 50% of affected dogs with ventricular tachycardia will die suddenly within the first year of life. Preliminary studies indicate that intravenous lidocaine and procainamide are effective antiarrhythmics, although controlled studies of oral therapy are not complete. However, therapy with oral procainamide in either the regular or slow-release form (15 and 20 mg/kg every 6 hr and every 8 hr, respectively) is recommended. Close monitoring for efficacy, ideally by Holter monitoring, is recommended. If 24-hr monitoring is not possible, long rhythm strips (10 to 15 min) should be recorded before therapy to establish the baseline frequency and severity of the arrhythmia and should be repeated after at least five doses of procainamide. The rhythm strips should be recorded approximately 3 to 4 hr after oral medication is given. If the frequency of ventricular ectopy has not decreased by 75 to 90%, the dosage of procainamide should be increased.* If the frequency of ventricular ectopy has increased substantially, a proarrhythmic effect should be considered and the medication changed to quinidine. Although this type of rhythm monitoring is less ideal when compared to repeated Holter monitoring, it provides a crude quantitation of drug efficacy. Preliminary data suggest that dogs that survive past 2 years of age have a decreased frequency of ectopy. When this is documented, antiarrhythmic therapy is not necessary.

ELECTROCARDIOGRAPHY

Electrocardiography and 24-hr, ambulatory Holter monitoring reveal variations in the frequency and type of ventricular ectopy. Some dogs have only a few premature complexes, others have frequent ventricular bigeminy and ventricular couplets, and others have rapid salvos of ventricular tachycardia (Figs. 3 and 4). Some dogs have occasional supraventricular premature complexes. Preliminary studies suggest that the ventricular ectopy is enhanced during sinus bradycardia and that dogs with ventricular tachycardia are at the greatest risk

References and Suggested Reading

Moise, N. S., Gilmour, R. F., Jr., and Meyers-Wallen, V.: Inherited ventricular ectopy and sudden death in young German shepherd dogs. J. Am. Coll. Cardiol. 15:152A, 1990.

Patterson, D. F., Detweiler, D. K., Hubben, K., et al.: Spontaneous abnormal cardiac arrhythmias and conduction disturbances in the dog. Am. J. Vet. Res. 22:355, 1961.

Sisson, D. D.: The clinical management of cardiac arrhythmias in the dog and cat. In Fox, P., (ed.): Canine and Feline Cardiology. New York: Churchill Livingstone, 1988, p. 289.

Tilley, L. P.: Essentials of Canine and Feline Electrocardiography. 2nd ed. Philadelphia: Lea & Febiger, 1985.

*Editors' Note. Evaluation of serum procainamide concentrations may be useful in dosage adjustment (therapeutic range is 4 to 10 µg/ml and in some cases up to 20 µg/ml).

UPDATE: INFECTIVE ENDOCARDITIS

WILLIAM P. THOMAS

Davis, California

Although the normal heart is quite resistant to infection by microorganisms, cardiac infections occasionally develop in bacteremic patients, especially when there are certain pre-existing cardiac defects. The term *infective endocarditis* is applied to such cardiac microbial infections, almost all of which occur as vegetative lesions on heart valves and are caused by bacteria in dogs and cats. The major clinical features of endocarditis in humans have been known for many years, although advances in antemortem diagnosis and in both medical and surgical therapy have markedly improved the survival rate compared with the preantibiotic era. The main changes in the human disorder over the past decade have involved improved understanding of pathogenesis, improved diagnosis by echocardiography, changes in patient populations (fewer congenital cardiac lesions, more infections of prosthetic valves, more infections caused by intravenous drug abuse), evolution of new antimicrobial therapy, and controversy over recommendations regarding risk and prophylactic therapy for patients with certain cardiac defects who are undergoing potentially bacteremic procedures. The clinical features of infective endocarditis have been reviewed in detail elsewhere (Finch et al., 1987; Weinstein, 1988; Woodfield and Sisson, 1989). It is important to understand that, although experimental endocarditis in animals has contributed to our understanding of the pathogenesis of this disorder, most of the information on diagnosis, therapy, and prevention that follows has been derived from extensive human patient studies and limited reports on dogs.

PATHOGENESIS

Factors in Establishing Vegetative Lesions

It is well established that bacteria enter the blood stream frequently, both during invasive (surgical) procedures and during seemingly more innocuous procedures, especially those involving trauma to mucosal surfaces (such as urinary catheterization and dental scaling). Such bacteremia is normally transient, asymptomatic, and readily cleared by the combined action of circulating antibodies and circulating or fixed phagocytic cells. Bacteremia may also result from a localized infection (e.g., abscess, metritis, pyoderma). The endocardial surfaces of the heart valves and walls are normally resistant to adherence and colonization by circulating bacteria. The primary site of microbial proliferation is usually on a platelet-fibrin thrombus caused by a pre-existing lesion of the endocardium. These lesions are usually produced by turbulent hemodynamic forces such as a regurgitant jet or Venturi effects around an abnormal heart valve or congenital lesion. Establishment of an infective vegetative lesion within the heart is believed to depend on a combination of the following factors: (1) bacteremia, which may be transient; (2) a previously damaged valve or abnormal hemodynamic setting (shunt, jet lesion, or other turbulence caused by congenital or acquired disease); (3) a small, sterile platelet-fibrin thrombus that forms at the site of endocardial disruption; and (4) a high titer of agglutinating antibodies against the infecting organism, which causes clumping and increases the inoculum. However, many cases in dogs (and probably cats) occur without an identifiable pre-existing congenital or acquired valvular lesion, and an obvious source of bacteremia may also be lacking.

Locations

In the dog and cat, as in most monogastric species, the mitral and aortic valves are most commonly affected. Infection of the tricuspid or pulmonary valves is rare, and mural (wall) endocarditis is considered extremely rare or nonexistent.

Common Organisms

Organisms reported to be most often recovered in dogs with endocarditis include *Staphylococcus aureus, Streptococcus, Corynebacterium, Pseudomonas aeruginosa, Erysipelothrix rhusiopathiae, Escherichia coli,* and *Aerobacter aerogenes.* The reported list, however, is long and includes both common and many uncommon organisms. Consequently, it is usually difficult to make an educated guess at the offending organism in the absence of culture confirmation.

752

Predisposing Conditions

Other factors predisposing to endocarditis include prolonged bacteremia caused by pathogenic organisms from other contaminated or infected sites (e.g., areas of metritis, periodontitis, or indwelling catheters) and decreased host resistance (e.g., concurrent disease, immunosuppressive therapy). The German shepherd and boxer dog breeds appear to be overrepresented in clinical reports, and large-breed male dogs older than 4 years of age are most often affected. Although pre-existing cardiac lesions are thought to be associated with infective endocarditis, no obvious relationship between myxomatous degeneration of the mitral valve and increased susceptibility to endocarditis of this valve has been established. However, a moderately strong association between congenital discrete subaortic stenosis and increased susceptibility to endocarditis of the aortic valve has been reported.

DIAGNOSIS

Other than direct histologic demonstration of bacteria within a vegetative lesion, there are no clinical findings that provide a definitive antemortem diagnosis of endocarditis. It is important to remember that each clinical sign exhibited by a patient with endocarditis is nonspecific and has many possible causes (hence the designation of the disease as the "great imitator"). The clinical diagnosis therefore usually results from a combination of clinical findings that, grouped together, define a syndrome that makes the probability of endocarditis very high. Clinical signs can be grouped into three major categories: (1) signs of infection or septicemia, (2) signs of cardiac involvement, and (3) signs of systemic complications due to embolization, metastatic infection, or immune phenomena. The most common clinical features of infective endocarditis follow.

Physical Examination

In the early stages the presence of fever and complaints of lethargy, depression, and anorexia may be the only findings, providing little to distinguish cardiac infection from many other febrile illnesses. Signs of infection include fever, which is often intermittent (cyclic) and temporarily responsive to antibiotic therapy. Occasionally there is evidence of a primary infection such as mastitis, metritis, prostatitis, or abscess. Signs of systemic organ involvement may include arthralgia/myalgia with lameness and poorly localized pain, often intermittent and shifting. Myocardial infarction or abscess may occur, and arrhythmias are common in endocarditis. Embolization or infarction of a variety of sites may result in a constellation of clinical signs, including:

1. Splenic infarction with splenomegaly (uncommon) or abdominal pain
2. Renal infarction or glomerulopathy causing hematuria or polyuria
3. Oral or cutaneous petechiae (uncommon)
4. Discospondylitis (dogs) or osteomyelitis with pain and weakness
5. Central nervous system and ocular embolization causing acute onset of seizures, paresis, blindness, or retinal hemorrhage
6. Gastrointestinal infarction with abdominal pain, vomiting and diarrhea
7. Major peripheral artery embolization leading to acute paralysis and loss of arterial pulse to the affected limb (uncommon)

Signs of heart failure usually include some combination of dyspnea, tachypnea, cough, fatigue, lethargy, and weight loss. Heart murmurs are usually the result of valve regurgitation and may change (usually becoming louder) during the course of the disease. Acquired murmurs of valvular stenosis are an uncommon result of endocarditis.

Auscultatory findings can be briefly summarized as follows:

1. Mitral valve: systolic regurgitant quality murmur over the affected valve. Remember that mitral regurgitation (due to myxomatous degeneration) is very common in older dogs and is not generally associated with endocarditis.
2. Aortic valve: early systolic and decrescendo diastolic murmurs over the affected valve and ventricle. Development of an aortic diastolic murmur in a dog is significant, because infective endocarditis is the most frequent cause of aortic regurgitation in dogs and usually results in congestive heart failure. Exaggerated (bounding) arterial pulses attend advanced aortic regurgitation.
3. Arrhythmias: very common, especially with aortic valve infection (dogs). Premature beats, tachycardia, and pauses due to atrioventricular (AV) block may cause syncope.
4. Signs of heart failure develop in advanced cases, and an S_3 gallop may be heard over the left ventricle.
5. Tricuspid, pulmonic valves: murmurs of valvular insufficiency accompanied by jugular vein distention and/or pulse, hepatomegaly, edema (ascites, pleural effusion, peripheral edema, depending on the species).

Electrocardiography/Radiography

In the early stages of endocarditis, the electrocardiogram (ECG) and chest radiographs are usually normal. Arrhythmias and conduction disorders are common in dogs, including ventricular premature contractions; ventricular tachycardia; atrial fibrillation; first-, second-, or third-degree AV block; and left bundle branch block (LBBB). Increased P-wave duration and QRS voltages from left atrial and ventricular enlargement occur in advanced aortic or mitral valve regurgitation. Radiography reveals variable and nonspecific cardiomegaly that is usually mild in acute cases.

Echocardiography

Multiple echoes from vegetative lesions are seen on the affected valve(s), usually during diastole. Secondary dilation of the atrium and/or ventricle subjected to the abnormal volume load from the regurgitating valve occurs. Aortic valve regurgitation commonly causes fine fluttering of the anterior mitral valve leaflet in diastole (M mode). Echocardiography is not diagnostic in all cases.

Laboratory Studies (Including Blood Culture/Sensitivity)

Laboratory abnormalities are variable and may include neutrophilic leukocytosis, anemia, elevated erythrocyte sedimentation rate, hematuria, pyuria, proteinuria, bacteremia, and increased total hemolytic complement. Other abnormalities depend on organ involvement and the presence of heart failure, and diffuse intravascular coagulopathy (DIC) is a common preterminal finding. Blood culture may be positive; the timing of blood sampling is not critical, because the bacteremia of endocarditis is usually continuous. Three venous samples (ideally 10 ml each) are obtained over 2 to 24 hr, depending on urgency, and aerobic and anaerobic cultures are taken for 7 to 14 days. Positive cultures are expected in 60 to 80% of cases, but individual laboratory results vary widely.

In summary, the diagnosis of infective endocarditis should be considered in any animal with unexplained fever, cardiac abnormalities, signs compatible with embolic phenomena, or unexplained multisystem disease. A positive antemortem diagnosis of infective endocarditis usually requires positive blood cultures associated with signs of cardiac involvement and embolic phenomena. A positive diagnosis can also be made with or without a positive blood culture by echocardiographic demonstration of a valvular vegetation associated with fever and signs of embolic phenomena. A *presumptive* diagnosis of infective endocarditis in the absence of a positive blood culture or echocardiographic vegetations may be warranted in an animal with fever, leukocytosis, previously diagnosed congenital or ac-

quired valvular or septal defect, a new or changing murmur, or signs of embolic phenomena.

The differential diagnosis of infective endocarditis includes other noncardiac viral or septicemic bacterial infections; generalized immunologic disease (e.g., systemic lupus erythematosus, noninfectious polyarthritis); neoplastic disease (lymphoma, leukemia); primary renal, neurologic, musculoskeletal, or other abdominal disease (depending on extracardiac complications); and other noninfective valvular or myocardial disorders.

THERAPY

The medical management of infective endocarditis requires treatment of the septicemic infection, including the cardiac infection and other sites of involvement, and management of cardiac and extracardiac complications. To be successful, therapy usually must be initiated early, must be aggressive, and requires careful monitoring, often for several weeks or months. It therefore should be understood at the outset that this is a comparatively expensive undertaking. The following principles are adapted from current recommendations for management of human infective endocarditis (Finch et al., 1987; Weinstein, 1988).

Treatment of Infection

First, establish a microbiologic diagnosis by blood culture. Whenever possible, blood culture identification of the infecting organisms should *precede* antimicrobial therapy. In most cases, the hours required to obtain two to three blood cultures will not adversely affect the course of the disease. Only when severe sepsis threatens to overwhelm the patient should antibiotic therapy be initiated prior to blood culture collection. Antimicrobial sensitivity testing by disk or broth dilution for minimal inhibitory concentration (MIC) or minimal bactericidal concentration (MBC) should be used to select one or more antibiotics (also see *CVT X*, pp. 1077–1081 and 1363–1364).

Second, administer bactericidal antibiotics parenterally in bactericidal doses. Ideally, drugs should be given intravenously for 4 to 6 weeks, but this is impractical in dogs and cats. More often, antibiotics are given parenterally for 7 to 10 days and continued orally at home for at least 6 weeks, well beyond the point of apparent clinical improvement. In culture-negative cases, consider administering a combination of penicillin, ampicillin, or oxacillin plus gentamicin or amikacin. Perform frequent physical examinations during treatment and repeat blood cultures after starting treatment and 1 to 2 months following completion of therapy.

Complications

CARDIAC COMPLICATIONS. Congestive heart failure requires medical treatment with cardiac glycosides, diuretics, and vasodilators. Arrhythmias should be managed as needed with appropriate pharmacotherapy or pacing.

SYSTEMIC COMPLICATIONS. Treat predisposing conditions and complications. Abscesses, periodontal disease, mastitis, or other sites of infection may require surgical treatment. Anticoagulant therapy is contraindicated except when DIC exists.

Although animals with pre-existing valvular or congenital heart disease may be at increased risk of endocarditis during spontaneous or induced bacteremia, the routine use of oral antibiotic prophylaxis immediately before and for 24 hours after dental or other invasive procedures, as recommended in humans, has not been studied. Such prophylaxis is probably advisable in selected patients (e.g., those with aortic stenosis). Parenteral ampicillin with or without gentamicin or cephalothin is often used.

Prognosis

The prognosis for animals with infective endocarditis depends on the virulence of the organism and its susceptibility to available antibiotics, the location and severity of valvular damage and resultant hemodynamic effects, and the nature and severity of extracardiac complications. Successful treatment often depends on early diagnosis and aggressive therapy before the development of severe cardiac or extracardiac complications. The prognosis in all cases is guarded, and is considered extremely guarded to poor in the presence of aortic valve endocarditis with regurgitation, congestive heart failure, renal failure, multisystemic complications, or a resistant organism.

References and Suggested Reading

Anderson, C. A., and Dubielzig, R. R.: Vegetative endocarditis in dogs. J. Am. Anim. Hosp. Assoc. 20:149, 1984.
A retrospective study of the clinical and pathologic features of infective endocarditis in 40 dogs.

Bennett, D., and Taylor, D. J.: Bacterial endocarditis and inflammatory joint disease in the dog. J. Small Anim. Pract. 29:347, 1987.
Clinical and pathologic features of 12 dogs with infective endocarditis and infective or noninfective joint disease.

Calvert, C. A.: Valvular bacterial endocarditis in the dog. J.A.V.M.A. 180:1080, 1982.
Clinical and pathologic features of 61 dogs with presumed (17 cases) or confirmed (44 cases) infective endocarditis.

Calvert, C. A.: Endocarditis and bacteremia. In Fox, P. R. (ed.): *Canine and Feline Cardiology.* New York: Churchill Livingstone, 1988, p. 419.
A review of the clinical features of dogs with bacteremia and/or infective endocarditis.

Finch, R. G., Shanson, D. C., and Littler, W. A. (eds.): Infective endocarditis. Based on a scientific meeting of the British Society for Antimicrobial Chemotherapy. J. Antimicrob. Chemother. 20, Suppl. A:1, 1987.
A review of current knowledge and recommendations concerning infective endocarditis in humans.

Harpster, N. K.: The cardiovascular system. In Holzworth, J. (ed.): *Diseases of the Cat. Medicine and Surgery,* Vol. 1. Philadelphia: W. B. Saunders, 1987, p. 820.
A review of current knowledge of cardiovascular disease in cats, with a brief review of limited available information on infective endocarditis.

Lombard, C. W., and Buergelt, C. D.: Vegetative bacterial endocarditis in dogs: Echocardiographic diagnosis and clinical signs. J. Small Anim. Pract. 24:325, 1983.
Clinical and echocardiographic features of infective endocarditis in 10 dogs.

Shouse, C. L., and Meier, H.: Acute vegetative endocarditis in the dog and cat. J.A.V.M.A. 129:278, 1956.
Clinical and pathologic features of infective endocarditis in 27 dogs and 13 cats.

Sisson, D., and Thomas, W. P.: Endocarditis of the aortic valve in the dog. J.A.V.M.A. 184:570, 1984.
A retrospective study of the clinical features of 24 dogs with infective endocarditis of the aortic valve.

Weinstein, L.: Infective endocarditis. In Braunwald, E. (ed.): *Heart Disease. A Textbook of Cardiovascular Medicine,* 3rd ed. Philadelphia: W. B. Saunders, 1988, p. 1093.
A review of current knowledge of infective endocarditis in humans.

Woodfield, J. A., and Sisson, D.: Infective endocarditis. In Ettinger, S. J. (ed.): *Textbook of Veterinary Internal Medicine,* 3rd ed. Philadelphia: W. B. Saunders, 1989, p. 1151.
A review of current knowledge of infective endocarditis in dogs and cats.

CARDIOVASCULAR COMPLICATIONS OF FELINE HYPERTHYROIDISM

GILBERT JACOBS
Athens, Georgia

and DAVID PANCIERA
Madison, Wisconsin

The diagnosis and treatment of uncomplicated hyperthyroidism in cats have been discussed in detail elsewhere (Feldman and Nelson, 1987; Peterson, 1989) and in this volume (p. 334). The cardiovascular manifestations of hyperthyroidism have attracted considerable attention because they can be dramatic. Fortunately, in feline hyperthyroidism, serious clinical cardiovascular manifestations are uncommon, and primary treatment of the hyperthyroid state may be conducted without significant delay or risk. In some cases, however, cardiac and circulatory abnormalities that develop require a clinician's specific attention. In this situation, definitive treatment of the hyperthyroid state is often delayed while intensive cardiovascular drug intervention is undertaken. Knowledge of the cardiovascular manifestations of hyperthyroidism and the role of the adrenergic nervous system in hyperthyroidism is important in the rational management of hyperthyroid cats.

CARDIOVASCULAR COMPLICATIONS

The explanations for the cardiac and circulatory changes in hyperthyroidism are exceedingly complex and are related to (1) the direct effects of thyroid hormone on cardiac muscle, (2) the effects of the interaction of the adrenergic nervous system with thyroid hormone on cardiac function, and (3) the indirect effects of hyperthyroidism, via altered cardiac function and adrenergic tone, on the peripheral vascular system.

Other biologic effects of thyroid hormone include increased thermogenesis, basal metabolic rate, and tissue oxygen demand. These effects add further to the complexity of hyperthyroidism's influence on the cardiovascular system because they impose an increased need for oxygen and metabolic substrate delivery to peripheral tissues and require removal of the increased heat that is liberated. It is clear that thyroid hormone has diverse and potentially profound effects on the cardiovascular system.

Hyperdynamic Circulation

In an effort to meet the increased metabolic demands of the body, one of the earliest and most consistent cardiovascular changes produced by excessive thyroid hormone is a hyperdynamic circulation. This situation is characterized by a decline in systemic vascular resistance, widened pulse pressure, and an increase in heart rate, cardiac contractility, cardiac output, blood volume (plasma volume and red blood cell mass), and oxygen consumption. Clinically, these changes may be detected as tachycardia, hyperdynamic femoral artery pulse and precordial impulse intensity, heart murmurs, and cardiac enlargement.

The hyperdynamic circulation is attributable, at least in part, to heightened sympathoadrenal activity. The exact mechanism involved in the interaction between thyroid hormone and sympathoadrenal activity in the heart and circulation has not been clarified. Increased cardiac beta-adrenergic receptor number and sensitivity to catecholamines and increased myocardial catecholamine levels have been proposed. Thyroid hormone also has direct tissue action on the heart, including direct positive chronotropic (increased heart rate) and inotropic (enhanced myocardial contractility) activities.

Systemic Hypertension

Increases in cardiac output and blood volume associated with hyperthyroidism may raise arterial pressure, and systemic hypertension appears to be a common sequela of feline hyperthyroidism. Retinopathies resembling those associated with hypertension have been observed occasionally in hyperthyroid cats.

Hypertrophic Cardiomyopathy

Excess thyroid hormone can lead to cardiac muscle hypertrophy. Remarkable concentric ventricular hypertrophy may develop, justifying the term *secondary hypertrophic cardiomyopathy* (Liu et al., 1984). Seemingly, based on ultrasonographic assessment, the degree of hypertrophy is modest in most instances. It is likely that the degree of hypertrophy depends largely on the duration and severity of the hyperthyroid state. Cardiac hypertrophy in hyperthyroid cats may be detectable electrocardiographically, usually as increased R-wave amplitudes consistent with left ventricular enlargement. Ultrasonography may reveal increased ventricular wall thickness. Although this has not been studied in cats, severe hypertrophy may impair diastolic function of the heart and contribute to atrial dilation and congestive heart failure (CHF). Distortion of the mitral valve apparatus, contributing to mitral regurgitation and cardiac murmurs, can also result from severe left ventricular hypertrophy.

Several mechanisms have been postulated to explain cardiac hypertrophy in hyperthyroidism. Tachycardia and increased contractility associated with hyperthyroidism impose an increased work load and metabolic demand on the heart. If sustained, this increase in cardiac work and metabolic demand activates synthetic processes, leading to hypertrophy. Thyroid hormone also stimulates cardiac hypertrophy directly by activation of protein-synthesizing processes.

Furthermore, it has been shown in hyperthyroidism that a greater fraction of the heart's adenosine triphosphate is consumed by heat production rather than for contractile purposes. This reduced efficiency combined with the increased work load may provide an explanation about why hyperthyroidism can lead to cardiac failure. Atrioventricular (AV) valvular regurgitation may contribute to the stimulus to hypertrophy and the tendency to develop CHF. Rate- and rhythm-related impairments in ventricular function probably also contribute to myocardial dysfunction in some patients.

Congestive Heart Failure

About 15% of cats with hyperthyroidism develop clinical signs and radiographic evidence of CHF. A term used to describe the hyperdynamic circulatory changes associated with hyperthyroidism, if congestion develops, is *high-output heart failure*. The circulatory changes may be manifested as cardiac dilation (particularly of the atria), pulmonary arterial and venous distention, and sometimes pulmonary edema on thoracic radiography. Ventricular hypertrophy may be observed by ultrasonography, and cardiac wall motion is often hyperdynamic. In some cases, pulmonary edema is severe and results in dyspnea.

Rarely, in cats with hyperthyroidism, a more ominous form of CHF develops and is characterized by severe generalized heart failure and poor contractile function that resembles dilated cardiomyopathy (Jacobs et al., 1986). Clinicians should be alert to this form of hyperthyroid heart disease, because the principal clinical problems do not resemble the classic description of feline hyperthyroidism. Affected cats may be brought to a veterinarian because of anorexia, lethargy, weakness, or respiratory distress. Physical examination often reveals weak femoral arterial pulses, dyspnea, hypothermia, and muffled heart and lung sounds if significant pleural effusion is present. Generalized cardiomegaly and pleural effusion are present on thoracic radiography, and hypodynamic ventricular wall motion is found on ultrasonographic examination.

Arrhythmias and Conduction Disorders

Sinus tachycardia is the most common rhythm disturbance in hyperthyroidism, but ectopic atrial and ventricular tachyarrhythmias are also important cardiac complications of thyrotoxicosis in cats (Peterson et al., 1982). Ectopic atrial and ventricular rhythm disturbances occur most frequently as single premature depolarizations and probably contribute little to a patient's clinical instability. Sustained and rapid tachyarrhythmias occasionally develop; they are of distinct clinical significance because they may contribute to signs of CHF. Various intraventricular conduction disturbances have been described in association with feline hyperthyroidism; most have no clinical significance. Rarely, AV heart block that leads to clinically significant bradyarrhythmia may be detected.

TREATMENT

Control Tachycardia

Although the exact interplay between the adrenergic nervous system and excessive thyroid hormone has not been elucidated, the hyperadrenergic state associated with hyperthyroidism lends itself to therapeutic intervention. Certainly, many cats with minimal cardiac complications can be stabilized with antithyroid medication alone. When needed, the use of beta-adrenergic blocking drugs can produce prompt short-term improvement in some of the cardiovascular manifestations of hyperthyroidism, particularly severe sinus tachycardia (> 250 beats/min at rest). Beta-adrenergic blocking drugs are also useful in the management of supraventricular or ventricular arrhythmias in hyperthyroidism. Propranolol (Inderal, Wyeth-Ayerst) is the most commonly recommended beta-adrenergic blocking drug, and the recommended dosage is 0.5 to 1.0 PO mg/kg every 8 hr. The hyperthyroid state may alter propranolol pharmacokinetics and, thus, dosages. However, preliminary studies from our laboratory suggest that the dosage is not markedly different from that in euthyroid cats. Calcium channel blocking drugs may also be helpful in controlling sinus tachycardia or atrial arrhythmias, particularly in cats with respiratory disease, when beta-adrenergic blocking agents are contraindicated; however, our experience with these drugs in hyperthyroid cats is limited.

Beta-adrenergic and calcium channel blocking drugs can impair contractile strength; thus, these two classes of drugs should generally not be used in combination. In cases in which tachyarrhythmias are complicated by CHF, beta-adrenergic or calcium channel blocking drugs should be used with extreme caution under vigilant observation. When accelerated heart rate is contributing to CHF, propranolol may be used cautiously.

Control Signs of Congestive Heart Failure

Patients with CHF can be categorized into those with normal to hyperdynamic wall motion and increased ventricular wall thickness (hypertrophy usually associated with left-side CHF and pulmonary edema) and those patients with hypodynamic wall motion and biventricular chamber dilation (usually associated with biventricular failure and pleural effusion). Patients with the hypertrophic form and CHF often benefit from judicious use of furosemide (Lasix, Hoechst-Roussel; Disal, Tech America) and beta-adrenergic blocking drugs, like propranolol. The recommended dosage of furosemide is 1 mg/kg PO every 12 to 24 hr. The decrease in heart rate and cardiac work associated with propranolol treatment appears to supersede the negative inotropic effect and leads to overall clinical improvement. It may be advisable to control CHF with furosemide (in conjunction with antithyroid medication) for 3 to 5 days before starting propranolol if a hyperdynamic state has not been documented echocardiographically.

Those patients with the *dilated* form usually require therapeutic thoracocentesis, furosemide, antithyroid medication, and inotropic therapy such as digoxin (Lanoxin, Burroughs-Wellcome). The initial recommended dosage of digoxin is 0.008 mg/kg every 24 hr if tablets are used. In cats under 5 kg, one fourth of a 0.125-mg tablet every other day has been used successfully. In cats that tolerate the elixir formulation (0.05 mg/ml), the dosage is 0.002 to 0.004 mg/kg every 12 hr (see this volume, p.

689). The pharmacokinetics of digoxin in hyperthyroid cats with CHF is difficult to predict; thus, dosage should be governed by serum digoxin assays. Because serious impairment in contractile strength exists in patients with the dilated form, beta-adrenergic blocking drugs are usually contraindicated. In cases with inadequate response to the described measures, captopril (Capoten, Squibb; 0.5 to 1.0 mg/kg PO every 8 hr) or enalapril (Vasotec, Merck Sharp & Dohme; 0.25 to 0.5 mg/kg PO every 12 to 24 hr) should be considered.

Antithyroid Treatment

Resolution of the hyperthyroid state requires normalization of serum thyroid hormone levels using antithyroid therapy; reversal of the hyperadrenergic signs alone with the use of beta-adrenergic blocking agents is inadequate. At present, antithyroid drugs, surgical thyroidectomy, and radioiodine are the available therapeutic modalities. The specifics of these therapeutic interventions are not reviewed here, because they are discussed in detail elsewhere (Feldman and Nelson, 1987; Peterson, 1989) (see this volume, p. 334). Important points related to management of cats with hyperthyroid heart disease are emphasized here.

In cats without signs of CHF or tachycardia and with minimal or no cardiac enlargement, use of cardiac drugs is unnecessary; treatment of the hyperthyroid state can proceed without delay. The routine use of cardiac drugs, such as propranolol, in all cases of hyperthyroidism is unjustified.

In patients with sustained tachycardia (> 250 beats/min) or CHF, definitive antithyroid treatment may need to be temporarily deferred. For example, if surgical thyroidectomy or radioiodine is to be used, then the cardiac complications should be stabilized, as described, before proceeding. Stabilization of cardiovascular problems is recommended because the risk of anesthetic complications is increased in surgical thyroidectomy and, in the case of radioiodine, because access to patients must be restricted to limit radiation exposure to personnel.

ANTITHYROID DRUGS

Antithyroid drugs like methimazole may be used as the primary therapeutic intervention or to establish euthyroidism when preparing patients for surgical thyroidectomy (see this volume, p. 338). Antithyroid drugs can be initiated at the same time as cardiovascular drugs in those patients with clinically important cardiovascular complications.

SURGICAL THYROIDECTOMY

Normalization of serum thyroid hormone levels before surgery is indicated. Cats should be treated with an antithyroid drug until euthyroidism is documented (usually 2 to 3 weeks). If persistent tachycardia is present, it should be controlled with propranolol before surgical thyroidectomy. Control of tachycardia can usually be accomplished within 3 to 5 days. Administration of propranolol should continue on the day of surgery and for approximately 3 to 5 days after surgery.* Propranolol can then be gradually discontinued by reducing the dose by 50% every 2 days. If severe cardiomegaly or CHF is present, furosemide and propranolol should be initiated preoperatively and continued for 5 to 7 days after surgery. More intensive preparation, as described, may be required for those patients with findings resembling dilated cardiomyopathy.

RADIOIODINE

Regarding cardiovascular drug intervention, similar patient preparation as for surgical thyroidectomy is recommended. However, because antithyroid drugs interfere with incorporation of iodine in the thyroid gland, recent use of these drugs can reduce the efficacy of radioiodine treatment. Thus, we do not recommend using antithyroid drugs before radioiodine treatment. If antithyroid drugs have been used, we recommend delaying radioiodine treatment for at least 7 days after discontinuing antithyroid drug therapy.

---

*Editor's Note: Some surgeons/anesthesiologists prefer the beta-blocker to be tapered off before surgery.

PROGNOSIS

Most of the cardiovascular manifestations of hyperthyroidism are reversible after normalization of serum thyroid hormone levels. Thus, the prognosis is favorable and cardiac drugs can usually be gradually discontinued within 1 to 3 weeks after normalization of serum thyroid hormone levels. Based on a limited number of cases, the prognosis for those cats with the form resembling dilated cardiomyopathy is guarded (though some totally recover), and cardiac drugs are often required despite normalization of serum thyroid hormone levels. In all cases, the need for continued cardiac drugs should be based on serial examinations including electrocardiography, thoracic radiography, and echocardiography.

References and Suggested Reading

Bond, B. R.: Hyperthyroidism and other high cardiac output states. In Fox, P. R. (ed.): Canine and Feline Cardiology. New York: Churchill Livingstone, 1988, p. 255.
  A review of the consequences of hyperthyroidism in cats with emphasis on the cardiovascular manifestations and treatment.
Feldman, E. C., and Nelson, R. W.: Canine and Feline Endocrinology and Reproduction. Philadelphia: W. B. Saunders, 1987, p. 91.
  A comprehensive review of the diagnosis and treatment of feline hyperthyroidism.
Jacobs, G., Hutson, C., Dougherty, J., et al.: Congestive heart failure associated with hyperthyroidism in cats. J.A.V.M.A. 188:52, 1986.
  Results of cardiac findings and treatment of four cats with CHF resembling dilated cardiomyopathy associated with hyperthyroidism.
Liu, S. K., Peterson, M. E., and Fox, P. R.: Hypertrophic cardiomyopathy and hyperthyroidism in the cat. J.A.V.M.A. 185:52, 1984.
  A retrospective study of pathologic findings in 23 cats with hypertrophic cardiomyopathy attributable to hyperthyroidism.
Peterson, M. E.: Treatment of feline hyperthyroidism. In Kirk, R. (ed.): Current Veterinary Therapy X. Philadelphia: W. B. Saunders, 1989, p. 1002.
  A concise, comprehensive review of therapeutic modalities in the management of feline hyperthyroidism.
Peterson, M. E., Keene, B., Ferguson, D. C., et al.: Electrocardiographic findings in 45 cats with hyperthyroidism. J.A.V.M.A. 180:934, 1982.
  A retrospective study of electrocardiographic changes associated with hyperthyroidism in 45 cats.

FIXED AND DYNAMIC SUBVALVULAR AORTIC STENOSIS IN DOGS

DAVID SISSON

Urbana, Illinois

Left ventricular outflow tract obstruction may be anatomically classified, in relation to the aortic valve, as supravalvular, valvular, or subvalvular and also may be functionally categorized as either fixed or dynamic. Supravalvular and isolated valvular aortic stenosis are uncommon heart defects in dogs (Patterson, 1971). In contrast, subvalvular aortic stenosis (SAS) is the second or third most common congenital heart defect of all dogs and the most common congenital heart defect of large breeds of dogs (Patterson, 1968; 1987). Breed predilections for SAS include boxer dogs, Newfoundland dogs, German shepherds, pointers, golden retrievers, and Rottweilers (Bonagura, 1989; Jones, 1989; Kersten, 1968; Lombard, 1990; Patterson, 1968; 1987; Patterson and Detweiler, 1963). According to Pyle and colleagues (1976), fixed SAS in Newfoundland dogs either results from a polygenic system or involves a major dominant gene with modifiers. A heritable basis for SAS is suspected in other breeds, but controlled breeding trials have not been performed.

In virtually all patients with valvular and supravalvular aortic stenosis and in most patients with SAS, the dimensions of the restrictive orifice are "fixed" by the morphologic characteristics of the obstructive lesion. The configuration of the obstruction does not change as systole progresses, nor does it vary from one heartbeat to the next. The severity of the obstruction in patients with fixed SAS can be reliably estimated by relatively simple clinical techniques. Within limits, the physiologic consequences of fixed obstructions can be predicted and an accurate prognosis offered. In comparison, the dimensions of the left ventricular outflow tract in dogs with a "dynamic" obstruction are labile, changing as systole progresses and sometimes varying conspicuously from one heartbeat to the next (Thomas et al., 1984). The most common mechanism of dynamic SAS is midsystolic apposition of the interventricular septum and the anterior leaflet of the mitral valve (Ross et al., 1966). The physiologic behavior of this uncommon disorder is complex, and the resulting physical findings are variable and therefore often confusing. The phenomenon of dynamic obstruction has been observed in humans and dogs with hypertrophic cardiomyopathy (HCM) and in patients with various congenital heart defects (Liu et al., 1979b; Shem-Tov et al., 1971; Sisson and Thomas, 1984a; Somerville and Becu, 1977).

PATHOLOGY

Fixed SAS

The left ventricular outflow tract is defined by the complex anatomy of the structures surrounding it: the muscular craniolateral portion of the left ventricular free wall, the membranous and muscular portions of the interventricular septum, and the anterior leaflet of the mitral valve and its associated structures. In adult dogs with fixed SAS, the obstructing lesion has been classically described as a discrete fibrous crescentic shelf or collar, partially or totally encircling the left ventricular outflow tract a variable distance below the aortic valve (Flickinger and Patterson, 1967; Muna et al., 1978; Patterson, 1968, 1971). Pathologic studies of dogs with SAS are complicated by well-documented evidence that the primary structural features of SAS are not fully developed at birth and that any obstruction may become progressively more severe over time (Jones et al., 1982b; Pyle et al., 1976). Pyle and colleagues (1976) described three grades of fixed SAS in Newfoundland dogs. The mildest lesions (grade I), consisting of small raised nodules of thickened endocardium on the interventricular septum below the aortic valve, were never observed in dogs over 3 months of age. The most advanced lesions (grade III), which encircled the outflow tract and consisted primarily of collagen, were predominantly found in dogs older than 6 months. In a colony of Newfoundland dogs with SAS, Jones and colleagues (1982) found evidence of outflow tract obstruction in 25% of dogs less than 1 year of age, 38% of dogs 13 to 24 months old, and 73% of dogs older than 24 months. The severity of obstruction was noted to be greater in older dogs. It is unclear to what extent increases in body size and compensatory left ventricular hypertrophy contribute to the progressive worsening of left ventricular obstruction in dogs with fixed SAS. It is also uncertain at what age an observed obstruction can be regarded as fully developed. It is certain that the pathology of SAS in dogs is even more variable and more complex than originally believed. Fixed SAS in dogs is often accompanied by other congenital heart defects, such as pulmonic stenosis, mitral valve dysplasia, and patent ductus arteriosus. In many dogs with fixed SAS, an asymmetric subvalvular fibromuscular shelf with a large septal muscular component is observed rather than a symmetric fibrous ring or collar. In some dogs, a hypertrophied, longitudinally oriented muscular ridge can be identified in the left ventricular outflow tract. In some dogs, the outflow tract is narrowed over a substantial distance by the formation of a long fibromuscular tunnel. In addition, the aorta is sometimes inclined horizontally as it exits the base of the left ventricle, and the upper portion of the hypertrophied septum projects at an odd angle into the left ventricular outflow tract. In my experience, this malformation can result in fixed or dynamic obstruction. The anatomic variability of fixed SAS in humans has also been emphasized in several reports (Hardesty et al., 1977; Somerville et al., 1980). A renewed perspective of the pathology of SAS in dogs should improve efforts to diagnose and treat this perplexing disorder.

A conglomeration of pathologic changes illustrate the consequences of fixed SAS. Concentric left ventricular hypertrophy develops in proportion to the magnitude of left ventricular systolic pressure. In the interventricular septum and left ventricular wall of dogs with fixed SAS and a pressure gradient greater than 35 mm Hg, remodeling of the intramural coronary arteries and arterioles is observed. These changes are characterized by luminal narrowing, intimal smooth-muscle proliferation, medial hypertrophy, and medial smooth-muscle disorganization (Flickinger et al., 1967; Muna et al., 1978; Pyle et al., 1976). Pyle and coworkers (1973) demonstrated retrograde blood flow during systole in the left circumflex coronary arteries of dogs with SAS. The coronary artery lesions are associated with focal ischemic areas of myocardial necrosis and fibrosis; these are most conspicuous in the anterior papillary muscle and inner half of the left ventricular wall (Flickinger et al., 1967; Levitt et al., 1989; Muna et al., 1978; Pyle et al., 1976). The cause of the vascular changes is uncertain, but they may result from the extraordinary compressive forces generated by the hypertrophied myocardium. Left atrial enlargement and pulmonary edema may result from declining left ventricular compliance, decreased myocardial contractility, or coexisting mitral regurgitation. Poststenotic dilatation of the aorta is also commonly but not invariably observed in dogs with fixed SAS. Thickening of the aortic valve leaflets, the presumed result of turbulent high-velocity blood flow, is observed in many affected

dogs. Although significant valvular stenosis does not result from these changes, various degrees of aortic insufficiency may develop (Carmichael et al., 1968; Eyster et al., 1976). Dogs with fixed SAS are also predisposed to bacterial endocarditis of the aortic valve, presumably as a result of flow-related damage to the endothelium (Muna et al., 1978; Sisson and Thomas, 1984b).

Dynamic SAS

Septal hypertrophy, a narrow left ventricular outflow tract, and a fibrous plaque on the interventricular septum at a location directly opposite a thickened and fibrotic anterior leaflet of the mitral valve are the reported pathologic findings in dogs with dynamic SAS (Liu et al., 1979b; Thomas et al., 1984). Evidence of mitral regurgitation, manifested by jet lesions and left atrial enlargement, may also be present as a consequence of abnormal coaptation of the mitral valve leaflets or secondary to coexisting mitral valve malformations (Swindle et al., 1984; Thomas et al., 1984). Coronary artery and myocardial changes, similar to those described in dogs with fixed SAS, are commonly observed in dogs and humans with dynamic SAS (Flickinger et al., 1967; Jones et al., 1982b; Liu et al., 1979b; Muna et al., 1978; Shem-Tov et al., 1971; Somerville and Becu, 1977; Thomas et al., 1984). Narrowing of the outflow tract appears to be a prerequisite for the development of dynamic subvalvular obstruction, whether it occurs as a consequence of septal hypertrophy, dextropositioning of the aorta, malformation of the mitral valve apparatus, or some combination of these changes. I have observed pathologic evidence of dynamic subvalvular obstruction in dogs with fixed SAS, pulmonic stenosis, tetralogy of Fallot, and idiopathic left ventricular hypertrophy. By inducing further hypertrophy of the interventricular septum, dynamic SAS appears to be a self-perpetuating aberration.

Dynamic SAS is most commonly observed in humans with HCM. In humans, HCM is regarded as a primary disease of the heart muscle in which diffuse or regional myocardial hypertrophy develops in the absence of any known precipitating condition (Maron and Epstein, 1980; Maron et al., 1978). Obstructive and nonobstructive forms of cardiomyopathy have been described (Maron and Epstein, 1980; Maron et al., 1978). HCM is thought to be a heritable condition in most but not all affected humans (Maron and Mulvihill, 1986; Powell, 1980). Disproportionate hypertrophy of the interventricular septum, defined in humans as a septal to left ventricular wall thickness ratio of 1.5:1.0, and evidence of dynamic SAS are distinctive findings in the obstructive form of HCM. Histologic examination of the myocardium demonstrates distinctive patterns of myocardial fiber disarray in the vast majority of humans with HCM (Maron and Epstein, 1980; Maron and Mulvihill, 1986; Maron et al., 1978; Powell, 1980). A disorder strikingly similar to HCM in humans has been reported in dogs, but the distinguishing features of disproportionate septal hypertrophy (without redefinition) and myocardial fiber disarray have been less consistent findings (Liu et al., 1979a,b; Maron et al., 1982; Swindle et al., 1984; Thomas et al., 1984). The relationship between SAS and HCM in dogs is uncertain. Many but not all of the dogs reported to suffer from HCM are breeds commonly affected by fixed SAS (Liu et al., 1979a,b; Maron et al., 1982; Swindle et al., 1984). It is not yet clear what percentage of dogs with isolated dynamic SAS suffer from an unusual muscular form of the same genetic disease usually expressed as fixed SAS and how many have a primary myocardial disease (HCM) unrelated to fixed SAS. Other explanations, not yet considered, are also possible. Such distinctions require additional clinical observations and, perhaps, additional and more extensive breeding trials.

CLINICAL ASSESSMENT

The systolic murmurs of fixed and dynamic SAS are typically crescendo-decrescendo in character and located at the left heart base or over the right cranial thorax. Marked beat-to-beat variation in the duration and intensity of the murmur, particularly when the murmur is accentuated after a premature beat, suggests dynamic outflow tract obstruction. However, similar findings can be observed in dogs with fixed SAS. The finding of slowly rising, weak femoral artery pulses may be detected in dogs with either form of obstruction, but abrupt pulses and varying pulse quality are more typical of dynamic obstruction. Electrocardiograms recorded in dogs with fixed or dynamic left ventricular obstruction may be normal or exhibit high-amplitude R waves, ST segment changes, and various arrhythmias, most commonly ventricular premature beats or atrial fibrillation (Bonagura, 1989; Jones, 1989; Kersten, 1968; Lombard, 1990; Patterson and Detweiler, 1963; Pyle et al., 1976). Thoracic radiographs are often normal but may suggest left ventricular enlargement or poststenotic dilatation of the aorta (Bonagura, 1989; Jones, 1989; Lombard, 1990; Pyle et al., 1976). Evidence of left atrial enlargement and pulmonary congestion may develop as a consequence of systolic (myocardial) or diastolic (compliance) pump failure or from mitral regurgitation.

Two-dimensional echocardiographic imaging of the aorta, outflow tract, and left ventricle, performed from right and left parasternal locations, permits visualization of most subvalvular obstructions, detection of poststenotic dilatation of the aorta, and assessment of the degree of left ventric-

ular hypertrophy (Cabrera et al., 1989; Wilcox et al., 1980). Diffuse, subtle narrowing of the outflow tract and mild focal lesions may, unfortunately, go undetected. In dogs with more serious obstructions, ischemia-induced myocardial fibrosis is evidenced by hyperechoic regions in the left ventricular myocardium, most apparent in the papillary muscles. The value of M-mode echocardiography resides in its ability to display the rapid movements of valvular structures. Premature midsystolic closure of the aortic valve can be observed in dogs with either fixed or dynamic SAS (Sisson and Thomas, 1984a; Thomas et al., 1984; Wingfield et al., 1983). Coexisting aortic insufficiency is often manifested by premature closure or diastolic fluttering of the mitral valve (Sisson and Thomas, 1984b). Detection of systolic anterior motion (SAM) of the mitral valve indicates probable dynamic SAS. Unfortunately, SAM is not always apparent in affected dogs at rest, and echocardiographic evidence of SAM does not always indicate significant dynamic obstruction (Maron and Epstein, 1980; Sisson and Thomas, 1984a). When dynamic obstruction is suspected, SAM may be provoked by exercise or the administration of positive inotropes or arterial vasodilators. The presence of obstruction can be verified by Doppler studies or invasively obtained pressure measurements. I have found acepromazine to be a safe and reliable agent for provoking or accentuating dynamic SAS in dogs. Evidence of dynamic obstruction should be diligently sought whenever the left ventricle is unexplainably and concentrically hypertrophied. Dynamic obstruction should also be suspected in dogs with fixed SAS when the severity of fixed obstruction appears mild in relation to the severity of left ventricular hypertrophy.

The severity of fixed SAS can be noninvasively estimated from spectral Doppler recordings by calculation of the peak pressure gradient (PG) across the stenotic lesion using the modified Bernoulli equation, $PG = 4 \times V^2$, where V is the maximum flow velocity across the stenotic orifice (Nishimura et al., 1985). Doppler-estimated pressure gradients have been shown to correlate closely with those obtained simultaneously by invasive methods (Thomas, 1990; Valdes-Cruz et al., 1983). Doppler estimates of PGs may be compromised by various technical errors, most significantly malalignment of the ultrasound beam with the stenotic jet (Nishimura et al., 1985). However, Doppler studies permit estimation of PGs in awake dogs and, by avoiding the depressant effects of anesthesia, are particularly useful for the identification of dogs with mild SAS and otherwise equivocal echocardiographic changes. In normal unsedated dogs, peak aortic flow velocities rarely exceed 1.7 m/sec. Velocities in excess of this value, particularly when accompanied by turbulent blood flow and aortic insufficiency, are suggestive of aortic stenosis. Thorough Doppler interrogation of the left ventricle and left atrium provides a sensitive means for detecting coexisting flow disturbances, such as aortic or mitral insufficiency (Ciobanu et al., 1982; Nishimura et al., 1985).

The presence and severity of fixed SAS can be confirmed by cardiac catheterization and contrast angiocardiography. The severity of obstruction can be estimated, in the presence of normal cardiac output, by direct measurement of left ventricular and aortic pressures and calculation of the peak-to-peak systolic PG (Lambert et al., 1971). However, an important consideration resides in the fact that the measured PG is roughly proportional to the square of the flow rate across the stenotic orifice, as evidenced by the hydraulic formula of Gorlin and Gorlin (Carabello and Grossman, 1986). By depressing myocardial function and decreasing stroke volume, general anesthesia can and often does diminish or even abolish hemodynamic evidence of obstruction. Infusion of isoproterenol, by increasing stroke volume, may provoke a measurable gradient in anesthetized dogs with mild fixed outflow tract obstruction.* Measurement of stroke volume and determination of the mean PG permit calculation of the area of the obstructive orifice and provide a theoretically more precise estimate of the severity of obstruction. Although these measurements are technically demanding and time-consuming to procure, they provide the most accurate estimate of the degree of obstruction and for documenting the success of an intervention (e.g., balloon valvuloplasty or surgery). After the hemodynamic measurements, contrast ventriculography is performed to demonstrate the site and morphology of the obstructing lesion, to confirm poststenotic dilatation of the aorta, and to detect mitral regurgitation (Buchanon and Patterson, 1965; Levitt et al., 1989; Pyle et al., 1976). Contrast injection into the aortic root should be routinely performed in dogs with SAS to detect and quantify aortic insufficiency (Bonagura, 1989; Carmichael et al., 1968; Eyster et al., 1976).

Hemodynamic documentation of dynamic obstruction requires comprehension of the pathophysiology of dynamic obstruction and meticulous technique (Brockenbrough et al., 1961). The use of catheters with two microtransducers at the tip is recommended for documenting the bisferious configuration of the arterial pressure tracing and for simultaneous measurement of left ventricular and aortic pressures. After resting intracardiac pressures are recorded, various interventions, designed to establish the presence of dynamic obstruction, are

implemented. Dynamic obstruction is accentuated by provocations that decrease the end-diastolic dimensions of the left ventricle or increase the velocity of circumferential shortening (Brockenbrough et al., 1961). With these changes, the anterior mitral valve leaflet is brought closer to the interventricular septum earlier in systole, resulting in more severe obstruction. Augmentation of the recorded PG can be achieved by rapid artificial cardiac pacing, by administration of positive inotropes or vasodilators, and by observation of the response to a spontaneously occurring or induced premature beat. As a consequence of increased contractility during the postextrasystolic beat, the PG is markedly enhanced, and aortic pulse amplitude usually remains constant or declines. Negative inotropes and hypertensive agents reduce or abolish dynamic obstructions. By decreasing contractility, general anesthetics can abolish echocardiographic evidence of SAM and the PG associated with it. This observation may explain why the phenomenon of dynamic SAS is only rarely mentioned in the veterinary literature. The importance of impaired diastolic function has been emphasized in human patients with HCM, but this aspect of the disease has been largely neglected in dogs with dynamic SAS (Powell, 1980; Sisson and Thomas, 1984a; Thomas et al., 1984).

NATURAL HISTORY

Information about the natural history of either fixed or dynamic SAS in dogs is meager. Development of congestive heart failure (CHF) and sudden death are the most commonly noted sequelae of fixed SAS. However, it is not known if affected dogs develop congestive signs as a result of systolic (myocardial) failure, diastolic (compliance) failure, or both. Most reports of the clinical course of fixed SAS in dogs were conducted before the availability of echocardiographic imaging. Patterson and Detweiler (1963) reported that 4 of 22 dogs with SAS died suddenly and 4 of 22 died of CHF. Flickinger and Patterson (1967) reported that of 19 dogs with fixed SAS, 12 had signs of CHF, 6 died of CHF, and 4 died suddenly. In this same report, 4 of 19 dogs experienced syncope, and 8 of 19 had ventricular arrhythmia. Jones and colleagues (1982b) reported sudden death in 16 of 66 Newfoundland dogs with SAS. Other documented clinical sequelae of SAS include aortic insufficiency and bacterial endocarditis (Carmichael et al., 1968; Eyster et al., 1976; Jones et al., 1982b; Muna et al., 1978; Pyle et al., 1976; Sisson and Thomas, 1984b).

Much less information is available about the natural history of dynamic SAS. Clinical or hemodynamic evidence of impaired diastolic function, commonly present in humans with HCM, has not yet been reported in affected dogs. Liu and colleagues

---

*Editors' Note: Caution is indicated in the performance and interpretation of isoproterenol-induced PGs, because intraventricular PGs can be induced in volume-depleted, otherwise normal dogs by this method.

(1979a) briefly described the clinical course of two dogs with the obstructive form of HCM; both dogs died suddenly. An additional dog with HCM, reported by Thomas and colleagues (1984), was asymptomatic when euthanized at 3 years of age. A pointer dog with isolated dynamic SAS, which was initially evaluated at 3 years of age and which I subsequently adopted, is asymptomatic at 8 years of age.

TREATMENT

Fixed SAS

In view of the limited knowledge of the natural history of fixed SAS in dogs, specific indications and recommendations for surgery are difficult to formulate. The documented progressive and catastrophic nature of its sequelae might suggest that surgical repair be attempted when fixed SAS is first diagnosed, preferably at 3 to 6 months of age and without regard for the severity of obstruction. In mature dogs, consideration should be given to the severity of obstruction, the presence of clinical signs, the intended use of the dog, and evidence of progression. Surgery, facilitated by cardiopulmonary bypass, is the only proven method to remedy fixed SAS, but it is very expensive and only available at a few referral centers. Surgical procedures that do not permit direct visualization of the outflow tract are contraindicated because of the complex and variable anatomy of the obstructive lesions and the dire consequences of unintentional damage to the mitral or aortic valves.

Reports describing the results of surgical correction of fixed SAS in dogs are scant (Baird and Duffell, 1974; Breznok et al., 1983), and advice regarding specific surgical techniques are, of necessity, based on studies of children with SAS. Good results are obtained in children when a discrete membranous lesion is identified and resected without damaging the aorta and mitral valves (Wright et al., 1983). However, this particular form of obstruction is uncommon in dogs. More variable results are obtained in children with fibromuscular rings or with muscular "tunnel" stenosis (Hardesty et al., 1977; Jones et al., 1982a; Newfeld et al., 1976; Somerville et al., 1980). Evidence of inadequate relief of obstruction, restenosis, and dynamic SAS following surgery in children with these malformations has prompted some investigators to perform a septal myectomy or to bypass the obstruction by implanting a valved conduit between the apex of the left ventricle and the descending aorta (Bernhard et al., 1975; Hardesty et al., 1977).

Balloon dilatation of fixed SAS is a possible alternative to surgery in some dogs. The short-term results of transluminal balloon dilatation for dis-

crete, membranous SAS in children are encouraging (De Lezo et al., 1986; Lababidi et al., 1987). However, the results of this technique are much less impressive when the obstruction is caused by a thick, fibromuscular ring, the most common type of obstruction found in dogs (De Lezo et al., 1986; Lababidi et al., 1987). Studies to determine the success of and indications for balloon dilatation in dogs with fixed SAS have been initiated (Thomas et al., 1990). Although still considered an experimental technique, balloon dilatation should be considered when the possibility of surgery is precluded by financial or other considerations.

When invasive procedures cannot be performed or are ineffective, other recommendations can be appropriately offered. Even in asymptomatic dogs with no arrhythmia, owners should promote a sedentary life-style for their pet and prevent opportunities for vigorous exercise and unnecessary excitement. Antiarrhythmic drug therapy is advisable but of uncertain benefit in affected dogs with unexplained syncope or when ventricular arrhythmias are observed on resting or postexercise electrocardiograms. Antiarrhythmic drug selection is an arbitrary choice because of the lack of studies reporting the efficacy of any agent for preventing sudden death in these circumstances. Continuously recorded 24-hr ambulatory electrocardiograms may be particularly useful to identify the cause of unexplained syncope, to detect infrequent arrhythmia, and to monitor the effects of antiarrhythmic therapy. The use of implanted defibrillators in dogs with SAS is an interesting possibility of unproven merit. Some investigators advise the use of beta receptor or calcium channel blocking drugs, based on their potential to enhance diastolic relaxation or to reduce myocardial oxygen demand (Bonagura, 1989; Pyle et al., 1976). The indications and value of these agents in dogs with fixed SAS have not been determined. As a result of the established risk of bacterial endocarditis in dogs with fixed SAS, antibiotic prophylaxis is advisable whenever dental or surgical procedures are performed.

Dogs with SAS should be re-evaluated every 3 months until 2 years of age and at least yearly thereafter. Echocardiography is the most practical method for detecting progressive obstruction, new or worsening valvular insufficiency, and myocardial dysfunction. Electrocardiography is indicated on a routine basis to detect arrhythmia and evidence of ischemia. If signs of heart failure develop, low-salt diets and diuretics can be used to control pulmonary edema. Digoxin may be efficacious in dogs with myocardial failure, particularly if atrial fibrillation develops. As a general rule, arterial vasodilators should be avoided, and venous vasodilators and angiotensin-converting enzyme inhibitors should be used with caution.

Dynamic SAS

Treatment of dynamic SAS in dogs has not been reported. Treatment recommendations are based on observations reported in humans with HCM. In some humans with dynamic SAS due to HCM, treatment with beta-blocking drugs or calcium channel blocking drugs has been shown to alleviate symptoms and to reduce or abolish dynamic obstruction (Flamm et al., 1968; Maron et al., 1987; Rosing et al., 1985). In patients refractory to medical therapy, septal myectomy has been shown to diminish the severity of obstruction and to alleviate symptoms in about 70% (Jones et al., 1982a; Maron et al., 1980). Regardless of the method of treatment, many patients die suddenly or develop progressive signs of CHF. Amiodarone has shown promise for control of ventricular and supraventricular arrhythmias in humans with HCM (McKenna et al., 1984; 1985), but this drug has not been evaluated in dogs. Positive inotropes, including digoxin, should not be administered to dogs with dynamic SAS unless they are needed to control supraventricular arrhythmias or to treat documented systolic pump failure. Congestive signs are managed by salt restriction and the use of diuretics.

PREVENTION

The heritability of fixed SAS in Newfoundland dogs has been established by controlled breeding trials. Until controlled breeding trials are conducted in other breeds, it is my opinion that fixed and dynamic SAS should be regarded as inherited diseases in all affected dogs and managed accordingly. Dogs with SAS should not be bred, regardless of the severity of the defect. This recommendation can be simply accomplished by not breeding any adult dog with a murmur of uncertain origin. Adult dogs that are 1 year of age or older and do not have a murmur are acceptable for breeding with no requirement for further evaluation. This recommendation is made for pragmatic reasons and it presupposes that "silent" defects in adult dogs are very infrequent, a conclusion I believe to be valid. If these recommendations are adhered to, some dogs with innocent or physiologic murmurs could be excluded from the breeding pool. If an owner is intent on breeding a dog with a murmur, I recommend performance of two-dimensional and Doppler echocardiography at 1 year of age. If the results are indicative of SAS or some other cardiac defect, the dog should not be bred. If results of these studies are equivocal, I recommend cardiac catheterization and angiocardiography. If these studies are indicative of SAS or some other defect, the dog should not be bred. If these studies are normal, the owner is advised that although a very mild form of SAS could be present, there is no conclusive evidence of heart disease. If the owner chooses to breed the dog, all offspring should be evaluated, by auscultation, for evidence of heart disease. Until the pattern of inheritance of SAS is established or a means to identify the carrier state developed, it will not be possible to make an informed recommendation about the intended use of normal dogs related to an SAS affected dog.

References and Suggested Reading

Baird, D. K., and Duffell, S. J.: Resection of a fibromuscular subaortic stenosis in a dog. J. Small Anim. Pract. 15:37, 1974.

Bernhard, W. F., Poirier, V., LaFarge, C. G., et al.: Relief of congenital obstruction to left ventricular outflow with a ventricular-aortic prosthesis. J. Thorac. Cardiovasc. Surg. 69:223, 1975.

Bonagura, J. D.: Congenital heart disease. In Ettinger, S. J. (ed.): Textbook of Veterinary Internal Medicine, 2nd ed. Philadelphia: W. B. Saunders, 1989, pp. 976–1030.

Breznock, E. M., Whiting, P., Pendray, D., et al.: Valved apico-aortic conduit for relief of left ventricular hypertension caused by discrete subaortic stenosis in dogs. J.A.V.M.A. 182:51, 1983.

Brockenbrough, E. C., Braunwald, E., and Morrow, A. G.: A hemodynamic technic for the detection of hypertrophic cardiomyopathy. Circulation 23:189, 1961.

Buchanon, J. W., Patterson, D. F.: Selective angiocardiography in dogs with congenital cardiovascular disease. J. Am. Vet. Radiol. Soc. 6:21, 1965.

Cabrera, A., Galdeano, J. M., Zumalde, J., et al.: Fixed subaortic stenosis: The value of cross-sectional echocardiography in evaluating different anatomic patterns. Int. J. Cardiol. 24:151, 1989.

Carabello, B. A., and Grossman, W.: Calculation of stenotic valve orifice area. In Grossman, W. (ed.): Cardiac Catheterization and Angiography, 3rd ed. Philadelphia: Lea & Febiger, 1986, pp. 143–145.

Carmichael, J. A., Liu, S. K., Tashjian, R. J., et al.: A case of subaortic stenosis and valvular insufficiency, with particular reference to diagnostic technique. J. Small Anim. Pract. 9:213, 1968.

Ciobanu, M., Abbasi, A. S., Allen, M., et al.: Pulsed Doppler echocardiography in the diagnosis and estimation of severity of aortic insufficiency. Am. J. Cardiol. 49:339, 1982.

De Lezo, J. S., Pan, M., Sanch, M., et al.: Percutaneous transluminal balloon dilatation for discrete subaortic stenosis. Am. J. Cardiol. 58:619, 1986.

Eyster, G. E., Anderson, L. K., and Cords, G. B.: Aortic regurgitation in the dog. J.A.V.M.A. 168:138, 1976.

Flamm, M. D., Harrison, D. C., and Hancok, E. W.: Muscular subaortic stenosis, prevention of outflow tract obstruction with propranolol. Circulation 38:846, 1968.

Flickinger, G. L., and Patterson, D. F.: Coronary lesions associated with congenital subaortic stenosis in the dog. J. Pathol. Bacteriol. 93:133, 1967.

Hardesty, R. L., Griffeth, B. P., Mathews, R. A., et al.: Discrete subvalvular aortic stenosis: An evaluation of operative therapy. J. Thorac. Cardiovasc. Surg. 74:352, 1977.

Jones, C. L.: Inheritable left ventricular outflow obstruction in the golden retriever. ACVIM Scientific Proceedings, 1989, pp. 851–853.

Jones, M., Barnhart, C. R., and Morrow, A. G.: Late results after operations for left ventricular outflow tract obstruction. Am. J. Cardiol. 50:569, 1982a.

Jones, M., Picone, A. L., Ferrans, V. J., et al.: Subaortic stenosis in Newfoundland dogs: An acquired congenital heart disease (abstract). Circulation 66(suppl. 2):II-317, 1982b.

Kersten, U.: Klinische Untersuchungen am herzkranken Hund. Thesis, Hanover, Germany, 1968.

Lababidi, Z., Weinhaus, L., Stoeckle, H., et al.: Transluminal balloon dilatation for discrete subaortic stenosis. Am. J. Cardiol. 59:423, 1987.

Lambert, E. C., Colombi, M., Wagner, H. R., et al.: The clinical outlook of congenital aortic stenosis (valvar and subvalvar) prior to surgery. In Langford, B. S., and Keith, J. D. (eds.): The Natural History and Progress in Treatment of Congenital Heart Defects. Springfield, IL: Charles C Thomas, 1971, pp. 205–213.

Levitt, L., Fowler, J. D., and Schuh, J. C. L.: Aortic stenosis in the dog: A review of 12 cases. J. Am. Anim. Hosp. Assoc. 25:357, 1989.

Liu, S.-K., Maron, B. J., and Tilley, L. P.: Canine hypertrophic cardiomyopathy. J.A.V.M.A. 174:708, 1979a.

Liu, S.-K., Maron, B. J., and Tilley, L. P.: Hypertrophic cardiomyopathy in the dog. Am. J. Pathol. 94:497, 1979b.

Lombard, C. W.: Subaortic stenosis in Rottweiler dogs. ACVIM Scientific Proceedings, 1990, pp. 893–896.

Maron, B. J., and Epstein, S. E.: Hypertrophic cardiomyopathy. Recent observations regarding the specificity of three hallmarks of the disease: Asymmetric septal hypertrophy, septal disorganization and systolic anterior motion of the anterior mitral leaflet. Am. J. Cardiol. 45:141, 1980.

Maron, B. J., and Mulvihill, J. J.: The genetics of hypertrophic cardiomyopathy. Ann. Intern. Med. 105:610, 1986.

Maron, B. J., Liu, S.-K., and Tilley, L. P.: Spontaneously occurring hypertrophic cardiomyopathy in dogs and cats: A potential model of a human disease. In Kaltenbach, M., and Epstein, S. E. (eds.): Hypertrophic Cardiomyopathy. The Therapeutic Role of Calcium Antagonists. New York: Springer-Verlag, 1982, pp. 73–87.

Maron, B. J., Bonow, R. O., Cannon, R. O., et al.: Hypertrophic cardiomyopathy: Interrelations of clinical manifestations, pathophysiology, and therapy. N. Engl. J. Med. 316:780, 1987.

Maron, B. J., Gottdiener, J. S., Roberts, W. C., et al.: Left ventricular outflow tract obstruction due to systolic anterior motion of the anterior leaflet in patients with concentric left ventricular hypertrophy. Circulation 57:527, 1978.

Maron, B. J., Koch, J.-P., Kent, K. M., et al.: Results of surgery for idiopathic hypertrophic subaortic stenosis. J. Cardiovasc. Med. 5:145, 1980.

McKenna, W. J., Harris, L., Rowland, E., et al.: Amiodarone for long-term management of patients with hypertrophic cardiomyopathy. Am. J. Cardiol. 54:802, 1984.

McKenna, W. J., Oakley, C. M., Krikler, D. M., et al.: Improved survival with amiodarone in patients with hypertrophic cardiomyopathy. Br. Heart J. 53:412, 1985.

Muna, F. T., Ferrans, V. J., Pierce, J. E., et al.: Discrete subaortic stenosis in Newfoundland dogs: Association of infective endocarditis. Am. J. Cardiol. 41:746, 1978.

Newfeld, E. A., Muster, A. J., Paul, M. H., et al.: Discrete subvalvular aortic stenosis in childhood. Am. J. Cardiol. 38:53, 1976.

Nishimura, R. A., Miller, F. A., Callahan, M. J., et al.: Doppler echocardiography: Theory, instrumentation, technique, and application. Mayo Clin. Proc. 60:321, 1985.

Patterson, D. F.: Epidemiologic and genetic studies of congenital heart disease in the dog. Circ. Res. 23:171, 1968.

Patterson, D. F.: Canine congenital heart disease: Epidemiology and etiological hypotheses. J. Small Anim. Pract. 12:263, 1971.

Patterson, D. F., and Detweiler, D. K.: Predominance of German shepherd and boxer breeds among dogs with congenital sub-aortic stenosis. Am. Heart J. 65:429, 1963.

Powell, W. J., Jr.: Hypertrophic nondilated cardiomyopathy: Idiopathic hypertrophic subaortic stenosis and its variants. In Johnson, R. A., Haber, E., and Austen, W. G. (eds.): The Practice of Cardiology. Boston: Little, Brown & Co., 1980, pp. 647–663.

Pyle, R. L., Patterson, D. F., and Chacko, S.: The genetics and pathology of discrete subaortic stenosis in the Newfoundland dog. Am. Heart J. 92:324, 1976.

Pyle, R. L., Lowensohn, H. S., Khouri, E. M., et al.: Left circumflex coronary artery hemodynamics in conscious dogs with congenital subaortic stenosis. Circ. Res. 33:34, 1973.

Rosing, D. R., Idanpaan-Heikkila, U., Maron, B. J., et al.: Use of calcium-channel blocking drugs in hypertrophic cardiomyopathy. Am. J. Cardiol. 55:185B, 1985.

Ross, J., Jr., Braunwald, E., Gault, J. H., et al.: The mechanism of the interventricular pressure gradient in idiopathic hypertrophic subaortic stenosis. Circulation 34:558, 1966.

Shem-Tov, A., Deutsch, V., Yahini, J. H., et al.: Cardiomyopathy associated with congenital heart disease. Br. Heart J. 33:782, 1971.

Sisson, D., and Thomas, W. P.: Dynamic subaortic stenosis in a dog with congenital heart disease. J. Am. Anim. Hosp. Assoc. 20:657, 1984a.

Sisson, D., and Thomas, W. P.: Endocarditis of the aortic valve in the dog. J.A.V.M.A. 184:570, 1984b.

Somerville, J., and Becu, L.: Congenital heart disease associated with hypertrophic cardiomyopathy. John Hopkins Med. J. 140:151, 1977.

Somerville, J., Stone, S., and Ross, D.: Fate of patients with fixed subaortic stenosis after surgical removal. Br. Heart J. 43:629, 1980.

Swindle, M. M., Huber, A. C., Kan, J. S., et al.: Mitral valve prolapse and hypertrophic cardiomyopathy in a pup. J.A.V.M.A. 184:1515, 1984.

Thomas, W. P.: Doppler echocardiographic estimation of pressure gradients in dogs with congenital pulmonic and subaortic stenosis. ACVIM Scientific Proceedings, 1990, pp. 867–869.

Thomas, W. P., DeLellis, L. A., and Sisson, D.: Balloon dilatation of congenital outflow obstructions in dogs: Mid-term results. ACVIM Scientific Proceedings, 1990, pp. 907–909.

Thomas, W. P., Mathewson, J. W., Suter, P. F., et al.: Hypertrophic obstructive cardiomyopathy in a dog: Clinical, hemodynamic, angiographic, and pathologic studies. J. Am. Anim. Hosp. Assoc. 20:253, 1984.

Valdes-Cruz, L. M., Pierce, J., Sahn, D. J., et al.: Prediction of the gradient in fibromuscular subaortic stenosis by continuous wave 2-D Doppler echocardiography: Animal studies (abstract). Circulation 68(suppl. III):366, 1983.

Wilcox, W. D., Seward, J. B., Hagler, D. J., et al.: Discrete subaortic stenosis: Two-dimensional echocardiographic features with angiographic and surgical correlation. Mayo Clin. Proc. 55:425, 1980.

Wingfield, W. E., Boon, J. A., and Miller, C. W.: Echocardiographic assessment of congenital aortic stenosis in dogs. J.A.V.M.A. 183:673, 1983.

Wright, G. B., Keane, J. F., Nadas, A. S., et al.: Fixed subaortic stenosis in the young: Medical and surgical course in 83 patients. Am. J. Coll. Cardiol. 52:830, 1983.

UPDATE: DILTIAZEM THERAPY OF FELINE HYPERTROPHIC CARDIOMYOPATHY

JANICE McINTOSH BRIGHT

Knoxville, Tennessee

Hypertrophic cardiomyopathy (HCM) is a common cause of heart failure, thromboembolism, and sudden death in cats. This disease is characterized by a hypertrophied, nondilated left ventricle in the absence of a cardiac or systemic disease that can produce left ventricular hypertrophy. A secondary form of the disease occurs in cats with excessive circulating levels of thyroxine or growth hormone.

Table 1. *Manifestations of Impaired Diastolic Function*

Prolonged isovolumic relaxation
Decreased rate of ventricular wall thinning
Decreased rate and extent of rapid filling
Shortening or abolition of diastasis
Enhanced active atrial filling

This chapter is intended to provide an updated view of the pathophysiology, clinical manifestations, and treatment of HCM and in particular will address the rationale, methods, and benefits of diltiazem therapy. Readers may wish to review previous texts for additional information concerning etiology, diagnosis, and management (*CVT IX*, p. 380; *CVT X*, p. 251 and p. 295; Fox, 1988).

PATHOPHYSIOLOGY

Diastolic Events

Impaired left ventricular (LV) diastolic function is the most important pathophysiologic mechanism in patients with HCM, and it is the major determinant of clinical signs in both humans and cats

with this disease. The abnormal diastolic filling is due to two factors: increased chamber stiffness (decreased compliance) and prolonged (incomplete) myocardial relaxation. Increased chamber stiffness in HCM is the result of increased mass, myocardial fibrosis and cellular disarray, and diminished chamber volume, and it is responsible for a disproportionate increase in diastolic pressure for a given increase in diastolic volume. Abnormal relaxation is manifested by a prolonged isovolumic relaxation period and a decreased rate of decline in LV pressure. Mechanisms contributing to this impairment of relaxation include altered contraction and relaxation loads, reduced inactivation of actomyosin formation, and asynchrony of the contraction and relaxation processes. The abnormalities in relaxation and distensibility reduce overall LV diastolic filling.

Impaired diastolic function has been documented in human HCM patients using echocardiographic, hemodynamic, radionuclide, and Doppler techniques (Table 1). Abnormal diastolic filling has been documented in cats hemodynamically (Golden and Bright, 1990), angiographically (Fox, 1988), and echocardiographically (Moise et al., 1986) (Fig. 1). Although diastolic dysfunction sufficient to cause clinical signs is usually associated with massive LV hypertrophy, clinically significant impairment of

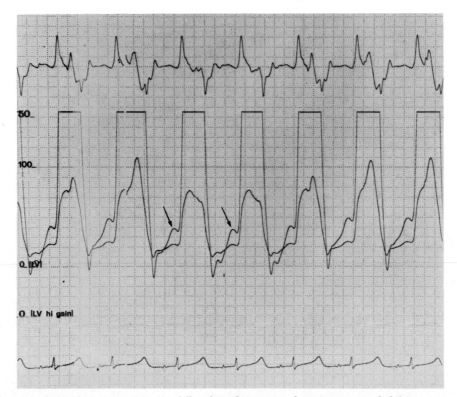

Figure 1. Left ventricular (LV) pressure tracing at full scale and at increased sensitivity recorded from a cat with hypertrophic cardiomyopathy. Note the abnormal increase in pressure *(arrows)* that follows the electrocardiographic P wave. This pressure rise results from a compensatory enhancement of active atrial contraction due to impaired ventricular relaxation and compliance (paper speed 50 mm/sec).

filling may occur in the presence of mild hypertrophy.

Systolic Events

In cats with HCM the left ventricle usually appears either normal or hyperdynamic on the echocardiogram, suggesting normal to increased myocardial contractility. Occasionally, however, the contractility is reduced as a result of the extensive myocardial fibrosis or ischemia associated with longstanding disease. In most patients with HCM, systolic abnormalities, if present, take the form of intraventricular pressure gradients rather than impaired contractility. The most common type of systolic pressure gradient in humans is a subaortic gradient due to contact of the anterior mitral valve leaflet with the septum. Controversy prevails as to whether this type of gradient represents actual obstruction to LV outflow. The significance and frequency of LV outflow tract gradients in feline patients are unknown, but intraventricular pressure gradients indicative of apical cavity obliteration are occasionally observed (Bright, 1990) (Fig. 2), and Doppler studies in unanesthetized cats may demonstrate systolic gradients. The presence of a gradient increases ventricular wall stress and myocardial oxygen demand. Systolic gradients also contribute to diastolic dysfunction because they cause asynchrony of contraction and relaxation. Finally, mitral regurgitation is relatively common and can reduce forward flow while raising left atrial pressure.

Ischemia

Myocardial ischemia contributes to the pathogenesis of HCM in many patients. The ischemia is believed to result from inadequate capillary density, narrowing of the intramural coronary arteries, microvascular spasm, decreased coronary perfusion pressure, and elevated LV diastolic pressure. Myocardial ischemia initiates a deleterious positive feedback cycle because it contributes to impaired active relaxation of the muscle leading to further elevation of the LV end diastolic pressure and further reduction in coronary flow (Fig. 3). Ischemia may contribute to malaise and lethargy in cats with HCM because it is responsible for chest pain in human patients. Myocardial ischemia has also been associated with lethal ventricular arrhythmias.

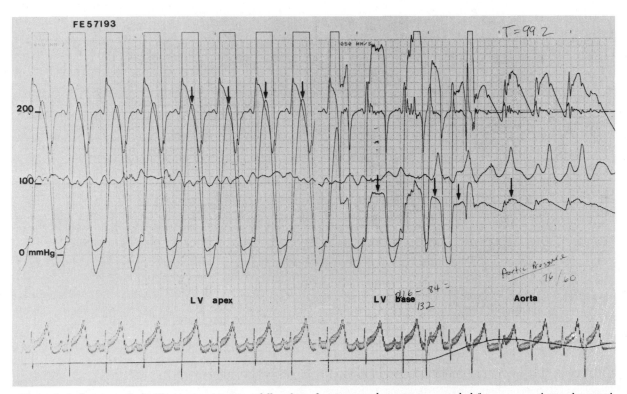

Figure 2. Left ventricular (LV) pressure tracing at full scale and at increased sensitivity recorded from an anesthetized cat with hypertrophic cardiomyopathy as the pressure transducer is being withdrawn from the apex to the base of the ventricle and then into the aortic root. Note the difference in peak systolic pressure *(arrows)* between the apex and the base (paper speed 50 mm/sec).

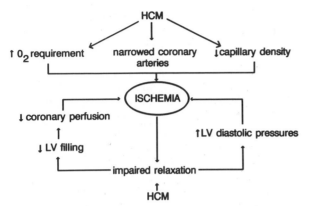

Figure 3. Deleterious interactions between ischemia and impaired myocardial relaxation in hypertrophic cardiomyopathy (HCM). Impaired relaxation is characteristic of the cardiomyopathic tissue. Ischemia results from inadequate capillary density, narrowing of intramural arteries, and increased oxygen (O_2) demand. Ischemia further impairs the active relaxation process, and impaired relaxation exacerbates ischemia by increasing left ventricular (LV) end diastolic pressure and reducing coronary blood flow. (Reprinted from Bright, J. M., and Golden, A. L.: Evidence for or against the efficacy of calcium channel blockers for management of hypertrophic cardiomyopathy in cats. Vet. Clin. North Am. Small Anim. Pract. 21:1025, 1991.)

Therapeutic Implications

Since all of these pathophysiologic processes (diastolic dysfunction, systolic pressure gradients [and mitral regurgitation], and myocardial ischemia) contribute to the clinical manifestations of feline HCM, medical management should be directed toward reversing each. The beta-adrenergic–blocking agents such as propranolol will reduce systolic gradients, decrease heart rate, and decrease myocardial oxygen demand; however, these agents have no direct beneficial effects on ischemia or relaxation. Beta-blockade may actually adversely affect active relaxation of the myocardium by slowing the rate at which calcium ions are transported from the sarcomere into the sarcoplasmic reticulum. In contrast, the calcium channel blocking agents have positive lusitropic and direct coronary vasodilating effects in addition to their negative chronotropic and negative inotropic properties. Thus, impaired LV relaxation and filling is improved in most patients with HCM by administration of these drugs. The calcium antagonists are believed to enhance diastolic performance by reducing myocardial ischemia and aschyronous myocardial relaxation and by reversing abnormal calcium handling in the hypertrophied myocytes.

CLINICAL PRESENTATION

Impaired diastolic function results in increased LV filling pressures, pulmonary edema, and dyspnea, as well as inadequate cardiac output, fatigue,

lethargy, and sudden death. Ischemia may contribute to malaise and clinically significant arrhythmias. Systemic arterial embolism is a common complication and is believed to occur as a result of circulatory stasis and platelet reactivity (Flanders, 1986; Fox, 1988). Although many feline patients have similar physical, radiographic, echocardiographic, and hemodynamic abnormalities, the spectrum of clinical findings is quite broad. Diagnosis must be based on echocardiographic or angiographic confirmation of LV hypertrophy in the absence of another disease that can produce cardiac hypertrophy.

Cats with HCM are most frequently presented for respiratory distress or rear limb paresis (Bright, 1990). Occasionally, lethargy and anorexia are the only presenting complaints. Some cats may experience recurrent syncopal attacks or sudden death without other clinical signs.

Abnormalities often noted on physical examination include cardiac auscultatory abnormalities such as gallops, systolic murmurs, or arrhythmias. The heart sounds are occasionally muffled due to the presence of pleural or pericardial effusion. Dyspnea as a result of pulmonary edema or pleural effusion is common. An occasional patient will have biventricular failure with venous distention and palpable hepatomegaly. Some affected animals appear normal on physical examination, especially those with paroxysmal arrhythmias.

Electrocardiographic abnormalities are common in cats with HCM and occur in 60% to 70% of affected animals (Bright, 1990; Harpster, 1986) (Table 2).

Table 2. *Electrocardiographic Findings From Two Clinical Studies of Cats With Hypertrophic Cardiomyopathy*

Abnormality	Frequency (n = 31)*	Frequency (n = 20)†
P wave		
>0.04 sec	10%	10%
>0.2 mV (lead II)	19%	5%
QRS >0.04 sec	36%	10%
LVH pattern‡	39%	10%
Arrhythmias (total)	71%	15%
Supraventricular	19%	20%
Ventricular	52%	20%
Conduction blocks (total)	48%	30%
Left anterior fascicular block	39%	30%
First-degree block	0%	10%
Sinus bradycardia	NR	10%
Sinus tachycardia	NR	20%

*Data from Harpster, N. K.: Feline myocardial diseases. *In* Kirk, R. W. (ed.): *Current Veterinary Therapy IX.* Philadelphia: W. B. Saunders, 1986, p. 383.

†Data from Bright, J. M., and Golden, A. L.: Feline hypertrophic cardiomyopathy: Variations on a theme. ACVIM Proceedings 1990, p. 293.

‡LVH pattern denotes presence of an increased R wave amplitude in one or more of the following leads: lead II >0.9 mV; lead V4 >1.0 mV; lead V6 >0.6 mV; lead base/apex >1.0 mV.

NR, not reported.

Prolongation of the P wave (>0.04 sec), a prolonged QRS duration (>0.04 sec), and an increase in P wave and R wave amplitude have been previously described as common electrocardiographic findings (Harpster, 1986). However, recent reports indicate that these changes in the P and R wave are less common than originally suggested (Bright, 1990). Atrial fibrillation, ventricular premature contractions, and paroxysmal ventricular tachycardia often occur and may cause deterioration in a patient's hemodynamic and clinical status. Intraventricular conduction abnormalities consistent with left anterior fascicular block are observed frequently (Bright, 1990; Harpster, 1986; Fox, 1988) (Fig. 4). Sinus bradycardia may be present, even in the presence of severe left heart failure (Bright, 1990; Moise et al., 1986).

Typical radiographic abnormalities associated with feline HCM include mild to moderate LV enlargement with more severe left atrial enlargement; however, variations may occur. Occasionally the radiographs will show generalized enlargement of the cardiac silhouette as a result of marked pericardial effusion. Whereas most cats have radiographic evidence of pulmonary edema, some have radiographic findings of biventricular heart failure as well (pleural effusion and hepatomegaly). Other feline patients have no radiographic evidence of circulatory congestion.

Echocardiography is the easiest and most sensitive method of determining the presence and severity of LV hypertrophy. Echocardiographic abnormalities usually noted in cats with HCM include symmetrical hypertrophy of the LV caudal wall and interventricular septum, reduced LV chamber dimensions, and left atrial enlargement (Bright, 1990; Moise et al., 1986). Some animals have significant right ventricular hypertrophy in addition to the characteristic LV hypertrophy (Fig. 5). Generally there is some correlation between the degree of LV hypertrophy and the severity of clinical signs, yet some severely symptomatic cats have mild hypertrophy and asymptomatic cats have been noted to have marked LV hypertrophy. The ventricle is usually hyperkinetic, but rarely systolic function is reduced owing to myocardial fibrosis associated with chronic disease. Systolic anterior motion of the mitral valve and asymmetric septal hypertrophy are common echocardiographic features of HCM in human patients but are uncommon in cats (Bright, 1990; Moise et al., 1986). Feline HCM secondary to either hyperthyroidism or hypersomatotropism cannot be reliably distinguished from primary HCM by echocardiography. Doppler echocardiography

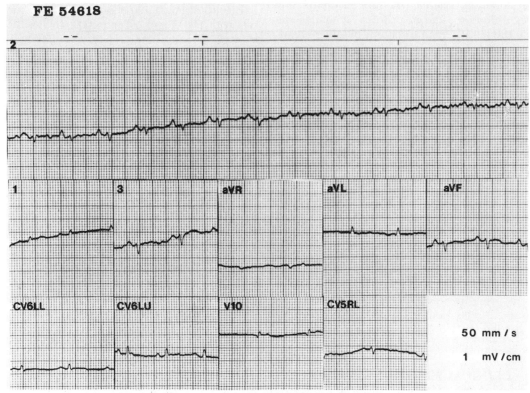

Figure 4. Electrocardiogram recorded from a cat with hypertrophic cardiomyopathy. Note the positive QRS complexes in leads I and aVL and S waves of greater amplitude than the r waves in leads II, III, and aVF. There is also a left axis deviation in the frontal plane. These findings are suggestive of a left anterior fascicular block, a common intraventricular conduction defect in cats with hypertrophic cardiomyopathy.

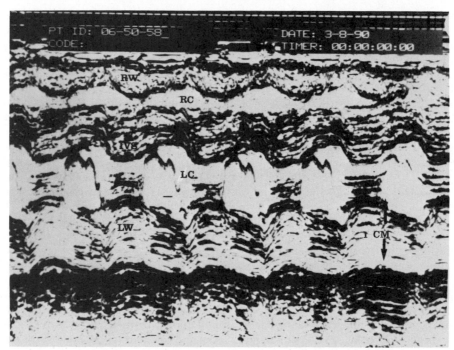

Figure 5. An M-mode echocardiogram recorded at the level of the mitral valve from a 4-year-old cat with hypertrophic cardiomyopathy. Note that this patient has hypertrophy of the right ventricular wall as well as the more typical findings of left ventricular free wall and septal hypertrophy (paper speed 100 mm/sec). IVS, interventricular septum; LC, left ventricular cavity; LW, left ventricular wall; RC, right ventricular cavity; RW, right ventricular wall.

demonstrates mitral regurgitation in the majority of cats with systolic murmurs.

TREATMENT OF HYPERTROPHIC CARDIOMYOPATHY

Medical management of HCM should be directed toward improving diastolic function, relieving myocardial ischemia, reducing LV systolic pressure gradients, eliminating circulatory congestion, and suppressing hemodynamically significant arrhythmias. In addition, therapy for acute and chronic management of thromboembolism should be considered. When possible, the underlying cause of myocardial hypertrophy should be identified and specifically treated.

Until recently, the treatment most often recommended for feline HCM has been beta-adrenergic blockade, usually with propranolol (Inderal, Wyeth-Ayerst Laboratories), and cautious use of diuretics to control pulmonary congestion. However, the clinical and hemodynamic benefits of propranolol have not been clearly documented in feline patients, and response to this drug is neither consistent nor always sustained. In humans with HCM, the beneficial effects of beta-blocking agents are primarily the result of drug-induced reduction of systolic outflow tract gradients. However, the importance of systolic pressure gradients, in feline patients is

uncertain (Bright, 1990). Furthermore, no consistent direct beneficial effects of beta-blockade on diastolic function have been demonstrated. In other words, beneficial effects of propranolol on diastolic LV volume and myocardial function occur indirectly through reduction of heart rate (prolonged filling and coronary perfusion time) and decreased myocardial oxygen demand (Lawson, 1987).

In contrast, the calcium channel blockers improve myocardial relaxation and increase ventricular filling. These drugs also reduce systolic gradients,* heart rate, and myocardial oxygen demand. Furthermore, calcium channel antagonists directly dilate the coronary vasculature, thereby relieving myocardial ischemia (Lawson, 1987).

Several calcium channel blocking agents are available, and these drugs have quite different cardiovascular effects (see this volume, p. 684; McCall et al., 1985). Nifedipine (Procardia, Pfizer Laboratories) and nicardipine (Cardene, Syntex Laboratories) are potent peripheral vasodilators that tend to produce reflex tachycardia, making them unsuitable for use in patients with HCM. Although verapamil (Isoptin, Knoll Pharmaceuticals) is the calcium channel blocking agent most widely used for treatment of humans with HCM, this drug has potent negative

---

Editors' Note: Calcium channel blockers may reduce systolic gradients if peripheral vasodilation and reduced afterload do not enhance ventricular shortening.

inotropic properties and a highly variable bioavailability in cats. Adverse effects including lethargy, inappetence, and acute pulmonary edema have occurred in cats receiving oral verapamil therapy (Bright et al., 1991).

Diltiazem (Cardizem, Marion Laboratories) is a calcium channel blocking agent that appears to be safe and effective for treatment of cats with HCM. Adverse effects are extremely rare when administered at a dose of 1.75 to 2.5 mg/kg orally t.i.d. Data from cats studied at the University of Tennessee suggest that diltiazem more consistently alleviates clinical signs and more effectively prolongs survival in cats with HCM than does either propranolol or verapamil. Radiographic, echocardiographic, and laboratory data indicate that orally administered diltiazem has sustained beneficial effects on LV filling and cardiac performance. In addition, long-term use of this drug may reverse myocardial hypertrophy in some patients (Bright et al., 1991).

Cats with HCM often present with life-threatening respiratory distress due to severe pulmonary edema or pleural effusion. In this situation, physical examination of the patient should be abbreviated to minimize stress and hasten therapeutic intervention. Immediate thoracocentesis is indicated when auscultation reveals muffled heart and lung sounds. The procedure is performed with the animal in the sternal position by introducing a sterile, 19- or 21-gauge butterfly needle (Abott Hospitals, Chicago, IL) into the seventh or eighth intercostal space at the level of the costochondral junction. Furosemide (Lasix, Hoechst-Roussel Pharmaceuticals) is immediately administered at a dosage of 2.2 mg/kg IM to cats with severe dyspnea due to pulmonary edema. The intramuscular route of administration is often preferred to intravenous administration in this situation because it causes less restraint-induced stress to the patient. At the same time, relief of circulatory congestion may be enhanced by administering 2% nitroglycerine ointment (Nitro-Bid, Marion Laboratories), 0.5 to 1.0 cm transdermally. Supplemental oxygen should be administered as well. These immediate interventions usually improve tissue oxygenation enough that a complete physical examination and diagnostic testing can be done safely.

Following stabilization of the patient's condition and confirmation of the diagnosis of HCM, furosemide administration is continued, usually at a dose of 1.1 mg/kg IM or PO t.i.d. to b.i.d. until edema has resolved radiographically. Aggressive diuretic therapy should be avoided because HCM patients need a higher than normal left atrial pressure to maintain adequate LV filling in the presence of reduced chamber compliance. Diltiazem administration is begun as soon as oral medication can be safely administered (1.75 to 2.5 mg/kg PO t.i.d.). It may take as long as 72 hours after initiating diltiazem to

detect a change in strength, appetite, and attitude in some animals. Following resolution of pulmonary edema, furosemide administration may be tapered and safely discontinued in many cats receiving diltiazem. Some cats may require chronic diuretic administration.

Although diltiazem has negative chronotropic effects, the drug does not appear to directly suppress sinoatrial nodal automaticity at the recommended dosage. Therefore, dosing should not be based on heart rate. With chronic diltiazem therapy, resting heart rate will decrease indirectly as cardiac performance improves. In cats with atrial fibrillation, propranolol may be cautiously administered in addition to diltiazem if needed to reduce the ventricular rate. However, cats receiving combined treatment with beta-blockade and calcium channel blockade should be closely monitored for the development of bradyarrhythmias and hypotension.

Certain drugs, including positive inotropic agents and arteriolar dilating drugs, are potentially harmful in patients with HCM. Cardiac glycosides, catecholamines, and phosphodiesterase inhibitors increase the myocardial oxygen demand and exacerbate systolic pressure gradients. Because patients with HCM have little preload reserve, inappropriate administration of afterload-reducing agents such as captopril (Capoten, E. R. Squibb & Sons) and hydralazine (Apresoline, CIBA Pharmaceuticals) can produce severe hypotension. These drugs as other vasodilating drugs (including some calcium-channel blockers) may also exacerbate intraventricular gradients if they are present. Any intervention that increases heart rate (e.g., catecholamines, hydralazine) is likely to have a deleterious effect on diastolic filling in cats with HCM.

Treatment of asymptomatic cats with HCM is predicated on the belief that medical intervention will either delay or prevent the onset of clinical signs or sudden death. Unfortunately, data are lacking to support this belief. Owners, therefore, may choose not to intervene medically. Trial therapy with diltiazem should perhaps be encouraged in this situation; in the author's experience, some cats considered normal by owners show an improvement in attitude and an increased level of activity when therapy is initiated. Furthermore, the drug is relatively inexpensive and has few, if any, side effects.

SYSTEMIC THROMBOEMBOLISM

Systemic arterial thromboembolism occurs frequently in cats with HCM and is often responsible for ischemic neuromyopathy or visceral organ dysfunction. A detailed discussion of the pathophysiology, diagnosis, and treatment of thromboembolism is available in other texts (Flanders, 1986; Fox,

1988) (see *CVT X*, p. 295). Administration of propranolol should be avoided, as this drug may reduce collateral circulation through beta$_2$-adrenergic antagonism. Arteriolar dilating agents such as acepromazine maleate (Prom Ace, Ayerst Laboratories) and hydralazine may have deleterious effects on cardiac performance in patients with HCM, and improved collateral flow following the use of these vasodilating drugs has not been demonstrated. Aspirin has been shown to inhibit the aggregation of feline platelets and to improve collateral circulation in cats with experimentally-induced aortic thrombosis. The recommended dose of aspirin is 25 mg/kg every third day (Flanders, 1986). No controlled clinical studies are available, however, to confirm the preventive effects of aspirin in cats with HCM. Aspirin administered at the recommended dose does not consistently prevent reoccurrence of thromboembolism (Fox, 1988).

Calcium channel blocking agents such as diltiazem inhibit platelet aggregation, which is theoretically beneficial in cats with HCM (Flanders, 1986). Diltiazem may, therefore, deter intravascular thrombus formation by this mechanism and also by improving cardiac performance.

PROGNOSIS

The prognosis for cats with hypertrophic cardiomyopathy is in general favorable. In many cats, even those refractory to diuretics, beta-adrenergic antagonists, and aspirin, signs of congestion, edema, and embolism may be eliminated with diltiazem therapy for a period of months to years. The presence of atrial fibrillation or severe biventricular heart failure confers a more guarded prognosis. Although some data are available to suggest that long-term administration of calcium channel antagonists such as diltiazem may reverse myocardial hypertrophy in patients with HCM, the results of these studies are inconclusive.

References and Suggested Reading

Bright, J. M., Golden, A. L., Gompf, R. E., et al.: Evaluation of the calcium channel blocking agents diltiazem and verapamil for treatment of feline hypertrophic cardiomyopathy. J. Vet. Intern. Med. 5(5), 1991.
A randomized, prospective study of calcium channel blocking agents and beta-adrenergic blocking agents in cats with hypertrophic cardiomyopathy.
Bright, J. M., and Golden, A. L.: Feline hypertrophic cardiomyopathy: Variations on a theme. Scientific Proceedings, ACVIM 1990, p. 293.
A descriptive study of the historical, physical, electrocardiographic, echocardiographic, radiographic, angiographic, and hemodynamic features of cats with idiopathic hypertrophic cardiomyopathy.
Flanders, J. A.: Feline aortic thromboembolism. Comp. Cont. Ed. Pract. Vet. 8:473, 1986.
A thorough discussion of the clinical presentation, pathogenesis, and treatment of aortic thromboembolism in cats.
Fox, P. R.: Feline myocardial disease. *In* Fox, P. R. (ed.): *Canine and Feline Cardiology.* New York: Churchill Livingstone, 1988, p. 435.
An exhaustive review of the various forms of feline myocardial disease, including hypertrophic cardiomyopathy.
Golden, A. L., and Bright, J. M.: Use of relaxation half-time as an index of ventricular relaxation in clinically normal cats and cats with hypertrophic cardiomyopathy. Am. J. Vet. Res. 51:1352, 1990.
A comparison of hemodynamic findings in cats with hypertrophic cardiomyopathy and normal cats.
Harpster, N. K.: Feline myocardial diseases. *In* Kirk, R. W. (ed.): *Current Veterinary Therapy IX.* Philadelphia: W. B. Saunders, 1986, p. 380.
A discussion of the various types of feline myocardial disease, including hypertrophic cardiomyopathy.
Lawson, J. W. R.: Southwest internal medicine conference: Hypertrophic cardiomyopathy: Current views on etiology, pathophysiology, and management. Am. J. Med. Sci. 294:191, 1987.
A thorough review of hypertrophic cardiomyopathy in human patients.
McCall, D., Walsh, R. A., Frohlick, E. D., et al.: Calcium entry blocking drugs: Mechanisms of action, experimental studies and clinical uses. Curr. Prob. Cardiol. 10:1, 1985.
A thorough review of the calcium channel antagonists.
Moise, N. S., Dietze, A. E., Mezza, L. E., et al.: Echocardiography, electrocardiography, and radiography of cats with dilatation cardiomyopathy, hypertrophic cardiomyopathy, and hyperthyroidism. Am. J. Vet. Res. 47:1476, 1986.
A prospective study of the echocardiographic, radiographic, and electrocardiographic findings in 35 cats with cardiomyopathy.

UPDATE: CANINE DILATED CARDIOMYOPATHY

CLAY A. CALVERT
Athens, Georgia

Idiopathic dilated cardiomyopathies are chronic diseases typically characterized by a protracted subclinical course terminating in end-stage, acute congestive heart failure (Calvert, 1986; Gooding et al., 1986; Harpster, 1983; Lunney and Ettinger, 1991). Ventricular dilation and dysfunction are insidious, gradual, and relentlessly progressive. Affected dogs may exhibit no overt abnormalities prior to the onset of congestive heart failure (CHF), after which the survival time is often very short. Sudden death may occur owing to ventricular tachyarrhythmias.

ETIOLOGY

The etiology of primary cardiomyopathies is unknown. It is possible that multiple etiologies exist among various breeds of dogs, and it is probable that genetic factors play a role in some breeds (e.g., Doberman pinschers, boxers, and cocker spaniels). Familial trends in some breeds seem to vary by country or geographic region. The author has observed familial clustering in lines of Doberman pinschers affecting as many as four consecutive generations. It is likely that some breeds carry one or more metabolic defects leading to deficiency of one or more enzymes or trophic factors necessary for myocardial biochemical integrity.

PREVALENCE

The incidence of cardiomyopathies is unknown. Dilated cardiomyopathy (DCM) primarily affects large dogs, although English bulldogs, cocker spaniels, Brittany spaniels, and bull terriers are also affected. During the past 10 years of the author's practice, the majority of cardiomyopathic dogs have been Doberman pinschers. During each of the past 5 years, clinical and electrocardiographic abnormalities consistent with CHF and DCM have been noted in approximately 1500 Doberman pinschers during transtelephonic consultation (Cardiopet, Floral Park, NY). Although partially explained by breed popularity, this prevalence far exceeds that of most other breeds. Boxers and cocker spaniels are also commonly affected.

TIME COURSE

Left ventricular (LV) dysfunction begins insidiously and progresses gradually over a period of several years. Serial echocardiographic monitoring of individual dogs indicates that LV dysfunction progresses gradually for approximately 2 to 2.5 years in the Doberman pinscher, after which LV dilation and decreasing contractility accelerate. After an additional year, CHF occurs (Fig. 1). Ventricular tachyarrhythmias are an inherent component of the disease throughout its course, and sudden death may intervene. A similar evolution exists in some affected boxers.

Typically, evidence of mild LV dysfunction and, in some breeds, cardiac arrhythmias are detectable by 4 to 5 years of age, and CHF most commonly

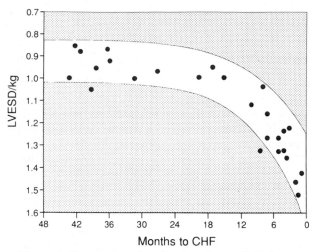

Figure 1. Time course of cardiomyopathy in 26 Doberman pinschers from the point of initial echocardiographic examination to the onset of congestive heart failure. The left ventricular end-systolic dimension (LVESD) normalized to body weight is plotted against time to onset of heart failure.

occurs between 6 and 9 years of age. However, the emergence and time course of the disease vary among individuals, and abnormalities may not be detected until 9 to 10 years of age. Some dogs develop CHF beyond these ages or die of intercurrent disease without manifesting cardiomyopathy, even though microscopic evidence of myocardial disease is found.

MANIFESTATIONS

Arrhythmias

Cardiac arrhythmias are inherent components of cardiomyopathy in Doberman pinschers, boxers, and American cocker spaniels. Both supraventricular and ventricular tachyarrhythmias develop early in the disease course. However, these arrhythmias are initially mild and paroxysmal and are often not readily apparent on physical examination or a brief, resting electrocardiogram (ECG).

SUDDEN DEATH. Sudden cardiac death is common among cardiomyopathic Doberman pinschers and boxers. It is generally believed, and has been documented in some instances, that these sudden deaths are the result of malignant ventricular tachycardia leading to fibrillation.

Congestive Heart Failure

Congestive heart failure is the end stage of the disease and is often the first overt manifestation, especially in breeds such as Great Danes, Irish wolfhounds, and others in which arrhythmias are less prevalent.

DIAGNOSIS

End-Stage Cardiomyopathy

The diagnosis of end-stage cardiomyopathy is not difficult and is characterized by ECG, radiographic, and echocardiographic evidence of cardiac enlargement (see *CVT X*, p. 240). Predominant left-sided CHF (pulmonary edema) occurs in Doberman pinschers, boxers, and cocker spaniels, while bilateral heart failure (ascites, pleural effusion, and pulmonary edema) is typical in most giant-breed dogs.

Occult Cardiomyopathy

Echocardiography and long-term ambulatory ECG (Holter) recording are useful in the diagnosis of occult cardiomyopathy. Echocardiography is a relatively sensitive test in all breeds; however, because there is often no overt evidence of the disease and one cannot examine all dogs, identification of affected dogs is difficult. Systolic heart murmurs may develop, but mitral or tricuspid regurgitation may be the result of endocardiosis rather than of cardiomyopathy.

Holter recording is useful in identifying affected Doberman pinschers, boxers, and American cocker spaniels because arrhythmias are inherent components of cardiomyopathy in these breeds (Fig. 2). Holter recording is less useful in other breeds owing to a lower incidence of arrhythmias. In any case, results of Holter recordings and echocardiography should be interpreted together. Holter recordings are indicated in dogs experiencing syncope and in those with arrhythmias detected during routine physical examination. Owing to the high prevalence of the disease in Doberman pinschers, routine

screening of these dogs may be justifiable. Screening tests are also justifiable in dogs with a familial history of cardiomyopathy.

THERAPY

Occult Cardiomyopathy

Diagnosis of cardiomyopathy is possible during the subclinical stage through the use of echocardiography and Holter recording. Left ventricular function and heart rhythm should be carefully evaluated and a surveillance schedule established so as to follow disease progression.

ARRHYTHMIAS. In the presence of potentially life-threatening ventricular arrhythmias such as ventricular tachycardia, antiarrhythmic therapy is recommended. In the author's experience, Holter recordings indicate that, compared with single-drug therapy, a Class I drug such as quinidine gluconate (Quinaglute, Berlex Laboratories) at a dosage of 8 to 10 mg/kg t.i.d., procainamide HCl (Procan SR, Parke-Davis) 15 to 20 mg/kg t.i.d., or tocainide HCl (Tonocard, Merck Sharp & Dohme) 15 to 20 mg/kg t.i.d. in combination with a Class II drug such as propranolol (Inderal, Wyeth-Ayerst Laboratories, 1 mg/kg t.i.d.) is more effective in terms of quantitative reduction of ventricular premature contractions and elimination of ventricular tachycardia.

In Doberman pinschers, the sequential use of Class I drugs indicates more effective quantitative control of arrhythmias by tocainide as compared with quinidine, procainamide, and moricizine HCl (Ethmozine, DuPont) in some dogs, particularly after several months of treatment. However, tocainide is significantly more expensive than quinidine and procainamide and may be associated with a higher incidence of gastrointestinal disturbances. Long-term use (longer than 4 months) of tocainide has also been associated with progressive corneal endothelial dystrophy and acute, hyposthenuric

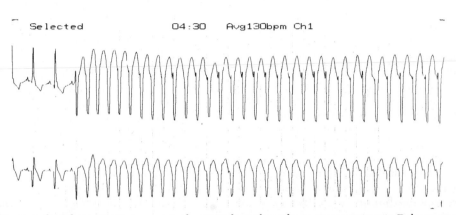

Figure 2. Holter recording demonstrating paroxysmal ventricular tachycardia in an asymptomatic Doberman pinscher. Sudden death occurred a few weeks later.

renal failure in a significant percentage of Doberman pinschers. A causal relationship to the drug is strongly suspected.

VENTRICULAR DYSFUNCTION. Whether early medical intervention can alter the progression of ventricular dysfunction remains to be proved. Angiotensin-converting enzyme (ACE) inhibitors, beta-adrenergic–blocking drugs, and L-carnitine have been variably prescribed. It is unlikely that ACE inhibitors will alter disease progression early in its course, since the renin-angiotensin-aldosterone system is not activated. When the disease progresses to the point where exercise intolerance, radiographic evidence of pulmonary lobar vein distention, or a gallop heart rhythm is present, drugs such as furosemide, an ACE inhibitor, and digoxin should be prescribed.

CONGESTIVE HEART FAILURE

Medical therapy is determined by the severity of CHF, presence and severity of ventricular tachyarrhythmias, and the presence or absence of atrial fibrillation.

Acute Life-Threatening Congestive Heart Failure

Immediately life-threatening CHF is most commonly encountered in Doberman pinschers, but cardiogenic stock may occur in any breed, particularly in dogs with atrial fibrillation and a ventricular response rate greater than 240/min. Affected dogs are extremely weak and dyspneic, have pale or gray oral mucous membranes and weak femoral pulses, are often hypothermic, and have excessive (>10°F) toe-web-to-rectal temperature differentials. Doberman pinschers and occasionally other breeds may exhibit a frothy, serosanguineous nasal discharge indicating the presence of florid pulmonary edema.

PRELOAD REDUCTION. Furosemide at a dosage of 2 to 8 mg/kg IV with re-evaluation and retreatment in 4 to 6 hr at a dosage of 2 to 4 mg/kg is the most effective initial treatment. Dosage reduction to 1 mg/kg t.i.d. after 1 day and b.i.d. after 2 days is desirable. Side effects of high-dose furosemide therapy are common and include dehydration, electrolyte depletion, azotemia, and aggravation of arrhythmias. Nitrate therapy such as with 2% nitroglycerin ointment (Nitrol, Adria Laboratories) at a dosage of 1 to 2 cm t.i.d. is also recommended and should be continued for 7 days.

POSITIVE INOTROPIC THERAPY. Even though the clinical signs of excess preload (dyspnea, orthopnea, coughing, crackles) may be improved with aggressive preload reduction therapy, a positive inotropic agent is indicated because cardiac output is severely embarrassed. Dobutamine (Dobutrex, Eli Lilly) (2

to 8 micrograms/kg/min, constant rate infusion) is recommended. Many dogs that do not receive a rapid-acting, potent, inotropic drug like dobutamine or amrinone succumb during the first 72 hr of therapy. Dobutamine causes direct myocardial stimulation with minimum effect on heart rate or vasoconstriction. Exacerbation or production of ventricular arrhythmias is a common complication associated with the use of these drugs; therefore, continuous monitoring of heart rhythm is recommended, especially in Doberman pinschers.

Digoxin is a modest cardiac stimulant that when given orally requires several days or longer to exert a positive inotropic effect. An increase in contractility may not develop in dogs with severe, global myocardial failure. Digoxin is not recommended for intravenous use because ventricular arrhythmias and vasoconstriction may be exacerbated. If the patient is in atrial fibrillation, digoxin may be initiated by an oral maintenance schedule (0.005 mg/kg b.i.d.). For hemodynamically unstable patients with heart rates above 240/min, a semiloading schedule (0.01 mg/kg given twice at 12-hr intervals) may be administered for the first 24 hr, followed by the maintenance schedule.

AFTERLOAD REDUCTION. Arteriolar dilator therapy is, in theory, indicated for patients with CHF due to dilated cardiomyopathy. However, afterload reducers such as hydralazine and ACE inhibitors may exacerbate pre-existing hypotension and are not recommended until systemic arterial blood pressure has been stabilized by a potent inotropic drug.

ARRHYTHMIA CONTROL. When complex, potentially life-threatening ventricular tachyarrhythmias are encountered, antiarrhythmic therapy is recommended. Such therapy is paramount and should be initiated immediately when dobutamine therapy is contemplated in dogs with ventricular arrhythmias.

Lidocaine is recommended at a dosage of 35 to 50 µg/kg/min constant rate infusion. Since steady-state levels are not achieved for several hours, periodic boluses of 1 mg/kg given over 30 sec are often necessary to suppress dangerous arrhythmias. Although arrhythmia severity may lessen with effective therapy of CHF, Doberman pinchers and some boxers usually continue to experience arrhythmias and maintenance antiarrhythmic therapy may be required.

SUPPORTIVE THERAPY. Oxygen therapy is vital in patients with florid pulmonary edema. Administration of 100% oxygen by face mask or transparent hood is recommended for the most severely affected patients. Intranasal oxygen administration is substituted when pulmonary function is improved. Myocardial oxygen perfusion may be improved and arrhythmias may lessen in severity. It is important to avoid exertion and stress. Unnecessary diagnostic tests should be postponed and even radiographs and echocardiography should sometimes be delayed under these circumstances. Morphine (0.05 to 0.1

mg/kg IM) may be indicated to reduce anxiety and dyspnea. One or two episodes of vomition may occur during the first 30 min after administration.

High-dose diuretic therapy coupled with decreased water intake frequently leads to dehydration, azotemia, and hyponatremia. Fluid therapy may be required but must be administered cautiously and is ideally guided by monitoring of pulmonary capillary wedge or at least central venous pressure (CVP). Lactated Ringer's solution or half-strength Ringer's and 2.5% dextrose is recommended at volumes not to exceed 30 to 40 ml/kg daily. The former is indicated in the face of hyponatremia, and potassium chloride supplementation of fluids is indicated at a rate of 20 to 40 mEq/L for hypokalemia. Fluid therapy is contraindicated if the CVP is greater than 12 to 15 cm of H_2O (or pulmonary wedge >2.0 mm Hg) and is administered very cautiously at CVPs between 8 and 12.

Pleural effusion and ascites are common sequelae of cardiomyopathy in giant-breed dogs but are less common in Doberman pinschers. Moderate to severe pleural effusion can significantly embarrass respiratory function and thoracocentesis is indicated for diagnostic and therapeutic purposes. Severe ascites can also embarrass respiration, cause the patient difficulty when lying down, and make resting or sleeping difficult. A volume of ascitic fluid should be removed sufficient to make the patient comfortable. Repeated or chronic paracentesis of this high-protein ascites will lead to fluid shifts, hypovolemia, and hypoalbuminemia.

Total restriction of activity must be enforced for several weeks after the onset of acute CHF, and thereafter only minimal activity should be allowed. Exercise places undue strain on the myocardium, may accelerate deterioration, and in Doberman pinschers can exacerbate ventricular arrhythmias, causing sudden death.

Maintenance Therapy

PRELOAD REDUCTION. Furosemide should be administered at a dosage of approximately 2 mg/kg b.i.d. With time, higher dosages are often required, and nitrate therapy may be necessary for refractory pulmonary edema. When nitrates are administered chronically, they should be given on alternate days to avoid drug resistance. Nitroglycerin ointment (2%) at a dosage of 1 to 2 cm t.i.d. or isosorbide dinitrate (Isordil, Wyeth-Ayerst Laboratories) 0.5 to 2.0 mg/kg, b.i.d. to t.i.d. is an acceptable regimen.

POSITIVE INOTROPIC TREATMENT. Digoxin (Lanoxin, Burroughs Wellcome) therapy is generally recommended for maintenance therapy of dogs with predominant sinus rhythm and is always recommended for dogs with atrial fibrillation, atrial tachycardia, or frequent atrial premature contractions. The maintenance dosage for large dogs is 0.005 mg/ kg b.i.d. However, because of uncertainties of the volume of distribution, renal excretion, and individual variation, measurement of serum digoxin concentrations is recommended at approximately 7 days of therapy and periodically thereafter. Acceptable serum concentrations are 1 to 2 ng/ml. Trough (12-hr postpill) values of 1 to 1.5 and peak values (4 to 6 hr postpill) of 1.5 to 2.0 are recommended. Serum digoxin concentrations must be interpreted in light of the patient's overall condition and treatment response because the therapeutic index is narrow.

AFTERLOAD REDUCTION. Peripheral arteriolar dilation therapy is usually recommended after the patient's blood pressure has been stabilized. The ACE inhibitors are recommended because they are the primary agents that block the neurohormonal mechanisms responsible for many of the symptoms of advanced CHF. Diuretics and direct-acting arteriolar dilators tend to enhance endocrine and sympathetic neural responses, producing reflex vasoconstriction, tachycardia, arrhythmias, fluid, and sodium retention.

Enalapril (Vasotec, Merck Sharp & Dohme) at 0.05 to 0.5 mg/kg b.i.d. is the author's first choice. Outpatient therapy should always begin conservatively and be gradually increased every 3 to 7 days. Diarrhea, lethargy, anorexia, and nausea may be encountered initially, and in such instances the drug should be withdrawn and reintroduced at a lower dosage, perhaps accompanied by a small meal. Diarrhea, anorexia, nausea, and hypotension may be encountered during dosage escalation, and the drug should then be withdrawn for 24 hr and reinstituted at the previous dosage. Captopril (Capoten, Squibb) at 0.5 to 1.0 mg/kg, t.i.d. is also an acceptable drug. Because anorexia and gastrointestinal disturbances are common side effects of both digoxin and ACE inhibitors, some clinicians prefer to establish the therapeutic dosage of one of the drugs before initiating the other. In the face of atrial fibrillation, digoxin therapy is initiated first.

INVESTIGATIONAL THERAPY. Although controversial, elective replenishment of catecholamines via the infusion of dobutamine (2 to 8 μg/kg/min) over a 72-hr period has produced sustained hemodynamic and clinical improvement (up to 6 months) in some cardiomyopathic human patients. Results have been inconsistent, sudden death is a potential complication, and long-term survival has not been improved. The author has administered this therapy to a number of Doberman pinschers with poorly controlled CHF. Some owners reported equivocal subjective improvement, but arrhythmias were exacerbated during infusion and survival times were not noticeably prolonged.

ANTIARRHYTHMIC THERAPY. Potentially life-threatening ventricular arrhythmias are commonly associated with cardiomyopathy in Doberman pinschers, boxers, possibly American cocker spaniels, and occasionally others. Complex ventricular tachyarrhythmias, particularly nonsustained or sustained ventricular tachycardia, are indications for therapy. A Class I drug such as procainamide (15 to 20 mg/kg t.i.d.) or tocainide (15 to 20 mg/kg t.i.d.) is recommended. In the author's experience, the latter is more effective in terms of quantitative reduction of arrhythmia, especially on a long-term basis, but cost is a limiting factor. Tocainide may have less proarrhythmic and negative inotropic activity than procainamide. Serum tocainide concentrations of 4 to 10 mg/L are considered as therapeutic but a range of 7 to 10 mg/L is recommended for optimum efficacy. A dose of 15 to 20 mg/kg t.i.d. usually produces peak (2-hr postpill) serum concentrations of 10 to 12 mg/L and trough (8-hr postpill) values of 6 to 8 mg/L. Holter recording data indicate that twice-daily administration and dosages less than 15 mg/kg t.i.d. are less effective. Anorexia, the most common adverse effect, may occur with peak serum concentrations not exceeding 10 mg/L but is most commonly associated with concentrations exceeding 12 mg/L. Weakness, head tremor, head bobbing, and ataxia may occur at concentrations above 14 mg/L. Quinidine is generally not recommended because of a drug interaction necessitating digoxin dosage reduction to avoid digoxin toxicity. Periodic Holter monitoring is recommended to confirm control of the arrhythmia.

ATRIAL FIBRILLATION WITH RAPID VENTRICULAR RESPONSE. Following adequate digitalization, as confirmed by serum concentrations and clinical signs, some dogs with atrial fibrillation maintain rapid ventricular responses (>180/min). Such rates are partially associated with increased sympathetic tone associated with CHF and the stress of hospitalization. Holter recording in the home environment is recommended. If rates above 160/min are common throughout the day, the prognosis is worse and additional therapy may be warranted. Adequately digitalized dogs that have responded well to therapy have heart rates below 160/min in the home environment during mild to moderate exertion. Severe exertion should not be permitted.

A beta-adrenergic–blocking drug such as Inderal (0.1 to 0.2 mg/kg t.i.d.) or a calcium entry-blocking drug such as diltiazem (Cardizem, Marion Laboratories) (0.4 to 0.5 mg/kg t.i.d.) may be cautiously employed. The dosage should be gradually increased every 2 to 3 days while the patient is observed for deterioration of cardiovascular function. Diltiazem produces peripheral vasodilation and significant negative inotropic effect in some cardiomyopathic humans. Dosages above 0.5 to 0.6 mg/kg of propranolol or 1.0 mg/kg of diltiazem are not recommended by the author. Whether blocking drugs exert a favorable long-term effect when used for this purpose remains to be demonstrated.

SUPPORTIVE THERAPY. A low-salt diet should be implemented as soon as is feasible; this can be accomplished immediately in dogs that have retained their appetites. However, anorexia is a common problem, and under such circumstances the patient should be offered more palatable food, although unnecessarily salty foods should be avoided. Most dogs lose 2 to 8 kg of weight within weeks of the onset of CHF, and cachexia becomes most severe in dogs exhibiting overt generalized CHF. Adequate protein and appropriate dietary supplements are recommended. Periodic monitoring of renal function and electrolytes is essential in the management of severe myocardial failure, particularly since diuretics and ACE inhibitors are known to predispose to renal dysfunction and electrolyte depletion. Both azotemia and electrolyte depletion predispose to digoxin toxicity and ventricular tachyarrhythmias.

PROGNOSIS

The prognosis for adult dogs is poor. In general, Doberman pinschers probably have the shortest survival times after the onset of CHF, while English cocker spaniels may have the longest survival times. The latter may survive several episodes of CHF if efficient and aggressive therapy is provided.

Occult Cardiomyopathy

Survival time following the diagnosis of occult cardiomyopathy is dependent upon the point of progression at which the diagnosis is made. In Doberman pinschers, if the LV shortening fraction is less than 20%, CHF usually occurs within 1 year. Radiographic evidence of left atrial enlargement is seen during the 9 months prior to CHF, wide and slurred R waves during the 6 months prior to CHF, and gallop heart rhythms up to 3 months prior to CHF. In breeds in which ventricular tachyarrhythmias are inherent problems sudden cardiac death may occur during the occult phase of the disease. Of 47 Doberman pinschers managed by the author, 10 (21%) died suddenly, and all had histories of ventricular tachyarrhythmias, including ventricular tachycardia in 7.

Congestive Heart Failure

Once CHF develops, the prognosis is extremely poor. Dogs with atrial fibrillation and peripheral edema have the shortest survival times. Six-month mortality of 75% to 85% is usual under these circumstances (Bohn et al., 1971; Bonagura and Ware, 1986; Thomas, 1984). The mean and median survival times of Doberman pinschers with pulmonary edema seen in the author's institution were 9.5 and 5 weeks, respectively (range, <1 to 64). Twenty-five percent died within 2 weeks. Of those surviving longer than 2 weeks, the mean and median survival times were 12 and 8 weeks, respectively. The cause of death after the onset of CHF in approximately 20% of the dogs was sudden death.

EFFECT OF MEDICAL THERAPY ON SURVIVAL

No rigorous, prospective clinical trials have been conducted in dogs. Although diuretic therapy is generally accepted as essential and the survival time of cardiomyopathic dogs in CHF not receiving diuretics is decreased, these drugs do not alter the progression of disease.

Occult Cardiomyopathy

The drugs that would most logically be expected to exert a favorable influence on disease progression are the ACE inhibitors and beta-adrenergic–blocking drugs. However, in the author's experience with Doberman pinschers, disease progression in a small group of dogs receiving these drugs was not different from that in a group without such treatment. Nonetheless, controlled clinical trials in this area are currently under way. Sudden cardiac death in Doberman pinschers, boxers, and possibly American cocker spaniels is a significant problem. Although antiarrhythmic therapy is probably effective in some dogs, in terms of prevention of sudden death, overall efficacy remains to be proved.

Congestive Heart Failure

Powerful positive inotropes such as dobutamine, amrinone, and milrinone exert rather impressive short-term effects in terms of clinical and hemodynamic improvement. Some patients will not survive acute CHF if they do not receive one of these drugs. In humans, it has been demonstrated that long-term therapy with milrinone is associated with increased mortality. Thus, the appropriate use of these agents is as short-term therapy in the face of severe, acute CHF. Dogs such as Doberman pinschers often cannot be stabilized without the use of powerful, rapid-acting inotropes.

Digoxin is most likely to exert a favorable influence on survival of dogs with atrial fibrillation (Kittleson et al., 1985). Improved contractility is not achieved in the majority of cardiomyopathic dogs and neither a favorable nor an unfavorable influence on long-term survival has been demonstrated in most dogs or in humans.

Enalapril, an ACE inhibitor, is the only drug convincingly proved by vigorous, placebo-controlled, prospective trials in humans to exert a favorable influence on disease progression in humans with advanced CHF, including dilated cardiomyopathy (The CONSENSUS Trial, 1987). It is not known whether these results can be duplicated in cardiomyopathic dogs.

Beta-adrenergic–blocking agents such as metoprolol and propranolol may exert a favorable influence on survival of humans with advanced cardiomyopathy (Swedberg et al., 1979). Even though vigorous prospective trials have not been completed, the use of low-dose beta-blockade with gradual dosage increase is gaining acceptance for the treatment of a not yet defined subset of cardiomyopathic humans. No data are available in dogs.

L-Carnitine appears to be an important treatment for some cardiomyopathic boxers, especially young dogs (Keene et al., 1991) (see this volume, p. 780).

References and Suggested Reading

Bohn, F. K., Patterson, D. F., and Pyle, R. L.: Atrial fibrillation in dogs. Br. Vet. J. 127:485, 1971.

Bonagura, J. D., and Ware, W. A.: Atrial fibrillation in the dog: Clinical findings in 81 cases. J. Am. Anim. Hosp. Assoc. 22:111, 1986.

Calvert, C. A.: Dilated cardiomyopathy in Doberman pinschers. Comp. Cont. Ed. Pract. Vet. 8:417, 1986.

Gooding, J. P., Robinson, W. F., and Mews, G. C.: Echocardiographic characterization of dilation cardiomyopathy in the English cocker spaniel. Am. J. Vet. Res. 47:1978, 1986.

Harpster, N.: Boxer cardiomyopathy. In Kirk, R. W. (ed.): Current Veterinary Therapy VIII. Philadelphia: W. B. Saunders, 1983, pp. 329–336.

Keene, B. W., Panciera, D. P., Atkins, C. E., et al.: Myocardial L-carnitine deficiency in a family of dogs with dilated cardiomyopathy. J.A.V.M.A. 198:647, 1991.

Kittleson, M. D., Eyster, G. E., Knowlen, G. G., et al.: Efficacy of digoxin administration in dogs with idiopathic dilated cardiomyopathy. J.A.V.M.A. 186:162, 1985.

Lunney, J., and Ettinger, S. F.: Canine dilated cardiomyopathies. Waltham International Focus. 1:16, 1991.

The CONSENSUS Trial Study Group: Effects of enalapril on mortality of severe congestive heart failure: Results of the Cooperative North Scandinavia Survival Study. N. Engl. J. Med. 316:1429, 1987.

Swedberg, K., Waagstein, F., Hjalmmarson, A., et al.: Prolongation of survival in congestive cardiomyopathy by beta-receptor blockade. Lancet 1:1374, 1979.

Thomas, R. E.: Atrial fibrillation in the dog: A review of eight cases. J. Small Anim. Pract. 25:421, 1984.

L-CARNITINE DEFICIENCY IN CANINE DILATED CARDIOMYOPATHY

BRUCE W. KEENE
Raleigh, North Carolina

This article briefly reviews the currently available scientific evidence and clinical experience regarding myocardial L-carnitine deficiency and its association with canine dilated cardiomyopathy. L-Carnitine (3-hydroxy, 4-*N*-trimethylaminobutyric acid) is a small (molecular weight 160), water-soluble quaternary amine found in high concentrations in mammalian heart and skeletal muscle. Although L-carnitine was discovered in 1905 and the chemical structure confirmed in 1927, extensive research into the functions of L-carnitine really began in the 1970's, and L-carnitine did not become commercially available until the 1980's.

SYNTHESIS AND DISPOSITION OF L-CARNITINE

In dogs, L-carnitine is synthesized from the amino acids lysine and methionine. The enzyme required for the final step in L-carnitine synthesis, gamma-butyrobetaine hydroxylase, is found primarily in the liver and is not present in mammalian heart or skeletal muscle. A poorly understood membrane transport mechanism concentrates L-carnitine in the cardiac and skeletal myocytes. In normal mammals, including normal dogs, plasma carnitine concentrations correlate closely with myocardial carnitine concentrations. This close correlation is often absent in the setting of dilated cardiomyopathy.

Commercially prepared L-carnitine administered orally to dogs is rapidly and completely absorbed, and plasma concentrations following a single oral dose remain elevated for approximately 8 hr. D-Carnitine (the other optical isomer) is not synthesized by mammals and renders mammalian L-carnitine–containing enzyme systems inactive when substituted for the L-isomer. Because of the biologic difference between the optical isomers of carnitine and the lack of any endogenous ability to convert D-carnitine to L-carnitine, neither D-carnitine nor the racemic mixture can be safely administered to mammals. In the rest of this article, the term *carnitine* refers to *L-carnitine only*.

FUNCTIONS OF L-CARNITINE

Adequate myocardial concentrations of free carnitine are required for fatty acid metabolism and serve an important detoxifying role in the mitochondria as well (Bremer, 1983). Although the heart utilizes various metabolic substrates to maintain the constant supply of energy needed to sustain effective contraction and relaxation, it is well established that long-chain free fatty acids are quantitatively the most important. Carnitine is a critical component of the mitochondrial membrane enzymes (carnitine acetyltransferase I and II), which transport activated fatty acids in the form of acylcarnitine esters across the mitochondrial membranes to the matrix, where beta-oxidation and subsequent high-energy phosphate generation occurs.

In addition to its role in fatty acid transport, free carnitine serves as a mitochondrial detoxifying agent by accepting (or "scavenging") acyl groups and other potentially toxic metabolites and transporting them out of the mitochondria as carnitine esters. Many defects in mitochondrial metabolism result in the toxic accumulation of these substances. For example, propionyl-CoA decarboxylase deficiency (one of the so-called organic acidurias) causes the toxic accumulation of propionyl-CoA in mitochondria unless free carnitine is available to form a propionyl-carnitine ester (which is excreted in the urine) and regenerate metabolically useful free CoA. Similarly, defects in mitochondrial medium-chain, long-chain, or multiple acyl-CoA dehydrogenase enzymes have been shown to cause the toxic accumulation of acyl-CoA unless the acyl group can be esterified to free carnitine, producing an acylcarnitine ester and regenerating free CoA. The excess carnitine esters generated when free carnitine is used in this capacity cannot be reabsorbed by the kidneys, and carnitine deficiency eventually results if large quantities of free carnitine are not supplied. Ideally, the buildup of metabolic toxins in the mitochondria can be prevented if adequate free carnitine is available. It is important to remember that the underlying mitochondrial defects are not corrected by carnitine supplementation in these situations, however, and carnitine therapy is at best palliative.

DIAGNOSIS OF CARNITINE DEFICIENCY

Carnitine deficiency states have been described since 1973 in humans. Various clinical signs have been reported in carnitine-deficient humans, including encephalopathy, muscle weakness, recurrent infections, failure to thrive, and congestive heart failure. Carnitine deficiency has been associated with primary myocardial diseases in humans, hamsters, and turkeys, and we have shown myocardial carnitine deficiency to be associated with dilated cardiomyopathy in a family of boxer dogs.

Normal canine values for total, free, and esterified carnitine concentrations in plasma and myocardium (Table 1) have been determined by constructing 95% confidence intervals based on measurements performed in a small (n=6) number of healthy dogs fed a standard commercial diet. These values are similar to those from larger, open-chest dog studies reported by other investigators (Rebouche and Engel, 1983).

Based on an accepted human classification system (Winter et al., 1987), an absolute decrease in the plasma free carnitine concentration is termed *plasma carnitine deficiency*. Similarly, myocardial carnitine deficiency is diagnosed when the myocardial carnitine concentration falls below the 95% confidence interval for normal. In humans, when the ratio of esterified to free carnitine in plasma exceeds 0.4 in the presence of normal plasma concentrations of free carnitine, carnitine insufficiency is said to exist. The utility of this ratio has not been extensively investigated in dogs. If both plasma and tissue free carnitine concentrations are decreased, affected animals can be said to have systemic carnitine deficiency. When endomyocardial biopsy specimens contain decreased free carnitine concentrations despite normal or even elevated plasma free carnitine concentrations, the term *myopathic carnitine deficiency* is often descriptive.

Tissue biopsy samples are needed to definitively document the presence of tissue carnitine deficiency. Plasma carnitine deficiency appears to be a specific but *insensitive* marker for myocardial car-

nitine deficiency in dogs with dilated cardiomyopathy. Most (80%) of the dogs in which myocardial carnitine deficiency has been identified in association with dilated cardiomyopathy fall into the classification of myopathic carnitine deficiency (i.e., decreased myocardial carnitine concentrations in the presence of normal or elevated plasma carnitine concentrations). Systemic carnitine deficiency accounts for approximately 20% of the cases.

A description of the technique for the measurement of plasma and tissue carnitine concentrations (Parvin and Pande, 1977) is beyond the scope of this article. Appropriate samples (1 ml of heparinized plasma that was immediately separated and frozen, two 5-mg endomyocardial biopsy specimens acquired by standard techniques [Keene et al., 1990], blotted dry, and frozen in liquid nitrogen within 15 sec of acquisition) may be sent to various commercial or research laboratories for analysis. The cost for plasma carnitine assays is approximately $40 to $100 per sample, depending on the provider. Tissue assays generally cost approximately twice as much because of the prolonged extraction procedure required.

Canine myocardial carnitine deficiency associated with dilated cardiomyopathy was first reported in a boxer dog that experienced dramatic clinical, echocardiographic, and functional improvement after carnitine supplementation and normalization of myocardial carnitine concentrations (Keene et al., 1991). Current investigations in our laboratory estimate (using a 95% confidence interval constructed from 20 consecutive, unrelated dogs) that myocardial free carnitine deficiency occurs in approximately 50 to 90% of dogs with dilated cardiomyopathy.

The mechanism by which carnitine deficiency occurs in dogs with dilated cardiomyopathy is unknown. Several potential causes of carnitine deficiency or contributors to its development exist, including decreased carnitine synthesis, decreased dietary intake (evidence now suggests that despite endogenous carnitine synthesis, dogs require a dietary carnitine source to maintain plasma carnitine concentrations at levels comparable to those found in other mammalian species because of their relatively limited renal capacity to reabsorb carnitine), intestinal malabsorption, increased renal loss, abnormally increased esterification of free carnitine, and membrane transport defects. Because approximately 80% of the dogs with dilated cardiomyopathy and myocardial carnitine deficiency have normal or elevated plasma carnitine concentrations, we have speculated that many of these dogs may suffer from a membrane transport defect that prevents adequate quantities of carnitine from moving into the myocardium from the plasma at normal plasma carnitine concentrations found in dogs fed commercial diets.

Table 1. *Normal Carnitine Concentrations in Plasma and Myocardium of Healthy Dogs Fed a Standard Commercial Diet**

Plasma Carnitine (μmol/L)			Myocardial Carnitine (nmol/mg Noncollagenous Protein)		
Total	Free	Esters	Total	Free	Esters
12–40	9–36	<7	4.5–14.0	3.5–11.5	<5.0

For any sample, the ratio of carnitine esters to free carnitine should not exceed 0.4.

*95% confidence intervals.

CARNITINE THERAPY IN CANINE DILATED CARDIOMYOPATHY

In dogs with myocardial carnitine deficiency associated with dilated cardiomyopathy, we have shown that high oral dosages of carnitine (50 to 100 mg/kg t.i.d.) elevate the plasma L-carnitine concentration 10 to 20 times above pretreatment values (Keene et al., 1991). These high levels of L-carnitine usually (but not always) increase myocardial L-carnitine concentrations into the normal range, as demonstrated by endomyocardial biopsy findings after 1 to 3 months of therapy. This finding, coupled with the results obtained in a few (primarily boxer) carnitine-treated dogs in which increased myocardial carnitine concentrations were associated with dramatic clinical and hemodynamic improvement, forms the basis for the use of carnitine as a therapeutic agent in dilated cardiomyopathy.

Supraphysiologic doses of carnitine have not been shown to produce serious adverse effects in any species studied (mild diarrhea has occasionally been reported in humans and one dog), and the compound is widely available in health-food stores without a prescription. Carnitine is classified by the Food and Drug Administration (FDA) as a "medicinal food," and it is widely added to carnitine-poor foods for human patients without an adequate source of carnitine and uncertain synthesizing capabilities (e.g., nearly all infant feeding formulas are now supplemented with carnitine).

Aside from the original report documenting the efficacy of carnitine supplementation in the therapy of two male boxer dogs with dilated cardiomyopathy, only anecdotal reports of carnitine therapy exist. Because the natural progression of dilated cardiomyopathy is variable and most clinicians prescribe multiple drugs to manage congestive heart failure and arrhythmias associated with the disease, the effects of carnitine supplementation on survival or any other objective parameter of myocardial function or clinical well-being are difficult to measure. As with any therapeutic intervention, a blinded, placebo-controlled, prospective clinical trial is needed to test efficacy.

In a prospective pilot study in which all of the dogs (18 Doberman pinschers with dilated cardiomyopathy and severe congestive heart failure) received carnitine supplementation regardless of their myocardial carnitine concentration at the outset of the trial, dogs with myocardial carnitine deficiency survived significantly longer than dogs that had normal carnitine concentrations (Keene et al., 1989). Although this study did not test the therapeutic efficacy of carnitine in this setting, the mean survival of Dobermans with myocardial carnitine deficiency treated with carnitine in addition to conventional pharmacotherapy was substantially longer than the average survival that has been reported in the veterinary literature for dilated cardiomyopathy in this breed.

My clinical impression is that carnitine is probably a useful adjunct to conventional pharmacotherapy in the treatment of heart failure for many but by no means all dogs suffering from myocardial carnitine deficiency associated with dilated cardiomyopathy. There is no evidence that high doses of carnitine have any effect in the absence of myocardial carnitine deficiency.

The relatively small percentage of dogs that appear to respond dramatically to carnitine therapy do so in a reasonably predictable manner. The first response noted is usually generalized clinical improvement (especially increased appetite and activity), often reported by the owner 1 to 4 weeks after the onset of oral carnitine supplementation. This improvement is noted in the majority of dogs treated with carnitine. Echocardiographic improvement is not generally demonstrable during the first 8 to 12 weeks of supplementation and may not occur at all. When observed, improvement in systolic time intervals and fractional shortening begin after 2 to 3 months of supplementation. Improvement may continue for about 6 to 8 months, when patients often reach a plateau at which they appear clinically well despite depressed echocardiographic ventricular function indices (fractional shortening rarely improves above the 15 to 25% range).

Although there are no prospective data evaluating the effect of carnitine on ventricular arrhythmias, my impression is that the frequency and severity of ventricular ectopy generally remain unaltered by carnitine therapy. As with conventional pharmacotherapy alone, a few of our patients with the most favorable response have died suddenly during carnitine therapy (presumably of ventricular fibrillation).

Conventional pharmacotherapy for heart failure can only occasionally be withdrawn from patients responding favorably to carnitine supplementation, and I do not believe this to be a worthwhile goal or reasonable expectation in a clinical setting. Because myocardial carnitine deficiency may represent only part of a spectrum of deleterious biochemical changes caused by many of the mitochondrial defects that may cause or contribute to dilated cardiomyopathy, it is not surprising that carnitine supplementation only imperfectly palliates many of those defects. This imperfect palliation may nevertheless be metabolically useful to the damaged myocardium, especially because it appears to be obtained without the potential metabolic or hemodynamic "penalties" often associated with the use of almost all conventional drugs.

Ideally, the decision to supplement with carnitine should be based on the documented presence of myocardial carnitine deficiency. Unfortunately, endomyocardial biopsy is technically demanding and relatively expensive. Plasma carnitine concentrations offer a relatively specific but insensitive indicator of myocardial carnitine deficiency, with limited usefulness in identifying carnitine-deficient patients. Using the most reliable available statistical extrapolations from a small sample population, it appears that at least half and possibly as many as 90% of dogs with heart failure secondary to dilated cardiomyopathy have associated myocardial carnitine deficiency. Presumably, most of these dogs would benefit at least marginally from L-carnitine supplementation. Carnitine appears to be extremely safe, and the risk of therapy is minimal, although the financial cost (approximately $80 to $200/month, depending on the source) may be prohibitive for some clients. If endomyocardial biopsy is unavailable and the owner is comfortable with the financial expenditure and aware of the uncertain benefits, L-carnitine supplementation is recommended. Large dogs (25 to 40 kg) in our practice receive 2 gm (approximately 1 teaspoonful of the commercially available pure substance) of carnitine mixed with food three times daily.

References and Suggested Reading

Bremer, J.: Carnitine metabolism and functions. Physiol. Rev. 63:1420, 1983.
Despite its age, this article provides a useful and extensively referenced review of carnitine metabolism and functions.
Keene, B. W., Kittleson, M. D., Atkins, C. E., et al.: Modified transvenous endomyocardial biopsy technique in dogs. Am. J. Vet. Res. 51:1769, 1990.
Description and clinical evaluation of a technique for acquiring endomyocardial biopsy specimens from dogs in heart failure.
Keene, B. W., Kittleson, M. D., Rush, J. E., et al.: Myocardial carnitine deficiency associated with dilated cardiomyopathy in Doberman pinschers. J. Vet. Intern. Med. 3:126, 1989.
Abstract documenting statistically increased survival in carnitine-deficient Doberman pinschers with dilated cardiomyopathy treated with carnitine versus non–carnitine-deficient Dobermans with cardiomyopathy receiving the same treatment.
Keene, B. W., Panciera, D. P., Atkins, C. E., et al.: Myocardial L-carnitine deficiency in a family of dogs with dilated cardiomyopathy. J.A.V.M.A. 198:647, 1991.
Clinical, hemodynamic, and biochemical findings, as well as response to carnitine therapy and its withdrawal, in a family of dogs with carnitine deficiency and dilated cardiomyopathy.
Parvin, R., and Pande, S. V.: Microdetermination of L-carnitine and carnitine acetyltransferase activity. Anal. Biochem. 79:190, 1977.
Detailed description of the biochemical assay procedures commonly used to measure plasma and tissue carnitine concentrations.
Rebouche, C. J., and Engel, A. G.: Kinetic compartmental analysis of carnitine metabolism in the dog. Arch. Biochem. Biophys. 220:69, 1983.
Description of carnitine kinetics in normal dogs.
Winter, S. C., Szabo-Aczel, S., Curry, C. J. R., et al.: Plasma carnitine deficiency: Clinical observations in 51 pediatric patients. Am. J. Dis. Child. 141:660, 1987.
Clinical signs, diagnostic criteria, and therapeutic responses are reviewed in the largest published series of carnitine-deficient children.

DOXORUBICIN CARDIOMYOPATHY

RODNEY L. PAGE
and BRUCE W. KEENE
Raleigh, North Carolina

SIGNIFICANCE OF DOXORUBICIN CARDIOMYOPATHY

Doxorubicin (Adriamycin, Adria) is the most active single antineoplastic agent used in veterinary oncology and as such forms the cornerstone of protocols used to control numerous canine and feline neoplasms (Helfand, 1989; Matus, 1989). The cardiotoxic effect of doxorubicin constitutes perhaps the most serious dose-limiting side effect of this drug, and many strategies have been studied in an attempt to overcome this problem.

The pattern of cardiac toxicity in older, tumor-bearing dogs appears to be similar to that observed in normal beagle dogs and humans (Herman et al., 1988). The hallmark of doxorubicin cardiotoxicity is progressive myocardial degeneration. Myocyte degeneration (myocytolysis, myofiber swelling, vacuolation, and fragmentation) and fibrosis are the histologic characteristics of early (within weeks) and late (usually >4 months) doxorubicin-induced lesions, respectively. The mechanisms by which doxorubicin results in cardiac toxicity are not yet clear, but free-radical generation and lipid membrane peroxidation have been suggested. The likelihood of congestive heart failure (CHF) increases with cumulative doxorubicin dose, although the onset may be delayed several weeks from the last dose. Arrhythmias and conduction disturbances occur frequently but are not necessarily associated with impending cardiac failure.

The true incidence of doxorubicin-induced cardiac toxicity in companion animals with neoplasia is unknown. In the largest published report, cardiac abnormalities were identified in 32 of 175 (18%) dogs receiving doxorubicin (Mauldin-Smith et al., 1987). Thirty-one dogs had electrocardiographic (ECG) changes, and seven dogs (4%) developed CHF. In two other reports, 3 of 37 dogs (8%) and 3 of 19 dogs (16%) receiving doxorubicin for lymphosarcoma developed CHF (Postorino et al., 1989; Price et al. [in press]). In these last two reports, four of the six dogs developing CHF were breeds potentially predisposed to cardiomyopathy. Although the 5 to 15% incidence of life-threatening cardiotoxicity seems high, the efficacy of doxorubicin warrants continued evaluation of methods to broaden its therapeutic index.

PREDICTIVE ASSESSMENT OF DOXORUBICIN CARDIOMYOPATHY

ECG and ultrasonography are not sufficiently sensitive to allow accurate decisions about continued doxorubicin administration in human patients. Radionuclide angiocardiography conducted before and after exercise has provided a more effective screening evaluation (McKillop et al., 1983). Radionuclide angiocardiography combined with endomyocardial biopsy currently provides sufficient specificity and sensitivity in the diagnosis of toxicity to eliminate the need for an empirical doxorubicin dose limit in humans.

ECG and ultrasonographic parameters have been examined prospectively in dogs with spontaneous lymphoma receiving doxorubicin alone or doxorubicin plus whole-body hyperthermia (Novotney et al [in press]; Page et al., 1991). Cardiac evaluation consisted of physical examination, ECG, and echocardiography before each doxorubicin treatment (30 mg/m^2 infused over 15 to 30 min every 3 weeks × 6; cumulative total = 180 mg/m^2) and, depending on clinical signs, as needed thereafter. Clinical evidence of cardiac failure was considered treatment limiting. In addition, ECG and echocardiographic criteria for cardiac dysfunction sufficient for discon-

tinuation were empirically established as follows: calculated cardiac ejection fraction less than 50%, left ventricular fractional shortening less than 27%, and new onset of frequent or multiform ventricular premature contractions.

Eleven of 52 dogs (21%) experienced doxorubicin cardiac toxicity as defined earlier. Four dogs (8%) developed clinical signs of heart failure despite having normal ECG and echocardiographic parameters. Failure occurred either before completion of the full treatment course (n = 2, both dogs had 150 mg/m^2 cumulative drug totals) or within 8 weeks after treatment completion (n = 2). The other seven dogs experienced subclinical "numeric toxicity" only (i.e., reduced echocardiographic fractional shortening). None of the dogs with subclinical toxicity developed clinical evidence of cardiac failure after treatment was discontinued (median follow-up of 240 days). Unlike studies reported in normal dogs, ECG abnormalities did not precede the onset of clinical cardiac failure or echocardiographic evidence of toxicity in any dog in this study. However, three dogs did develop ECG changes compatible with doxorubicin toxicosis (ventricular premature contractions, n = 2; right bundle branch block, n = 1) after completion of treatment.

This study suggests that, as in humans, ECG and echocardiographic monitoring in dogs provides a useful but not a highly accurate indicator of doxorubicin-induced cardiac toxicity.

CONCLUSIONS

Breeds with increased risk of cardiomyopathy and dogs with pre-existing cardiac abnormalities (murmurs, arrhythmias) should be considered at greater risk of doxorubicin-induced cardiotoxicity. Despite the acknowledged lack of sensitivity, treatment should be monitored using ECG and echocardiographic techniques.

Table 1 details suggested diagnostic criteria for three general levels of cardiotoxicity. Pretreatment ECG and two-dimensional guided echocardiographic measurements should be established on dogs undergoing doxorubicin treatment. Re-evaluation of the two-dimensional echocardiogram is recommended before the fourth, fifth, and sixth

Table 1. Recommendations for Grading Cardiotoxic Effects of Cancer Chemotherapy in Dogs

	Normal Range	Mild Toxicity	Moderate Toxicity	Severe Toxicity
Left ventricular fractional shortening	28–50%	25–28% or 20% reduction from pretreatment value	20–25%	<20%
ECG changes	None	Rare ventricular/ supraventricular ectopia	Ventricular/ supraventricular premature complexes (5–20/min)	Frequent/complex arrhythmias Atrioventricular block or conduction disturbance

doxorubicin treatments. Earlier evaluation is recommended if any indication of toxicity is identified (arrhythmia, gallop, or new/changed murmur). Treatment should be continued if no toxicity is observed. If signs of mild toxicity are observed, doxorubicin should be delayed 1 to 2 weeks and cardiac function re-evaluated. If the cardiac function is stable at re-examination, clinical judgment regarding risk versus benefit must dictate future treatment. In dogs that have reached the standard cumulative dose without evidence of toxicity and in dogs with ECG or echocardiographic evidence of mild or moderate toxicity, endomyocardial biopsy should be helpful in patient assessment. Treatment should be discontinued if severe toxicity develops.

FUTURE CONSIDERATIONS

If available, radionuclide angiography or Doppler-derived indices of ventricular function may provide more sensitive methods for evaluating doxorubicin cardiotoxicity.

Endomyocardial biopsy can accurately predict the likelihood of cardiac failure in human patients treated with doxorubicin (Bristow et al., 1978). Endomyocardial biopsy techniques have been developed and refined in veterinary medicine, and their predictive value for the identification of doxorubicin-induced cardiotoxicity is being prospectively evaluated in dogs. Incorporating endomyocardial biopsy into the clinical monitoring regimen (pretreatment and at the sixth treatment or at the first indication of abnormal performance) should result in improved ability to deliver the maximally tolerable dose of doxorubicin to the greatest number of dogs.

Several strategies to reduce doxorubicin cardiotoxicity have been successful in preclinical studies. Doxorubicin-induced cardiac toxicity can be reduced by prolonging the infusion time to greater than 6 hr or by using a low-dose weekly schedule (Anders et al., 1986; Shapira et al., 1990). Concern about this infusion method on tumor response has not yet been fully investigated. ICRF-187 is a compound that purportedly chelates intracellular iron, making it unavailable for doxorubicin-generated oxygen free radicals. This compound has been shown to significantly reduce cardiac toxicity while enhancing antitumor activity (Wadler et al., 1986). Anthracycline analogues with reduced cardiac toxicity have also been developed and are being evaluated in dogs and cats with neoplasia (e.g., mitoxantrone [see this volume, p. 399], epirubicin).

In summary, doxorubicin-induced cardiotoxicity is a relatively frequent and potentially life-threatening complication of this useful antineoplastic agent. Toxicity is progressive and somewhat unpredictable. Improved screening evaluation of cardiac performance or cardiac ultrastructure during therapy may increase our ability to determine an individual's maximally tolerable dose of doxorubicin.

References and Suggested Reading

Anders, R. J., Shanes, J. G., and Zeller, F. P.: Lower incidence of doxorubicin-induced cardiomyopathy by once-a-week low-dose administration. Am. Heart J. 111:755, 1986.
Literature review of various doxorubicin administration regimens and correlation of functional and histologic criteria to clinical toxicity.
Bristow, M. B., Mason, J. W., Billingham, M. E., et al.: Doxorubicin cardiomyopathy: Evaluation by phonocardiography, endomyocardial biopsy, and cardiac catheterization. Ann. Intern. Med. 88:168, 1978.
Prospective evaluation of endomyocardial biopsy for prospectively quantifying the risk of doxorubicin-induced cardiotoxicity.
Helfand, S. C.: Chemotherapy of solid tumors. In Kirk, R. W. (ed.): Current Veterinary Therapy X. Philadelphia: W. B. Saunders, 1989, p. 489.
Review of chemotherapeutic principles and current results of chemotherapy clinical trials in solid tumors of dogs and cats.
Herman, E. H., Ferrans, V. J., Young, R. S. K., et al.: Effect of pretreatment with ICRF-187 on the total cumulative dose of doxorubicin tolerated by beagle dogs. Can. Res. 48:9618, 1988.
Detailed study of clinical parameters and histologic changes in normal dogs given multiple courses of doxorubicin with or without ICRF-187 as a cardioprotector.
Matus, R. E.: Chemotherapy of lymphoma and leukemia. In Kirk, R. W. (ed.): Current Veterinary Therapy X. Philadelphia: W. B. Saunders, 1989, p. 482.
Review of diagnosis, treatment, and prognosis of canine and feline lymphoproliferative disorders.
Mauldin-Smith, G. E., Matus, R. E., Bond, B. R., et al.: Doxorubicin cardiotoxicity in thirty-two dogs. Proceedings of the 7th Annual Veterinary Cancer Society Conference, Madison, WI, 1987, p. 41.
Retrospective analysis of dogs experiencing cardiac abnormalities as a result of doxorubicin administration.
McKillop, J. H., Briwtos, M. R., Goris, M. L., et al.: Sensitivity and specificity of radionuclide ejection fractions in doxorubicin cardiotoxicity. Am. Heart J. 106:1048, 1983.
Evaluation of radionuclide angiography as a screening tool in 37 patients receiving doxorubicin with endomyocardial biopsy confirmation of cardiotoxicity risk.
Novotney, C. A., Page, R. L., Macy, D. W., et al.: Phase I evaluation of doxorubicin and whole body hyperthermia in dogs with lymphosarcoma. J. Vet. Intern. Med. (in press).
Dose determination and toxicity characterization of doxorubicin administered concurrently with whole-body hyperthermia.
Page, R. L., Macy, D. W., Ogilvie, G. K., et al.: Phase III evaluation of doxorubicin and whole body hyperthermia in dogs with lymphoma. Int. J. Hyperthermia (in press).
Randomized prospective evaluation of doxorubicin administered with or without whole-body hyperthermia.
Postorino, N. C., Susaneck, S. J., Withrow, S. J., et al.: Single agent therapy with Adriamycin for canine lymphosarcoma. J. Am. Anim. Hosp. Assoc. 25:221, 1989.
Efficacy and toxicity of doxorubicin alone administered to 37 dogs with lymphoma.
Price, G. S., Page, R. L., Fischer, B. M., et al.: Efficacy and toxicity of doxorubicin/cyclophosphamide maintenance therapy in dogs with multicentric lymphosarcoma. J. Vet. Intern. Med. (in press).
Clinical trial with doxorubicin-based maintenance protocol in dogs with lymphosarcoma.
Shapira, J., Gotfried, M., Lishner, M., et al.: Reduced cardiotoxicity of doxorubicin by a 6-hour infusion regimen. Cancer 65:870, 1990.
Randomized study comparing toxicity of doxorubicin given as a standard (15- to 20-minute) infusion or a 6-hr infusion.
Wadler, S., Green, M. D., and Muggia, F. M.: Synergistic activity of doxorubicin and the bisdioxopiperazine (+)-1,2-bis(3,5-dioxopiperazinyl-1-yl) propane (ICRF-187) against the murine sarcoma S180 cell line. Cancer Res. 46:1176, 1986.
In vitro evaluation of ICRF-187 as a doxorubicin modifier.

PERSISTENT ATRIAL STANDSTILL (ATRIOVENTRICULAR MUSCULAR DYSTROPHY)

MICHAEL S. MILLER
LARRY P. TILLEY
Floral Park, New York

and CLARKE E. ATKINS
Raleigh, North Carolina

Atrial standstill is an electrocardiographic diagnosis characterized by an absence of P waves and by a regular escape rhythm with a supraventricular type of QRS complex. It may be temporary, terminal, or persistent (Bloomfield and Sinclair-Smith, 1965; Tilley, 1992). Atrial standstill can develop with digitalis toxicity, hyperkalemia, hypothermia, and as a terminal event. Atrial standstill has also been reported in humans with certain types of muscular dystrophy, amyloidosis, coronary heart disease, and other long-standing cardiac diseases (Wooliscroft and Tuna, 1982).

In humans, numerous progressive neuromuscular disorders are associated with cardiac disease (Perloff, 1988). These neuromuscular disorders include progressive muscular dystrophy, myotonic muscular dystrophy, and Friedreich's ataxia. The muscular dystrophies are a group of genetically determined, primary, degenerative myopathies. The well-known human muscular dystrophies and many of their associated cardiac disorders are listed in Table 1 (Moise, 1990; Perloff, 1988; Stevenson et al., 1990). The most common varieties are the Duchenne type, Becker's X-linked dystrophy, the autosomal recessive limb-girdle type, and the autosomal dominant facioscapulohumeral form. In all of the muscular dystrophies, the primary degenerative process affects the muscle fibers (myopathy) in specific topographic muscle groups, and no primary abnormality can be found in the motor nerves supplying the muscle groups. Cardiac disease that occurs with the different varieties of muscular dystrophy may include myocardial dysfunction (e.g., cardiomyopathy) or disorders of impulse formation and conduction. Although the clinical presentations among the different types of muscular dystrophy vary from asymptomatic to complete inability to use the affected muscle groups, progressive muscular weakness often occurs. There is no correlation between the extent of skeletal muscle disease and the severity of cardiac signs. Several articles describing the Duchenne type of muscular dystrophy that occurs in purebred dogs with associated cardiac pathology have recently been reviewed (Moise, 1990).

A recent report characterized electrocardiographic changes and echocardiographic lesions in 13 purebred or mixed-breed golden retriever dogs with X-linked Duchenne's muscular dystrophy and 11 female carrier dogs (Moise et al., 1991). Compared with control dogs, affected dogs had significantly increased Q-R ratios because of deep and narrow Q waves in electrocardiogram (ECG) leads II-III-aVF, CV6LL (V2), and CV6LU (V4). Carrier dogs had significantly increased Q-R ratios in leads V2 and V4. Other ECG changes in affected dogs included shorter P-R intervals and also ventricular arrhythmias in some dogs. This study, which also documented consistent echocardiographic changes in affected and carrier dogs and progressive cardiomyopathy in affected dogs, concluded that the dog affected with Duchenne-type muscular dystrophy is an animal model for Duchenne-type cardiomyopathy in humans.

In both the veterinary and human literature, facioscapulohumeral muscular dystrophy has been reported to be associated with persistent atrial standstill. Initially, the atrial standstill may be regional with focal atrial areas inactive while other areas trigger atrial arrhythmias such as atrial tachycardia or atrial flutter. A recent publication (Stevenson et al., 1990) concludes that the reported human cases of persistent atrial standstill, thought to be due to facioscapulohumeral muscular dystrophy, are actually associated with a phenotypically similar Emery-Dreifuss variety of muscular dystrophy (see Table 1) in which there is no facial muscle dysfunction. This finding may be similar in the dog, as no facial muscle involvement was reported in the

Table 1. Classification of Heredofamilial Muscular Dystrophy and Associated Cardiac Disease in Humans

Common Muscular Dystrophies	Selected Cardiac and ECG Abnormalities*
Duchenne (early onset), X-linked	Dilated cardiomyopathy Tall R waves in right precordial lead V_1 (local posterior wall disease); deep Q waves in left precordial leads V_4, V_5, V_6; deep Q waves in I and aVL (lateral wall disease mimics myocardial infarction); sinus tachycardia, short P-R interval, mean electrical axis deviation, atrial and ventricular arrhythmias
Becker's (late onset), X-linked	Cardiomyopathy (four chambers) Atrial arrhythmias Fascicular block Complete AV block
Erb's, Limb-girdle, Autosomal recessive	Cardiomyopathy Bradycardia, tachycardia (atrial flutter) First-degree AV block, bundle branch block, complete AV block
Landouzy-Déjérine, Facioscapulohumeral	P wave abnormalities; electrophysiologically induced atrial flutter or atrial fibrillation Sinus node dysfunction AV nodal or intranodal conduction abnormalities
Emery-Dreifuss, Scapulohumeral	Atrial standstill Atrial flutter or fibrillation Junctional rhythm Complete AV block

*Listed cardiac abnormalities for a specific muscular dystrophy are not found in all patients.

AV, atrioventricular; ECG, electrocardiographic.

pathologic reports of dogs with persistent atrial standstill associated with facioscapulohumeral muscular dystrophy (Liu et al., 1989). Cardiac involvement in the human facioscapulohumeral variety of muscular dystrophy was found via electrophysiologic studies to be characterized by a high susceptibility to induced atrial fibrillation or flutter, abnormalities of atrioventricular (AV) nodal conduction, and abnormalities of sinus node function, rather than persistent atrial standstill. Further clarification of the two diseases may be required to differentiate between these human forms of muscular dystrophy and the persistent atrial standstill associated with apparent facioscapulohumeral muscular dystrophy in the dog.

CLINICAL PRESENTATION

Spontaneous persistent atrial standstill is a rare cardiac arrhythmia in the dog and cat. There ap-

pears to be a breed predisposition for atrial standstill in English springer spaniels and Siamese cats. Thirty-one cases of persistent atrial standstill in the dog and cat have been reviewed (Tilley and Liu, 1983). The twenty dogs included 14 English springer spaniels, four mixed breeds, one Shih tzu, and one Old English sheepdog; the 11 cats included eight Siamese, one Burmese, and two domestic short-hair. The Old English sheepdog had persistent standstill of only the left atrium, with no skeletal muscle involvement.

Clinical signs of persistent atrial standstill include weakness, fainting, dyspnea; physical and radiographic examination may reveal ascites, pulmonary edema, and pleural effusion. Extreme enlargement of the atria is evident on radiographic, angiocardiographic, and echocardiographic studies (Fig. 1). The atria are immobile when viewed fluoroscopically, and no atrial motion ("atrial kick") or typical mitral valve response (A point) is seen echocardiographically. Ventricular hypokinesis (reduced shortening fraction) may be evident echocardiographically (Fig. 1). A normal left ventricular shortening fraction may, however, be found early in the disease course or when severe mitral insufficiency permits enhanced left ventricular shortening. Doppler echocardiography reveals atrioventricular valvular insufficiency in the majority of cases. Persistent atrial standstill must be distinguished from the atrial standstill of hyperkalemia (e.g., hypoadrenocorticism, acute renal failure, urinary tract obstruction, diabetic ketoacidosis, and oral or iatrogenic potassium intoxication), hypothermia, and downward depression of the pacemaker that is part of a terminal event, as with the dying heart or with extreme hyperkalemia. Serum electrolytes are normal, ruling out hyperkalemia as a cause of the atrial standstill.

ELECTROCARDIOGRAPHIC FEATURES

Persistent atrial standstill is clinically diagnosed by the following features (Figs. 2 and 3):

1. The heart rate is slow, usually 60 beats/min or less (160 beats/min or less for the cat), and the rhythm is often regular.

2. No P waves are observed in any lead, including intracardiac electrograms. Low-voltage atrial activity may be found. Extremely small P waves were found in the Old English sheepdog with persistent standstill of the left atrium.

3. The QRS complex is of nearly normal configuration with supraventricular-type escape QRS complexes, or of increased duration typical of bundle branch block or ventricular enlargement.

4. There is no increase in heart rate, nor are P waves evident after injection of atropine sulfate or exercise (Fig. 4).

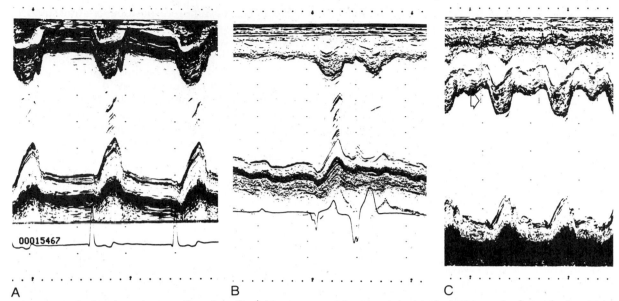

Figure 1. M-mode echocardiograms from three English springer spaniels with atrioventricular (AV) muscular dystrophy (persistent atrial standstill). Time scale: 1 sec between each large dot; distance scale: 1 cm between each dash. *A*, Eighteen-month-old female with bilateral AV valvular insufficiency and right heart failure. Note the lack of P waves with an enhanced junctional escape rhythm of 83 beats/min and left bundle branch block. The left ventricle (LV) is dilated (end-diastolic volume index [EDVI]: 136 ml/m²; [normal: <100 ml/m²]), but performance appears to be normal (fractional shortening [FS]: 47%; end-systolic volume index [ESVI]: 21 ml/m²; [normal: <30 ml/m²]). *B*, Three-year-old male with syncope and AV valvular insufficiency. The electrocardiogram (ECG) reveals complete AV block, ventricular escape rhythm, and ventricular premature complexes (VPCs). Despite prolonged filling time and volume load (EDVI: 283 ml/m²), LV performance is diminished (ESVI: 82 ml/m²). The VPC was followed by at least 3.5 sec of asystole, demonstrating failure of subsidiary pacemakers. Syncope was most likely due to asystole or ventricular tachycardia complicated by diminished myocardial performance. *C*, One-year-old female presented with left heart failure, AV valvular incompetence, and complete AV block with barely discernible P waves and an enhanced ventricular escape rhythm. This ECG and echocardiogram, recorded 8 months later, demonstrate an artificially paced rhythm of 90 beats/min (*arrow* denotes pacemaker spike), atrial standstill, and volume overload (FS: 38%; ESVI: 32 ml/m²; EDVI: 137 ml/m²).

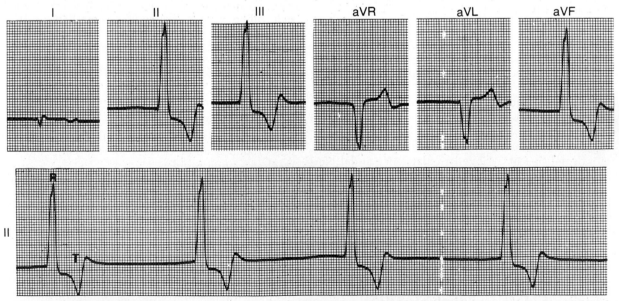

Figure 2. Persistent atrial standstill in an English spaniel. No P waves are present on any of the leads (including chest leads and intracardiac electrocardiograms [*not shown here*]). The regular bradycardia is junctional in origin with left bundle branch block, left ventricular enlargement, or diffuse ventricular conduction disease (wide, positive QRS complexes). (Reprinted with permission from Tilley, L. P.: *Essentials of Canine and Feline Electrocardiography.* Philadelphia: Lea & Febiger [in press].)

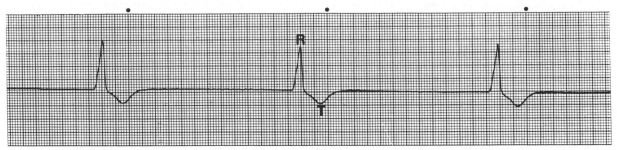

Figure 3. Persistent atrial standstill in a 4-year-old Siamese cat with clinical signs of dyspnea. Pleural effusion and cardiomegaly were found on thoracic radiographs. No P waves are present; the QRS complexes are increased in voltage and duration, indicating left bundle branch block, diffuse conduction disease, or left heart enlargement. The heart rate is only 40 beats/min. An idioventricular rhythm should also be considered. (Reprinted with permission from Tilley, L. P.: *Essentials of Canine and Feline Electrocardiography.* Philadelphia: Lea & Febiger [in press].)

5. The atria cannot be stimulated electrically or mechanically (Fig. 5).

Other dogs with AV muscular dystrophy have shown advanced AV block (Bonagura and O'Grady, 1983; Tilley and Liu, 1983), some with small P waves or sinus rhythm with very small P waves rather than persistent atrial standstill. Rarely, atrial fibrillation with intact AV conduction is seen in dogs with atrial muscular dystrophy.

PATHOLOGY

Gross inspection shows the atria to be greatly enlarged, paper-thin, pinkish white, and transparent. Affected cats suffer from extremely dilated hearts with hypoplasia of the atrial myocardium. Histologic findings include marked fibrosis, chronic mononuclear inflammation, fibroelastosis, and steatosis throughout the atria and interatrial septum. In 30% of the affected dogs (Liu et al., 1989), there is

marked muscle wasting involving the skeletal muscles of the upper forelimbs and scapula. Histologic changes of the skeletal muscles include hyalinized, degenerated muscle fibers with occasional regenerative activity and mild to moderate steatosis. Localized or generalized skeletal muscle wasting is not a feature in cats.

Based on the pathologic findings, AV muscular disease can be divided into two clinical groups:

1. Long-standing cardiac disease. Diffuse involvement of the atria from the increased hemodynamic load due to valvular dysfunction, congenital heart disease, myocarditis, or cardiomyopathy can result in fibrous replacement of normal atrial muscle cells. The dilated form of cardiomyopathy was found most often in the cat with persistent atrial standstill. At necropsy, greatly enlarged and paper-thin atria were observed. At microscopic examination, little atrial myocardium was present.

2. Neuromuscular disease associated with cardiomyopathy. In humans, Emery-Dreifuss disease is associated with persistent atrial standstill (Stevenson

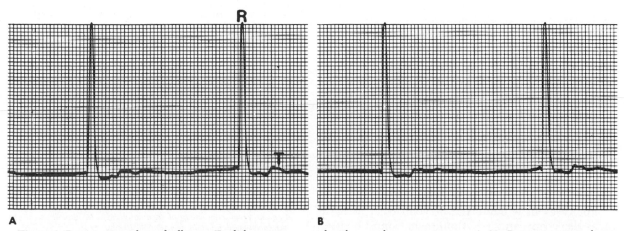

A   **B**

Figure 4. Persistent atrial standstill in an English springer spaniel with normal serum potassium. *A,* No P waves present, heart rate 70 beats/min, and QRS complexes of a probable junctional focus. *B,* After atropine the heart rate is still close to 70 beats/min with no P waves. (Reprinted with permission from Tilley, L. P.: *Essentials of Canine and Feline Electrocardiography.* Philadelphia: Lea & Febiger [in press].)

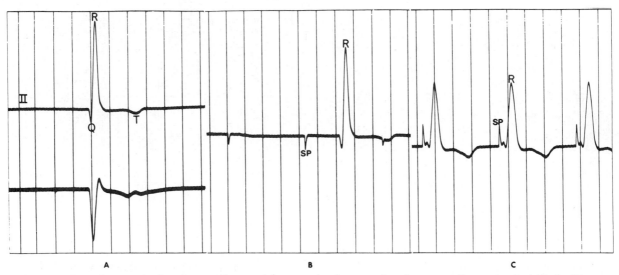

Figure 5. *A,* Simultaneous lead II electrocardiogram *(top tracing)* and intracardiac electrogram *(bottom tracing).* Lack of P waves is confirmed by the electrogram; the electrode catheter is located in the right atrium. *B,* Electrical pacing at high milliamperes from the right atrium at multiple sites under fluoroscopy did not elicit either an atrial or a ventricular response. SP, pacemaker spike. *C,* In contrast to *B,* electrical pacing from within the right ventricle easily produced ventricular activation. (Reprinted with permission from Tilley, L. P.: *Essentials of Canine and Feline Electrocardiography.* Philadelphia: Lea & Febiger [in press].)

et al., 1990). Neuromuscular disease associated with persistent atrial standstill probably represents a genetically determined disease in most dogs.

THERAPY

A guarded prognosis is always present with AV muscular dystrophy because myocardial failure is a common, life-threatening sequela. Death may be sudden (presumably due to failure of impulse formation, conduction, or other fatal arrythmia), or the animal may eventually succumb to heart failure. Traditional medical therapy for heart failure (e.g., digitalis, diuretics, vasodilators, and a low-salt diet) is indicated for managing signs of heart failure secondary to myocardial disease.

The only reliable method of treatment for dogs and cats with persistent atrial standstill is implantation of a permanent artificial cardiac pacemaker (Sisson, 1989). Adrenergic drugs can be used to temporarily increase the heart rate by increasing the discharge rate of the ventricular or AV junctional escape pacemaker. Of the available drugs, terbutaline (2.5 to 5 mg b.i.d. to t.i.d.) appears to be the most useful oral agent. Vagolytic drugs are typically ineffective for this purpose, although an atropine response test is generally performed (atropine 0.04 mg/kg SC 20 min before repeating the ECG).

For cases in which atrial or ventricular arrhythmias also occur, antiarrhythmic agents must be used judiciously as these agents may suppress escape rhythms and affect skeletal muscle membranes and electrolytes and worsen muscle weakness.

References and Suggested Reading

Bloomfield, D. A., and Sinclair-Smith, B. C.: Persistent atrial standstill. Am. J. Med. 39:335, 1965.
A review study of persistent atrial standstill in humans.

Bonagura, J. D., and O'Grady, M.: ECG of the month. J.A.V.M.A. 183:658, 1983.
An ECG case study report of persistent atrial standstill in a dog.

Jeraj, K., Ogburn, P. N., Edwards, W. D., et al.: Atrial standstill, myocarditis, and destruction of cardiac conduction system. Clinicopathologic correlation in a dog. Am. Heart J. 99:185, 1980.
An excellent case study of one dog with persistent atrial standstill.

Liu, S. K., Hsu, F. S., and Lee, R. C. T.: *An Atlas of Cardiovascular Pathology.* Taiwan: Wonder Enterprise, 1989, p. 283.
A pictorial review of the cardiac pathology of persistent atrial standstill in the dog and cat.

Moise, N. S.: Duchenne cardiomyopathy in a canine model. ACVIM Proceedings, 1990.
A review of human Duchenne muscular dystrophy and a possible canine model for this disease.

Moise, N. S., Valentine, B. A., Brown, C. A., et al.: Duchenne's cardiomyopathy in a canine model: Electrocardiographic and echocardiographic studies. J. Am. Coll. Cardiol. 17:812, 1991.
A recent report establishing X-linked Duchenne's muscular dystrophy in the dog.

Perloff, J. K.: Neurological disorders and heart disease. *In* Braunwald, E. (ed.): *Heart Disease: A Textbook of Cardiovascular Medicine,* 3rd ed., Philadelphia, W. B. Saunders, 1988, p. 1782.
This chapter deals with the varied and complex interplay between cardiology and neurology.

Sisson, D. D.: Bradyarrhythmias and cardiac pacing. *In* Kirk, R. W. (ed.): *Current Veterinary Therapy X:* Philadelphia: W. B. Saunders, 1989, p. 286.
A review of the pacemaker implantation approach to treating atrial standstill.

Stevenson, W. G., Perloff, J. K., Weiss, J. N., and Anderson, T. L.: Facioscapulohumeral muscular dystrophy: Evidence for selective genetic electrophysiologic cardiac involvement. J. Am. Coll. Cardiol. 15:292, 1990.
A recent prospective study of cardiac changes in humans associated with facioscapulohumeral muscular dystrophy.

Tilley, L. P.: *Essentials of Canine and Feline Electrocardiography: Interpretation and Treatment.* Philadelphia: Lea & Febiger (in press).
A review of the electrocardiographic aspects of persistent atrial standstill in the dog and cat.

Tilley, L. P., and Liu, S. K.: Persistent atrial standstill in the dog and cat. ACVIM Proceedings, New York, 1983, p. 43.
A review of 31 cases of persistent atrial standstill in the dog and cat.

Wooliscroft, J., and Tuna, N.: Permanent atrial standstill: The clinical spectrum. Am. J. Cardiol. 49:2037, 1982.
A review of the causes of permanent atrial standstill in humans.

MYOCARDIAL ISCHEMIA AND INFARCTION

SI-KWANG LIU
and PHILIP R. FOX
New York, New York

CAUSES OF MYOCARDIAL ISCHEMIA AND NECROSIS

Acute myocardial infarction from coronary artery disease is responsible for approximately one quarter of human mortalities in the United States. More than 60% of these deaths occur within 1 hour of the event, usually attributable to ventricular arrhythmias. When coronary arterial thrombosis, plaque, or occlusion reduces blood supply, myocardial ischemia results. Prolonged, severe ischemia causes irreversible necrosis known as myocardial infarction (MI).

Little clinical attention has been directed to the evaluation and treatment of myocardial ischemia and infarction in veterinary medicine. There are at least two explanations for this. One is the difficulty in antemortem recognition and lack of validated therapy. The other is that coronary artery disease *per se* in companion animals does not cause morbidity and mortality on a scale comparable to that observed in humans.

Myocardial Infarction in Dogs and Cats

The necropsy register of The Animal Medical Center indicates that ischemic-related myocardial necrosis is evident in a wide variety of disorders associated with cardiovascular diseases. Because some affected pets experience sudden or premature death, antemortem clinical identification of these conditions is important. Infarction can develop secondary to extramural coronary obstruction—the typical situation in humans—or secondary to small or microscopic intramural coronary disease. The clinical consequences of myocardial ischemia and infarction depend on the magnitude of myocardial injury, pre-existent heart disease, and the electrophysiologic consequences of the insult.

In small animals, necropsy evidence of MI is especially common in cats with left ventricular hypertrophic disorders and with coronary thromboembolic complications accompanying decompensated heart failure. In the dog, areas of MI are observed with severe aortic and pulmonic stenosis, advanced, uncorrected, patent ductus arteriosus, atherosclerosis, idiopathic hypertrophic cardiomyopathy, primary coronary amyloidosis, coronary thrombosis associated with renal disease, and coronary vasculitis and thrombosis. Vegetative endocarditis and septic coronary thromboembolism, especially associated with *Serratia marcescens*, cause myocardial infarction in the dog and cat.

Interactions between coronary blood flow physiology and anatomy are complex. A brief review may be beneficial to aid in clinical recognition of myocardial ischemia and infarction and provide a basis for therapeutic intervention.

Coronary Blood Flow

Anatomic, mechanical, hydraulic, neurohumoral, and metabolic factors all interact to regulate coronary blood flow. Major coronary arteries at the epicardial surface (extramural, conductance vessels) give rise to smaller, penetrating, intramural "resistance" vessels. The dog has an extensive epicardial collateral network that is absent in pigs and primates. These collaterals may have functional significance in preventing infarction from coronary occlusion, but their clinical relevance in dogs and cats is unclear.

Coronary perfusion pressure depends on the gradient between coronary arteries and diastolic right atrial or left ventricular pressures. Coronary vascular resistance is regulated by intramyocardial pressure, which directly compresses vessels, and by conditions intrinsic to the coronary bed, including metabolic, neural, and humoral factors. Myocardial blood flow is greatly reduced during systole, especially in the left ventricle, and extravascular compressive forces are higher in subendocardial than in subepicardial zones. Thus, 'most left ventricular coronary blood flow occurs during diastole, and subendocardial perfusion reserves are smaller than those in the rest of the myocardium.

Factors that decrease diastolic perfusion pressure gradients (e.g. systemic arterial hypotension, coronary artery obstruction, elevated left ventricular end-diastolic pressure, and tachycardia) further reduce the subepicardial to subendocardial flow ratio and may cause subendocardial ischemia. Tachycardia may compromise coronary perfusion by decreasing total diastolic time per min while increasing myocardial oxygen demands. This is especially true in the setting of severe ventricular hypertrophy, which impairs coronary reserve.

Coronary arteries are innervated by sympathetic and parasympathetic nerves. Alpha$_1$ and alpha$_2$ stimulation by norepinephrine causes coronary vasoconstriction. Beta$_1$ and beta$_2$ stimulation causes vasodilation. However, neuronal effects on coronary vascular resistance are complex.

Myocardial perfusion is generally maintained within a relatively narrow range by autoregulatory mechanisms. Myogenic, extravascular, compressive forces and metabolic factors are responsible for autoregulation of coronary blood flow. Metabolic control involves several mediators including oxygen, carbon dioxide, and vasodilator metabolites such as adenosine.

DETERMINANTS OF MYOCARDIAL OXYGEN CONSUMPTION

Although disruption of coronary blood flow is the cause of myocardial ischemia, myocardial blood flow, oxygen delivery, and oxygen consumption are balanced depending upon prevailing physiologic conditions. Determinants of myocardial oxygen demand modify these factors and set the threshold for ischemia. The most important of these determinants are heart rate, myocardial systolic wall tension, and contractility. Thus, ischemia is more likely to occur at high heart rates or in settings of increased wall tension (e.g., high pressures, chamber enlargement, wall thinning) or endogenous or exogenous contractile stimulation.

MYOCARDIAL ISCHEMIA AND INFARCTION

Myocardial ischemia results from fixed or transient disruption of coronary blood flow whenever myocardial oxygen consumption exceeds the coronary reserve. When ischemia is prolonged, irreversible myocellular damage and cell death may occur. Resultant myocardial tissue necrosis (myocardial infarction) represents a temporal and three-dimensional geomorphic event. The size and microscopic characteristics of an MI are shaped by collateral coronary blood flow and underlying metabolic tissue demands. Coronary microanatomy is organized into an end-vessel system in which separately derived microcirculations generally do not anastomose. This causes infarcted regions to be sharply delineated by the anatomic limit of affected capillary beds supplied by each coronary artery.

Myocardial cell death results not only from oxygen deprivation *per se* but also from biochemical changes initiated by ischemia. Ischemic injury has been associated with phospholipid degradation from the generation of free radicals and activation of endogenous phospholipases. Phospholipid depletion in addition to lysophosphatide generation can alter membrane function within ischemic tissue, inhibit mitochondrial oxidative phosphorylation, and be arrhythmogenic. Thus, phospholipid degradation may play a role in the transition from reversible to irreversible ischemic cell injury.

Gross and Histologic Characterization

GROSS FINDINGS. Gross evidence of MI has been observed in relation to a number of cardiovascular diseases in the dog and cat. In canine atherosclerosis, permanent yellow-white, dilated, and tortuous coronary arteries are associated with adjacent irregular foci of pale, dull patches of myocardium. With acute renal failure, focal or diffuse irregular patches of necrosis have been observed. Vegetative endocarditis and coronary vasculitis cause focal coronary thromboembolism and hemorrhagic necrosis in the adjacent myocardium. In severe ventricular hypertrophy from congenital canine aortic or pulmonic stenosis, circular myocardial necrosis may occur as concentric, pale, dull or dark purple regions involving the subepicardial region of the ventricular myocardium, including papillary muscles and trabeculae carneae. Gross changes with coronary amyloidosis and myocardial necrosis are not specific. The left ventricle is usually hypertrophic, with focal diffuse pale areas associated with various degrees of coronary arterial occlusion.

In feline hypertrophic cardiomyopathy with thromboembolism, extensive ventricular hypertrophy with focal, dark gray or pale myocardium and occasional thrombosis in adjacent coronary arteries may be detected in the papillary muscles and left ventricular apex (Fig. 1). Intraluminal coronary arteries are frequently thickened.

HISTOLOGIC FINDINGS. Histologically, infarcted myocardium reveals myocyte streaking and waviness with sarcoplasmic coagulation, granulation,

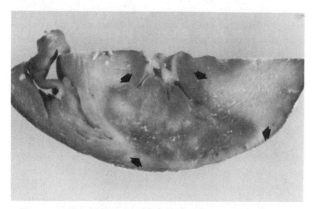

Figure 1. Cross section of left and right ventricle from a cat with acute sudden death. There is severe left ventricular hypertrophy of the interventricular septum and left ventricular caudal wall; myocardial infarction is evident as darkened areas *(arrows)* relative to the normal tissue in these segments.

contraction bands, sarcoplasmic vacuolization, fragmentation, and lysis. There are extracellular, edematous ground substances and occasional extravasation of erythrocytes separating the affected myocytes. Atherosclerotic, thromboembolic, amyloid, or vasculitic coronary arteries are usually enclosed in adjacent necrotic myocardium. Contraction bands, fragmentation, and vacuolization of sarcoplasm with or without extravasation of erythrocytes in and around the affected myocytes are observed in circular myocardial necrosis with minimal coronary artery changes. Vacuolar necrosis with focal islands of coagulative change is often detected in juvenile (large) animals with acute vitamin E deficiency. Affected myocytes reveal vacuolar sarcoplasmic changes or displacement of myofilaments by sarcoplasmic vacuoles. Myocytolytic myofibers are widely separated by extracellular, edematous ground substances or extravasation of erythrocytes. Fibrinoid necrosis of arteriolar walls, leukocytic infiltration, cellular debris, and extravasation of erythrocytes are evident in coronary arteries from the adjacent myocardium. Focal interstitial or massive myocardial fibrosis and acute vacuolar or coagulative necrosis are observed in the feline myocardium with severe hypertrophic cardiomyopathy. Abnormal coronary arteries characterized by thickening of vessel walls and decreased luminal size occur in approximately one third of affected hearts.

EFFECTS OF ISCHEMIA ON MYOCARDIAL FUNCTION

Myocardial ischemia is associated with regional myocardial dysfunction resulting in dyssynergic contraction. Absent or paradoxic motion in the central ischemic zone, reduced motion of adjacent myocar-

dium, and hyperfunction of surrounding normal myocardium may all be seen.

The severity of ventricular dysfunction relates in part to the exent and duration of the ischemic insult. Global ventricular function may be maintained by hyperfunctioning residual myocardium if damage is limited. Repeated or transient ischemic episodes may impair systolic and diastolic function. Postischemic depression (myocardial "stunning") may be prolonged for days from brief coronary occlusion. In contrast, widespread impairment of contractility may reduce overall left ventricular function, cause severe ventricular dyssynergy, and lead to heart failure.

Diastolic properties of the heart may also be altered by ischemia and infarction impairing ventricular relaxation. Together with reduced ventricular emptying (systolic failure), ventricular filling pressures may rise, resulting in pulmonary edema.

DIAGNOSIS

Clinical signs with severe MI include sudden depression and dyspnea, especially in cats with acute pulmonary edema or thromboembolism. Underlying cardiovascular disease will often be demonstrated through physical examination, radiography, and electrocardiography. Sudden death without premonitory signs of cardiovascular disease is sometimes encountered. This has been observed in cats with compensated severe hypertrophic cardiomyopathy and sometimes occurs in perioperative settings.

ECHOCARDIOGRAPHY. Two-dimensional echocardiography may reveal regional left ventricular wall motion abnormalities (hyperkinesis, hypokinesis, akinesis, dyskinesis), regional wall thinning (especially left apex in the parasternal long-axis view), aneurysms, left heart thrombi, and ventricular dysfunction. Long-standing injury with fibrosis may be evident as focal areas of endocardial hyperechogenicity. Doppler echocardiography helps detect and assess severity of valvular regurgitation and evaluate diastolic function.

ELECTROCARDIOGRAPHY. Standard electrocardiography may be valuable in certain cases, but results often appear normal, especially in cases of intramural coronary insufficiency. Despite experimental data from canine coronary occlusion models, we are not aware of clinical reports correlating electrocardiographic patterns of ischemia and infarction with natural diseases in dogs and cats. The resting electrocardiogram (ECG) may reveal abnormalities of the QRS complex, ST segment, or T wave and display arrhythmias and conduction disturbances. However, many of these changes may be recorded in a variety of disorders and may not be recognized as dynamic events. Endocardial ischemia may cause delayed repolarization (QT prolongation), ST-T depression, and T-wave inversion. Transmural MI may cause ST-segment elevation and tall T waves in leads facing the electrical activity of the affected myocardium. Abnormal Q waves and ST-segment depression may occur early in acute subendocardial MI. Microscopic intramural MI in dogs has been associated with a "notched" R-wave descent. At times the ECG will display abnormalities during and after exercise when the resting ECG is normal. Such ST-T changes have been seen following exercise in dogs with subaortic stenosis.

The roles of radionuclide angiography, perfusion imaging, and stress echocardiography have not been sufficiently explored in veterinary practice. Presumably, serum muscle enzymes (MB-CK) could be useful for detecting cardiac injury.

The diagnosis of myocardial ischemia and MI can only be made if the clinician understands predisposing causes and maintains a high level of suspicion for these problems. In the dog or cat with substantial hypertrophy of the left ventricle, as in cases of subaortic stenosis or idiopathic hypertrophic cardiomyopathy, subendocardial ischemia and associated myocardial injury are likely; prevention of further injury may be a reasonable therapeutic goal. Ischemia further stiffens the poorly compliant left ventricle and may potentiate diastolic dysfunction and congestive heart failure in some pets. MI, which has been observed in some cats with hypertrophic cardiomyopathy, may prompt sudden left ventricular failure, or fatal ventricular arrhythmia. Patients with bacterial endocarditis or other conditions with thromboembolic potential may demonstrate pain or cardiac arrhythmias related to coronary occlusion. MI should be considered in the dog with acute tachypnea, anxiety, and significant ST-segment elevation. The possibility of acute MI leading to ventricular fibrillation should be considered during the necropsy of any animal that dies suddenly and unexpectedly.

MANAGEMENT

Acute MI is a dynamic process that may evolve slowly. Therapeutic interventions are intended to limit ischemia, preserve myocardium, restore perfusion, reduce myocardial oxygen requirements, remove or inhibit toxic metabolites, augment energy substrates, and inhibit or blunt mediators of cellular injury (e.g., free oxygen radicals, calcium). Unfortunately, proof of clinical efficacy in spontaneous animal diseases is lacking. Therefore, management emphasizes principles derived from treating human conditions. General care should include: (1) hospitalization and cage rest, (2) pharmacologic efforts to limit infarct size, establish reperfusion of ischemic tissue, and treat life-threatening arrhyth-

mias, (3) treatment of the underlying disease, (4) management of congestive heart failure, (5) correction of acid-base and electrolyte imbalances, and (6) treatment of thromboembolic complications.

Hospitalization and cage rest are recommended to facilitate diagnosis and therapy, reduce cardiac work load, and minimize myocardial oxygen consumption. Management of associated medical disorders should begin immediately according to the underlying disease process. Hypoxemia must be reversed with oxygen-enriched air when associated with chronic respiratory disease, pneumonia, or left heart failure. Severe anemia and causes of fever should be corrected, and congestive heart failure treated. Diuretics may be used, but cardiotonics like digoxin should be avoided if there is clear-cut evidence of ischemia and infarction. Electrocardiographic monitoring and management of severe arrhythmias are important.

Beta-adrenergic receptor-blocking drug therapy has been shown to reduce the risk of mortality and nonfatal reinfarction in humans surviving acute MI. It has been used to reduce ischemic injury during early hours of acute MI. Patients with sinus tachycardia and hypertension in which beta-blockers lower heart rate and blood pressure (reducing myocardial oxygen consumption) are particularly suited for this therapy. There are currently no conclusive data suggesting that any beta-blocking drugs are more beneficial than others in decreasing mortality. The use of beta-blocking drugs in the cardioprotection of dogs with left ventricular hypertrophy and intramural coronary narrowing may have merit. This empirical approach is often used in dogs with severe subaortic stenosis. Similarly, beta-blocking drugs might reduce myocardial oxygen demand in cats with hypertrophic cardiomyopathy.

Unlike beta-blocking drugs, calcium entry antagonists have not been shown to reduce human mortality from MI. Even though they are potent antiischemic agents, they have no effect on reducing sudden death. In fact, they may actually cause a slight increase in mortality when given prophylactically to human survivors of acute MI. Because hypotension may develop, these and other arterial dilating drugs must be used with great care, if at all. Whether calcium channel blockers are beneficial for chronic treatment and prevention of further myocardial injury in animals prone to chronic left ventricular ischemia is unknown. There is, however, clinical evidence that calcium channel blockers like diltiazem may be helpful in management of feline hypertrophic cardiomyopathy. This benefit may be related to improvement of myocardial perfusion, decrease in oxygen demand, or facilitation of ventricular relaxation.

Other interventions have been described to protect the ischemic myocardium. Nitroglycerin administered intravenously may affect infarct size in humans treated early. Careful dose titration is required. Topical nitrates may theoretically benefit dogs or cats with myocardial ischemia. In dogs with experimental fixed coronary artery ligation, administration of the phospholipase inhibitor quinacrine reduced the extent of myocardial necrosis. This lends support to the premise that inhibition of phospholipase activation or biochemical events triggered by ischemia may be of therapeutic benefit.

References and Suggested Reading

Bradley, A. J., and Alpert, J. S.: Coronary flow reserve. Am. Heart J. 122:1116, 1991.

Chiariello, M., Ambrosio, G., Cappelli-Bigazzi, M., et al.: Reduction in infarct size by the phospholipase inhibitor quinacrine in dogs with coronary artery occlusion. Am. Heart. J. 120:819, 1990.

Fox, P. R.: Feline myocardial disease. In Fox, P. R. (ed.): Canine and Feline Cardiology. New York: Churchill Livingstone, 1988, p. 435.

Hampton, J. R.: Secondary prevention of acute myocardial infarction with beta-blocking agents and calcium antagonists. Am. J. Cardiol. 66:3C, 1990.

Jonsson, L.: Coronary arterial lesions and myocardial infarcts in dogs: A pathologic and microangiographic study. ACTA Vet. Scand. (suppl 38):1, 1972.

Liu, S-K., and Tilley, L. P.: Animal models of primary myocardial diseases. Yale J. Biol. Med. 53:191, 1980.

Liu, S-K., Hsu, F. S., and Lee, C. T.: An atlas of cardiovascular pathology. Taiwan: Wonder Enterprise, 1989.

Liu, S-K., Tilley, L. P., Tappe, J. P., et al.: Clinical and pathologic findings in dogs with atherosclerosis: 21 cases (1970–1983). J.A.V.M.A. 189:227, 1986.

Pasternak, R. C., Braunwald, E., and Sobel, B. E.: Acute myocardial infarction. In Braunwald, E. (ed.): Heart Disease. 3rd ed. Philadelphia: W. B. Saunders, 1988, pp. 1222–1314.

Singh, B. N.: Advantages of beta-blockers versus antiarrhythmic agents and calcium antagonists in secondary prevention after myocardial infarction. Am. J. Cardiol. 66:9C–20C, 1990.

Tilley, L. P., Liu, S-K., Gilbertson, S. R., et al.: Primary myocardial disease in the cat: A model for human cardiomyopathy. Am. J. Pathol. 87:493, 1977.

TRACHEAL WASH AND BRONCHOALVEOLAR LAVAGE IN THE MANAGEMENT OF RESPIRATORY DISEASE

ELEANOR C. HAWKINS
Raleigh, North Carolina

Tracheal wash and bronchoalveolar lavage (BAL) are valuable tools for the diagnostic evaluation of dogs and cats with lower respiratory tract disease. In this article, *lower respiratory tract* refers to the trachea, bronchi, and lungs. Localization of disease to the lower respiratory tract is achieved through taking a history and by performing a physical examination and thoracic radiography in nearly all cases. Narrowing and prioritization of the differential diagnosis are also possible with this information; however, few cases can be definitively diagnosed without further testing.

Tracheal wash and BAL are minimally invasive procedures that provide specimens from the lower respiratory tract. These specimens can be evaluated cytologically and microbiologically for evidence of inflammation, malignancy, and infectious agents. Based on this information, the differential diagnosis can be further prioritized, and in some cases a definitive diagnosis can be made. Specific ancillary tests can be selected based on the refined differential diagnosis. Appropriate treatment and accurate prognostication can be offered once a definitive diagnosis is made.

Tracheal wash and BAL specimens are also useful for the diagnosis of concurrent or secondary problems in animals with known respiratory disease, such as bacterial infections in animals with tracheal collapse or chronic bronchial disease. These procedures can be performed repeatedly in the same animal, making it possible to monitor response to treatment or progression of disease.

INDICATIONS FOR TRACHEAL WASH AND BRONCHOALVEOLAR LAVAGE: WHICH PROCEDURE TO PERFORM

Tracheal Wash

Tracheal wash fluid is collected through a small-diameter catheter with the tip positioned at the carina. Contamination of the specimen with pharyngeal cells and flora is minimized by passing the catheter transtracheally or through a sterile endotracheal tube. Small volumes of saline are injected and withdrawn by syringe to collect cells, organisms, and proteins. Complications are extremely rare; however, the procedure is contraindicated in animals with severe respiratory compromise, because any additional stress can easily precipitate a crisis in such cases.

Tracheal wash specimens are representative of disease processes involving the trachea and large airways. The procedure is indicated for animals with historical, physical, or radiographic evidence of airway disease. Diseases of the pulmonary parenchyma resulting in coughing, sputum production, and alveolar flooding often involve the major airways as well. Tracheal wash specimens are generally representative of these processes.

Localized diseases of the pulmonary parenchyma or those that involve only the pulmonary interstitium (leading to tachypnea and minimal or nonproductive coughing) are much less likely to be identified by tracheal wash. Generally, because it is safe, simple, and inexpensive, tracheal wash is indicated even in animals with interstitial or localized disease before performing more invasive tests including BAL. Animals with pulmonary mass lesions located adjacent to the body wall that can be directly aspirated with few complications and high diagnostic yield are an exception to this generalization.

Ideally, tracheal wash or BAL should be performed before initiating any specific treatment such as antibiotics, because diagnostic findings can be obscured by therapy even if clinical signs have not resolved.

Bronchoalveolar Lavage

BAL is the injection of saline into an airway in large enough volumes to flood the alveoli dependent on that airway, followed by removal of the fluid to collect cells, organisms, and proteins lining the epithelial surfaces of the alveoli and small airways. General anesthesia is required for BAL in animals, increasing the potential for complications. It is contraindicated in animals with severe respiratory compromise. The procedure is usually performed through a flexible fiberoptic bronchoscope, increasing the cost of the procedure but allowing for directed sampling from a specific lung lobe (see CVT X, p. 219).

BAL fluid is representative of processes involving the deep lung: the bronchioles, alveoli, and in some cases the interstitium. In healthy animals, the predominant cell type is the alveolar macrophage rather than respiratory epithelial cells. The many alveoli dependent on the subsegmental bronchus in which the scope is lodged are sampled, and several differ-

ent lung lobes can be lavaged in the same animal; therefore, a large volume of lung tissue is represented. Large numbers of cells are retrieved for examination. Any mucus present in the specimen is greatly diluted by the saline, and excellent quality slides can be prepared without the clumping of cells and organisms commonly seen in cytologic preparations of tracheal wash fluid.

BAL is particularly indicated in animals with undiagnosed pulmonary disease in which tracheal wash fluid analysis does not provide adequate information. It is much less expensive and invasive than obtaining pulmonary biopsy samples by thoracotomy. Compared with lung aspiration, BAL provides specimens representative of a greater area of lung, provides more material for examination, and is not associated with pneumothorax or hemothorax.

PROCEDURES AND SPECIMEN HANDLING

Tracheal Wash

Tracheal wash is a commonly used clinical procedure. The performance of transtracheal and endotracheal techniques has been reviewed in several articles (Creighton and Wilkins, 1974; Moise and Blue, 1983; Moise and Dietze, 1989; Schaer et al., 1989).

Fluid collected by tracheal wash is placed on ice or refrigerated immediately after collection, and slides are ideally prepared within 30 min. If a clinical pathologist is to be consulted, prepared slides rather than fluid are submitted. Several drops of fluid are cultured for aerobic bacteria. Antibiotic sensitivity testing is performed on any isolates. In cases that are poorly responsive to therapy, cultures for Mycoplasma may be helpful, especially in cats with chronic bronchial disease.

The remaining fluid is evaluated cytologically. Direct and sediment smears are made. If mucus is present in the specimen, it is helpful to remove the mucus and make slides of it using the squash technique. The mucus can be a site of cell or organism clumping. Removing the mucus also improves the quality of slide that can be prepared from the remaining fluid. Clumping can interfere with the creation of a monolayer of cells for qualitative examination. Slides are stained with standard Romanovsky's stains such as Wright's stain or with quick Romanovsky's stains such as Diff-Quik.*

All slides are evaluated for quality and evidence of oropharyngeal contamination. Adequate specimens are examined thoroughly for increased numbers of inflammatory cells, abnormal cell populations, and infectious agents (Table 1). Tracheal wash fluid from normal animals contains respiratory epi-

---

*American Scientific Products, McGaw Park, IL 60085.

Table 1. *Infectious Agents That May Be Recovered From Tracheal Wash or Bronchoalveolar Lavage Fluid*

Viruses
    Distemper
    Adenovirus
Bacteria
Protozoa
    Toxoplasma gondii
    Pneumocystis carinii
Fungi
    Histoplasma capsulatum
    Blastomyces dermatitidis
    Cryptococcus neoformans
    Coccidioides immitis
Parasites
    Capillaria aerophila eggs
    Aleurostrongylus abstrusus larvae or larvated eggs
    Paragonimus kellicotti eggs
    Filarioidea larvae or larvated eggs
    Dirofilaria immitis microfilaria

thelial cells, a few macrophages, and occasional inflammatory cells. Bacterial cultures are usually negative. Bacteria are present in the trachea of some healthy animals, presumably from minor aspiration of oropharyngeal flora. Growth of bacteria in conjunction with supportive cytologic abnormalities is considered to be significant.

Bronchoalveolar Lavage

BAL is most commonly performed through a bronchoscope. A technique for BAL in cats that does not require endoscopic equipment has been described (Hawkins and DeNicola, 1989; Hawkins et al., 1990) (see this volume, p. 803). Summaries of two techniques are provided in Tables 2 and 3.

Fluid is cultured for aerobic bacteria and, in some cases, *Mycoplasma*. Antibiotic sensitivity testing is performed on all isolates. For economic reasons, several drops of fluid from each syringe can be pooled for culture.

Cytologic evaluation of BAL fluid includes performing total nucleated cell counts and examining smears. Cell counts and slide preparation are ideally performed within 30 min of BAL. As with tracheal wash fluid, if a clinical pathologist is to be consulted, prepared slides rather than fluid are submitted. If cost allows, fluid from each lobe should be evaluated independently because variation can exist between lobes even in animals with apparently diffuse disease. Individual aliquots collected from the same location can also be evaluated independently. The first syringe collected from each location has a higher number of cells from the larger airways than do subsequent lavages. Clinical benefit from evaluating individual aliquots from the same lobe has not been proved in veterinary medicine.

Table 2. *Bronchoalveolar Lavage in Dogs and Cats Through a Fiberoptic Bronchoscope*

1. Anesthetize as for routine bronchoscopy, including premedication with atropine.
2. Perform bronchoscopic examination of all airways.
3. Select lobes to lavage based on radiographic or bronchoscopic abnormalities. If no localization, arbitrarily select two to four lobes.
4. Pass scope peripherally into a lobe until a snug fit is achieved between scope and airway wall.
5. Inject 25 ml of warmed sterile saline through biopsy channel.
6. Immediately aspirate saline by syringe with gentle suction.
7. Disconnect syringe to discharge air, then repeat aspiration attempts until no more fluid is retrieved; 40 to 80% recovery of fluid should be achieved.
8. Repeat using another 25 ml of saline without moving the scope.
9. Place collected fluid on ice.
10. Repeat lavage procedure for each lobe.
11. Allow animal to breath 100% oxygen until extubation is required. Inflate lungs with gentle positive-pressure ventilation several times.
12. Monitor for signs of hypoxemia.* Treat with oxygen supplementation if it occurs. Bronchodilators may be helpful in nonresponsive cases.

*Hypoxemia occurs immediately after BAL. Arterial oxygen tensions gradually increase to prelavage values during the next 2 hr. Hypoxemia responds dramatically to oxygen supplementation in nearly all cases. Supplementation is usually unnecessary after extubation and even in compromised animals is rarely required for more than 15 min.

Table 3. *Bronchoalveolar Lavage Through an Endotracheal Tube in Cats*

1. Premedicate with atropine and anesthetize with intravenous ketamine or other rapidly acting agent.
2. Intubate with sterilized, cuffed endotracheal tube. Place lidocaine on larynx and use laryngoscope to minimize pharyngeal contamination of tube. Inflate cuff.
3. Place syringe adapter on end of tube in place of anesthetic tube adapter.
4. Place cat in lateral recumbency. If disease is not diffuse, place most diseased side of chest against table.
5. Gently inject 5 ml/kg body weight warmed, sterile saline by syringe through endotracheal tube.
6. Immediately apply gentle suction.
7. Disconnect syringe to discharge air, then repeat aspiration attempts until no more saline is retrieved; 40 to 80% recovery should be achieved.
8. Recovery of fluid is facilitated by elevating the caudal half of the cat a few centimeters off the table.
9. Repeat lavage two more times, with 5 ml/kg of saline each time.
10. Place fluid on ice.
11. Connect endotracheal tube to oxygen source. Inflate lungs with gentle positive-pressure ventilation several times and allow cat to breathe oxygen until extubation is necessary.
12. Monitor for signs of hypoxemia.* Treat with oxygen supplementation if it occurs. Bronchodilators may be helpful in nonresponsive cases.

*Hypoxemia occurs immediately after BAL. Arterial oxygen tensions gradually increase to prelavage values during the next 2 hr. Hypoxemia responds dramatically to oxygen supplementation in nearly all cases. Supplementation is usually unnecessary after extubation and even in compromised animals is rarely required for more than 15 min.

Total nucleated cell counts are performed with a hemocytometer using undiluted fluid. Differential cell counts are performed on smears prepared by sedimentation or cytocentrifugation. Direct smears can be made from highly cellular specimens. Slides are stained with Wright's or other Romanovsky's stains.

Qualitative evaluation is also performed. Inflammatory cells are examined for phagocytosis of organisms or debris, activation, and degenerative changes. Cells are examined for criteria of malignancy. Infectious agents may be present in extremely low numbers, and exhaustive examination of all slides for organisms is necessary (see Table 1).

A wide range of cytologic values can be found in BAL fluid from clinically normal animals. In general, total nucleated cell counts are less than 500/μl in normal dogs and less than 400/μl in normal cats. Seventy-five to ninety-five per cent of normal BAL cells are macrophages. Lymphocytes, neutrophils, and eosinophils each account for less than 10% of nucleated cells, and mast cells and epithelial cells represent only 1 to 2%. In addition to relative differential cell counts, consideration is given to absolute counts in BAL fluid with extremely high or low total cell counts. Clinically normal cats and dogs can have high relative or absolute eosinophil counts.

ABNORMALITIES AND THEIR EFFECT ON MANAGEMENT

Cytologic characterization of inflammation, identification of cellular criteria of malignancy, and organism identification for specimens from the lower respiratory tract resemble those of other organ systems. Diagnostic and therapeutic implications for the lower respiratory tract based on general categories of cytologic abnormalities are discussed later. In addition to these guidelines, the source of the specimen and all other available diagnostic information must be considered when modifying the differential diagnosis or making a diagnostic or treatment plan. The source of the specimen is the airways with tracheal wash and the deep lung and specific lung lobes with BAL. Other diagnostic information minimally should include findings from history taking, physical examination, funduscopic examination, thoracic radiographs, and complete blood count.

Neutrophilic Inflammation

Neutrophilic inflammation is most often a result of bacterial infection. Cytologic findings supporting this diagnosis include the presence of degenerative changes within the neutrophils and intracellular

bacteria. Bacterial cultures are often positive. Appropriate antibiotic therapy is initiated. Selection of antibiotic can be made pending culture results based on cytologic morphology of organisms. Follow-up evaluation of these animals is indicated to assess response to therapy. If clinical and radiographic signs fail to improve during the next 3 to 5 days, a change in therapy or collection of additional specimens or both are considered.

Bacterial infections can occur secondary to various diseases including tracheal collapse, chronic bronchitis, neoplasia, allergic disease, and viral, mycotic, or parasitic infections. Cases with bacterial infection are further evaluated after resolution of infection for the presence of underlying disease obscured by the inflammatory response to infection.

Not all animals with neutrophilic inflammation resulting from bacterial infection have cytologic evidence of toxicity or visible bacteria present in tracheal wash or BAL specimens, particularly if antibiotic therapy was initiated before specimen collection. Unless other information is suggestive of a different diagnosis, treatment with a broad-spectrum antibiotic is initiated after specimen collection. Other differential diagnoses are pursued if there is no response to therapy and cultures result in no growth.

Other diseases that can cause neutrophilic inflammation include viral, mycoplasmal, protozoal, and fungal infection; neoplasia; foreign bodies; acute aspiration pneumonia; and inhaled toxins or irritants. Lower respiratory tract specimens are scrutinized for fungal or protozoal organisms, which can be present in extremely low numbers. Allergic and parasitic disease can cause neutrophilia, but eosinophilia is usually present as well. Neutrophilic inflammation can be present in animals with chronic bronchitis or pulmonary alveolitis-fibrosis with no identifiable etiology (see *CVT X*, p. 361).

In most cases, clinical and radiographic signs are supportive of one of these diagnoses and can be used in formulating a plan even if a causative agent is not apparent in tracheal wash or BAL fluid. If signs are nonspecific, specimen collection from any abnormal superficial tissues, such as peripheral lymph nodes, can be performed in search of infectious agents or neoplasia. Fungal antibody titers are measured in dogs. If a definitive diagnosis is not possible, a decision based on all available information must be made about whether to perform lung aspiration or biopsy or to evaluate response to anti-inflammatory therapy with corticosteroids. Corticosteroids are contraindicated if infectious disease is still a consideration, and close monitoring of the animal is essential if a therapeutic trial is elected.

Eosinophilic Inflammation

Lower respiratory tract specimens demonstrating apparent eosinophilic inflammation have been noted in clinically normal cats and dogs. Despite this fact, the presence of increased numbers of eosinophils is generally considered significant in cats and dogs being evaluated for respiratory disease. A concurrent nonseptic neutrophilic or chronic inflammatory response is frequently present. Increased numbers of mast cells may also be present but are a nonspecific finding.

Eosinophilic inflammation is most common in animals with allergic bronchitis. Major differential diagnoses include pulmonary parasites and heartworm disease in both dogs and cats. Specimens are examined closely for the presence of parasitic organisms or ova. Organisms are frequently absent even in cases with parasitic disease, and whole blood microfilarial examination, adult *Dirofilaria* antigen testing, and appropriate fecal examinations for pulmonary parasites are always performed. The diagnosis of allergic bronchitis is made if the minimum database is supportive of the disease and test results for the major differential diagnoses are negative.

A hypersensitivity response can occur secondary to other antigens as well. Bacterial, protozoal, and fungal infections and neoplasia are considered in animals in which the minimum database or other information is either not consistent with allergic bronchitis or is supportive of one of these other diseases. These diseases are also considered more possible if the eosinophilic inflammation is a minor abnormality compared with other changes present in the lower respiratory specimens. Bacterial cultures, serologic tests, or more invasive respiratory specimen collection is considered.

More rare causes of eosinophilic inflammation are pulmonary infiltrates with eosinophils (PIE) (see *CVT X*, p. 369) or eosinophilic granulomatosis (see this volume, p. 813). Thoracic radiographs may demonstrate a patchy interstitial or alveolar pattern or may mimic neoplasia or mycotic disease when large nodules or hilar lymphadenopathy is present. Other differential diagnoses, particularly infectious and parasitic diseases, must be ruled out before initiating therapy. Histopathologic examination of tissues may be necessary for a definitive diagnosis. Corticosteroids, initially at immunosuppressive doses, are recommended for treatment. More potent immunosuppressive drugs are usually necessary in cases of eosinophilic granulomatosis.

Chronic and Chronic-Active Inflammation

Chronic inflammation refers to a mixed inflammatory response with the predominant cell type being the activated macrophage. Activated macrophages are distinguished from normal alveolar macrophages by increased cytoplasm and many cytoplasmic vacuoles. *Chronic-active inflammation* is used to describe a similar response, with the predominant cell types being activated macrophages and neutrophils. Care must be taken in evaluating BAL specimens, because fluid from normal animals has up to 95% macrophages. Increased total cell counts, macrophage activation, and increased numbers of inflammatory cells support an interpretation of inflammation. Anthracosis, phagocytosis of dark granules, may be seen in animals chronically exposed to smoke or soot.

These types of inflammatory responses are nonspecific, and differential diagnoses are numerous. Active chronic or atypical bacterial infection, resolving bacterial infection, fungal or parasitic infection, heartworm disease in both dogs and cats, neoplasia, lung lobe torsion, lipid aspiration, aspiration pneumonia, and thromboembolic disease can cause chronic or chronic-active inflammation. All slides are carefully examined for organisms or atypical cells. BAL fluid is more likely to demonstrate organisms or atypical cells of interstitial diseases than is tracheal wash fluid. Heartworm tests and serologic tests for infectious diseases are performed if an etiology is not apparent. If other information is not highly suggestive of a particular disease, lung biopsy is indicated.

Hemorrhage with Inflammation

Hemorrhage with inflammation is characterized by a chronic or chronic-active inflammatory response with erythrophagocytosis, hemosiderin-laden macrophages, and increased numbers of red blood cells. Systemic clotting disorders must be considered. Many diseases of the respiratory tract can potentially cause hemorrhage with inflammation. Common differential diagnoses are dirofilariasis, neoplasia, fungal infection, foreign body, thromboembolic disease, and lung lobe torsion. Traumatically induced hemorrhage is usually diagnosed presumptively based on other information. Congestive heart failure can cause intrapulmonary hemorrhage, but heart failure is usually diagnosed before the collection of respiratory specimens.

Selection of further diagnostic tests is based on the minimum database or other information. Microfilarial and occult heartworm tests, fungal titers, and angiography are considered. If a diagnosis cannot be made, more invasive collection of respiratory specimens (fine-needle aspiration, open lung biopsy) is indicated.

Lymphoid Reactivity

Increased numbers of lymphocytes and the presence of reactive lymphocytes and plasma cells are nonspecific indicators of immune stimulation. The presence of a monotonous population of lymphoid cells demonstrating increased amounts of basophilic cytoplasm and large or multiple nucleoli is supportive of a diagnosis of lymphoma, particularly in the absence of other inflammatory cells.

Neoplasia

Neoplastic cells are sometimes identifiable in lower respiratory tract specimens. BAL fluid is more likely to have identifiable cells than tracheal wash fluid, because most pulmonary tumors in animals are metastatic or multicentric and involve primarily the interstitium rather than the major airways. Cells from primary or metastatic carcinoma or malignant lymphocytes may be present.

It can be dangerous to make a definitive diagnosis of carcinoma based solely on cytologic specimens. Differentiation of criteria for malignancy in epithelial cells from hyperplastic change is often difficult or impossible, especially in the setting of marked inflammation. Slides can be referred to a clinical pathologist for consultation. Histologic evaluation of lung tissue may be necessary to confirm a diagnosis. In the absence of inflammation and with other information supportive of neoplastic disease, a presumptive diagnosis can be made. Evaluation of lymphoid cells was discussed previously.

Etiologic Agents

In some cases of infectious disease involving the lower respiratory tract, organisms are apparent cytologically and a definitive diagnosis can be made. Possible underlying or concurrent diseases are also considered. Treatment is initiated against the identified agent.

The absence of visible organisms does not eliminate infectious disease from the differential diagnosis. Even in specimens in which infectious agents are present, their low concentration can make identification difficult. Regardless of collection technique, all slides must be examined carefully. When performing BAL, multiple lobes are lavaged. Identification and characterization of specific organisms may be enhanced by culturing techniques or special staining procedures. Other specimens, such as feces or blood, are evaluated for parasites. If infectious disease is highly suspected but organisms cannot be identified, more invasive collection of respiratory specimens is indicated.

Organisms that may be present in tracheal wash or BAL fluid are listed in Table 1.

Acknowledgment

The author acknowledges Dennis B. DeNicola, D.V.M., Ph.D., Dipl., A.C.V.P., for his contribution in the evaluation and interpretation of cytologic abnormalities in bronchoalveolar lavage fluid.

References and Suggested Reading

Cowell, R. L., Tyler, R. D., and Baldwin, C. J.: Transtracheal and bronchial washes. *In* Pratt, P. W. (ed.): *Diagnostic Cytology of the Dog and Cat.* Goleta, CA: American Veterinary Publications, 1989, p. 167.
Review of techniques for tracheal wash and interpretation of cytologic responses.

Creighton, S. R., and Wilkins, R. J.: Transtracheal aspiration biopsy: Technique and cytologic evaluation. J. Am. Anim. Hosp. Assoc. 10:219, 1974.
Description of the technique of transtracheal wash.

Hawkins, E. C., and DeNicola, D. B.: Collection of bronchoalveolar lavage fluid in cats, using an endotracheal tube. Am. J. Vet. Res. 50:855, 1989.
Description of a technique for nonbronchoscopic performance of BAL for use in cats.

Hawkins, E. C., DeNicola, D. B., and Kuehn, N. F.: Bronchoalveolar lavage in the evaluation of pulmonary disease in the dog and cat. J. Vet. Intern. Med. 4:267, 1990.
Review of BAL including performance of lavage and interpretation of cytologic abnormalities.

King, R. R., Zeng, Q. Y., Brown, D. J., et al.: Bronchoalveolar lavage cell populations in dogs and cats with eosinophilic pneumonitis. Proceedings of the 7th Veterinary Respiratory Symposium. Chicago: The Comparative Respiratory Society, 1988.
Cytologic parameters of BAL fluid from normal cats and from cats and dogs with allergic or parasitic disease.

Moise, N. S., and Blue, J.: Bronchial washings in the cat: Procedure and cytologic evaluation. Comp. Cont. Ed. Pract. Vet. 5:621, 1983.
Description of tracheobronchial wash through an endotracheal tube in cats.

Moise, N. S., and Dietze, A. E.: Bronchopulmonary diseases. *In* Sherding, R. G. (ed.): *The Cat: Diseases and Clinical Management.* New York: Churchill Livingstone, 1989, p. 775.
Performance of lower respiratory diagnostic procedures and discussion of lower respiratory diseases in cats.

Rebar, A. H., DeNicola, D. B., and Muggenburg, B. A.: Bronchopulmonary lavage cytology in the dog: Normal findings. Vet. Pathol. 17:294, 1980.
Cytologic results of BAL fluid analysis in normal dogs.

Schaer, M., Ackerman, N., and King, R. R.: Clinical approach to the patient with respiratory disease. *In* Ettinger, S. J. (ed.): *Textbook of Veterinary Internal Medicine,* 3rd ed. Philadelphia: W. B. Saunders, 1989, p. 747.
General approach to animals with respiratory disease including a description of diagnostic procedures.

ACQUIRED NASOPHARYNGEAL STENOSIS IN CATS

RUSSELL W. MITTEN
Victoria, Australia

Chronic upper respiratory disease is common in feline practice, and successful resolution of these cases is often difficult. Correct identification of the type of problem in each case is essential if the practitioner is to maximize the chances of resolution. Acquired nasopharyngeal stenosis is a relatively recently recognized cause of ongoing upper respiratory distress in cats but is one that can be successfully treated.

ANATOMIC CONSIDERATIONS

The nasal conformation of cats is considerably foreshortened compared with the dog, and some feline breeds such as the Persian are considered to be brachycephalic. Despite this foreshortening, relatively few cats appear to suffer from the respiratory difficulties experienced by brachycephalic dogs. Stenosis of the external nares resulting in chronic respiratory distress has been reported in a Persian cat, with successful surgical resolution (Harvey, 1986).

Because of its conformation, the nose of the cat is not easy to examine thoroughly. A small otoscope cone is useful for inspecting the nose rostrally. While improved visualization both rostrally and caudally may be achieved with a small-bore, flexible fiberoptic endoscope, the view with these instruments is frequently obscured by secretions or bleeding, and relatively few practitioners have access to such instruments.

The caudal nares of the cat form the rostral boundary of the nasopharynx. This area is examined with the patient under general anesthesia. The mouth is held wide open and the soft palate is retracted rostrally to reveal the nasopharynx. Use of a dental mirror at this stage will improve visualization. The caudal nares are seen at approximately the level of the hard palate and form an ovoid orifice measuring about 6 mm dorsoventrally and 5 mm laterally in the adult cat (Fig. 1A). Inspection of this area should be part of the diagnostic workup of feline chronic upper respiratory disease.

ETIOLOGY AND PATHOGENESIS

In acquired nasopharyngeal stenosis, the normal ovoid opening of the caudal nares is reduced to a pinhole-sized orifice by the presence of a thin but tough membrane (see Fig. 1B). Histologic examination of tissue excised from this area has revealed evidence of chronic inflammation, with submucosal fibrosis and infiltration with cells suggesting either an infectious or allergic stimulus for formation of the membrane. The cats seen with this condition are all known to have had normal respiration earlier in life and to have acquired a chronic upper respiratory obstruction. It is likely that some of these cats initially had a chlamydial or viral upper respiratory infection. In these conditions, particularly in herpes virus rhinotracheitis, severe mucosal ulcerations occur, and it is possible that the initiating stimulus for development of the stenotic membrane in the nasopharynx was herpes-associated ulceration.

A condition described as nasopharyngeal cicatrix occurs in horses and is described as weblike strands of scar tissue across the nasopharynx forming as part of a chronic nasopharyngeal inflammatory process (Schumacker and Hanselka, 1987). Nasopharyngeal cicatrix also occurs in humans, again developing after acute and chronic ulcerative pharyngitis due to caustic burns and a range of infectious diseases (Stevenson, 1969).

CASE HISTORY AND PRESENTATION

Cats with acquired nasopharyngeal stenosis usually present with a history of nasal obstruction of several months' duration. There may be an underlying history of an initial acute upper respiratory tract infection. There may be snuffling and mucopurulent discharge, but the nasal discharge is not profuse. The most characteristic sign is obstruction, recognized as a stertorous or wheezing upper respiratory noise. When the cat's mouth is held open, the respiratory noise and distress are relieved, thus indicating their nasal origin. There is no external nasal or sinus swelling, and external palpation of the pharynx, larynx, and trachea is normal.

DIAGNOSIS

Cats should be anesthetized and intubated for further investigation. Lateral and open-mouth ven-

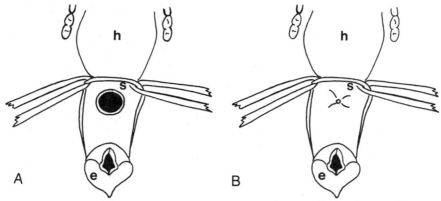

Figure 1. Line diagrams depicting the nasopharynx in a normal cat *(A)* and a cat with nasopharyngeal stenosis *(B)*. The cat is in sternal recumbency with the mouth held wide open. *A* shows the normal ovoid opening of the nasopharynx, approximately 5 mm in diameter; *B* shows the stenotic opening with a thin membrane covering the nasopharynx and a central pinpoint orifice. e, epiglottis with adjacent laryngeal opening; h, hard palate and upper dental arcade; s, soft palate with its margins retracted rostrolaterally (use of a dental mirror enhances visualization). (Reprinted with permission from Mitten, R. W.: Nasopharyngeal stenosis in four cats. J. Small Anim. Pract. 29:343, 1988.)

trodorsal radiographs of the nose will appear normal or will reveal evidence of minimal soft-tissue thickening and accumulation of some exudate around the turbinate bones. With the cat in sternal recumbency and the mouth held wide open, the nasopharynx is examined as described earlier. It may be necessary to swab away secretions to see the structures clearly. It is very useful at this point to pass a narrow tube (e.g., a feline urinary catheter) from the external nares through the ventral meatus on each side to ascertain patency. In the normal cat the catheter will pass readily into the pharynx, but in the case of nasopharyngeal stenosis the catheter cannot be passed and can be seen impinging on the acquired nasopharyngeal membrane. The membrane is quite tough, and it does not appear to be possible to force the catheter through it (Mitten, 1988).

Differential Diagnosis

Several other conditions have a similar clinical appearance and should be considered at this time (Lane, 1982).

CHRONIC RHINITIS/SINUSITIS. Cats with this condition are often termed "snufflers" and usually exhibit bouts of sneezing with persistent and often profuse nasal discharge, which is usually mucopurulent and at times may be flecked with blood. Although histologically there is submucosal proliferation and epithelial hyperplasia, it is still possible to pass a catheter through the nasal passage. An obvious soft-tissue/fluid density is seen radiographically in the nasal chambers or sinuses, and in the more chronic cases there may be thinning and distortion of the overlying facial bones. Nasal mucosal biopsy and culture from nasal washings are part of the diagnostic workup.

NASAL MYCOSES. *Cryptococcus neoformans* is the fungal agent most frequently identified, with *Aspergillus fumigatus* and *Penicillium* occurring very rarely (Goodall et al, 1984). The presenting signs are similar to severe chronic rhinitis. Occasionally, granulomatous lesions may be visible at the external nares or may invade through the overlying nasal bones or extend through the cribriform plate into the brain. *Cryptococcus* organisms may be identified in direct smears, from nasal washes, or from nasal biopsies. In both chronic sinusitis/rhinitis and mycoses one should consider the possibility of an underlying immunosuppressive disease process such as feline immunodeficiency virus infection.

FOREIGN BODIES. These are much less common in the cat than in the dog. The resulting discharge is likely to be unilateral and mucopurulent, with the foreign object or the associated turbinate damage identified radiographically.

INTRANASAL NEOPLASIA. These also appear to be less common than in the dog. Lymphosarcoma is the most common tumor identified; most others are carcinomas. Nasal tumors are characterized by unilateral obstruction with mucopurulent or sometimes bloody discharge, with some cases showing facial distortion and protrusion of the mass from the external nares. Radiographs assist in the diagnosis, and a nasal biopsy is definitive.

NASOPHARYNGEAL POLYPS. This condition is very similar in clinical presentation to acquired nasopharyngeal stenosis, as there is upper respiratory obstruction and purulent nasal discharge. The polyps, which are inflammatory in origin, arise in the middle ear and extend into the nasopharynx via the auditory tube. In some cases they may also extend through the tympanic membrane and fill the external ear canal. The polyps are readily identified as discrete soft-tissue masses in lateral radiographs of the nasopharynx and are easily seen when visually inspecting the nasopharynx, particularly when the soft palate is retracted rostrally. Polyps are treated by severing their stalklike attachment at the opening of the auditory tube. In a few instances there may be recurrence, and involvement of the tympanic bullae has been reported (Stanton et al, 1985).

LARYNGEAL DISEASES. Abnormalities in the larynx should be easily distinguished by the lack of signs of nasal discharge or obstruction and by the presence of abnormal findings in the larynx. Differential diagnoses here include laryngeal trauma and foreign bodies, laryngeal paralysis, lymphocytic-plasmacytic laryngopharyngitis, and laryngeal neoplasia.

TREATMENT

Acquired nasopharyngeal stenosis is treated surgically. The occluding membrane appears to be too tough to puncture with an intranasal catheter. To gain adequate access to the area, the anesthetized cat is placed in dorsal recumbency and the mouth is held wide open. A midline incision is made through the soft palate from its free border rostrally toward the hard palate, and the cut edges are retracted. The stenotic nasopharyngeal opening is then enlarged to the normal size (approximately 5

mm × 6 mm) by excising the membrane. Fine iris scissors are useful for this purpose. The soft palate is then sutured with fine absorbable suture material (e.g., PDS 1.5 metric). Broad-spectrum antibiotics in oral drop form, such as amoxicillin (Amoxil, Beecham Laboratories), 10 mg/kg every 12 hr are given for 5 to 7 days. This treatment has proven satisfactory in all cases treated to date, although one cat required minor repair of a partial breakdown of the suture line in the soft palate. Although recurrence of stenosis is reported in humans after excision of nasopharyngeal cicatrices, this has not occurred in the cats, which have been followed up over several years.

References and Suggested Reading

Goodall, S. A., Lane, J. G., and Warnock, D. W.: The diagnosis and treatment of a case of nasal aspergillosis in a cat. J. Small Anim. Pract. 25:627, 1984.

Harvey, C. E.: Surgical correction of stenotic nares in a cat. J. Am. Anim. Hosp. Assoc. 22:31, 1986.

Lane, J. G.: *ENT and Oral Surgery of the Dog and Cat.* Bristol: J. Wright. 1982, p. 65.

Mitten, R. W.: Nasopharyngeal stenosis in four cats. J. Small Anim. Pract. 29:341, 1988.

Schumacker, J., and Hanselka, D. V.: Nasopharyngeal cicatrices in horses: 47 cases. J.A.V.M.A. 191:239, 1987.

Stanton, M. E., Wheaton, L. G., Render, J. A., et al.: Pharyngeal polyps in two feline siblings. J.A.V.M.A. 186:1311, 1985.

Stevenson, E. W.: Cicatrical stenosis of the nasopharynx. Laryngoscope 79:2035, 1969.

FELINE BRONCHIAL DISEASE

JANICE A. DYE
Urbana, Illinois

and N. SYDNEY MOISE
Ithaca, New York

Bronchial disease in the cat describes an abnormality (e.g., inflammation, bronchoconstriction, infection) of the airways distal to the tracheal bifurcation, excluding disease originating in or primarily involving the alveoli, interstitium, vasculature, or pleura. Feline bronchial disease is a common problem; however, clinical signs and presentations, diagnostic findings, therapeutic responses, and prognoses may vary tremendously (Moise et al., 1989). To eliminate the confusion caused by this diversity,

clinically descriptive categories of feline bronchial disease have been proposed. These categories may refine and direct the diagnostic and therapeutic approach and more accurately predict the outcome of individual cats. Further understanding of the etiologies involved in feline bronchial disease, objective methods of measuring lung function and treatment response, and conscientious follow-up will be required to solidify these classifications. This chapter describes the etiopathogenesis, clinical features, diagnosis, and therapeutic management of cats with bronchial disease.

ETIOPATHOGENESIS

The precise pathophysiologic processes of feline bronchial disease have yet to be defined. Clues can be gained by studying the pathologic changes in cats that died as a result of lung disease. Histologic findings often include some degree of bronchial smooth muscle hypertrophy and bronchoconstriction (Fig. 1). This may occur in combination with airway mucosal inflammation and edema, epithelial cell desquamation, airway mucous plugs, or intraluminal inflammatory exudate. Varying degrees of emphysema, submucosal gland hyperplasia, or increased numbers of airway goblet cells may also be found.

These diverse pathologic changes all contribute to the development of airway obstruction. This obstruction, in turn, results in increased airflow resistance in affected airways. In simple terms, increased airway resistance can be due to changes inside the bronchial lumen, changes in the bronchial wall, or changes in the tissues surrounding the airways (West, 1987). In humans with chronic bronchitis, airway obstruction is primarily due to the presence of excessive intraluminal secretions. Bronchial wall thickening results from various conditions including bronchial smooth muscle hypertrophy and constriction (as occurs in humans with asthma), mucosal gland hyperplasia (as in chronic bronchitis), or mucosal edema and inflammation (as occurs in either asthma or chronic bronchitis). Finally, increased lung resistance can also occur in emphysema, as destruction of the structural support of the lung parenchyma results in loss of the normal radial traction surrounding the airway.

How can these types of airway disease be differentiated? Part of the answer is to assess reversibility of the airway obstruction, although this may be difficult when overlapping conditions exist. In cases of excessive bronchial smooth muscle constriction (e.g., asthma), treatment with a bronchodilator will result in nearly complete reversal of the airway obstruction. If the increased resistance is primarily due to mucosal edema and inflammation or to emphysema, bronchodilator therapy (which primarily relaxes bronchial smooth muscle) will yield minimal changes in lung function. If both bronchoconstriction and bronchial wall thickening are present, partial improvement in pulmonary function would be expected following administration of a bronchodilator. Although bronchodilator therapy is considered an important component in the management of cats with bronchial disease, the efficacy of such treatment depends on the dynamic nature of the underlying pathologic processes. Without the ability to measure lung function changes in the feline patient, this can be difficult to assess.

In addition to assessing reversibility, one can assess how easily bronchoconstriction is induced. In humans, airway reactivity is determined through bronchoprovocation testing. If a predetermined reduction in pulmonary function occurs at very low concentrations of inhaled methacholine, the patient is said to have hyperreactive airways. In humans,

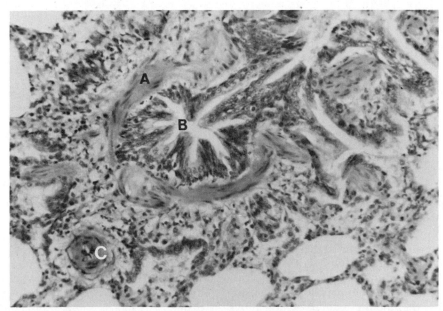

Figure 1. Photomicrograph of an airway from a cat with bronchial disease. Note the bronchial smooth muscle hypertrophy (A) and constriction with narrowing of the lumen (B). Peribronchial inflammatory cells and medial artery hypertrophy (C) are also present. (Courtesy of W. Haschek-Hock, Urbana, Illinois.)

asthma is defined as a state of reversible airway obstructive disease in patients *with* airway hyperreactivity. The phenomenon of airway hyperreactivity is clinically important. Just as inhalation of relatively low concentrations of methacholine induces bronchoconstriction, inhalation of tiny amounts of nonspecific irritants (dusts, sprays, cigarette smoke) can also trigger significant bronchoconstriction (i.e., an asthmatic attack). In the authors' experience, some cats with seemingly mild bronchial disease may worsen acutely following a change in the environment such as introduction of a scented litter or carpet freshener. Although definitive proof would require provocation testing, these observations suggest that some cats with bronchial disease may also exhibit airway hyperreactivity.

Airway inflammation appears to play a key role in the development and maintenance of a state of airway hyperreactivity in humans. Regardless of the initiating event, once inflammatory cells are in the airway, they release a variety of mediators that augment and perpetuate the inflammatory response. These mediators include histamine, the peptidoleukotrienes (LTC_4, LTD_4, LTE_4), and platelet activating factor. Through complex interactions of these and other mediators, the early and late phases of bronchoconstriction are induced. Drugs like corticosteroids are of benefit in controlling asthmatic symptoms because they decrease mediator production and influence inflammatory cell activity. Relatively little is known of the mediators involved in the development of bronchial disease in the cat. Because inflammatory cells are typically present in feline airways, corticosteroid therapy is considered a mainstay in the management of feline bronchial disease.

Normal airway smooth muscle tone in humans is thought to be the result of a balance between excitatory cholinergic nerves inducing bronchoconstriction and the inhibitory arm of the nonadrenergic, noncholinergic system (NAINS) that maintains bronchodilation. One of the purported neurotransmitters for the NAINS is vasoactive intestinal peptide (VIP). It is thought that certain asthmatic patients have a defective NAINS. Thus, while nonasthmatics have both circulating catecholamines and a functional NAINS to counteract episodes of bronchoconstrictor tone, these asthmatic patients would rely primarily on circulating catecholamines. They would be expected to be particularly sensitive to the effects of beta-blocking medications, and in fact some asthmatics develop severe bronchoconstriction if beta-antagonists are used. For reasons not entirely understood, about 20% of human asthmatics are also sensitive to aspirin. Therefore it has been recommended that beta-blocking medications and aspirin therapy be avoided in cats with bronchial disease (Moses and Spaulding, 1985).

The NAINS may also have an excitatory arm. Substance P is one of several putative neurotransmitters for this system. Although the importance of this system in the pathophysiology of asthma is still debated, a small study involving clinically ill asthmatic humans demonstrated decreased airway concentrations of VIP while substance P concentrations were increased. The NAINS and excitatory system have also been demonstrated in the airways of normal cats. In cats with serotonin-induced bronchoconstriction, VIP is a potent bronchial smooth muscle relaxant when given intravenously but not when given via airway nebulization (Diamond et al., 1983). Although the relevance of this finding has yet to be determined for cats with naturally acquired airway disease, it demonstrates that the airways of cats may closely resemble those of humans.

CLINICAL PRESENTATION

Cats with bronchial disease may be of all ages, with the Siamese breed perhaps overrepresented. The most common clinical sign is coughing, followed in decreasing order of frequency by dyspnea, wheezing, occasional sneezing, and vomiting. Cats may exhibit more than one sign, and the severity of clinical signs is variable. Approximately 25% of the cats have paroxysms of severe coughing while in a squatted position with the neck extended. This type of coughing can be confused with the vomiting or gagging action of a cat attempting to expel a hairball. Some owners report seasonal exacerbation of signs; however, the peak seasonal incidence is variable. Careful history taking may reveal that signs developed or were exacerbated following changes in the environment, such as exposure to smoke (fire places, cigarettes), sprays (flea control products, hair spray, household cleaners, spray starch), dusts (litter, flea powder, carpet fresheners), or unusual scents and fragrances (scented litter, odor neutralizers, perfumes, air fresheners, Christmas trees). The duration of clinical signs may vary from less than 24 hr to several years. Although some cats may have coughing or dyspnea for months or years, the clinical signs may be widely separated by asymptomatic periods. Other cats have relentless persistent coughing or dyspnea. Owners may report periodic dyspnea that cannot be appreciated during the physical examination. This notation should be taken seriously because some cats will have an exacerbation of clinical signs when stressed during diagnostic procedures.

On auscultation, most affected cats have some degree of abnormal lung sounds ranging from subtly increased bronchial sounds to severe crackles and wheezes. One third of cats have noticeable dyspnea or tachypnea (>60 breaths/min). Because the airways normally narrow during expiration, signs of lower airway obstruction are most evident then. Expiratory dyspnea is classic, though not absolute. The breathing pattern may be slow and deliberate with marked abdominal heaving, or it may be tachypneic with an expiratory push. The severity of the dyspnea is variable, ranging from detectable only with careful observation to severe and life-threatening. In the latter situation the cat is often cyanotic and may exhibit sinus bradycardia and excessively quiet lung fields owing to the absence of significant airflow into and out of the airways. Mild hyperthermia is present in about 25% of the cats. Percussion of the thorax or tracheal palpation will frequently elicit a cough. Posttussively, lung sounds may be more abnormal. With chronic or severe bronchial disease, cats may develop weight loss and generalized debility.

DIAGNOSTIC EVALUATION

The thoracic radiograph is essential in evaluating the cat with bronchial disease. A prominence of the bronchial walls (bronchial pattern) is the classic abnormality identified. The severity of the bronchial pattern present does not necessarily correlate with the severity of the coughing, dyspnea, or prognosis. A mild to moderate pulmonary interstitial pattern may be seen concurrently. A few cats may have mild, patchy alveolar infiltrates as well. Collapse of the right middle lung lobe is seen in about 10% of the cats. Since the main bronchus of this lobe deviates ventrally, it is more easily plugged with excessive bronchial mucus, resulting in atelectasis. Less commonly, the caudal portion of the left cranial lobe may be collapsed. Either of these findings indicate chronic disease. Overinflation of the lungs (Fig. 2) is identified in about 15% of cats and is characterized by a flattened, caudally displaced dia-

phragm, increased distance between the heart and diaphragm, ventral bowing of the caudal vena cava and sternum, increased radiolucency of the lungs, and extension of the lungs to the first lumbar vertebra with hypaxial muscle between the vertebra and lung border. Depending on the type of underlying bronchial disease, overinflation of the lungs may be temporary, with total resolution after therapy; permanent, but with partial resolution after therapy; or permanent with no resolution despite therapy. In the last case, cats typically have emphysema. Mild right heart enlargement may be identified in a few cats, and some may have aerophagia because of dyspnea.

Alterations in the complete blood count are not diagnostic for a particular type of bronchial disease. Although circulating eosinophilia is detected in about 20% of the cats, this does not always correlate with an eosinophilic inflammatory response in the airway. Hyperproteinemia (plasma protein concentration >7.5 gm/dl) is present in approximately 30% of the cats. Multiple fecal examinations may be required to detect underlying parasitic infections such as ascarids (which may undergo lung migration), lungworms (*Aelurostrongylus abstrusus*, *Capillaria aerophilia*), and lung flukes (*Paragonimus kellicotti*). An occult heartworm test for the serologic detection of adult *Dirofilaria immitis* should also be performed.

Bronchial cytology is an important diagnostic test in the evaluation of the cat with bronchial disease. It is used to characterize the bronchial inflammatory response present and to detect underlying parasitic or infectious agents. Bronchial secretions may be obtained from an endotracheal tube bronchial washing procedure (Fig. 3) or during bronchoalveolar lavage (see this volume, p. 795). Collected bronchial secretions should be suspended in sterile saline for cytologic evaluation and bacterial culture. (Alter-

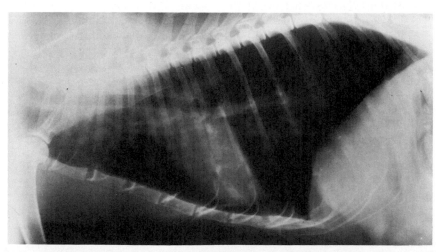

Figure 2. Lateral radiograph from a cat demonstrating a prominent bronchial pattern and overinflation of the lungs (flattened diaphragm, increased air space between the heart and diaphragm).

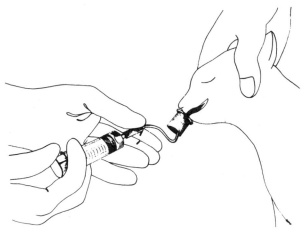

Figure 3. Endotracheal tube bronchial washing procedure. Using sterile technique, a 14-gauge catheter (without a metal stylet) is passed through a sterilized endotracheal tube to the level of the bronchi. Gentle aspiration is applied with or without instillation of 1 to 3 ml of sterile saline. The catheter is then withdrawn into the endotracheal tube. The catheter and tube are removed together as the cat is extubated, thereby protecting the sample from contamination by oral flora. The sample is placed into a sterile tube for culture and cytologic analysis. The endotracheal tube should be inspected for mucus, which may also be examined cytologically.

natively, to avoid oral contamination, a guarded catheter brush may be used to obtain material for culture. In this case, a second sample using washing techniques should be obtained for cytologic analysis.) Normal cats may have macrophages in the bronchial secretions, but the numbers are not excessive and the amount of mucus is minimal. On the other hand, cats with bronchial disease typically have abundant mucus and increased numbers of inflammatory cells. Suspended secretions may appear as small flecks of thick, white or yellow material. Bronchial secretions may be classified according to the predominant inflammatory cell type present. Mixed inflammatory cells, particularly eosinophils and neutrophils, can also be present. Mast cells, clusters of hyperplastic columnar epithelial cells, and goblet cells can be seen in all types of exudates. Calcospherites and coiled mucinous fibrils are seen occasionally. Bacteria can be isolated from about 25% to 40% of cats with bronchial disease, and cats with positive bacterial cultures frequently exhibit a neutrophilic inflammatory response. A variety of organisms may be isolated, the most common being *Pasteurella multocida* and *Moraxella*. Cats should also be cultured for *Mycoplasma*, as this has been isolated in a few cases.

Differential Diagnosis

The most common diseases to be excluded in the evaluation of the cat with bronchial disease are hypertrophic cardiomyopathy, pulmonary parasitic infections, heartworm disease, and neoplasia, primarily bronchoalveolar carcinoma. Of interest is the finding that cats with bronchial disease almost always cough while cats with hypertrophic cardiomyopathy rarely do. Cats with hypertrophic cardiomyopathy commonly have either a gallop rhythm or heart murmur. Hypertrophic cardiomyopathy can be ruled out more definitively by echocardiography or radiography. *A. abstrusus* is the most common symptomatic pulmonary parasite, usually infecting cats less than 1 year of age. The larvae may be found on fecal examination or bronchial cytology, and radiographically there tends to be a more prominent interstitial/patchy alveolar pattern with a caudal lung lobe distribution. Radiographic evidence of feline heartworm disease may include enlarged pulmonary arteries and parenchymal lung disease, with a lobar distribution and patchy, perivascular changes. Alternately, only a peribronchial and linear interstitial pattern may be present. Serologic detection of adult heartworm antigen should assist in the differentiation. In the aged cat with radiographic evidence of predominantly bronchial disease, bronchoalveolar carcinoma should be considered in the differential diagnosis, especially if follow-up radiographs demonstrate progression of disease. Neoplastic cells may be detected by bronchial cytology. Metastatic mammary adenocarcinoma may also occasionally have a similar appearance.

Additional diagnostics may be required if the cat fails to respond to treatment or the clinical signs change. Laryngoscopy and tracheobronchoscopy may be used to detect gross airway mucosal changes, intraluminal masses, collapsing airways, or laryngeal paralysis. If interstitial lung disease predominates, fine-needle lung aspirates may be necessary to obtain inflammatory cells, neoplastic cells, or fungal organisms. Although not indicated in uncomplicated bronchial disease, an open lung biopsy may provide a definitive histologic diagnosis in an atypical case.

Categories of Bronchial Disease

Variability in the duration and type of clinical signs and physical, radiographic, and cytologic findings, as well as differences in response to treatment and disease progression, illustrates the need to divide feline bronchial disease into more clinically useful categories. Examination of one variable, such as the type of bronchial exudate present, is often inadequate to characterize the disease process in a given cat. Therefore, all clinical features must be considered. Although still formative, the following classifications are suggested: bronchial asthma, acute bronchitis, chronic bronchitis, chronic asthmatic bronchitis, and chronic bronchitis with emphysema.

Cats with bronchial asthma are often young adults, although they may be of any age. Episodes of dyspnea occur sporadically and may be associated with mild to marked coughing. Between episodes, the cats are asymptomatic. Clinical response to bronchodilator therapy is often dramatic. During episodes of dyspnea (i.e., clinical airway obstruction), air trapping may result in radiographic evidence of lung overinflation. This may resolve during clinical remission or following treatment; however, a prominent bronchial pattern usually persists. Eosinophilia (airway or peripheral) is not uncommon. Prognosis is good to excellent if the acute exacerbations can be controlled. Intermittent therapy during respiratory distress may be sufficient.

Coughing of relatively short duration is the chief complaint in cats with acute bronchitis. Radiographs may reveal a mild to moderate bronchial pattern, and bronchial cytology is variable. Cats tend to recover completely and usually do not exhibit recurrent episodes.

Cats with chronic bronchitis are often middle-aged to old. Siamese cats are commonly affected. The chief complaints include coughing, with or without dyspnea. Radiographically, a marked bronchial pattern is seen, frequently with an interstitial and mild, patchy alveolar pattern. The middle lobe of the right lung may be collapsed. Neutrophilic or mixed inflammatory cells are often present. Bronchial bacterial cultures may be positive and plasma protein concentrations may be elevated, a finding consistent with chronic inflammation. Prognosis for complete recovery is poor, although the severity of clinical signs may be reduced by constant treatment. Some cats with chronic coughing also exhibit episodes of severe dyspnea (i.e., chronic asthmatic bronchitis), and others have permanent overinflation of the lungs, presumably due to the development of emphysema and chronic air trapping.

Newer Methods of Diagnostic Evaluation

At the University of Illinois, investigators are using tidal breathing flow-volume loop (TBFVL) analysis and lung resistance measurements to evaluate cats with bronchial disease. In awake, untrained cats, TBFVL testing can provide objective information on expiratory flow rate limitations occurring in cats with bronchial disease. Although determination of lung resistance is a more direct method of assessing airway obstruction, anesthesia is required to place an endotracheal tube and esophageal balloon. Preliminary findings indicate that some cats with bronchial disease have increased lung resistance measurements. As discussed earlier, some of these cats appear to have reversible airway

obstruction (i.e., bronchial asthma), while others have only partially reversible obstruction.

Techniques to objectively measure lung function changes in individual cats could provide better understanding and documentation of the types of bronchial disease occurring in the cat. Furthermore, the coupling of these techniques with drug administration (i.e., drug efficacy studies) will help to develop better treatment strategies for managing feline bronchial disease.

THERAPEUTIC CONSIDERATIONS

In general, treatment may be specific, supportive, or both. Ideally, treatment of lower airway disease is based on the identification of a specific disease process. Diagnostic efforts in the cat with bronchial disease are mostly directed toward identifying a known disease in the hope that a specific therapy can be instituted. When ascarid ova are found in the feces of a cat with chronic coughing and respiratory distress, appropriate anthelminthic therapy to eliminate the parasites may be combined with short-term corticosteroid therapy to suppress the pulmonary inflammatory response due to ascarid migration. Antibiotic selection is based on sensitivity results, and treatment should be continued for 2 to 3 weeks whenever significant bacterial growth is obtained from a tracheobronchial culture. If clinical signs fail to improve, the bronchi should be recultured to detect the development of resistant strains. Antibiotic therapy may be more efficacious when combined with bronchodilators to enhance clearance of retained bronchial secretions.

In most cats with bronchial disease, however, a specific underlying disease process cannot be identified. Depending on the severity of the clinical and diagnostic findings, supportive therapy often includes corticosteroids to suppress airway inflammation and bronchodilators to reverse bronchoconstriction; bronchodilation is often maintained. Recent advances in the treatment of human asthmatics have relied upon the use of aerosol therapy with beta$_2$-adrenergic agents, anticholinergic medications, and anti-inflammatory agents (e.g., beclomethasone and cromolyn). Aerosolized drug administration allows sufficient drug concentrations to reach the airways and achieve a local response, while avoiding most of the adverse side effects associated with other routes of administration that require achievement of systemic drug concentrations. Owing to the degree of patient cooperation necessary for proper use of these inhalers, it is unlikely that these new products will be very useful in veterinary medicine.

TREATMENT

The following is a general guideline for the management of feline bronchial disease. Because there is no single effective treatment regimen, each cat should be treated as a unique case.

In cats with infrequent or very mild clinical signs, a conservative approach may be all that is necessary. This includes avoidance of trigger events and appropriate weight reduction if obesity is present. Caloric restriction should be carefully instituted to avoid rapid weight loss, which may induce hepatic lipidosis. If clinical signs persist or worsen to the point that the cat is having two to three bouts of coughing per day, the next step is to institute a 2-week therapeutic bronchodilator trial. At the end of the trial, medication is discontinued for several days. If clinical improvement is noted during these 2 weeks or if signs worsen when medication is stopped, the bronchodilator is continued for up to several months. If there was only partial improvement during the trial, corticosteroids are added to the treatment regimen.

If the presenting signs are more severe (more than three to five periods of coughing per day) or include evidence of respiratory distress and wheezing, the initial therapy will include both corticosteroids and a bronchodilator. Depending on the cat's response, tapering of the corticosteroid dose over weeks to months is usually possible. The bronchodilator is continued indefinitely. Owners, not unlike human asthmatic patients, may become frustrated when the doctor cannot "make the disease go away." Appropriate management of the cat with bronchial disease requires patience and astute reevaluation by the attending veterinarian to avoid under- or overtreatment.

Theophylline, a widely used bronchodilator in human medicine, may also improve airway function by enhancing mucociliary transport and decreasing respiratory muscle fatigue (see this volume, p. 660). It is available as aminophylline in injectable and immediate-release tablet formulations or as sustained-release theophylline products. The goal in human medicine is to maintain constant plasma theophylline concentrations within a therapeutic range of 5 to 20 μg/ml. Assuming a similar therapeutic range in the cat, the recommended dosage regimen for immediate-release aminophylline in the cat is 5 mg/kg (equivalent to 4 mg/kg of theophylline) given every 8 to 12 hr. Many owners find it difficult to administer medication this frequently on a long-term basis.

The pharmacokinetics of two sustained-release theophylline products were recently determined in the cat (Dye et al., 1990). Sustained-release products allow longer dosage intervals while maintaining stable plasma concentrations. Administration of either Slo-bid Gyrocaps (Rorer Pharmaceuticals) or Theo-Dur Tablets (Key Pharmaceuticals) at 25 mg/kg once a day in the evening maintains therapeutic plasma concentrations. Slo-bid Gyrocaps are available in 50-, 100-, and 200-mg capsules, and Theo-Dur is available as 100- and 200-mg scored tablets. During the 2-week trial period, it is advisable to begin treatment with the lower dosage capsule or tablet. If there is minimal clinical improvement but no evidence of toxic effects (vomiting, diarrhea, muscle tremors, hyperactivity, or seizures) the dose may be increased to the next larger dose size. Therapeutic monitoring of plasma theophylline concentrations can ensure that the correct dose is being administered. With either product, the sample to determine the peak theophylline concentration should be taken 12 hours after the previous evening dose after steady-state concentrations are reached (i.e., after five dosages). The plasma should be separated and frozen until analysis. Peak concentrations should remain within the 5 to 20 μg/ml range. Other sustained-release formulations should *not* be substituted, as they may have very different pharmacokinetic characteristics. The most common side effect is vomiting, most likely due to gastrointestinal irritation. Muscle tremors or seizures appear to be uncommon and are associated with excessively high doses.

Alternatively, terbutaline, a beta$_2$-agonist, may be used as a bronchodilator. Terbutaline (Brethine, Geigy Pharmaceuticals) is available in injectable and oral (2.5- and 5-mg tablets) forms. A recent study determined that the currently recommended dose (1.25 to 2.5 mg every 8 to 12 hr PO) resulted in peak plasma concentrations approximately 30 times those shown to induce bronchodilation in humans (Dye et al., 1990). Furthermore, profound hypotension can result when an intravenous dose of 1 mg (also recommended in recent veterinary literature) is given. Until more complete studies are available in the cat, the authors suggest using terbutaline at smaller doses initially (approximately one eighth to one quarter of a 2.5-mg tablet twice a day) along with monitoring for potential adverse effects. If the cat fails to improve at this dose and assuming no adverse effects are evident, the dose may be gradually increased up to a maximum of 1.25 mg twice a day. The primary side effects—tachycardia and hypotension—may be difficult for the owner to appreciate. The drug should be discontinued if gastrointestinal upset, weakness, general inactivity, or depression develops.

Anti-inflammatory therapy primarily involves the administration of corticosteroids. Depending upon the severity of disease present, short-acting steroids (e.g., prednisolone, prednisone) are used initially and are given orally at dosages ranging from 0.5 to 2.0 mg/kg divided into two daily doses. As clinical signs abate, the dose is tapered over a 2- to 3-week period to approximately 0.5 to 1.0 mg/kg once a day. Attempts at further reduction should be gradual. Alternate- or every-third-day therapy of 0.5 mg/kg for several months may be necessary to prevent exacerbation of signs. When corticosteroids are combined with bronchodilators, the steroid dose necessary to control signs may often be reduced. These sustained-release theophylline products are ideally given once daily in the evening, and some authors recommend evening administration of corticosteroids in the cat as well. Thus, the owner can conveniently give both medications together at night.

The same therapeutic principles can be applied to cats presenting in acute respiratory distress or with an acute exacerbation of long-standing bronchial disease. Wasting no time, the respiratory pattern should be observed without directly handling the cat. Then, with as little restraint as possible, the cat is examined, percussed, and auscultated to rule out obvious thoracic trauma, pleural effusion, and cardiac abnormalities and to confirm that the lung sounds present are consistent with significant airway obstructive disease. All other diagnostic steps are delayed until the cat (preferably in a cage or box) is stabilized with supplemental oxygen and bronchodilators. In the cat, oral absorption for both immediate-release aminophylline and terbutaline is rapid, with peak plasma concentrations occurring within 0.5 to 1.5 hr. Therefore, in most cats, the bronchodilator can be given orally, and while it takes effect the patient should receive supplemental oxygen. This route entails less physical restraint (and stress to the cat) than an intravenous injection and avoids the potential cardiac disturbances associated with rapid intravenous injection of these products. If, however, the cat appears cyanotic and is in severe respiratory distress, terbutaline can be given subcutaneously at an approximate dose of 0.01 mg/kg. If no improvement is noted within 5 to 10 min, the dose should be repeated once. Alternatively, isoproterenol (Isuprel Hydrochloride, Winthrop Pharmaceuticals) may be given initially (0.1 to 0.2 ml SC of a 1:5000 solution). If there is no improvement with 5 min, a second dose should be given. If additional therapy is still needed, anticholinergics (atropine, 0.04 mg/kg SC or IM) may be used on a short-term basis to block vagal input and decrease bronchial secretions. In the extremely stressed, hypoxic cat, all of these drugs cause tachycardia and can potentially lead to the development of arrhythmias. Intravenous glucocorticoids (Solu-Cortef, Upjohn; Azium, Schering) are often recommended during acute distress. However, the acute response seen with these drugs is most likely due to the relatively weak bronchodilator effect of glucocorticoids; significant decreases in airway inflammation could not be achieved this quickly. It is usually possible to stabilize the cat with the other steps discussed. When diagnostic evaluation is more complete, corticosteroids can be given if still indicated.

Some cats respond well to treatment and remain asymptomatic when medication is discontinued. Other cats' clinical signs will be controlled only through continuous drug administration. Treatment efficacy can be difficult to assess because clinical signs tend to wax and wane over time regardless of treatment. All alterations in therapy should be based on follow-up examinations. Significant weight gain may occur during corticosteroid therapy and can compound underlying respiratory difficulties. Again, appropriate weight reduction should be instituted. Tactful questioning of compliance with medication administration should be conducted before changing the therapeutic regimen. Additional history taking may reveal new trigger situations. If a new kitten was introduced to the household, both cats may have gone through a bout of upper respiratory viral disease. In cats with signs of upper as well as lower airway disease, treatment efforts may require controlling nasal discharge and rhinitis/sinusitis as part of overall management.

In humans with chronic bronchitis or emphysema, mucociliary tract clearance mechanisms are often impaired owing to decreased efficiency of the cough reflex and alterations in the viscoelastic properties of airway mucus. It is likely that chronic bronchial disease also alters airway defense mechanisms in the cat. Therefore, cultures should be reevaluated in cats with clinical exacerbations to detect secondary bacterial colonization of airways.

If no complicating conditions can be identified, determination of peak theophylline concentrations may be performed to ensure that a therapeutic theophylline dose is being administered. If one type of bronchodilator is ineffective, an alternate type can be tried. If this fails, the corticosteroid dose should be increased. If no improvement is achieved, combinations of bronchodilators can be tried. Be aware that these drug interactions have not been studied in the cat. Some authors report improved control of clinical signs with repository steroid injections. This therapy may be reserved for particularly fractious cats or those with refractory disease.

Physiotherapy is important for the removal of retained secretions in humans with chronic bronchitis and emphysema, but this aspect of treatment has often been ignored in the feline patient. Although objective evidence is lacking, the completely sedentary feline could also perhaps benefit from regular periods of active play. This not only would induce deep respirations to open previously plugged airways and enhance clearance of retained secretions, but could also maintain general muscle tone and help to control obesity. Light coupage followed by postural drainage could also be performed after allowing the cat to breathe moisturized air.

Unfortunately, some cats will fail to improve despite aggressive treatment. They may die during severe bouts of respiratory distress or owing to chronic debility from the development of advanced lung pathology. Much remains to be learned about bronchial disease in the cat.

References and Suggested Reading

Diamond, L., Szarek, J. L., Gillespie, M. N., et al.: *In vivo* bronchodilator activity of vasoactive intestinal peptide in the cat. Am. Rev. Respir. Dis. 128:827, 1983.
Airway responses in cats with experimentally induced bronchoconstriction.

Dye, J. A., McKiernan, B. C., Neff-Davis, C. A., et al.: Chronopharmacokinetics of theophylline in the cat. J. Vet. Pharmacol. Ther. 13:278, 1990.
A summary of the dosing influences related to time of day on theophylline pharmacokinetics in the cat.

Dye, J. A., McKiernan, B. C., Rozanski, E. A., et al.: Pharmacokinetics of terbutaline in two cats. (Abstract). Eighth Annual ACVIM Proceedings, Blacksburg, VA, 1990, p 1120.

McKiernan, B. C., Dye, J. A., Rozanski, E. A., et al.: Lung resistance and dynamic lung compliance in normal cats. (Abstract). Proceedings of the Eighth Annual Veterinary Respiratory Society Symposium, 1989.

Moise, N. S., Wiedenkeller, D., Yeager, A. E., et al.: Clinical, radiographic, and bronchial cytologic features of cats with bronchial disease: 65 cases (1980–1986). J.A.V.M.A. 194(10):1467, 1989.
An extensive retrospective review of clinical findings in cases of feline bronchial disease.

Moses, B. L., and Spaulding, G. L.: Chronic bronchial disease of the cat. Vet. Clin. North Am. 15(5):929, 1985.
A review of the pulmonary anatomy and physiology of the cat, with discussion of immunologic and other aspects of feline chronic bronchial disease.

West, J. B.: *Pulmonary Pathophysiology: The Essentials.* Baltimore: Williams & Wilkins, 1987, p. 59.
A review of the relationships between structure and function in the diseased lung.

PRIMARY CILIARY DYSKINESIA

WALLACE B. MORRISON
West Lafayette, Indiana

Primary ciliary dyskinesia (PCD) is a congenital respiratory disorder that is characterized by absent or deficient mucociliary clearance in the respiratory tract (Wilsman et al., 1987). The central feature of this disorder is a failure of respiratory cilia to function normally. Ineffective clearance of mucus from the airways results in clinical signs that are secondary to rhinosinusitis, bronchitis, bronchiectasis, and bronchopneumonia. Although there is one report of this disorder occurring in an aged dog (Killingsworth et al., 1987), the typical presentation is a young, purebred (frequently inbred) dog with a history of bilateral purulent nasal discharge since very early in life. Chronic cough and bronchopneumonia are common findings. A leukocytosis (neutrophilia and monocytosis) is common, but findings of serum chemistries and urinalysis are usually normal.

Other organs with ciliated epithelia may be affected, and symptoms of otitis media and male sterility secondary to immotile spermatozoa (spermatozoa flagella are modified cilia) may occur (Edwards et al., 1983, 1989b). Other abnormalities associated with PCD in dogs include renal fibrosis; dilated distal renal tubules; abnormal sternebrae, vertebrae, and ribs; and hydrocephalus (Edwards et al., 1989b; Morrison et al., 1987).

In the respiratory tract, mucociliary clearance has a crucial role in host defense of the airways. The clearance of mucus is achieved by the sequential, coordinated movement of mucus and adherent particles toward the pharynx. Mucus is directed posteriorly from the nasal airways and upward from the lung and converges in the pharynx by the metachronous movement of respiratory cilia (Umeki, 1988).

In most cases, various defects in ciliary ultrastructure combine to reduce ciliary motility (Table 1). Ciliary ultrastructure has been reviewed by Morrison and colleagues (1987) and by Wilsman and associates (1987).

The term *immotile cilia syndrome* has been used to describe a condition in which functionally immotile respiratory cilia have been identified as the basis of the disorder. Respiratory cilia from affected patients may have random orientation, asynchronous motion, and normal beat frequency (Edwards et al., 1989a). Although the cilia may be capable of motility, the configuration of the waveform and the orientation of the cilia make mucus transport ineffectual.

Specific ultrastructural defects have been correlated to specific motility abnormalities in humans. Immotile or hypomotile cilia are associated with partial or complete absence of the outer dynein arms, whereas numerous other ultrastructural lesions such as microtubular and radial spoke abnormalities are associated with an asynchronous ciliary beat of normal frequency (Edwards et al., 1989a).

Table 1. Common Ciliary Defects in Dogs With Primary Ciliary Dyskinesia

Random orientation of cilia
Short or absent outer dynein arms
Electron dense material in basal bodies
B microtubule abnormalities
Central microtubular abnormalities
Radial spoke defects
Compound or giant cilia

In a few cases in both humans and dogs, ciliary ultrastructure is normal but ciliary function is abnormal. In humans with abnormal mucociliary clearance, ultrastructurally normal cilia were reported to have synchronous hyperfrequent trembling. One dog with decreased mucociliary clearance and ultrastructurally normal cilia was reported to have a normal beat frequency (Edwards et al., 1989a). The cause of the abnormal mucociliary clearance in this dog was not determined.

Frequently observed radiographic changes include evidence of bronchitis, bronchiectasis, and bronchopneumonia. Approximately 50% of affected humans and dogs have situs inversus (transposition of normal visceral orientation) of the thorax, abdomen, or both. Situs inversus of the thorax is not apparent on a lateral radiographic image alone. A dorsal-ventral or ventral-dorsal image allows the apex of the heart to be seen pointing to the right instead of to the left. An interesting aspect of situs inversus of the thorax is the electrocardiographic diagnosis of dextrocardia that is reflected by inversion of lead I and transposition of leads II and III. Situs inversus of the abdomen can be detected when either the gastric air bubble is seen on the right side instead of the left or when the left kidney is found anterior to the right kidney. The triad of the clinical features of situs inversus, rhinosinusitis, and bronchiectasis is known as *Kartagener's syndrome*. Although a striking feature and an important clinical clue for approximately half of dogs affected with PCD, situs inversus itself is not associated with clinical signs.

Clinicians are cautioned to evaluate all cases of bronchopneumonia and chronic purulent nasal discharge in young dogs to search for PCD. The similarity of the respiratory disease of PCD to canine distemper viral infection may result in misdiagnosis and euthanasia. The definitive diagnosis of this disorder is based on finding characteristic ultrastructural defects by electron microscopy or by documenting decreased mucociliary transport. However, the hallmark clinical features of this disease (bilateral purulent nasal discharge, bronchiectasis, bronchopneumonia), when they occur in well-vaccinated, young, purebred dogs, should alert a clinician to include PCD in the differential diagnosis. Finding the hallmark clinical features of this disease in combination with situs inversus is highly suggestive of PCD.

Thus far, PCD has been reported primarily in humans and dogs. The breeds of dogs in which PCD has been diagnosed include the border collie, English setter, Dalmatian, Doberman pinscher, Chihuahua, English springer spaniel, golden retriever, Old English sheepdog, English pointer, chow chow, and bichon frise.

The disorder has also been identified in pigs that were initially evaluated because of infertility (Roperto et al., 1991). It is likely that PCD will in time be identified in additional species.

THERAPY

Even though PCD is not a curable respiratory disorder, it can frequently be managed for many years. A key element in the successful management is the monitoring of infecting microorganisms and the use of antibiotics to which the microorganisms are sensitive. Over time there is considerable variation in the types of microorganisms that can be isolated from patients with PCD. *Streptococcus, Staphylococcus,* and various gram-negative rod microorganisms are common. *Pseudomonas* species frequently become established and may be difficult to control. *Mycoplasma* species are also often isolated from the respiratory tract of affected dogs. Regular culture and sensitivity testing of transtracheal washings is important to identify the changing populations of respiratory flora. Culture and sensitivity testing of nasal exudate does not adequately identify infecting microorganisms from the lung, because the flora of the upper and lower respiratory tract may be different.

Even in patients with little mucociliary transport, coughing is an effective method of mucus removal. Daily coupage and vigorous exercise help to clear mucus from the airways. Because coughing is the primary defense mechanism of the respiratory tract in dogs with PCD, the use of cough suppressants to control clinical signs is contraindicated. The long-term prognosis for many patients with PCD can be favorable with diligent medical care.

References and Suggested Reading

Edwards, D. F., Kennedy, J. R., Toal, R. I., et al.: Kartagener's syndrome in a chow chow dog with normal ciliary ultrastructure. Vet. Pathol. 26:338, 1989a.
A case report of a male chow chow dog with infertility and normal respiratory ciliary ultrastructure but decreased mucociliary clearance.
Edwards, D. F., Kennedy, J. R., Patton, C. S., et al.: Familial immotile-cilia syndrome in English springer spaniel dogs. Am. J. Med. Genet. 33:290, 1989b.
This excellent review article includes analysis of mucociliary clearance, ciliary ultrastructure, semen quality, and hydrocephalus in a colony of dogs with this disorder.
Edwards, D. F., Patton, C. S., Bemis, D. A., et al.: Immotile cilia syndrome in three dogs from a litter. J.A.V.M.A. 183:667, 1983.
A case report and general review of this subject.
Killingsworth, C. R., Slocumbe, R. F., and Wilsman, N. J.: Immotile cilia syndrome in an aged dog. J.A.V.M.A. 190:1567, 1987.
The only canine report of this disorder in an aged individual.
Morrison, W. B., Wilsman, N. J., Fox, L. E., et al.: Primary ciliary dyskinesia in the dog. J. Vet. Intern. Med. 1:67, 1987.
A case report and review of the veterinary literature of this disorder.
Roperto, F., Galati, P., Troncone, A., et al.: Primary ciliary dyskinesia in pigs. J. Submicroscop. Cytol. Pathol. 23:233, 1991.
A report of infertility and primary ciliary dyskinesia in pigs.
Umeki, S.: Primary mucociliary transport failure. Respiration 54:220, 1988.
A general review of disorders that result in failure of mucociliary transport.

Wilsman, N. J., Morrison, W. B., Farnum, C. E., et al.: Microtubular protofilaments and subunits of the outer dynein arm in cilia from dogs with primary ciliary dyskinesia. Am. Rev. Respir. Dis. 135:137, 1987.

A detailed review of the ultrastructure of cilia from dogs with this disorder.

EOSINOPHILIC PULMONARY GRANULOMATOSIS

CLAY A. CALVERT

Athens, Georgia

Eosinophilic granulomatosis manifesting primarily as a pulmonary disease was first reported by Confer et al. in 1983. Subsequent reports described lesions in additional organs as well (Calvert et al., 1988; Neer et al., 1985). Eosinophilic pulmonary granulomatosis is a nodular lung disease that must be differentiated from pulmonary neoplasia, systemic mycoses, and lymphomatoid granulomatosis. Although some features of eosinophilic pulmonary granulomatosis in dogs are shared by eosinophilic pulmonary syndromes in humans, all of these syndromes, including pulmonary eosinophilic granuloma, differ in one or more significant aspects. Notably, eosinophilic pulmonary granulomatosis in dogs is not characterized by vasculitis.

There is a high incidence of occult heartworm infection in dogs with eosinophilic pulmonary granulomatosis, which suggests a causal relationship in many cases. True occult heartworm infection is due to antibody-dependent leukocyte adhesion to microfilariae in the pulmonary circulation and results in entrapment of microfilariae in the capillaries. Microfilaria-granulocyte complexes are engulfed by phagocytic cells of the pulmonary reticuloendothelial system, and granulomatous inflammation occurs around the entrapped microfilariae. In some cases of occult infection, the granulocyte reaction is dominated by eosinophils and allergic pneumonitis results (Calvert and Losonsky, 1985). In some instances the granulomatous inflammation may progress uncontrollably, leading to eosinophilic pulmonary granulomatosis that behaves in a fashion similar to that of malignant pulmonary histiocytosis. Microfilariae have not been detected at the center of these granulomas, and adult *Dirofilaria immitis* fragments are only occasionally seen. As eosinophilic and eosinophil granulomatous inflammation are often found in various tissues and organs, a soluble antigen or immune complex would seem to be the inciting agent.

CLINICAL FINDINGS

History

Eosinophilic pulmonary granulomatosis is usually manifested as progressive coughing and dyspnea of variable duration. Affected dogs are typically medium to large in size, spend considerable time outside, and are not receiving heartworm prophylaxis. If the patient has been examined previously for respiratory complaints diuretics or antibiotics may have been prescribed. Respiratory signs, often present for 1 to 5 weeks prior to diagnosis, are sometimes present for 2 to 3 months and occasionally for as long as 6 to 12 months. As the disease progresses, decreased appetite, weight loss, exercise intolerance, and lethargy often develop. Occasionally, fever and hemoptysis occur.

Physical Examination

Coughing, dyspnea, and auscultatable pulmonary crackles are the most common physical abnormalities. Fever, harsh lung sounds, muffled heart and lung sounds, and limited peripheral lymphadenopathy are occasionally detected. Weight loss may be obvious.

DIAGNOSIS

Thoracic Radiography

Radiographic abnormalities are characterized by multiple pulmonary masses of various sizes (Fig. 1). Some nodules are only 1 cm in diameter, others may be as large as 20 cm, and nodules of intermediate size are often also present. Mixed interstitial-alveolar or interstitial, alveolar, and bronchial lung

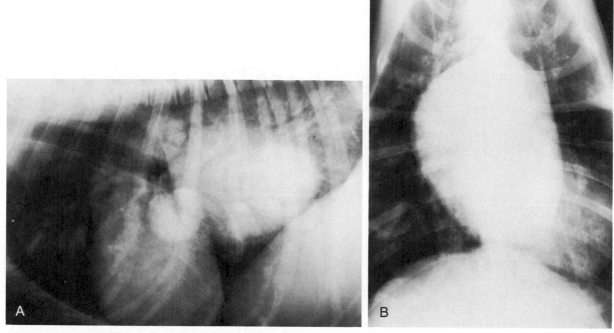

Figure 1. *A*, Lateral thoracic radiograph of a dog with multiple large pulmonary granulomas in the caudal and cranial lung lobes. Diffuse interstitial disease is also present in the caudal lobes. *B*, Ventrodorsal thoracic radiograph of a dog with a large eosinophilic granuloma in the left caudal lobe. Smaller nodules are present in the right middle and caudal lobes.

disease may be present in addition to the pulmonary nodules. Hilar lymphadenopathy is common, pleural fissure lines are often present, and pleural mediastinal masses or intratracheal masses are seen occasionally. Lobar pulmonary arterial enlargement may be detected, as many affected dogs are heartworm infected.

DIFFERENTIAL DIAGNOSIS. Pulmonary nodules with hilar lymphadenopathy are suggestive of the pulmonary manifestations of systemic mycoses. Primary and metastatic pulmonary neoplasia, along with lymphomatoid granulomatosis, must also be considered. Large lesions in the caudal lung lobe may bear a striking radiographic resemblance to bronchogenic carcinoma.

Clinical Pathology

Eosinophilia and neutrophilia are the most common hematologic abnormalities. Both were present in 13 of 19 dogs (68%) seen by the author. Absolute eosinophil counts are often between 1000 and 6000/μl and may be over 20,000/μl. Basophilia occurs in approximately 50% of affected dogs. Hyperglobulinemia occurs occasionally.

An eosinophilic exudate is occasionally obtained by transtracheal lavage. Pleural effusion, when present, usually contains a high percentage of eosinophils. Although peripheral lymphadenopathy is uncommon, cytology obtained by fine-needle aspiration of enlarged lymph nodes is characterized by eosinophils.

Seroimmunodiagnostic tests for heartworm infection are indicated, as 15 of 19 dogs (79%) with eosinophilic pulmonary granulomatosis seen by the author have had evidence of heartworm infection. Microfilariae concentration tests are usually negative but adult *D. immitis* antigen tests are usually positive.

LUNG BIOPSY. Although the clinical, radiographic, and clinical pathologic findings in affected dogs are usually suggestive of eosinophilic pulmonary granulomatosis, a fine-needle aspiration biopsy of a large, accessible lung nodule is recommended.* Cytologic characteristics are typified by eosinophils and basophils with fewer numbers of plasma cells, histocytes, neutrophils, and lymphocytes.

Histopathology

Although eosinophilic granulomas primarily affect the lungs, infiltration of the intrathoracic lymph nodes, trachea, peripheral lymph nodes, liver, spleen, abdominal lymph nodes, small intestine,

---

Editors' Note: Extreme caution is advised when performing fine-needle aspiration in patients with pulmonary arterial hypertension.

and kidney with either eosinophils or eosinophilic granulomas has occurred in 6 of 12 dogs (50%) necropsied.

Lung Histology. Diffuse changes are consistently present. Interalveolar septa are often thickened owing to fibrous connective tissue, lymphocytes, and plasma cells. Alveoli often contain eosinophilic granular material and some macrophages. The granulomas consist of dense accumulations of large epitheloid cells, macrophages, and eosinophils that tend to obliterate the normal architecture. A few plasma cells, lymphocytes, and mast cells are also present. Areas of necrosis are occasionally observed. Some pulmonary arteries and arterioles have a mild eosinophilic infiltrate. At the periphery of granulomas, alveoli can be identified and are characterized by proliferation of type II pneumocytes and infiltrations of eosinophils and macrophages. A mixed eosinophilic-neutrophilic inflammation occurs in zones surrounding the granulomas. Bronchial smooth muscle hypertrophy is prominent in granulomatous areas. Perivascular lymphocytic-eosinophilic infiltration is inconsistently present around small arterioles.

THERAPY

Surgery

Although an open lung biopsy may be required for definitive diagnosis, experience with surgical excision of pulmonary granulomas as a definitive treatment has been unfavorable. There are usually multiple small granulomas present in multiple lung lobes that are not visualized on thoracic radiographs. When a lobectomy is performed for apparently localized disease, occult lesions in additional lobes may subsequently develop. Some patients are poor anesthetic risks. Extensive exudate that may embarrass pulmonary function is sometimes found in bronchioles and bronchi, and perioperative death has occurred. Nonetheless, considering the limited success associated with medical therapy, lobectomy may be a reasonable option when the disease appears to be limited to one lung lobe. Follow-up chemotherapy should be administered if the disease is discovered at surgery to involve more than one lung lobe. Whether extrathoracic disease, which may exist undetected in some instances, will persist or progress following lobectomy is unknown.

Thiacetarsamide sodium treatment is administered after surgical convalescence in dogs with evidence of heartworm infection.

Chemotherapy

Eosinophilic pulmonary granulomatosis responds to immunosuppressive and cytotoxic drug therapy.

Unfortunately, most patients treated have experienced only partial remissions or have relapsed within weeks of the initiation of therapy. It may be that previous treatment regimens for this syndrome have not been sufficiently aggressive. Although prednisone (1 to 2 mg/kg PO once daily) has produced partial and occasionally complete remission, relapse invariably occurs when the dosage is reduced, when the interdosage interval is prolonged, and even when the dosage and interval are not altered.

Complete remission is more likely with combination therapy such as prednisone at a dosage of 4 mg/kg PO or IM once daily (or an equivalent regimen of an alternate corticosteroid) plus cyclophosphamide (Cytoxan, Bristol-Myers) at a dosage of 250 to 300 mg/m^2 IV once weekly. The induction regimen should be continued until the maximum response is obtained. Thiacetarsamide sodium treatment is administered after induction chemotherapy in those dogs with evidence of heartworm infection.

Maintenance therapy is required and is initiated immediately following the induction regimen. Drugs such as prednisone (2 mg/kg PO on alternate days) plus either cyclophosphamide (200 to 300 mg/m^2 IV on alternate weeks) or azathioprine (Imuran, Burroughs Wellcome, 50 mg/m^2 PO once daily for 7 days on alternate weeks) are recommended.

Chemotherapy sometimes produces only partial remission, and relapse following complete remission occurs in most patients within 1 to 3 months. When relapse or disease progression occurs, additional chemotherapy has been ineffective. Three- and four-drug combination therapies may prove to be more effective but clinical trials have not been performed.

Toxicity. When cytotoxic drugs are employed, anorexia, vomiting, diarrhea, and lethargy may occur. Myelosuppression will occur, and weekly complete blood counts (CBCs) must be performed before treatment. In general, if the neutrophil count is less than 2500/μl or the platelet count is less than 50,000/μl, chemotherapy is delayed for 3 to 4 days and the CBC is then repeated.

Hemorrhagic cystitis is a common complication of cyclophosphamide therapy. Weekly and even biweekly treatment at the aforementioned dosages, particularly in dogs weighing less than 12 to 15 kg, carries a significant risk of this side effect. To reduce the risk of cyclophosphamide cystitis, the drug should be administered in the morning and diuresis encouraged by fluid administration or by adding salt to the diet on the day prior to, the day of, and the day following treatment. If cyclophosphamide-related cystitis develops, either azathioprine or chlorambucil (Leukeran, Burroughs Wellcome, 12 to 15 mg/m^2 PO once weekly or on alternate weeks during maintenance treatment) is administered.

Heartworm Treatment

In dogs with confirmed or suspected *D. immitis* infection, thiacetarsamide sodium (Caparsolate, Abbott Laboratories) should be administered at the standard adulticide protocol (0.22 ml/kg IV twice daily for 2 days) as soon as the patient's condition is suitable for therapy. If lobectomy is the initial treatment, adulticide treatment can be safely administered after 1 to 2 weeks. When chemotherapy is employed as the initial therapy, adulticide treatment is initiated when a partial (greater than 50% reduction of granulomatous mass) or complete remission is achieved and clinical signs are largely or totally eliminated. Such responses usually take 1 to 6 weeks depending on the severity of disease at presentation. Ivermectin (Ivomec) is recommended by the author at the microfilaricide dosage (50 μg/kg orally) 3 weeks after the adulticide regimen, whether or not microfilaremia is detected.

PROGNOSIS

Most patients have received corticosteroids as the initial treatment, and a complete remission rate of less than 25% has been achieved. Regardless of the degree of response, relapse has invariably occurred, usually within a few weeks. Combination therapy has resulted in complete remission in over 50% of patients, but relapse has occurred within 3 months in all but two dogs treated by the author.

One dog has been in remission for 6 months at the time of this writing. The other dog experienced a complete remission that was maintained for 5 months, at which time diffuse histiocytic lymphoma was discovered. An association between chronic eosinophilic pneumonia and histiocytic lymphoma has been reported in humans (Bremmer and Thorgeirsson, 1977).

References and Suggested Reading

Bremmer, B. E., and Thorgeirsson, G.: An association between chronic eosinophilic pneumonia and histiocytic lymphoma. Am. J. Med. Sci. 278:83, 1977.

Calvert, C. A., and Losonsky, J. M.: Occult heartworm disease associated allergic pneumonitis. J.A.V.M.A. 1986:1097, 1985.

Calvert, C. A., Mahaffey, M. B., Lappin, M. R., et al.: Pulmonary and disseminated eosinophilic granulomatosis in dogs. J. Am. Anim. Hosp. Assoc. 24:311, 1988.

Confer, A. W., Qualls, C. W., MacWilliams, P. S., et al.: Four cases of pulmonary nodular eosinophilic granulomatosis in dogs. Cornell Vet. 73:41, 1983.

Neer, T. M., Waldron, D. R., and Miller, R. I.: Eosinophilic pulmonary granulomatosis in two dogs and literature review. J. Am. Anim. Hosp. Assoc. 22:593, 1986.

Section
10

URINARY DISORDERS

JEANNE A. BARSANTI

Consulting Editor

SOLUTE FRACTIONAL EXCRETION RATES

DELMAR R. FINCO,
JEANNE A. BARSANTI,
and SCOTT A. BROWN
Athens, Georgia

DEFINITIONS AND SIGNIFICANCE

Homeostasis is defined as the maintenance of a steady state in the body. The kidneys are important organs in the process of homeostasis, being responsible for maintaining normal concentrations of several plasma solutes including sodium, potassium, chloride, inorganic phosphate, bicarbonate, and protons (H^+). The kidneys also are important in excretion of urea and creatinine, but they do not modify their function to regulate plasma concentration of these materials.

Materials passing from blood through the filter of the renal glomeruli are potentially lost from the body. The rate of glomerular filtration (GFR) in mammals is far higher than needed for excretion of the major plasma electrolytes, even when large excesses are consumed. Renal regulation of plasma electrolyte concentrations is relegated to the renal tubules. The tubules selectively reabsorb components of filtrate or they secrete solutes delivered to them by the peritubular circulation, in order to maintain a normal, stable plasma composition.

Fractional excretion (FE) is defined as the fraction of filtered solute that is not reclaimed as it passes through the renal tubular system. Numerically, it is the urinary excretion of a solute, per unit time, divided by the amount of that solute filtered during the same amount of time.

Dietary intake of a nonmetabolized solute is normally matched by its excretion, in order for body balance to be maintained. It follows that even in normal animals, FE values are not fixed but vary as needed to maintain homeostasis. For example, if an animal were switched from a diet containing 0.4% phosphorus (P) to a diet containing 1.2% P, then FE would markedly increase, all other things being equal, in order for body P balance to be maintained.

METHODS OF MEASUREMENT OF FRACTIONAL EXCRETION RATES

The classic method of determining FE is to measure GFR and plasma concentration of the solute in question. Multiplying GFR times plasma concentration gives the amount filtered, assuming unimpeded passage through the glomerular filtration barrier. Urine collected during the interval of GFR measurement is analyzed for the solute, and excretion is calculated as the product of urine volume times urine solute concentration. Dividing the amount excreted by amount filtered gives FE. These procedures are expressed mathematically in the two following formulas:

$$(1) \qquad FE = \frac{U_c \times U_v \ (ml/min)}{GFR \times P_c}$$

$$(2) \qquad GFR = \frac{U_{inulin\ conc} \times U_v}{P_{inulin\ conc}}$$

In conducting the measurement by classic procedures, GFR usually is measured by determining inulin clearance, as indicated in Equation 2, or by exogenous creatinine clearance.

The laborious nature of determining FE by classic procedures makes it impractical for clinical use. Consequently, alternatives have been sought. One alternative is to use the clearance of endogenous creatinine as a marker for GFR, obviating the need for constant infusions of inulin or creatinine. A further simplification is to dispense with timed urine collections (U_{volume}) and use "spot" samples of both plasma and urine. The spot sample method has mathematical validity according to the following formulas:

$$(3) \qquad FE = \frac{U_{c(solute)} \times U_{volume}}{GFR \times P_{c(solute)}}$$

$$(4) \qquad FE = \left(\frac{\dfrac{U_{c(solute)} \times U_{volume}}{\dfrac{U_{c(creatinine)} \times U_{volume}}{P_{c(creatinine)}}} \right) \times P_{c(solute)}$$

$$(5) \qquad FE = \frac{U_{c(solute)} \times P_{c(creatinine)}}{U_{c(creatinine)} \times P_{c(solute)}}$$

As indicated in Equation 5, the need for measuring GFR as well as for collecting timed urine specimens is eliminated by the spot procedure.

LIMITATIONS AND ERRORS OF METHODS OF MEASUREMENTS

Several factors must be considered in evaluating the accuracy of FE measurements:

1. Accuracy of measurement of amount of solute filtered.
2. Effect of diet and food intake on plasma concentration or urinary excretion of solutes.
3. Effect of diurnal rhythms on plasma concentration or urinary excretion of solutes.

Reliability of Measurements of Filtered Solute

Both inulin and exogenous creatinine clearance are reliable methods of measuring GFR in dogs and cats (Finco et al., 1982, 1991), and their use to measure the amount of solute that is filtered is reliable.

Endogenous creatinine clearance and spot measurements of plasma and urine creatinine usually are not accurate methods of quantifying the amount of solute filtered. With either the kinetic or the regular Jaffe method for measurement of plasma creatinine concentration, values are spuriously elevated by as much as 100% because of the presence of noncreatinine chromogens in plasma. These noncreatinine chromogens do not pass into the urine, so urine creatinine measurements are not affected. Thus, whether endogenous creatinine clearance or Equation 5 is used to measure FE, an error exists because of the inaccurate measurement of plasma creatinine concentration.

Effects of Diet and Food Intake

Determining FE by any procedure requires a knowledge of plasma concentration of solute, over the interval of collection or production of urine.

The form of inorganic solutes in food and their pharmacokinetics once absorbed from the gut affect plasma concentration and FE of the solute. For example, inorganic P is more readily absorbed from the intestines of cats than organic forms, resulting in a marked increase in plasma concentration during the postprandial period (Finco et al., 1989). With forms of P that are readily absorbed, urinary excretion of P is markedly increased for about 8 hr postprandially but diminishes thereafter. Under these circumstances, FE values for P may not reliably reflect renal homeostatic activities under several conditions of FE measurement.

1. During spot FE determinations, plasma P concentration represents the value at that instant in time, whereas urine collected at the same time usually represents a pooling of excretion over several hours. Depending on the interplay between time of eating and sampling, measured plasma P concentration may underestimate or overestimate the mean plasma P concentration existing during excretion of the urine pool.

2. Even when classic FE measurements are made with short-term collections of urine, FE values for P may differ in the fasted state compared with the postprandial state.

Effects of diet may not be so important for other solutes as for P, but studies are needed to determine how diet affects plasma concentrations and urinary excretion rates in dogs and cats.

Effects of Circadian Rhythm in Solute Excretion

Rhythmic fluctuations in plasma concentration and renal excretion of some solutes have been noted in humans and several other species of animals. Although these fluctuations are usually subtle, they could have minor effects on FE measurements. Studies are needed to determine the magnitude of fluctuations in dogs and cats, to determine if they could lead to errors in interpretation of FE values.

USE OF FRACTIONAL EXCRETION DETERMINATIONS IN SMALL ANIMAL PRACTICE

Applications

The motive in use of FE measurements is to detect an abnormality in renal homeostatic responses for solute excretion. The abnormality could be an unusual message to the tubules (hormone imbalance) or an abnormality in the tubules themselves. Some examples of application are as follows:

1. Fanconi's syndrome is suspected in a Basenji—generalized proximal tubule dysfunction, and renal wasting, particularly of P, potassium, and bicarbonate is expected. The FE values for these solutes should be increased.
2. A cat has a urolith composed of calcium oxalate—there could be an increased rate of calcium excretion in the urine as a result of either a renal leak or intestinal hyperabsorption. With either category of abnormality, an increase in FE for calcium would be expected.
3. A dog has mild, chronic renal failure, and it is desirable to restrict P in order to avoid or minimize renal secondary hyperparathyroidism. The FE would be expected to decrease if there were compliance with P restriction.

Implementation

The spot method of sampling is probably the only method practical in veterinary practice. As previously indicated, several compromises and variables are inherent in its use. Although values for FE are easily generated by analyzing plasma and urine, the interpretation of the results requires standardization of conditions of collection and of sample analysis for both normal animals and those with suspected abnormalities. When these data are available, clinical use can be reliably implemented.

References and Suggested Reading

Finco, D. R., and Barsanti, J. A.: Mechanism of urinary excretion of creatinine by the cat. Am. J. Vet. Res. 43:2207, 1982.
Finco, D. R., Barsanti, J. A., and Brown, S. A.: Influence of dietary source of phosphorus on fecal and urinary excretion of phosphorus and other minerals by male cats. Am. J. Vet. Res. 50:263, 1989.
Finco, D. R., Brown, S. A., Crowell, W. A., et al.: Exogenous creatinine clearance as a measure of glomerular filtration rate in dogs with reduced renal mass. Am. J. Vet. Res. 52:1029, 1991.

RENAL DISEASE IN CATS: THE POTASSIUM CONNECTION

STEVEN W. DOW
and MARTIN J. FETTMAN
Fort Collins, Colorado

Renal disease is the second leading cause of death in cats, surpassed only by feline leukemia virus infection. Despite the frequency of chronic renal disease, its pathogenesis in cats is poorly understood, and there are few effective treatments for improving or stabilizing renal function in affected animals. A series of studies have focused attention on the role of potassium in the pathogenesis of chronic renal disease in cats. These studies have also provided preliminary evidence that dietary potassium supplementation may interrupt the typical downward spiral in renal function characteristic of cats with chronic renal disease.

STUDIES LINKING RENAL DISEASE AND POTASSIUM DEPLETION

A link between hypokalemia and renal disease in cats first emerged from studies of cats with severe neuromuscular weakness associated with persistent hypokalemia (Dow et al., 1987a). The most consistent abnormality besides myopathy in these cats was chronic renal disease, as documented by persistent, moderate elevations in serum urea nitrogen and creatinine concentrations (Dow et al., 1987b). Most of the cats also had persistent metabolic acidosis. The concurrence of hypokalemia and metabolic acidosis in these animals suggested whole-body potassium depletion rather than transient potassium redistribution. When urinary potassium excretion (as assessed by fractional excretion of potassium) was measured in an attempt to explain the potassium depletion, abnormally and inappropriately high excretion indices were found. Thus, it

appeared that excessive renal potassium losses were largely responsible for inducing severe potassium depletion in these cats, because other sources of potassium loss (especially gastrointestinal disease) had been ruled out. These studies also implicated dietary potassium deficiency as a contributing factor in at least some of these cats (Dow et al., 1987b). Additional studies have provided further evidence associating hypokalemia and chronic renal disease in cats (DiBartola et al., 1987; Dow et al., 1989).

RENAL REGULATION OF POTASSIUM BALANCE

Renal excretion is the major route by which potassium from dietary sources and cellular breakdown is eliminated from the body. Although a large amount of potassium is present in the glomerular filtrate, most of this is absorbed in the proximal nephron, irrespective of body potassium balance. Regulation of renal potassium excretion is accomplished primarily via potassium secretion by the principal cells of the cortical collecting tubule in the distal nephron. Secretion increases after high potassium intake and decreases during potassium restriction.

Potassium secretion into the tubular cell lumen is largely a passive event, dependent primarily on changes in tubular membrane permeability as well as concentration and electrical gradients across the luminal membrane. Aldosterone and plasma potassium concentrations are the two primary physiologic regulators of renal potassium secretion. Aldosterone increases potassium secretion by increasing tubular elecronegativity (via increased sodium reabsorption), activating a sodium-potassium adenosine triphosphatase pump that increases intracellular potassium concentration as sodium is pumped out, and by opening potassium channels on the luminal side of the tubular membrane. Increased plasma potassium concentration augments the effects of aldosterone and alone can reproduce most of the same effects on potassium secretion. Distal nephron potassium secretion can be greatly reduced during potassium depletion, mediated by both decreased aldosterone and plasma potassium concentrations. Tubular flow rate also affects potassium secretion by altering the sodium concentration in the distal nephron; if tubular flow rate is increased while aldosterone concentration remains normal or elevated, excessive potassium loss will ensue. The luminal negative potential difference, maintained largely by sodium reabsorption, also affects potassium secretion; the higher the luminal negative potential, the more potassium secreted.

DISORDERS ASSOCIATED WITH INCREASED URINARY POTASSIUM EXCRETION

Increased urinary potassium losses may be the result of primary renal functional impairment or may be secondary to other disease processes that affect renal potassium handling. One cause is increased plasma aldosterone concentrations, which may occur in primary hyperaldosteronism, adrenal cortical tumors, magnesium depletion, and persistent vomiting due to high intestinal obstruction. Bartter's syndrome, a primary renal defect in chloride absorption that may be mediated by abnormal elevations in renal prostaglandin synthesis, occurs in humans, dogs, and cats and leads to hypokalemia as a result of excessive urinary potassium losses. In the preceding disorders of increased renal potassium excretion, metabolic alkalosis is typically observed. The renal tubular acidoses (proximal and distal) are the two most important hyperkaliuric states associated with metabolic acidosis.

In our series of hypokalemic cats, we attempted to determine the cause of excessive urinary potassium losses. Plasma aldosterone and renin concentrations in affected cats were normal, compared with age-matched controls. To determine whether renal tubular acidosis might account for hyperkaliuria in these cats, proximal and distal nephron function were evaluated. A bicarbonate challenge test was administered to assess proximal nephron function because proximal tubular acidosis is characterized by a defect in proximal tubular absorption of bicarbonate. Urine bicarbonate concentrations were not significantly different from those in control cats, indicating normal proximal nephron function.

At the same time, urine proton excretion (as assessed by urine pH) was similar in control and hypokalemic cats. Thus, renal tubular acidosis was excluded as a cause of excessive urinary potassium losses in this group of cats.

POTASSIUM DEPLETION AND RENAL FAILURE: A VICIOUS CYCLE

At present, the exact mechanism underlying the apparent association between renal disease and increased urinary potassium losses in cats remains unexplained. Renal lesions in several cats examined at necropsy were variable and nonspecific, consisting of chronic interstitial nephritis, along with papillary necrosis and glomerulonephritis in individual cases. Vacuolar degeneration of distal tubular epithelial cells, as has been described in potassium-depleted rats and humans, was not observed. Increasing urinary potassium losses may represent a basic renal physiologic response to decreased renal function in cats. However, other factors must be considered, including the role of diet. Feline diets that induce chronic metabolic acidosis (to prevent urolithiasis) have been shown in experimental studies to induce net negative potassium balance in cats, at least in part by reducing gastrointestinal potassium resorption (Ching et al., 1989).

Chronic potassium depletion in turn has a deleterious effect on renal function in cats (Dow et al., 1990). Experimentally, cats fed a potassium-deficient diet plus a dietary acidifier (0.8% ammonium chloride) for a period of 8 weeks experienced significant declines in glomerular filtration rate. This decline was reversed by potassium supplementation. Furthermore, potassium depletion induced metabolic acidosis in cats; metabolic acidosis in turn increases potassium losses. Thus, it seems likely that some forms of chronic renal disease in cats, by accelerating urinary potassium losses and inducing potassium depletion and metabolic acidosis, may eventually lead to a self-perpetuating cycle of worsening renal function and continued potassium losses.

RESPONSE TO TREATMENT

Further evidence of the key role that potassium depletion has in feline chronic renal disease comes from clinical studies of the response to potassium supplementation (Dow et al., 1987b). Of the cats treated in the original group, all experienced either improved renal function (persistent declines in serum urea nitrogen and creatinine concentration) or at least stabilization of renal function during a period of months. Prolonged dietary potassium supplementation was the only treatment given these cats. In addition to improved renal function, these cats also had improvements in other clinical abnormalities associated with chronic renal failure, including anemia, poor haircoat, and weight loss. Despite the improved clinical status, however, excessive urinary potassium losses persisted in the older adult cats. In several young cats that had potassium depletion and renal insufficiency and that received potassium supplementation, renal function returned to normal, as did urinary potassium excretion. Therefore, in older cats with chronic renal disease, hyperkaliuria is likely to persist for the life of the animal or as long as renal function remains impaired.

TREATMENT RECOMMENDATIONS

A careful assessment of potassium balance should constitute part of the initial assessment of cats with renal disease. In cats with low or borderline serum potassium concentration (and metabolic acidosis), urinary potassium excretion should be evaluated. The urinary fractional excretion of potassium should be less than 5% in cats that are concurrently hypokalemic (Dow et al., 1987b). For more accurate assessment of urinary potassium losses, determination of 24-hr urinary potassium losses is recommended. In addition, it may be prudent to determine urinary potassium losses in cats with chronic renal disease and normal serum potassium, because total body potassium depletion may be present despite normal serum levels.

Potassium gluconate, as either an elixir (Kaon elixir, Adria) or a powder (Tumil-K, Daniels), is currently the recommended potassium supplement for hypokalemic cats. Potassium chloride supplements should not be used, because they are very unpalatable in cats and also contribute to metabolic acidosis. An initial starting dosage of potassium gluconate is given empirically, generally 2 to 6 mEq per cat per day. The dosage is based on the estimated severity of depletion and the cat's size. The final maintenance dosage is determined on the basis of serial measurements of serum potassium concentration at weekly intervals. Development of hyperkalemia has not been a problem in cats treated thus far but may be a concern in cats with advanced renal disease and reduced urine output. Lifelong treatment will probably be necessary for older cats with chronic renal disease.

The routine supplementation of all cats with chronic renal disease, regardless of their potassium balance status, has not been evaluated clinically in controlled studies. There may be merit to this approach in normokalemic cats, however, using a low maintenance dose (2 mEq/day) as a preventive measure to stabilize renal function before potassium depletion exacerbates the disease. We have observed positive responses in several normokalemic cats that had chronic renal disease and were treated with potassium supplementation.

Treatments that may exacerbate metabolic acidosis should be avoided. Therefore, cats with renal disease should not be fed diets that contain a dietary acidifier. In addition, drugs that induce renal potassium wasting, such as furosemide, should be administered cautiously and potassium balance monitored closely. This is especially true during fluid diuresis for management of renal failure. If possible, potassium balance should be restored by oral administration of potassium *before* beginning fluid loading, and parenteral potassium supplementation continued during fluid therapy. A number of cats have died of complete muscle paralysis resulting from fluid diuresis and lowering of already critically depleted body potassium stores. Close attention to serum potassium concentration during the period of fluid administration is essential; potassium concentration should be measured daily and supplementation adjusted accordingly.

Potassium depletion and metabolic acidosis have also been shown to induce potentially fatal reductions in plasma taurine concentration in cats. Therefore, determination of plasma taurine concentration may be useful in the management of patients with chronic renal failure, especially those with abnormalities of cardiac or platelet function, both of which are manifestations of taurine depletion in cats.

References and Suggested Reading

Ching, S. V., Fettman, M. J., Hamar, D. W., et al.: The effect of chronic dietary acidification using ammonium chloride on acid-base and mineral metabolism in the adult cat. J. Nutr. 119:902, 1989.
DiBartola, S. P., Rutgers, H. C., Zack, P. M., et al.: Clinicopathologic findings associated with chronic renal disease in cats: 74 cases (1973–1984). J.A.V.M.A. 190:1196, 1987.
Dow, S. W., Fettman, M. J., Curtis, C. R., et al.: Hypokalemia in cats: 136 cases (1984–1987). J.A.V.M.A. 194:1604, 1989.
Dow, S. W., Fettman, M. J., LeCouteur, R. A., et al.: Potassium depletion in cats: Renal and dietary influences. J.A.V.M.A. 191:1569, 1987a.
Dow, S. W., Fettman, M. J., Smith, K. R., et al.: Effect of dietary acidification and potassium depletion on acid-base balance, mineral metabolism, and renal function in adult cats. J. Nutr. 120:569, 1990.
Dow, S. W., LeCouteur, R. A., Fettman, M. J., et al.: Potassium depletion in cats: Hypokalemic polymyopathy. J.A.V.M.A. 191:1563, 1987b.

RENAL AMYLOIDOSIS
IN DOGS AND CATS

STEPHEN P. DIBARTOLA
Columbus, Ohio

Amyloidosis is characterized by the extracellular deposition of fibrils formed by polymerization of protein subunits with a specific biophysical conformation called the beta-pleated sheet. This conformation is responsible for the unique optical and tinctorial properties of amyloid deposits (i.e., green birefringence under polarized light after Congo red staining).

Reactive (secondary) amyloidosis is a systemic syndrome characterized by tissue deposition of amyloid A (AA) protein, which is an amino terminal fragment of an acute-phase reactant called *serum amyloid A protein* (SAA). Congo red–stained amyloid deposits from patients with reactive amyloidosis lose their affinity for Congo red after permanganate oxidation. This feature is useful in the preliminary differentiation of reactive from other types of amyloidosis. Naturally occurring systemic amyloidosis in domestic animals is reactive amyloidosis. Among the domestic animals, reactive amyloidosis is most common in dogs and appears to occur as a familial disease in the Shar pei. Amyloidosis is uncommon in domestic cats, with the exception of Abyssinian cats, in which reactive systemic amyloidosis is a familial disease.

Chronic inflammation and a prolonged increase in the concentration of SAA are prerequisites for development of reactive amyloidosis. However, only a small percentage (< 10%) of individuals with chronic inflammatory disease develop amyloidosis. Thus, other factors must also be important in development of reactive amyloidosis.

Monocytes contain cell surface–associated serine proteases that initially degrade SAA to AA-like intermediates and then to soluble peptides. The second stage of the degradative process may be defective in some individuals and may be a constitutional factor predisposing to amyloidosis. Normal serum also has AA-degrading activity, which may be decreased in serum from patients with chronic inflammatory disease and from those with amyloidosis. Chronic inflammation also may contribute to amyloidosis by increasing the concentration of other acute-phase proteins that are protease inhibitors and by providing a persistent increase in SAA concentration.

There is no discernible associated inflammatory or neoplastic disease in most dogs and cats with reactive systemic amyloidosis at the time of diagnosis. However, various diseases have been observed in some dogs with reactive amyloidosis, including systemic mycoses, chronic bacterial infections, dirofilariasis, neoplasia, and cyclic hematopoiesis (gray collies).

SIGNALMENT

Most dogs and cats with renal amyloidosis are old at the time of presentation. The mean age is 9 years (range, 1–15 years) in dogs and 7 years (range, 1–17 years) in cats. On the other hand, most Abyssinian cats with familial amyloidosis are 5 years of age or younger at the time of death or euthanasia (mean, 4 years; range, < 1 to 13 years). The mean age of 14 Shar pei dogs with familial amyloidosis was also 4 years (range, 1.5 to 6 years) at the time of death or euthanasia. Beagles, collies, pointers, and Walker hounds may be at increased risk and German shepherds and mixed-breed dogs at decreased risk for renal amyloidosis. Glomerular amyloidosis has been reported in families of older beagle dogs, and diabetes mellitus and hypothyroidism may occur concurrently. Amyloidosis occurs in both male and female dogs, possibly with a slight predilection for females. The female:male ratio for 119 Abyssinian cats with familial amyloidosis was 1.6 (73 females, 46 males), and of 14 Shar pei dogs with familial amyloidosis, 10 were female and 4 were male.

CLINICAL FINDINGS

The clinical findings in amyloidosis depend on the organs affected, the amount of amyloid present, and the reaction of the affected organs to the presence of the amyloid deposits. In dogs and cats, amyloid deposits in the kidneys lead to progressive renal disease, and the observed clinical signs are those of chronic renal failure and uremia. Amyloid deposits in other tissues usually do not cause clinical signs.

Patients most commonly have no history of a predisposing disorder, and the clinical findings are those of chronic renal failure. Anorexia, lethargy, and weight loss are commonly observed in both dogs and cats. Polyuria and polydipsia are more commonly detected by owners of dogs than cats but occur in both species. Vomiting is more often observed in dogs than cats. Diarrhea is relatively uncommon in both species.

The presenting clinical signs may result from thromboembolic phenomena, which occur in up to 40% of affected dogs. This complication is rare in cats. Dyspnea due to pulmonary thromboembolism is most common. Caudal paresis with thromboembolism of the iliac or femoral arteries also occurs. Other less common sites of thromboembolism include the coronary arteries, renal artery, mesenteric artery, portal vein, splenic arteries, and brachial artery.

If ascites or subcutaneous edema develops as a result of hypoalbuminemia, the animal may be presented for abdominal distention or swelling of the distal extremities. This is a relatively uncommon presentation in dogs and cats with renal amyloidosis. Asymptomatic proteinuria occasionally is detected on urinalysis during clinical evaluation of another medical problem. Rarely, dogs with amyloidosis may be presented for signs compatible with uremia of apparently acute onset and may have oliguria. This presentation mimics acute renal failure.

Physical examination findings are variable and are usually related to the presence of chronic renal failure. Emaciation and dehydration are commonly observed. The kidneys usually are small, firm, and irregular in affected cats but may be of normal size or even slightly enlarged in affected dogs. The presence of slightly enlarged kidneys in some affected dogs occasionally causes confusion with acute renal failure. Other physical findings may be related to primary inflammatory or neoplastic disease processes. Some affected Shar pei dogs have had a previous history of episodic joint swelling (usually of the tibiotarsal joints) and high fever that resolve within a few days, regardless of treatment. This syndrome resembles familial Mediterranean fever in humans. Ascites or subcutaneous edema occasionally is found if classic nephrotic syndrome is present. Signs of thromboembolism are dependent on the site of the thrombus, but some dogs with thromboembolism have no detectable clinical signs.

LABORATORY FINDINGS

Complete blood count findings in dogs and cats with renal amyloidosis are those of chronic renal failure and include lymphopenia and nonregenerative anemia. Neutrophilic leukocytosis may indicate an underlying inflammatory disease or the stress of chronic disease. Hypoproteinemia (< 6 gm/dl) is more commonly observed in dogs with amyloidosis than is hyperproteinemia (> 8 gm/dl). When pres-

ent, hyperproteinemia may result from dehydration or chronic inflammatory disease. Hyperproteinemia due to hyperglobulinemia is more common in cats with amyloidosis.

Azotemia may be absent or mild at presentation in approximately 50% of dogs with renal amyloidosis but commonly is observed at presentation in cats with amyloidosis. Azotemia reflects prerenal (i.e., dehydration) and renal (i.e., chronic progressive renal disease with destruction of ≥ 75% of functional nephrons) factors when present. Hyperphosphatemia parallels azotemia, is due to decreased GFR, and indicates loss of ≥ 85% of functional nephrons.

Hypercholesterolemia is common in dogs and cats with renal amyloidosis but is also noted in other types of renal diseases. Hypoalbuminemia occurs in most dogs and cats with renal amyloidosis. In dogs, severe loss of protein via the glomeruli probably is the most important contributing factor. The mechanism of hypoalbuminemia may be somewhat different in affected cats, because cats with medullary amyloidosis do not have large urinary losses of protein. The chronic inflammatory pattern observed on protein electrophoresis (i.e., polyclonal gammopathy) in affected cats indicates that the hypoalbuminemia may be reactive in character.

Increased creatine kinase activity may be observed in some dogs with renal amyloidosis, possibly as a result of thromboembolism. Hypocalcemia occurs in 50% of dogs with renal amyloidosis and is attributed to hypoproteinemia and a decreased protein-bound fraction of calcium. Mild hyperglycemia occurs in some dogs with renal amyloidosis and is attributed to the insulin resistance of uremia. Metabolic acidosis characterized by decreased serum bicarbonate concentration, high anion gap, and normal serum chloride concentration occurs in some dogs with amyloidosis and is attributed to uremia. Hyperkalemia occasionally is observed, but the specific cause is not known.

Proteinuria in the absence of remarkable sediment findings is the hallmark of glomerular disease. Moderate to marked proteinuria is common in dogs with amyloidosis because of the predominant glomerular location of the deposits. Proteinuria is mild or absent in animals that have medullary amyloidosis without concurrent glomerular involvement (e.g., most domestic cats with amyloidosis, at least 25% of Abyssinian cats with familial amyloidosis, and up to 33% of Shar pei dogs with familial amyloidosis). Thus, the absence of proteinuria does not rule out a diagnosis of amyloidosis, especially in Abyssinian and other domestic cats and in Shar pei dogs. Proteinuria usually is more severe in dogs with glomerular amyloidosis than in dogs with glomerulonephritis, but there is much individual variation.

Isosthenuria is observed in most dogs and cats with amyloidosis. It reflects the osmotic diuresis typical of renal disease that has progressed to destruction of 67% or more of the renal parenchyma. Severe medullary amyloid deposits may contribute to defective concentrating ability by their physical presence and lead to early interference with urine-concentrating ability. Isosthenuria without proteinuria is common in cats with medullary amyloidosis.

Glucosuria may be observed in some affected animals in the presence of normal blood glucose concentration, but this is a nonspecific finding and probably reflects altered proximal tubular function. Casts are observed in the urine of many dogs with renal amyloidosis. Hyaline cylindruria classically is considered typical of glomerular disease, but studies of dogs with glomerulonephritis and amyloidosis have shown that granular casts may be observed more commonly than hyaline casts. Hematuria and pyuria are uncommon unless there is concurrent urinary tract infection.

Twenty-four-hour urinary protein excretion tends to be higher in dogs with glomerular amyloidosis than in dogs with glomerulonephritis, but there is much individual variation. In one study, a mean value of 481.7 mg/kg/day (range, 350.8 to 533.7 mg/kg/day) was observed in 6 dogs with amyloidosis, whereas a mean value of 116 mg/kg/day (range, 7.5 to 526.1 mg/kg/day) was observed in 26 dogs with glomerulonephritis. In an earlier study, a mean value of 506.9 mg/kg/day (range, 150.3 to 959.6 mg/kg/day) was observed in 6 dogs with amyloidosis, whereas a mean value of 164.7 mg/kg/day (range, 81.2 to 387.1 mg/kg/day) was observed in 11 dogs with glomerulonephritis. One study of dogs with amyloidosis showed urinary protein losses greater than 150 mg/kg/day in nine dogs, 91 to 150 mg/kg/day in four dogs, and less than 30 mg/kg/day (normal) in only one dog.

Urine protein:creatinine ratios also tend to be higher in dogs with glomerular amyloidosis compared with dogs with glomerulonephritis. A mean urine protein:creatinine ratio of 22.5 (range, 11.17 to 46.65) was observed in 6 dogs with amyloidosis compared with 5.73 (range, 0.47 to 43.39) in 26 dogs with glomerulonephritis. Urine protein:creatinine ratio was greater than 10 in eight dogs, 2.0 to 9.9 in seven dogs, and 0.41 to 1.9 in only one dog with amyloidosis in a retrospective study.

In one study, urinary tract infection was documented in almost 40% of 18 dogs with amyloidosis. Urinary tract infection should be ruled out, especially if there is pyuria. Urinary tract infection in dogs with amyloidosis may be incidental or may reflect chronic cystitis or pyelonephritis, either of which could contribute to development of reactive amyloidosis.

Renal size typically is small in affected cats (< 2 times the length of the second lumbar vertebra). Renal size may be small (< 2.5 times the length of the second lumbar vertebra), normal, or increased (> 3.5 times the length of the second lumbar vertebra) in affected dogs.

PATHOLOGIC FINDINGS

A renal biopsy is necessary to differentiate glomerular amyloidosis from glomerulonephritis. In dogs other than Shar peis, amyloidosis primarily is a glomerular disease and can be diagnosed by renal cortical biopsy. In Abyssinian and other domestic cats, medullary amyloidosis may occur without glomerular involvement, and renal cortical biopsy specimens will be negative for amyloid. Medullary amyloidosis without glomerular involvement also occurs in some Shar pei dogs with familial amyloidosis. In these cases, amyloidosis can be difficult to document clinically unless sufficient medullary tissue is obtained at the time of renal biopsy.

In routine hematoxylin and eosin sections, substantial amounts of renal medullary amyloid can be missed. It is important that the clinician request a Congo red stain when amyloidosis is suspected. Renal papillary necrosis may occur in cats and Shar pei dogs with medullary amyloidosis. This lesion is thought to be due to direct interference with blood flow to the inner medulla via the vasa recta by medullary amyloid deposits.

TREATMENT

Clinicians should identify and treat any underlying inflammatory or neoplastic predisposing disease process. It is unlikely, however, that such treatment will alter the course of the disease in animals with uremia secondary to renal amyloidosis. Dehydration should be corrected by appropriate fluid therapy, and renal failure should be managed according to established principles of conservative medical treatment (see this volume, p. 842).

Administration of dimethyl sulfoxide (DMSO) during the rapid phase of amyloid deposition results in resolution of the deposits and a persistent decrease in SAA concentration. Unfortunately, dogs and cats with renal amyloidosis typically are presented much later in the course of their disease. DMSO may benefit patients with established renal amyloidosis by three potential mechanisms: (1) solubilizing amyloid fibrils and allowing urinary excretion of subunit proteins, (2) reducing SAA concentration, and (3) reducing renal interstitial inflammation and fibrosis. The first of these effects is unlikely because the amount of amyloid in the kidneys of human patients who improve clinically after DMSO therapy is unchanged. The last of these effects may result in improvement of renal function and reduction in proteinuria.

Administration of DMSO results in nausea (in human patients) and an unpleasant garlic-like odor. These factors may lead to failure of owner compliance and anorexia with decreased water consumption in the affected animal, thus worsening prerenal azotemia. Intravenous administration of DMSO can lead to transient hemoglobinuria, presumably as a result of intravascular hemolysis. Perivascular inflammation and local thrombosis may occur if undiluted DMSO is administered intravenously. Subcutaneous administration of undiluted DMSO also may cause pain. The standard 90% DMSO solution may be diluted 1:4 with sterile water before subcutaneous administration.

Whether or not DMSO actually is beneficial in treatment of renal amyloidosis in dogs and cats is controversial. In one report, 80 mg/kg DMSO was administered subcutaneously three times a week for 1 year and then topically for another year to a dog with glomerular amyloidosis. The magnitude of proteinuria decreased, and serum albumin concentration increased to normal. In another report, two dogs with renal amyloidosis were treated with a 10% DMSO solution, 125 mg/kg PO b.i.d. Renal function and clinical condition improved for 9 months, but the magnitude of proteinuria did not change. In another study of four dogs with renal amyloidosis, DMSO was given on a daily basis, 300 mg/kg PO, and three of the four dogs died of renal failure within 9 months of beginning therapy. The severity of amyloid deposition in the kidneys of these dogs was not affected by treatment. I have observed 14- and 20-month survival times in two dogs with renal amyloidosis treated with DMSO, 90 mg/kg SC three times per week. Renal function and magnitude of proteinuria did not improve in these dogs, and both were in renal failure at the time of death. The minimal toxicity of DMSO suggests that a therapeutic trial be instituted in dogs and cats with stable renal amyloidosis, but its effectiveness in this situation is uncertain.

Colchicine impairs the release of SAA from hepatocytes by binding to microtubules and preventing secretion. During the predeposition phase of amyloidosis, SAA concentration is increased but no amyloid deposits are observed. Colchicine administered during this phase may prevent the formation of amyloid-enhancing factor. This glycoprotein product of chronic inflammation appears in the spleen 48 hr before amyloid deposits are detected histologically and greatly shortens the time required for development of amyloidosis in experimental animals. The deposition phase of amyloidosis is characterized by an initial rapid accumulation of amyloid deposits in tissues, followed by a plateau during which the amount of amyloid in the tissues remains relatively stable. Colchicine given during the rapid portion of the deposition phase delays but does not prevent tissue deposition of amyloid and decreases SAA concentration. Neither colchicine nor DMSO is thought to be beneficial if given during the plateau portion of the deposition phase. Colchicine prevents the development of amyloidosis in patients with familial Mediterranean fever and promotes stabilization of renal function in those patients with nephrotic syndrome but without overt renal failure. There is no evidence, however, that it is beneficial once amyloidosis has resulted in renal failure. Colchicine is somewhat toxic to human patients, and its side effects include vomiting, diarrhea, and nausea. To my knowledge, there has been no experience with this drug in the treatment of dogs and cats with amyloidosis.

References and Suggested Reading

Center, S. A., Smith, C. A., Wilkinson, E., et al.: Clinicopathologic, renal immunofluorescent, and light microscopic features of glomerulonephritis in the dog: 41 cases (1975–1985). J.A.V.M.A. 190:81, 1987.

Center, S. A., Wilkinson, E., Smith, C. A., et al.: 24-Hour urine protein/creatinine ratio in dogs with protein-losing nephropathies. J.A.V.M.A. 187:820, 1985.

Chew, D. J., DiBartola, S. P., Boyce, J. T., et al.: Renal amyloidosis in related Abyssinian cats. J.A.V.M.A. 181:139, 1982.

Cowgill, L. D.: Diseases of the kidney. In Ettinger, S. J. (ed.): *Textbook of Veterinary Internal Medicine*, 2nd ed. Philadelphia: W. B. Saunders, 1983, p. 1843.

DiBartola, S. P., and Benson, M. D.: Pathogenesis of reactive systemic amyloidosis. J. Vet. Intern. Med. 3:31, 1989.

DiBartola, S. P., Spaulding, G. L., Chew, D. J., et al.: Urinary protein excretion and immunopathologic findings in dogs with glomerular disease. J.A.V.M.A. 177:73, 1980.

DiBartola, S. P., Tarr, M. J., Parker, A. T., et al.: Clinicopathologic findings in dogs with renal amyloidosis: 59 cases (1976–1986). J.A.V.M.A. 195:358, 1989.

DiBartola, S. P., Tarr, M. J., Webb, D. M., et al.: Renal amyloidosis in related Chinese Shar pei dogs. J.A.V.M.A. 197:483, 1990.

Gruys, E., Sijens, R. J., and Biewenga, W. J.: Dubious effect of dimethylsulfoxide (DMSO) therapy on amyloid deposits and amyloidosis. Vet. Res. Comm. 5:21, 1981.

Slauson, D. O., and Gribble, D. H.: Thrombosis complicating renal amyloidosis in dogs. Vet. Pathol. 8:352, 1971.

Slauson, D. O., Gribble, D. H., and Russell, S. W.: A clinicopathological study of renal amyloidosis in dogs. J. Comp. Pathol. 80:335, 1970.

Spyridakis, L., Brown, S., Barsanti, J., et al.: Amyloidosis in a dog: Treatment with dimethylsulfoxide. J.A.V.M.A. 189:690, 1986.

Zemer, D., Pras, M., Sohar, E., et al.: Colchicine in the prevention and treatment of amyloidosis of familial Mediterranean fever. N. Engl. J. Med. 314:1001, 1986.

COAGULATION DISORDERS IN
GLOMERULAR DISEASES

ROBERTA L. RELFORD
and ROBERT A. GREEN
College Station, Texas

The clinical presentations of glomerular disease are variable, ranging from mild asymptomatic proteinuria to nephrotic syndrome and acute or chronic renal failure. Coagulation disorders occur at two phases of glomerular disease: during the nephrotic stage and during the uremic stage of acute or chronic renal failure. Nephrotic animals are predisposed to thromboembolism (Rasedee et al., 1986). When glomerular damage is severe, marked reduction in glomerular filtration may lead to acute or chronic renal failure. With reduced glomerular filtration, the degree of proteinuria decreases, eliminating many of the factors contributing to hypercoagulability. However, the resultant uremia impairs platelet function and causes prolongation of bleeding times.

NEPHROTIC SYNDROME

Nephrotic syndrome results from markedly increased permeability of the glomerulus to selected plasma proteins. The consistent tetrad of clinical and laboratory features accompanying nephrotic syndrome includes hypoalbuminemia, marked proteinuria, hypercholesterolemia, and third-space fluid accumulation (i.e., ascites or subcutaneous edema). One of the serious complications of nephrotic syndrome is thromboembolism.

Plasma alterations in nephrotic syndrome that contribute to thrombotic tendencies include urinary loss of albumin and antithrombin-III (AT-III) (Greco and Green, 1987). Hypoalbuminemia permits increased availability of potent arachidonic acid metabolites (e.g., thromboxane B$_2$), promoting increased platelet aggregation. Decreased levels of AT-III, an important serine protease inhibitor, allow increased activation of the serine-containing coagulation factors (factors IX, X, XI, and XII), resulting in increased thrombin generation. Thrombin, in turn, causes further stimulation of the platelet release reaction.

Other consistent findings include increased fibrinogen, factor V, and factor VIII. Increased fibrinogen production has been found to be proportional to urinary protein loss and the degree of concurrent hypercholesterolemia. Elevated fibrinogen levels enhance platelet-fibrinogen interactions and alter plasma viscosity, which may have an important role in hypercoagulability. It has been hypothesized that the increase in factors V and VIII results from increased protein synthesis by the liver in response to decreased plasma oncotic pressure resulting from the hypoalbuminemia. The high molecular weight of factors V and VIII prevents their loss in the urine of nephrotic patients. It is doubtful whether increased levels of these cofactors have an important role in hypercoagulability because they are normally present in great excess in circulation. Furthermore, they are increased during many acute inflammatory responses that are not associated with thromboembolism.

Normal fibrinolysis involves adherence of plasminogen to fibrin and subsequent conversion of plasminogen into the active protease, plasmin. The end result is dissolution of the fibrin clot. Reduced fibrinolysis may contribute to the thrombotic tendency associated with nephrotic syndrome (Llach, 1985). Factors causing reduced fibrinolysis and persistence of thromboemboli in nephrotic syndrome include decreased levels of inhibitors of fibrinolysis, plasminogen, and alpha-1 antitrypsin. Plasminogen and alpha-1 antitrypsin are lost in the urine along with albumin. The primary plasmin inhibitor, alpha-2 antiplasmin, is increased in nephrotic syndrome. Alpha-2 antiplasmin binds to plasmin and interferes with the binding of plasminogen to fibrin. The urinary loss of plasminogen along with the binding of alpha-2 antiplasmin to plasmin results in decreased availability of plasmin. Additionally, interference with plasminogen incorporation into the fibrin clot by excess alpha-2 antiplasmin results in resistance to lysis.

Platelet abnormalities in nephrotic syndrome include hyperaggregability, enhanced platelet adhesiveness, thrombocytosis, and increased platelet turnover rate (Walter et al., 1981). *In vivo* evidence of increased platelet activation is based on increased plasma levels of platelet factor IV and beta-thromboglobulin, platelet-specific proteins that are released from cytoplasmic alpha granules only during platelet activation. Hypercholesterolemia in nephrotic syndrome contributes to altered platelet

827

function by enhancing expression of platelet surface membrane receptors for active hemostatic enzymes or by increasing prostaglandin endoperoxide synthesis. Aggregation studies have shown platelets to be more sensitive to agonists, although there is no definitive evidence about the level of platelet activation in nephrotic syndrome.

UREMIA

The multifactorial pathophysiologic mechanisms of uremic bleeding are controversial (Harris and Krawiec, 1990). Briefly, several compounds that potentially affect platelet function accumulate in the blood of uremic patients. These compounds include urea, guanidinosuccinic acid, phenolic acid, middle molecules, and parathyroid hormone. It has been shown in humans that reduction of these toxins by dialysis reduces the frequency and severity of bleeding. Other reported abnormalities involve the factor VIII–von Willebrand complex and eicosanoid synthesis, resulting in impaired platelet-plug formation.

DETECTION OF COAGULATION DISORDERS

Precise documentation of a hypercoagulable state is difficult and often is largely based on the presence of contributing pathophysiologic factors (i.e., hypoalbuminemia, hypercholesterolemia). Furthermore, detection of thromboemboli usually requires procedures not routinely available to practitioners, such as nuclear imaging, Doppler ultrasonography, and contrast angiography. The remarkable collateral circulation in dogs often minimizes clinical signs, resulting in subclinical thrombosis. Laboratory results suggesting a hypercoagulable state are lowered AT-III and increased fibrinogen levels. Elevated fibrin degradation products usually imply active secondary fibrinolysis. Coagulation test times (one-stage prothrombin time, activated partial thromboplastin time, thrombin time) are occasionally shortened, but these findings are inconsistent. Activated clotting times and bleeding times offer a qualitative evaluation of the coagulation cascade and platelet function; alterations in results of these tests can be noted in both uremia and nephrotic syndrome. *In vitro* platelet aggregation studies may show increased responsiveness of platelets to subthreshold levels of agonists (i.e., adenosine diphosphate, collagen, epinephrine). Increased levels of plasma beta-thromboglobulin and thromboxane also indicate increased platelet activation.

MANAGEMENT

Treatment of glomerular disease is directed toward eliminating the initiating factors and slowing the progression of the glomerular lesion. Discussions of the medical management of glomerulopathies and renal failure are addressed elsewhere in this section. If a hypercoagulable state is suspected because of alterations in the coagulation profile, anticoagulants (heparin, warfarin) or antiplatelet drugs (aspirin) should be incorporated into the therapeutic plan to prevent thromboembolic disease. It has been shown that aspirin at a dosage of 5 mg/kg every 24 hr is effective in preventing formation of arterial thrombi in dogs (Escudero-Vela et al., 1989). In an attempt to correct factors predisposing to hypercoagulability, low-protein diets have been found to maintain albumin mass by decreasing urinary protein loss and to lower elevated serum cholesterol in humans (Kaysen, 1988). When dehydration is present, maintaining adequate tissue perfusion with appropriate fluid therapy is essential to prevent sludging of blood and accumulation of procoagulant substances that promote thrombosis.

Once thrombosis has occurred, treatment with thrombolytic drugs is advocated but is not without risk. The prevention and treatment of thrombosis in animals have been reviewed by Feldman (1986). In humans, thrombolytic compounds currently used or under clinical investigation include thrombolytic agents such as streptokinase, urokinase, recombinant tissue plasminogen activator, single-chain urokinase, and anisoylated plasminogen streptokinase activator complex. The major disadvantages of these agents are expense and uncontrollable bleeding due to hyperfibrinolysis. The safety and efficacy of these drugs are not established in animals.

References and Suggested Reading

Escudero-Vela, M. C., Alvarez, L., Rodriguez, V., et al.: Prevention of the formation of arterial thrombi using different antiplatelet drugs: Experimental study in dogs. Thromb. Res. 54:187, 1989.
   A study evaluating the prophylactic efficacy of several drugs against experimentally induced arterial thrombosis.
Feldman, B. F.: Thrombosis—diagnosis and treatment. *In* Kirk, R. W. (ed.): *Current Veterinary Therapy IX.* Philadelphia: W. B. Saunders, 1986, pp. 505–508.
   A review of current diagnostic and therapeutic approaches to thromboembolism of dogs.
Greco, D. S., and Green, R. A.: Coagulation abnormalities associated with thrombosis in a dog with nephrotic syndrome. Comp. Cont. Ed. Pract. Vet. 9:653, 1987.
   A case report and discussion of coagulation abnormalities associated with nephrotic syndrome in dogs.
Harris, C. L., and Krawiec, D. R.: The pathophysiology of uremic bleeding. Comp. Cont. Ed. Pract. Vet. 12:1294, 1990.
   A review of the pathophysiology of coagulation disorders associated with uremia.
Kaysen, G. A.: Albumin metabolism in nephrotic syndrome: The effect of dietary protein intake. Am. J. Kidney Dis. 12:461, 1988.
   A study of albumin homeostasis in patients with nephrotic syndrome and the effect of dietary protein.

Llach, F.: Hypercoagulability, renal vein thrombosis, and other thrombotic complications of nephrotic syndrome. Kidney Int. 28:429, 1985.
An in-depth review of the pathophysiology of the hypercoagulable state associated with nephrotic syndrome.
Rasedee, A., Feldman, B. F., and Washabau, R.: Naturally occurring canine nephrotic syndrome is a potentially hypercoagulable state. Acta Vet. Scand. 27:369, 1986.

An article discussing pathomechanisms associated with platelet hyperaggregability in nephrotic syndrome.
Walter, E., Deppermann, D., Andrassy, K., et al.: Platelet hyperaggregability as a consequence of the nephrotic syndrome. Thromb. Res. 23:473, 1981.
An article discussing the impact of nephrotic syndrome on the platelet population.

ACUTE RENAL FAILURE ASSOCIATED WITH SYSTEMIC INFECTIOUS DISEASE

S. DRU FORRESTER
Blacksburg, Virginia

and GEORGE E. LEES
College Station, Texas

Acute renal failure (ARF) is a clinical syndrome associated with sudden deterioration of renal function and characterized by abnormalities arising from inability of the kidneys to adequately regulate fluid and electrolyte balance and excrete catabolic waste products. In small animal patients with ARF, the renal lesion may be either nephrosis or nephritis. Nephrotoxins and ischemic insults are frequent causes of nephrosis, whereas nephritis may be due to infectious or noninfectious conditions. Although nephritis causes ARF infrequently, systemic infectious diseases such as leptospirosis, Rocky Mountain spotted fever, ehrlichiosis, and bacterial endocarditis sometimes produce ARF. Renal failure is a part of the clinical illness; other organ systems (e.g., liver, coagulation) often are affected concurrently.

PATHOPHYSIOLOGY

The pathophysiology of ARF associated with systemic infectious disease varies with the underlying cause. Renal failure associated with *bacterial endocarditis* usually is associated with renal infarction. Other renal lesions may include thrombosis secondary to disseminated intravascular coagulation, renal abscesses, toxic tubular changes, pyelonephritis, and glomerulonephritis (Toboada and Palmer, 1989). Decreased renal perfusion from either dehydration or congestive heart failure may contribute to declining renal function in dogs with endocarditis by causing additional ischemic injury.

Leptospires apparently produce a toxin that causes functional and morphologic capillary damage. The organisms replicate and persist in renal tubular epithelial cells. Interstitial swelling and decreased renal perfusion may lead to decreased glomerular filtration and ARF (Greene and Shotts, 1990). Clinically, leptospirosis manifests either as a hemorrhagic syndrome, icterus, or renal failure. There is some correlation between the serovar involved and the clinical syndrome; *Leptospira canicola* primarily causes renal disease in dogs (see this volume, p. 260).

Rickettsial organisms invade and replicate in capillary endothelial cells, causing a necrotizing vasculitis; the kidneys are especially vulnerable because of their endarterial circulation (Greene and Breitschwerdt, 1990). Acute renal failure may occur secondary to Rocky Mountain spotted fever, especially in the terminal stages. We have observed ARF in a dog with acute ehrlichiosis; an immune-mediated vasculitis was suspected as the cause.

DIAGNOSIS

History and Clinical Signs

Historical complaints often include sudden onset of lethargy, depression, anorexia, vomiting, lameness, icterus, and discolored urine. Physical examination findings may include dehydration, oral ulcerations, abdominal pain, cardiac murmur, petechial and ecchymotic hemorrhages, pale or icteric mucous membranes, splenomegaly, hepatomegaly, lymphadenopathy, and fever.

Laboratory Findings

Laboratory abnormalities associated with ARF are due mainly to decreased excretion of catabolic wastes and include increased serum urea nitrogen and creatinine, hyperphosphatemia, and metabolic acidemia. Hypocalcemia may be observed in some patients. Hyperkalemia reflects acidemia and oliguria. The urinalysis reveals inadequately concentrated urine regardless of the type or cause of renal failure. Other findings may include pyuria, hematuria, proteinuria, bilirubinuria, and increased numbers of casts. Indeed, finding indicators of inflammation (pyuria, proteinuria, hematuria, and sometimes leukocyte casts) in the urine of patients with ARF often is an important aid in differentiating nephritis from nephrosis, which mainly produces renal epithelial cellular debris and granular casts. Therefore, thorough analysis of a fresh urine specimen is a crucial part of the clinical investigation of ARF.

Differentiating between ARF and chronic renal failure is important because ARF is potentially reversible. Oliguria and hyperkalemia are more typical of ARF, although both may occur in the terminal stages of chronic renal failure. In general, the greater the degree of renal injury, the greater the likelihood of oliguric renal failure. Nonoliguric ARF occurs in small animals; however, it is most often associated with nephrotoxicity due to aminoglycoside antibiotics. A normocytic, normochromic nonregenerative anemia suggests chronic renal failure; however, as ARF progresses, anemia may occur as a result of gastrointestinal hemorrhage, hemodilution, and hemolysis. Also, nonregenerative anemia often occurs in Rocky Mountain spotted fever and ehrlichiosis.

Depending on the cause of renal failure, other abnormalities may include hyperbilirubinemia, increased serum activities of hepatic enzymes, hypoalbuminemia, leukocytosis, and thrombocytopenia. Prolonged clotting times (e.g., one-stage prothrombin time, activated partial thromboplastin time), increased fibrin degradation products, hypofibrinogenemia, and decreased antithrombin-III may be observed in patients with disseminated intravascular coagulation.

Diagnosis of Underlying Disease

When ARF exists in a patient exhibiting clinical signs and laboratory abnormalities listed earlier, an infectious etiology should be suspected. Most infectious diseases associated with ARF are diagnosed by serology, except for bacterial endocarditis, which is confirmed by positive blood cultures. Urine culture also may be positive in animals with bacterial endocarditis. Bacteremia or septic renal infarction can lead to bacteriuria; however, bacterial infection of the urinary tract or prostate gland also can be the origin of septicemia or bacterial endocarditis.

TREATMENT

The goals of treatment are to minimize further renal injury, promote diuresis, and combat metabolic consequences of uremia. With time, the damaged kidneys may be able to repair lesions sufficiently to regain adequate function. To minimize additional renal injury, all potentially nephrotoxic drugs should be discontinued, if possible, or the dose should be modified appropriately. In addition, the animal should be rehydrated to establish adequate renal perfusion. If oliguria persists despite appropriate fluid therapy, additional treatment to increase urine production is indicated. Although increased urine formation does not necessarily indicate improved renal function, clinical management of nonoliguric patients is usually also facilitated by diuresis. Medical management of ARF and its complications (e.g., oliguria, hyperkalemia, metabolic acidemia, hypocalcemia, hyperphosphatemia, and vomiting) is discussed in greater detail elsewhere (Low and Cowgill, 1983).

In addition to general supportive care, specific treatment of the associated infectious disease is indicated. These patients also may have other life-threatening conditions (e.g., coagulopathies, hepatic failure) that require therapeutic intervention.

The initial treatment of choice for leptospirosis is penicillin. Other drugs (e.g., chloramphenicol, tetracycline) are considered less effective for eliminating leptospiremia (Greene and Breitschwerdt, 1990). Because penicillins are eliminated primarily by the kidneys, their dose should be adjusted in patients with renal failure. Precise adjustments usually are unnecessary, and in general the dose is either halved or the dosing interval is doubled (Riviere, 1981). Once serum urea nitrogen and creatinine levels return to normal, dihydrostreptomycin is administered to eliminate leptospires from the kidneys and terminate the carrier state. In human patients with leptospirosis, treatment with doxycycline (Vibramycin, Pfizer) effectively terminates leptospiremia and leptospiruria (McClain et al., 1984). Doxycycline may be an alternative treatment for canine leptospirosis; however, its effectiveness needs to be evaluated.

Most rickettsial infections respond to treatment with tetracyclines or chloramphenicol. In general, tetracyclines should be avoided in renal failure because of their extensive renal elimination and potential to cause acute tubular necrosis. Doxycycline is an exception; it undergoes less renal elimination than other tetracyclines and therefore does not accumulate in renal failure. In addition, doxycycline can be administered parenterally, an important consideration in vomiting, uremic patients. Chloramphenicol (Chloromycetin, Parke-Davis) also is an effective treatment for both Rocky Mountain spotted fever and ehrlichiosis. The dose should be decreased by 10% in uremic patients because of the catabolic effects of chloramphenicol on protein synthesis (Greene and Ferguson, 1990). Imidocarb dipropionate is effective for treatment of ehrlichiosis, and relapses occur less frequently than in dogs treated conventionally (Troy and Forrester, 1990). However, its use in renal failure has not been evaluated, and the drug is not commercially available in the United States.

Bacterial endocarditis is treated initially with parenteral antibiotics (5 to 10 days), followed by long-term oral treatment (4 to 8 weeks). Ideally, antibiotic selection is based on results of blood culture. However, when culture results are pending or when endocarditis is suspected in the absence of a positive culture, empirical treatment with broad-spectrum bactericidal antibiotics is recommended. A combination of an aminoglycoside and a beta-lactamase–resistant penicillin or cephalosporin is effective against most bacterial species that cause endocarditis; however, aminoglycosides should be avoided in patients with renal failure. Cephalosporins are effective against gram-positive and gram-negative bacteria and can be used alone while awaiting results of culture and susceptibility. Alternatively, one of the fluorquinolones can be administered. With the exception of anaerobes, quinolones are effective against most bacteria that cause endocar-ditis. When aminoglycosides must be used in patients with renal failure (e.g., organism susceptible only to an aminoglycoside), serum drug concentrations should be monitored to avoid additional renal damage. Ideally, a clinical pharmacologist should be consulted to plan a monitoring regimen.

References and Suggested Reading

Greene, C. E., and Breitschwerdt, E. B.: Rocky Mountain spotted fever and Q fever. In Greene, C. E. (ed.): Infectious Diseases of the Dog and Cat. Philadelphia: W. B. Saunders, 1990, p. 419.
A review of the pathogenesis, diagnosis, treatment, and prevention of Rocky Mountain spotted fever.

Greene, C. E., and Ferguson, D. C.: Antibacterial chemotherapy. In Greene, C. E. (ed.): Infectious Diseases of the Dog and Cat. Philadelphia: W. B. Saunders, 1990, p. 461.
A review of the classes of antibacterial agents including spectrum of activity, indications, and toxicities.

Greene, C. E., and Shotts, E. B.: Leptospirosis. In Greene, C. E. (ed.): Infectious Diseases of the Dog and Cat. Philadelphia: W. B. Saunders, 1990, p. 498.
A review of the pathogenesis, diagnosis, and clinical management of leptospirosis.

Low, D. G., and Cowgill, L. D.: Emergency management of the acute uremic crisis. In Kirk, R. W. (ed.): Current Veterinary Therapy VIII. Philadelphia: W. B. Saunders, 1983, p. 981.
A review of the diagnosis and treatment of uremia and other metabolic consequences of acute and chronic renal failure.

McClain, B. L., Ballou, W. R., Harrison, S. M., et al.: Doxycycline therapy for leptospirosis. Ann. Intern. Med. 100:696, 1984.
A prospective study describing doxycycline treatment of leptospirosis in 29 human patients.

Riviere, J. E.: Dosage of antimicrobial drugs in patients with renal insufficiency. J.A.V.M.A. 178:70, 1981.
A review of the effect of renal disease on antimicrobial drug disposition and how to modify dosage regimens in these patients.

Toboada, J., and Palmer, G. H.: Renal failure associated with bacterial endocarditis in the dog. J. Am. Anim. Hosp. Assoc. 25:243, 1989.
A retrospective study of the diagnosis, treatment, and pathologic findings in four dogs with ARF and bacterial endocarditis.

Troy, G. C., and Forrester, S. D.: Canine ehrlichiosis. In Greene, C. E. (ed.): Infectious Diseases of the Dog and Cat. Philadelphia: W. B. Saunders, 1990, p. 404.
A review of the pathogenesis, diagnosis, and treatment of canine ehrlichiosis.

EFFECTS OF VASOACTIVE
AGENTS ON KIDNEY FUNCTION

SCOTT A. BROWN,
JEANNE A. BARSANTI,
and DELMAR R. FINCO
Athens, Georgia

OVERVIEW

In the normal animal, the contribution of the kidneys to the maintenance of health is dependent upon the presence of adequate levels of renal blood flow (RBF) and glomerular filtration rate (GFR). Though many factors contribute to stable levels of kidney function, control of RBF and GFR rests mainly with pre- and postglomerular vascular segments: the afferent and efferent arterioles (Fig. 1). Conceptually, the formation of glomerular filtrate is controlled through adjustments in vascular resistance at the inflow (afferent arteriole) and outflow (efferent arteriole). Vasoconstriction of either arteriole segment will decrease glomerular blood flow, and arteriolar vasodilation will increase glomerular blood flow. If generalized to all nephrons, arteriolar vasodilation increases RBF and vasoconstriction reduces RBF. Similarly, GFR is enhanced by generalized dilation of both arterioles and reduced when both are constricted.

In animals with disease, the veterinary clinician frequently encounters conditions or employs therapeutic agents with effects on the vascular system. Often the effects go unnoticed despite the fact that

Table 1. *Agents or Conditions That Reduce RBF and GFR Directly Through Effects on Renal Arterioles*

Conditions
Septicemia
Myoglobinemia
Intravascular hemolysis
Hypercalcemia
Hypokalemia
Hepatic failure
Therapeutic agents
Angiotensin-converting enzyme inhibitors
Nonsteroidal anti-inflammatory agents
Amphotericin B
Dopamine antagonists (e.g., metoclopramide)
Propranolol
Radiographic contrast material

changes in GFR and RBF may be detrimental to the animal, producing azotemia or renal injury.

Commonly encountered causes of reductions in GFR and RBF include a wide variety of conditions and therapeutic agents that act directly upon the renal arterioles (Table 1). Although the extent of effects will vary, these agents may produce azotemia or uremia in susceptible animals. Prompt removal of the offending agent or condition will generally result in a rapid return of kidney function to normal.

Conversely, many agents or conditions enhance RBF and GFR through vascular effects (Table 2). Although an increase in RBF and GFR may be viewed as beneficial, some of these stimuli produce marked increases in glomerular capillary pressure that could theoretically be deleterious to the kidney. The consequences of glomerular capillary hypertension have not been established in dogs and cats.

Although a single stimulus usually affects both arteriole segments (afferent and efferent) in the same manner, some agents will preferentially affect one or the other. Vasodilation of the afferent arteriole will increase inflow to the glomerulus, resulting in an increase in glomerular blood flow and pressure and enhancing GFR. On the other hand, afferent arteriolar constriction will tend to lower GFR. Because of its postglomerular location, effer-

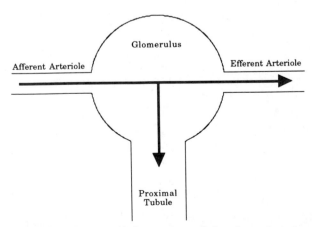

Figure 1. Because of the anatomy of the glomerulus, the formation of glomerular filtrate is under the control of the afferent and efferent arterioles.

Table 2. *Agents or Conditions That Increase RBF and GFR Directly Through Effects on Renal Arterioles*

Conditions
  Protein ingestion
  Pregnancy
  Diabetes mellitus
Therapeutic agents
  Amino acid solutions (hyperaminoacidemia)
  Glucose solutions (hyperglycemia)
  Alpha₁-antagonists (e.g., prazosin, phenoxybenzamine)
  Calcium channel blockers (e.g., verapamil, nifedipine, diltiazem)
  Dopamine
  Vasodilators (e.g., nitroprusside, hydralazine)

ent arteriolar dilation increases outflow from the glomerulus and will generally produce a dramatic fall in glomerular pressure, causing GFR to decrease. In contrast, GFR may be increased by selective efferent arteriolar constriction.

Although few agents have these preferential effects on one arteriole type, two important classes of therapeutic agents are in this category: angiotensin-converting enzyme (ACE) inhibitors (e.g., captopril, enalapril, lisinopril) and nonsteroidal anti-inflammatory drugs (NSAIDs) (e.g., aspirin, flunixin meglumine, ibuprofen). The former produce efferent arteriolar dilation, and the latter cause afferent constriction. Although the effect of these agents in normal kidneys is minimal, they can have disastrous consequences in animals with renal disease or congestive heart failure. In the acutely or chronically diseased kidney, compensatory hyperfunction in surviving nephrons is dependent upon the maintenance of efferent resistance coincident with afferent vasodilation. In these nephrons, efferent tone is maintained by angiotensin II and preglomerular dilation by vasodilatory prostaglandins. The administration of ACE inhibitors will block angiotensin II production and cause vasodilation of the efferent arteriole, which may cause a precipitous fall in GFR. The administration of NSAIDs reduces local production of vasodilatory prostaglandins, effectively causing afferent constriction and a reduction in GFR.

Some conditions or therapeutic agents have important effects on the ability of the kidney to maintain constancy of RBF and GFR despite variations in mean arterial pressure. This is an inherent property of the normal kidney and is known as renal autoregulation. This autoregulatory capacity lies within the afferent arteriole. It not only maintains

constancy of renal function (GFR and RBF) but also protects the susceptible glomerular capillaries from injury when systemic blood pressure becomes elevated (i.e., systemic hypertension) and maintains adequate levels of GFR when systemic blood pressure falls (i.e., systemic hypotension).

Several conditions and therapeutic agents disrupt renal autoregulation, predisposing the animal to renal injury when systemic hypertension is present and to prerenal azotemia when systemic hypotension develops. These may include acute and chronic renal failure, chronic ingestion of high-protein diets, hyperglycemia, hyperaminoacidemia, and calcium channel blockers.

THERAPY

The key to successful therapy of problems that occur secondary to these agents and conditions is to recognize and alter or remove the causative factor wherever possible. It is apparent that agents that reduce RBF and GFR have the potential to produce undesirable clinical sequelae, specifically uremia. Enhancement of RBF and GFR or alterations of the renal autoregulatory capability may also be harmful to dogs and cats, although the effects of these changes are likely to be gradual and may go unrecognized until significant, irreversible renal parenchymal injury has occurred. Fluid therapy and reduction of diuretic dose will be beneficial to animals that develop acute renal failure from ACE inhibitors.

References and Suggested Reading

Brown, S. A., Finco, D. R., Crowell, W. A., et al.: Single-nephron adaptations to partial renal ablation in the dog. Am. J. Physiol. 258:F495, 1990.
  A report of the physiologic response of remnant nephrons to renal dysfunction in dogs, including a consideration of the role of renal arterioles in controlling the glomerular filtration process.
Brown, S. A., Finco, D. R., Crowell, W. A., et al.: Single-nephron responses to systemic administration of amino acids in dogs. Am. J. Physiol. 259:F739, 1990.
  A report of the response of renal arterioles to hyperaminoacidemia, including a discussion of changes in renal autoregulatory capability.
Carmines, P. K., Perry, M. D., Hazelrig, J. B., et al.: Effects of preglomerular and postglomerular vascular resistance alterations on filtration fraction. Kidney Int. 31:S229, 1987.
  A discussion of the theoretical effects of changes in the resistance in the afferent and efferent arterioles that includes data from dogs.
Maddox, D. A., and Brenner, B. M.: Glomerular ultrafiltration. In Brenner, B. M., and Rector, F. C. (eds.): The Kidney, 4th ed. Philadelphia: W. B. Saunders, 1991, p. 205.
  A general discussion of the renal microcirculation and the glomerular filtration process.

USE OF BLOOD PRESSURE MONITORS

MICHAEL PODELL

Columbus, Ohio

Systemic arterial blood pressure (ABP) has been measured in animals since first reported by Stephen Hales in 1733. The first direct measurements of arterial pressure were recorded in dogs in the early 1800's by Poiseuille. Indirect blood pressure measurement was not advanced until Korotkoff enhanced the occlusive cuff technique of Riva-Rocci in 1905 by using an auscultatory method that associated specific changes in sound with changes in ABP. Despite the use of animals as an integral part of the development of blood pressure monitoring in medicine, the overall prevalence of routine monitoring in veterinary medicine is still low. Today's technologic advances allow for easier accessibility to blood pressure measurements in human and veterinary medicine. These current monitoring instruments, however, still use the basic biophysical concepts that have been developed during the past century.

In clinical situations, ABP monitoring is useful in the diagnosis of systemic hypertension secondary to renal or endocrine disorders (e.g., hyperthyroidism, hyperadrenocorticism). Blood pressure monitoring also aids in monitoring critical care patient status, the effects of surgery, anesthesia, and cardiovascular and antihypertensive vasodilator therapy.

BIOMECHANICS OF BLOOD PRESSURE

To use the information obtained in blood pressure monitoring, one must have a basic understanding of the components of ABP. Blood pressure is defined as the lateral force per unit area of vascular wall. Blood flow is the amount of motion provided by blood pressure working against vascular resistance. The arterial vasculature is a high-pressure branching system whose energy is generated by the left ventricle. As a result of the cardiac cycle, systemic ABP oscillates about a mean pressure (pulsatile pressure). Systolic pressure is the maximum height of the oscillation; diastolic pressure is the minimum height of the oscillation. Pulse pressure, the major determinant of peripheral pulse strength, is just the difference between systolic and diastolic pressures.

Systolic pressure is determined by left ventricular stroke volume, peak rate of ejection, and arterial compliance. Determinants of diastolic pressure are end-systolic arterial pressure, diastolic duration, peripheral vascular resistance, and blood volume (Kittleson and Olivier, 1983). Mean ABP (MAP), responsible for major organ perfusion, can be approximated by the following formula:

$$MAP = \text{diastolic pressure} + \frac{\text{systolic} - \text{diastolic pressure}}{3}$$

A more accurate assessment of MAP is achieved through direct or indirect blood pressure monitoring.

Differences in systolic and diastolic blood pressure changes can be attributed to their respective determinants. In veterinary medicine, diastolic hypertension is usually associated with systolic hypertension, whereas the latter also can occur alone. Elevations or reductions in either systolic or diastolic pressure can concomitantly change MAP.

DIRECT BLOOD PRESSURE MEASUREMENT

Direct ABP measurement reflects the intravascular pressure at the site of monitoring. This method offers the potential advantages of a more accurate and consistent representation of systemic pressure, constant monitoring for anesthesia and critical care cases, measurement of central, inaccessible arteries, and a standard for comparison of indirect methods.

The disadvantages of direct monitoring are that specific technical skills are required; the procedure is invasive; restraint without chemical sedation can be difficult; the equipment is expensive; and the measurements are vulnerable to error if basic hydraulic principles are not followed.

ABP can be directly monitored with one of three main techniques. First, needle puncture of the femoral artery can provide brief recordings, especially in small dogs and cats (Scully et al., 1983). Second, percutaneous catheterization of the femoral or dorsal metatarsal artery can be used for continuous monitoring for anesthesia or for critical care monitoring (Haskins, 1989). Finally, central arterial monitoring can be performed by catheter advancement into the abdominal aorta.

The needle puncture technique requires puncture of the femoral artery with a needle (26 gauge, 1½ in.) connected to a nylon catheter. Animals can be lightly restrained in lateral or dorsal recumbency. A constant infusion of sterile saline from a syringe infusion pump keeps the catheter patent. The nylon catheter tubing from the needle is connected to a reservoir (Intraflo Reservoir System).* This reservoir is directly attached to a blood pressure transducer (1290C universal quartz pressure transducer),† whose output can be recorded on an oscilloscope or multichannel polygraph. The magnitude or deflection is compared with that produced by a previously calibrated scale. Direct mean and pulsatile ABP then can be determined.

Percutaneous catheterization requires sterile preparation over the desired artery. The dorsal metatarsal artery is easy to stabilize and readily accessible over the dorsolateral aspect of the metatarsal region. A semiflexible over-the-needle catheter (20 to 22 gauge, 2½ in.) is inserted with the bevel up just above the artery. While palpating the pulse, the artery is penetrated, the catheter rotated slowly into the artery, and the needle stylet removed. The catheter is then flushed with heparinized saline and capped.

A transducer monitoring device as previously described can be attached, or an aneroid manometer can be used. Extension tubing is placed between the catheter and manometer to prevent backflow of blood or water into the manometer. A three-way stopcock is attached between the manometer and the catheter. Saline is injected toward the manometer until the compressed air increases the manometer pressure to a level above mean pressure. The system is then allowed to equilibrate with the MAP (Haskins, 1989).

INDIRECT BLOOD PRESSURE MEASUREMENT

All indirect blood pressure techniques are dependent on detection of flow beneath an occluding cuff. Only the sensor differs between methods. Indirect measurements offer general advantages over the direct technique: they are noninvasive, easier to perform, require relatively minimal technical expertise, and can be performed during a short time interval. Indirect techniques are least accurate when blood pressure is low, vessels are constricted, or excessive movement occurs. The indirect techniques used in human medicine are the palpatory, flush, auscultatory, oscillometric, and ultrasonic techniques (Geddes, 1970). The occlusive cuff position varies with the technique used.

With the palpatory method, the sensor is the reader's fingers, and the return of palpable beats with cuff deflation is equal to systolic pressure. The technique does not provide for measurement of diastolic pressure or MAP and is not reliable in veterinary medicine.

The auscultatory method is the most widely used technique in human medicine. This method of arterial occlusion followed by gradual arterial expansion through cuff deflation produces low-energy acoustic phenomena that are divided into specific phases called Korotkoff's sounds. Systolic pressure is the maximal pressure at which the first tones appear (phase I). Phases II through IV represent turbulent flow of blood through the artery with progressive muffling of sounds. Diastolic pressure is measured at the cessation of sounds (phase V).

Indirect auscultatory systolic and diastolic pressures can be monitored in anesthetized dogs with the use of piezoelement amplification of Korotkoff's sounds (Wessale et al., 1985). Compared with direct pressure readings in the same dogs, this indirect method provided correlation coefficients of 0.98 for systolic pressure and 0.99 for diastolic pressure. The main disadvantages of this technique are the need for anesthesia or sedation for a patient's complete cooperation, increased chance for error with conditions that result in moderate to severe peripheral vasoconstriction (e.g., hemorrhage), difficulty in applying the apparatus to short-legged dogs, and difficulty associated with precise determination of diastolic pressures.

Oscillometric Method

The oscillometric method of blood pressure determination is based on the detection of changes in oscillations of the occluded artery during cuff deflation. The oscillations are produced by changes in arterial diameter secondary to changes in pulsatile pressure. Systolic pressure is equal to a sudden increase in the amplitude of oscillations; the lowest point of maximum oscillations indicates the diastolic pressure. MAP is the lowest cuff pressure at which the oscillations reach their highest amplitude.

The advent of microprocessor technology has permitted precise identification of the change in oscillation amplitude. Several oscillometric recording instruments designed initially for human neonatal and pediatric use are available for veterinary use. Dinamap* monitors (Critikon) automatically regulate cuff inflation and deflation, determine systolic and diastolic pressures and MAP, and record pulse rate. Previous models (845, 847, 1255) require that sensitivities be adjusted externally according to expected pressures; only models 847 and 1255 can

---

*Sorenson Research Co., Salt Lake City, UT.
†Hewlett Packard, Andover, MA.

*Johnson and Johnson, Tampa, FL.

be used in animals weighing less than 20 kg. The newer models (8100, 1846SX) have internal monitoring for sensitivity, can be run manually or automatically, provide digital readings within a maximum of 120 sec, monitor for limb movement artifact, provide alarm limits, and may be purchased with an adjoining printer.

Using the oscillometric method is relatively easy but requires adherence to specific guidelines. Foremost is the need to use the proper cuff width. In dogs, the proper width is 40% of the limb circumference (Geddes et al., 1980). Cuffs that are too narrow give falsely elevated values, and wide cuffs give falsely lower values. Cuff length is not as critical as long as the cuff is secured well. Second, the limitations of the instrument used must be realized. The Dinamap units in the neonatal mode have limitations in determinations for systolic pressure of 190 mm Hg, diastolic pressure of 160 mm Hg, MAP of 170 mm Hg, and pulse rate of 220 bpm. If pediatric cuffs can be used in larger dogs, these limitations increase an average of 50 mm Hg. These limitations prevent accurate assessment of severe hypertension in smaller animals (<20 kg) and recordings in cats with rapid heart rates. Third, as with all blood pressure measurements, animals must be kept quiet and still. The accuracy of oscillometric measurements has been shown to increase with serial readings over a short time. Five sequential readings are recommended.

System failures can occur in animals with lower heart rates, cardiac arrhythmias, abrupt limb movement, or poor positioning of the cuff. Reliable measurements have been reported with cuff placement over the antebrachium, tarsus, or tail base to occlude the underlying respective artery. I have found that tail base placement over a small clipped area is well tolerated by most dogs. To correct for distance from the heart, 1.8 mm Hg is added to each pressure measurement for every inch the cuff is above the heart level, whereas 1.8 mm Hg is subtracted for every inch the cuff is below the heart level.

Monitoring blood pressure with the oscillometric method in awake and anesthetized animals has yielded reliable and reproducible results. In awake normal dogs in a clinical setting, the mean pressure readings were 144, 110, and 91 mm Hg for systolic, mean, and diastolic pressures, respectively (Coulter and Keith, 1984). For dogs, the upper limits of normal are 180, 140, and 125 mm Hg, respectively. In my opinion, oscillometric recordings from awake cats are not consistently reproducible because of the nature of the species and the limitations of the instrument. One report, however, published upper limit normal values of 149, 124, and 102 for systolic, mean, and diastolic pressures (Edwards, 1990).

Concerning the reliability and reproducibility of this technique, the Dinamap oscillometric method has been shown to yield correlation coefficients of 0.908, 0.925, and 0.908 for systolic, mean, and diastolic pressures in anesthetized dogs (Hamlin et al., 1982). As with any blood pressure monitoring, excitement with resultant sympathetic stimulation changes pressure readings. I have found that the large majority of hospitalized dogs adapt well to being monitored if kept recumbent in a quiet room and allowed a 5-min adaptation period. Recordings are then taken every minute for five sequential readings. This method provides reproducible measurements to allow for an accurate assessment of blood pressure trends. The emphasis on following trends is a crucial factor of the merits of indirect blood pressure monitoring.

Another disadvantage of the oscillometric method is the expense. Dinamap units cost from $3000 to $6500, depending on the model. Less expensive oscillometric instruments have been evaluated in anesthetized dogs (Hunter et al., 1990). One monitor (Model 1091)* was less accurate (correlation coefficients of 0.77, 0.87, and 0.87) but sells at a significantly lower cost.

Ultrasonic Method

Ultrasound kinetoarteriography involves the detection of arterial wall motion by the use of ultrasonic waves. With gradual deflation of suprasystolic cuff pressure, the underlying artery initially opens and then closes when the arterial pulse falls below cuff pressures. As cuff pressure is further reduced, the time between the opening and closing signals increases. Finally, the closing and opening signals merge and disappear as the vessel remains open throughout the pulse. The wall opening and closing motion associated with systolic and diastolic pressures produces an ultrasound frequency shift that can be detected as Doppler sounds and recorded visually or reproduced acoustically. Electronic detection of these signals can be incorporated to trigger indicators at the appropriate systolic and diastolic pressures.

Various ultrasonic Doppler sensing devices to monitor blood pressure can be used in cats and dogs (Arteriosonde†; Model 1022A‡). The cranial tibial artery is compressed with an inflatable cuff with an attached transducer (8 MHz). The transducer must be flush with the cuff surface. Coupling gel is applied to the shaved area over the medial aspect of the distal limb where the pulse is palpable. The cuff must be secured tightly, usually with tape. The cuff is then inflated to a pressure approximately 30 mm Hg higher than needed to obliterate the

*Lumiscope Co., Inc., Edison, NJ.
†Roche-Medical Co., Cranbury, NJ.
‡Kantron Medical Instruments, Everett, MA.

pulse and is then slowly deflated. Systolic pressure is recorded as the first audible sound; diastolic pressure is recorded when the sounds abruptly decrease or become muffled. Reconstruction of the whole arterial pressure wave is possible with the proper instrumentation. No evidence exists to document the necessity for specific cuff widths.

Ultrasonic sphygmomanometry offers the advantages of being adaptable to all sizes of animals, providing measurements during wide fluctuations of high and low blood pressure situations, and being portable. The disadvantages are similar to those of the oscillometric method. Abrupt body movements change measurements. The effects of autonomic stimulation are still prevalent. Determination of the actual systolic and diastolic cutoff points is operator dependent. Systolic pressure can be identified too early, thereby giving an erroneously high value as a result of emission infrasonics (Garner et al., 1975). Finally, MAP cannot be determined with this method.

The values reported with ultrasound recordings in dogs are very similar to those of the oscillometric method. Correlation coefficients are higher for anesthetized dogs, however, with values of 0.99 and 0.97 reported for systolic and diastolic pressures, respectively (Garner et al., 1975). Values for lightly sedated cats were slightly less, 0.94 and 0.82, respectively, with the upper limits of systolic and diastolic pressures being 129 and 96 mm Hg (Kobiyashi et al., 1990).

Much controversy exists in the comparison of direct and indirect methods of blood pressure. Because the energy measured differs between the two techniques (direct measures pressure; indirect measures flow), there is no biophysical reason to expect their values to be identical. What is important to realize is that blood pressure is a function of the way it is measured. Many years of monitoring in people have led to precise, established protocols for indirect methods. Veterinary medicine is just starting to develop this information. Clinicians need to be aware of the value of monitoring blood pressure trends in animals with underlying diseases or those receiving medications or surgical manipulations predisposing them to pressure fluctuations. Although information is needed to validate further the different techniques in clinical situations, the methodology is currently available for clinicians to add this vital piece of clinical datum to every patient's examination.

References and Suggested Reading

Coulter, D. B., and Keith, J. C.: Blood pressures obtained by indirect measurement in conscious dogs. J.A.V.M.A. 184:1375, 1984.
Results of indirect oscillometric blood pressure measurements in normal and renal failure in awake dogs in a hospital setting.

Edwards, N. J.: Non-invasive blood pressure measurements in the clinical setting. ACVIM Scientific Proceeding, 1990, p. 273.
Results of oscillometric blood pressure measurements in awake normal cats and dogs using a Dinamap monitor.

Garner, H. E., Hahn, A. W., Hartley, J. W., et al.: Indirect blood pressure measurement in the dog. Lab. Anim. Sci. 25:197, 1975.
Results of ultrasound blood pressure measurements in normal, awake dogs.

Geddes, L. A.: The Direct and Indirect Measurement of Blood Pressure. Chicago: Year Book Medical Publishers, 1970.
A monograph reviewing the scientific development and methodology of all known types of blood pressure monitoring techniques.

Geddes, L. A., Combs, W., Denton, W., et al.: Indirect mean arterial pressure in the anesthetized dog. Am. J. Physiol. 238:H664, 1980.
Results of experiments that document the validity of oscillometric measurements when the cuff width is 40% of the limb circumference in the dog.

Hamlin, R. L., Kittleson, M. D., Rice, D., et al.: Noninvasive measurement of systemic arterial pressure in dogs by automatic sphygmomanometry. Am. J. Vet. Res. 43:1271, 1982.
Results of the comparison of oscillometric to direct blood pressure measurements in anesthetized dogs.

Haskins, S. C.: Monitoring the critically ill patient. Vet. Clin. North Am. Small Anim. Pract. 19:1059, 1989.
Review of the methodology of percutaneous arterial catheterization to record direct ABP.

Hunter, J. S., McGrath, C. J., Thatcher, C. D., et al.: Adaptation of human oscillometric blood pressure monitors for use in dogs. Am. J. Vet. Res. 51:1439, 1990.
Results of comparing two inexpensive oscillometric monitoring devices to direct measurements in anesthetized dogs.

Kittleson, M. D., and Olivier, N. B.: Measurement of systemic arterial blood pressure. Vet. Clin. North Am. Small Anim. Pract. 13:321, 1983.
A review of the biophysics and methodology of blood pressure monitoring in small animal medicine.

Kobiyashi, D. L., Peterson, M. E., Graves, T. K., et al.: Hypertension in cats with chronic renal failure or hyperthyroidism. J. Intern. Vet. Med. 4:58, 1990.
Results of Doppler ultrasound blood pressure measurements in normal, hyperthyroid cats and in cats with chronic renal failure.

Scully, P. S., Chan, P. S., Cervani, P., et al.: A method of measuring direct arterial blood pressure. Canine Pract. 10:24, 1983.
Results and methodology of needle puncture direct ABP monitoring in awake dogs.

Wessale, J. L., Smith, L. A., Reid, M., et al.: Indirect auscultatory systolic and diastolic pressures in the anesthetized dog. J.A.V.M.A. 46:2129, 1985.
Results of piezoelement amplification of Korotkoff's sounds for indirect blood pressure measurement in anesthetized dogs.

UPDATE: TREATMENT OF HYPERTENSION IN DOGS AND CATS

MERYL P. LITTMAN

Philadelphia, Pennsylvania

Spontaneous systemic hypertension (HT) in dogs and cats is being documented with increasing frequency. This is in part because clinicians are beginning to measure blood pressure (BP) in clinical settings and they have become aware of the common clinical signs of HT, of underlying diseases that predispose animals to HT, and of target organ damage due to HT (see "References and Supplemental Reading"). Although many review articles about HT have appeared in the veterinary literature in the past decade, much of the material concerning treatment is derived from studies of humans. Double-blind prospective studies to prove that antihypertensive therapy in dogs and cats improves prognosis have not been done. It seems prudent, however, to treat animals that have clinical signs due to hypertensive damage to target organs. It is more nebulous whether to treat animals with mild HT when no clinical signs of the HT exist but when mild HT is discovered during routine examination for one of the common predisposing diseases (e.g., renal disease, hyperadrenocorticism, or hyperthyroidism).

This article reviews the history, physical examination, and diagnostic test results commonly encountered in dogs and cats with HT that has caused clinical signs due to target organ damage at the Veterinary Hospital of the University of Pennsylvania (VHUP). Available treatment modalities that seem to help decrease morbidity and mortality due to such HT are reviewed.

HISTORY

Most animals that were presented with clinical signs due to HT at VHUP were male (76.7% of 30 dogs, 63% of 24 cats). Hypertensive dogs were younger (mean age 8.9 ± 3.6 years, range 2 to 14 years) than hypertensive cats (mean age 15.1 ± 3.8 years, range 7 to 20 years). No breed predilections were noted. The common clinical signs (Table 1) were acute (1 day) or chronic (up to 1 year; mean, 2 months). Signs were related to the primary dis-

eases that caused secondary HT or to target organ damage to the eyes, kidneys, or cardiovascular or cerebrovascular system. Polyuria/polydipsia may have been due to renal insufficiency (cause or effect of HT), hyperadrenocorticism, hyperthyroidism, or pressure diuresis. Seizures, syncope, or decerebrate posture was encountered in hypertensive cats more often than in hypertensive dogs.

PHYSICAL EXAMINATION

Bilateral ocular changes were most common; retinal hemorrhages were more frequent than retinal detachments. Hyphema, glaucoma, corneal ulcers, and hyper-reflectivity were less commonly encountered.

Small kidneys were palpated in many of the hypertensive cats. It is not known whether renal disease is the main cause of HT in cats, whether HT is primary and causes renal disease, or whether renal disease and HT are coincident and common in elderly cats.

Low-grade mitral murmurs were auscultated in the hypertensive dogs (57%) and cats (42%). Chronic HT is most often associated with increased total peripheral resistance (TPR). The increased afterload is thought to cause ventricular hypertrophy, dilation, and mitral valve insufficiency.

Three of 24 hypertensive cats had hyperthyroidism. Cats with thyroid enlargement should be screened for HT.

Table 1. *Common Clinical Signs* Seen in Dogs and Cats with Spontaneous Systemic Hypertension*

Dogs	Cats
Blindness	Blindness
Polyuria, polydipsia	Polyuria, polydipsia
Vomiting, anorexia	Weight loss
Signs of hyperadrenocorticism	Neurologic signs
Epistaxis	Labored breathing
Neurologic signs	Epistaxis

*In decreasing order of frequency as seen at VHUP.

838

DIAGNOSTIC TEST RESULTS

BP measurements can be done either directly by arterial puncture or indirectly with a cuff device (see this volume, p. 834). At VHUP, we have relied most heavily on direct BP measurements with awake, nonsedated animals in lateral recumbency. A 25-gauge needle connected to a physiologic pressure transducer and an oscilloscope/recorder is used (Littman et al., 1988). Normal values for untrained animals are less than 160/100 mm Hg systolic/diastolic. Care should be taken when interpreting data, because excitement and labile sympathetic activity may increase heart rate (HR) and BP. Repeated measurements over several days and assessment of HR and attitude of the animal during measurements are important observations that help to determine if HT really exists. The BP measurements in hypertensive animals at VHUP ranged from 135 to 390/105 to 200 mm Hg systolic/diastolic. Hypertensive animals presenting with ocular damage most often had BP measurements on the order of 235/145 mm Hg systolic/diastolic.

Indirect BP measurements using the Doppler cuff were done on hypertensive cats, many of which also had direct BP measurements. Although the values did not always predict direct BP measurements within 10 mm Hg, I believe that indirect measurements correlate reasonably well with direct measurements and can be used as a screening tool. The indirect BP measurements on the VHUP hypertensive cats ranged from 155 to greater than 300 mm Hg systolic (mean 220 ± 42 mm Hg).

Common abnormal diagnostic test results in hypertensive animals included urine specific gravity of 1.020 or less, mild azotemia, proteinuria, left ventricular hypertrophy, and cardiomegaly. The degree of azotemia did not correlate with the degree of HT. Many of the cats had elevated total solids and serum sodium concentration. The most common renal biopsy finding was glomerulosclerosis (cause or effect of hypertension). A few dogs had immune-mediated glomerulonephritis, amyloidosis, or chronic interstitial nephritis. Necropsy in two hypertensive cats with seizures showed multifocal cerebral hemorrhages, arteriosclerosis, and nephrosclerosis.

About 30% of the hypertensive VHUP dogs had hyperadrenocorticism (either pituitary dependent or due to adrenal tumor), which was thought to be causing HT. Another 30% had various renal diseases. A few dogs were diagnosed as having essential (primary) HT (Bovée et al., 1989; Littman et al., 1988). Most of the hypertensive VHUP cats had renal disease. Few hypertensive cats also had hyperthyroidism.

Investigators have found HT in dogs with glomerular diseases (80%), other renal diseases (61%), hyperadrenocorticism (59%, Kallett and Cowgill, 1982), and pheochromocytoma (50%, Ross, 1989) and in cats with renal diseases (61%, Kobayashi et al., 1990; 65%, Ross, 1989) and hyperthyroidism (87%, Kobayashi et al., 1990). However, it is not apparent how many of these animals had target organ damage from HT (i.e., it is unknown whether mild hypertension is clinically important in dogs and cats). Target organ damage was found in hypertensive cats with renal disease, anemia, or hyperthyroidism (Littman, 1990a; Morgan, 1986).

TREATMENT

Management of HT in dogs or cats begins with dietary restriction of salt (0.1 to 0.3% sodium by dry weight, Cowgill and Kallett, 1983, 1986), a careful weight reduction plan for obese animals (Rocchini et al., 1987), and management of any primary disease that may be causing the HT. Some but not most dogs with essential HT were salt-sensitive (Bovée, 1990). Animals with renal disease or hyperadrenocorticism may not be able to excrete salt (NaCl) and fluid normally. The use of other sodium salts (e.g., sodium bicarbonate for hypertensive animals with renal failure and acidosis) does not seem to increase BP (Kurtz and Morris, 1983). Treatment of hyperthyroidism in cats may eliminate HT (Kobayashi et al., 1990); however, at VHUP, treatment of hyperadrenocorticism in dogs with target organ damage usually was not adequate to control HT. The mechanism of perseverant HT after treatment for hyperadrenocorticism may be arteriolar damage causing permanent changes in TPR or increased adrenocorticotropic hormone levels, which may alter BP.

Monitoring of BP should be done every 1 to 2 weeks. If HT continues, drug therapy is given (Table 2). Because BP is related to cardiac output (CO) and TPR (BP = CO × TPR) and CO is related to blood volume (extracellular fluid volume [ECFV]) and HR, antihypertensive management can be used to decrease ECFV (low-salt diet, diurctics), decrease HR (beta-blockers, central alpha-2 agonists), and decrease TPR (alpha-1 blockers, alpha-2 agonists, angiotensin-converting enzyme [ACE] inhibitors, and calcium channel blockers).

The choice of drug or combination of drugs is individualized and depends on an animal's hydration status, renal function, HR, cardiac function, underlying primary disease process, and response to therapy (see this volume, p. 309).

Diuretics

At VHUP, hydrochlorothiazide is the most commonly used antihypertensive diuretic for dogs without azotemia. Cases with renal disease do not re-

Table 2. Oral Antihypertensive Drugs Commonly Used at VHUP

Drug	Dose for Dogs	Dose for Cats
Diuretics		
Hydrochlorothiazide	1–5 mg/kg q 12 hr	2–4 mg/kg q 12 hr
(HydroDIURIL, Merck Sharp & Dohme)		
Furosemide	0.55—2.2 mg/kg q 8–24 hr	Same as for dogs
(Lasix, Hoechst-Roussel)		
Beta-blockers		
Propranolol	5–80 mg q 8–12 hr or	2.5–5.0 mg q 8–12 hr
(Inderal, Wyeth-Ayerst)	up to 200 mg/day	
Atenolol	2 mg/kg q 24 hr	Same as for dogs
(Tenormin, ICI Pharma)		
Alpha-blockers		
Prazosin	1 mg q 8–24 hr	
(Minipress, Pfizer)		
ACE inhibitors		
Captopril	1–10 mg/kg q 8–12 hr	6.25–12.5 mg q 8–12 hr
(Capoten, Squibb)		
Enalapril	0.5–3.0 mg/kg q 12–24 hr	
(Vasotec, Merck Sharp & Dohme)		
Lisinopril	0.4–2.0 mg/kg q 24 hr	
(Prinivil, Merck Sharp & Dohme)		

spond as well, and furosemide is given. Care must be used lest the animal become dehydrated. A starting dose may be low and increased to effect, or a second drug is added.

Beta-Blockers

Atenolol (a cardioselective beta-blocker) is now more often used at VHUP for dogs and cats with HT than is propranolol because of its once-a-day dosage regimen and relative lack of side effects. Propranolol, a nonselective beta-blocker, can potentially cause bronchospasm or glucose intolerance. Hyperthyroid cats are treated with beta blockade for 2 weeks while methimazole (Tapazole, Lilly) begins to bring them to a euthyroid state. Continued monitoring of elderly cats is important because renal disease may be concomitant with HT or hyperthyroidism. In hypertensive dogs, the dose of beta-blockers has a broad range. Monitoring of BP and HR is important. Doses may be increased, another type of antihypertensive drug can be added to the regimen, or beta-blockers may be discontinued while another class of drug is tried. Beta-blockers are not used in combination with calcium channel blockers, because both are negative inotropes.

Vasodilators

The alpha-1 blocker prazosin has been effective in some dogs with resistant HT. It may be used in conjunction with other drugs or as a primary drug. There is scant experience in clinical veterinary medicine with direct vasodilators (hydralazine) or centrally acting alpha-2 agonists (guanabenz, guanfacine, clonidine) for treatment of HT. Clonidine worked well as an intravenous bolus in one dog

with HT but was not effective even at high doses when given orally. Cessation of clonidine therapy in humans has been associated with a dangerous rebound effect in which HT rapidly worsens with a missed dose.

Angiotensin-Converting Enzyme Inhibitors

ACE inhibitors act by inhibiting ACE and kininase. The result is decreased TPR due to decreased angiotensin II (a vasoconstrictor), increased kinin (a vasodilator), and decreased aldosterone causing decreased ECFV. These drugs are helpful even in cases of non–renin-dependent HT and may help decrease proteinuria. ACE inhibitors were effective in dogs and cats (alone or with diuretics or beta-blockers or both) with HT due to renal disease, hyperadrenocorticism, and essential HT. Neutropenia developed in one cat; this adverse side effect was reversed when captopril therapy ceased. The antihypertensive dose is much higher than for cardiac failure. This is because renal perfusion is already poor when CO is low. Doses of more than 6 mg/kg/day of captopril in cardiac cases have caused increased azotemia and can potentially damage renal function permanently. However, doses as high as 30 mg/kg/day have been used in dogs with essential HT, with no apparent side effects (Bovée et al., 1989; Littman et al., 1988).

Calcium Channel Blockers

I have not yet evaluated diltiazem, nicardipine, nifedipine, and verapamil. These drugs cause vasodilation by inhibiting calcium transport into vascular smooth-muscle cells. Evidence suggests that left ventricular hypertrophy in humans can be reversed. Verapamil at 2 mg/kg every 8 hr caused anorexia, lethargy, and vomiting in two dogs; 0.5 to 1.0 mg/kg every 12 hr was not effective in lowering BP (see this volume, p. 832; Paulsen et al., 1989).

True hypertensive emergencies requiring intravenous drugs to lower BP within minutes to hours are rare in veterinary medicine. Intravenous drugs such as nitroprusside, labetalol, and diazoxide are used in humans requiring emergency therapy (Calhoun and Oparil, 1990). In the few cases in which nitroprusside was given to critically ill animals at VHUP, the renal function deteriorated rapidly (possibly as a result of the primary disease process, the HT, or the decreased renal perfusion induced by overzealous therapy).

Monitoring of BP, HR, hydration, renal status, cardiac status, ophthalmic changes, and neurologic status is important follow-up for hypertensive dogs and cats. In our experience at VHUP, acute ophthalmologic changes can improve rapidly with antihypertensive treatment (retinas reattach, hemorrhages clear) and vision can return. However, renal function usually does not improve and often deteriorates in dogs that were presented with renal azotemia. This may be because the primary renal disease process may not respond to therapy or because of overly aggressive antihypertensive therapy. Alternatively, hypertensive cats that were presented with mild renal azotemia often could be maintained for years without further deterioration of renal function. Dogs with essential HT were maintained for years without renal compromise (Bovée et al., 1989; Tippett et al., 1987).

References and Suggested Reading

Bovée, K. C.: Variance of blood pressure response to oral sodium intake in hypertensive dogs. J. Vet. Intern. Med. 4:126, 1990.

Bovée, K. C., Littman, M. P., Crabtree, B. J., et al.: Essential hypertension in a dog. J.A.V.M.A. 195:81, 1989.

Calhoun, D. A., and Oparil, S.: Treatment of hypertensive crisis [in humans]. N. Engl. J. Med. 323:1177, 1990.

Cowgill, L. D., and Kallett, A. J.: Recognition and management of hypertension in the dog. In Kirk, R. W. (ed.): Current Veterinary Therapy VIII. Philadelphia: W. B. Saunders, 1983, p. 1025.

Cowgill, L. D., and Kallett, A. J.: Systemic hypertension. In Kirk, R. W. (ed.): Current Veterinary Therapy IX. Philadelphia: W. B. Saunders, 1986, p. 360.

Dimski, D. S., and Hawkins, E. C.: Canine systemic hypertension. Comp. Cont. Ed. Pract. Vet. 10:1152, 1988.

Houston, M. C.: New insights and new approaches for the treatment of essential hypertension: Selection of therapy based on coronary heart disease risk factor analysis, hemodynamic profiles, quality of life, and subsets of hypertension [in humans]. Am. Heart J. 117:911, 1989.

Kallett, A. J., and Cowgill, L. D.: Hypertensive states in the dog. ACVIM Scientific Proceedings, 1982, p. 79.

Kobayashi, D. L., Peterson, M. E., Graves, T. K., et al.: Hypertension in cats with chronic renal failure or hyperthyroidism. J. Vet. Intern. Med. 4:58, 1990.

Kurtz, T. W., and Morris, R. C., Jr.: Dietary chloride as a determinant of "sodium-dependent" hypertension. Science 222:1139, 1983.

Littman, M. P.: Naturally occurring hypertension in the dog. ACVIM Scientific Proceedings, 1986. Section 13, p. 45.

Littman, M. P.: Spontaneous systemic hypertension in cats. ACVIM Abstract 82, 1990. J. Vet. Intern. Med. 4:126, 1990a.

Littman, M. P.: Chronic spontaneous systemic hypertension in dogs and cats. ACVIM Scientific Proceedings, 1990b, p. 209.

Littman, M. P., Robertson, J. L., and Bovée, K. C.: Spontaneous systemic hypertension in dogs: Five cases (1981–1983). J.A.V.M.A. 193:486, 1988.

Morgan, R. V.: Systemic hypertension in four cats: Ocular and medical findings. J. Am. Anim. Hosp. Assoc. 22:615, 1986.

1988 Joint National Committee: The 1988 report of the Joint National Committee on detection, evaluation, and treatment of high blood pressure [in humans]. Arch. Intern. Med. 148:1023, 1988.

Paulsen, M. E., Allen, T. A., Jaenke, R. S., et al.: Arterial hypertension in two canine siblings' ocular and systemic manifestations. J. Am. Anim. Hosp. Assoc. 25:287, 1989.

Rocchini, A. P., Moorehead, C., Wentz, E., et al.: Obesity-induced hypertension in the dog. Hypertension 9(suppl. 3):III-64, 1987.

Ross, L. A.: Hypertensive disease. In Ettinger, S. J. (ed.): Textbook of Veterinary Internal Medicine, 3rd ed., Vol. 2. Philadelphia: W. B. Saunders, 1989, p. 2047.

Ross, L. A., and Labato, M. A.: Use of drugs to control hypertension in renal failure. In Kirk, R. W. (ed.): Current Veterinary Therapy X. Philadelphia: W. B. Saunders, 1989, p. 1201.

Tippett, F. E., Padgett, G. A., and Eyster, G.: Primary hypertension in a colony of dogs. Hypertension 9:49, 1987.

MEDICAL MANAGEMENT OF CANINE CHRONIC RENAL FAILURE

SCOTT A. BROWN,
JEANNE A. BARSANTI,
and DELMAR R. FINCO
Athens, Georgia

OVERVIEW

In the healthy animal, the kidney controls the composition of extracellular fluid while serving as an excretory and endocrine organ. In fulfilling these diverse roles, the kidney actually behaves as the sum of the functions of hundreds of thousands of individual nephrons. For illustrative purposes, renal functions may be segregated on the basis of the anatomic site of the nephron primarily responsible for performance of the individual function. The excretion of phosphate and nitrogenous wastes occurs primarily through the process of filtration at the glomerulus. The proximal tubule is responsible for the final step in the activation of vitamin D, the production of erythropoietin, and the reabsorption of sodium and bicarbonate. The urine-concentrating mechanism allows the production of concentrated (and dilute) urine in accordance with the animal's needs for water conservation. Distal tubular functions include proton and potassium secretion.

In most renal diseases, some nephrons are destroyed entirely while others, termed remnant nephrons, remain intact and functional. If enough nephrons are destroyed, the remnant nephrons will no longer be able to collectively fulfill the functional demands placed upon them. Because the kidney serves such a diverse set of functions, organ failure can (and generally does) disrupt a wide variety of homeostatic functions simultaneously.

The consequences of altered glomerular function (Fig. 1) include retention of nitrogenous wastes with resulting uremia and retention of phosphates leading to hyperphosphatemia that subsequently contributes to the genesis of renal secondary hyperparathyroidism. Diseased glomeruli often lose their permselectivity, causing proteinuria. If severe, proteinuria can lead to hypoalbuminemia or hypercoagulability. The consequences of the aggregate loss of functional proximal tubules include reduced erythropoietin production, decreased activation of vitamin D, and reduced bicarbonate reabsorption. These abnormalities lead, respectively, to the de-velopment of nonregenerative anemia, renal secondary hyperparathyroidism (with or without renal osteodystrophy), and metabolic acidosis. Disruption of the renal concentrating mechanism is frequently present in animals with advanced, chronic renal failure. Consequently, urine-diluting and -concentrating ability is compromised, predisposing the animal to volume overload or dehydration. Potassium and proton secretion occurs in normal distal tubules, and the loss of this capacity in chronic renal failure may result in hyperkalemia or acidosis. In some animals with polyuric renal disease, potassium secretion may actually be enhanced in the diseased distal tubule, contributing to hypokalemia. Reduced glomerular perfusion coupled with disorders in renal handling of sodium and water contributes to the development of systemic hypertension in dogs with renal failure.

In remnant nephrons that remain initially free of disease, compensatory processes result in enhancement of structure and function, referred to as compensatory hypertrophy and hypertension. It has been proposed that these responses are maladaptive, causing nephron injury and progressive renal disease (Brenner et al., 1982; Polzin et al., 1983). Some nephrologists have discounted the importance of this phenomenon in dogs (Bovée et al., 1979). Currently available clinical and experimental data do not allow resolution of this issue.

Treatment of an animal with chronic renal failure presents the clinician with two distinct challenges that may be successfully met. First, the veterinarian must recognize the presence of treatable complications or abnormalities. This requires the early institution of a system for routine, thorough patient evaluation (Table 1) and an understanding of the causes and consequences of all the abnormalities identified. The second challenge facing the clinician is to institute effective treatment that minimizes or resolves the identified problem without harming the patient. The purpose of this chapter is to address these two challenges and suggest medical therapy for the management of dogs with chronic renal failure.

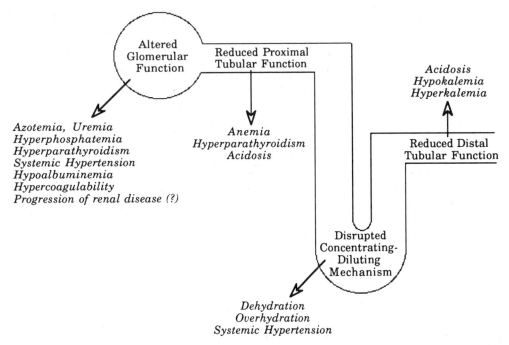

Figure 1. Abnormalities associated with disruption or loss of function at various nephron sites. A disease must destroy many or most nephrons to produce these clinically detectable abnormalities.

PROBLEM IDENTIFICATION

Problems are generally identified by a combination of history, physical examination, and clinical laboratory evaluation of blood and urine. Most abnormalities can be present in a dog with chronic renal failure for weeks or months before they result in symptoms that the owner will recognize. Consequently, the veterinarian should try to schedule routine evaluations that will identify these problems (see Table 1).

Anemia

The severity of anemia in dogs with chronic renal failure varies markedly. It will contribute to the clinical signs of uremia in some animals, specifically leading to inappetence and lethargy. The cause of the anemia should be addressed prior to institution of therapy. Anemia caused by reduced renal production of erythropoietin is characterized by lack of both regenerative response and adequate bone marrow iron stores. It should not be assumed that all anemic dogs with renal failure suffer only from a lack of erythropoietin. If erythropoietin production is marginally reduced, malnutrition or the burden of ectoparasites or endoparasites can contribute to the severity of anemia. In a patient with mild or moderate anemia, these contributory factors should be eliminated and the hematocrit monitored monthly for 1 to 2 months prior to the institution

of further therapy. Therapy for dogs with marked nonregenerative anemia (hematocrit <20) might include the administration of anabolic steroids, but these do not usually produce any beneficial increment in the hematocrit. Recombinant human erythropoietin (Epogen, Amgen, Thousand Oaks, CA; Marogen, Chugai-Upjohn, Rosemont, IL) is currently being employed successfully in dogs with severe anemia caused by chronic renal failure. Although results are often dramatic, it is expensive in larger dogs and requires thrice weekly subcutaneous administration for the life of the animal. Concurrent administration of iron may enhance the response. Few adverse reactions have been noted to date, and these agents offer a great deal of promise (see

Table 1. *Clinical Evaluation of the Dog With Chronic Renal Failure**

History, physical examination (including body weight)
Serum albumin and total protein
Serum creatinine
Blood urea nitrogen (BUN)
Calcium, phosphorus
Sodium, potassium, and bicarbonate (or total carbon dioxide measurement)
Hematocrit
Urinalysis and urine culture
Other tests may include measurement of parathyroid hormone, blood pressure, urinary fractional excretion of phosphate, and a plasma lipid profile

*Routine tests for all dogs with chronic renal failure should be conducted at least every 3 months.

this volume, p. 484). However, allergic or immunologic reactions to the human albumin in the Epogen vehicle solution or to the recombinant human erythropoietin molecule itself could produce adverse effects.

Glomerular Hypertension

Although veterinary textbooks have frequently noted the presence of glomerular capillary hypertension and hyperfiltration in remnant nephrons of dogs with renal disease, these parameters have only recently been measured. While surviving nephrons in kidneys from dogs with chronic renal failure most likely exhibit glomerular hypertension and hyperfiltration, it is possible to define the magnitude of these changes only through the use of specialized micropuncture studies that are not available clinically. The efficacy of therapy designed to limit glomerular capillary hypertension (e.g., dietary protein restriction) remains to be clearly established in dogs (Brown et al., 1991b). For further discussion of this topic, see the later section "Progressive Loss of Renal Function."

Hypercoagulability

Alterations in glomerular permeability causing severe proteinuria may lead to hypoalbuminemia and other changes in plasma composition or platelet function that contribute to the genesis of hypercoagulability. This may lead to thromboses in pulmonary or systemic vessels. The pathogenesis, treatment, and prevention of this complication of proteinuric renal diseases are discussed elsewhere in this volume (p. 827).

Hyperparathyroidism, Hyperphosphatemia, Hypocalcemia, and Renal Osteodystrophy

Secretion of parathyroid hormone (PTH) is stimulated by hypocalcemia, reduced circulating levels of $1,25(OH)_2$ vitamin D, and (possibly) hyperphosphatemia. The stimulation of PTH secretion by hypocalcemia and hypovitaminosis D is apparently due to direct effects on the parathyroid gland. An independent role for phosphate retention is that it is hypothesized to act either directly on the parathyroid gland or indirectly through a mass action effect to lower plasma calcium concentration. In dogs with chronic renal failure, hyperphosphatemia and reduced renal conversion of $25(OH)$ vitamin D to $1,25(OH)_2$ vitamin D are frequently present and contribute to the development of renal secondary hyperparathyroidism.

Consequences that may theoretically result from chronic, severe renal secondary hyperparathyroidism include osteodystrophy, glucose intolerance, anemia, acidosis, hyperlipidemia, encephalopathy, and progressive renal dysfunction. Only the first two have been well documented in dogs. The long-term sequelae of renal secondary hyperparathyroidism and the potential benefits of its suppression in dogs with chronic renal failure are poorly understood. However, in addition to reducing the degree of hyperparathyroidism, dietary restriction of phosphorus intake has been demonstrated to reduce the rate of decline of renal function in dogs with induced renal disease (see the later section "Progressive Loss of Renal Function").

In animals exhibiting an abnormality attributable to excess PTH (e.g., osteodystrophy), the degree of hyperparathyroidism should be documented through determination of the plasma concentration of PTH or urinary fractional excretion of phosphate (see this volume, p. 820). Further efforts to reduce the degree of hyperparathyroidism may include oral calcium supplementation (e.g., calcium carbonate) and the administration of active vitamin D metabolites (Rocaltrol, Roche Laboratories).

In addition to dietary calcium supplementation, several of the calcium salts (e.g., calcium carbonate, calcium lactate, calcium citrate) can be utilized as alkalinizing and intestinal phosphorus–binding agents. Intestinal phosphorus binding is favored when calcium salts are given with meals. In contrast, intestinal calcium absorption is enhanced when these agents are given between meals. A significant risk with these agents is their potential to lead to hypercalcemia, and appropriate monitoring should include weekly calcium determinations when dietary calcium supplementation is first instituted.

Because reduced circulating levels of $1,25(OH)_2$ vitamin D may stimulate PTH secretion, the administration of activated vitamin D analogues (e.g., 3 ng Rocaltrol/lb body weight orally once daily or 6.6 ng Rocaltrol/kg body weight orally once daily) may reduce the degree of hyperparathyroidism. However, most of the currently available vitamin D analogues will enhance intestinal absorption of calcium and phosphate and should not be given with meals. Activated vitamin D metabolites should be avoided in animals with pre-existent hyperphosphatemia until after the successful institution of dietary phosphorus restriction or intestinal phosphorus binders, and these agents should rarely, if ever, be used in conjunction with dietary calcium supplementation. Plasma concentrations of calcium and phosphate should be monitored weekly upon initiation of $1,25(OH)_2$ vitamin D therapy and the agent discontinued if hypercalcemia or marked hyperphosphatemia should occur.

Malnutrition

Malnutrition is frequently encountered in dogs with chronic renal failure. Inadequate energy intake can lead to a catabolic state, causing an elevation of plasma levels of urea and uremic toxins. Although little precise information is available on the caloric requirements of dogs with renal failure, a reasonable initial goal is 75 to 100 kcal/kg body weight per day. Weekly measurement of body weight and daily assessment of caloric intake can be performed at home by the owner. These measurements provide an accurate assessment of caloric intake and a barometer for the early detection of many of the complications of chronic renal failure.

Metabolic Acidosis

In dogs, dietary intake usually provides a net acid load to the animal. Ammoniagenesis in the proximal tubules consumes these hydrogen ions, contributing to acid-base homeostasis. When functional renal mass is reduced, dietary acid load may exceed the renal ability to consume acid by limiting the renal capacity to generate ammonia. In particular, diets containing egg protein may have a high content of sulfur-containing amino acids, which are acidifying. In contrast, diets containing vegetable-source proteins often provide very little acid load to the animal with renal failure. Diagnosis of metabolic acidosis usually relies upon measurement of plasma concentrations of total carbon dioxide or bicarbonate. Animals with a total carbon dioxide concentration above 15 mmol/L are usually not treated. Appropriate therapy for more acidemic animals is 1 to 9 mEq of alkali/kg of body weight. Alkalinizing agents (e.g., potassium citrate, sodium bicarbonate, calcium carbonate) should be initiated at the lower end of the dosage range and increased as necessary. The choice of alkalinizing agent will depend upon the presence or absence of other problems in the animal. For example, sodium-containing agents such as sodium bicarbonate should be avoided in animals with systemic hypertension. Calcium carbonate should be used cautiously in dogs with hyperphosphatemia, as the coexistence of hyperphosphatemia and hypercalcemia may lead to the mineralization of soft tissues.

Progressive Loss of Renal Function

Even when the primary renal disease is resolved or effectively controlled, a frequent cause of death in dogs with chronic renal failure is uremia secondary to declining renal function. To explain this progressive loss of renal function, it has been proposed that the kidneys of animals with renal disease

Table 2. *Factors That May Contribute to Progressive Loss of Renal Function*

Nephrocalcinosis
Hyperphosphatemia
Hyperparathyroidism
Glomerular hypertension
Loss of intrinsic control of renal hemodynamics
Glomerular hypertrophy
Systemic hypertension
Metabolic acidosis with enhanced renal ammoniagenesis
Hyperlipidemia
Diabetes mellitus

have an inherent tendency for renal function to decline until terminal uremia is reached. While many factors that could contribute to this tendency have been identified (Table 2), few have been studied in dogs. Many recommendations for dietary therapy in dogs with renal disease can be made on the basis of results of studies in the remnant kidney model of renal failure in rats (Table 3). However, the results of experimental or clinical studies in dogs do not support the contention that renal disease in dogs is identical to that in rats. Fortunately, results of recent, ongoing, and future studies in the dog may help to clarify some of these issues. In particular, some evidence is available on the role of dietary phosphate and protein restriction in dogs with renal failure (see *CVT X*, p. 1198).

Prior to initiation of therapy to slow the progressive decline of renal function, the temporal pattern of renal function should be carefully evaluated (Allen et al., 1987). It should not be assumed that all

Table 3. *Maneuvers That May Slow the Progressive Decline of Renal Function in Animals With Renal Failure*

Dietary therapy
Phosphorus restriction to reduce the degree of hyperphosphatemia and hyperparathyroidism
Protein restriction to prevent glomerular capillary hypertension, hypertrophy, and hyperparathyroidism*
Calcium supplementation to reduce the degree of hyperphosphatemia†
Sodium restriction to limit systemic hypertension†
Alkalinization to reduce renal ammoniagenesis†
Saturated fatty acid restriction to limit hyperlipidemia†
Fish oil (eicosapenataenoic fatty acids) supplementation to lower plasma cholesterol†
Calorie restriction to prevent glomerular capillary hypertension and hypertrophy†

Pharmacologic therapy
Angiotensin-converting enzyme inhibitors to limit glomerular capillary hypertension and hypertrophy†
Nonsteroidal anti-inflammatory agents to limit glomerular capillary hypertension and hypertrophy†
Lipid-lowering agents (e.g., mevinolin) to lower plasma cholesterol†

*Controversial.
†Not yet studied in dogs.

dogs with renal failure have declining renal function. Some dogs with chronic renal failure have stable renal function and are not candidates for therapy designed to slow progressive decrements in renal function. Documentation of the pattern of renal function requires at least three determinations of serum creatinine concentration. A plot of time (x-axis) versus serum creatinine or 1/serum creatinine may provide an identifiable pattern of change in renal function in some patients. The rate of change in renal function should be noted and can be subsequently compared to the rate of change in renal function following therapy.

Potential causes of declining renal function should be identified (see Table 2). A thorough evaluation including urinalysis and urine culture, determination of systemic blood pressure, and measurement of plasma PTH concentration or urinary fractional excretion of phosphate (see this volume, p. 818) should be performed. While a plasma lipid profile would identify dogs with hypercholesterolemia or hypertriglyceridemia, little is known about the long-term effects of these metabolic aberrations on the kidney or about the effectiveness of maneuvers intended to reduce the degree of hyperlipidemia in dogs with renal failure.

Dietary restriction of phosphorus intake has been shown to benefit dogs (and cats) with induced renal disease (Brown et al., 1991a). The degree of dietary restriction necessary to achieve this effect and the mechanism of the protection remain unknown. Nevertheless, dietary phosphorus restriction is recommended, and a reasonable goal for this therapy is normophosphatemia. Dietary phosphorus restriction should be at least in proportion to the degree of reduction of glomerular filtration rate, which means reduction of phosphorus intake to 25% or less of normal. The National Research Council minimum requirement for phosphorus intake in adult dogs has recently been defined as 89 mg/kg body weight per day, roughly equivalent to a dry matter phosphorus content of 0.5%. Low-phosphorus diets (e.g., Hill's Prescription Diet k/d, Hill's Pet Products) contain approximately 0.25 to 0.5% phosphorus, supplying 45 to 90 mg/kg body weight per day. Very low-phosphorus diets (e.g., Hill's Prescription Diet u/d) contain <0.25% phosphorus on a dry matter basis, supplying less than 45 mg/kg body weight per day. Although most commercially available preparations for dogs with renal failure are reduced in both phosphorus and protein content, it is not necessary to reduce dietary protein intake to obtain the beneficial effects of phosphorus restriction.

If normophosphatemia is not achieved by dietary phosphorus restriction alone, further benefit may be derived by the administration of intestinal phosphorus binders (e.g., aluminum hydroxide or calcium carbonate). These agents should be added to the therapeutic regimen only when hyperphosphatemia is not resolved by dietary restriction of phosphorus intake, and they should be dosed to effect. As indicated earlier, dietary phosphorus restriction or the use of phosphorus binders may also reduce the degree of renal secondary hyperparathyroidism, which may benefit the patient.

The possibility that reduced-protein diets will slow the progression of renal failure in dogs has been investigated (Bovée et al., 1979; Polzin et al., 1983, 1988). The rationale for this therapy is based upon results of studies in rats that demonstrate that low-protein diets limit the adaptive increases in glomerular capillary pressure (glomerular hypertension) in remnant nephrons. Only two studies have reported values for glomerular capillary pressure in dogs with chronic renal dysfunction (Brown et al., 1990, 1991b). Dogs with reduced renal function exhibit glomerular hypertension, and moderate protein restriction does not prevent the development of glomerular capillary hypertension. The level of dietary protein restriction necessary to prevent the development of glomerular capillary hypertension in dogs with chronic renal disease is undetermined, however, and appropriate studies are needed. Consequently, most of the critical issues pertaining to the effects of glomerular hypertension on the canine glomerulus also remain unanswered.

Beyond dietary restrictions of phosphate, protein, and sodium (see this volume, pp. 834 and 838), the effects of other strategies to preserve kidney function in dogs with chronic renal failure (see Table 3) have yet to be studied. These other strategies cannot be routinely recommended at this time.

Systemic Hypertension

Adequate characterization of systemic arterial pressure is difficult in the dog (see this volume, p. 834). However, systemic hypertension is a frequently reported observation in dogs with chronic renal failure. Because of the potential for systemic hypertension to produce secondary injury of the kidneys, eyes, or the cardiovascular system, dietary and pharmacologic management of systemic hypertension should be attempted in animals with chronic renal failure and an established diagnosis of systemic hypertension (see this volume, p. 838).

Uremia

When the production of uremic toxins exceeds renal excretion, toxins accumulate and can produce the characteristic clinical signs of uremia (e.g., inappetence, vomiting, lethargy). The most important determinant of the rate of excretion of uremic toxins is the glomerular filtration rate (GFR). Since the kidneys of dogs with chronic renal disease have generally already undergone the maximal degree of compensatory hyperfunction, further increases in GFR are unlikely and maneuvers to reduce the production of uremic toxins should be considered. As the by-products of protein metabolism include uremic toxins, dietary restriction of protein intake is routinely recommended in azotemic dogs with clinical signs attributable to uremia. Restriction of dietary protein intake should remain within the limits of 2 to 3 gm protein/kg body weight (approximately 13% to 17% protein on a dry matter basis). Further limitation of protein intake may lead to malnutrition, hypoalbuminemia, and hypercoagulability (Barsanti and Finco, 1985; Polzin et al., 1983).

Urinary Tract Infections

Because the normal defenses of the urinary tract against microbes are compromised in animals with renal failure, the potential for the development of a urinary tract infection is always present. Urinalysis and urine culture should be routinely performed (see Table 1). While the role of pyelonephritis in progressive renal failure remains unclear in dogs, the potential exists for a bacterial infection to lead to serious consequences in the urinary tract of a dog with pre-existing renal insufficiency. These infections should be treated with 3 to 6 weeks of antibiotic therapy based upon antibiotic sensitivity testing. Dogs with renal failure usually have a reduced urinary excretion of antibiotics and an increased urine volume; thus, the concentration of antibiotics in the urine is low in such dogs. Therapy should be evaluated by urinalysis 2 to 4 days following the institution of antibiotics and by follow-up evaluation with a urine culture immediately following the completion of therapy and 2 to 4 weeks later.

References and Suggested Reading

Allen, T. A., Jaenke, R. S., and Fettman, M. J.: A technique for estimating progression of chronic renal failure in the dog. J.A.V.M.A. 190:866, 1987.
  A report of the use of the inverse of serum creatinine concentration to monitor progression of renal failure in dogs.
Barsanti, J. A., and Finco, D. R.: Dietary management of chronic renal failure in dogs. J. Am. Anim. Hosp. Assoc. 21:371, 1985.
  A clinical study of the use of dietary therapy in the management of renal failure in dogs.
Bovée, K. C., Kronfeld, D. S., Ramberg, C., et al.: Long-term measurement of renal function in partially nephrectomized dogs fed 56, 27, or 19% protein. Invest. Urology 16:378, 1979.
  A report suggesting that protein restriction is not of benefit to dogs with renal dysfunction.
Brenner, B. M., Meyer, T. W., and Hostetter, T. H.: Dietary protein intake and the progressive nature of renal disease: The role of hemodynamically mediated glomerular injury in the pathogenesis of progressive glomerular sclerosis in aging, renal ablation, and intrinsic renal disease. N. Engl. J. Med. 307:652, 1982.
  A discussion of the hypothesis that glomerular capillary hypertension is injurious to remnant nephrons.
Brown, S. A., Crowell, W. A., Barsanti, J. A., et al.: Beneficial effects of dietary mineral restriction in 15/16 nephrectomized dogs. J. Am. Soc. Nephr. 1:1169, 1991a.
  A study of the beneficial effects of dietary phosphorus restriction in dogs with reduced renal function fed a low-protein diet.
Brown, S. A., Finco, D. R., Crowell, W. A., et al.: Single-nephron adaptations to partial renal ablation in the dog. Am. J. Physiol. 258:F495, 1990.
  A report of the physiologic response of remnant nephrons to renal dysfunction in dogs.
Brown, S. A., Finco, D. R., Crowell, W. A., et al.: Dietary protein intake and the glomerular adaptations to partial nephrectomy in dogs. J. Nutr. 1991b (in press).
  A limited study of the effects of protein restriction on glomerular hypertension in remnant nephrons of dogs.
Finco, D. R., Brown, S. A., Groves, C., et al.: The effect of dietary phosphate restriction in dogs with induced renal disease maintained on a high protein diet. Am. J. Vet. Res. 1991 (in press).
  A study of the beneficial effects of dietary phosphorus restriction in dogs with reduced renal function fed a high-protein diet.
Polzin, D. J., Leininger, J. R., Osborne, C. A., et al.: Development of renal lesions in dogs after 11/12 reduction of renal mass. Laboratory Invest. 58:172, 1988.
  A morphologic study documenting the occurrence of glomerular lesions in dogs with renal dysfunction.
Polzin, D. J., Osborne, C. A., Hayden, D. W., et al.: Influence of reduced protein diets on morbidity, mortality, and renal function in dogs with induced chronic renal failure. Am. J. Vet. Res. 45:506, 1983.
  A study documenting some adverse effects in animals with renal dysfunction of diets with either a very high or a very low protein content.

MEDICAL MANAGEMENT OF FELINE CHRONIC RENAL FAILURE

DAVID J. POLZIN,
CARL A. OSBORNE,
LARRY G. ADAMS,
and JODY P. LULICH
St. Paul, Minnesota

Chronic renal failure (CRF) is a common finding in middle-aged and older cats (Fig. 1). In our hospital, the prevalence of CRF in aged cats from 1984 to 1989 was three times greater than in aged dogs. In its earliest stages, CRF often remains clinically silent for extended periods in cats. At the time of diagnosis, renal dysfunction is often more severe in cats than in dogs, perhaps because of owners' delayed recognition of relatively subtle early signs of CRF in cats. Mild to moderate polyuria, polydipsia, and nocturia are often among the earliest signs observed in dogs with CRF. However, such evidence of altered fluid balance may be less prominent in cats with renal failure. In a recent study, polyuria was reported in only 26 of 73 cats (35.6%) with spontaneous CRF (DiBartola et al., 1987). This finding may have been related to own-

ers' poor attention to the micturition habits of their cats or to the apparently greater intrinsic urine-concentrating ability of cats with CRF. However, urine specific gravity values were less than 1.015 in 42 of 74 cats and exceeded 1.025 in only 8 of 74 cats in this study. In this same study, 67.2% of 64 cats had serum creatinine concentrations in excess of 3.6 mg/dl, and 34.4% had serum creatinine concentrations in excess of 7.2 mg/dl. These findings emphasize the need to routinely screen middle-aged and older cats for evidence of subclinical renal dysfunction.

Cats with CRF often survive for months to years with a good quality of life. Although no therapy can eliminate the irreversible renal lesions of CRF, the clinical and biochemical consequences of reduced renal function can be minimized by symptomatic

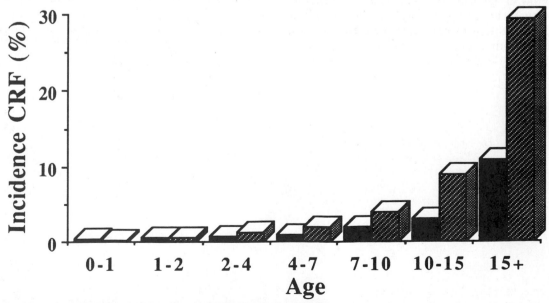

Figure 1. Bar graph illustrating the prevalence of chronic renal failure (CRF) for various age groups at the University of Minnesota Veterinary Medical Teaching Hospital between 1984 and 1989. Black bars represent canine data and stippled bars represent feline data. CRF was not necessarily the only or primary diagnosis in these patients.

848

and supportive therapy (conservative medical management of renal failure). In addition, recent advances in our understanding of the spontaneously progressive nature of CRF provide clues about how this self-perpetuating deterioration of renal function may be slowed or stopped.

DIAGNOSTIC EVALUATION OF CATS WITH CHRONIC RENAL FAILURE

Diagnosis of feline CRF is usually confirmed by demonstrating concurrent azotemia and inadequate urine-concentrating ability (i.e., urine specific gravity < 1.035). In order to optimize their interpretation, serum and urine samples should be obtained concurrently and before initiating treatment. Diagnosis of renal failure in nonazotemic cats requires determination of glomerular filtration rate (e.g., creatinine clearance).

On confirming the diagnosis of renal failure, its severity and the need for immediate therapeutic intervention should be assessed. Indications for immediate therapeutic intervention include dehydration, hyperkalemia or hypokalemia, severe metabolic acidosis (serum total carbon dioxide concentrations less than 10 mEq/L), retinal detachment, and intractable uremic manifestations. Additional diagnostics may be required to differentiate acute from chronic renal failure, to determine the etiology of renal failure, and to identify treatable complications of CRF (Table 1). Chronicity of renal failure may be confirmed by evidence that primary renal failure has been present for an extended period. Renal osteodystrophy, reduced kidney size, and historic or serial laboratory confirmation of persistent primary renal failure over several months are unequivocal evidence of chronicity.

TREATMENT OF FELINE CHRONIC RENAL FAILURE

Conservative medical management of CRF consists of supportive and symptomatic therapy designed to minimize the clinical and pathophysiologic consequences of reduced renal function (Table 2) by correcting deficits and excesses in fluid, electrolyte, acid-base, endocrine, and nutritional balance. This type of therapy will not halt, reverse, or eliminate renal lesions responsible for CRF. Therefore, conservative medical management is most beneficial when combined with specific therapy directed at correcting the primary cause of renal disease.

Specific therapy of renal disease consists of therapy designed to slow or stop development of renal lesions by influencing the underlying etiopathogenic processes. Examples of specific treatment include

correction of hypercalcemia that has caused calcium nephropathy, administration of antibiotics to eliminate bacterial pyelonephritis, administration of antimycotic agents to eliminate mycotic pyelonephritis, removal of lesions causing obstructive uropathy (e.g., tumors or uroliths), and correction of abnormal renal perfusion that has caused ischemic renal lesions. Although determining the initiating disease process in cats with CRF is frequently difficult or impossible, the value of formulating specific therapy based on an etiologic/pathologic diagnosis should not be overlooked. Because renal lesions responsible for CRF are irreversible, they cannot be completely reversed or eliminated by specific therapy. Nonetheless, progression of renal lesions and thus progression of renal failure may be slowed or stopped by therapy designed to eliminate the underlying causes of active renal diseases. Therefore, diagnostic efforts directed especially at detecting treatable renal diseases should be performed before formulating plans for conservative medical management. In addition, nonrenal conditions that may aggravate or precipitate uremic crisis (e.g., dehydration) should be sought and corrected.

Table 1. *Problem-Specific Database for Cats with Renal Failure**

1. Medical history, physical examination, and accurate body weight
2. Urinalysis including urine sediment examination
3. Quantitative urine culture (or screening urine culture)
4. Complete blood count
5. Serum urea nitrogen concentration
6. Serum creatinine concentration
7. Serum (or plasma) electrolyte and acid-base profile
   a. Sodium, potassium, and chloride concentrations
   b. Bicarbonate or total carbon dioxide concentrations
   c. Calcium and phosphorus concentrations
8. Serum albumin and total protein concentrations
9. Kidney-bladder-urethra survey radiographs
   a. Kidneys—size, shape, location, number
   b. Uroliths or masses affecting ureters or urethra
   c. Urinary bladder—size, shape, location, uroliths
10. Consider:
    a. Freezing aliquots of serum (or plasma) and urine for additional diagnostic determinations that may be desired later
    b. Renal ultrasonography (rule out: urinary obstruction, nephroliths, renal cystic disease, renal neoplasia, or other infiltrative disease)
    c. Intravenous urography (rule out: urinary obstruction, nephroliths, pyelonephritis, renal cystic disease, renal neoplasia)
    d. Blood pressure determination (rule out systemic hypertension)
    e. Renal biopsy (may provide etiologic diagnosis; primarily indicated when kidneys are of normal size or enlarged)

*Reprinted with permission from Polzin, D. J., Osborne, C. A., and O'Brien, T. D.: Diseases of the kidneys. *In* Ettinger, S. J. (ed.): *Textbook of Veterinary Internal Medicine*, 3rd ed. Philadelphia, W. B. Saunders, 1989, p. 1969.

Table 2. Conservative Medical Management of Chronic Renal Failure in Cats*

Treatable Complication	Clinical or Laboratory Abnormality	Treatment Options
Progression of chronic renal failure	Progressively increasing serum creatinine concentrations	Dietary modification Minimize acidosis Minimize hypokalemia Control hypertension
Uremic manifestations	Azotemia, clinical signs of uremia	Diet therapy Antiemetics Appetite stimulants
Dehydration and negative fluid balance	Polyuria, polydipsia, nocturia, dehydration	Avoid stress Free access to water Consider diet therapy Adequate dietary salt intake Supplemental fluid therapy
Metabolic acidosis	Reduced total carbon dioxide or bicarbonate concentration	Therapeutic alkalization
Hypokalemic myopathy	Hypokalemia, muscle weakness	Oral or parenteral potassium supplementation
Anemia of chronic renal failure	Reduced hematocrit (normocytic, normochromic)	Androgen therapy Transfusion therapy Erythropoietin therapy (?)
Divalent ion imbalances: Hyperphosphatemia	Elevated serum phosphorus concentration	Diet therapy Intestinal phosphate-binding agents
Hypocalcemia	Reduced serum calcium concentrations	Oral calcium supplements Vitamin D therapy†
Renal osteodystrophy	Radiographic evidence of skeletal lesions	Correct hyperphosphatemia Vitamin D therapy† Oral calcium supplements
Systemic hypertension	Increased arterial blood pressure, retinopathy, retinal detachment	Sodium restriction Antihypertensive drug therapy
Drug reactions/overdose	Varies according to drug and type of reaction	Adjust drug doses according to renal function Avoid nephrotoxic drugs
Urinary tract infection	Pyuria, positive urine culture	Antibiotic therapy Monitor for urinary infection

*Adapted with permission from Polzin, D. J., Osborne, C. A., and O'Brien, T. D.: Diseases of the kidneys. *In* Ettinger, S. J. (ed.): *Textbook of Veterinary Internal Medicine*, 3rd ed. Philadelphia: W. B. Saunders, 1989, p. 1986.

†Vitamin D therapy should be used only after serum phosphorus concentrations have been normalized.

Diet Therapy

The rationale for restricting protein intake of cats with CRF is based on the premise that controlled reduction of nonessential proteins will result in decreased production of nitrogenous wastes with consequent amelioration of clinical signs. By formulating diets that contain a reduced quantity of high-quality protein and adequate nonprotein calories, many of the signs associated with uremia may be reduced in severity or eliminated, even though renal function is not improved.

Although the principal benefit ascribed to dietary protein restriction in CRF is amelioration of clinical signs of uremia due to reduced retention of nitrogenous waste products, protein restriction may also benefit renal failure patients in various other ways, such as by (1) minimizing spontaneous, progressive renal damage by modifying renal hemodynamics or renal hypertrophy; (2) reducing phosphate intake, thereby ameliorating hyperphosphatemia, renal secondary hyperparathyroidism, and renal osteodystrophy, as well as potentially minimizing progression

of CRF; and (3) minimizing severity of polyuria and polydipsia by reducing protein-related urinary solute excretion. Studies performed in our laboratory indicate that unrestricted intake of a high-protein diet may promote proteinuria and glomerular injury in cats with CRF (Adams et al., 1990). Reducing protein and calorie intake limited these effects. Studies by Ross and colleagues (1982) indicate that consumption of diets containing normal dietary phosphate concentrations may promote microscopic evidence of renal mineralization, fibrosis, and mononuclear cell infiltration in cats with CRF. Reducing dietary phosphorus intake limited these effects. Thus, restriction of dietary protein, phosphorus, and perhaps calories may prove useful in limiting progressive renal injury in cats with spontaneous CRF, thereby prolonging patients' survival. An important implication of these findings is that some form of dietary therapy should probably be considered for all cats with CRF, regardless of severity of renal dysfunction.

Dietary protein restriction presents a unique problem in cats because they have significantly higher dietary protein requirements than dogs. Dietary protein requirements for normal adult cats have been estimated to be approximately three times greater than for adult dogs. The higher protein requirement for cats is not solely the result of a higher requirement for one or more essential amino acids. Rather, it appears to reflect reduced efficiency of anabolic utilization of dietary protein in cats compared with other species. A significant portion of the protein in their diets is used as a source of calories. Thus, the extent to which dietary protein intake can be restricted is limited. Diets designed for dogs with CRF should not be fed to cats because of the lower protein content of canine diets.

We currently recommend that cats with CRF be fed diets containing approximately 20% of calories as protein (equivalent to 3.3 to 3.5 gm/kg/day of high-biologic value protein when consuming 70 to 80 kcal/kg/day). Protein intake should be individualized by monitoring response to therapy. However, caution is advised in reducing dietary protein intake below 20% protein calories.

The need for intestinal phosphorus-binding agents should be evaluated by determining serum phosphorus concentrations 10 to 14 days after restricting dietary protein and phosphorus intake. If hyperphosphatemia continues despite dietary restriction, intestinal phosphate-binding agents should be considered (see this volume, p. 853).

Cats may resist efforts to reduce dietary protein intake, presumably because they find protein-restricted diets less palatable. Therefore, it is important to introduce new diets gradually by progressively adding a small quantity to the regular diet. It may require several weeks to completely convert to the new diet. Although it may not be possible to convert all cats completely from their usual diet to a protein-restricted diet, benefits afforded by even partial protein restriction may be significant.

Although inadequate intake of reduced-protein diets is often ascribed to poor palatability, other factors may also affect appetite. Patients with anorexia should be evaluated for metabolic acidosis, hypokalemia, anemia, or dehydration. Uremic nausea and vomiting may also be associated with anorexia. Nausea and vomiting resulting from uremic gastritis may respond to oral or parenteral cimetidine therapy. Metoclopramide also appears to be an effective antiemetic for cats with CRF and may prove useful in cats that fail to respond to cimetidine therapy.

Therapy of Metabolic Acidosis

Metabolic acidosis is a common finding in feline CRF. In a recent study of feline chronic renal disease, 37 of 59 (62.7%) cats had laboratory evidence of metabolic acidosis (DiBartola et al., 1987). Acidosis may promote anorexia, nausea, vomiting, weight loss, muscle weakness, lethargy, hypokalemia, and skeletal demineralization. In addition, the body's ability to compensate for increased acid intake (e.g., a high-protein meal) or production (e.g., lactate) may be limited during metabolic acidosis because of reduced buffer reserve.

Therapy for metabolic acidosis is usually indicated when serum bicarbonate (or total carbon dioxide) concentrations decline below normal values established for the laboratory in which they were determined. Sodium bicarbonate is the alkalizing agent used most often to correct metabolic acidosis. It may be administered as tablets, powder (added to food), or solution. A solution containing 1 mEq/mL of bicarbonate can be prepared by adding one third of an 8 oz. box of baking soda to 1.0 L of distilled water. This solution will remain stable up to 3 months if kept in a capped container and refrigerated. Sodium bicarbonate therapy is initially administered at about 10 mg/kg (1 ml of solution per 8.5 kg) PO every 8 to 12 hr. However, the dose of sodium bicarbonate required to reverse acidosis varies greatly and must be determined by evaluating a patient's response to therapy. The goal is to return serum bicarbonate concentrations to the normal range. Alternatively, potassium citrate or calcium carbonate, acetate, or citrate may be used when additional sodium intake is deemed undesirable.

Because urinary acidifiers and diets designed to produce acid urine may promote metabolic acidosis, they are not appropriate for cats with CRF. The need for alkalization in cats receiving such therapy should be evaluated after withdrawing the drug or diet.

Therapy of Hypokalemia

Hypokalemia occasionally develops as a complication of feline CRF. Although the precise mechanism of hypokalemia has not been determined, it may result when urinary loss exceeds dietary intake of potassium. Studies performed in our laboratory have confirmed that renal failure is a risk factor for development of hypokalemia in cats. Preliminary evidence suggests that chronic ingestion of a potassium-deficient diet may induce primary renal failure in cats (Buffington et al., 1990). Despite these findings, it is our opinion that hypokalemia is most often secondary to CRF in cats.

The cardinal sign of hypokalemia is generalized muscle weakness. Cats with hypokalemia often have profound cervical ventroflexion and difficulty ambulating. Mild cardiac rhythm disturbances and generalized flaccid muscle weakness occasionally severe enough to cause respiratory failure may occur.

Muscle weakness usually resolves within 1 to 5 days after initiating parenteral or oral potassium supplementation. Oral administration is the safest route of administration for potassium because parenteral administration is more likely to induce iatrogenic hyperkalemia, and fluid therapy may actually decrease serum potassium. Therefore, parenteral therapy is generally reserved for patients requiring emergency reversal of hypokalemia or for patients that cannot or will not accept oral therapy (see this volume, p. 820). Potassium may be given orally at the rate of approximately 2.2 mEq/100 kcal of required energy intake. Potassium dose may be adjusted based on the clinical response of the patient and daily serum potassium determinations during the initial phase of therapy. Potassium may be administered orally as potassium gluconate in a palatable powder form (Tumil-K, Daniels), potassium gluconate elixir (Kaon Elixir, Adria), or potassium citrate solution (Polycitra-K, Willen). Oral potassium supplements may cause gastrointestinal irritation, ulceration, nausea, and vomiting. They should be used with caution in older and debilitated patients. Gastrointestinal irritation may be lessened in patients receiving oral liquid potassium supplements by diluting the preparation at least 1:2 with water. We have not recognized gastrointestinal irritation in patients receiving the oral powdered product.

Some cats require chronic potassium supplementation of approximately 2 to 4 mEq/day to prevent recurrent hypokalemia (Dow et al., 1987). Although dietary potassium deficiency is unlikely to be the sole cause of hypokalemia in these patients, inadequate potassium intake appears to be a contributing factor. There is reason to suspect that diets that are acidifying and restricted in magnesium content may promote hypokalemia. Therefore, it is prudent to avoid feeding such diets to cats with CRF.

Intensive fluid therapy during uremic crises, particularly with potassium-deficient fluids, may promote hypokalemia even in cats that have not previously experienced hypokalemia. Attention to the potassium needs of these patients is necessary to prevent hypokalemia. Serum potassium concentrations should be monitored during fluid therapy, and maintenance fluids should be supplemented with potassium chloride to a concentration of approximately 13 to 20 mEq/L. Fluids should generally be administered such that potassium is delivered intravenously at a rate no greater than 0.5 mEq/kg/hr.

Therapy of Hypoproliferative Anemia

In one study of feline CRF, nonregenerative anemia was detected in 30 of 73 (41.1%) cats (DiBartola et al., 1987). The severity of anemia varies widely in cats with CRF. Although mild anemia is not of therapeutic concern, moderate to severe anemia (e.g., packed cell volume [PCV] <20 vol%) promotes lethargy, weakness, and anorexia. Correlations between severity of anemia, magnitude of renal dysfunction, and cause of renal failure have not been determined, but empirically, severe anemia appears to occur most often in cats with advanced renal dysfunction.

Treatment of the anemia of CRF may encompass administration of androgens, transfusion therapy, and hormone replacement. The only satisfactory treatments for anemia of CRF in humans are renal transplantation or hormone replacement therapy with recombinant human erythropoietin (rHuEpo [Epogen], Amgen). Because hormone replacement therapy with rHuEpo is expensive and has not been approved for use in cats and because renal transplantation is not currently available for most feline patients with CRF, androgen therapy is often used. However, the efficacy of androgen therapy of anemia of CRF has not been critically evaluated in cats. Our clinical impression is that response to androgen therapy is usually disappointing. Nonetheless, a therapeutic trial with androgens may be indicated for patients with moderate to severe anemia of CRF, because serious adverse side effects have not been recognized.

We have observed a beneficial response to administration of rHuEpo to cats with anemia of CRF. In most cats we have treated, PCV began to increase within the first 7 to 10 days of treatment. Improvement in PCV in our patients was associated with improved appetite, weight gain, and improved clinical well-being. These findings are similar to those reported by Cowgill and colleagues (1990). However, rHuEpo is a recombinant human hormone that is suspended in a solution containing human albumin, which may promote immunogenic and allergic reactions in cats (see this volume, p. 484).

Therapy of Arterial Hypertension

Arterial hypertension occurs in about two thirds of cats with CRF (Ross and Labato, 1989). Ocular complications of arterial hypertension in cats are apparently common. Ocular lesions may include retinal vascular changes, retinal hemorrhages, hyphema, papilledema, and retinal exudates with retinal detachment and acute blindness.

In humans, arterial hypertension is a major risk factor for progressive renal injury. Preliminary studies in our laboratory have suggested that increased arterial pressures may be related to progressive renal injury in cats as well. However, these findings must be confirmed before a definite link between arterial hypertension and progressive renal injury can be established for cats.

Treatment of hypertension should be considered after persistent elevation of arterial pressure has been documented on three separate occasions. In addition, the ability to monitor response to therapy is a prerequisite for therapy. Although the drug of choice for management of arterial hypertension in feline CRF has not been established, we typically begin therapy with a combination of dietary sodium restriction and propranolol (see this volume, p. 838, for additional information on management of arterial hypertension).

MONITORING PATIENTS

Response to treatment should be monitored at appropriate intervals so that treatment can be individualized to the specific and often changing needs of the patient. The problem-specific database obtained before initiation of conservative medical management should be used as a baseline for comparison of the patient's progress. This evaluation should be repeated at appropriate intervals; monthly evaluations are suggested for the first several months. However, the frequency of evaluation may vary depending on the severity of renal dysfunction, complications affecting a patient, and response to treatment. Patients undergoing certain forms of therapy, such as administration of rHuEpo, may also necessitate more frequent monitoring.

References and Suggested Reading

Adams, L. G., Polzin, D. J., and Osborne, C. A.: Effects of reduced dietary protein in cats with induced chronic renal failure. J. Vet. Intern. Med. 4:125(A), 1990.
An abstract summarizing data that indicate that unrestricted intake of a high-protein diet promotes proteinuria and glomerular injury, whereas reducing protein and calorie intake prevented these adverse effects.

Buffington, C. A., DiBartola, S. P., and Chew, D. J.: Effect of low potassium commercial diet on renal function of adult cats. Proceedings of the Waltham International Symposium on the Nutrition of Small Companion Animals, Davis, CA, 1990, pp. 28A.
An abstract that presents preliminary evidence that low potassium intake may promote renal dysfunction.

Cowgill, L. D., Feldman, B., Levy, J., et al.: Efficacy of recombinant human erythropoietin for anemia in dogs and cats with renal failure. J. Vet. Intern. Med. 4:126(A), 1990.
An abstract summarizing preliminary findings on the clinical use of recombinant human erythropoietin for treatment of anemia of canine and feline CRF.

DiBartola, S. P., Rutgers, H.C., Zack, P. M., et al.: Clinicopathologic findings associated with chronic renal disease in cats: 74 cases (1973–1984). J.A.V.M.A. 190:1196, 1987.
A review of the clinical and pathologic findings in feline CRF.

Dow, S. W., Fettman, M.J., LeCouteur, R. A., et al.: Potassium depletion in cats: Renal and dietary influences. J.A.V.M.A. 191:1569, 1987.
A report documenting the clinical syndrome of potassium depletion in cats with spontaneous CRF.

Polzin, D. J., Osborne, C. A., and O'Brien, T. D.: Diseases of the kidneys. In Ettinger, S.J. (ed.): Textbook of Veterinary Internal Medicine, 3rd ed. Philadelphia: W.B. Saunders, 1989, p. 1962.
A comprehensive review of the diagnosis and treatment of chronic renal failure.

Ross, L. A., Finco, D. R., and Crowell, W. A.: Effect of dietary phosphorus restriction on the kidneys of cats with reduced renal mass. Am. J. Vet. Res. 43:1023, 1982.
A report of the effects of varying dietary phosphorus intake on renal structure and function in cats with induced CRF.

Ross, L. A., and Labato, M. A.: Use of drugs to control hypertension in renal failure. In Kirk, R. W. (ed.): Current Veterinary Therapy X. Philadelphia: W.B. Saunders, 1989, p. 1201.
A review of the therapy of systemic hypertension in dogs and cats with CRF.

PHOSPHORUS RESTRICTION IN THE TREATMENT OF CHRONIC RENAL FAILURE

DENNIS J. CHEW,
STEPHEN P. DiBARTOLA,
LARRY A. NAGODE,
and ROBERT J. STARKEY
Columbus, Ohio

Phosphorus retention in the course of chronic progressive renal disease is important in the development and maintenance of renal secondary hyperparathyroidism (2-HPTH) and also contributes by mass action to soft-tissue mineral deposits. Compensatory increases in the serum concentration of biologically active parathyroid hormone (PTH) maintain serum phosphorus concentrations within the normal range until advanced stages of nephron loss (less than 20% of normal glomerular filtration rate [GFR]). Serum phosphorus concentration increases progressively when serum creatinine concentration exceeds 3.5 mg/dl in most dogs and cats that have chronic renal failure (CRF) and that remain well hydrated. Dehydration can increase the magnitude of hyperphosphatemia.

The magnitude of PTH increase during renal 2-HPTH in dogs is variable, but most affected dogs have increases above the normal range when serum creatinine concentration exceeds 2 mg/dl. Increased PTH in dogs with serum creatinine concentration in the range of 1 to 2 mg/dl may occur but not be recognized because the increase resulted in a serum PTH concentration that was within the normal range. Some animals with renal 2-HPTH have serum PTH concentrations 10 to 20 times above normal. Normally hydrated dogs and cats with CRF and increased serum phosphorus concentrations can safely be assumed to have renal 2-HPTH. They have completely expended the normal renal compensatory mechanisms for maintaining normal external balance for phosphorus (i.e., increased fractional urinary excretion of phosphorus mediated by increased PTH).

BENEFITS OF PHOSPHORUS RESTRICTION

Phosphorus restriction decreases serum PTH concentration by increasing calcitriol production and increasing serum ionized calcium concentration when initial serum phosphorus concentrations are markedly increased. A direct decrease in PTH that is independent of either serum ionized calcium concentration or calcitriol has been proposed, but proponents did not fully consider "trade-off" aspects of calcitriol-PTH, which explain their results without need for invoking a new mechanism (Slatopolsky et al., 1990). Proportional reduction of phosphorus intake designed to match the degree of decrease in GFR can prevent or reverse renal 2-HPTH in dogs with experimental CRF (Kaplan et al., 1979; Slatopolsky et al., 1972). Phosphorus restriction may preserve GFR, renal histology, or both in animals with severe reduction in renal mass. Renal histologic changes but not functional changes were prevented by phosphorus restriction in experimental cats with approximately 80% reduction in renal mass (Ross 1982). Moderate dietary phosphorus restriction resulted in higher survival, higher GFR, and lower serum PTH concentration in experimental dogs with 90% reduction in renal mass when studied after 1 year (Brown et al., 1987). These observations form the basis for phosphorus restriction in the prevention or reversal of renal 2-HPTH in clinical patients.

MEASUREMENT OF SERUM PHOSPHORUS

Normal fasting serum phosphorus concentrations in adult dogs and cats range from 2.5 to 6.0 mg/dl and largely reflect the balance between intestinal absorption of dietary phosphorus, uptake by tissues, and renal excretion. Metabolic acidosis and excess PTH concentrations may contribute to increased serum phosphorus concentrations following bone mobilization in addition to effects from reduced renal mass and lack of calcitriol-induced renal factors required for phosphaturic effects. Protein feeding transiently increases serum phosphorus concentrations by as much as 1 to 2 mg/dl over fasting concentrations, whereas lipemia falsely increases serum phosphorus measurements by several milligrams per deciliter, depending on its extent. It is recommended that animals be fasted for 12 hr and that samples be taken at the same time of day for serial evaluations in order to minimize the possible effects of diurnal variation, feeding, and lipemia on serum phosphorus concentrations.

METHODS OF PHOSPHORUS RESTRICTION

Control of serum phosphorus concentrations by dietary phosphorus restriction and intestinal phosphate binders is important because increased phosphorus concentration and resulting reduced calcitriol concentration are central in the pathogenesis of renal 2-HPTH. This can be achieved to a minimal extent by feeding normal foods with phosphate binders, to a greater extent with phosphorus-restricted foods, and to the largest extent with phosphorus-restricted diets and phosphate binders. The approach varies depending on the severity of the 2-HPTH and hyperphosphatemia. In some instances, it is possible to normalize both serum phosphorus and PTH concentrations with this approach, but PTH is not normalized by serum phosphorus correction alone in animals with more advanced CRF. For example, feeding normal diets with phosphorus binders may be helpful in managing 2-HPTH when serum creatinine concentration is 3.5 mg/dl or less (Finco, 1983). However, serum phosphorus concentrations remained above the normal range in experimental dogs with 90% reduction in renal mass despite the administration of an aluminum-containing intestinal phosphate binder during feeding of high- or moderate-protein diets containing an excess of 1% phosphorus (Finco et al., 1985). The sequential prescription of a phosphorus-restricted diet followed by the addition of intestinal phosphate binders at a later point in the progression of renal disease is a realistic clinical approach to patients with CRF.

Most commercial dog and cat foods contain in excess of 1% phosphorus on a dry weight basis in order to meet requirements for all life stages (growth, maintenance, pregnancy, and lactation). Dietary phosphorus originates from proteins and amino acids, bone meal, and sodium tripolyphosphate added to some formulations. Dietary phosphorus content expressed as a percentage of dry weight or calories does not necessarily predict availability of phosphorus for intestinal absorption. Availability of phosphorus from commercial formulations may vary from approximately 30 to 90%. This variability is accounted for by differences in the source of phosphorus (animal versus plant), form (organic versus inorganic phosphorus), cation composition, and digestibility.

The minimal dietary requirement for phosphorus in normal dogs has been estimated as 89 mg/kg/day for adult maintenance and 240 mg/kg/day for growth, but requirements during CRF are not known. Normal dogs and cats often ingest phosphorus in excess of 200 mg/kg/day from commercial foods.

Dietary phosphorus restriction is accomplished primarily by protein restriction because diets that are low in protein also are low in phosphorus. There is a practical limit to which foods can be restricted in phosphorus, however, because severe restriction results in unpalatable formulations. A range of phosphorus intake can be achieved using special commercial diets such as Hill's Prescription Diet Canine gd, kd, and ud, which provide 0.42%, 0.26%, and 0.13% phosphorus on a dry matter basis, respectively. Alternatively, homemade diets can be formulated. Additional measures usually are necessary to control serum phosphorus concentration and renal 2-HPTH in patients with advanced renal failure.

Intestinal Phosphate Binders

Intestinal phosphate binders reduce the absorption of phosphorus and thereby increase phosphorus excretion in feces. Nonabsorbable salts of phosphate form during chemical reactions between the cation of the phosphate binder, dietary phosphate, and phosphate in intestinal secretions. Additionally, binder particles may adsorb phosphate ions on their surfaces (Sheikh et al., 1989). The most widely used oral phosphorus-binding agents are aluminum and calcium salts of hydroxide, carbonate, and acetate. Magnesium-containing compounds should be avoided in renal failure because of limited ability to excrete magnesium, with risk of hypermagnesemia.

The timing of administration of phosphate binders in relation to feeding strongly influences their efficacy in binding phosphate. Phosphate binders are most effective when given with meals. In one study of human patients, calcium acetate was most potent in reducing gastrointestinal absorption of phosphate

when ingested just before or after a meal and was much less effective when given 2 hr after a meal (Schiller et al., 1989). Ingestion of a meal also decreased the absorption of calcium from calcium acetate.

Aluminum Salts

Aluminum salts (aluminum hydroxide and aluminum carbonate) are considered potent intestinal phosphate binders and have been commonly administered to dogs and cats. Aluminum can be absorbed from these salts, however, by both normal and uremic human patients. Concern has thus been raised about the role of aluminum accumulation in metabolic bone disease and encephalopathy during uremia. Experimental dogs with 90% nephrectomy treated with aluminum salts for 3 months did not develop aluminum toxicity as determined by aluminum content of brain and kidney (Finco et al., 1985). The role, if any, of aluminum toxicosis in the development of metabolic bone disease or encephalopathy during CRF has not been explored clinically in dogs or cats. Aluminum-containing salts are preferred over calcium salts in patients presenting with hypercalcemia or in those that develop hypercalcemia while receiving calcium-containing phosphate binders. Aluminum-containing phosphate binders are available as gels, tablets, or capsules. The aluminum-containing binders are better tolerated by many dogs and cats when given as tablet or capsule, but the desiccated form has a lower capacity than the liquid gel for binding phosphate (Rutherford et al., 1973).

Calcium Salts

Calcium salts (calcium carbonate and calcium acetate) have been advocated as replacements for aluminum salts. Calcium carbonate is not as potent a phosphorus binder as the aluminum salts, however, and hypercalcemia occasionally occurs. Calcium acetate binds between two and three times more phosphorus than does calcium carbonate in human beings when given in doses containing an equivalent amount of elemental calcium, and it is nearly as efficient in binding phosphorus as aluminum carbonate (Sheikh et al., 1989). Hypercalcemia should occur less frequently during use of calcium acetate because less calcium is absorbed from calcium acetate as compared with calcium carbonate. Calcium acetate (Phos-Ex, Vitaline Formulas) is available for use in human beings as a nutritional supplement, or as a prescription drug (PhosLo, Braintree). Although advocated as a phosphate binder (Cushner, 1988), calcium citrate is not recommended because it is not an efficient intestinal phosphate binder and also has the deleterious effect of enhancing aluminum absorption from the intestine in humans (Nolan et al., 1990). Calcium-containing phosphate binders should be given with meals to maximize phosphorus binding and to reduce the risk of hypercalcemia.

Combination of Aluminum and Calcium Salts

It may be preferable to administer aluminum-containing phosphate binders initially to decrease serum phosphorus concentration when it exceeds the normal range, before calcium-containing phosphate binders are used. This approach aims to maintain the product of serum calcium and serum phosphorus concentration at less than 70, which presumably reduces the risk of soft-tissue mineralization. Combination of an aluminum-containing phosphate binder and calcium acetate may reduce a patient's risk of aluminum toxicity while promoting maximal intestinal binding of phosphorus. Aluminum salts bind phosphorus in the acid environment of the stomach. Less total phosphorus is thus left for calcium acetate to bind in the intestine, where it exerts its effect at a more alkaline pH. This combination also may limit the development of hypercalcemia.

Dose

The appropriate dose of phosphate binder must be determined by monitoring individual patient response, but approximately 100 mg/kg/day divided b.i.d. or t.i.d. and administered with meals is a starting dosage for both aluminum- and calcium-containing phosphate binders when serum phosphorus concentration is greater than 6.0 mg/dl. Lower dosages (30 to 90 mg/kg/day) may suffice during early CRF, characterized by normal serum phosphorus concentration. The dose is increased if serum phosphorus concentration increases, and dose should be decreased if serum phosphorus concentration falls below 3.5 mg/dl. More than 150 mg/kg of aluminum carbonate was tolerated by experimental dogs with reduced renal mass (Finco et al., 1985), and greater than 300 mg/kg calcium acetate given at the time of feeding was well tolerated by dogs with experimentally reduced renal mass in a study that we conducted. Because calcium acetate is more efficient than calcium carbonate in binding intestinal phosphorus on a basis of phosphorus bound/calcium absorbed (Mai et al., 1989), lower doses may be considered. Based on its higher molecular weight and higher phosphorus-binding ratio, it appears that a dose of calcium acetate at approximately 60 mg/kg/day will provide the same amount of intestinal phosphorus binding as 100 mg/

kg/day of calcium carbonate. On the basis of calcium, this acetate dose is about two fifths of the dose of calcium carbonate. Doses of calcium salts must be decreased if hypercalcemia develops.

Toxicity

Nausea and constipation can occur with most formulations of intestinal phosphorus binders. Hypophosphatemia may occur after overzealous intestinal phosphorus binding but is unlikely in patients with severe hyperphosphatemia at the time treatment is initiated. Hypercalcemia is an occasional side effect of calcium-containing phosphate binders.

Monitoring the Patient

It is desirable to reduce fasting serum phosphorus concentration to less than 6 mg/dl in patients presented with hyperphosphatemia. Fasting serum phosphorus concentrations from 3.5 to 5.5 mg/dl are the goal. Concurrently, fasting serum total calcium concentrations should remain less than 12 mg/dl in dogs and less than 11 mg/dl in cats. The initial response to phosphate binders may be slow, because the pool of accumulated phosphate is large. Nevertheless, if a patient will eat a phosphorus-restricted diet and tolerates the phosphate binder, fasting serum phosphorus concentration often can be returned to the normal range within a few weeks.

Measurement of fractional urinary excretion of phosphorus or serum PTH (amino terminal or intact molecule) is helpful in making further dose adjustments when serum phosphorus concentration is within the normal range. One investigator suggested that values for fractional urinary excretion of phosphorus less than 30% are indicative of adequate phosphate restriction (Finco, 1983), but another has found this to be a relatively insensitive indicator of the degree of 2-HPTH in dogs (Hansen et al., 1991). Decreased serum PTH concentration after phosphorus restriction provides definitive evidence of the effectiveness of phosphorus restriction in blunting renal 2-HPTH. Calcitriol supplementation may be required to further reduce serum PTH concentrations in patients in which PTH concentrations remain increased despite maximal phosphorus restriction (see this volume, p. 857).

References and Suggested Reading

Brown, S., Finco, D., Crowell, W., et al.: Beneficial effect of moderate phosphate(phos) restriction in partially nephrectomized dogs on a low protein diet (abstract). Kidney Int. 31:380, 1987.

Cushner, H. M., Copley, J. B., Lindberg, J. S., et al.: Calcium citrate, a non–aluminum containing phosphate binding agent for treatment of CRF. Kidney Int. 33:95, 1988.

Finco, D. R.: The role of phosphorus restriction in the management of chronic renal failure in the dog and cat. Proceedings of the Seventh Annual Kal Kan Symposium for the Treatment of Small Animal Diseases, 1983, pp. 131–133.

Finco, D. R., Crowell, W. A., and Barsanti, J. A.: Effects of three diets on dogs with induced chronic renal failure. Am. J. Vet. Res. 46:646, 1985.

Hansen, B., DiBartola, S. P., Chew, D. J., et al.: Clinical and metabolic findings in dogs with spontaneous renal failure fed two different diets. Am. J. Vet. Res. (in press).

Kaplan, M. A., Canterbury, J. M., Bourgoignie, J. J., et al.: Reversal of hyperparathyroidism in response to dietary phosphorus restriction in the uremic dog. Kidney Int. 15:43, 1979.

Mai, M. L., Emmett, M. E., Sheikh, M. S., et al.: Calcium acetate, an effective phosphorus binder in patients with renal failure. Kidney Int. 36:690, 1989.

Nolan, C. R., Califano, J. R., and Butzin, C. A.: Influence of calcium citrate on intestinal aluminum absorption. Kidney Int. 38:937, 1990.

Ross, L. A., Finco, D. R., and Crowell, W. A.: Effect of dietary phosphorus restriction on the kidneys of cats with reduced renal mass. Am. J. Vet. Res. 43(6):1023, 1982.

Rutherford, E., King, S., Perry, B., et al.: Use of a new phosphate binder in chronic renal insufficiency. Kidney Int. 17:528, 1980.

Rutherford, E., Mercado, A., Hruska, K., et al.: An evaluation of a new and effective phosphorus binding agent. Trans. Am. Soc. Artif. Intern. Organs 19:446, 1973.

Schiller, L. R., Santa Ana, C. A., Sheikh, M. S., et al.: Effect of the time of administration of calcium acetate on phosphorus binding. N. Engl. J. Med. 320:1110, 1989.

Sheikh, M. S., Maguire, J. A., Emmett, M., et al.: Reduction of dietary phosphorus absorption by phosphorus binders, a theoretical, in vitro, and in vivo study. J. Clin. Invest. 83:66, 1989.

Slatopolsky, E., Caglar, S., Gradowska, L., et al.: On the prevention of secondary hyperparathyroidism in experimental chronic renal disease using "proportional reduction" of dietary phosphorus intake. Kidney Int. 2:147, 1972.

Slatopolsky, E., Lopez-Hilker, S., Delmez, J., et al.: The parathyroid-calcitriol axis in health and chronic renal failure. Kidney Int. 38 (suppl. 29):S41, 1990.

CALCITRIOL IN THE TREATMENT OF CHRONIC RENAL FAILURE

DENNIS J. CHEW
and LARRY A. NAGODE
Columbus, Ohio

Calcitriol (1,25-dihydroxycholecalciferol) is the final, most potent, and only significant biologically active form of vitamin D. Calcitriol therapy can safely be prescribed in low doses to prevent or reverse renal secondary hyperparathyroidism (2-HPTH) in dogs and cats with chronic renal failure (CRF).

Chronic renal 2-HPTH is a clinical and subclinical syndrome characterized by increased concentrations of biologically active parathyroid gland hormone (PTH) as a result of progressive decline in functional nephron mass. Increased concentrations of PTH commonly develop in dogs and cats with CRF to a magnitude roughly proportional to increases in serum phosphorus and serum creatinine, but PTH increases may start before blood urea nitrogen and serum creatinine levels become elevated. Deficits of ionized calcium, decreased intestinal absorption of calcium, increased skeletal resistance to the effects of PTH, and an increased set-point for calcium to inhibit the secretion of PTH are changes that may occur during renal 2-HPTH. All of these changes can be caused by a relative or absolute deficiency of calcitriol. Excess serum PTH is a result of decreased plasma calcitriol production and de-creased ionized calcium (Fig. 1). Actions of plasma phosphorus to lower ionized calcium by mass action have traditionally been emphasized, but calcitriol deficits following increased serum phosphorus and loss of proximal tubular mass occur earlier and are more important. Decreased ionized calcium concentration in blood is thus largely the result of decreased intestinal calcium absorption due to calcitriol deficiency, although very high serum phosphorus concentrations also contribute via mass action. Serum calcitriol and calcium levels return toward normal as a result of the activating influence of the newly increased serum PTH, but these levels remain normal only at the expense of a continuously elevated serum PTH level. Finding normal serum total calcium and even normal serum ionized calcium levels in uremic animals is therefore common even when 2-HPTH is advanced.

RATIONALE FOR USE

Injury to many tissues including the kidney can occur in the presence of excess PTH. Binding of PTH to its receptor increases a calcium channel

Calcitriol "Trade-Off" Hypothesis
EARLY CHRONIC RENAL FAILURE

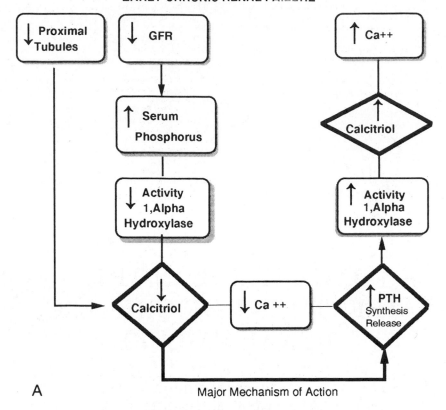

A   Major Mechanism of Action

Calcitriol "Trade-Off" Hypothesis
LATE CHRONIC RENAL FAILURE

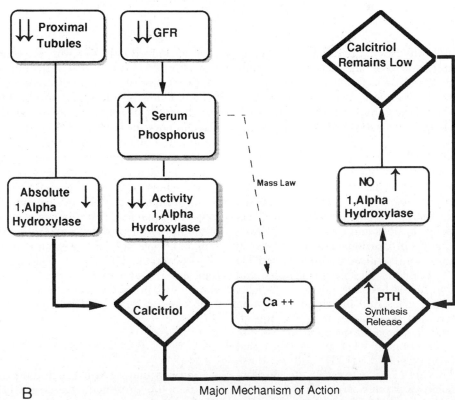

B   Major Mechanism of Action

Figure 1 *See legend on opposite page*

opening, allowing intracellular influx of calcium. Excess PTH can thus cause necrosis of soft tissues as a consequence of excess intracellular calcium (calciphylaxis). This change occurs early in the proximal tubules of the kidneys and when present contributes to the progression of chronic renal disease. Soft-tissue mineralization may be enhanced from increased serum phosphorus.

Calcitriol treatments during CRF result in decreased serum PTH concentrations. The most important mechanism is attributed to the ability of calcitriol to block PTH synthesis directly after binding to specific receptors within the parathyroid secretory cells; calcitriol also blocks PTH secretion. Calcitriol supplementation restores a lower setpoint for calcium to inhibit PTH secretion and additionally prevents or reverses parathyroid gland hyperplasia. Increased ionized calcium results from increased gastrointestinal absorption after calcitriol treatment. This increased ionized calcium contributes synergistically with calcitriol to decrease serum PTH levels by lowering both secretion and synthesis of PTH. In this synergism, calcitriol is the dominant and earlier acting factor. Bone sensitivity to lowered PTH concentrations is restored in the presence of calcitriol.

PTH-induced phosphaturia is enhanced in the presence of acute calcitriol supplementation in rats with reduced renal mass (Rubinger et al., 1990). If operative in dogs and cats, this effect may contribute to an ability to maintain serum phosphorus concentrations at closer to normal concentrations than might otherwise occur. Calcitriol-induced reductions in PTH may also contribute to reduced serum phosphorus concentrations by reducing phosphorus mobilization from bone.

Calcitriol treatments have traditionally been advocated in veterinary medicine only for those patients with symptomatic metabolic bone disease or hypocalcemia, but these represent advanced stages of CRF and 2-HPTH. External manifestations attributable to early renal 2-HPTH are not obvious, but excess PTH may act as a uremic toxin.

Conservative recommendations for vitamin D metabolite supplementation to patients with CRF were initially valid because of concern about vitamin D toxicity resulting in hypercalcemia and soft-tissue mineralization (including the kidneys). Advances in the clinical use of intestinal phosphate binders and the advent of new vitamin D metabolites with a short half-life and high receptor activity now minimize these dangers. Previous studies in dogs that showed toxicity with calcitriol supplementation used about 10 times greater doses than we now recommend for dogs and cats with CRF.

The magnitude of renal 2-HPTH often increases as CRF progresses. The PTH concentration that is critical for tissue toxicity has not been determined in clinical cases, but our assumption has been that patients with the greatest elevations are most likely to suffer the greatest consequences. There is a limit to the extent that restriction of dietary phosphorus intake and the use of intestinal phosphorus binders can successfully diminish PTH concentrations. Calcitriol treatments provide an additional method to control renal 2-HPTH.

STARTING CALCITRIOL SUPPLEMENTATION

It is absolutely necessary to serially measure serum calcium and phosphorus levels during calcitriol treatments. If this cannot be done, do not start calcitriol treatment. A 12-hr fast should precede collection of serum samples to eliminate postprandial changes in serum phosphorus and calcium concentrations. Before calcitriol treatment, the patient is medically stabilized with fluids, antibiotics, antiemetics, H2 receptor blockers, dietary protein and phosphorus restriction, and intestinal phosphorus binders as needed. It is important to ensure that the serum phosphorus concentration be within the normal range (< 6 mg/dl) before and throughout calcitriol treatments to minimize the risk for soft-tissue mineralization from calcium and phosphorus mass-law interactions that could otherwise occur if serum calcium increased after calcitriol (see this volume, p. 853). One guideline is to keep the [calcium $\times$ phosphorus] product less than 70. The dose of calcitriol that suppresses PTH synthesis is lower than needed to raise blood calcium levels.

We have used calcitriol doses from 1.5 ng/kg to 3.5 ng/kg, with an average dose of 2.5 ng/kg PO once daily to dogs and cats with clinical CRF. One nanogram is the equivalent of 1×10^{-6} mg or $1 \times$

Figure 1. A, This theory emphasizes the role for calcitriol deficits in initiating and perpetuating excess parathyroid hormone (PTH) concentrations. Insufficient calcitriol binding in parathyroid glands allows this to occur directly. Low levels of ionized calcium (Ca^{++}) due to calcitriol deficits also stimulate PTH release. Excess PTH is able to restore calcitriol concentrations in early stages of chronic renal failure when enough proximal tubular mass is preserved. GFR, glomerular filtration rate.

B, As GFR is further decreased, greater increases in serum phosphorus of sufficient magnitude occur such that mass law interactions contribute to lowering of ionized calcium. Greater reductions in the activity of 1,alpha-hydroxylase also occur in the proximal tubules as a consequence of the increased serum phosphorus. Additionally, absolute loss of proximal tubules leads to further decrease in calcitriol. PTH increase, which occurs as described in A, is no longer able to restore calcitriol concentrations to normal because of lack of 1,alpha-hydroxylase enzyme.

10^{-3} µg. Commercial capsules of calcitriol for human prescription contain far too much calcitriol for use in small animal medicine (0.25 µg or 0.50 µg per capsule equivalent to 250 ng and 500 ng, respectively). One of the 0.25-µg capsules provides enough calcitriol for 10 daily doses for a 10-kg animal. Microliter aspirates of various volumes from liquid capsules designed for humans (Rocaltrol, Roche) can be performed to make individual gelatin capsule doses suitable for small animals. We have made different doses for animals in 10-lb weight ranges up to 40 lb and in 20-lb ranges above 40 lb. Commercial formulations of calcitriol may become available in doses appropriate for small animals. Custom-made capsules containing doses of calcitriol appropriate for use in small animals are available upon prescription (Island Pharmacy Services, Inc., P.O. Box 23124, Hilton Head Island, SC 29925-3124; telephone 1-800-328-7060).

ADJUSTMENTS DURING CALCITRIOL TREATMENTS

Supplementation with calcitriol to dogs and cats with CRF is designed as a daily therapy for life. The average dose of calcitriol at 2.5 ng/kg PO once daily has in our experience resulted in the return of PTH concentrations to normal or almost normal in most dogs and cats. It is necessary for proving that renal 2-HPTH has been controlled to measure PTH by a method that determines biologically active PTH (intact molecule or amino-terminal PTH). The Allegro (Nichols Institute Diagnostics, San Juan Capistrano, CA) intact PTH molecule measurement is available at reasonable cost through some commercial laboratories and has been found in dogs to correlate highly with amino-terminal (biologically active end) methods for PTH measurement. Some dogs and cats require at least 1 week of calcitriol treatment before PTH enters the normal range, but others respond more rapidly. Decreases in PTH usually occur without a concomitant change in serum total calcium concentration. If serum PTH level remains elevated, the dose should be cautiously increased until the serum PTH concentration is reduced without production of hypercalcemia. It has rarely been necessary to use higher doses,

except for animals with severe hypocalcemia. Increases in PTH occur soon after calcitriol treatments are discontinued.

Hypercalcemia is an uncommon development during calcitriol treatments at these doses, but when hypercalcemia does occur, it has been associated with the simultaneous use of calcium carbonate phosphate binders. Reduction of the dose of calcium carbonate, a change to calcium acetate, or substituting an aluminum salt phosphate binder often restores serum calcium levels to normal. Reduction of the dose of calcitriol could be necessary if serum calcium concentrations remain elevated despite these modifications. Hypercalcemia can also develop in animals with CRF for reasons other than excessive dose of calcitriol, in which case the hypercalcemia persists after discontinuation of calcitriol treatment. Calcitriol should be discontinued in cases with persistent increases in serum calcium levels above the normal range, unless direct measurement of ionized calcium shows it to be low.

We have successfully reduced the magnitude of serum PTH elevation to normal or almost normal concentrations in some dogs and cats with CRF after treatment with calcitriol for as long as 2 years. Further studies are needed to determine whether calcitriol treatments result in an improved quality and length of life, as well as whether renal function and histology are preserved to a greater degree than without treatment.

References and Suggested Reading

Coburn, J. W.: Use of oral and parenteral calcitriol in the treatment of renal osteodystrophy. Kidney Int. 38(Suppl. 29):S54, 1990.
Coburn, J. W., and Slatopolsky, E.: Vitamin D, parathyroid hormone, and the renal osteodystrophies. In Brenner, B. M., and Rector, F. C. (eds.): The Kidney, 4th ed. W.B. Saunders, 1991, pp. 2036–2120.
Finco, D. R.: The role of phosphorus restriction in the management of chronic renal failure in the dog and cat. Proceedings of the Seventh Annual Kal Kan Symposium for the Treatment of Small Animal Diseases, Columbus, OH, 1983, pp. 131–133.
Nagode, L. A., and Chew, D. J.: The use of calcitriol in treatment of renal disease of the dog and cat. Purina International Symposium, 1991, pp. 39–49.
Rubinger, D., Wald, H., and Popovtzer, M. M.: 25-hydroxycholecalciferol and 1,25-dihydroxycholecalciferol enhance phosphaturia in rats with reduced renal mass: Evidence for a PTH-dependent mechanism. Miner. Electrolyte Metab. 16:348, 1990.
Slatopolsky, E., Lopez-Hilker, S., Delmez, J., et al.: The parathyroid-calcitriol axis in health and chronic renal failure. Kidney Int. 38(Suppl. 29):541, 1990.

MEDICAL MANAGEMENT OF CANINE GLOMERULONEPHRITIS

SHELLY L. VADEN

Raleigh, North Carolina

and GREGORY F. GRAUER

Fort Collins, Colorado

Glomerulonephritis in dogs results from a reaction to immune complexes that have accumulated in the glomerulus either as a result of deposition of circulating immune complexes or by *in situ* formation. Both exogenous and endogenous antigens have been implicated in eliciting immune complex formation (Table 1). As the body attempts to clear itself of these complexes, complement is activated, initiating cell membrane damage and leukocyte accumulation. Neutrophils, monocytes, platelets, lysosomal enzymes, reactive oxygen species, platelet-activating factor, leukotriene B4, thromboxane, vasoactive amines, and the coagulation system all have been implicated as important factors in this cyclic process that culminates in glomerular injury. The glomerulus responds to this injury by cellular proliferation (proliferative glomerulonephritis), thickening of the glomerular basement membrane (membranous glomerulonephritis), and eventually hyalinization and sclerosis. Damage to the glomerular basement membrane and loss of anionic sialoproteins lead to increased filtration of plasma proteins. Cellular proliferation, mesangial cell contraction, and glomerular obliteration reduce the surface area available for filtration, thereby reducing the glomerular filtration rate. Tubular atrophy and fibrosis eventually occur because of insufficient blood flow through the postglomerular peritubular capillaries. Glomerular hyperfiltration develops as intact nephrons compensate for reduced nephron mass. Unfortunately, sustained increases in glomerular capillary pressure and flow may result in glomerulosclerosis of the remaining nephrons.

Medical management of a disease like glomerulonephritis, which has multiple factors involved in its pathogenesis, is often frustrating. More than one therapeutic modality may be necessary. Theoretically, pharmacologic interventions directed against factors involved in the pathogenesis of glomerulonephritis should reduce further damage to the glomerulus, and those aimed at reducing glomerular hyperfiltration and hypertension should slow the progression of the disease. Unfortunately, experimental studies have neither proved (nor disproved) the existence of glomerular hyperfiltration and hypertension nor determined the responsiveness of the various histologic classifications of the disease in dogs. Prospective clinical trials are currently in progress to evaluate the effects of specific drugs (cyclosporine, thromboxane synthetase inhibitors) against factors that are presumed to be important in the pathogenesis of immune-mediated glomerulonephritis in dogs. However, until the results of well-controlled clinical trials in dogs are available, information must be drawn from the current body of knowledge gained in laboratory animal and human studies.

Dogs with glomerulonephritis should be managed individually, as determined by their stage of disease and response to therapy. Animals with transient proteinuria may not require therapy. In dogs with biopsy-proven glomerulonephritis and persistent proteinuria, specific therapy (Table 2) should be considered when (1) an underlying disease process cannot be identified, (2) the suspected underlying disease is not reversible, or (3) the suspected underlying disease has been appropriately treated but proteinuria has not resolved. Because glomerular

Table 1. *Diseases That Have Been Associated With Glomerulonephritis in Dogs*

Infectious
  Canine adenovirus I
  Bacterial endocarditis
  Brucellosis
  Dirofilariasis
  Ehrlichiosis
  Leishmaniasis
  Pyometra
  Borreliosis
  Chronic bacterial infections
Neoplasia
Inflammatory
  Pancreatitis
  Systemic lupus erythematosus
  Other immune-mediated diseases
Other
  Idiopathic
  Familial

861

Table 2. *Treatment Guidelines for Glomerulonephritis*

1. Identify and correct any underlying disease processes
2. Immunomodulation
   a. cyclophosphamide,* 2.2 mg/kg or 50 mg/m² q 24 hr for 3–4 days per week
   b. azathioprine,* 2 mg/kg q 24 hr
   c. cyclosporine,† 15 mg/kg q 24 hr
   d. corticosteroids: immunosuppressive, tapering dosage protocol
   e. chlorambucil, 0.1–0.2 mg/kg q 24 or 48 hr
   f. levamisole (?), 0.5–2.0 mg/kg q 48 hr
3. Platelet-hypercoagulability treatment
   a. aspirin,* 0.5–5 mg/kg q 12 hr
   b. thromboxane synthetase inhibitors or receptor antagonists
   c. warfarin
   d. dipyridamole, 4–10 mg/kg q 24 hr
4. Supportive care
   a. dietary: sodium and phosphorus restriction, high-quality–low-quantity protein (e.g., Hill's Prescription Diet Canine k/d)
   b. hypertension: dietary sodium restriction
      captopril, 1–2 mg/kg q 12 hr
      enalapril
      other vasodilators
   c. edema/ascites: dietary sodium restriction
      furosemide, 2.2 mg/kg as needed for ascites

*Interval extension may be required in the face of severe renal failure (see *CVT VIII*, pp. 1036–1041).
†Dose should be adjusted to maintain blood or serum concentrations within the therapeutic range determined by the reference laboratory.

lesions generally worsen with time, it seems reasonable that the earlier patients are treated, the more likely they are to respond favorably. Whenever treatment is initiated, dogs should be closely monitored for disease progression. As the disease progresses and glomerular filtration rate declines, urinary protein excretion usually decreases. Therefore, clinical monitoring should include repeated biochemical panels, endogenous creatinine clearance tests, and urine protein quantitation (frequent urine protein:creatinine ratios, occasional 24-hr urine protein excretion tests). If a treatment regimen does not slow the rate of disease progression, it should be discontinued and another treatment strategy used; however, months of therapy may be required before improvement is noted.

IMMUNOMODULATION

Although it is clear that the immune system is involved in the pathogenesis of glomerulonephritis, it is unclear whether the immune system is overactive and in need of suppression or defective and in need of stimulation. Nonspecific immunosuppression would be expected to inhibit T-cell responses, inhibit antibody formation, and, in the case of corticosteroids, have an anti-inflammatory effect and modify the activity of complement. Some of these effects would be expected to benefit patients with glomerulonephritis. In fact, many human patients with glomerulonephritis are treated primarily with immunosuppressive agents (mostly corticosteroids). Recent retrospective studies have suggested little or no benefit associated with glucocorticoid treatment in dogs. However, prospective trials are needed to adequately assess the response of dogs with different histologic grades of glomerulonephritis to corticosteroids as well as other immunosuppressive agents. It is interesting to note that corticosteroid treatment of glomerulonephritis has been reported to be more efficacious in cats.

When prednisolone is administered every other day to persons with glomerulonephritis, a fluctuating pattern of proteinuria may be noted, with increased proteinuria observed on days when prednisolone is given. Therefore, if corticosteroids are administered to dogs with glomerulonephritis, proteinuria should be assessed on days when corticosteroids have not been administered.

The human patients that consistently respond to immunosuppressive therapy are those with minimal change disease. In this group of patients, 80 to 90% have complete disappearance of proteinuria when treated with corticosteroids alone. The responses of patients with other forms of glomerulonephritis are more variable. Although some studies report beneficial responses to corticosteroid treatment in humans with membranous glomerulonephritis, other studies do not. Humans with membranous glomerulonephritis that does not respond to corticosteroid treatment may have a more favorable response when cytotoxic agents (chlorambucil or cyclophosphamide) are added to the treatment regimen.

At high doses, corticosteroids have some immunosuppressive and anti-inflammatory properties that cannot be obtained with standard doses. Clinical trials in humans have recently used short-term high-dose methylprednisolone pulse therapy followed by long-term low-dose oral prednisolone. This therapy appears to be better tolerated and induces faster remission than does standard prednisolone therapy. The effectiveness and appropriate dosing strategies of methylprednisolone pulse therapy have yet to be determined in dogs. It should also be noted that the catabolic effects of corticosteroids may cause or worsen azotemia.

Chlorambucil, cyclophosphamide, azathioprine, and cyclosporine have been used with various results in the treatment of human and veterinary patients that have failed to respond or have developed unwanted side effects when given corticosteroids. Preliminary results suggest that dogs with canine glomerulonephritis do not predictably respond to cyclosporine. The antiproteinuric effects of cyclosporine may be mediated not only by the drug's immunosuppressive effects but also through reductions in glomerular filtration rate and changes in glomerular permselectivity.

Enhancement of antigen removal by increasing antibody formation or reticuloendothelial system activity through immunostimulation is an alternative to immunosuppression that has been advocated by some investigators. The use of immunostimulants has not been evaluated in dogs with glomerulonephritis.

If immunomodulatory drugs are used, biochemical panels and degree of proteinuria should be evaluated frequently to assess the effects of treatment. In some instances, immunomodulatory treatment may exacerbate glomerular lesions and proteinuria.

ANTICOAGULANT TREATMENT

Increasing evidence suggests that platelets and their arachidonic acid metabolites (thromboxanes) are integrally involved in the pathogenesis of glomerulonephritis. Beneficial responses to antiplatelet therapy including aspirin, indomethacin, dipyridamole, and platelet-activating factor antagonists have been demonstrated in several studies. Dose appears to be important when nonspecific cyclo-oxygenase inhibitors such as aspirin are used. Low-dose aspirin therapy (0.5 to 5.0 mg/kg PO b.i.d.) may selectively inhibit platelet cyclo-oxygenase without preventing prostacyclin (vasodilator and platelet aggregation antagonist) formation. In several studies with mice, rats, rabbits, and dogs, thromboxane synthetase inhibitors and thromboxane receptor antagonists have attenuated experimental glomerulonephritis as evidenced by decreased proteinuria, decreased glomerular cell proliferation and infiltration, decreased fibrin deposition, and preservation of glomerular filtration rate.

Hypercoagulability and thrombus formation associated with proteinuria occur secondary to several abnormalities in the clotting system. In addition to a mild thrombocytosis, hypoalbuminemia-related platelet hypersensitivity increases platelet adhesion and aggregation proportional to the magnitude of hypoalbuminemia. Loss of antithrombin-III in urine also contributes to hypercoagulability. Antithrombin-III works in concert with heparin to inhibit serine proteases (clotting factors II, IX, X, XI, XII) and normally has a large role in modulating thrombin and fibrin production. Finally, altered fibrinolysis and increases in the concentration of high-molecular-weight clotting factors (fibrinogen, V, VII, VIII, X) lead to a relative increase in clotting factors versus regulatory proteins. The pulmonary arterial system is the most common location for thromboembolism. Dogs with pulmonary thromboembolism are usually dyspneic and hypoxic but show minimal pulmonary parenchymal radiographic abnormalities. Treatment of pulmonary thromboembolism is difficult, often expensive, and frequently unrewarding; therefore, early prophylactic treatment is important. Measurement of antithrombin-III and fibrinogen concentrations may be helpful in determining which patients should be treated with anticoagulant therapy. Dogs with antithrombin-III concentrations less than 70% of normal and fibrinogen concentrations greater than 300 mg/dl are candidates for therapy.

Warfarin and heparin, in addition to being anticoagulants, have been used in an attempt to slow the progression of glomerulonephritis. Heparin failed to offer protection from the disease, and in some cases the histologic appearance of the kidney was actually worse in treated animals. This is not surprising inasmuch as heparin requires normal antithrombin-III concentrations to inhibit coagulation, and plasma antithrombin-III concentrations are often decreased in animals with glomerulonephritis. Warfarin has, however, protected animals against fibrin deposition and glomerular epithelial crescent formation, although there was no apparent effect on proteinuria.

Low-dose aspirin is easily administered on an outpatient basis and does not require extensive monitoring as does warfarin treatment. Because fibrin accumulation within the glomerulus is a frequent consequence of glomerulonephritis, anticoagulant treatment may serve a dual purpose. Recent clinical trials in humans have focused on the combination of immunosuppressive, antiplatelet, and anticoagulant agents. More prospective studies are needed to identify an effective therapy for glomerulonephritis in dogs.

SUPPORTIVE CARE

Dietary Factors

The effects of dietary protein and mineral content on the progression of renal disease have been investigated in dogs. Restriction of dietary phosphorus and calcium improves survival and decreases the rate of decline of glomerular filtration rate in dogs with partial renal ablation and may be of benefit in dogs with progressive glomerulonephropathies. It is generally accepted that reduction of dietary protein reduces nausea associated with uremia. However, it remains controversial whether diets with reduced protein retard the progression of renal disease in dogs. High-protein diets have been implicated in contributing to hyperfiltration, glomerular capillary hypertension, and glomerular pathology in rats. In dogs with partial renal ablation, disease progression was not altered by feeding low-protein diets, although other factors implicated in glomerular capillary hypertension were not controlled in these studies. Dietary protein reduction did limit increases in proteinuria associated with experimentally induced chronic renal failure in dogs.

Although it was once recommended that dietary protein intake be increased with high-quality protein to approximate daily urine protein excretion, this practice has now been questioned. When patients with glomerulonephritis are fed a high-protein diet, albumin synthesis increases but renal excretion of albumin also increases. The net result of increased protein intake is frequently decreased serum albumin concentrations. Conversely, when dietary protein is severely restricted, albumin synthesis cannot be increased in response to hypoalbuminemia. In rats, the use of angiotensin-converting enzyme inhibitors often blunts the increased albuminuria caused by dietary protein supplementation, allowing albumin stores to be increased. Research has not determined if the same is true for dogs. A diet of moderately reduced protein, with reduced sodium and phosphorus content (e.g., Hill's Prescription Diet Canine k/d) should be fed to dogs with glomerulonephritis until the results of a well-controlled dietary study are available.

Control of Hypertension

Systemic hypertension has been identified in up to 80% of canine patients with glomerulonephritis. Hypertension probably occurs in association with glomerulonephritis as a result of a combination of sodium retention, glomerular capillary and arteriolar scarring, decreased renal production of vasodilators, and increased responsiveness to pressor mechanisms. The morbidity and mortality of hypertensive patients may be reduced by lowering systemic arterial blood pressures.

Systemic hypertension may also contribute to the progression to chronic renal failure by causing hyalinization and fibrinoid degeneration of small renal vessels and contributing to glomerular hyperfiltration. Limiting capillary hypertension through control of arterial hypertension is an important consideration in preventing progressive loss of nephron mass in humans and laboratory animals with glomerulonephritis, although this has not been specifically evaluated in dogs. Unfortunately, reduction in arterial pressure is not always accompanied by similar reductions in glomerular capillary pressures in rats, and glomerular capillary hypertension is not always associated with arterial hypertension. Whereas thiazide diuretics and peripherally acting vasodilating agents have little effect on glomerular capillary pressure, angiotensin-converting enzyme inhibition frequently results in pronounced decline in glomerular capillary pressure even with only modest decreases in systemic arterial pressure. However, angiotensin-converting enzyme inhibitors should be used cautiously in dogs with glomerulonephritis, because high doses can in some cases cause proteinuria, glomerulonephropathies, and decreased renal function (see this volume, p. 838).

References and Suggested Reading

Cameron, J. S.: The treatment of glomerulonephritis with inhibitors of coagulation. In Kluthe, R., Vogt, A., Batsford, S. R., et al. (eds.): Glomerulonephritis: International Conference on Pathogenesis, Pathology and Treatment. New York: John Wiley & Sons, 1977, pp. 154–164.

Cameron, J. S.: Treatment of primary glomerulonephritis using immunosuppressive agents. Am. J. Nephrol. 9:33, 1989.

Finco, D. R., and Brown, S. A.: Newer concepts and controversies on dietary management of renal failure. In Kirk, R. W. (ed.): Current Veterinary Therapy X. Philadelphia: W. B. Saunders, 1989, pp. 1198–1201.

Glassock, R. J.: The kidney: Therapeutic implications of angiotensin-converting enzyme inhibition. Prevention of renal disease: Where do we go from here? Am. J. Hypertens. 1:389S, 1988.

Kaysen, G. A.: Albumin metabolism in nephrotic syndrome: The effect of dietary protein intake. Am. J. Kidney Dis. 12:461, 1988.

Ross, L. A., and Labato, M. A.: Use of drugs to control hypertension in renal failure. In Kirk, R. W. (ed.): Current Veterinary Therapy X. Philadelphia: W. B. Saunders, 1989, pp. 1201–1204.

PERITONEAL DIALYSIS: AN UPDATE ON METHODS AND USEFULNESS

INDIA F. LANE,
LESLIE J. CARTER,
and MICHAEL R. LAPPIN
Fort Collins, Colorado

Peritoneal dialysis is a method of removing excess solutes or water from one solution (plasma) to another (dialysate) via osmotic gradients. The large surface area of the peritoneum serves as a semipermeable membrane for the exchange. Substances that can pass through the small intercellular channels between endothelial and mesothelial cells include urea, creatinine, phosphorus, and electrolytes. The actual clearance times of these and larger solutes such as proteins are affected by their molecular size, the dwell time (period of time the dialysate is in the peritoneal cavity), the dialysate composition, and an individual patient's membrane characteristics.

The most common indications for peritoneal dialysis are acute renal failure, acute decompensation of chronic renal failure, and the presurgical management of uremia due to uroabdomen or urinary tract obstruction. Other conditions in which peritoneal dialysis may be beneficial include metabolic emergencies such as hyperkalemia, hypercalcemia, resistant metabolic acidosis, hepatic encephalopathy, severe fluid overload, and congestive heart failure. Management of intra-abdominal diseases such as acute hemorrhagic pancreatitis or peritonitis may also be augmented by peritoneal flushing.

Peritoneal dialysis is an alternative to hemodialysis in humans and has proved to be more adaptable to small animals than hemodialysis. Various regimens have been used, including intermittent peritoneal dialysis, continuous cycling peritoneal dialysis, and continuous ambulatory peritoneal dialysis (CAPD). The continuous ambulatory method is used most frequently in animals and is discussed here.

METHODS

Patient Selection

Patients should be selected primarily on the basis of need for CAPD, but consideration also should be given to the owner's dedication to the financial and time commitment, the hospital staff's ability to attend to the extensive demands of peritoneal dialysis, and the animal's tolerance of intensive procedures. Optimal performance of CAPD requires 24-hr care. The total cost for CAPD varies with body size, dialysate used, dialysis cycle selected, complications incurred, and duration of hospitalization. Excluding the initial diagnostic evaluation, catheter placement and start-up costs usually average $250 in our hospital, with additional costs averaging $250 per day of dialysis, depending on the source of dialysate and supplies (Table 1).

In small animals, CAPD is used most frequently for the control of clinical signs of uremia by reducing plasma concentrations of urea, creatinine, and other uremic wastes. Previously reported poor survival rates for dogs receiving CAPD are related to the severity of the primary disease being treated (Crisp et al., 1989). The use of CAPD in the presurgical management of postrenal obstruction or uroabdomen has the best chance for success, because underlying renal function is often normal or the renal pathology is reversible. However, uremia in these cases can often be managed with other techniques. Anuric or oliguric acute renal failure due to conditions such as toxin ingestion, drug overdoses, hypotensive crises, or pyelonephritis has a variable prognosis. Anuric or oliguric uremic crises that develop as a result of decompensation of chronic polyuric renal insufficiency carry the most guarded prognosis because of previous reduction in functional nephron numbers, and the use of CAPD in these cases is questionable. In cases of anuric or oliguric renal failure, medical management protocols such as aggressive rehydration with diuretic administration, osmotic diuresis, and dopamine administration should be attempted before initiating CAPD. If attempts to induce diuresis fail, CAPD should be initiated promptly to maximize potential benefits.

The primary considerations in electing CAPD should be whether the initiating condition is reversible and whether adequate renal tissue remains.

865

Table 1. Comparison of Dialysate Solutions Available for Peritoneal Dialysis

	1.5% Dextrose*	4.25% Dextrose†	LRS/1.5% Dextrose‡
Sodium (mEq/L)§	141	141	130
Potassium (mEq/L)§	0	0	4
Calcium (mEq/L)	3.5	3.5	3
Magnesium (mEq/L)	1.5	1.5	0
Chloride (mEq/L)	101	101	109
Lactate (mEq/L)	45	45	28
Dextrose (gm/L)	15	42.5	15
Osmolality (mOsm/L)	366	505	356

*Dianeal with 1.5% dextrose (Baxter Health Care, Travenol, Deerfield, IL). The approximate cost per exchange for a 15-kg dog is $3 to $12.
†Dianeal with 4.25% dextrose (Baxter Health Care, Deerfield, IL). The approximate cost per exchange for a 15-kg dog is $3 to $12.
‡Lactated Ringer's solution (Sanofi, Overland Park, KS) with 1.5% dextrose added. The approximate cost per exchange for a 15-kg dog is $3.
§Sodium and potassium can be added to dialysate solution as indicated. Initial exchanges are usually completed with potassium-free dialysate, then 4 to 5 mEq/L potassium chloride can be added to supply adequate potassium.

Renal biopsy samples for histopathologic study should be obtained from cases being considered for CAPD in order to help predict the likelihood for return of renal function. We generally obtain biopsy specimens of one or both kidneys when placing the peritoneal dialysis catheter.

CAPD is contraindicated in patients with intra-abdominal conditions that prevent safe dialysate exchange, such as abdominal wall trauma and peritoneal infections or adhesions that lead to the loss of more than 50% of the peritoneal surface. Severe ascites, obesity, bowel distention, or abdominal masses may interfere with catheter placement or adequate volume exchanges and are relative contraindications for CAPD.

Catheter Placement

Peritoneal dialysis is most commonly performed using straight or curled fenestrated tubing or column disk catheters. The column disk catheter* is less likely to develop outflow obstruction, especially when combined with partial omentectomy (Birchard et al., 1988). The column disk, composed of two Silastic sheets separated by multiple pillars, is placed directly against the peritoneum (Fig. 1). Two Dacron cuffs provide seals at the preperitoneum and the subcutis. The catheter should be surgically placed using strict sterile technique. The surgical approach and technique for catheter placement are described elsewhere (Birchard et al., 1988).

After surgical placement of the dialysis catheter, the tail of the catheter tubing is connected to a transfer tubing set† (Figs. 1 and 2) that has previously been attached to and primed with a prewarmed bag of dialysate. This connection is made using a special adapter* supplied with the column disk catheter, and strict sterile technique should be maintained throughout all manipulations. Connections should be protected with connection shields† or povidone-iodine–soaked sponges. The exit site should be dressed with antiseptic ointment and sterile 4 × 4 gauze squares. A roller clamp on the transfer tubing controls the flow of dialysate to and from the peritoneal cavity.

Dialysate Solutions

Commercially prepared dialysate solutions containing various concentrations of dextrose are available (see Table 1). CAPD for removal of solutes is generally performed using 1.5% dextrose. Dialysates containing 2.5% and 4.25% dextrose are used in mild to severely overhydrated patients. Heparin (250 to 1000 U/L) is added to the dialysate for the first few days after catheter placement to help prevent occlusion of the catheter by fibrin deposition.

Alternatively, a suitable dialysate can be prepared by adding dextrose to lactated Ringer's solution or other balanced electrolyte solution (Parker, 1984). Osmolality should closely approximate that of the patient, and the dextrose concentration should be at least 1.5% (see Table 1). Patient magnesium levels should be monitored if lactated Ringer's solution is used, because the solution does not contain this element (Crisp et al., 1989). The use of acetate-based dialysis solutions leads to progressive decreases in ultrafiltration over time and should be avoided.

In addition to various dextrose concentrations, dialysate composition can be altered according to individual needs and situations. For example, the

*Lifecath or Vetcath, Quinton Instrument Company, Seattle, WA.

†CAPD solution transfer set, Baxter Health Care Corporation, Deerfield, IL.

*Beta-Cap Adapter, Quinton Instrument Company, Seattle, WA.

†Connection Shield, Baxter Health Care Corporation, Deerfield, IL.

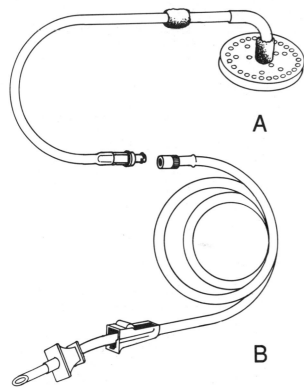

Figure 1. Schematic representation of the column disk catheter (*A*) and standard CAPD solution transfer tubing set (*B*) for straight single-spike systems.

bicarbonate concentration in the dialysate can be adjusted to help correct persistent severe metabolic acidosis. Many patients on CAPD become hyponatremic, and additional sodium may be required,

particularly if lactated Ringer's solution is used as the primary dialysate, because this solution has a lower sodium concentration than the commercial dialysate solutions (see Table 1). Potassium may be added to commercial solutions used for hypokalemic patients at doses up to 5 mEq/L of dialysate.

The recommended infusion volume for small animals is 30 to 40 ml/kg. For small patients, wastage of a large dialysate bag can be avoided by using multiple small-volume exchanges with a single bag (Carter et al., 1989). The approximate volume for each exchange is determined by weight.

The Exchange Procedure

For the first 12 to 24 hr after catheter placement, exchange volumes should be half the calculated ideal volume in order to assess the degree of abdominal distention, the effect on respiratory function, and the potential for dialysate leakage. After instillation, the empty dialysate bag is rolled up and taped to the animal's side. The following is a brief description of our standard exchange procedure using a straight single-spike system (see Fig. 1; see *CVT VIII*, p. 1028):

1. After a fresh bag of dialysate is prepared, the collapsed empty dialysate bag is unrolled and placed below the level of the animal for drainage.

2. The roller clamp on the transfer tubing is opened to allow slow drainage of fluid from the peritoneal cavity. The time required for drainage is variable but usually is less than 15 min. The roller clamp is closed when drainage is complete.

3. Following careful aseptic procedure (Table 2), the fresh dialysate bag is connected to the transfer set spike, and dialysate is infused by hanging the bag above the animal and opening the roller clamp to allow infusion of the appropriate volume over approximately 10 min. The volume of dialysate can

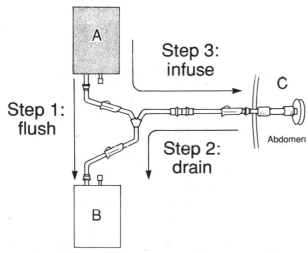

Figure 2. The Y-set connector system (Baxter Health Care Corporation, Deerfield, IL) for CAPD. Step 1: Fresh dialysate (*A*) is flushed from the dialysate bag to the empty container (*B*). Step 2: The peritoneal cavity (*C*) is drained into the empty container (*B*). Step 3: The fresh dialysate (*A*) is then infused into the peritoneal cavity.

Table 2. Tips for Preventing Infection

Define a clean work space in a low traffic area.
Wash hands thoroughly.
Wear examination gloves and a surgical mask when handling dialysis supplies and exchanges.
Open bag ports on the edge of the work space and do not allow them to touch any surfaces.
Use protective "clamshells" or povidone-iodine–soaked dressings covered with sterile gauze to cover all connections.
Scrub injection ports with povidone-iodine solution for 2 min before making any injections or connections.
Avoid multiple-dose vials (e.g., for heparin or antibiotic additives) or scrub their injection caps before repeated use.
Change the catheter dressing and abdominal bandage daily or more frequently if leakage is a problem.
Visually examine each bag of dialysate for cloudiness or discoloration before and after use.

be increased to 30 to 40 ml/kg/exchange after the first 12 to 24 hr if no leakage exists.

4. The dialysate is left in the peritoneal cavity for an appropriate dwell time. Exchanges are generally completed hourly in a uremic crisis. The dwell times are adjusted as the patient stabilizes and are gradually extended to 4 to 6 hr.

A Y-set system for catheter connection and exchanges (see Fig. 2) has been developed as an alternative to the conventional straight single-spike systems. Directions for its use follow:

1. The Y-set tubing, with a fresh dialysate bag and drainage container attached to either segment, is connected to the catheter tubing or transfer set.

2. First, a small amount of fresh dialysate is flushed to the drainage bag (open roller clamps for about 5 sec), then the peritoneal cavity is drained, so that any contaminants introduced during the connection procedures are flushed into the drainage bag and not into the peritoneal cavity.

3. After drainage, the fresh dialysate is infused.

4. If the Y-segment is disconnected from the catheter tubing between exchanges, the catheter tubing may be infused with disinfectant, depending on the tubing type and manufacturer. A disinfectant-filled cap is applied to the catheter segment.

This drain first/infuse later principle has significantly reduced the incidence of peritonitis in human patients on CAPD as compared with the infuse first/drain later principle used in the straight single-spike system. The Y-set system is also beneficial when administering multiple small-volume exchanges with a single large dialysate bag.

Monitoring Therapy

Careful records of the dialysate volumes infused and recovered during each exchange period should be maintained. Less fluid may be recovered from the abdomen than was delivered for the first few exchanges. As dialysis proceeds, outflow should approximate or exceed inflow if the patient is adequately hydrated (the excess being true ultrafiltrate).

Body weight and hydration status should be monitored frequently, with body weight recorded consistently, either with or without dialysate in the abdomen. Measurement of central venous pressure through a jugular catheter is a sensitive method for detecting overhydration. Packed cell volume and plasma total protein determinations should be made at least twice daily. Serum electrolytes and other blood chemistries including blood urea nitrogen, creatinine, albumin, and acid-base determinations initially should be completed daily and then as needed based on an animal's clinical condition. A

select few animals can receive maintenance CAPD at home with careful training of a dedicated client.

The objectives of peritoneal dialysis are to reduce azotemia and resolve clinical signs of uremia as well as to help correct fluid, electrolyte, and acid-base imbalances until a patient's renal function can maintain these objectives alone. Conversion of anuric or oliguric patients to a polyuric state and stabilization or improvement of azotemia are the primary indications for discontinuation of CAPD.

MANAGEMENT OF PATIENTS ON CAPD

A number of metabolic aberrations may occur in patients on CAPD, including alterations in sodium, potassium, magnesium, and glucose levels as well as acid-base status. Frequent monitoring and adjustment of dialysate and supplemental fluid composition may be necessary. Several other conditions commonly require special attention in patients on CAPD.

Nonregenerative anemia is a common sequela of chronic renal failure and may be exacerbated by dialysis. The use of recombinant human erythropoietin administered subcutaneously in humans improves the efficiency of peritoneal dialysis, resulting in increased ultrafiltration and improved urea and creatinine clearances (Steinhauer et al., 1989). Similar benefits may occur in small animals (see this volume, p. 484).

Protein losses are significant with CAPD. Losses may increase dramatically (50 to 100%) when peritonitis is present. Hypoalbuminemia was the most common complication in a recent review of peritoneal dialysis cases in dogs and cats, with 41% of the patients affected (Crisp et al., 1989). Severe hypoalbuminemia can be attenuated with adequate protein intake and plasma transfusions. We generally administer supplemental plasma when the total plasma protein level declines to 3.5 gm/dl or less. Complete correction of hypoalbuminemia with plasma alone is unlikely because of the large volumes of plasma required to supply significant amounts of albumin.

Dialysis dysequilibrium may occur during or shortly after early dialysis exchanges, especially in animals with extreme azotemia, acidosis, hypernatremia, or hyperglycemia. It is suspected that rapid removal of urea and other osmotic products from the blood creates an osmotic gradient with subsequent movement of water into cells in the brain. This syndrome is manifested by restlessness, vomiting, dementia, seizures, or death (Parker, 1984). Although this is a rare complication, it can be prevented by slowly reducing azotemia in dialysis patients. Temporary discontinuation of dialysis or reduced exchange frequencies may help reverse the condition once it has occurred.

Increased intraperitoneal pressure following dialysate infusion may affect respiratory function. Atelectasis and hypoxemia may result. These changes are magnified in uremic patients with concurrent pneumonia, pulmonary edema, or anemia, and the infusion volume should be reduced accordingly.

Acute pleural effusion is another uncommon complication of CAPD in dogs, usually occurring early in the course of dialysis. Although shunts between the peritoneal and pleural cavities cannot always be documented, small pleuroperitoneal connections may exist or fluid may move through lymphatic channels. Thoracocentesis or thoracostomy drainage is used to relieve the pleural pressure, and reduced dialysate volumes and dwell times may help prevent recurrence (Carter et al., 1989).

Maintaining adequate nutritional intake in patients on peritoneal dialysis is compounded by the anorexia and vomiting that are often present in uremic patients, as well as by protein loss in the dialysate. Nutritional requirements should be estimated by establishing basal metabolic needs (70 × body weight (kg)$^{0.75}$ = kcal/day required) and multiplying by a factor of 2 to account for severe catabolic needs and protein loss. Dextrose present in the dialysate supplies approximately 8 kcal/kg/day in energy sources toward this total. Protein intake should be approximately 1.8 gm/kg/day, and water-soluble vitamins should be supplemented. When possible, caloric needs should be met with oral intake or enteral methods. However, surgical placement of gastrostomy or jejunostomy tubes may result in compromised dialysis catheter function and leakage.

Nasogastric and pharyngostomy tubes are enteral feeding alternatives that do not require penetration of the peritoneum. Total parenteral nutrition may be indicated when persistent vomiting is present, gastrointestinal function is poor, or feeding tubes are not feasible (see *CVT X*, p. 25).

DRUG THERAPY IN PATIENTS ON CAPD

The presence of renal failure alone affects the biotransformation and clearance of drugs that are primarily excreted by the kidneys. In CAPD, a number of factors influence the elimination of drugs given systemically, including composition and flow rate of the dialysate, properties of the drug, and permeability and blood flow of the peritoneal membrane. However, peritoneal clearance is minimal for most drugs compared with plasma clearance, and dosage adaptations for patients on CAPD, other than those recommended in renal failure, are not necessary.

In contrast, uptake of drugs given intraperitoneally can be significant and rapid. This phenomenon is mainly due to the concentration gradient created between the dialysate volume and the much larger plasma distribution volume as well as higher protein binding that may occur in plasma versus dialysate. The absorption of drugs increases with peritonitis and should be anticipated when potentially toxic antibiotics are used intraperitoneally. Strongly charged cationic drugs or poorly soluble drugs are not transported well across the peritoneum. Heparin, for instance, is not absorbed when added to the dialysate and thus is unlikely to affect systemic coagulation when used to prevent catheter occlusion.

COMPLICATIONS OF PERITONEAL DIALYSIS

Although the column disk catheter has reduced the frequency of catheter obstruction, complications with peritoneal catheters still present a frustrating problem in peritoneal dialysis. Dialysate retention due to catheter obstruction of inflow or outflow, exit site and tunnel infections, and leakage of dialysate remain the most common complications. Careful surgical placement of the catheter and attention to aseptic technique will reduce the possibility of infection. Mild infections can be controlled with local treatment and appropriate parenteral antibiotics. Povidone-iodine or hydrogen peroxide soaks can be used at the exit site. If the infection does not respond to adequate therapy, catheter removal should be considered.

If subcutaneous leakage of dialysate occurs, decreased exchange volumes and frequencies may help resolve the problem. If leakage is severe or persists, surgical exploration and correction are indicated. Omentectomy and the addition of heparin to the dialysate for the first few days help prevent catheter occlusion with omentum or fibrin. Aggressive sterile flushing may be attempted to alleviate catheter obstruction. Replacement of the catheter may be necessary if resistant obstruction occurs.

Peritonitis is a serious complication of peritoneal dialysis. Reported incidence rates in veterinary patients are 22% and 40%, with the likelihood of infection increasing the longer dialysis is continued. Bacterial penetration may occur around or through the exit site of the peritoneal catheter or as a result of touch contamination of tubing or bag spikes. Bowel perforation or hematogenous spread of bacteria may infrequently lead to peritonitis in patients on CAPD.

The diagnosis of peritonitis is based on the presence of at least two of the following three criteria: (1) cloudy dialysate effluent; (2) detection of greater than 100 inflammatory cells per microliter or organisms in Gram's stains or cultures of the effluent; (3) clinical signs of peritonitis. To facilitate early detection of peritonitis, each bag of drained dialysate should be examined for cloudiness, which if present mandates cytologic examination of a sample of the fluid. The fluid should be cultured if any evidence of peritonitis exists. It should initially be cultured for aerobes; if samples are negative, samples for anaerobic culture should be obtained. Organisms isolated from veterinary patients in one review included *Mycoplasma, Acinetobacter, Klebsiella, Escherichia coli, Proteus, Providencia,* and *Pseudomonas* (Crisp et al., 1989).

Treatment of peritonitis should begin as soon as cytologic findings suggest infection. Cephalosporins are usually used systemically or intraperitoneally before the availability of culture results (Thornhill, 1984). Heparin should be added to the dialysate during episodes of peritonitis. Treatment should be continued for 7 days after cultures become negative.

Prevention of peritonitis can be accomplished by strict adherence to aseptic technique, because seemingly minor contaminations can lead to peritonitis in patients on CAPD. The guidelines listed (see Table 2) are helpful in preventing infection.

References and Suggested Reading

Birchard, S. J., Chew, D. J., Crisp, M. S., et al.: Modified technique for placement of a column disc peritoneal dialysis catheter. J. Am. Anim. Hosp. Assoc. 24:663, 1988.
A description of the column disk catheter and the surgical technique for placement.
Carter, L. J., Wingfield, W. E., and Allen, T. A.: Clinical experience with peritoneal dialysis in small animals. Comp. Cont. Ed. Pract. Vet. 11:1335, 1989.
An overview of peritoneal dialysis techniques and potential complications.
Crisp, M. S., Chew, D. J., DiBartola, S. P., et al.: Peritoneal dialysis in dogs and cats: 27 cases. J.A.V.M.A. 195:1262, 1989.
A retrospective analysis of peritoneal dialysis in 25 dogs and 2 cats, including methods, complications, and results.
Parker, H. R.: Peritoneal dialysis and hemofiltration. *In* Bovée, K. C. (ed.): *Canine Nephrology.* New York: Harwal, 1984, p. 723.
A complete review of the theory, methods, and complications of peritoneal dialysis in small animals.
Steinhauer, H. B., Lubrich-Birkner, I., Dreyling, K. W., et al.: Increased ultrafiltration after erythropoietin-induced correction of renal anemia in patients on continuous ambulatory peritoneal dialysis. Nephron 53:91, 1989.
Comparison of ultrafiltration, creatinine, and urea clearances in human patients on CAPD after the initiation of recombinant human erythropoietin injections.
Thornhill, J. A.: Therapeutic strategies involving antimicrobial treatment of small animals with peritonitis. J.A.V.M.A. 185:1181, 1984.
A review of the diagnosis, management, and antibiotic therapy of peritonitis in patients on CAPD.

RENAL TRANSPLANTATION IN CLINICAL VETERINARY MEDICINE

CLARE R. GREGORY
and IRA M. GOURLEY
Davis, California

Three major factors have led to the successful performance of renal transplantation in veterinary practice: (1) introduction of the immunosuppressive agent cyclosporine, (2) a better understanding of the immune response to foreign organs and tissue (rejection), and (3) the development of microsurgical techniques (Gregory et al., 1987). Introduction of the immunosuppressive agent cyclosporine started a new era in successful immunotherapy for organ transplantation in human medicine. When compared with traditional antirejection therapies, cyclosporine resulted in superior graft and patient survival in heart and liver transplantation and improved graft survival in renal transplantation. Cyclosporine was the first potent immunosuppressive agent to act on specific T-lymphocyte responses without concomitant myelotoxicity (Gregory, 1989). Cyclosporine did not inhibit migration of leukocytes and had no significant effect on the viability of nonstimulated lymphocytes. This specific, reversible mechanism of action spared nonspecific host resistance and resulted in a lower incidence of viral and bacterial infections when compared with other immunosuppressive agents.

The recognition of foreign tissue antigens by sensitized cells or antibodies marks the beginning of the active effort of rejection by the recipient's immune system. The primary mechanism of destruction is by generation of T lymphocytes that are cytotoxic for the allograft. Graft cell lysis is accomplished through the direct action of T-cytotoxic cells and by the activation of cascading enzyme systems, including the complement, clotting, and probably the kinin pathways. Other cellular mediators such as B lymphocytes, plasma cells, macrophages, platelets, and polymorphonuclear leukocytes have both a direct and an indirect role in allograft rejection.

Three overlapping "types" of organ rejection are recognized clinically. Hyperacute rejection is an accelerated form of rejection that is associated with preformed circulatory antibody in the serum of the recipient that reacts with donor cells, particularly the endothelium of vessel walls. Polymorphonuclear leukocytes line the capillary walls, and most capillaries and arterioles are blocked by microthrombi, resulting in tissue necrosis. In hyperacute rejection, the recipient has been sensitized to the allograft antigens by previous blood transfusions, pregnancy, or transplantation. Pre-existing antibody can be identified before transplantation by testing leukocytes of the potential donor with serum of the recipient in the presence of complement. However, this assay is only available at major hospitals or universities. Fortunately, we have not experienced this type of rejection in a clinical patient. Most recipients have not borne litters or previously received a transplant. As discussed later, blood transfusions may have a protective effect on the transplanted organ.

Acute rejection typically occurs 7 to 21 days after transplantation or when effective immunosuppression is terminated. Pathologic studies of the rejected organ reveal a predominant pattern of mononuclear leukocyte infiltration in the tissue.

Chronic rejection is characterized by gradual loss of organ function over months to years, often without any clear-cut clinical rejection episode. Kidneys undergoing chronic rejection show severe narrowing of numerous arteries and thickening of the glomerular capillary basement membrane. The lesions are formed by adherence of platelets and fibrin aggregates to the vessel walls. These deposits become covered by endothelium and incorporated in the intima, which often contains IgM and complement.

Without the use of immunosuppressive agents, matching the donor and recipient for similar or identical cell surface histocompatibility antigens will prolong allograft survival. Approximately half of the genetic information that codes for cell surface histocompatibility antigens is inherited from each parent. Therefore, siblings may be matched (25%), partially matched (50%), or mismatched (25%). For canine transplant recipients, therefore, siblings and parents constitute the best source of donor organs, but many will be incompatible. If related canine organ donors can be found, an estimate of histocompatibility between the donor and recipient can be made using a microcytotoxicity assay or mixed-lymphocyte response assay (Stevenson and Schwartz, 1985). Although these tests are performed only at major hospitals or university laboratories, blood samples can be shipped, using special handling techniques, over long distances.

It was initially hoped that the immunosuppressive effects of cyclosporine would allow organ transplantation across major histocompatibility barriers (i.e., between unrelated canine pairs). Initial reports were encouraging, showing renal allograft survival of greater than 100 days without rejection episodes (Homan et al., 1980, 1981). A beagle dog recipient of a nonmatched renal allograft survived 805 days (Gregory et al., 1986). However, we performed renal allograft transplantation on three dogs using unrelated donors. Cyclosporine and prednisolone were used to suppress the host immune response. The average survival time before loss of the grafts to rejection was approximately 70 days. Combination daily and alternate-day treatment using cyclosporine and azathioprine has been studied in dogs receiving kidneys from unrelated donors (Davies et al., 1989). Seventy-seven per cent of the dogs survived less than 275 days.

With cyclosporine and prednisolone as immunosuppressant agents, cats can tolerate renal allografts from unrelated donors. We have performed 23 renal transplants in cats using kidneys from unrelated donors (Gregory et al., 1990). The average survival period was 12 months, with the longest surviving a period of 31 months. Only two of the 23 cats experienced a recognizable rejection episode. One occurred 30 days after surgery, and the other occurred 15 months following surgery. The second episode was caused by an unexplained decrease in whole blood levels of cyclosporine. Once blood levels of cyclosporine were increased, renal function returned to normal.

RENAL TRANSPLANTATION IN CATS

Criteria for a Suitable Renal Recipient

Renal transplantation is one method of treatment for renal insufficiency. It cannot be regarded as an emergency treatment or last-ditch effort to save the life of a critically ill, malnourished patient (Gregory et al., 1987). Surgical intervention has to take place before all medical means of therapy have been exhausted.

We consider body weight to be a very important indication of the status of the renal transplant candidate. If a cat has been in compensated renal failure and starts to lose weight or presents in renal failure with a history of chronic weight loss, transplantation should be considered as an option before further weight loss occurs. Our previous attempts to alter the course of physical deterioration due to decompensated renal failure via enteral or parenteral alimentation before transplantation have failed. Age, plasma creatinine levels, blood urea nitrogen concentration, and other clinical pathologic assessments of renal function cannot in themselves select a suitable patient for transplantation.

Candidates for renal transplantation should be free of bacterial urinary tract infection (UTI). If the candidate has had several negative urine cultures but has a past history of UTI, a renal biopsy should be considered. In our experience, dogs or cats with a previous history of UTI will become bacteriuric after transplantation and immunosuppression. In two cases, UTI recurred despite removal of the recipient's native kidneys and ureters. Bacterial UTI in a transplant recipient causes direct morbidity and mortality as a result of the infection itself and may also activate the rejection process (Rubin et al., 1981).

Feline candidates for renal transplantation should be free of feline leukemia virus infection and other complicating diseases. Renal insufficiency can produce systemic hypertension in feline patients, leading to congestive heart failure (Ross and Labato, 1989). Cats in renal failure often have systolic murmurs secondary to anemia; these may not represent significant cardiac disease. Cardiac enlargement determined by ultrasonographic examination, gallop rhythms, and electrocardiographic abnormalities all are indications to decline a candidate for transplantation.

The feline renal donor/recipient pair do not have to be related or tissue matched, but they must be blood crossmatched. The antigens present on red blood cells are also present on the endothelium of the graft blood vessels. Preformed antibodies to these antigens will cause clotting of the graft vessels and infarcts of the organ at the time of surgery.

Feline renal recipients must also be blood crossmatched to two to three blood donor cats. The primary reason for this is the anemia that accompanies chronic renal failure. Following rehydration of a patient before surgery, packed red blood cell volumes may fall to as low as 12 to 15%. As much as 180 to 250 ml of whole blood may be required to attain a packed red blood cell volume of 30% in the renal recipient before surgery. Also, in our experience, some cats in chronic renal failure are not transfusible (i.e., all crossmatch assays show agglutination of donor red cells, even in cats of the same blood type; all agglutinated samples should undergo saline dispersion to rule out rouleaux formation). This is an important consideration if a transplant patient is traveling a great distance to the transplant clinic. Crossmatching should be done locally to ensure that transfusions can be given before surgery.

Progressive renal disease in cats has been attributed to membranous glomerulonephropathy, chronic interstitial nephritis, amyloidosis, feline infectious peritonitis, lymphosarcoma, polycystic renal disease, bacterial nephritis, and systemic lupus erythematosus. The majority of the cats pre-

sented to us for transplantation had a histopathologic diagnosis of chronic interstitial nephritis. Two cats received renal transplants for renal failure secondary to bacterial pyelitis, two cats for polycystic kidney disease, and one cat for ethylene glycol toxicosis.

Criteria for the Renal Donor

Renal donors should be in excellent health and have no evidence of renal insufficiency based on clinical pathologic testing, complete blood count, serum chemistry panel, and urinalysis. An intravenous pyelogram is performed to assure that the donor has two normally shaped, well-vascularized kidneys. The feline donor should be free of feline leukemia virus infection and be blood crossmatch–compatible with the recipient. Unilateral renal donation should not reduce normal life expectancy.

Preoperative Preparation of the Recipient

Before surgery, the renal recipient is given balanced electrolyte solutions (Lactated Ringer's Injection USP, Travenol) subcutaneously or intravenously at 1.5 to 2 times daily maintenance requirements. Transfusions of whole blood are administered until a packed red cell volume of 30% is achieved. Twenty-four to 48 hr before surgery, cyclosporine oral solution (Sandimmune, Sandoz) is administered at a dosage of 7.5 mg/kg every 12 hr. The cyclosporine oral solution should be placed in gelatin capsules before administration. Capsule sizes 0 or 1 work well for most cats. Cyclosporine oral solution has a very unpleasant taste that causes some cats to salivate profusely, resulting in partial loss of the dose.

On the morning of surgery, a blood sample is taken from the recipient 12 hr after the last oral dose of cyclosporine to determine a 12-hr trough blood level. We monitor whole blood levels of cyclosporine assayed by high-pressure liquid chromatography (Kabra and Wall, 1985). In cats, a level of 500 ng/ml is maintained for the first 30 postoperative days, reducing to 250 ng/ml by 3 months after transplantation. Prednisolone, 0.25 mg/kg/12 hr PO, is also started the morning of surgery and is reduced to 0.25 mg/kg/24 hr by 1 month postoperatively.

Surgery

Two teams perform renal transplantation; one team harvests the donor kidney and closes the abdominal wound, and one team prepares the recipient vessels and receives the kidney (Gregory and Gourley, in press). The two-team approach minimizes the warm ischemia time of the donor kidney, which should be kept to less than 60 min.

Anastomosis of the renal vessels and the ureter in small dogs and in cats requires 3× to 10× magnification. The higher magnification is necessary to stent the ureter in the bladder. We use an operating microscope.* The renal vein of the autograft is anastomosed end to side with the recipient's external iliac vein. The renal artery is anastomosed end to end with the external iliac artery. The ureter is then implanted into the bladder (Gregory and Gourley, in press).

Unless we see evidence of bacterial nephritis, we do not remove the recipient's native kidneys at the time of transplantation. These kidneys are available to provide some support if the transplanted organ should fail and can be removed at a later date if indicated.

Postoperative Care of Renal Recipients

Recipients receive balanced electrolyte solutions intravenously at a daily maintenance rate until eating and drinking resume. Cyclosporine is administered at levels necessary to achieve trough whole blood levels of 500 ng/ml. Prednisolone is administered at 0.25 mg/kg/12 hr PO and is tapered to 0.25 mg/kg/24 hr by 4 weeks postoperatively.

Urine specific gravity is monitored twice daily by free catch of the urine. Urine specific gravity is usually greater than 1.020 by the third postoperative day. Approximately every second day, packed blood cell volume, total plasma protein level, and the plasma creatinine level are assessed. During the early postoperative period, needless venipuncture, blood sampling, and patient handling should be avoided. If the surgery is a technical success, the urine specific gravity will be increased, and the plasma creatinine will be decreased by the third postoperative day. The recipient will look clinically improved, and normal appetite usually returns by postoperative day 3 to 5. If the graft has failed, the recipient will be depressed and anorexic. The urine will remain isosthenuric.

Approximately 10 days after surgery, an ultrasonographic examination of the transplanted kidney and ureter can be performed for evidence of hydronephrosis or hydroureter secondary to obstruction. Obstruction of the ureter is usually accompanied by a urine specific gravity of 1.015 or less. If all signs indicate that the graft is functioning well at this point postoperatively, the recipient is discharged from the hospital.

*Operation Microscope OPMI 6 C, Carl Zeiss, Inc., Thornwood, NY.

Long-Term Management of Feline Renal Recipients

Management of transplant patients must be coordinated with the client, the local veterinarians, and the transplant center (Gregory et al., 1987). Examinations are initially performed weekly by a local veterinarian. Packed blood cell volume, total serum protein level, plasma creatinine level, whole blood cyclosporine level, and a urinalysis are performed. Periods between examinations are gradually extended to 3 or 4 weeks. We recommend that a complete blood count, a serum chemistry panel, and cardiac examination be performed three times a year.

PROTOCOL FOR CANINE RENAL TRANSPLANTATION

There are only a few differences in the technical aspects of renal transplantation between dogs and cats. Most dogs, because of their size, do not require magnification for anastomosis of the vessels, although 2× to 3× magnifying loupes are very helpful. Ureteroneocystostomy is technically much simpler in dogs.

The primary difference in transplantation between dogs and cats is selection of the donor. Using cyclosporine and prednisolone to achieve immunosuppression, we use only mixed-lymphocyte response-matched related donors.

COMPLICATIONS ENCOUNTERED AFTER RENAL TRANSPLANTATION IN CATS

Technical failure of the graft due to thrombosis of the renal artery or vein can occur up to 72 hr after surgery. Ureteral obstruction was encountered in four cats (Gregory, C. R., and Gourley, I. M., unpublished data, 1991). Falling urine specific gravity and rising creatinine levels caused by ureteral obstruction may be confused with graft rejection. Diagnosis of ureteral obstruction is made by ultrasonographic examination of the ureter and kidney or by exploratory laparotomy. Obstruction usually occurs at the junction of the ureter and the bladder wall. The ureter is freed from the bladder, and the stenotic section is excised. Ureteroneocystostomy is then performed at a new site. Mucosa-to-mucosa anastomosis between the bladder and the ureter can often be achieved by dilation of the ureter. Despite what may appear to be severe hydronephrosis, the kidney can return to normal function.

The most common form of bacterial infection affecting human renal transplant recipients is UTI (Rubin et al., 1981). Treatment should be based on proper antibiotic sensitivity testing and a knowledge of the antibiotics that can be toxic when administered with cyclosporine. All aminoglycoside antibiotics should be avoided (Gregory et al., 1987). Trimethoprim alone or combined with sulfamethoxazole may produce nephrotoxicity (Gregory et al., 1987). We have successfully used cephalosporin and fluoroquinolone antibiotics to treat UTI in transplant recipients (Gregory, C. R., and Gourley, I. M., unpublished data, 1991).

Two of 23 cats died at 5 and 11 months after transplantation as a result of systemic bacterial infections caused by an *Actinobacillus* and *Actinomyces* (Gregory, C. R., and Gourley, I. M., unpublished data). Despite a lower reported incidence of post-transplantation infections, this and other studies indicate that cyclosporine and prednisolone immunosuppression can permit the development of lethal bacterial and fungal infections (Gregory et al., 1986, 1987). However, both of these cats were maintained on at least twice the currently recommended trough whole blood levels of cyclosporine. Further experience in clinical transplantation will better define the minimum trough whole blood levels of cyclosporine necessary to maintain renal allografts in cats.

Acute renal rejection can occur at any time but is most common within the first 30 days after transplantation (Stevenson and Schwartz, 1985). Clinical signs of malaise, vomiting, and severe depression ("hangdog look") precede elevations in serum creatinine and blood urea nitrogen (Gregory et al., 1987). If acute allograft rejection is suspected, it must be treated aggressively. Delay in treatment may result in loss of the graft. To treat acute allograft rejection, cyclosporine intravenous solution is administered daily at 6 to 8 mg/kg over a 4- to 6-hr period. Initially, prednisolone is administered at 5 mg IV, followed by 2 to 3 mg/kg SC every 12 hr. Parenteral administration of cyclosporine and prednisolone is continued until oral intake of food and water is tolerated by the patient. Oral administration of cyclosporine is then resumed at a level that achieves higher trough whole blood levels than those before the rejection episode.

Three of 23 cats developed signs of mild to lethal congestive heart failure after transplantation. Ultrasonographic evaluation of the heart in one case revealed mild hypertrophic enlargement of the left ventricle. This cat responded to symptomatic treatment with diuretics. One cat died of congestive heart failure 14 days after surgery and the other 22 months after surgery. Heart failure in these cats could have been a primary problem or secondary to hypertension caused by renal failure or administration of cyclosporine (Civati et al., 1989; Joss et al., 1982). The native kidneys, via effects on both the local circulation and the renin-angiotensin system, can provide a chronic source of hypertension leading to heart failure (Linas et al., 1978; Popovtzer

et al., 1973). The relationship of renal disease, hypertension, and heart disease in cats has to be more fully understood before strong recommendations for treatment are made. After the maintenance of a functioning graft for a period of 2 to 3 months, we recommend removal of the native kidneys if an indication arises. Native kidneys have been removed from feline transplant patients because of recurrent UTI and polycystic kidney disease.

Cyclosporine and prednisolone are used in combination for their synergistic effects. In addition to other mechanisms of action, together they have an additive inhibitory effect on T-cell proliferation and interleukin-2 production (Manfro et al., 1989). Blood levels of cyclosporine can be reduced during the first several months of treatment without development of acute graft rejection, because a degree of graft tolerance appears to be achieved by the host and the bioavailability of cyclosporine increases over time (Klintmalm et al., 1984). However, if blood levels become too low, a rejection episode will occur.

There is little correlation between the oral dose of cyclosporine and the trough whole blood level that will be achieved in a particular patient. Because of interpatient and intrapatient variability in the absorption of oral cyclosporine and its metabolism during chronic therapy, cyclosporine blood levels should be regularly monitored to maintain therapeutic concentrations and minimize toxic side effects. Fortunately, unlike the situation in human beings, cyclosporine rarely produces nephrotoxicity or hepatotoxicity in dogs and cats (Gregory, 1989; Gregory et al., 1987, 1990).

Pretransplant blood transfusions have been shown to improve graft survival in both human and animal renal allograft recipients. The mechanism of this beneficial effect is not clearly understood, but evidence suggests that blood transfusions are immunosuppressive. Most chronic renal failure patients undergoing transplantation require blood transfusions to correct anemia before anesthesia and surgery; immunosuppression is a secondary benefit.

References and Suggested Reading

Civati, G., Busnach, G., Perrino, M. L., et al.: Early and late complications of cyclosporine treatment in a 5-year follow-up of 250 renal transplant recipients. Transplant. Proc. 21:1571, 1989.

Davies, H. S., St. John Collier, D., Thiru, S., et al.: Long-term survival of kidney allografts in dogs after withdrawal of immunosuppression with cyclosporin and azathioprine. Eur. Surg. Res. 21:65, 1989.

Gregory, C. R.: Cyclosporine. *In* Kirk, R. W. (ed.): *Current Veterinary Therapy X.* Philadelphia: W. B. Saunders, 1989, pp. 513–515.

Gregory, C. R., and Gourley, I. M.: Organ transplantation in clinical veterinary practice. *In* Slatter, D. H. (ed.): *Textbook of Small Animal Surgery.* Vol II. Philadelphia: W. B. Saunders (in press).

Gregory, C. R., Gourley, I. M., Broaddus, T. W., et al.: Long-term survival of a cat receiving a renal allograft from an unrelated donor. J. Vet. Intern. Med. 4:1, 1990.

Gregory, C. R., Gourley, I. M., Taylor, N. J., et al.: Experience with cyclosporin-A after renal allografting in two dogs. Vet. Surg. 15:441, 1986.

Gregory, C. R., Gourley, I. M., Taylor, N. J., et al.: Preliminary results of clinical renal allograft transplantation in the dog and cat. J. Vet. Intern. Med. 1:53, 1987.

Homan, W. P., French, M. E., Millard, P., et al.: Studies on the effects of cyclosporin A upon renal allograft rejection in the dog. Surgery 88:168, 1980.

Homan, W. P., French, M. E., Millard, P. R., et al.: A study of eleven drug regimens using cyclosporine-A to suppress renal allograft rejection in the dog. Transplant. Proc. 13:397, 1981.

Joss, D. V., Barrett, A. J., Dendra, J. R., et al.: Hypertension and convulsions in children receiving cyclosporin A. Lancet 1:906, 1982.

Kabra, P. M., and Wall, J. H.: Solid-phase extraction and liquid chromatography for improved assay of cyclosporine in whole blood or plasma. Clin. Chem. 31:1717, 1985.

Klintmalm, G., Sawe, J., von Bahr, C., et al.: Optimal cyclosporine plasma levels decline with time of therapy. Transplant. Proc. 16:1208, 1984.

Linas, S. L., Miller, P. D., McDonald, K. M., et al.: Role of the renin-angiotensin system in post-transplantation hypertension in patients with multiple kidneys. N. Engl. J. Med. 298:1440, 1978.

Manfro, R. C., Pohanka, S., Tomlanovich, S., et al.: Cyclosporin A and prednisolone: An additive inhibitory effect of cell proliferation and interleukin-2 production. Transplant. Proc. 21:1457, 1989.

Popovtzer, M. M., Pinnggera, W., Katz, F. H., et al.: Variations in arterial blood pressure after kidney transplantation. Circulation 47:1297, 1973.

Ross, L. A., and Labato, M. A.: Use of drugs to control hypertension in renal failure. In Kirk, R. W. (ed.): Current Veterinary Therapy X. Philadelphia: W. B. Saunders, 1989, pp. 1201–1204.

Rubin, R. H., Wolfson, J. S., Cosimi, A. B., et al.: Infection in the renal transplant recipient. Am. J. Med. 70:405, 1981.

Stevenson, S., and Schwartz, A.: Transplantation immunology. In Slatter, D. H. (ed.): Textbook of Small Animal Surgery. Vol. 1. Philadelphia: W. B. Saunders, 1985, pp. 199–212.

RELATIONSHIP OF INCONTINENCE TO NEUTERING

SUSI ARNOLD

Zurich, Switzerland

Spaying of bitches can result in various side effects, such as an increase in body weight, coat changes, and pyoderma of the vulvar fold. However, none of these side effects is as troublesome as urinary incontinence. It has been well known that spayed bitches may become incontinent (Pearson, 1973), but a positive association between acquired urinary incontinence and spaying has now been confirmed statistically (Thrusfield, 1985). A retrospective study has shown that a fairly high percentage of spayed bitches are affected (Arnold et al., 1989).

ETIOLOGY

The relationship between urinary incontinence and neutering is at present poorly understood. Lack of ovarian hormones seems to have an important role in the etiology. Because many affected bitches respond well to the administration of estrogen, the term *estrogen-responsive incontinence* has been used to describe this type of incontinence (Finco et al., 1974). However, for the following reasons, it seems unlikely that estrogen deficiency alone accounts for urinary incontinence: (1) Serum concentrations of ovarian hormones do not vary between spayed bitches with urinary incontinence and intact continent bitches in anestrus (Richter and Ling,

1985). (2) Not all bitches with acquired urinary incontinence respond to estrogen replacement therapy. (3) Most spayed bitches are continent. (4) The time interval between surgery and the occurrence of incontinence can be many years.

Incontinence in bitches has also been attributed to adhesions between the uterine stump and the bladder after oophorohysterectomy (Finco et al., 1974). However, this theory fails to explain the onset of incontinence years after the surgery, a response to estrogen therapy, similar incidence in oophorectomized compared with oophorohysterectomized bitches, or occurrence of urinary incontinence in neutered male dogs.

PATHOPHYSIOLOGY

Urine is passed if bladder pressure exceeds urethral closure pressure. In continent bitches, this combination is only achieved during the emptying phase of the bladder (micturition), whereas in incontinent bitches it also occurs during the filling phase, resulting in urinary leakage. Generally, two different pathophysiologic mechanisms are responsible for urinary leakage. Either bladder function is normal but urethral closure pressure is reduced (sphincter incompetence), or urethral closure pressure is normal but is exceeded by an abnormally elevated bladder pressure during the filling phase.

By means of urethral pressure profilometry, it has been consistently shown that sphincter incompetence accounts for urinary incontinence after spaying (Richter and Ling, 1985). The cause and pathophysiologic mechanisms for this acquired sphincter incompetence remain obscure, however.

INCIDENCE, CLINICAL SIGNS, AND DIAGNOSIS

Urinary incontinence can develop at any time after surgery, but in 75% of cases, incontinence develops within 3 years (Arnold et al., 1989).

Incidence and Breed Predisposition

A retrospective study of 412 spayed bitches revealed an incidence of 20.1%. There appears to be a strong correlation between body weight and the incidence of incontinence (Fig. 1). Of bitches with a body weight of less than 20 kg, only 9.3% were incontinent, whereas in bitches with a body weight of more than 20 kg, the incidence was 30.9%. Boxers showed the highest incidence (65%).

Clinical Signs and Diagnosis

A thorough history should be taken because it provides important clues about incontinence and may help decide what further procedures are necessary to reach a diagnosis (Table 1). The dog is

Table 1. *Routine Workup of Bitches With Urinary Incontinence*

Examinations	Rule Out
Performed in all dogs	
Physical examination	Polyuria/polydipsia,
Blood biochemistry	urinary tract infection
Urinalysis	
Bacterial culture of urine	Urinary tract infection
Neurologic examination	Neurologic causes of incontinence
Performed in young bitches	
Intravenous pyelogram	Genitourinary abnormality (i.e., ectopic ureters)
Performed in bitches with incontinence < 1 month after surgery	
Intravenous pyelogram	Iatrogenic ureterovaginal fistula

typically presented with a complaint of urinary incontinence that is mainly observed during sleep. Micturition and frequency of urination are normal. If incontinence was present *before* surgery, congenital malformation of the genitourinary tract (ectopic ureters, patent urachus, intersexuality) has to be considered. If incontinence occurred *immediately* after surgery, it may be caused by an iatrogenic ureterovaginal fistula. Information should be gained about the daily water intake. Because of a necessity to urinate during the night, dogs with polyuria and polydipsia sometimes are falsely presented as incontinent when they are actually conscious of urination. Diseases resulting in polyuria and polydipsia may predispose to sphincteric incontinence by increasing the volume of urine that the bladder must store. Urine collected by cystocentesis should be processed for bacteriologic culture to rule out a urinary tract infection. Because sphincter incompetence predisposes a bitch to urinary tract infection, a bitch may remain incontinent after successful treatment of cystitis.

If a dog is very young, an intravenous pyelogram should be performed to assess the possibility of congenital malformations such as ectopic ureters. A neurologic examination should also be included to rule out neurogenic causes of incontinence. In patients that have become incontinent immediately after surgery, a contrast study of the lower urinary tract should be considered to rule out an iatrogenically created ureterovaginal fistula.

If none of the procedures just mentioned reveals any abnormality, sphincter incompetence is suggested and medical treatment is indicated.

The diagnosis of sphincter incompetence can be confirmed only by urodynamic examination (Fig. 2). A recording catheter is mechanically withdrawn from the bladder, measuring pressure over the

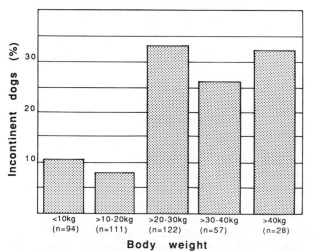

Figure 1. Occurrence of incontinence in relation to body weight. (Reprinted with permission from Arnold, S., et al.: Incontinentia urinae bei der kastrierten Hündin: Häufigkeit und Rassedisposition. Schweiz. Arch. Tierheilkd. 131:259, 1989.)

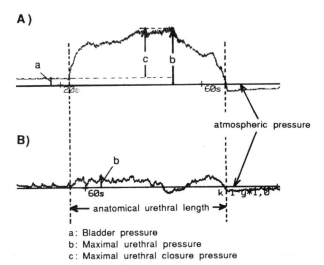

A)

a

c b

20s   60s

atmospheric pressure

B)

b

60s   k·1·g*1,0

← anatomical urethral length →

a: Bladder pressure
b: Maximal urethral pressure
c: Maximal urethral closure pressure

Figure 2. Typical urethral pressure profiles of a continent bitch (*A*) and a bitch with sphincter incompetence (*B*). (Pressure profile was recorded with a Microtip Transducer Catheter, Model No. SUPC 780 B, Millar Instruments, Houston, TX.)

entire urethral length (a urethral pressure profile). Parameters such as functional urethral length, bladder pressure, and maximal urethral pressure can be obtained from this test. The most important parameter is maximal urethral closure pressure, which is calculated as the difference between bladder pressure and maximal urethral pressure. The maximal urethral closure pressure usually occurs in the middle third of the urethra and provides valuable information about urethral sphincter function (Holt, 1988). In continent bitches, the maximal urethral closure pressure is significantly higher than in bitches with sphincter incompetence (Holt, 1988; Richter and Ling, 1985).

Table 2. *Response to Drug Therapy in 57 Bitches With Sphincter Incompetence**

	Estrogen (n = 17)	Alpha-Adrenergic Drugs (n = 38)	Others (n = 2)
Good results	11 (64.7%)	28 (73.7%)	—
Improvement	2 (11.8%)	9 (23.7%)	2†
No response	4 (23.5%)	1 (2.6%)	—

*Reprinted with permission from Arnold, S., et al.: Incontinentia urinae bei der kastrierten Hündin: Häufigkeit und Rassedisposition. Schweiz. Arch. Tierheilkd. 131:259, 1989.

†Homeopathic therapy.

THERAPY

Alpha-adrenergic drugs (phenylpropanolamine or ephedrine) are most appropriate for the treatment of sphincter incompetence. Stimulation of alpha receptors in the urethral wall increases urethral closure pressure, resulting in relief of incontinence. Alternatively, estrogens can also be used. The minimum dose and frequency of administration to control incontinence should be determined for each dog to minimize the risk of bone marrow toxicity. Estrogens most likely act by increasing the sensitivity of the alpha receptors for adrenergic transmitters. However, the results with adrenergic drug therapy are superior to those with estrogen therapy (Table 2) (see *CVT X*, p. 1214).

In incontinent bitches that fail to respond to drug therapy, surgical procedures can be performed. Good results have been achieved by colposuspension (Holt, 1985) or by endoscopic injection of Teflon into the submucosa of the urethral wall (Arnold et al., 1989).

References and Suggested Reading

Arnold, S., Arnold, P., Hubler, M., et al.: Incontinentia urinae bei der kastrierten Hündin: Häufigkeit und Rassedisposition. Schweiz. Arch. Tierheilkd. 131:259, 1989.
A retrospective study of 412 bitches 3 to 10 years after spaying: occurrence, extent of urinary incontinence and response to medical treatment.
Arnold, S., Jäger, P., DiBartola, S. P., et al.: Treatment of urinary incontinence in dogs by endoscopic injection of Teflon. J.A.V.M.A. 195:1369, 1989.
Description of the Teflon injection technique and follow-up study in 22 incontinent dogs.
Finco, D. R., Osborne, C. A., and Lewis, R. E.: Nonneurogenic causes of abnormal micturition in the dog and cat. Vet. Clin. North Am. 4:501, 1974.
Description of diseases resulting in urinary incontinence.
Holt, P. E.: Urinary incontinence in the bitch due to sphincter mechanism incompetence: Surgical treatment. J. Small Anim. Pract. 26:237, 1985.
Description of the method of surgical treatment and results obtained in 33 bitches.
Holt, P. E.: Simultaneous urethral pressure profilometry: Comparison between continent and incontinent bitches. J. Small Anim. Pract. 29:761, 1988.
A study of 50 continent and 50 incontinent bitches.
Pearson, H.: The complications of ovariohysterectomy in the bitch. J. Small Anim. Pract. 14:257, 1973.
Description of the complications in 72 bitches after oophorohysterectomy.
Richter, K. P., and Ling, G. V.: Clinical response and urethral pressure profile changes after phenylpropanolamine in dogs with primary sphincter incompetence. J.A.V.M.A. 187:605, 1985.
Clinical investigation of 8 male and 11 female dogs.
Thrusfield, M. V.: Association between urinary incontinence and spaying in bitches. Vet. Rec. 116:695, 1985.
An observational study conducted on a clinic population to assess the risk of developing urinary incontinence in spayed compared with entire bitches.

USE OF CYSTOSCOPY

DAVID F. SENIOR

Gainesville, Florida

New techniques in human endourology can often eliminate the need for open surgery of the urinary tract. Many procedures can also be performed via cystoscopy in small animals (Brearley and Cooper, 1987; Senior and Sundstrom, 1988). The rigid human cystoscope is well suited for use in female dogs weighing more than 7 kg. Rigid cystoscopes have been used experimentally in male dogs via a perineal urethrostomy incision, but clinical application of this technique has not been reported. In large male dogs, a long flexible fiber-optic bronchoscope or choledocoscope can be passed into the bladder through the urethra. Prepubic percutaneous cystoscopy can be performed in small dogs and cats using a needle endoscope introduced with the aid of an endoscopic trocar and cannula (McCarthy and McDermaid, 1986). Although a wide variety of procedures can be performed using a rigid endoscope, all the techniques just described allow for direct visualization, biopsy, and photography. Light sources used for other endoscopic equipment are adaptable to most cystoscopes.

Cystoscopy is performed using general anesthesia. For rigid cystoscopy, a dog is positioned in dorsal recumbency. Introduction of the cystoscope and examination are easiest when a dog is positioned so that the hindquarters extend slightly beyond the end of the examination table and the animal is elevated caudally. Perivulval hair should be clipped and the perineum prepared with a surgical scrub before draping. For flexible and prepubic cystoscopy, a patient can remain in lateral recumbency and the prepuce or lateral abdomen can be prepared as just described.

All equipment for cystoscopy should be sterilized and organized on a sterile drape. Rigid cystoscopes are made in two lengths, adult and pediatric, by many instrument manufacturing companies including Olympus, Storz, Wolf, and ACMI. In dogs weighing more than 10 to 15 kg, a 17 to 21 French adult length cystoscope is suitable. In smaller dogs, a 14 to 15 French pediatric length cystoscope can be used. A rigid cystoscope set consists of an outer sheath through which all instruments are passed; an obturator designed to make the leading end of the cystoscope smooth and rounded so that passage of the cystoscope through the urethra is nontraumatic; an Albarran operating bridge designed to deflect instruments such as catheters, biopsy forceps, or electrocautery electrodes as they are passed

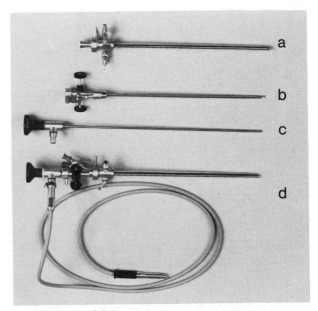

Figure 1. An adult-length rigid cystoscope: sheath with obturator in place (*a*), Albarran operating bridge (*b*), telescope (*c*), and fully assembled cystoscope with light cable attached (*d*).

through the sheath so they can be directed and manipulated at various angles within the urinary tract; and various telescopes with several different viewing angles (Fig. 1). Telescopes with 5° and 70° lenses enable visualization of the entire bladder and urethra and are suitable for most operative procedures.

The cystoscope can be fully assembled and introduced through the urethra into the bladder guided by direct visualization. This procedure is assisted by maintaining a constant flow of irrigation fluid from the front of the cystoscope. Urethral trauma associated with passage of relatively large cystoscopes may be minimized by balloon dilation* of the urethra for 30 to 60 sec before passage of the cystoscope sheath. After dilation, the cystoscope sheath with an obturator in place can be gently advanced into the bladder. For introduction of the balloon dilator and the cystoscope sheath, the urethral os can be visualized using a 3-in. Killian nasal

---

*Diaflex Urethral Dilator Catheter, Model #7500-01, Female, American Medical Systems, Minnetonka, MN.

speculum* and head lamp.† All urethral dilators and cystoscopic instruments should be liberally coated with sterile lubricant before passage through the urethra.

Once the cystoscope sheath is passed through the urethra into the bladder, the obturator can be withdrawn and the Albarran bridge and telescope can be locked in place to complete the assembly (see Fig. 1). Irrigation lines, drainage lines, and the light cable can be connected and examination of the bladder can begin.

The bladder must initially be rinsed several times with irrigation fluid to allow clear visualization and for photography. This is particularly necessary when there is inflammation with abundant cellular debris and hemorrhage. Any physiologic salt solution is a satisfactory irrigant for routine examination. For electrocautery, a nonelectrolyte solution such as 1.5% glycine is preferable; the osmolality of this solution prevents osmolar damage of tissue samples taken for histologic examination. For electrohydraulic shock-wave lithotripsy, 0.01% saline allows better spark generation and hence more powerful transmission of shock waves.

The mucosal surface of the bladder should be observed both when the bladder is partially contracted and again when distended. Small lesions may become flattened and less obvious once the bladder wall is stretched. Overdistention of the bladder should be avoided because it induces iatrogenic submucosal petechial hemorrhages. Bladder rupture is also a possibility, particularly if the bladder wall is weakened by the presence of an infiltrative neoplasm. During placement of the cystoscope, a small quantity of air is always introduced into the bladder. When a dog is in dorsal recumbency, the air bubble remains at the ventral (uppermost) region of the bladder. The entire bladder wall should be examined systematically by successively advancing and retracting the cystoscope followed by partial rotation. In this way, even small lesions will not be missed. Useful landmarks include the cranial pole of the bladder, the trigone and neck of the bladder, the air bubble, and the location of the ureteral orifices. Urine can be observed intermittently flowing out of the ureteral orifices. The bladder neck and urethra are best examined by slowly advancing or withdrawing the cystoscope with the irrigation fluid running.

When distended, the normal bladder has a flat, pale, blanched appearance and the submucosal vascular pattern becomes apparent. When contracted, the mucosa develops irregular folds and appears more red. Abnormalities such as uroliths, inflam-

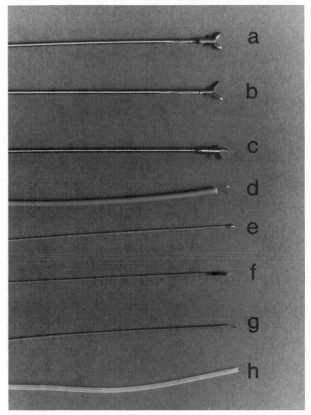

Figure 2. Instruments for procedures performed through a cystoscope: biopsy forceps (*a*), grasping forceps (*b*), scissors (*c*), various electrocautery electrodes (*d* through *g*), and laser fiber (*h*).

matory polyps, neoplasms, and the location of ectopic ureters are easily seen.

Various instruments are available for passage through the cystoscope, including forceps for grasping, biopsy, and cutting; stone baskets for recovery of small uroliths; laser fibers and electrocautery electrodes for tissue resection; electrohydraulic shock-wave electrodes for lithotripsy; and needles for making submucosal injections (Fig. 2).

Several procedures can be performed by means of cystoscopy, including direct visual examination and biopsy of lesions in the bladder and urethra; resection of superficial polyps and tumors by electrocautery or laser; identification of the presence and location of ectopic ureters; catheterization of ectopic ureters as an aid to subsequent surgical correction; ureteral catheterization to perform differential renal function studies, to collect urine for urinalysis, and for retrograde pyelography (Senior and Newman, 1986); electrohydraulic shock-wave lithotripsy (Senior, 1984); and periurethral injection of polytetrafluoroethylene paste* to treat urinary incontinence due to urethral incompetence (Arnold et al., 1989).

---

*Killian Nasal Speculum, American Hospital Supply, McGaw Park, IL.

†Welch Allyn Headlamp, American Hospital Supply, McGaw Park, IL.

---

*Polytef Paste for injection, Mentor, Nowell, MA.

Contraindications to cystoscopy in human patients are few, although acute inflammatory processes such as cystitis, prostatitis, or urethritis should be resolved before performing the procedure.

References and Suggested Reading

Arnold, S., Jäger, P., DiBartola, S. P, et al.: Treatment of urinary incontinence in dogs by endoscopic injection of Teflon. J.A.V.M.A. 195:1369, 1989.
A description of the technique for injecting Teflon paste submucosally into the urethra via cystoscopy to treat urethral incompetence and documentation of the clinical outcome in 22 dogs.

Brearley, M. J., and Cooper, J. E.: The diagnosis of bladder disease in dogs by cystoscopy. J. Small Anim. Pract. 28:75, 1987.
A description of cystoscopic technique in dogs, including the photographic appearance of commonly observed structures and lesions.

McCarthy, T. C., and McDermaid, S. L.: Prepubic percutaneous cystoscopy in the dog and cat. J. Am. Anim. Hosp. Assoc. 22:213, 1986.
A description of the technique for performing prepubic percutaneous cystoscopy.

Senior, D. F.: Electrohydraulic shock-wave lithotripsy in experimental canine struvite bladder stone disease. Vet. Surg. 13:143, 1984.
A description of electrohydraulic shock-wave lithotripsy performed by means of cystoscopy in two dogs.

Senior, D. F., and Newman, R. C.: Retrograde ureteral catheterization in female dogs. J. Am. Anim. Hosp. Assoc. 22:831, 1986.
An illustrated description of ureteral catheterization via cystoscopy in female dogs.

Senior, D. F., and Sundstrom, D. A.: Cystoscopy in female dogs. Comp. Cont. Ed. Pract. Vet. 10:890, 1988.
An illustrated guide to setting up and performing cystoscopy in female dogs.

URETHRAL DILATION

DAVID F. SENIOR

Gainesville, Florida

Urethral dilation is indicated to treat urethral strictures and to facilitate urethral passage of cystoscopes. The dilators most useful in small animal urology include urethral and esophageal balloon dilators, metal urethral sounds, nephrostomy tract fascial dilators, and the Otis urethrotome.

In human medicine, balloon dilation procedures have been used in angioplasty to reopen arteriosclerotic cardiac vessels, for dilation of esophageal strictures, for nephrostomy tract dilation, for dilation of the intramural portion of the ureter, and more recently for dilation of the prostatic urethra in men with benign prostatic hyperplasia. In dogs, a urethral balloon dilator* (Fig. 1) has been used to dilate the urethra before cystoscopy so that large rigid cystoscope sheaths can be passed through the urethra with less risk of trauma. Balloon dilators have also been used to dilate urethral strictures. A series of esophageal balloon dilators* were used to dilate the proximal urethra in a dog when urethral stricture developed after surgical resection of a botryoid rhabdomyosarcoma arising from the neck of the bladder (Fig. 2). Balloon dilators are advanced through the urethra in the deflated state and positioned so that the balloon spans the region to be dilated. Care should be taken to ensure that the balloon does not migrate away from the stricture site during inflation, and the position is best checked under fluoroscopy during inflation of the balloon or radiographically after the balloon is inflated. When inflated, the balloon adopts a fixed shape with a known diameter. To dilate surrounding tissue, high pressure must be maintained in the balloon for a brief period of time; 1 min is usually adequate. The pressure level required to achieve dilation varies with the type of stricture and the degree of dilation needed; however, the manufacturers' recommended maximum pressure level should not be exceeded. Urethral dilators are intended for single use, but in our experience they can be used many times with gas sterilization between uses. There are several advantages in using balloons for dilation. Balloon dilation minimizes unnecessary trauma to the urethral mucosa because the dilator is passed through the urethra deflated, when the outer diameter is relatively small. Thus, repeated scraping of oversized instruments against

---

*Diaflex Urethral Dilator Catheter, Model #7500-01, Female, American Medical Systems, Minnetonka, MN.

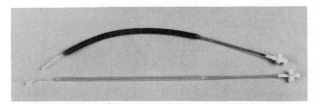

Figure 1. Urethral balloon dilator deflated and inflated with a colored solution.

---

*Rigiflex TTS Dilators, Microvasive, Milford, MA.

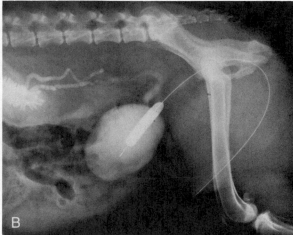

Figure 2. *A*, Retrograde urethrogram demonstrating stricture of the proximal urethra in a male dog. *B*, Balloon dilation of the urethral stricture using an esophageal dilator.

the urethral mucosa is avoided. When using balloon dilators for dilating strictures, perforation of the urethral mucosa and development of a false tract are much less likely than with rigid instruments. There are disadvantages to balloon dilation. The precise location of strictures may not be apparent by simple passage of the dilator, and urethrography and fluoroscopy may be required to locate the stricture and place the dilator accurately. Also, when strictures are very dense as a result of large amounts of organized fibrous tissue, balloon dilators may not provide sufficient pressure to achieve adequate dilation.

Metal urethral sounds are available in a series of graduated sizes for sequential passage through the urethra (Fig. 3).* Straight and curved urethral sounds are made for use in human females and males, respectively. Only straight metal sounds should be used in female dogs because the curved sounds cause superficial lacerations and tears in the mucosa of the proximal urethra and neck of the bladder. Dilation is performed by sequentially advancing well-lubricated sounds of progressively larger diameter through the stricture. The diameter and location of single strictures are easily determined with urethral sounds, which may also be

*Urethral Bougies, Olympus Corporation, Lake Success, NY.

used to calibrate the effective maximum diameter of strictures as well as the diameter of the urethra in normal dogs. Metal urethral sounds are more effective than balloon dilators in breaking down very dense organized fibrous strictures because more force can be applied to induce dilation. However, the risk of perforating the urethra and creating a false passage is also more likely.

Nephrostomy tract fascial dilators* (Fig. 4) have been used experimentally to establish and dilate a urethrotomy site so that rigid cystoscopy can be performed in male dogs (Brearley et al., 1988). However, there have been no reports of this procedure being performed on clinical patients at this time. In the experimental studies, the urethrotomy was established by making an incision over the urethra just ventral to the anus. The perineal urethra was distended with saline infused through a urethral catheter, and a needle was placed directly into the urethra. A flexible guide wire was then

*Amplatz renal dilator set and dilators, Cook Urological, Spoencer, IN.

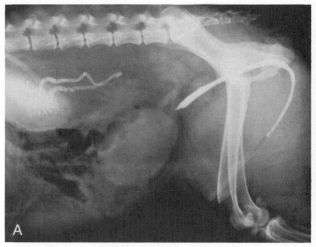

Figure 3. Straight metal urethral sound.

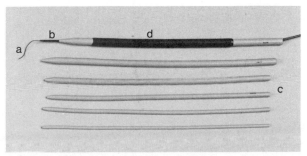

Figure 4. Nephrostomy tract fascial dilator system: guide wire (*a*), thin dilating catheter (*b*), fascial dilator catheters (*c*), and Amplatz sheath (*d*).

passed through the needle via the urethra into the bladder. The needle was then withdrawn, leaving the wire in place, and a thin dilating catheter was passed over the wire into the urethra. To complete the dilation procedure, progressively larger fascial dilators were passed sequentially to dilate the urethrotomy site up to as much as 26 French. Finally, an Amplatz sheath was passed over the last dilating catheter, and the catheters were withdrawn. The wire can be left in place to ensure that the tract is not inadvertently lost during the procedure. Once the open sheath is in place, a rigid cystoscope can be passed through the sheath and urethra into the bladder. Spontaneous healing of the urethrotomy site was uneventful and rapid. Our preliminary experience with this technique suggests that it may be applicable to clinical patients. We have used small over-the-wire concentric dilator systems in a similar manner to dilate urethral strictures in cats with a history of urethral obstruction and traumatic catheterization.

The Otis urethrotome* (Fig. 5) has been used to dilate the distal urethra in male dogs before cystoscopy with a flexible endoscope (Cooper et al., 1984). The urethrotome was used without the cutting blade in place so that the urethral os was stretched rather than incised. An Otis urethrotome is used to incise strictures in human patients; the blunt nature of the blade tends to separate submucosal fibrous tissue without cutting through the urethral mucosa. We have not used the Otis urethrotome in our clinic. One disadvantage of the urethrotome in human patients is the tendency of incised strictures to recur.

In human patients, excessive stretching of urethral strictures at a single dilation procedure can lead to perforation and rapid return of an even denser or longer stricture. For this reason, increases in lumen diameter are limited to 2 to 4 French at

*Otis Urethrotome, Olympus Corporation, Lake Success, NY.

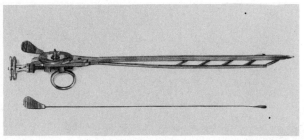

Figure 5. Otis urethrotome.

each dilation, and the dilation procedure is repeated several times at weekly intervals until the desired degree of dilation is achieved. Placement of an indwelling Foley catheter for several days before dilation serves to establish bladder drainage to relieve obstruction and may soften the stricture, making subsequent dilation more successful.

In human patients, stricture dilation is more difficult when the stricture is long or very dense, because both factors tend to result in early recurrence. Also, difficult strictures may require repeated dilation from time to time on a regular basis. In our experience, strictures due to tumors have proved refractory to dilation, whereas granulomatous urethritis can respond to a combination of dilation and treatment with corticosteroids.

References and Suggested Reading

Brearley, M. J., Milroy, E. J., and Rickards, D.: A percutaneous approach for cystoscopy in male dogs. Res. Vet. Sci. 44:380, 1988.
Describes the establishment of a temporary perineal urethrostomy using fascial dilators to enable rigid cystoscopy in male dogs.
Cooper, J. E., Milroy, E. J., Turton, J. A., et al.: Cytoscopic examination of male and female dogs. Vet. Rec. 115:571, 1984.
Describes the use of the Otis urethrotome to dilate the distal urethra in preparation for passage of a flexible endoscope into the bladder.
Lange, P. H.: Diagnostic and therapeutic urologic instrumentation. In Walsh, P. C., Gittes, R. F., Perlmutter, A. D., et al. (eds.): Campbell's Urology, 5th ed. Philadelphia: W.B. Saunders, 1986, p. 510.
A comprehensive description including uses of some of the human urologic instruments referred to in this article.

FELINE URETHRAL OBSTRUCTION: MEDICAL MANAGEMENT

JEANNE A. BARSANTI,
DELMAR R. FINCO,
and SCOTT A. BROWN
Athens, Georgia

Feline urethral obstruction defines a medical problem rather than a specific disease. With urethral obstruction, a cat senses bladder fullness and unsuccessfully attempts to void. If the cat cannot void any urine, uremia will result within 48 to 72 hr and normal functional abilities of the bladder and urethra may be compromised.

Etiology, pathophysiology, and diagnosis of obstructive uropathy have been reviewed by Osborne and colleagues (1989) (see *CVT IX*, pp. 1164 and 1196; and *CVT X*, p. 1209). This article focuses on symptomatic management of urethral obstruction.

Symptomatic treatment consists of two aspects: instituting fluid therapy to reverse uremia and removing or bypassing the urethral obstruction to reestablish urine output. Such therapy has been fairly well defined in cats through research, although some controversy still exists.

Management of urethral obstruction in cats varies with the severity of the resultant clinical signs, which in turn vary with the degree and duration of the obstruction. If the obstruction is recognized and treated promptly (within 24 hr and before development of azotemia), relief of obstruction may be sufficient therapy. In cats with clinical signs of uremia, both relief of obstruction and fluid therapy are essential for survival (Finco and Cornelius, 1977). Whether fluid therapy or relief of obstruction should be attempted first depends on the condition of the cat. If the cat is depressed and weak, we usually start fluid therapy first and may use cystocentesis to temporarily relieve bladder distention. If the cat is alert, we try to relieve obstruction first.

FLUID THERAPY

Cats that are uremic at the time of presentation are usually hyperkalemic and acidemic (Burrows and Bovée, 1978). The major goals of fluid therapy are to reduce hyperkalemia and azotemia, to improve acid-base balance, and to correct dehydration. Alkalizing electrolyte solutions, such as lactated Ringer's, reverse acidemia and hyperkalemia in experimentally induced urethral obstruction, even though these fluids do contain a small amount of potassium (Finco, 1976). Adding sodium bicarbonate to the treatment regimen more rapidly reverses acidemia (Burrows and Bovée, 1978), but no benefit in survival over cats treated with alkalizing electrolyte solutions has been shown (Finco, 1976). We usually infuse only a balanced, alkalizing electrolyte solution such as lactated Ringer's; however, some clinicians also administer sodium bicarbonate or calcium salts when severe electrocardiographic changes are observed.

The amount of fluids administered is based on the severity of dehydration, uremic signs, and hyperkalemia. Approximately 5% body weight should be given if the signs are mild, 8% if moderate, and 12% if severe (1 lb equals approximately 500 ml, and 1 kg equals 1000 ml). This amount should be administered over approximately 2 hr. These are only general guidelines. Actual volume must be individualized for each cat based on vital signs, changes in hydration status, mental attitude, and urine output. Hyperkalemia, acidemia, and uremia will not be rapidly reversed if the rate of fluid administration is too slow. Pulmonary edema may result from too rapid fluid replacement (>60/kg/hr) (Finco, 1976).

After the initial fluid amount is given, a cat's mental attitude usually is improved, urine output is sustained, and severe hyperkalemia is reversed (as shown by biochemical measurement or reversal of cardiac and electrocardiographic abnormalities). When a cat's condition has improved, the rate of fluid administration can be reduced, but sufficient volume should be given over 24 hr to provide insensible water losses (estimated at 20 ml/kg/day) and replace urine losses. If urine output is not measured, sufficient fluids should be given to provide maintenance needs (estimated at 66 ml/kg/day) and correct any dehydration, which is detected by changes in skin turgor or moisture of the mucous membranes. Food and water can be offered as soon as vomiting stops, which is usually within the first 24 hr.

Fluid therapy is continued until azotemia is resolved or minimal. Subcutaneous fluids can be substituted for intravenous fluids once the uremic signs abate and serum potassium level is normal (usually within 4 to 24 hr).

Cats with partial or total anorexia and a postobstructive diuresis may become hypokalemic a few days after obstruction is relieved. Recurrent or worsening weakness and lethargy may be the only clinical signs. Hypokalemia was a problem within 24 hr in clinical cases treated with potassium-free fluids and sodium bicarbonate (Burrows and Bovée, 1978) but was not a problem in experimental cats treated with isotonic, balanced electrolyte solutions (Finco, 1976). If hypokalemia is suspected, it should be confirmed by measurement of serum potassium concentration and treated. Potassium supplementation can be given orally if the cat is not vomiting (2 to 4 mEq/day), or 20 mEq potassium chloride can be added to each liter of balanced electrolyte solution. If hypokalemia is severe (<3 mEq/L), additional potassium supplementation may be needed (see *CVT X*, p. 37).

RELIEF OF URETHRAL OBSTRUCTION

Retrograde Flushing of the Urethra

In all cats with urethral obstruction, the obstruction must be relieved. This is most often accomplished by retrograde flushing of the urethra with a sterile solution through a lubricated urethral catheter. This procedure has been reviewed elsewhere (see *CVT IX*, p. 1196).

Catheterization of the Urethra/Bladder

After the obstruction is relieved or bypassed, a flexible no. 3.5 French rubber feeding tube type catheter* should be inserted into the bladder. Flexible catheters are preferred because they are longer and produce less bladder and urethral trauma (Lees et al., 1980). The catheter should be inserted just into the bladder by determining the point at which urine is aspirated. Inserting the catheter too deeply can result in trauma to the bladder. If large quantities of crystalline material or blood are evident in the urine, the bladder is repeatedly flushed with a sterile isotonic solution.

Whether the catheter is removed or sutured in place should be based on the characteristics of each individual case. Leaving the catheter in place pre-

---

*Sovereign Sterile Disposable Feeding Tube and Urethral Catheter, Sherwood Medical Industries, St. Louis, MO 63103.

vents immediate reobstruction and facilitates monitoring of urine output, but it also leads to bacterial urinary tract infection and urethral irritation (Lees et al., 1981; Smith et al., 1981). If the urethral catheter is left in place, a closed drainage system should be established by connecting the urethral catheter via extension tubing to an empty, sterile fluid bottle or bag. The catheter system should be opened as infrequently as possible and only with careful attention to cleanliness. The cat is fitted with an Elizabethan collar to prevent it from removing the urethral catheter or disconnecting the drainage system.

At present, our recommendation is to leave the catheter in place only if one of the following four conditions is present: (1) the obstruction was relieved or bypassed with difficulty; (2) the urine stream is weak and small after relief of obstruction; (3) the cat is uremic; (4) detrusor dysfunction is present secondary to overdistention. To avoid catheter-induced complications, the catheter should be left in place as short a time as possible. Because uremic signs abate within 24 hr in most appropriately treated cats, the urinary catheter is usually removed within 1 to 2 days.

Unless clinical signs of bacterial infection develop, antimicrobial therapy is not recommended while the urinary catheter is in place. Urinary tract infection is unusual in cats presenting for urethral obstruction. Use of antibiotics while the catheter is in place can result in infection with resistant organisms (Barsanti et al., 1985; Lees et al., 1981; Lippert, et al., 1988). We prefer to collect a urine sample for urinalysis and culture when the catheter is removed. Any bacteria isolated should be considered significant as long as the sample was collected from the catheter or by cystocentesis and aseptic technique was used. Antibiotic treatment is directed specifically to any organism detected (see *CVT IX*, p. 1174) and continued for at least 10 days. A urine culture is performed again 3 to 5 days after the antibiotic regimen is completed, to ensure that the infection was eliminated.

Anti-inflammatory agents, such as glucocorticoids, have been advocated to reduce inflammation secondary to obstruction and to catheterization. However, we found that experimental cats with indwelling catheters had a significantly increased risk of renal infection if treated with prednisolone. Renal infection could occur even if an antibiotic (amoxicillin) was given in addition to the prednisolone. Cats with renal infection had a higher mortality rate than cats with only lower tract infection. In addition, because of the severity of the urinary infections that developed, no anti-inflammatory benefit of prednisolone was found. On the basis of this study, we strongly recommend that anti-inflammatory doses of glucocorticoids *not* be given to cats while indwelling urinary catheters are in place.

Intravesicular dimethyl sulfoxide (DMSO) has also been recommended as an anti-inflammatory agent in cats with urethral obstruction. We found no benefit to the use of 45% DMSO in experimental studies of cats with induced cystitis and indwelling urethral catheters. There was no reduction in the severity of inflammation or the incidence of infection.

MANAGEMENT OF BLADDER/URETHRAL DYSFUNCTION

A potential consequence of urethral obstruction is damage to the bladder detrusor muscle by prolonged overdistention. Loss of the tight junctions between muscle fibers prevents spread of motor nerve impulses that permit bladder contraction. Thus, even after relief of obstruction, affected cats cannot voluntarily void, although the bladder can be manually expressed to produce a strong urine stream, indicating that no outflow obstruction exists. Treatment entails keeping the bladder empty so that the tight junctions can reform. This can be done by frequent manual expression or by use of an indwelling urinary catheter. Bethanechol (1.25 to 5.0 mg PO every 8 hr) can be tried after a few days of keeping the bladder empty. Response to bethanechol should occur within a few hours of administration. Because bethanechol can increase urethral resistance, it should be administered with a urethral relaxant such as phenoxybenzamine (0.5 mg/kg PO every 24 hr or 0.25 mg/kg PO every 12 hr) (see *CVT X*, p. 1214). The urethra must be patent during administration of parasympathomimetic drugs, or rupture of the bladder could theoretically occur. The time required for return of bladder function varies with degree of injury.

Another reason for inability to urinate after relief of obstruction is outflow resistance. Physical examination shows that even with adequate manual compression, the urine stream is weak. Causes of outflow resistance include recurrence of intraluminal obstruction, extraluminal obstruction, inflammatory swelling of the urethra, and urethral spasm. Physical obstructions should be ruled out by passage of a catheter or by contrast radiography. If urethral spasm is present, drug therapy may be of benefit, but it has not been evaluated in cats. Extrapolating from other species, drugs to consider would include phenoxybenzamine to block urethral alpha-adrenergic receptors or diazepam (1.25 to 2.5 mg PO every

8 to 12 hr) to relieve skeletal muscle spasm (see *CVT X*, p. 1214). One side effect of phenoxybenzamine is hypotension, related to alpha-adrenergic blockade. The drug should not be used in cats with cardiovascular disease. Side effects of diazepam include sedation and unusual behavior.

References and Suggested Reading

Barsanti, J. A., Blue, J., and Edmunds, J.: Urinary tract infection due to indwelling bladder catheters in dogs and cats. J.A.V.M.A. 187:384, 1985.
This prospective study found a high incidence of infection associated with indwelling urinary catheters in a teaching hospital intensive care unit.

Bovée, K. C., Reif, J. S., Maguire, T. G., et al.: Recurrence of feline urethral obstruction. J.A.V.M.A. 174:93, 1979.
A retrospective review of clinical cases of urethral obstruction to determine recurrence rate and possible associations with therapy advised.

Burrows, C. F., and Bovée, K. C.: Characterization and treatment of acid-base and renal defects due to urethral obstruction in cats. J.A.V.M.A. 172:801, 1978.
A study of the laboratory abnormalities found in cats presented for urethral obstruction and the changes in these abnormalities with fluid therapy.

Finco, D. R.: Induced feline urethral obstruction: Response of hyperkalemia to relief of obstruction and administration of parenteral electrolyte solution. J. Am. Anim. Hosp. Assoc. 12:198, 1976.
An experimental study of the efficacy of fluid therapy in cats with urethral obstruction.

Finco, D. R., and Cornelius, L. M.: Characterization and treatment of water, electrolyte, and acid-base imbalances of induced urethral obstruction in the cat. Am. J. Vet. Res. 38:823, 1977.
An experimental study that documented the clinical and laboratory abnormalities that develop after urethral obstruction and the response of these abnormalities to fluid therapy.

Lees, G. E., Osborne, C. A., Stevens, J. B., et al.: Adverse effects caused by polypropylene and polyvinyl feline urinary catheters. Am. J. Vet. Res. 41:1836, 1980.
An experimental study in cats that examined the effects of indwelling urinary catheters on the urethra.

Lees, G. E., Osborne, C. A., Stevens, J. B., et al.: Adverse effects of open indwelling urethral catheterization in clincally normal male cats. Am. J. Vet. Res. 42:825, 1981.
An experimental study in normal cats that found that urinary tract infections commonly developed in cats with indwelling urinary catheters that were left open.

Lippert, A. C., Fulton, R. B., and Parr, A. M.: Nosocomial infection surveillance in a small animal intensive care unit. J. Am. Anim. Hosp. Assoc. 18:627, 1988.
A prospective clinical study that found that urinary tract infections were not uncommon in animals with indwelling urinary catheters, even if antibiotics were given.

Osborne, C. A., Kruger, J. M., Johnston, G. R., et al.: Feline lower urinary tract disorders. In Ettinger, S. J. (ed.): *Textbook of Veterinary Internal Medicine*, 3rd ed. Philadelphia: W. B. Saunders, 1989, p. 2057.
An excellent review of all the potential causes of lower urinary tract signs (hematuria, dysuria, urethral obstruction) in cats.

Smith, C. W., Schiller, A. G., Smith, A. R., et al.: Effects of indwelling urinary catheters in male cats. J. Am. Anim. Hosp. Assoc. 17:427, 1981.
An experimental study of open indwelling urinary catheters in cats that found that infection and inflammation were not infrequent, especially when perineal urethrostomy and catheterization were combined.

NONSURGICAL RETRIEVAL OF UROLITHS FOR MINERAL ANALYSIS

CARL A. OSBORNE,
JODY P. LULICH,
and LISA K. UNGER
St. Paul, Minnesota

Medical protocols have been developed to promote the dissolution of uroliths composed of struvite, ammonium urate, and cystine, as well as to prevent all major types of uroliths in cats and dogs. However, because the causes of different types of uroliths vary, medical protocols for their dissolution and prevention also vary. Therefore, detection of uroliths is only the beginning of the diagnostic process. Determination of the composition of the uroliths and the associated underlying causes of urolith formation are essential prerequisites to selection of medical protocols designed to promote their dissolution and prevention.

Medical dissolution of uroliths poses the problem of formulating therapy without the availability of surgically removed uroliths for analysis. To overcome this problem, we follow a checklist that facilitates "guesstimation" of urolith composition (see *CVT X,* p. 1189). However, quantitative mineral analysis of representative portions of uroliths by polarizing light microscopy, x-ray diffractometry, infrared spectroscopy, or energy dispersive x-ray spectroscopy remains the diagnostic gold standard.

COLLECTION OF UROLITHS DURING THE VOIDING PHASE OF MICTURITION

Small uroliths located in the urinary bladder or urethra are commonly voided during micturition by female dogs and cats; they are occasionally voided by male dogs and cats (Fig. 1). Uroliths with a smooth surface (such as those composed of ammonium urate or calcium oxalate monohydrate) are more likely to pass through the urethra than uroliths with a rough surface (such as those composed of calcium oxalate dihydrate or silica). Commercially manufactured tropical fish nets designed for household aquariums facilitate retrieval of uroliths during voiding (Fig. 2). They are much less expensive than collection cups with wire mesh bottoms designed for humans and available from medical supply houses.

CATHETER-ASSISTED RETRIEVAL OF UROCYSTOLITHS

Detection of Uroliths

The size, number, and location of uroliths in all portions of the urinary tract should be evaluated by survey abdominal radiography. Detection of small uroliths (less than approximately 3 mm in diameter), especially those with a low degree of radiodensity, typically requires double-contrast cystography. Urocystoliths detected by survey radiography may be too large to be removed with the aid of a urethral catheter. However, large urocystoliths are often associated with small ones that can be detected by double-contrast cystography (Fig. 3).

Equipment

Small urocystoliths may be retrieved for analysis by aspirating them through a urethral catheter into a syringe. The diameter of uroliths retrieved is limited by the size of openings or "eyes" located in the proximal portion of the catheter and by the diameter of the catheter lumen. Therefore, it is best to select the largest-diameter catheter that can be advanced into the bladder lumen without causing

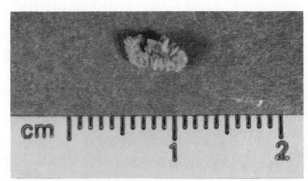

Figure 1. Photograph of a calcium oxalate dihydrate urolith voided by a 7-year-old female domestic short-hair cat.

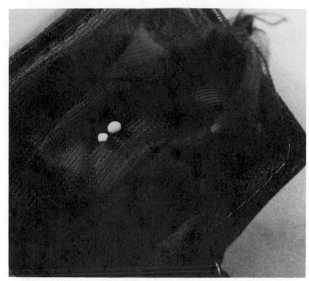

Figure 2. Struvite uroliths caught in a tropical fish net placed in a stream of urine voided by a 5-year-old female miniature schnauzer.

trauma to the urethral mucosa. Well-lubricated soft, flexible catheters are preferable to less flexible ones. To facilitate retrieval of urocystoliths, the size of openings in the proximal portion of the catheter may be enlarged with a scalpel, razor blade, or scissors. However, care must be used not to weaken the catheter to the point where it could break while being inserted into or removed from the urethra and urinary bladder.

Technique

With the patient in lateral recumbency, a well-lubricated sterilized catheter should be advanced through the urethra into the bladder lumen (Fig. 4A). The tip of the catheter should be positioned so that it will not interfere with movement of the bladder wall as fluid is aspirated from the bladder lumen.

If the urinary bladder is not distended with urine, it should be moderately distended with physiologic (0.9%) saline solution. As a rule of thumb, a normal empty canine or feline urinary bladder can be moderately distended by injecting 6 ml of fluid per kilogram of body weight. However, palpation of the urinary bladder per abdomen during the time it is distended with saline should be used as the primary method to ensure that it is not overdistended.

The next step is crucial to successful retrieval of urocystoliths. During aspiration of urine (and saline) into the syringe, an assistant should vigorously and repeatedly move the patient's abdomen in an

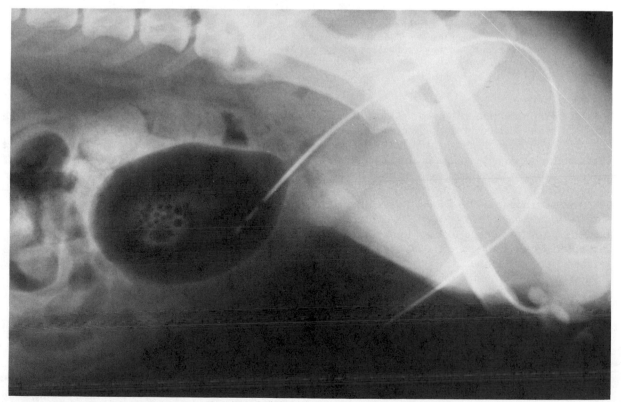

Figure 3. Lateral view of a double-contrast cystogram of a year-old male English bulldog with numerous urocystoliths of various sizes. Analysis of small urocystoliths aspirated through the urinary catheter revealed that they were composed of 100% cystine.

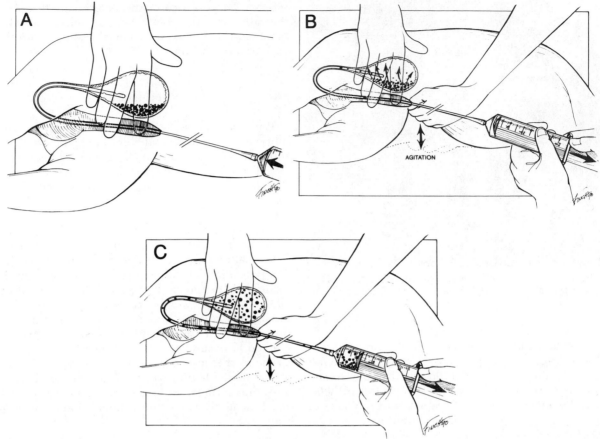

Figure 4. *A*, Schematic illustration of catheter-assisted retrieval of urocystoliths. With the patient in left lateral recumbency, uroliths have gravitated to the dependent portion of the urinary bladder. The bladder lumen has been distended by injection of 0.9% saline solution. *B*, Vigorous movement of the abdomen in an up-and-down direction results in dispersion of uroliths throughout fluid in the bladder lumen. *C*, Aspiration of fluid from the urinary bladder during movement of the abdominal wall may result in the movement of one or more small uroliths into the catheter and syringe. (Reprinted with permission from Lulich, J.P.E. and Osborne, C.A.: J.A.V.M.A. [in press].)

up-and-down direction (**Fig. 4***B*). This maneuver causes uroliths located in the dependent portion of the bladder urine to disperse throughout fluid in the bladder lumen. Small uroliths in the vicinity of the catheter tip may then be sucked into the catheter along with the urine-saline mixture (**Fig. 4***C*).

It may be necessary to repeat this sequence of steps several times before a sufficient number of uroliths is retrieved. The bladder lumen should be distended with saline each time. Difficulty in aspirating urine and saline into the syringe may be caused by poor positioning of the catheter tip or by partial occlusion of the catheter lumen with one or more uroliths. Uroliths that have occluded the catheter lumen can readily be retrieved by flushing saline through the catheter after it has been removed from the patient.

Precautions

Care must be used not to overdistend the urinary bladder with saline. Because patients with uroliths are predisposed to catheter-induced bacterial urinary tract infections, antimicrobial therapy should be considered immediately before this procedure and for an appropriate duration afterward. Proper selection, insertion, and positioning of urethral catheters minimize iatrogenic trauma to the lower urinary tract.

COLLECTION AND ANALYSIS OF CRYSTALLINE SEDIMENT

If available data do not indicate the probable mineral composition of uroliths and if uroliths cannot be retrieved with the aid of a urethral catheter, consider preparing a large pellet of urine crystals by centrifugation of urine in a conical-tip centrifuge tube. The quantity of crystalline sediment available for analysis may be increased by repeatedly removing the supernatant after centrifugation, adding additional noncentrifuged urine to the tube containing sediment, and again centrifuging the preparation.

If the conditions that caused urolith formation are still present, evaluation of the crystalline pellet of sediment by quantitative methods designed for urolith analysis may provide meaningful information about the mineral composition of a patient's uroliths. However, crystals identified by this method may only reflect the outer portions of compound uroliths. Therefore, results of quantitative urine crystal analysis should be interpreted in conjunction with other pertinent clinical data (see *CVT X*, p. 1189).

NEPHROLITHS: APPROACH TO THERAPY

THERESE M. DIERINGER
and GEORGE E. LEES
College Station, Texas

Nephrolithiasis is uncommon in dogs and cats. Fewer than 4% of canine and feline uroliths are found in the kidneys; the remainder are discovered in the lower urinary tract (i.e., bladder and urethra) (Osborne et al., 1986a). In contrast, most uroliths in humans (> 90%) are found in the kidneys. The true prevalence of canine and feline nephrolithiasis may be higher than indicated by published data. Many nephroliths are discovered incidentally on abdominal radiographs, suggesting that the condition is often subclinical and therefore underdiagnosed in small animals. Approximately 25% of canine and feline nephroliths are composed of calcium oxalate (Osborne et al., 1990); however, struvite, urate, silica, xanthine, calcium phosphate, mixed, and compound nephroliths have also been found in dogs and cats (Osborne et al., 1990).

HISTORY AND CLINICAL SIGNS

The history and clinical signs of animals with nephrolithiasis depend on the degree of renal pelvic obstruction and associated hydronephrosis and on the presence or absence of infection. When obstruction and infection are absent, the animal is often asymptomatic and nephroliths are incidentally discovered only when survey abdominal radiographs are taken for an unrelated reason. Other animals may exhibit intermittent or persistent hematuria or have recurrent urinary tract infection if the nephrolith is infected. Obstruction of one renal pelvis without infection often causes few clinical signs if the opposite kidney is functioning normally. However, progressive destruction of the obstructed kidney accompanied by functional deterioration will occur. Unilateral renal pelvic obstruction together with infection may produce acute generalized pyelonephritis, septicemia, and possibly death (Osborne and Polzin, 1986). Bilateral renal calculi often eventually cause renal failure, a process that is accelerated by renal pelvic obstruction.

The most common symptom in humans with nephroliths is severe, intense, acute abdominal pain (renal colic) associated with passage of the urolith to the ureter (Stewart, 1988). Clinical signs suggesting such an event are rarely recognized in small animals. Humans with free renal calculi or calculi lodged in the calyces may be asymptomatic or may experience dull flank pain. If this occurs in small animals, it is unlikely to be recognized.

LABORATORY FINDINGS

Laboratory findings associated with nephrolithiasis depend on the degree of renal compromise, the amount of physical injury to adjacent tissues, and the presence or absence of infection. Some patients have normal laboratory values, whereas others exhibit only microscopic hematuria or proteinuria. Findings indicative of urinary tract infection (pyuria, hematuria, proteinuria, bacteriuria, leukocyte casts) or renal failure (impaired urine-concentrating ability and azotemia) may be observed in some animals with nephrolithiasis.

RADIOGRAPHIC AND ULTRASONOGRAPHIC FINDINGS

Canine and feline nephroliths are commonly detected incidentally when the abdomen is radiographed for another reason. Nephroliths discovered in this manner must be radiopaque and sufficiently large. Small calculi are easily missed, radiolucent calculi are impossible to visualize, and overlying gas and feces often at least partially obscure the area of the kidneys and ureters (Stewart, 1988).

The intravenous pyelogram (IVP) is a more accurate method for diagnosis of nephro- and ureterolithiasis. Even small calculi and radiolucent calculi can be detected with this technique when renal blood flow and function are adequate to permit imaging of the renal pelves and ureters. The IVP may also provide useful functional information about both kidneys and may demonstrate dilation of the renal pelves (hydronephrosis), which implies some degree of obstruction.

Renal ultrasonography can also be used to detect small calculi as well as obstruction. This technique is especially useful when renal blood flow and function are compromised, causing difficulty in evaluation of an IVP. Aging cats frequently develop renal mineralization, which should not be confused with renal calculi (Lucke and Hunt, 1967). Radiographically, nephrocalcinosis appears as diffuse mineralization of the kidney or renal pelves, whereas renal calculi are usually more discrete and reside in the renal pelves. However, calculi that reside in the renal calyces may be confused with mineralization of the renal pelvis. These possibilities are impossible to differentiate with either IVP or ultrasonography.

THERAPY

Therapeutic options available for treatment of renal calculi include medical dissolution, surgical removal, and disintegration by lithotripsy. The optimal therapeutic choice depends on a patient's status and on the availability of specialized equipment and expertise.

Patient Considerations

Several variables should be considered before choosing a therapeutic approach. The entire upper urinary tract should be evaluated with an IVP to determine number, location, and size of uroliths as well as to determine the extent of renal pelvis obstruction and associated hydronephrosis. Renal calculi may be unilateral or bilateral and may be located either within the renal pelvis or within the renal parenchyma. Radiographic lucency or opacity of calculi should be evaluated as an aid in identifying their mineral composition.

Laboratory studies that are needed include a complete blood count (CBC), serum chemistry profile and electrolytes, urinalysis, and urine culture.

Results of these tests aid evaluation of renal function (blood urea nitrogen, serum creatinine and electrolytes, urine specific gravity) and assessment of anesthetic risk. Results of the CBC, urinalysis, and urine culture help identify concomitant pyelonephritis. Presence of infection aids presumptive identification of stone composition because struvite calculi are most often associated with urinary tract infection due to urease-producing organisms (staphylococci, *Proteus*). Stone composition may also be suggested by urine pH and crystal identification (Osborne et al., 1989b).

Where available, nuclear scintigraphy can be used to further evaluate renal function. Technetium-99m–labeled diethylenetriaminepentaacetic acid (DTPA) is the radiopharmaceutical used most often to determine glomerular filtration rate (GFR). Total GFR can be measured, and the proportional contribution of each kidney to total renal function can be estimated.

Therapeutic Options

MEDICAL MANAGEMENT

Before choosing medical management, renal function should be evaluated and absence of renal pelvis obstruction should be confirmed with an IVP. If renal function is compromised or if obstruction exists, a more aggressive therapeutic plan should be used to minimize the further progression of renal dysfunction. A nephrolith may occasionally be so large that surgical removal would be extremely difficult and potentially harmful. In such instances, temporary use of medical management may be indicated to decrease the size of the urolith, making it more amenable to surgical removal.

Conservative medical management of nephroliths may be considered when struvite urolithiasis (alkaline urine pH, urinary tract infection, radiopaque stone, struvite crystalluria), cystine urolithiasis (acidic urine pH, radiopaque stone, cystine crystalluria), or urate urolithiasis (acidic urine pH, radiolucent stone, urate crystalluria, Dalmatian dog) is suspected. Feeding of a calculolytic acid-residue diet (e.g., Hill's Prescription Diet s/d) and antibiotic treatment of urinary tract infection may produce dissolution of struvite stones (Osborne et al., 1986b). Cystine stone dissolution may be achieved by combining a low-protein diet (e.g., Hill's Prescription Diet u/d) and administration of *N*-(2-mercaptopropionyl)-glycine (2-MPG) (Osborne et al., 1989a). Urate stone dissolution may be achieved with a low-purine diet (e.g., Hill's Prescription Diet u/d) and administration of allopurinol (Senior, 1989).

SURGICAL MANAGEMENT

Surgical removal of nephroliths is recommended in several instances. As indicated previously, surgery should be considered when further deterioration of renal function might occur during the time required for medical dissolution or when obstruction (partial or complete) is present. Surgery is also indicated when nephroliths are suspected to be composed predominantly of calcium crytalloids; effective dissolution protocols for these stone types have not been developed. Young animals with all types of nephroliths should be considered for surgery because the safety of low-protein and low-magnesium diets for growing animals is not proven. Animals with urate stones complicating portacaval shunts are also candidates for surgery because allopurinol may require liver metabolism to be effective in stone dissolution. Males with uroliths in multiple sites that require abdominal surgery and cystotomy to correct obstruction of the lower urinary tract are also candidates for removal of nephroliths.

Three surgical procedures are used for nephrolith removal: nephrolithotomy, pyelotomy, and nephrectomy. Because some recovery of renal function after stone removal is likely even in obstructed kidneys (Osborne and Polzin, 1986), every effort should be made to salvage the affected kidney. Nephrectomy should be reserved for cases complicated by severe pyelonephritis or hydronephrosis when the opposite kidney is functional. The choice of nephrolithotomy versus pyelotomy can be made during surgery. Pyelotomy is preferred over nephrolithotomy because occlusion of renal blood supply and incision into the renal parenchyma are not required for pyelotomy. Thus, further nephron destruction and loss of renal function are minimized with pyelotomy. Unfortunately, this technique is only feasible when the nephrolith is contained within a dilated proximal ureter and the extrarenal portion of the renal pelvis (Greenwood and Rawlings, 1981). When the nephrolith is surrounded by renal parenchyma, nephrotomy is required for stone removal.

Bilateral nephrolithiasis requires further decisions regarding timing of stone removal. If azotemia is absent and urine-concentrating ability is adequate, both kidneys may be operated during one surgery. However, when renal dysfunction is present, only one kidney should be operated initially. After recovery from surgery, renal function should be re-evaluated as a basis for planning the second procedure. Nephrolithotomy produces additional renal dysfunction; therefore, the two operations should be separated by at least several weeks if this procedure is used.

Percutaneous nephrolithotomy is an established procedure for nephrolith removal in humans. It is used more commonly than either pyelotomy or nephrotomy because it is minimally invasive and results in less renal damage than other surgical techniques. The procedure involves fluoroscopy-guided introduction of a series of Teflon dilating tubes of gradually increasing diameter through a keyhole incision into the renal parenchyma to the renal pelvis. The calculi are then removed using an endoscope. This procedure has not been routinely used in veterinary medicine because canine kidneys are considered too mobile and the renal pelvis too small. However, it has been used successfully in an experimental situation (Donner et al., 1987).

EXTRACORPOREAL SHOCK-WAVE LITHOTRIPSY

Extracorporeal shock-wave lithotripsy (ESWL) is the treatment of choice for more than 80% of human patients with nephrolithiasis (Wilson and Preminger, 1990). The technique involves subjecting uroliths to repeated shock waves, resulting in their disintegration. Patients must be submerged in water, which would require anesthesia in veterinary patients. For this reason and because of the limited availability of shock-wave lithotriptor units, as well as the expense involved, ESWL is not routinely used in veterinary medicine.

References and Suggested Reading

Donner, G. S., Ellison, G. W., Ackerman, N., et al.: Percutaneous nephrolithotomy in the dog: An experimental study. Vet. Surg. 16:411, 1987.
A description of percutaneous nephrolithotomy in dogs.
Greenwood, K. M., and Rawlings, C. A.: Removal of canine renal calculi by pyelolithotomy. Vet. Surg. 10:12, 1981.
A description of pyelolithotomy in dogs.
Lucke, V. M., and Hunt, A. C.: Renal calcification in the domestic cat. Pathol. Vet. 4:120, 1967.
Description of renal mineralization in aging cats.
Osborne, C. A., Clinton, C. W., Banman, L. K., et al.: Prevalence of canine uroliths. Vet. Clin. North Am. Small Anim. Pract. 16:27, 1986a.
A review of the composition and location of canine uroliths.
Osborne, C. A., Hoppe, A., and O'Brien, T. D.: Medical dissolution and prevention of cystine uroliths. In Kirk, R. W. (ed.): *Current Veterinary Therapy X*. Philadelphia: W. B. Saunders, 1989a, p. 1189.
A description of a medical dissolution protocol for cystine uroliths.
Osborne, C. A., Lulich, J. P., Bartges, J. W., et al.: Medical dissolution and prevention of canine and feline uroliths: Diagnostic and therapeutic caveats. Vet. Rec. 127:369, 1990.
A review of various medical dissolution protocols for canine and feline uroliths.
Osborne, C. A., O'Brien, T. D., Davenport, M. P., et al.: Crystalluria: Causes, detection and interpretation. In Kirk, R. W. (ed.): *Current Veterinary Therapy X*. Philadelphia: W. B. Saunders, 1989b, p. 1127.
A description of various urine crystals and what they indicate.
Osborne, C. A., and Polzin, D. J.: Nonsurgical management of canine obstructive urolithopathy. Vet. Clin. North Am. Small Anim. Pract. 16:333, 1986.
A review of nonsurgical techniques used to relieve obstruction in the urinary tract.
Osborne, C. A., Polzin, D. J., Kruger, J. M., et al.: Medical dissolution and prevention of canine struvite uroliths. In Kirk, R. W. (ed.): *Current Veterinary Therapy X*. Philadelphia: W. B. Saunders, 1986b, p. 1177.
A review of a medical dissolution protocol for canine struvite uroliths.

Senior, D. F.: Medical management of urate uroliths. *In* Kirk, R. W. (ed.): *Current Veterinary Therapy X.* Philadelphia: W. B. Saunders, 1989, p. 1178.
  A description of a medical dissolution protocol for canine urate uroliths.
Stewart, C.: Nephrolithiasis. Emerg. Med. Clin. North Am. 6:617, 1988.

A review of human nephrolithiasis.
Wilson, W. T., and Preminger, G. M.: Extracorporeal shock-wave therapy: An update. Urol. Clin. North Am. 17:231, 1990.
  A review describing extracorporeal shock-wave therapy in human medicine.

CANINE CALCIUM OXALATE UROLITHIASIS: RISK FACTOR MANAGEMENT

JODY P. LULICH
CARL A. OSBORNE
St. Paul, Minnesota

and CHARLES L. SMITH
Minneapolis, Minnesota

Calcium oxalate urolithiasis is not a specific disease but the sequela of a group of underlying disorders that result in precipitation of calcium oxalate in urine. Alterations in the balance between urine concentrations of calculogenic minerals (calcium and oxalate) and crystallization inhibitors (including citrate, phosphorus, magnesium, sodium, potassium) have been associated with initiation and growth of calcium oxalate uroliths (Smith, 1990). The fact that urolith formation is erratic and unpredictable emphasizes that several inter-related physiologic and pathologic factors are often involved. Identification of one or more risk factors promoting urolith formation may aid in their management (Table 1).

ETIOLOGIC RISK FACTORS

Hypercalciuria

In order for uroliths to form, urine must be supersaturated with respect to that crystal system (Smith, 1990). For example, increasing urinary concentrations of calcium promote calcium oxalate crystal formation. Hypercalciuria has been a significant finding in dogs with calcium oxalate uroliths (Lulich, 1991a).

Calcium homeostasis is principally achieved through the actions of parathyroid hormone (PTH) and 1,25-cholecalciferol (1,25-vitamin D) on bones, intestines, and kidneys. Hypercalciuria can result from increased renal clearance of calcium due to (1) excessive intestinal absorption of calcium, (2) impaired renal conservation of calcium, and (3) excessive skeletal mobilization of calcium.

In dogs, normocalcemic hypercalciuria is thought to result from either intestinal hyperabsorption of calcium (called *absorptive hypercalciuria*) or decreased renal tubular reabsorption of calcium (called *renal leak hypercalciuria*). Hypercalcemic hypercalciuria results from increased glomerular filtration of mobilized calcium, which overwhelms normal renal tubular reabsorptive mechanisms (called *resorptive hypercalciuria* because excessive bone resorption is associated with increased serum calcium concentrations).

Absorptive hypercalciuria is characterized by increased urine calcium excretion, normal serum calcium concentration, and normal or low serum PTH concentration. Because absorptive hypercalciuria is dependent on dietary calcium, urine calcium excretion during food fasting is normal or significantly reduced when compared with urine calcium excretion during nonfasting conditions. Mean 24-hr urine calcium excretion in 33 normal beagles was 0.32 ± 0.2 mg/kg/24 hr during fasting and 0.51 ± 0.3 mg/kg/24 hr when dogs consumed a standard diet (Prescription Diet Canine k/d, Hill's Pet Products) (Lulich, 1991b). By comparison, mean urine calcium excretion in five miniature schnauzers with calcium oxalate urolithiasis and absorptive hypercalciuria was 1.0 ± 0.5 mg/kg/24 hr during fasting and 2.84 ± 0.9 mg/kg/24 hr during nonfasting urine collections (Lulich, 1991a).

Primary intestinal abnormalities in calcium absorption, disorders of 1,25-vitamin D production, and hypophosphatemia-induced hypervitaminosis D have been recognized as causes in humans. A single pathogenic mechanism for absorptive hypercalciuria has not been identified in dogs we have evaluated. However, we did not observe hypophosphatemia or

Table 1. Management of Calcium Oxalate Urolith Risk Factors

Risk Factor	Etiopathologic Disorder	Therapeutic Management	
		Goal	*Method*
Hypercalciuria	*Intestinal Hyperabsorption*		
	Idiopathic	Dietary calcium reduction	Provide diets with reduced calcium (Prescription Diet u/d)
	Hypophosphatemia	Normalize vitamin D production by sustaining a normal serum phosphorus concentration	Provide phosphorus supplementation (Neutra-Phos-K; Willen)
	Vitamin D excess	Limit excessive intestinal calcium absorption	Avoid oral vitamin D supplementation
	Renal Leak		
	Idiopathic	Promote renal calcium reabsorption	Consider thiazide diuretic?
	Renal tubular acidosis	Increase renal tubular reabsorption of bicarbonate to enhance calcium reabsorption	Provide oral alkali therapy (potassium citrate)
	Dietary protein excess	Increase renal tubular reabsorption of bicarbonate to enhance calcium reabsorption and promote adequate citrate excretion	Provide diets with reduced protein (Prescription Diet u/d)
	Dietary sodium excess	Minimize renal sodium and calcium excretion	Provide diets with reduced sodium (Prescription Diet u/d)
	Glucocorticoid excess	Decrease glucocorticoid-enhanced bone resorption and urine calcium excretion	Control hyperadrenocorticism, avoid glucocorticoid supplementation
	Excessive Skeletal Resorption		
	Primary hyperparathyroidism	Normalize skeletal calcium resorption, serum calcium concentration, and renal calcium filtration	Parathyroidectomy
	Pseudohyperparathyroidism	Control paraneoplastic parathyroid hormone–like activity	Neoplasm eradication or remission
	Osteolytic lesions	Minimize release of excessive skeletal calcium	Correct underlying bone disorder
Hyperoxaluria	Dietary oxalate excess	Avoid foods of high oxalate content	Provide diets low in oxalate (Prescription Diet u/d)
	Fat malabsorption	Decrease intestinal fat	Provide diets with reduced fat
	Vitamin C excess	Minimize precursor of oxalate	Avoid vitamin C supplementation
	Vitamin B_6 deficiency	Permit conversion of glyoxylate (an oxalate precursor) to glycine	Provide adequate vitamin B_6
	Primary hyperoxaluria	Minimize oxalate synthesis	Provide excess vitamin B_6?
Hypocitraturia	Idiopathic	Promote citrate excretion	Provide oral potassium citrate (Urocit-K Mission Pharmacal)
	Acidosis	Minimize acidosis	Provide oral alkali therapy (potassium citrate)
Defective macromolecular inhibitors	Inherited disorder?	Restore urinary concentration of effective inhibitors	Unknown

elevated levels of 1,25-vitamin D in five dogs with absorptive hypercalciuria.

In our studies of dogs, *renal leak hypercalciuria* has been recognized, but less frequently than excessive intestinal absorption of calcium. In these dogs, renal leak hypercalciuria was characterized by normal serum calcium concentration, increased urine calcium excretion, and increased serum PTH concentration. Unlike patients with absorptive hypercalciuria, these dogs did not show a decline in urinary calcium loss during food fasting. As a result, urinary calcium excretion during fasting was similar to calcium excretion during nonfasting conditions. The underlying cause was not established. The defect in human patients with renal leak hypercalciuria is associated with impaired tubular reabsorption of calcium. The resulting decline in serum calcium concentration causes enhanced secretion of PTH, which in turn increases synthesis of 1,25-vitamin D. The resulting increase in intestinal calcium absorption further contributes to hypercalciuria. In humans, disorders altering the kidneys' ability to appropriately conserve calcium include distal renal tubular acidosis, acquired and congenital Fanconi's syndrome, chronic metabolic acidosis, glucocorticoid excess, and excess dietary sodium or protein consumption.

Resorptive hypercalciuria is characterized by excessive filtration and excretion of calcium in urine as a result of hypercalcemia. In our experience, hypercalcemic disorders have been infrequently recognized causes of calcium oxalate uroliths in dogs.

Hyperoxaluria

Oxalic acid is the end-product of metabolism of ascorbic acid and amino acids (glycine and serine) derived from both endogenous and dietary sources. Oxalic acid forms soluble salts with sodium and potassium ions but a relatively insoluble salt with calcium ions. Increases in urine oxalate concentration promote calcium oxalate urolith formation to a greater degree than comparable increases in urine calcium concentration.

Hyperoxaluria has not been documented in dogs with calcium oxalate uroliths. However, lack of recognition of canine hyperoxaluria is related to the unavailability of a reproducible method of determining the concentration of oxalate in urine. In humans, hyperoxaluria has been associated with inherited abnormalities of excessive oxalate synthesis (primary hyperoxaluria), increased consumption of foods containing high quantities of oxalate or oxalate precursors, pyridoxine deficiency, and disorders associated with fat malabsorption (Williams and Smith, 1983).

Hypocitrituria

Hypocitrituria is a common physiologic disturbance in human patients with calcium oxalate urolithiasis; however, the role of low urine citrate concentration in the etiology of calcium oxalate uroliths is not completely resolved. Nonetheless, urine citrate has been recognized as one inhibitor of calcium oxalate urolith formation. By complexing with calcium ions to form the relatively soluble salt of calcium citrate, citrate reduces the quantity of calcium available to bind with oxalate.

Hypocitrituria has been observed in dogs with calcium oxalate uroliths; however, mechanisms responsible for decreased urinary citrate excretion are unknown. It is known that acid-base homeostasis influences the quantity of citrate excreted in urine (Simpson, 1983). In normal dogs, acidosis is associated with decreased urinary citrate excretion, whereas alkalosis promotes urinary citrate excretion.

Defective Macromolecular Crystal Growth Inhibitors

In addition to urinary concentration of calculogenic minerals and other ions, large-molecular-weight proteins in urine have a profound ability to enhance solubility of calcium oxalate. One such protein, called *nephrocalcin,* minimized calcium oxalate crystal growth in human urine (Nakagawa et al., 1983). Nephrocalcin found in urine of human patients with calcium oxalate urolithiasis was structurally different from nephrocalcin found in healthy human urine. Nephrocalcin from urolith-forming patients lacked appropriate quantities of carboxyglutamic acid residues and was unable to effectively prevent crystal growth. Preliminary studies of urine obtained from dogs with calcium oxalate uroliths have revealed that nephrocalcin also lacked appropriate numbers of carboxyglutamic acid residues compared with nephrocalcin isolated from normal dog urine.

DIAGNOSTIC FACTORS

Prevalence

Detection of calcium oxalate in canine uroliths submitted to the University of Minnesota Urolith Center has been increasing. Ten years ago, canine calcium oxalate uroliths were uncommonly detected (4%). However, as of 1990, uroliths composed primarily of calcium oxalate accounted for 20.7% of canine uroliths submitted (n = 5051) to our urolith center. Because surgical removal remains the most reliable short-term treatment for calcium oxalate uroliths, presurgical differentiation of calcium oxalate uroliths from uroliths amenable to medical dissolution (struvite, ammonium urate, and cystine) is essential (Osborne et al., 1989).

Patient Signalment and Clinical Signs

Although calcium oxalate uroliths have been recognized in many breeds of dogs, miniature schnauzers, Lhasa apsos, Shih tzus, Yorkshire terriers, and miniature poodles have been most commonly af-

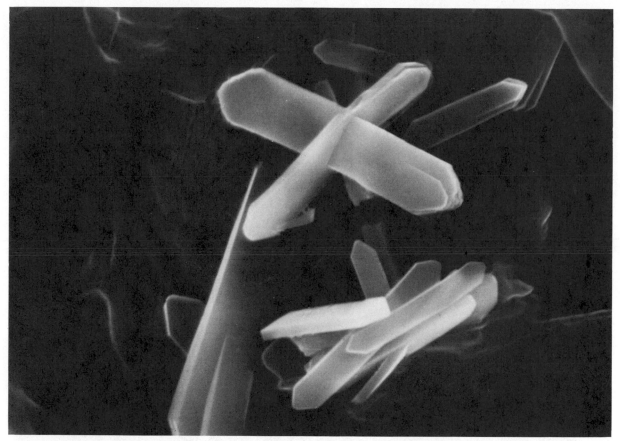

Figure 1. Scanning electron micrograph of calcium oxalate monohydrate crystals in canine urine (original magnification × 10,800). (Reprinted with permission from Osborne, C. A., Davis, L. S., Sanna, J., et al.: Identification and interpretation of crystalluria in domestic animals: A light and scanning electron microscopic study. Vet. Med. 85:18, 1990.)

fected. Infrequently affected breeds include the boxer, English bulldog, golden retriever, and Labrador retriever. Approximately 70% of calcium oxalate uroliths have affected male dogs. Most were detected in adults (mean age = 8 to 9 years).

Clinical signs associated with uroliths are not specific for their mineral composition; however, signs referable to hypercalcemia (e.g., polydipsia, polyuria, and muscle weakness) may be observed in dogs with hypercalcemia and calcium oxalate uroliths.

Urinalysis

Calcium oxalate crystals may or may not be detected in urine of dogs with calcium oxalate uroliths. Two types of calcium oxalate crystals have been recognized: calcium oxalate monohydrate and calcium oxalate dihydrate (Figs. 1 and 2). Detection of calcium oxalate crystals indicates that the urine is supersaturated with calcium oxalate; therefore, they represent a risk factor for calcium oxalate urolith formation.

Although urine pH is an important determinant for struvite and urate crystal formation, calcium oxalate solubility changes minimally within the physiologic range of urine pH values of dogs (5.0 to 7.5). Nonetheless, urine pH values of most dogs with calcium oxalate uroliths have been slightly acid to neutral.

Radiographic Characteristics

Calcium oxalate uroliths can be located anywhere in the urinary tract but most commonly are detected in the bladder and urethra. Analysis of uroliths submitted to our laboratory has revealed a slightly higher percentage of nephroliths composed of calcium oxalate (24%, n = 80) compared with those analyzed from the lower urinary tract (20.6%, n = 4971).

Compared with soft tissue, uroliths composed of calcium oxalate are radiodense. Calcium oxalate uroliths may be single or multiple and vary in size from a millimeter to several centimeters in diameter. Uroliths composed primarily of calcium oxalate monohydrate are usually round (sometimes elliptical) with a smooth surface (Fig. 3). By comparison,

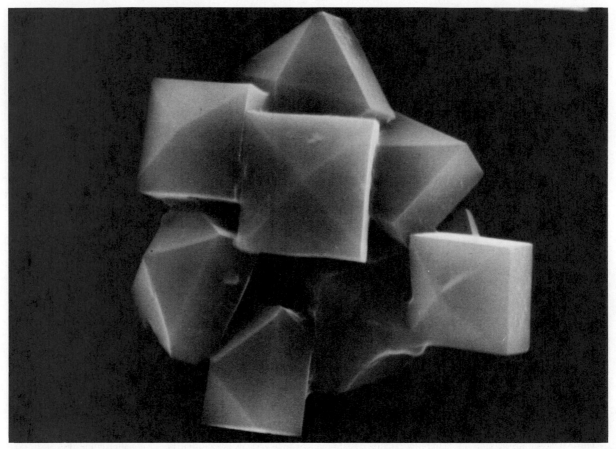

Figure 2. Scanning electron micrograph of calcium oxalate dihydrate crystals in canine urine (original magnification × 7040). (Reprinted with permission from Osborne, C. A., Davis, L. S., Sanna, J., et al.: Identification and interpretation of crystalluria in domestic animals: A light and scanning electron microscopic study. Vet. Med. 85:18, 1990.)

uroliths composed primarily of calcium oxalate dihydrate or a mixture of calcium oxalate monohydrate and calcium oxalate dihydrate are usually round to ovoid and have an irregular surface caused by protrusions of sharp-edged crystals (see Fig. 3).

Serum Chemistry Values

In most dogs with calcium oxalate uroliths, serum concentrations of calcium, phosphorus, magnesium, and electrolytes have been normal. However, in some patients with primary hyperparathyroidism and calcium oxalate uroliths, increased serum calcium concentrations, low to normal concentrations of phosphorus, and increased serum PTH concentrations were observed.

Elevated serum alkaline phosphatase activity has been recognized in approximately 54% of dogs (33 of 63) with calcium oxalate urolithiasis evaluated at our veterinary teaching hospital. The relationship between elevated serum alkaline phosphatase activity and calcium oxalate urolithiasis (if any) has not been evaluated. Further studies are needed to

determine if increased serum alkaline phosphatase activity originates from bone, coincides with the onset of hyperadrenocorticism, or merely results from other unrelated increases in this enzyme.

Urine Chemistry Values

Evaluation of urine often provides information about specific abnormalities associated with urolith formation. For best results, 24-hr urine samples should be collected. Determination of fractional excretion of many metabolites in "spot" urine samples does not accurately reflect 24-hr metabolite excretion. Urine concentrations of potentially calculogenic metabolites are also influenced by the amount and composition of diet consumed and by whether urine was collected during conditions of fasting or food consumption.

Analysis of Voided or Retrieved Uroliths

Quantitative analysis of uroliths voided during micturition or retrieved via urethral catheters pro-

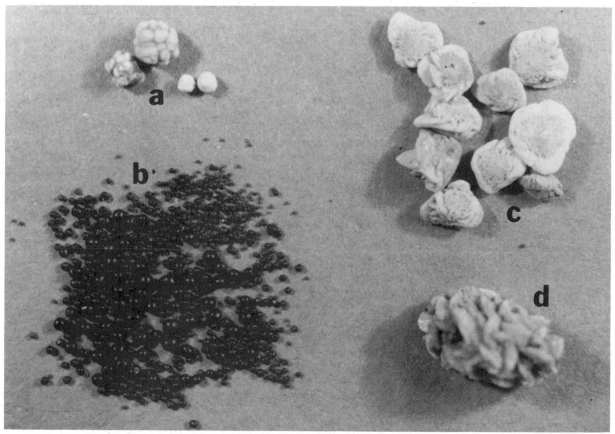

Figure 3. Comparison of the smooth contour of uroliths composed of calcium oxalate monohydrate (*a* and *b*) to sharp-edged surface protrusions typical of uroliths composed of calcium oxalate dihydrate (*c* and *d*).

vides the most reliable information about the composition of uroliths remaining in the urinary tract (see this volume, p. 886).

MANAGEMENT CONSIDERATIONS

In contrast to our experience with struvite, urate, and cystine uroliths, which dissolve when oversaturation of urine with calculogenic substances is abolished (Osborne et al., 1989), we have been unable to dissolve calcium oxalate uroliths in dogs. Therefore, surgery currently remains the most effective method to remove calcium oxalate uroliths in dogs. However, medical protocols may be considered to prevent further growth of uroliths remaining in the urinary tract or to minimize urolith recurrence after removal.

In general, medical therapy should be formulated in a step-wise fashion, with the initial goal of reducing urine concentration of calculogenic substances. Medications that have the potential to induce a sustained alteration in body composition of metabolites, in addition to urine concentration of metabolites, should be reserved for patients with active or frequently recurrent calcium oxalate uroliths.

Caution must be used so that side effects of treatment are not more detrimental than the effects of uroliths.

In patients with hypercalcemia and resorptive hypercalciuria, the cause of hypercalcemia (e.g., primary hyperparathyroidism) should be corrected. Whether calcium oxalate uroliths remaining in the patient after parathyroidectomy will subsequently dissolve is unknown; however, calcium oxalate urolith growth or recurrence is unlikely.

In patients with normal serum calcium concentrations, an attempt should be made to identify risk factors for urolith formation. Amelioration or control of the consequences of risk factors (urine oversaturation with calculogenic minerals) should minimize urolith growth and recurrence.

Dietary Considerations

Although reduction of urine calcium and oxalate concentrations by decreasing dietary calcium and oxalate appears to be a logical therapeutic goal, it is not necessarily a harmless maneuver. Reducing consumption of only one of these constituents (such as calcium) may increase the availability of the other (such as oxalate) for intestinal absorption and subsequent urinary excretion (Goldfarb, 1988). In general, reduction in dietary calcium should be accompanied by an appropriate decrease in dietary oxalate.

Humans with calcium oxalate uroliths are often cautioned to avoid milk and milk products to reduce calcium intake, and because the carbohydrate component (lactose) of these products may augment intestinal absorption of calcium from any dietary source. Likewise, they are often discouraged from consuming foods containing relatively high quantities of oxalate (chocolate, nuts, beans, sweet potatoes, wheat germ, spinach, and rhubarb). Although there is agreement that excessive consumption of calcium and oxalate should be avoided, the general consensus of urologists is that it is inadvisable to restrict dietary calcium unless absorptive hypercalciuria has been documented. Even then, only moderate restriction is advocated in order to prevent negative balance of calcium in the body.

Consumption of high levels of sodium may augment renal excretion of calcium. Twenty-four-hour urinary calcium excretion of normal dogs consuming diets with 0.8% sodium (dry weight analysis) was comparable to calcium excretion observed in dogs with calcium oxalate uroliths. Therefore, moderate dietary restriction of sodium (<0.3% sodium) is recommended for calcium oxalate stone formers.

Studies of laboratory animals, dogs, and humans suggest that dietary phosphorus should not be restricted in patients with calcium oxalate urolithiasis because reduction in dietary phosphorus is often associated with augmentation of hypercalciuria. If calcium oxalate urolithiasis is associated with hypophosphatemia and normal serum calcium concentration, oral phosphorus supplementation should be considered. However, caution must be used because excessive dietary phosphorus may predispose to formation of calcium phosphate uroliths.

Although supplemental dietary magnesium contributes to formation of magnesium ammonium phosphate uroliths in some species (cats and ruminants), urine magnesium apparently impairs formation of calcium oxalate crystals. For this reason, supplemental magnesium has been used in an attempt to minimize recurrence of calcium oxalate uroliths in humans. However, we observed increased urinary excretion of calcium by normal dogs given supplemental magnesium. Pending further studies, we do not recommend dietary magnesium restriction or supplementation for treatment of canine calcium oxalate uroliths.

Ingestion of foods that contain high quantities of animal protein may contribute to calcium oxalate urolithiasis by increasing urinary calcium excretion and decreasing urinary citrate excretion. Some of these consequences result from obligatory acid excretion associated with protein metabolism. We have observed hypercalciuria in normal dogs fed high-protein diets (40% dry weight analysis). Therefore, excessive dietary protein consumption should be avoided in dogs with active calcium oxalate urolithiasis.

A diet moderately restricted in protein, calcium, oxalate, and sodium (such as Prescription Diet Canine u/d, Hill's Pet Products) may be considered to help prevent recurrence of active calcium oxalate uroliths in dogs. Ideally, diets should not be restricted or supplemented with phosphorus or magnesium. Excessive levels of vitamin D (which promotes intestinal absorption of calcium) and ascorbic acid (a precursor of oxalate) should also be avoided. A deficiency of pyridoxine should be avoided, because vitamin B_6 deficiency promotes endogenous production of oxalate.

Thiazide Diuretics

Thiazide diuretics have been recommended to reduce recurrence of calcium-containing uroliths in humans because of their ability to reduce urine calcium excretion. The exact mechanisms by which thiazide diuretics reduce urinary calcium excretion are unknown; however, several factors appear to be involved. For instance, studies of rats revealed that thiazide diuretics directly stimulated distal renal tubular resorption of calcium. Although results of studies in humans suggest that thiazide diuretics potentiate the action of PTH, effects of thiazide diuretics on urinary calcium excretion were not altered in parathyroidectomized rats or dogs. Because the hypocalciuric response to thiazide diuretics was blocked when volume depletion was prevented by sodium chloride administration in humans, it was hypothesized that thiazide diuretics promote mild extracellular volume contraction and thereby promote proximal tubular reabsorption of several solutes, including sodium and calcium.

In dogs, urinary calcium excretion may increase, decrease, or remain unchanged after thiazide diuretic administration. In one canine study, fractional clearance of calcium increased after intravenous administration of chlorothiazide. In contrast, infusion of thiazide diuretics into left renal arteries of dogs resulted in a significant reduction in calcium clearance compared with calcium clearance by right kidneys. In another canine study, distal tubular concentrations of calcium did not change after intravenous administration of chlorothiazide. These results suggest that the effect of thiazide diuretics on urinary excretion of calcium in dogs is variable. When we evaluated the effect of chlorothiazide (21, 42, and 65 mg/kg every 12 hr) in six normal dogs, a hypocalciuric effect was not observed. In fact, the opposite occurred. As the dose of chlorothiazide was increased, daily urinary calcium excretion also increased. Pending studies evaluating the effect of thiazide diuretics in calcium oxalate urolith–forming dogs, we do not recommend thiazide diuretics for treatment or prevention of canine calcium oxalate uroliths.

Citrate

Citrate inhibits calcium oxalate crystal formation because of its ability to form soluble salts with calcium. This may explain why some humans with abnormally low quantities of urine citrate are at risk for development of calcium oxalate uroliths. Oral administration of potassium citrate (approximately 90 mg/kg/day) to human patients has been associated with marked increases in urinary citrate excretion. However, administration of up to 150 mg/kg/day of potassium citrate to normal dogs was not associated with a consistent increase in urine citrate concentration. Nonetheless, a dose-dependent rise in urine pH did occur. These results suggest that metabolism and excretion of potassium citrate in dogs may differ from that in humans. Although 10 to 35% of filtered citrate is excreted in urine by humans, only 1 to 3% of filtered citrate is excreted by dogs (Simpson, 1983). Even though administration of potassium citrate orally may not be associated with a sustained increase in urine citrate concentration, potassium citrate may be beneficial in management of calcium oxalate because of its alkalizing effect. In dogs, chronic metabolic acidosis inhibits renal tubular reabsorption of calcium, whereas metabolic alkalosis enhances tubular reabsorption of calcium. Potassium citrate is preferred to sodium bicarbonate as an alkalizing agent because oral administration of sodium enhances urine calcium excretion. A commercially available diet for the dissolution or prevention of urate, cystine, and calcium oxalate uroliths in dogs (Prescription Diet Canine u/d, Hill's Pet Products) contains potassium citrate. If hypocitrituria is recognized in dogs (mean urinary citrate excretion of 33 normal beagles was 2.57 ± 2.31 mg/kg/24 hr, median urinary citrate excretion of 33 normal beagles was 1.88 mg/kg/24 hr), wax matrix tablets of potassium citrate (Urocit-K, Mission Phar-

macal) may be considered. We currently recommend a dose of 150 mg/kg/day (divided into two subdoses); tablets should be crushed and then mixed with food.

Other Agents

Various other agents have been suggested for management of calcium oxalate uroliths in humans. They include allopurinol to minimize heterogeneous nucleation of calcium oxalate on uric acid crystals, sodium cellulose phosphate to bind intestinal calcium, and orthophosphates to minimize calcium excretion. Consult the reference list for details and applications to veterinary medicine (Goldfarb, 1988; Osborne, et al., 1986; Smith, 1990).

References and Suggested Reading

Goldfarb, S.: Dietary factors in the pathogenesis and prophylaxis of calcium nephrolithiasis. Kidney Int. 34:544, 1988.
Review of dietary factors important in human calcium oxalate urolithiasis.

Lulich, J. P., Osborne, C. A., Nagode, L. A., et al.: Evaluation of urine and serum analytes in miniature schnauzers with calcium oxalate urolithiasis. Am. J. Vet. Res. 52:1583, 1991a.

Lulich, J. P., Osborne, C. A., Parker, M. L., et al.: Urine chemistry values in nonfasted and fasted normal beagle dogs. Am. J. Vet. Res. 52:1573, 1991b.

Nakagawa, Y., Veronika, A., Kezdy, F. J., et al.: Purification and characterization of the principal inhibitor of calcium oxalate monohydrate crystal growth in human urine. J. Biol. Chem. 258:12594, 1983.
Methods of nephrocalcin identification and function assay.

Osborne, C. A., Poffenbarger, E. M., Klausner, J. S., et al.: Etiopathogenesis, clinical management of canine calcium oxalate urolithiasis. Vet. Clin. North Am. Small Anim. Pract. 16:133, 1986.

Osborne, C. A., Polzin, D. J., Lulich, J. P., et al.: Relationship of nutritional factors to the cause, dissolution, and prevention of canine uroliths. Vet. Clin. North Am. Small Anim. Pract. 19:583, 1989.
Review of dietary considerations for dissolution and prevention of common canine uroliths.

Simpson, D. P.: Citrate excretion: A window on renal metabolism. Am. J. Physiol. 244:F223, 1983.
Review of citrate metabolism in many species including dogs.

Smith, L. H.: The pathophysiology and medical treatment of urolithiasis. Semin. Nephrol. 10:31, 1990.
Review pertains to urolithiasis in humans.

Williams, H. E., and Smith, L. H.: Primary hyperoxaluria. *In* Stanbury, J. B., Wyngaarden, J. B., Fredrickson, D. S., et al. (eds.): *The Metabolic Basis of Inherited Disease,* 5th ed. New York: McGraw-Hill, 1983, pp. 204–228.
Discusses normal and abnormal oxalate synthesis and excretion in relation to human disorders.

CANINE XANTHINE UROLITHS: RISK FACTOR MANAGEMENT

JOSEPH W. BARTGES,
CARL A. OSBORNE,
and LAWRENCE J. FELICE
St. Paul, Minnesota

As of 1986, only one report of a xanthine urolith in small animals was found in the English literature. In 1968, bilateral renoliths discovered at necropsy in a 2 ½-year-old male King Charles spaniel were considered to be composed of xanthine on the basis of chemical and spectrophotometric analysis (Kidder and Chivers, 1968). The renoliths were small, greenish brown, ovoid, and hard. Unfortunately, no clinical or laboratory data were included with this case report.

Our first encounter with xanthine uroliths occurred in 1987 during medical management of multiple urocystoliths in a 1-year-old male English bulldog. Quantitative analyses of several uroliths voided during micturition revealed that they were composed of 100% ammonium urate. Medical therapy consisted of a purine-restricted alkalizing diet (Prescription Diet Canine u/d, Hill's Pet Products) and orally administered allopurinol (10 mg/kg every 8 hr). During the following 12 weeks, there was a dramatic reduction in the number and size of uroliths. However, coincidental with supplementation of the diet with protein by the owner, one urocystolith became refractory to dissolution during the next 5 months. Evaluation of the stone after surgical removal revealed that it was ovoid, bright yellow-orange, and had an irregular surface. Quantitative analysis of the urocystolith by optical crystallography and x-ray diffraction revealed an outer shell composed of 100% xanthine surrounding a nucleus of 100% ammonium urate (Fig. 1).

Since 1987, 13 canine uroliths submitted to the University of Minnesota Urolith Center were found to contain various quantities of xanthine (Table 1). All were obtained from dogs given allopurinol orally for at least 3 months. In several instances, owners supplemented their dogs' purine-restricted diet (Prescription Diet Canine u/d, Hill's Pet Products) with various types of protein.

The apparent rarity of recognition of xanthine uroliths in dogs may be related, at least in part, to widespread use of chemical qualitative methods of urolith analysis. In addition, one cannot reliably differentiate ammonium urate from xanthine by polarizing light microscopy. Confirmation of xanthine as a component of uroliths can be obtained

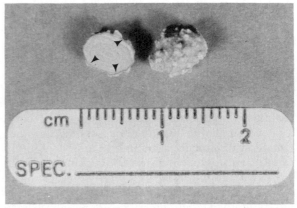

Figure 1. Urocystolith removed from the urinary bladder of a 1-year-old male English bulldog and sectioned with a diamond saw. The nucleus was composed of 100% ammonium urate, and the shell *(arrowheads)* was composed of 100% xanthine.

by high-pressure liquid chromatography and infrared spectroscopy.

APPLIED BIOCHEMISTRY

Hereditary xanthinuria is a rarely recognized disorder of humans characterized by a deficiency of xanthine oxidase, the enzyme that catalyzes the oxidation of hypoxanthine to xanthine and xanthine to uric acid (Holmes and Wyngaarden, 1989) (Fig. 2). As a consequence, abnormal quantities of xanthine are excreted in urine as a major end-product of purine metabolism. Because xanthine is the least soluble of the purines naturally excreted in urine, xanthinuria may be associated with formation of uroliths. Naturally occurring xanthinuria has not yet been reported in dogs or cats.

Allopurinol (4-hydroxypyrazolo(3,4-D)-pyrimidine) is a synthetic isomer of hypoxanthine (Hande et al., 1978). It rapidly binds to and inhibits the action of xanthine oxidase and thereby decreases production of uric acid by inhibiting conversion of hypoxanthine to xanthine and xanthine to uric acid (Fig. 3). The result is a reduction in serum and urine uric acid

Table 1. Summary of Findings From 13 Dogs With Uroliths Containing Xanthine

Breed	Sex	Age (Years)	Uroliths Obtained Before Therapy*		Uroliths Obtained During Allopurinol Therapy*	
			Location	*Analysis†*	*Location*	*Analysis†*
Malamute	Male, castrate	8	Voided	100% ammonium urate	Bladder	nucleus: 100% ammonium urate / shell: 100% xanthine
Miniature schnauzer	Male, intact	3	Bladder	100% ammonium urate	Kidney (necropsy)	100% xanthine
English bulldog	Male, intact	2	Bladder	100% ammonium urate	Bladder	90% sodium urate / 5% ammonium urate / 5% xanthine
English bulldog	Male, intact	1	Voided	100% ammonium urate	Bladder (cystotomy)	nucleus: 100% ammonium urate / shell: 100% xanthine
English bulldog	Male, intact	4	Bladder	100% ammonium urate	Bladder	60% sodium urate / 35% ammonium urate / 5% xanthine
English bulldog	Male, castrate	6	Bladder	80% sodium urate / 20% ammonium urate	Bladder	100% xanthine
English bulldog	Female, spay	4	Bladder	100% ammonium urate	Bladder	100% xanthine
Yorkshire terrier	Female, spay	4		Unknown	Kidney (necropsy)	65% ammonium urate / 35% xanthine
Dalmatian	Male, castrate	3.5	Bladder	100% ammonium urate	Voided	100% xanthine
Dalmatian	Male, castrate	5	Bladder	100% ammonium urate	Bladder	70% ammonium urate / 30% xanthine
Dalmatian	Male, castrate	6	Bladder	100% ammonium urate	Bladder	100% xanthine
Dalmatian	Male, castrate	9	Bladder	80% ammonium urate / 20% magnesium ammonium phosphate	Bladder	80% ammonium urate / 15% magnesium ammonium phosphate / 5% xanthine
Dalmatian	Male, castrate	2		Unknown	Voided	70% ammonium urate / 30% xanthine

*Uroliths voided during micturition or aspirated from the bladder through a transurethral catheter.
†Analysis performed by x-ray diffraction or infrared spectroscopy.

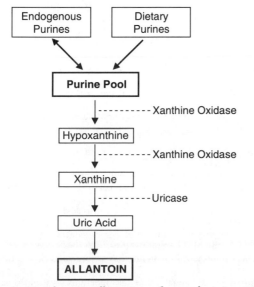

Figure 2. Schematic illustration of normal canine purine metabolism.

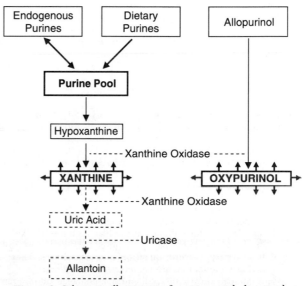

Figure 3. Schematic illustration of purine metabolism in dogs consuming a normal diet and given allopurinol.

concentration within approximately 2 days (Foreman, 1984). Although allopurinol has a short half-life in humans with normal renal function (approximately 90 min), its metabolic derivative oxypurinol is also a xanthine oxidase inhibitor and has a half-life of approximately 12 to 16 hr. The biologic half-lives of allopurinol and oxypurinol in dogs are unknown to us. Increased reutilization of hypoxanthine during allopurinol therapy contributes substantially to decreased purine excretion. Nonetheless, decreased urinary excretion of uric acid is associated with an increase in urine xanthine concentration.

Administration of allopurinol (at a dosage of 15 mg/kg/12 hr) to two nonfasting dogs with ammonium urate urocystoliths was associated with a 5- to 10-fold decrease in plasma uric acid concentration and a 10-fold decrease in urine uric acid concentration. Xanthine was undetectable in plasma (< 0.02 mg/dl) and urine (< 0.5 mg/dl) by high-pressure liquid chromatography before allopurinol therapy. After administration of allopurinol, plasma xanthine concentration was approximately 0.3 mg/dl, and the 24-hr urinary excretion of xanthine was approximately 5.6 mg/kg (200 mg). Although the formation of xanthine uroliths by humans treated with allopurinol is uncommon (O'Sullivan, 1974), our recent experience indicates that this risk may be higher in dogs than previously recognized.

MINIMIZING FORMATION OF XANTHINE UROLITHS

Our current recommendations for medical dissolution of ammonium urate uroliths include a combination of (1) low-purine diets, (2) administration of xanthine oxidase inhibitors (allopurinol), (3) alkalization of urine, and (4) eradication or control of secondary urinary tract infections (Table 2) (Osborne et al., 1989). Using this protocol, we have induced dissolution of nine episodes of ammonium urate urocystoliths in six dogs in a mean of 14.2 weeks (range = 4 to 40 weeks) (Figs. 4 and 5). However, it is apparent that this regimen may be associated with a therapeutic dilemma. A desired reduction in urine uric acid concentration may be accompanied by an undesired rise in urine xanthine concentration. Formation of a shell of xanthine around existing ammonium urate uroliths may reduce their rate of dissolution or prevent further dissolution (see Fig. 1).

The magnitude of allopurinol-induced xanthinuria may be influenced by several variables, including (1) the dosage of allopurinol, (2) the quantity of purine precursors in the diet (Figs. 6 and 7), (3) the rate of production of endogenous purine precursors, (4) the rate and completeness of endogenous and exogenous purine degradation, and (5) the status of

Table 2. Summary of Recommendations for Medical Dissolutions of Canine Ammonium Acid Urate Uroliths

1. Perform appropriate diagnostic studies, including complete urinalyses, quantitative urine culture, and diagnostic radiography. Determine precise location, size, and number of uroliths. The size and number of uroliths are not a reliable index of probable efficacy of therapy.
2. If available, determine mineral composition of uroliths. If unavailable, "guesstimate" their composition by evaluation of appropriate clinical data.
3. Consider surgical correction if uroliths are obstructing urine outflow.
4. Determine baseline pretreatment serum uric acid concentrations (and if possible fractional excretion of urine uric acid).
5. Initiate therapy with calculolytic diet (Prescription Diet Canine u/d, Hill's Pet Products). No other food supplements should be fed to the patient. Compliance with dietary recommendation is suggested by reduction in serum urea nitrogen concentration (usually < 10 mg/dl).
6. Initiate therapy with allopurinol at a dosage of 30 mg/kg/day divided into two equal subdoses (a lesser dose will be required in azotemic patients).
7. If necessary, administer sodium bicarbonate or potassium citrate orally in order to eliminate aciduria. Strive for a urine pH of approximately 7.
8. If necessary, eradicate or control urinary tract infections with appropriate antimicrobial agents. Maintain antimicrobial therapy during urate urolith dissolution and for an appropriate period afterward.
9. Devise a protocol to monitor efficacy of therapy:
   a. Try to avoid diagnostic follow-up studies that require urinary catheterization. If they are required, give appropriate pericatheterization antimicrobial agents to prevent iatrogenic urinary tract infection.
   b. Evaluate serial urinalyses. Urine pH, specific gravity, and microscopic examination of sediment for urate crystals are especially important. Remember, crystals formed in urine stored at room or refrigeration temperatures may represent *in vitro* artifacts.
   c. Serially evaluate the serum uric acid concentrations and (if possible) fractional excretion of urine uric acid.
   d. Evaluate urolith locations, number, size, density, and shape at approximately monthly intervals. Intravenous urography may be used for radiolucent uroliths located in the kidneys, ureters, or urinary bladder. Retrograde contrast urethrocystography may be required for radiolucent uroliths located in the bladder and urethra.
   e. If necessary, perform quantitative urine cultures. They are especially important in patients that are infected before therapy and in patients that are catheterized during therapy.
10. Continue calculolytic diet, allopurinol, and alkalizing therapy for approximately 1 month after disappearance of uroliths as detected by radiography.

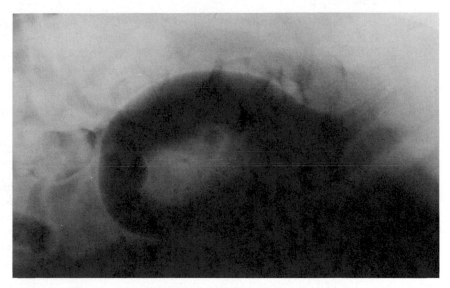

Figure 4. Double-contrast cystogram of a 3-year-old male English bulldog illustrating multiple radiolucent uroliths. Analysis of a spontaneously voided urolith revealed that it was composed of 100% ammonium urate.

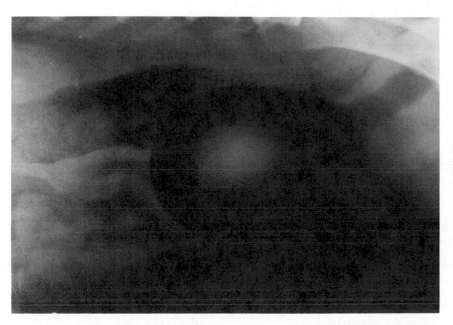

Figure 5. Double-contrast cystogram of the English bulldog described in Figure 4 obtained 10 weeks after initiation of therapy with a purine-restricted diet and allopurinol. There are no uroliths in the bladder lumen.

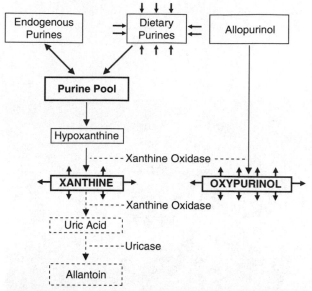

Figure 6. Schematic illustration of purine metabolism in dogs consuming a purine-restricted diet and given allopurinol.

hepatic function (biotransformation of allopurinol to oxypurinol requires adequate hepatic function). Because allopurinol and its metabolites are eliminated from the body primarily by the kidneys, the status of renal function also influences the quantity of allopurinol and its metabolites available to inhibit xanthine oxidase. Because these variables affect the safety and efficacy of allopurinol, studies are needed to evaluate them in normal dogs and dogs that form purine uroliths. Pending results of such studies, xanthine should be suspected as a component of all uroliths obtained from dogs given allopurinol, especially at high doses or for long periods.

To reduce the likelihood of inducing xanthine urolithiasis, simultaneous consumption of purine-rich or purine-supplemented diets and administration of allopurinol should be avoided (Figs. 6 and 7). Foods that contain large quantities of purine precursors include liver, brain, kidneys, intestines, seafood, meat extracts, spinach, beans, lentils, and peas. Foods low in purines include cereals, fruits, most vegetables, milk, and eggs (Pyrah, 1979). Purine-restricted commercial diets are also available (Prescription Diet Canine u/d, Hill's Pet Products). We compared plasma and urine concentrations of uric acid in six normal adult female beagle dogs fed a low-purine diet (Prescription Diet Canine u/d) and a nonrestricted purine diet (Prescription Diet Canine p/d) using a crossover design. Plasma and urine uric acid concentrations were measured by high-pressure liquid chromatography (Felice et al., 1990). Although no statistical differences were noted in plasma concentrations of uric acid during consumption of either diet, the urine concentration of uric acid during consumption of the normal purine diet was three times greater than during consump-

tion of the purine-restricted diet. Differences in urine xanthine concentration were not detected.

Further studies are in progress to evaluate the relationship between allopurinol dosage, dietary purines, and urinary uric acid and xanthine excretion in normal dogs and dogs that form ammonium urate uroliths. The goal is to determine dosages of allopurinol that will reduce urine uric acid concentration sufficiently to promote ammonium urate urolith dissolution while minimizing excessive xanthinuria. Pending results of these studies, prolonged administration of allopurinol at dosages exceeding 15 mg/kg/12 hr should be avoided. Even this dosage may predispose some dogs to xanthine urolithiasis. Initial reduction in the size and number of ammonium urate uroliths in dogs given allopurinol, followed by a period during which uroliths remain refractory to further dissolution, should arouse suspicion that remaining uroliths have been coated with xanthine. In addition, the possibility that new uroliths have formed composed primarily of xanthine should be considered. This suspicion may be verified by analysis of voided uroliths or analysis of urocystoliths retrieved with the aid of a urethral catheter (see this volume, p. 886). On two occasions when we encountered this situation, withdrawal of allopurinol (but not Prescription Diet Canine u/d) for 8 weeks, followed by resumption of allopurinol and continued dietary therapy for 4 additional weeks, resulted in dissolution of remaining uroliths.

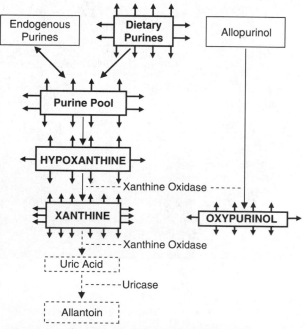

Figure 7. Schematic illustration of hypothesis of purine metabolism in dogs consuming a purine-supplemented diet and given allopurinol.

References and Suggested Reading

Felice, L. J., Dombrovskis, D., Lafond, E., et al.: Determination of uric acid in canine serum and urine by high performance liquid chromatography. Vet. Clin. Pathol. 19:86, 1990.

Foreman, J. W.: Renal handling of urate and other organic acids. *In* Bovée, K. C. (ed.): *Canine Nephrology*. Media: Harwall, 1984, p. 135.

Hande, K. R., Reed, E., and Chabner, B.: Allopurinol kinetics. Clin. Pharmacol. Ther. 23:598, 1978.

Holmes, E. D., and Wyngaarden, J. B.: Hereditary xanthinuria. *In* Scriver et al. (eds.): *The Metabolic Bases Of Inherited Disease*. New York: McGraw-Hill, 1989, p. 1085.

Kidder, D. E., and Chivers, P. R.: Xanthine calculi in a dog. Vet. Rec. 83:228, 1968.

Osborne, C. A., Oldroyd, N. O., and Clinton, C. W.: Etiopathogenesis of uncommon canine uroliths: Xanthine, carbonate, drugs, and drug metabolites. Vet. Clin. North Am. Small Anim. Pract. 16:217, 1986.

Osborne, C. A., Polzin, D. J., Johnston, G. R., et al.: Canine urolithiasis. *In* Ettinger, S. J. (ed.): *Textbook of Veterinary Internal Medicine*, 3rd ed. Vol. 2. Philadelphia: W. B. Saunders, 1989, p. 2083.

O'Sullivan, W. J.: Metabolic side-effects of oxypurinol. *In* Edwards, K. D. G. (ed.): *Drugs and the Kidney*. Progress in Biochemical Pharmacology. New York: S. Karger, 1974, p. 174.

Pyrah, L. N.: Uric acid calculi. *In* Pyrah, L. N. (ed.): *Renal Calculus*. New York: Springer-Verlag, 1979, p. 334.

FELINE METABOLIC UROLITHS: RISK FACTOR MANAGEMENT

CARL A. OSBORNE,
JODY P. LULICH,
JOSEPH W. BARTGES,
and DAVID J. POLZIN

St. Paul, Minnesota

HOW COMMON ARE DIFFERENT TYPES OF FELINE UROLITHS?

Feline uroliths and urethral plugs have physical and probable etiopathogenic differences (Osborne et al., 1989a). Therefore, the terms *uroliths* and *urethral plugs* should not be used as synonyms. Uroliths are polycrystalline concretions composed primarily of minerals (inorganic and organic crystalloids) and small quantities of matrix. In contrast, feline urethral plugs commonly are composed of large quantities of matrix mixed with lesser quantities and types of minerals. This discussion pertains to uroliths, although those portions of the discussion related to different types of minerals (rather than matrix) have application to the crystalline components of urethral plugs.

Although the most commonly encountered type of mineral in feline uroliths has been struvite (Ling et al., 1990; Osborne et al., 1984; Osborne et al., 1989b), in recent years the frequency with which struvite has been identified as the primary mineral in feline uroliths has been declining. As of October, 1990, about 65% of naturally occurring feline uroliths submitted to the University of Minnesota Urolith Center were composed primarily of struvite (Table 1). In 1989, the frequency of naturally occurring feline struvite uroliths was 70% (Osborne et al., 1989b), whereas in 1984, it was 88% (Osborne

et al., 1984). Note that uroliths tabulated in 1990 include those analyzed as part of the 1989 and 1984 reports. The frequency of feline uroliths composed of ammonium urate and uric acid was slightly higher in 1990 (6.3%; see Table 1) than in 1989 (5.6%) (Osborne et al., 1989b) and 1984 (2%) (Osborne et al., 1984). Likewise, the frequency of feline uroliths composed of calcium oxalate rose from 2.4% in 1984 to 10.6% in 1989 and 19.0% in 1990 (see Table 1).

The decline in detection of feline struvite uroliths during the past several years may be explained in part by the widespread use of a calculolytic diet designed to dissolve them and modification of maintenance and prevention diets designed to minimize struvite crystalluria (Osborne et al., 1990). However, data submitted to our urolith laboratory indicate that diets known to be effective in dissolving and preventing struvite uroliths and struvite crystalluria are being inappropriately used in an attempt to manage other types of uroliths. Likewise, it appears that once a protocol for dietary management is selected, follow-up evaluation of efficacy by urinalysis is performed too infrequently.

Causes, detection, and management of feline struvite uroliths have been extensively described elsewhere (Osborne et al., 1989a, 1990). The primary purpose of this article is to summarize available information about feline uroliths, other than those composed primarily of struvite, and to provide recommendations for their management.

URINARY DISORDERS

Table 1. *Mineral Composition of 1800 Feline Uroliths Evaluated by Quantitative Methods*

Predominant Mineral Type		Number of Uroliths	%
Magnesium ammonium phosphate 6H₂O		1170	65.0
	100%	(855)	(47.5)
	70–99%*	(315)	(17.5)
Magnesium hydrogen phosphate 3H₂O		5	0.3
	70–99%*	(5)	(0.3)
Calcium oxalate		345	19.2
Calcium oxalate monohydrate			
	100%	(114)	(6.3)
	70–99%*	(118)	(6.6)
Calcium oxalate dihydrate			
	100%	(28)	(1.6)
	70–99%*	(38)	(2.1)
Calcium oxalate monohydrate and dihydrate			
	100%	(30)	(1.7)
	70–99%*	(17)	(0.9)
Calcium phosphate		40	2.2
Calcium phosphate			
	100%	(16)	(0.9)
	70–99%*	(12)	(0.7)
Calcium hydrogen phosphate 6H₂O			
	100%	(5)	(0.3)
	70–99%*	(5)	(0.3)
Tricalcium phosphate			
	100%	(1)	(0.1)
	70–99%*	(1)	(0.1)
Uric acid and urates		112	6.2
Ammonium acid urate			
	100%	(79)	(4.4)
	70–99%*	(26)	(1.4)
Sodium urate			
	70–99%*	(1)	(0.1)
Uric acid			
	100%	(3)	(0.2)
	70–99%*	(3)	(0.2)
Cystine		2	0.1
Silica		0	0
Mixed†		63	3.5
Compound‡		22	1.2
Matrix		41	2.3
	Total	1800	100%

*Urolith composed of 70–99% of mineral type listed; no nucleus and shell detected.
†Uroliths did not contain at least 70% of mineral type listed; no nucleus or shell detected.
‡Uroliths contained an identifiable nucleus and one or more surrounding layers of a different mineral type.

DIAGNOSIS

Uroliths are usually suspected on the basis of typical findings obtained by history and physical examination. Urinalyses, quantitative urine cultures, radiography, and ultrasonography may be required to differentiate uroliths from other causes of clinical signs such as idiopathic disease, urinary tract infections, and neoplasia.

Most uroliths in cats cannot be detected by abdominal palpation. For example, in one study of 30 urocystoliths in cats, stones were detected by palpation in only three patients (Osborne et al., 1990). Likewise, it is not possible to detect uroliths located in the renal pelves by palpation through the abdominal wall. Therefore, radiographic or ultrasonographic evaluation of the urinary tract is re-quired to consistently detect feline uroliths. In a prospective diagnostic study of feline lower urinary tract disease, radiographic evidence of uroliths was observed in 32 of 143 (22%) cats with hematuria or dysuria (Osborne et al., 1989a).

Medical dissolution of uroliths detected by radiography or ultrasonography poses the problem of formulating therapy without the availability of surgically removed uroliths for analysis. Recommendations to resolve this diagnostic problem are discussed elsewhere (see *CVT X*, p. 1189).

AMMONIUM URATE UROLITHS

Etiopathogenesis

In our feline urolith series, ammonium urate and uric acid accounted for approximately 6% of the total (see Table 1). All were located in the urethra or urinary bladder; five were voided through the urethra. However, ammonium urate and uric acid uroliths have been reported in the kidneys and ureters of cats. In our most recent studies, males were affected (48.6%) about as often as females (45.9%) (the gender of 5.5% was unknown). The mean age of affected cats was 5.5 ± 3 years.

There have been isolated case reports of uric acid and ammonium urate uroliths in cats during the past 20 years (Osborne et al., 1989a). Although a renal tubular reabsorptive defect and portovascular anomalies have been incriminated as causes in a few cases, the cause of formation of most feline urate uroliths has not been established (Osborne et al., 1989). We have not been able to determine the precise cause of feline urate uroliths in our stone series. This problem has been compounded by the difficulty of reproducibly measuring the concentration of uric acid in serum and urine by methods commonly used in clinical laboratories. Nonetheless, formation of highly acidic and highly concentrated urine associated with consumption of diets high in purine precursors (especially liver) appears to be a risk factor in some cases (Kruger and Osborne, 1986).

Management

Medical protocols that consistently promote dissolution of ammonium urate uroliths in cats have not yet been developed. Surgery remains the most reliable method to remove active uroliths from the urinary tract. Prevention should encompass consumption of diets that are low in purine precursors (e.g., low in liver) and that promote formation of less acid urine (pH ± 7) that is not highly concentrated. We induced dissolution of an ammonium urate urocystolith affecting a 3-year-old male castrated domestic short-hair cat with a combination of allopurinol (30 mg/kg/day divided into two equal subdoses) and a diet relatively low in purine precursors (Hill's Prescription Diet Feline k/d). Although allopurinol may be considered to reduce formation of uric acid, additional studies of the

efficacy and potential toxicity of allopurinol in cats are required before meaningful generalities are established. Of particular concern is the potential of inducing xanthine uroliths (see this volume, p. 900).

CALCIUM OXALATE UROLITHS

Etiopathogenesis

In our most recent studies, calcium oxalate uroliths accounted for approximately 19% of the total (see Table 1). They were detected in the kidneys, ureters, urinary bladder, or urethra. Nine calcium oxalate uroliths were voided through the urethra. Calcium oxalate was the most common mineral identified in feline nephroliths submitted to our laboratory (Table 2). In our series, males were more commonly affected (55%) than females (42%). The gender of 3% of the cats with calcium oxalate uroliths was not specified. The mean age of affected cats was 6.7 ± 3.4 years.

The underlying causes of naturally occurring feline calcium oxalate uroliths are unknown. Detectable hypercalcemia has not been common, although available pretreatment data are scanty. The mean pretreatment serum calcium concentrations of eight affected cats evaluated at our Veterinary Teaching Hospital was 10.4 ± 1.3 mg/dl. Affected cats typically had concentrated urine (mean pretreatment urine specific gravity of eight affected cats was 1.038 ± 0.015). The urine of eight affected cats was acid (mean pH = 6.4 ± 0.3). Mean pretreatment blood pH was 7.3 ± 0.1; mean blood bicarbonate concentration was 18.7 ± 2.2 mEq/L.

Although experimentally induced vitamin B_6 deficiency resulted in oxalate nephrocalcinosis in kittens (Osborne et al., 1989a), a naturally occurring form of this syndrome has not been observed. It is noteworthy that magnesium has been reported to be a calcium oxalate crystallization inhibitor in rats and humans. For this reason, orally administered magnesium sometimes is recommended to prevent recurrence of calcium oxalate uroliths. It also is of interest that use of urine acidifiers or supplemental

Table 2. *Mineral Composition of 62 Nephroliths Evaluated by Quantitative Methods*

Composition of Nephrolith		Number of Nephroliths	%
Magnesium ammonium phosphate 6H$_2$O	70–99%*	5	8.1
Calcium phosphate	70–99%	11	17.7
Tricalcium phosphate	70–99%	1	1.6
Calcium oxalate	70–99%	18	29.0
Mixed†		10	16.1
Matrix		17	27.4

*Urolith composed of 70–99% of mineral type listed; no nucleus and shell detected.
†Uroliths did not contain at least 70% of one mineral type; no nucleus or shell detected.

sodium (usually sodium chloride) or both has been associated with hypercalciuria in some species. Because therapy of feline sterile struvite uroliths often encompasses restriction of magnesium, sodium chloride-induced diuresis, and acidification of urine, the relationship of these factors to feline calcium oxalate uroliths deserves further study.

Management

Medical protocols that will promote dissolution of calcium oxalate uroliths in cats are not available as yet. Surgery remains the only alternative for removal of clinically active calcium oxalate uroliths. However, some calcium oxalate uroliths, especially those located in the kidneys, may remain clinically silent for months to years. Because of the unavoidable destruction of nephrons during nephrotomy, this procedure is not recommended unless it can be established that the stones are a cause of clinically significant disease. Serially performed urinalyses, renal function tests, serum electrolyte evaluations, or radiographic studies may be indicated to evaluate the clinical activity of calcium oxalate uroliths.

No controlled studies designed to evaluate the efficacy of protocols for calcium oxalate urolith prevention have been reported. Procedures recommended for prevention of calcium oxalate uroliths in dogs therefore should be considered (see this volume, p. 892). Pending further studies, we recommend consumption of nonacidifying, protein-restricted, and sodium-restricted diets (e.g., Hill's Prescription Diet Feline k/d). Recommendations pertaining to the relationship of dietary magnesium to management of feline calcium oxalate uroliths must await further study.

CALCIUM PHOSPHATE UROLITHS

Etiopathogenesis

In our current series, calcium phosphate accounted for 2.2% of naturally occurring feline uroliths. They were located in the kidneys (n = 12), urinary bladder (n = 21), and urinary bladder and urethra (n = 1) (the location of uroliths removed from six patients was not recorded). As was the situation with nephroliths composed of calcium oxalate, calcium phosphate nephroliths were more commonly encountered than struvite nephroliths (see Table 2). Calcium phosphate uroliths affected 14 males and 20 females (the gender of 6 affected patients was not recorded). The mean age of affected cats was 8.8 ± 2.9 years.

We have documented nephroliths composed of blood clots mineralized with calcium phosphate. Such mineralized blood clots may be found in renal pelvic diverticula in addition to the renal pelvis. Formation of highly concentrated urine in patients with gross hematuria may favor formation of blood clots. In one persistently hematuric patient, such nephroliths remained inactive (did not increase in number or size, or cause outflow obstruction, or predispose to bacterial urinary tract infection) during a 3-year period of evaluation.

Although calcium phosphate uroliths may occur in association with primary hyperparathyroidism in humans and dogs, this association has not been noted in cats. One 3-year-old male castrated domestic short-hair cat with multiple calcium hydrogen phosphate (brushite) urocystoliths and urethroliths consumed large quantities of spinach, according to the owner. Spinach contains large quantities of oxalate salts.

Management

Protocols designed to dissolve or prevent calcium phosphate uroliths in cats have not been studied. Surgery is the most reliable way to remove active uroliths from the urinary tract. We emphasize that surgery may be unnecessary for clinically inactive calcium phosphate uroliths. Based on results of studies in other species, avoiding excessive dietary protein and sodium may minimize hypercalciuria (see this volume, p. 892).

OTHER UROLITHS

We have encountered two urocystoliths composed of cystine (see Table 1). One was removed from a 6-year-old male Korat, and the other was removed from a 3-year-old spayed female domestic short-hair cat. Neither patient was available for further diagnostic evaluation.

Compound uroliths (nucleus composed of one mineral type and shells of a different mineral type) accounted for approximately 1% of uroliths analyzed in our series (see Table 1). Examples include a nucleus of 100% calcium oxalate monohydrate surrounded by a shell of 80% magnesium ammonium phosphate and 20% calcium phosphate; and a nucleus composed of 95% magnesium ammonium phosphate and 5% calcium phosphate surrounded by a shell of 95% ammonium acid urate and 5% magnesium ammonium phosphate. Sulfadiazine composed 30% of the shell of one compound urocystolith removed from a 7-year-old female domestic short-hair cat. Because risk factors that predispose to precipitation (nucleation) of different minerals vary, the development of compound uroliths poses a unique challenge in terms of prevention of recurrence. In absence of clinical evidence to the contrary, it seems logical to recommend management protocols designed primarily to minimize recurrence of nucleation of minerals composing the nucleus (rather than those in shells) of compound uroliths. Follow-up studies designed to evaluate efficacy of preventive protocols should include complete urinalyses, radiography, and, if available, evaluation of the urine concentrations of calculogenic metabolites.

References and Suggested Reading

Kruger, J. M., and Osborne, C. A.: Etiopathogenesis of uric acid and ammonium urate uroliths in nondalmatian dogs. Vet. Clin. North Am. Small Anim. Pract. 16:87, 1986.

Ling, G. V., Franti, C. E., Ruby, A. L., et al.: Epizootic evaluation and quantitative analysis of urinary calculi from 150 cats. J.A.V.M.A. 196:1459, 1990.

Osborne, C. A., Clinton, C. W., Brunkow, H. C., et al.: Epidemiology of naturally occurring feline uroliths and urethral plugs. Vet. Clin. North Am. Small Anim. Pract. 14:481, 1984.

Osborne, C. A., Kruger, J. M., Johnston, G. R., et al.: Feline lower urinary tract disorders. In Ettinger, S. J. (ed.): Textbook of Veterinary Internal Medicine, 3rd ed. Vol. 2. Philadelphia: W. B. Saunders, 1989a, pp. 2063–2069.

Osborne, C. A., Lulich, J. P., Kruger, J. M., et al.: Medical dissolution of feline struvite urocystoliths: Prospective clinical study of 30 cases. J.A.V.M.A. 196:1053, 1990.

Osborne, C. A., Sanna, J. J., Unger, L. K., et al.: Mineral composition of 4500 uroliths from dogs, cats, horses, cattle, sheep, goats, and pigs. Vet. Med. 84:750, 1989b.

UPDATE: BACTERIAL URINARY TRACT INFECTIONS

GEORGE E. LEES

College Station, Texas

and S. DRU FORRESTER

Blacksburg, Virginia

Urinary tract infection (UTI) is microbial colonization of any portion of the urinary system that is normally sterile. The great majority of urinary infections are caused by aerobic bacteria; therefore, this discussion focuses on bacterial UTI. Treatment of fungal UTI is described in the next article.

Methods for diagnosis and treatment of UTI have changed little in recent years. Consequently, several detailed discussions of these topics in previous volumes of *Current Veterinary Therapy* remain relevant. Some basic principles are repeated here for emphasis (see *CVT IX*, p. 1118, for a more complete review of diagnosis and localization of UTI; see *CVT X*, p. 1204, for principles of antimicrobial therapy for UTI).

Recent developments in the management of UTI in dogs and cats have had two main themes. First, the inherent difficulty of accurately localizing UTIs has led to increased emphasis on careful monitoring of response to therapy as a means of assuring appropriate treatment. Second, development and introduction of new antibacterial products have added to the pharmaceutical armamentarium available for treating UTI.

CLINICAL DIVERSITY OF URINARY TRACT INFECTION

In dogs, UTI is a common clinical problem that can be manifested in various ways. Although UTI is less common in cats than in dogs, UTI nonetheless is a diverse and sometimes troublesome problem in cats. Existence of UTI may be suspected because of clinical signs (e.g., pollakiuria, dysuria, visibly abnormal urine), laboratory abnormalities (e.g., hematuria, pyuria), or diagnosis of other urinary disorders (e.g., urolithiasis, abnormal micturition). However, a definitive diagnosis of UTI is established by a positive urine culture. Demonstrating abundant bacteria in a urine specimen that was obtained and processed with care to preclude extraurinary sources of bacteria in such abundance proves existence of UTI.

Labeling patients with positive urine culture results as having UTI is accurate, but using this diagnostic designation alone places all affected patients in a single group. Numerous factors operate to make instances of UTI substantially different from one another in different patients and sometimes at different times in the same patient. Such factors influence the course of disease and response to treatment; therefore, accurate prognosis, effective therapy, and appropriate follow-up depend on diagnostic subcategorization of patients with UTI according to these factors.

Infecting Organisms

Seven genera of bacteria (*Escherichia, Staphylococcus, Streptococcus, Proteus, Klebsiella, Pseudomonas,* and *Enterobacter*) account for most episodes of UTI in dogs and cats. Most episodes of UTI are caused by a single strain of bacteria, but dual infections account for about one fifth of all episodes. Pathogenesis of disease caused by UTI can be influenced by traits of the infecting organisms. For example, when bacteria that produce urease (e.g., staphylococci and *Proteus*) cause UTI, formation of uroliths composed of magnesium ammonium phosphate (struvite) may occur as a complication of infection.

With respect to treatment of UTI, important traits of infecting organisms are those that govern susceptibility to antimicrobial agents. Bacterial susceptibility or resistance to antibiotics is influenced by inherent as well as acquired traits. Because of inherent traits, the antimicrobial drug susceptibility of certain organisms is highly predictable. Bacteria also can acquire resistance to antimicrobial drugs because of antibiotic therapy. When animals with UTI have been given antibiotics for any reason in recent months, the infecting organisms are more likely to be resistant to antimicrobial drugs.

Anatomic Extent of Infection

In animals with UTI, extent of infection within the urinary tract is one of the most influential factors affecting biologic behavior of the condition and its response to treatment. Most episodes of UTI are caused by ascending colonization of the tract from more distal sites. That is, the proximal part of the urethra and the urinary bladder usually become infected with bacteria from the distal urethra or epithelial surfaces surrounding the external urethral orifice. The usual source of bacteria that cause infections of the ureters, renal pelves, or renal parenchyma is the urinary bladder. In noncastrated males with UTI, bacterial colonization of prostatic parenchyma probably occurs routinely.

At any site in the urinary tract, extent of infection also can vary with respect to depth of tissue involvement. Ascending UTI not only works its way up the tract through the urinary space but extends out from the urinary space into surrounding tissues.

Bacteria in the urine generally must adhere to the epithelial lining of the urinary space to successfully colonize a portion of the urinary tract. Some infections may remain superficial (i.e., involving only the urinary space and uroepithelial surface), whereas others penetrate the mucosa to involve the submucosa and possibly deeper tissues. When bacteria or their products penetrate to tissues containing vessels and nerves (i.e., beneath the uroepithelial surface), inflammation and discomfort are induced in various degrees. Depending on the severity of associated pain and inflammation, normal functions of the affected portions of the urinary tract may be impaired.

Extent of infection has great influence on manifestations of UTI and on response to treatment. Because manifestations of UTI are produced mainly by infection-induced inflammation, variations in clinical signs and laboratory abnormalities produced by UTI in different patients are attributable mainly to differences in the distribution and depth of inflammation due to infection. However, variations in extent of infection in different patients are not reflected by detectable manifestations with sufficient consistency to permit accurate localization of UTI using criteria based on clinical signs and diagnostic test results. In addition, noninfectious diseases of the urinary tract often mimic UTI by causing many of the same clinical and laboratory manifestations (e.g., signs of inflammation), which further confounds diagnosis. Nonetheless, few factors influence response to treatment of UTI more than does extent of infection. For example, superficial infection of the mucosa of the urinary bladder may be so easily cured that a single dose of an appropriate drug will be effective, whereas an infection that extends into the medullary portions of the kidneys may be impossible to cure even with administration of an appropriate drug for a protracted period.

Extent of infection and of infection-induced alterations in urinary tract tissues also influences the rate at which the normal mechanisms that defend the urinary system against infection are restored. Duration of treatment for UTI must not only be long enough to eradicate bacteria from the urinary tract; it must prevent reinfection until normal defenses have recovered sufficiently to meet this goal. Chronic infections often induce tissue changes that subside more slowly than those caused by acute infections; therefore, duration of treatment usually must be extended for chronic UTI.

Concomitant Urinary Abnormalities

A healthy urinary tract is quite difficult to infect with bacteria, and UTI is fundamentally an opportunistic type of infection. Organisms ordinarily succeed in colonizing the urinary tract only when normal host defenses against infection are impaired for some reason. Thus, integrity of host defenses must be questioned and possible existence of other disorders that predispose to infection must be considered whenever UTI is discovered.

In dogs (but very rarely in cats), UTI sometimes occurs as the initial and only demonstrable cause of urinary disease in affected patients. That is, UTI develops in an otherwise healthy subject, nothing besides UTI can be found to be wrong with the subject, appropriate antimicrobial therapy returns the subject to normal, and the subject remains healthy after treatment is stopped. Such episodes of UTI are labeled as simple (i.e., uncomplicated). An undetected and transient impairment of host defenses presumably permitted UTI to develop, but an identifiable underlying urinary disease predisposing to development of UTI does not exist. Production of lasting cure by antibacterial therapy alone is an important hallmark of uncomplicated episodes of UTI.

In dogs and cats, development of UTI often complicates other urinary tract disorders because such disorders commonly impair defenses against UTI. Virtually all other urinary diseases can predispose to development of UTI, but common examples include urolithiasis, urinary tract obstruction, renal failure, urinary catheterization, neoplasia, developmental anomalies, urethral incompetence, neurogenic disorders of micturition, and prostatic diseases. Episodes of UTI associated with additional urinary abnormalities such as these are labeled as complicated. The crucial concept for management of complicated UTI is that antimicrobial treatment of the infection must be coupled with correction of the underlying abnormality to obtain lasting cure and sometimes even to obtain favorable initial results. Of course, some abnormalities that predispose to UTI cannot be corrected, and management must focus on rational strategies to prevent UTI or minimize its effects in affected patients.

DIAGNOSTIC EVALUATION

To provide a basis for planning effective therapy, diagnostic evaluation of animals with UTI must assess each of the major factors producing clinical diversity among episodes of UTI. Infecting organisms should be identified and characterized, especially regarding their susceptibility to antimicrobial drugs. The probable anatomic extent of infection should be appraised, and presence of underlying abnormalities predisposing to UTI should be considered.

Bacteria causing UTI are isolated, identified, and characterized by performing urine cultures. Methods of urine collection, specimen storage, laboratory processing, and susceptibility testing are important considerations bearing on proper interpretation and application of urine culture results. Detailed recommendations for performing and interpreting urine cultures are provided elsewhere (see *CVT IX*, p. 1118). Antimicrobial drug susceptibility testing should use minimum inhibitory concentration (MIC) values determined *in vitro* for comparison with expected urine concentrations of drug during treatment (see *CVT X*, p. 1204).

Accurate localization of UTI (identification of the anatomic extent of infection) is an elusive goal. Uncomplicated episodes of UTI usually are localized on the basis of clinical signs, urinalysis findings, and sometimes survey abdominal radiographs; however, localization based on such evidence often is incorrect. Sublumbar pain, fever, leukocytosis, leukocyte casts in the urine, or an abnormal radiographic renal silhouette can indicate pyelonephritis in an animal with UTI, but these criteria may yield false-positive and false-negative conclusions. When pollakiuria, dysuria, or strangury accompanies UTI, involvement of the urinary bladder (cystitis) or urethra (urethritis) is suspected. Because cystitis and urethritis seem clinically inseparable, *urethrocystitis* probably is a more accurate term to use when these abnormal patterns of micturition are displayed by animals with UTI.

Many dogs and cats with UTI do not exhibit any clinical signs referable to UTI. Such animals are said to have subclinical UTI; however, lack of clinical signs should not lessen concern about the importance of the infection to the animal's health. Animals with subclinical bacteriuria are presumed to have bladder infections, but other portions of the urinary tract might or might not be involved as well. Data regarding the prevalence of various possible distributions of infection in dogs and cats with subclinical UTI are not available.

Episodes of complicated UTI are subclassified according to the nature of the underlying disease. Knowledge of an associated condition that justifies diagnosis of complicated UTI when the infection is first discovered can arise in many ways. A thorough history and careful physical examination coupled with routine diagnostic testing (e.g., hemogram, urinalysis, and serum chemistry profile) often provide compelling or highly suggestive evidence of the problem. Appropriate steps for further diagnostic investigation generally are defined by the nature of the suspected disease. Discovery that an episode of UTI is complicated becomes more problematic when the previously mentioned methods of investigation fail to indicate existence of underlying disease. Evaluation of survey abdominal radiographs is a noninvasive, relatively inexpensive, and fairly sensitive way to screen for undetected urolithiasis, and other important abnormalities are found occasionally. Mature, noncastrated males with UTI should be presumed to have prostatic infection as well, and a careful search for any complicating prostatic disease (e.g., hypertrophy, abscess, cyst, tumor) often is indicated for such patients.

Unless UTI is a recurrent problem, invasive diagnostic testing such as contrast radiography is unwarranted. Animals that seem to have uncomplicated UTI should be treated accordingly, and their response to treatment should be carefully defined, preferably using urine culture results but at least using urinalysis findings. Because of the prevalence of subclinical UTI, relying entirely on clinical signs to indicate treatment outcome is not recommended. Animals with uncomplicated UTI, if properly classified and treated, will have rapid eradication of bacteriuria, prompt and complete resolution of their clinical and laboratory abnormalities, and lasting cure of their infections. Animals that are misclassified or improperly treated will be troubled by recurrent UTI, which should be detected promptly by appropriate follow-up evaluation.

In animals with recurrent UTI, the pattern of bacteriuria that emerges as response to treatment is monitored also gives clear indications of the most likely source of diagnostic or therapeutic error. Indeed, post-treatment evaluations are more cost-effective and probably more accurate than extensive pretreatment testing, especially when initial historical and physical examination findings seem innocuous. When UTI is recurrent, one of three outcomes of treatment will emerge, each one having its own special implications. *Persistence* of original bacteriuria during treatment indicates incorrect drug therapy. If the prescribed drug was given correctly (proper dose and treatment schedule), persistence means that the pathogens are resistant to the chosen drug and that antimicrobial drug susceptibility test results should be used to select a more appropriate drug to administer. *Relapse* is identified by finding that bacteriuria resolves during drug treatment and then rapidly (within 2 weeks) reappears after treatment stops. Relapse indicates recrudescence of the original infection, which was suppressed but not eradicated by treatment, and organisms recovered from follow-up cultures always are the same bacterial strain that was cultured before treatment. Relapse of UTI generally means that duration of antimicrobial drug therapy was insufficient; eradication of bacteriuria during treatment is reliable evidence that the bacteria were intrinsically susceptible to the chosen drug. Usual causes of relapse are penetration of the infection into the renal or prostatic parenchyma and forms of complicated UTI that provide a nidus of infection where antimicrobial drugs cannot penetrate (e.g., infected urolith, abscess). Unless previous diagnostic studies have excluded it, the possibility of complicated UTI should be investigated when relapse is observed. Finally, *reinfection* is identified by finding a new type of bacteriuria (i.e., different bacteria) after treatment of an episode of UTI. Entirely satisfactory choices of drug, dosage, and duration of treatment for previous episodes of UTI are indicated by cure of those infections, but a new UTI developed. Unusually frequent reinfection means that the animal has an abnormal predisposition to developing UTI, and a search should be conducted for conditions that might impair normal defenses against UTI, especially abnormalities of the bladder or urethra or immunosuppressive diseases.

Regardless of other considerations, complicated UTI should be suspected and thoroughly investigated when bacteriuria is eradicated by antimicrobial drug treatment while evidence of urinary disease (e.g., clinical signs, abnormal urinalysis findings) fails to resolve completely during therapy. Treatment of UTI complicating another urinary tract disease often substantially improves the patient's clinical condition at least temporarily. Nonetheless, an astute clinician in this instance should be concerned by persistence of abnormalities even if they are subtle (e.g., occult hematuria) rather than being reassured by the clinical or laboratory improvements that are attained.

ANTIMICROBIAL THERAPY

Patients with UTI can be properly treated by following the seven steps outlined in Table 1. Therapeutic efficacy depends on maintaining adequate urine concentration of an antimicrobial drug; therefore, agents that are most useful in treating UTI are excreted in their active form by the kidneys. A rational first choice of antibiotic often can be based on knowledge of the identity of the infecting organisms because susceptibility of common pathogens to certain antimicrobial drugs is highly predictable (Table 2). Results of *in vitro* susceptibility tests are most useful when antimicrobial therapy must be selected for organisms with unpredictable susceptibility, including pathogens causing complicated infections and those found in patients previously treated with antimicrobial drugs. Antimicrobial drug susceptibility testing based on determination

Table 1. *Seven Steps in Treatment of Urinary Tract Infection*

1. Select appropriate candidates for treatment.
2. Select an appropriate antimicrobial drug.
3. Select an appropriate dosing regimen.
4. Select an appropriate duration of treatment.
5. Select appropriate ancillary treatment, when needed.
6. Perform appropriate follow-up evaluations.
7. Select appropriate prophylactic or suppressive treatment, when needed.

Table 2. *Drugs Recommended for Treating Uncomplicated Urinary Tract Infection Based on Identity of the Pathogens*

	Susceptibility	
Organism	Approaching 100%	Approximately 80%
Escherichia		Trimethoprim-sulfa
Staphylococcus	Ampicillin	
Proteus		Ampicillin
Streptococcus	Ampicillin	
Klebsiella		Cephalexin
Pseudomonas		Tetracycline
Enterobacter		Trimethoprim-sulfa

of MIC values is preferred. A drug is highly likely to be effective for treatment of UTI when the MIC for the infecting organisms is one fourth or less of the average concentration of drug expected in the urine during therapy.

Ampicillin, trimethoprim-sulfa, cephalexin, and tetracycline have been well-established mainstays for treatment of UTI in dogs and cats for more than a decade. Recommendations (Table 3) for using these drugs were promulgated primarily by Ling (1986) initially, but they have been reiterated many times subsequently (see *CVT X*, p. 1204). These recommendations have stood the test of time and continue to be appropriate because they are safe, effective, and economical. Rather than replacing or superseding available drugs, newly developed antimicrobial drugs with efficacy for treating UTI mainly have just increased treatment options. Having more drug choices, however, is valuable when treating more resistant infections and for treating patients that develop adverse reactions to certain drugs.

Two new classes of drugs have found prominent roles in the management of UTI. The first of these are products in which a compound that inhibits beta-lactamase activity is mixed with a beta-lactam antibiotic (Kilgore, 1989). A combination of amoxicillin trihydrate and clavulanate potassium is the most widely used veterinary product of this class.

Inclusion of the beta-lactamase inhibitor (clavulanic acid) increases the chances that some common urinary pathogens will be more susceptible to the combination compared with amoxicillin alone. Most importantly, the high likelihood that UTI caused by *Escherichia coli* is susceptible to amoxicillin-clavulanic acid makes this combination a reasonable alternative to using trimethoprim-sulfa, especially when there is concern about adverse effects caused by trimethoprim-sulfa products. Particularly with prolonged or repeated use, administration of trimethoprim-sulfa combinations may lead to keratoconjunctivitis sicca, immune-mediated polyarthritis or vasculitis, and possibly nonregenerative anemia. In contrast, amoxicillin–clavulanic acid is unlikely to produce adverse effects except in the rare animals that are allergic to penicillin. For treatment of susceptible UTI in noncastrated males, however, trimethoprim-sulfa has the advantage of better penetration into prostatic fluid.

The second important new class of drugs with efficacy in treatment of UTI is the fluoroquinolones (Neer, 1988). Enrofloxacin is the fluoroquinolone most widely used by veterinarians, but use of norfloxacin (Budsberg et al., 1989) and ciprofloxacin (Aucoin et al., 1990) has been reported as well. Fluoroquinolones are bactericidal antimicrobial agents that have a wide margin of safety and a broad spectrum of activity, particularly for common urinary pathogens. Bacteria that are resistant to numerous other drugs often are susceptible to fluoroquinolones. Besides attaining high urinary drug concentrations, fluoroquinolones may penetrate prostatic fluid. For these reasons and because they can be given orally, fluoroquinolones often are especially useful for treating UTI that is difficult to treat otherwise.

Treatment for 7 to 10 days cures most episodes of acute uncomplicated bacterial urethrocystitis. Chronic but otherwise uncomplicated bladder infections may require treatment for 14 to 21 days or occasionally longer to permit pathologic changes in urinary tract tissues to subside completely. Most episodes of pyelonephritis that are diagnosed in dogs and cats are chronic conditions, and they often are complicated infections. Therefore, pyelonephri-

Table 3. *Guidelines for Antimicrobial Therapy of Urinary Tract Infection*

Drug	Suggested MIC Cutoff for Susceptibility	Recommended Treatment Regimen	
		Dosage	Frequency
Ampicillin	≤ 64 µg/ml	25 mg/kg	q 8 hr
Trimethoprim-sulfa	≤ 16 µg/ml	15 mg/kg	q 12 hr
Cephalexin	≤ 32 µg/ml	18 mg/kg	q 8 hr
Tetracycline	≤ 32 µg/ml	18 mg/kg	q 8 hr
Amoxicillin with clavulanic acid	≤ 32 µg/ml	16.5 mg/kg	q 8 hr
Enrofloxacin	≤ 8 µg/ml	2.5 mg/kg	q 12 hr

tis usually should be treated for 4 to 6 weeks. The appropriate duration of treatment for complicated UTI, however, is greatly influenced by the time course and efficacy of treatment to correct the underlying urinary abnormality. Treatment of UTI combined with other therapeutic strategies to produce dissolution of uroliths, for example, must continue until all calculi have completely dissolved—a process that often requires several months. Episodes of UTI in noncastrated males should be treated for at least a month because of the high probability of prostatic colonization.

References and Suggested Reading

Aucoin, D. P., Hardie, L., Cohn, L., et al.: Clinical study of ciprofloxacin in 67 canine patients with multiresistant bacterial infections (abstract). ACVIM Scientific Proceedings, 1990, p. 1112.
A brief report of frequently successful use of ciprofloxacin to treat dogs with multiresistant bacterial infections in organ systems that were unstated but probably included instances of UTI.
Budsberg, S. C., Walker, R. D., Slusser, P., et al.: Norfloxacin therapy in infections of the canine urogenital tract caused by multiresistant bacteria. J. Am. Anim. Hosp. Assoc. 25:713, 1989.
A report of successful use of norfloxacin to treat six dogs with UTI, including two dogs with concomitant prostatic infections, due to multiresistant pathogens.
Kilgore, R. W.: Clavulanate-potentiated antibiotics. In Kirk, R. W. (ed.): *Current Veterinary Therapy X.* Philadelphia: W. B. Saunders, 1989, pp. 78–81.
A general review of the use of clavulanic acid to improve the antimicrobial activity of the beta-lactam antibiotics amoxicillin and ticarcillin.
Ling, G. V.: Management of urinary tract infections. In Kirk, R. W. (ed.): *Current Veterinary Therapy IX.* Philadelphia: W. B. Saunders, 1986, pp. 1174–1177.
A review of diagnosis and treatment of urinary tract infections in dogs and cats.
Neer, T. M.: Clinical pharmacologic features of fluoroquinolone antimicrobial drugs. J.A.V.M.A. 193:577, 1988.
A general review providing fundamental information about fluoroquinolones for individuals who are unfamiliar with this class of antimicrobial drugs.

FUNGAL URINARY TRACT INFECTIONS

JODY P. LULICH
and CARL A. OSBORNE
Saint Paul, Minnesota

DEFINITIONS

Bacteriuria and its clinical implications are well known. The implications of funguria are less well understood because they have been less extensively studied. Of the myriad fungi present in nature, only a few are known to be pathogenic for animals, and many of these cause infection only under conditions of impaired cellular immunity or disruption of local host defenses.

PREVALENCE

Fungal infections of the urinary tract have been uncommonly recognized in dogs and cats (Wooley and Blue, 1976). Their rarity may be partly because of the infrequency with which fungi have been considered as urinary tract pathogens. Because bacteria are commonly associated with urinary tract disorders, fungal cultures are often overlooked. Suspicions of funguria may be assuaged by the insensitivity of urine sediment analysis in detection of yeast or hyphae. Likewise, the inconspicuous nature of asymptomatic fungal urinary tract infections (UTIs) may dampen efforts to detect fungi in patients with predisposing illnesses. As a result, the true incidence of fungal urinary tract infections may be higher than reported.

Candida albicans appears to be the most commonly recognized urinary fungal pathogen. In one study of 851 canine urine cultures, five of six fungal isolates were *C. albicans* (Wooley and Blue, 1976). *Candida, Torulopsis, Cryptococcus,* and *Blastomyces* species have been most commonly identified in our hospital. However, urinary invasions by *Trichosporon, Aspergillus,* and *Histoplasma* species have also been reported (Clinkenbeard et al., 1989; Doster et al., 1987; Neer, 1988).

PATHOGENESIS

Fungal UTIs are often associated with impaired systemic or local host defenses (Ehrensaft et al., 1979). Phagocytosis of fungi by neutrophils is an important defense against fungal colonization. Immune inadequacies may account for increased susceptibility of patients receiving corticosteroids or cytotoxic chemotherapy, as well as those with diabetes mellitus or leukopenia (Table 1).

Candida and *Torulopsis* are normal saprophytic inhabitants of the gastrointestinal tract of dogs and cats (Greene and Chandler, 1990). Because *Candida* and *Torulopsis* are rarely found in soil or plants, the majority of infections caused by *Candida* and *Torulopsis* are considered to originate from a patient's indigenous flora. The commensal relationship between bacteria and fungi in the gastrointestinal tract minimizes excessive proliferation of either microorganism. However, by reducing intestinal bacterial numbers, antibiotic administration may increase the quantity of intestinal fungi and thus enhance the likelihood of their dissemination to the urinary tract.

Altered local host defenses of the urinary tract are also important in the development of funguria. Glucosuria, indwelling urinary catheters, urethrostomy, and urolithiasis have been associated with fungal UTI of dogs and cats admitted to our hospital.

DIAGNOSIS

The diagnosis of funguria is based on results of urinalyses and urine cultures. Because several fungal species commensally inhabit several organ systems and may transiently affect the urinary tract, laboratory findings must be interpreted in association with clinical findings.

Clinical Syndromes

ASYMPTOMATIC FUNGURIA. Fungi are not found in the urine of healthy animals. Therefore, fungi identified in properly collected urine samples should be considered as pathogens. In fact, unexplained funguria should prompt evaluation of a patient's local and systemic host defenses (see Table 1). Although asymptomatic funguria may spontaneously resolve if predisposing risk factors are eliminated, symptomatic infections or bezoar (fungal ball) formation may also develop.

SYMPTOMATIC FUNGURIA. Symptomatic fungal UTI may be associated with signs of urethrocystitis, pyelonephritis, and septicemia. Clinical signs of urethrocystitis and pyelonephritis are similar to those observed with bacterial urethrocystitis and pyelonephritis with the exception of potential bezoar formation. In patients with poorly controlled diabetes mellitus, pneumaturia may occur, reflecting fungal fermentation of glucose in urine.

BEZOAR FORMATION. Bezoars (fungal balls) are clusters of intertwined fungal hyphae, which may further aggregate to form even larger bezoars. In humans, bezoars have ranged from 1 mm to 10 cm in diameter. Most yeastlike fungi (e.g., *Torulopsis* and *Cryptococcus*) lack the ability to form bezoars because they do not form hyphae. However, in addition to forming budding yeasts, *Candida* also forms elongated filamentous structures (pseudohyphae) capable of coalescing into bezoars. Other fungi

Table 1. Risk Factors That May Predispose to Funguria

Risk Factor	Human	Dog	Cat
Impaired cell-mediated immunity			
Leukopenia	+	+	?
Defective granulocyte function	+	+	?
Cytotoxic and immunosuppressive therapy (corticosteroids, cyclophosphamide)	+	+	?
Some diseases impairing cell-mediated immunity			
Feline leukemia virus infection	−	−	?
Feline immunodeficiency virus infection	−	−	?
Hyperadrenocorticism	+	?	?
Hypothyroidism	+	?	?
Diabetes mellitus	+	+	+
Increased numbers of commensal fungi			
Antibacterial therapy	+	+	+
Defects of urinary tract			
Structural abnormalities			
Urogenital fistula	+	?	?
Urorectal fistula	+	?	?
Urethrotomy	?	?	?
Urethrostomy	?	+	?
Nephrostomy	+	?	?
Foreign material in urinary tract			
Catheters	+	+	?
Stents	+	?	?
Uroliths	+	+	+
Blood clots	+	?	?
Urine stasis/obstruction	+	+	+
Renal transplant	+	?	?

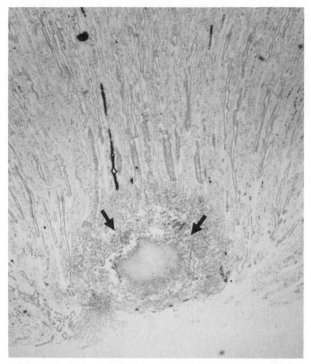

Figure 1. Bezoar (fungal ball) of *Cephalosporium* organisms (*arrows*) in the pelvis of a feline kidney. The cat had diabetes mellitus. (Hematoxylin and eosin stain; original magnification × 4.)

capable of forming hyphae also have potential for bezoar formation (Fig. 1).

Bezoars may be present in patients with asymptomatic or symptomatic fungal UTI and are analogous to infected uroliths. They are sources of persistent funguria and potential fungemia and may obstruct urine flow. Therefore, acute onset of abdominal pain, oliguria, or anuria in patients with funguria may result from bezoar formation. If these signs develop, intravenous urography or other diagnostic imaging should be considered to rule out this possibility. Small bezoars may pass spontaneously; however, larger bezoars may require mechanical disruption or surgical removal.

Urinalysis

Examination of urine sediment facilitates a diagnosis of fungal UTI. Budding yeasts or elongated hyphae are typically observed. Yeasts may be difficult to distinguish from red blood cells in urine. Yeasts can be identified by their oval shape, lack of color, variable size, budding growth, and failure to stain with eosin. Gram's stain and new methylene blue can be used to highlight their appearance.

In past years, yeasts identified in urine sediment have been commonly considered to be contaminants. However, clinically significant funguria

should be considered in patients with fungal organisms observed in serial urinalyses, with risk factors predisposing to fungal UTI (see Table 1), or with bacteriologically "sterile" pyuria.

In addition to fungal organisms, white blood cells and red blood cells may be observed in urine sediment. Pyuria may occur in patients with asymptomatic or symptomatic fungal UTI. Absence of pyuria is not synonymous with nonpathogenic fungi; fatal renal candidiasis has been observed in the absence of pyuria in humans (Dreetz and Fetchick, 1988). In this situation, lack of pyuria may have been associated with impaired immune defenses.

Urine Culture

A definitive diagnosis of fungal UTI must be based on results of urine culture. Most common fungal culture media, including Sabouraud's dextrose agar, are satisfactory for fungal isolation; however, media that contain cycloheximide inhibit growth of some fungal species.

Unlike bacteriuria, the clinical significance of funguria in humans could not be reliably predicted by counting the number of colony-forming units per milliliter of urine. Although significant bacteriuria is often defined as more than 10^5 colony-forming units per milliliter of urine, fewer than 10^5 fungal organisms per milliliter of urine are commonly observed in human patients with clinically significant fungal infections. Because the appearance of fungal organisms is abnormal in properly collected and processed urine samples, funguria should be initially regarded as pathologic, regardless of colony count; however, demonstration of fungal tissue invasion remains the standard by which pathogenic colonization cannot be disputed (Figs. 2 and 3). Because several fungi normally inhabit the genital and gastrointestinal tracts of animals, cystocentesis facilitates differentiation of true fungal UTI from genital or fecal contaminants. Isolation and growth of fungal organisms from two properly collected serial urine specimens should be considered as significant.

PROGNOSIS

The prognosis for asymptomatic funguria in dogs and cats is not known. In humans, asymptomatic fungal UTIs may resolve spontaneously or persist for years without discernible harm. We have observed asymptomatic funguria (*Torulopsis glabrata*) persist for 2 years in an English bulldog with ammonium urate urolithiasis. Dysuria was not recognized, and pyuria was an infrequent finding. Based on such limited empirical observations in dogs and cats, the long-term prognosis for asymp-

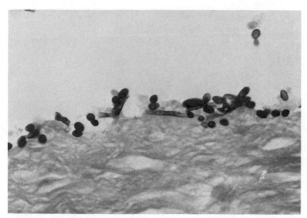

Figure 2. Photomicrograph of a section of urinary bladder of the cat described in Figure 1 illustrating colonization of the luminal surface with *Cephalosporium*. (Gomori's methenamine silver stain; original magnification × 100.)

tomatic funguria may be favorable. However, asymptomatic funguria has the potential to progress to symptomatic disease, especially if a patient's general condition deteriorates as a result of other disease processes or after administration of cytotoxic or antibacterial therapy. Because the kidneys appear to be a principal target organ in systemic mycoses, funguria may be an early indication of fungal infection in other organ systems. The prognosis for renal fungal infection or disseminating fungemia is less favorable. Early detection and treatment may enhance successful management of these cases.

THERAPY

Therapy of fungal UTI should be based on a patient's clinical history, physical examination, and laboratory findings. Because funguria may be transient and benign, aggressive therapy should be reserved for cases with clinical evidence of symptomatic infection (Fig. 4).

In patients with asymptomatic funguria, allowing a patient to spontaneously clear fungi from the urinary tract should precede antifungal therapy. First, strive to correct identifiable predisposing risk factors (see Table 1). Urinary catheters should be removed or, if needed, used intermittently. If possible, antibacterial and immunosuppressive (corticosteroids) agents should be discontinued.

Results of *in vitro* studies indicate that *Candida* species survived poorly at extremes of pH and that pseudohyphae formation was restricted in alkaline urine (Taola et al., 1970). Based on results of these studies, alkalization of urine continues to be recommended. However, we have not been successful in eradicating fungal UTIs with alkalization of urine alone, although alkalization may be helpful. Urine alkalization may be induced by oral administration

of sodium bicarbonate (12 mg/kg every 8 hr) or potassium citrate (50 mg/kg every 12 hr) in a dose sufficient to increase urine pH to 7.5 or greater. Dosage should be adjusted to maintain the desired pH.

A more aggressive therapeutic approach may be indicated for patients with symptomatic funguria, asymptomatic patients with debilitating disease, or asymptomatic patients requiring cytotoxic chemotherapy. In addition to correcting predisposing risk factors, consideration may be given to treatment with 5-fluorocytosine (flucytosine) or amphotericin B. Flucytosine has a narrow range of antifungal activity, limited primarily to yeastlike fungi such as *Candida*, *Torulopsis*, and *Cryptococcus*. Flucytosine is deaminated to 5-fluorouracil in fungal cells; 5-fluorouracil is incorporated into fungal messenger RNA, resulting in faulty protein synthesis with subsequent cell death. One disadvantage of flucytosine is development of resistance, especially when low doses are administered. The likelihood of development of resistance has limited the use of flucytosine to adjunctive therapy for most mycoses. However, because flucytosine is excreted unchanged in urine in high concentrations, it has achieved popularity as a single agent in the treatment of *Candida* in humans. A dose of 200 mg/kg/day (divided into three or four subdoses) has been empirically recommended for dogs. Flucytosine should be continued at least 2 to 3 weeks beyond clinical resolution of fungal UTI. Because this drug is almost exclusively excreted by the kidneys, the dose should be reduced in patients with compromised renal function in order to minimize toxicity. Adverse effects include reversible bone marrow depression, hepatic toxicity, and dermatitis.

Amphotericin B is also effective in the treatment of fungal infections; however, it is associated with substantial nephrotoxicity. The vulnerability of most

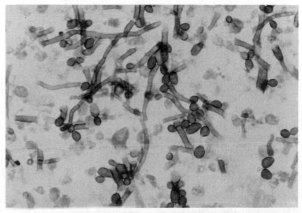

Figure 3. *Candida albicans* in the kidney parenchyma of a Springer spaniel given chemotherapy (1,3-bis (2-chloroethyl)-1-nitrosourea) to treat cerebral neoplasia. (Gomori's methenamine silver stain; original magnification × 100.)

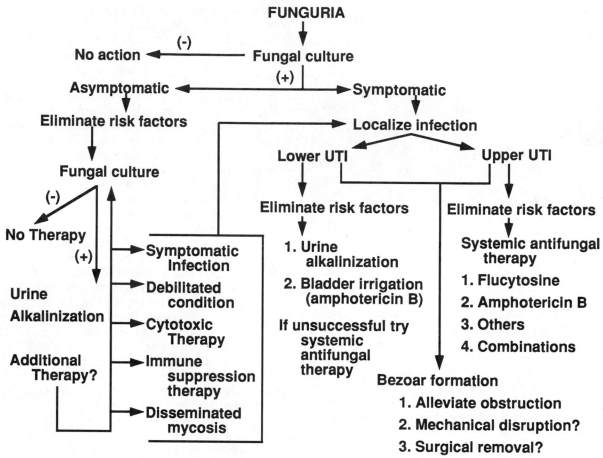

Figure 4. Algorithm designed for management of fungal urinary tract infection.

fungi to amphotericin B is explained by its ability to disrupt fungal cell membranes and the infrequency with which fungal resistance develops. Although only approximately 20% of amphotericin B is eliminated in canine urine (Craven et al., 1979), urine concentration appears adequate to kill most fungi. For example, most *Candida* organisms are susceptible to concentrations less than 1 μg/ml.

Amphotericin B should be considered for use in patients with systemic mycoses, fungal septicemia, or fungal UTI unresponsive to treatment with flucytosine. Amphotericin B must be administered intravenously (see *CVT X*, p. 1101) or as a local irrigant. The lower dose range of amphotericin B may be used if flucytosine is simultaneously administered. Amphotericin B and flucytosine appear to be synergistic when used in combination.

For irrigation of the urinary bladder of humans, a concentration of 200 mg of amphotericin B per liter of sterile water has been recommended (Dreetz and Fetchick, 1988). This solution is infused (5 to 10 ml/kg) into the urinary bladder lumen daily for 5 to 15 days. Duration of administration may vary with persistence of underlying risk factors, degree of tissue invasion, and existence of bezoars.

Ketoconazole and itraconazole are less toxic fungistatic agents that, like amphotericin B, disrupt cell wall synthesis. Although these imidazole derivatives are gaining in popularity for control of systemic mycoses, their role in the treatment of urinary tract mycoses is limited because little active drug is excreted in urine (Wise et al., 1985). Therefore, ketoconazole and itraconazole have been reserved for patients in whom fungi may be resistant to flucytosine and for azotemic patients at increased risk for amphotericin B–induced toxicity. However, fluconazole may provide a viable alternative to the use of flucytosine and amphotericin B (Grayhill, 1989). This imidazole is smaller, more water-soluble, and less protein-bound than ketoconazole and itraconazole. As a result, active fluconazole is cleared primarily by renal excretion. Although a dosage of 200 to 400 mg/day has been recommended for humans, prospective clinical trials are needed to accurately define the dose and effectiveness of antifungal imidazoles for the treatment of fungal UTI in dogs and cats.

Response to treatment should be monitored by serially performed urine fungal cultures. Treatment should be continued until two successive negative urine cultures are obtained at 1- to 2-week intervals (Polzin and Klausner, 1983).

References and Suggested Reading

Clinkenbeard, K. D., Wolf, A. M., Cowell, R. L., et al.: Feline disseminated histoplasmosis. Comp. Cont. Ed. Pract. Vet. 11:1223, 1989.

Craven, P. C., Ludden, T. M., Drutz, D. J., et al.: Excretion pathways of amphotericin B. J. Infect. Dis. 140:329, 1979.

Doster, A. R., Erickson, E. D., and Chandler, F. W.: Feline trichosporonosis. J.A.V.M.A. 190:1184, 1987.

Dreetz, D. J., and Fetchick, R.: Fungal infections of the kidney and urinary tract. In Schrier, R. W., and Gottschalk, C. W. (eds.): Diseases of the Kidney, 4th ed. Boston: Little, Brown & Co., 1988, pp. 1015–1045.

Ehrensaft, D. V., Epstein, R. B., Sarpel, S., et al.: Disseminated candidiasis in leukopenic dogs. Proc. Soc. Exp. Biol. Med. 160:6, 1979.

Grayhill, J. R.: New antifungal agents. Eur. J. Clin. Microbiol. Infect. Dis. 8:402, 1989.

Greene, C. E., and Chandler, F. W.: Candidiasis. In Greene, C. E. (ed.): Infectious Diseases of the Dog and Cat. Philadelphia: W. B. Saunders, 1990, pp. 723–727.

Neer, T. M.: Disseminated aspergillosis. Comp. Cont. Ed. Pract. Vet. 10:465, 1988.

Polzin, D. J., and Klausner, J. S.: Treatment of urinary tract candidiasis. In Kirk, R. W. (ed.): Current Veterinary Therapy VIII. Philadelphia: W. B. Saunders, 1983, pp. 1055–1057.

Taola, P., Schroeder, S. A., Dayl, A. K., et al.: Candida at Boston City Hospital. Arch. Intern. Med. 126:983, 1970.

Wise, G. J., Goldberg, P. E., and Kozinn, P. J.: Do the imidazoles have a role in the management of genitourinary fungal infections? J. Urol. 133:61, 1985.

Wooley, R. E., and Blue, J. L.: Bacterial isolates from canine and feline urine. Mod. Vet. Pract. 57:535, 1976.

THERAPY OF TRANSITIONAL CELL CARCINOMA OF THE CANINE BLADDER

KENITA S. ROGERS
and MICHAEL A. WALKER
College Station, Texas

Although important advances have been made in the therapy of bladder cancer in humans, the treatment of transitional cell carcinoma (TCC) in veterinary patients has been frustrating in terms of developing methods that result in adequate tumor control and an acceptable quality of life. The difference in response can be attributed to several factors that ultimately result in a more advanced and less treatable disease in dogs. First, owners often do not recognize the clinical signs associated with bladder neoplasia in their pets, so the diagnosis is frequently delayed. In addition, when an animal with chronic hematuria and stranguria presents to the hospital, the veterinarian may continue to treat the animal for more common causes of these signs, such as urinary tract infection, and delay definitive diagnostic testing. This approach may be reinforced because the hemorrhage in early cases is intermittent and can spontaneously diminish. Antibiotic therapy may also appear to be effective if there is a secondary urinary tract infection subsequent to abnormal urinary tract defense mechanisms associated with the tumor. The clinical signs of TCC of the bladder can be easily confused with infectious or inflammatory cystitis because the signs are not specific for neoplasia and patients often appear healthy in all other respects. Signs of local disease include hematuria, stranguria, pollakiuria, and urinary incontinence. Signs of systemic disease such as vomiting, anorexia, and lethargy may be apparent if the tumor has resulted in urinary obstruction due to a large trigonal mass. Specific clinical signs such as respiratory difficulty or bone pain may occasionally be related to metastatic disease.

For these reasons, the disease is often advanced at the time of definitive diagnosis. The precise stage of the disease is important when making decisions about appropriate therapy. The World Health Organization staging scheme has been adapted for veterinary patients (Table 1). Most cases of TCC are T2 or T3, making effective management more difficult. The metastatic pattern is generally via both lymphatics and blood to regional lymph nodes, lung, bone, and liver. The depth of bladder wall invasion, with involvement of muscle and fat, tends to correspond with the chance of distant metastasis, although distant metastasis is often not recognized at the time of primary tumor diagnosis.

Because of the advanced nature of the disease in most patients, curative therapy is often an unattainable goal, but clinical signs may be minimized for a period of time in many cases. The approach should

Table 1. *Clinical Stages of Canine Tumors of the Urinary Bladder As Approved by the World Health Organization in 1980*

T: Primary tumor
    Tis Carcinoma *in situ*
    T0 No evidence of tumor
    T1 Superficial papillary tumor
    T2 Tumor invading bladder wall, with induration
    T3 Tumor invading neighboring organs (prostate, uterus, vagina, anal canal)
    The symbol (m) added to the appropriate T category indicates multiple tumors.
N: Regional lymph nodes
    N0 No evidence of regional lymph node involvement
    N1 Regional lymph nodes involved
    N2 Regional lymph nodes and juxtaregional lymph nodes involved
    Regional lymph nodes are the internal and external iliac nodes. The juxtaregional lymph nodes are the lumbar nodes.
M: Distant metastasis
    M0 No evidence of distant metastasis
    M1 Distant metastasis detected—specify site(s)

STAGE GROUPING: No stage grouping is at present recommended.

be to stage each case as accurately as possible and to choose the therapy or combination of therapies most likely to locally control the tumor, maintain urinary continence, and prevent or treat metastatic disease. The therapeutic plan must also recognize that each form of treatment has potential complications; it is important to maintain the goal of improving the overall quality of life. The purpose of this article is to outline current knowledge and experience about the treatment of TCC of the canine urinary bladder.

SURGERY

The goals of any operation designed to treat TCC are to alleviate clinical signs while maintaining urinary continence and to prevent secondary complications such as hydroureter and hydronephrosis. The surgical procedure should also be used to stage the neoplasm more accurately, with collection of regional lymph nodes for histopathologic evaluation.

TCC tends to have poorly defined borders and often involves the bladder trigone, with variable involvement of the ureters and urethra. In the few instances in which the tumor is located at the bladder apex, complete excision may be possible with maintenance of continence, because 80% of the bladder can be excised with full return to function (Withrow, 1989). The excision should attempt to include a 2-cm border of healthy tissue and the entire depth of the bladder wall. Complete excision of tumor in other locations is usually not possible unless a total cystectomy is performed. Obviously, total cystectomy necessitates a urinary

diversion technique. Although cytoreductive (debulking) surgery may temporarily relieve clinical signs, tumor regrowth is usually rapid. This type of surgery may be very useful, however, when used as a complement to radiation therapy, with the goal being to reduce the thickness of the irradiated tissue to 1.5 cm to ensure more uniform and adequate penetration (Withrow et al., 1989). It is imperative that proper oncologic surgical principles be strictly followed because carcinomas of the urinary tract are one of the neoplasms most commonly associated with surgically induced tumor seeding.

Although other procedures such as gastrocystoplasty, ureteroileostomy, ureterohysterostomy, and trigonal colostomy have been attempted, the most commonly performed urinary diversion has been ureterocolonic anastomosis (Stone et al., 1988). This procedure involves preparing submuscular flaps in the distal portion of the colon and performing an end-to-side anastomosis of the ureter to the colonic mucosa. Urinary and fecal continence is usually maintained with this operation, but there are numerous other important complications, including diarrhea, hyperchloremic acidosis, hyperammonemia, pyelonephritis, and uremia, with subsequent gastrointestinal and neurologic dysfunction.

Proper postoperative management of these patients often includes allowing elimination every 3 to 4 hours, administration of oral sodium bicarbonate and appropriate antibiotics, and supportive measures if renal dysfunction develops. The procedure is rarely curative, and most animals have metastatic disease at the time of death. The procedure has been performed in both dogs and cats, but in general, ureterocolonic anastomosis has been unsatisfactory for tumor control and for providing an acceptable quality of life.

RADIATION THERAPY

Radiation is an important additional form of therapy for local neoplastic disease; it can be used as an adjunct to other types of therapy or as a solitary modality. It has been used to complement surgery preoperatively, intraoperatively, and postoperatively. Problems encountered with the use of radiation therapy are twofold. First, by the time a TCC is diagnosed, the tumor often has extensive local invasion, lymph node involvement, or distant metastasis. Each of these conditions makes it quite unlikely that the tumor can be cured by radiation alone. Second, the tumoricidal dose can potentially cause temporary or permanent damage to the surrounding normal tissues. Thus, the total radiation dose must be within acceptable radiation injury levels for the involved tissues yet be at least palliative if not curative.

The focus of study in veterinary medicine has been on the effects of radiation on healthy urinary tracts, but some studies have used radiation in the treatment of TCC of the canine bladder.

Two studies evaluated the use of radiation in a substantial number of dogs with spontaneously occurring TCC (Walker and Breider, 1987; Withrow et al., 1989). Both studies used intraoperative radiation therapy, with the additional use of postoperative irradiation in some patients in one study (Withrow et al., 1989). Both groups of workers found intraoperative therapy to be a technically feasible procedure, but several important complications were noted. Although cystotomy incisions healed without complications, the ureters often became stenotic and fibrotic, with secondary hydroureter and mild to moderate hydronephrosis. These changes became evident by 1 month after surgery and appeared to remain stable. It has been our experience that although secondary hydronephrosis is a common sequela, it usually does not result in clinically apparent signs of renal dysfunction and is not a common reason for euthanasia. The investigators concluded that the dose to the ureters should be less than 25 Gy to minimize serious ureteral damage and secondary renal complications. It has been estimated that at least 25 to 35 Gy as a single dose is necessary to be cancericidal (Craig et al., 1985). When the whole bladder was included in the radiation field, the wall became thickened, fibrotic, and clinically nondistensible within 1 to 2 months. Urinary incontinence and pollakiuria were common sequelae, and local tumor control was usually incomplete; however, one protocol appeared to improve survival, with mean and median survival times following irradiation of 16.8 and 15 months, respectively (Walker and Breider, 1987).

The degree of radiation damage to the tissues is of major concern in the outcome, because many of the resultant complications make a patient unacceptable as a house pet or are indeed life-threatening. The advantage of intraoperative radiation is the ability to expose the tumor surgically, exclude radiosensitive structures, and selectively deliver large doses of radiation to the tumor. The most effective way to use intraoperative radiation and the effect of the addition of preoperative or postoperative radiation therapy or other forms of anticancer treatment remain to be determined. Radiation therapy as a solitary modality should be withheld if metastases are recognized beyond the regional lymphatics.

CHEMOTHERAPY

Chemotherapy, administered both systemically and intravesicularly, is an important part of the therapeutic strategy in human medicine. This is true because of the high percentage of cases with only superficial disease and a lower tumor burden. Compared with research on other treatment modalities, information on the role of chemotherapy in the treatment of canine TCC is sparse.

Emphasis has been placed on the role of cisplatin in the management of canine TCC. Two studies have investigated the efficacy of this chemotherapy agent in treating bladder neoplasia in dogs (Moore et al., 1990; Shapiro et al., 1988). The results with cisplatin alone for tumor control have been disappointing. Several of the patients had stable disease for short periods of time, and a few achieved partial remission, but complete responses were not seen. Moore and colleagues' work showed a median survival of 180 days for 12 dogs with TCC. Cisplatin chemotherapy given to animals with concurrent or pre-existing renal dysfunction was found to pose an additional risk factor that may negatively affect the outcome of treatment. In addition, two dogs ruptured their bladders at the tumor site after the onset of drug administration (Moore et al., 1990). Rupture was thought to result from restricted urinary outflow, increased urine volume due to diuresis, and increased intra-abdominal pressure associated with vomiting. It was recommended that the bladder be emptied frequently in patients receiving cisplatin, particularly those with persistent vomiting.

SUPPORTIVE CARE

Because of the invasive characteristics of the tumor, disruption of the normal urinary tract defense mechanisms, and the often ulcerated and necrotic surface of the neoplasm, patients with TCC are susceptible to secondary bacterial cystitis. Mucosal damage caused by the neoplasm can be further compounded by the effects of therapy such as radiation. Thus, it may be possible to partially relieve some of the clinical signs by recognition and control of secondary disease processes such as urinary tract infection.

SUMMARY

It is apparent that TCC is not generally amenable to curative treatment with a single modality. Future efforts should be directed at determining what combinations of therapy most effectively control the tumor while decreasing the incidence of severe, irreversible damage to normal urinary tissues. In addition, new treatment methods such as photodynamic therapy (Beck et al., 1990) and piroxicam (Knapp et al., 1991) are being investigated and may have a role in the treatment of TCC in canines.

References and Suggested Reading

Beck, E. R., Hetzel, F. W., Morris, K., et al.: Response of canine transitional cell carcinomas to photodynamic therapy. Proc. A.C.V.I.M., 1990, p. 1121. *Results of a study of 10 dogs with advanced stage transitional cell carcinoma treated with photodynamic therapy as a solitary modality.*

Craig, J. A., Sigler, R., and Walker, M.: Effects of intraoperative irradiation on gastric and urinary bladder incisions in the dog. Am. J. Vet. Res. 46:1647, 1985. *A study of the clinical and histologic effects of whole-bladder intraoperative irradiation with and without surgery in normal dogs.*

Knapp, D. W., Richardson, R. C., Chan, T. C., et al.: Piroxicam therapy in twenty-four dogs with transitional cell carcinoma of the bladder. Proc. A.C.V.I.M., 1991, p. 896. *An evaluation of the results of a phase I and a phase II trial using piroxicam as therapy for transitional cell carcinoma of the canine urinary bladder.*

Moore, A. S., Cardona, A., Shapiro, W., et al.: Cisplatin (cisdiammine dichloroplatinum) for treatment of transitional cell carcinoma of the urinary bladder or urethra. J. Vet. Intern. Med. 4:148, 1990. *A retrospective study of the results of cisplatin treatment in 15 dogs with TCC of the bladder or urethra.*

Shapiro, W., Kitchell, B. E., Fossum, T. W., et al.: Cisplatin for treatment of transitional cell and squamous cell carcinomas in dogs. J.A.V.M.A. 193:1530, 1988. *An evaluation of the results of cisplatin therapy of eight dogs with TCC and five dogs with head and neck squamous cell carcinoma.*

Stone, E. A., Withrow, S. J., Page, R. L., et al.: Ureterocolonic anastomosis in ten dogs with transitional cell carcinoma. Vet. Surg. 17:147, 1988. *Discussion of the surgical procedure, complications, and follow-up of ten dogs treated with ureterocolonic anastomosis because of TCC of the bladder trigone or urethra.*

Walker, M., and Breider, M.: Intraoperative radiotherapy of canine bladder cancer. Vet. Radiol. 28:200, 1987. *Evaluation of the clinical results in 13 dogs that received partial surgical extirpation and whole-bladder intraoperative radiotherapy for urinary bladder cancer.*

Withrow, S. J.: Tumors of the urinary system. *In* Withrow, S. J., and MacEwen, E. G. (eds.): Clinical Veterinary Oncology. Philadelphia: J. B. Lippincott, 1989, p. 312. *A review of the incidence, biologic behavior, clinical presentation, diagnosis, treatment, and prognosis of tumors of the urinary system of the dog and cat.*

Withrow, S. J., Gillette, E. L., Hoopes, P. J., et al.: Intraoperative irradiation of 16 spontaneously occurring canine neoplasms. Vet. Surg. 18:7, 1989. *A review of the results in 16 dogs treated with intraoperative radiation therapy and surgical debulking with the addition of fractionated external beam radiotherapy in 11 dogs.*

TUMOR MARKERS FOR DIAGNOSIS OF URINARY TRACT NEOPLASMS

STEPHEN D. GILSON

Phoenix, Arizona

and ELIZABETH A. STONE

Raleigh, North Carolina

Treatment of malignant urinary tract neoplasms is often unsuccessful because animals have large tumor burdens and distant metastases at the time of diagnosis. In our practices, animals typically are presented with prolonged (weeks to months) histories of hematuria, dysuria, and various symptomatic therapies. Greater clinical acumen and improved diagnostic test methods such as tumor markers are needed for early detection of urologic cancers.

WHAT IS A TUMOR MARKER?

Tumor markers are biologic substances that are produced uniquely or in excess amounts by malignant neoplasms. Markers can be various biologic molecules, including oncofetal gene products, hormones, enzymes, proteins, and tumor-associated antigens. Other potential tumor markers include chromosomal markers, nucleolar antigens, cellular metabolites, and flow cytometric characteristics. Tumor markers are generally detected clinically in conveniently sampled body fluids, such as blood, urine, and cerebrospinal fluid.

Oncofetal gene products are biologic substances produced only by embryonal or cancer cells. In tumors, they reflect dedifferentiation and expression of genes normally suppressed in mature cells. Primitive cell types are similar for most species. Hence, most oncofetal gene products are not species-specific and may have application in veterinary medicine in the future.

Hormones, proteins, and enzymes are used as markers when they are produced in excess or ectopically. Production of these substances can reflect tumor cell burden or degree of gene expression and is often recognized clinically as a paraneoplastic syndrome. Excess production of these substances is often not specific for malignancy and can be associated with benign tumors (e.g., excess T_4 production by thyroid adenoma). Hormones, proteins, and enzymes are frequently species-specific.

Tumor-associated antigens are highly specific cell surface antigens that are eluted into body fluids. Their identification and clinical usefulness have greatly increased with the advent of monoclonal antibody technology. Tumor-associated antigens have been identified for various cell types. They are highly cell-specific and thus are virtually always species-specific.

THE IDEAL TUMOR MARKER

The ideal tumor marker has a high sensitivity and specificity for a particular malignancy, is readily secreted into easily obtained body fluids, and can be simply and consistently measured in the laboratory. Tumor marker concentrations should correlate directly with tumor burden and have a short half-life in sample fluids so that changes following treatment can be monitored. The ideal tumor marker is exemplified by use of human chorionic gonadotropin (hCG) for detection and monitoring of gestational trophoblastic neoplasia in women (Bast et al., 1987). Assays of hCG are sensitive enough to detect as few as 10,000 viable cells, with a specificity of greater than 98%. The hormone is measured using routine serum immunoassays, marker values correlate with tumor burden, and serum half-life is short (36 hr).

USE OF TUMOR MARKERS IN URINARY TRACT NEOPLASMS

The use of tumor markers in animals has had limited investigation, particularly in the urinary tract (Bell et al., 1990; Feldman et al., 1988; Kloppel et al., 1978; Poli et al., 1986). Serum concentrations of prostatic acid phosphatase and prostate-specific antigen (PSA) are routinely used to monitor recurrence of prostatic carcinoma after prostatectomy in men. However, in dogs, serum acid phosphatase is not specific for prostatic carcinoma and serum PSA does not appear to increase with carcinoma (Bell et al., 1990; Weaver, 1981). Other tumor markers that are valuable for the diagnosis of urinary tract tumors in humans include serum and urine concentrations of fibrinogen degradation products and carcinoembryonic antigen, as well as urine concentrations of lactate dehydrogenase isoenzymes. Evaluation of these tumor markers in dogs is inconclusive at this time.

References and Suggested Reading

Bast, R. C., Hunter, V., and Knapp, R. C.: Pros and cons of gynecologic tumor markers. Cancer 60:1984, 1987.

Bell, F. W., Klausner, J. S., Hayden, D. W., et al.: Serum markers in prostatic carcinoma. Vet. Cancer Soc. Newsletter 14:13, 1990.

Feldman, B. F., Brummerstedt, E., Larsen, L. S., et al.: Plasma fibronectin concentration associated with various types of canine neoplasia. Am. J. Vet. Res. 49:1017, 1988.

Kloppel, T. M., Franz, C. P., Morre, D. J., et al.: Serum sialic acid levels increased in tumor-bearing dogs. Am. J. Vet. Res. 39:1277, 1978.

Lange, P. H., and Wingfield, H. N.: Biologic markers in urologic cancer. Cancer 60:464, 1987.

Poli, A., Arispici, M., Camillo, F., et al.: Increase of serum lipid-associated sialic concentrations in dogs with neoplasms. Am. J. Vet. Res. 47:607, 1986.

Weaver, A. D.: Fifteen cases of prostatic carcinoma in the dog. Vet. Rec. 100:71, 1981.

Section

11

REPRODUCTIVE DISORDERS

VICKI N. MEYERS-WALLEN
Consulting Editor

DIFFERENTIAL DIAGNOSIS OF CANINE ABORTION

B.J. PURSWELL

Blacksburg, Virginia

Abortion in the bitch is rare, but when it does occur, it is a diagnostic challenge. Information on the incidence of canine abortion is limited, and data on early abortion (early embryonic death) are almost nonexistent. Even though canine abortion is less common than in larger domestic species, the same approach can be used to determine the cause (Table 1).

Following canine abortion, it is essential to perform a necropsy of the aborted fetus or fetuses as soon as possible. The client should be advised to refrigerate, not freeze, both the fetuses and placentas and to present them promptly for necropsy. If a pathologist is available, the entire fetus and placenta can be submitted. Otherwise, all organs (liver, lung, spleen, heart, segments of intestine, kidney, and placenta) should be placed in formalin and submitted to a diagnostic laboratory. Stomach contents should be handled appropriately and submitted for bacterial culture. A necropsy of all fetal structures should be performed in all cases (including those late-term abortions that present as apparently stillborn puppies). A definitive diagnosis may not be possible in all cases, but no answers will be obtained if a necropsy is not performed.

A thorough medical history should be taken at the initial examination. The reproductive history should include data on previous matings, resulting pregnancies, *Brucella canis* serology status, and any genital problems such as estrous cycle abnormalities or vulvar discharges. Take a detailed account of the present breeding, including complete information about the male dog. It is important to know his fertility rate, frequency of use, *B. canis* serology status, contact with other dogs, and data about his general health. Additional important historical information includes vaccination status of both the bitch and the dog and, for the bitch, data about travel and contact with other dogs during the pregnancy; nutritional information, including any supplements; and general environmental conditions.

Examination of the bitch should be performed at the earliest possible time following an abortion. A thorough physical examination should be done, and laboratory tests should include a complete blood count, urinalysis, serum thyroid hormone levels, and a serum chemistry profile. Vaginal cytology should be performed to determine the existence and extent of uterine inflammation. A guarded swab culture should be made from the anterior vagina. In evaluation of the culture, the laboratory should be advised to screen for *B. canis* in addition to performing routine aerobic bacterial culture and sensitivity tests. Serology for *B. canis*, canine herpesvirus, and *Toxoplasma gondii* should be performed (Table 1).

INFECTIOUS CAUSES OF CANINE ABORTION

Brucellosis

The first and most important differential diagnosis for abortion in the bitch is *B. canis*, which typically causes abortion at 45 to 59 days' gestation (see *CVT X*, p. 1317). The aborted pups will be partially autolyzed. Less commonly, a bitch may experience "infertility," which is actually undetected embryonic resorption, or delivery of live pups that die shortly after birth. The vaginal discharge accompanying the abortion will be brown or greenish-gray. The discharge contains large numbers of organisms; therefore, extreme caution should be taken to avoid contact with the discharge by people or dogs. The primary mode of transmission is by oronasal contact with the organism. The majority of human cases of *B. canis* occur following contact with an aborting bitch.

Diagnosis of *B. canis* as the causative agent in a canine abortion is usually fairly straightforward and is accomplished by culturing the vaginal discharge for the organism. This requires special culture media. Isolation of the organism confirms the diagnosis. Alternatively, serologic testing can be conducted with the rapid slide agglutination test (RSAT) (D-Tec CB, Pitman-Moore, Washington Crossing, NJ) and the tube agglutination test (TAT), available through most state diagnostic laboratories. All negative serology tests should be repeated in 30 days to decrease the possibility of false-negative results. Serologic tests are often negative in the first 4 weeks post infection, and therefore, recent infection can be missed by a single test. Further diagnostic confirmation by serology can be accomplished by the agar-gel immunodiffusion (AGID) test. The

Table 1. *Causes and Methods of Diagnosis of Canine Abortions*

Causative Agent	Clinical Findings	Necropsy Findings	Tests
Bacteria			
Brucella canis	Third-trimester abortion	Autolyzed fetuses	Culture (special media): vaginal discharge and blood Serology: RSAT, TAT, and AGID
B. abortus, B. suis, or B. melitensis	History of contact with infected livestock Third-trimester abortion	Autolyzed fetuses	Serology: specific for organism
Salmonella spp.	Systemic disease in bitch Purulent vaginal discharge	Fetal septicemia Placentitis	Culture: vaginal discharge and fetal tissues
Campylobacter spp.	History of diarrhea in bitch or contact humans	Fetal septicemia	Culture (special media): vaginal discharge and fetal tissues
Escherichia coli or Streptococcus spp.	Purulent vaginal discharge Systemic disease in bitch	Fetal septicemia	Culture: vaginal discharge and fetal tissues
Viruses			
Canine herpesvirus	Third-trimester abortion Bitch asymptomatic Vaginal vesicles Stillbirth Infertility	Multifocal petechiae and necrosis in fetal adrenal glands, kidney, liver, and lung	Serology in bitch: paired samples 2 wk apart, run together
Canine distemper or canine adenovirus	Systemic involvement in bitch	Depends on virus involved	Depends on virus involved
Other Organisms			
Mycoplasmataceae (Mycoplasma or Ureaplasma spp.)	Asymptomatic bitch housed in overcrowded conditions Vaginal discharge Infertility	Fetal septicemia	Culture: vaginal discharge and fetal tissues
Toxoplasma gondii	May be asymptomatic bitch or have multisystemic involvement	Placentitis Multiorgan involvement in fetus	Serology: paired samples 2 wk apart, run together (fourfold increase significant)
Endocrine Causes			
Progesterone deficiency	Infectious causes ruled out	None	Serial progesterone assays during luteal phase
Hypothyroidism	Obesity Lethargy Symmetric hair loss	None	TSH stimulation test

AGID, agar-gel immunodiffusion test; RSAT, rapid slide agglutination test; TAT, tube agglutination test; TSH, thyroid-stimulating hormone.

AGID test is particularly helpful in ruling out false-positive results, which are common with both the RSAT and TAT. False-positive tests are particularly confusing in asymptomatic animals. Blood culture of suspect animals also may confirm the extent of spread of the organism within a kennel. Negative blood cultures should be followed by serology testing before declaring an animal free of infection. Negative results by RSAT or TAT in paired samples 30 days apart confirms that the animal is free of infection. Positive serology by RSAT or TAT that is unconfirmed by culture results should be validated by AGID tests before declaring the animal to be infected with *B. canis*.

MANAGEMENT

Recommendations made to the client should be flexible. The traditional advice has been to euthanize all infected animals. This is still a common option. Therapy with antibiotics is uncertain because of the intracellular location of *B. canis* organisms. Treatment can be considered for pet dogs if they can be neutered and placed on long-term multiple antibiotic protocols (e.g., minocycline 25 mg/kg PO, s.i.d. for 2 weeks followed by 12.5 mg/kg PO, b.i.d. for 2 weeks in conjunction with dihydrostreptomycin 5 mg/kg IM, b.i.d. for 1 week) (see also Nicolleti, 1989). Retesting by blood culture and serology should be done at least 6 months following the cessation of antibiotic therapy to evaluate the therapy. Practically speaking, infected animals should not be used for breeding and should be removed from breeding kennels.

Other *Brucella* organisms (*B. abortus, B. suis,* and *B. melitensis*) have been shown to cause abortion in the bitch. Exposure to potentially infected livestock is usually a key part of the history when these infections are considered in the differential diagnoses. If these organisms are suspected, culture and serology specific for them should be performed.

The serology tests for *B. canis* do not provide diagnostic information for the other *Brucella* organisms, so specific screening for these organisms must be done. Human infection is possible from contact with dogs infected with any of the *Brucella* organisms.

Canine Herpesvirus Infection

Canine herpesvirus infection should be considered as a differential diagnosis in any canine abortion (Evermann, 1989). Canine herpesvirus is fairly ubiquitous in dogs, and 80 to 100% of certain segments of the canine population have been exposed. Dogs exposed to many other dogs, as in dog shows or multidog facilities, are at highest risk. As with other herpesvirus infections, lifelong states of latency occur with canine herpesvirus. Although canine herpesvirus stimulates both T-cell and B-cell immunity, humoral responses are minimal and short-lived. Therefore any serum-neutralizing antibody titer is considered significant, especially if coupled with clinical signs.

The period of greatest risk for abortion and neonatal mortality from canine herpesvirus is the last 3 weeks of gestation and the first 3 weeks of life, since the fetuses and neonatal puppies are most susceptible then. Isolation of the bitch and her puppies during this 6-week period is an essential part of preventing losses caused by canine herpesvirus.

Experimentally, canine herpesvirus has been shown to cause abortion in the bitch, so it must be considered in the differential diagnosis. Neonatal septicemia is the most well-known form of canine herpesvirus infection and is almost always fatal. Even surviving neonates may have permanent nervous, renal, or lymphoid tissue damage, making the prognosis poor for infected neonatal puppies. Experimentally induced infections suggest that natural canine herpesvirus infections may cause fetal death, mummification, premature birth, or abnormal parturition in the bitch (Hashimoto and Hirai, 1986).

Aborted fetuses and fetal membranes should be submitted for virus isolation and histopathology. Tissues must be refrigerated, but not frozen. If submitted separately, fetal liver, lung, kidney, adrenal gland, and spleen are essential for diagnosis. Serology of the bitch should be run immediately because of the short-lived nature of the antibody response. Any antibody titer concurrent with clinical signs is considered significant (1:2 to 1:8). Paired serum samples will be helpful in identifying the time frame of the infection.

As with all viral infections, therapy is extremely limited. The maternal immune status plays an important role in the progression of the disease, particularly when neonatal losses are the problem. With few exceptions, bitches will subsequently have normal litters after having a canine herpesvirus–affected litter. The key to dealing with canine herpesvirus infections is prevention. However, no vaccine is currently available. Pregnant bitches should be isolated from other dogs, particularly during the last 3 weeks of gestation, and puppies should be isolated for their first 3 weeks of life. Infections occurring after 3 weeks of age are usually asymptomatic or mild.

Toxoplasmosis

Toxoplasmosis is not a common cause of canine abortion but must be considered in the differential diagnosis. The dog is considered an intermediate host. Cats or other felidae are the only definitive hosts. There are three major routes of transmission to the dog: (1) congenital infection, (2) ingestion of oocysts excreted in cat feces, and (3) ingestion of infected meat.

The most common form of canine toxoplasmosis is generalized toxoplasmosis seen in dogs less than 1 year of age. Clinical signs depend on the location and degree of tissue damage. Signs can be multisystemic or localized to the neurologic, respiratory, or gastrointestinal systems. Congenital transmission is thought to occur only when the dam is initially infected while pregnant, as in other species.

Diagnosis of toxoplasmosis is accomplished by paired serum samples taken 2 weeks apart. The paired samples should be assayed on the same day to reduce test variability. A fourfold increase in the titer is considered significant. However, previous exposure can produce titers as high as 1:2024 and not be indicative of an acute infection.

Prevention is the key to controlling losses associated with toxoplasmosis. A pregnant bitch should not have access to cat feces or raw meat products. Cats shed infective oocysts for only a short time following initial exposure to toxoplasma organisms. Cats with titers to toxoplasma are not likely to be a source of infection. Raw meat products should never be fed to dogs or cats if toxoplasmosis is a concern.

Mycoplasma and *Ureaplasma* Infections

Mycoplasma and *Ureaplasma* are two genera in the family Mycoplasmataceae. Both organisms are considered normal flora in the canine vagina (urogenital tract) as well as the nasopharyngeal cavity. Information obtained from other species (humans and cattle) and studies that show an increased percentage of isolation of these organisms from infertile dogs and bitches has caused much interest recently in their role in canine reproductive problems. Canine *Mycoplasma* and *Ureaplasma* isolates have been associated with infertility, early embryonic death, abortion, stillbirths or weak newborns, and neonatal mortality. As in cattle, these problems have been associated with overcrowded (kennel) operations. Under such conditions, these organisms multiply beyond normal levels. Individuals in single-dog households are rarely affected.

Diagnosis of abortion associated with *Mycoplasma* and *Ureaplasma* is supported by positive cultures from the anterior vagina, using a guarded swab and a sterile speculum. Swabs should be placed in Amies transport medium (Difco Laboratories, Detroit, MI) and transported on ice overnight to a laboratory capable of culturing the organisms. If an aborted fetus and placenta are available, they should be transported on ice as well for similar cultures. Vaginal cytology should be performed to confirm the presence of inflammatory cells in the vaginal discharge.

Treat affected individuals with parenteral antibiotics (chloramphenicol or tetracycline) for 10 to 14 days. Erythromycin, though not as effective, can be used safely in pregnant bitches. Long-term control measures must center on reducing the number of animals housed together. Without correction of the overcrowding, problems are likely to recur.

Miscellaneous Bacterial Infections

Bacterial abortions may be caused by a variety of opportunistic bacteria. Many are in the normal vaginal flora of the bitch. *Escherichia coli* and *Streptococcus* (usually groups G and L) are the most common organisms. Organisms that can cause abortion less frequently in the bitch include *Salmonella* and *Campylobacter*. Predisposing factors are usually present to enable these bacteria to cause infection during pregnancy. Older bitches whose endometrium has been compromised by cystic endometrial hyperplasia are prime candidates for bacterial abortions. Uterine infection, which may vary in severity between the uterine horns, can occur concurrently with pregnancy. Death of the puppies will usually result in an abortion. Parturition accompanied by a purulent discharge is indicative of this kind of uterine bacterial infection. Some puppies may actually survive, but they may have septicemia, neonatal conjunctivitis, or other postpartum complications.

Diagnosis of bacterial abortion is based on clinical signs and vaginal cultures. Vaginal cytology will reveal a pronounced inflammatory process with massive numbers of degenerative neutrophils. The bitch may show signs of systemic involvement, such as neutrophilia with a left shift and fever. Antibiotics should be administered immediately after cultures are obtained and the medication changed if dictated by culture and sensitivity results. Uterine evacuation is important and can be accomplished with

prostaglandin F_2-alpha (Lutalyse, Upjohn, Kalamazoo, MI) given at a dose of 0.05 to 0.1 mg/kg SC, s.i.d. to t.i.d. until the discharge stops. *Campylobacter* sp. should be considered if there is a history of diarrhea in either the bitch or in the humans in contact. Because of special growth requirements, *Campylobacter* culture must be specifically requested from the laboratory.

Miscellaneous Viruses

Unlike the larger domestic species, viral abortion in the bitch is relatively rare. Abortion following infections of canine distemper virus and canine adenovirus has been reported (Roberts, 1986). These viruses, along with canine herpesvirus, have been isolated from aborted fetuses, placentas, and neonatal puppies. Breeding bitches should be vaccinated for canine distemper virus and canine adenovirus prior to the onset of proestrus. Modified-live vaccines should not be administered to pregnant bitches.

NONINFECTIOUS CAUSES OF CANINE ABORTION

Progesterone Insufficiency

Progesterone insufficiency as a cause of canine abortion is possible because of the bitch's dependence on luteal progesterone for the maintenance of pregnancy. Care must be taken to rule out all other causes, especially infectious causes, before making the diagnosis. Serum progesterone levels should be monitored in order to document a premature drop in progesterone. This now can be accomplished in practice with progesterone enzyme-linked immunosorbent assay (ELISA) kits (ICG-Target, Malvern, PA). This ELISA kit is available commercially and is marketed for breeding management of the bitch (see this volume, p. 943). The minimum serum progesterone concentration necessary to maintain pregnancy may be difficult to determine because of variation among individual bitches. However, Concannon (1977) reported data showing that bitches in late gestation aborted when serum progesterone was less than 2 ng/ml in response to prostaglandin F_2-alpha injections. Progesterone levels coupled with the timing of previous abortions will help determine when exogenous progesterone therapy is needed. Progesterone in oil, administered at 2 mg/kg IM every 48 hours will maintain the progesterone level above 2 ng/ml and should maintain the pregnancy (Scott-Moncrief, 1990). Parturition can be expected 72 hours after the last injection. Parturition should be planned for 57 days after the first day of diestrus, determined by vaginal cytology (Concannon, 1977).

should be avoided to prevent other problems, such as uterine inertia and prolonged gestation.

Miscellaneous Causes

Fetal defects are reported to be a cause of spontaneous abortion in women. It is possible that similar problems may affect canine pregnancies. Multiple fetuses would have to be affected in a litter for an abortion to occur. Chromosome analysis of aborted fetuses can be done to support this diagnosis.

Endocrine abnormalities other than progesterone insufficiency may also play a role in canine abortions. Hypothyroidism has been reported to occur in bitches that abort, but a cause-and-effect relationship has not been established. Other endocrine diseases should be considered and ruled out as part of an overall physical examination of the bitch. Bitches with any endocrine abnormality should probably not be used as breeding stock.

Nutritional causes of abortion in the bitch are rare. Manganese deficiency has been reported to cause early embryonic death. As long as the bitch has been fed a balanced commercial dog food, without supplements, nutritional causes can be ruled out as a cause of abortion (p. 971). Vitamin and mineral supplements (especially calcium)

References and Suggested Reading

Carmichael, L. E., and Greene, C. E.: Canine herpesvirus infection. In Greene, C. E. (ed.): Infectious Diseases of the Dog and Cat. Philadelphia: W. B. Saunders, 1990, pp. 252–258.

Carmichael, L. E., and Greene, C. E.: Canine brucellosis. In Greene, C.E. (ed.): Infectious Diseases of the Dog and Cat. Philadelphia: W.B. Saunders, 1990, pp. 573–584.

Concannon, P. W., and Hansel, W.: Prostaglandin F_2 alpha luteolysis, hypothermia and abortions in beagle bitches. Prostaglandins. 13:533, 1977.

Evermann, J. F.: Diagnosis of canine herpetic infections. In Kirk, R. W. (ed.): Current Veterinary Therapy X. Philadelphia: W.B. Saunders, 1989, pp. 1313–1316.

Hashimoto, A., and Hirai, K.: Canine herpesvirus infection. In Morrow, D. A. (ed.): Current Therapy in Theriogenology, Vol. 2. Diagnosis, Treatment, and Prevention of Reproductive Diseases in Small and Large Animals. Philadelphia: W. B. Saunders, 1986, pp. 516–520.

Lein, D. H.: Infertility and reproductive diseases in bitches and queens. In Roberts, S. J. (ed.): Veterinary Obstetrics and Genital Diseases (Theriogenology). Woodstock, VT: S. J. Roberts, 1986, pp. 728–734.

Johnston, S. D.: Spontaneous abortion. In Morrow, D. A. (ed.): Current Therapy in Theriogenology. Philadelphia: W. B. Saunders, 1980, pp. 606–608.

Nicoletti, P.: Diagnosis and treatment of canine brucellosis. In Kirk, R. W. (ed.): Current Veterinary Therapy X. Philadelphia: W. B. Saunders, 1989, pp. 1317–1320.

Roberts, S. J.: Diseases and accidents during the gestation period. In Roberts, S. J. (ed.): Veterinary Obstetrics and Genital Diseases (Theriogenology). Woodstock, VT: S. J. Roberts, 1986, pp. 206–210.

Scott-Moncrief, J. C., Nelson, R. W., Bill, R. L., et al.: Serum disposition of exogenous progesterone after intramuscular administration in bitches. Am. J. Vet. Res. 51:893, 1990.

FELINE SEMEN ANALYSIS AND ARTIFICIAL INSEMINATION

JOGAYLE HOWARD
Washington, D.C.

The domestic cat is an important animal model for biomedical, genetic, and zoologic research. Serving as a model for 36 human anomalies, cats demonstrate anatomic, chromosomal, immunologic, cardiovascular, oncologic, and metabolic defects that are analogous to the disorders observed in humans. Because of similarities in chromosomal linkage homology with humans, cats also are studied as a model for human genetic analysis. In the field of conservation biology, domestic cats are valuable for comparative research of rare felid species. Thirty-six species of wild Felidae exist, all of which are listed as threatened or endangered. Many of these nondomestic felids reproduce poorly in captivity

and exhibit abnormal semen characteristics, including a high percentage (range, 36 to 84%) of morphologically abnormal spermatozoa in the ejaculate (Howard et al., 1984; Wildt et al., 1983). Available data suggest that a compromised genotype adversely affects reproductive potential and spermatozoal integrity of nondomestic felids (Wildt et al., 1987).

The propagation of laboratory cat colonies maintained as feline animal models often is complicated, and reproductive performance may be compromised by behavioral incompatibility, physical handicaps, and infertile matings. Similar difficulties also are observed in the breeding of purebred cat colonies, a finding that may be associated with a decrease in genetic variation resulting from inbreeding. Because a male's reproductive characteristics may influence feline propagation, evaluation of male fertility is a prerequisite to determining the cause of reproductive failures.

Male fertility in cats is traditionally assessed by the production of a viable pregnancy and live offspring following natural breeding. Direct evaluation of a male, however, may be a more practical approach for assessing potential fertility and sperm fertilizing ability. Evaluation of seminal and hormonal traits is important, in addition to a complete physical examination and testing for diseases such as toxoplasmosis, feline infectious peritonitis, feline immunodeficiency virus, and feline leukemia. Specific information on sperm function is beneficial, and various *in vitro* procedures have been developed in cats for examining sperm motility profiles and ovum penetration. In addition to assessing fertility, a fundamental understanding of semen characteristics and sperm fertilizing ability also is critical when considering artificial breeding techniques such as *in vitro* fertilization and artificial insemination. These techniques may be useful and perhaps necessary for propagating feline models and nondomestic felids.

SPERM COLLECTION

Puberty in domestic cats generally occurs within 8 to 12 months of birth, coincident with the appearance of sperm in the ejaculate. Numerous methods of sperm collection have been used in cats. Viable spermatozoa have been obtained by flushing the ductus deferens or cauda epididymidis immediately after castration. Postmortem retrieval of spermatozoa, also involving flushing the ductus deferens or epididymis, has been used to salvage germ plasm from valuable animals. A more practical approach is to recover spermatozoa using an artificial vagina (AV) (Sojka et al., 1970) or electroejaculation (Howard et al., 1990; Platz et al., 1978). The AV approach requires a "teaser" or estrous queen and a training period of at least 3 weeks for the male to ejaculate into the semen collection device. Electroejaculation requires anesthesia, an electroejaculator, a rectal probe, and no prior training of the animal. For electroejaculation, food is withheld for 12 hr, and males are anesthetized with either an intramuscular injection of ketamine hydrochloride (HCl) (Vetalar, Parke-Davis; 25 mg/kg) or tiletamine-zolazepam (Telazol, Robins; 7 mg/kg). Certain anesthetics relax the musculature surrounding the urethra, and urine contamination of the semen and rapid loss of sperm motility can result. These drugs include xylazine (Rompun, Haver-Lockhart), diazepam (Valium, Roche), phenothiazine derivatives such as acepromazine maleate, and inhalation anesthetics including halothane and isoflurane. Various designs of electroejaculators delivering either alternating current (AC) or direct current (DC) are effective for semen collection. Our laboratory uses a commercially available AC 60-Hz sine-wave electroejaculator with a variable transformer and a Teflon rectal probe (1 cm in diameter and 13 cm long) with three longitudinal electrodes (2.6 mm in width and 3.75 cm in length) to deliver the electrical stimuli (P.T. Electronics, Boring, OR). The probe is lubricated and inserted 7 to 9 cm into the rectum with the electrodes positioned ventrally. A standardized electroejaculation regimen, in which each male receives the same number of electrical stimuli at the same voltage increments, is beneficial for comparison of males and ejaculate traits. Our laboratory uses a total of 80 electrical stimuli divided into three series consisting of 30 (10 stimulations at 2, 3 and 4 volts: series 1), 30 (10 stimulations at 3, 4 and 5 volts: series 2), and 20 (10 stimulations at 4 and 5 volts: series 3) stimuli, respectively (Howard et al., 1990). The stimulus cycle is composed of approximately 1 sec from 0 to the desired voltage, 2 to 3 sec at the desired voltage, and an abrupt return to 0 volts for 3 sec. Males are rested for 2 to 3 min between series.

SEMEN EVALUATION

Semen analysis is a critical part of the fertility evaluation in male felids. Immediately after collection, semen is transferred to a 1.5-ml conical tube and evaluated microscopically at 37°C for percentage of sperm motility (range, 0 to 100%) and progressive motility (scale of 0 to 5). Criteria for assessing progressive motility are based on the following:

0 = no motility or movement.
1 = slight side-to-side movement with occasional slow forward progression.
2 = moderate side-to-side movement with occasional slow forward progression.
3 = side-to-side movement with slow forward progression.
4 = steady forward progression.
5 = rapid, steady forward progression.

At least four separate fields at 250× are examined, and an average sperm per cent motility and progressive motility rating are calculated. To determine an overall sperm assessment rating with equal emphasis on both sperm per cent motility and progressive motility, a sperm motility index (SMI) is calculated: SMI = (sperm progressive motility × 20) + (% sperm motility) divided by 2. Ejaculate volume and pH are measured, and sperm concentration is determined using a hemocytometer and a commercially available erythrocyte determination

Table 1. *Characteristics of Semen Obtained from Domestic Cats by Artificial Vagina or Electroejaculation*

	Artificial Vagina*	Electroejaculation†
Ejaculate volume (μl)	34–40	124–224
Sperm concentration ($\times 10^6$/ml)	1730–1795	133–168
Total number of sperm/ejaculate ($\times 10^6$)	57–61	21–30
Sperm motility (%)	78–83	70–84

*Data from Sojka and associates (1970) and Platz and associates (1978).
†Data from Platz and associates (1978) and Howard and associates (1990).

kit (Unopette, Becton-Dickinson, Rutherford, NJ). The capillary pipette of the latter is filled with 10 μl of semen, which is mixed with the reservoir solution, resulting in a 1:200 dilution ratio. Both hemocytometer chambers are filled with the diluted semen, and the number of sperm in the four large (1 mm²) corner squares of each chamber is counted. The number of sperm cells counted in each chamber is divided by two to obtain a sperm count in millions per milliliter of ejaculate. The procedure is repeated for the second hemocytometer chamber, and an average concentration is calculated. Total number of sperm per ejaculate ($\times 10^6$) is calculated by multiplying ejaculate volume times sperm concentration per milliliter.

Ejaculates obtained by an AV generally contain less volume and more total sperm per ejaculate than semen collected by electroejaculation (Table 1). High ratings of sperm motility are detected in cats, which are unaffected by the method of semen collection (see Table 1). The pH of cat semen ranges from 7.0 to 8.6, and the osmolality of seminal plasma is approximately 330 mOsm/kg.

Sperm morphology is evaluated by fixing ejaculate aliquots (20 μl) in 1% glutaraldehyde (0.5 ml) followed by phase-contrast microscopic examination of 200 sperm per aliquot at 1000×. The linear dimensions of cat spermatozoa are distinguished from those of other carnivores by the comparatively small length of the spermatozoon (total sperm length, approximately 60 μm). Classification of sperm morphology includes categorizing sperm as either being normal or having one of the following anomalies: macrocephalic, microcephalic, bicephalic, tricephalic, mitochondrial sheath aplasia (including partial or complete aplasia of mitochondrial sheath), tightly coiled flagellum, bent midpiece with or without a cytoplasmic droplet, bent flagellum with or without a cytoplasmic droplet, proximal or distal cytoplasmic droplet (Fig. 1). Assessment of the ultrastructure of cat spermatozoa including visualization of the acrosome is difficult by light microscopy because of the small configuration of the acrosome (Fig. 2).

The proportion of structurally abnormal sperm in the ejaculate (teratospermia) of most cats ranges from 2 to 29% (Sojka et al., 1970; Wildt et al., 1983). However, certain males maintained in a laboratory cat colony have now been observed to routinely produce more than 60% aberrant sperm forms (Howard et al., 1990) (Table 2). The most prevalent abnormalities include spermatozoa with a bent midpiece with a laterally displaced cytoplasmic droplet positioned within the bent angle (Fig. 1g), a residual cytoplasmic droplet (Fig. 1l), and a bent flagellum (Fig. 1j). The cause of teratospermia in domestic cats is unknown; however, structurally defective sperm observed in the cheetah (Wildt et al., 1983) and geographically isolated lion (Wildt et al., 1987) have been related to diminished genetic variation and decreased circulating testosterone concentrations.

ENDOCRINE EVALUATION

Control of testicular function is a complex feedback system involving the hypothalamic production of gonadotropin-releasing hormone (GnRH) and pituitary secretion of follicle stimulating hormone (FSH) and luteinizing hormone (LH). The interstitial or Leydig's cells in the testes produce testosterone under the influence of LH, whereas actual spermatogenesis is controlled by FSH and testosterone acting directly on the seminiferous tubular epithelium. After release from the seminiferous tubules, spermatozoa are transported into the epididymis for further maturation and storage. Spermatozoal transit through the epididymis is accompanied by critical androgen-dependent changes that ultimately result in the acquisition of sperm motility and the capacity to fertilize ova. In assessing male reproductive status, hormonal evaluation is useful in identifying gonadotropin deficiencies and profound Leydig's cell dysfunction.

Systemic FSH, LH, and testosterone concentrations have been measured in male cats (see Table 2). Serum FSH and LH profiles vary among intact males (ranges, 18 to 55 ng/ml, 0.5 to 7.0 ng/ml, respectively); however, little variation is observed within individual males. FSH and LH pulsatility has not been determined in intact toms; however,

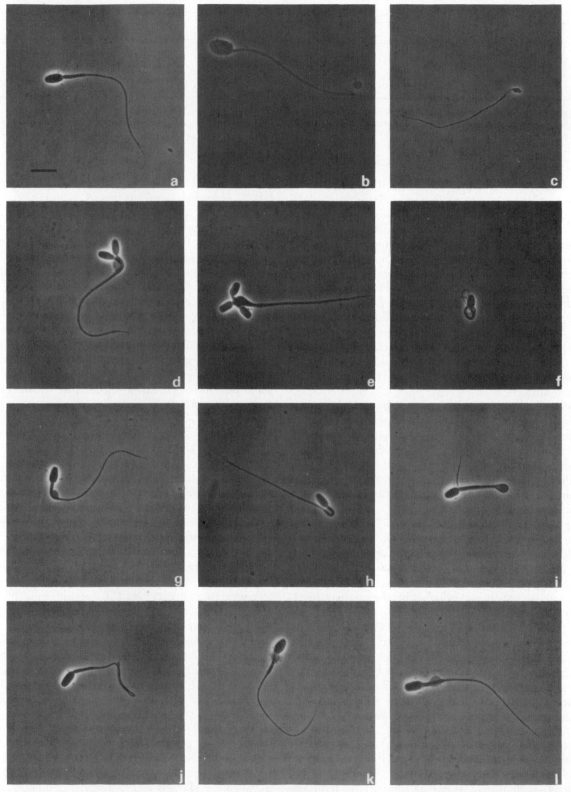

Figure 1. Sperm forms detected in the cat electroejaculate. *a*, Normal. *b*, Macrocephalic. *c*, Microcephalic with mitochondrial sheath aplasia. *d*, Bicephalic. *e*, Tricephalic. *f*, Tightly coiled flagellum. *g*, Bent midpiece with cytoplasmic droplet. *h*, Bent midpiece without cytoplasmic droplet. *i*, Bent flagellum with cytoplasmic droplet. *j*, Bent flagellum without cytoplasmic droplet. *k*, Proximal cytoplasmic droplet. *l*, Distal cytoplasmic droplet. *Scale bar* on photomicrograph in *a* represents 10 μm.

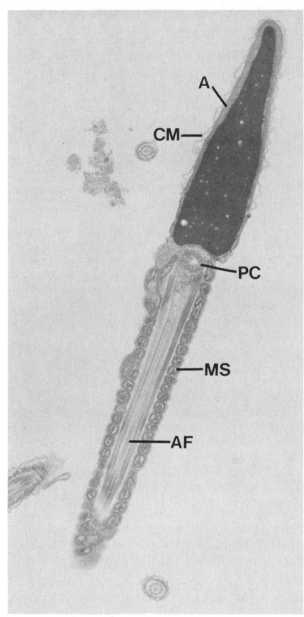

Figure 2. Transmission electron micrograph of a cat spermatozoon showing the head, neck, and midpiece region. The head is composed of the acrosome (A), nucleus (N), and cell membrane (CM). The ruptured CM was presumed to be an artifact of the fixation process. The neck region contains proximal centriole (PC), and the midpiece consists of the axial filament (AF) surrounded by the mitochondrial sheath (MS). (×18,000.)

episodic LH activity has been observed in immature and mature gonadectomized males, with pulses occurring every 20 to 30 min. Marked increases in LH occur within 5 days and often within 24 hr after castration, apparently because of a loss in negative feedback by gonadal steroids.

Systemic testosterone concentrations fluctuate widely in male cats and are influenced by the time of collection within a given sampling interval (0.1 to 5.9 ng/ml) (Howard et al., 1990). Serum testos-

terone level tends to decrease in individual cats sampled over a 90-min period, either while fully conscious or under ketamine-induced anesthesia. The cornified papillae (spines) on a cat's penis appear to be androgen-dependent. Corresponding to the presence or absence of testosterone, the spines are detected first at 6 to 7 months of age and diminish in size after castration. Of particular interest is the apparent relationship between sperm structural morphology and gonadal androgen production in cats (Howard et al., 1990). Although FSH and LH concentrations are similar, teratospermic males produce lower circulating levels of testosterone than normospermic cats (see Table 2).

ENHANCEMENT OF SPERM MOTILITY AND MORPHOLOGY

Cat spermatozoa are sensitive to environmental and culture conditions. Sperm motility is observed for only 60 min when semen is maintained at 37°C in room atmosphere, whereas longevity is increased to 140 min by reducing the temperature to 23°C (Goodrowe et al., 1989). The duration of sperm motility is prolonged significantly by diluting raw semen with either 200 µl Biggers-Whitten-Whittingham (BWW) medium or modified Krebs-Ringer bicarbonate (mKRB) medium. After simple dilution and maintenance in a 5% carbon dioxide in air, humidified environment, high ratings of sperm motility are observed for more than 6 hr (Fig. 3). Processing methods such as low-speed centrifugation (i.e., 300 g) are not detrimental to cat sperm motility, as demonstrated by similar motility profiles between diluted raw aliquots and samples centrifuged for either swim-up sperm separation or seminal plasma removal (see Fig. 3).

The swim-up technique has been used in numerous species including humans to improve a spermatozoal population by separating spermatozoa on the basis of motility and structural morphology. This processing method consists of seminal dilution, centrifugation (300 g, 8 min), removal of the supernatant, and layering of fresh medium (50 to 150 µl) onto the sperm pellet without disturbing the pellet. Spermatozoa are allowed to migrate into the fresh layer of medium. After a 1- to 2-hr incubation, the swim-up suspension is recovered and evaluated for sperm motility and morphology. The swim-up approach is very effective in cats for recovering high proportions of motile, structurally normal spermatozoa from males prone to producing an extremely high incidence of pleomorphic spermatozoa. Compared with diluted seminal aliquots, a greater sperm motility index and percentage of normal spermatozoa are detected in aliquots subjected to the swim-up separation technique (Fig. 4). Longevity of sperm motility also is influenced and improved by

Table 2. *Spermatozoal Morphology and Serum Follicle-Stimulating Hormone, Luteinizing Hormone, and Testosterone Concentrations in Normospermic and Teratospermic Domestic Cats**

	Normospermic† Cats	Teratospermic‡ Cats
Spermatozoal morphology		
Normal spermatozoa (%)	71.6 ± 2.3§	33.8 ± 2.3‖
Abnormal spermatozoa (%)		
Macrocephalic	0.1 ± 0.04	0.2 ± 0.04
Microcephalic	0.1 ± 0.03	0.2 ± 0.03
Bicephalic	0.2 ± 0.2	2.1 ± 0.2
Tricephalic	0.0	0.8 ± 0.1
Mitochondrial sheath aplasia	0.0	0.4 ± 0.1
Coiled flagellum	2.1 ± 0.8	5.3 ± 0.8
Bent midpiece with droplet	9.3 ± 1.8	24.1 ± 1.8
Bent midpiece without droplet	1.0 ± 0.5	2.3 ± 0.5
Bent flagellum with droplet	0.9 ± 1.5	5.4 ± 1.5
Bent flagellum without droplet	5.8 ± 1.8	8.2 ± 1.8
Proximal cytoplasmic droplet	2.2 ± 0.3	5.1 ± 0.3
Distal cytoplasmic droplet	6.7 ± 1.6	12.1 ± 1.6
Serum hormones		
Follicle stimulating hormone (ng/ml)	32.4 ± 6.4§	21.7 ± 6.4§
Luteinizing hormone (ng/ml)	2.5 ± 0.3§	1.9 ± 0.3§
Testosterone (ng/ml)	1.2 ± 0.1§	0.4 ± 0.1‖

*Data from Howard and associates (1990).
†Normospermic cats produce >60% morphologically normal spermatozoa per ejaculate.
‡Teratospermic cats produce <40% morphologically normal spermatozoa per ejaculate.
§,‖Within rows, means (± SEM) with different superscript symbols differ ($P<.05$).

swim-up processing, as evidenced by a greater 6-hr sperm motility index compared with diluted raw and seminal plasma removal treatments (see Fig. 3).

SPERM CAPACITATION

Domestic cat spermatozoa must undergo capacitation before ovum penetration can occur. Capacitation, defined as the physiologic process by which a spermatozoon achieves the ability to fertilize an ovum, involves removal or alteration of components associated with the sperm surface. Freshly ejaculated, nonincubated cat spermatozoa fail to fertilize ovulated oocytes *in vitro*, whereas penetration occurs if spermatozoa are incubated in the uterus of estrous females for 0.5 to 24 hr.

Capacitation of ejaculated cat spermatozoa can be induced *in vitro* after dilution and incubation of semen in culture medium. Cat spermatozoa begin interacting with oocytes after 30 min of co-culture,

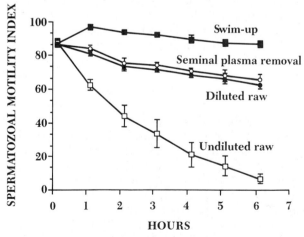

Figure 3. Influence of semen processing on longevity of cat sperm motility *in vitro*. Aliquots of raw semen (undiluted raw) were compared with aliquots diluted in Biggers-Whitten-Whittingham or modified Krebs-Ringer bicarbonate medium (diluted raw) or centrifuged for either swim-up sperm separation (swim-up) or resuspension in medium following removal of seminal plasma (seminal plasma removal). Data are from a study by Howard and associates (1990).

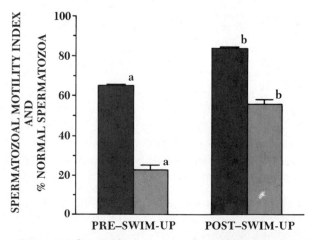

Figure 4. Influence of swim-up separation technique on sperm motility index *(solid bars)* and structural morphology *(lighter bars)* in teratospermic cat ejaculates. Within each sperm trait, means with different lettered superscripts differ ($P<.05$). Data are from a study by Howard and associates (1990).

and moderate penetration rates (70%) into the outer one half of the zona pellucida are observed at culture intervals ranging from 1.5 to 2.5 hr. The highest incidence of outer zona penetration (90 to 100%) occurs after 3 hr of co-incubation. Cat spermatozoa collected from the cauda epididymidis are capable of penetrating oocytes as early as 20 min after insemination. After 30 min in culture, 100% of the oocytes are penetrated, suggesting a physiologic difference between ejaculated spermatozoa and epididymal spermatozoa. As suggested for other species, cat epididymal spermatozoa may be in a capacitated condition in the cauda epididymidis and become decapacitated when exposed to seminal plasma components binding to the sperm plasma membrane. Interestingly, however, removal of seminal plasma from cat spermatozoa is not a prerequisite for sperm-oocyte interaction. Penetration of oocytes *in vitro* is not enhanced by centrifuging the semen and decanting the seminal plasma (Howard et al., 1991[a]).

ASSESSMENT OF SPERM FUNCTION

Conventional semen analysis provides general information on a male's ability to produce motile, normally shaped cells; however, the basic semen traits fail to evaluate the sperm's ability to penetrate and fertilize an ovum (i.e., functional competence). Largely as a result of human infertility and *in vitro* fertilization (IVF) research, sophisticated procedures have been developed to assess sperm function and the events associated with fertilization.

Zona-Free Hamster Ovum Assay

One popular procedure for testing sperm fertilizing ability has been the zona-free hamster ovum penetration assay, commonly referred to as the sperm penetration assay. This method measures the capability of a spermatozoon to penetrate an ovum and undergo nuclear decondensation within the ooplasm. This bioassay is based on the unique ability of zona pellucida–free hamster ova to be penetrated by heterologous spermatozoa. Ultrastructural observations reveal that the heterologous binding and fusion of spermatozoa to zona-free hamster ova is similar to homologous fertilization. This assay has been used extensively to assess functionality of human spermatozoa. Hamster ova also can be penetrated *in vitro* by spermatozoa from numerous domestic and laboratory species including the guinea pig, mouse, rabbit, cattle, pig, horse, goat, sheep, and several species of primates.

The zona-free hamster ovum assay has been used in our laboratories to assess sperm function in domestic cats and, specifically, to determine the

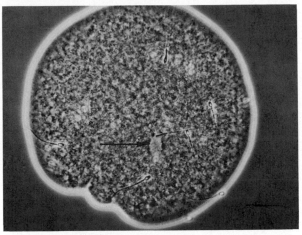

Figure 5. Penetration of zona-free hamster ovum by a domestic cat spermatozoon. One swollen sperm head *(arrow)* with attached flagellum is visible in the vitellus of the ovum. *Scale bar* on photomicrograph represents 30 μm.

impact of teratospermia on ovum penetration (Howard et al., 1991[a]). To obtain ova for this assay, the oviducts of hormonally stimulated hamsters are flushed, and ova are treated with hyaluronidase and trypsin to remove the cumulus cells and zonae pellucidae, respectively. Zona-free hamster ova are placed in a culture dish containing cat spermatozoa and are later evaluated for penetration. Spermatozoa from normospermic and teratospermic cats are capable of penetrating hamster ova, as demonstrated by the presence of a decondensed sperm head within the ooplasm (Fig. 5). The penetration rate (defined as the percentage of ova with a decondensed sperm head) for normospermic males, however, is five times greater than for teratospermic males (Fig. 6). Although swim-up processing improves sperm per cent motility, progressive motility, and normal morphology in teratospermic ejaculates, penetration rates are not increased using swim-up spermatozoa. Because increasing the proportion of normal spermatozoa or enhancing sperm motility has no effect on hamster ovum penetration, it is possible that some other factor inherent in the teratospermic ejaculate may be compromising sperm function.

The hamster ovum assay is effective for studying the influence of culture media on sperm-ovum interaction (Howard et al., 1991[a]). In normospermic ejaculates, ovum penetration is enhanced when cat spermatozoa are incubated with hamster ova in the presence of mKRB (13.5%) compared with BWW (7.6%) medium. This bioassay also has been particularly valuable for studying basic sperm physiology in nondomestic felids. Spermatozoa from the leopard cat *(Felis bengalensis)*, Siberian tiger *(Panthera tigris altaica)*, and cheetah *(Acinonyx jubatus)* have been shown to penetrate zona-free hamster ova. Using this heterologous hamster ovum

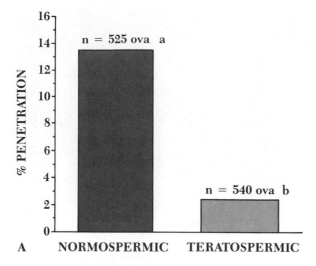

A   NORMOSPERMIC   TERATOSPERMIC

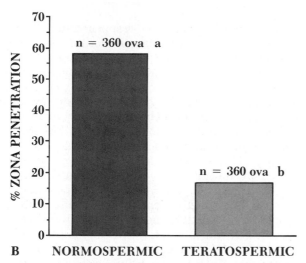

B   NORMOSPERMIC   TERATOSPERMIC

Figure 6. Penetration of zona-free hamster ova *(A)* and zona-intact domestic cat oocytes *(B)* by normospermic and teratospermic domestic cat spermatozoa. Within each assay, means with different lettered designations differ *(P<.05)*. Data are from a study by Howard and associates (1991[a]).

assay, the influence of various sperm processing methods and *in vitro* culture conditions on ovum penetration can be determined in nondomestic felids (Howard and Wildt, 1990).

Zona-Intact Cat Oocyte Assay

The zona-free hamster ovum assay does not assess the ability of a spermatozoon to bind and penetrate the zona pellucida, which is a serious limitation because defective sperm-zona interaction is one cause of infertility. Therefore, inclusion of the zona barrier is important for assessing certain sperm functions including zona binding and penetration.

Homologous immature oocytes collected from ovarian antral follicles have been useful for assessing fertilization in numerous species including humans. This strategy is feasible for cats because zona-intact oocytes can be recovered easily from readily available ovaries after ovariohysterectomy. To obtain oocytes for this assay, cat ovaries are punctured repeatedly with a 22-gauge needle to release cumulus-oocyte complexes. Cumulus cells are removed using hyaluronidase, and oocytes are placed in a culture dish containing a processed sperm suspension. After incubation, each oocyte is evaluated for sperm binding and zona penetration.

In our laboratories, immature cat oocytes have been used to determine the impact of teratospermia on sperm function and zona penetration in domestic cats (Howard et al., 1991[a]). Spermatozoa from normospermic and teratospermic cats are capable of zona binding and penetration (Fig. 7); however, sperm-zona interaction (defined as the percentage of ova with spermatozoa binding to or penetrating into the zona pellucida) is more than twice as great in the normospermic group. A fivefold increase is noted in the number of bound spermatozoa/ovum as well as a threefold increase in percentage of zona penetration (defined as the percentage of ova with spermatozoa penetrating into the zona) for normospermic compared with teratospermic males (see Fig. 6). There appears to be a fundamental functional defect in sperm from teratospermic cats, which is expressed as a diminished ability of the sperm to interact, bind, and penetrate the zona pellucida. The compromised sperm function observed in these androgen-deficient cats may be related to a developmental or maturational anomaly resulting from defective spermatogenesis or epididymal dysfunction.

Zona-intact domestic cat oocytes also are useful for studying the mechanisms controlling ovum pen-

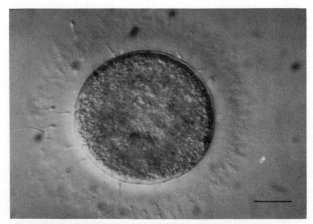

Figure 7. Homologous penetration of a zona-intact domestic cat oocyte. Cat spermatozoa are visible within the zona pellucida. *Scale bar* on photomicrograph represents 30 μm.

etration in nondomestic felids (Howard and Wildt, 1990). Leopard cat spermatozoa are capable of penetrating domestic cat oocytes *in vitro*, and penetration rates are almost identical to that observed in normospermic domestic cats. Unlike most nondomestic felids, leopard cats generally produce a high proportion of structurally normal spermatozoa (65% normal sperm/ejaculate), which is similar to the incidence observed in normospermic domestic cats. In the context of the cat oocyte assay, this observation suggests that mechanisms controlling sperm-ovum interaction between these two species are extremely conserved.

The zona-free hamster ovum and zona-intact cat oocyte bioassays provide two important tools for studying fertilization in cats. When combined with conventional seminal analyses data, an improved assessment of potential fertility is possible while providing a detailed understanding of the events controlling reproductive success in felids.

SPERM PROCESSING FOR ARTIFICIAL BREEDING

Sperm Processing for *In Vitro* Fertilization

The first successful IVF of cat oocytes was reported in 1970 using ovulated oocytes and ejaculated spermatozoa capacitated *in utero*. Ductus deferens spermatozoa suspended in a modified BSW or a modified Ham's F-10 medium also have been used for IVF of ovulated oocytes. The early events of IVF including the formation of the male pronucleus have been studied with epididymal spermatozoa. Spermatozoa from the caudae epididymides were diluted in mKRB medium and placed with ova in a 5% carbon dioxide in air, humidified environment at 37°C and allowed to culture for 0.25 to 5 hr. Under these conditions, ovum penetration occurred within 30 min, followed by decondensation of sperm heads and male pronucleus formation 3 to 4 hr after insemination.

In our laboratories, we have demonstrated the developmental competence of unovulated, follicular oocytes fertilized with electroejaculated spermatozoa processed by the swim-up procedure (Goodrowe et al., 1989). Follicular development and oocyte maturation were induced by a single injection of pregnant mare's serum gonadotropin (PMSG, Sigma Chemical) and human chorionic gonadotropin (hCG, Sigma Chemical), respectively. Oocytes were collected by laparoscopic transabdominal aspiration of ovarian follicles. Following dilution of spermatozoa in mKRB medium, centrifugation, and a 1-hr swim-up incubation at 25°C, gametes were mixed and co-cultured at 37°C for 24 to 30 hr. The results of this study indicated that fertilization rates are influenced by the interval between PMSG and hCG

injections, apparently because of intrafollicular maturation before oocyte recovery. Two- and four-cell embryos, transferred surgically into the oviducts of oocyte donors, are biologically competent as demonstrated by the births of live young.

Sperm Processing for Artificial Insemination

Pregnancies have resulted in domestic cats after artificial insemination (AI) with fresh and frozen-thawed semen. Vaginal insemination of 100 μl of fresh saline-diluted semen containing 1.25 to 50×10^6 spermatozoa has been performed in natural estrous queens induced to ovulate with 50 IU hCG (Sojka et al., 1970). Single inseminations coincident with the hCG injection result in a 50% conception rate, and the rate is increased to 75% if a second insemination follows 24 hr later.

Platz and colleagues (1978) demonstrated that cat spermatozoa are capable of surviving freezing and of producing live young after AI. Semen collected by electroejaculation or the use of an AV was mixed with a cryodiluent at room temperature using a 1:1 semen-to-diluent (v/v) ratio. The diluent consisted of 20% (v/v) egg yolk, 11% (v/v) lactose, and 4% (v/v) glycerol in distilled water. After a 20-min equilibration at 5°C, additional diluent was added and the sample was equilibrated (5°C) for an additional 10 min before pellet freezing. The pellet method of freezing involved pipetting single drops of the diluted semen into 3 × 4-mm indentations in a block of solid carbon dioxide, followed by deposition of pellets into a bath of liquid nitrogen. For AI, pellets were thawed in saline (37°C) and deposited (50 to 100×10^6 motile sperm per inseminant) into the vagina of anesthetized queens either in natural or gonadotropin-induced estrus. Ovulation was stimulated by mating with a vasectomized male or by administering hCG (250 to 500 IU). Although post-thaw motility ratings ranged from 54 to 71%, conception rate was low (10.6%), perhaps as a result of gonadotropin-induced ovarian hyperstimulation, asynchrony between insemination and ovulation, or the use of an anesthetic during insemination.

In our laboratories, the timing of insemination with respect to ovulation has been evaluated in anesthetized, gonadotropin-stimulated females. Queens were administered 100 IU PMSG and 75 or 100 IU hCG to stimulate follicular development and induce ovulation, respectively. A laparoscopic intrauterine AI technique, developed for carnivores (Howard et al., 1991[b,c]), was used to compare conception rates in cats inseminated either before or after ovulation. Each female was anesthetized with ketamine HCl and acepromazine 25 to 50 hr after hCG for assessment of ovulation (presumed to occur 28 to 30 hr after hCG) and insemination. Preovulatory females produced an average of 10.5

± 1.1 follicles and no corpora lutea (CL), compared with 1.9 ± 0.5 follicles and 7.5 ± 0.9 CL for the postovulatory females. Six days later, assessment of ovarian activity and embryo development revealed that cats in the preovulatory group produced significantly fewer CL (2.8 ± 1.5) and embryos (0.4 ± 0.3) than postovulatory females (18.9 ± 3.3 CL; 4.6 ± 1.2 embryos). In queens allowed to complete gestation, a 14% pregnancy rate resulted in cats inseminated before ovulation, whereas a 50% pregnancy rate was achieved in females inseminated after ovulation. These data indicate that the preovulatory administration of anesthesia compromises ovulation in cats subjected to AI. Performing laparoscopic AI after ovulation results in embryos capable of developing into live young.

CONCLUSION

An understanding of reproductive traits in cats including semen characteristics, hormonal traits, and gamete physiology is a prerequisite for developing reproductive techniques potentially useful for fertility assessment and enhanced reproduction. Procedures developed for assessing sperm function using heterologous and homologous ova are useful for studying factors influencing fertilization in domestic cats.

References and Suggested Reading

Goodrowe, K. L., Howard, J. G., Schmidt, P. M., et al.: The reproductive biology of the domestic cat with special reference to endocrinology, sperm function and in vitro fertilization. J. Reprod. Fertil. 39:73, 1989. *A review of the reproductive biology of cats, including sperm function and IVF.*

Howard, J. G., Barone, A. M., et al.: Preovulatory anesthesia compromises ovulation in laparoscopically inseminated domestic cats. J. Reprod. Fertil. 1991(c).

Howard, J. G., Brown, J. L., Bush, M., et al.: Teratospermic and normospermic domestic cats: Ejaculate traits, pituitary-gonadal hormones, and improvement of spermatozoal motility and morphology after swim-up processing. J. Androl. 11:204, 1990. *Reproductive traits in teratospermic and normospermic domestic cats.*

Howard, J. G., Bush, M., Hall, L. L., et al.: Morphological abnormalities in spermatozoa of 28 species of non-domestic felids. Proceedings of the 10th International Congress of Animal Reproduction and Artificial Insemination 2:57, 1984. *Incidence of structurally abnormal spermatozoa in 28 species of non-domestic felids.*

Howard, J. G., Bush, M., and Wildt, D. E.: Teratospermia in domestic cats compromises penetration of zona-free hamster ova and cat zonae pellucidae. J. Androl. 12:36, 1991(a). *Influence of teratospermia on ovum penetration in domestic cats.*

Howard, J. G., Bush, M., Morton, C., et al.: Comparative semen cryopreservation in ferrets and pregnancies after laparoscopic intrauterine insemination with frozen-thawed spermatozoa. J. Reprod. Fertil. 92:109, 1991(b). *Description of laparoscopic intrauterine AI technique.*

Howard, J. G., Wildt, D. E.: Ejaculate-hormonal traits in the leopard cat (Felis bengalensis) and sperm function as measured by in vitro penetration of zona-free hamster ova and zona-intact domestic cat oocytes. Mol. Reprod. Devel. 26:163, 1990. *Use of zona-free hamster ova and zona-intact domestic cat oocytes to assess sperm function in the leopard cat.*

Platz, C. C., Wildt, D. E., and Seager, S. W. J.: Pregnancy in the domestic cat after artificial insemination with previously frozen spermatozoa. J. Reprod. Fertil. 52:279, 1978. *Characteristics of cat semen collected by AV and electroejaculation are described, as well as pregnancy in cats with frozen-thawed spermatozoa.*

Sojka, N. J., Jennings, L. L., and Hamner, C. E.: Artificial insemination in the cat (Felis catus). Lab. Anim. Care 20:198, 1970. *Characteristics of cat semen collected by an AV.*

Wildt, D. E., Bush, M., Goodrowe, K. L., et al.: Reproductive and genetic consequences of founding isolated lion populations. Nature 329:328, 1987. *Influence of reduced genetic variation on reproductive traits in male lions.*

Wildt, D. E., Bush, M., Howard, J. G., et al.: Unique seminal quality in the South African cheetah and a comparative evaluation in the domestic cat. Biol. Reprod. 29:1019, 1983. *A comparison of seminal traits in the cheetah and domestic cat.*

COLLECTION AND EVALUATION OF CANINE SEMEN

PATRICIA N. OLSON

St. Paul, Minnesota

The World Health Organization has published a manual for the examination of human semen (WHO, 1987). Although some of the published guidelines are not applicable for evaluating canine semen, many suggested procedures can be standardized and used in a small animal practice. By adhering to a standardized procedure, consistency may be achieved in collecting and evaluating semen samples from dogs, allowing for meaningful interpretation of results. Reproductive dysfunction should never be diagnosed on the basis of an incomplete ejaculate, poor collection techniques, or improper handling of the sample.

SAMPLE COLLECTION

The length of sexual abstinence prior to collection should be recorded. Because daily sperm output decreases with frequent ejaculation (Olar et al., 1983), total numbers of sperm in the ejaculate can vary with length of abstinence.

At least two semen samples should be obtained before suggesting a dog has abnormal semen quality. Ideally, the samples should be obtained at least 48 hours apart.

The semen sample should be collected in a quiet room. The presence of a teaser bitch may facilitate the collection process. Anestrous bitches frequently serve as excellent teasers, especially if methylparaben is applied to the vulvar region (Goodwin et al., 1979). Owners should be allowed to observe the collection procedure, especially if the dog is apprehensive when the owner is absent. Conversely, other dogs may give a better sample when the owner is absent.

The sample should be obtained by using a latex or polystyrene artificial vagina attached to a glass or plastic tube. All equipment used for the collection process should be evaluated for toxic effects on spermatozoa. Lubricants are generally not necessary for semen collection; some lubricants are spermatocidal to canine spermatozoa (Froman and Amann, 1983). All equipment should be sterile or disinfected. Methods of sterilization or sanitization should be evaluated for possible deleterious effects on sperm.

Incomplete samples should not be evaluated or overinterpreted if evaluated. Spermatozoa may be absent in semen samples obtained from dogs that ejaculate only the presperm fraction (i.e., frightened dogs, dogs with pain).

For complete evaluation, a semen sample should consist of one tube (T-1) that contains the presperm and sperm-rich fraction and a second tube (T-2) that contains prostatic fluid. Prostatic fluid can be easily collected from most dogs by maintaining pressure over the bulbus glandis after the first two fractions have passed. By replacing the first tube with a second collection tube, prostatic fluid can be collected and evaluated separately. A third tube (T-3) can be attached and an additional 1 ml of prostatic fluid collected for culturing, if deemed necessary, for evaluating prostatic disorders.

The sample should be protected from temperature extremes during the collection process. Ideally, equipment should be warmed to 37°C before use to avoid temperature extremes.

The sample should be labeled with the dog's name, the date, and time of collection.

HANDLING AND EVALUATION OF SAMPLES

Handling

Laboratory technicians should be informed that semen samples present a possible biohazard. Although unlikely, samples containing various *Brucella* spp. could pose a human health hazard.

Evaluation

APPEARANCE

The semen sample is first evaluated by simple visual inspection. The T-1 sample should be cream to white in color and homogenous in appearance. A clear or slightly cloudy sample may indicate azoospermia or oligozoospermia. Hematospermia frequently suggests prostatic disease or traumatic collection. A yellow sample may imply contamination of semen with urine. The T-2 sample should appear clear (i.e., have the appearance of water). The presence of blood in T-2 frequently suggests prostatic disease.

VOLUME

The volume of the T-1 sample should be measured. This is easily accomplished if the attached collection tube is graduated. The volume of T-1 will be necessary to calculate the total number of spermatozoa in the ejaculate. Volume need not be recorded for the T-2 sample, since the volume of prostatic fluid varies depending on length of collection. Only 1 to 2 ml of prostatic fluid need be collected for evaluation.

pH

A drop of the T-1 sample is spread evenly onto pH paper (range of pH paper to use: 5.5 to 8.5). Likewise, a drop of the T-2 sample is evaluated for pH.

MOTILITY

A drop from the T-1 sample is placed on a precleaned and warmed microscope slide. A precleaned and warmed coverslip is placed on the drop of sample. Progressive motility should be evaluated immediately by using a phase-contrast microscope with ×20 and ×40 objective lenses. If a phase-contrast microscope is unavailable, progressive motility can be estimated if the light passing through the condenser of a conventional microscope is decreased enough that spermatozoa can be adequately visualized. Progressive motility should be estimated to the nearest 10%. Progressively motile spermatozoa should move along a straight path. Spermatozoa merely rotating or circling in a field with a small radius are not progressively motile. The sample may need to be diluted 1:1 with phosphate-buffered saline at 37°C (pH of 7.5) to estimate the percentage of progressively motile spermatozoa in concentrated samples.

Spermatozoa should also be evaluated for agglutination. Agglutination means that motile spermatozoa stick to each other (head to head, midpiece to midpiece, tail to tail, midpiece to tail, and so forth). The adherence of immotile or motile spermatozoa to mucous threads, cells other than spermatozoa, or debris is not considered agglutination and should not be recorded as such.

CONCENTRATION

The T-1 sample should be gently mixed. A fixed volume of semen (20 μl) should be placed into 1.98 ml of diluent (Unopette-TM for WBC, Becton Dickinson). After mixing, a hemocytometer chamber is loaded with the diluent that contains the sample. The number of spermatozoa in one primary square of a hemocytometer grid containing nine primary squares is counted; this number equals the number of spermatozoa (in millions) per 1.0 ml of sample.

TOTAL SPERM NUMBER

The total number of spermatozoa in T-1 can be determined by multiplying the concentration by the volume (see earlier).

SPERM MORPHOLOGY

Sperm morphology can be evaluated by using various stains and conventional light microscopy or phase-contrast microscopy without prior staining. Using conventional light microscopy, one method of evaluating morphology is to place a small drop of the T-1 sample and a small drop of an eosin-nigrosin stain (Hancock's stain, Lane Manufacturing, Denver, CO) on one edge of a microscope slide. Then, with a second slide, the two drops are gently mixed and spread across the first slide. A second method

is to prepare semen smears similar to blood films, letting the smear air dry after preparation. The smear is then placed for 5 minutes into each of the three components (fixative, solution 1, and solution 2) of a rapid Wright's-Giemsa's stain (Diff-Quik, Scientific Products). The smear is then rinsed gently with water and allowed to air dry, or it can be blotted dry. Both methods described allow for adequate staining of spermatozoa to evaluate morphology. One hundred sperm cells should be evaluated and categorized using at least 1000 × magnification (oil immersion).

OTHER CELLS

Using a protocol similar to that for preparing and staining blood films, smears can be made from T-1 and T-2 samples and stained with a rapid Wright's-Giemsa's stain (Diff-Quik, Scientific Products). Smears should be evaluated for erythrocytes, inflammatory cells, epithelial cells, and bacteria. Samples that appear to be acellular can be centrifuged so that the sediment can be smeared, stained, and evaluated.

OPTIONAL TESTS

Semen Culture

Semen samples (T-1) collected aseptically can be cultured for various microorganisms. Because bacteria and mycoplasma are normal inhabitants of the canine prepuce and urethra, positive cultures must be interpreted cautiously.

Prostatic Fluid Culture

Prostatic fluid (T-2) can be collected aseptically and cultured if septic prostatitis or prostatic dysfunction seems likely based on physical examination and cytologic evaluation of prostatic fluid.

Epididymal Markers

There are various biochemical markers that can be measured to differentiate secretory azoospermia (gonadal dysfunction) from obstructive azoospermia (bilateral blockage of epididymides or ductus deferens). Two such markers are carnitine and alkaline phosphatase.

Measuring Immunoglobulins in Semen

Various methods for evaluating the presence of sperm antibodies in seminal fluid have been used

Table 1. Influence of Body Weight on the Reproductive Capacity of Adult Dog†*

Characteristic	Body Weight (lb)		
	10–34	35–39	60–84
Total scrotal testes width (mm)	36 ± 2‖	50 ± 1¶	56 ± 1**
Paired testes weight (gm)	16 ± 1‖	31 ± 1¶	44 ± 2**
DSP/gm parenchyma (10^6)	20 ± 2	17 ± 1	20 ± 3
DSP/dog (10^6)	287 ± 33	472 ± 32	750 ± 111
Extragonadal spermatozoal reserves (10^9) at sexual rest			
Caput epididymidis	0.07 ± 0.01	0.23 ± 0.04	0.23 ± 0.05
Corpus epididymidis	1.10 ± 0.18	1.85 ± 0.16	2.27 ± 0.24
Cauda epididymidis	2.06 ± 0.31	3.30 ± 0.36	4.68 ± 0.39
Ductus deferens‡	0.06 ± 0.02	0.21 ± 0.03	0.23 ± 0.04
Semen ejaculated after sexual rest			
Volume (ml)§	2.4 ± 0.3	3.9 ± 0.5	5.4 ± 1.3
Concentration (10^6/ml)§	209 ± 42	359 ± 72	228 ± 58
Total sperm (10^9)	0.4 ± 0.11	1.12 ± 0.13	1.43 ± 0.46

*Reprinted with permission from Amann, R. P.: Reproductive physiology and endocrinology of the dog. *In* Morrow, D. A. (ed.): *Current Therapy in Theriogenology* 2. Philadelphia: W. B. Saunders, 1986, p. 536.

†Mean (± SEM) for 30, 53, and 32 dogs in the 10–34, 35–59, and 60–84 lb groups, but data on extragonadal spermatozoal reserves are for 17, 32, and 14 dogs and data for characteristics of a single ejaculate collected after ≥ 7 days of sexual rest are for 12, 14, and 11 dogs, respectively. DSP = daily spermatozoal production. For a characteristic, means without a superscript symbol (§, ‖, ¶,**) or with the same superscript symbol are not different (p>.05).

‡Not all of the ductus deferens was available for dogs castrated rather than euthanized.

§The presperm and sperm-rich fractions were collected together, but ejaculation was terminated when ejaculation of the postsperm prostatic fluid started.

for evaluating human semen samples. Unfortunately, similar methods have not been critically evaluated for dogs.

NORMAL VALUES OF SEMEN VARIABLES

Presperm + Sperm-Rich Fraction (T-1)

Appearance: cream to white, opaque
Volume: varies, depending on breed and contribution of prostatic fluid
pH: 6.0 to 7.0
Motility: ≥ 70%
Concentration: varies, depending on contribution of prostatic fluid
Total sperm: ≥ 250 million spermatozoa; increased numbers with large breeds (Table 1)
Morphology: ≥ 200 million spermatozoa with normal morphology (5)
Semen culture: variable
Epididymal markers: carnitine > 100 nmol/ml for T-1; alkaline phosphatase > 1000 IU/L for T-1 (Note: presperm fraction has low concentration of alkaline phosphatase, as can be seen in Table 2.)
Immunoglobulins: ?

Prostatic Fraction (T-2)

Appearance: clear
Volume: varies, depending on length of collection time

pH: 6.5 to 7.0
Cytology: acellular
Culture: < 100 CFU/ml if aseptically collected and fractionated (T-3)

NOMENCLATURE FOR SOME SEMEN VARIABLES

Normozoospermia—normal ejaculate

Oligozoospermia—sperm number < 100 million/ejaculate

Asthenozoospermia—abnormal, reduced, or absent motility

Teratozoospermia—< 50% spermatozoa with normal morphology

Oligoasthenoteratozoospermia—signifies disturbance

*Table 2. Concentrations of Alkaline Phosphatase in Seminal Fluid (IU/L)**

Presperm	Sperm-rich	Prostatic
15	31,510	4,337
79	17,140	18
84	15,720	934
48	94,310	113
10	10,780	1,658
16	14,370	141
3	251	8
67	30,120	799

*Reprinted with permission from Olson, P.N. Exfoliative cytology of the canine reproductive tract. Proc. Soc. Theriogenology, Coeur d'Alene, ID, 1989, p. 274.

n = 8 samples/8 dogs.

Evaluation Form for Canine Semen

Name of owner _____ Date _____

Address _____

Name of dog _____ Reg # _____

Date of birth _____ Breed _____

Previous litters sired and date(s) _____
_____

Pedigree available _____ Libido (0–4) _____

Reason for evaluation _____

Brucella canis status _____ Previous evaluation _____

Method of collection: _____ AV _____ Other _____ Teaser bitch

Progressive motility: _____ % Diluent used _____

Volume: pH

    Fraction 1 + 2 (T-1) _____ ml   _____

    Fraction 3 (T-2) _____ ml   _____

Concentration:
    Fraction 1 + 2 (T-1) _____ /ml

Total sperm number/ejaculate _____

Morphology (100-cell differential)
  Percent
    Normal _____

    Macrocephalic head _____

    Microcephalic head _____

    Pyriform head _____

    Amorphous head _____

    Detached head _____

    Duplicate head _____

    Abnormal acrosome _____

    Tapered head _____

    Multiple tails _____

    Abaxial attachment _____

    Thickened midpiece _____

    Cytoplasmic droplet
      Proximal _____

      Distal _____

    Bent principal piece _____

    Coiled principal piece _____

    Midpiece reflex _____

    Dag defect _____

    Bowed midpiece _____

Cytologic findings/culture results

  Fraction 1 + 2 (T-1): _____
_____
_____

  Fraction 3 (T-2): _____
_____

Comments : _____
_____

Figure 1. Sample form for evaluating canine semen.

of all three variables (combination of only two prefixes may also be used)

Azoospermia—no spermatozoa in the ejaculate

Aspermia—no ejaculate

DEFINING SOME SEMEN VARIABLES

The *sperm structure* consists of the sperm head and tail. The sperm tail includes the midpiece, the principal piece, and the end piece.

Abnormal spermatozoa have malformations of either the head or tail. Head abnormalities include duplicate head, macrocephalic head, microcephalic head, pyriform head, tapered head, amorphous head, detached head, and abnormal acrosome (knobbed acrosome). Tail abnormalities include midpiece reflex, bent principal piece, the Dag defect, thickened midpiece, bowed midpiece, coiled principal piece, abaxial tail, multiple tail, proximal droplet, and distal droplet. (Note: Although abnormal spermatozoa can be identified and quantitated, correlation of fertility with specific defects has not been critically studied in the dog.)

Other abnormal cells include immature germ cells, neutrophils, lymphocytes, plasma cells, and erythrocytes. (Note: Numbers of inflammatory cells anticipated in normal canine semen have not been determined.)

EVALUATION FORM FOR CANINE SEMEN

Figure 1 presents a sample form for evaluating canine semen. A standardized form for evaluating canine semen is currently being prepared by the Society for Theriogenology and the American College of Theriogenologists. Readers' suggestions for the standardized form would be appreciated.

References and Suggested Reading

Froman, D. P., and Amann, R. P.: Inhibition of motility of bovine, canine, and equine spermatozoa by artificial vagina lubricants. Theriogenology 20:357, 1983.

Goodwin, M., Gooding, K. M., and Regnier, F.: Sex pheromone in the dog. Science 203:559, 1979.

Mickelsen, W. D.: Relationship of total morphologic normal spermatozoa to fertility with artificial insemination in the bitch. Proc. Soc. Theriogenology, Orlando, FL, 1988, p. 387.

Olar, T. T., Amann, R. P., and Pickett, B. W.: Relationships among testicular size, daily production and output of spermatozoa, and extragonadal spermatozoal reserves of the dog. Biol. Reprod. 29:1114, 1983.

World Health Organization: Collection and examination of human semen. *In WHO Laboratory Manual for the Examination of Human Semen and Semen-Cervical Mucus Interaction.* Cambridge: Cambridge University Press, 1987.

USE OF SERUM PROGESTERONE ELISA TESTS IN CANINE BREEDING MANAGEMENT

REBECCA L. HEGSTAD
and SHIRLEY D. JOHNSTON
St. Paul, Minnesota

Two days before ovulation in a bitch, at the time of the luteinizing hormone (LH) surge, serum progesterone concentrations increase from nondetectable levels to approximately 2 ng/ml (6.36 nmol/L) (Concannon et al., 1989). When progesterone concentration is measured frequently during proestrus, this increase can be identified and used to predict day of ovulation. Knowledge about ovulation date provides important information for several aspects of canine breeding management. Conception rate and litter size using natural or artificial insemination with fresh or frozen semen can be optimized when ovulation date is known, and insemination can then be achieved 2 to 3 days after ovulation. Gestation length in a bitch is 62 to 64 days from ovulation, so parturition date can be predicted accurately when ovulation data is known. Proestrus or estrus onset is not a reliable predictor of ovulation date, and methods other than serum progesterone assay (laparoscopy or serum LH measurement) are not readily available to clinicians.

Measurement of canine serum progesterone concentration by radioimmunoassay (RIA) may be limited by laboratory access, expense, and long turnaround times. Rapid enzyme-linked immunosorbent assays (ELISA) are now available for in-house measurement of canine serum progesterone concentration. These assays typically require 0.5 ml of serum, involve six to eight simple steps, and can be completed in 15 to 60 min. Use of these ELISA kits will enhance opportunities for small animal clinical practices to become more actively involved in the canine breeding management concerns of their clients.

ELISA TEST KITS

ELISA Test Principles

ELISA, like RIA, is based on competitive absorption of endogenous serum progesterone and exogenous enzyme-labeled progesterone to progesterone-specific antibody. In most ELISA kits, progesterone antibody is coated on tubes, cups, or microtiter plate wells. Progesterone in the sample (standard, control, or unknown) and a constant amount of enzyme-labeled progesterone compete for antibody-binding sites in proportion to their concentration during a short incubation period (typically 1 to 30 min). The greater the progesterone concentration in the test sample, the lower the antibody binding of enzyme-labeled progesterone. A series of washing steps removes unbound enzyme-labeled hormone, and a substrate solution, specific for the enzyme label, is added. After a second short incubation (1 to 30 min), a substrate-induced change in color or color intensity occurs; it is proportional to the amount of (antibody-bound) enzyme-labeled progesterone and inversely proportional to progesterone concentration in the sample. Test samples that contain high progesterone concentration show little or no color change, and samples with low progesterone concentration produce a deep color result. Quantitative ELISA tests require a microtiter plate reader and spectrophotometer to determine absorbency levels of reference standards and samples, which are then translated into exact progesterone concentration. Qualitative ELISA assays use visual comparison of color intensity between sample and control sera results to determine general concentration ranges of progesterone (low, medium, or high) in each sample. Blue end points are frequently used. Control sera (included in qualitative kits) contain low progesterone concentrations and result in bright blue end points. When compared with a low progesterone control (blue result), samples producing light blue or white (or clear) results indicate medium or high progesterone concentration ranges, respectively. Sample results that are as blue as or darker blue than control results are interpreted as containing low concentrations of progesterone.

ELISA Kits Available for Use in Dogs

Qualitative and quantitative ELISA kits that currently are available for progesterone determinations in a bitch are listed in Table 1. Cost per sample depends on the test used and the number of tests performed at one time. Kits shown have a shelf life of approximately 1 year. All three kits are affected by temperature, and it is important that reagents and samples be at room temperature when samples are tested. Strict adherence to assay protocols is necessary for optimal results. Incubation intervals that are longer or shorter than those recommended may cause errors, and improper washing or reagent contamination may produce nonspecific color development.

With the ICAGEN-Target Kit (International Canine Genetics, Malvern, PA), an aliquot of serum or low-progesterone control is dispensed into the center of a small cup that contains a disk treated with monoclonal progesterone antibody. Results are determined after addition of reagents and incubations as directed in the kit instructions. After a final 9-min incubation period, progesterone concentration range is denoted by color of the cup disk; samples producing a strong blue, light blue, or white end point mean "low" (between 0.0 and 1.0 ng/ml [0.0 and 3.18 nmol/L]), "medium" (approximately 2.0 ng/ml [6.36 nmol/L]), or "high" (5.0 ng/ml [15.9 nmol/L] or greater) progesterone concentration, respectively. For determination of the LH surge, the first appearance of a sample producing a distinct fading of color from a strong blue to a light blue end point signals the initial progesterone rise from less than 1.0 ng/ml (3.18 nmol/L) to about 2.0 ng/ml (6.36 nmol/L), which is coincident with and indicative of the LH surge.

The Estrucheck kit (Synbiotics, San Diego, CA) contains individually detachable clear acrylic microtiter wells that have been coated with a monoclonal progesterone antibody and arranged in strips. A holder is included for well manipulation, and a maximum of five tests (including the control) can be run at one time. A low-progesterone control included in the kit produces a deep blue test result. Samples with similar blue results contain low progesterone, and samples with little or no color contain intermediate or high progesterone concentrations, respectively. Presence of the LH surge is determined by first occurrence of a sample well that is lighter in color than the progesterone control well.

The Ovusure Plasma/Serum Progesterone 96-Well Kit (Cambridge Veterinary Sciences, Littleport, Ely, U.K.) contains a microtiter plate consisting of a plastic frame with six plastic strips, each containing 16 wells coated with a polyclonal progesterone antibody. Included is a set of four progesterone standards (0.5, 1.0, 5.0, and 10.0 ng/ml [1.59

Table 1. Characteristics of ELISA Kits Available for Measurement of Canine Serum Progesterone Concentrations

	ICAGEN—Target	Estrucheck	Ovusure Plasma/Serum Progesterone 96-Well Kit
Assay type	Qualitative	Qualitative	Quantitative
Sample	Serum, plasma	Serum	Serum, plasma
Time requirement	15–30 min	20 min	60 min
Number of steps	6	6	6
Test interpretation	Color comparison with low-progesterone control	Color comparison with low-progesterone control	Spectrophotometer reading of optical density of samples and standards
Maximum number of tests	12	10	16–92
Suggested retail kit price	$72	$85.50	$155
Extra items needed	None	Wash bottle, saline, or distilled or deionized water	10, 200 μl pipettes Spectrophotometer, plate reader
Storage and maximum shelf life	Refrigeration, 1 year	Refrigeration, 1 year	Refrigeration, 1 year
Special instructions	Kit and sample must be at room temperature before use	Kit and sample must be at room temperature before use	Kit and sample must be at room temperature before use
Manufacturer	International Canine Genetics, Inc. 271 Great Valley Parkway Malvern, PA 19355 (215) 640-1244 (800) 248-8099	Synbiotics Company 11011 Via Frontera San Diego, CA 92127 (619) 451-3770 (800) 247-1725	Cambridge Veterinary Sciences Henry Crabb Row Littleport, Ely Cambridgeshire, England CB6-1SE 011-44-353-861-911

to 31.8 nmol/L]) used for constructing a standard curve of optical absorbance versus concentration value. Precise progesterone concentration (nanograms per milliliter) in the unknowns is determined from this standard curve. The assay can be completed within about an hour and requires precision pipettes, a plate reader, and a spectrophotometer.

ACCURACY OF ELISA KITS COMPARED WITH RIA

Progesterone results from canine serum samples reported using ELISA kits developed for measurement of bovine plasma progesterone (Dieleman and Blankenstein, 1988; Eckersall and Harvey, 1987; England et al., 1989) and preliminary data from our laboratory using a canine progesterone ELISA kit (Hegstad and Johnston, 1989) indicate that these kits are fairly reliable for determining the preovulatory rise in progesterone in canine serum.

Significant correlations between canine progesterone concentration measured by RIA and by quantitative bovine progesterone ELISA kits have been reported (Eckersall and Harvey, 1987; England et al., 1989), and in one study, mean recovery of progesterone added to canine plasma and measured by quantitative ELISA was 97% (Eckersall and Harvey, 1987).

Manufacturers of the ICAGEN-Target ELISA test suggest in the kit instructions that estimation of the LH surge has an accuracy of ± 1 day when samples are tested using their kit every other day.

Accuracy information related to use of Estrucheck or Ovusure ELISA kits with canine samples is not included in kit documentations, and data using these techniques have not been reported in the literature.

Preliminary data comparing the qualitative ICAGEN-Target ELISA kit and samples measured by RIA have been reported. Known concentrations of progesterone (0.5 to 15.0 ng/ml [1.59 to 47.7 nmol/L]) were added to canine serum and measured using both techniques. At all concentrations tested, ELISA results accurately estimated progesterone concentration (Hegstad and Johnston, 1989).

In addition, progesterone concentration in 100 canine serum samples measured by RIA and ICAGEN-Target ELISA agreed in 89 of 100 samples (Johnston, S. D., Manothaiudom, K., and Hegstad, R. L., unpublished data, 1990). Results measured by RIA were not significantly different from those measured using the ELISA kit. Eleven errors occurred when ELISA test color indicated a higher (false-positive) or lower (false-negative) progesterone concentration than was measured by RIA. All errors occurred in categories one level above or below the true value. No samples determined by ELISA to be high (> 5.0 ng/ml [15.9 nmol/L]) were really low (between 0 and 1 ng/ml [0.0 and 3.18 nmol/L]), and vice versa. Frequencies of false-positive (6 of 11) and false-negative (5 of 11) errors were similar, and the highest error rate of 20% (15% false-positives + 5% false-negatives) occurred in the group of samples classified by ELISA as containing medium progesterone concentration. Successful use of this ELISA for detecting rising

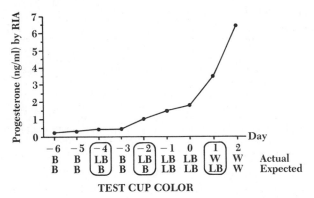

Figure 1. Serial serum progesterone concentrations in one bitch before and after progesterone rise to approximately 2 ng/ml as detected by the ICAGEN-Target ELISA kit. Day 0, defined by the kit manufacturer as the first day progesterone is approximately 2 ng/ml, is indicated by the first appearance of a light blue ELISA result. ELISA results not in agreement with radioimmunossay (RIA) results (errors) are highlighted. *B*, strong blue (0.0 to 1.0 ng/ml); *LB*, light blue (approximately 2.0 ng/ml); *W*, white (>5.0 ng/ml).

progesterone concentration at the time of the LH surge depends on the change in test cup color from blue (low) to light blue (medium). The error rate in samples known to contain progesterone concentrations between 1 and 5 ng/ml (3.18 and 15.9 nmol/L) indicates that use of this technique on a single sample at the time of the LH surge may result in 20% error. Such error may result in decisions to breed a bitch too early (based on a false-positive error) or too late (based on a false-negative error). A similar error rate has been reported in a study of 28 bitches; 74.3% agreement occurred between breeding decisions based on RIA and an ELISA kit developed for use in cows. It was determined that 18.9% of the dogs may have been bred too late based on the ELISA results (Dieleman and Blankenstein, 1988).

Reagent contamination, failure to follow method protocol, temperature (environment, reagents, sample) considerations, or use of expired reagents may contribute to ELISA errors. Frequency and impact of errors may be minimized by serial testing (every day or every other day), as recommended by kit manufacturers.

Daily ICAGEN-Target test results and true progesterone concentration in serum from an intact bitch near time of ovulation are shown in Figure 1. Day 0 was defined as the first day progesterone concentration was greater than or equal to 2 ng/ml (6.36 nmol/L) when measured by RIA. In this example, light blue test results occurred 4 and 2 days before the true day 0 and were false-positive errors. Daily testing may enhance the user's ability to detect errors and increase accuracy but is also more expensive for the client.

HOW TO USE CANINE PROGESTERONE ELISA KITS TO TIME OVULATION IN CLINICAL PRACTICE

Progesterone determination by RIA, if available, is more accurate and precise than by ELISA. However, when RIA technology is not readily available or convenient, ELISA kits provide a useful tool for detecting progesterone concentration in a bitch. The following steps are recommended for detecting the serum progesterone increase indicative of the preovulatory LH surge in a bitch using the qualitative in-house ELISA kits (see Table 1).

1. Determine when to start testing.
   a. Based on proestrus onset: Test at least one serum sample early in proestrus (3 to 4 days after onset of bloody vaginal discharge) to confirm low progesterone concentration. Continue testing every other day (or daily) until a color change is observed.
   b. Based on vaginal cytologic examination: Begin testing serum progesterone concentration every other day (or daily), starting when exfoliated vaginal epithelial cells become 50 to 60% cornified.
   c. Based on previous cycle information: If day of ovulation of a previous cycle is known (from previous pregnancy, vaginal cytologic diestrus onset, or previous serum progesterone concentration), begin testing serum progesterone concentration 2 to 4 days before the expected day of ovulation.
2. Continue testing and identify the day of the LH surge.
   a. Test daily or every other day.
   b. Compare the low-progesterone control (blue) result with the sample result.
   c. Look for a distinct fading of color from blue to light blue in the sample.
   d. The first occurrence of a definite decrease in sample color intensity is an indicator of the LH surge.
   e. Count the day of the LH surge as day 0.
3. Use ELISA results to estimate ovulation date and optimal breeding period based on the day of LH surge (day 0).
   a. From day 0, count forward 2 days to estimate ovulation date.
   b. From ovulation date, count forward 2 to 4 days to determine optimal breeding dates.
4. To confirm the presence of postovulatory progesterone concentration (white or clear results), test on at least one breeding day.

OTHER USES OF CANINE ELISA PROGESTERONE TESTS

In addition to using rising serum progesterone concentration as an indicator of the coincident LH surge and subsequent ovulation, changing progesterone concentration is a useful monitor of other reproductive events involved in small animal breeding management issues.

Progesterone concentrations exceeding 2 ng/ml (6.36 nmol/L) are required for pregnancy maintenance; progesterone ELISA kits provide a simple method for monitoring progesterone concentration in bitches with impaired ability to maintain pregnancy.

Prediction date of parturition is more accurate when gestation length is timed from day of ovulation (based on progesterone concentration as described earlier) than from breeding date. In a study of 12 bitches, actual gestation lengths from ovulation date were 61 to 64 days, whereas gestation lengths from first breeding were 58 to 69 days (Johnston, S.D., Manothaiudom, K., and Hegstad, R.L., unpublished data, 1990).

Progesterone concentration, which exceeds 2 ng/ml (6.36 nmol/L) during pregnancy, declines to less than 2 ng/ml (6.36 nmol/L) 36 to 48 hr before whelping (Concannon et al., 1989). This decline or an absolute concentration in the low range using ELISA kits may, with other clinical information, provide support for a decision that parturition is imminent, that parturition is overdue, or that elective cesarean section can be performed safely.

Finally, serum progesterone concentration can be used to choose appropriate time for prostaglandin treatment or to monitor its effectiveness for pregnancy termination in a bitch. Within 24 to 48 hr of prostaglandin treatment, progesterone concentration should decrease from greater than 5 ng/ml (15.9 nmol/L) to less than 2 ng/ml (6.36 nmol/L). Prostaglandins have been reported to be effective at inducing luteolysis as early as the fifth day after onset of cytologic diestrus (Johnston, 1990; Oettle, et al., 1988). When time of breeding is unknown, progesterone measurement before prostaglandin treatment indicates whether ovulation has occurred, and measurement after treatment can be used to confirm the expected decline in progesterone concentration.

SUMMARY

Measurement of serum progesterone in a bitch enables a clinician to determine day of ovulation and make appropriate breeding management decisions. The ELISA kits currently available for measurement of progesterone in canine serum or plasma are fairly reliable, quick, and convenient. Skills needed to perform the assays are easily learned. The kits have a long shelf life and require very few extra materials to use. When available, RIA is the method of choice for progesterone assay because of its accuracy and precision. Although not as accurate as RIA, ELISA kits can provide a useful tool for in-house progesterone determinations, which can be incorporated into any small animal clinical setting.

References and Suggested Reading

Concannon, P. W., McCann, J. P., and Temple, M.: Biology and endocrinology of ovulation, pregnancy and parturition in the dog. J. Reprod. Fertil. 39(Suppl.):3, 1989.

Dieleman, S. J., and Blankenstein, D. M.: Determination of the time of ovulation in the dog by estimation of progesterone in blood: Applicability of an EIA method in comparison to RIA. Proceedings of the 11th International Congress on Animal Reproduction and Artificial Insemination. Dublin, Ireland, June 26–30, 1988, p. 21.

Eckersall, P. D., and Harvey, M. J. A.: The use of a bovine plasma progesterone ELISA kit to measure progesterone in equine, ovine and canine plasmas. Vet. Rec. 120:5, 1987.

England, G. C. W., Allen, W. E., and Porter, D. J.: A comparison of radioimmunoassay with quantitative and qualitative enzyme-linked immunoassay for plasma progestogen detection in bitches. Vet. Rec. 125:107, 1989.

Hegstad, R. L., and Johnston, S. D.: Use of a rapid, qualitative ELISA technique (Biometallics, Inc.) to determine serum progesterone concentrations in the bitch. Proc. Soc. Theriogenology Annual Meeting, Coeur d'Alene, ID, September 29–30, 1989, pp. 277–287.

Johnston, S. D.: Canine pregnancy termination with prostaglandin F2 alpha. Proc. Soc. Theriogenology Annual Meeting, Toronto, Ontario, Canada, August 10–11, 1990, pp. 264–269.

Oettle, E. E., Bertschinger, H. J., Botha, A. E., et al.: Luteolysis in early diestrous beagle bitches. Theriogenology 29:757, 1988.

INFERTILITY IN THE QUEEN

ALICE M. WOLF
College Station, Texas

It is important to be familiar with normal reproductive activity in the queen in order to evaluate reproductive performance and determine if infertility really exists. Estrus activity in queens can begin as early as 4 months of age; however, the domestic queen of mixed breeding usually begins estrus cycling at 7 to 9 months, and purebred queens often begin cycling from 9 to 12 months of age. Birman, Colorpoint, and some other long-hair queens tend to mature late and may not exhibit estrus until 18 months of age (Jemmett and Evans, 1977).

Optimal reproductive fertility in the queen occurs between 1 and 8 years of age. Younger cats often have irregular cycles and unpredictable breeding behavior. Older queens have reduced reproductive capacity and may have irregular estrus cycles, fewer litters per year, fewer kittens per litter, and more kittens with congenital defects.

Domestic cats are seasonally polyestrus, with the light cycle having a controlling effect on estrous cycling activity. Under natural lighting conditions in North America, most queens cycle from late winter to early fall. Artificial lighting conditions, with controlled exposure to 12 to 14 continuous hours of light per day, can be used to keep most queens cycling all year (Lein, 1986).

Cats are induced ovulators, and ovulation usually occurs within 48 hours postcoitus. The vaginal stimulation threshold required to stimulate luteinizing hormone release and induce ovulation in queens is quite variable. One breeding may be sufficient for some; other cats will require several breedings for induction of ovulation. Alternatively, spontaneous ovulation has been observed in a few queens.

Because of seasonal estrous cycling and induced ovulation, the estrous cycle of the queen is different from that of the bitch. Anestrus is the period of no ovarian activity that occurs only between estrous seasons usually from late fall to early winter. Proestrus may be difficult to detect because most queens do not show physical changes during this phase of the cycle. Some queens will have pollakiuria or a small amount of mucoid vaginal discharge during proestrus. Some proestrual queens will exhibit estrus-like behavior (see later) but will not be sexually receptive if placed with a male. The duration of proestrus is 1 to 3 days.

Estrus is the period of sexual receptivity and is detected primarily by behavioral changes such as vocalization ("calling"), rolling and rubbing against the owner or inanimate objects, and lordotic posturing. When an estrual queen is stroked over the back and tailhead, she may elevate her hindquarters, deviate the tail, and tread with her hind feet. Temporary anorexia or urine spraying also occurs in some estrual queens. Estrus lasts 1 to 21 days with an average of 7 to 10 days (Feldman and Nelson, 1987). Estrus activity ceases within 72 hours of ovulation in most queens.

Ovulation will alter the ovarian follicular activity and hormonal patterns that occur following estrus. In nonovulatory queens, the ovarian follicles degenerate, and follicular activity ceases for 3 to 15 days (interestrus). If the cat has ovulated but is not pregnant (pseudopregnancy), progesterone pro-duced by the corpora lutea also results in a period of reproductive inactivity (diestrus). The duration of diestrus ranges from 35 to 70 days with an average of 45 days (Feldman and Nelson, 1987). Interestrus or diestrus will be followed by proestrus (during the breeding season) or anestrus.

Monitoring vaginal cytology to follow estrous cyclic activity is more difficult in the queen than in the bitch because vaginal stimulation may cause ovulation. A saline-moistened, cotton-tipped swab can be used to gently collect cells from the vaginal vault. Alternatively, a short, round-tip medicine dropper filled with a few drops of sterile saline can be used to perform a vaginal flush (Lein, 1986). Vaginal cytology slides are air dried and stained with new methylene blue or Wright's hematologic stains. The epithelial cell changes in feline vaginal cytology specimens under the progressive influence of estrogen are similar to those of the dog; however, leukocytes and red blood cells are found only in low numbers. Clearing (reduction in mucus and background debris) of the smear and increasing cornification of epithelial cells are the best cytologic indicators of estrus cycling activity (Feldman and Nelson, 1987). Because estrous cycling is a dynamic activity, following changes in sequential cytologic samples is more valuable than examining an isolated specimen.

DEFINITION AND GENERAL CAUSES OF INFERTILITY

Definition

Infertility in the queen is the inability to be bred by a male, the inability to conceive following successful breeding, or the inability to carry a pregnancy to term.

General Causes of Infertility

The major causes of infertility include inbreeding, poor husbandry or management, infectious diseases, anatomic and functional reproductive defects, and the complex emotional nature and territorial and dominance hierarchy of cats.

Although human beings have not had as long to alter the genetic makeup of cats as they have that of dogs, some purebred cat breeders have made significant inroads in undermining the natural vigor and health of this species. Some cat "breeds" have been developed from a single mutant individual, and these breeds have a limited gene pool. Some mutant genes (e.g., lack of a tail in the Manx) are lethal in the homozygous state, and fetal deaths contribute to small litter sizes in the breed. By inbreeding for a desired facial "look" that produced show ring winners, breeders of Burmese cats had early fetal deaths and produced kittens with severe congenital deformities or cardiac anomalies. Cats that are difficult to breed tend to beget difficult breeders; therefore, inbreeding should always be considered when evaluating poor reproductive performance.

Poor husbandry and poor cattery management is often the result of breeder ignorance and fads among cat fanciers. The current trend of raising cats "under foot" (i.e., cats of all ages running around together in the household) does produce more socialized cats but reduces the efficacy of sanitation and strategies for control of parasites and infectious diseases. Improper or unbalanced nutrition, often fostered by fads and nutritional misconceptions among cat breeders, also causes poor reproductive performance. A high-quality commercial maintenance food is recommended for nonpregnant queens; pregnant and nursing queens should be fed a growth type of ration. The overall health status of cats is very important because reproduction is not essential for survival of the individual and is one of the first systems to "shut down" to conserve energy needed to preserve the life of the adult. Further reproductive failures occur because breeders lack knowledge about the reproductive cycle of the cat and the sensitivity of the cat to stress.

Infectious diseases seriously affect reproductive performance and kitten viability. The feline retroviruses, feline leukemia virus, and feline immunodeficiency virus cause significant morbidity and mortality among cats. Feline leukemia virus has been associated with infertility, abortion, fetal resorption, and thymic atrophy resulting in early neonatal mortality. Many breeding catteries have successfully eliminated feline leukemia virus by testing and removing affected cats. Feline immunodeficiency virus is currently under extensive study and has been associated with reproductive failure. Fortunately, the incidence of feline immunodeficiency virus seems to be very low in purebred cats and catteries. The upper respiratory viruses, herpesvirus and calicivirus, are endemic in many cattery populations. Herpesvirus can cause abortion, but, more important, both viruses cause chronic recurring disease among adult cats, early postpartum kitten mortality ("fading kittens"), and the development of more chronic carrier cats in breeding populations. Feline infectious peritonitis virus is endemic in many cattery populations and causes sporadic disease among cats and kittens. Reproductive disorders associated with feline infectious peritonitis virus include infertility, repeat breeding, stillbirths, endometritis, abortion, fetal resorption, and "fading kitten" syndrome. Test and removal procedures to eliminate this virus from a cattery are not practical because a reliable test to identify cats affected by feline infectious peritonitis virus and carrier cats is not available. Infection of pregnant queens with feline parvovirus (panleukopenia) can cause abortion, stillbirths, and fetal cerebellar hypoplasia.

Mycoplasma and *Ureaplasma* are endemic in many catteries, and these organisms have been associated with abortion, poor fetal development, and early postpartum kitten deaths (Pedersen, 1988). Cats in catteries where *Chlamydia* is endemic may experience abortions, stillbirths, infertility, and fatal neonatal pneumonia (Pedersen, 1988). *Toxoplasma gondii* has been reported to cause abortion and congenital infection in cats, but the incidence of this disease is rare among cattery populations (Troy and Herron, 1986). Numerous bacterial agents have been associated with endometritis and pyometra in cats (Kenney et al., 1987).

Anatomic defects of the feline reproductive tract are relatively uncommon, although persistent hymen, vulvar and vaginal atresia and strictures, and abnormal uterine development have been reported (Herron, 1986). Various anomalies have also been seen in hermaphrodite and pseudohermaphrodite individuals. Functional defects of the reproductive tract (e.g., gonadal dysgenesis) in the queen are suspected to be of endocrine origin but have been poorly defined (Cline et al., 1981).

Modern husbandry of cats, particularly in purebred colonies, is vastly different from the solitary, territorial lifestyle of feral cats. High population density subjects these very individualistic animals to tremendous social stress. Social dominance, territorial behavior, and mate selection can inhibit reproductive performance. Shipping stress and stressful environmental conditions also cause reproductive failures.

CLINICAL EVALUATION FOR INFERTILITY

History

A thorough history is essential in determining whether infertility actually exists. It is important to know if the queen produced viable litters in the past but is now apparently infertile or whether it has never been successfully bred. Other questions include the breeding history of parents and relatives, the pedigree of this cat, and its relationship to toms to which it was bred. Record the age of onset of the first estrus, number and duration of estrus periods during each season, and the duration of the anestrus interval. Determine if the queen was receptive to the tom for breeding, whether the owner/breeder actually observed mating, and if these people are knowledgeable about feline reproduction. Evaluate the proven reproductive performance of the queen (previous pregnancies and their outcome) and the tom (recent history of viable litters). Determine the general health status of the cat, and record any medications being given or applied to the cat.

Inquire carefully into the cattery's husbandry practices, including (but not limited to) method of housing, light regulation, nutrition, sanitation; general health management procedures, including vaccination; and infectious disease and parasite control. Discuss breeding management procedures, including whether animals are shipped in or out for breeding. It may be helpful to visit the cattery to examine the facilities and other individuals in the colony.

Physical Examination

A thorough physical examination will help determine if systemic disease is the cause of reproductive failure. All body systems should be evaluated carefully before attention is directed to specific evaluation of the reproductive tract.

Noninvasive evaluation of the reproductive tract is difficult because of the small size of the queen. The vulva should be examined for evidence of discharge, erythema, vesicles, or ulcers. The uterus may be palpable in the pelvic canal and abdominal cavity and its size, consistency, and location should be evaluated. Sedation or anesthesia is required for rectal or vaginal examination. The body of the uterus may be palpable by digital rectal examination. Vaginal examination is best accomplished with an otoscope or rhinoscope. The cervix should be examined for patency and the presence of hemorrhage or discharge originating in the uterus.

Laboratory Evaluation

The routine laboratory evaluation includes a complete blood count and biochemistry profile to detect the presence of inflammatory or infectious disease or systemic abnormalities. A urine sample should be collected by cystocentesis for routine urinalysis, sediment examination, and bacteriologic culture. Serum should be tested for feline leukemia virus antigen and feline immunodeficiency virus antibodies. The coronavirus antibody test is not specific for feline infectious peritonitis virus and is not recommended because of difficulty in interpreting test results. Other selected serologic or specialized diagnostic tests can be performed, depending on the results of the physical examination and routine laboratory evaluation.

Specimens for cytologic evaluation can be obtained during vaginal examination. Bacteriologic cultures can be obtained from the vagina or cervix if there is evidence of vaginitis or uterine discharge. These culture results must be interpreted cautiously, however, because the normal vaginal flora contains many organisms that could be considered potential pathogens (Clemetson and Ward, 1990). Special transport and culture media are needed if specimens are to be cultured for *Mycoplasma, Ureaplasma,* or *Chlamydia.*

Abdominal radiography is rarely helpful unless gross abnormalities are present in the reproductive tract. Ultrasonography is a much more sensitive tool for evaluating uterine wall thickness and fluid retention. Laparoscopy can be used to determine the status of ovarian function. Exploratory laparotomy is a procedure of last resort that can be used to examine for acquired or congenital abnormalities, and uterine biopsy can be performed to detect occult cystic endometrial hyperplasia. The measurement of reproductive hormones may be useful in selected cases and will be discussed in the following section. Hormone levels should always be interpreted in conjunction with observed behavior, vaginal cytology, and physical evaluation of the queen.

DIFFERENTIAL DIAGNOSIS OF INFERTILITY

Failure to Cycle

If the history is incomplete, the possibility of previous ovariohysterectomy must be considered. Silent heat (failure to exhibit behavioral signs of estrus) occurs in young, aged, and shy queens. Estrus can be detected in these cats by examining sequential vaginal cytologic specimens. These queens may be receptive and will breed if placed with a male at the appropriate time.

Prolonged anestrus is often a management problem. The general health and nutritional status of the queen should be evaluated and any problems corrected. Attaching cattery lights to a timer can assure exposure of the queen to 14 hours of light per day. Visual and auditory stimuli and pheromones play a significant role in estrus induction and behavior. Solitary queens failing to exhibit estrus in a single-cat household may cycle when housed with other estrual queens ("dormitory effect") or in the continual presence of a tom. Stressful environmental changes, such as shipping to a new cattery, can result in cessation of estrous cycling activity for days to months.

If these problems have been thoroughly investigated and a physical cause for prolonged anestrus is not apparent, hormonal induction of estrus can be attempted. Follicle-stimulating hormone-P (FSH-P, Schering) is given at a dose of 2.0 mg/cat IM every 24 hr for up to 5 days until behavioral signs of estrus occur (Lein, 1986). Cats should be allowed to mate at least four times; a single dose of human chorionic gonadotropin (chorionic gonadotropin—Carter-Glogau) 500 IU/cat IM can be given following breeding to ensure that ovulation occurs. This protocol should not be used in cats less than 1 year or more than 5 years of age and should not be used merely for the convenience of the owner. Possible side effects of FSH-P treatment include the development of cystic ovaries, cystic endometrial hyperplasia endometritis, or pyometra. This regimen will induce estrus in about 75% of queens, and the estrus will be fertile in about 75% of these (Feldman and Nelson, 1987).

Failure to Breed

Failure of an apparently estrual queen to breed may be caused by inexperience on the part of the queen, the tom, or both. Ideally, a gentle, congenial, and experienced tom should be selected for neophyte queens. Misinterpretation of proestrus behavior for estrual behavior may cause a queen to reject a tom. Faulty timing can be detected by vaginal cytology.

Queens exhibit considerable mate selectivity, and they may reject a carefully selected mate, yet breed willingly with another tom. Social dominance over a particular tom can also lead to rejection by the queen. Finding an acceptable tom for these queens will correct this problem. Some queens may show strong estrual behavior and have appropriate vaginal cytologic changes, yet reject any male that attempts to breed. These queens may have an innate behavioral aversion to breeding, or they may have had an adverse previous breeding experience. Physical restraint of queens resistant to breeding can be attempted but is not without hazard to the holders. Artificial insemination is possible in cats but requires a trained tom (not usually available outside research settings) or anesthetizing of the tom for electroejaculation.

Queens with cystic ovaries may exhibit prolonged obvious estrual behavior but are frequently ill-tempered and resist breeding by a tom. These cats have persistently elevated (greater than 20 pg/ml) serum estrogen levels (Feldman and Nelson, 1987). An attempt can be made to induce ovulation by repeated vaginal stimulation or with exogenous hormones (see section on "Failure to Conceive Following Breeding"). However, this treatment is often unsuccessful. Exploratory laparotomy with manual removal of follicles and corpora lutea can be used as a salvage procedure for valuable queens. If cycling is resumed, the queen should be bred during its first estrus period. Unfortunately, prolonged exposure to estrogen produced by the cystic follicles may have caused endometrial hyperplasia and rendered the uterus unsuitable for embryonic implantation.

Physical incompatibility can occur with a long-bodied tom and a short-bodied queen or vice versa. Most cats are quite acrobatic and can assume an appropriate breeding posture if given sufficient time. Dental disease in the tom may cause oral pain or tooth loss and result in failure to maintain an appropriate neck grasp on the female to allow positioning for intromission.

Failure to Conceive Following Breeding

First, it is important to determine that intromission and ejaculation actually occurred. The classical behavioral after-reaction of the queen to intromission (jumping away, hissing and swatting at the tom, licking the vulva, rolling) can occur without complete intromission or ejaculation (Lein, 1986). The tom should be examined for a penile hair ring or anomalies that might have prevented complete intromission. Finding sperm on a postbreeding vaginal swab or wash can confirm ejaculation. The recent (past 6 months) fertility history of the male should also be investigated.

Assuming that insemination occurred, the sequence of estrous cycling activity should be monitored to determine if ovulation occurred following breeding. A short interestrus interval suggests the possibility of ovulation failure. The queen should be allowed as many breeding attempts as it will accept to provide maximal stimulation for release of luteinizing hormone. Repeated ovulation failure can be treated with a single dose of one of the following agents postbreeding: human chorionic gonadotropin 500 IU IM; luteinizing hormone (P.L.H.; Chromalloy) 50 IU IM, or gonadotropin-releasing hormone (Cystorelin; Ceva) 25 μg IM (Feldman and Nelson, 1987).

A long interestrus interval without pregnancy suggests ovulation with pseudopregnancy. If ovulation has occurred, serum progesterone levels should be higher than 2.0 ng/ml for 40 days (Feldman and Nelson, 1987). The queen should be examined carefully for vaginitis, cervicitis, persistent hymen, or other obstructive disorders. The presence of uterine disease, including anatomic abnormalities, cystic endometrial hyperplasia, endometritis, or pyometra should also be suspected in these cats.

Failure to Carry the Pregnancy to Term

In these cases it is important to establish that the cat was, in fact, pregnant. How was the diagnosis made and by whom? Breeders often use external signs such as weight gain and changes in nipple color to assess queens for pregnancy. These same physical changes can occur in pseudopregnant cats. The accuracy of manual palpation for pregnancy depends on the skill and experience of the palpator and is most reliable at about days 17 to 25 of gestation. Routine radiographs cannot confirm pregnancy until fetal skeletons become calcified at about days 43 to 45 of gestation. Ultrasonography has recently been shown to be a very useful tool in confirming pregnancy as early as 15 days; fetal hearts can be seen beating by 22 to 24 days of gestation (Feldman and Nelson, 1987). Ultrasound can also be used to assess fetal viability and development and to predict the expected date of parturition (Beck et al., 1990). The only limitation of ultrasonography is that it cannot answer our most frequently asked clinical question: "How many kittens are there?"

If the cat has been confirmed as pregnant, the next step is to classify the gestational failure as fetal resorption, abortion, or stillbirth. All of these problems can be caused by poor general health, reproductive tract disorders, systemic diseases, lethal fetal defects, or stress (e.g., shipping, environmental change), particularly in the last trimester of pregnancy. Aborted fetuses or stillborn kittens should be necropsied promptly and examined for congenital defects, and tissues should be submitted for histopathologic examination and bacteriologic culture.

A syndrome of chronic abortion in otherwise healthy queens is thought to be caused by failure of extraovarian progesterone support for the pregnancy. Abortion in these cats usually occurs between days 50 to 58 of gestation. This condition is rare and is diagnosed by ruling out other causes of abortion and documenting low progesterone levels (less than 1.0 ng/ml) in the presence of confirmed pregnancy (Feldman and Nelson, 1987). Following diagnosis, an attempt can be made to sustain a subsequent pregnancy with once-weekly doses of repositol progesterone (Depo-Provera, Upjohn) 1.1 to 2.2 mg/kg IM or medroxyprogesterone acetate (Ovaban, Schering) 10 mg/cat PO, starting 1 to 2 weeks prior to the date of previous abortions. Because progesterone inhibits cervical relaxation, treatment should be discontinued 7 to 10 days prior to the expected date of parturition. Prolonged gestation occurs in some progestin-treated cats, and a cesarean section may be required in some of these. Progestin treatment may also predispose the cat to the development of pyometra and cause masculinization of female fetuses (Feldman and Nelson, 1987).

SELECTED REPRODUCTIVE DISORDERS

Cystic Endometrial Hyperplasia

Cystic endometrial hyperplasia results from prolonged progesterone stimulation of the uterine lining. These changes occur in apparently normally cycling queens and queens treated with exogenous progesterone compounds. There are usually no external signs of the disease, but failure of implantation results in small litters or infertility. In many cases, confirmation of the diagnosis can be made only by histologic examination following uterine biopsy or ovariohysterectomy (Cline et al., 1981). There is no effective treatment for cystic endometrial hyperplasia and affected cats should be removed from the breeding program.

Endometritis and Pyometra

Endometritis and pyometra are degrees in a continuum of uterine infection. Any cat may be affected, but endometritis and pyometra are more likely to occur in middle-aged and older cats because ascending bacterial infection becomes more easily established in the abnormal uterine environment created by cystic endometrial hyperplasia. *Escherichia coli* is the most common organism isolated from queens with uterine infection, but numerous other bacteria have been found (Feldman and Nelson, 1987; Kenney et al., 1987).

Endometritis is often low grade and smoldering, and infertility is the only sign. The amount of uterine discharge is usually small and may go unnoticed until internal vaginal and cervical examination is performed. Hematology and biochemistry profiles are usually normal. Ultrasonography may reveal mild to modest uterine enlargement caused by thickening of the uterine wall or fluid retention. Because queens with endometritis often progress to pyometra, ovariohysterectomy is the treatment of choice. Valuable breeding cats can be treated for 2 to 4 months with an antibiotic selected on the basis of uterine culture and sensitivity results.

Pyometra, severe endometrial infection, is a diestrual or interestrual disease usually characterized by systemic signs of illness such as depression, malaise, anorexia, and fever (Kenney et al., 1987). Vomiting, diarrhea, polyuria, polydipsia, and dehydration can occur as the disease progresses. Vaginal discharge is usually present but may be difficult to observe in the fastidiously grooming queen. Closed cervix pyometra in the queen quickly leads to severe illness, abdominal distention, and life-threatening toxemia.

Most cats with pyometra will have elevated leukocyte counts; a degenerative left shift suggests severe infection and toxemia. Biochemistry profiles may demonstrate azotemia, hyperproteinemia, hyperglobulinemia, and electrolyte abnormalities (Kenney et al., 1987). Abdominal radiographs reveal a moderately to markedly enlarged uterus; ultrasonography can confirm the diagnosis.

Treatment includes supportive care to replace fluid deficits, correct electrolyte imbalances, and maintain hydration, and antibiotic therapy to combat the infection. A bacteriologic culture should be performed, and parenteral broad-spectrum antibiotic therapy is instituted while culture results are pending. Because *E. coli* is the most common uterine isolate, trimethoprim-sulfadiazine (Tribrissen, Wellcome) 15 mg/kg every 12 hr, SC is an excellent first-choice antibiotic. If toxemia is suspected, a combination of a penicillin or cephalosporin with an aminoglycoside may provide better antibacterial coverage.

Ovariohysterectomy is the treatment of choice for the majority of cats with pyometra. Medical therapy with dinoprost tromethamine-prostaglandin $F_2\alpha$ (Lutalyse, Upjohn) can be used to evacuate the uterus of young, valuable breeding queens with open cervix pyometra. This drug acts to relax the cervix and stimulate myometrial contractions, but it should not be used in queens that are seriously ill. In queens with advanced pyometra, myometrial contraction can rupture the thin, diseased uterine wall, causing septic peritonitis.

Prostaglandin $F_2\alpha$ is given at a dose of 0.1 to 0.25 mg/kg every 24 hr SC for 5 days (Davidson et al., 1990). The amount of vaginal discharge will increase after the first dose and should decrease with successive doses. Concurrent antibiotic therapy is given as previously described. The queen should be observed carefully during treatment because the side effects of prostaglandin $F_2\alpha$ are dramatic, begin within 15 minutes of administration, and can include collapse with tachycardia, vocalization, intense grooming activity, restlessness, ptyalism, urination, panting, defecation, vomiting, and pupillary dilatation (Davidson et al., 1990; Feldman and Nelson, 1987). These side effects usually subside within 60 minutes and become less intense with each day of treatment (Davidson et al., 1990). Prostaglandin $F_2\alpha$ is not approved for use in the cat, and the owner should be so advised prior to its use.

Following prostaglandin therapy, queens should be re-examined weekly for 2 weeks after the last treatment. An additional 5-day course of therapy can be given if vaginal discharge or clinical signs of pyometra persist. Most cats exhibit estrus within 6 weeks of treatment. Queens should be bred during their first post-treatment estrus because recurrence of pyometra is likely. About 75% of queens can have successful pregnancies and normal litters following prostaglandin $F_2\alpha$ therapy for pyometra (Davidson et al., 1990).

Reproductive Tract Neoplasia

Neoplasms of the reproductive tract of the queen are rare and usually occur in animals beyond the age of optimal fertility (Herron, 1986). Ovarian tumors are usually unilateral, but they often attain considerable size and have metastasized by the time they are detected. The clinical signs associated with ovarian tumors can include abdominal distention and discomfort, ascites, vomiting, intestinal obstruction, and weight loss. Granulosa cell tumors may produce sufficient estrogens to cause signs of persistent estrus and dermatologic changes. Dysgerminomas may also cause persistent estrus or masculinization. Ovarian teratomas may occur in younger animals and often contain mineralized areas that are apparent on routine radiographs. Other ovarian tumors include cystadenoma and adenocarcinoma, leiomyoma, and metastatic tumors from other primary sources.

Endometrial adenocarcinoma is the most frequently reported tumor of the uterus. Other tumors include leiomyoma, leiomyosarcoma, fibroma, and lipomas. The clinical signs associated with these neoplasms often result from the size and location of the tumors and impingement on other intra-abdominal organs. These signs include anorexia, constipation, dyschezia, and abdominal enlargement. Vaginal discharge and irregularities of the estrous cycle have also been observed in queens with uterine tumors (Herron, 1986).

Vaginal tumors, including fibroma and leiomyoma, have been reported. The most common clinical sign associated with these masses is constipation caused by rectal obstruction. These masses could also physically prevent successful breeding.

Surgical removal is the treatment of choice for neoplasms of the reproductive tract. Complete ovariohysterectomy is recommended to remove hormone stimulation that might enhance tumor growth. A thorough evaluation for metastasis should be performed before and during surgery. The prognosis for cats with solitary, apparently nonmetastatic tumors is fair. The prognosis for cats with metastatic disease is poor, but adjunctive chemotherapy may be helpful in reducing the tumor burden and delaying tumor recurrence in selected patients.

References and Suggested Reading

Beck, K. A., Baldwin, C. J., and Bosu, W. T. K.: Ultrasound prediction of parturition in queens. Vet. Radiol. 31:32, 1990.
Eight pregnancies in five queens were followed with serial ultrasound examination, and parturition dates were accurately predicted within 2 days in seven of the eight pregnancies.
Clemetson, L. L., and Ward, A. C. S.: Bacterial flora of the vagina and uterus of healthy cats. J.A.V.M.A. 196:902, 1990.
Results of aerobic and anaerobic bacterial culture of the vagina and uterus in 53 clinically healthy cats.
Cline, E. M., Jennings, L. L., and Sojka, N. J.: Feline reproductive failures. Feline Pract. 11(3):10, 1981.
The results of gross and histologic examination of the reproductive tracts of 33 cats culled from a breeding colony because of chronic infertility.
Davidson, A., Feldman, E., and Nelson, R.: Treatment of feline pyometra with prostaglandin F2-alpha. Proceedings of ACVIM Forum, 8:1126, 1990.
Clinical signs and successful treatment of 20 cats with open pyometra;

14 out of 18 of these were successfully bred after treatment and gave birth to live kittens.

Feldman, E. C., and Nelson, R. W.: Feline reproduction. In Feldman, E. C., and Nelson, R. W. (eds.): Canine and Feline Endocrinology and Reproduction. Philadelphia: W. B. Saunders, 1987, p. 525.
An excellent review of normal feline reproduction and abnormalities of the feline reproductive tract.

Herron, M. A.: Infertility from noninfectious causes. In Morrow, D. A. (ed.): Current Therapy in Theriogenology 2. Philadelphia: W. B. Saunders, 1986, p. 829.
Review of psychogenic and physiologic causes of infertility in the queen.

Jemmett, J. E., and Evans, J. M.: A survey of sexual behavior and reproduction of female cats. J. Small Anim. Pract. 18:31, 1977.
Survey of onset of estrus, estrous cycling activity, and duration of pregnancy in purebred cats.

Kenney, K. J., Matthiesen, D. T., Brown, N. O., et al.: Pyometra in cats: 183 cases (1979–1984). J.A.V.M.A. 191:1130, 1987.
The clinical, hematologic, biochemical, radiographic findings, and response to ovariohysterectomy in 183 cats with pyometra.

Lein, D. H.: Feline reproduction. Cornell Feline Health Center Information Bulletin, 7:1, 1986.
Overview of normal reproductive physiology and vaginal cytology in the queen.

Pedersen, N. C.: Feline Infectious Diseases. Goleta, CA: American Veterinary Publications. 1988, p. 21.
Excellent review of feline infectious diseases.

Troy, G. C., and Herron, M. A.: Infectious causes of infertility, abortion, and stillbirths in cats. In Morrow, D. A. (ed.): Current Therapy in Theriogenology 2. Philadelphia: W. B. Saunders, 1986, p. 834.
Review of viral, bacterial, and protozoal agents associated with infertility in the queen.

INFERTILITY IN THE BITCH

SHIRLEY D. JOHNSTON

St. Paul, Minnesota

The first step in an infertility workup in the bitch is remembering the millions of dogs put to death every year because of the pet overpopulation problem and discussing with the client the suitability of breeding the bitch at all.

Infertility may be the presenting complaint for bitches that fail to show external signs of estrus prior to (primary anestrus) or after (secondary anestrus) the pubertal estrus, for bitches that show signs of estrus that the owner interprets as abnormal, for bitches that show normal signs of estrus but do not accept copulation by the male, and for bitches that show normal signs of estrus and undergo mating but do not conceive and maintain a normal pregnancy.

NORMAL REPRODUCTIVE CYCLE

The normal reproductive cycle in the intact female dog consists of the stages of proestrus, estrus, diestrus, and anestrus. Proestrus, also called the follicular phase, begins with the onset of bloody vaginal discharge and vulvar swelling and ends with receptivity of the female to mating by the male. This stage lasts 9 days in the average bitch and ranges from 3 to 17 days in populations of normal bitches. During proestrus, ovarian follicles increase in size and secrete increasing concentrations of estradiol, which can be detected by measuring this hormone in daily serum samples or by noting a progressive increase in the percentage of cornified cells in the vaginal epithelium. The vaginal smear of the proestrous bitch also contains erythrocytes and, for the first part of proestrus, neutrophils. Because estradiol is secreted in pulsatile bursts and because peak concentrations vary greatly among individual animals, measurement of this steroid in serum often is less useful diagnostically than detecting the presence of vaginal cornification, which is a bioassay of estrogen activity. The stage of estrus is defined as the time of receptivity to mating. This stage generally is characterized by a vaginal smear composed predominantly of cornified squamous epithelial cells, with some cornified superficial cells, and variable presence of erythrocytes. Estrus lasts 9 days in the average bitch and ranges from 3 to 21 days in populations of normal bitches. Ovulation occurs about 2 days after estrus onset in the average bitch and may occur a few days before to as many as 11 days after estrus onset in normal bitches. The hormone progesterone increases to serum concentrations of about 2 ng/ml (6.4 nmol/L) 2 days prior to ovulation and continues to rise thereafter, peaking about 2 to 3 weeks after ovulation. Measurement of progesterone by radioimmunoassay in a laboratory or by enzyme-linked immunosorbent assay using an in-house test kit (see this volume, p. 943) is a very useful clinical tool for timing ovulation and managing breeding, characterizing the stage of the cycle in bitches showing ambiguous signs of heat, documenting maintenance of the normal luteal phase, checking the effectiveness of luteolytic mismating regimens, and documenting the end of the progesterone-dominated luteal phase. Best reproductive performance (conception rate and litter size) occurs when the bitch is bred 2 days after ovulation. The stage of diestrus, also called the luteal phase, begins with an abrupt shift in the vaginal smear from a cornified to a noncornified state. This shift, defined as the first day of diestrus, occurs about 6 days after ovulation. Diestrus ends when progesterone declines to concentrations less than 1 ng/ml (3.2 nmol/L), which occurs just prior to whelping in the pregnant bitch or about 2 months after ovulation in the nonpregnant one. Anestrus begins with the drop in serum progesterone concentrations and ends with onset of proestrual bleeding. Anestrus may be quite variable in length but is typically 4 to 4½ months. In general, the use of vaginal cytology to detect cornification is the clinician's best way to detect estradiol secretion and follicular activity; and measurement of serum progesterone is the best way to detect luteal activity. Select use of these tools over time permits understanding of the ovarian function in most bitches.

INITIAL WORKUP

Initial workup for infertile bitches should include a complete history of past breeding attempts, if any, with information about the age and previous reproductive success of the male. Dates of proestrus onset, estrus onset, and breeding, and dates of whelping at previous pregnancies, if any, should be recorded. General physical examination should include careful abdominal palpation to try and identify presence and size of the uterus and digital examination of the vestibule and vagina to confirm presence of normal anatomy and adequate size to permit normal copulation. Blood should be collected to detect the presence of *Brucella canis* and canine herpesvirus antibodies, and to perform a screening hemogram and chemistry profile. The patient should be negative for antibodies to *B. canis* and have a positive canine herpesvirus titer. Vaccinations and parasite control, if indicated, should be administered prior to the onset of the estrous cycle.

The importance of retrospectively, and prospectively, evaluating the fertility of the male when managing infertility in the bitch cannot be overemphasized. Whether historical infertility followed mating with a proven or unproven male, the first step in the bitch's workup almost always should be to evaluate the male's semen quality, even if he has recently sired litters in other bitches. Unproven males of any age may be sterile. The great majority of male dogs over 6 years of age show some degree of prostatic hypertrophy, often with superimposed ascending bacterial infection with normal urethral flora. Dogs with chronic prostatitis may intermittently shed bacteria in the semen, failing to sire litters in some bitches and, intermittently, doing so successfully in others. Therefore, a history of siring a recent litter does not necessarily mean that fertility of the male is normal. Because dog semen is easy to collect and culture and is a good indicator of fertility, this step should not be overlooked. Similarly, if a new male is identified for future use as part of an infertility management plan, which may be costly in time and money for the owner of the bitch, semen should be demonstrated normal before he is used.

APPROACH TO THE BITCH WITH PRIMARY OR SECONDARY ANESTRUS

Possible causes of failure to cycle in the bitch include abnormalities of sexual differentiation, thyroid insufficiency, lymphocytic oophoritis, luteal ovarian cyst, pituitary insufficiency, and ovarian aplasia. In addition, some dogs with severe metabolic disease (hyperadrenalcorticism, renal failure, metastatic neoplasia) may fail to show normal estrous cycles. These animals usually are not presented for complaints of prolonged anestrus. Therapy with mibolerone, progestogens, or glucocorticoids may suppress estrus pharmacologically. Management strategy is to confirm the presence of anestrus and to perform diagnostic tests that best fit each patient.

Confirm the Problem

The client's history of the bitch's failing to cycle usually is the basis on which the diagnosis is made, especially if the bitch is observed closely, or is housed with or near a male dog that might detect female pheromones secreted because of ovarian activity. For bitches that are not observed closely and that would not have access to males should estrus occur, blood may be drawn monthly for 6 months for measurement of serum progesterone. Progesterone exceeds concentrations of 2 ng/ml, (6.4 nmol/L) for 2 months after each estrus in the normal bitch. Alternatively, blood may be drawn once for measurement of serum luteinizing hormone and follicle-stimulating hormone concentrations. These are elevated in bitches with ovarian aplasia and hypoplasia, after ovariohysterectomy, and in some cases of premature ovarian failure, when ovarian hormones fail to exert the normal negative feedback inhibition effect on the pituitary gland. Commercial measurement of canine luteinizing hormone and follicle-stimulating hormone is not always available but may be possible at some commercial or institutional veterinary endocrine laboratories.

Diagnostic Approach

ABNORMALITIES OF SEXUAL DIFFERENTIATION

Abnormalities of sexual differentiation may occur in dogs at the time of establishment of chromosomal sex (at or near fertilization), at the time of translation of chromosomal sex to gonadal sex, and at the time of development of the internal tubular tract of the bitch and of the external genitalia into phenotypic sex. These disorders are irreversible causes of primary/secondary anestrus. Companion animals have been described that appear female externally, have primary or secondary anestrus, and have sex chromosome monosomy (XO), trisomy (XXX or XXY), or chimerism (XX chromosomes in some cells and XY cells in others). These animals that have errors in the establishment of chromosomal sex may have gonads that are small, lack oocytes, or are composed of both ovarian and testicular tissue (true hermaphrodites). Some true hermaphrodites have been shown to demonstrate estrous cycles.

A few animals have been described with errors in the establishment of gonadal sex, in which histologic appearance of the gonad does not agree with chromosomal sex of the animal. In phenotypic females, these include animals with an XX or XY sex chromosome complement and ovotestes or testes (with XX) or ovaries (with XY). These gonads usually do not function normally.

Animals with errors in phenotypic sex have gonadal sex that matches chromosomal sex but fail to develop the appropriate internal tubular tract or external genitalia for the genotype. These include male pseudohermaphrodites, which may appear female externally but contain the XY sex chromosome complement and abdominal testes; such animals do not show signs of estrus.

Diagnostic approach to all categories of abnormality of sexual differentiation is to draw a 10-ml heparinized blood sample or a small skin biopsy sample for karyotyping. Commercial karyotyping service is available at several colleges of veterinary medicine and will reveal abnormalities of chromosomal sex and categories of defects in which chromosomal and phenotypic sex do not agree.

THYROID INSUFFICIENCY

Thyroid insufficiency is a common endocrinopathy in many breeds of dog, and it has been associated, in some bitches, with primary or secondary anestrus, mild signs of heat (minimal bleeding, minimal vulvar swelling), prolonged proestrus, and ovulation failure. Ovarian histology in one hypothyroid bitch with primary anestrus showed the presence of degenerating follicles with infiltration of plasma cells, which may suggest the presence of immune-mediated disease. Most hypothyroid bitches with primary or secondary anestrus show normal reproductive cycling and fertility within 3 to 6 months of administration of adequate replacement therapy. Thyroid insufficiency may be a hereditary disorder, and the value of breeding affected bitches should be weighed against perpetuating the trait in the gene pool. Diagnostic approach to thyroid insufficiency is to measure thyroid hormones in serum; a thyroid-stimulating hormone response test or measurement of antithyroid antibodies may be indicated in bitches with ambiguous results.

LYMPHOCYTIC OOPHORITIS

Lymphocytic oophoritis has been reported in bitches with primary anestrus. One of these animals had other evidence of immune-mediated disease (keratoconjunctivitis sicca and polyarthritis). The ovaries contained degenerating follicles with infiltration of lymphocytes, oocyte degeneration, and thickening and collapse of the zonae pellucidae. Diagnosis of lymphocytic oophoritis is by ovarian histology.

LUTEAL OVARIAN CYST

Ovarian cysts composed of luteinized cells have been reported in pathologic surveys of canine ovaries; their incidence and role in patients with primary/secondary anestrus is unknown. Tentative diagnosis is based on detection of serum progesterone concentrations exceeding 2 ng/ml (6.4 nmol/L), which persist for more than the normal 2-month luteal phase. Ovarian ultrasound is indicated, if available, to detect ovarian enlargement. Diagnosis is confirmed by ovarian histology or response to luteolytic treatment, described later.

PITUITARY INSUFFICIENCY

Pituitary insufficiency is very rare in the dog but has been reported, most frequently in German shepherds with hereditary dwarfism. Affected animals retain the physical stature, haircoat, and dentition of puppies and have variable thyroid and adrenal gland function. Some of these animals have shown reproductive cycling. Diagnosis is based on history and physical examination findings, endocrine evaluation of some of the glands controlled by the pituitary (thyroid, adrenal, ovary), and computed tomographic scan, if available, of the region of the pituitary to look for cystic dilatation and absence of the gland.

OVARIAN APLASIA/HYPOPLASIA

Ovarian aplasia has been reported in necropsy/pathology surveys of the dog, but antemortem case histories have not. Diagnosis is suggested by elevation in serum concentrations of luteinizing hormone and follicle-stimulating hormone and confirmed by exploratory laparotomy.

Treatment

The only cause of primary or secondary anestrus in the bitch that is known to be reversible is thyroid insufficiency, which usually responds to administration of 0.01 mg/kg thyroxine every 12 hr PO. Affected bitches usually will show improvement in coat and skin quality in 4 to 6 weeks and onset of a fertile estrus in 3 to 6 months. A potentially reversible cause of primary/secondary anestrus in the bitch is a luteal ovarian cyst, which may respond to the luteolytic action of prostaglandin F_2-alpha (dose in normal diestrus is 0.25 mg/kg prostaglandin F_2-alpha THAM salt every 12 hr SC [Lutalyse, Upjohn]) or to surgical excision.

APPROACH TO THE BITCH WITH ABNORMAL ESTROUS CYCLES

The key approach to the bitch with a history of abnormal estrus is to use serial vaginal cytology and serum progesterone measurements to determine true ovarian function. Some historical accounts of dogs cycling every 1 to 2 months occur because owners misinterpret a split heat (mild manifestation of vulvar bleeding that may occur 4 to 5 weeks before a normal heat), or attraction of males at the end of diestrus, or attraction of males to a bitch with vulvar discharge as evidence of ovarian follicular activity. Some bitches with premature luteolysis will cycle frequently. Some bitches may have mild or irregular heats or extended proestrual bleeding because they are hypothyroid. Some normal bitches may have minimal bleeding throughout their cycle, may clean the vulvar discharge regularly, and, if not observed carefully by the owner or housed with other dogs, may appear to be anestrous during a normal cycle. Because the canine endometrium is known to slough and regenerate during a 3½ to 4-month period of anestrus, bitches that have been documented to have normal follicular and luteal phases and abnormally short anestrous periods may benefit from estrous suppression with mibolerone (Cheque Drops, Upjohn; 2.6 μg/kg daily PO, started more than 30 days before the next proestrus), to permit time for complete endometrial regeneration.

APPROACH TO THE BITCH THAT DOES NOT ACCEPT NATURAL MATING

Female causes of copulation failure include presence of a vaginal/vestibular barrier to breeding, attempting breeding at the wrong time of the cycle, and mate preference on the part of the female. In addition, copulation failure may be a result of prostatic disease in the male which makes ejaculation painful or lumbosacral or hip disorders in the male or female which make mounting uncomfortable.

Diagnostic Approach

PRESENCE OF A VAGINAL/VESTIBULAR BARRIER TO BREEDING

The two major categories of obstruction to natural breeding include vaginal/vestibular anomalies and vaginal prolapses. Vaginal/vestibular anomalies include persistent hymenal remnants, annular strictures, vaginal hypoplasia, and vertical septa bifurcating part or all of the vagina. Presumptive diagnosis is based on digital and vaginoscopic examination of the vagina, followed by retrograde vaginography to demonstrate extent or multiplicity of the problem. Type I vaginal prolapses are those that arise from the ventral midline of the vagina, cranial to the external urethral orifice, and fill part of the vagina without prolapsing through the vulva. These prolapses may be diagnosed by digital or vaginoscopic examination during proestrus, estrus, or early diestrus only and may not be present in mid- to late diestrus or in anestrus. Vaginal prolapses are most common in young, large breed dogs and recur in at least two thirds of affected animals.

ATTEMPTING BREEDING AT THE WRONG TIME

A major cause of refusal of mating by the bitch is attempting breeding far from her time of ovulation. Although the average bitch ovulates 12 days after the onset of proestrual bleeding, some normal bitches may ovulate as early as 3 to 4 days or as late as 24 to 26 days after proestrus onset. In these animals, mating around day 12 may be refused. Diagnosis and management of timing problems rely on a combination of observed behavior, vaginal cytology, and serum progesterone concentrations throughout the course of the estrous cycle.

MATE PREFERENCE

Some bitches appear to exhibit a mate preference, accepting mating by one male and refusing another. If the desired male is not one that she will accommodate, a single artificial insemination, performed 2 days following ovulation as determined by serial serum progesterone assay, is indicated.

Treatment

Some vaginal/vestibular anomalies are surgically correctable, using electrocautery via an episiotomy incision. Vaginal hypoplasia is not correctable, and affected bitches must be managed with artificial insemination, as must bitches with particular mate preference. Bitches with vaginal prolapse may be managed by excising the prolapsed tissue in early diestrus (to minimize bleeding at a time when the mass is regressing but is still present to indicate region to excise) using episiotomy. Alternatively, artificial insemination may be used and the owner advised that, if the prolapse recurs at delivery, cesarean section may be necessary.

APPROACH TO THE BITCH THAT DOES NOT CONCEIVE FOLLOWING MATING

The most common cause of conception failure in bitches that have undergone natural copulation with a fertile male or artificial insemination with good quality canine semen and failed to conceive is improper timing of insemination. There is great individual variation among bitches as to when in their cycle they ovulate. The average bitch ovulates about 12 days after proestrus onset and should be bred 2 days later. The normal bitch, however, may ovulate as soon as day 3 or as late as day 26 after proestrus onset and needs to be bred 2 days following ovulation, regardless of when it occurs. Even when other causes of infertility have been identified and corrected, determination of ovulation day is essential for successfully managing the next breeding. Other causes of conception failure in the mated bitch include presence of intrauterine infection, impatency of the female tubular tract, and an insufficient luteal phase.

Diagnostic Approach

TIMING OF OVULATION

Timing problems should be suspected in bitches with a history of infertility that were bred only one or a few times, over a small number of days, during their cycle. This cause is less likely in the bitch bred every other or every third day during her period of receptivity. Day of ovulation is best determined retrospectively by collecting daily vaginal smears and counting back 6 days from the first diestrous smear or, prospectively, by collecting serial blood samples for progesterone assay and counting forward 2 days from the first rise to a concentration of about 2 ng/ml (6.4 nmol/L). The client can be taught to collect daily vaginal smears to be brought in for staining and examination after the end of the season. Serum progesterone assays should be planned based on what is known of the bitch. If she has never conceived, samples from early (days 3 to 5), middle (days 10 to 14), and later (days 20 to 22) parts of the cycle may be submitted. If the seasons have been short and early ovulation is suspected, multiple early samples may be preferred. If the bitch has had a previous pregnancy and dates of proestrus onset, breeding, and whelping are known, ovulation day at that cycle may be calculated as 63 days prior to whelping, and the number of days from proestrus onset to that day may be used as a rough indicator of when in her cycle she ovulates. The pubertal estrus is not an average one for most bitches, but, at most seasons thereafter, most bitches will ovulate at about the same time after onset of proestrus.

UTERINE INFECTION

Infectious causes of infertility in the bitch include uterine infection with B. canis or with any of the bacteria that constitute normal vaginal flora of the bitch, including Escherichia coli, Staphylococcus spp., Streptococcus spp., Proteus mirabilis, Pseudomonas aeruginosa, or Mycoplasma canis. Presumptive diagnosis of infection with B. canis is made using a commercially available card agglutination test kit. Because false positives are not uncommon with this kit, positive animals should be evaluated further by tube agglutination or radial immunodiffusion procedures. Although canine brucellosis is thought of as a predominant cause of abortion in the dog, early embryonic death and apparent conception failure may also occur.

Risk of ascending uterine infection with bacteria that are part of the normal vaginal flora increases as the bitch ages and as the incidence of cystic endometrial hyperplasia, a sequel to the recurrent 2-month progesterone-dominated luteal phases, rises. Because the small intraluminal diameter and the abdominal location of the cervix of the bitch preclude cannulation for uterine culture, this diagnosis is best confirmed by exploratory laparotomy, at which time a full-thickness uterine biopsy sample and culture sample of the lumen of the uterus can be collected. Alternatively, and especially in infertile patients over age 6, a cranial vaginal culture can be collected in early proestrus, per vagina. Use a long guarded swab so that bacteria shed from an infected endometrium and present in the bloody proestrual vulvar discharge may be collected, identified, and treated specifically. The owner should be advised, however, that a positive proestrual vaginal culture does not confirm the presence of uterine infection, since normal vaginal bacteria may be collected.

Uterine infection with canine herpesvirus during

pregnancy is a potential cause of infertility in the bitch. This virus was incriminated in an early report as being associated with male and female infertility as well as neonatal deaths. At present, because of the ubiquitous nature of the virus in canine populations and the danger to normal fertility if the virus is encountered by the pregnant or early postpartum female, some virologists recommend exposing all intact bitches to the virus and breeding only those that are seropositive.

IMPATENCY OF THE FEMALE TUBULAR TRACT

Segmental aplasia of the tubular reproductive tract derived from the müllerian duct system has been observed in the bitch and, though rare, is a potential cause of conception failure. Impatency of the tract also may occur following trauma at whelping or cesarean section. Diagnosis may be made by exploratory laparotomy and distention of the uterus with saline or by retrograde hysterography performed during proestrus or estrus when the cervix is patent, permitting infusion of aqueous contrast medium. Uterine tube patency cannot be demonstrated by such infusions in the postpubertal bitch and may not be identifiable except by histologic examination following removal.

INSUFFICIENT LUTEAL PHASE

A small number of infertile bitches have been observed to show premature luteolysis or decline in serum progesterone concentrations to less than 1 ng/ml (3.2 nmol/L) 2 to 4 weeks following breeding. The bitch requires progesterone concentrations greater than 2 ng/ml (6.4 nmol/L) to maintain pregnancy. Diagnosis of an insufficient luteal phase requires documentation of progesterone drop during this time.

OTHER CAUSES

Poorly documented but possible exclusion diagnoses for infertility in the bitch following mating include presence of antisperm antibodies, implantation failure, early embryonic death, and adverse effect of stress on maintenance of pregnancy. Current lack of appropriate diagnostic tests, including an early pregnancy detection test, hampers diagnosis of these potential causes. In patients in which other causes of infertility have been excluded, diagnostic and therapeutic strategy may include breeding attempts (following determination of ovulation day) to an outcross or genetically dissimilar male, at the bitch's home, to remove stress of shipping or unfamiliar environments.

Treatment

Management strategy for all infertile cycling bitches of all categories includes timing of ovulation to accomplish insemination 2 days later. This is best done using progesterone measurement by radioimmunoassay (most accurate) or in-house, semiquantitative enzyme-linked immunosorbent assay kits. The kits are less accurate but provide rapid turnaround time and low cost when other assay is not available. Progesterone measurement dates should be determined by the clinician and owner at the time the bitch enters proestrus, based on her previous history and the number of assays the owner can afford. In general, if the history provides no information on timing of ovulation, blood samples should be collected at 2- to 5-day intervals from time of proestrus onset until the bitch goes out of heat. Sampling can stop once a rise in the preovulatory progesterone to concentrations of 2 ng/ml (6.4 nmol/L) is detected. Natural or artificial insemination should be accomplished 2 days following ovulation.

Although bitches with canine brucellosis have been reported to reproduce successfully while on antibacterial therapy, the low rate of cure of this disease suggests that *B. canis*–positive bitches not be bred. Some bitches with bacterial uterine infection have conceived and maintained a normal pregnancy when treated with a 3-week course of antibiotics, starting in early estrus. Mycoplasma infection of the uterus probably is best treated with enrofloxacin (2.5 mg/kg every 12 hr PO for 2 weeks). Treatment is not recommended during pregnancy; affected bitches should be treated at time of diagnosis and should not be bred until the next cycle.

Some impatencies of the female tubular tract have been corrected surgically in bitches that subsequently conceived and experienced a normal pregnancy.

References and Suggested Reading

Concannon, P. W., Hansel, W., and Visek, W. J.: The ovarian cycle of the bitch: Plasma estrogen, LH and progesterone. Biol. Reprod. 13:112, 1975.
A description of canine ovarian function with circulating concentrations of reproductive hormones.
Evermann, J.: Comparative clinical and diagnostic aspects of herpesvirus infections of companion animals with primary emphasis on the dog. Proc. Soc. Theriogenology Annual Meeting, Cocur d'Alene, ID, 1989, p. 335.
A review of current knowledge of canine herpesvirus, its transmission, and its effects on reproduction in the bitch.
Holst, P. A., and Phemister, R. D.: Onset of diestrus in the Beagle bitch: Definition and significance. Am. J. Vet. Res. 35:401, 1974.
A study documenting the relationship between the diestrous vaginal smear and other parameters of reproductive performance in the bitch; documentation of the value of breeding bitches 2 days following ovulation.
Johnston, C. A., Bennett, M., Jensen, R. K., et al.: Effect of combined antibiotic therapy on fertility in brood bitches infected with *Brucella canis*. J.A.V.M.A. 180:1330, 1982.

Description of successful reproduction in B. canis–infected dogs on antibacterial therapy.

Johnston, S. D.: Vaginal prolapse. *In* Kirk, R. W. (ed.): *Current Veterinary Therapy X.* Philadelphia: W. B. Saunders, 1989, p. 1302.
A review of incidence, types, presenting complaints, and treatment options for vaginal prolapse in the bitch.

Johnston, S. D.: Premature gonadal failure in female dogs and cats. J. Reprod. Fertil. Suppl. 39:65, 1989.
A review of documented types and causes of gonadal failure in phenotypic female companion animals.

Olson, P. N. S., and Mather, E. C.: Canine vaginal and uterine bacterial flora. J.A.V.M.A. 172:708, 1978.
A review of bacteria found in the reproductive tracts of normal bitches.

Wykes, P. M., and Soderberg, S. F.: Congenital abnormalities of the canine vagina and vulva. J. Am. Anim. Hosp. Assoc. 19:995, 1983.
A retrospective study of types and clinical signs of vaginal/vulvar anomalies in the dog.

METHODS FOR RAPID INDUCTION OF FERTILE ESTRUS IN DOGS

PATRICK W. CONCANNON
Ithaca, New York

Reported methods for induction of estrus in anestrus bitches fall into two main categories (Table 1). One category involves the administration of exogenous gonadotropic hormones that induce the development or ovulation of ovarian follicles. The other category involves the administration of synthetic gonadotropin-releasing hormone peptides that release endogenous gonadotropic hormones from the pituitary gland. The gonadotropins that have been commercially available and used in dogs include follicle-stimulating hormone (FSH), pregnant mare serum gonadotropin (PMSG; eCG, equine chorionic gonadotropin), luteinizing hormone (LH), and human chorionic gonadotropin (HCG). Methods for estrus induction using these exogenous gonadotropins have included (1) the serial administrations of FSH or PMSG to induce development of follicles and proestrus, (2) the same followed by an injection of LH or HCG to cause ovulation of the induced follicles, and (3) similar protocols preceded by estrogen treatments intended to "estrogen prime" the pituitary-ovarian axis.

In general, most protocols using PMSG appear to have used supraphysiologic doses for longer than necessary. Arnold et al. (1989) reported that PMSG injected IM at doses of 20 IU/kg daily for 10 days, followed immediately by a terminal injection of an ovulating dose of HCG (500 IU/dog) resulted in abnormally high levels of estrogen, abnormal ovulations producing short luteal phases, and estrogen toxicity resulting in uterine disease, thrombocytopenia, and loss of pregnancies. In contrast, the same PMSG doses given for only 5 days and followed immediately by injection of HCG resulted in more physiologic elevations in estrogen, continued follicle growth following the HCG injection, spontaneous ovulations about 1 week after the HCG injection, and a fertility rate of 50%. The same protocol studied by England et al. (1991) induced higher than normal levels of estrogen in some bitches, but fertility was not evaluated. Differences among studies may also relate to variation in biopotency among different PMSG preparations. Unfortunately, there have been no detailed reports on the potential to use even lower doses of PMSG or fewer days of PMSG administration, the effects of varying the timing or dosage of HCG, or the use of a second administration of HCG to facilitate ovulation during the induced estrus. Until such information is available, it would appear that application of the method should consider PMSG doses of 20 IU/kg, or less, daily for 5 days or less, followed immediately by 500 IU HCG, and breeding at the induced estrus about 5 to 9 days after the HCG injection.

Protocols using FSH alone as the folliculotropin stimulus have been less successful than those using PMSG in terms of ovulation induction and pregnancy (Olson et al., 1981; Shille et al., 1984). However, the use of serial injections of FSH or LH following an estrogen-priming regimen of diethylstilbestrol (DES) has had reasonable success at inducing estrus and fertile ovulations (Moses and Shille, 1988). In this study, DES was administered orally at a dose of 5 mg/dog, daily for 7 or more days, to induce proestrus signs. Then at 5, 9 and 11 days of the induced proestrus, bitches were given, respectively, LH (5 mg, IM), FSH (10 mg, IM), and FSH. All bitches became pregnant at the

Table 1. Methods Reported for the Hormonal Induction of Estrus in Anestrous Bitches

Category and Methods	Estrus (%)	Ovulation (%)	Litters (%)	References
Gonadotropin injections				
Weekly PMSG (100 IU)	80	60	—	Chakraborty et al. (1982)
Daily PMSG followed by HCG (500–1000 IU)	0–50	0–50	0	
PMSG (2–50 IU/kg) for 9–14 days	50–100	50–100	0–20	Archbald et al., 1980; Arnold et al., 1989; Baker et al., 1980; Chaffaux et al., 1984; Nakao et al., 1985; Thun et al., 1977; Wright, 1982
PMSG (20 IU/kg) for 5 days	80–90	80–100	50	Arnold et al., 1989; England and Allen, 1991
Daily FSH (1–10 mg/day)	0–50	0–50	0	Olson et al., 1981; Shille et al., 1984
Oral DES followed by FSH, then HCG	90	30	—	Olson et al., 1981
Oral DES (5 mg/day) to induced proestrus				
Followed by LH, then FSH	100	100	100	Moses and Shille, 1988
Followed by HCG, then FSH	40	20	0	Shille et al., 1989
Followed by FSH (10 mg) at 2–4 day intervals	70	50	30	Bouchard et al., 1991
Gonadotropin-releasing hormone therapy				
GnRH pulses, IV, every 90 min	60–100	50–80	40–80	Cain et al., 1988; Vanderlip et al., 1987
GnRH agonist SC infusion for 14 days	90	75	25–50	Concannon, 1989
GnRH agonist injections, every 8 hr	80	80	80	Cain et al., 1990

induced estrus. In a second study in which HCG was substituted for LH in the protocol, fertility and the incidence of behavioral estrus were poor (Shille et al., 1989). For clinical application, a more recent modification of the protocol might be considered. This approach, which uses injections of only FSH following the DES priming, was reported to have reasonable success by Bouchard et al. (1991). In that study, 13 bitches received DES doses of 5 mg/dog, daily for 4 to 10 days, that is, until day 3 of the DES-induced proestrus. Then, on days 5, 9, and 11, after the start of the induced proestrus, FSH-P doses of 10 mg/dog were injected IM. As a result, 70% showed estrus after 5 to 10 days of treatment, 46% ovulated based on increased progesterone, and 30% became pregnant and had normal litters. Ovulations in some dogs occurred as early as 1 day after the end of DES treatment and as late as 14 days afterward in others. Unfortunately, there are no reports on the potential of DES use alone, the effects of alternate doses of DES and FSH, or the potential to facilitate ovulation by administration of HCG during the induced estrus. Nevertheless, reports to date show that the use of DES to induce proestrus followed by FSH injections can result in fertile estrus and merits clinical consideration as outlined earlier.

The second main category of methods for estrus induction involves the administration of exogenous gonadotropin-releasing hormone (GnRH) or GnRH agonist to cause the release of endogenous gonadotropins from the pituitary, which, in turn, causes follicle growth and estrus. Ovulation in such instances has apparently occurred spontaneously as a result of an endogenous surge of gonadotropins triggered by the induced wave of follicle growth and estrogen secretion. However, there are no reports on the potential for using properly timed administration of LH or HCG to facilitate ovulation of the induced follicles. The reported protocols have included (1) pulsatile intravenous administration of GnRH every 90 min for 6 to 12 days (Cain et al., 1988; Vanderlip et al., 1987), (2) constant subcutaneous infusion of a GnRH agonist for 14 days (Concannon, 1989), and (3) injections of a GnRH agonist, subcutaneously, three times a day for 14 days (Cain et al., 1990).

Administration of native GnRH in pulses of 40 to 400 ng/kg every 90 min induced proestrus in 3 to 6 days, resulted in estrus and fertile ovulation within 1 to 2 weeks of treatment, and provided fertility rates of 37 to 85% in anestrus bitches (Cain et al., 1988; Vanderlip et al. 1987). However, the effort and expense in using portable, battery-operated pulsatile infusion pumps makes the method impractical for routine or clinical application. The subcutaneous infusion of a potent GnRH agonist also caused a rapid induction of proestrus and estrus, with fertility rates of 25% when given after the end of lactation and 50% when given during anestrus following nonpregnant cycles (Concannon, 1989). Although the method shows promise, the agonist used is not commercially available, and the small, inexpensive osmotic pumps require minor surgery for subcutaneous placement and removal. The continuous intravenous infusion of native GnRH was also reported to cause a rapid induction of estrus, but any ovulations that occurred were apparently very delayed (Cain et al., 1988). The subcutaneous injection of a GnRH agonist (D-Trp-6 GnRH), at a dose of 1 µg/kg, every 8 hr, for 11 days, and 0.5 µg/kg, every 8 hr, for 3 days, resulted in estrus within 9 to 11 days in 80% of dogs, all of which became pregnant (Cain et al., 1990). Despite the inconvenience of three-times-a-day injections, this protocol appears to present the best combination of efficacy and clinical utility among approaches involving gonadotropin-releasing hormone.

Unfortunately, whichever approach is considered, there are the problems of availability, quality, consistency, and dependability of hormone preparations. Different synthetic hormone agonists, such as those of GnRH, may have different potencies. Different commercial preparations of PMSG, and probably other hormones, may have different biopotencies because of differences in assay methods or because of questionable assay reliability. Some preparations of gonadotropins used experimentally are either no longer marketed or are sold in countries other than the United States. At present, there are no GnRH agonists commercially available at prices feasible for animal studies, but the situation should change over the next few years. However, preparations that have been available in recent years include those for PMSG (Gestyl, Diosynth, Inc., Chicago; Equinex, Ayerst Laboratories, Montreal; and Folligon, Intervet Ltd., Cambridge, U.K.); those for HCG (Chorulon, Intervet, Ltd., Cambridge, U.K.; Chorionic Gonadotropin for Injection, Burns Biotech, Omaha, NE); for FSH (FSH-P, Schering Corp, Kennilworth, NJ); and for DES (Eli Lilly and Co., Indianapolis).

References and Suggested Reading

Archbald, L. F., Baker, B. A., Clooney, L. L., et al.: A surgical method for collecting canine embryos after induction of estrus and ovulation with exogenous gonadotrophins. Vet. Med. Small Anim. Clin. 75:228, 1980.
Reports on embryos recovered from uteri in six of eight dogs in which estrus and ovulation was induced by nine daily injections of PMSG followed by HCG on day 10 or on second day of estrus.
Arnold, S., Arnold, P., Concannon, P. W., et al.: Effect of duration of PMSG treatment on induction of oestrus, pregnancy rates and the complications of hyperoestrogenism in dogs. J. Reprod. Fertil. Suppl. 39:115, 1989.
Reports pathophysiology and hyperestrogenism caused by daily treatment with PMSG for 10 days and the more physiologic responses and 50% fertility rate for 5 days of PMSG treatment, prior to injection of HCG.
Baker, B. A., Archbald, L. F., Clooney, L. L., et al.: Luteal function in the hysterectomized bitch following treatment with prostaglandin F2α (PGF2α). Theriogenology 14:195, 1980.
Suggests that corpora lutea induced by exogenous gonadotropins may have a shorter than normal life span based on studies in which bitches were hysterectomized after ovulation induction.
Bouchard, G., Youngquist, R. S., Clark, B., et al.: Estrus induction in the bitch using a combination diethylstilbestrol and FSH-P. Theriogenology 36:51, 1991.
Reports vaginal cytology and hormone profiles for study in which four of 13 bitches became pregnant at estrus induced by giving DES daily

until third day of signs of proestrus, and then giving FSH on days 5, 9, and 11 after start of proestrus. Includes 44 references.*
Cain, J. L., Cain, G. R., Feldman, E. C., et al.: Use of pulsatile intravenous administration of gonadotropin-releasing hormone to induce fertile estrus in bitches. Am. J. Vet. Res. 49:1993, 1988.
Reports timing of estrus and pregnancy, progesterone levels, and shortening of anestrus in seven of eight bitches administered 140 ng pulses of GnRH IV every 90 min for 11 or 12 days.
Cain, J. L., Davidson, A. P., Cain, G. R., et al.: Induction of ovulation in bitches using subcutaneous injection of gonadotropin-releasing hormone analog. ACVIM Scientific Proceedings, 1990, p. 1126.
Subcutaneous injections of a GnRH analogue every 8 hr for 11 to 14 days resulted in rapid fertile estrus in four of five anestrus adults and in delayed but synchronous estrus and ovulation in four of five prepubertal bitches.
Chaffaux, S., Locci, D., Pontois, M., et al.: Induction of ovarian activity in anoestrous Beagle bitches. Br. Vet. J. 140:191, 1984.
Reports the induction of proestrus in each of 24 bitches injected with 500 IU PMSG daily for 10 days followed by an injection of HCG or GnRH, a short estrus in 16 of them, and the occurrence of pregnancy in three bitches that were in late anestrus at the start of treatment.
Chakraborty, P. K., Wildt, D. E., and Seager, S. W. J.: Induction of estrus and ovulation in the cat and dog. Vet. Clin. North Am. 12:85, 1982.
Reviews several methods of estrus induction, including weekly injections of PMSG favored by the authors.
Concannon, P. W.: Induction of fertile oestrus in anoestrous dogs by constant infusion of GnRH agonist. J. Reprod. Fertil. Suppl. 39:149, 1989.
Reviews canine estrus induction (39 references) and reports a 38% pregnancy rate for 24 bitches in which estrus induction was attempted using 14 days of constant subcutaneous release of a GnRH agonist.
England, G. C. W., and Allen, W. E.: A comparison of events during spontaneous and gonadotrophin induced oestrus in bitches. J. Reprod. Fertil. (in press), 1991.
Compares vaginal cytology, plasma estrogen and progesterone levels, and ultrasound appearance of ovaries between normal cycles and cycles induced by five daily injections of PMSG followed by an injection of HCG.
Moses, D. L., and Shille, V. M.: Induction of estrus in Greyhound bitches with prolonged idiopathic anestrus or with suppression of estrus after testosterone administration. J.A.V.M.A. 192:1541, 1988.
Reports 100% pregnancy rate for seven bitches in which estrus was induced with a protocol that included 9 to 15 days of DES to induced proestrus, LH on day five of induced proestrus, and FSH on days 9 and 11.
Nakao, T., Aoto, Y., Fukushima, S., et al.: Induction of estrus in bitches with exogenous gonadotrophins and pregnancy rate and blood progesterone profiles. Jap. J. Vet. Sci. 47:17, 1985.
Reports 64% estrus induction rate and 36% fertility rates in 11 bitches administered PMSG for 9 days and HCG on the tenth day and the occurrence of insufficient luteal phases in most nonpregnant bitches.
Olson, P. N., Bowen, R. A., and Nett, T. M.: Induction of estrus in the bitch. Proc. Am. Vet. Med. Assoc. Annual Meeting, St Louis, 1981, p. 96.
Reports the failure of estrus and ovulation following induction of proestrus with ten daily injections of FSH and the failure of ovulation in most bitches in which estrus was induced by injection of FSH after administration of DES and then injection of HCG.
Shille, V. M., Thatcher, M. J., Lloyd, M. L., et al.: Gonadotrophic control of follicular development and the use of exogenous gonadotrophins for induction of oestrus and ovulation in the bitch. J. Reprod. Fertil. Suppl. 39:103, 1989.
A review (43 references) of several methods and report of negative results for a protocol involving DES, HCG and FSH in greyhounds in which contraception was recently accomplished using testosterone.
Shille, V. M., Thatcher, M. J., and Simmons, K. J.: Efforts to induce estrus in the bitch, using pituitary gonadotrophins. J.A.V.M.A. 184:1469, 1984.
Reports use of a single injection of FSH, of increasing daily doses of FSH for 10 days, or of increasing doses of FSH and LH every other day for 11 days, in a total of 14 bitches, and a single resulting pregnancy, as well as a review of other studies (28 references).
Takeishi, M., Kodama, Y., Mikami, T., et al.: Studies on reproduction in the dog XI. Induction of estrus by hormonal treatment and results of the following insemination. Jap. J. Anim. Reprod. 22:71, 1971.
Reports pregnancy at induced estrus for six of seven bitches in which proestrus was induced by 3 to 9 days of estrone injections, followed by injection of PMSG together with HCG after the onset of proestrus and again after completion of vaginal cornification (in Japanese).
Thun, R., Watson, P., and Jackson, G. L.: Induction of estrus and

ovulation in the bitch using exogenous gonadotrophins. Am. J. Vet. Res. 38:483, 1977.
Reports occurrence of estrus, ovulation, and elevated plasma progesterone levels in 14 of 25 bitches treated with 20 to 500 IU PMSG daily for 10 days and then one injection of 500 IU HCG.
Vanderlip, S. L., Wing, A. E., Felt, P., et al.: Ovulation induction in anestrous bitches by pulsatile administration of GnRH. Lab. Anim. Sci. 27:459, 1987.

Reports on the incidence of estrus and ovulation, estrogen and progesterone levels, and three pregnancies obtained in eight bitches administered intravenous pulses of GnRH every 90 minutes for 6 to 12 days.
Wright, P. J.: The induction of oestrus in the bitch using daily injection of pregnant mare serum gonadotrophin. Aust. Vet. J. 59:123, 1982.
Reports variation in follicle development and ovulation in eight bitches given 250 IU PMSG daily for the 14 to 20 days required to induced estrus, and then given an injection of 500 IU HCG.

PERSISTENT ESTRUS IN THE BITCH

VICKI N. MEYERS-WALLEN

Ithaca, New York

THE NORMAL ESTROUS CYCLE

Serum estrogen concentrations rise to peak levels during proestrus and decrease to baseline levels in early estrus (Fig. 1). Peak serum estrogen concentrations are followed by a serum luteinizing hormone (LH) peak, which is followed approximately 2 days later by ovulation (Concannon and Lein, 1989). Serum progesterone concentrations are low during proestrus, rise rapidly on the day of the LH peak, and continue to rise until early diestrus. The average duration of both proestrus and estrus is 9 days, although each can vary from 3 days to 3 weeks. However, definition of proestrus or estrus based on external or behavioral signs can be unreliable. Estrous behavior in normal bitches usually occurs during cytologic estrus but can begin 4 days before or 6 days after the serum LH peak (Concannon et al., 1977). Cornification of vaginal epithelial cells is a reliable bioassay for estrogens in a bitch. In a normal cycle, the estrogen peak induces vaginal cornification, which persists for several days. Cytologic estrus is reliably defined as the presence of 90% or more cornified epithelial cells on a vaginal cytologic study (see Fig. 1). The first day of diestrus is defined as the first day in which 50% or less cornified epithelial cells are present in the vaginal smear (Holst and Phemister, 1974).

DIAGNOSIS OF PERSISTENT ESTRUS

When any one of the following is observed for 21 days or longer, evaluation for persistent estrus is warranted:

1. Ninety per cent or greater cornification of epithelial cells in vaginal smears.

2. Standing behavior with tail deviation or allowing coitus.
3. Edematous vulvar swelling.

Vaginal cytologic examination is the first diagnos-

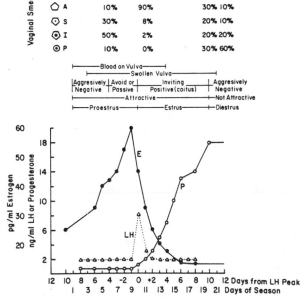

Figure 1. Relationship of vaginal cytology, physical signs, and behavioral signs to serum hormone concentrations during normal proestrus, estrus, and early diestrus. Vaginal epithelial cells: A, anuclear squames; S, superficial cell; I, intermediate cells; P, parabasal cells. Abbreviations in graph: E, follicular estrogen; LH, luteinizing hormone; P, postovulatary luteal progesterone. (Reprinted with permission from Shille, V. M., and Stabenfeldt, G. H.: 1980. Clinical reproductive physiology in dogs. *In* Morrow, D. A. [ed.]: *Current Therapy in Theriogenology.* Philadelphia: W. B. Saunders, 1980, p. 572, as originally adapted from Concannon, P. W., et al.: Biol. Reprod. 13:112, 1975, with permission of authors.)

tic test. Cornification of 90% or more of the vaginal epithelial cells is conclusive evidence that elevated serum estrogen concentrations were recently present. Although the cause of persistent estrus may vary among dogs, the common factor is elevated serum estrogen concentrations from an exogenous or endogenous source.

Exogenous Estrogen

Parenteral estrogen therapy to terminate unwanted pregnancy is frequently accompanied by prolonged estrus, which should subside with clearance of the hormone. A complete history including the type and dose of estrogen therapy is necessary. Pyometra, bone marrow aplasia, and formation of abnormal ovarian cysts are frequently associated with such estrogen therapy. As a guideline, prolongation of estrus beyond 21 days after a single estrogen injection should lead to investigation of endogenous estrogen sources (Olson et al., 1989).

Endogenous Estrogen

Ovarian structures, including developing follicles, abnormal follicular cysts, and functional ovarian tumors, are the most likely source of estrogen in intact and spayed bitches. Rarely, serum estrogen concentrations may be elevated as a result of pathology in other organs.

DEVELOPING FOLLICLES

In young bitches, developing follicles may produce estrogen concentrations sufficient to induce vaginal cornification but insufficient to provoke LH release. Alternatively, ovulation and luteinization may fail to follow the LH peak. In either case, follicular estrogen secretion might continue for an abnormally long period. Bitches treated with gonadotropins, for the purpose of inducing estrus, could also exhibit this pattern.

ABNORMAL FOLLICULAR CYSTS

Estrogen-secreting follicular cysts, reported to cause persistent estrus in young and old dogs (Olson et al., 1989), are likely to be those containing a granulosa cell lining and are likely to be anovulatory. Luteinized follicular cysts are more likely to secrete progesterone than estrogen and thus are unlikely to cause vaginal cornification or persistent estrus. Cystic endometrial hyperplasia has been associated with both types of cysts, and pyometra may be a sequela.

FUNCTIONAL OVARIAN TUMORS

Although the mean age for ovarian tumors is 8 years, ovarian neoplasia can also cause persistent estrus in young dogs. Olson and colleagues (1989) reported persistent estrus (range, 6 weeks to 3 months) in five bitches with ovarian tumors. Granulosa cell tumors, the most common steroid-secreting ovarian tumors, may be bilateral or unilateral and can vary tremendously in size and consistency (Withrow and Susaneck, 1986). Common sequelae to these tumors are cystic endometrial hyperplasia, metritis, pyometra, and hematopoietic disorders (Olson et al., 1989).

PATHOLOGY IN OTHER ORGANS

Functional tumors of the hypothalamus or pituitary could cause abnormal patterns of ovarian estrogen secretion. Severe liver disease, such as portosystemic shunt, could cause persistently elevated estrogen levels, because this hormone is normally metabolized by the liver (Olson et al., 1989). Adrenal disorders resulting in persistent estrus have not been reported in dogs.

Diagnostic Tests

SERUM HORMONE CONCENTRATIONS

Because vaginal cornification persists for days after peak estrogen concentrations have occurred in the normal cycle (see Fig. 1), it is not surprising that bitches presented for persistent estrus and confirmed to be in cytologic estrus may not have elevated serum estrogen concentrations (Olson et al., 1989). Similarly, normal serum estrogen concentrations at the time of presentation do not rule out persistent estrus.

Serum progesterone enzyme-linked immunoassay (ELISA), available for use in veterinary practice, in conjunction with vaginal cytology, can aid in diagnosis (see this volume, p. 943). In one report (Olson et al., 1989), serum progesterone was 2 ng/ml or less in the majority of dogs presented with persistent estrus (16 of 18).

ULTRASOUND EXAMINATION

Ultrasonographic detection of anechoic circular regions in the ovary of a bitch with persistent estrus is suggestive of an estrogen-secreting cyst but not diagnostic. Abnormal ovarian cysts can appear as anechoic circular areas but can vary greatly in diameter (<5 mm to >190 mm) (Olson et al., 1989). Normal preovulatory follicles (diameter 4 to 9 mm)

(Wildt et al., 1977), ovarian cysts that do not secrete steroids, such as subsurface epithelial cysts or cysts of the rete ovarii (Olson et al., 1989), and follicles induced by exogenous gonadotropins (5 mm diameter) (Inaba et al., 1984), may also appear as anechoic regions. The antra of normal corpora lutea may also be visible as anechoic regions for 2 to 3 weeks after ovulation but should be accompanied by elevated serum progesterone concentrations ($\geq$10 ng/ml) (Olson et al., 1989). Normal ultrasonographic ovarian appearance does not rule out ovarian tumor, because these can vary widely in size and consistency. Functional ovarian tumors may have a mixed ultrasonographic appearance, and larger tumors may displace the ovary in a caudal direction (Wrigley and Finn, 1989). Exploratory laparotomy with biopsy or excision is frequently necessary for definitive diagnosis of estrogen-secreting abnormal cysts or ovarian tumor. A complete blood count and platelet count should be evaluated before surgery because anemia, leukopenia, thrombocytopenia, and pyometra have been reported to occur with prolonged estrogen exposure (Olson et al., 1989).

TREATMENT

In some bitches, persistent estrus ceases without treatment, implying that some estrogen-secreting follicles or follicular cysts undergo spontaneous atresia or luteinization. In such cases, elevated serum progesterone concentrations should accompany luteinization, and vaginal cytology indicative of diestrus or anestrus should occur within 2 to 3 weeks.

Administration of progestins is not recommended unless such treatment is followed within 3 weeks by ovariohysterectomy (Shille, 1986). In bitches in which breeding is undesirable, megestrol acetate (Ovaban, Schering; 2 mg/kg PO for 8 days) has been given to reduce clinical signs of estrus. Ovariohysterectomy is mandatory after treatment, because cystic endometrial hyperplasia and pyometra are sequelae of progestin therapy. Examination of ovarian histopathologic findings is recommended.

In breeding bitches, various regimens using gonadotropin-releasing hormone (GnRH) or human chorionic gonadotropin (hCG) have been recommended, but few have been extensively evaluated. Although ovulation may follow either therapy, it is unlikely, and mating is not recommended at this time (Larsen and Johnston, 1980). To induce luteinization, Olson and colleagues (1989) recommend one to three injections of GnRH (Cystorelin, Ceva) at 50 to 100 μg IM per bitch, separated by 24 to 48 hr, or one to three injections of hCG (Follutein, Solvay Veterinary) at 22 units/kg IM, separated by 24 to 48 hr. It is uncertain whether multiple injections of either are necessary for success. Vaginal

cytologic findings and serum progesterone levels are monitored weekly, and cytologic findings indicative of diestrus or anestrus should be observed in 2 to 3 weeks with successful treatment. Serum progesterone concentrations of 10 ng/ml or greater indicate that a bitch has entered diestrus. Pyometra or recurrence of persistent estrus has been reported in some bitches after gonadotropin therapy.

If estrus persists or recurs soon after GnRH or hCG therapy, increased suspicion of neoplasia is warranted. Ultrasound examination and surgical exploration are helpful. Unilateral ovarian tumors may be removed and fertility preserved (Olson et al., 1989). However, the gross appearance of ovarian tumors can be deceptive, so ovariohysterectomy with histopathologic examination of the ovaries and uterus may be necessary for both diagnosis and treatment.

DIFFERENTIAL DIAGNOSIS

Three conditions may resemble persistent estrus: persistent proestrus, split estrus, and recurrent estrus.

Persistent Proestrus

In persistent proestrus, only 50 to 90% cornified epithelial cells are observed on vaginal cytologic examination, and preovulatory serum progesterone concentrations (<2 ng/ml) are present (see Fig. 1). Serial vaginal cytologic study and serum progesterone determinations will document that progression from proestrus to estrus, and diestrus fails to occur. Treatment is as outlined for persistent estrus.

Split Estrus

In split estrus, a bitch has an apparently normal proestrus but fails to enter estrus or has only a short estrus (1 to 2 days). As early as 3 to 4 weeks later, external signs of proestrus return (a second proestrus), and the bitch proceeds through a normal cytologic proestrus and estrus. If the owner fails to notice the change in signs between the first and second proestrus, the history will resemble that of persistent estrus. Split estrus is commonly encountered at the first cycle of young bitches but may also occur in adults. No treatment is necessary. Progression to diestrus, as documented by vaginal cytologic study and serum progesterone determinations, differentiates this condition from persistent estrus.

Recurrent Estrus

In recurrent estrus, also called *shortened inter-estrous intervals* or *polyestrus*, estrus periods of normal length are separated by intervals of less than 4 months. It is likely that because of failure of ovulation or luteinization, serum progesterone concentrations are insufficient to be recognized by the hypothalamus, leading to the premature initiation of another estrous cycle. Reports suggest that infertility coincides with extended periods of recurrent estrus but that normal, fertile cycles can subsequently occur (Phemister, 1980). One case report linking recurrent estrus with shortened luteal phase, shortened interestrous intervals, and functional follicular cysts (Shille et al., 1984) suggests that some cases may respond to gonadotropin therapy, as suggested for persistent estrus. Others have recommended mibolerone therapy (Cheque Drops, Upjohn) to lengthen interestrus intervals (Larsen and Johnston, 1980).

Neoplasia within the hypothalamic-pituitary-ovarian axis should be considered when persistent estrus follows recurrent estrus, as reported in a 4-year-old malamute with a unilateral granulosa cell tumor (Olson et al., 1989).

References and Suggested Reading

Concannon, P. W., Hansel, W., and McEntee, K.: Changes in LH, progesterone and sexual behavior associated with preovulatory luteinization in the bitch. Biol. Reprod. 17:604, 1977.
A study correlating serum LH and progesterone concentrations, ovarian histologic findings, and mating behavior with the time of ovulation in bitches.

Concannon, P. W., and Lein, D. H.: Hormonal and clinical correlates of ovarian cycles, ovulation, pseudopregnancy, and pregnancy in dogs. *In* Kirk, R. W., and Bonagura, J. D. (eds.): *Current Veterinary Therapy X.* Philadelphia: W. B. Saunders, 1989, pp. 1269–1282.

Holst, P. A., and Phemister, R. D.: Onset of diestrus in the beagle bitch: Definition and significance. Am. J. Vet. Res. 35:401, 1974.
A description of vaginal cytologic study, its use in estimating ovulation and whelping date, and the effect of the time of breeding on conception rate and litter size.

Inaba, T., Matsui, N., Shimizu, R., et al.: Use of echography in bitches for detection of ovulation and pregnancy. Vet. Rec. 115:276, 1984.
An ultrasonographic study of ovarian changes associated with ovulation in four anestrous bitches in which estrus was induced with gonadotropins.

Larsen, R. E., and Johnston, S. J.: Management of canine infertility. *In* Kirk, R. W. (ed.): *Current Veterinary Therapy VII.* Philadelphia: W. B. Saunders, 1980, pp. 1226–1231.

Olson, P. N., Wrigley, R. H., Husted, P. W., et al.: Persistent estrus in the bitch. *In* Ettinger, S. J. (ed.): *Textbook of Veterinary Internal Medicine,* 3rd ed. Vol 2. Philadelphia: W. B. Saunders, 1989, p. 1792.
A review of the causes and treatment of persistent estrus in bitches, with a tabulation of the characteristics of individual cases.

Phemister, R. D.: Abnormal estrous activity. *In* Morrow, D. A. (ed.): *Current Therapy in Theriogenology.* Philadelphia: W. B. Saunders, 1980, p. 620.
A review of the causes and treatment of abnormal estrous cycles in bitches.

Shille, V. M.: Management of reproductive disorders in the bitch and queen. *In* Kirk, R. W. (ed.): *Current Veterinary Therapy IX.* Philadelphia: W. B. Saunders, 1986, pp. 1225–1229.

Shille, V. M., Calderwood-Mays, M. B., and Thatcher, M. J.: Infertility in a bitch associated with short interestrous intervals and cystic follicles: A case report. J. Am. Anim. Hosp. Assoc. 20:171, 1984.
A description of a bitch with recurrent estrus, abnormal follicular cysts, and cystic endometrial hyperplasia.

Shille, V. M., and Olson, P. N.: Dynamic testing in reproductive endocrinology. *In* Kirk, R. W., and Bonagura, J. D. (eds.): *Current Veterinary Therapy X.* Philadelphia, W. B. Saunders, 1989, pp. 1282–1288.

Wildt, D. E., Levinson, C. J., and Seager, S. W. J.: Laparoscopic exposure and sequential observation of the ovary of the cycling bitch. Anat. Rec. 189:443, 1977.
A description of the gross characteristics of ovarian follicles before, during, and after ovulation as observed through a laparoscope after surgical alteration of the ovarian bursa.

Withrow, S. J., and Susaneck, S. J.: Tumors of the canine female reproductive tract. *In* Morrow, D. A. (ed.): *Current Therapy in Theriogenology,* 2nd ed. Philadelphia: W. B. Saunders, 1986, pp. 521–528.
A review of clinical signs, diagnosis, treatment, and pathology of reproductive tract tumors in bitches.

Wrigley, R. H., and Finn, S. T.: Ultrasonography of the canine uterus and ovary. *In* Kirk, R. W., and Bonagura, J. D. (eds.): *Current Veterinary Therapy X.* Philadelphia: W. B. Saunders, 1989, pp. 1239–1242.

OVARIAN REMNANT SYNDROME

MELISSA S. WALLACE
New York, New York

The ovarian remnant syndrome is the presence of functional ovarian cortex in the abdomen following an ovariohysterectomy. The ovarian tissue subsequently produces sex hormones (estrogens and progesterone), which results in signs of proestrus and estrus and, occasionally, clinical false pregnancy. In a retrospective study of 72 dogs referred for complications of ovariohysterectomy, 12 (17%) were for recurrent estrous cycles (Pearson, 1973). This complication occurs in both dogs and cats and is, in my experience, more frequent in the cat.

ETIOLOGY

The ovarian remnant syndrome occurs in women following ovariohysterectomy for benign inflammatory diseases of the ovaries. The complication arises because local inflammation and adhesions prevent the surgeon from successfully removing all of the ovarian tissue. In canine and feline ovarian remnant syndrome, there is seldom a pathologic condition, and most cases follow routine ovariohysterectomies. Failure to remove all of the ovarian cortex may result from poor visualization of the surgical field and improper placement of clamps or ligatures. A small piece of ovary left in the abdomen can revascularize and exhibit hormonal activity similar to that of an intact ovary. It is conceivable that a piece of ovary inadvertently dropped into the abdominal cavity may vascularize and become functional. This theory is supported by a study in which ovarian cortex was sutured to the parietal peritoneum of four cats, who later exhibited estrus and had viable ovarian tissue at a repeated laparotomy (Shemwell and Weed, 1970). Most ovarian remnants are found at the ovarian pedicle, making the second hypothesis less likely.

CLINICAL PRESENTATION

Queens with ovarian remnant syndrome will exhibit cyclic signs of estrus, such as vocalization, treading, and lordosis, as well as attraction of male cats. Bitches will show proestrus and estrus with vulvar swelling, sanguineous to serosanguineous vaginal discharge, flagging and standing behavior, and attraction of male dogs. Once the estrous cycles reappear, they show the normal periodicity for that species. The first observed estrus after ovariohysterectomy may occur within days of the surgery or years later. False pregnancy with lactation, an indication that serum progesterone concentrations were elevated and subsequently declined, is occasionally observed. In rare cases it may be the only sign of ovarian remnant syndrome reported by the owner. Signs of false pregnancy are more often noted in the bitch than in the queen, since elevated serum progesterone concentrations normally follow each estrus in the bitch. Induced ovulation is necessary for elevation of serum progesterone concentrations in the queen; therefore, false pregnancy will not occur after an anovulatory estrus.

DIAGNOSTIC METHODS

The easiest and least expensive way to diagnose the presence of functional ovarian cortex is to perform vaginal cytology during proestrus or estrus. Cornification of vaginal epithelial cells in a properly collected vaginal smear is consistent with an elevated serum concentration of estrogen. The owner should be questioned regarding possible administration of exogenous estrogenic compounds such as diethylstilbestrol. If no exogenous source of estrogen was administered, estrogen secretion from an ovarian remnant is probable. Estrogen secretion by the adrenal glands may cause signs of estrus in some species, but this has not been reported in the dog or cat.

Resting hormone assays are performed by many laboratories and may be useful in some cases of ovarian remnant syndrome. Resting serum estradiol concentrations can be assayed. Timing of the sample collection and proper interpretation of the result are critical to the diagnosis. The best time to collect the sample in the bitch is during proestrus, since estradiol levels peak toward the end of proestrus and then rapidly fall. A serum estradiol concentration above 20 pg/ml (73 pmol/L) is consistent with follicular activity. It is sometimes difficult, even with vaginal cytology, to distinguish proestrus from estrus. Therefore, a low estradiol level could mean that the sample was collected too late, rather than that the diagnosis was in error. In the queen, the sample should be drawn during estrus behavior. However, some queens will continue to exhibit estrus behavior for a few days after the estradiol level has fallen, making interpretation of a low concentration difficult. Other drawbacks to the use of resting estradiol assays are that they are affected by serum lipids, the rise may be transient, and the low concentrations found in dogs and cats are below the sensitivities of some assays. In general, the use of vaginal cytology as a bioassay for estrogen is more accurate than a single serum sample.

Serum progesterone is more easily measured in the dog and cat and more useful as a single sample than serum estradiol concentration. Like estradiol, knowledge of when to draw the sample is necessary for meaningful interpretation of the result. In the bitch with ovarian remnant syndrome, the follicles that develop during proestrus become luteinized and secrete progesterone during estrus and diestrus. Therefore, the best time to draw a serum progesterone sample in the bitch suspected of ovarian remnant syndrome is in early diestrus or 1 to 3 weeks after cessation of estrus. An elevation of serum progesterone above 2 ng/ml (6.4 mmol/L) is evidence of functional luteal tissue, which confirms the presence of an ovarian remnant. This technique will not be diagnostic in most cats with ovarian remnant syndrome because they may not be induced to ovulate and will therefore not have a rise in serum progesterone.

The best way to use a serum progesterone assay to confirm the presence of ovarian tissue, especially in the queen, is with a hormone challenge or response test. The queen with an ovarian remnant exhibiting estrous behavior and the bitch in late proestrus have mature ovarian follicles. The administration of a gonadotropin that mimics the luteinizing hormone surge will cause the follicles to ovulate, luteinize, and secrete progesterone that can be measured (Shille and Olson, 1989). Human chorionic gonadotropin has luteinizing hormone activity and can be given at a dose of 44 IU/kg IM for bitches and 250 IU for queens. An alternative protocol is to use gonadotropin-releasing hormone, which stimulates endogenous luteinizing hormone release, at a dose of 2.2 µg/kg for bitches and 25 µg/queen IM. With either drug, the hormone should be administered during behavioral and cytologic estrus, and the poststimulation progesterone assay should be drawn 1 to 3 weeks later. A serum progesterone above 2 ng/ml (6.4 mmol/L) confirms functional ovarian luteal tissue.

THERAPY

The treatment of choice for ovarian remnant syndrome is exploratory laparotomy with removal of the remnant tissue. Histology of the excised tissue and elimination of cyclic estrous activity postoperatively confirms the diagnosis. The ovarian remnant may be difficult to find during anestrus. Some surgeons prefer to perform the surgery when the animal is in estrus because ovarian follicles make the remnant tissue easier to locate. Corpora lutea are also easily visualized, so performing the surgery during diestrus in the bitch or after the previously discussed hormone stimulation tests in the queen is just as successful. The surgeon should fully explore the abdomen from the caudal poles of each kidney to the uterine stump. Any suspicious tissue should be removed, taking care to identify and avoid the ureters. Remnant ovarian tissue is usually found at one or both ovarian pedicles, with the right pedicle being the most common site. Other structures such as uterine tubes or horns and paraovarian cysts are occasionally found. Any uterine remnants should be removed to decrease the chance of a future segmental pyometra or uterine stump pyometra. If ovarian tissue cannot be identified, it is wise to remove the granulation tissue at each ovarian pedicle and submit the tissue for histopathology.

If exploratory laparotomy is unsuccessful, referral to a surgical specialist who has experience with this syndrome is recommended. Usually the signs can be resolved surgically, but it is not unusual for these cases to undergo one or more negative laparotomies prior to referral and resolution. If the client refuses surgery, medical management may be considered.

In the dog, the use of mibolerone to prevent estrous cycle activity is recommended. Megestrol acetate will interrupt or delay proestrus in the bitch but should not be used continuously for prevention of estrous cycles. There is no FDA-approved drug for estrous cycle prevention in the cat. Both megestrol acetate and mibolerone have been reported for this use. Endocrinologic side effects of megestrol acetate, such as suppression of the adrenocortical axis and insulin resistance leading to diabetes mellitus, must be considered. I have no experience with the use of mibolerone in the cat and cannot advise its use at present. Early trials with this drug in cats indicated that severe toxic effects, including death, could be expected with misuse or overdose, and a minimal effective dose for estrus prevention was not established (Burke, 1978). An animal can be left untreated, keeping in mind the increased incidence of mammary neoplasia in the bitch and the possibility of uterine stump pyometra in both species.

References and Suggested Reading

Burke, T. J.: Mibolerone studies in the cat. Proceedings of the symposium on Cheque for canine estrous prevention. Brooklodge, Augusta, MI, 1978, pp. 61–64.
A description of drug trials using mibolerone for estrus prevention in the cat.
Johnston, S. D.: Reproductive disorders: Diagnostic endocrinology. Proc. Am. Anim. Hosp. Assoc. Annual Meeting, Phoenix, 1987, p. 184.
A discussion of the interpretation and assay limitations of various sex hormone assays and a protocol for an HCG and GnRH challenge test.
Pearson, H.: The complications of ovariohysterectomy in the bitch. J. Small Anim. Pract. 14:257, 1973.
A review of 72 canine cases of complications of ovariohysterectomy, including a description of the symptoms and surgical therapy of ovarian remnant syndrome in 12 of the cases.
Shemwell, R. E., and Weed, J. C.: Ovarian remnant syndrome. Obstet. Gynecol. 36:299, 1970.
A discussion of the pathogenesis and treatment of ovarian remnant syndrome in women and a small study of surgically implanted ovarian remnants in four cats.
Shille, V. M., and Olson, P. N.: Dynamic testing in reproductive endocrinology. In Kirk, R. W. (ed): Current Veterinary Therapy X. Philadelphia: W. B. Saunders, 1989, p. 1282.
An overview of the use of reproductive hormone assays to aid in timing of reproductive events and diagnosis of reproductive disorders, including a discussion and protocol for diagnosis of the ovarian remnant syndrome using hormone challenge testing.
Wallace, M. S.: The ovarian remnant syndrome in the bitch and queen. Vet. Clin. North Am. (Small Anim. Pract.) 21:501, 1991.
This article discusses signs, diagnostic tests, and treatment of the ovarian remnant syndrome in the dog and cat and includes a retrospective study of 11 cases of the syndrome in the cat.
Wildt, D. E.: Estrous cycle control—Induction and prevention in cats. In Morrow, D. A. (ed.): Current Therapy in Theriogenology, 2nd ed. Philadelphia: W. B. Saunders, 1986, p. 808.
A discussion of protocols to induce estrus and ovulation in the cat, including the dosages of HCG and GnRH to induce ovulation and a discussion of drugs useful in the prevention of estrus.

MEDICAL MANAGEMENT OF FELINE PYOMETRA

CHERI A. JOHNSON

East Lansing, Michigan

Cystic endometrial hyperplasia-pyometra is one of the few life-threatening disorders of the reproductive tract. It is a result of an abnormal response to progesterone stimulation of the uterus. The normal uterine responses to progesterone are an increase in the number and secretory activity of endometrial glands and a decrease in myometrial activity, both of which are beneficial for pregnancy. An exaggerated, prolonged, or inappropriate response to progesterone results in cystic endometrial hyperplasia with accumulation of fluid within the glands and the uterine lumen (mucometra or hydrometra). The abnormal uterine contents then become infected, presumably by ascension of vaginal bacteria, resulting in pyometra. Although the bacterial infection is not the inciting cause of pyometra, it is the cause of most of the morbidity and mortality associated with cystic endometrial hyperplasia–pyometra.

In cats, ovulation occurs as a result of a neuroendocrine reflex initiated by mechanical stimulation of the vagina and cervix. This sensory input causes the pituitary to release luteinizing hormone, which in turn causes mature ovarian follicles to ovulate. Following ovulation, the corpora lutea produce progesterone. Unless the cat is induced to ovulate, progesterone is not produced. Since progesterone initiates the pathogenesis of cystic endometrial hyperplasia–pyometra, the disorder is seen in cycling females following nonfertile matings or drug-induced ovulation, and following treatment with exogenous progestins. Corpora lutea are found on the ovaries of 40 to 70% of cats with pyometra. Approximately 10 to 20% have ovarian cysts (Dow, 1962; Kenney et al., 1987). Less commonly, pyometra occurs in the uterine stump of ovariohysterectomized cats after progestin administration.

DIAGNOSIS

Affected cats range in age from 1 to 20 years, with an average of about 7 years. Most are known to have experienced an estrous cycle within 1 week to 2 months before the onset of clinical signs. Many are known to have been bred. The abnormality most often reported by the owners is the presence of a vulvar discharge. Additional historical findings are lethargy, vomiting, polydipsia and polyuria, and weight loss. Less commonly, there is a history of infertility. Vulvar discharge, abdominal distention, enlargement of the uterus, and dehydration are the most common physical findings. Most cats do not have a fever. Some may be extremely ill from septicemia or endotoxemia.

The diagnosis is strongly suggested by the history of the onset of clinical signs during a time of potential progesterone stimulation and the characteristic findings of uterine enlargement and a septic vulvar discharge. Approximately one third of cats with pyometra have no detectable vulvar discharge, indicating that the cervix is not patent, the uterine contents are extremely viscous, or the queen grooms fastidiously. The most important differential diagnosis, especially for animals without a discharge, is pregnancy.

Radiology will almost always confirm the uterine enlargement that was found by abdominal palpation during the physical examination. However, the radiographic appearance of pyometra and the gravid uterus are essentially identical until fetal calcification is detectable at approximately 40 days' gestation. Ultrasonography will distinguish fetal structures from intraluminal fluid as the cause of uterine enlargement. Abnormalities of the uterine wall, such as cystic endometrial hyperplasia, may also be identified by ultrasonography. Ascitic fluid, suggesting possible uterine rupture, can be identified in a small percentage of cats with pyometra.

A biochemical profile, complete blood count, and urinalysis are necessary to detect the metabolic abnormalities associated with sepsis and to evaluate renal function. A sample of the uterine exudate should be submitted for culture and susceptibility testing so that the most appropriate antibiotic can be chosen. Aerobic bacteria are recovered from approximately 80% of the animals. *Escherichia coli* is by far the most common organism. Hemolytic *Streptococcus, Staphylococcus, Klebsiella, Pasteurella,* and *Moraxella* have also been reported.

The complete blood count is almost always abnormal. A leukocytosis with a regenerative left shift is the most common finding. Leukopenia with a degenerative left shift occurs in some animals. The remainder of the hemogram is usually normal, although a small percentage of cats will have a non-regenerative anemia. Fewer than one third of the animals have abnormalities in the biochemical profile. These include hyperproteinemia, azotemia, hypokalemia, increased activity of alanine aminotransferase, and hyperbilirubinemia.

TREATMENT

Treatment of cystic endometrial hyperplasia–pyometra must be prompt and aggressive because septicemia or endotoxemia can develop at any time, if they do not already exist. Intravenous fluid therapy is indicated to correct existing deficits, to maintain adequate tissue perfusion, and to improve renal function. Antibiotic therapy should begin immediately after specimens are collected for microbiologic examination. A broad-spectrum, bactericidal antibiotic with efficacy against *E. coli,* such as ampicillin (20 mg/kg, IV, IM, SC, or PO, every 8 hr), trimethoprim-sulfonamide (15 to 30 mg/kg, PO, SC, or IV, every 12 hr), or a cephalosporin (cephalexin, 20 to 40 mg/kg, PO, every 8 hr; or cephalothin, 15 to 25 mg/kg, IV, IM, or SC, every 8 hr), should be administered, pending the culture and susceptibility results. Other antibiotics (tetracycline, chloramphenicol, quinolones, aminoglycosides) are also efficacious in the treatment of *E. coli* infections of the genital tract, but they are poorly tolerated by some cats. Antibiotics are administered for 2 to 3 weeks. As soon as the fluid deficits are corrected and antibiotic therapy is initiated, further surgical or medical treatment for pyometra can begin.

The treatment of choice for feline pyometra is ovariohysterectomy. It is the only reasonable choice for animals that are critically ill because surgical extirpation has an immediate effect, whereas medical therapy does not. It is the most reasonable therapy for animals that are not going to breed in the future. Medical management of pyometra with prostaglandin $F_2\alpha$ (Lutalyse, Upjohn) could be considered for valuable brood stock that are not critically ill. Prostaglandins are not approved for use in small animals in the United States. Prostaglandins of the F series cause myometrial contractions that can evacuate the uterine contents if the cervix is patent. The cervix normally dilates in response to pressure against it, but there is some risk that cervical dilation will not be as rapid as necessary to allow the uterine contents to escape. Uterine rupture or leakage of the intraluminal contents into the abdomen via the uterine tubes is possible. This may be of greater concern in cats than in dogs for several reasons. First, uterine rupture with generalized peritonitis is found in about 4% of cats with pyometra before therapy (Kenney et al., 1987). Second, on rare occasions, feline pyometra is seen in conjunction with uterine torsion, a condition that would greatly increase the chance of rupture. Finally, the uterine exudate found in cats with pyometra is occasionally so viscous and tenacious that it seems unlikely to be expelled.

Prostaglandins also cause luteolysis, which would be beneficial in the treatment of pyometra since the source of progesterone might then be removed. The sensitivity of the corpus luteum to the effects of prostaglandin depends on the age of the corpus luteum, the dosage of prostaglandin, and the duration of treatment. Early in the luteal phase, sublethal doses of prostaglandin do not cause luteolysis in cats. Luteolysis may or may not occur during treatment, depending on each of these variables for each individual cat.

The dose-dependent effects of prostaglandins are certainly not limited to the reproductive tract. The LD_{50} for prostaglandin $F_2\alpha$ is 5.13 mg/kg in dogs. The LD_{50} has not been reported for cats, but cats given 5 mg/kg developed severe respiratory distress and ataxia, although none died. (The more potent prostaglandins, such as cloprostenol and fluprostenol, have not been adequately studied for safety in cats.) All cats can be expected to show some of the adverse reactions, which include vocalization, panting, restlessness, salivation, grooming, kneading, diarrhea, urination, mydriasis, emesis, and lordosis. The effects are seen within 15 minutes of injection of prostaglandin $F_2\alpha$ and usually subside within an hour. The severity seems to diminish with subsequent injections (Davidson et al., 1990).

To treat pyometra in cats with cervical patency, prostaglandin $F_2\alpha$, 0.1 to 0.25 mg/kg, SC, every 12 hr or every 24 hr, is administered until the uterus is empty. This usually requires 3 to 5 days. The volume of vulvar discharge should increase as the uterus empties. The discharge usually becomes less purulent and more mucoid or hemorrhagic as treatment continues. Uterine size should return to normal. The size of the feline uterus can usually be easily assessed by abdominal palpation. This could be confirmed with abdominal radiographs or ultrasonography, if necessary. Treatment can be continued for more than 5 days if the uterus is not yet empty. However, there is some evidence to suggest that animals needing longer treatment are less likely to fully recover.

OUTCOME

Pregnancy rates of 71 to 88% are reported for queens after prostaglandin $F_2\alpha$ therapy for open-cervix pyometra (Davidson et al., 1990; Nelson and Feldman, 1986). Successful medical management of closed-cervix pyometra in the cat has yet to be reported, but only 25% of bitches treated with prostaglandin $F_2\alpha$ for closed-cervix pyometra recovered (Nelson and Feldman, 1986). Pyometra can be expected to recur in at least 15% of cats within 2 years of medical therapy (Davidson et al., 1990). Given the prevalence of ovarian pathology in cats with pyometra, the fact that many have passed the reproductive prime of 1 to 5 years of age (Schmidt, 1986), and the expected eventual recurrence of pyometra, pregnancy should be achieved as soon as possible. Breeding during the next estrous cycle, to a male that is known to be fertile, using optimal breeding management (three copulations per day for 3 days) is strongly recommended. Although there are a few reports of successful medical treatment of recurrent pyometra, ovariohysterectomy is usually suggested.

References and Suggested Reading

Davidson, A., Feldman, E., and Nelson, R.: Treatment of feline pyometra with prostaglandin $F_2\alpha$. ACVIM Scientific Proceedings, 1990, p. 1126.
A prospective study of prostaglandin $F_2\alpha$ therapy for 20 queens with open-cervix pyometra
Dow, C.: The cystic endometrial hyperplasia-pyometra complex in the cat. Vet. Rec. 74:141, 1962.
The classic study of historical, physical, histopathologic, microbiologic, and hematologic abnormalities associated with pyometra in 91 cats.
Kenney, K. J., Matthiesen, D. T., Brown, N. O., et al.: Pyometra in cats: 183 cases (1979–1984). J.A.V.M.A. 191:1130, 1987.
A retrospective study of the historical, physical, laboratory, and radiologic findings and the morbidity and mortality associated with the surgical treatment of pyometra in 183 cats.
Nelson, R. W., and Feldman, E. C.: Pyometra. Vet. Clin. North Am. 16:561, 1986.
A discussion of the pathophysiology, diagnosis, and treatment of pyometra in the bitch and queen.
Schmidt, P. M.: Feline breeding management. Vet. Clin. North Am. 16:435, 1986.
A comprehensive discussion of the behavioral-gonadal-endocrine interrelationships necessary for the effective management of a feline breeding program.

NUTRITIONAL RECOMMENDATIONS FOR REPRODUCTIVE PERFORMANCE

SUSAN DONOGHUE

Pembroke, Virginia

Essential nutrients and calories have been implicated individually and collectively in reproductive failure under experimental conditions. Reproductive failure from malnutrition under clinical conditions is suspected often but verified rarely. In my experience of nutrition consulting in a teaching hospital and in a private specialty practice, two situations concerning reproduction in dogs and cats are most prevalent: (1) veterinarians requesting consultations for periparturient dogs and cats that are malnourished and (2) breeders requesting consultations to improve reproductive efficiency in relatively well-nourished dogs and cats. The former situation requires provision of diets with improved nutrient quality, whereas in the latter clients seek advice on potential benefits and risks of changing diets and of nutrient supplementation.

ASSESSMENT OF NUTRITIONAL STATUS

Nutritional status is assessed by diet history, by direct and indirect measurements of body composition and metabolic rate, and by morphometrics, such as measurements of skinfold thickness and body mass index, often combined with serum biochemistry evaluations, such as transthyretin concentrations. Such assessments are not well developed for dogs and cats. For now, diet history and body condition scores serve to assess nutritional status of dogs and cats.

Diet History

Malnutrition due to a failure to provide adequate calories and nutrients can occur at any time during the reproductive cycle but presents clinically most commonly during early lactation. This is the time of greatest nutritional need, and a bitch or queen with marginal nutrient intake depletes her nutrient stores during gestation, predisposing her to failed lactation. The most typical presentation is a bitch or queen that is in the first 4 weeks of lactation and is nursing offspring that are suffering from inadequate milk intake. If malnutrition is detected early in the course of the disorder, the offspring will have failed to grow. If it is noticed later, the offspring will have died from dehydration, starvation, or secondary problems such as infection. Diet history reveals inadequate calorie intake, most often because inadequate or inappropriate food was offered.

Breeders' animals with reproductive inefficiency often appear well nourished. Detailed nutritional evaluation is undertaken to assess the influence of nutrition on the problem. Complete dietary histories include actual recording of intakes for up to 7 days if possible; detailed offerings of commercial products, homemade diets, table foods, snacks, and supplements; and frequencies and amounts of purchases of commercial products fed free choice. If several different foods are consumed, nutrient intake is calculated most conveniently by means of commercial software programs.

Body Condition Scores

Traditionally, nutritionists recommended that the body condition of females of mammalian domestic species should be lean and increasing slightly at the time of conception. This idea was challenged by equine theriogenologists, who found progressively lower conception rates in quarter horse mares as condition diminished below a score of 4.5 on a scale of 1 to 10 (Henneke et al., 1984). The most appropriate body condition for successful conception in dogs and cats has not been determined rigorously but is usually accepted as approximating a midpoint in conditions score and moderate weight, neither declining. In practice, it will depend in part on management. A bitch bred every year, for example, has high nutritional demands from repeated lactations. A young queen bred unintentionally has high nutritional needs from the additive demands of growth and pregnancy. These animals may be expected to perform better (higher litter birth weights, greater milk production) when their body condition is slightly heavier than moderate.

I use a five-point body condition score in which 1 represents cachexia, 5 represents obesity, and 3 represents optimal condition for each breed type; for example, a Saluki with a score of 3 is leaner than a bulldog scoring 3. For bitches and queens managed as brood animals with successive pregnancies, body condition scores of 3 to 4 are recommended. In contrast, a lower score, 2.5, may be tolerated for a house pet that is to be bred only once.

The body condition score primarily reflects past energy balance and present fat stores. Pets with high calorie intake and low calorie expenditure tend to have higher scores. Malnourished dogs and cats tend to have lower scores.

Body condition also relates importantly to lean body mass, however. Assessment of lean body mass in dogs and cats is relatively subjective at this time, although various techniques, such as calculated body mass index, bioelectrical impedance, and double-labeled water, are used by nutritionists for most species, including humans, large animals, and non-domestics. When body conditions of dogs and cats are assessed, attention is given to the degree of musculature in sites related to activity, such as muscle groups associated with long bones, and to those muscles that readily reveal muscle wasting, such as those over the cranium. Malnourished bitches and queens usually score between 1 and 1.5 by the fourth week of lactation, and muscle wasting is evident on visual inspection and palpation.

NUTRITIONAL NEEDS FOR PREGNANCY AND LACTATION

Calories

Energy intakes and requirements are measured in kilocalories, usually referred to as simply *calories* or abbreviated as *kcal*. Calories are derived from the metabolism of dietary carbohydrate, protein, and fat via glucose, amino acids, and fatty acids, respectively. Fatty acids and ketone bodies from fat depots and amino acids from tissue protein are used when insufficient fuels are consumed.

Energy requirements for pets increase during gestation and lactation, but at different rates for dogs and cats. Pregnant bitches require approximately maintenance levels of calories for the first two trimesters (Fig. 1). Requirements increase gradually, starting in the sixth week, and reach about 60% over maintenance by the eighth week (National Research Council [NRC], 1985). In contrast, pregnant queens require extra calories early, starting in the second week and reaching 70% over maintenance by week 8 (Loveridge and Rivers, 1989; NRC, 1986) (see Fig. 1).

The differences in energy metabolism between dogs and cats are apparent in weight changes during gestation. Weight of dogs increases by 6 to 10% of the total gain by week 4 of gestation, whereas the weight of cats has already increased 28% of the total gain by this time (Loveridge and Rivers, 1989). Slight differences are noted in relative growth rates between fetal kittens and puppies (Noden and deLahunta, 1986) (Fig. 2), however, and weight gains by queens in the first two trimesters do not relate to the number of fetal kittens (Loveridge and Rivers, 1989). A queen's unique weight gains in early gestation may represent a combination of embryonic growth and increased extrauterine adipose tissue (fat) or, less likely, lean tissue (protein); both would be used during early lactation.

Weight loss in healthy queens at parturition re-

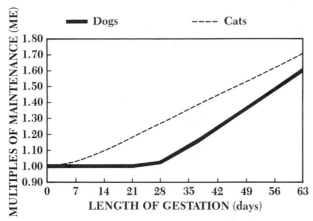

Figure 1. Energy requirements in pregnant bitches increase above maintenance by the last trimester. Energy requirements for pregnant queens increase linearly from week 2 until parturition. ME, metabolizable energy.

lates to litter size: WL = 159.1 + 108.1(N), where WL is weight loss in grams and N is the number of kittens (Loveridge and Rivers, 1989). Bitches tend to lose all gained weight at parturition, but healthy queens should retain weight and average about 20% above their prebreeding weight.

Queens require 58 to 118 kcal/kg/day during the first week of lactation, when litter size ranges from one to five, respectively, and require 97 (one kitten) to 354 (five kittens) kcal/kg/day by week 6. Kittens will be consuming some of these calories directly from food by week 3 (Loveridge and Rivers, 1989).

Kittens average about 106 gm at birth (Loveridge and Rivers, 1989) and require about 60 kcal/day (NRC, 1986). Kittens from unplanned pregnancies of still-growing queens may have to be hand-fed if growth is inadequate and may be tube-fed milk replacer when young and, when older, high-quality canned cat foods blended with milk replacer or liquid enterals (Donoghue, 1989).

Energy requirements of lactating bitches and queens increase from parturition and peak at two to four times maintenance by week 4. The magnitude of increase depends on litter size and factors that affect metabolic rate, such as environmental temperature and activity of the dam.

Estimates of average caloric requirements for gestation and lactation use standard equations derived from experimental data. These averages for various body weights and various multiples of maintenance are tabulated here to facilitate their use (Tables 1 and 2).

These averages are useful guidelines but often need adjustment for individuals. About one of seven healthy individuals may require up to 20% more calories, and another one from the same seven will require 20% less calories than the estimates provided (see Tables 1 and 2). Further adjustments may be needed for patients suffering from disease and stress (Donoghue, 1989).

Fuel Sources and Essential Nutrients

INTAKE VERSUS REQUIREMENTS

Knowledge of recommended intakes of the fuel sources (protein, fat, and carbohydrate) and essential nutrients (amino acids, fatty acids, vitamins, and minerals) is of little value if the nutrient contents of the consumed foods are unknown. Nutrient contents of table foods, including commercial preparations for humans, are relatively well studied and published widely. Nutrient contents of commercial pet foods, on the other hand, are less well known, occasionally secret, and often available only on request to the manufacturer. The task for veterinarians may be to ascertain if a particular diet is at fault when available dietary information is inadequate.

Although minimal requirements have been determined experimentally for nitrogen, essential amino acids, and many vitamins and minerals for growth and maintenance, much work remains to be directed at pregnancy and lactation in bitches and

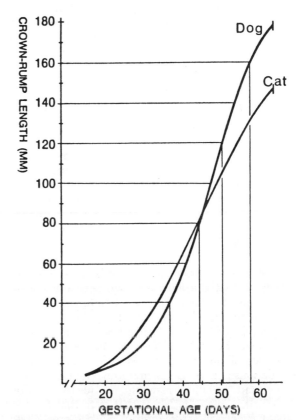

Figure 2. Comparative fetal growth rates in dogs and cats. (Reprinted with permission from Noden, D., and DeLahunta, A.: *The Embryology of Domestic Animals.* Baltimore, Williams & Wilkins, 1986.)

Table 1. *Average Daily Calories Required by Pregnant and Lactating Bitches*

Body Weight		Multiples of Maintenance (kcal ME/Day)						
lb	*kg*	*1.0*	*1.5*	*2.0*	*2.5*	*3.0*	*3.5*	*4.0*
2.5	1.1	145	218	290	363	436	508	581
5	2.3	244	366	487	611	733	855	977
7.5	3.4	331	497	662	828	994	1159	1325
10	4.5	411	616	822	1027	1233	1438	1644
15	6.8	557	835	1114	1392	1671	1949	2228
20	9.1	691	1037	1382	1728	2073	2419	2764
25	11.4	817	1225	1634	2042	2451	2859	3268
30	13.6	937	1405	1873	2342	2810	3278	3747
40	18.2	1162	1743	2324	2906	3487	4068	4649
50	22.7	1374	2061	2748	3435	4122	4809	5496
60	27.3	1575	2363	3151	3938	4726	5514	6301
70	31.8	1768	2652	3537	4421	5305	6189	7074
80	36.4	1955	2932	3909	4887	5864	6841	7819
90	40.9	2135	3202	4270	5338	6405	7473	8541
100	45.4	2311	3466	4622	5777	6932	8088	9243
120	54.5	2649	3974	5299	6623	7948	9273	10597
140	63.6	2974	4461	5948	7435	8922	10409	11896
160	72.7	3287	4931	6575	8218	9862	11506	13149

Columns were calculated as multiples of maintenance (M) energy.

$M = 132(BW_{kg}^{0.75})$ where M = maintenance energy requirement of metabolizable energy, kcal/day and BW = body weight in kilograms. This is an average for healthy dogs; one dog in seven needs 20% more, and another from the same seven needs 20% less. Data derived from National Research Council: *Nutrient Requirements of Dogs.* Washington, D. C.: National Academy Press, 1985.

queens. The existing experimental data concern minimal requirements, useful in the work of nutritional scientists but often less relevant in clinical situations when recommending feeding programs for pets. Successful breeding programs result from optimal, not minimal, nutrition.

PETFOOD LABELS

In general, commercial dog foods have relatively wide ranges of nutrient content. Labels may state that the food meets or exceeds recommendations established by the NRC. The latest NRC publication tabulates recommended nutrient intakes for growth and maintenance, but not for pregnancy and lactation. These recommendations are for available nutrients, but bioavailabilities of nutrients are not well determined in commercial pet foods (Kronfeld, 1989).

Labels on commercial pet foods may contain a statement that the food meets or exceeds recommendations for growth and maintenance (only). Foods with such labels should not be fed during pregnancy or lactation. Other labels claim that the food meets or exceeds NRC recommendations for all stages of the life cycle. Whether these recommendations genuinely reach optimal levels for pregnancy and lactation remains in question. More assurance is given by labels that state that the food passed American Association of Feed Control Officials (AAFCO) feeding trials for the entire life cycle; these pet foods should meet needs for reproduction.

The minimal contents of protein and fat and the maximal contents of water and fiber are provided in the guaranteed analysis. Further information in this panel on the label is at the manufacturer's discretion. Some manufacturers provide recent average analyses in pamphlets or on request. This is the information—up-to-date average nutrient composition—needed to evaluate a commercial pet food.

During the past decade, a few small companies have sold dry dog foods containing 27 to 30% protein and 15 to 25% fat (as fed, on the label). These foods are sold regionally, with brand names often referring to performance or protein, and appear, from their labels, to mimic the original superior dense-dry products. In my experience, the quality of these new products is highly variable. Some appear to be excellent, and others appear to be questionable (associated with diarrhea, flatulence, poor acceptability, and "blown coats"). These latter products are unacceptable.

PROTEIN AND FAT

Commercial dog foods that I recommend for bitches in the last 4 weeks of gestation and first 4 weeks of lactation contain at least 27% protein and 20% fat (metabolizable energy [ME] basis); corresponding numbers for dry dog foods are 27% protein and 10% fat and for canned foods are about 8% protein and 3% fat by weight as fed according to the label. These products should have at least half of the first six ingredients of animal origin (to ensure adequate digestibility, bioavailability, and palatabil-

Table 2. *Average Daily Calories Required by Pregnant and Lactating Queens*

Body Weight		Multiples of Maintenance (kcal ME/Day)						
lb	*kg*	*1.0*	*1.5*	*2.0*	*2.5*	*3.0*	*3.5*	*4.0*
4.0	1.8	127	191	254	318	382	445	509
4.5	2.0	143	215	286	358	430	501	573
5.0	2.3	159	239	318	398	477	557	636
5.5	2.5	175	262	350	438	525	612	700
6.0	2.7	191	286	382	477	573	668	764
6.5	3.0	207	310	414	517	620	724	827
7.0	3.2	223	334	445	557	668	780	891
7.5	3.4	239	358	477	596	716	835	954
8.0	3.6	254	382	509	636	764	891	1018
8.5	3.9	270	406	541	676	811	946	1082
9.0	4.1	286	430	573	716	859	1002	1145
10.0	4.5	318	477	636	795	954	1114	1273
10.5	4.8	334	501	668	835	1002	1169	1336
11.0	5.0	350	525	700	875	1050	1225	1400
11.5	5.2	366	549	732	915	1098	1281	1464
12.0	5.4	382	573	764	954	1145	1336	1527
13.0	5.9	414	620	827	1034	1241	1448	1654
14.0	6.4	445	668	891	1114	1336	1559	1782
15.0	6.8	477	716	954	1193	1432	1670	1909
16.0	7.3	509	764	1018	1273	1527	1782	2036

Columns were calculated as multiples of maintenance (M) energy.

M = 70(BW$_{kg}$) where M = maintenance energy requirement of metabolizable energy (kcal/day) and BW = body weight in kilograms. Data derived from National Research Council: *Nutrient Requirements of Cats.* Washington, D. C.: National Academy Press, 1986.

ity) and should include label claims for the dog's entire life cycle demonstrated by AAFCO feeding trials. Certain dense-dry dog foods (also called super premiums) sold in specialty shops and certain canned dog foods meet these criteria. Many commercial canned cat foods also meet the criteria and are useful foods for toy and miniature breeds of dogs as well as cats.

Most generic brands and many of the senior or reducing brands of dog foods are too low in protein (16 to 22% of ME) and fat for gestation and lactation. Dietary protein content is a major determinant of milk production. This was demonstrated in bitches 60 years ago, but today the most common dietary association with inadequate lactation is limited protein.

Dog foods with plant-based ingredients tend to be lower in digestibility and bioavailability and to have a less desirable amino acid profile, so that protein quality is lower than in meat-based dog foods. They may be less palatable, although flavoring agents may be used to mask unpalatable ingredients. Palatability becomes a major concern when feeding bitches with large litters in early lactation.

Low dietary fat is contraindicated in late pregnancy and early lactation because it limits caloric density. Vegetable oils provide essential fatty acids and, usually, vitamin E. Animal fats provide high palatability. Both contain 9 kcal/gm, thus helping to achieve the high energy density needed late in gestation and early in lactation.

Cats require commercial foods with 30 to 40% protein (ME basis) throughout the life cycle. They are unable to down-regulate hepatic metabolism of amino acids and have specific requirements for arginine, taurine, retinol, niacin, and arachidonic acid. Cats require the essential fatty acids and taurine for successful reproduction. Cats relish foods with high levels of animal-based protein and fat.

Commercial cat foods recommended for pregnancy and lactation are those containing at least 30% protein and 30% fat (ME basis); corresponding numbers on an as-fed label basis are 30% protein and 14% fat for dry food and 8.5% protein and 4% fat for canned cat food. They should be made up primarily of animal-based ingredients (at least four of the first six listed on the label) and should state on the label that the food was tested for the entire life cycle by AAFCO feeding trials. Exceptions are made for individual finicky cats that refuse to change brands, because pregnancy and lactation are not appropriate times for a queen to engage in self-imposed starvation because a new food is unacceptable. In these cases, the accepted food is modified progressively if nutrient quality needs improvement.

Protein, Calories, and Puppies

Proposals that too much dietary protein may be harmful to puppies, especially those of large breeds, have not been supported by sound experimental or clinical evidence. Dietary protein does confer palatability and thus may increase intake if food is allowed free choice. Both protein and energy intakes directly influence growth rate; therefore, highly palatable products containing abundant protein are best fed "by hand and by eye" to achieve desired growth rates in puppies.

One nutritional study found that pups of large breeds (Briards, Labrador retrievers, Great Danes, and Newfoundlands) grew at a slower percentage rate than pups of small breeds (miniature dachshunds, Cairn terriers) (Rainbird, 1987). The age at which 50% of mature weight was reached approximated 16 to 20 weeks for all breeds, but age when mature weight was reached varied with feeding regimen, especially calories consumed (Rainbird, 1987). Preliminary data from this study suggested that large-breed dogs also required more energy per $kg^{0.75}$ than small breeds, but this finding may have been confounded by differences in activity (e.g., by sizes of cages and runs).

In my experience, owners tend to oversimplify the role of dietary protein and overemphasize the minimum as-fed percentage of crude protein on commercial pet food labels. Protein should be considered within the context of its role as a fuel source (per cent protein, ME basis) and its balance with the other fuel sources, fat and carbohydrate, as well as its role as the provider of essential amino acids—protein quality. The latter is determined in part by the protein source, animal generally better than plant.

A level of 30% crude protein (as fed, guaranteed minimum) may be too low, too high, or just right, depending on the rest of the diet. For example, a diet of salmon and caribou mixed with minerals and fed to Alaskan village sled dogs contains up to 75% fat. It would be better balanced if more protein could temper the high intake of "fat calories." Alternatively, a dog food containing minimal fat, say 5%, and using soy as the main ingredient to attain 30% crude protein will be poorly utilized by bitches and puppies because of low digestibility and a less than optimal amino acid profile. More fat and less soy protein would improve this diet.

Another neglected area concerns associations (i.e., possible therapeutic responses) that may be confused with causation by owners. Association is not causation. Recovery from disease during slowed growth and calorie restriction does not prove that calorie excess caused a disease. Calorie restriction may mitigate specific nutrient deficiencies that are difficult to verify. Recovery from disease may occur parallel to but independent of diet changes. In my experience, management factors other than feeding, such as exercise programs and use of drugs, are rarely evaluated by concerned owners. Also, possible adverse genetic (pedigree) influences are usually de-emphasized.

Veterinarians should not be too quick to dismiss the nutritional suspicions of breeders, but anecdotal testimonials do not advance our knowledge of canine nutrition. Multifactorial diseases involving interactions of genetic, nutritional, and environmental influences are difficult to comprehend. Such diseases are considered the challenge of the 1990's in human medicine (Marx, 1990). Nutritional influences on skeletal growth of large-breed dogs remain a challenge in veterinary medicine.

In my experience, breeding kennels with musculoskeletal problems in pups often have management problems, such as poorly designed and inadequate exercise programs, and goals that are inconsistent with selection for sound conformation. Nutritional problems then arise from diet changes made after the onset of disease or in efforts to prevent disease. Many imbalances occur from additions of large volumes of one ingredient, such as rice, chicken, cottage cheese, or corn oil, and from additions of a vitamin or mineral supplement.

Table foods are not intended to be complete or balanced. (Balance is derived through variety.) Most table foods have imbalanced fuel sources, high phosphorus, and deficient calcium, iodine, and many vitamins (Kronfeld, 1989).

Every survey of dog feeding practices that I know of in U.S. homes finds significant use of table foods. Food sharing appears to be a normal part of dog-human relationships. Rather than prescribe a diet of only commercial pet foods—a prescription unlikely to be followed—table foods may be included in diet formulations for breeders desiring such programs. Fortunately, a vast array of table foods is readily available, so that appropriate food lists can be provided to owners, along with guidance about their use and upper limits designed to retain balanced nutrition for specific situations.

Table foods such as rice and cottage cheese can be added to commercial dog foods up to a point before imbalances occur. If more is added, other supplementation may be necessary to achieve balance. Texts of table food values provide the needed nutrient data to custom design diets for bitches and puppies (Pennington and Church, 1985).

CARBOHYDRATE

The last of the three fuel sources, carbohydrate, provides no essential nutrients for cats and probably dogs. Glucose precursors are provided by dietary protein and fat (contributing amino acids and glycerol, respectively). Carbohydrate in commercial pet foods originates from plant ingredients. Diets high in carbohydrate thus tend to have other characteristics associated with plant-based foods, such as low caloric density, low digestibility, and low palatability. For these reasons, plant-based diets are not recommended during pregnancy and lactation.

Dogs also do not require carbohydrate during most of their life cycle, with the possible exception of bitches in the last week of gestation and first week of lactation. Bitches fed diets of 26% protein and 74% fat (energy basis)—levels not found commercially or fed practically—developed low blood concentrations of glucose, lactate, and alanine (Romsos et al., 1981). Puppy survival was reduced in the first postparturient week. However, when dietary protein was increased from 26% to 48% of digestible energy, the untoward effects just described, including puppy mortality, were ameliorated or eliminated (Kienzle and Meyer, 1989). Presumably, the higher protein intakes supported more gluconeogenesis.

Diets containing no carbohydrate are impractical commercially and usually expensive and thus are fed only in special circumstances. For example, dogs in remote northern villages may be fed local meat or fish that is more available and less expensive than commercial dog foods. Bitches in racing sled dog kennels have whelped and raised pups successfully while fed no carbohydrate. Nevertheless, a form of pregnancy toxemia marked by hypoglycemia has been observed clinically in bitches of large breeds carrying large litters. The contribution of diet to this clinical condition has not been determined. It is prudent to avoid overfeeding bitches early in pregnancy or underfeeding late in pregnancy.

VITAMINS AND MINERALS

Many vitamins and minerals have been shown experimentally to affect reproduction in laboratory animals through fetal resorption, testicular degeneration, and fetal malformations. Experimental deficiencies of calcium, zinc, and vitamin E, as well as toxicity of vitamin A, are reported to affect canine reproduction (NRC, 1985). Experimental deficiencies of iodine, zinc, and riboflavin reportedly affect feline reproduction (NRC, 1986).

The concentrations of vitamins and minerals in commercial pet foods are not listed on most labels. Pet owners may be aware of substantial losses that occur in the processing and storage of pet foods and thus may elect to feed supplements. However, a major manufacturer of vitamins in the United States has determined vitamin losses and has published appropriate overages for typical dry, moist, and canned pet foods. Use of these overages by manufacturers should ensure adequacy of vitamins in pet foods.

Reservations persist. Not all pet foods are typical, and not all micronutrient suppliers provide appropriate overages. Changes in pet food ingredients affect availability of micronutrients (Kronfeld, 1989). Acidogenic cat foods, for example, have induced conditioned deficiencies of taurine and potassium. Acidogenic cat foods that induce mild, persistent acidosis might be expected to impair reproduction.

Judicious use of balanced, broad-spectrum vitamin-mineral supplements does not imbalance nutrient intake in dogs and cats. Injudicious use may occur, however, during pregnancy, lactation, or early growth. The most common abuses of supplements in bitches, queens, and offspring in my practice involve calcium, especially with vitamin D.

Calcium

Breeders may be concerned about calcium because of eclampsia in bitches and skeletal problems in pups. Owners of large breeds appear to oversupplement more than others.

There is no documentation that calcium supplementation of diets of pregnant bitches prevents eclampsia. Indeed, pregnant ruminants susceptible to hypocalcemia benefit from low-calcium diets prepartum. In dairy cows, excessive dietary calcium prepartum tends to retard homeostatic responses to the calcium drain at the initiation of lactation. Prepartum calcium supplementation thus is not considered an appropriate means of preventing periparturient hypocalcemia. The value of postpartum calcium supplementation is unknown. Increased intake of a high-quality commercial dog food should suffice. Food intake, weight changes, voluntary exercise, and attitude should be monitored closely in bitches prone to eclampsia.

Calcium supplementation is given commonly to puppies of large breeds. It may have been advantageous more than 30 years ago, before current calcium levels in dry dog foods were adopted, but it is not recommended today. Great Dane puppies were fed low (0.55% dry matter [DM]), normal (1.1% DM), or high (3.3% DM) quantities of calcium from 6 to 26 weeks of age (Hazewinkel, 1989). The puppies on the low-calcium diet grew most rapidly and developed limb deviations, lordosis, and painful locomotion. Bone calcium turnover was high, and calcium balance was low. Bones showed generalized osteoporosis with greenstick and compression fractures. The pups fed a high-calcium diet developed curved radii and posterior paresis. Calcium absorption and balance were high. Bones contained more calcium and showed lesions of osteochondrosis. Pups fed diets containing normal amounts of calcium developed mild osteochondrosis and myelin degeneration.

The normal calcium intake in this study approximated the 1974 NRC guidelines; the low calcium intake approximated the 1985 NRC guidelines (Hazewinkel, 1989). Most puppies grow well and have no musculoskeletal abnormalities when fed diets approximating either of these NRC guidelines. The relevance of Hazewinkel's experimental data to clinical feeding systems for puppies is confounded by likely interactions of calcium with other nutrients. Other studies using similar calcium intakes in puppies have found no abnormalities or bone lesions, and these other diets presumably contained calcium in sound proportions with phosphorus, vitamin D, zinc, copper, and manganese.

Well-formulated commercial dog foods should contain adequate but not excessive minerals and vitamins. The current NRC recommendations of 1.6 gm calcium and 1.2 gm phosphorus per 1000 kcal serve as a guideline to assess these minerals in commercial foods and in homemade diets (NRC, 1985). Some manufacturers use meat and bone meal as a primary protein source; this ingredient contains very high calcium levels, about 35 gm/1000 kcal. Use of commercial pet foods containing high levels of a poor-quality meat and bone meal will result in extremely high calcium intakes during times of high calorie intake, such as in late pregnancy and early lactation.

High intake of dietary calcium inhibits the absorption of zinc, copper, and iodine. It is the putative genesis of the "generic dog food disease" of conditioned zinc deficiency. The prevalence of conditioned and subclinical deficiencies of copper and iodine is not well documented clinically in dogs but could potentially affect bitches and pups.

Dog owners may believe that calcium supplementation with products containing phosphorus and vitamin D is safe because an appropriate calcium:phosphorus ratio is maintained. When calcium is supplemented with vitamin D, however, a major homeostatic control is bypassed, and much more of the calcium is absorbed from the gastrointestinal tract. Calcium supplemented with vitamin D is more dangerous than calcium supplemented alone.

Until more is known about calcium requirements in puppies, calcium should not be supplemented when commercial dog foods are fed. The highest-quality commercial dog foods should be offered to puppies of large breeds. On the other hand, calcium must always be supplemented, following NRC guidelines, when table foods *only* are fed, for both cereals and meat are deficient in calcium.

Micronutrients

Several nutrients, notably vitamin A, vitamin D, and iodine, may be toxic if supplemented excessively. Others, such as zinc and copper, are also toxic, but clinical poisonings are less common. Zinc and copper affect each other's metabolism, and supplementation with only one thus imbalances the other.

Under practical conditions, supplementation with a multiple vitamin-mineral product manufactured by a nationally known company and fed according to label instructions will be safe for bitches, queens, and offspring. Under certain management regimens and with certain disorders, supplementation is warranted. A recent monograph details vitamin and

mineral supplementation for all stages of canine and feline life cycles (Kronfeld, 1989).

Non-Nutrients in Food

FIBER

High fiber intake is contraindicated during pregnancy and lactation because it limits caloric density and nutrient bioavailability. In other words, large amounts of dietary fiber prevent the intake of above maintenance levels of calories and nutrients that are necessary for successful reproduction. Crude fiber should not exceed about 5% of dry matter.

ANTIOXIDANTS

Most pet foods contain non-nutrients such as flavoring agents (e.g., beef digest), coloring agents, and antioxidants. The latter include butylated hydroxytoluene (BHT), butylated hydroxyanisole (BHA), and ethoxyquin. Pet foods without antioxidants added at the time of processing often contain ingredients (such as animal tallow) preserved with antioxidants. Naturally occurring antioxidants (such as vitamin E and vitamin C) may be added to pet foods; they are ineffective outside the body and usually require protection themselves by synthetic antioxidants.

At the time of writing, there is concern among breeders about reproductive failure (and other problems) possibly due to ethoxyquin alone or in interaction with drugs, such as anthelmintics. Pet food manufacturers use ethoxyquin because of its excellent antioxidant qualities, high stability, and safety (Hilton, 1989). Ethoxyquin is readily absorbed, metabolized, and excreted in urine and feces (Gosselin et al., 1984).

Many synthetic and naturally occurring substances are toxic when ingested in large quantities. Ethoxyquin is assigned a toxicity rating of 3 or "moderately toxic," indicating the probable oral lethal human dose is 0.5 to 5.0 gm/kg (between 1 oz and 1 pint in a 150-lb human) (Gosselin et al., 1984). The LD_{50} in laboratory rats is 1 gm/kg. Toxicity signs in laboratory rats and mice include depression, reversible liver changes, and inhibited cytochrome P450 in liver microsomes. Safety studies of dogs in the 1950's might not be regarded as adequate today.

For human consumption, ethoxyquin is permitted only in paprika. Ethoxyquin is permitted in pet foods, fats, and oils in levels not to exceed 0.015% (Hilton, 1989). At the present time, ethoxyquin appears to be an effective and safe pet food ingredient when used according to regulations. If future studies of safety become warranted, consideration should be given to modern toxicologic techniques, appropriate medical and epidemiologic assessment of cases and complaints, and multifactorial causation in highly inbred lines of dogs.

In my nutrition practice, dog owners wishing to omit synthetic additives from their pet's diet are counseled about their options. Canned pet foods may contain coloring and flavoring agents but no added antioxidants (some are present in fat). Balanced homemade diets can be prepared using wholesome ingredients intended for human consumption. In my practice, such diets, when balanced and prepared properly, provide optimal nutrition that supports pregnancy and lactation.

SPECIAL CONSIDERATIONS FOR CATS

In many respects, cats are much easier to manage nutritionally during pregnancy and lactation than dogs. Their strict nutrient requirements constrain diet formulations of commercial pet foods. Most of

the better national brands thus support reproduction, although some are labeled for growth and maintenance only. Owners seem less inclined to manipulate cats' diets, and cats are less inclined to indulge their owners by eating peculiar diets.

The primary clinical nutrition problem during reproduction arises from unplanned breedings. Owners may not know when or if their cats are bred, so meal sizes and frequencies are not increased during gestation. Also, some queens are bred (unintentionally) very early in life, while still kittens themselves, so energy must be partitioned for growth as well as pregnancy and lactation. These circumstances place heavy demands on queens, and it is remarkable that so many raise kittens successfully.

When pregnancy is first noticed in the last trimester (or sometimes at parturition), feeding management is critical during lactation. Much of the thought and effort given to feeding during pregnancy is to prepare the queen nutritionally for lactation. Without this preparation and thus without

Table 3. *Nutrient Content of Foods From Groceries That Are Frequently Added to Pet Foods During Pregnancy and Lactation**

Item	Amount	Weight (g)	Water (%)	kcal	Protein	Fat (% kcal)	Carbohydrate
Cottage cheese							
Creamed	1 cup	210	79	213	49	40	11†
Low fat	1 cup	226	82	158	71	13	16†
Cheddar cheese	1 oz	28	37	115	25	74	1†
Milk							
Whole	1 cup	244	88	151	21	49	30†
Low-fat, 2%	1 cup	244	89	122	26	35	38†
Low-fat, 1%	1 cup	244	90	102	31	23	46†
Yogurt, plain							
Whole milk	1 cup	227	88	141	22	47	30†
Low-fat milk	1 cup	227	85	143	33	22	45†
Egg, whole	1 item	50	75	77	32	65	3
Vegetable oil	1 tbsp	14	0	125	0	100	0
Liver, beef	3.5 oz	100	70	135	59	25	16
Chicken							
With skin, stewed	3.5 oz	100	64	212	47	53	0
No skin, stewed	3.5 oz	100	67	170	64	35	0
Hamburger, cooked	1 patty	85	—	218	40	60	0
Rice, cooked	1 cup	188	73	199	8	1	91
Baby foods							
Cereal							
High-protein, dry	1 tbsp	2	4	9	40	10	50
Oatmeal, dry	1 tbsp	2	4	10	12	18	68
Beef and rice	1 jar	177	82	144	6	32	43
Lamb, strained	1 jar	99	79	107	56	44	0
Enterals							
Ensure	8 oz	240	83	250	14	32	54
Isocal	8 oz	240	83	250	13	37	50

*Data derived from Pennington, J.A. T., and Church, H. N.: *Bowes and Church's Food Values of Portions Commonly Used*, 14th ed. Philadelphia: J. B. Lippincott, 1985. Also see Appendices.
†Carbohydrate in dairy products is primarily lactose.

adequate fat deposition, the energy drain of milk production will result in huge losses of body weight.

In practice, such cats are offered free-choice high-quality canned cat food. Daily food and water are available throughout 24 hr and are freshened at least four times daily. The food may be warmed and may be top-dressed with tasty tidbits such as fish, crab, chicken, or cheese. Kittens are encouraged to share the queen's food from 3 weeks of age.

PRACTICAL CONSIDERATIONS FOR BITCHES AND QUEENS

The high calorie intakes needed for pregnancy, lactation, and early growth cannot be met by simply increasing meal size. Meal frequency is also increased, usually from one to two meals daily during midpregnancy, then to three or four meals daily by peak lactation. Water may be added and food may be warmed to increase food intake.

Caloric density is increased as well by changing to a higher-fat product or by additions of animal fat. When fat is added, care is taken that the proportions of protein, fat, and carbohydrate remain optimal. For example, if 2 tablespoons of bacon fat (28 gm; 250 kcal) are added to 1 8-oz cupful of dry dog food containing 430 kcal composed of 30% protein, 30% fat, and 40% carbohydrate, the food now contains 680 kcal and only 19% protein but 56% fat. Additions of a mixture of animal protein and fat, such as from skeletal muscle or from eggs, may be more desirable than additions of fat only. A table of protein and fat contents of selected table foods is provided (Table 3).

Household constraints may preclude the feeding of premium or super-premium dog foods. Most limitations arise from economic restrictions or, especially in the elderly, limited access to specialty pet food outlets. One company has a superior pet food line available for delivery to the door by private carrier, an advantage for handicapped or house-bound owners. Alternatively, lower-quality pet foods may be improved by judicious additions of highly digestible table foods such as eggs and meats (see Table 3), as noted earlier. As upper limits of table foods are approached, a broad-spectrum vitamin-mineral supplement may become desirable. The total cost of supplements and low-price pet food may compare with that of unsupplemented high-quality pet food.

The simplest plan is for a high-quality diet, suitable for peak lactation, to be introduced gradually during midpregnancy. Daily intakes are first selected by use of calorie charts (see Tables 1 and 2), then modified to adapt to individual variation in calorie needs. The daily intake is divided into two meals. The animal's feeding program thus becomes established at the time of low to moderate demand and well before the peak demand that occurs 3 or 4 weeks into lactation. After parturition, food intake is increased by increasing the size and frequency of meals.

References and Suggested Reading

Donoghue, S.: Nutrition support of hospitalized patients. Vet. Clin. North Am. Small Anim. Pract. 19:475, 1989.
A review of nutrition support for sick dogs and cats.
Gosselin, R. E., Smith, R. P., and Hodge, H. C.: *Clinical Toxicology of Commercial Products*, 5th ed. Baltimore: Williams & Wilkins, 1984, pp. II–406.
A clinical toxicology reference text.
Hazewinkel, H. A. W.: Calcium metabolism and skeletal development of dogs. *In* Burger, I. H., and Rivers, J. P. W. (eds.): *Nutrition of the Dog and Cat.* Cambridge: Cambridge University Press, 1989, p. 293.
A report on several research studies on calcium in Great Dane puppies.
Henneke, D. R., Potter, G. D., and Kreider, J. L.: Body condition during pregnancy and lactation and reproductive efficiency of mares. Theriogenology 21:897, 1984.
The first report that mares in lean body condition had lower conception rates.
Hilton, J. W.: Antioxidants: Function, types and necessity of inclusion in pet foods. Can. Vet. J. 30:682, 1989.
A short review on ethoxyquin in pet foods.
Kienzle, E., and Meyer, H.: The effects of carbohydrate-free diets containing different levels of protein on reproduction in the bitch. *In* Burger, I. H., and Rivers, J. P. W. (ed.): *Nutrition of the Dog and Cat.* Cambridge: Cambridge University Press, 1989, p. 243.
Results from research studies of dietary carbohydrate in bitches and puppies.
Kronfeld, D. S.: *Vitamin and Mineral Supplementation for Dogs and Cats.* Santa Barbara: Veterinary Practice Publishing Co., 1989.
A monograph on vitamin and mineral supplementation.
Loveridge, G. G., and Rivers, J. P. W.: Bodyweight changes and energy intakes of cats during gestation and lactation. *In* Burger, I. H., Rivers, J. P. W. (eds.): *Nutrition of the Dog and Cat.* Cambridge: Cambridge University Press, 1989, p. 113.
A review of the authors' nutrition studies on queens and kittens.
Marx, J.: Dissecting the complex disease. Science 247:1540, 1990.
A review of common diseases with complex causes, including nutrition-genetic interactions.
National Research Council: *Nutrient Requirements of Dogs.* Washington, D.C.: National Academy Press, 1985.
A summary of experimental data and committee recommendations regarding canine nutrition.
National Research Council: *Nutrient Requirements of Cats.* Washington, D.C.: National Academy Press, 1986.
A summary of experimental data and committee recommendations regarding feline nutrition.
Noden, D., and deLahunta, A.: *The Embryology of Domestic Animals.* Baltimore, Williams & Wilkins, 1986.
Pennington, J. A. T., and Church, H. N.: *Bowes and Church's Food Values of Portions Commonly Used*, 14th ed. Philadelphia: J. B. Lippincott, 1985.
A compilation of nutrient and calorie values for table foods and commercial foods for humans.
Rainbird, A. L.: Growth and energy requirements of dogs. *In* Edney, A. T. B., and English (eds.): *Nutrition, Malnutrition and Dietetics in the Dog and Cat*, 1987, p. 44.
A summary of research studies on energy requirements.
Romsos, D. R., Palmer, H. J., Muiruri, K. L., et al.: Influence of a low carbohydrate diet on performance of pregnant and lactating dogs. J. Nutr. 111:678, 1981.
A study of dietary carbohydrate in bitches and puppies.

PEDIATRIC NORMAL BLOOD VALUES

MARJORIE L. CHANDLER

Fort Collins, Colorado

HEMATOLOGY

At birth, the packed cell volume of a puppy or kitten is approximately that of the adult dog or cat. The mean corpuscle volume and mean corpuscle hemoglobin are above the normal adult range because of the presence of fetal red blood cells, which are larger than the adult corpuscle. The packed cell volume of the neonate begins to decrease within several days after birth. The physiologic anemia that results is an adaptation to the extrauterine environment, which has a higher oxygen tension than the intrauterine environment. Several factors contribute to the physiologic anemia, including an increased rate of destruction of red blood cells, decreased red blood cell production, and rapid growth of the neonate. Growth of the neonate causes an expansion of the blood volume without a similar increase in the number of red blood cells, resulting in hemodilution. The packed cell volume is lowest in kittens at 3 to 4 weeks of age and in puppies at 4 to 5 weeks of age. The number of red blood cells shows a similar pattern. In puppies less than 2 months of age, the percentage of reticulocytes is about 7%, compared with less than 2% in the normal adult dog. The packed cell volume, number of red blood cells, and hemoglobin concentration increase to normal adult values at approximately 3 to 4 months of age in both puppies and kittens.

The total and differential white blood cell counts of puppies less than 3 months of age are generally in the high normal range for adult dogs. Kittens less than 2 months of age are also in the high normal range for adult cats but may be slightly higher at 3 months of age. Kittens, like adult cats, exhibit an emotional or physiologic leukocytosis when excited. (Tables 1 and 2 present the hematologic values for healthy puppies and kittens.)

SERUM CHEMISTRY

Normal values of several serum chemistry tests differ among young dogs and cats and their adult counterparts (Tables 3 and 4). The differences in normal ranges are frequently a result of the growth process.

Because of bone growth serum phosphorus and calcium concentrations are higher in young, growing animals than in adults. Serum phosphorus concentration may be as high as 11 to 12 mg/dl in a puppy or kitten. Serum calcium concentrations are approximately 2 mg/dl higher in growing animals than in adults.

Serum alkaline phosphatase activity can be 20 to 25 times adult activity in 1- to 3-day-old puppies, possibly because of ingestion of alkaline phosphatase–rich colostrum. The activity decreases by 1 week of age but will remain two to three times adult values during the period of growth. This elevation is due to an increase in the bone alkaline phosphatase isoenzyme derived from the high osteoblast activity in rapidly growing bones. Serum alkaline phosphatase activity will decline in parallel with serum phosphorus concentration as the growth rate decreases.

Serum bilirubin concentrations in puppies less than 3 days old and kittens less than 10 days old may be as high as 1 mg/dl. These concentrations usually decrease to adult concentrations by 10 to 14 days.

Concentrations of total serum protein in puppies and kittens are generally below adult values until 4 to 5 months of age. Concentrations of serum albumin reach adult values at about 2 months of age, but total globulin concentration increases more slowly in response to antigenic stimulation.

Serum creatinine concentration is usually low in puppies and kittens. Creatinine is derived primarily from muscle creatine. Young animals have a lower proportion of muscle relative to total body mass and therefore produce less creatine and creatinine.

Blood urea nitrogen concentration is influenced by the length of the presample fast and by the diet. Fasted puppies will generally have a lower blood urea nitrogen than nonfasted puppies. Caution must be used, however, in fasting young animals to avoid dehydration or hypoglycemia, especially if the animals are sick or stressed. Fasted kittens will generally have a lower blood urea nitrogen than adult cats, but the blood urea nitrogen will not be as low as that for puppies because of the cat's inability to regulate nitrogen catabolism in response to dietary change. If a large proportion of the caloric intake is of protein origin, the cat or dog is likely to have a higher blood urea nitrogen concentration than if the

Table 1. *Hematologic Values of Growing Healthy Puppies**

	Age in Weeks					
Test	*Birth†*	*1†*	*3†*	*6†*	*12‡*	*Adult§*
PCV (%)	47.5	40.5	31.7	32.5	40.9	
	(45.0–52.5)	(33.0–52.0)	(27.0–37.0)	(26.5–35.5)		37–55
Red blood cell count ($\times 10^6/\mu l$)	5.1	4.6	3.8	4.7	6.34	
	(4.7–5.6)	(3.6–5.9)	(3.5–4.3)	(4.3–5.1)		5.5–8.5
Hemoglobin (gm/dl)	15.2	12.9	9.7	10.2	14.3	
	(14.0–17.0)	(10.4–17.5)	(8.6–11.6)	(8.5–11.3)		12–18
Mean corpuscle volume (fl)	93.0	89.0	83.0	69.0	64.6	60–72
Mean corpuscle hemoglobin (pg)	30.0	28.0	25.0	22.0	35.5	—
Reticulocytes (%)	6.5	6.9	6.9	4.5	—	0–2
	(4.5–9.2)	(3.8–15.2)	(5.0–9.0)	(2.6–6.2)		
Total white blood cell count	12.0	14.1	11.2	16.3	17.1	
($\times 10^6/\mu l$)	(6.8–18.4)	(9.0–23.0)	(6.7–15.1)	(12.6–26.7)		6.0–17.0
Band neutrophils	0.23	0.50	0.09	0.05	0.08	
	(0–1.5)	(0–4.8)	(0–0.05)	(0–0.3)		0–0.3
Segmented neutrophils	8.6	7.4	5.1	9.0	9.8	
	(4.4–15.8)	(3.8–15.2)	(1.4–9.4)	(4.2–17.6)		3.0–11.5
Lymphocytes	1.9	4.3	5.0	5.7	5.7	
	(0.5–4.2)	(1.3–9.4)	(2.1–10.1)	(2.8–16.6)		1.0–4.8
Monocytes	0.9	1.1	0.7	1.1	0.9	
	(0.2–2.2)	(0.3–2.5)	(0.1–1.4)	(0.5–2.7)		0.2–1.4
Eosinophils	0.4	0.8	0.3	0.5	0.4	
	(0–1.3)	(0.2–2.8)	(0.07–0.9)	(0.1–1.9)		0.1–1.2
Basophils	0.0	0.01	0.0	0.0	0.0	rare
		(0–0.2)				

*Reprinted with permission from Hoskins, J. D. (ed.): *Veterinary Pediatrics*. Philadelphia: W. B. Saunders, 1990, p. 294. Original data from:
†Earl, F. L., Melvegar, B. A., and Wilson, R. L.: The hemogram and bone marrow profile of normal neonatal and weanling beagle dogs. Lab. Anim. Sci. 23:630, 1973.
‡Anderson, A. C., and Gee, W.: Normal blood values in the beagle. Vet. Med. 53:135, 1958.
§Normal canine adult ranges. Veterinary Pathology Laboratory, Veterinary Teaching Hospital, Colorado State University, Ft. Collins, CO, 1990.
—, Values not available.

Table 2. *Hematologic Values of Growing Healthy Kittens**

	Age in Weeks					
Test	*0–2* Mean (SD‡)	*2–4* Mean (SD)	*4–6* Mean (SD)	*6–8* Mean (SD)	*12–13* Mean (SD)	*Adult†* (Range)
Packed cell volume (%)	35.3 (1.7)	26.5 (0.8)	27.1 (0.8)	29.8 (1.3)	33.1 (1.6)	24–45
Red blood cell count ($\times 10^6/\mu l$)	5.29 (0.24)	4.67 (0.10)	5.89 (0.23)	6.57 (0.26)	7.43 (0.23)	5–11
Hemoglobin (gm/dl)	12.1 (0.6)	8.7 (0.2)	8.6 (0.3)	9.1 (0.3)	10.1 (0.3)	8–15
Mean corpuscle volume (fl)	67.4 (1.9)	53.9 (1.2)	45.6 (1.3)	45.6 (1.0)	44.5 (1.8)	39–50
Mean corpuscle hemoglobin (pg)	23.0 (0.6)	18.8 (0.8)	14.8 (0.6)	13.9 (0.3)	13.7 (0.4)	—
Total white blood cell count	9.67 (0.57)	15.31 (1.21)	17.45 (1.37)	18.07 (1.94)	23.20 (3.36)	5.5–19.5
($\times 10^6/\mu l$)						
Band neutrophils	0.06 (0.02)	0.11 (0.04)	0.20 (0.06)	0.22 (0.08)	0.15 (0.07)	0–0.3
Segmented neutrophils	5.96 (0.68)	6.92 (0.77)	9.57 (1.65)	6.75 (1.03)	11.0 (1.77)	2.5–12.5
Lymphocytes	3.73 (0.52)	6.56 (0.59)	6.41 (0.77)	9.59 (1.57)	10.46 (2.61)	1.5–7.0
Monocytes	0.01 (0.01)	0.02 (0.02)	0	0.01 (0.01)	0	0–0.8
Eosinophils	0.96 (0.43)	1.40 (0.16)	1.47 (0.25)	1.08 (0.20)	1.55 (0.35)	0–1.5
Basophils	0.02 (0.01)	0	0	0.02 (0.02)	0.03 (0.03)	rare

*Modified from Meyers-Wallen, V. N., Haskins, M. E., and Patterson, D. F.: Hematologic values in healthy neonatal, weanling, and juvenile kittens. Am. J. Vet. Res. 45:1322, 1984.
†Normal feline adult ranges. Veterinary Pathology Laboratory, Veterinary Teaching Hospital, Colorado State University, Ft. Collins, CO, 1990.
‡ST, standard deviation; —, value not available.

Table 3. Serum Chemistry Values of Growing Healthy Puppies

Test	3–8 days*† (n = 10)	3 weeks*† (n = 12)	5 weeks* (n = 18)	8–12 weeks*† (n = 10)	12–24 weeks‡ (n = 200)	Adult§
Glucose (mg/dl)	123 (104–132)	126 (109–140)	131 (110–146)	114 (88–131)	111 (85–133)	(65–122)
Blood urea nitrogen (mg/dl)	30 (22–37)	23 (15–23)	15 (10–21)	24 (21–30)	13 (7–19)	(7–28)
Creatinine (mg/dl)	0.5 (0.4–0.6)	0.4 (0.3–0.5)	0.4 (0.3–0.5)	0.5 (0.5–0.6)	0.6 (0.3–0.9)	(0.9–1.7)
Calcium (mg/dl)	12.4 (11.9–13.1)	11.4 (10.7–12.3)	11.1 (10.3–12.6)	11.5 (10.5–12.1)	11.0 (9.8–12.4)	(9.8–12.4)
Phosphorus (mg/dl)	10.4 (8.7–11.8)	9.1 (7.8–10.1)	8.8 (7.0–9.8)	10.5 (10.1–11.3)	9.0 (7.2–10.1)	(2.8–6.1)
Total protein (gm/dl)	4.2 (3.8–4.7)	4.1 (3.6–4.6)	4.7 (3.9–5.3)	4.6 (3.9–5.0)	5.1 (4.6–5.8)	(5.4–7.4)
Albumin (gm/dl)	2.6 (2.3–2.9)	2.7 (2.1–3.2)	3.3 (2.4–4.3)	2.9 (2.0–3.3)	2.8 (2.4–3.1)	(2.7–4.5)
Cholesterol (mg/dl)	223 (160–283)	249 (210–270)	248 (147–322)	111 (86–159)	174 (105–255)	(130–370)
Bilirubin (mg/dl)	1.0 (0.5–1.8)	0.4 (0.2–0.5)	0.5 (0.2–0.7)	0.2 (0.1–0.5)	0.4 (0.2–0.9)	(0.0–0.4)
Alkaline phosphatase (IU/L)	706 (371–1297)	378 (249–512)	355 (150–539)	569 (411–705)	117 (77–199)	(35–280)
Alanine aminotransferase (IU/L)	45 (25–82)	18 (10–24)	24 (6–61)	38 (26–56)	19 (9–30)	(10–120)
Sodium (mEq/L)	144 (143–145)	144 (142–148)	142 (138–145)	149 (146–153)	152 (138–160)	(145–158)
Potassium (mEq/L)	5.6 (5.1–6.5)	4.8 (4.2–5.5)	5.7 (4.0–6.8)	5.5 (5.2–6.6)	5.3 (4.3–6.2)	(4.1–5.5)
Chloride (mEq/L)	102 (99–105)	105 (102–108)	108 (102–117)	106 (104–109)	105 (103–114)	(106–127)

*Chandler, ML and Miller, EV: Unpublished data, means and ranges. Colorado State University, Ft. Collins, CO, 1990.

†Puppies not fasted prior to sampling.

‡Data used with permission from: Lawler, D. F.: Reference intervals for canine blood values: Medians and 95th percentiles. St. Louis, MO: Ralston Purina Co., 1986.

§Normal canine adult range. Veterinary Pathology Laboratory, Veterinary Teaching Hospital, Colorado State University, Ft. Collins, CO, 1990.

Table 4. Serum Chemistry Values of Growing Healthy Kittens

Test	Age in Weeks					
	0–2*	2–4†	4–6†‡	7–12†‡	12–20§	Adult‖
Glucose (mg/dl)	117 (76–129)	110 (99–112)	—	—	82 (59–102)	(67–124)
Blood urea nitrogen (mg/dl)	39 (22–54)	23 (17–30)	25 (15–36)	31 (25–38)	26 (19–34)	(17–34)
Creatinine (mg/dl)	0.4 (0.2–0.6)	0.4 (0.3–0.5)	0.7 (0.2–1.2)	0.6 (0.4–1.0)	0.7 (0.4–0.9)	(0.9–2.1)
Calcium (mg/dl)	—	—	9.7 (8.4–11.0)	9.9 (8.8–11.2)	9.9 (8.9–10.9)	(8.9–10.9)
Phosphorus (mg/dl)	8.0 (6.9–9.3)	8.5 (7.5–9.5)	8.7 (7.6–9.8)	8.6 (7.7–9.5)	8.2 (6.9–10.9)	(3.3–7.8)
Total protein (gm/dl)	4.1 (3.5–4.7)	4.4 (4.1–4.7)	5.0 (4.1–5.9)	5.4 (5.1–5.7)	6.0 (5.4–6.8)	(5.9–8.1)
Albumin (gm/dl)	2.1 (2.0–2.4)	2.3 (2.2–2.4)	—	—	3.1 (2.5–3.6)	(2.3–3.9)
Cholesterol (mg/dl)	229 (164–443)	361 (222–434)	—	—	91 (63–132)	(60–270)
Bilirubin (mg/dl)	0.3 (0.1–1.0)	0.2 (0.1–0.2)	—	—	0.7 (0.4–1.2)	(0 0.3)
Alkaline phosphatase (IU/L)	123 (68–269)	111 (90–135)	—	—	71 (39–124)	(11–210)
Alanine aminotransferase (IU/L)	21 (10–38)	14 (10–18)	25 (9–41)	36 (23–50)	33 (18–58)	(30–100)
Sodium (mEq/L)	140 (134–145)	145 (142–148)	147 (143–151)	150 (147–152)	156 (143–162)	(146–160)
Potassium (mEq/L)	4.7 (4.0–5.4)	5.4 (4.7–6.1)	5.3 (4.7–5.9)	5.6 (5.0–6.2)	5.0 (4.1–5.9)	(3.7–5.4)
Chloride (mEq/L)	—	—	122 (118–127)	122 (113–128)	115 (107–121)	(112–129)

*Data used with permission from Hoskins, J. D. (ed.): *Veterinary Pediatrics*. Philadelphia: W. B. Saunders, 1990, p. 206. Medians and ranges Original data from: Center, S. A., and Hornbuckle, W. E.: New York State College of Veterinary Medicine, 1987, Cornell University, Ithaca, NY.

†Data from Meyers, V. N., Haskin, M. E., and Patterson, D. F.: Unpublished data. University of Pennsylvania, School of Veterinary Medicine, 1984. Means and standard deviations.

‡Data used with permission from Hoskins, J. D.: *Veterinary Pediatrics*. Philadelphia: W. B. Saunders, 1990, p. 274. Means and ranges. Original data from: Hoskins, J. D., and Turnwald, G. H.: Louisiana State University.

§Data used with permission from Lawler, D. F.: Reference intervals for feline blood values: Medians and 95th percentiles. St. Louis, MO: Ralston Purina Co., 1980.

‖Normal feline adult range. Veterinary Pathology Laboratory, Veterinary Teaching Hospital, Colorado State University, Ft. Collins, CO, 1990.

—, Values not available.

major caloric content of the diet is not of protein origin.

Puppies and kittens cannot be viewed as small adult dogs and cats. Blood values for pediatric patients must be evaluated with consideration for the age of animals and the differences present in young animals.

References and Suggested Reading

Bounous, D. I., Hoskins, J. D., and Boudreaux, M. K.: The hematopoietic system. *In* Hoskins, J. D. (ed.): *Veterinary Pediatrics.* Philadelphia: W. B. Saunders, 1990, p. 293.

Center, S. A., Hornbuckle, W. E., and Hoskins, J. D.: The liver and pancreas. *In* Hoskins, J. D. (ed.): *Veterinary Pediatrics.* Philadelphia: W. B. Saunders, 1990, p. 205.

Crawford, M. A.: The urinary system. *In* Hoskins, J. D. (ed.): *Veterinary Pediatrics.* Philadelphia: W. B. Saunders, 1990, p. 274.

Jain, N. C.: *Schalms Hematology.* Philadelphia: Lea & Febiger, 1986, pp. 104–106.

Jezyk, P. F.: Assessment of the sick pediatric patient. *Viewpoints in Veterinary Medicine—Canine Pediatrics.* Allentown, PA: ALPO Pet Center, 1985.

Meyers-Wallen, V. N., Haskins, M. E., and Patterson, D. F.: Hematologic values in healthy neonatal, weanling, and juvenile kittens. Am. J. Vet. Res. 45(7):1322, 1984.

Section
12

NEUROLOGIC AND NEUROMUSCULAR DISORDERS

JOE N. KORNEGAY

Consulting Editor

MANAGEMENT OF REFRACTORY SEIZURES

DOROTHEA SCHWARTZ-PORSCHE

Berlin, Germany

The goal of anticonvulsant therapy is freedom from seizures or at least a significant reduction in seizure frequency with negligible side effects. This goal is not always achieved, however, and some seizure disorders are poorly responsive or refractory to usual anticonvulsant therapy.

In humans with epilepsy, 20 to 30% of the cases are intractable (Schmidt, 1986). This figure may be even higher in affected dogs. Seizures in 20% (Schwartz-Porsche et al., 1985) to 52% (Farnbach, 1984) of dogs are refractive to phenobarbital (PB); between 40% (Schwartz-Porsche et al., 1985) and 48% (Farnbach, 1984) are refractive to primidone (PRM). Similar results have been noted in cats (Schwartz-Porsche and Kaiser, 1989).

Investigations in humans have clearly shown that therapeutic failures are often due to factors other than pharmacoresistance. Patients treated optimally and promptly are resistant to therapy far less often. Therefore, other factors must contribute to the failure of therapy and ultimately pharmacoresistance. Generally, the longer seizures continue after the start of treatment, the less likely they are to be controlled (Schmidt, 1986). In animals, too, and especially in dogs, inappropriate therapeutic management may be partially responsible for refractory seizures (Table 1).

FACTORS RESPONSIBLE FOR INADEQUATE CONTROL OF SEIZURES

Choice of Medication and Dosage

The success of anticonvulsant therapy is definitely dependent on the selection of the antiepileptic drug (Schmidt, 1986). Although human medicine offers drugs of first and second choice for control of different types of seizures, drug selection in dogs is determined less by the type of seizure than by pharmacokinetics, loss of efficacy, and side effects. Most conventionally used antiepileptics for humans are quickly metabolized by dogs, so that even extremely high doses do not maintain therapeutic serum concentrations. Only PB and PRM have proved effective. In cats, diazepam (DZP) and PB are the anticonvulsants of first choice. In both

Table 1. Factors Responsible for Inadequate Control of Seizures

Medication and dosage
  Improper choice of drug
  Insufficient drug dosage
  Delayed increase in dosage
  Inadequate increase in dosage
  Too rapid change of medication
  Too rapid reduction of dosage
  Excessive fluctuations in serum concentrations
  Inappropriately combined drugs
Noncompliance
Drug-drug interactions
Other precipitating factors
  Additional medications
  Additional diseases
  Physical or psychologic stress
Diagnostic failures
  Extracerebral causes of seizures
  Progressive brain lesions

species, however, far less suitable drugs are unfortunately still used by some veterinarians.

The efficacy of an anticonvulsant drug is determined, in large part, by its serum concentration. The most common reason for a lack of therapeutic success is a dose that is too low, resulting in an ineffective serum concentration. The dose is often set too low and then in the course of further therapy not increased quickly enough. When adjusting the dose, it should be raised incrementally by 10 to 30% of the previous amount until seizures do not recur or the limit of drug tolerance is reached. During this process, the serum concentration should be monitored. The therapeutic effect cannot be evaluated until a steady-state concentration has been reached—that is, after approximately five half-lives. This is also true after each increase in dose. Until then, there is no point in measuring the concentration or in increasing the dose; for the anticonvulsants of first choice in dogs and cats, this point is reached after 2 to 3 weeks of therapy.

Serum concentration is determined not only by dose but also by bioavailability, resorption, and elimination of the drug. The same dose can lead to very different serum concentrations in different animals. For this reason alone, blood levels must be critically monitored. Concentrations should be measured in various circumstances: before and after

986

increases in dose; when seizures recur; if behavior or mood changes develop; in conjunction with other diseases; to check an owner's compliance; and routinely at 3- to 6-month intervals. In our judgment, the lowest (trough) serum concentration should be determined immediately before administration of the next dose, because that is when protection is at its lowest. The serum concentration should be measured during or right after a seizure only when seizures recur. The therapeutic serum concentration varies among individual animals. The therapeutic range of PB is from 20 to 40 µg/ml in dogs and from 10 to 30 µg/ml in cats. In animals with persistent seizures that have a concentration in the upper range but tolerate the drug well, even higher doses can be given. In *humans,* the therapeutic range varies somewhat with seizure type; focal seizures with or without secondary generalization require higher concentrations of anticonvulsants than do generalized tonic-clonic seizures (GTCS) (Schmidt, 1986). In *dogs,* there seems to be a relationship between the intensity and frequency of the seizures and the serum concentration; the most difficult seizures to treat are clusters of GTCS and generalized tonic seizures. In cats, complex focal seizures are the most difficult to treat.

The more rapidly the therapeutic serum concentration is reached, the greater the success of therapy may be. We attain the best therapeutic success in animals that are treated without regard to initial side effects. Owners may otherwise become frustrated and request euthanasia prematurely. Initially, higher than normal doses (PB, 3 to 6 mg/kg), are given. In some cases, a loading dose is used. We subsequently raise the dose by greater increments (up to a dose of 10 to 15 mg/kg, or in rare cases 20 mg/kg). Most animals with violent and frequent serial seizures treated in this way—generally as inpatients—became seizure-free within a few weeks, and most remain seizure-free. In outpatients, especially with PRM, the initial dose should be low (PRM, 15 to 30 mg/kg), raised gradually to avoid sedation, and later increased in a stepwise manner (up to a dose of 50 to 70 mg/kg, or in rare cases 100 mg/kg) to avoid the risk of an owner's noncompliance due to unacceptable side effects.

Medication is usually changed too quickly (i.e., before the upper limit of the therapeutic serum concentration range has been reached). An antiepileptic of first choice should only be changed once it has proved unsuccessful after the highest possible serum concentration has been reached. Because monotherapy is superior to polytherapy (Schmidt, 1986), another drug of first choice should be used (e.g., PB [3 to 5 or 10 mg/kg] substituted for DZP [0.5 to 1.0 or 2.0 mg/kg] in cats). Only after the second antiepileptic has also proved ineffective should an additional drug be added. Also, an ap-

parently ineffective anticonvulsant should be changed or discontinued gradually rather than abruptly; otherwise, withdrawal symptoms, seizures, or even status epilepticus may occur. The only exception is a change from PRM to PB: *5 mg PRM is equivalent to 1 mg PB.*

Once therapeutic success has been achieved, a rapid reduction in dose can lead to a serious relapse. After 6 to 12 seizure-free months, the dose may be reduced by about 10 to 20% of the immediately preceding dose at 6-month intervals, while the serum concentration is monitored. If seizures recur, the dose should be raised again to the level at which the animal became free of seizures. To achieve this, even higher doses than were initially necessary may be needed.

Fluctuations in the serum concentration can also lead to failure. If the intervals between doses are too long or the daily dose is not evenly distributed, the serum concentration can vary between ineffective and toxic. Intervals between doses should be substantially shorter than the half-life of elimination, because the shorter the interval, the less the concentration fluctuates. The daily doses should be distributed as follows: in dogs—PB at least twice a day, PRM at least three times a day; in cats on DZP and PB at least three times a day, given at regular intervals. At shorter intervals, the serum concentration declines less if a dose is missed.

Frequent mistakes in an inappropriate combined therapy are as follows: (1) the dose of the first drug is not increased sufficiently before the second drug is added; (2) the doses of both drugs are too low; (3) a drug that is inappropriate because of its pharmacokinetics, the development of tolerance, or the indication (absence seizures) is added; or (4) both drugs are unsuitable.

Noncompliance

Apparent resistance to therapy or relapses are often due to noncompliance, which may or may not be intentional. Noncompliance may arise because of the relationship between the veterinarian and an animal's owner. Insufficient education of an owner about seizure incidence and therapy, unrealistically high expectations of therapy, anxiety about initial side effects, and potential organ damage from medication can cause an owner to reduce the dose, to medicate irregularly, and to change veterinarians repeatedly.

We try to involve the owners intensively in the therapy. They are asked to keep a notebook in which all seizures are recorded with the date, time of day, and description of the event. The daily administration of medication, drug serum concentrations (which are monitored periodically), the animal's condition, additional illnesses (even trivial

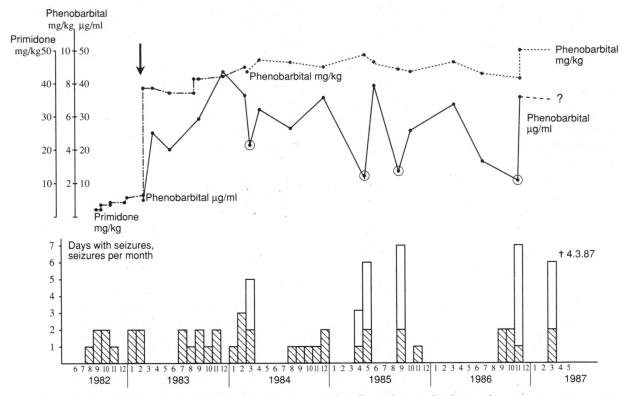

Figure 1. Therapeutic failure as a result of noncompliance in a male collie with generalized tonic-clonic seizures. Age at onset was 8 years. The dog was initially treated with primidone in very low doses. After referral to our clinic (*arrow*), we raised the dose twice and switched over to phenobarbital because of an increase in liver enzymes. During this therapy, the dog suffered repeated relapses with clusters of seizures, at which point we checked the serum concentration of the phenobarbital four times (circled on the graph). The low concentrations were due to forgotten medication. At the last relapse, the dog died without access to emergency treatment. *Shaded areas* represent number of seizure days per month; *shaded* plus *unshaded areas* represent number of seizures per month.

ones), and physical and psychologic stress the animal suffers are also recorded. Keeping this notebook contributes to the regular administration of the medication. At the same time, factors responsible for relapses come to light.

Figure 1 shows that especially when the seizures have stopped or been reduced, anticonvulsants are easily forgotten or given irregularly. In the case pictured, the relapse was not due to drug resistance but rather to a decrease in serum concentration. By filling a drug dispenser each evening, one can draw attention to a forgotten dose that can then be administered.

Drug-Drug Interactions

Anticonvulsants can influence each other's effects, either intensifying them (increase in serum concentration) or reducing them (reduction in serum concentration). Interaction can occur with other drugs, too. In many cases, interaction depends on the amount of the drug involved, because the quantity of the added drug determines the extent and direction of enzyme induction or enzyme inhibition.

Nonanticonvulsants with which interactions are encountered include antibiotics, antacids, cardiac medications, theophylline and its derivatives, antirheumatics, steroids, and other drugs. Because interactions and their effects are not always known and predictable, the concentration of the anticonvulsant should be determined before beginning combined therapy. Additional medication should be noted. If relapses or sedation appear with co-medication, the blood level of the anticonvulsant must be checked. This way, over time, we may be able to collect more information about drug interactions and avoid therapeutic failures.

Other Precipitating Factors

Administration of other drugs may precipitate seizures by lowering the seizure threshold. Phenothiazines, especially acepromazine, are known to have this effect. Other drugs can have similar side effects. It may not be possible to predict deleterious drug interactions. For example, we have encountered seizure relapses with anthelmintics (piperazine, mebendazol) and metoclopramide in dogs that had been seizure-free for months, but not all of our epileptic dogs that received these medications have had seizures.

Additional diseases can contribute to the incidence of seizures. With gastroenteritis, the concentration of anticonvulsants can quickly decline to subtherapeutic levels. Animals that repeatedly vomit or need to fast should be given PB or DZP (cats) parenterally from the first day. Other diseases that do not cause a reduction in the concentration of anticonvulsants (e.g., pneumonia, metabolic disturbances) may increase seizure activity.

Physical and psychologic stress also infrequently provoke seizures. When seizures have repeatedly occurred in animals subsequent to the same events, such as long trips, the absence of the owner, or loud parties, we increase the dose of the anticonvulsant for a short time in advance of the situation.

Diagnostic Failures

If the number of seizures persists or increases despite a constant serum concentration in the upper therapeutic range of an antiepileptic of first choice, diagnosis should be re-evaluated. Intractable seizures can also be brought about by extracerebral causes (e.g., hypoglycemia and hypocalcemia) and by progressive brain lesions (e.g., brain tumors).

COMBINED THERAPY

Combined therapy for refractory seizures is only suitable when the antiepileptic of first choice has been given to the limits of its tolerance without success and when the following factors have been ruled out: other mistakes in therapy, noncompliance, drug interactions, precipitating factors, and diagnostic failures.

Only a few antiepileptics are suitable for combined therapy in dogs. Phenytoin, carbamazepine, and valproate are so quickly metabolized that effective serum concentrations cannot be reached, even with extremely high doses. With the exception of clonazepam (saturation kinetics), the benzodiazepines exhibit a short half-life, and central tolerance develops. Two drugs have been successfully used as adjuvants in dogs: potassium bromide (KBr) and mephenytoin (MHT).

Bromide was first used in 1957 by Locock for the treatment of epilepsy. Interest in bromide waned rapidly with the development of modern antiepileptic drugs, and it has only recently been reintroduced for the treatment of intractable epilepsy, especially in children (Boenigk et al., 1985; Ernst et al., 1988).

Bromide is quickly absorbed in the small intestine and is neither metabolized nor bound to serum protein. In contrast to other antiepileptics, it does not lead to enzyme induction and does not react with any other drugs. Its elimination, which is almost exclusively renal, is very slow.

The average half-life of elimination for bromide in dogs is nearly 25 days, which is about twice as long as in humans. The statistically estimated half-life during the accumulation phase, 16.5 days on the average, proved to be shorter than the half-life calculated during the subsequent elimination phase. Therefore, the steady-state concentration of bromide is reached before five half-lives of elimination (Schwartz-Porsche et al., 1990).

We achieved a marked reduction in seizure frequency with the addition of KBr in 58% of the dogs that had proved absolutely therapy-resistant to PB or PRM or both. This result was reached primarily in dogs that had only suffered GTCS with an onset between 1 and 4 years of age. In evaluating only these animals, 85% showed more than a 50% reduction in seizures; of these, 31% became seizure-free. We had no success in dogs with different seizure types and generalized tonic seizures (Schwartz-Porsche et al., 1990; Schwartz-Porsche and Jürgens, 1991). These results correspond to those in children with intractable epilepsy who were given KBr as a second drug. Again, the best results were noted in children suffering only GTCS. In 64 to 79% of these patients, the frequency of seizures fell by more than 50%, and of these, 18 to 32% became seizure-free (Boenigk et al., 1985; Ernst et al., 1988). In some animals, we were gradually able to reduce somewhat the PB and KBr doses, as a case example in Figure 2 shows.

The therapeutic serum concentration of bromide in humans is 0.5 to 1.9 mg/ml (Boenigk et al., 1985), which is about the same as in dogs. As in humans, dogs show individual sensitivity differences. Most dogs can tolerate a concentration of bromide up to 1.5 mg/ml quite well. In older animals and those with additional diseases, concentrations of 1.5 to 2.0 mg/ml cause distinct and in some cases intolerable side effects, whereas young and otherwise healthy dogs may tolerate concentrations of even 2.0 to 2.5 mg/ml.

Adjunctive therapy should begin with daily doses of 30 to 40 mg/kg of KBr. Pure KBr salt can be measured into capsules or dissolved in water to be given orally.* KBr can be obtained as a reagent-grade chemical from chemical suppliers. The plasma concentration can be elevated more rapidly with a double or triple loading dose on the first day of therapy. In urgent cases, Sisson (1990) begins bromide therapy in dogs on the first day with a loading dose of 400 to 600 mg/kg of KBr in a water solution administered over 30 to 60 min. He thus achieves an immediate bromide concentration of 1.0 to 1.5 mg/ml.

---

*Editors' Note: Client's permission should be obtained before initiating this therapy.

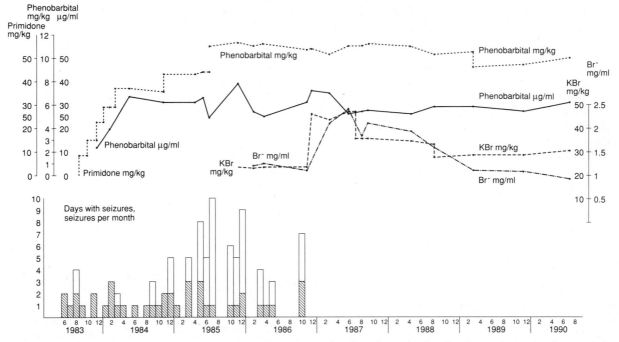

Figure 2. Therapeutic success with postassium bromide (KBr) in a female cocker spaniel with refractory generalized tonic-clonic seizures. Age at onset was 1.9 years. Therapy began with primidone; because of increasing liver enzymes, therapy was changed to phenobarbital. Only after the addition of bromide and an increase in the dose to 46 mg/kg did the dog become free of seizures, at an average concentration of 2.2 mg/ml. After that, both doses were gradually decreased. The dog remained free of seizures at about 1 mg/ml of bromide. *Shaded areas* represent number of seizure days per month; *shaded* plus *unshaded areas* represent number of seizures per month.

We have not yet given this high a dose, for fear of powerful sedative side effects as well as stomach irritation resulting in nausea and vomiting. Because serum concentrations differ from dog to dog given the same dose, the dose must be individually adapted during the course of the therapy. This involves monitoring serum levels, taking into account the length of time required for bromide to reach a steady state. The therapy cannot be evaluated before the steady state is reached, so the dose should not be increased before then. Variations in the bromide concentration can be caused by changing the intake of table salt. A higher intake of chloride leads to an increase in renal excretion and a reduction in the serum concentration of bromide.

At the beginning of combined therapy, some animals show transient sedation. This may continue for up to 3 weeks in older animals or those with additional diseases. We have not encountered chronic bromide intoxication even after several years of administration of doses up to 60 mg/kg. In hematologic and biochemical tests carried out at irregular intervals, there were no changes that could be attributed to the bromide, and the chloride concentration was always in the normal range.

Combination anticonvulsant therapy that includes KBr has been associated with the development of pancreatitis in some of our patients. Since monotherapy with PB and PRM also has been related to

development of pancreatitis, we cannot be certain of the role, if any, played by KBr. Accordingly, the clinician should be aware of this possible adverse effect and consider drug-associated pancreatitis in epileptic animals that develop clinical signs consistent with this response.

As an additional drug in adjunctive therapy, Sisson (1990) recommends *MHT*, which works through its main metabolite, nirvanol. He controlled seizures with this compound in several dogs that had been refractory to PB and KBr. As an initial dosage, he recommends 10 mg/kg PO every 8 hr, with the dosage increased as needed to achieve a therapeutic blood level of nirvanol of 25 to 40 μg/ml. A steady-state blood level should be achieved in 6 days. Because of its various side effects, especially on the hematopoietic system, this substance is generally not used in humans. Dogs should therefore be carefully monitored when the drug is used, although the only observed reaction thus far has been sedation. I have had no experience with this drug.

Chlorazepate, which is quickly metabolized to desmethyldiazepam, may be valuable as an adjuvant drug. Therapeutic concentrations of desmethyldiazepam were reached in experiments with 2 mg/kg PO every 8 hr. Less tolerance seems to develop than with DZP and clonazepam. An abrupt discontinuation of the drug, however, led to severe withdrawal symptoms and even lethal seizures (Scherkel et al., 1989). I am not aware of any clinical experience with chlorazepate in dogs.

Combined antiepileptic therapy has rarely been used in *cats*. I have only combined DZP with phenytoin in prolonged therapy. A daily dose of 1 to 2 mg/kg resulted in a phenytoin concentration of 5 to 17 μl/ml. Over time, concentrations of greater than 10 μg/ml were not tolerated very well. In two of three animals, more than a 50% reduction in seizure frequency was achieved.

PARENTERAL AND RECTAL ADMINISTRATION OF ANTIEPILEPTICS

In animals that continue to suffer from clusters of seizures despite all therapeutic efforts, we try to achieve a breakthrough with parenteral or rectal administration of antiepileptics. We have owners give these dogs PB, about 10 mg/kg IM or SC, immediately after a seizure occurs. If necessary, the dose can be repeated. We have been able to reduce the number of seizures significantly or avoid the transition to status epilepticus in some animals. We have had less success with DZP in dogs. With the same indication in cats, however, we have had good success with DZP, which we apply at the rate of 1 mg/kg SC or 1 to 2 mg/kg rectally with a solution commercially available for babies.

CONCLUSION

The number of animals who suffer from refractory seizures should be significantly reduced with the selection of a truly appropriate antiepileptic, a gradual increase in the dose of this drug to the limits of its tolerance, and the avoidance or limitation of all factors that might have a negative effect on the therapy. If seizures still occur, adjunctive therapy with KBr or MHT is an option. With GTCS, KBr may give especially good results.

References and Suggested Reading

Boenigk, H.-E., Lorenz, J.-H., and Jürgens, U.: Bromide—heute als antiepileptische Substanzen noch nützlich? Nervenarzt 56:579, 1985.
One of the first uses of bromide showing success in the treatment of intractable epilepsy in children.

Ernst, J. P. E., Doose, H., and Baier, W. K.: Bromides were effective in intractable epilepsy with generalized tonic-clonic seizures and [sic] onset in early childhood. Brain Dev. 10:385, 1988.
Report on the efficacy of KBr in children with different intractable seizure types, which could not be controlled with conventional anticonvulsants at the highest tolerable doses.

Farnbach, G. C.: Serum concentrations and efficacy of phenytoin, phenobarbital, and primidone in canine epilepsy. J.A.V.M.A. 184:1117, 1984.
Comparison of the effectiveness of phenytoin, PB, and PRM, relating dosage to serum concentration in dogs with epilepsy.

Scherkel, R., Kurudi, D., and Frey, H.-H.: Chlorazepate in dogs: Tolerance to the anticonvulsant effect and signs of physical dependence. Epilepsy Res. 3:144, 1989.
Comparison of experimental results in six dogs given chlorazepate for 5 to 6 weeks.

Schmidt, D.: Diagnostic and therapeutic management of intractable epilepsy. In Schmidt, D., and Morselli, P. L. (eds.): *Intractable Epilepsy.* L.E.R.S. Monograph Series. Vol. 5, New York: Raven Press, 1986, p. 237.
Discussion of factors that can cause intractable epilepsy and of diagnostic and therapeutic assessments.

Schwartz-Porsche, D., and Jürgens, U.: Die Wirksamkeit von Bromid bei den therapieresistenten Epilepsien des Hundes. Tierärztl. Prax. 19:395, 1991.
Report on the efficacy of bromide depending on seizure type, dose, and serum concentration in intractable canine epilepsy.

Schwartz-Porsche, D., and Kaiser, E.: Feline epilepsy. Probl. Vet. Med. 1:628, 1989.
A detailed review of the etiology and diagnostic and therapeutic management of feline epilepsy, including the authors' investigation results.

Schwartz-Porsche, D., Löscher, W., and Frey, H.-H.: Therapeutic efficacy of phenobarbital and primidone in canine epilepsy: A comparison. J. Vet. Pharmacol. Ther. 8:113, 1985.
Comparison of the effectiveness of PB and PRM in a prospective study of a minimum of 6 months with routine monitoring of serum concentrations.

Schwartz-Porsche, D., Jürgens, U., May, T., et al.: Pharmacokinetics of bromide and bromide therapy in canine epilepsy. Proceedings of the 4th Annual Symposium of the ESVN, Bern, 1990, p. 32.
Report on the accumulation and elimination of bromide and the efficacy of KBr in the treatment of intractable canine epilepsy.

Sisson, A.: Diagnosis and treatment of seizure disorders of dogs and cats. ACVIM Scientific Proceedings, 1990, p. 349.
Overview of diverse diagnostic and therapeutic possibilities.

PSYCHOMOTOR SEIZURES IN DOGS

D. C. SORJONEN

Auburn, Alabama

The occurrence of bizarre behavioral activity with or without motor seizures is most appropriately termed psychomotor seizures (PMS). The clinician managing dogs with PMS is faced with many frustrations. First, confusion exists regarding the nosology and resulting terminology in PMS. In addition, the clinician must differentiate PMS from other forms of bizarre, frequently stereotyped behavioral abnormalities of non-neurologic origins or from neurologic lesions in locations remote from the cerebral cortex (e.g., tail chasing with lumbosacral lesions) (see this volume, pp. 995 and 1020). Finally, the diagnostic tests and treatment modalities currently available often are inadequate to sufficiently diagnose and treat dogs with PMS. This report will review pertinent literature regarding PMS from veterinary and human medicine and discuss current acceptable and experimental diagnostic and therapeutic modalities.

NOMENCLATURE

Seizures have been classified according to cause, location, clinical signs, frequency, and electroencephalographic (EEG) correlates. As a result, a profusion of terms have been used synonymously with PMS, including temporal lobe, pyriform lobe, hippocampal, automatic, autonomic, behavioral, and rhinencephalic seizures. Recently, a classification based on clinical signs and EEG correlates has been internationally adopted for humans with seizures; this classification also appears useful for affected animals (Gastaut, 1970). Using this classification, PMS would be considered a partial complex seizure. A partial seizure indicates involvement of a focal area of the brain (compared with generalized brain involvement). Complex symptomatology indicates impairment of consciousness. Humans are diagnosed as having partial complex seizures based on sophisticated electrodiagnostic, neuroimaging, and neuropsychologic evaluations not available in veterinary medicine. Until more sensitive techniques for animal evaluation become available, the use of the term psychomotor seizure in veterinary medicine appears most appropriate.

CLINICAL FEATURES

In PMS, a clear predilection for age and breed is not apparent. Of 82 reported cases of PMS, 27 different breeds of dogs were affected (Breitschwerdt et al., 1979; Carithers, 1973; Cash and Blauch, 1979; Holliday et al., 1970). Clinical signs began between 6 months and 12 years of age. In one report (Breitschwerdt et al., 1979), eight of ten dogs were males; however, in another study involving a large number of dogs (Holliday et al., 1970), data regarding a sexual bias were not reported. From the sample population available for review, a predilection by gender for PMS cannot be determined.

The "psychic" or behavioral changes precede any motor component that may occur with PMS. The events that constitute the behavioral abnormalities are extremely varied and can include apparent blindness or staring into space, viciousness, attacking inanimate objects, restlessness, somnolence, inappetence or voracious appetite, vomiting, diarrhea, terror-stricken behavior, trembling, walking in circles, jaw champing, and inappropriate howling, barking, running, and licking. Dogs are often nonresponsive during these episodes. These changes may last from minutes to hours. The behavioral sign may be the only abnormality or may be followed by a generalized (tonic-clonic) motor seizure.

The clinical signs associated with PMS in dogs and humans are similar. In humans, PMS are not peculiar to any period of life but show an increased incidence in adolescence and adult years. The aura (a simple partial seizure) can include illusions (objects or persons in the environment shrink or recede into the distance), hallucinations (visual, auditory, gustatory, or olfactory), states of disordered cognition (déjà vu or jamais vu), or affective experiences (fear and anxiety). As in dogs, the psychic changes may constitute the entire seizure or may be followed by a motor phase. The motor component principally contains stereotypic (automatistic) inappropriate behavior, including lip smacking, chewing or swallowing, walking in circles, running, and laughing. During this phase, patients may have periods of intense rage or blind fury. Seizures of this type may proceed to tonic spasms or generalized (tonic-clonic) motor seizures. Although at times it is illogical to anthropomorphize, the psychic and motor events recorded in humans with PMS appear to have similar manifestations in dogs.

PATHOPHYSIOLOGY

Experimentally, PMS can be produced in cats by destruction of the pyriform lobe or hippocampus. The affected structures in animals with experimental PMS are located in the temporal lobe and are part of the limbic system, which serves to modulate emotional expression such as eating, rage, sexual activity, fear, and drinking. All or some of these experimentally induced activities have been noticed in dogs with spontaneous PMS.

Diseases that produce PMS in humans principally affect structures in the temporal lobe. In most cases, lesions occur in the medial portion of the temporal lobe. The hippocampus and amygdala also may be affected. Focal lesions arise from tumors, tuberous sclerosis, parasitic cysts, hemorrhagic foci, hematomas, and post-traumatic scars. Nonfocal lesions are mainly observed in the anteromedial part of the temporal lobe, the anterior insular lobe, and the orbital area of the frontal lobe. The most common etiopathologic causes are ischemic anoxia secondary to birth trauma, inflammatory vascular lesions, or the seizures themselves.

Although focal lesions secondary to traumatic scars and neoplasia reportedly may produce spontaneous PMS in dogs, most cases involve diffuse lesions. Inflammatory diseases, notably canine distemper virus encephalomyelitis (see this volume, p. 1003), have produced disseminated demyelination in the pyriform lobe and polioencephalomalacia in the pyriform lobe, hippocampus, and ventromedial structures of the temporal lobe. Ischemic anoxia (secondary to vascular lesions and seizures) was the proposed mechanism for the polioencephalomalacia (Braund and Vandevelde, 1979). Unassisted parturition that occurs in most dogs also can produce traumatic ischemic lesions that can result in PMS, seemingly more frequently than in human neonates.

DIAGNOSIS

A diagnosis of PMS may be suspected in dogs with paroxysmal bizarre behavior alterations that are often accompanied by generalized motor seizures. Causes of PMS include, but are not limited to, canine distemper virus encephalomyelitis, thromboembolic disease, trauma, lead poisoning, and idiopathic causes. Selection of diagnostic tests to confirm an intracranial cause for the clinical signs is predicated on evidence from the neurologic examination for a focal versus multifocal localization.

Although not intended to detect an etiologic cause, scalp recordings of the EEG can help determine an intracranial origin for the abnormalities noticed in dogs and humans with PMS and may suggest a focal versus multifocal localization. Most dogs have generalized slow waves with synchronous spindles (Breitschwerdt et al., 1979); however, in dogs with lead toxicosis, the EEG contains paroxysmal high voltage–medium frequency waves (Knecht et al., 1979). EEG recordings during a PMS event have not been reported. In humans, ictal EEG recordings can identify the temporal lobe as the site of the seizure focus, thus providing a clinicopathologic correlation for the diagnosis of PMS. In dogs, definitive antemortem evidence for a temporal lobe origin for PMS is uncommon. This may result from the multifocal nature of most causes of PMS or from the insensitivity of scalp electrodes to detect focal electrical discharges in deep brain structures like the temporal lobe. The EEG recordings from subdural electrodes or electrodes implanted into the brain of humans diagnosed with PMS have greatly improved the ability to detect the initial seizure onset and have provided a more precise indication that the temporal lobe is the origin of the seizure focus. It is hoped that with the increased availability in veterinary medicine of the advanced imaging techniques required for electrode placement, these newer EEG recording techniques will also benefit companion animals with PMS.

Cerebrospinal fluid analysis can help establish an etiologic diagnosis. In canine distemper virus infection, cerebrospinal fluid analysis typically reveals 15 to 60 white blood cells per cubic millimeter that are predominantly mononuclear (lymphocytes and macrophages) (see this volume, p. 1003). Mature dogs with canine distemper virus may have elevated gamma globulin levels. The presence of neutralizing antibody to canine distemper virus or canine distemper virus–specific IgG titers in cerebrospinal fluid, especially without evidence of blood-brain barrier disturbance, is the most definitive evidence of a patent canine distemper virus infection (Thomas, 1990).

In most cases of PMS, hematologic and biochemical analyses are normal. In lead poisoning, dogs usually have circulating nucleated red blood cells and basophilic stippling without marked anemia. Blood lead levels normally should not exceed 0.35 ppm. Radiopaque densities may be present in the intestinal tract, and immature dogs may also have radiopaque lines just proximal to the epiphyseal plates of long bones.

Trauma, tumor, and thromboembolism of the brain are focal conditions that less frequently produce PMS. Neuroimaging techniques such as computed tomography, magnetic resonance imaging, and single photon emission computed tomography are ideal for the detection of focal brain lesions and are routinely used to confirm the diagnosis of PMS in humans. Computed tomography and magnetic resonance imaging can directly image intraparenchymal abnormalities such as tumors and atrophy (secondary to vascular necrosis or trauma). Single photon emission computed tomography provides information that can indicate a region of nonspecific dysfunction. A large percentage of the cases of PMS reported in dogs is idiopathic. Adaptation of these technologies to veterinary neurology will greatly increase the veterinarian's ability to definitively diagnose these intracranial conditions.

DIFFERENTIAL DIAGNOSIS

Non-neurogenic abnormal stereotypical behaviors are common in dogs (Dodman et al., 1988). Some of the clinical signs include self-licking, fly-biting, staring, destructive behavior, vicious behavior, aggression, pacing or circling, and hypersexuality. These changes are thought to be attention-getting behaviors or *psychosomatic* disturbances (Breitschwerdt et al., 1979) (see this volume, p. 995) and may be difficult to differentiate from a PMS event. In general, if the neurologic examination is normal, if the abnormal behavior ceases when the dog is placed in an unfamiliar environment, and if it is easy to distract the dog from the abnormal behavior with auditory or visual stimuli, a psychosomatic or inappropriate behavior, as opposed to a PMS, must be considered.

Lumbosacral lesions or peripheral neuropathies may produce compulsive tail chasing or self-licking and chewing of affected areas that can mimic a PMS. Lumbosacral disease or peripheral neuropathy is suspected if there is pain or gait and reflex abnormalities not attributable to PMS.

PROGNOSIS

Currently, there is not a permanent cure for PMS. If the underlying cause can be determined and successfully treated, the prognosis can be upgraded. However, in many instances, the pathologic brain changes induced by the inciting cause persist after treatment and continue to act as a seizural focus.

TREATMENT

Every reasonable effort should be made to discover and treat the underlying cause for the PMS. However, anticonvulsants are the cornerstone of therapy for PMS. Results of anticonvulsant therapy in dogs with PMS range from unrewarding to nearly 100% success. This variability in results may reflect the diagnostic index (see earlier discussion of EEG sensitivity). The principles of anticonvulsant therapy have previously been discussed (Bunch, 1986) (see this volume, p. 986).

Phenobarbital remains the drug of choice for dogs with generalized motor seizures and PMS. Effective dosages range from 5 to 16 mg/kg/day, divided twice or three times daily. Effective steady-state serum and tissue concentrations of phenobarbital are achieved after 7 to 10 days of oral administration. Serum phenobarbital levels should be determined after steady state is achieved, and then every 6 months. Effective levels range from 10 to 45 μg/ml. Anticipated side effects include sedation, ataxia, polydipsia, and polyuria.

Primidone (5 to 15 mg/kg every 8 hr PO) is metabolized to phenobarbital and phenylethylmalonamide. The side effects and recommendations for therapeutic serum concentrations are similar to those for phenobarbital. Phenytoin is an effective anticonvulsant in humans but is unsuitable in dogs because of its short half-life, which necessitates high doses administered three times daily, making it expensive and inconvenient. Several newer anticonvulsants that act on the γ-aminobutyric acid inhibitory systems, inhibit release of excitatory amino acids, or interact with neuronal membranes and change ion flow are available to treat seizures in humans. Therapeutic studies to establish effective dosages of these newer drugs have not been done in veterinary medicine.

A surgical option exists for humans with intractable PMS. The seizure focus is located electrically with depth or subdural electrode EEG recordings, anatomically by computed tomography and magnetic resonance imaging, and metabolically with single photon emission computed tomography. Surgical procedures include lobectomy for focal lesions and hemispherectomy or corpus callosotomy for diffuse lesions. Approximately 40% of all cases in humans with PMS are candidates for surgical therapy. Approximately one third of these patients became seizure-free and one third have a marked reduction in seizures after surgery. The mortality rate is approximately 0.2%. The advent of newer diagnostic and surgical techniques in veterinary medicine should allow a similar response in the dog.

References and Suggested Reading

Braund, K. G., and Vandevelde, M.: Polioencephalomalacia in the dog. Vet. Pathol. 16:661, 1979.
Clinical and histopathologic features in 25 dogs with polioencephalomalacia.
Breitschwerdt, E. B., Breazile, J. E., and Broadhurst, J. J.: Clinical and electroencephalographic findings associated with ten cases of suspected limbic epilepsy in the dog. J. Am. Anim. Hosp. Assoc. 15:37, 1979.

A review of the anatomy and physiology, clinical features, and medical treatment of limbic epilepsy.

Bunch, S. E.: Anticonvulsant drug therapy in companion animals. *In* Kirk, R. D. (ed.): *Current Veterinary Therapy IX.* Philadelphia: W. B. Saunders, 1986, p. 836.
A review of the diagnostic rationale and medical therapy of seizures in the dog and cat.

Carithers, R. W.: Psychomotor episode of a poodle. Iowa State University Veterinarian 35:48, 1973.
A report involving aggression that responded to anticonvulsant medications.

Cash, W. C., and Blauch, B. S.: Jaw snapping syndrome in eight dogs. J.A.V.M.A. 175:709, 1979.
Clinical and histopathologic features of dog with bizarre behavior.

Dodman, N. H., Shuster, L., White, S. D., et al.: Use of narcotic antagonists to modify stereotypic self-licking, self-chewing, and scratching behavior in dogs. J.A.V.M.A. 193:815, 1988.
A review of the pathophysiology, pharmacokinetics, and effects of two narcotic antagonists for the treatment of spontaneous stereotypic behavior in 11 dogs.

Gastaut, H.: Clinical and electroencephalographical classification of epileptic seizures. Epilepsia 11:281, 1970.
Results of a 20-year clinical and electrophysiologic study in humans that served as a basis for a classification of epileptic seizures.

Holliday, T. A., Cunningham, J. G., and Gutnick, M. S.: Comparative clinical and electroencephalographic studies of canine epilepsy. Epilepsia 11:281, 1970.
Results of the clinical and electroencephalographic features of 70 dogs with spontaneous seizures.

Knecht, C. D., Crabtree, J., and Katherman, A.: Clinical, clinicopathologic and electroencephalographic features of lead poisoning in dogs. J.A.V.M.A. 175:196, 1979.
A review of the clinical features and results of diagnostic tests and treatment in 11 dogs with suspected lead poisoning.

Thomas, W. B.: Diagnostic findings in confirmed CNS distemper viral infections. ACVIM Scientific Proceedings, 1990, p. 109.
A review of the clinical features and results of diagnostic tests in 38 dogs with histopathologic evidence of canine distemper encephalomyelitis.

TAIL CHASING IN DOGS

SHARON L. CROWELL-DAVIS

Athens, Georgia

Tail chasing is a normal component of play behavior in dogs, perhaps more so in those without another dog available as a playmate (Houpt and Wolski, 1982). It becomes a problem when it occurs excessively, when the dog injures itself in the process of chasing its tail, and when the dog cannot be distracted from tail chasing for other activities.

PATHOGENESIS

There are three primary etiologies of excessive tail chasing: it can be an entirely learned behavior, it can be due to central nervous system lesions, or it can be due to peripheral lesions. One or all of these factors can contribute to the behavior in a given case.

Learned Behavior

A variety of normal and abnormal behaviors can increase in frequency and duration as a result of operant conditioning. Operant conditioning is the process by which a behavior is affected by its consequences. Because the dog is a social animal, owner attention is often a positive reinforcer and causes the frequency of a behavior to increase even if the owner does not intend for this to happen. Under certain circumstances, even adversive stimulation by the owner can serve as a positive rein-forcer. For example, the dog that receives little owner attention may experience any kind of owner attention as highly rewarding. Behavior problems that result from increased frequency of a given behavior as a result of owner attention have been referred to as "attention-getting behavior" by Hart and Hart (1985).

It is possible for attention-seeking behavior to appear suddenly as a severe problem subsequent to a single learning incident. However, more typically it has a gradual onset, progressively worsening over at least several days. Once the problem is established, it will be maintained by even occasional owner attention when the behavior occurs. Tail chasing may occur in isolation as a learned attention-seeking behavior, or it may be part of a complex of behaviors (e.g., jumping and barking).

Central Nervous System Pathology

Severe tail chasing has previously been described as a subepileptic episodic behavior (Pemberton, 1980). Psychomotor epilepsy is discussed in detail in this volume, p. 992.

Tail chasing, as well as various other stereotypic behaviors, has been successfully treated using narcotic antagonists (Brown et al., 1987; Dodman et al., 1988; Marder, 1987). Therefore, endogenous, morphine-like substances must be involved in the manifestation of the behaviors in these cases. One possibility is that the behaviors cause a release of endogenous opioids that stimulate the pleasure center. In cases involving self-mutilation, the endogenous opioids would also protect the animal from the perception of pain. This and other theories are discussed in detail by the authors noted.

Peripheral Disease or Injury

A variety of peripheral lesions resulting in pain, itching, or other irritating sensations on the tail or hindquarters can cause a dog to run in circles. These include but are not limited to diseases or injury of the peripheral nervous system (Komarek, 1988) and skin (Pemberton, 1983).

MANAGEMENT

Evaluation

The severity of pathologic tail chasing ranges from occasional and moderately excessive tail chasing without injury (which owners may find distracting but which otherwise causes no harm) to persistent tail chasing with self-mutilation, anorexia, and adipsia. In the severest type of case, the dog will stop chasing its tail only when exhaustion causes it to sleep briefly.

When a client initially complains of a dog's tail-chasing problem, several questions are important in initially assessing the severity of the problem (Table 1). These questions are designed to ascertain the extent and duration of the tail chasing per se, and to determine whether the problem is most likely learned or medical. A dog that can easily be distracted from tail chasing, that exhibits such behavior only under certain circumstances, and that engages in various other behaviors in conjunction with the tail chasing has probably learned the behavior. Conversely, a dog that cannot be distracted, that chases its tail persistently in a wide variety of circumstances, and that mutilates itself probably has a medical problem. However, there are exceptions even to these extreme examples (Crowell-Davis et al., 1989), and many histories have mixed evidence supporting both medical and learned problems.

Treatment

Treatment of tail chasing as a learned behavior caused by positive reinforcement requires removal of the positive reinforcer. When this is done, extinction will occur. Extinction is the process by which a behavior that has previously been re-

***Table 1.** Anamnestic Questions for Tail Chasing**

1. What is the duration of the problem?
2. Did the behavior begin suddenly at its current intensity, or has the problem increased gradually?
3. How frequently does tail chasing occur?
4. How long is a typical bout of tail chasing?
5. How many hours per day does the dog engage in tail chasing?
6. Is it easy/moderately difficult/very difficult/impossible to distract the dog?
7. Does tail chasing occur only under certain circumstances (e.g., when the owner first comes home or while the family is eating)?
8. Does the dog chase its tail at night?
9. Does the dog engage in other active behaviors in close temporal sequence to the tail chasing (i.e., jumping, barking)?
10. Was there a visible injury on the hindquarters, hindlimbs, or tail prior to the time the dog began chasing its tail?
11. Does the dog mutilate itself on the hindquarters, hindlimbs, or tail?
12. Does the dog run into objects (e.g., walls and furniture) as it chases its tail? Does it appear to be aware of doing so? Does it injure itself by running into objects?
13. Does the dog engage in normal maintenance behaviors (i.e., eating, drinking, and sleeping)?

*Questions 1–5 are designed to ascertain extent and duration; remaining questions are designed to determine whether behavior is learned or medical in nature.

inforced gradually decreases in frequency when the reinforcement no longer occurs.

It is also important to provide positive reinforcement for alternative, acceptable behaviors. While this may seem simple and straightforward, numerous nuances of the learning process and logistical problems often confound treatment. Some of the more common confounding problems will be discussed here.

Extinction procedures produce strong emotional effects coupled with behavioral arousal (i.e., there is a general increase in activity). As the animal becomes aroused owing to the absence of the expected reward, tail chasing may initially increase dramatically.

The dog will have learned to chase its tail on one or more of a variety of reinforcement schedules. These can be broadly categorized as continuous reinforcement, in which every occurrence of the behavior is rewarded, and partial or intermittent reinforcement. In general, if an animal has received continuous reinforcement, there will be greater emotional arousal when the extinction process is initiated. If the animal has received intermittent reinforcement, there will be less arousal but extinction will take longer. This phenomenon is reviewed in detail in various texts on learning (Domjan and Burkhard, 1986).

Consequently, the dog's owner may be confronted with an initial increase in tail chasing or with persistence of tail chasing even after several days of nonreinforcement. This can be very frustrating for the client and may lead to a resumption of partial rewards in an attempt to calm the dog or for other reasons. Resumption of rewards after they have been withdrawn for a period does not merely end treatment. It can exacerbate the problem and makes future attempts at treatment even more difficult.

Thus, in advising clients regarding treatment, it is important to make sure they understand the difficulties they may encounter. The entire family must be involved in the program, as noncompliance by one family member can nullify the efforts of the others. Whenever the dog engages in tail chasing, it must be totally ignored. The family also needs to decide what alternative behaviors are desirable and reinforce these with attention. Jumping up and initiation of tail chasing always cause an immediate removal of any form of attention. If the owners are persistent and consistent with this treatment, the nonreinforced behavior (tail chasing) will gradually occur less and less frequently and will be replaced by the behaviors that are being reinforced.

The treatment of psychomotor epilepsy and peripheral pathologies that can cause tail chasing are discussed extensively elsewhere in this book and in other veterinary literature.

Whether a case of tail chasing will respond to a narcotic antagonist can be determined only by assessing the current extent of tail chasing, administering an antagonist, and then reassessing the behavior. This can be done in the clinic with a subcutaneous injection of 0.01 mg/kg of naloxone (Brown et al., 1987). If the dog responds, home treatment with oral naltrexone at 1 to 2 mg/kg daily, such as has also been used with excessive licking (Marder, 1987), may alleviate the problem.

Use of narcotic antagonists for the treatment of tail chasing is still experimental. Criteria for determining duration of treatment do not yet exist. Some dogs remain free of clinical signs after short-term treatment of 2 to 4 weeks (Marder, 1987); others resume the behavior when medication is withdrawn after longer treatment. A bull terrier with severe, persistent tail chasing was successfully treated with a combination product containing 50 mg of pentazocine and 0.5 mg of naloxone every 12 hr PO (Brown et al., 1987). It was maintained on this dosage without side effects for 2 years, after which medication was withdrawn. Tail chasing then only occurred during excitement, and the dog could be distracted.

References and Suggested Reading

Brown, S. A., Crowell-Davis, S., Malcolm, T., et al.: Naloxone-responsive compulsive tail chasing in a dog. J.A.V.M.A. 190:884, 1987. (Published erratum appears in J.A.V.M.A. 190:1434, 1987.)
  A case report on tail chasing in a bull terrier that responded to naloxone.
Crowell-Davis, S. L., Lappin, M., and Oliver, J. E.: Stimulus-responsive psychomotor epilepsy in a Doberman pinscher. J. Am. Anim. Hosp. Assoc. 25:57, 1989.
  Case report of a Doberman pinscher that exhibited abnormal stereotypical behavior that could be ameliorated temporarily by environmental stimuli but which had an abnormal electroencephalogram and responded to treatment with anticonvulsants alone.
Dodman, N. H., Shuster, L., White, S. D., et al.: Use of narcotic antagonists to modify stereotypic self-licking, self-chewing, and scratching behavior in dogs. J.A.V.M.A. 193:815, 1988.
  The effects of naltrexone and nalmefene on dogs' stereotypical self-licking, chewing, and scratching were evaluated.
Domjan, M., and Burkhard, B.: *The Principles of Learning and Behavior.* Pacific Grove: Brooks/Cole, 1986, p. 148.
  A review of research on extinction of operantly learned behaviors.
Hart, B. L., and Hart, L. A.: *Canine and Feline Behavioral Therapy.* Philadelphia: Lea & Febiger, 1985, p. 82.
  A discussion of diagnosis and therapy for attention-getting behavior in dogs.
Houpt, K. A., and Wolski, T. R.: *Domestic Animal Behavior for Veterinarians and Animal Scientists.* Ames, Iowa: Iowa State University Press, 1982, p. 196.
  A discussion and review of characteristics of play behavior in the dog.
Komarek, J. V.: Fallbericht: Verfolgung der Rute beim Hund-Cauda-equina-Syndrom. (Case report: Tail chasing in a dog with cauda equina syndrome.) Kleintierpraxis 33:25, 1988.
  Tail chasing in a German shepherd caused by compression of the cauda equina was treated by decompression with dorsal laminectomy.
Marder, A. R.: Naltrexone for the treatment of acral lick dermatitis in dogs. Newsletter of American Veterinary Society of Animal Behavior 10:8, 1987.
  Six dogs with acral lick dermatitis were treated with 1 to 2 mg/kg of naltrexone.
Pemberton, P. L.: Canine and feline behavior control: Progestin therapy. In Kirk, R. W. (ed.): *Current Veterinary Therapy VIII.* Philadelphia: W. B. Saunders, 1983, p. 62.
  A descriptive summary of the different types of behavior problems seen by the author, with information on the use of progestins to treat these problems.
Pemberton, P. L.: Feline and canine behavior control: Progestin therapy. In Kirk, R. W. (ed.): *Current Veterinary Therapy VII.* Philadelphia: W. B. Saunders, 1980, p. 845.
  A descriptive summary of the types of behavior problems seen by the author, with information on the use of progestins and other medications in their treatment.

METABOLIC ENCEPHALOPATHIES

DENNIS P. O'BRIEN,
and ROBERT A. KROLL
Columbia, Missouri

Metabolic encephalopathy (ME) refers to a disturbance of brain function and resulting neurologic deficits caused by disorders of metabolism. The brain is one of the most metabolically demanding organs in the body. The maintenance of the resting membrane potential and the synthesis, transport, release, and termination of neurotransmitters require a large percentage of the body's energy production. Metabolic diseases can interfere with normal central nervous system (CNS) function through a number of different processes, such as interference with energy metabolism, alterations of fluid and electrolyte balance, or production of endogenous toxins.

Energy deficiencies produce the most rapid and severe disturbances. The brain has few endogenous substrates for energy metabolism and relies almost exclusively on blood glucose for its energy needs. Likewise, the brain has little capacity for anaerobic metabolism and requires a constant supply of oxygen. As the available oxygen or glucose diminishes, brain activity decreases, resulting in depression of function. A large percentage of the energy consumed by the brain is devoted to the maintenance of the resting membrane potential by the Na^+-K^+ pump. As this pump fails, membrane potential will decay toward threshold, producing discharge and seizures. With further decreases in energy metabolism, electrical activity ceases, cell loss occurs, and, when vital areas of the brain are affected, death ensues.

Calcium, sodium, and potassium are the electrolytes most directly involved in normal neurologic function, although others such as magnesium and zinc also play a role. Calcium is essential for a variety of functions in the nervous system, including release of neurotransmitters from synaptic vesicles and the generation of dendritic potentials. Thus, alterations of calcium can profoundly influence CNS function. Interference with neurotransmission can result in either decreased or increased CNS activity, depending on whether predominantly excitatory or inhibitory neurotransmitters are involved. Changes in potassium and sodium concentrations primarily affect muscle strength and osmolality, respectively.

Changes in serum osmolality and water balance can have a dramatic effect on the brain. Acute hyperosmolar syndromes cause dehydration and shrinkage of brain cells. If the onset of hyperosmolality is gradual, the brain cells increase intracellular osmolality by incorporating plasma solutes and by producing other, unknown (idiogenic) osmoles. Thus, if a chronic hyperosmolar state is corrected too rapidly, the brain may become hypertonic in relation to the serum, resulting in cerebral edema. Similar cerebral edema occurs in cases where the serum becomes hypo-osmolar because of metabolic disturbances such as hyponatremia.

Normally, the blood-brain barrier serves to tightly regulate the internal milieu of the brain by excluding unwanted compounds while selectively transporting in necessary ones. Osmolality changes may disrupt the integrity of the blood-brain barrier by shrinking endothelial cells, thus allowing compounds that are normally excluded access to the CNS.

Endogenous toxins may alter neurotransmission by interfering with neurotransmitter synthesis or through the synthesis of "false neurotransmitters," compounds that act like neurotransmitters but not in a normal fashion. Toxins can also interfere with energy metabolism in the brain, producing cellular hypoxia. Seizures may occur as the result of this hypoxia or direct excitatory effects of the endogenous toxins on the cerebral cortex.

CLINICAL SIGNS OF METABOLIC ENCEPHALOPATHY

The onset of signs in ME can be either peracute, as in abrupt hypoxia, or chronic and insidious, as in gradual liver failure. Since metabolic diseases will diffusely affect the CNS, signs will generally be bilaterally symmetric. Although occasionally some asymmetry may be present, it is generally not as dramatic as that seen with focal CNS disease. The cerebral cortex has the greatest metabolic requirements; thus, clinical signs seen with ME usually reflect cortical dysfunction. The primary signs will be behavioral changes, alterations in consciousness, motor deficits, and seizures. Signs of brainstem dysfunction (especially nystagmus) may develop later in the course of ME, and in some cases (such as thiamine deficiency) brainstem signs may predominate.

Signs of Cerebral Cortical Dysfunction

Early in the course of ME, behavior changes will predominate. The animal will often be depressed and lethargic and may demonstrate confusion and disorientation. Alternatively, the animal may show excitability, hyperactivity, and irritability. Loss of housebreaking and other learned behaviors indicate failure of memory functions. Signs may be intermittent and may be associated with feeding (hepatic encephalopathy) or exercise (hypoglycemia, hypoxia). As the disease progresses, further depression of consciousness will occur. Aimless pacing, circling, and head pressing are common findings. When circling is present, the animal generally walks in large, irregular circles which may vary in direction, in contrast to the tight, unidirectional circles seen with brainstem or vestibular disease. Visual deficits may present as reluctance to move or bumping into objects. If untreated, ME can progress to stupor and coma in the terminal stages of the disease.

Motor deficits in ME are relatively mild early in the disease, since cortical control is not critical for generating locomotion in animals. With progression toward stupor and coma, ataxia, paresis, and eventually paralysis become apparent.

Seizures, myoclonus, and tremors occur commonly with certain metabolic diseases. While seizures usually occur with other signs of cortical disease, they may be the only sign of ME. The seizures are usually generalized because of the diffuse effects of the metabolic disturbances. When focal muscle twitching occurs, it is usually bilaterally symmetric and often affects the facial muscles more severely than other muscle groups. Myoclonus may also occur, especially in hypoxic and uremic encephalopathies. It tends to be diffuse, symmetric, and induced by stimulation as opposed to the focal, spontaneous myoclonus of canine distemper.

DIAGNOSTIC APPROACH

Since numerous metabolic disturbances can cause ME and since signs are nonspecific, a thorough workup is essential in a patient showing signs of encephalopathy. Ancillary tests such as cerebrospinal fluid analysis, serology, skull radiographs, and brain imaging may be necessary to rule out some of the other causes of encephalopathy.

History and Physical Examination

A careful history in ME cases will usually reveal other signs of metabolic disturbances (anorexia, polyuria/polydypsia, vomiting, diarrhea, dyspnea, and so forth). If the case has progressed to stupor or coma, physical and neurologic exam findings become similar to those of many other diseases. An accurate history then becomes critical to limiting differential diagnoses and providing direction for testing and therapy. Many signs of cortical dysfunction, such as seizures, incontinence, and behavior changes, are best identified in the history as are certain cranial nerve signs such as dysphagia, regurgitation, and voice change. Physical examination, like the history, may reveal signs of the systemic disease responsible for the ME.

Neurologic Examination

A patient with suspected ME should receive a complete neurologic examination to rule out multifocal diseases, such as canine distemper (see this volume, p. 1003), and to provide a baseline from which to judge progression of the disease. The neurologic findings in ME will reflect the diffuse cortical dysfunction. Early in the disease, the behavior changes may be episodic and may not be evident on examination; however, obvious depression of consciousness or inappropriate behavior will generally be evident. Gait will often be relatively normal but not appropriately directed. Postural reactions will often be affected, especially visual placing and sensitive tests of coordination such as hemiwalking. Failure to respond to visual stimuli, such as cotton balls tossed through the air, may indicate blindness or depressed consciousness. The response to visual menace is often lost. The pupillary light reflex will distinguish central blindness from lesions of the retina, optic nerve, and chiasm. Along with the doll's eye reflex, the pupillary light reflex is important for assessing midbrain and pontomedullary function. This aids in determining whether the altered consciousness is caused by diffuse cortical disease or a brainstem reticular activating system lesion. Segmental reflexes and extensor tone may be increased or normal, depending on the degree of motor involvement. In some cases, such as hypermagnesemia, they may be depressed because of effects at the neuromuscular junction or spinal cord.

Clinical Pathology

In any animal with signs of ME, a minimum database consisting of a complete blood count, urinalysis, and serum chemistry profile (including electrolytes) is essential (Table 1). With hepatic failure caused by cirrhosis or portosystemic shunts, liver enzymes may be normal, and the only abnormalities on routine serum chemistries may be decreased

Table 1. Database in Metabolic Encephalopathies

Minimum Database	Ancillary Tests
Physical exam	Blood gases
Neurologic exam	pH
Complete blood count	Po_2
Urinalysis	Pco_2
Serum chemistries	Serum magnesium
Glucose	Serum osmolality
Blood urea nitrogen	Thyroid function tests
Alanine aminotransferase	Serum bile acids
Alkaline phosphatase	Resting ammonia/ammonia
Albumin	challenge
Cholesterol	Electrocardiogram
Total CO_2	Chest and abdominal
Amylase/lipase	radiographs
Electrolytes	Electrodiagnostics
Sodium	(electroencephalogram and
Potassium	brainstem auditory-evoked
Calcium	responses)
Phosphorus	

blood urea nitrogen, glucose, albumin, or cholesterol. Thus liver function tests, such as serum bile acids, fasting ammonia, or ammonia challenge, are necessary to rule out hepatic encephalopathy. An ammonia challenge may be necessary if the fasting blood ammonia level is near normal. Exogenous ammonia may decompensate borderline hepatic failure, and a challenge test is unnecessary and contraindicated if the fasting blood ammonia level is unequivocally elevated.

In cases where hypoxia is suspected, an electrocardiogram, chest radiographs, and blood gases will be necessary. Blood gases are also useful to assess acid-base status. If hyperosmolar coma is possible (e.g., diabetes mellitus or hypernatremia), serum osmolality should also be measured directly, if possible. Alternatively, effective osmolality can be calculated by the formula:

$$osmolality = 2Na + glucose/18 + BUN/2.8$$
$$(normal = 285 \text{ to } 310 \text{ mOsm}).$$

Thyroid function tests should be considered in all cases of undiagnosed encephalopathy, particularly if other signs of hypothyroidism are present (see this volume, p. 330).

Electrodiagnostic Tests

Electrodiagnostic evaluation of patients with stupor or coma can aid in determining which level of the nervous system is affected. The electroencephalogram provides a means of assessing cortical function. With depressed cortical function there is diffuse slowing of the electroencephalographic frequency. Early in the course of disease, the changes may be minimal and indistinguishable from normal drowsiness or sedation. As the disease pro-

gresses to coma, slowing intensifies, and eventually flattening of the electroencephalogram occurs as cortical activity ceases. In some cases, such as hypoglycemia, epileptic discharges may also be apparent. The changes in the electroencephalogram reflect the alteration of cortical activity and tend to be similar regardless of the cause. Brainstem auditory-evoked responses are useful in assessing brainstem function and, thus, rule out reticular activating system lesions as a cause of the altered mental status.

GENERAL CONSIDERATIONS IN THERAPY

Therapy in ME always centers on correcting the underlying metabolic disturbance. In mild cases, diagnostic testing should be used to direct appropriate therapy. In an animal that has progressed to coma, the ABCs of emergency medicine (Airway, Breathing, Circulation) are the highest priority. If the animal is in status epilepticus, an anticonvulsant drug should be used to control the seizures, pending definitive diagnosis and treatment. (Hypoglycemia should also be ruled out.) The benzodiazepines, such as diazepam, are the drugs of choice in suspected metabolic disease, since they have a wide margin of safety and minimal hepatotoxicity. If barbiturates are necessary, they must be administered cautiously, since metabolism may be compromised. Also, acidosis decreases ionization of barbiturates, allowing better penetration of the blood-brain barrier. In some cases, seizures will be poorly responsive to anticonvulsant drugs, and correction of the underlying metabolic disturbance is the only way to stop the seizures.

SPECIFIC ENCEPHALOPATHIES

It is beyond the scope of this discussion to review in depth all the different metabolic diseases associated with signs of encephalopathy (Table 2). We will limit our discussion to selected aspects of pathophysiology and therapy as they relate to the encephalopathy. The reader is referred to the references that follow for more detailed discussions.

Hypoxia

Diminished oxygen tension will quickly interfere with major brain functions. An acute drop in arterial Po_2 below 40 to 50 mm Hg will cause diminished cerebral function. At levels below 20 to 30 mm Hg, consciousness is lost. Permanent brain damage ensues very rapidly unless adequate oxygenation is restored.

Table 2. Metabolic Diseases Associated with Signs of Encephalopathy

Hypoglycemia (insulinoma, sepsis, insulin overdose, liver failure)
Hyperglycemia (hyperosmolar diabetes mellitus)
Hyponatremia (Addison's disease, water intoxication, syndrome of inappropriate antidiuretic hormone)
Hypernatremia (dehydration, diabetes insipidus, hyperaldosteronism)
Hypocalcemia (eclampsia, hypoparathyroidism)
Hypercalcemia (paraneoplastic, rodenticide toxicity, hyperparathyroidism)
Hypothyroidism
Hepatic insufficiency (hepatic cirrhosis, portosystemic shunts)
Uremia
Pancreatitis
Hypoxia (heart failure, respiratory disease, toxins)
Acidosis
Alkalosis
Thiamine deficiency

Hypoglycemia

The severity of signs associated with hypoglycemia depends on the degree of hypoglycemia and how rapidly it developed. The earliest signs associated with hypoglycemia are behavior changes. Lethargy and depression or hyperexcitability and irritability may be present; some animals will fluctuate between these states. Muscle tremors and focal twitching, especially of the facial muscles, can be a prominent feature. The hypoglycemia stimulates catecholamine secretion, which contributes to the muscle tremors and behavior changes. Syncopy or seizures will occur if the glucose drops rapidly or the ability of the brain to adapt to lower glucose levels is exceeded. If the condition is not corrected, permanent damage to the CNS or peripheral nervous system can result as neurons die from lack of energy substrates.

Treatment with intravenous glucose (2 to 4 ml/kg of 50% glucose diluted to 25% concentration to avoid phlebitis) will quickly reverse the signs of encephalopathy in all but the most severe cases. An aggressive search for, and correction of, the underlying cause must accompany symptomatic therapy (see this volume, p. 368).

Hepatic Encephalopathy

Hepatic encephalopathy is probably one of the most intensely studied metabolic encephalopathies; yet the precise pathogenesis of the CNS signs remains unclear. Various endogenous toxins normally cleared by the liver (amino acids, mercaptans, ammonia, γ-aminobutyric acid, and false neurotransmitters) have been implicated and undoubtedly all contribute to some degree. Clinical signs are predominantly depression of consciousness and altered behavior (pacing, circling, head pressing). Seizures sometimes occur, especially late in the disease. Therapy is directed toward decreasing production or absorption of toxins generated by bacterial activity in the lower gastrointestinal tract (see this volume, p. 639).

Uremic Encephalopathy

Renal failure is often associated with deterioration of mental functions, terminating in coma and death. As in hepatic failure, numerous endogenous toxins contribute to the cerebral dysfunction, but parathormone elevation in response to renal failure may be a primary cause of the encephalopathy. In experimental uremia in dogs, brain calcium is elevated to twice normal levels. The elevation in brain calcium, electroencephalographic changes, and neurologic signs are prevented by parathyroidectomy prior to inducing uremia. Thus, therapy in renal failure should include decreasing phosphorus uptake through the use of low phosphate diets and phosphate binders, as well as directly antagonizing parathormone action with drugs such as cimetidine.

Hypothyroidism

Hypothyroidism can produce encephalopathic signs through several mechanisms. Chronic hypothyroidism may result in cerebral atherosclerosis and ischemic damage to the brain. In addition, hypothyroidism has direct effects on the nervous system, causing diminished brain activity. Both changes can be reversed by thyroid supplementation (see this volume, p. 330).

Electrolyte Abnormalities

HYPOCALCEMIA

In addition to the muscle twitching and tetany characteristic of the disease, there are often signs of profound CNS dysfunction, including hyperactivity, irritability, and seizures. Treatment consists of intravenous 10% calcium gluconate (0.5 to 1.5 ml/kg up to 10 ml) diluted in 5% dextrose and given slowly while monitoring the heart for bradycardia or electrocardiographic changes. This quickly reverses muscle twitching and tremors. The behavioral changes, however, may take considerably longer to reverse, presumably because of the slow equilibration of calcium through the blood-brain barrier.

HYPERCALCEMIA

With hypercalcemia, signs of gastrointestinal disturbances, renal failure, and cardiac dysrhythmias predominate, but weakness, hyporeflexia, and depression are also common. In severe cases, stupor, coma, and seizures may be present. Therapy consists of diuresis with intravenous 0.9% NaCl and furosemide. If necessary, glucocorticoids are used to decrease gastrointestinal absorption of calcium and as specific therapy for lymphoma (a common cause of hypercalcemia of malignancy). In extreme cases, intravenous sodium bicarbonate or sodium ethylenediaminetetraacetic acid may be needed to decrease serum ionized calcium; diuresis lowers total serum calcium.

HYPONATREMIA

Hyponatremia occurs in primary polydypsia, hypoadrenocorticism, severe congestive heart failure, and the syndrome of inappropriate antidiuretic hormone. The decreased serum osmolality in hyponatremia can cause cerebral edema and signs of depression, weakness, seizures, and eventually coma. Since the syndrome of inappropriate antidiuretic hormone can occur secondary to a variety of neurologic diseases, it is important to establish whether the neurologic signs are caused by a primary brain lesion. In mild cases, water restriction may be sufficient to restore normal sodium concentrations. In more severe cases, intravenous normal saline or hypertonic saline administration may be necessary. Sudden correction of hyponatremia can lead to lysis of myelin in the thalamus and brainstem, causing progressive, spastic quadriplegia and death beginning 3 to 5 days after instituting therapy. Consequently, serum sodium concentrations should not be increased more than 10 mEq/L/day (see this volume, p. 301).

HYPERNATREMIA

Sodium is a major osmole in serum. Therefore, hypernatremia can result in hyperosmolality and intracellular dehydration. This effect on brain cells produces typical encephalopathic signs of depression, weakness, seizures, coma, and eventually death. In cases with prolonged or severe hypernatremia (>170 mEq/L), it is critical to correct the hypernatremia very slowly, since compensatory increases in intracellular osmolality could cause cerebral edema if serum osmolality is decreased too rapidly. It is best to administer half-strength or normal saline (which will still be hypo-osmolar in relation to the patient's serum) for the first 24 to 48 hours. As serum sodium concentrations approach normal, 5% dextrose may be used to correct the remaining water deficits.

HYPERMAGNESEMIA

Magnesium imbalances are not common in small animals. Hypermagnesemia will interfere with calcium utilization and cause signs similar to those of hypocalcemia. We have seen neurologic signs associated with hypermagnesemia following the administration of a magnesium sulfate cathartic to a cat.

Acid-Base Imbalances

ACIDOSIS

Since carbon dioxide diffuses readily across the blood-brain barrier, respiratory acidosis produces significant acidosis in the CNS. In cases of metabolic acidosis, cerebrospinal fluid pH drops more slowly and seldom reaches blood pH levels. Decreased cerebrospinal fluid pH is associated with diminished cerebral function, although the exact mechanism is unclear. Seldom is acidosis the sole metabolic disturbance affecting the brain. Hypoxia may complicate cases of respiratory disease, while most causes of metabolic acidosis (uremia, diabetes, and so forth) can also cause ME independent of acidosis.

When bicarbonate is given to correct acidosis, paradoxical CNS acidosis may result. The bicarbonate combines with hydrogen ions to produce carbon dioxide and water. The carbon dioxide diffuses across the blood-brain barrier much more readily than bicarbonate and combines with water, thereby liberating carbonic acid and lowering CNS pH. This effect is usually transient, but it can temporarily worsen the encephalopathy.

ALKALOSIS

Hypocapnia seen with respiratory alkalosis will decrease cerebral blood flow, thereby decreasing brain oxygenation. In addition, alkalosis will alter serum phosphorus and ionized calcium levels. Since hyperventilation may be caused by CNS disease, primary brain disease needs to be considered as a cause of abnormal neurologic signs and alkalosis.

CONCLUSION

Metabolic encephalopathies represent a diagnostic challenge in that numerous diseases may present with similar clinical signs. However, with a thorough neurologic evaluation and appropriate diagnostic tests, an accurate diagnosis can be made. With proper attention to some of the details discussed earlier, many of the neurologic complications of metabolic disease can be completely reversed.

References and Suggested Reading

Adams, R. D., and Victor, M.: The acquired metabolic disorders of the nervous system. *In* Adams, R. D. (ed.): *Principles of Neurology.* 3rd ed. New York: McGraw Hill, 1985, pp. 787–808.
  An overview of metabolic encephalopathies in human neurology.
Asbury, A. K., McKhann, G. M., and McDonald, W. I.: *Diseases of the Nervous System: Clinical Neurobiology.* Philadelphia: W. B. Saunders, 1986.
  Several good chapters devoted to human metabolic encephalopathies.
Fraser, C. L., and Arief, A. I.: Nervous system complications in uremia. Ann. Int. Med. 109:143, 1988.
  A review of neurologic signs and treatment of human uremic encephalopathy and a discussion of relevant animal experiments.
Kornegay, J. N., and Mayhew, I. G.: Metabolic, toxic, and nutritional diseases of the nervous system. *In* Oliver, J. E., Hoerlein, B. F., and

Mayhew, I. G. (eds.): *Veterinary Neurology.* Philadelphia: W. B. Saunders, 1987, p. 255.
Kruger, J. M., Osborne, C. A., and Polzin, D. J.: Treatment of hypercalcemia. *In* Kirk, R. W. (ed.): *Current Veterinary Therapy IX.* Philadelphia: W. B. Saunders, 1986, p. 75.
Laureno, R.: Central pontine myelinolysis following rapid correction of hyponatremia. Ann. Neurol. 13:232, 1983.
  Experimental study showing myelinolysis in dogs with too rapid correction of hyponatremia.
Martin, R. A. (ed.): Portosystemic shunts. Semin. Vet. Med. Surg. 5, 1990.
  Contains reviews of the pathophysiology of hepatic encephalopathy, surgical treatment of shunts, and medical management of the encephalopathy.
McCandless, D. W.: *Cerebral Energy Metabolism and Metabolic Encephalopathies.* New York: Plenum Press, 1985.
Mikicuik, M. G., and Thornhill, J. A.: Control of parathyroid hormone in chronic renal failure. Comp. Cont. Ed. 11:831, 1989.
  A review of the role of parathyroid hormone in renal failure and recommendations for therapy.
Ross, L. A.: Disorders of sodium metabolism. ACVIM Scientific Proceedings, 1986, p. 2/111.
Schaer, M.: The diagnosis and treatment of metabolic and respiratory acidosis. *In* Kirk, R. W. (ed.): *Current Veterinary Therapy IX.* Philadelphia: W. B. Saunders, 1986, p. 59.
Wheeler, S. L.: Emergency management of the diabetic patient. Semin. Vet. Med. Surg. 3:265, 1988.
  Management of ketoacidosis and hyperosmolar syndrome.

THE NEUROLOGIC FORM OF CANINE DISTEMPER

M. VANDEVELDE
and M. CACHIN
Berne, Switzerland

PATHOGENESIS

Canine distemper virus (CDV) is a morbillivirus that enters its host usually by way of an aerosol infection (Appel et al., 1981). The virus replicates first in the lymphoid tissues and 10 to 14 days postinfection invades various epithelial tissues and the central nervous system (CNS). The virus has been shown to cross the blood-brain barrier by way of infected lymphoid cells and can also enter the brain parenchyma through the cerebrospinal fluid pathways. CDV replicates in neurons and glial cells and induces gray and white matter disease. The lesions in the white matter are characterized by demyelination (selective loss of the myelin sheaths with preservation of axons) and occur in predilection sites such as the cerebellum, optic system, and spinal cord. Involvement of the gray matter is also possible, though less frequent, and includes not only cerebellar and cerebral cortex but also the gray matter of the spinal cord.

Most research on distemper pathogenesis has focused on the mechanisms of demyelination in this disease. To understand lesion development in the brain and the neurologic signs, it is important to consider the severe immunosuppressive effect of CDV in the acute stage of the infection (Krakowka et al., 1980). Dogs that are unable to mount a quick effective antiviral immune response develop a rapidly progressive disease and die. Those that are able to respond early to CDV will recover with little or no clinical signs. A third group shows a delayed or intermediary immune response and tends to develop a chronic neurologic disease (Appel et al., 1982). The early demyelinating lesions are associated with viral replication in glial cells of the white matter (Vandevelde et al., 1985). There is little evidence that oligodendrocytes, the cells producing the myelin sheaths, are infected, but *in vitro* and *in vivo* studies have shown that these cells are severely damaged by some mechanism that is still not well understood. In the chronic stage of the infection, an inflammatory response occurs in the areas of demyelination. The inflammation is often associated with worsening of the tissue damage and progression of the neurologic signs. Thus, immune-mediated mechanisms appear to be involved. The inflammatory infiltrate consists of lymphocytes and monocytes and many immunoglobulin-secreting cells. Indeed, the intrathecal humoral immune response is reflected in the composition of the cerebrospinal fluid, with marked elevation of IgG content. These antibodies, which are produced in the brain, are directed against CDV, as well as against myelin antigens (mainly myelin basic protein) (Vandevelde et al., 1986). The presence of antimyelin antibodies both in serum and cerebrospinal fluid in distemper suggests that autoimmunity could be involved in lesion formation. However, neither occurrence nor titer of these antimyelin antibodies correlates with the course of the disease; in fact the highest titers are found in recovering animals (Krakowka et al., 1973). In addition, comparative morphologic studies between distemper encephalitis and experimental allergic encephalitis, a defined autoimmune demyelinating disease, did not provide support for autoimmunity in distemper. It is likely that the intrathecal antiviral immune response plays an important role in the formation of the chronic lesion. We found that addition of serum or cerebrospinal fluid from dogs with distemper to brain cell cultures infected with CDV resulted in stimulation of the brain macrophages that are present in large number in these cultures. Stimulation of the macrophages resulted in secretion of free radicals of oxygen (Griot et al., 1989). In subsequent experiments, it was shown that such oxygen radicals are highly toxic for oligodendrocytes, the myelin-producing cells. These observations *in vitro* are probably applicable to the lesions *in vivo*, where the necessary ingredients, including virus-infected glial cells, macrophages, and antiviral antibody, are all available. Thus, these experiments showed how the antiviral immune response could be responsible for the severe tissue damage seen in chronic demyelinating lesions. It is clear that such macrophage reactions are damaging to the virus as well and that, in this sense, they are beneficial for the host. Indeed, it has been shown that the inflammatory response is associated with clearance of CDV from the chronic lesions. However, despite the presence of an apparently effective intrathecal immune response, CDV manages to persist in the central nervous system, providing a continuous source of viral antigen to maintain tissue-damaging reactions. Viral persistence is probably the key to the pathogenesis of the chronic disease (Summers et al., 1983). The mechanisms by which CDV is able to persist in the central nervous system must be further investigated.

CLINICAL SIGNS

The classic clinical presentation of distemper is seen in a puppy that develops signs of a systemic illness with respiratory and gastrointestinal stress, fever, emaciation, and lymphopenia. These signs are followed, 2 or 3 weeks later, by neurologic signs. In our cases, systemic signs occurred in about half of the animals, either prior to or accompanying the neurologic signs. When present, the most common extraneural stress are gastrointestinal or upper respiratory stress, conjunctivitis, hyperkeratosis of the footpads (hard pad disease) or the nose, fever, and lymphopenia. However, the clinical presentation varies widely, and neurologic distemper can occur at any age. Systemic signs are often very mild or remain subclinical and unnoticed. Many dogs with distemper are presented with neurologic signs only. The type of neurologic signs depends on the distribution of virus in the central nervous system and localization of the lesions. A clinical pathologic correlation is often lacking; in fact, experimental studies have shown a very high incidence of subclinical lesions. The lesions are multifocal, but one localization can often clinically dominate. Common signs include blindness and seizures and signs of central vestibular, cerebellar, and spinal cord disease.

Myoclonus, rhythmic jerking of single muscles or muscle groups, is a common sign of distemper, often involving muscles of the head and the limbs. It occurred in about one third of the cases we have evaluated. It is thought that myoclonus in dogs is a pathognomonic sign for distemper; however, we have observed myoclonus in other conditions as well. The mechanism of myoclonus in distemper is not well understood. Experimental studies have shown that focal spinal cord lesions may be responsible for this sign. It is also possible that a basal nuclei lesion may initiate myoclonus by establishing a "pacemaker" in the cord or brainstem (De Lahunta, 1983). Hyperkeratosis of the footpads or nose, which may be related to viral persistence in epidermal cells, occurs in our experience in about 8% of dogs with neurologic distemper.

Ocular changes may also be present. Optic tracts are often affected by CDV, producing optic neuritis characterized by unilateral or bilateral blindness with fixed, dilated pupils. In some animals, mild swelling of the optic disk may be evident on fundic examination. Retinitis can also occur. In the acute stage, ill-defined gray to pink densities in the tapetal or nontapetal area can be seen, whereas well-lineated hyper-reflexic retinal densities occur in inactive chronic stages.

CDV infection in young puppies during development of their permanent teeth causes enamel hypoplasia of the permanent dentition. Such lesions in adult dogs are a sure indicator of a previous infection with CDV. Transplacental infection with CDV can cause neurologic signs in 4- to 6-week-old puppies. Abortions, stillbirths, and birth of weak puppies have also been reported (Greene, 1990).

The onset of signs is mostly acute to subacute and, in most instances, rapidly progressive. A protracted course over weeks and months is also possible. Because of the poor prognosis and because severe neurologic signs are often present, most animals with distemper affecting the central nervous system are euthanized early during the course of the disease. Experimental studies have rarely lasted for more than 2 months. Therefore, the total course of distemper is not really well known. In our own experience, a relapsing course is very rare, and it cannot be excluded that such spontaneously occurring relapses are the result of reinfection.

DIAGNOSIS

A clinical diagnosis of distemper is often difficult when a typical course with systemic signs preceding or accompanying the neurologic disease is lacking. In addition, the neurologic presentation of distemper varies widely. When signs of multifocal disease are found, which is generally suggestive of an infectious disease in the central nervous system, distemper should be considered in the differential diagnosis. In many instances, only signs of focal disease are apparent.

Distemper can also occur together with other infectious diseases in the central nervous system, mostly with protozoan infections such as toxoplasmosis or *Neospora caninum* infection (see this volume, p. 263).

LABORATORY FINDINGS

Hematologic findings include lymphopenia and thrombocytopenia. Dogs with marked lymphopenia usually have a rapidly progressive, fatal form of the disease. Inclusion bodies may be occasionally found on stained peripheral blood films and, more rarely, in monocytes, neutrophils, and erythrocytes. Serum biochemical findings are nonspecific and rarely contribute to the diagnosis of the disease.

Cerebrospinal Fluid Findings

Examination of the cerebrospinal fluid can be very useful in distemper. However, it should be kept in mind that during the acute demyelinating stage of the disease, inflammatory reactions are lacking. Therefore, protein content and cell count in these animals are often entirely normal. In inflammatory distemper, both protein content and

cell count are elevated. The cell count rarely exceeds 30 cells/μl. The pleocytosis consists only of mononuclear cells, including lymphocytes, plasma cells, and monocytes. Such a finding in cerebrospinal fluid is highly suggestive of viral encephalitis but not typical for distemper. By determining albumin and immunoglobulin content, both in serum and in cerebrospinal fluid (using, for example, rocket immunoelectrophoresis or a quantitative enzyme-linked radioimmunosorbent assay [ELISA]), an intrathecal production of IgG can be demonstrated, even in cases in which the cell counts are normal. Intrathecal IgG synthesis is diagnostic for encephalitis but not specific for distemper. More work is needed to determine whether electrophoretic patterns of cerebrospinal fluid proteins can be used to differentiate between distemper and other encephalitides. Isoelectrofocusing of cerebrospinal fluid immunoglobulins can reveal oligoclonal bands (restricted heterogeneity) in chronic cases of distemper, but is hardly a diagnostic tool.

Demonstration of Viral Antigens

The ultimate diagnosis is based on demonstration of viral antigens in scrapings and body fluids such as conjunctival smears, transtracheal washings, urine sediment, and cerebrospinal fluid. In our experience, viral antigen is difficult to find in extraneural tissues of dogs with neurologic involvement. We have searched for viral antigen in cerebrospinal fluid cells, using highly sensitive and specific monoclonal antibodies in an indirect fluorescent antibody test. The cells were collected by cytocentrifugation. This technique has the disadvantage that the cell yield is relatively small in cases of normal cell counts or a modest pleocytosis. We found distemper antigen in cerebrospinal fluid cells in 80% of the cases examined.

Antiviral Antibodies

Anticanine distemper virus antibody is found in the serum of dogs with distemper. Both serum neutralization assays on CDV-infected cultures and ELISA techniques using purified CDV antigen have been used to demonstrate antiviral antibody. The ELISA allows detection of IgM antibodies that occur in the early stages of the active disease. However, animals that have had no prior exposure to CDV and are severely immunosuppressed in the early stages of the disease may not have any detectable antibody. In addition, antibodies are found in vaccinated animals. Therefore, the demonstration of anti-CDV antibodies in serum is of limited diagnostic value. The finding of intrathecally produced anti-CDV IgG by comparing the serum with cerebrospinal fluid titers is probably diagnostically significant in dogs with nervous involvement.

PROGNOSIS

The prognosis of dogs with neurologic involvement caused by distemper is generally considered to be guarded. This is undoubtedly so in severely immunosuppressed animals with rapidly progressive neurologic signs. Seizures in distemper are very difficult to control and are a serious threat to the animal. If subacute or chronic focal signs occur (e.g., spinal ataxia or blindness), animals may recover, especially when immune function is restored. We believe that the decision to euthanize a dog, once a clinical diagnosis of distemper is established, is often taken too early. If the animal is not severely incapacitated, it should be kept under supportive treatment for at least 1 or 2 weeks to study the course of the disease.

THERAPY

It is clear that prevention of the disease is possible through active immunization. Vaccinations for CDV should be performed every 3 to 4 weeks between 6 to 16 weeks of age, followed by periodic boosters (Greene, 1990) (see this volume, p. 202). However, in our own experience, vaccination breakthroughs may occur. In addition, we have observed several cases of postvaccinal encephalitis. There is at present no effective antiviral treatment against CDV, and therapy is mainly supportive and symptomatic.

Patients should be kept clean, warm, and quiet. Intravenous or subcutaneous fluid therapy, including polyionic isotonic fluid such as Ringer's solution, should be given to dogs with vomiting and diarrhea. Parenterally administered antiemetics may be necessary if vomiting persists. B vitamins should be given intramuscularly or added to the intravenous fluid to counteract anorexia and diuresis and to stimulate appetite. Dogs with respiratory signs should be given antibiotics if evidence of secondary bacterial bronchopneumonia exists. Bacterial infections are mostly caused by *Bordetella bronchiseptica*, which requires the use of broad-spectrum antibiotics such as ampicillin or chloramphenicol. Tetracycline should be avoided in puppies because of dental staining (Greene, 1990).

If a dog is having seizures, anticonvulsant therapy, such as phenobarbital (2 mg/kg every 12 hr PO), should be given.

Many drugs, such as procainamide or clonazepam, have been tried for the treatment of myoclonus without much success. Myoclonus is likely to be an irreversible condition. We have seen one dog with distemper in which marked myoclonus in one forelimb recovered spontaneously.

Since the antiviral antibody response is very important in the dog's defense against CDV, passive administration of canine hyperimmune sera has been advocated in distemper. While such antibodies may be beneficial in combating viremia and perhaps viral replication in extraneural tissues, it is very doubtful that significant amounts of these IgGs can cross the blood-brain barrier. Therefore, passive administration of anti-CDV antibodies is probably of little use, once the infection has been established in the central nervous system.

Therapeutic Outlook

It is clear that a more specific therapy for dogs with neurologic involvement will only become possible when we understand more about the molecular mechanisms involved in lesion formation. Based on our recent research, it appears that macrophages and their products are important in the induction of tissue damage. Therefore, anti-inflammatory agents can be beneficial. Glucocorticosteroids can also be used in inflammatory distemper because of their potential to combat brain edema. The immunosuppressive effect of steroids, however, can be a serious disadvantage, in view of the fact that the immunologic inflammatory response also clears the virus. Antioxidants such as vitamin E, vitamin C, superoxidedismutase, and iron chelators should perhaps be used more systematically in inflammatory distemper, since it has been shown that free radicals of oxygen, very powerful mediators of tissue damage, are probably involved (Griot et al., 1989). However, clinical trials with such drugs have not been performed. Vitamin C treatment, which has been advocated previously and criticized recently (Greene, 1990), should perhaps be re-evaluated.

Virus persistence, despite the presence of a vigorous antiviral immune response, is the key in the chronic progression of the disease. Specific antiviral agents against CDV are not available today. Research in our laboratory will be directed at elimination of persistent infection using molecular biologic methods *in vitro*. Even if these attempts are successful, it will take some time to apply such methods *in vivo*.

References and Suggested Reading

Appel, M. J. G., Shek, W. R., and Summers, B. A.: Lymphocyte-mediated immune cytotoxicity in dogs infected with virulent canine distemper virus. Infect. Immunol. 37:592, 1982.
An experimental study on the role of the cell-mediated antiviral immune response in distemper.
Appel, M. J. G., Gibbs, E. P. J., Martin, S. J., et al.: Morbillivirus diseases of animals and man. Comp. Diag. Viral Dis. 6:235, 1981.

A review of virologic, clinical, and pathologic aspects of canine distemper and related viral diseases.

De Lahunta, A.: Upper motor neuron system. *In* De Lahunta, A. (ed.): *Veterinary Neuroanatomy and Clinical Neurology,* 2nd ed. Philadelphia: W. B. Saunders, 1983, p. 146.
  A discussion on the mechanism of myoclonus in canine distemper.

Greene, C. E., and Appel, M. J. G.: Canine distemper. *In* Greene, C. E. (ed.): *Infectious Diseases of the Dog and Cat.* Philadelphia: W. B. Saunders, 1990, p. 226.
  A comprehensive review on the microbiology, pathology, clinical features, and treatment of canine distemper.

Griot, C., Bürge, T., Vandevelde, M., et al.: Antibody-induced generation of reactive oxygen radicals by brain macrophages in canine distemper encephalitis: A mechanism for bystander demyelination. Acta Neuropathol. (Berlin) 78:396, 1989.
  An experimental study in brain tissue cultures that shows how antiviral antibodies can contribute to tissue damage by stimulating macrophages.

Krakowka, S., Higgins, R. J., and Koestner, A.: Canine distemper virus: Review of structural and functional modulations in lymphoid tissues. Am. J. Vet. Res. 41:284, 1980.

A review on the effects of CDV on the lymphoid tissues, resulting in a variety of immunologic defects in this disease.

Krakowka, S., McCullough, B., Koestner, A., et al.: Myelin specific autoantibodies associated with central nervous system demyelination in canine distemper virus infection. Infect. Immunol. 8:819, 1973.
  An initial report on the occurrence of antimyelin antibodies in distemper suggesting the presence of autoimmune mechanisms in this disease.

Summers, B. A., Greisen, H. A., and Appel, M. J. G.: Does virus persist in the uvea in multiple sclerosis, as in canine distemper encephalomyelitis? Lancet 2:372, 1983.
  An experimental study showing how CDV can persist in its host.

Vandevelde, M., Zurbriggen, M., Higgins, R. J., et al.: Spread and distribution of viral antigen in nervous canine distemper. Acta Neuropathol. (Berlin) 67:211, 1985.
  An experimental study showing the correlation between the replication of CDV in glial cells and occurrence of demyelination.

Vandevelde, M., Zurbriggen, A., Steck, A., et al.: Studies on the intrathecal humoral immune response in canine distemper encephalitis. J. Neuroimmunol. 11:41, 1986.
  Antibody produced in the inflammatory brain lesions is directed against CDV as well as against myelin antigens.

BREED-SPECIFIC MENINGITIS IN DOGS

SUSAN M. MERIC

Saskatoon, Saskatchewan

Canine meningitis and meningoencephalomyelitis may occur as a result of infection with bacterial, viral, protozoal, mycotic, rickettsial, or parasitic pathogens. Syndromes of canine meningitis that have no identifiable infectious etiology and are thought to have an immunologic basis have also been recognized. These are being diagnosed with increasing frequency and include granulomatous meningoencephalomyelitis (GME) and a steroid-responsive aseptic suppurative meningitis of young dogs. In addition to these clinical syndromes a group of breed-specific meningitis disorders have been recognized. This article will discuss the breed-specific meningitis syndromes that have been identified in beagles, Bernese Mountain Dogs, and pugs.

BEAGLE PAIN SYNDROME

In 1978 a severe form of meningitis and polyarteritis causing cervical pain was reported in a colony of research beagles (Harcourt, 1978). Since that time, the disorder has been recognized occasionally in pet beagles and in beagles in research kennels. This disorder has been called beagle pain syndrome or canine pain syndrome. Recently, an additional

five beagles with this syndrome have been examined and studied (Scott-Moncrieff et al., 1990).

Most affected beagles are from 5 to 10 months of age when they first become symptomatic. Males and females are affected with equal frequency. Clinical findings include fever, depression, reluctance to move, and intense cervical hyperesthesia. Affected dogs stand with their head, neck, and spine held in a straight line and the nose elevated or directed toward the ground. Proprioceptive deficits are variable but may be present in one or both forelimbs. The clinical signs and laboratory abnormalities often have a remitting and relapsing course, with signs recurring every 2 to 4 weeks in untreated dogs. Some dogs develop a more constant syndrome of pain that does not resolve without treatment.

Clinicopathologic abnormalities are consistently demonstrated during clinical expression of disease. Complete blood counts reveal a nonregenerative anemia and leukocytosis with neutrophilia. A mild neutrophilic pleocytosis is found in the synovial fluid of some affected dogs. Cerebrospinal fluid analysis reveals a neutrophilic pleocytosis (15 to 10,000 cells/μl) with mild to moderate increases in protein. A single sample of cerebrospinal fluid collected early in the course of the disease or during a period of relapse may be normal. Culture of urine, cerebrospinal fluid, and blood for aerobic and anaerobic bacteria and mycoplasma has been negative.

Serologic tests for *Ehrlichia canis*, Rocky Mountain spotted fever, borreliosis, *Brucella canis*, chlamydia, and toxoplasma have all been negative, and no organisms have been visualized cytologically in the cerebrospinal or synovial fluid. Transmission studies using whole blood and cerebrospinal fluid have been unsuccessful.

A genetic predisposition for this syndrome is suspected, and breeding studies are under way. Although serologic markers for immune-mediated disease such as positive antinuclear antibody tests and lupus erythematosus cell tests have not been demonstrated, the disorder is thought to have an immunologic basis.

Therapy with broad-spectrum antibiotics such as ampicillin, amoxicillin, potentiated sulfonamides, chloramphenicol, and tetracycline has not produced clinical improvement. Prednisone at an initial dose of 2 to 4 mg/kg/day has been associated with complete resolution of clinical signs. Long-term control of clinical signs in most dogs has been accomplished by the administration of 0.50 to 1.0 mg/kg of prednisone every other day. Response to other immunosuppressive and anti-inflammatory therapy is uncertain. In some dogs, prednisone has been discontinued after 2 to 6 months without relapse. Even without continued therapy, episodes of pain may become less frequent as affected dogs mature, with complete resolution of the clinical signs in some dogs after 18 months of age (Harcourt, 1978; Scott-Moncrieff, personal communication, 1990).

Postmortem examinations have revealed massive perivascular infiltration by inflammatory cells with fibrinoid necrosis and thrombosis of the small and medium-size arteries of the meninges. Similar pathologic changes are consistently observed in the coronary vessels. Amyloidosis and lymphocytic thyroiditis, recognized in some of the dogs previously reported, have not been present in any of the recently studied dogs.

BERNESE MOUNTAIN DOG ASEPTIC MENINGITIS

Severe necrotizing vasculitis of the central nervous system resulting in signs of meningeal inflammation has been recognized in Bernese Mountain Dogs. Young dogs 3 to 12 months of age are most commonly affected. There is no apparent sex predilection.

Affected dogs experience a sudden onset of the classic signs of meningitis, including fever, cervical rigidity, spinal pain, and stilted gait. The signs may be episodic initially, resolving without treatment in mildly affected dogs with pain-free intervals lasting days to months. Most dogs, however, are severely affected and require treatment. Progression to signs of parenchymal nervous system involvement, including paralysis, blindness, and seizures, has occurred in some dogs in which therapy was not instituted. Most affected dogs have peripheral neutrophilia. Cerebrospinal fluid analysis reveals moderately increased protein and an extreme neutrophilic pleocytosis of 50 to 2000 cells/μl. No infectious agents have been isolated.

Immunosuppressive treatment with prednisone at 2 to 4 mg/kg/day results in rapid resolution of clinical signs in most dogs. After 2 weeks the corticosteroid dosage should be decreased slowly until the dog is maintained on 1 mg/kg of prednisone every other day. Long-term therapy is necessary to maintain remission of clinical signs. Resolution of the disorder after 4 to 6 months of treatment without the need for continuing medication is common. Some dogs, however, have had relapses when the corticosteroid dose was reduced, requiring prolonged high-dose corticosteroid treatment or the addition of a more potent immunosuppressive drug. Although experience is limited, administration of azathioprine (Imuran) at a dosage of 2 mg/kg every 24 hr in these cases has met with some success. Approximately 10% of dogs require lifelong treatment (Presthus, personal communication, 1990). In spite of aggressive therapy, a few dogs have been euthanized because of recurrences and progressive parenchymal involvement.

At necropsy an extensive suppurative leptomeningitis is found in association with severe arteritis and fibrinoid necrosis of vessel walls. Tissue ischemia and hemorrhage account for the neurologic signs. The etiology of the central nervous system vasculitis in these dogs has not been determined. No underlying concurrent disease process has been uncovered, and there is little evidence for a systemic or generalized immune disorder.

This aseptic suppurative meningitis syndrome is common in the Bernese Mountain Dog breed, with an estimated 1 to 2% of the breed affected (Presthus, personal communication, 1990). Many affected dogs have been closely related, and in most affected litters, approximately one quarter of the pups will be affected. Test mating of affected dogs has produced affected puppies. A syndrome with very similar clinical and pathologic features has been described as a rare disorder in young German shorthaired pointers (Meric, 1988).

PUG MENINGOENCEPHALITIS

A breed-specific encephalitis was first recognized in pug dogs in the 1960's in California. This disease has now been diagnosed throughout the United States, Australia, and Europe and appears to be common in the breed. Affected dogs will first show clinical signs between 9 months and 7 years of age. There is no apparent sex predilection.

Affected dogs may have an acute or chronic course. Dogs with acute disease are usually presented with a sudden onset of seizures and neurologic signs referable to the cerebrum and meninges. Abnormalities of behavior, gait, and posture usually persist between seizures. Affected dogs may have difficulty walking, may be weak or uncoordinated, may circle, may have a head tilt, may head press, may exhibit blindness with normal pupillary light reflexes, or may show signs of cervical rigidity and pain. These neurologic signs progress rapidly, and within 5 to 7 days, the dogs develop uncontrollable seizures or become recumbent, unable to walk, and comatose. Some acutely affected dogs are initially presented in status epilepticus that cannot adequately be controlled, resulting in euthanasia (Holliday, personal communication, 1990).

Dogs with a more slowly progressive form of this disease will also commonly present with a generalized or partial motor seizure but are usually neurologically normal following the seizure. Seizures then recur at varying intervals of a few days to a few weeks. Recurrent seizures and the development and progression of other cerebrocortical neurologic signs (blindness, incoordination, screaming, circling) ultimately have led to euthanasia (de Lahunta, personal communication, 1990). Dogs generally survive only a few weeks, with a maximum survival of less than 6 months from the time of initial presentation.

Diagnosis should be based on the signalment and on characteristic clinical and laboratory features. Hematologic and serum biochemical findings have been unremarkable. In one study, the mean cerebrospinal fluid nucleated cell count was 374 cells/μl, 71 to 98% of the cells were small lymphocytes, and protein averaged 122 mg/dl (Cordy and Holliday, 1989). Aerobic and anaerobic bacterial culture of the cerebrospinal fluid has been negative, and attempts at viral isolation have been unsuccessful. The preponderance of small lymphocytes in the cerebrospinal fluid is an important diagnostic feature, since this would be an unusual finding in dogs with granulomatous meningoencephalitis or toxoplasmosis. Definitive diagnosis requires autopsy or brain biopsy.

There is no specific treatment for this disease. Treatment with phenobarbital may decrease the severity and frequency of the seizures for a short period of time. As the disease progresses, anticonvulsant therapy may be ineffective, or the interictal signs may become too severe, necessitating euthanasia. Corticosteroids are commonly administered but do not alter the course of the disease.

Pathologically, there is a nonsuppurative necrotizing meningoencephalitis, primarily affecting the cerebral hemispheres. Extensive cerebral necrosis often is present without evidence of concurrent inflammation. Leptomeningitis, characterized by perivascular accumulations of lymphocytes, plasma cells, and macrophages, is widespread. The extensive necrosis and the affinity for the cerebral hemispheres are features suggestive of alpha-type herpesvirus encephalitides of humans and other animals. It has been speculated that pug dog meningoencephalitis could result from activation of a latent canine herpesvirus type I infection after an initial neonatal infection (Cordy and Holliday, 1989). Further studies are under way to investigate a possible viral etiology for this disease.

This disorder has been recognized only in pugs and commonly occurs in certain pug lineages. More than one animal in a litter has often been affected, with the onset of clinical signs weeks to months apart. A genetic predisposition is likely. This may represent a genetically programmed neurologic disorder or a genetically determined abnormality of the immune system, making affected dogs susceptible to an infectious agent such as a herpesvirus.

References and Suggested Reading

Cordy, D. R., and Holliday, T. A.: A necrotizing meningoencephalitis of pug dogs. Vet. Pathol. 26:191, 1989.
 A review of the clinical and pathologic features of pug dog meningoencephalitis in 17 dogs.
de Lahunta, A.: Personal communication. New York State College of Veterinary Medicine, Department of Anatomy, October 1990.
de Lahunta, A.: *Veterinary Neuroanatomy and Clinical Neurology.* Philadelphia: W. B. Saunders, 1983, p. 384.
 A description of the clinical features of pug dog meningoencephalitis.
Harcourt, R. A.: Polyarteritis in a colony of beagles. Vet. Rec. 102:519, 1978.
 A review of the clinical and pathologic features of beagle pain syndrome in 20 dogs.
Holliday, T.: Personal communication. University of California at Davis College of Veterinary Medicine, Department of Surgery, October 1990.
Meric, S. M.: Canine meningitis: A changing emphasis. J. Vet. Int. Med. 2:26, 1988.
 A review of the diagnosis and treatment of infectious and idiopathic meningitis syndromes in the dog.
Meric, S. M., Child, G., and Higgins, R. J.: Necrotizing vasculitis of the spinal pachyleptomeningeal arteries in three bernese mountain dog littermates. J. Am. Anim. Hosp. Assoc. 22:459, 1986.
 A description of the clinical and pathologic features and response to treatment of Bernese mountain dog aseptic meningitis in three littermates.
Presthus, J.: Personal communication. Norwegian College of Veterinary Medicine, Department of Small Animal Clinical Sciences, October 1990.
Scott-Moncrieff, J. C., Snyder, P. W., Glickman, L. T., et al.: Systemic vasculitis (canine pain syndrome) in young laboratory beagles. J. Vet. Int. Med. 4:112, 1990.
 A review of the clinical and pathologic features of beagle pain syndrome in five dogs.
Scott-Moncrieff, J. C.: Personal communication. Purdue University School of Veterinary Medicine, Department of Veterinary Clinical Sciences, October 1990.

NEUROLOGIC DISEASE ASSOCIATED WITH FELINE RETROVIRAL INFECTION

STEVEN W. DOW
and EDWARD A. HOOVER
Fort Collins, Colorado

Clinical and experimental evidence indicates that most if not all retroviruses are neurotropic and potentially neurovirulent. Lentiviruses are arguably the most important retroviral neuropathogens in terms of their neuroinvasiveness and neuropathogenicity. The original neuropathologic models employed lentivirus-induced neurologic disease in ungulates, particularly visna virus in sheep and caprine arthritis-encephalitis virus in goats (Cork et al., 1974; Nathanson et al., 1985). Soon after the human immunodeficiency virus (HIV) was linked to the acquired immunodeficiency syndrome (AIDS) epidemic, it became apparent that neurologic dysfunction occurred early and was one of the most important consequences of infection with this human lentivirus. HIV infection is linked to several neurologic syndromes, including AIDS encephalopathy, vacuolar myelopathy, and peripheral neuropathies (McArthur, 1987; Price et al., 1988). Simian immunodeficiency virus infection induces similar neurologic diseases in Asian macaques (Ringler et al., 1988). There are also reports of neurologic disease in horses infected with equine infectious anemia virus and in bovine immunodeficiency virus–infected cattle.

Human T-lymphotropic virus type 1 (HTLV-1), a human oncornavirus, has been linked to a distinct spinal cord degenerative syndrome, HAM/TSP (HTLV-associated myelopathy/tropical spastic paraparesis) (Bhagavati et al., 1988; Ceroni et al., 1988). Several murine oncornaviruses also induce specific neurologic syndromes in susceptible mice (Gardner, 1985). In general, oncornavirus infections are associated with diseases of the spinal cord and peripheral nerves, whereas lentivirus neuropathologic effects are more widespread, involving brain, spinal cord, and peripheral nerves.

Since feline immunodeficiency virus (FIV), a lentivirus of domestic cats, was first discovered in 1986, there have been reports of neurologic abnormalities in infected animals (Pedersen et al., 1987). The authors have investigated a series of ten naturally infected cats (with and without neurologic abnormalities) and found evidence of viral central nervous system (CNS) infection in nine of ten (Dow et al., 1990). Experimental studies have also demonstrated FIV infection of the feline CNS (Dow et al., 1990; Yammamoto et al., 1989).

There are reports that FeLV, a feline oncornavirus, is associated with neurologic syndromes in cats, including anisocoria and myelopathy (Brightman et al., 1977; Haffer et al., 1987). Experimentally, FeLV infection has been shown to infect the CNS and induce spinal cord dysfunction in cats (Gasper et al., 1989). Thus, there is growing evidence that both FIV and FeLV are neurotropic retroviruses associated with neurologic diseases in infected cats.

Clinical Neurologic Disease: FIV Infection

The most common neurologic abnormalities in FIV-infected cats appear to involve cortical or subcortical functions and include primarily behavioral and mood changes. Pedersen and colleagues (1987) described signs resembling rage and hysteria in the cat from which the original FIV was isolated. The authors have observed neurologic abnormalities in over one third (8 of 22) of FIV-positive cats studied over a 3-year period. Abnormalities included depression, social withdrawal, persistent staring, and inappropriate elimination; focal neurologic deficits and motor dysfunction have not been observed. However, electrophysiologic evidence of both neuropathy and myelopathy has been reported recently in FIV-infected cats (Wheeler et al., 1990). In these studies, abnormal impulse transmission through the spinal cord was the most consistent abnormality detected. Obvious neurologic abnormalities have not been observed to date in a number of experimentally inoculated cats, despite serologic and virologic evidence of CNS infection (Dow et al., 1990). Neurologic abnormalities including immunodeficiency and weight loss seem to occur most often in cats with advanced FIV-related disease. It is not presently clear whether FIV-associated neurologic disease in cats develops as a result of opportunistic CNS infection (e.g., CNS toxoplasmosis), increase in the overall virus burden in the CNS,

Table 1. Cerebrospinal Fluid (CSF) Antibody and Virus Isolation Data From Cats Naturally Infected With Feline Immunodeficiency Virus (FIV)*

Cat	Disease	Virus Isolation PBL	Virus Isolation CSF	FIV Antibody CSF	IgG† Index
CSU-Sa	Gingivitis	+	−	−	0.53
CSU-Sp	Rhinitis	+	−	+	nd
CSu-T	None	+	+	+	2.75
1731	None	+	+	+	1.31
1729	None	+	+	+	0.34
AK	Neurologic	nd	−	+	nd
CSU-F	Neurologic, polyarthritis	+	+	+	3.51
1831	None	+	+	+	1.83
DL	Neurologic	nd	nd	+	2.53
963	Immunodeficiency disease	+	−	+	0.85

*Reprinted with permission from Dow, S. W., et al.: Feline immunodeficiency virus: A neurotropic lentivirus. J. Acquir. Immune Defic. Syndr. 3:658, 1990.
†Normal CSF IgG index (95% CI) in six control SPF cats was .61–1.65.
nd, not done.
PBL = peripheral blood lymphocytes; SPF = specific pathogen-free.

emergence of increasingly neurovirulent FIV during the course of infection, or as an indirect consequence of systemic immune dysfunction.

Clinical Neurologic Disease: FeLV Infection

FeLV infection has been incriminated in several neurologic diseases of cats. Infected cats occasionally develop anisocoria, which may persist or spontaneously resolve and recur (Brightman et al., 1977). The pathogenesis is poorly understood and may result from FeLV infection of ciliary ganglia or more central structures involved in pupillary contraction. Unexplained paraparesis and paraplegia have also been reported in FeLV-infected cats (Haffer et al., 1987). Experimentally, FeLV infection has been reported to induce abnormalities in spinal cord and peripheral nerve conduction velocities in cats, although the cats remained clinically normal (Gasper et al., 1989).

Diagnosis of CNS Infection

Currently, diagnosis of FIV CNS infection relies primarily on demonstration of an intrathecal antiviral antibody response. FIV-specific antibodies can be demonstrated in the cerebrospinal fluid (CSF) of infected cats by either enzyme-linked immunosorbent assay (ELISA), immunoprecipitation, or immunoblot (Table 1). Of these assays, immunoprecipitation is the most specific for demonstrating FIV antibodies, especially antibodies to FIV envelope proteins. By means of an FIV-antibody ELISA, CSF antibody titers ranging from 1:4 to 1:64 have been detected in naturally and experimentally infected cats. By contrast, serum FIV antibody titers in chronically infected cats generally range from

1:1000 to 1:10,000 (Dreitz, M., unpublished data). However, to interpret the results of CSF antibody analysis, it is imperative that the CSF specimen not be contaminated with blood. Blood contamination (>50 red blood cells/μl) introduces serum FIV antibodies into CSF, and the peripheral or intrathecal origin of these antibodies cannot be differentiated. Leukocyte counts in CSF of naturally infected cats have usually been mildly elevated (5 to 10 leukocytes/μl), consisting primarily of lymphocytes, some of which are large and apparently activated. Culture of freshly collected CSF also yields FIV in the majority of infected cats; interestingly, most positive isolations are obtained when CSF is cultured with feline glial cells rather than with lymphocytes (Dow, S., unpublished data). An increase in CSF IgG index, a measure of intrathecal immunoglobulin synthesis, has also been found in most FIV-infected cats with neurologic disease (Dow et al., 1990) (Table 1). CSF total protein concentrations have been normal in infected cats evaluated to date.

In FeLV-infected cats CSF FeLV-specific antibodies have not been detected by either immunoblot or immunoprecipitation (Dow, S., unpublished observations). However, FeLV has been recovered by culture of CSF from three cats with neurologic disease (Dow, S., unpublished data).

Experimental FIV Infection

Cats have been inoculated with FIV experimentally to evaluate viral neuropathogenesis. After either intrathecal or intravenous inoculation, FIV antibodies appeared in CSF within 8 to 14 weeks (Dow et al., 1990). CSF leukocytes (primarily lymphocytes) also increased, preceding the appearance of FIV antibodies in CSF by several weeks (Fig. 1).

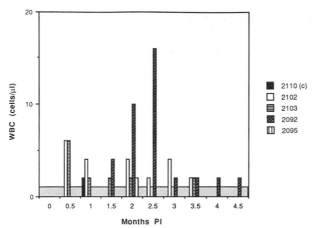

Figure 1. Changes in cerebrospinal fluid (CSF) leukocyte counts of four cats inoculated with feline immunodeficiency virus (FIV) (2102, 2103, 2092, and 2095) and a sham-inoculated cat (2110) evaluated over a 4.5-month period. CSF leukocytes consisted primarily of lymphocytes, some of which were enlarged and apparently activated. The *shaded region* represents normal CSF leukocyte counts as determined in ten uninfected cats. (PI = postinoculation.) (Reprinted with permission from Dow, S.W., et al.: Feline immunodeficiency virus: A neurotropic lentivirus. J. Acquir. Immune Defic. Syndr. 3:658, 1990.)

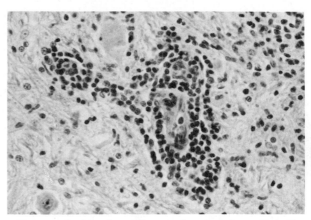

Figure 2. Perivascular infiltration of mononuclear cells in the brainstem of a cat 15 months after experimental FIV inoculation. Diffuse gliosis is also present. FIV was isolated from primary brain culture. (H & E stain; × 200.)

CSF IgG index also increased transiently at approximately the time that FIV antibodies appeared in CSF. Intrathecal inoculation apparently shortens the time to appearance of FIV antibodies but does not increase the intensity of the antibody response; intrathecally inoculated animals also develop systemic virus infection. Thus, FIV infects the CNS regardless of the route of inoculation and results in intrathecal synthesis of FIV antibodies.

FIV was recovered by primary regional brain culture of three experimentally infected cats (Dow et al., 1990). Virus was most often recovered from regions that also had histologic lesions. Brain lesions in both naturally and experimentally FIV-infected cats have consisted primarily of perivascular mononuclear cell infiltrates, glial nodules, and diffuse gliosis. Lesions have been confined primarily to several brain regions, including subcortical gray-matter structures (basal nuclei and thalamus) and brainstem and cervical spinal cord gray matter (Fig. 2). Obvious white-matter lesions have not been observed. Studies to locate viral antigen and nucleic acid within brain tissues are in progress.

In vitro experiments have determined that the primary CNS target cells for FIV are astrocytes and brain macrophages. Cultured astrocytes are readily infected; infection leads rapidly to syncytium formation and eventually to cell death (Fig. 3). By contrast, FIV infection of brain macrophages is relatively noncytopathic. Thus, persistently infected brain macrophages may serve as a reservoir for FIV infection within the CNS.

Diagnosis and Treatment

At present, a presumptive diagnosis of FIV-induced neurologic disease may be based on suggestive clinical signs (primarily behavioral changes), positive FIV serology, and exclusion of other diseases that might cause similar neurologic symptoms (e.g., toxoplasmosis, feline infectious peritonitis). Demonstration of FIV antibodies in CSF would strengthen a diagnosis of FIV encephalopathy. A conclusive diagnosis of FeLV-induced neurologic disease is more difficult, although demonstration of FeLV antigen in CSF or tissue biopsy material or FeLV culture from CSF would provide strong supportive evidence.

At present, an effective treatment for FIV has not been developed. Of currently available anti-retroviral drugs, the acyclic adenosine derivative phosphonomethoxyethyl adenine (PMEA) has

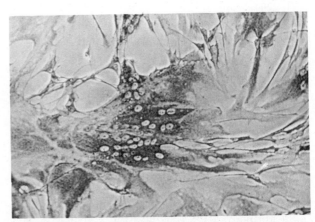

Figure 3. Syncytium formation in cultured feline astrocytes 3 days after FIV infection. Dark peroxidase reaction product indicates the presence of viral antigens in infected cells. (Immunoperoxidase technique; × 400.)

shown the most promise in cats and is currently undergoing experimental and clinical trials (Egberink et al., 1990). CNS penetration by this drug has not been studied in cats. Azidothymidine (AZT) in combination with human recombinant interferon-α (see this volume, p. 211) has been shown to be an effective prophylactic treatment for experimental FeLV infection in cats. After oral administration, AZT appears to reach therapeutic concentrations in feline CSF (Zeidner, N., unpublished data). In humans with AIDS encephalopathy, AZT has been shown to significantly reduce the severity of neurologic impairment. AZT effectively inhibits FIV replication *in vitro* and may therefore potentially benefit cats with either FIV- or FeLV-induced neurologic disease.

References and Suggested Reading

Bhagavati, S., Ehrlich, G., Kula, R. W., et al.: Detection of human T-cell lymphoma/leukemia virus type 1 DNA and antigen in spinal fluid and blood of patients with chronic progressive myelopathy. N. Engl. J. Med. 318:1141, 1988.

Brightman, A. H., Macy, D. W., and Gosselin, Y.: Pupillary abnormalities associated with the feline leukemia complex. Feline Pract. 5:23, 1977.

Ceroni, M., Piccardo, P., Rodgers-Johnson, P., et al.: Intrathecal synthesis of IgG antibodies to HTLV-1 supports an etiologic role for HTLV-1 in tropical spastic paraparesis. Ann. Neurol. 23(suppl):S188, 1988.

Cork, L. C., Hadlow, W. J., Crawford, T. B., et al.: Infectious leukoencephalomyelitis of young goats. J. Infect. Dis. 129:134, 1974.

Dow, S. W., Poss, M. L., and Hoover, E. H.: Feline immunodeficiency virus: A neurotropic lentivirus. J. Acquir. Immune Defic. Syndr. 3:658, 1990.

Egberink, H., Borst, M., Niphiuis, H., et al.: Suppression of feline immunodeficiency virus infection in vivo by 9-(2-phosphonomethoxyethyl)adenine. Proc. Natl. Acad. Sci. USA 87:3087, 1990.

Gardner, M. B.: Retroviral spongiform polioencephalomyelopathy. Rev. Infect. Dis. 7:99, 1985.

Gasper, P. W., Whalen, L. R., Orbaugh, J., et al.: Isolation and preliminary characterization of a neurotropic strain of feline leukemia virus. Fifth International AIDS Conference, Montreal, 1989.

Haffer, K. N., Sharpee, R. L., Beckenhauer, W., et al.: Is the feline leukemia virus responsible for neurologic abnormalities in cats? Vet. Med. Aug:802, 1987.

McArthur, J. C.: Neurologic manifestations of AIDS. Medicine 66:407, 1987.

Nathanson, N., Georgsson, G., Palsson, P. A., et al.: Experimental visna in Icelandic sheep: The prototype lentiviral infection. Rev. Infect. Dis. 7:75, 1985.

Pedersen, N. C., Ho, E. W., Brown, M. L., et al.: Isolation of a T-lymphotropic virus from domestic cats with an immunodeficiency-like disease. Science 235:790, 1987.

Price, R. W., Brew, B., Sidtis, J., et al.: The brain in AIDS: Central nervous system HIV-1 infection and AIDS dementia complex. Science 239:586, 1988.

Ringler, D. J., Hunt, R. D., Derosiers, R. C., et al.: Simian immunodeficiency virus–induced meningoencephalomyelitis: Natural history and retrospective study. Ann. Neurol. 23(suppl):S101, 1988.

Wheeler, D., Whalen, L. R., Gasper, P. W., et al.: A feline model for AIDS dementia complex (ADC)? Sixth International AIDS Conference, San Francisco, 1990.

Yammamoto, J. K., Sparger, E., Ho, E. W., et al.: Pathogenesis of experimentally induced feline immunodeficiency virus infection in cats. Am. J. Vet. Res. 49:1246, 1989.

INTERVERTEBRAL DISK DISEASE: TREATMENT GUIDELINES

JOE N. KORNEGAY
Raleigh, North Carolina

Treatment of intervertebral disk disease remains controversial. Few prospective studies have contrasted results of medical and surgical management. Moreover, although specialists have increasingly tended to recommend surgery for affected dogs, they have disagreed as to whether laminectomy, fenestration, or a combination of these procedures is indicated. In an attempt to define therapeutic guidelines for dogs with varying clinical involvement (Table 1), results of studies using different treatments have been compared. Results of these previous studies, and my own experience, form the basis for this review.

CONSERVATIVE VERSUS SURGICAL THERAPY

Conservative therapy generally includes strict confinement, manual bladder compression or catheterization at least three times daily, and judicious use of analgesics and glucocorticoids (see section on pharmacologic management later). Surgical management involves laminectomy, fenestration, or both. The few studies that have contrasted results of medical and surgical therapy have understandably been conducted at universities, where a disproportionate number of dogs that had failed to respond

Table 1. *Classification of Dogs with Thoracolumbar Disk Disease*

Group 1. Hyperesthesia with no neurologic deficits
Group 2. Ambulatory paraparesis (incomplete loss of voluntary motor function in the pelvic limbs). Urinary/fecal continence and pain sensation are intact.
Group 3. Nonambulatory paraparesis. Urinary/fecal continence and pain sensation are intact.
Group 4. Paraplegia (complete loss of voluntary motor function in the pelvic limbs). Urinary/fecal continence is generally lost and pain sensation is intact.
Group 5. Paraplegia with loss of urinary/fecal continence and pain sensation.

Reprinted with permission from Kornegay, J. N.: Intervertebral disk disease: Treatment guidelines. Texas Vet. Med. J. 48:29, 1986.

to conservative therapy might be evaluated. One such study, conducted at Auburn University, suggested that the prognosis for dogs with intervertebral disk disease is considerably better when they are treated by hemilaminectomy and fenestration than when managed conservatively, regardless of the degree of neurologic dysfunction (Table 2) (Hoerlein, 1978). In another study from Sweden, only 36.9% of dogs corresponding to groups 3 to 5 (see Table 1) became ambulatory after conservative therapy, whereas 81.8% of those treated by dorsal laminectomy regained the ability to walk (Funkquist, 1962). A later study by this same author showed the success rate of conservative therapy in groups 3 to 5 (51.2%) was again considerably less than that of dogs managed by dorsal laminectomy (89.0%) (Funkquist, 1970). Funkquist relied heavily in her classification system on whether there was muscle tone in the pelvic limbs of affected dogs, thus making extrapolation to the groups discussed

here difficult. However, it appeared that the greatest benefit of laminectomy was gained in group 5.

The success rate of other surgeons using laminectomy alone as a treatment for clinical intervertebral disk disease has varied from 61.5 to 89.5% (Brown et al., 1977; Gambardella, 1980; Henry, 1975; Knecht, 1972). One study suggested that some severely affected dogs improved immediately after surgery (Funkquist, 1962), but no cumulative data were given. Another study found that nonambulatory dogs walked, on an average, at 32.6 days after surgery (Brown et al., 1977). Factors affecting the success rate, such as severity and duration of neurologic involvement, are addressed later.

Others have compared conservatively managed dogs with thoracolumbar disk disease with those treated by fenestration. One study showed no difference in recovery rate between group 1 and 2 dogs that were fenestrated (76 of 80; 95%) or managed conservatively (104 of 117; 88.9%) (Funkquist, 1978). However, some of the conservatively managed dogs deteriorated, while none of those in the fenestrated group did. Similar results were also obtained in group 1 and 2 dogs in another comparative study (Davies and Sharp, 1983). This same study also found no difference in the recovery rate of group 3 dogs managed conservatively (13 of 16; 81.3%) versus those that were fenestrated (13 of 16; 81.3%). In addition, neither study identified a definite difference in speed of recovery between fenestrated and conservatively managed dogs, although there was a tendency for more severely affected dogs to respond more rapidly to fenestration. Group 1 and 2 dogs required an average of 4 to 6 weeks to recover whether they were fenestrated or managed conservatively, and dogs in groups 3 and 4

Table 2. *Results of Treatment of Dogs with Intervertebral Disk Extrusions Observed 6 Months or Longer in 1184 Cases (Hoerlein, 1950–1975)*

	Surgical Therapy						Nonsurgical Therapy					
	6 mo–1 yr	1–2 yr	3–5 yr	6 yr & over	Total	Per Cent	6 mo–1 yr	1–2 yr	3–5 yr	6 yr & over	Total	Per Cent
Paralysis												
Good	56	141	214	58	479	87.0	1	5	4	1	11	22.4
Fair	17	12	8	6	43	8.0	6	0	2	1	9	18.4
Poor	22	1	3	1	27	5.0	25	2	2	0	29	59.2
Total	95	154	225	65	539	100.0	32	7	8	2	49	100.0
Paresis												
Good	60	84	115	18	277	90.5	6	5	7	1	19	29.7
Fair	8	4	9	0	21	6.9	4	13	6	1	24	37.5
Poor	6	1	1	0	8	2.6	19	0	2	0	21	32.8
Total	74	89	125	18	306	100.0	29	18	15	2	64	100.0
Pain												
Good	44	29	44	17	134	82.7	9	3	10	2	24	37.5
Fair	3	5	3	2	13	8.0	11	10	7	1	29	45.3
Poor	6	3	3	3	15	9.3	6	2	2	1	11	17.2
Total	53	37	50	22	162	100.0	26	15	19	4	64	100.0
Total	222	280	400	105	1007		87	40	42	8	177	

Reprinted with permission from Hoerlein, B. F. (ed.): *Canine Neurology*, 3rd ed. Philadelphia: W. B. Saunders, 1978, p. 547.

required 6 to 12 weeks. While a definite therapeutic value of fenestration over conservative management was not shown, both did suggest a significant prophylactic role for fenestration (see later).

Other studies have addressed the outcome of dogs with disk disease managed by fenestration, without discussion of results from dogs managed conservatively. Success rates between 90 and 98.1% have been reported (Denny, 1978; Flo, 1975; Knapp et al., 1990). One gave little data regarding duration or severity of neurologic involvement (Flo, 1975). All clinical groups were included in the other studies. Only one considered rapidity of recovery. Group 3 to 5 dogs generally did not become ambulatory until 4 to 6 weeks postoperatively (Denny, 1978).

RECURRENT INTERVERTEBRAL DISK DISEASE EXTRUSION AND THE ROLE OF PROPHYLACTIC FENESTRATION

Clinical signs of intervertebral disk disease may recur because of further extrusion of the same disk or involvement of an additional disk. The degree to which each contributes to recurrence is not clear. In one study, clinical signs recurred in 29 of 187 (15.5%) dogs with thoracolumbar disk extrusions treated by dorsal laminectomy, but these recurrences were attributed to involvement of a second disk in only five (2.7%) (Brown, 1977). Recurrences in the other 24 cases were thought to be caused by an assortment of other factors. Other studies have suggested that the risk of disk extrusion at a site different from the original lesion is considerably greater. An overall recurrence rate of 21.3% was noted in 155 dogs with thoracolumbar disk disease treated with a variety of methods (Levine and Caywood, 1984). Of the 33 dogs that had recurrences, only 13 had survey radiography, myelography, additional surgery, or a necropsy to confirm the cause of the second episode. The recurrence was attributed to a second disk extrusion in 12 of the 13 (92.3%). Another study found the recurrence rate of clinical signs caused by intervertebral disk disease was 41.7% in dogs treated by dorsal laminectomy (Funkquist, 1970). Relatively few had recurrences within 6 months of the surgery, during which time perioperative complications would seem most likely. This suggests that many of the recurrences were caused by extrusion of a second disk, but data to definitely confirm this were not presented by the author.

Studies contrasting rates of recurrence in dogs managed conservatively (34 to 48%) with those that were fenestrated (0 to 17%) have shown a clear prophylactic value (Davies and Sharp, 1983; Funkquist, 1978; Levine and Caywood, 1984). The prophylactic value of fenestration in these studies appeared to be directly related to the number of disks that were fenestrated. Most surgeons advocating fenestration recommend that the six disks from T11-T12 through L3-L4 should be fenestrated. Since approximately 70% of thoracolumbar disk extrusions occur at either T12-T13, T13-L1, or L1-L2, a considerable prophylactic effect could presumably be gained if these three disks alone were fenestrated. However, a more recently published study showed that 24.4% of dogs that were fenestrated between T9-T10 and L5-L6, nevertheless, subsequently had generally mild and, for the most part unexplained, clinical signs (Knapp et al., 1990). Presumably, in many such cases in which dogs are fenestrated without myelography or concomitant laminectomy, clinical signs recur because of persistent intervertebral disk extrusion. Fenestration also has been shown to significantly reduce the rate of recurrence of clinical signs in dogs with cervical disk disease. In one study, the rate of recurrence was 5.6% in fenestrated dogs and 36.3% in those that were managed conservatively (Russell and Griffiths, 1968).

EFFECT OF SEVERITY AND DURATION OF NEUROLOGIC INVOLVEMENT ON CLINICAL OUTCOME

Regardless of the method of treatment for dogs with intervertebral disk disease, the prognosis is considerably better in those with lesser neurologic involvement (see Table 2). The single most important factor in establishing a prognosis is whether or not pain sensation is intact caudal to the lesion. However, the actual effect that loss of pain sensation has on the rate of recovery of affected dogs is not clear. Only 1 of 14 (7.1%) conservatively managed group 5 dogs regained the ability to walk in one study (Davies and Sharp, 1983). In contrast, 53 of 75 (70.7%) dogs with intact pain sensation in this study recovered after conservative therapy. Nineteen of 52 (36.5%) dogs with no pain sensation and good muscle tone in the pelvic limbs were eventually able to walk after conservative therapy in another report, but only four of them walked normally (Funkquist, 1962). In this same study, none of the 44 conservatively managed dogs with neither pain sensation nor muscle tone in the pelvic limbs walked. When the data from these two groups are combined, 19 of 96 (19.8%) recovered the ability to walk, but only four (4.2%) walked normally. In contrast, 8 of 9 (88.9%) group 5 dogs walked when treated by dorsal laminectomy and 7 (77.8%) walked normally (Funkquist, 1962). From 7 to 50% of group 5 dogs have regained the ability to walk subsequent to dorsal laminectomy in other studies (Brown et al., 1977; Gambardella, 1980; Henry, 1975; Knecht,

1972). The duration of loss of pain sensation appeared to be the most important predictor of recovery. Dogs without pain sensation operated within 24 to 36 hours had a considerably better chance for recovery than those in which surgery was more delayed.

Fenestration has also been evaluated in group 5 dogs. Six of nine (55.6%) group 5 dogs that were fenestrated regained the ability to walk in one study (Denny, 1978). The three dogs that failed to improve had acute clinical signs, whereas four of the six that improved had gradually progressive neurologic dysfunction. The prognosis for recovery seemed to be better when the surgery was done within 24 hours of the onset of signs in acutely affected dogs.

The effect of the degree of motor impairment on prognosis in dogs with intervertebral disk disease is less clear. Thirty-two of 38 (84.2%) group 2 and 3 dogs managed conservatively regained the ability to walk in one study (Davies and Sharp, 1983). The recovery rate of group 4 dogs was similar; 13 of 16 (81.3%) became ambulatory. Results of another study differed considerably in that only 40.8% of paraplegic dogs regained the ability to walk after conservative therapy, whereas 67.2% of paraparetic dogs became ambulatory (see Table 2). However, this study did not subdivide the paralyzed group into those with and without pain sensation, so it may have misrepresented the importance of voluntary function. In a study of dogs with disk extrusions treated by dorsal laminectomy, the rate of recovery of ambulation of paraplegic dogs (52 of 58; 89.7%) was essentially identical to that of paraparetic dogs (16 of 18; 88.9%) (Gambardella, 1980). Another study, in which hemilaminectomy was used, found that 36 of 37 (97.3%) dogs with paraparesis regained the ability to walk versus 37 of 42 (88.1%) that were paraplegic with intact pain sensation (Knecht, 1972). In this series, all of the dogs that failed to respond had surgery after 3 or more days, again indicating the potential benefit of acute surgery. However, the need for immediate surgery seemed considerably less critical in these dogs than in group 5 dogs. Sixteen of 21 (76.2%) group 4 dogs recovered ambulation when operated between 3 and 10 days after the onset of signs. Twenty-nine of 30 (96.7%) paraparetic dogs recovered when operated beyond 3 days after the onset of clinical signs.

OVERALL RECOMMENDATIONS

Groups 1 and 2

Dogs with initial episodes of hyperesthesia alone (group 1) or with mild ataxia (group 2) appear to have up to a 75 to 85% chance of recovery when managed conservatively. For this reason, I do not initially recommend surgery in such cases, preferring instead conservative management, as outlined earlier. The average time for recovery, however, is 4 to 6 weeks, so some owners may prefer that surgery be done either early in the course of the disease or after a few weeks of unsuccessful conservative therapy. That fenestrated and conservatively managed dogs recover over a similar time frame suggests that fenestration has little actual therapeutic value. Moreover, group 1 and 2 dogs I have studied have consistently had moderate, to often dramatic, spinal cord compression on myelography. For this reason, I recommend that dogs with persistent or recurrent hyperesthesia or ataxia should have a myelogram and laminectomy to remove an extruded disk, if indicated. Fenestration should be done in conjunction with the laminectomy to reduce the risk of recurrence. The disks from T11-12 through L3-L4 ideally should be fenestrated. At a minimum, those from T12-T13 through L1-L2 should be removed.

Groups 3 and 4

The prognosis for group 3 and 4 dogs that are managed conservatively has not been well defined. Recovery rates have varied from 55 to 85% versus rates of up to 95% with laminectomy. Furthermore, some dogs that are managed conservatively recover only after a lengthy time and have residual deficits. Most important, others deteriorate to the group 5 level, further degrading the prognosis. While conclusive data are lacking, removal of extruded disk material compressing the spinal cord should speed recovery. In addition, fenestration of the affected disk should prevent further extrusion, thus reducing the risk of continued deterioration. For these reasons, I recommend concomitant laminectomy and fenestration of disks in the T11 to L4 area in group 3 and 4 dogs. While dogs operated acutely appear to have a slightly better prognosis for recovery, the time interval between the onset of clinical signs and surgery is not as critical as with group 5 dogs.

Group 5

Dogs that are paraplegic and have lost pain sensation have only a 5 to 10% chance of recovery if managed conservatively or operated on a delayed basis. However, when they are operated within 24 to 36 hours of the onset of signs, the recovery rate has been up to 50% in some studies. For this reason, I recommend that group 5 dogs have a laminectomy combined with fenestration as soon as possible after the onset of their clinical signs. Durotomy should be considered if the spinal cord is extensively swollen.

OTHER CONSIDERATIONS

Pharmacologic Therapy

Acute disk extrusions often cause pronounced intramedullary hemorrhage and edema not directly amenable to surgery. Undoubtedly, removal of disk fragments and extradural hemorrhage, together with durotomy in some cases, lessens the degree of spinal cord ischemia by relieving pressure on both intramedullary and extradural vessels. However, the removal of pre-existing spinal cord hemorrhage and edema and the reversal of further progression of these lesions must be accomplished through intrinsic body systems or by the administration of pharmacologic agents. Numerous studies have reached conflicting conclusions regarding the beneficial effects of glucocorticoids, dimethyl sulfoxide, cholinergic blockers, endorphin antagonists (naloxone), antifibrinolytic agents, and hyperosmolar solutions (mannitol) in experimental spinal cord trauma. As a result, there is no clear consensus as to the role of these agents in the treatment of acute intervertebral disk extrusions. Nevertheless, most veterinary surgeons and neurologists continue to give glucocorticoids (methylprednisolone, 30 mg/kg, IV; then either give ¼ to ½ of this dose every 6 hr for as long as 48 hours or give up to 5.4 mg/kg IV hourly by continuous slow IV perfusion) to affected group 3 to 5 dogs (Rucker, 1990) (also see section on complications later).

Rehabilitation

Whether dogs with intervertebral disk extrusions are managed conservatively or with surgery, there is often an extended recovery phase. Most dogs that are ambulatory retain control of urination and recover motor function without need for significant rehabilitation. However, dogs that become paraplegic often retain urine, which necessitates either manual expression or catheterization of the bladder at least three times daily. Indwelling urinary catheters should be avoided, if at all possible, because they predispose to urinary tract infections. Dogs usually regain the micturition reflex concomitant with voluntary motor function. However, urinary tract infections caused by prolonged urine retention may require additional antibiotic therapy.

Several forms of exercise seem useful in speeding recovery of voluntary motor function. Closely supervised "swimming" in a tub of warm, soapy water, with or without a whirlpool, is particularly beneficial. This encourages movement of the limbs and also fosters cleanliness. Manual extension and flexion of the paralyzed limbs at least twice daily also helps retain muscle tone and mass.

Complications

Urinary tract infections, urine scalding, and decubitus are the most common complications of paralysis, regardless of cause. As discussed earlier, bladder expression or catheterization reduces urine retention. However, urinary tract infections still occur frequently and must be managed according to established principles. The potential for urine scalding can be reduced to some extent by placing affected dogs on a grate through which urine can drain. Decubitus is not a frequent complication in smaller dogs but occurs commonly in larger breeds. Accordingly, large recumbent dogs should be kept on padded surfaces whenever possible.

The frequent use of glucocorticoids in dogs with intervertebral disk extrusions has resulted in several problems. The most severe potential problem is the risk of gastrointestinal bleeding and even perforation from increased gastrin production and decreased proliferation of gastric epithelium (Toombs et al., 1980). While dexamethasone, in particular, has been incriminated, the severity of neurologic involvement and use of surgery appear to be additional potentiating factors. In one study of dogs with gastrointestinal complications, neither the dose of dexamethasone nor the duration of therapy seemed significant (Toombs et al., 1980). Nevertheless, the judicious use of glucocorticoids seems indicated. In dogs with gastrointestinal complications, intestinal protectants (kaolin-pectin, 1 to 2 ml/kg, PO, every 6 hr) and cimetidine (Tagamet, 10 mg/kg, PO, every 8 hr) are indicated.

References and Suggested Reading

Brown, N. O., Helphrey, M. L., and Prata, R. G.: Thoracolumbar disc disease in the dog: A retrospective analysis of 187 cases. J. Am. Anim. Hosp. Assoc. 13:665, 1977.
A retrospective review of 187 dogs that had undergone dorsal laminectomy for treatment of intervertebral disk disease.

Davies, J. V., and Sharp, N. J. H.: A comparison of conservative treatment and fenestration for thoracolumbar disc disease in the dog. J. Small Anim. Pract. 24:721, 1983.
A comparison of the outcome of dogs with intervertebral disk disease managed conservatively and by fenestration.

Denny, H. R.: A lateral fenestration of canine thoracolumbar disc protrusions: A review of 30 cases. J. Small Anim. Pract. 19:259, 1978.
A review of the basic surgical technique for thoracolumbar disk fenestration using a lateral approach and the results of this technique in 30 affected dogs with varying degrees of clinical involvement.

Flo, G. L., and Brinker, W. L.: Lateral fenestration of thoracolumbar discs. J. Am. Anim. Hosp. Assoc. 11:619, 1975.
A review of the outcome of 67 dogs with thoracolumbar disk disease of varying clinical severity managed by lateral fenestration.

Funkquist, B.: Thoraco-lumbar disk protrusion with severe cord compression in the dog. Acta Vet. Scand. 3:256, 1962.
A systematic overview of thoracolumbar disk disease divided into three parts, discussing clinical effects and results of treatment by both conservative means and dorsal laminectomy.

Funkquist, B.: Decompressive laminectomy in thoraco-lumbar disc protrusions with paraplegia in the dog. J. Small Anim. Pract. 11:445, 1970.
A retrospective review comparing results of dogs with thoracolumbar disk disease managed conservatively and by dorsal laminectomy.

Funkquist, B.: Investigations of the therapeutic and prophylactic effects

of disc evacuation in cases of thoraco-lumbar herniated discs in dogs. Acta Vet. Scand. 19:441, 1978.
A review of the comparative effects of fenestration and conservative therapy in dogs with thoracolumbar disk disease.

Gambardella, P. C.: Dorsal decompressive laminectomy for treatment of thoracolumbar disc disease in dogs: A retrospective study of 98 cases. Vet. Surg. 9:24, 1980.
A study of the outcome of 98 dogs with thoracolumbar disk disease treated by dorsal laminectomy.

Henry, W. B.: Dorsal decompressive laminectomy in the treatment of thoraco-lumbar disc disease. J. Am. Anim. Hosp. Assoc. 11:627, 1975.
A retrospective review of the results of dogs with thoracolumbar disk disease, often operated on a delayed basis, in which the author stresses the merits of acute surgery.

Hoerlein, B. F.: Intervertebral disks. In Hoerlein, B. F. (ed.): Canine Neurology, 3rd ed. Philadelphia: W. B. Saunders, 1978, p. 470.
An overview comparing the outcome of a large number of dogs with thoracolumbar disk disease managed either by hemilaminectomy and fenestration or by conservative therapy.

Knapp, D. W., Pope, E. R., Hewett, J. E., et al.: A retrospective study of thoracolumbar disk fenestration in dogs using a ventral approach: 160 cases (1976–1986). J. Am. Anim. Hosp. Assoc. 26:543, 1990.
A retrospective review of 160 generally mildly affected dogs with thoracolumbar disk disease managed by ventral fenestration.

Knecht, C. D.: Results of surgical treatment for thoracolumbar disc protrusion. J. Small Anim. Pract. 13:449, 1972.
A review of the outcome of 99 dogs with thoracolumbar disk disease with varying clinical severity and duration managed by hemilaminectomy.

Levine, S. H., and Caywood, D. D.: Recurrence of neurological deficits in dogs treated for thoracolumbar disk disease. J. Am. Anim. Hosp. Assoc. 20:889, 1984.
A retrospective review of the recurrence rate of dogs with thoracolumbar disk disease managed by various surgical methods and conservative means.

Rucker, N. C.: Management of spinal cord trauma. Prog. Vet. Neurol. 1:397, 1990.
A review of the clinical features, pathogenesis, and pharmacologic management of spinal cord trauma.

Russell, S. W., and Griffiths, R. C.: Recurrence of cervical disc syndrome in surgically and conservatively treated dogs. J.A.V.M.A. 11:1412, 1968.
A retrospective review of 110 dogs with cervical disk disease in which approximately equal numbers were managed by fenestration and conservative means.

Toombs, J. P., Caywood, D. D., Lipowitz, A. J., et al.: Colonic perforation following neurosurgical procedures and corticosteroid therapy in four dogs. J.A.V.M.A. 177:68, 1980.
A review of dogs with colonic perforation subsequent to intervertebral disk disease managed surgically and with glucocorticoids.

CHYMOPAPAIN CHEMONUCLEOLYSIS

CLETA SUE BAILEY

Davis, California

THE DEVELOPMENT OF CHEMONUCLEOLYSIS

Chemonucleolysis ("diskolysis") is the dissolution of the nucleus pulposus of the intervertebral disk by injection of a chemical (usually a protease enzyme) into the nucleus. The development of chemonucleolysis as a treatment for intervertebral disk herniation began serendipitously with Lewis Thomas (Ford et al., 1985). Thomas, an experimental pathologist, was working on the Shwartzman reaction, an allergic phenomenon that causes death by the precipitation of protein in the kidney tubules. Looking for a proteolytic enzyme that would reduce serum protein when injected intravenously, Thomas injected the protease papain into rabbits. He was amazed to find that within 4 hr of injection, the rabbit's ears began to wilt. The ears reached their peak of collapse by 24 hr and by 5 days after injection had recovered their tone. Thomas' histologic studies showed that the collapse of ear cartilage was associated with a loss of the extracellular ground substance of the cartilage and that all cartilaginous tissue in the body was similarly affected (Thomas, 1956).

Lyman Smith, an Illinois orthopedist, came across Thomas' paper and was intrigued. Smith had also read a paper on low back pain in which the author theorized that a chondrolytic enzyme might be found that could be injected into a degenerating disk, transforming it to dense connective tissue. Smith and his colleagues injected crude papain into the intervertebral disks of rabbits and found that, when the animals were killed a few days later, much of the nucleus pulposus had been removed with no apparent effect on the surrounding tissues (Smith et al., 1963). Wishing to study the enzyme effect on diseased disks, Smith collaborated with E. C. Saunders, a veterinarian. One to seven thoracolumbar disks of 75 dogs presumed to have disk disease were injected with chymopapain; 71% of the dogs improved clinically following treatment (Saunders, 1964).

The researchers were impressed with these results, and clinical trials in people were begun in 1963. In 1967, Smith and Brown reported the results of chemonucleolysis in 75 patients; two of these patients developed serious neurologic deficits (quadriplegia, paraplegia). Smith and Brown did not believe the complications were a result of the chymopapain injection, but others did not agree with them. As a result of these two cases, cervical disk injections were forbidden, and the technique for lumbar disk injection was altered. The physician who subsequently treated Smith and Brown's quadriplegic patient spearheaded a campaign against chemonucleolysis, and the medical-political controversy began (Ford et al., 1985).

Despite heated debate over the next decade, the Food and Drug Administration scheduled chymopapain for release for phase IV clinical studies in 1975. However, just prior to the scheduled release, the Food and Drug Administration canceled the release, awaiting the results of a multicenter double-blind study. The study was completed within a few months, and the researchers concluded that chymopapain was almost as effective as its diluent. With this, Baxter-Travenol, the producer of chymopapain, withdrew its new drug application. Within the same year, chymopapain was approved in Canada, and thousands of patients were referred there for treatment. Meanwhile, the double-blind study had been reviewed and criticized on a number of points, and additional double-blind studies were performed. The Food and Drug Administration was subjected to a great deal of political pressure, and, finally, in 1982, chymopapain was released for phase IV clinical use (Ford et al., 1985).

MECHANISM OF ACTION OF CHYMOPAPAIN

Chymopapain is a protease that depolymerizes the protein-disaccharide ground substance of the nucleus pulposus. This chondrolytic action is dose dependent; only with large quantities of the enzyme are macroscopic lesions of the annulus fibrosus or vertebral end-plate found. The destruction of the normally hygroscopic ground substance releases water molecules, which then diffuse out of the disk (Benoist, 1986). Destruction begins immediately and proceeds quickly; collapse of the disk space is evident radiographically within 48 hr. Because chymopapain is a chondrolytic enzyme, calcified disk material is not dissolved.

Although the biochemical action of chymopapain has been well demonstrated, the mode of action of chemonucleolysis in relief of radicular pain is not completely understood. Theories advanced are that the diminution of the water content decreases the intradiskal pressure and that disk height and the volume of the herniated portion are also decreased, relieving compression and tension on the adjacent nerve root. An anti-inflammatory effect of the enzyme has also been theorized. Interestingly, if intact chondrocytes survive the chemonucleolysis, the disk may be reconstituted with normal tissue (Benoist, 1986). No scientific evidence exists that chy-

mopapain chemonucleolysis is useful prophylactically.

CHEMONUCLEOLYSIS IN VETERINARY MEDICINE

Despite the extensive activity in human medicine, chemonucleolysis has received little attention in veterinary medicine, and no controlled clinical studies have been published. Two early reports of clinical studies (Saunders, 1964; Widdowson, 1967) had inadequate pretreatment diagnosis and no clinical control groups. More recently, Biggart (1988) reported an uncontrolled study of disk herniation and suggested that chemonucleolysis may be efficacious.

I have completed a 3-year pilot study of chymopapain (Discase, Travenol Laboratories) chemonucleolysis of type II cervical disk protrusion using a ventral surgical approach (Atilola et al., 1988) in ten large breed dogs (Bailey et al., 1988). This study was also uncontrolled (no untreated or other treatment comparison groups), but the results indicated that chymopapain chemonucleolysis can be performed safely and may be effective for treatment of painful type II cervical disk protrusion in dogs with minimal or no neurologic deficit. For dogs with significant myelopathy (obvious gait deficit), chymopapain chemonucleolysis may not be any more effective than surgery. If this is the case, the advantage of chemonucleolysis over surgery would be that the injection procedure is less risky than decompressive surgery. Chemonucleolysis probably does not have a monetary advantage because of the enzyme cost. A pilot study of chymopapain chemonucleolysis of type II lumbosacral disk protrusion is currently in progress, and initial results are promising. This condition resembles the one in humans for which chemonucleolysis is advocated, i.e., selected patients with lumbosacral radiculopathy caused by a single, contained disk herniation. In human medicine, chemonucleolysis is contraindicated in patients with myelopathy, cauda equina syndrome (including bowel or bladder dysfunction), or other severe, progressive neurologic deficit (Batson, 1989). Currently, chemonucleolysis in veterinary medicine must be considered an experimental procedure, awaiting controlled clinical studies to further test its safety and efficacy.

References and Suggested Reading

Atilola, M. A. O., Bailey, C. S., and Morgan, J. P.: Cervical chemonucleolysis in the dog: Surgical technique. Vet. Surg. 17:135, 1988.
A description of the surgical technique for cervical chemonucleolysis and results of chemonucleolysis in 16 healthy dogs.
Bailey, C. S., Kasper, J. B., and Morgan, J. P.: Chemonucleolysis in Type II disk disease. ACVIM Scientific Proceedings, 1988, p. 75.

A preliminary report of a prospective study of chymopapain chemonucleolysis using a ventral surgical approach for treatment of type II cervical disk protrusion in ten large breed dogs.

Batson, E.: Diagnostic and therapeutic technology assessment (DATTA): Chemonucleolysis for herniated lumbar disk. J.A.M.A. 18:953, 1989.
A report reflecting the views of a panel of physicians and reports in the scientific literature as of June 1989.

Benoist, M.: Principles of chemonucleolysis using chymopapain. *In* Bonneville, J-F. (ed.): *Focus on Chemonucleolysis.* New York: Springer-Verlag, 1986, p. 9.
A review of the composition of the intervertebral disk, the action of chymopapain on diskal and surrounding tissues, and proposed action in relief of radicular pain.

Biggart, J. F.: Results of diskolysis in the treatment of 125 patients with herniated disks. Vet. Surg. 17:29, 1988.
A report of the clinical results in 125 dogs treated for disk herniation.

Ford, L. T., Brown, J. E., and Smith, L.: The investigation and approval of chymopapain chemonucleolysis. *In* Brown, J. E., Nordby, E. J., Smith, L. (eds.): *Chemonucleolysis.* Thorofare, NJ: Slack, 1985, p. 1.

A historical review of the discovery and development of chymopapain chemonucleolysis.

Saunders, E. C.: Treatment of the canine intervertebral disc syndrome with chymopapain. J.A.V.M.A. 145:893, 1964.
First description of clinical use of chymopapain chemonucleolysis in veterinary medicine.

Smith, L., Garvin, P. J., Gesler, R. M., et al.: Enzyme dissolution of the nucleus pulposus. Nature 198:1311, 1963.
The original article describing chymopapain chemonucleolysis of intervertebral disks.

Thomas, L.: Reversible collapse of rabbit ears after intravenous papain, and prevention of recovery by cortisone. J. Exp. Med. 104:245, 1956.
The original article describing the chondrolytic effect of papain.

Widdowson, W. L.: Effects of chymopapain in the intervertebral disc of the dog. J.A.V.M.A. 150:608, 1967.
A prospective study of the effects of chymopapain injected into experimental dogs, and a brief description of nine dogs with disk herniation treated by chemonucleolysis.

LUMBOSACRAL DEGENERATIVE STENOSIS

JONATHAN N. CHAMBERS

Athens, Georgia

Lumbosacral spinal disease is much more common in the dog than was previously recognized. The predominant affliction is a degenerative disease analogous to the most common lower back problem in humans. The disorder has been known by several terms including cauda equina and lumbosacral syndrome, but the term lumbosacral degenerative stenosis (LDS) more properly designates the location, anatomic sequela, and common pathophysiologic pathway (Chambers, 1989).

SIGNALMENT, CLINICAL SIGNS, AND DIFFERENTIAL DIAGNOSIS

One of the reasons that the extent of LDS has been unappreciated is that the condition mimics other notorious problems that affect the pelvic limbs, particularly degenerative hip disease. Most but not all of the patients affected are of middle age and represent the popular large breeds (retrievers, German shepherds, Rottweilers) commonly associated with hip dysplasia. The diagnostic difficulty is compounded because many of the affected individuals harbor one or more of these other diseases in a mildly clinical or subclinical state. Thus, the challenge is not in finding disease, but discovering which disease is presently most significant.

The clinical signs shared by LDS and its impostors include pelvic limb pain, lameness, and weakness. The dysfunction associated with LDS is usually of relatively recent onset (days to weeks), and the owner will often describe the animal's reluctance to rise, jump, or climb stairs. The pain is typically intermittent and excruciating and the lameness severe. Pain specifically localized to the lumbosacral area may be described historically and is usually found on physical examination. Severe compression of associated nerve roots may produce pelvic limb proprioceptive deficits, urinary or fecal incontinence, or a weak tail or pelvic limbs. However, these signs are present in only a minority of cases.

The common differential diagnoses for LDS are listed in Table 1 along with historical or physical clues that tend to exclude them. Other rare causes of spontaneous pelvic limb dysfunction, such as lumbosacral spine or nerve root neoplasia, polyneuropathies, or polymyopathies, are possible.

LESION DEVELOPMENT AND CHARACTERIZATION

Like most degenerative diseases, the lesion or lesions of LDS are thought to develop in response to cumulative strain of the connective tissues that extends beyond physiologic limits and causes micro-

Table 1. *Differential Diagnoses for Lumbosacral Degenerative Stenosis (LDS)*

Differential	Contrast With LDS
Coxofemoral degenerative joint disease and hip dysplasia (CHD)	Slower, more subtle onset (weeks to months with CHD versus days to weeks with LDS)
Degenerative myelopathy (DM)	Slow, subtle onset (months to years); consistent and profound neurologic deficits; painless if DM is singular problem
Thoracolumbar type II disk herniation (TL disk)	Similar in onset but consistent neurologic deficits
Lumbosacral diskospondylitis* (Gilmore, 1987)	Similar in onset and signs to LDS; other clinical signs of infectious disease may be present but not consistently
Cranial cruciate disease	Constant unilateral lameness with signs localized to the stifle (instability, pain, swelling, crepitus, etc.)

*Based on Gilmore, 1987.

trauma. The process appears to begin in the normally elastic tissues of the intervertebral disk, which are replaced by stiff, inelastic, fibrous tissue. The now inferior constraining tissue (annulus fibrosus) tears, allowing herniation of the disk. There may be a brief period of local instability, but this is rapidly supplanted by rigidity as surrounding bone, ligaments, and joint capsules hypertrophy. The herniated disk and hypertrophic tissues encroach on the nerve roots, causing radicular pain and dysfunction. Although dramatic degenerative change is often seen on survey radiographs, the most common and often singular lesion actually compressing the nerve roots is the disk herniation (Chambers et al., 1988; Selcer et al., 1988).

DIAGNOSTIC PATHWAY

After a complete general, neurologic, and routine laboratory examination, the dog should be anesthetized for electromyography (EMG) and radiographic imaging. The EMG is not compulsory to establish the diagnosis, but it may help substantiate the diagnosis and it is the most sensitive (but not specific) indicator of denervation of muscles supplied by involved nerve roots (Sisson et al., in press). It will also prevent a misdiagnosis in cases of polyneuropathy or polymyopathy in which more diffuse changes would be expected and may be valuable in correlative localization and prognosis (Chambers, 1989).

Radiographic imaging should begin with survey radiographs (Selcer, 1989). They will neither confirm nor refute the diagnosis but may provide indirect evidence of lumbosacral disease and will usually detect other causes of lumbosacral pain, such as diskospondylitis, vertebral neoplasia, and trauma. *Epidurography* (Fig. 1) is a relatively easy and reliable (93%) technique for demonstrating space-occupying masses and compression at the lumbosacral junction and is presently the method of choice for imaging LDS (Hathcock et al., 1988; Selcer et al., 1988). Diskography has also been studied and shows promise (Sisson et al., in press). Computerized tomography and magnetic resonance imaging are also being evaluated in this setting. Although the dural sac terminates cranial to the lumbosacral area in some dogs and fails to fill the epidural space in most dogs, it may be helpful in delineating compressive lesions in some cases (Lang, 1988). Myelography should be performed if there are neurologic deficits and spinal cord disease (thoracolumbar disk herniation, degenerative myelopathy) is suspected as a primary or additional problem, especially in predisposed dogs such as German shepherds. With either epidurography or myelography, compressive lesions may be dynamic. Compression is typically most pronounced when the pelvic limbs are extended caudally, thus causing lumbar lordosis (Fig. 1).

THERAPY

Nonoperative

Conservative therapy consisting of strict rest and nonsteroidal anti-inflammatory drugs (NSAIDs) can be tried in patients with suspected or confirmed LDS if there has been a single episode and the clinical signs are limited to pain or lameness. Aggravating life-style factors such as strenuous activity or obesity must be eliminated.

No large-scale retrospective or prospective study has been conducted to evaluate the effectiveness of conservative therapy; two reports suggest disappointing results. Regardless, surgery is strongly recommended for dogs with recurrent signs, severe unrelenting pain, or neurologic deficits.

Surgical

Two fundamentally different surgical techniques have been advocated: exploratory laminectomy and excision of encroaching tissues (diskectomy with or without foraminotomy) (Chambers et al., 1988; Chambers, 1989) or traction, internal fixation, and fusion (Slocum and Devine, 1986 and 1989). The former technique will be briefly described here.

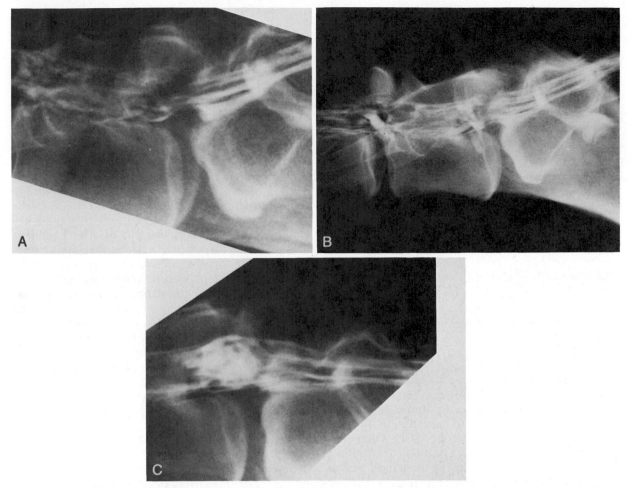

Figure 1. Lateral epidurogram views made with the pelvic limbs, *A*, extended caudally, *B*, in neutral position, and *C*, flexed cranially. An intervertebral disk herniation is usually most apparent on the extension view. (Reprinted with permission from Selcer, B.A.: Radiographic imaging in canine lumbosacral disease. Veterinary Medicine Report 1:289, 1989.)

EXPLORATORY LAMINECTOMY

General anesthesia with tracheal intubation and ventilatory support is used. The dog is placed in sternal recumbency with the pelvic limbs forward, and sandbags are placed under the tuber ischia to lessen the pressure on the abdomen; this aids in ventilation and assists venous drainage.

The skin incision is from the tip of the L6 spinous process to the sacrocaudal junction on the dorsal midline. The subcuticular fat layer is divided to the level of the lumbar fascia. The fascia is released from the tip of the L7 spinous process and incised to the S2 level. The paravertebral muscles are subperiosteally elevated from the spinous processes and laminae of L7–S2 and the L7–S1 facets. Exposure is maintained with Gelpi retractors. The L7–S1 interspinous ligament is excised, allowing exposure of the interarcuate ligament (Fig. 2A).

The interarcuate ligament is carefully excised over the interlaminar space to gain access to the vertebral canal (see Fig. 2B). The caudal half of the L7 spinous process and the S1 dorsal spine are removed with a bone cutter, and a conservative laminectomy* (sparing the pedicles and facets) is performed, removing approximately 1 cm of bone from the caudal margin of L7 and cranial margin of S1 (see Fig. 2C). The nerve roots are inspected and carefully retracted with blunt nerve hooks to expose the floor of the vertebral canal and herniated disk (see Fig. 2D). The bulging disk is sharply excised and the disk space curetted. The L7 nerve roots are inspected for encroaching tissues, and foraminotomies are performed if necessary. Facetectomy, especially bilaterally, should be avoided. Wound closure is performed routinely in multiple layers after copious crystalloid lavage.

Editors' Note: Laminectomy is considerably facilitated in larger dogs by use of a power drill.

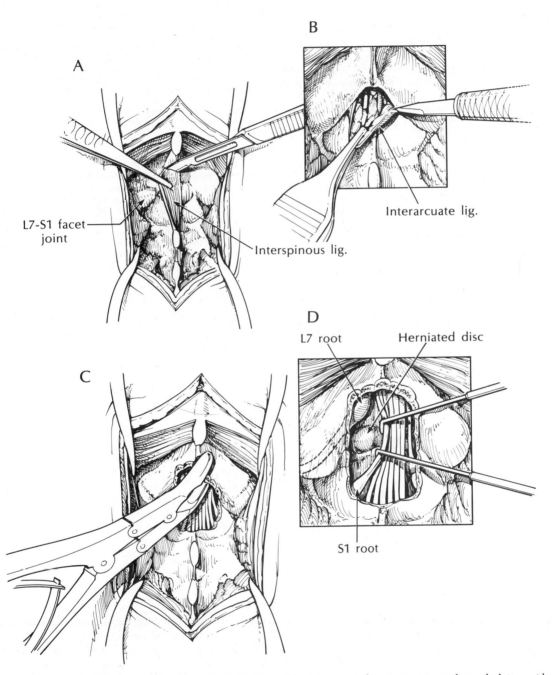

Figure 2. *A*, Excision of the interspinous ligament. *B*, Excision of the interarcuate ligament exposing the underlying epidural fat and nerve roots. *C*, Laminectomy of L7 and S1 to gain wider access to the epidural space. *D*, Exposure of the L7 nerve root and disk herniation. (Reprinted with permission from Chambers, J.N.: Degenerative lumbosacral stenosis in dogs. Veterinary Medicine Report 1:175, 1989.)

POSTOPERATIVE CARE

The dog's activity should be strictly confined to short leash walks for 6 weeks. NSAIDs can be used as needed for early postoperative pain.

PROGNOSIS

Dogs with pain or lameness as the only clinical sign usually improve rapidly and sometimes dramatically after surgery (Chambers et al., 1988). Dogs with chronic neurologic deficits take substantially longer to improve, and the recovery may be incomplete.

References and Suggested Reading

Chambers, J. N.: Degenerative lumbosacral stenosis in dogs. Veterinary Medicine Report 1:166, 1989a.
A comprehensive review of degenerative lumbosacral stenosis in dogs, including anatomy, pathophysiology, diagnosis, and treatment.
Chambers, J. N.: Optimal treatment for lumbosacral stenosis: Surgical exploration and excision of tissue. Veterinary Medicine Report 1:248, 1989b.
A referenced monograph explaining the rationale for the routine use of conventional decompressive surgery as opposed to spinal fusion for degenerative lumbosacral stenosis.
Chambers, J. N., Selcer, B. A., and Oliver, J. E.: Results of treatment of degenerative lumbosacral stenosis in dogs by exploration and excision. Vet. Comp. Orthoped. Trauma 1:130, 1988.
A retrospective clinical study reporting the results of conventional decompressive surgery in 26 dogs with degenerative lumbosacral stenosis.
Gilmore, D. R.: Lumbosacral diskospondylitis in 21 dogs. J. Am. Anim. Hosp. Assoc. 23:57, 1987.
A retrospective study describing the clinical findings in 21 dogs with diskospondylitis and describing its similarity to degenerative lumbosacral stenosis.
Hathcock, J. T., Pechman, R. D., Dillon, A. R., et al.: Comparison of three radiographic contrast procedures in the evaluation of the canine lumbosacral spinal cord. Vet. Radiol. 29:4, 1988.
A laboratory study comparing epidurography, myelography, and sinus venography for the detection of lumbosacral masses, with the investigators concluding epidurography offered the most potential.
Lang, J.: Flexion-extension myelography of the canine cauda equina. Vet. Radiol. 29:242, 1988.
A review of myelographic findings at the lumbosacral junction in normal dogs and in those with pathologic lesions in this area.
Selcer, B. A.: Radiographic imaging in canine lumbosacral disease. Veterinary Medicine Report 1:282, 1989.
A review of the various radiographic techniques available for diagnosing lumbosacral spinal disease, including advantages and disadvantages.
Selcer, B. A., Chambers, J. N., Schwensen, K., et al.: Epidurography as a diagnostic aid in canine lumbosacral compressive disease: 47 cases (1981–1986). Vet. Comp. Orthoped. Trauma 1:97, 1988.
A retrospective study describing the epidurographic findings in a large series of dogs with degenerative disease of the lumbosacral spine.
Sisson, A. F., LeCouteur, R. A., Ingram, J. T., et al.: Diagnosis of cauda equina abnormalities in dogs using electromyography, diskography and epidurography. J. Vet. Intern. Med. (in press).
A laboratory and prospective clinical study comparing diagnostic techniques, with the investigators concluding that electromyography is most sensitive and that diskography rivals epidurography.
Slocum, B., and Devine, T.: L7-S1 fixation fusion for treatment of cauda equina compression in the dog. J.A.V.M.A. 188:31, 1986.
Report of a surgical alternative to conventional decompressive surgery (see following reference), including its use in a series of 14 clinical cases.
Slocum, B., and Devine, T.: Optimal treatment for degenerative lumbosacral stenosis: Traction, internal fixation, and fusion. Veterinary Medicine Report 1:249, 1989.
Report of a surgical alternative to conventional decompressive surgery, utilizing traction, dorsal internal fixation, and bone graft to induce fusion.

FELINE NEUROMUSCULAR DISEASES

PAUL A. CUDDON
Madison, Wisconsin

Feline neuromuscular diseases can be broadly categorized into those involving peripheral nerves/nerve roots, the neuromuscular junction, and muscle. Although all will produce lower motor neuron (LMN) disease, significant variation in clinical signs occurs. Both peripheral nerve and muscle disorders usually involve varying degrees of paresis, muscle atrophy, hyporeflexia, and hypotonia, although the severity of the latter two signs is usually much greater in peripheral nerve disease. Ataxia and proprioceptive deficits are also more characteristic of peripheral nerve involvement. Muscle hypertrophy rather than atrophy may be a characteristic of some primary muscle disorders. Clinical signs of neuromuscular junction diseases are variable, ranging from exercise-induced weakness to flaccid paralysis.

Accurate diagnosis of feline neuromuscular disease requires careful neurologic examination, selected blood work, electrophysiologic evaluation, and muscle/peripheral nerve biopsies. Muscle biopsies are usually evaluated by routine hematoxylin and eosin stains, histochemical analysis, and electron microscopy (EM). Peripheral nerve biopsies are usually immersion fixed in 2.5% glutaraldehyde and embedded in plastic for light and electron microscopy. Single nerve fiber teasing can also be extremely informative.

INHERITED POLYNEUROPATHIES

Feline Niemann-Pick Disease–Associated Polyneuropathy

Niemann-Pick disease, an autosomal-recessive lysosomal storage disease characterized by a deficiency of sphingomyelinase, may be associated with a primary polyneuropathy. Three Siamese cats between 2 and 5 months of age with this disease have been described (Cuddon et al., 1989). Neurologic signs included progressive tetraparesis and ataxia, a palmigrade/plantigrade stance, fine generalized tremors, and hypo- or areflexia. Hepatosplenomegaly was also present.

The primary demyelinating nature of this polyneuropathy is supported diagnostically by a dramatic slowing of sensory and motor nerve conduction velocities (NCVs) and diffuse myelin degeneration surrounding largely intact axons on peripheral nerve biopsy. A lysosomal storage disease should be suspected with the finding of large vacuolated Schwann cells and macrophages lining axons on nerve biopsy, foamy macrophages on bone marrow aspirate, and activated Kupffer cells on liver biopsy. Definitive diagnosis of Niemann-Pick disease, however, can be made only via lysosomal enzyme and lipid analysis of either cultured skin fibroblasts, liver, spleen, kidney, or brain. Negligible quantities of sphingomyelinase with accumulation of sphingomyelin and unesterified cholesterol in these tissues characterize this disease. Associated increases in brain GM_2 and GM_3 gangliosides also occur. This disease is progressive and fatal, with no treatment available.

Inherited Primary Hyperchylomicronemia–Associated Peripheral Neuropathy

This suspected autosomal-recessive disease is characterized by fasting hyperlipemia, lipemia retinalis, and peripheral neuropathy (Jones et al., 1986). There is a uniform decrease in lipoprotein lipase with resultant increases in triglycerides, cholesterol, and very low-density lipoproteins. Clinical signs usually are not seen until 8 months of age. Lipid granulomas, thought to form secondary to trauma, are consistently found in abdominal organs and often in the skin. Neurologic involvement, although not seen in all cases, is due to compression of peripheral, cranial, and cervical sympathetic nerves by these granulomas, especially at the level of intervertebral foramina. The development of multiple peripheral and cranial nerve signs with possible

Horner's syndrome is usually slow and often unilateral. Total paralysis does not usually occur.

Treatment consists solely of a low-fat diet. Following 2 to 3 months of dietary management, resolution of neurologic signs and a decrease in blood lipid levels occurred in the reported cats.

Primary Hyperoxaluria–Associated Peripheral Neuropathy

This suspected autosomal-recessive disease has been seen primarily in related domestic short-hair cats in Britain and appears analogous to primary hyperoxaluria type II in man (McKerrell et al., 1989). Cats between 5 and 9 months of age develop signs of acute renal failure due to renal tubular deposition of oxalate crystals in combination with profound generalized LMN weakness. Weakness is attributed to accumulation of neurofilaments in ventral nerve roots, proximal axons, and intramuscular nerves.

Electromyography (EMG) shows spontaneous activity, and muscle biopsy demonstrates the classic changes of denervation. L-glyceric aciduria and intermittent hyperoxaluria accompany the classic biochemical changes of acute renal failure. Disease confirmation is made through measurement of hepatic D-glycerate dehydrogenase (<5% of normal). All of the reported cats died before 1 year of age despite symptomatic therapy for acute renal failure. The pathogenesis of the peripheral nerve lesions is not known.

Hypertrophic Polyneuropathy

A possibly inherited hypertrophic polyneuropathy has been described in two unrelated 1-year-old cats (Dahme et al., 1987). Both cats showed intention tremor, decreased postural reactions, hyporeflexia, and mild sensory loss. Sensory, motor, and autonomic nerves showed demyelination and incomplete remyelination with resultant "onion-bulb" formation. Axonal changes were rare.

ACQUIRED POLYNEUROPATHIES

Diabetic Polyneuropathy

Cats with uncontrolled or poorly controlled diabetes mellitus may develop a distal polyneuropathy that initially affects the pelvic limbs (Kramek et al., 1984). Initial neurologic abnormalities include a plantigrade stance, progressive paraparesis, muscle atrophy, and patellar hyporeflexia (Fig. 1). Forelimbs also eventually demonstrate LMN involve-

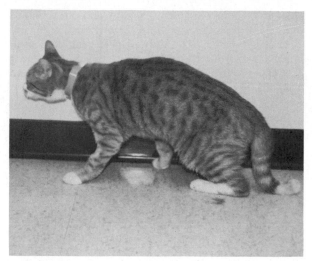

Figure 1. The classic plantigrade stance of a cat with a distal polyneuropathy secondary to uncontrolled diabetes mellitus.

ment. The etiopathogenesis of this polyneuropathy is not fully understood.

Diagnostically, these cats demonstrate polyuria/polydypsia, hyperglycemia, glycosuria, spontaneous activity on EMG, and a decrease in motor NCVs. A fascicular tibial nerve biopsy will demonstrate the typical changes seen with this polyneuropathy (myelin ballooning, axonal degeneration, and demyelination), and muscle biopsy will show classic denervation atrophy (types I and II angular fibers).

If early, well-controlled insulin therapy is instituted (see this volume, p. 364), many cats will show marked improvement in neurologic function with consistent increases in NCVs. In particular, wide blood glucose swings should be avoided. Some cats will return to normal following weeks to months of proper insulin regulation. The use of aldose reductase inhibitors to decrease peripheral nerve sorbitol accumulation is controversial.

Ischemic Neuromyopathy

This possible sequela to feline myocardial disease is the result of arterial thromboembolism. The terminal aortic trifurcation is most commonly affected (>90% of all cases), followed by the brachial artery. The ischemic injury to both muscle and peripheral nerve is produced by collateral circulation vasoconstriction induced by substances such as serotonin and thromboxane A_2 released by platelets trapped in the thrombus. Cats of all ages can be affected, with male cats having a higher incidence. Persians and domestic short-hair cats are overly represented (Fox, 1987).

Clinically, cats present with variably lateralized paraparesis or paraplegia; painful, firm gastrocnemius and cranial tibial muscles; cold extremities with cyanosis of the nail beds and absence of femoral pulses; anesthesia distal to the tarsus; and an inability to flex or extend the hocks.

Diagnosis is based on clinical signs, documentation of cardiac dysfunction, and elevations in serum creatine kinase (CK) and lactate dehydrogenase levels. Spontaneous activity on EMG, decreased action potential amplitudes, and slowed or absent sciatic/tibial motor and sensory NCVs provide confirmation but are generally unnecessary for diagnosis. Histopathologically, areas of focal muscle necrosis and phagocytosis are seen, especially in the cranial tibial muscle, as well as severe necrosis and myelinated fiber loss in the central areas of each fascicle of the mid to distal sciatic nerve and its branches.

Treatment centers on management of the underlying heart failure. Antiplatelet-aggregating drugs such as aspirin (one fourth of a 5-grain tablet PO every 2 to 3 days) might help prevent future emboli by decreasing thromboxane A_2 synthesis. (Details of therapy can be found in *CVT X*, p. 295.)

Although improvement in pelvic limb motor function may occur within days or weeks following the return of collateral circulation, complete recovery may take as long as 6 months, if it occurs at all. Prognosis remains guarded owing to the high rate of disease recurrence.

Feline Dysautonomia (Key-Gaskell Syndrome)

This syndrome of autonomic denervation has been seen primarily in Britain and Europe (Griffiths et al., 1982), although single cases have recently been reported in the United States. Affected cats are usually young adults with no apparent breed or sex predilection. Most show an acute onset of signs related to both sympathetic and parasympathetic nervous system dysfunction. Depression, anorexia, constipation, a dry rhinarium, reduced tear production, megaesophagus, and dilated, fixed pupils are seen in over 90% of cases. Other signs may include vomiting, prolapse of the nictitating membranes, xerostomia, constant bradycardia (<120 beats/min), urinary and fecal incontinence, anal areflexia, and occasional paresis. Some cats will collapse during stressful periods owing to their lack of autonomic reserve.

Thoracic and abdominal radiography will demonstrate megaesophagus, gastric dilation, urinary bladder distention, and, with the help of contrast, delayed gastric emptying and intestinal ileus. Pharmacologic testing of eye function demonstrates denervation hypersensitivity indicative of ganglionic involvement. Plasma catecholamine levels are significantly decreased. Electrophysiologic studies are usually normal.

Treatment consists primarily of intravenous fluid

therapy, nasogastric feeding or total parenteral nutrition, artificial tears, laxatives, and antibiotics for possible aspiration pneumonia. Metoclopramide (Reglan, Robins) at 0.2 to 0.4 mg/kg every 6 to 8 hr SC or PO may be helpful in enhancing gastric emptying. Pilocarpine (0.1%) or physostigmine (0.5%) eye drops will help alleviate some of the ocular signs. Bethanechol (Urecholine, Merck Sharp & Dohme), a systemic parasympathomimetic, at 2.5 to 5 mg every 8 hr PO may improve bladder and colon function, although side effects (bradycardia, colic, ptyalism) are common. Systemic and ophthalmic cholinergic preparations should not be used together. If cats survive, initial improvement should be seen within 7 to 10 days, with recovery taking up to 1 to 2 months. Megaesophagus and pupillary dilation may persist in many cats. Overall prognosis, however, is poor, with only a 22 to 30% survival rate. Persistent vomiting usually indicates a poor prognosis.

The primary pathologic changes relate to a profound decrease in the number of neurons and an increase in non-neuronal cells within the parasympathetic and sympathetic ganglia. However, dorsal root and cranial nerve ganglia as well as ventral horn cells may be involved to a lesser degree. The ganglionic neurons that remain show signs of degeneration (Nissl substance depletion and vacuolation).

Trauma

Brachial plexus avulsion produced by severe forelimb abduction with secondary stretching or tearing of nerve roots is probably one of the more common peripheral nerve injuries in cats, although it has rarely been addressed. The forelimb neurologic deficits produced will depend on whether the entire plexus or just the cranial (C6–C7) or caudal (C8–T1/T2) nerve roots are involved. Injury to C8–T1 or T1–T2 nerve roots can also result in an ipsilateral panniculus reflex loss or a partial Horner's syndrome, respectively.

Ilial fractures with craniomedial displacement of bone fragments or sacroiliac fracture/dislocation can damage the sixth and seventh lumbar and first two sacral ventral nerve roots. With nerve entrapment, extreme pain is usually present at the injury site. If there is nerve severance, there will be anesthesia distal to the stifle.

Caudal thigh intramuscular injections of especially irritant substances in the vicinity of the sciatic nerve also can result in varying severity of neurologic dysfunction distal to the stifle in the affected limb (Fig. 2).

Complete investigation of the severity of injury incorporates gait analysis, neurologic examination with autonomous zone testing, EMG, nerve con-

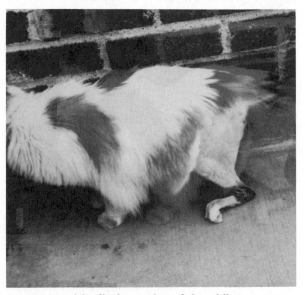

Figure 2. Left hindlimb neurologic deficits following an injection injury to the left proximal sciatic nerve. Note the loss of conscious proprioception, the dropped hock, and the muscle atrophy of the semitendinosus, cranial tibial, and gastrocnemius muscles (the limb has been shaved for exploratory surgery).

duction studies, and assessment of dorsal and ventral nerve root function.

Surgical exploration of the brachial plexus is usually unrewarding because the main area of injury is usually associated with the nerve roots between the dorsal root ganglia and the spinal cord. However, surgical intervention may be warranted in other injuries, especially when nerve entrapment is suggested or the injury is acute with moderate to severe LMN limb deficits present. If the peripheral nerve injury is mild, surgery does not appear to change the rate or degree of function recovery. Any possible return of neurologic function in the limb should be followed sequentially via neurologic and electrophysiologic examinations. Supportive care and intensive physiotherapy should be performed to prevent secondary limb contracture. A poor prognosis should be given if no improvement occurs in 4 to 6 months. Amputation or tendon transplantation/joint fusion may be a viable option in such patients.

Neoplasia

Feline lymphosarcoma, usually associated with FeLV infection, can involve nerve roots or peripheral nerves via metastatic spread. Unlike other peripheral nerve tumors, lymphosarcoma spreads rapidly, so there is little chance that removal of one or more nerve roots or even limb amputation will contain the tumor spread. The tumor may diffusely and widely infiltrate nerves in multiple body regions, producing a mononeuropathy multiplex. It may invade the brain and spinal cord as well. Prognosis in virtually all cases of nervous system lymphosarcoma is poor despite attempts at systemic or intrathecal chemotherapy.

Miscellaneous Peripheral Neuropathies

Single case reports of a variety of peripheral neuropathies have been described. These include two cases of histologically confirmed inflammatory polyneuropathy (a chronic relapsing polyradiculoneuritis [Flecknell and Lucke, 1978] and an acute polyneuritis [Lane and deLahunta, 1984]), an idiopathic chronic relapsing polyneuropathy responsive to immunosuppressive steroid therapy (Shores et al., 1987), and an acute brachial plexus neuropathy with a suspected relation to previous vaccination (Bright et al., 1978).

Laryngeal paralysis with presenting signs of dysphonia, absence of purring, and progressive inspiratory dyspnea has also been reported in the cat (Hardie et al., 1981).

INHERITED MYOPATHIES

Feline X-linked Muscular Dystrophy

A rare suspected X-linked muscular dystrophy has been reported separately in three different groups of male cats (Siamese, European, and domestic short-hairs). For a discussion of this disorder see this volume, p. 1042.

Nemaline Myopathy

A suspected inherited myopathy has been described in five related cats between 6 and 18 months of age with an onset of reluctance to walk and a forced, rapid, abrupt, hypermetric gait (Cooper et al., 1986). Other signs included muscle tremors, hyporeflexia, and muscle atrophy, which was more pronounced in the proximal limb musculature. Despite continued muscle atrophy, all other clinical signs did not appear progressive. Only mild elevations in CK occurred, and all EMG studies were normal.

This myopathy is characterized by large but variable numbers of nemaline rods within myofibers, with marked fiber size variation, fiber splitting, myofiber atrophy, and sarcolemmic infolding. Multiple biopsies may be required because some muscle sections in the described cats lacked rods completely. The pathogenesis of this condition is un-

known. A Z-band or other cytoskeletal abnormality has been suggested. There is no known specific therapy for this condition.

Generalized Ossifying Myositis

Generalized ossifying myositis, a non-neoplastic form of heterotopic ossification affecting skeletal muscle and fibrous connective tissue, has been described in two young cats with a history of progressive weakness, stiffness, difficulty in jumping, decreased range of limb motion, and pain on forced movement (Norris et al., 1980; Waldron et al., 1985). Calcified masses were palpated initially in the cervical and thoracic paraspinal muscles, with eventual incorporation of all proximal thoracic and pelvic limb musculature.

Diagnosis of this disease is based on radiography, which reveals extensive soft-tissue mineralization, and muscle biopsy, which demonstrates a noninflammatory muscle ossification with well-differentiated cartilage and bone.

Palliative treatment with diphosphonate disodium etidronate (Didronel, Norwich Eaton), an inhibitor of further mineralization, at 10 mg/kg every 24 hr PO has been suggested. Eventual prognosis, however, is poor with relentless progression of calcification. Clinical signs are not alleviated by corticosteroid therapy. This is an inherited disease in humans.

ACQUIRED MYOPATHIES

Hypokalemic Polymyopathy

This acute feline polymyopathy, produced by a severe total body K^+ depletion, is usually secondary to a concurrent decreased K^+ intake and increases in the fractional excretion of K^+ in urine (due to renal dysfunction) (see this volume, p. 1042). A similar syndrome with a suspected hereditary basis has been reported in young Burmese cats (Mason, 1988). Classic signs include muscle weakness, cervical ventroflexion, stiff, stilted gait, and muscle pain.

Biochemical confirmation of this disease includes a significantly elevated CK and a serum K^+ <3.5 mEq/L. Although EMG changes are variably present, muscle biopsies are usually normal.

Most cats can be successfully treated with oral supplementation of a K^+ gluconate elixir (Kaon Elixir, Adria Laboratories) and dietary changes, with a dramatic response occurring within 24 hr. Parenteral K^+ therapy should be reserved only for cats with severe hypokalemia. (A detailed description of this syndrome is found in *CVT X*, p. 812.)

Polymyositis

Although cats are the only known definitive hosts for *Toxoplasma gondii* and up to 64% of all cats in certain areas of the United States have serum antibodies to this organism, *Toxoplasma* infections are usually not clinically evident in this species. In clinically affected cats, lesions are most frequently related to the lungs, liver, gastrointestinal tract, eyes, and brain. Muscle involvement is not an outstanding feature (Burridge, 1980).

Experimental inoculation of cats with the protozoon *Neospora caninum* can produce fatal, necrotizing encephalomyelitis, polymyositis, pneumonia, and hepatitis (see this volume, p. 263). Prenatally and neonatally infected kittens and immunosuppressed adults are most susceptible. Natural feline neosporosis, however, has not been reported (Dubey et al., 1990).

Suspected immune-mediated polymyositis also has been reported in cats and may be associated with thymoma (Carpenter and Holzworth, 1982).

Cats with polymyositis clinically resemble those with hypokalemic polymyopathy, with dysphagia often accompanying the weakness. Serum creatine kinase and other muscle-associated enzymes will be elevated, generalized spontaneous activity will be seen on EMG, and multifocal infiltration of muscle fascicles with primarily lymphocytes, macrophages, and neutrophils will be present on muscle biopsy. The absence of either *Toxoplasma* or *Neospora* cysts on muscle biopsy does not rule out these etiologies; therefore, definitive diagnosis relies on a strongly positive or fourfold increase in antibody titer to these organisms on paired serum samples. Serologic testing for concurrent FeLV or FTLV infection should also be performed in suspected protozoal polymyositis, due to the increased predisposition of immunosuppressed cats to these infections. Serum ANA may be positive in cases of immune-mediated polymyositis.

Recommended therapy for *T. gondii* and *N. caninum* infection consists of either clindamycin (Antirobe, UpJohn) at 25 to 50 mg/kg/day divided every 8 to 12 hr PO or IM or trimethoprim/sulfadiazine (Tribrissen, Coopers) at 30 mg/kg every 12 hr PO alone or with the addition of pyrimethamine (Daraprim, Burroughs Wellcome) at 0.5 mg/kg/day PO for 7 to 10 days. Pyrimethamine is unpalatable and cats are very susceptible to its toxic effects, so therapy should not extend past 2 weeks. Supplementation with folinic acid (Leucovorin Calcium, Lederle) at 1 mg/kg every 24 hr PO is recommended. Treatment for immune-mediated polymyositis consists of immunosuppression with corticosteroids (prednisone, 1.5 to 2 mg/kg every 12 hr PO). If a thymoma is present, thymectomy is also indicated. Despite aggressive therapy, prognosis is very poor in cases of protozoal infection but is fair in immune-mediated polymyositis.

Miscellaneous Muscle Diseases

A number of single case reports of other muscle-related diseases have been described in cats. They include nutritional myopathy secondary to vitamin E deficiency (Dennis and Alexander, 1982); myositis secondary to *Clostridium chauvoei* and *Clostridium septicum* infections (Poonacha et al., 1982); fibrotic myopathy of the semitendinosus muscle (Lewis, 1988); and quadriceps contracture secondary to trauma (Carberry and Flanders, 1986).

DISEASES OF THE NEUROMUSCULAR JUNCTION

Myasthenia Gravis

Unique features of this disease that pertain to the cat will be addressed here. (For a review of the general pathophysiologic mechanisms of myasthenia gravis, see this volume, p. 1039.)

Feline myasthenia gravis is a relatively rare syndrome with a total of twelve cases now documented. Ten have been acquired, and two were assumed to be the congenital form (Cuddon, 1989). Two of the acquired cases were associated with a thymoma (Scott-Moncrieff et al., 1990) and another with a cystic thymus (O'Dair et al., 1991). Abyssinians and Somalis, a close relative of the former breed, constitute the majority of cats with acquired myasthenia, which may suggest a possible association with the major histocompatibility complex, as in humans.

The most consistent signs in cats include tremors, initial stiffness with progression to generalized weakness on exercise, cervical weakness, dysphagia, dysphonia, ptyalism, facial weakness, and dyspnea (Fig. 3). Overt megaesophagus or esophageal hypomotility is common.

Confirmation of the disease in cats is identical to that in dogs. Cats, however, do not react as predictably to the ultra–short-acting anticholinesterase edrophonium chloride (Tensilon, Roche). A single IV injection of 0.5 to 1 mg is used by the author. The classic decremental response to supramaximal repetitive nerve stimulation is also observed in cats with both congenital and acquired myasthenia. All cases of acquired myasthenia tested for the presence of circulating antiacetylcholine-receptor antibodies had strongly positive results. The direct immunocytochemical localization of immune complexes at the motor end-plate using staphylococcal protein A

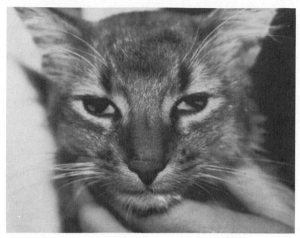

Figure 3. Bilateral facial weakness and protrusion of the nictitating membranes in a Somali cat with acquired myasthenia gravis.

conjugated with horseradish peroxidase, originally described in dogs, can also be performed in cats with acquired myasthenia gravis.

Cats with the acquired form of the disease appear to be more therapeutically challenging compared with dogs. However, with careful use of immuno-suppressive corticosteroid therapy (prednisone, 1.5 to 2 mg/kg every 12 hr PO) alone or in initial combination with the anticholinesterase pyridostig-mine (Mestinon, Roche) at a starting dose of 0.5 mg/kg every 12 hr PO, successful treatment, often with complete remission, can be achieved. Gradual corticosteroid dosage reduction and eventual cessation of therapy may take months. Although a specific dosage of anticholinesterase is mentioned here, therapy must always be tailored to the cat's individual response. Thymectomy will be an integral part of therapy if a thymoma is present. The number of cases of feline congenital myasthenia gravis is too small to comment on prognosis with appropriate anticholinesterase therapy. Corticoste-roids would not be indicated in this form of myas-thenia, owing to its nonimmune etiology.

References and Suggested Reading

Bright, R. M., Crabtree, B. J., and Knecht, C. D.: Brachial plexus neuropathy in the cat: A case report. J. Am. Anim. Hosp. Assoc. 14:612, 1978.
A case report and discussion of brachial plexus neuropathy including a description of the clinical and electrophysiologic findings of the syndrome in man.

Burridge, M. J.: Toxoplasmosis. Comp. Cont. Ed. Pract. Vet. 2:233, 1980.
A review of the life cycle, clinical signs, diagnosis, treatment, and public health significance of toxoplasmosis in small animals.

Carberry, C. A., and Flanders, J. A.: Quadriceps contracture in a cat. J.A.V.M.A. 189:1329, 1986.
A case report.

Carpenter, J. L., and Holzworth, J.: Thymoma in 11 cats. J.A.V.M.A. 181:248, 1982.
A retrospective study of the clinical signs, paraneoplastic effects, diagnosis, treatment, and histopathology of thymomas in 11 cats.

Cooper, B. J., deLahunta, A., Gallagher, E. A., et al.: Nemaline myopathy of cats. Muscle and Nerve 9:618, 1986.
A detailed pathologic description of this myopathy in five cats with a brief discussion of clinical signs and diagnostic findings.

Cuddon, P. A.: Acquired immune-mediated myasthenia gravis in a cat. J. Small Anim. Pract. 30:511, 1989.
A case report of a Somali with myasthenia, with discussion of the other reported cases and new methods of diagnosis and treatment.

Cuddon, P. A., Higgins, R. J., Duncan, I. D., et al.: Polyneuropathy in feline Niemann-Pick disease. Brain 112:1429, 1989.
A detailed clinical, diagnostic, and biochemical investigation of NPD-associated polyneuropathy in three cats.

Dahme, E., Kraft, W., and Scabell, J.: Hypertrophische polyneuropathie bei der katze. J. Vet. Med. A. 34:271, 1987.
A description of the clinical and pathologic findings in two cats with hypertrophic polyneuropathy.

Dennis, J. M., and Alexander, R. W.: Nutritional myopathy in a cat. Vet. Rec. 111:195, 1982.
A case report of a myopathy secondary to vitamin E deficiency.

Dubey, J. P., Lindsay, D. S., and Lipscomb, T. P.: Neosporosis in cats. Vet. Pathol. 27:335, 1990.
A paper on the successful experimental transmission of Neospora caninum to immunosuppressed adult cats and resultant clinical signs and pathology.

Flecknell, P. A., and Lucke, V. M.: Chronic relapsing polyradiculoneuritis in a cat. Acta. Neuropathol. (Berl.) 41:81, 1978.
A case report concentrating on the pathology of this disease.

Fox, P. R.: Feline cardiomyopathy. In Bonagura, J. D. (ed.): Contemporary Issues in Small Animal Practice: Cardiology. Vol. 7. New York: Churchill Livingstone, 1987, p. 453.
A general review of feline myocardial diseases, including a discussion of thromboembolic disease.

Griffiths, I. R., Nash, A. S., and Sharp, N. J. H.: The Key-Gaskell syndrome: The current situation. Vet. Rec. 111:532, 1982.
A general discussion of the knowledge concerning this disease in Britain soon after its initial recognition.

Hardie, E. M., Kolata, R. J., Stone, E. A., et al.: Laryngeal paralysis in three cats. J.A.V.M.A. 179:879, 1981.
A clinical description of three cases of acute laryngeal paralysis in the cat, with discussion of EMG findings, possible etiology, and surgical correction.

Jones, B. R., Johnstone, A. C., Cahill, J. I., et al.: Peripheral neuropathy in cats with inherited primary hyperchylomicronemia. Vet. Rec. 119:268, 1986.
A detailed study of the clinical signs, biochemical alterations, treatment, and histopathology of this inherited disease in 20 cats.

Kramek, B. A., Moise, N. S., Cooper, B., et al.: Neuropathy associated with diabetes mellitus in the cat. J.A.V.M.A. 184:42, 1984.
A retrospective study of seven diabetic cats with associated polyneuropathy incorporating clinical signs, electrophysiologic studies, nerve pathology, and treatment.

Lane, J. R., and deLahunta, A.: Polyneuritis in a cat. J. Am. Anim. Hosp. Assoc. 20:1006, 1984.
A case report including peripheral nerve pathology.

Lewis, D. D.: Fibrotic myopathy of the semitendinosus muscle in a cat. J.A.V.M.A. 193:240, 1988.
A case report with discussion of surgical treatment options and possible etiologies.

Mason, K.: A hereditary disease in Burmese cats manifested as an episodic weakness with head nodding and neck ventroflexion. J. Am. Anim. Hosp. Assoc. 24:147, 1988.
A retrospective study of seven Burmese cats with a suspected autosomal-recessive condition similar to cats with hypokalemic polymyopathy.

McKerrell, R. E., Blakemore, W. F., Heath, M. F., et al.: Primary hyperoxaluria (L-glyceric aciduria) in the cat: A newly recognized inherited disease. Vet. Rec. 125:31, 1989.
A retrospective study of 16 related cats with peripheral neuropathy associated with primary hyperoxaluria, including clinical findings, detailed biochemical investigations, and histopathology.

Norris, A. M., Pallett, L., and Wilcock, B.: Generalized myositis ossificans in a cat. J. Am. Anim. Hosp. Assoc. 16:659, 1980.
A case report with details on pathology and possible etiology.

O'Dair, H. A., Holt, P.E., Pearson, G. R., et al.: Acquired immune-mediated myasthenia gravis in a cat associated with a cystic thymus. J. Small Anim. Pract. 32:198, 1991.
A case report of thymic related feline myasthenia gravis with total resolution of signs following thymectomy and initial corticosteroid therapy.

Poonacha, K. B., Donahue, J. M., and Leonard, W. H.: Clostridial myositis in a cat. Vet. Pathol. 19:217, 1982.
A very brief case report.

Scott-Moncrieff, J. C., Cook, J. R., and Lantz, G. C.: Acquired myasthenia gravis in a cat with thymoma. J.A.V.M.A. 196:1291, 1990.
A case report of thymoma-associated myasthenia gravis in a cat with a discussion of the possible association between the thymus and this disease.
Shores, A., Braund, K. G., and McDonald, R. K.: Chronic relapsing polyneuropathy in a cat. J. Am. Anim. Hosp. Assoc. 23:569, 1987.

A case report of an acquired polyneuropathy with details on sequential neurologic examinations, electrophysiology, and treatment.
Waldron, D., Pettigrew, V., Turk, M., et al.: Progressive ossifying myositis in a cat. J.A.V.M.A. 187:64, 1985.
A case report with descriptions of the clinical presentation, radiographic findings, treatment options, and theories of etiology.

CANINE VENTRAL HORN CELL DISEASES

LINDA C. CORK

Baltimore, MD

Motor neuron diseases compose the group of degenerative disorders that selectively affect the motor neuron without involvement of other neuronal populations (e.g., sensory or cerebellar neurons). Motor neuron diseases are relatively common in humans (Tandan and Bradley, 1985a and 1985b), but reports of motor disease in dogs are rare. To date, motor neuron disease has been reported in Rottweiler pups (Shell et al., 1987) and Brittany spaniels (Cork et al., 1979; Lorenz et al., 1979). This report will use the latter disease, hereditary canine spinal muscular atrophy (HCSMA), to illustrate disturbances in the function of motor neurons and processes that might be involved in other motor neuron diseases.

CLINICAL FEATURES

The first clinical features of motor neuron disease are muscle weakness and atrophy, with an accompanying gait abnormality. Because gait abnormalities may accompany common skeletal disorders such as hip dysplasia, the coexisting neurologic disease may be overlooked and incorrectly attributed to skeletal deformities. In the same fashion, myopathies may cause gait abnormalities, but these can be distinguished from motor neuron disease on the basis of muscle enzyme and biopsy studies and electromyography (see this volume, p. 1042). It is important to note, however, that affected muscles must be examined in these studies.

In Brittany spaniels, the muscle weakness initially involves proximal muscles and progresses in a caudal-to-rostral fashion that leads to a characteristic posture and gait (Fig. 1). Weakness of the hip and thigh muscles reduces the extension of the proximal

limb, so dogs have a crouched stance, and the "top line" is not straight but drops at the rump. Palpation of the muscle mass along the vertebral column and proximal thigh reveals muscle atrophy. The weakness and instability of the pelvic girdle lead to a rolling, waddling gait when dogs are observed from the rear. When observed from the front, the stifle joints "wing out" away from the body. Many dogs take short, jerky steps, with the hindlimbs exhibiting an almost rabbit-like hopping gait in the rear. To distribute the body weight more evenly, dogs typically thrust the body weight forward over the shoulders and place the forelimbs more caudally under the rib cage. As the disease progresses, the neck muscles typically weaken, and the head is carried low; in advanced disease, it dangles in a limp fashion. The tail is paralyzed and droops.

Although the dog may appear active, careful observation will show that it spends a disproportionate amount of time sitting or lying, and activity is brief. Because the disease involves the intercostal muscles, breathing is impaired and may be quite labored; this further decreases stamina and the ability to thermoregulate via panting. Brief periods of activity and excitement have led to temperatures of 108°F in severely affected dogs. The costal rib margins are flared when viewed from above, and the normal tapering to the flank is absent. With time, the muscles of swallowing and mastication are involved and the dog will have difficulty in prehension and deglutition of food. Careful observation of the tip of the tongue may reveal fasciculations. Reflexes may or may not be depressed, depending on the stage of disease.

As the disease progresses, the unequal opposition of the facial musculature leads to a wrinkled brow and quizzical expression. The ears are drawn dor-

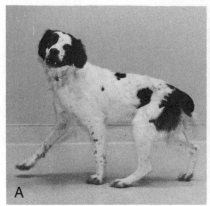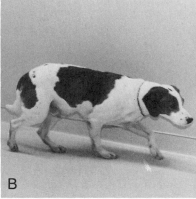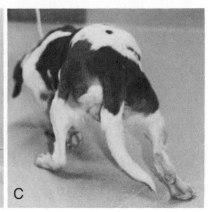

Figure 1. *A,* This 1-year-old Brittany spaniel is in the early stage of motor neuron disease. Neck muscles are still strong, but hindlimbs are weak and the hip and stifle are not well extended. Note the atrophy of the upper hindlimb and pelvic girdle. The dog has a short-stepped, rabbit-like gait in the hindlimbs, and the forelimbs are placed slightly more caudally than normal. *B,* This Brittany beagle shows more advanced disease. Proximal muscles of both forelimbs and hindlimbs are weak and cannot be fully extended, so that the dog has a crouched posture. The intercostal muscles are also atrophied. Note that the forelimbs are placed well back under the body and the head is carried low because of weakness of the neck muscles. The tail is also paralyzed. *C,* In this view of the same Brittany beagle, the instability of the pelvis is demonstrated. The stifle is not held close to the body but moves laterally owing to weakness of the pelvic girdle, giving a broad-based waddling gait.

sally and medially, and the medial canthus of the eye may be widened.

Electromyography of affected muscles reveals positive sharp waves and fibrillations. Nerve conduction is normal. The most definitive diagnostic technique in dogs over 6 months of age is a muscle biopsy of affected muscles in which denervation atrophy without fiber-type grouping is noted. In some cases with slowly progressive disease, a second biopsy several months later is needed to confirm the diagnosis (Tandan and Bradley, 1985b).

INHERITANCE

HCSMA is inherited as an autosomal dominant, and the progression of clinical disease varies with the genotype (Sack et al., 1984). Pups homozygous for the trait develop weakness between 6 to 8 weeks and typically progress to tetraparesis by 3 to 4 months of age. Heterozygous individuals usually appear weak during the first year of life, often during the first 6 months, but weakness may be quite mild. Muscle biopsies of lumbar paraspinous muscles can reveal abnormalities even when clinical weakness is questionable or quite mild. The course of disease in heterozygotes is variable, presumably owing to differences in penetrance. Some cases will progress and become severely incapacitated between 2 and 5 years; others have a chronic form and simply appear languid and may or may not have a low tolerance for exercise. Individuals heterozygous for the dominant trait are probably responsible for maintaining the trait because they transmit the disease to their offspring. When two heterozygous individuals are mated, 25% of their progeny will be

homozygous with rapidly progressive disease. If heterozygous individuals are mated to normal individuals, 50% of their progeny will be heterozygous and may or may not manifest the trait (Sack et al., 1984). Homozygous individuals are so severely affected that they have not been maintained until puberty.

The incidence of HCSMA in the canine population is unknown, but it has been identified in Brittany spaniels, which are widely separated geographically. One of the difficulties of determining the incidence and genetic etiology of late-onset, degenerative diseases like HCSMA is that even breeders of purebred dogs often lose contact with purchasers of puppies after a few months, and thus may be unaware of the incidence of disease within a litter when disease is manifest months or years later. Some breeders may also be resistant to the idea that a disease may have a genetic basis in their breeding stock.

PATHOLOGIC FEATURES

The most dramatic changes in the spinal cord are seen in homozygous pups with accelerated disease. Within the ventral horn of these pups, motor neurons are pale, chromatolytic, and in later stages are undergoing phagocytosis. In addition, there are pale, eosinophilic, axonal swellings equal in size or larger than the largest motor neurons. Ultrastructurally, these swollen axons are internodes that are distended by massive accumulations of maloriented neurofilaments. The myelin sheath over many of these distended axonal segments has either become extremely attenuated or has disappeared completely, leaving the distended internode encompassed by astroglial processes. The perikarya and dendrites of some motor neurons also contain increased numbers of neurofilaments (Cork et al., 1982). In dogs heterozygous for HCSMA that have more slowly progressive disease, axonal swellings are not as prominent. Axonal swellings and chromatolytic neurons are present in the spinal cord and motor nuclei of the brainstem. Lesions have not been recognized in the motor cortex.

Morphometric and immunocytochemical studies of dogs with mild, clinical HCSMA revealed that early in the disease ventral horn neurons in the cervical enlargement have not been lost. On the contrary, affected dogs had 26% more neurons in the ventral horn than age-matched controls. However, the ventral horn neurons in HCSMA were smaller than in control dogs, and approximately 5% of putative motor neurons did not express immunoreactivity for choline acetyl transferase, a marker for cholinergic neurons (Cork et al., 1989a).

Morphometric analysis of the ventral roots from homozygous and heterozygous animals with HCSMA complemented these findings. Ventral roots in HCSMA were smaller and more densely packed than in age-matched controls, and there was no evidence early in disease that axons were lost. Comparisons of myelin sheath thickness and axon caliber between the two groups showed that in HCSMA axons did not reach normal caliber (i.e., there was growth arrest). In addition, the reduced circularity of axons and increased thickness of the myelin sheath relative to the diameter of the axon suggested that the axons in heterozygous, adult dogs with HCSMA had not only failed to attain their normal caliber but had undergone atrophy as well. To determine whether these changes primarily affected large (i.e., motor) axons, the axons were ranked by size, and the greatest changes in axon caliber, myelin thickness, and circularity were observed in the largest axons (Cork et al., 1989b). These observations suggest a protracted effect of disease on the caliber of the axon and its neurofilament content.

MECHANISMS OF MOTOR NEURON INJURY

The cytoskeleton appears to be at risk in HCSMA, as well as in other motor neuron diseases, perhaps because the large size of the perikarya of these neurons and the great length of their processes may render them uniquely susceptible to disruptions of the cytoskeleton. Pathologic changes in HCSMA include alterations in the caliber of the axons and in accumulations of neurofilaments, so it is pertinent to consider the role of neurofilaments in normal neurons. Neurofilaments are composed of a triplet of polypeptides that are assembled in the perikarya

and transported constitutively down the axon at a rate of approximately 1 to 2 mm/day. The caliber of the axon is determined by the number of neurofilaments (i.e., large axons have more neurofilaments than small axons) (Hoffman et al., 1984 and 1987). In HCSMA, the rate of transport of neurofilaments is approximately half of normal (Griffin et al., 1982), but this decrease in transport is unlikely to account for the smaller caliber of axons seen in HCSMA. A more likely possibility is that synthesis of neurofilament polypeptides is reduced, but whether this is a primary or secondary phenomenon is not yet clear.

Investigations of the simplest model of motor neuron injury, axotomy, have shown that following axotomy synthesis of neurofilaments and neurotransmitter is reduced, while proteins essential for repair are increased (Hoffman et al., 1985 and 1987). Thus, in HCSMA the decreases in axon size and caliber and in immunoreactivity for the neurotransmitter may represent a response to injury. The nature of the injury is unknown.

During development, the nervous system remodels itself into its final configuration by pruning back excessive neurons that have failed to establish appropriate contacts with their targets (Hamburger and Oppenheim, 1982). The fact that early in disease dogs with HCSMA have more neurons than age-matched controls suggests the possibility that this developmental period of cell death is abnormal. The corollary of this hypothesis would be that appropriate interactions with the motor neuron target (i.e., the neuromuscular junction) do not occur. The result would be survival of excessive numbers of neurons. The factors that control the plasticity of the nervous system during development are poorly understood in mammalian systems, but considerable progress has been made in avian and invertebrate species. As the factors that control these processes are elucidated, it may be possible to identify strategies (e.g., administration of trophic factors) that will restore the function of diseased neurons; at present, there is no therapy for this condition.

References and Suggested Reading

Cork, L. C., Altschuler, R. J., Bruha, P. J., et al.: Changes in neuronal size and neurotransmitter markers in hereditary canine spinal muscular atrophy. Lab. Invest. 61:69, 1989a.

Cork, L. C., Griffin, J. W., Choy, C., et al.: Pathology of motor neurons in accelerated hereditary canine spinal muscular atrophy. Lab. Invest. 46:89, 1982.

Cork, L. C., Griffin, J. W., Munnell, J. F., et al.: Hereditary canine spinal muscular atrophy. J. Neuropathol. Exp. Neurol. 38:209, 1979.

Cork, L. C., Struble, R. G., Gold, B. G., et al.: Changes in the size of motor axons in hereditary canine spinal muscular atrophy. Lab. Invest. 61:333, 1989b.

Griffin, J. W., Cork, L. C., Adams, R. J., et al.: Axonal transport in hereditary canine spinal muscular atrophy (HCSMA). J. Neuropathol. Exp. Neurol. 41:370, 1982.

Hamburger, V., and Oppenheim, R. W.: Naturally occurring neuronal death in vertebrates. Neurosci. Comment. 1:39, 1982.

Hoffman, P. N., Cleveland, D. W., Griffin, J. W., et al.: Neurofilament gene expression: a major determinant of axonal caliber. Proc. Natl. Acad. Sci. USA 84:3472, 1987.

Hoffman, P. N., Griffin, J. W., and Price, D. L.: Control of axonal caliber by neurofilament transport. J. Cell. Biol. 99:705, 1984.

Hoffman, P. N., Thompson, G. W., Griffin, J. W., et al.: Changes in neurofilament transport coincide temporally with alterations in the caliber of axons in regenerating motor fibers. J. Cell. Biol. 101:1332, 1985.

Lorenz, M. D., Cork, L. C., Griffin, J. W., et al.: Hereditary spinal muscular atrophy in Brittany Spaniels: clinical manifestations. J.A.V.M.A. 175:833, 1979.

Sack, Jr., G. H., Cork, L. C., Morris, J. M., et al.: Autosomal dominant inheritance of hereditary canine spinal muscular atrophy. Ann. Neurol. 15:369, 1984.

Shell, L. G., Jortner, B. S., and Lieb, M. S.: Familial lower motor neuron disease in Rottweiler dogs: Neuropathological studies. Vet. Pathol. 24:139, 1987.

Tandan, R., and Bradley, W. G.: Amyotrophic lateral sclerosis: Part I. Clinical features, pathology, and ethical issues in management. Ann. Neurol. 18:271, 1985a.

Tandan, R., and Bradley, W. G.: Amyotrophic lateral sclerosis: Part 2. Etiopathogenesis. Ann. Neurol. 18:419, 1985b.

CANINE INFLAMMATORY POLYNEUROPATHIES

J. F. CUMMINGS

Ithaca, New York

The inflammatory polyneuropathies in dogs include acute idiopathic polyradiculoneuritis, ganglioradiculitis, protozoan polyradiculoneuritis, chronic polyradiculoneuritis, and brachial plexus neuritis. The last two are rarer than the others, and because there is little new to add to their descriptions in *CVT VI*, they are not included. The distinctive clinicopathologic features of the first three disorders are presented in updated form.

ACUTE IDIOPATHIC POLYRADICULONEURITIS

In my experience, acute idiopathic polyradiculoneuritis is the most frequent inflammatory disease of the canine peripheral nervous system, and coonhound paralysis is the most common form of this disorder.

Clinical Findings

As first observed by Kingma and Catcott in 1954, coonhound paralysis is a rapidly progressive paralytic syndrome that develops 7 to 12 days after an encounter with a raccoon. Typically, weakness develops first in the hindlimbs and ascends. The clinician is frequently presented with a paraparetic or quadriparetic coonhound or rural dog bearing telltale scars about the head from a recent battle with a raccoon. Usually paralysis peaks within 10 days of onset. Rapid progression to flaccid quadri-

plegia (i.e., in 3 days) is cause for concern because of attendant weakening of respiration. A severely affected dog is quadriplegic, areflexic in the limbs, and incapable of raising its head or wagging its tail. The voice is lost, and there may be facial weakness. Paralyzed dogs maintain their appetites and are afebrile. While *motor* signs always predominate, dogs often seem to experience discomfort when the limbs are palpated lightly.

Electromyography, when performed 6 or more days after onset, in most cases reveals denervation potentials. Motor nerve conduction studies may reveal mild to marked delays. In some quadriplegic dogs, supramaximal nerve stimulation may fail to evoke a recordable muscle response. Albuminocytologic dissociation has been demonstrated more commonly in cerebrospinal fluid samples taken by lumbar puncture than in samples from the cerebellomedullary cistern.

Pathologic Findings

The pathologic changes in coonhound paralysis usually are most marked in the ventral roots and spinal nerves and decrease distally. Despite variable dorsal root involvement, changes have not been found in sensory nerve biopsies. Changes in ventral roots and spinal nerves consist of leukocytic infiltration of varying intensity and composition, paranodal and segmental demyelination, and wallerian degeneration (Cummings et al., 1982). In acutely fatal coonhound paralysis, leukocytic infiltrates contain neutrophils and mononuclear cells. In cases with longer survival, infiltrates include lymphocytes, mononuclear cells, and macrophages. Ultrastructural studies suggest a role for serum factors in that demyelination is initiated without direct cellular participation. Macrophages found within degenerating myelin sheaths appear to be responding to myelin degeneration rather than causing it. The prevalence of axon degeneration in coonhound paralysis varies. It has been marked in dogs dying acutely with respiratory paralysis and in animals with protracted paralysis and marked muscle atrophy.

Prognosis and Treatment

Although dogs with coonhound paralysis may succumb to respiratory failure or intercurrent disease, recovery is usual. The speed and completeness of recovery vary. A quadriplegic dog with generalized denervation potentials and rapidly developing muscle atrophy is likely to have a prolonged recovery that may be marred by residual weakness. Good nursing care is essential for quadriplegic dogs. They should be maintained on soft bedding (e.g., a water bed) and turned often to prevent decubital ulcers. The limbs should be manipulated to prevent contractures. Water and food have to be presented to quadriplegic animals; in spite of cervical weakness, these dogs will drink and eat if their head and neck are supported.

The cause of coonhound paralysis remains unknown. One severe bout of coonhound paralysis, however, was produced experimentally by injecting a 1 ml dose of pooled raccoon saliva into a Walker hound that had recovered fully from two spontaneous bouts of this paralysis (Holmes et al., 1979). Cuddon (1990) recently demonstrated circulatory antibodies to raccoon saliva in dogs with coonhound paralysis and in recovered dogs, but not in normal controls or dogs with other neurologic diseases. My experiences with dogs with five and six separate bouts of coonhound paralysis indicate that animals that have sustained one episode of coonhound paralysis are at increased risk to redevelop this paralysis on subsequent encounters with raccoons.

On this basis, I advise the owners of recovering dogs to prevent recurrences by keeping their dogs from encounters with raccoons. This avoidance is obviously difficult for working coonhounds. Perhaps, the persistence of circulating antibodies in recovered dogs explains their inclination to redevelop this syndrome (Cuddon, 1990). Coonhound paralysis, like Guillain-Barré syndrome in humans, is suspected to be an immune-mediated disorder. As in this form of idiopathic polyradiculoneuritis in humans, corticosteroid treatment of paralyzed dogs has not proved beneficial. Plasmapheresis, which

has been effective in many patients with Guillain-Barré syndrome, may be equally efficacious when it is applied to cases of coonhound paralysis.

While coonhound paralysis is well recognized by virtue of its unique antecedent, acute idiopathic polyradiculoneuritis also develops in dogs with no access to raccoons and no identified antecedent (Northington et al., 1981; Vandevelde et al., 1981). Since the clinical and pathologic features reported in many of these dogs are very similar to those of coonhound paralysis, the general nursing care provided for these cases should be comparable.

CANINE GANGLIORADICULITIS

This nonsuppurative inflammatory disease of the cranial and spinal ganglia and roots was considered in *CVT X* under the heading of acquired sensory neuropathy in an article by Duncan and Cuddon. Since the initial descriptions (Cummings et al., 1983; Wouda et al., 1983), additional reports of this disorder have appeared (Duncan and Cuddon, 1989; Steiss et al., 1987). The cases of sensory neuronopathy recorded by Braund (1986) also may belong in this category.

Clinical Findings

Adult dogs of both sexes and various breeds present with largely *sensory* deficits that evolve acutely or subacutely. To date, Siberian huskies seem to be overrepresented among affected dogs (Duncan and Cuddon, 1989). Clinical findings have included ataxia, hypermetria, base wide stance, head tilt, depressed or absent tendon reflexes, impaired proprioceptive positioning, facial hypalgesia, difficulty in grasping food, dysphagia, and masticatory muscle atrophy. Impairments increase in both number and severity with time. Near the onset, the patellar reflex may be depressed unilaterally, but soon thereafter, there may be bilateral reflex loss. Other findings in affected dogs have included megaesophagus, dysphonia, and unilateral Horner's syndrome. Self-inflicted injuries seen in some dogs are thought to be in response to dysesthesias. Cerebrospinal fluid findings have ranged from normal to increases in both cells and protein. Electrodiagnostic findings have also varied. Electromyography has demonstrated scattered denervation potentials in some, but not all, dogs. Similarly, motor nerve conduction delays have been recorded but have not been a consistent finding. Sensory nerve conduction delay was demonstrated in one of two dogs tested. Examination of sensory nerve biopsy specimens in two dogs has revealed axon degeneration.

Pathologic Findings

On gross inspection, the dorsal roots in some cases have appeared discolored. Microscopic studies have consistently demonstrated that nonsuppurative inflammatory changes concentrate in the spinal ganglia, dorsal roots, and the ganglia and fascicles of the cranial nerves. The ventral or motor roots are spared or mildly affected. In some dogs inflammatory infiltrates have been found also in sympathetic and myenteric ganglia. In the sensory ganglia, infiltrates of nongranular leukocytes have formed perineuronal, perivascular, and diffuse arrays. In all cases these inflammatory changes have been attended by substantial degeneration of neurons. The loss of ganglionic neurons results in wallerian degeneration in both sensory and mixed nerves. Centrally, ganglioradiculitis produces axonal degeneration in the spinal and bulbar projections of the primary sensory neurons, i.e., the dorsal funiculus of the spinal cord, the spinal tract of the trigeminal nerve, and the solitary tract.

Electron microscopic studies of inflamed ganglia reveal that perineuronal lymphocytes and macrophages abut satellite cells and displace these encapsulating cells from the surface of the neuronal cell bodies. These images of leukocytes displacing the satellite cells are reminiscent of those depicting cellular stripping of the myelin sheath in experimental allergic neuritis. The changes in this ganglioradiculoneuritis, however, are not so benign in that they eventuate in neuronal destruction rather than myelin loss around intact axons.

Etiologic and Therapeutic Considerations

The cause of this neuronitis is unknown. No consistent antecedent has been identified. In humans, similar ganglioradiculitis occurs together with central inflammatory changes in association with carcinoma, usually of the lung. Demonstration in some human patients of an antibody that crossreacts with the tumor and neuron nucleoprotein suggests that this paraneoplastic syndrome has an immunopathogenesis. In our most recent case, ganglioradiculitis occurred together with brainstem inflammatory changes in a 10-year-old male Weimaraner with two neoplasms, a squamous cell carcinoma, and an adrenal adenocarcinoma. Neoplasms, however, have not been a usual finding in dogs with ganglioradiculitis. Attempts to isolate virus from the spinal ganglia of this Weimaraner after corticosteroid treatment were unsuccessful. In humans an acutely developing sensory neuropathy has been reported in patients receiving antibiotic therapy for febrile illnesses. In addition, dorsal root ganglionitis, remarkably similar to the canine variety in its pathologic appearance, has occurred in humans in association with Sjögren's syndrome (Griffin et al., 1990).

Despite indications that canine ganglioradiculitis may have an immunogenic basis, attempts at immunosuppressive therapy with corticosteroids have been unrewarding. In our experience, corticosteroid administration has been associated with accelerated deterioration of the animal's condition. Similarly, the idiopathic forms of ganglioradiculitis in humans have proved to be generally refractory to immunosuppressive therapy.

PROTOZOAN POLYRADICULONEURITIS

Until recently, *Toxoplasma gondii* was considered as the sole cause of protozoan radiculoneuritis in the dog. The recent identification of a "new" protozoan, *Neospora caninum*, has led to the revision of many earlier diagnoses of toxoplasmosis through retrospective immunocytochemical studies (Dubey et al., 1988a) (see this volume, p. 263). Thus, the subject of canine protozoan radiculoneuritis has become more complicated.

Clinical Findings

The classic radiculoneuritic form of toxoplasmosis has been described in pups usually under 3 months of age that became acutely monoparetic or paraparetic, with the limbs fixed in rigid extension. Hindlimb muscles are firm and contracted and undergo atrophy. Patellar and withdrawal reflexes are lost. Pain sensation persists as palpation of the hindlimbs evokes evidence of discomfort. Electromyography reveals denervation potentials in the hindlimb musculature. Delayed motor nerve conduction has been recorded in some pups. After the progressive stage of the infection, the signs stabilize. There is no remission, and muscle wasting becomes more pronounced. Many pups presenting with these findings were assumed to have toxoplasmosis without confirming serologic studies being done. In some cases, however, the diagnosis was confirmed by immunohistochemical demonstration of the organisms in tissues (Suter et al., 1984). Recently, I have seen pups with remarkably similar clinical signs and findings. These were negative for *T. gondii* on serologic testing. Immunohistochemical procedures performed on sections of spinal cord and roots subsequently indicated *N. caninum* infection. Thus, it appears that the clinical manifestations of *Toxoplasma* and *Neospora* in pups may be indistinguishable.

In addition to the monoparetic or paraparetic form of protozoan disease, I have also observed a fulminating form of protozoan polyradiculoneuritis in an unweaned litter of Labrador retriever puppies.

These pups suddenly developed asymmetric paraparesis, which quickly became symmetric, and within 3 days had evolved into a flaccid quadriplegia with cervical paralysis and dysphagia. Death ensued quickly, presumably caused by respiratory failure. An indirect hemagglutination test for *T. gondii* was negative. In a second affected litter from the same bitch, Dubey and coworkers (1988b) recovered *Neospora* organisms. Tachyzoites grown in cell cultures produced widespread disease when they were inoculated into a control dog. In a subsequent study (Dubey and Lindsay, 1989), injection of a 35-day-pregnant bitch with *Neospora* tachyzoites resulted in transplacental infection of the pups.

Pathologic Findings

In both the paraparetic and the more aggressive quadriplegic forms of protozoan disease, the radiculoneuritic lesions were accompanied by myositis and meningoencephalomyelitis. In the acutely quadriplegic pups, especially, the central nervous system changes were overshadowed by polyradiculoneuritis that was intense and pervasive. Dense leukocytic infiltrates in the roots and nerves consisted largely of lymphocytes, macrophages, and plasma cells. In some infiltrates, neutrophils and eosinophils were abundant. Elongated parasitophorous vacuoles were frequent in some areas. Ultrastructural inspection of these acute lesions revealed large numbers of tachyzoites that differed in several morphologic aspects from those of *T. gondii* (Cummings et al., 1988). Through their invasion and proliferation, the tachyzoites participated directly in inducing degenerative changes in Schwann cells and axons. While many demyelinated axons were distended by maloriented neurofilaments, even greater numbers were undergoing wallerian degeneration. The nature of the lesions in these quadriplegic, unweaned pups appeared histologically indistinguishable from the less extensive changes in the paraparetic form of *Neospora* infection and from the lesions found in confirmed cases of the radiculoneuritic form of toxoplasmosis.

Prophylaxis and Treatment

Unlike *T. gondii*, the life cycle of *N. caninum* is unknown as is its possible public health significance.

Because it poses a hazard as a zoonosis, treatment of toxoplasmosis in animals other than humans has been discouraged. Although treatment with pyrimethamine (0.5 to 1.0 mg/kg, PO, every 24 hr) and sulfadiazine (60 mg/kg, PO, divided every 24 hr) may suppress proliferation of the organisms, in my experience, the radiculoneuritic forms of protozoan infection have evolved rapidly and resulted in unremitting paralysis and contractures. It is this crippling that has compelled owners to request euthanasia for affected pups.

References and Suggested Reading

Braund, K. G.: *Clinical Syndromes in Veterinary Neurology.* Baltimore: Williams & Wilkins, 1986, p. 163.

Cuddon, P. A.: Electrophysiological and immunological evaluation in coonhound paralysis. ACVIM Scientific Proceedings, 1990, p. 1009.

Cummings, J. F., de Lahunta, A., Holmes, D. F., et al.: Coonhound paralysis. Further clinical studies and electron microscopic observations. Acta Neuropathol. (Berlin) 56:167, 1982.

Cummings, J. F., de Lahunta, A., and Mitchell, W. J., Jr.: Ganglioradiculitis in the dog. A clinical, light- and electron-microscopic study. Acta Neuropathol. (Berlin) 60:29, 1983.

Cummings, J. F., de Lahunta, A., Suter, M. M., et al.: Canine protozoan polyradiculoneuritis. Acta Neuropathol. (Berlin) 76:46, 1988.

Dubey, J. P., Carpenter, J. L., Speer, C. A., et al.: Newly recognized fatal protozoan disease of dogs. J.A.V.M.A. 192:1269, 1988a.

Dubey, J. P., Hattel, A. L., Lindsay, D. S., et al.: Neonatal *Neospora caninum* infection in dogs. Isolation of the causative agent and experimental transmission. J.A.V.M.A. 193:1259, 1988b.

Dubey, J. P., and Lindsay, D. S.: Transplacental *Neospora caninum* infection in dogs. Am. J. Vet. Res. 50:1578, 1989.

Duncan, I. D., and Cuddon, P. A.: Sensory neuropathy. *In* Kirk, R. W. (ed.): *Current Veterinary Therapy X.* Philadelphia: W. B. Saunders, 1989, p. 822.

Griffin, J. W., Cornblath, D. R., Alexander, E., et al.: Ataxia sensory neuropathy and dorsal root ganglionitis associated with Sjögren's syndrome. Ann. Neurol. 27:304, 1990.

Holmes, D. F., Schultz, R. D., Cummings, J. F., et al.: Experimental coonhound paralysis: Animal model of Guillain-Barré syndrome. Neurology 29:1186, 1979.

Kingma, F. J., and Catcott, E. J.: A paralytic syndrome in coonhounds. North Am. Vet. 35:115, 1954.

Northington, J. W., Brown, M. J., Farnbach, G. C., et al.: Acute idiopathic polyneuropathy in the dog. J.A.V.M.A. 179:375, 1981.

Steiss, J. E., Pook, H. A., Clark, E. G., et al.: Sensory neuropathy in a dog. J.A.V.M.A. 190:205, 1987.

Suter, M. M., Hauser, B., Palmer, O. G., et al.: Polymyositis polyradiculitis due to toxoplasmosis in the dog: Serology and tissue biopsy as diagnostic acids. Zbl Vet. Med. A 31:792, 1984.

Vandevelde, M., Oettli, P., and Rohr, M.: Polyradikuloneuritis beim Hund. Klinische, histologische und ultrastrukturelle Beobachtungen. Schweiz. Arch. Tierheilk. 123:201, 1981.

Wouda, W., Vandevelde, M., Oettli, P., et al.: Sensory neuronopathy in dogs: A study of four cases. J. Comp. Pathol. 93:437, 1983.

HEREDITARY POLYNEUROPATHY
OF ALASKAN MALAMUTES

LARS MOE

Oslo, Norway

Peripheral neuropathies are usually seen as single cases, but some inherited conditions involving several individuals from the same litter have been described. This report of peripheral polyneuropathy of Alaskan malamutes is based on a study of eight spontaneous cases and four cases produced from a test mating. The first clinical cases were recognized in Norway from 1977 to 1979. They all were offspring from one male dog, and an inherited disease was suspected. Pedigree studies showed that both the father and the four mothers of four affected litters could be traced back to one common ancestor. All the parents were clinically normal. Some of them had produced litters without clinical signs of disease in other combinations. Evidence gathered from pedigree studies and the results of a test mating performed in 1983 strongly suggests that this polyneuropathy is inherited in an autosomal recessive way, but the pathogenetic mechanisms responsible for the changes are unknown.

CLINICAL SIGNS

The condition is characterized by slowly progressive limb weakness that might result in tetraparesis, coughing, dyspnea, and regurgitation. Both sexes can be affected, and the age of onset of signs varies. In some cases, clinical signs can be recognized at 7 months of age, but owners usually recognize the problems between 12 and 18 months. Posterior ataxia, reduced exercise tolerance and hindlimb strength, and difficulties climbing stairs are the first signs. Frequent coughing may in some cases be an additional feature. After short periods of running or walking, the dog may stop and rest, sometimes falling down on its chest. After a few minutes of rest, it can, sometimes with great effort, stand and walk again. Heavy breathing and panting are observed during such activity. There is no clinical improvement after intravenous injection of edrophonium chloride (Tensilon, Roche). Although the disease is slowly progressive, an acute worsening is common. Most dogs develop paraparesis or less often tetraparesis during the course of the disease. Muscle atrophy varies from moderate to severe and is most easily recognized in the muscles of the shoulder and thigh. Reduced muscle strength and hypotonia are typical in all limbs but are always more prominent in the hindlimbs. The patellar, anterior tibial, and panniculus reflexes are bilaterally depressed or absent depending on stage of the disease, whereas proprioceptive function, pedal reflexes, and pain sensation usually are preserved. Chronic regurgitation of a mixture of foamy saliva, mucus, and frequently undigested food may be a serious problem in some cases. A dilated esophagus is a common finding on chest radiographs of dogs given contrast media orally. The peristaltic contractions of the esophagus during swallowing are depressed or absent.

ELECTROPHYSIOLOGY

Spontaneous activity, such as fibrillation potentials and positive sharp waves, is found bilaterally in the proximal and distal skeletal muscles of the forelimbs and hindlimbs. In cases with mild clinical signs, spontaneous activity may be noted only in the interosseous muscles, but such activity is not found before 7 months of age. A moderate reduction in motor nerve conduction velocity (MNCV) of the ulnar nerve is found after 8 months. Affected dogs have an MNCV of 25 to 50 m/sec, whereas clinically normal Alaskan malamutes have values of 55 to 70 m/sec. The MNCV remains reduced even when the clinical condition improves.

PATHOLOGY

Typical necropsy findings are atrophy of skeletal muscles, prominent megaesophagus, and in some dogs marked atrophy of the laryngeal muscles. The changes of the skeletal muscles consist of grouped atrophy and fiber-type grouping, necrotic muscle fibers in severely affected areas, and, particularly in older dogs, an infiltration of fibrous and fatty tissue. Nerve fiber degeneration is found at all levels of peripheral nerves, including spinal roots and intramuscular nerves. Both motor and sensory fibers are affected. A marked loss of affinity for myelin staining is noted in some nerves. Scattered nerve fiber degeneration is demonstrated in white matter of the brainstem and spinal cord. Splitting and fragmentation, particularly of the inner lamellae of myelin sheaths, are common findings in peripheral nerves. Fragments of degenerated myelin frequently accumulate between the axon and the remaining dilated myelin lamellae and also in macrophages and Schwann cells. Swollen axons, with increased amounts of neurofilament and membranous material, are not uncommon, and necrotic axons are occasionally found. There is evidence of remyelination and nerve fiber regeneration.

CONTROL

There is currently no known treatment of peripheral polyneuropathy of Alaskan malamutes. Various forms of medication (e.g., prednisolone, neostigmine, vitamin E, selenium) have been tried without significant effect. The disease as a population problem can, however, be controlled by breeding measures. Since 1980, the Breed Council of the Alaskan Malamute Breed Club has lessened disease occurrence by breeding restrictions and information. Club members were advised to report all suspicious cases to the breed council. Because there is no way to detect heterozygous carriers, known carriers or highly probable carriers were not approved for breeding. Consequently, all affected animals, their parents, and their siblings were rejected. Other dogs with high probabilities of being carriers (e.g., dogs in normal litters in which one of the parents had produced affected dogs in other combinations) were likewise not recommended for breeding. The

rewarding result of this effort is that the last known spontaneous case was diagnosed in 1982.

PROGNOSIS

If an afflicted dog is nursed properly and not euthanatized in the recumbent stage, it will survive and improve after some weeks. During this time, it is important to feed, clean, and handle the paralyzed dog with care to avoid decubitus ulcers and other problems. Several dogs have regained the ability to walk or run short distances. They cannot work or serve as sled dogs but may be acceptable house pets. After several years, deterioration is commonly seen, either as recurrence of severe paresis or as chronic coughing or regurgitation. The majority of dogs that survived the initial paretic state of the disease were later euthanatized because of these problems.

References and Suggested Reading

Cummings, J. F., Cooper, B. J., de Lahunta, A., et al.: Canine inherited hypertrophic neuropathy. Acta Neuropathol. (Berl.) 53:137, 1981.
A histopathologic description of 10 Tibetan Mastiff pups with a demyelinating neuropathy.
Moe, L., Bjerkås, I., Nóstvold, S. O., et al.: Hereditær polyneuropathi hos Alaskan malamute. Proceedings of 14th Nordic Veterinary Congress, 1982, p. 172.
Moe, L., and Bjerkås, I.: Hereditary Polyneuropathy in the Alaskan Malamute. Proceedings of 3rd Annual Symposium of the European Society of Veterinary Neurology, 1989, p. 28.
Northington, J. W., Brown, M. J., Farnbach, G. C., et al.: Acute idiopathic polyneuropathy in the dog. J.A.V.M.A. 179:375, 1981.
A retrospective study of clinical signs, electrophysiologic, and pathologic findings in 10 dogs (including one Alaskan malamute) with peripheral nerve disorder.

CANINE MYASTHENIA GRAVIS

G. DIANE SHELTON
La Jolla, California

Myasthenia gravis (MG) is a disorder of neuromuscular transmission characterized by muscular weakness and excessive fatigability (Lindstrom et al., 1988). Transmission failure at the neuromuscular junction (NMJ) results from structural or functional abnormalities of nicotinic acetylcholine receptors (AChRs) in the congenital form of MG and from autoantibody-mediated destruction of AChRs and postsynaptic membranes in the acquired form of MG. While congenital MG is rare, acquired MG is being recognized with increasing frequency and has

recently been shown to take on many varied clinical presentations.

ROLE OF ACETYLCHOLINE RECEPTORS IN NEUROMUSCULAR TRANSMISSION

In order to fully understand MG, it is necessary to understand the basic features of neuromuscular transmission and the function of AChRs. When an action potential reaches the nerve terminal of the

NMJ, a decrease in membrane potential leads to transient opening of presynaptic Ca^{++} channels. Ca^{++} flux into the nerve terminal stimulates the release of acetylcholine (ACh), which binds to AChRs on the postsynaptic membrane. AChRs are cation channels, permeable to Na^+ and K^+ that transiently open as a result of ACh binding. The net flux of Na^+ into the muscle fiber results in a wave of depolarization (muscle action potential) that spreads in all directions along the muscle fiber sarcolemma, resulting ultimately in muscle contraction. In MG, insufficient AChRs are available for activation, a muscle action potential cannot be triggered, and contraction does not occur. Transmission failure may be immediately evident or occur following successive nerve firings as the number of readily releasable ACh quanta decreases and remaining AChRs become desensitized.

CONGENITAL MYASTHENIA GRAVIS

A congenital familial form of MG, inherited as an autosomal-recessive trait, has been described in Jack Russell terriers (Palmer and Goodyear, 1978), springer spaniels (Johnson et al., 1975), and smooth fox terriers (Miller et al., 1983). Clinical signs become evident at about 6 to 8 weeks of age. Generalized muscle weakness has been described with the variable presence of megaesophagus. Failure of neuromuscular transmission has been demonstrated to be the result of a deficiency in muscle AChR content in the absence of autoantibodies to AChR. A presumptive diagnosis can be made by the demonstration of increased muscle strength in response to an intravenous dose of the short-acting anticholinesterase drug edrophonium chloride (Tensilon, Roche Laboratories) at a dosage of 0.1 to 0.2 mg/kg, a decremental response of the compound muscle action potential upon repetitive nerve stimulation, and a negative serum AChR antibody titer. The definitive diagnosis is made by the demonstration of a quantitative decrease in muscle AChR content. Anticholinesterase drugs are the cornerstone of treatment for congenital MG (see discussion on treatment of acquired MG).

ACQUIRED MYASTHENIA GRAVIS

Classically described as an exercise-related muscle weakness that progressively worsens with exercise and improves with rest, it is now evident that there is a spectrum of clinical presentations in MG in which weakness may be restricted to specific muscle groups in its mildest form (esophagus, pharyngeal or laryngeal muscles, ocular muscles) to a marked generalized weakness that may mimic botulism in its most severe form. For a discussion of

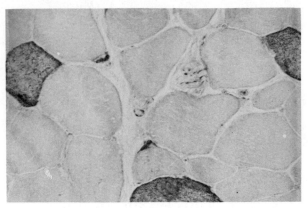

Figure 1. Immunocytochemical detection of immunoglobulin binding to neuromuscular junctions and myofibers. Dilutions of patient's serum are incubated with control cryostat sections of canine muscle. Subsequently, the sections are incubated with the immunoreagent staphylococcal protein A-horseradish peroxidase (SPA-HRPO) and stained for peroxidase. Alternatively, patient's muscle biopsy sections may be directly incubated with SPA-HRPO for *in situ* localization of immune complexes within the biopsy specimen. (Courtesy of Dr. G. H. Cardinet, III.)

the diagnosis and management of the focal forms of MG, see this volume, page 580.

Diagnosis

Myasthenia gravis should be considered in all cases of adult onset megaesophagus and generalized muscle weakness. A presumptive diagnosis of acquired MG may be made by the demonstration of increased muscle strength following the administration of intravenous edrophonium chloride (0.1 to 0.2 mg/kg) or the demonstration of a decremental response of the compound muscle action potential by repetitive nerve stimulation that partially or completely reverses following intravenous edrophonium chloride. Problems, however, are associated with both of these procedures. With edrophonium chloride, a positive response is not necessarily specific for MG. Some dogs with MG may not show an increase in strength, while dogs with other neuromuscular disorders may be somewhat responsive. In cases of focal MG, weakness associated with specific muscle groups (i.e., esophageal or pharyngeal weakness) may not be amenable to subjective evaluation. Problems associated with repetitive nerve stimulation testing include availability to the practitioner, variability in testing methods that could result in a false-positive evaluation, and potential risks associated with anesthesia required for the testing procedure.

Immunocytochemical tests that provide a presumptive diagnosis of acquired MG and require only a serum sample are available at some institutions (Fig. 1). Using these assays, patient's serum is incubated with cryostat sections of normal dog muscle. Antibodies in the patient's serum that bind to end-plates within the muscle section are detected with either an enzyme- or fluorescence-linked secondary reagent. This method, while providing an adequate screening test for antibodies against end-plate proteins, is not specific for AChR and may also detect antibodies against proteins other than AChR present at the NMJ. Though a positive result using these methods should be confirmed with an AChR-specific assay, a negative result is probably reliable. An advantage to this testing method is the concurrent detection of antibodies against other muscle components such as striational proteins, muscle nuclei, and sarcolemma.

The definitive diagnosis of acquired MG is made by quantitating the presence of serum AChR antibodies by radioimmunoassay (RIA) using ^{125}I alpha-bungarotoxin–labeled canine AChR obtained from near-term fetal muscle extracts. This provides a sensitive, AChR-specific assay that demonstrates an antigen-specific autoimmune response. In rare cases, serum AChR antibody titers may be within the normal range. In some of these cases AChR antibodies may be detected in an intercostal muscle biopsy with a decreased AChR content. These cases possibly represent situations in which a low titer of very high affinity antibodies is present. It is important in both the immunocytochemical assay and the RIA that serum samples are collected for evaluation *prior to any corticosteroid treatment.*

Chest radiographs should be performed in all suspected cases of canine MG due to the high incidence of megaesophagus and resulting aspiration pneumonia. Further, the radiograph should also be evaluated for the presence of a cranial mediastinal mass, because MG associated with thymoma is well documented. There are also recent reports of possible paraneoplastic-associated MG in isolated cases of cholangiocellular carcinoma (Krotje et al., 1990), anal sac adenocarcinoma (Shelton, 1989), and in two dogs with osteosarcoma (Moore et al., 1990).

A thorough examination should also be made for other autoimmune and endocrine disorders. In some seropositive dogs with acquired MG, thyroglobulin autoantibodies and concurrent hypothyroidism, Addison's disease, and positive serum antinuclear antibody titers have been demonstrated. Polymyositis may occur in some MG cases, particularly in association with a thymoma.

Treatment

Acquired MG is a treatable disorder and should not always be associated with a poor prognosis. Early diagnosis and proper management of a megaesophagus is essential to a successful outcome. If megaesophagus is radiographically apparent, *do not* perform a barium swallow just for confirmation.

While megaesophagus due to MG has a favorable prognosis in the absence of an aspiration pneumonia, a barium aspiration pneumonia carries a very poor prognosis.

Initial treatment should be supportive and aimed at reducing the risk of possible aspiration pneumonia. As with other cases of megaesophagus, food and water should be elevated when the dog eats, and the animal should remain in a standing position for 5 to 10 min following feeding. In severe cases in which regurgitation and aspiration are still a problem or if pharyngeal dysfunction is also present, a percutaneous gastrostomy tube may be placed for delivery of nutrients, fluids, and medications. Treatment of other concurrent problems should also be initiated.

The cornerstone of therapy for generalized MG is administration of anticholinesterase drugs. These drugs inhibit enzymatic hydrolysis of ACh at the neuromuscular junction, prolonging the interaction of ACh released at the nerve terminus with remaining AChRs and thereby increasing the effective concentration and duration of the effect of ACh in the synaptic cleft. If oral medication can be tolerated, pyridostigmine bromide syrup (Mestinon Syrup, Roche Laboratories) may be initiated at 1 to 3 mg/kg every 8 to 12 hr PO beginning at the low end of the scale with gradual increases. The dose should be adjusted based on duration of increased muscle strength. If megaesophagus is severe and drug delivery is compromised by the oral route, injectable neostigmine (Prostigmin, Roche Laboratories) has been recommended at a dosage of 0.04 mg/kg every 6 hr IM. In the treatment of MG it is important that dosages be titrated to each animal's needs because requirements may vary from day to day in response to activity levels and stress.

Immunosuppressive doses of corticosteroids are recommended in cases that do not respond adequately to anticholinesterase therapy but only in the absence of aspiration pneumonia. Although acquired MG is a true autoimmune disorder, the clinical signs in most cases can be controlled with anticholinesterase drugs, minimizing the necessity for generalized immunosuppression and its side effects. Since a significant proportion of dogs experience spontaneous remission, with AChR antibody titers returning to normal range in a few weeks to months, corticosteroids cannot be recommended for all cases. In addition, in some cases muscle weakness is exacerbated by corticosteroids. Other immunosuppressive drugs, such as azathioprine and cyclophosphamide, have not been fully evaluated in canine MG, but may not be indicated due to the natural course of the disorder.

Problems in Treatment

While a more favorable prognosis can now be given for MG than previously, there are still two critical areas that may result in death of the animal. The first is aspiration pneumonia. Early recognition of megaesophagus, careful management, and *judicious* use of barium studies should considerably reduce these problems. If pharyngeal paralysis is concurrently present, the prognosis must be guarded. Second, establishing and maintaining an optimal dosage of anticholinesterase drugs may be difficult. Worsening muscle weakness and possible death due to paralysis of intercostal muscles can result from underdosing (myasthenic crisis) or overdosing (cholinergic crisis). In a myasthenic crisis, rapid improvement usually follows intravenous administration of edrophonium chloride. In a cholinergic crisis, no change or transient deterioration occurs after administration. Muscarinic side effects (bradycardia, airway obstruction), if present, can be controlled with atropine.

Several drugs have been shown to reduce the safety margin of neuromuscular transmission when given parenterally or in cathartics. These include aminoglycoside antibiotics, antiarrhythmic agents, phenothiazines, methoxyflurane, and magnesium. Such drugs may worsen or unmask pre-existing disorders of neuromuscular transmission and should be used with caution, if at all, in suspected MG cases.

Monitoring the Course of Myasthenia Gravis

A pretreatment serum AChR antibody titer should be determined, and the titer repeated approximately 4 to 6 weeks following an initial positive result. Spontaneous remissions occur in a large percentage of dogs with MG, which necessitates alterations in therapeutic regimens. There is usually a good correlation between the serum AChR antibody titer and the clinical course of the disease in an individual animal. The serum AChR antibody titer will decrease or return to normal range as the animal goes into a clinical remission. The owner should be informed that clinical signs could recur. Medication may be discontinued, however, during periods of remission. Recently, a recurrence of clinical signs and positive AChR antibody titers was documented in two dogs that had been in clinical remission for periods of 1 to 2 years (Shelton, unpublished data).

References and Suggested Reading

Johnson, R. P., Watson, A. D. J., Smith, J., et al.: Myasthenia in Springer Spaniel littermates. J. Small Anim. Pract. 16:641, 1975.
Diagnosis and clinical management of clinical myasthenia gravis in springer spaniels.
Krotje, L. J., Fix, A. S., and Potthoff, A. D.: Acquired myasthenia gravis and cholangiocellular carcinoma in a dog. J.A.V.M.A. 197:488, 1990.
Case report of acquired myasthenia gravis and cholangiocellular carcinoma in a dog.
Lindstrom, J., Shelton, G. D., and Fujii, Y.: Myasthenia gravis. Adv. Immunol. 42:233, 1988.
In-depth review of the pathophysiology, diagnosis, and treatment of myasthenia gravis.
Miller, L. M., Lennon, V. A., Lambert, E. H., et al.: Congenital myasthenia gravis in thirteen smooth fox terriers. J.A.V.M.A. 182:694, 1983.
In-depth study of congenital myasthenia gravis in the smooth fox terrier.
Moore, A. S., Madewell, B. R., Cardinet, G. H., III, et al.: Osteogenic sarcoma and myasthenia gravis in a dog. J.A.V.M.A. 197:226, 1990.
Case presentations and discussion of possible association of neoplasia and myasthenia gravis.
Palmer, A. C., and Goodyear, J. V.: Congenital myasthenia in the Jack Russell terrier. Vet. Rec. 103:433, 1978.
Clinical description of congenital myasthenia gravis in the Jack Russell terrier.
Shelton, G. D.: Disorders of neuromuscular transmission. Semin. Vet. Med. Surg. (Small Anim.) 4:126, 1989.
General overview of acquired and congenital canine myasthenia gravis.

THE X-LINKED MUSCULAR DYSTROPHIES

JOE N. KORNEGAY
Raleigh, North Carolina

The term muscular dystrophy refers collectively to a group of primary myopathies that are inherited and are characterized by progressive degeneration of skeletal muscle. Several distinct forms have been recognized in human beings. These conditions are distinguished by a number of factors, including the pattern of inheritance, distribution of muscular involvement, and pathologic features. Duchenne muscular dystrophy (DMD), the most severe form of the human dystrophies, and its less clinically

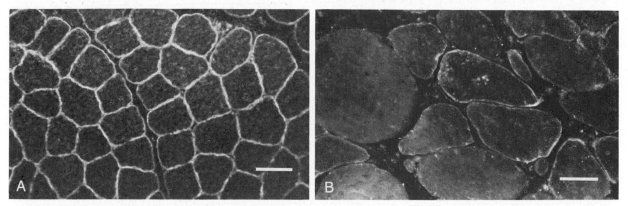

Figure 1. Characteristic subsarcolemmal staining pattern of dystrophin in a normal dog *(A)* and relative absence of staining in a littermate affected with golden retriever muscular dystrophy (GRMD) *(B)*. Several myofibers show focal peripheral staining (in *B*). Marked variation in myofiber size is also noted in the affected dog. *Bar* = 75 μm in *A* and 38 μm in *B*. (Immunofluorescence; C-terminal domain antibody provided by Dr. Zubrzycka-Gaarn.)

severe allele, Becker muscular dystrophy (BMD), have long been known to be inherited through an X-linked mode. Both conditions principally cause clinical disease in males, with females serving as carriers. More recently, analogous X-linked forms of muscular dystrophy have been described in dogs, mice, and cats. These conditions have considerable potential value as animal models and may be encountered in patients of practicing veterinarians.

ETIOLOGY AND PATHOGENESIS

Several theories have been suggested through the years to explain the devastating clinical disease seen in boys with DMD. Much attention focused on potential membranal defects that not only could allow efflux of muscle enzymes such as creatine kinase (CK) (see later section "Diagnosis") but also might lead to influx of deleterious compounds such as calcium. However, although apparent membranal defects, termed delta lesions, were recognized in DMD patients, other investigators suggested that neural and vascular mechanisms might be involved. Proponents of the membranal theory were undoubtedly gratified when DMD patients were recently shown to lack a membrane-associated protein termed dystrophin (Hoffman et al., 1987) (Fig. 1). Simultaneous with the discovery that dystrophin was deficient in DMD patients, its absence was also shown in a genetically homologous murine form of muscular dystrophy referred to as the mdx mouse. X-linked, dystrophin-deficient conditions were subsequently identified in dogs (Cooper et al., 1988b) (Fig. 1) and cats (Carpenter et al., 1989).

The exact function of dystrophin remains somewhat enigmatic. Its subsarcolemmal location suggests a role in maintenance of membranal integrity, presumably through poorly defined interactions with other membrane-associated proteins such as

spectrin and alpha-actinin. Given the fact that DMD patients and animals with X-linked dystrophies have greater myofiber mineralization than most other myopathies (Fig. 2), interest has focused specifically on whether dystrophin is involved in calcium homeostasis.

Presumed X-linked forms of muscular dystrophy were recognized in Irish terriers (Wentink et al., 1972) and golden retrievers (Kornegay et al., 1988) well before dystrophin was identified as the deficient protein in DMD. Although parallels between these conditions and DMD were drawn because both shared an apparent X-linked pattern of inheritance and other clinicopathologic features, definition of true genetic homology was impossible until the DMD defect was defined. Studies in Irish terriers initially suggested that oxidative phosphorylation was defective, and analogies were drawn to the mitochondrial myopathies, as well as DMD. Several golden retrievers with clinical fea-

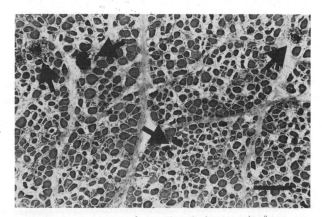

Figure 2. Overview of cranial sartorius muscle from a 7-month-old dog with GRMD. There is marked variation in myofiber size. Myofibers are separated by increased endomysial connective tissue. Scattered myofibers are necrotic, and several are mineralized *(arrows)*. *Bar* = 400 μm. (H & E stain.)

tures similar to those seen in Irish terriers were subsequently described, and deLahunta noted that this condition was analogous to the Irish terrier myopathy (deLahunta, 1977). Two additional affected golden retrievers were subsequently evaluated by the author beginning in 1981 (Kornegay et al., 1988). One of these dogs was later used by Cooper and colleagues to develop a colony of affected dogs at Cornell University. Pedigree analysis showed that the condition was indeed X-linked (Cooper et al., 1988a). Furthermore, dystrophin transcript and protein were absent on Northern and Western blot analysis, respectively (Cooper et al., 1988b). Using progeny from Cornell, a second colony was subsequently established at North Carolina State University, and additional colonies are now being developed at several other sites around the world.

This condition was initially termed golden retriever myopathy (Kornegay, 1984 and 1986) and has more recently been termed canine X-linked muscular dystrophy (CXMD) (Cooper et al., 1988b) and golden retriever muscular dystrophy (GRMD) (Kornegay et al., 1988). Additional, presumably X-linked forms of muscular dystrophy have also been characterized in Samoyeds (Presthus and Nordstoga, 1989), Rottweilers (Cooper, B.J., personal communication, 1990), and Belgian Shepherds (Van-Han, L., personal communication, 1991). Several cats with an apparently similar form of muscular dystrophy have also been described (Hulland, 1970; Vos et al., 1986). An additional two cats that had essentially identical clinical features to those previously described and lacked dystrophin were subsequently reported (Carpenter et al., 1989).

Approximately 65% of DMD patients have deletions in the coding sequence (exonic DNA) of the dystrophin gene. As a result, dystrophin is either not produced or truncated; dysfunctional forms are synthesized. Defects in exonic DNA are not identified in the remaining 35% of DMD patients. Mechanisms responsible for dystrophin deficiency in these patients are not clear. Defects in the DMD gene also lead to Becker muscular dystrophy. Clinical symptoms are less pronounced, presumably because truncated, partially functional dystrophin molecules are produced. A point mutation in exonic DNA has been identified in the mdx mouse. Genomic DNA appears to be intact in both dogs and cats with forms of X-linked muscular dystrophy thus far studied (Cooper et al., 1988b; Carpenter et al., 1989), suggesting that defects in these animals may be analogous to those of the 35% of DMD patients mentioned above. A defect in RNA processing, which leads to skipping of exon 7, has been identified in GRMD (Sharp, N.J.H. et al., unpublished data, 1991).

CLINICAL FINDINGS

Half of the boys with DMD fail to walk until 18 months of age (Gardner-Medwin, 1980). Most develop a characteristic waddling gait by 4 years (Gardner-Medwin, 1980) and experience a relatively rapid decline in motor function beginning at 6 to 7 years of age (Brooke et al., 1989). By this age, the calf muscles are characteristically enlarged due to deposition of connective tissue and fat (pseudohypertrophy). Affected boys are usually confined to wheelchairs by the time they are 12 to 13 years old (Brooke et al., 1989). During this same general period, scoliosis often develops. With improved supportive care, DMD patients now survive longer, but most die before they reach 25 years of age (Brooke et al., 1989; Gardner-Medwin, 1980). Death generally occurs due to pneumonia arising because of respiratory muscle involvement and reduced pulmonary vital capacity. Some patients also die subsequent to cardiomyopathy and cardiac failure (Brooke et al., 1989). BMD patients have a considerably slower course of disease, with a mean age of 11 years at clinical onset, 27 years at inability to walk, and 42 years at death (Gardner-Medwin, 1980). Females carrying either the Duchenne or Becker defect may develop lesser symptoms, depending on the degree to which the normal X chromosome is inactivated. Manifesting DMD carriers typically have enlarged calf muscles and slowly progressive weakness over a period of 5 or more decades (Gardner-Medwin, 1980).

Understanding of the clinical features of GRMD in dogs has been facilitated by colony studies at Cornell and North Carolina State University. The character and rapidity of progression of clinical signs vary. In a colony setting, homozygous females can also be produced by breeding affected males to obligate female carriers. Studies at Cornell have suggested that homozygous females and smaller affected dogs may inexplicably be less severely affected (Valentine et al., 1988a). Affected dogs are stunted compared to normal littermates, perhaps due to negative nitrogen balance that has been demonstrated in DMD patients. In the author's experience, affected pups remain stunted even when supplemented daily by stomach tube. Failure to gain weight could relate directly to malabsorption because of dystrophin deficiency, given the fact that DMD patients may have severe gastrointestinal complications due presumably to smooth muscle dysfunction.

Clinical signs of GRMD other than stunting are noted as early as 6 weeks of age, when simultaneous advancement of the pelvic limbs and partial trismus may be noted (Kornegay et al., 1988; Valentine et al., 1988a). Dogs subsequently develop a progressively more stilted gait, atrophy of particularly the

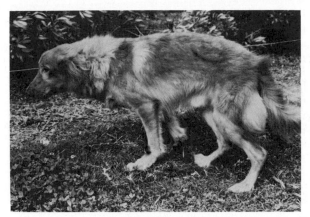

Figure 3. Dog with GRMD at approximately 18 months of age with characteristic kyphosis, plantigrade stance, and temporalis/masticatory muscle atrophy. (Reprinted with permission from Sharp, N.J.H., et al.: The muscular dystrophies. Semin. Vet. Med. Surg. (Small Anim.) 4:133, 1989.)

truncal and temporalis muscles, a plantigrade stance, excessive drooling due apparently to pharyngeal muscle involvement, initial lumbar kyphosis and later lordosis, and exercise intolerance (Fig. 3). Somewhat paradoxically, certain muscles (especially the tongue) appear to hypertrophy. Spinal reflexes are preserved initially but later become hypoactive, apparently due to fibrosis. Clinical signs tend to stabilize after 6 months (Valentine et al., 1989a). Aspiration pneumonia may develop due to pharyngeal or esophageal muscle involvement (Kornegay et al., 1988). Cardiac failure due to cardiomyopathy may also occur terminally (Valentine et al., 1989a). Peritoneopericardial, diaphragmatic hernias may occur, although it is not clear whether this is related to dystrophin deficiency (Valentine et al., 1988b).

Clinical features described in Irish terriers parallel those seen in GRMD (Wentink et al., 1972). No clinical abnormalities were noted during the first 8 weeks of life. Dysphagia and difficulty in walking were seen at 8 and 13 weeks of age, respectively. By 6 months of age, lumbar kyphosis, muscle atrophy and hypertonia, a stilted gait, partial trismus, glossal hypertrophy, soiling of the face with saliva and food, and resistance to dorsal cervical flexion were noted. One of the dogs had a peritoneopericardial, diaphragmatic hernia at necropsy. Samoyeds with a similar condition were evaluated initially at 10 to 12 weeks of age because of drooling, vomiting, and weight loss (Presthus and Nordstoga, 1989). Radiographic and pathologic evidence of megaesophagus was noted in one dog. Other signs were similar to those seen in Irish terriers.

Clinicopathologic features of two cats of unspecified gender with an apparent form of muscular dystrophy were described in 1970 (Hulland, 1970). Marked weakness in these cats resulted in a peculiar gait characterized by "laborious, back-humping",

sternal locomotion. Two additional male cats with muscle disease were later characterized (Vos et al., 1986). Vomiting, believed due to megaesophagus, and a "kangaroo-like" gait were the principal signs in one cat; similar signs were noted in two littermates of unspecified gender. The other cat was presumably unrelated and had nonspecific, slowly progressive gait abnormalities from at least 3 months of age. The cats described in these two studies shared certain clinicopathologic features with two dystrophin-deficient cats (Carpenter et al., 1989), suggesting that they might have the same disease. One of the cats described by Carpenter and colleagues was normal until approximately 21 months, when bilateral symmetrical enlargement of most muscles was noticed. Cervical rigidity, adduction of the hocks, exercise intolerance, and a "falling down technique" to assume lateral recumbency were noted over the next 2 months. Similar signs developed more acutely in the other cat, with a swaggering gait first noted at 6 months of age.

That both the canine and feline X-linked conditions are characterized by progressive clinical dysfunction distinguishes these diseases from the mdx mouse. Affected mice have a period of marked muscle necrosis around 3 weeks of age followed by active regeneration but remain essentially normal clinically. Because of the relative absence of clinical disease, some researchers have questioned the value of the mdx model, particularly with regard to evaluation of potential therapies.

DIAGNOSIS

Clinical signs of the X-linked muscular dystrophies suggest a diagnosis but are nonspecific. Because it occurs in affected individuals of all species, dramatic elevation of serum muscle enzymes, most notably CK, is the most straightforward diagnostic feature. Serum CK values in pups with GRMD are often in excess of 30,000 units/L at 1 to 2 days of age. These values then decrease somewhat but stabilize at a similar level by 6 weeks of age (Valentine, 1988a). Further increases are noted subsequent to exercise in dogs with GRMD or DMD. Serum muscle enzyme levels in these animals tend to decrease somewhat in more chronically affected individuals. Although serum muscle enzymes are also dramatically elevated in the other X-linked canine and feline conditions, data on effects of age and exercise are not available. Serum CK values were not as dramatically elevated in affected Irish terriers (Wentink et al., 1972).

As with other myopathies, serum muscle enzyme levels do not necessarily correlate with disease severity. However, results from the Cornell colony have suggested that more severely affected dogs and pups that die during the neonatal period may have greater serum CK values (Valentine et al., 1988a). Serum CK values also are elevated to a lesser degree in both DMD and GRMD carrier females.

In all canine and feline conditions thus far characterized, there have been dramatic, complex repetitive discharges on electromyographic (EMG) evaluation (Kornegay et al., 1988; Valentine et al., 1989b). Discharges noted in GRMD-affected dogs contain frequency components of up to 2000 Hz on power spectral analysis (Kornegay et al., 1988). Other forms of spontaneous activity, such as fibrillation potentials and positive sharp waves, are not commonly noted but may occur.

Even considering the stereotypic way in which muscle reacts to disease histologically, certain features distinguish the X-linked dystrophies (Kornegay et al., 1988). Grouped muscle fiber necrosis and regeneration with additional and at times dramatic myofiber mineralization (see Fig. 2) characterize all conditions. DMD patients have progressive fibrosis and lipid deposition resulting in characteristic gross muscle pseudohypertrophy. These changes are not as pronounced in the canine and feline conditions. Myofiber hypertrophy has been noted in some muscles of dogs with GRMD (Kornegay et al., 1988) and affected cats (Carpenter et al, 1989). Cardiac changes mirror and, to some extent, exceed those seen in skeletal muscle; fibrosis and lipid infiltration are perhaps more pronounced in GRMD dogs (Valentine et al., 1989b). Dystrophin deficiency but not necessarily absolute absence, demonstrated either immunocytochemically or by Western blot analysis, substantiates the diagnosis of X-linked muscular dystrophy (see Fig. 1). Of the canine and feline conditions thus far characterized, only the GRMD genomic defect has been identified.

TREATMENT

Despite recognition of the basic molecular defect of DMD and subsequent elucidation of appropriate animal models, little progress has been made toward developing effective therapy. Glucocorticoids have provided unexplained and relatively minor benefits (Mendell et al., 1989). Most other therapies, including use of the antioxidant selenium, allopurinol to potentially increase high-energy phosphate compounds, calcium channel blockers such as nifedipine and flunarizine, leucine to potentially promote positive protein balance, and the nerve growth stimulant isaxonine, have had no benefit in DMD. In part because of the ineffectiveness of these therapies, several investigators have pursued transplantation of muscle precursor cells (myoblasts) from normal to dystrophic individuals. Based on evidence that such transplanted myoblasts may actually result

in clinical improvement in a poorly understood neuromuscular disease of mice termed the dy mouse and are capable of producing dystrophin in the mdx mouse, preliminary trials are now being conducted in DMD patients (Law et al., 1990). However, before myoblast transplantation can be offered as a truly plausible therapeutic option for DMD, numerous potential technical problems and limitations must be addressed. Further studies conducted in animal models such as GRMD should be valuable in addressing these concerns, as well as in defining merits of other treatments.

References and Suggested Reading

Brooke, M. H., Fenichel, G. M., Griggs, R. C., et al.: Duchenne muscular dystrophy: Patterns of clinical progression and effects of supportive therapy. Neurology 39:475, 1989.
A review of sequential clinical parameters of almost 300 Duchenne and Becker muscular dystrophy patients.

Carpenter, J. L., Hoffman, E. P., Romanul, F. C. A., et al.: Feline muscular dystrophy with dystrophin deficiency. Am. J. Pathol. 135:909, 1989.
A study defining clinicopathologic features of two cats with dystrophin-deficient muscular dystrophy.

Cooper, B. J., Valentine, B. A., Wilson, S., et al.: Confirmation of X-linked inheritance of canine muscular dystrophy. J. Hered. 79:405, 1988a.
A study defining the X-linked pattern of muscular dystrophy in dogs with X-linked muscular dystrophy.

Cooper, B. J., Winand, N. J., Stedman, H., et al.: The homologue of the Duchenne locus is defective in X-linked muscular dystrophy of dogs. Nature 334:154, 1988b.
A study defining dystrophin deficiency in dogs with X-linked muscular dystrophy.

deLahunta, A.: Veterinary Neuroanatomy and Clinical Neurology. Philadelphia: W. B. Saunders, 1977, p. 84.
A review that notes similarities between progressive forms of muscular dystrophy in Irish terriers and golden retrievers.

Gardner-Medwin, D.: Clinical features and classification of the muscular dystrophies. Brit. Med. Bull. 36:109, 1980.
A review of the classification and clinical features of the human muscular dystrophies.

Hoffman E. P., Brown, R. H., Kunkel, L. M.: Dystrophin: the protein product of the Duchenne muscular dystrophy locus. Cell 51:919, 1987.
A study identifying dystrophin as the deficient protein in both Duchenne muscular dystrophy and the mdx mouse.

Hulland, T. J.: Muscle. In Jubb, K. V. F., and Kennedy P. C. (eds.): Pathology of Domestic Animals. 2nd ed. New York: Academic Press, 1970, p. 474.
A brief review of clinicopathologic features of two cats with a progressive form of muscular dystrophy.

Kornegay, J. N.: Golden retriever myopathy. Proceedings of ACVIM Annual Forum, Washington, D.C., 1984, p. 193.
A review of the clinicopathologic features of two golden retrievers with progressive muscular dystrophy.

Kornegay, J. N.: Golden retriever myopathy. In Kirk, R. W., (ed.): Current Veterinary Therapy IX. Philadelphia: W. B. Saunders, 1986, p. 792.
A review of the clinicopathologic features of golden retrievers with progressive muscular dystrophy.

Kornegay, J. N., Tuler, S. M., Miller, D. M., et al.: Muscular dystrophy in a litter of golden retriever dogs. Muscle Nerve 11:1056, 1988.
A review of the clinicopathologic features of two golden retrievers with muscular dystrophy studied until 27 and 40 months of age.

Law, P. K., Bertorini, T. E., Goodwin, T. G., et al.: Dystrophin production induced by myoblast transfer therapy in Duchenne muscular dystrophy. Lancet 336:114, 1990.
A discussion of preliminary results of myoblast transfer in Duchenne muscular dystrophy.

Mendell, J. R., Moxley, R. T., Griggs, R. C., et al.: Randomized, double-blind six-month trial of prednisone in Duchenne's muscular dystrophy. N. Engl. J. Med. 320:1592, 1989.

A study of the effects of prednisone over a 6-month period on 103 boys with Duchenne muscular dystrophy.

Presthus, J., and Nordstoga, K.: Probable X-linked myopathy in a Samoyed litter. Proceedings of the European Society of Veterinary Neurology, Bern, Switzerland, 1989, p. 52.
A study of the clinicopathologic features of three male Samoyed littermates with a progressive form of apparently X-linked muscular dystrophy.

Valentine, B. A., Cummings, J. F., and Cooper, B. J.: Development of Duchenne-type cardiomyopathy: Morphologic studies in a canine model. Am. J. Pathol. 135:671, 1989a.
A study of cardiac lesions in dogs with X-linked muscular dystrophy.

Valentine, B. A., Kornegay, J. N., and Cooper, B. J.: Clinical electromyographic studies of canine X-linked muscular dystrophy. Am. J. Vet. Res. 50:2145, 1989b.
A review of characteristic electromyographic features noted in golden retrievers with muscular dystrophy.

Valentine, B. A., Cooper, B. J., deLahunta, A., et al.: Canine X-linked muscular dystrophy: An animal model of Duchenne muscular dystrophy: Clinical studies. J. Neurol. Sci. 88:69, 1988a.
A review of the sequential clinical features of dogs with X-linked muscular dystrophy.

Valentine, B. A., Cooper, B. J., Dietze, A. E., et al.: Canine congenital diaphragmatic hernia. J. Vet. Intern. Med. 2:109, 1988b.
A study of a form of congenital diaphragmatic hernia noted in golden retrievers with muscular dystrophy.

Vos, J. H., van der Linde-Sipman, J. S., and Goedegebuure, S. A.: Dystrophy-like myopathy in the cat. J. Comp. Pathol. 96:335, 1986.
A study of two cats with a form of muscular dystrophy similar to that seen in cats with dystrophin deficiency.

Wentink, G. H., van der Linde-Sipman, J. S., Meijer, A. E. F. H., et al.: Myopathy with possible recessive X-linked inheritance in a litter of Irish terriers. Vet. Pathol. 9:328, 1972.
A study of the clinicopathologic features of Irish terriers with a progressive, X-linked form of muscular dystrophy.

Section
13

OPHTHALMOLOGIC DISEASES

THOMAS J. KERN
Consulting Editor

OCULAR THERAPEUTICS

MICHAEL DAVIDSON
Raleigh, NC

Despite the fact that pharmaceutical therapeutic agents are administered for the majority of ocular disease processes in animals, well-designed, controlled clinical studies investigating their efficacy are, unfortunately, almost nonexistent in the veterinary literature. Much of the available information about veterinary ocular therapeutics is therefore derived from studies in nondomestic laboratory animal species, clinical trials in humans, or subjective impressions of experienced clinicians. Although in many cases this extrapolated information proves to be correct, caution should be exercised if these data are used to evaluate the efficacy of a specific ocular therapeutic agent. Differences in drug metabolism, anticipated side effects of the drug, specific ocular pathogens, pathogenic mechanisms of ocular disease, and ocular anatomy in different animal species all must be considered when predicting the outcome of a specific treatment. Additionally, the natural course of a disease process or placebo effect on the owner must be discounted before ascribing a therapeutic effect to a drug.

With the exception of a number of topical antibiotic or corticosteroid preparations, most of the ophthalmic preparations available to veterinarians are products labeled for use by humans. Even in the case of products marketed specifically for veterinary use, the quality and composition of the formulation and bioavailability of the drug often have significant disadvantages. In many instances, the added expense of ophthalmic agents for humans is cost-effective because of a superior therapeutic effect. During the course of treatment, they may prove to be less expensive. Because of the higher quality and the difficulty of veterinary access to some of these drugs, practicing veterinarians are strongly encouraged to establish a working relationship with a licensed pharmacist so they can be obtained.

ROUTE OF ADMINISTRATION

Drugs are generally delivered to ocular tissues by one of three methods: topical administration, injection in periocular tissues, or systemic administration. Topically administered medications are most common and often the most effective means of delivering a drug to the ocular surface and anterior segment. High concentrations of drugs in the ocular surface are generally possible with frequent administration. However, the potential for local or systemic side effects may limit frequency of administration. Deep corneal and intraocular penetration of a topically administered drug is generally limited by its lipid- and water-soluble properties. Drugs (or more specifically, the carrier state of the drug) capable of existing in a biphasic state reach higher levels within the eye. The absence of corneal epithelium usually greatly facilitates passage of a drug through the cornea and into anterior intraocular tissues. Topically applied drugs do not reach adequate therapeutic levels in the posterior ocular segment (ocular tissues posterior to the ciliary body).

Topical ointments, solutions, or suspensions are usually equivalent in efficacy and side effects if administered at appropriate intervals. Most owners find solutions easier to administer to animals. Ointments are often more expensive because of waste (owners have difficulty applying only a small amount). The potential for damage to the cornea and contamination of the container tip during owner administration are also greater with tubes of ointment. Ointments do provide a longer contact time with the eye and thus a longer protective effect from physical irritation as compared with solutions. Because the canine conjunctival sac volume is smaller than the volume of one drop of a solution, more than one drop of a medication is not necessary because it simply spills over the lids onto the face. Administration of multiple drops of different solutions should be spaced over a several-minute interval to prevent drug washout. Vasodilation of the conjunctival and scleral vessels and lacrimation from a painful eye condition may limit the amount of a topically applied medication in contact with the eye.

Subconjunctival administration of medications is generally used in situations in which frequent administration of topical medications is not possible. In theory, frequent topical therapy can achieve as high or higher therapeutic levels than subconjunctival administration for those medications capable of crossing the intact cornea. Subconjunctival therapy is also useful for certain antibiotics, when high, deep corneal stromal or intraocular levels are needed—especially in cases with an intact corneal epithelium. Although some of a subconjunctivally administered drug reaches the ocular tissue by

1049

direct penetration across the sclera, much of the drug is absorbed into the cornea and intraocularly through drug leakage at the needle hole through which it is delivered. Subconjunctivally administered medications have the disadvantage of the inability to discontinue the drug should complications arise. Additionally, the depot forms of corticosteroids often leave a subconjunctival plaque, which may be permanent. Dosages of subconjunctival drugs are usually limited by the volume of the medication (0.15 to 0.25 ml is typically administered to small animals).

Retrobulbar administration of drugs for delivery to the posterior segment is dangerous and *not recommended*. Intraocular injection of a medication is rarely indicated, with the exception of intravitreal injection of gentamicin for cycloablation.

Systemic (oral or parenteral) administration of drugs is necessary when intraocular sepsis or prophylaxis of sepsis is needed, for treatment of eyelid diseases, for moderate to severe inflammatory conditions of the anterior segment, and for treatment of any posterior segment disease process. The main obstacle to penetration of a systemically administered drug into the eye is the blood-ocular barrier, which consists of tight junctions around strategic epithelial and vascular components. Lipid-soluble, non–protein-bound drugs penetrate this barrier most efficiently. Most systemically administered drugs reach adequate intraocular levels during intraocular inflammation (which usually produces disruption of the blood-ocular barrier).

ANTIBIOTICS

Topically administered antibiotics are generally used for treatment of bacterial surface infection of the tissues of the eye (eyelids, conjunctiva, or cornea) or for prophylaxis when the surface integrity of the conjunctiva or cornea is disrupted (e.g., a traumatic corneal ulcer). When treating a surface bacterial infection of the eye, the initial choice of the antibiotic should be based on cytologic findings from eyelid, conjunctival, or corneal scrapings. The overwhelming majority of bacterial infections of these tissues can be managed with one of a few antibiotics, such as a triple antibiotic preparation or chloramphenicol if gram-positive organisms (usually cocci) are present, or an aminoglycoside (e.g., gentamicin) if gram-negative organisms (usually rods) are present. Only rarely are other antibiotics necessary for antibiotic-resistant bacteria (e.g., tobramycin or fortified cephalosporins). The choice of antibiotic may also be facilitated by bacterial culture and sensitivity test results. However, because much higher levels may be achieved with topical administration when compared with serum levels of systemically administered drugs, the minimum inhib-

itory concentrations or Kirby-Bauer test results usually overestimate the importance of resistance of an ocular infection. As a result, response to therapy, based on cytology, is generally much more helpful as an indication of efficacy. Although resistant strains of bacteria rarely develop, if they do, the progression of the disease is usually quite rapid. Poor response to seemingly appropriate therapy often indicates a misdiagnosis or persistence of an underlying cause of the disorder.

Topical preparations containing tetracycline are generally recommended for cats with conjunctivitis because the drug is effective against *Chlamydia* and *Mycoplasma*, two common feline pathogens, and as prophylaxis in cats with feline herpesvirus (FHV) conjunctivitis. Medication is usually applied four to six times daily, and therapy markedly shortens the course of chlamydial or mycoplasmal conjunctivitis.

All topically administered antibiotics have some degree of cytotoxicity to corneal epithelium; therefore, the frequency of administration should be decreased and discontinued commensurate with response to therapy. For prophylaxis of corneal or conjunctival injury, medication given three to four times daily is generally adequate. Deep, progressive, or necrotic corneal infection may require application as often as every hour. Most topically applied antibiotics only reach low levels in the deep corneal stroma and intraocular tissues when the corneal epithelium is intact. Removal or debridement of epithelium from a deep or progressive healing corneal ulcer greatly facilitates antibiotic penetration of the stroma. Fortified topical solutions may be formulated by adding antibiotics to artificial tear preparations. These are generally reserved for serious or progressive corneal ulcers, when perforation of the eye is possible. Topical hypersensitivity to aminoglycosides (particularly neomycin) is well documented and probably occurs more frequently than generally recognized. Progression or worsening of conjunctival inflammation despite topical aminoglycoside therapy should alert the clinician to the possibility of this condition.

Systemic antibiotics have no role in treating conjunctival or corneal infections because only very low levels reach the tear film. Intraocular administration of antibiotics is dangerous and is used only in very low levels when intraocular infection is confirmed and loss of the globe is imminent (see *CVT IX*, p. 684, for a complete listing of commonly used topical and subconjunctivally administered antibiotics, antibiotic spectra, and susceptibility of common ocular pathogens to antibiotics).

ANTIVIRAL AGENTS

Several topical antiviral agents are available commercially, because they are commonly used to treat

Table 1. *Commonly Used Topical Antiviral Agents*

Agent	Trade Name	Preparation	Mechanism of Action
Idoxuridine	Herplex (Allergan)	0.1% solution	Inhibits thymidine incorporation into viral DNA (pyrimidine analogue)
	Stoxil (Smith Kline & French)	0.1% solution	
Vidarabine (adeninine arabinoside)	Vira-A (Parke-Davis)	3% ointment	Inhibits viral DNA polymerase
Trifluridine	Viroptic (Burroughs Wellcome)	1% solution	Nucleoside analogue, subsequently inhibits messenger RNA

herpes simplex keratitis in humans. The only common indication for use of an antiviral agent in veterinary ophthalmology is feline herpetic keratoconjunctivitis. Topical antivirals generally are not used for cats with only herpetic conjunctivitis but are reserved for cats with active corneal lesions. Of the available antiviral agents (Table 1), trifluridine has been shown to have the greatest *in vitro* activity against FHV type 1 (FHV-1). Topical administration of the solution every 2 to 3 hr for the first 24 to 48 hr, followed by four to five times daily, is generally necessary for cats with active epithelial or stromal keratitis caused by FHV-1. Idoxuridine represents an effective alternative to trifluridine and is sometimes preferred because of the high cost and occasional difficulty obtaining trifluridine. Administration of idoxuridine solution (0.1%) five to six times daily is recommended. Antiviral agents have a moderate host cellular toxicity and delay corneal wound healing. Therefore, the clinician should decrease frequency of administration on improvement of clinical signs and avoid prolonged (several weeks) duration of therapy. Acyclovir, an antiviral agent commonly used in humans, has only limited *in vitro* activity against FHV-1 and appears to be a poor choice for antiviral therapy in cats with herpetic lesions. Topically applied corticosteroids should be used with great caution in cats with nonulcerative herpetic stromal keratitis. However, they have been advocated in some instances when an immune-mediated component to FHV-1 keratitis is suspected. Concurrent antiviral therapy and referral of the case to a veterinary ophthalmologist are recommended under these circumstances.

ANTIFUNGAL AGENTS

Fungal infections of the cornea and conjunctiva are rarely encountered in small animals. Although several antifungal agents are available for use with fungal keratitis (Table 2), only two agents are widely available, natamycin (Natacyn, Alcon) and miconazole (Monistat IV, Janssen). Other topically applied antifungal medications offer little or no advantages over these two agents. Natamycin has a wider fungal spectrum when compared with miconazole (which occasionally is ineffective against *Fusarium*, a common equine fungal keratitis pathogen). Miconazole has the advantage of superior drug penetration and is therefore preferred for keratitis with deep corneal involvement. Both drugs should be used frequently (every 1 to 2 hr) for the first 24 hr of therapy, then decreased in frequency to four to five times daily as the case responds. Prolonged therapy (3 to 4 weeks following cessation of clinical signs and demonstration of fungal elements in cytologic specimens) is generally recommended for horses with fungal keratitis, as well as for small animals. Concurrent topical antibiotic therapy (three to four times daily) is recommended for prophylaxis. Small animal patients with concurrent ocular involvement of systemic mycosis require systemic antifungal therapy. If anterior uveal inflammation is present, judicious use of topical corticosteroids is recommended.

ANTIRICKETTSIAL AGENTS

Rickettsia rickettsii (causative agent of Rocky Mountain spotted fever), *Ehrlichia canis*, and *Ehrlichia platys* all may be associated with intraocular inflammatory lesions such as anterior uveitis, retinal vasculitis, and chorioretinitis. Systemically administered tetracycline hydrochloride (15 mg/kg t.i.d. for 14 days) is the currently recommended therapy for both of these diseases. Both agents also show sensitivity to systemically administered chloramphenicol, and dogs with *R. rickettsii* infection have recently been shown to respond to standard dosages of enrofloxacin (Baytril, Haver Lockart). Topically administered corticosteroids (1% prednisolone acetate [Econopred Plus 1%, Alcon] three to six times daily, depending on severity of lesions) is indicated for animals with anterior uveal inflammation due to rickettsial agents.

ANTIPROTOZOAL AGENTS

Toxoplasma gondii infection causes ocular anterior and posterior segment inflammatory lesions in both dogs and cats. Orally administered clindamycin

Table 2. Properties of Commonly Used Antifungal Agents

Drug	Classification	Available Form	Recommended Topical Concentration	Spectrum	Comments
Amphotericin B	Polyene antibiotic	Fungizone, desiccated for intravenous use with sodium deoxycholate	2–5 mg/ml	Broad spectrum against filamentous fungi and *Candida*, variable sensitivity among *Fusarium*	Topical irritation and pain Poor corneal and aqueous penetration Subconjunctival use not recommended because of pain
Miconazole	Imidazole	Monistat, 10 mg/ml for intravenous use	10 mg/ml	Broad spectrum against yeast, filamentous fungi, and dermatophytes	Good corneal and aqueous penetration 5 mg for subconjunctival use
Natamycin	Polyene antibiotic	Natacyn, 5% ophthalmic suspension	5% suspension	Similar to amphotericin B. More effective against *Fusarium*	Limited cornea and aqueous penetration with subconjunctival use
Flucytosine	Pyrimidine	Ancobon, 250- and 500-mg capsules	1% solution	*Candida, Cryptococcus.* Some strains of *Aspergillus* and *Penicillium*	Ineffective against many filamentous fungi
Clotrimazole	Imidazole	Investigational compound	1% solution in peanut oil	*Candida, Fusarium, Aspergillus*	Not widely available Available solution, cream, or lotion not for ophthalmic use
Ketoconazole	Imidazole	Nizoral 200 mg tablets	2% solution	Broad spectrum	Systemic and topical use reported in humans
Silver sulfadiazine		Silvadene topical cream	1% cream	Broad spectrum	Early clinical trials in humans indicate low toxicity potential

hydrochloride (12.5 mg/kg b.i.d. for 21 days) (Antirobe, Upjohn) may be effective in ameliorating the lesions associated with ocular toxoplasmosis, although no clinical trials have been performed in domestic animals. This antibiotic has been shown to be effective in the treatment of ocular toxoplasmosis in clinical trials in humans. It also reduces the number of replicating organisms in ocular tissues in rabbits with experimental infection. Trimethoprim-sulfa (Tribrissen, Pitman Moore) (30 mg/ kg b.i.d.) is also widely used in the treatment of systemic toxoplasmosis in cats but has not been specifically investigated for its effect on ocular lesions. The most common clinical manifestation of ocular toxoplasmosis in cats is anterior uveitis, which may be the result of a hypersensitivity reaction, not due to the presence of the organism. Topical prednisolone acetate is therefore indicated in cats with suspected toxoplasmosis with anterior uveitis.

ANTI-INFLAMMATORY AGENTS

Nonsteroidal Anti-Inflammatory Drugs

Prostaglandins are mediators of certain types of intraocular inflammation and may induce disruption of the blood-ocular barrier, increased vascular permeability within the eye, leukocytosis, and changes in intraocular pressure. They also are as-sociated with intraoperative miosis during intraocular surgical procedures by mechanisms independent of cholinergic stimulation of the iris sphincter muscle. Because of these properties, systemic and topical nonsteroidal anti-inflammatory drugs (NSAIDs) often have beneficial effects on intraocular inflammation (Krohne and Vestre, 1989). They are most useful for mild intraocular inflammation when systemic corticosteroid therapy is considered unnecessary or when topical or systemic corticosteroid therapy is contraindicated or undesirable (e.g., in diabetic patients).

The recommended dosage of buffered aspirin (in dogs only) for treatment of mild uveitis or before cataract surgery is 20 mg/kg b.i.d. Flunixin meglumine (Banamine, Schering) is also helpful in the treatment of intraocular inflammation, especially as prophylaxis before intraocular surgery. The routine dosage in dogs before surgery (if no contraindications exists, e.g., pre-existing renal insufficiency) is a one-time dose of 0.5 mg/kg IV. Phenylbutazone is not recommended for use in small animals.

Two topical NSAIDs are available (0.03% flurbiprofen sodium [Ocufen, Allergan] and 1% suprofen [Profenal, Alcon]); these are most useful before cataract surgery to prevent miosis and disruption of the blood-aqueous barrier. Topical NSAIDs and topical corticosteroids have been shown to have a synergistic, though not additive effect on suppressing intraocular inflammation. Topical NSAIDs are occasionally also helpful in moderate to severe cases of anterior uveitis, in conjunction with topical or systemic steroid therapy. Topical NSAIDs are contraindicated in the presence of a septic corneal ulcer, because in experimental animals with bacterial corneal ulceration they cause potentiation of stromal necrosis and melting. They also have been shown to have some detrimental effect on corneal wound healing, although not to the same degree as topical corticosteroids.

Corticosteroids

Systemic corticosteroid therapy is often beneficial for the treatment of anterior and posterior segment inflammatory conditions not caused by an infectious disease. I generally reserve the use of systemic corticosteroids for moderate to severe intraocular inflammatory disease or for inflammatory scleral diseases that have been unresponsive to topical therapy (see *CVT X*, p. 54, for discussion of appropriate dose and systemic side effects of corticosteroids).

Topical corticosteroid therapy is indicated for the treatment of eyelid, conjunctival, scleral, corneal, and anterior uveal inflammatory diseases that are nonseptic. The detrimental effects on corneal wound healing, inhibition of normal tear film immune responses, and activation of collagenase enzymes contraindicated topical corticosteroid therapy in the presence of corneal ulceration. The integrity of the corneal epithelium should always be determined by the fluorescein dye test before topical corticosteroid use.

Topical corticosteroids used as infrequently as four times daily have been shown to be associated with signs of adrenocortical dysfunction, including alterations in adrenocorticotropic hormone response tests and hepatic glycogen accumulation. In general, the least potent corticosteroid that is effective should be used for surface ocular inflammation.

For treatment of anterior uveal inflammation, the efficacy of a topical corticosteroid is dependent not only on the relative potency of the drug but also on its bioavailability, including intraocular penetration properties inherent to the drug and drug carrier. Compounds that are formulated in an acetate or alcohol carrier usually penetrate the intact corneal epithelium, the major physical barrier to drug penetration into the eye (Table 3). Because it penetrates well, 1% prednisolone acetate (Econopred Plus, Alcon) is the topical corticosteroid preferred by most ophthalmologists for treatment of intraocular inflammation. One per cent dexamethasone solutions or ointments are also efficacious and widely used.

ANTIBIOTIC/CORTICOSTEROID COMBINATION PRODUCTS

Combination topical products with antibiotics and corticosteroids (Wyman, 1986) are the most widely misused and overprescribed medications in veterinary ophthalmology. Ocular conditions that are septic or have the potential to be septic (e.g., a traumatic corneal ulcer) require topical antibiotic therapy. Ocular conditions that are inflammatory

Table 3. Ophthalmic Corticosteroid Preparations*

Generic Name	Trade Name	Manufacturer	Strength (%)
Hydrocortisone			
acetate	Hydrocortone Acetate	Merck Sharp & Dohme	2.5
acetate	Hydrocortone Acetate	Merck Sharp & Dohme	1.5
	Optef drops	Upjohn	0.2
Prednisolone			
acetate	Pred Mild/Pred Forte	Allergan	0.12/1.0
acetate	Econopred/Econopred Plus	Alcon	0.125/1.0
acetate	Ak-Tate	Akorn	1.0
sodium phosphate	Inflamase, Inflamase Forte	Iolab	0.12/1.0
sodium phosphate	B-H(TM) Prednisolone	Barnes-Hind	0.125/1.0
sodium phosphate	Ak-Pred	Akorn	0.125/1.0
phosphate	Hydeltrasol	Merck Sharp & Dohme	0.5
phosphate	Metreton	Schering	0.5
phosphate	Hydeltrasol	Merck Sharp & Dohme	0.25
Dexamethasone			
phosphate	Decadron	Merck Sharp & Dohme	0.1
phosphate	Decadron	Merck Sharp & Dohme	0.05
suspension	Maxidex	Alcon	0.1
Progesterone-like compounds			
Medrysone	HMS Liquafilm	Allergan	1.0
Fluorometholone	FML S.O.P.	Allergan	0.1/0.25

*Copyright © Physicians' Desk Reference for Ophthalmology, 1991 Edition. Published by Medical Economics Co. Inc., Oradell, NJ 07649. Reprinted with permission.

and nonseptic or have little potential to become septic should be treated with a topical corticosteroid. In few ocular conditions are both an antibiotic and corticosteroid concurrently indicated (e.g., allergic conjunctivitis with secondary bacterial infection). Topical antibiotic therapy should be based on cytologic or microbiologic findings from eyelid, conjunctival, or corneal specimens. Unnecessary use of a topical antibiotic may alter the normal bacterial flora and establish a milieu for other surface ocular diseases. Topical corticosteroid therapy should not be instituted without first eliminating the possibility of an infectious agent or the presence of corneal ulceration. Indiscriminate use of these combination products in animals with corneal ulceration (even very small ulcers) is a leading cause of ulcer progression, ocular perforation, and loss of the globe and is indefensibly negligent. Likewise, use of these combination products as nonspecific therapy, without an etiologic diagnosis, often results in temporary masking of clinical signs and ultimate progression of the disease process, occasionally with disastrous results. Combination products are widely used because of their widespread availability and their tendency to improve the clinical signs of surface ocular disease that would probably resolve with no therapy.

IMMUNOSUPPRESSIVE AGENTS

Immunosuppressive agents are occasionally useful in the management of refractory inflammatory conditions, such as inflammatory scleral nodules (nodular granulomatous episclerokeratitis [NGE]). Their use should be reserved for cases failing to respond to traditional anti-inflammatory therapy, and the risk:benefit ratio should be carefully considered and discussed with the owner. Azathioprine (Imuran, Burroughs Wellcome; 2 mg/kg/day, but taper the dose on response) has been the most widely used immunosuppressive agent with refractory NGE. Periodic monitoring of complete blood counts is recommended to monitor for leukopenia. Cyclophosphamide (Cytoxan, Mead Johnson, Oncology) is rarely used to treat severe, vision-threatening, recalcitrant anterior uveitis in humans. Its use in humans is controversial, and practicing veterinarians are encouraged to consult with a veterinary ophthalmologist and internist when contemplating its use. Cyclosporin A (CSA) as a topical agent is ineffective for the treatment of intraocular inflammation because of its poor ocular penetration. Low intraocular levels are also obtained with systemic use in normal eyes, but measurable levels can be achieved in inflamed eyes. It may prove useful for select cases of intraocular inflammatory diseases in which corticosteroid therapy is precluded. Potential toxicity precludes its systemic use in veterinary ophthalmology.

OCULAR HYPOTENSIVE AGENTS

Several pharmacologic agents are used in the management of primary glaucoma in dogs and cats. The most effective agents inhibit or lower aqueous humor production rather than reverse the underlying defect in this condition, which is inadequate aqueous humor drainage. Therefore, long-term medical management is often unsuccessful (Martin and Ward, 1989). These agents are used predominantly for acute glaucoma cases to lower intraocular pressure to acceptable levels. They are also used in conjunction with surgical intervention for long-term management.

Parasympathomimetics

Constriction of the iris sphincter and contraction of the ciliary muscle facilitate conventional outflow of aqueous humor and are the mechanisms of action of the topical agents in this class. The latter mechanism is probably not as important in small animals (when compared with humans) because they have relatively poorly developed smooth ciliary muscle. All miotics should be avoided in cases of secondary glaucoma, when intraocular inflammation already acts to cause miosis and ciliary muscle spasm.

Pilocarpine, a direct-acting, acetycholine-like miotic, is the most widely used. It is generally given every 15 to 20 min during acute congestive glaucoma, and then three times daily after miosis occurs. Although many concentration are available, 1 to 2% concentrations (usually supplied as a combination 1 to 2% pilocarpine and 1% epinephrine [E-Pilo-1, E-Pilo-2, Iolab]) have been shown experimentally to be as effective as higher concentrations, which have a higher likelihood of side effects. Topical application often results in iris and ciliary muscle spasm, so the patient may appear to be in pain. This effect is usually transient and lasts only several days. Persistence of discomfort occasionally necessitates discontinuation of the drug. A 4% pilocarpine gel is available (Pilopine HS Gel, Alcon) and has been shown to effectively lower intraocular pressure in dogs with administration once or twice times daily. The 4% gel is more irritating to many dogs and therefore is not recommended for routine use. Pilocarpine inserts (Ocusert, Alza), placed in the lower conjunctival cul-de-sac once daily, are also available. Because of possible displacement from the conjunctival sac and, therefore, unreliable dosing, their use is not recommended.

Several indirect-acting miotics are available (Wyman, 1986), including physostigmine (0.25) (eserine sulfate, Iolab), demecarium bromide (0.125, 0.25%) (Humorsol, Merck Sharp & Dohme), and echothiophate (0.3, 0.06, 0.125, 0.25%) (Phospholine Iodide, Wyeth-Ayerst). These agents are cholinesterase inhibitors and cause miosis by blocking the action of acetylcholinesterase at the sphincter muscle receptor. As a result, they are often more powerful miotics than pilocarpine, with the advantage of administration frequencies of once every other day to twice daily. However, because of their potency, they are more likely to cause painful miosis and ciliary muscle spasm, and the potential for systemic toxicity is present, particularly with concurrent use of organophosphate flea control products. As a result, they should be used cautiously and only in cases in which topical administration of pilocarpine two to three times daily is undesirable or impossible.

Adrenergics

Topical 1% epinephrine is available alone or in combination with various concentrations of pilocarpine. The specific mechanism of action is poorly defined; however, most of its therapeutic effect is derived from an increased facility of outflow of aqueous humor from the eye. The concentration of epinephrine commonly used to treat glaucoma has no significant mydriatic effect and therefore can effectively be used in combination with miotics. Dipivefrin (Propine, Allergan), a prodrug comprised of two molecules of epinephrine, has superior intraocular penetration and therefore greater therapeutic effect when compared with epinephrine alone. High costs prohibit its routine use. Side effects with the adrenergic agents are extremely rare.

Beta-Blockers

Three beta-adrenergic blocking agents are currently available for treatment of primary glaucoma: timolol maleate (0.25, 0.5%) (Timoptic, Merck Sharp & Dohme), betaxalol (0.25, 0.5%) (Betoptic, Alcon), and levobunolol (0.25, 0.5%) (Betagan, Allergan). They function by lowering aqueous humor production, probably by blocking specific receptors in the ciliary body that facilitate its production. Beta-blockers may be used in conjunction with beta-adrenergic agents in the same patient and have been shown to be synergistic but not additive in humans with primary glaucoma. Both are extremely effective and widely prescribed for treatment of primary open-angle glaucoma in humans. Clinical trials documenting their efficacy in dogs or cats are not available. Subjectively, they appear to lower intraocular pressure in some cases of primary glaucoma in dogs and secondary glaucoma in cats, but

Table 4. Carbonic Anhydrase Inhibitors

Drug	Strength	Recommended Dosage (Dogs)*†
Diclorphenamide (Daranide, Merck Sharp & Dohme)	50 mg tablets	2–4 mg/kg b.i.d.–t.i.d.
Methazolamide (Neptazane, Lederle)	50 mg tablets	4–6 mg/kg b.i.d.–t.i.d.
Ethoxzolamide (Cardrase, Upjohn)	125 mg tablets	4 mg/kg b.i.d.–t.i.d.
Acetazolamide* (Diamox, Lederle)	125, 250, 500 mg; 500 mg/vial (as sodium)	20 mg/kg b.i.d.

*Not recommended for routine use in dogs.
†Dosages should be decreased in proportion to development of signs compatible with metabolic acidosis.

not to the same degree as in humans. This variation probably reflects a species difference in the number and concentration of beta-1 receptors within the eye and different mechanisms for glaucoma in different species. These agents are more expensive than other antiglaucomatous agents. I use them twice daily for cases requiring long-term medical management when miotics are not tolerated or as an additional form of therapy in glaucoma refractory to other forms of medical or surgical therapy.

Carbonic Anhydrase Inhibitors

Carbonic anhydrase (CA) inhibitors lower intraocular pressure by decreasing aqueous humor production by the ciliary epithelia. The mechanism of action at this site may relate either to a direct effect of this enzyme inhibitor on the production of aqueous humor or to a secondary local acidosis that lowers aqueous humor production. Oral CA inhibitors are widely used in the long-term medical management of primary glaucoma in dogs (Table 4). All of the available agents may cause systemic side effects, including vomiting and diarrhea from an irritative effect and clinical findings associated with metabolic acidosis (gastrointestinal effects, lethargy, panting, and exercise intolerance). They also may induce polyuria/polydipsia through their diuretic effect. Methazolamide (4 to 6 mg/kg b.i.d. to t.i.d.) and dichlorphenamide (2 to 4 mg/kg b.i.d. to t.i.d.) appear to have similar clinical efficacy. Both are available in 50-mg tablets, with the choice of product usually based on the size of the animal (smaller dogs are more conveniently dosed with methazolamide). Acetazolamide, although the most readily available CA inhibitor from local pharmacies, appears to be associated with a higher percentage of adverse side effects in dogs, and its use is not recommended. Acetazolamide is the only agent widely available in parenteral form and is sometimes useful as an initial intravenous agent for rapidly lowering intraocular pressure in dogs with acute congestive glaucoma. Topical CA inhibitors to lessen the potential side effects from metabolic acidosis associated with oral medications may become available within the next several years.

Osmotic Agents

Mannitol (0.5 to 1 gm/kg IV) (Mannitol Injection, Astra) and glycerol (1 to 2 mg/kg PO) (Osmoglyn, Alcon) both acutely lower intraocular pressure through an osmotic effect on the aqueous humor and vitreous humor. Glycerol may induce emesis in dogs and may therefore be ineffective; its use is not recommended. Mannitol should be administered intravenously over a 20- to 30-min interval to avoid rapid changes in blood osmolality. Time of onset of action is 20 to 30 min after administration, with peak action being 2 to 3 hr later. Water should be withheld from the animal for 2 to 3 hr after administration. The dose of mannitol may be repeated once or twice after 8 hr, but tachyphylaxis usually develops quickly, and subsequent doses are rarely effective if a poor response to initial administration is noted. Osmotic agents are less effective in animals with disruption of the blood-aqueous barrier (i.e., from anterior uveitis) because of leakage of the drug intraocularly. A rebound effect, with an initial lowering followed by elevation in intraocular pressure after several hours, is occasionally encountered. Mannitol should be used with extreme caution in patients with cardiovascular disease, because volume overload, congestive heart failure or compromise, and pulmonary edema can occur in these patients.

Topical osmotic agents (2 to 5% sodium chloride solution [Adsorbonac, Alcon]) or 5% ointment (Muro 128 [Muro Pharmaceutical, Tewksbury, MA]) are recommended by some clinicians for management of corneal edema resulting from corneal endothelial cell degeneration or dystrophy. I have found topical use of these compounds to be irritating because of their hypertonicity, and the duration of action of corneal edema clearing is quite transient. Definitive therapy of corneal edema by other means is recommended. The osmotic effect of topically applied 50% USP glycerol facilitates intraocular examination (e.g., gonioscopy) when corneal edema precludes visualization, by temporarily clearing corneal edema.

TEAR FILM SUPPLEMENTS AND LACRIMOGENIC AGENTS

Artificial Tear Preparations

A wide variety and number of artificial tear preparations (Wyman, 1986) are available for primary or adjuvant therapy in animals with tear film abnormalities such as keratoconjunctivitis sicca (KCS) or qualitative (mucin-deficient) tear film disorders. Qualitative tear film disorders are best treated with a trilaminar tear film supplement, which mimics the composition of the normal tear film (Tears Naturale, Alcon). Artificial tears are generally composed of methylcellulose, polyvinyl alcohol, or polyvinylpyrrolidone polymers, often with thimerosal or benzalkonium chloride as a preservative. I have no preference for any of these formulations because most appear to have similar clinical efficacy. Animals with low Schirmer's tear test values need frequent administration of artificial tears (up to every 2 hr) to totally supplement or replace their tear film and maintain corneal surface health. This is obviously impractical for most pet owners. Following artificial tear solution with an ophthalmic lubricating ointment (usually containing white petrolatum, mineral oil, and lanolin [Duratears Naturale, Alcon]) prolongs contact time and is recommended when a longer interval between administration of tears is anticipated (e.g., before bedtime). Collyria (eye washes, saline) may be effective to cleanse the characteristic excessive mucus from the eyes of animals with KCS but are not suitable as tear film replacements.

Tear film supplements are also available as inserts (Lacrisert, Merck Sharp & Dohme) that are placed in the conjunctival cul-de-sac and allowed to slowly dissolve during the day. These inserts theoretically could alleviate the necessity for frequent administration of artificial tear preparations. However, they frequently become dislodged by the nictitating membrane in animals. In addition, they are occasionally irritating, are unreliable, and therefore are not recommended.

Hyaluronic Acid

Formulated hyaluronic acid solution of 0.1 to 0.2% has been used as a tear film supplement in humans with tear film disorders. Because of its viscous properties, it theoretically has a longer contact time. Blinded, controlled clinical studies in humans suggest that most patients benefit as much from artificial tear preparations. Concerns of product sterility and appropriate formulation also limit routine use.

Pilocarpine

Use of oral 1 to 2% pilocarpine or 0.25% pilocarpine in formulated topical solutions (see CVT IX, p. 684, concerning Severin's solution formula) as a lacrimogenic agent has virtually been replaced since the advent of topical CSA for KCS. Unpalatability of pilocarpine when placed in the food, occasional side effects (usually gastrointestinal), and unpredictable and variable efficacy currently make this drug a poor choice for use as a lacrimogenic agent.

Acetylcysteine

Tear film supplements formulated with 1% acetylcysteine have been widely advocated and used as a mucolytic agent to dissolve the mucoid discharge in patients with KCS (see *CVT X*, p. 684, concerning Severin's solution). Indeed, this agent appears to effectively reduce the amount of discharge in dogs with KCS, a major concern for owners. Long-term topical administration of acetylcysteine may alter the remaining tear film adversely, however, resulting in a qualitative tear film disorder superimposed on a tear film deficiency. I recommend using acetylcysteine only when excessive mucus production is a major concern and when CSA therapy has been unsuccessful.

Cyclosporin A

Since its advent in 1988, topical use of CSA has revolutionized treatment of idiopathic, breed-related KCS in dogs. Through an incompletely understood mechanism, CSA increases tear production in 70 to 80% of dogs with KCS. It also appears to alleviate associated clinical signs including excessive mucus production, corneal pigmentation, corneal granulation tissue, and corneal vascularization. These effects may be independent of its lacrimogenic properties. Its use has greatly reduced the need for corrective surgery (parotid duct transposition) and the impractical frequent use of artificial tear preparations.

CSA is currently formulated in a 1 or 2% solution, prepared from the oral elixir form of the medication (Sandimmune, Sandoz) and diluted in olive oil or corn oil. Clinical trials have suggested that the 1% concentration is as efficacious as 2%; however, an occasional patient responds to 2% solution after no response to 1% solution. The oral elixir contains 12.5% ethyl alcohol, which is generally removed before formulating. The shelf life of this product is currently not known; it is recommended that it be stored in a light-proof container to prevent oxidation of the carrier. The likelihood of systemic toxicity of CSA appears to be very low in concentrations currently used. However, owners should be aware that this therapy, although widely used, is still in the investigational stages in animals. Local side effects appear to be uncommon and usually are related to topical hypersensitivity to the olive oil carrier. This may require use of another carrier. Because of the necessity of ensuring product steril-

ity and proper formulation, the expense of the oral elixir, and the investigational nature of the product at this time, practicing veterinarians are strongly advised to have the product formulated by a licensed pharmacist. CSA will probably be available in a commercial veterinary form within the next several years.

The currently recommended dosage frequency of CSA is twice daily. Most animals require therapy indefinitely, and KCS usually recurs immediately on cessation of therapy. Initial Schirmer's tear test values less than 2 mm are a possible indicator of poor responsiveness. Duration of KCS before therapy appears not to influence responsiveness. At least 10 weeks of therapy is recommended before assuming a negative response, although onset of CSA's lacrimogenic effect typically takes 1 to 3 weeks. Concurrent supplementation with artificial tears is recommended until a response to therapy is documented (i.e., an improved Schirmer's tear test result). Following a positive response, some animals can be maintained on therapy once daily or once every other day, though most continue to require therapy twice daily. Efficacy of CSA in KCS with etiologies other than breed-related lacrimal degeneration (e.g., neurogenic, traumatic, drug-induced, virus-related) has not been investigated (see this volume, p. 1092).

MYDRIATICS/CYCLOPLEGICS

Mydriatics and cycloplegics are used for diagnostic purposes to evaluate the crystalline lens or ocular posterior segment or to prevent posterior synechiae and iris and ciliary body spasm due to activation of the axonal and oculopupillary reflexes induced by corneal, scleral, or anterior uveal lesions. They have their effect by blocking acetylcholine receptors in the iris sphincter muscle and ciliary body muscle. One per cent tropicamide is the standard diagnostic mydriatic, with an onset of mydriasis in 15 to 25 min and a duration of 4 to 5 hr. One per cent atropine is generally used therapeutically as a mydriatic/cycloplegic. Its onset of action and duration are dependent on the magnitude of the causative ocular reflexes (which generally correlates with the severity of the ocular disease). In a normal eye, mydriasis with atropine typically lasts 4 to 5 days, but residual effects may be seen for 10 to 14 days. Atropine is generally used to effect (i.e., frequently enough to maintain mydriasis. This may vary from once every other day to six to eight times daily). Four per cent atropine is also available for use to disrupt synechia or to counteract profound stimulation of causative ocular reflexes. Frequent administration (six to eight times daily) may be associated with systemic adverse effects, including but not limited to dry mucous membranes, tachycardia,

Table 5. Mydriatics/Cycloplegics†

Drug	Peak (min)†	Duration (days)	Available %
Atropine sulfate 1% (Isopto Atropine, Alcon)	60	4–5	0.5–3
Homatropine 2% (Isopto-Homatropine, Alcon)	40–60	1–3	2–5
Scopolamine 0.25% (Isopto Hyoscine, Alcon)	20–30	4–5	0.25
Cyclopentolate 1% (Ak-Pentolate, Akorn)	30–60	2–3	0.5–2
Tropicamide 1% (Tropicacyl, Akorn)	20–40	4–12 hr	0.5–1

*Reprinted with permission from Rubin, L. F., Wolfes, R.L.: Mydriatics for canine ophthalmoscopy. J.A.V.M.A. 140:137, 1962.

†Times listed are for effects in normal dogs; variation may be noted dependent on pigmentation of irides.

ataxia, and dementia. The potential for toxicity is greatest with higher concentrations and in small dogs or cats. Both of these mydriatics have a slower onset of action and longer duration in animals with darkly pigmented irides, because melanin binding of the drugs occurs in the iris. Systemically administered atropine, at commonly used preanesthetic doses, has little effect on pupillary function.

Several other mydriatic/cycloplegics are commercially available (Table 5), but they offer very few advantages when compared with atropine and are not commonly used in veterinary ophthalmology. Phenylephrine (2.5%, 10%) (Ak-Dilate, Akorn) has mydriatic but no cycloplegic effect through direct stimulation of adrenergic receptors on the iris dilator muscle. It is generally ineffective as a sole mydriatic agent because the sphincter muscle is more powerful than the iris dilator muscle. Phenylephrine is occasionally used in combination with atropine for eyes with posterior synechia or when full mydriasis is necessary (i.e., before intraocular surgery). Cardiac arrhythmias and even cardiac arrest while under anesthesia have been documented in children with topical phenylephrine use before ophthalmic surgery.

TOPICAL ANESTHETICS

Topical anesthetics provide anesthesia to the corneal and conjunctival surface for routine diagnostic or minor surgical procedures. These agents are *contraindicated* for the *treatment* of corneal ulcers or other painful ocular conditions, owing to their ability to inhibit corneal epithelial wound healing and normal blink reflex mechanisms, as well as rapid development of tachyphylaxis with their repeated use. Proparacaine hydrochloride (Ophthaine, Squibb; Ophthetic, Allergan; Alcaine, Al-

con; all in 0.5% solution) is the most widely used preparation, although tetracaine hydrochloride (Bausch and Lomb, 0.5% solution) is also available (Wyman, 1986). The time of onset of action following administration is 15 to 20 sec, with a duration of 15 to 20 min. Repeated applications may be necessary for animals with painful eye conditions and blepharospasm, and the efficacy and duration of action are lessened when conjunctival or scleral vascular injection or excessive lacrimation is present. Local anesthetic action on the conjunctival surface (e.g., before subconjunctival injections) may be facilitated by placing a drop of solution on a cotton swab and applying it to the desired area for 30 sec. Perform a Schirmer's tear test and collect samples for microbiologic isolation before using a topical anesthetic.

Local anesthetics are occasionally injected into the retrobulbar space to fix the globe in a central position for surgical procedures (Wyman, 1986). Retrobulbar anesthetics also help prevent elicitation of the oculocardiac reflex during globe manipulation. Damage to the retrobulbar tissues, particularly the optic nerve, is the primary danger in this use. Although providing no known protective effect against the oculocardiac reflex, neuromuscular blocking agents provide a more reliable and a safe method to paralyze extraocular muscles and manipulate the globe for corneal, conjunctival, and intraocular surgical procedures.

ANTIENZYME AGENTS

Rapid corneal stromal necrosis, lysis, and liquefaction are frequent clinical features of septic corneal ulcers. Degradative enzymes released from the bacteria, necrotic corneal stromal cells, and polymorphonuclear inflammatory cells all contribute to the stromal loss, through dissolution of corneal intercellular ground substances and collagen lamellae during this process. Because of its anticollagenase activity, N-acetylcysteine 10% solution (Mucomyst, Bristol; every 2 to 4 hr topically) is frequently used in the management of melting corneal ulcers. Because zinc is a necessary element for many collagenases activated in septic corneal ulcers, chelators of zinc ions (e.g., disodium ethylenediaminetetraacetic acid and dimethylcysteine [Wyman, 1986]) also have been advocated for use with these ulcers. Additionally, the anticollagenolytic action of homologous fresh serum has led clinicians to use this topically in melting corneal ulceration. Although topical anticollagenolytic therapy appears subjectively to be helpful in select cases and although the use of these agents is widely advocated, controlled clinical studies supporting their efficacy are lacking in both human and veterinary ophthalmology. Frequent debridement of necrotic tissue and, with rapidly progressive ulceration, placement of a conjunctival graft usually are more appropriate therapy for collagenolytic ulcers than use of anticollagenolytic agents alone.

CAUTERANTS

Although several topically applied cautery agents (e.g., trichloroacetic acid crystals, liquid phenol, silver nitrate sticks, or undiluted iodine preparations) have traditionally been used to manage refractory superficial ulcers, their topical use (particularly the first three agents) is unpredictable and dangerous and is not recommended (see this volume, p. 1081, for more appropriate means of therapy).

VITAL STAINS

Two vital stains, sodium fluorescein (NaFl) and rose bengal, are commonly used for diagnostic purposes in veterinary ophthalmology. Individually packaged NaFl-impregnated strips (Fluori-Strip, Wyeth-Ayerst) are recommended, rather than preprepared solutions, because the disastrous potential for bacterial contamination exists with solutions. The end of the strip is moistened and touched to the upper bulbar conjunctival; excess fluorescein is rinsed from the eye with collyrium. Retention of the brilliant green dye on the corneal surface indicates loss of (lipid-soluble) epithelium. NaFl is also retained in areas of corneal epithelial degeneration as a faint, more diffuse granular stain. This staining pattern may be seen after instillation of a topical anesthetic, tonometry, or use of Schirmer's tear test strips, which contact the cornea. Diffuse, granular staining of the corneal epithelium may also indicate a pathologic process that causes corneal epithelial degeneration but not overt ulceration. NaFl also stains the tear film and tear meniscus and can be used to evaluate tear film breakup time. Conjunctival or corneal cytologic specimens for immunofluorescent antibody testing should be collected before fluorescein administration to avoid causing false-positive results.

Ten per cent NaFl solution (Fundescein 10% Injection, Iolab) is used intravenously to evaluate and photograph the ocular posterior segment by a technique termed *fluorescein angiography*. The dose of 10% NaFl is 25 mg/kg for dogs and cats; anaphylaxis is a well-documented though rare complication in humans, and I have observed it in a cat. Therefore, an emergency tray including intravenous epinephrine solution and an endotracheal tube should be readily available.

Rose bengal dye (Rose Bengal 1%, Akorn) stains necrotic tissue, degenerative conjunctival or corneal

cells, and mucus. It is occasionally useful in facilitating an early diagnosis of KCS* with marginal Schirmer's tear test values and is very useful in detecting dendritic lesions associated with FHV-1 corneal infection in cats. Some *in vitro* antiviral effect has been documented, and as a result, samples for viral isolation should be collected from cats with suspected FHV-1 infections before administration.

TISSUE ADHESIVES

Cyanoacrylate glue (Nexaband, CRX Medical) is a tissue adhesive with selected indications for ophthalmic use, including management of select refractory ulceration and temporarily sealing a small corneal or scleral defect until definitive surgical correction can be performed. It is also used when anesthetic concerns make surgery impractical. Healing of the refractory ulcers occurs by migration of corneal epithelium under the applied cyanoacrylate. Cyanoacrylate is not useful or indicated when necrotic corneal tissue is present or in the presence of corneal bacterial infections. It is toxic to intraocular tissues. Application generally requires heavy sedation or anesthesia and immobilization of the eye and lid margins. The affected area is thoroughly dried with a cotton swab, and a small amount of glue is placed in the defect. I use a sterile, wooden-tip applicator. I apply a small amount of glue to the broken end of the stick and gently touch it to the defect. The most common error is use of excessive glue, because only minute amounts are necessary. Excessive amounts lead to early glue separation from the wound and a rough, uncomfortable surface that irritates the lids. The cyanoacrylate is spontaneously sloughed by growth of epithelium under it in several days to several weeks.

CONTACT LENSES AND COLLAGEN SHIELDS AS BANDAGES

Collagen corneal shields (Opti-Cor, Pitman Moore) have recently been marketed for the treatment of corneal ulceration and corneal incisional wounds in dogs. Potential benefits include improved epithelial wound healing and increased comfort for the patient. Some experimental studies indicated a positive effect on corneal wound healing, whereas other studies have failed to show significant differences compared with control groups. Clinical trials in humans suggest increased comfort from the bandaging effect, which is often preferred to eye patching. The shields are composed of collagen,

---

*Rose bengal dye retention is not pathognomonic for KCS in animals.

Table 6. *Viscoelastic Substances in*
*Ophthalmology**

Substance	Trade Name	Manufacturer
1% sodium hyaluronate	Healon	Pharmacia
1% sodium hyaluronate	Amvisc	Iolab
1.6% sodium hyaluronate	Amvisc Plus	Iolab
20% and 50% chondroitin sulfate	Chondroitin sulfate	Cooper Vision/Cilco
3% sodium hyaluronate and 4% sodium chondroiton sulfate	Viscoat	Cooper Vison/Cilco
2% hydroxypropyl-methycellulose	Occucoat	Storz
0.5% polyacrylamide	Orcolon	Optical Radiation Corporation

*Modified with permission from Liesegang, T. J.: Viscoeleastic substances in ophthalmology. Surv. Ophthalmol. 34:268, 1990.

which is dissolved by the tear film within 24 to 72 hr, depending on the shield type. Application involves applying a wetting agent to the shield and to the eye, placing it on the corneal surface, then holding the animal's lids closed for 60 sec. I currently consider the cost:benefit ratio of collagen shields to be too high for routine use after corneal surgical procedures or superficial corneal ulceration, although in select cases, when increased patient comfort is of concern to the owner, their use may be warranted. Soft contact lenses may be used in a similar manner as a temporary bandage to improve patient's comfort.

Soft contact lenses have also been used in the management of refractory corneal ulcers (Hermann, 1989), with the primary benefits probably being protection of the epithelial margin of the ulcer from the action of the eyelids and improved comfort for patients. Soft contact lenses should not be left in for prolonged periods (more than 2 to 3 days) because of the possibility of inducing a bacterial corneal infection (especially in patients with insufficient tear production).

VISCOELASTIC COMPOUNDS

Viscoelastic compounds (Table 6) are used during intraocular surgery to maintain anterior chamber integrity, to protect the corneal endothelium from contact with instruments or intraocular lenses, and to act as a lubricant to protect delicate uveal tissues. They are extremely beneficial and, in many surgeons' opinion, essential during surgical procedures to remove cataracts and implant intraocular lenses. Their use is also helpful to maintain or re-establish anterior chamber depth during repair of a perforating corneal or scleral wound complicated by uveal prolapse. I routinely remove the viscoelastic substance at the conclusion of the surgical procedure and replace it with balanced salt solution. However, no detrimental effects on intraocular pressure or intraocular structures have been documented in experimental dogs when the compound was not removed. A transient elevation in intraocular pressure following their use has been documented in humans, presumably from obstructive effects of the viscous substance. My preference, for both its viscoelasticity and other rheologic properties, is 1% sodium hyaluronate.

References and Suggested Reading

Hermann, K.: Therapeutic use of hydrophilic contact lenses. *In* Kirk, R. W., and Bonagura, J. D. (eds.): *Current Veterinary Therapy X.* Philadelphia, W. B. Saunders, 1989, p. 640.
 A brief review of therapeutic soft contact lenses, including fitting and cleaning, indications, and complications of use.
Krohne, S. G., and Vestre, W. A.: Ophthalmic usage of nonsteroidal anti-inflammatory agents. *In* Kirk, R. W., and Bonagura, J. D. (eds.): *Current Veterinary Therapy X.* Philadelphia, W. B. Saunders, 1989, p. 642.
 A brief summary of the role of prostaglandin in ocular inflammation and the use of topical and systemic NSAIDs for the treatment of ocular inflammation.
Martin, C. L., and Ward, D. A.: Medical therapy for glaucoma. *In* Kirk, T. W., and Bonagura, J. D. (eds.): *Current Veterinary Therapy X.* Philadelphia, W. B. Saunders, 1989, p. 647.
 A review of the commonly used medications of the treatment of primary glaucoma in dogs, including notes on emergency and prophylactic medical therapy and salvage surgical procedures.
Regnier, A.: Ocular pharmacology and therapeutic modalities. *In* Gelatt, K. N. ed.: *Veterinary Ophthalmology*, 2nd ed. Philadelphia, Lea & Febiger, 1991, pp. 167–194.
 An overview of veterinary ocular pharmacology and therapeutic techniques.
Walsh, J. B., and Gold, A. (eds.): *Physician's Desk Reference for Ophthalmology.* Oradell, NJ, Medical Economics, 1991.
 A complete listing of currently available ophthalmic medications for use in humans, with extensive description of pharmacokinetics and metabolism, indications for use, complications and side effects, dosages, and manufacturers for each drug.
Wyman, M.: Contemporary ocular therapeutics. *In* Kirk, R. W., and Bonagura, J. D. (eds.): *Current Veterinary Therapy IX.* Philadelphia, W. B. Saunders, 1986, p. 684.
 A review of contemporary (1986) classes of veterinary ophthalmic medications, with particular emphasis on antimicrobial agents.

OCULAR MANIFESTATIONS OF SYSTEMIC DISEASE

MARY B. GLAZE

Baton Rouge, Louisiana

Early reviews of ocular manifestations of systemic disease were limited to discussions of diabetic cataracts, herpetic keratoconjunctivitis, and hepatitis "blue eye." Today, hundreds of reports document the impact of systemic disease on the eyes of companion animals, and consideration must now be given to a myriad of infectious, metabolic, neoplastic, immunologic, nutritional, and toxicologic etiologies.

Why should the eyes receive such scrutiny in the presence of potentially life-threatening diseases? The eyes can be conveniently examined using noninvasive diagnostic techniques. Important clues to neurologic disease may be found by examining the optic nerve or another of the six cranial nerves accessible in an ocular examination. The ease of evaluating retinal and conjunctival vessels also makes the eyes an important source of information in vascular and hematologic disorders. The highly vascular uveal tract can act as a filter for infectious agents or neoplastic cells, and the lens and cornea are potential targets of metabolic disease.

The eyes may be the first organs noticeably affected by a systemic disorder. Because exudative or infiltrative ocular lesions generally dictate the need for physical examination, clinicians have the opportunity to document concurrent systemic abnormalities and institute appropriate therapy early in the course of a disease. Sequential examinations of ocular lesions also give a firsthand view of treatment efficacy as the lesions alter their size and character.

The growing list of systemic diseases with ocular manifestations is most easily managed by grouping diseases into basic etiologic categories. A familiar scheme for recalling such broad classifications is the acronym DAMNIT (Table 1), on which the remaining section headings are based.

DEVELOPMENTAL DISORDERS

Tetralogy of Fallot

Rarely does an animal demonstrate an ophthalmic abnormality attributable to a systemic developmental defect. An exception has been reported in dogs and cats with tetralogy of Fallot. Affected animals may be presented for evaluation of decreasing visual acuity or sudden blindness. Increased blood viscosity in response to compensatory polycythemia gives rise to swollen, tortuous retinal vessels and retinal detachment. Concurrent clinical signs include cyanosis, dyspnea, and exercise intolerance. Transient ocular improvement has been reported following phlebotomy, but prognosis is generally poor.

Mucopolysaccharidosis

Ocular and skeletal abnormalities have been described in dogs and cats with mucopolysaccharidoses (MPS), rare hereditary disorders characterized by defective degradation and abnormal deposition of glycosaminoglycans in body tissues. Dogs with MPS-I demonstrate degenerative joint disease and corneal opacification by 1 year of age. Cats with MPS-VI are stunted, with broad faces and widely separated palpebral fissures. Corneal clouding occurs by 10 weeks and increases in severity with age. Although glycosaminoglycans also accumulate in the retinal pigment epithelium, retinal degeneration has only been reported in dogs with MPS-VII. A decrease in corneal clouding and slowed progression of joint disease has followed bone marrow transplantation in dogs with MPS-I and in cats with MPS-VI.

AUTOIMMUNE DISEASES

Several dermatologic conditions are characterized by changes that may begin, or at least be noticed

Table 1. Etiologic Categories of Disease

D	Developmental
	Degenerative
A	Autoimmune
	Allergic
M	Metabolic
N	Neoplastic
	Nutritional
I	Iatrogenic
	Idiopathic
	Immune-mediated
	Infectious
T	Toxic
	Traumatic

first, at the eyelid margins. Included in this group are pemphigus foliaceous and systemic lupus erythematosus (SLE). Periocular ulceration, depigmentation, and crust formation are usually accompanied by similar cutaneous lesions on the face, nasal planum, ears, trunk, and footpads. Multisystemic involvement is suggestive of SLE. Diagnosis is based on histopathology and immunofluorescence testing. Immunosuppressive therapy with glucocorticoids or azathioprine (Imuran, Burroughs Wellcome) or both is recommended, though dosage and duration vary with the disease and its severity.

METABOLIC DISEASES

Endocrine Disorders

DIABETES MELLITUS

Rapidly developing cataracts are a well-known consequence of canine diabetes. The accumulation of sorbitol as a by-product of glucose metabolism creates an osmotic gradient leading to lens fiber rupture. The cataracts begin as equatorial vesicles, progressing to prominent suture lines, cortical rays, scattered focal opacities, and finally complete opacification. The rapidity of the changes varies, but mature cataracts developed within 90 days in a study of 6-month-old beagles. Owners are unlikely to notice the lens changes until the final stages, explaining reports of rapid progression over a 2- to 3-week period. Concurrent clinical signs of polyuria, polydipsia, and weight loss are often overshadowed by the rapid onset of blindness.

Although proliferative retinopathy is the leading cause of vision loss in humans with diabetes, the same retinal vascular changes do not appear to be clinically significant in dogs. Capillary aneurysms and retinal hemorrhages have been reported, but progression to the proliferative stage is rare.

Treatment is directed at controlling blood glucose levels with insulin supplementation and dietary restriction. Cataract surgery can be performed with good results in dogs with well-regulated diabetes.

HYPOTHYROIDISM

Various ocular lesions secondary to hyperlipidemia can occur in hypothyroid dogs. Corneal lipidosis is most common and appears as central oval or peripheral arciform opacities, typically free of vascularization. Thyroid supplementation halts progression but does not significantly reverse the opacification.

Occasional changes in retinal vessel color and in aqueous clarity also occur. Creamy pink retinal vessels typify lipemia retinalis. Reduction of plasma lipid levels resolves the retinal changes. If uveal inflammation compromises the selective barrier that normally excludes large lipid molecules, the aqueous can also assume a milky character. Symptomatic treatment of the anterior uveitis prevents further influx of lipid. The remainder exits with the aqueous through the iridocorneal angle.

Vascular hypertension has been documented in hypothyroid dogs. Lipid deposition in the vessel walls increases vascular resistance; subsequent ischemia is incriminated in the pathogenesis of retinal detachment and hemorrhage. Thyroid supplementation and antihypertensive agents must be instituted soon after the detachment occurs to minimize secondary retinal degeneration. Prognosis for vision is poor if detachments are chronic or extensive.

Nystagmus and dysfunction of the facial, trigeminal, and oculomotor nerves can occur in hypothyroid dogs. Reported ocular abnormalities include ptosis, decreased corneal sensation, and ventral positional strabismus. Clinical signs are at least partially reversible with thyroid hormone supplementation. Retrospective studies of dogs with facial neuropathy or Horner's syndrome have investigated an association with low serum T_3 or T_4 concentrations but were unable to confirm a relationship to hypothyroidism documented by response to testing with thyroid-stimulating hormone.

HYPERADRENOCORTICISM

Rapidly developing corneal calcification has been reported in association with canine Cushing's disease. The lesion appears as a white plaque in the superficial cornea, with or without corneal ulceration. Debridement of the plaque, followed by frequent topical application of 3 to 5% calcium disodium ethylenediaminetetraacetic acid (Versenate, Sterling) to chelate the remaining mineral, may be beneficial in ulcerated lesions.

Corneal ulcers occurring in an affected animal may be difficult to resolve. High levels of endogenous corticosteroid have the potential not only to delay corneal healing but also to potentiate the rapid enzymatic degradation of the corneal stroma by collagenases and proteinases.

HYPOPARATHYROIDISM

Hypocalcemia and hyperphosphatemia accompany the clinical signs of restlessness, muscle fasciculations, and convulsions that occur in parathyroid dysfunction. A unique cataract may develop, characterized by small punctate to linear white opacities in the anterior and posterior cortical subcapsular regions of the lens. Vision is unaffected.

Hypertension

Hypertension exists when the systolic blood pressure is sustained above 180 mm Hg or the diastolic pressure is sustained above 95 mm Hg. Idiopathic hypertension, chronic renal disease, hypothyroidism, hyperadrenocorticism, and pheochromocytoma are thought to contribute to blood pressure elevations in dogs. Chronic renal disease, chronic anemia, and hyperthyroidism have been incriminated in cats.

Retinal changes can be the first indication of hypertension in both species. Acute blindness often is the presenting complaint. Ophthalmoscopic lesions include increased tortuosity of retinal arterioles, retinal hemorrhage, retinal detachment, and papilledema.

Treatment with diuretics and beta-blocking agents has proved beneficial, although prognosis for vision is poor when retinal detachments are extensive or of long standing. Oral captopril (Capoten, Squibb; 1 to 2 mg/kg every 8 to 12 hr) appears to be an effective antihypertensive agent in dogs, but treated dogs have remained blind. Retinal hemorrhages and detachments have resolved in cats receiving 2.5 mg oral propranolol (Inderal, Wyeth-Ayerst) twice daily, but as in their canine counterparts, functional vision seldom improves.

NEOPLASTIC DISEASE

Lymphosarcoma

The most common metastatic tumor of the eyes in dogs and cats is lymphosarcoma. Solitary intraocular masses are rare in contrast to diffuse uveal infiltration. Concurrent uveitis is a prominent feature, often characterized by iris thickening, hypopyon, or hyphema. Retinal detachment and optic nerve infiltration occur but may be obscured by the anterior segment changes. Exophthalmos suggests orbital infiltration. In dogs, lymphoma most commonly causes a painless, generalized lymphadenopathy, whereas specific organ dysfunction is more common in cats.

Histopathologic examination of nonocular biopsy specimens is the preferred method of confirmation and should be relied on in animals with vision. Cytologic evaluation of anterior chamber aspirates may support a diagnosis of lymphosarcoma but should be reserved for animals with significant cellular accumulations within the eye. A test for feline leukemia virus (FeLV) should be performed in cats.

Once the diagnosis has been established, an oncologist should be consulted regarding systemic therapy. Topical ocular therapy to decrease uveal inflammation combines corticosteroids and mydri-

atics. The potential for secondary glaucoma due to infiltration or obstruction of the iridocorneal angle necessitates periodic assessment of intraocular pressure. One study in dogs indicated decreased survival times in animals with ocular disease.

Multiple Myeloma

Changes in the concentration of serum immunoglobulins occurs in association with multiple myeloma, a neoplastic proliferation of plasma cells. Distended, sacculated, or tortuous retinal venules, retinal hemorrhages, retinal detachments, and papilledema may be early signs of increased serum viscosity. One study reported a 35% incidence of ocular lesions in dogs. The mechanisms responsible for the changes are not clear, but overdistention of the vasculature secondary to expanded plasma volume, tissue hypoxia secondary to hypoperfusion, and impaired hemostasis all may play a part.

Response to therapy is promising. One study reported 90% of the dogs treated with a combination of melphalan (Alkeran, Burroughs Wellcome), cyclophosphamide (Cytoxan, Bristol-Myers), and prednisone had a major clinical response, with a median survival time of 540 days (Matus et al., 1986). Prognosis for vision in patients with retinal detachments is initially guarded but may be upgraded based on therapeutic response.

Other Metastatic Tumors

Ocular metastasis of various sarcomas and carcinomas occurs in both dogs and cats, usually late in the course of the neoplastic disease. The vascular nature of the uveal tract makes it a preferential site for tumor embolization. Although obvious masses may develop, ocular signs are often nonspecific and include uveitis, intraocular hemorrhage, secondary glaucoma, retinal detachment, and papilledema. Metastases distant to the eye can also affect ocular function. Ophthalmoplegia has been reported after invasion of the cavernous sinus by thyroid adenocarcinoma in dogs and by squamous cell carcinoma in cats.

If an animal's long-term prognosis is good, enucleation of the affected eye is recommended. Symptomatic therapy for uveitis may be palliative in terminal cases. Evisceration and implantation of a silicone sphere are contraindicated in cases of metastatic ocular neoplasia.

NEUROLOGIC DISORDERS

Feline Dysautonomia (Key-Gaskell Syndrome)

Striking systemic and ocular consequences have been reported in young cats with generalized loss of autonomic innervation. Affected animals are often acutely blepharospastic, with prominent third eyelids and markedly decreased tear production. Intraocular structures are normal with the exception of widely dilated, nonresponsive pupils. Vision is unaffected. Multisystemic signs include bradycardia, constipation, urine retention, and regurgitation due to megaesophagus. The disease has been reported primarily in the United Kingdom.

The etiology of the disorder is unknown. Treatment is primarily supportive. Artificial tear solutions or ointments are used to lubricate the ocular surface. One drop of 2% ophthalmic pilocarpine solution (Isopto Carpine, Alcon) can be applied to the food twice daily to directly stimulate tear production. Unfortunately, cats often refuse medicated meals even without the pre-existing gastrointestinal abnormalities that characterize dysautonomia. The mortality rate is high. Megaesophagus, mydriasis, and keratoconjunctivitis sicca persist in survivors.

Horner's Syndrome

Ocular sympathetic denervation is characterized by an array of clinical signs: miosis, ptosis, narrowing of the palpebral fissure, enophthalmos, and protrusion of the nictitans. Lesions may occur anywhere along the long, three-neuron sympathetic chain that originates in the hypothalamus and traverses the cervical spinal cord, anterior thorax, vagosympathetic trunk, middle ear, and orbit to enter the eye. Systemic disorders that have been associated with Horner's syndrome include thoracic, cervical, and intracranial neoplasia; otitis media/interna; ischemic spinal cord disorders; brachial plexus avulsion; hypothyroidism; and vascular, infectious, or traumatic lesions of the brainstem.

Pharmacologic differentiation of central and peripheral Horner's syndrome may be useful prognostically. Dilation of the miotic pupil following topical application of 1% hydroxyamphetamine (Paredrine Solution, Smith Kline & French) is consistent with a central lesion and generally denotes a poorer prognosis for resolution of both the underlying cause and the ocular signs. Failure to dilate with hydroxyamphetamine but mydriasis within 20 min of 10% phenylephrine (Ak-Dilate, Akorn) application is consistent with peripheral Horner's and implies a favorable prognosis for eventual recovery. Topical phenylephrine may be used to minimize nictitans protrusion in peripheral Horner's.

NUTRITIONAL DEFICIENCIES

The association between *taurine deficiency* and feline retinal degeneration has been known for more than a decade. Because myocardial and reproduc-

tive diseases have also been linked to inadequate dietary taurine, retinal evaluation should be routine in cats with cardiomyopathy or infertility.

The classic disorder was described in cats fed only dog food, but recent investigation would seem also to dispute the adequacy of taurine levels in some feline products. The earliest lesions are bilateral focal hyper-reflective areas temporal to the optic disc. As the deficiency persists, bilaterally symmetric, horizontal bands of hyper-reflectivity develop across the tapetal fundus. Prolonged deficiency results in complete retinal atrophy and blindness. Restoration of taurine to the diet will arrest progression of the retinal abnormality, but blindness is permanent in cats with generalized retinal atrophy.

IMMUNE-MEDIATED DISEASES

Canine Uveodermatologic Syndrome

Thought to result from an immune-mediated destruction of uveal and dermal melanocytes, canine uveodermatologic syndrome resembles a human uveomeningoencephalitic disease known as Vogt-Koyanagi-Harada (VKH) syndrome. Akitas and Arctic breeds such as the Siberian husky, Samoyed, and malamute appear predisposed, although all breeds are probably susceptible. Most patients are presented for sudden onset of blindness or with a history of chronic uveitis. Bilateral uveitis, granulomatous choroiditis, and retinal detachment are accompanied by alopecia, loss of skin pigmentation, and whitening of the hair. Ocular complications related to the inflammation include posterior synechiae, cataracts, glaucoma, and retinal degeneration. Exacerbations are common.

Because granulomatous ocular lesions also occur in bacterial and mycotic diseases, it is important to rule out infectious etiologies before instituting aggressive systemic therapy. Topical or subconjunctival corticosteroids and topical mydriatics are indicated in patients with anterior uveitis. Immunosuppressive doses of oral prednisone (1 to 2 mg/kg/day) are essential in the management of posterior uveitis and retinal detachment. If treatment with corticosteroids is not effective, oral azathioprine (1 to 2 mg/kg) may be administered daily or every other day as an alternative immunosuppressive agent. Complete blood and platelet counts should be monitored biweekly for the first 8 weeks, then monthly for potential azathioprine-induced bone marrow suppression.

Long-term prognosis is generally poor, but anterior uveitis and retinal detachment might respond to therapy instituted early in the course of the disease. Despite chronic therapy, recurrences can still occur with lower doses or after therapy is discontinued.

Canine Adenovirus Type 1 Infection

The ocular lesions of canine adenovirus are attributed to an Arthus-type hypersensitivity, initiated by the formation of virus-antibody complexes. The subsequent activation of complement damages the uveal and corneal endothelium and produces an anterior uveitis with profound corneal edema. The majority of cases are unilateral. Ocular complications include persistent corneal edema, keratoconus, and secondary glaucoma.

Twenty per cent of dogs recovering from infectious canine hepatitis develop ocular signs. Vaccination with a modified live virus vaccine may also produce ocular signs within 10 to 14 days. Postvaccinal reactions have been reduced but not completely eliminated with the use of the adenovirus type 2 product.

Topical 1% prednisolone acetate (Pred Forte, Allergan) and atropine (Atropine Care, Akorn) may minimize uveal inflammation in the early stages. A topical hypertonic agent (5% sodium chloride ointment, AK-NaCl, Akorn) may temporarily reduce corneal edema but requires frequent, often irritating applications. Because endothelial reparative properties are limited, prognosis is guarded. A low percentage of dogs will have permanent corneal opacification. The Afghan hound, Siberian husky, Samoyed, and Norwegian elkhound appear predisposed to secondary glaucoma and are generally given a poorer prognosis.

INFECTIOUS DISEASES

Although the eyes are commonly affected in pansystemic diseases, they rarely serve as the primary site of infection. More likely routes of dissemination are by hematogenous spread of organisms to the uvea and retina or by direct extension to the eye from adjacent tissues.

Bacterial Infections

BRUCELLOSIS

A history of intermittent or relapsing uveitis characterizes *Brucella canis* infection. Hypopyon is a common feature. Concurrent clinical signs are often vague, although classic findings of testicular enlargement, scrotal dermatitis, and reproductive failure may be present.

Definitive diagnosis is based on serologic testing.

Positive results using a rapid slide agglutination test should be confirmed using a second method such as agar-gel immunodiffusion or tube agglutination. Samples of aqueous humor may demonstrate titers above serum concentrations owing to local antibody formation within the uveal tract. The organism also has been cultured from the vitreous.

Elimination of the systemic infection is hampered by the organism's intracellular location. High-dose oral minocycline (Minocin, Lederle) or generic doxycycline therapy (12.5 mg/kg every 12 hr for 2 weeks) combined with intramuscular streptomycin (Roerig; 5 mg/kg every 12 hr for 1 week) or gentamicin (Gentocin, Schering; 2 mg/kg every 12 hr for 1 week) has given the highest rate of success in experimental infections. Treatment is expensive, and bacteremia may reoccur weeks to months after therapy has been discontinued. Conventional treatment of the uveitis combines topical corticosteroids and atropine. Prognosis is guarded; the exudative and recurrent nature of the inflammatory disease predispose the eye to endophthalmitis and secondary glaucoma.

BACTEREMIA

The uveal tract may respond to the presence of any bacterial organism in the circulating blood. Anterior uveitis and choroiditis have been associated with pyometra, endocarditis, anal sacculitis, pancreatitis, prostatitis, and dental disease. In addition to the effects of direct bacterial invasion, the inflammatory disease may also reflect the presence of bacterial toxins or the patient's own immunologic response to the organism. Ocular prognosis is usually favorable with symptomatic treatment of the uveitis and specific treatment of the primary infection.

Chlamydial Infections

Conjunctivitis and mild respiratory signs accompany *Chlamydia psittaci* infection in cats. Initially unilateral, the infection involves the second eye within a few days. In addition to nonspecific conjunctival hyperemia and chemosis, the conjunctival surface and nictitating membrane may appear roughened as a result of lymphoid hyperplasia and vesicle formation. An early serous discharge becomes mucopurulent within 3 to 5 days.

Basophilic intracytoplasmic inclusions within conjunctival epithelial cells may be found early in the disease. Immunofluorescent antibody tests of conjunctival scrapings are also available through many diagnostic laboratories. Response to treatment has also been used to differentiate the ocular disease from that caused by herpesvirus infection.

Topical tetracycline ointment (Achromycin, Lederle) is the treatment of choice. Application three times daily can be irritating but produces rapid improvement in acute cases. Chronic infections may require several weeks of therapy. Treatment should be continued for 1 week after resolution of clinical signs.

Mycotic Diseases

BLASTOMYCOSIS

Blastomyces dermatitidis is indigenous to regions of the Mississippi and Ohio rivers and the central Atlantic states. Ocular lesions are a common consequence of canine blastomycosis and have also been reported in feline infections. Patients may be presented for evaluation of vision loss or assessment of a red, cloudy eye even before signs of systemic illness are noted. One or both eyes may be affected. Off-white granulomatous choroidal exudates cause elevation of the overlying retina. Vitreal exudates or bullous retinal detachments obscure fundic detail as the disease progresses. A nonspecific anterior uveitis persists despite conventional anti-inflammatory therapy. Panophthalmitis may develop rapidly, with pronounced corneal edema, deep corneal vascularization, and secondary glaucoma. Advanced cases often appear exophthalmic as a result of scleral and episcleral inflammation and swelling. Concurrent clinical signs include dry, harsh lung sounds, fever, and lymphadenopathy. Early diagnosis and appropriate treatment are essential to preserve vision. In endemic areas, dogs with nonresponsive anterior uveitis, vision loss associated with leukokoria, or pronounced scleral/episcleral inflammation should be suspected of having systemic blastomycosis. Organisms may be demonstrated in subretinal or vitreal aspirates but are rarely found in the anterior chamber.

Ocular blastomycosis is notoriously difficult to eradicate. Early lesions can be successfully treated by combining intravenous amphotericin B (Fungizone, Squibb; 0.5 mg/kg for dogs, 0.25 mg/kg for cats, three times weekly until the cumulative dose reaches 4 mg/kg) with oral ketoconazole (Nizoral, Janssen; 30 mg/kg/day for dogs, 10 mg/kg/day for cats, for a minimum of 2 months). Based on preliminary studies, oral itraconazole (5 mg/kg every 12 to 24 hr) may be less toxic and equally efficacious when used alone in a 60-day regimen. Conventional topical management of anterior uveitis is also recommended.

Ocular prognosis is poor in blind animals with long-standing retinal detachments, secondary glaucoma, or panophthalmitis. Approximately 20% of animals will suffer a relapse after treatment. Ocular tissues may serve as a nidus for reinfection after therapy is discontinued.

COCCIDIOIDOMYCOSIS

Coccidioides immitis is limited to the southwestern United States. The respiratory disease that characterizes canine coccidioidomycosis may develop several months before signs of ocular infection. Common ophthalmic complaints include photophobia, redness, cloudiness, or acute loss of vision. Ocular lesions are more often unilateral than bilateral. Granulomatous subretinal exudates are similar to those of blastomycosis and may lead to retinal detachment. Extension into the anterior segment produces keratitis, corneal vascularization, anterior uveitis, and secondary glaucoma. Concurrent systemic signs include weight loss, lethargy, a harsh dry cough, and lameness associated with painful bone swelling or joint enlargement.

In vivo diagnosis is based on serologic testing rather than attempts at histopathologic documentation of the organism within the retina and choroid. A complement fixation titer of 1:8 is suspicious but should be repeated within 3 to 4 weeks to document a rising titer.

Treatment with oral ketoconazole (5 to 10 mg/kg every 12 hr) for a minimum of 12 months is recommended. Symptomatic topical treatment of anterior uveitis is also indicated. The eye should be enucleated if it is the only site of active infection or does not respond to antifungal therapy.

CRYPTOCOCCOSIS

Anterior uveitis has been described in canine and feline infections, but the ocular lesions of cryptococcosis are more often localized within the posterior segment. Signs of chorioretinitis range from small serous retinal detachments to fluffy gray-white choroidal exudates with pigmented centers. Meningeal inflammation may lead to optic neuritis, with clinical signs of blindness, mydriasis, and optic disc swelling. Upper respiratory signs are usually evident in cats, whereas central neurologic disease is more typical of the disease in dogs.

The thickly encapsulated budding yeasts may be demonstrated in subretinal or vitreal fine-needle aspirates. Serologic testing using latex agglutination to detect cryptococcal antigen can be used when ocular centesis is impractical or unrewarding.

Cryptococcosis has been successfully treated with amphotericin B, flucytosine, and ketoconazole, alone or in combination. Chorioretinitis resolved within 3 months in a cat treated with intravenous amphotericin B (0.5 mg/kg three times weekly to a cumulative dose of 4 mg/kg) and oral flucytosine

(Ancobon, Roche; 50 mg/kg every 8 hr). Low-dose combination therapy using oral ketoconazole (10 mg/kg once daily) and oral flucytosine (125 mg once daily) has proved successful in the treatment of feline nasal cryptococcosis, but its efficacy in ocular infections is unproven. Decreasing antigen titers are used to document response to therapy. Therapy is recommended for 2 months after resolution of clinical signs.

HISTOPLASMOSIS

Histoplasma capsulatum is more common in the midwestern and southern river valleys and plains. The posterior segment lesions of histoplasmosis rarely demonstrate the granulomatous appearance associated with other ocular fungal infections. The disease more often is characterized by multiple areas of abnormal pigment proliferation and retinal edema within the tapetal fundus. Anterior uveitis is less commonly described. Weight loss and diarrhea are common clinical signs in dogs. Cats are more likely to demonstrate anemia and dyspnea.

Definitive diagnosis can be made by cytologic examination of rectal scrapings or fine-needle aspirates of bone marrow or lung. No reliable immunodiagnostic test currently exists.

Ketoconazole (10 to 15 mg/kg every 12 hr) is currently the drug of choice in early pulmonary infections. Itraconazole (5 to 10 mg/kg every 24 hr) may be less toxic to cats and shows a high affinity for affected tissues. Duration of treatment is determined by the severity of the infection and the clinical response of the patient. Prognosis with disseminated histoplasmosis is guarded.

MISCELLANEOUS FUNGI

Chorioretinitis has been described in dogs with disseminated aspergillosis and paecilomycosis. Anterior uveitis and granulomatous chorioretinitis have also been reported in a cat with systemic candidiasis. None of the animals were treated successfully.

ALGAE

Prototheca is a colorless alga that contaminates soil and water. Protracted bloody diarrhea is the most common clinical sign of infection; two thirds of infected dogs also have ocular lesions. Blindness is common owing to bilateral granulomatous panuveitis and secondary retinal detachment. Vitreous exudates produce a characteristic leukocoria and obscure fundic detail.

Protothecosis is confirmed by demonstrating the organism in the vitreous, cerebrospinal fluid, or rectal mucosa. No effective therapy has been reported.

Parasitic Diseases

Migratory stages of *Toxocara canis* may invade the eye on rare occasion and induce a multifocal granulomatous chorioretinitis. Small, raised gray-white nodules can be easily visualized in the nontapetal fundus. Postinflammatory retinal atrophy and blindness have been attributed to larval migrans in a group of border collies.

Protozoal Diseases

TOXOPLASMOSIS

Ocular inflammation secondary to *Toxoplasma gondii* infection may be the result of direct parasitism of ocular tissues or a consequence of immunologic responses to the organism. The most common ocular lesion is multifocal retinochoroiditis. Exudative retinal detachments and optic neuritis represent more serious manifestations of infection; affected animals are usually blind. Anterior uveitis ranges from inconsequential to severely exudative in character. Ocular lesions are seen more commonly in cats than in dogs and may occur without systemic illness. Respiratory, neuromuscular, or gastrointestinal signs occur in both species.

Definitive diagnosis of ocular toxoplasmosis is often complicated by the absence of systemic disease. A single elevated immunoglobulin G (IgG) titer cannot be equated with active toxoplasmosis. Instead, tests that measure IgG must document a fourfold rise in titer in blood samples taken 2 to 3 weeks apart. Simultaneous measurement of immunoglobulin M (IgM) and IgG antibodies offers the most reliable means of determining the presence of toxoplasmosis in cats and dogs. Recent documentation of antibody production in the aqueous humor also shows diagnostic promise.

Clindamycin (Antirobe, Upjohn) is the drug of choice for treating clinical toxoplasmosis in cats (12.5 to 25 mg/kg every 12 hr) and dogs (10 to 20 mg/kg every 12 hr) and may be administered orally or intramuscularly with equal efficacy. Anterior uveitis and retinochoroiditis often improve within 1 week. Conventional topical treatment of anterior uveitis is recommended concurrently.

LEISHMANIASIS

Once limited to Mediterranean, Asian, and South American countries, infections by protozoa of the genus *Leishmania* are now recognized in the United States and Canada. Isolated foci of infection have been found in Texas, Oklahoma, and Ohio.

Almost 90% of dogs with leishmaniasis have skin disease. Periocular scaling occurs as part of a generalized hyperkeratosis, with an affinity for the face and footpads. Weight loss, lameness, and lymphadenopathy are other prominent systemic findings. The ocular lesions include nodular blepharitis, keratoconjunctivitis, anterior uveitis, retinitis, and retinal detachment.

Diagnosis is usually confirmed by demonstration of the organism in bone marrow or lymph node aspirates. Parenteral meglumine antimonate is the preferred leishmanicidal agent, but relapses usually occur within months. With the possibility of direct transmission of the protozoa to humans and between dogs, the public health significance must be considered.

Rickettsial Diseases

EHRLICHIOSIS

Three disease phases are recognized in *Ehrlichia canis* infections. The acute phase is characterized by fever, lymphadenopathy, and thrombocytopenia. Although most dogs recover, some progress to a subclinical stage in which hematologic abnormalities persist but clinical signs resolve. Chronically infected dogs are pancytopenic and often die as a result of hemorrhage and secondary infections.

Acutely infected dogs may exhibit retinal vessel engorgement and perivascular edema before the onset of anterior uveitis. Uveitis ranges from inconsequential to severe. The most common is a low-grade inflammatory process characterized by gradually progressive corneal edema, keratic precipitates, and subtle iridocyclitis. Intraocular and retrobulbar hemorrhages reflect the animal's thrombocytopenia. Severe ocular manifestations include serous retinal detachment and optic neuritis. Anterior uveitis has also been described in association with *Ehrlichia platys*, the causative agent of canine infectious cyclic thrombocytopenia.

Diagnosis of ehrlichiosis is based on clinical signs, hematologic findings, and serologic testing. A 2- to 3-week regimen of oral tetracycline (22 mg/kg every 8 hr) or a 10-day regimen of oral doxycycline (5 to 10 mg/kg every 12 hr) is recommended, in addition to conventional topical therapy for anterior uveitis. Dogs treated with doxycycline have had a lower incidence of relapse or reinfection than have dogs treated with oxytetracycline.

ROCKY MOUNTAIN SPOTTED FEVER

The acute stages of ehrlichiosis and Rocky Mountain spotted fever are impossible to differentiate on the basis of ocular and clinical signs. Anterior uveitis, retinal edema, and perivascular inflammatory cell infiltration are generally mild in *Rickettsia rickettsii* infections. Thrombocytopenic dogs are predisposed to subconjunctival hemorrhage, hyphema, and petechiae within the iris and retina.

An IgG titer increase of fourfold or greater is required to definitively document active infection. Treatment is as described for ehrlichiosis; systemic antibiotic therapy need only be continued for 1 to 2 weeks.

Viral Diseases

CANINE DISTEMPER

Conjunctivitis is a common extraocular feature of canine distemper virus infection, often accompanied by acute decreases in tear production. Specific immunofluorescence testing of conjunctival scrapings may document the infection. A serous ocular discharge usually becomes mucopurulent within 7 to 10 days. Indistinct grayish foci within the tapetal and nontapetal fundus characterize the active retinopathy. If the dog survives, chorioretinal scars may persist as well-defined areas of tapetal hyperreflectivity and foci of altered pigment within the nontapetum. Blindness may occur with optic neuritis or cortical disease.

No specific antiviral therapy is available. Secondary bacterial infections and corneal ulcers can be prevented with topical antibiotics and lubricants.

FELINE CORONAVIRUS

Feline infectious peritonitis is most often diagnosed in young adult cats. Ocular abnormalities occur in both the effusive and noneffusive forms of the disease but are more common in the latter. The ocular changes are similar to those attributed to FeLV infection and include bilateral anterior uveitis, exudative chorioretinitis, and retinal hemorrhages and detachments. Perivascular sheathing of retinal vessels is commonly described. Blindness may accompany optic neuritis.

The clinical diagnosis is based on history, clinical signs, routine hematologic tests, analysis of thoracic and abdominal fluids, and serum protein electrophoresis. A coronavirus antibody titer in a diseased cat should be used only as an aid in diagnosis. In cats with prolonged illness, a fourfold or greater increase in titer during a 4- to 6-week period is highly suggestive of active coronavirus infection. Symptomatic treatment of ocular inflammation is indicated but rarely attempted because of the terminal nature of the systemic illness.

FELINE HERPESVIRUS

Feline herpesvirus (FHV) targets surface epithelial cells and produces various ocular lesions as part of the upper respiratory complex. Acute bilateral conjunctivitis develops in kittens and young cats in association with upper respiratory signs of disease. Adult cats typically exhibit conjunctivitis without respiratory signs and are more likely to develop keratitis. Dendritic corneal erosions are considered pathognomonic for FHV infection, but large ulcers and deep keratitis do occur.

The acute ocular-respiratory disease is usually self-limiting, requiring only prophylactic topical antibiotic therapy to control secondary invaders. The major indication for topical antiviral agents is keratitis; their use in conjunctivitis is typically unrewarding. Trifluridine (Viroptic, Burroughs Wellcome) is the drug of choice. Prognosis in acute cases is favorable, although up to 80% of the animals will become chronic carriers. The prognosis for cure in cases of chronic conjunctivitis and keratitis is guarded.

FELINE IMMUNODEFICIENCY VIRUS

Original reports of this lentiviral infection described only a persistent or cyclic exudative conjunctivitis in the terminal stages of feline immunodeficiency virus (FIV) infection. Since that time, intraocular disease has been described in FIV-positive cats with anterior uveitis, glaucoma, and retinal perivasculitis. Pars planitis, a distinctive lesion characterized by anterior vitreal cellular infiltrates, was described in four of nine cats (English et al., 1990).

Serologic testing should document FIV antibodies and rule out infections by FeLV, feline coronavirus, and *T. gondii*. Continued low-frequency topical corticosteroid administration may be required to control anterior uveitis in affected cats.

FELINE LEUKEMIA VIRUS

Anterior uveitis is reported as the most common ocular manifestation of FeLV infection. Acute inflammation is characterized by corneal edema, aqueous flare, keratic precipitates, iridal hyperemia, and various degrees of miosis. Iridal thickening or isolated iris masses may develop with FeLV-associated lymphoma. Recurring or chronic episodes of inflammation lead to alterations in pupillary shape as a result of synechiae. Intraocular pressure may decrease owing to ciliary body atrophy or may increase with iris bombé or iridocorneal angle adhesions. Posterior segment lesions include retinal hemorrhages, retinal detachments, and focal cellular infiltrates within the vitreous, retina, and choroid.

Diagnosis is based on serologic testing. Despite the often exudative nature of the uveitis, aqueous aspirates are nondiagnostic, with the exception of FeLV-associated lymphosarcoma. Symptomatic treatment of anterior uveitis is warranted to reduce the likelihood of secondary glaucoma.

FELINE PANLEUKOPENIA VIRUS

With its affinity for rapidly dividing cells, panleukopenia virus may cause developmental ocular abnormalities following prenatal or neonatal infection. Well-defined hyper-reflective foci in the tapetal fundus, focal areas of nontapetal depigmentation, and optic nerve hypoplasia may occur in conjunction with cerebellar hypoplasia. No ocular therapy is indicated.

IDIOPATHIC DISEASE

An idiopathic disease of the central nervous system, granulomatous meningoencephalitis (GME) may cause acute blindness due to reticuloendothelial cell infiltration of the optic nerve, retina, and choroid. The optic disc appears swollen, often accompanied by peripapillary retinitis and hemorrhage. Concurrent neurologic signs vary depending on the area of brain or spinal cord affected; ataxia, tetraparesis, and cervical hyperesthesia are common.

Diagnosis is based on clinical signs and the demonstration of lymphocytes, undifferentiated mononuclear cells, and elevated protein in the cerebrospinal fluid. Prognosis for permanent recovery in dogs with GME is poor. A decreasing regimen of oral prednisone is recommended, beginning at 1 to 2 mg/kg/day and tapering to an alternate-day dosage. Too rapid a reduction in corticosteroid dose may cause acute exacerbation of clinical signs.

TOXICITIES

Ethylene Glycol

Anterior uveitis and severe retinal edema have been described in cases of ethylene glycol intoxication. Dramatic retinal folds may be the result of vascular damage caused by calcium oxalate embolization. Ocular abnormalities resolve without specific therapy as the animal's clinical status improves.

Ivermectin

Blindness, pupillary dilation, and focal retinal edema have occurred in dogs after ivermectin overdose. Concurrent clinical abnormalities include stupor, localized muscle fasciculations, and hypermetria. Ocular signs are transient and are apparently responsive to parenteral corticosteroid therapy.

References and Suggested Reading

Bovee, K. C., Littman, M. P., Crabtree, B. J., et al.: Essential hypertension in a dog. J.A.V.M.A. 195:81, 1989.
  A case report describing the ocular manifestations of canine hypertension and the response to treatment during a 4-year period.
English, R. V., Davidson, M. G., Nasisse, M. P., et al.: Intraocular disease associated with feline immunodeficiency virus infection in cats. J.A.V.M.A. 196:1116, 1990.
  A description and comparison of intraocular lesions attributed to FIV with those of FeLV and feline infectious peritonitis.
Martin, C. L.: Ocular infections. *In* Green, C. E. (ed.): *Infectious Diseases of the Dog and Cat.* Philadelphia: WB Saunders, 1990, p. 197.
  A review of the ocular manifestations of systemic infectious diseases.
Matus, R. E., Leifer, C. E., MacEwen, E. G., et al.: Prognostic factors for multiple myeloma in the dog. J.A.V.M.A. 188:1288, 1986.
  A discussion of treatment regimens and prognostic criteria in 60 cases of canine multiple myeloma.
Sorjonen, D. C.: Clinical and histopathological features of granulomatous meningoencephalomyelitis in dogs. J. Am. Anim. Hosp. Assoc. 26:141, 1990.
  A review of the clinical features, diagnostic criteria, and response to therapy in canine GME.
Swanson, J. F.: Ocular manifestations of systemic disease in the dog and cat. Vet. Clin. North Am. 20:849, 1990.
  A review of the pathophysiologic mechanisms and ocular lesions that accompany systemic disease in companion animals.

FELINE OPHTHALMIC DISORDERS

THOMAS J. KERN
Ithaca, New York

The ocular disorders that afflict cats parallel those of other species. Diagnosis of feline ocular disorders is facilitated by the application of accessory diagnostic tests, including Schirmer's tear test (STT), fluorescein dye tests, tonometry, culture, and exfoliative cytologic techniques, which are indicated by specific ocular signs. In certain instances, pathogenic agents or disease processes peculiar to cats are involved. In general, though, diagnosis and therapy of feline ocular problems are similar to management of ocular disorders of other companion animal species.

The numerous ocular disorders that affect domestic cats include congenital malformations; genetic disorders; inflammatory, infectious, and neoplastic disorders; and traumatic and degenerative conditions. Problems involving the conjunctiva, cornea, and anterior uvea seem especially prevalent. Feline glaucoma, with more subtle manifestations than in dogs, may be inadvertently overlooked.

CONGENITAL DISORDERS

Microphthalmos, anophthalmos, nanophthalmos, and cyclopia occur, though rarely. Burmese cats with a genetic craniofacial malformation are especially at risk. Esotropia, or medial strabismus, most commonly afflicts breeds with the Siamese (partially albinotic) coat color pattern. In these animals, it is due to disorganization of the lateral geniculate body and other subcortical centers controlling ocular position resulting from aberrantly increased decussation of optic nerve fibers. Vision appears reduced in proportion to the degree of esotropia and for the same reason. Surgical correction of eye position is not warranted. Nystagmus frequently accompanies esotropia as well as microphthalmos and nanophthalmos.

Dermoids occasionally involve the cornea, conjunctiva, or eyelids; Burmese cats appear at increased risk. Excision by keratoconjunctivectomy or *en bloc* eyelid resection is usually curative. Eyelid agenesis appears to be a sporadic nongenetic defect (see later). Punctal and nasolacrimal duct atresia or malformation occurs most commonly in the brachycephalic breeds.

Iris colobomas are infrequent. Persistent pupillary membranes cause focal corneal or lens opacities where they attach. Colobomas of the posterior segment occur; autosomal dominant inheritance has been suggested. Treatment is neither available nor necessary.

Congenital cataract occurs uncommonly as a result of genetic or teratogenic influences. Retinal dysplasia results from *in utero* or neonatal infection with panleukopenia virus and, experimentally, from feline leukemia virus infection. Cerebellar hypoplasia may accompany the condition.

Optic nerve hypoplasia and coloboma occur uncommonly, either alone or associated with other ocular defects (e.g., microphthalmos). Treatment is not available. Vision in affected eyes is poor to absent.

ACQUIRED DISORDERS

Orbit

INFLAMMATION

Clinical signs include periocular swelling, chemosis, nictitans prolapse, exophthalmos, pain on opening the mouth, fever, and anorexia, often of acute onset. Differential diagnosis includes primary versus secondary inflammation of the orbit (occurring by extension from a sinus or the oral cavity) as well as septic versus nonseptic inflammation. The diagnostic plan should include physical and ocular examinations, hemogram, and skull radiography to rule out unsuspected fracture, sinus, or dental disease. Because infection is the predominant cause, broad-spectrum antibiotic therapy (ampicillin, 10 to 20 mg/kg every 6 hr PO or 5 to 10 mg/kg every 6 hr IV, IM, or SC) should be initiated; parenteral administration is advised for the first 1 to 2 days pending improvement that would facilitate treatment per os. If improvement does not occur within 24 hr of treatment initiation, drainage of the orbit through the soft palate should be considered (see this volume, p. 1081). Anti-inflammatory dosages of prednisolone (0.22 mg/kg once daily) may be indicated if antibiotic therapy is incompletely effective.

NEOPLASIA

The clinical signs of orbital neoplasia parallel those of inflammation (exophthalmos, membrana nictitans prolapse, chemosis), except that pain, periocular swelling, and fever are absent. The onset of signs is usually gradual, often not apparent until exophthalmos or nictitans prolapse is marked. Middle-aged and older cats are at greater risk than young adults. Like canine orbital neoplasia, malignant tumor types predominate; both primary and secondary tumors (from local extension or distant metastasis) occur. Prognosis for life is poor, although palliative orbital exenteration may be worthwhile.

TRAUMATIC PROPTOSIS

Proptosis of the globe requires prompt emergency treatment to optimize prognosis for survival of the globe and, less likely, preservation of vision. Brachycephalic cats are predisposed; significantly greater trauma is required to cause proptosis in a cat with normal facial conformation. Emergency assessment and treatment are the same as for dogs (see this volume, p. 1081). Assessment should include complete physical, ocular, and neurologic examinations and skull radiography as soon as possible.

Eyelids

INFLAMMATION

Eyelid inflammation develops secondary to infections with bacteria, especially *Staphylococcus* (pyoderma, cellulitis, abscess), dermatophytes, or parasites (focal demodicosis, notoedric mange, cuterebriasis, other myiases) as well as primarily a manifestation of allergy (food allergy, atopy) or other immune-mediated disorders (pemphigus). Specific therapy should be directed toward elimination of infection (with antibiotics, antifungal drugs, parasiticides, surgical removal when appropriate), removal of offending allergens, or immunosuppressive therapy (Angarano, 1989; Scott, 1987).

NEOPLASIA

Unlike in dogs, eyelid neoplasia in cats is almost invariably *malignant*. Squamous cell carcinoma (especially in predominantly white-faced cats), basal cell carcinoma, mast cell tumor, fibrosarcoma, neurofibrosarcoma, hemangiosarcoma, adenocarcinoma, papilloma, fibroma, and hemangioma have been reported (Szymanski, 1987). Early wide excision of all eyelid masses in cats is strongly recommended. Distant metastases occasionally occur from eyelid masses.

ANATOMIC ABNORMALITIES

Entropion develops spontaneously in brachycephalic cats as well as secondarily in many other cats as a result of conjunctival or eyelid scarring (cicatricial entropion). Surgical correction of the anatomic component of the entropion (defined as that which remains following topical anesthesia of the eye in an unsedated animal) is usually curative. Cicatricial ectropion may follow healing of facial wounds. Surgical correction is indicated if exposure keratitis or conjunctivitis develops.

Ankyloblepharon, failure of neonatal eyelid separation, may be corrected in young kittens by gentle manual separation or careful separation with blunt scissors. The neonatal ophthalmia that is sometimes present should be treated by instillation of broad-spectrum topical antibiotic ointment four times daily for at least 1 week.

Eyelid lacerations should promptly be surgically repaired to minimize postoperative scarring and dysfunction. After two-layer closure with fine suture material, systemic and topical broad-spectrum antibiotic prophylaxis is indicated.

Eyelid agenesis, segmental failure of development of all layers of the eyelid (usually the lateral portion of both upper eyelids), is a sporadic, probably nongenetic malformation most commonly of mixed-breed cats. If it remains uncorrected, chronic corneal ulceration, vascularization, and scarring invariably develop secondary to exposure, dryness, and trichiasis. Functional surgical correction is challenging; aspiring surgeons are referred to veterinary ophthalmic and general surgical texts for details (see this volume, p. 1085).

Membrana Nictitans

PROLAPSE OF THE NICTITANS GLAND

Idiopathic nictitans gland prolapse ("cherry eye") occurs much less commonly in cats than dogs; Burmese cats are at greatest risk, with Siamese cats less so. Prolapsed glands should not be surgically excised (especially in Burmese), because keratoconjunctivitis sicca (KCS) almost invariably develops. Instead, surgical tacking of the gland to the orbital rim, to the ventral rectus muscle, or (less desirably) to the sclera should be performed (Szymanski, 1987).

MEMBRANA NICTITANS PROTRUSION

Causes of nictitans prolapse include Horner's syndrome, orbital masses, dehydration, cachexia, microphthalmos, phthisis bulbi, autonomic polyganglionopathy (Key-Gaskell syndrome), and tetanus. Idiopathic protrusion (haw syndrome) occurs primarily in young cats and usually resolves spontaneously. If vision is impaired, palliative therapy with topical 1 or 2% epinephrine (L-epinephrine Solution, Pharmafair) or 2.5% phenylephrine (Mydfrin Ophthalmic 2.5%, Alcon) twice a day may be prescribed.

NEOPLASIA

Primary neoplasia of the third eyelid is rare in cats. Fibrosarcoma, lymphosarcoma, squamous cell carcinoma, and adenocarcinoma have been encountered. Early complete excision of the nictitans is

the best potentially curative treatment; orbital extension (or origin) or distant metastasis may be complications. Exenteration may be required.

Lacrimal System

KERATOCONJUNCTIVITIS SICCA

Uncommon in cats, KCS is more commonly secondary to conjunctival swelling or scarring from acute or chronic inflammation or infection rather than primary secretory failure (the most common cause in dogs). Primary secretory failure does occur, however, especially as a potentially genetic disorder in Burmese, Abyssinian, and other purebred cats; KCS is occasionally associated with facial neuropathy, orbital inflammation, or traumatic injury. Much more commonly, clinicians mistakenly assess the finding of low STT values (wetting < 10 mm/min) in cats *in the absence of* corneal or conjunctival disease as KCS. The normal feline STT value is lower than a dog's (< 16 mm vs. > 20 mm).

Treatment objectives for KCS include (1) tear replacement, (2) infection control, and (3) lacrimation improvement. Aggressive tear replacement should be initiated and maintained as long as necessary; aqueous tear replacement (six or more times daily) and petrolatum ointment administration (at least every 6 hr) are recommended. Topical antibiotic therapy at least every 6 hr directed by results of periodic exfoliative conjunctival cytology should be used *intermittently*, for periods of 10 to 14 days, as needed. Continuous topical antibiotic therapy is counterproductive because of its propensity for promoting overgrowth of resistant bacterial strains. The safety and efficacy of topical 2% cyclosporine for KCS in cats are uncertain (see this volume, p. 1092).

Cornea

ULCERATION

The causes of superficial and deep corneal ulceration in cats include traumatic injury with or without foreign body (due to entropion or facial fold trichiasis, exogenous trauma); infection (bacterial, viral; rarely, mycotic, protozoal); lagophthalmos (due to orbital disorders, facial neuropathy); and KCS. The diagnostic plan should include a careful, *complete* ophthalmic examination that includes STT (*first!*), corneal culture collection and scraping for cytologic study (if ulceration is deep or progressive), and inspection of the bulbar surface of the nictitans after topical anesthesia.

Management of traumatic corneal perforation usually involves surgical wound closure; small self-sealing wounds may be allowed to heal with medical therapy and careful observation. Topical broad-spectrum antibiotic therapy (ointment every 6 hr), topical 1% atropine to maintain mydriasis, and systemic antibiotic therapy should be prescribed for at least 3 weeks. Deep stromal ulcers and descemetoceles should be supported by conjunctival flaps or free grafts or cyanoacrylate tissue adhesive.*

Infection with feline herpesvirus type 1 should be (at least) suspected to be the cause of most nontraumatic ulcers. The earliest lesion is a subtle dendritic erosion; focal to geographic superficial or deep ulcers occur also. Confirmation by viral culture or conjunctival fluorescent antibody testing (FABT) is ideal but inconsistent; negative test results probably do not preclude the diagnosis. Because fluorescein might cause a false-positive FABT result, samples should be collected before fluorescein instillation. Antiviral drug therapy for presumptive and confirmed infections should be instituted. *In vitro* experimental data confirm that trifluridine (Viroptic, Burroughs Wellcome), vidarabine (Vira-A Ophthalmic Ointment, Parke-Davis), and idoxuridine (Stoxil, Smith Kline & French) are effective against feline herpesvirus type 1; trifluridine was clearly superior to the other two agents (see this volume, p. 1049). No *in vivo* efficacy studies have been reported. Because of the high cost of trifluridine, I recommend initial therapy for presumptive herpesvirus keratitis with vidarabine or idoxuridine ointment six or more times daily. Trifluridine is reserved for persistent confirmed or presumptive infections.

Bacterial keratitis is suggested by extensive corneal edema, a yellow infiltrate surrounding the ulcer margins, progressive deepening or widening of the ulcer, or inappropriately severe anterior uveitis, often with hypopyon (Kern, 1990). Following cytologic examination of a corneal scraping and culture/sensitivity sample submission, intensive antibiotic therapy should be initiated and sustained until progression stops and the serious signs of ulceration resolve. Both fortified topical and subconjunctival antibiotic administration should be considered, as well as topical atropinization to effect; antiprotease agents may be indicated if "melting" is evident (see this volume, p. 1101; Kern, 1990).

SEQUESTRA

A uniquely feline abnormality, corneal sequestrum formation follows chronic epithelial erosion; the stroma develops a pale amber discoloration that progresses to a discrete brown or black opacity. Corneal neovascularization usually develops. Experimentally, some cats with chronic herpetic ker-

atitis developed sequestra (Nasisse, 1990). Lagophthalmos, entropion, tear film abnormalities, and genetic predisposition (brachycephalic cats) have been postulated to be promotional factors.

Treatment may be either medical or surgical. During several weeks or months, most sequestra slough from the cornea, associated with chronic corneal neovascularization. Prophylactic topical broad-spectrum antibiotic therapy and atropinization to effect are indicated if observation is elected. Keratectomy may expedite resolution, though all areas of affected stroma frequently cannot be safely excised. Sequestra may recur or develop in contralateral eyes. If present, anatomic entropion should be corrected or KCS should be treated.

EOSINOPHILIC/PROLIFERATIVE KERATOPATHY

Another uniquely feline abnormality, eosinophilic/proliferative keratopathy is an idiopathic keratopathy that appears as unilateral or bilateral, usually symmetric corneal neovascularization involving any corneal quadrant. Chronic lesions often have a white granular surface. The margin of a lesion may occasionally be ulcerated. A corneal scraping shows eosinophils, lymphocytes and plasma cells, and mast cells.

Therapy is topical corticosteroid administration on a regimen of decreasing frequency (e.g., six to eight times daily initially, reduced to one to three times daily over 4 to 6 weeks). Subconjunctival administration of a few milligrams of a repositol corticosteroid at initial presentation greatly improves the outcome. After 4 to 8 weeks of decreasing frequency, topical corticosteroid treatment is discontinued if lesions are inactive. If recurrences develop, long-term topical therapy may become necessary. Megestrol acetate (Ovaban, Schering) has been recommended by others as the initial treatment of choice; I prefer to avoid this drug for all except corticosteroid-nonresponsive cats because of its potentially serious side effects (e.g., diabetes mellitus and mammary hyperplasia).

Conjunctiva

INFLAMMATION

Primary conjunctivitis in cats results from infectious agents (bacteria, *Chlamydia*, *Mycoplasma*, viruses; rarely fungi or parasites), chemical irritation from environmental insults (smoke, soap, fumes), and possibly from allergy. Signs of conjunctivitis from these causes are generic; causation can rarely be inferred from clinical signs. Unilateral or bilateral chemosis (said to be most remarkable with *Chlamydia* infection), conjunctival hyperemia, and se-

---

*Ophthalmic Nexaband, CRX Medical, Raleigh, NC.

rous to mucopurulent discharge are present to various degrees. *Mycoplasma* is classically incriminated in conjunctival pseudomembrane formation. Calicivirus reputedly has a predilection for causing oral but not corneal ulceration. Herpesvirus may cause ulcerative keratitis. These distinctions are imperfect in clinical practice; documentation of etiology is difficult and expensive to achieve. The diagnostic plan for conjunctivitis should always include exfoliative conjunctival cytology examination for categorization of cellular response (relative neutrophil versus mononuclear cell response) and for inclusions and intracellular bacteria. Chlamydial inclusions in epithelial cells are large, sparse, intracytoplasmic, and near the nucleus. Mycoplasmal inclusions on the cell membrane are numerous and minute in size. Viral infection may be documented by FABT (herpesvirus) or viral isolation. Bacteria may be noted in the cytoplasm of neutrophils.

Treatment for chlamydial infection is topical tetracycline or chloramphenicol ointment every 6 hr for at least 1 month. Oral therapy with the same antibiotics is indicated at least in the presence of respiratory signs; note that tetracycline administered to kittens may result in dental discoloration and is best avoided. *Mycoplasma* is sensitive to most antibiotics except neomycin and penicillins. Presumed or proven herpesvirus conjunctivitis should be treated with an antiviral agent. Bacterial conjunctivitis, present alone or concurrent with infection by another agent, should be treated with broad-spectrum topical antibiotics. Secondary conjunctivitis may result from mechanical irritation (eyelid defects, foreign bodies), KCS, or periocular extension of intraocular, orbital, or eyelid inflammation. Careful complete ocular examination, including STT, *must* be performed every time! Identification and specific treatment for the offending cause are potentially curative.

Symblepharon, a pathologic adhesion between the conjunctiva and cornea, nictitans, or other conjunctival surfaces, may follow extensive conjunctival ulceration, presumably as a result of herpesvirus or *Mycoplasma*. Surgical treatment is difficult and frequently ineffective. KCS may result.

NEOPLASIA

Squamous cell carcinoma of the conjunctiva may appear as a chronic ulcerative or proliferative lesion; early excision is recommended. Limbal melanomas, rare in cats, appear to be benign; early excision or cryotherapy is probably indicated.

Uvea

INFLAMMATION

Anterior uveitis is a predictable sequela of corneal ulceration. Its severity and resolution parallel that of the keratitis. Iridocyclitis without corneal ulceration or choroiditis is usually a manifestation of obvious or occult systemic disease. Cats commonly are not presented for examination until anterior or posterior uveitis is chronic and advanced. Unlike in dogs, conjunctival hyperemia is often subtle or absent, ocular pain is not evident, and vision loss may be inapparent. Signs of anterior uveitis include keratic precipitates, dyscoria, rubeosis iridis, hypopyon, posterior and anterior synechiae, lens subluxation, and secondary glaucoma. Signs of choroiditis include multifocal retinal edema, hemorrhage, or detachment.

The diagnostic plan should include complete physical and ocular examinations (including *tonometry*), hemogram, serum chemistry panel, testing for feline viral infections (feline infectious peritonitis, leukemia, immunodeficiency viruses) and *Toxoplasma* serology. In endemic areas, systemic mycoses should be considered; serology and vitreocentesis may confirm the diagnosis. Specific therapy is available only for toxoplasmosis and the mycoses (see this volume, p. 1061). Nonspecific therapy should include topical corticosteroids and 1% atropine to effect. Glaucoma should be managed (see this volume, p. 1125).

NEOPLASIA

Primary uveal neoplasms are diffuse or solitary iris melanomas, ciliary body adenomas or adenocarcinomas, or sarcomas. Enucleation is strongly recommended; diffuse iris melanoma, especially, metastasizes early. Multicentric or secondary neoplasia has a grave prognosis; lymphosarcoma is the most common. Uveal neoplasia may masquerade as anterior or posterior uveitis and should be suspected if palliative treatment for uveitis fails.

Glaucoma

Primary glaucoma is uncommon in cats. Elevated intraocular pressures (IOP) without evidence of significant inflammation, hemorrhage, or neoplasia suggest this diagnosis. The iridocorneal angle (visible without a goniolens because of the cat's deep anterior chamber and large cornea) may appear normal, narrow, or closed. Unlike in dogs, corneal edema and episcleral injection are not necessarily present, even with very high IOP.

Secondary glaucoma is probably more common than primary. Chronic anterior uveitis due to infection, neoplasia, or occult causes is usually responsible. Diagnosis is substantiated by increased IOP with vision loss in the presence of signs of uveitis or neoplasia. Extensive hyphema or vitreous hemorrhage due to trauma or coagulopathy is occasionally responsible.

Therapy for glaucoma includes oral carbonic anhydrase inhibitors (especially methazolamide [Neptazane, Lederle; ≤2 to 4 mg/kg every 12 hr]), topical sympathomimetics, and beta-blocking drugs (see this volume, p. 1125). When glaucoma is not responsive to medical therapy, enucleation is indicated. Evisceration with intrascleral silicone prosthesis implantation may be used for eyes unlikely to harbor neoplasms or bacterial or fungal infections. *The evisceration specimen must be examined histologically to rule out these conditions..*

Lens

LUXATION/SUBLUXATION

Unilateral or bilateral lens subluxation in the absence of obvious uveitis or elevated IOP occurs in cats (especially nonpurebred), in which its natural history parallels that of the canine condition. Affected cats typically develop chronic glaucoma, more likely due to a physiologic predisposition than to a simple effect of lens displacement; glaucoma is often well established even before lens subluxation is severe. Retinal detachment may develop. Medical therapy for glaucoma, including treatment with miotic drugs, is indicated; tonometry should be performed regularly. Referral for removal of anteriorly luxated lenses may become necessary. With or without lensectomy, long-term prognosis for vision retention is guarded to poor.

CATARACT

Cataracts are distinctly uncommon in cats. Inherited cataracts have been described in Persians (with and without Chédiak-Higashi syndrome) and Himalayans. Unlike dogs, cats with diabetes mellitus rarely develop significant cataracts. The most common cause of cataract in cats is chronic uveitis; focal lens opacities develop from synechiae, whereas mature cataracts develop after chronic inflammation. Such cats are not candidates for lens extraction because other uveitis sequelae have probably rendered affected eyes permanently blind. Penetrating injury that involves the lens may cause focal or complete cataract formation. Lens injury predictably results in chronic severe lens protein–associated uveitis that threatens permanent blindness.

Retina

DEGENERATION

Nutritional retinal degeneration is associated with taurine deficiency. Lesions typically begin focally in the area centralis (hence the term *feline central retinal degeneration*) then expand into a band above the tapetal/nontapetal junction. Generalized degeneration ensues. Plasma taurine levels may be low or normal. The diet of affected cats should be investigated; taurine supplementation may be indicated.

Inherited retinal degeneration occurs uncommonly in cats. Abyssinians have retinopathies of both early (8 to 12 weeks of age, dominantly inherited) and later onset (1.5 to 2 years, recessively inherited). Early onset (4 months of age) of recessively inherited retinal degeneration has been encountered in Persians.

Postinflammatory retinal degeneration, usually focal or multifocal rather than generalized, follows retinitis or chorioretinitis due to various infections (parasitic [e.g., toxoplasmosis, migrating nematode or dipterous larvae]; mycotic, bacterial, viral [e.g., feline infectious peritonitis, panleukopenia, possibly feline immunodeficiency virus]).

DETACHMENT

Retinal detachment occurs because the retina is pushed off, pulled off, or perforated. Traction from vitreal inflammation (a common complication of anterior uveitis) or hemorrhage; choroidal or retinal effusion from inflammation, infection, or hypertension; or injury may be involved. If the underlying disorder is treatable (e.g., hypertension, systemic mycosis), retinal reattachment may occur; degeneration of the affected retina usually ensues (see this volume, p. 1061).

Optic Nerve

INFLAMMATION

Optic neuritis is usually a manifestation of intraocular infection such as cryptococcosis (or other systemic mycosis), feline infectious peritonitis, toxoplasmosis; orbital inflammation; or traumatic proptosis. Treatment should be directed toward the suspected or proven etiology. Optic atrophy is a likely sequela.

NEOPLASIA

Primary (meningiomas, astrocytomas), multicentric (lymphosarcoma), and metastatic (from any site) optic nerve neoplasms occasionally occur. Exenteration with histopathologic evaluation is necessary for diagnosis. With rare exceptions, prognosis is grave.

Neuro-Ophthalmic Disorders

HORNER'S SYNDROME

Horner's syndrome (ptosis, miosis, apparent enophthalmos, nictitans prolapse) occurs secondary to interruption of the sympathetic innervation of the eye and adnexa. Interruption of the pathway anywhere between the hypothalamus and the eye produces signs of variable prominence and duration. Cranial, cervical, orbital, thoracic, or middle/inner ear traumatic injury, infection, or neoplasia must be ruled out. In many instances, no cause is apparent. The prognosis for resolution is generally favorable, though dependent on the prognosis for the inciting cause, if discovered (Kern et al., 1989; Morgan and Zanotti, 1989).

FACIAL NEUROPATHY

Facial nerve dysfunction leading to lagophthalmos may develop after surgical or nonsurgical trauma or otitis media/interna associated with infection or neoplasia (Kern and Erb, 1987). Horner's syndrome or KCS may be present. Facial neuropathy was idiopathic in 25% of cases (Kern and Erb, 1987). Treatment is directed toward eliminating the cause (e.g., otitis media/interna) and protecting the eye with lubricants. Prognosis for resolution is fair.

FELINE DYSAUTONOMIA (KEY-GASKELL SYNDROME)

The ocular manifestations of this idiopathic, often fatal condition primarily encountered in the United Kingdom include KCS, mydriasis, blepharospasm, and nictitans prolapse. Tear replacement is required. Prognosis is poor.

References and Suggested Reading

Angarano, D. W.: Dermatologic disorders of the eyelid and periocular region. In Kirk, R. W. (ed.): Current Veterinary Therapy X. Philadelphia: W. B. Saunders, 1989, p. 678.
A discussion of the differential diagnosis and treatments of eyelid dermatologic disorders.
Kern, T. J.: Ulcerative keratitis. Vet. Clin. North Am. Small Anim. Pract. 20:643, 1990.
A detailed review of diagnostic and therapeutic management of corneal ulceration in small animals.
Kern, T. J., Aromando, M. C., and Erb, H. N.: Horner's syndrome in dogs and cats: 100 cases (1975–1985). J.A.V.M.A. 195:369, 1989.
An epidemiologic review and analysis of the relationship between Horner's syndrome and signalment, potential causes, and associated clinical signs in 74 dogs and 26 cats.
Kern, T. J., and Erb, H. N.: Facial neuropathy in dogs and cats: 95 cases (1975–1985). J.A.V.M.A. 191:1604, 1987.
An epidemiologic review and analysis of the relationship between facial nerve dysfunction and signalment, potential causes, and associated clinical signs in 79 dogs and 16 cats.
Morgan, R. V., and Zanotti, S. W.: Horner's syndrome in dogs and cats: 49 cases (1980–1986). J.A.V.M.A. 194:1096, 1989.
A tabulation of the causes and outcomes of Horner's syndrome in 33 dogs and 16 cats.
Nasisse, M. P.: Feline herpesvirus ocular disease. Vet. Clin. North Am. Small Anim. Pract. 20:667, 1990.
A comprehensive review of the natural history, clinical syndromes, and current treatments of ocular feline herpesvirus type 1 infection.
Nasisse, M. P.: Feline opthalmology. In Gelatt K. N. (ed.): Veterinary Ophthalmology, 2nd ed. Philadelphia: Lea & Febiger, 1991, pp. 529–575.
An extensively referenced comprehensive review of feline ophthalmology.
Scott, D. W.: The skin. In Holzworth, J. (ed.): Diseases of the cat. Medicine and Surgery. Vol. 1. Philadelphia: W. B. Saunders, 1987, p. 619.
An extensive review of diagnosis and treatment of feline skin disorders.
Slatter, D. H.: Fundamentals of Veterinary Ophthalmology, 2nd ed. Philadelphia: W. B. Saunders, 1990.
A comprehensive contemporary text that details practical medical and surgical ophthalmology in all species of veterinary interest.
Szymanski, C.: The eye. In Holzworth J. (ed.): Diseases of the Cat. Medicine and Surgery. Vol. 1. Philadelphia: W. B. Saunders, 1987, p. 676.
A comprehensive review of feline ophthalmic disorders with extensive literature citations.

GERIATRIC OPHTHALMIC DISORDERS

STEPHANIE L. SMEDES

Madison, Wisconsin

Few ophthalmic disorders are unique to geriatric patients. However, several disease states and senile changes occur with increased frequency in older dogs and cats.

EYELID DISORDERS

Lagophthalmos

Partial or complete lagophthalmos due to facial neuropathy has an increased incidence in dogs 7 years or older and cats 6 years or older. It may be idiopathic or secondary to otitis media/interna. The relationship between facial neuropathy and hypothyroidism is unclear. Its occurrence had been statistically associated with low resting serum T_4 levels, but not with thyroid-stimulating hormone (TSH) response test–confirmed hypothyroidism (Kern and Erb, 1987). Animals with facial paralysis/paresis may have concurrent keratoconjunctivitis sicca (KCS), vestibular signs, a propensity for indolent or recurrent ulcers, or dryness of the axial cornea with associated keratitis. These animals may benefit from permanent lateral tarsorrhaphy, in addition to treatment for their concurrent or secondary disorders.

Older animals, including those without lagophthalmos due to facial neuropathy or facial conformation, may sleep with their eyes partially open. These animals may also benefit from permanent lateral canthal closures or the application of artificial tear ointments (Lacrilube, Allergan; Duratears, Alcon) before periods of sleep.

Entropion

Entropion may manifest itself in older animals as a result of masticatory muscle atrophy, dehydration, or debilitating disease, with resultant loss of retrobulbar tissue. Depending on the expected duration of the condition, temporary eyelid tacking or permanent surgical repair may be indicated to decrease the likelihood of corneal irritation, keratitis, and ulcer formation.

Eyelid Tumors

Eyelid tumors occur frequently in geriatric patients. Most tumors in dogs are meibomian (sebaceous) gland adenomas, melanomas, and papillomas. Almost all are benign, although histologically the melanomas may appear malignant. Eyelid tumors in dogs cause problems by local invasion of adjacent tissues, contact irritation of the cornea, or interference with eyelid function. Early removal by wedge or pentagonal resection is recommended when excision still can be accomplished by removal of one fourth to one third or less of the eyelid margin. (The amount that can be removed depends on the degree of laxity of the lid margin and therefore is a function of the breed.) Larger masses may require reconstructive blepharoplasty techniques for complete excision (Barrie and Gelatt, 1980). All excised tumors should be submitted for histopathologic examination. Cryosurgery can be used successfully with large or small eyelid tumors. This is an especially desirable technique in aged animals, because it can often be adequately accomplished with sedation and local anesthesia (Roberts et al., 1986). The tumor should be debulked initially, allowing more adequate freezing of tissues and making available a sample for histopathologic examination.

Unlike in dogs, eyelid masses in cats are usually malignant. Squamous cell carcinomas are the most common feline eyelid tumors. They can be very invasive, causing eyelid ulceration, thickening, and destruction. Basal cell carcinomas have also been reported in cats. Metastases are rare, but local invasiveness is common. Early and complete treatment of feline eyelid tumors by surgical resection or cryosurgery is recommended. Histopathologic examination is indicated.

CONDITIONS OF THE LACRIMAL SYSTEM AND CORNEA

Keratoconjunctivitis Sicca (KCS)

KCS, inadequate tear production, occurs with significantly increased frequency in older animals. Clinical signs include a tenacious, ropey, mucopurulent ocular discharge; blepharospasm, lackluster appearance of the cornea; conjunctivitis; and melanosis and neovascularization of the cornea. Not all animals exhibit each of these signs, and the degree of reduction in tear quantity is not necessarily related to the severity of signs. Any animal with the previously mentioned signs, recurrent conjunctivitis, or corneal ulceration should be evaluated for KCS and treated appropriately (see this volume, p. 1092).

Persistent Corneal Ulcers

Persistent corneal ulcers or erosions (boxer ulcers, indolent ulcers, and chronic corneal erosions) are epithelial erosions that have an abnormally prolonged rate of healing or that appear to heal adequately, only to recur a short time later. Redundant or loose edges of corneal epithelium are characteristically noted at the ulcer margins. After ruling out predisposing conditions (e.g., KCS, lagophthalmos, eyelid tumors, chalazia, infectious keratoconjunctivitis, ectopic cilia, or foreign body), corneal endothelial dystrophies, corneal epithelial/basement membrane diseases, and neurotrophic keratitis should be considered in older animals. Treatment is aimed at controlling the underlying disease, removing nonadherent epithelium, and promoting more normal epithelial adhesion (see this volume, p. 1101).

Corneal Endothelial Dystrophy

Corneal endothelial dystrophy is due to loss and incomplete replacement of normal endothelium. It presents clinically as diffuse corneal edema. Epithelial and stromal bullae and keratoconus are potential sequelae. If the bullae rupture, a chronic corneal erosion can result.

Clinical cure is difficult. Topical 5% sodium chloride ointments or drops (Muro 128, Bausch & Lomb; AK-NaCl, Akorn), applied one to four times a day, are used topically as hyperosmotic, dehydrating agents to reduce the amount of edema. The edema usually requires treatment indefinitely and only partially resolves. Animals occasionally develop chronic conjunctival irritation from the medications, necessitating discontinued use.

Corneal Degeneration

Corneal degenerations occur more commonly in older dogs and, rarely, in elderly cats. Animals present with opacification of the corneal epithelium or stroma due to lipid or calcium deposition. The superficial layers of the cornea are more frequently involved than the deep layers. Lipid degenerations are usually spicule-like in appearance, whereas calcium is likely to appear as bright white specks within the cornea. A biomicroscope may be necessary to make this differentiation. The degenerations may occur primarily or be associated with chronic ocular inflammation, corneal irritation or ulceration, lagophthalmos, or systemic diseases causing hypercholesterolemia, hyperlipidemia, or hypercalcemia. Measurement of serum levels of cholesterol, triglyceride, or calcium may prove useful.

Degenerations do not usually require specific treatment unless their severity precludes useful vision or unless they are associated with a chronic nonhealing ulcer. Superficial keratectomy may be performed to remove the affected layers of cornea, but the regenerated epithelial and subepithelial tissues often rapidly become reinvolved with the degenerative process. Alternatively, topical ethylenediaminetetraacetic acid (EDTA) has been advocated for dissolution of calcium; its application is quite painful, and general anesthesia is required. Treatment two to four times daily with an artificial tear ointment (Lacrilube, Allergan; Duratears, Alcon) may decrease the occurrence of chronic irritation with secondary superficial erosions.

DISORDERS OF THE UVEA

Iris Atrophy

Iris atrophy is a common aging change in both cats and dogs and is the single most common cause of incomplete pupillary light reflexes. If the iridal sphincter muscle atrophies, the pupillary margin will have an irregular edge. Strands of iris occasionally remain and span across portions of the pupil. Less commonly, the iris stroma or iris dilator muscle atrophies, leaving large holes that resemble multiple pupillary openings.

Uveal Cysts

Uveal cysts can form off the pigmented epithelium of the iris or ciliary body epithelium. They may be attached or free-floating in the anterior or posterior chamber or in the pupillary space and can be transilluminated, an important characteristic distinguishing them from intraocular melanomas. They usually require no treatment but can be aspirated with a 27- or 30-gauge needle if excessively large. Golden and Labrador retrievers appear to be affected more commonly than other breeds.

CONDITIONS OF THE LENS

Senile and pathologic changes in the lenses of domestic dogs and cats are quite common. Nuclear sclerosis, cataract formation, and lens luxation/subluxation are the most frequent changes. Nuclear sclerosis begins to occur at 5 to 6 years of age and can become quite marked by 11 to 12 years of age. This opacification of the central portion of the lens is secondary to compaction of nuclear lens fibers. Direct illumination through this is possible, and the fundus should be visible. However, when trying to view the fundus through dense nuclear sclerosis, it may be more easily seen with indirect than with direct ophthalmoscopy. A tapetal reflex can be elicited, and retroillumination reveals a pearlescent ring in the center of the lens. On retroillumination of the lens, a cataract appears as an opacity within the tapetal reflex; if extensive, it may interfere with direct examination of the fundus. An important distinction between nuclear sclerosis and a cataract is that nuclear sclerosis does not interfere appreciably with vision or visual evaluation of the fundus, whereas a cataract may, depending on the stage of development and location within the lens. Nuclear sclerosis requires no treatment. Because it does not interfere with vision, the eyes of animals with nuclear sclerosis and visual deficits should be further evaluated. Removal may be considered for senile cataracts (nonhereditary, noninflammatory, nondiabetic cataracts occurring in older animals with concurrent nuclear sclerosis) if they interfere significantly with vision and the animal's quality of life (see this volume, p. 1119).

DISORDERS OF THE VITREOUS

Four changes commonly occur within the vitreous of geriatric patients: vitreal liquefaction, vitreal floaters, asteroid hyalosis, and synchysis scintillans.

Vitreal Liquefaction

As an animal ages, the vitreous may undergo degenerative liquefaction (syneresis). The change is not detectable unless vitreal floaters or synchysis scintillans is visible.

Vitreal Floaters

Vitreal floaters are focal condensations of collagenous vitreal remnants that remain after liquefaction or inflammation. They appear as strands of white or pigmented tissue within the vitreous, where they may shadow the retina. Uncommonly they occur in the anterior chamber. Rarely they are associated with fly-catching behavior. This behavior usually has a neurologic origin, however.

Asteroid Hyalosis

Asteroid hyalosis is a collection of minute calcium-lipid opacities suspended within the vitreous. The opacities move slightly with eye movement and return to their former positions when the eye is at rest. Little or no evidence of vitreal liquefaction is present. Asteroid hyalosis usually does not interfere with an animal's vision, although it may make fundus examination difficult.

Synchysis Scintillans

In patients with synchysis scintillans, cholesterol crystals are present within a liquefied vitreous. They settle ventrally when the animal is at rest, resembling the glass-encased scenes of snowstorms that swirl around when shaken.

All four vitreal changes are irreversible. No treatment is necessary unless an ongoing hyalitis or chorioretinitis is present. Therapy is then aimed at discovering and treating the primary or secondary disorder.

DISORDERS OF THE RETINA

Progressive Retinal Atrophy

Progressive retinal atrophy (PRA) has an increased incidence in many breeds of dogs and most often afflicts young or middle-aged animals. Certain breeds (e.g., miniature and toy poodles) are more prone to PRA in later years. Signs include progressive vision loss, first occurring in dim light settings, eventually resulting in complete blindness. The rate of progression is variable. The tapetal fundus appears variably hyper-reflective, with vascular attenuation and optic nerve atrophy. No treatment is available.

Sudden Acquired Retinal Degeneration

Sudden acquired retinal degeneration (SARD) is reported to occur most commonly in dogs 6 to 11 years old. Affected dogs become blind within 24 hr to 1 month. The retina initially appears normal but with time becomes identical to a retina with end-stage PRA. Sudden blindness due to SARD must be differentiated from optic neuropathy. A definitive diagnosis is based on electroretinogram results. The cause is unknown, and the changes are irreversible (see *CVT X*, p. 644).

Peripheral Cystoid Retinal Degeneration

Peripheral cystoid retinal degeneration is characterized by the presence of single or multiple nonpigmented cystic structures within the peripheral sensory retina. These structures are most easily observed by indirect ophthalmoscopy following maximal mydriasis. They cause no discernible problem.

Retinal Detachment

Retinal detachments occur more commonly in older than in younger cats. They may be the result of the retina being pushed off by a subretinal or choroidal mass or exudate. Of particular importance in aged cats is *hypertensive retinopathy*, with retinal detachment or retinal hemorrhage, which may be idiopathic or secondary to hyperthyroidism or kidney disease. I routinely evaluate cases of retinal detachment in older cats with a hemogram, serum biochemical profile, urinalysis, baseline thyroid hormone level, and blood pressure measurement.

Older dogs do not appear to be at increased risk for retinal detachment as compared with younger dogs. When detachments occurs, I recommend evaluation of a routine hemogram, serum biochemical profile, urinalysis, and blood pressure measurement. Because dogs can develop hypertensive retinopathy secondary to hypothyroidism, evaluation of thyroid function (e.g., TSH response test, when available) may be indicated.

Treatment in both dogs and cats is aimed at correcting the underlying disease when possible (see *CVT IX*, p. 360). If an animal's state of health does not preclude their use, diuretics and corticosteroids can be used to encourage reattachment.

Feline Central Retinal Degeneration

Feline central retinal degeneration (FCRD) is a bilateral, symmetric, horizontally oval-shaped region of hyper-reflectivity initially located temporal to the optic disk in the region of the area centralis. The nasal portion of the retina may become involved later. At end stage, the entire tapetal fundus is hyper-reflective. FCRD is due to taurine deficiency. The retinal changes are irreversible but no longer progress once the cat is placed on a diet that is adequately supplemented with taurine. Because all commercial cat foods are now supplemented with taurine, it is likely that the only cats found to have this disease will be older cats affected at a young age, cats on noncommercial feline diets, or those with malabsorptive or maldigestive disorders.

INTRAOCULAR TUMORS

Uveal Neoplasms

The most common primary intraocular neoplasms in dogs and cats are uveal melanomas. Most are benign in dogs, but still warrant close follow-up examinations; malignancies are possible, and even benign tumors can cause glaucoma if tumor cells infiltrate the iridocorneal angle. Aggressive-appearing tumors may warrant early enucleation to decrease the risk of distant metastases.

In contrast to dogs, in cats, uveal tumors are not usually solid masses but rather present as diffuse infiltrations of the iris. They must be differentiated from the normal age-related pigmentary changes of the feline iris. Tumors are raised off the iridal surface and may cause irregular pupillary margins or secondary glaucoma. Pigmentary changes are flattened areas within the iris that do not disrupt the iridal contours.

Histopathologic studies of feline uveal melanomas show a high prevalence of malignancy. Therefore, they warrant close observation. I currently recommend removal of all feline eyes that have unquestionable iridal pigmentary masses, if the cat can be shown to be free of biochemical and radiographic evidence of metastases. Distant metastases may become evident as late as 2 years after enucleation (Dubielzig, 1990).

Other primary and secondary intraocular tumors can occur. The presence of any intraocular mass merits the performance of a complete physical examination to look for evidence of distant involvement.

ORBITAL DISEASE

Animals with orbital masses present with prolapse of the third eyelid, episcleral injection, variable pain when the mouth is opened, exophthalmos, or less commonly enophthalmos. In general, tumors are less painful than infections, have a slower and more insidious onset, and are more common in older animals (see this volume, p. 1081).

References and Suggested Reading

Barrie, K. P., and Gelatt, K. N.: Diseases of the eyelids, Part I. Comp. Cont. Ed. Pract. Vet. 1:405, 1980.
A review of eyelid disorders including descriptive techniques for surgical removal of eyelid masses.
Dubielzig, R. R.: Ocular neoplasia in small animals. Vet. Clin. North Am. Small Anim. Pract. 20:837, 1990.
A review of the clinical presentation and histopathologic characteristics of tumors in the canine and feline globe.
Fischer, C. A.: Geriatric ophthalmology. Vet. Clin. North Am. Small Anim. Pract. 19:103, 1989.
A comprehensive review of disorders and normal aging changes found in the eyes and related structures of geriatric dogs and cats.
Kern, T. J., and Erb, H. N.: Facial neuropathy in dogs and cats: 95 cases (1975–1985). J.A.V.M.A. 191:1604, 1987.
A retrospective study of the potential association between facial neuropathy and other disorders.
Roberts, S. M., Severin, G. A., and Lavach, J. D.: Prevalence and treatment of palpebral neoplasms in the dog: 200 cases (1975–1983). J.A.V.M.A. 189:1355, 1986.
A retrospective study of the type, treatment and recurrence of palpebral neoplasias, including a description of the protocol for cryosurgical removal of such masses.

DISORDERS OF THE ORBIT

DENISE M. LINDLEY

West Lafayette, Indiana

Orbital disease is relatively common in dogs and cats and is caused by a wide spectrum of abnormalities. Clinicians should be aware of the differential diagnosis for orbital disease. Accurate diagnosis is essential for the selection of correct treatment. Disorders of the orbit can be divided into those causing exophthalmos due to space-occupying disease and those causing enophthalmos due to decreased orbital contents. The challenge lies in the fact that orbital disorders are evident only indirectly, and signs involve changes in surrounding structures.

FUNCTIONAL ANATOMY OF THE ORBIT

Lesions affecting orbital contents or structures adjacent to the orbit may cause orbital disease; therefore, an understanding of orbital anatomy is important.

The orbit is a conical cavity with its apex located posteriorly at the orbital fissure. In dogs and cats, only the orbital roof and medial wall are osseous. The orbital floor and lateral wall are soft tissue. The ventral floor is composed of zygomatic salivary gland, medial pterygoid muscle, and fat. The orbital ligament forms the lateral aspect of the otherwise bony anterior orbital margin, whereas the ramus of the mandible, masseter muscle, and zygomatic arch contribute to form the posterior orbital margin. The frontal sinus is located dorsal to the orbit, and the maxillary sinus is ventral to it. Between the bony medial orbital walls is the nasal cavity. The ventral floor of the orbit is close to the oral cavity and alveoli of the upper premolar and molar teeth. The orbital cavity contains the second, third, and fourth cranial nerves, the ophthalmic branch of the fifth cranial nerve; the sixth cranial nerves, arteries, and veins; smooth muscle; and extraocular muscles ensheathed by periorbita. The lacrimal gland lies dorsolateral to the globe. Orbital fat supports the orbital contents and allows for movement of the globe.

SPACE-OCCUPYING ORBITAL DISEASE

Because the orbit is a finite space and the globe is mobile, the location and volume of a space-occupying lesion determine the direction and amount of displacement of the globe. Skeletal conformation, enlargement of normal structures due to inflammation, and mass lesions result in exophthalmos, the hallmark of space-occupying orbital disease. Because the orbital space is cone-shaped and has a wide anterior base, each additional increment of exophthalmos requires a greater volume of space-occupying orbital disease. Assessment of position of the exophthalmic globe may help determine the position of the mass. Decreased ocular motility and retropulsion are found on ophthalmic examination. Tonometric readings in exophthalmic globes are usually normal. Glaucoma is not a cause of exophthalmos; therefore, buphthalmos must be differentiated from exophthalmos. Exophthalmos can be congenital or acquired, caused by retrobulbar cellulitis or abscess, eosinophilic myositis, zygomatic mucocele, orbital neoplasia, craniomandibular osteopathy (hyperostosis), or proptosis secondary to trauma or severe buphthalmos.

Congenital (Relative) Exophthalmos

Shallow orbits in brachycephalic breeds result in decreased orbital space and prominent, protruding globes. Bilateral, symmetric exophthalmos may be accompanied by divergent strabismus and is a brachycephalic breed-related condition. The anterior placement of the globes and the large palpebral fissures in brachiocephalic breeds cause lagophthalmus. These brachycephalic dogs may sleep with their eyelids partially open. The inability to adequately distribute tear film, especially over the central cornea, results in exposure keratitis, which may lead to ulcerative and pigmentary keratitis. The exposure keratitis may be further aggravated by keratoconjunctivitis sicca, which also commonly occurs in brachycephalic breeds. Corneal sequestrum is more common in cats with exophthalmos. Use of ophthalmic lubricant ointments provides corneal protection for both cats and dogs. Lateral canthoplasty is the permanent treatment of choice for lagophthalmos in dogs. It preserves tear film and provides better eyelid coverage for the globe. Lateral canthoplasty also decreases the likelihood of traumatic proptosis. The lateral canthus is surgically moved medially, usually requiring 25 to 30% closure of the eyelid fissure. The lateral limbus is a useful surgical landmark for the amount of lateral eyelid fissure closure necessary for each animal.

Congenital arteriovenous fistulas have been reported rarely in dogs and cats. Diagnosis is made by auscultation of a bruit over the orbit. It is confirmed by orbital angiography. No specific therapy is recommended, because circulatory embarrassment to the globe is possible even after successful surgical correction. Exenteration may be necessary in patients with severe exophthalmos.

Retrobulbar Cellulitis and Abscess

Inflammatory orbital diseases include orbital cellulitis, retrobulbar abscess, and myositis. Presenting signs can be similar. The animal may show pain when opening its mouth. The pain may be evidenced by a reluctance to eat, especially hard food. Most animals with inflammatory orbital disease continue to drink. Early clinical signs of orbital cellulitis or abscess and acute myositis include asymmetry of globe position, decreased globe motility, serous to mucopurulent ocular discharge, chemosis secondary to decreased venous return from the orbit, conjunctival hyperemia, prolapse and congestion of the third eyelid, acute onset of periocular pain, pain when opening the mouth, lethargy, and fever. Corneal ulceration may be present secondary to lagophthalmos caused by exophthalmos and exposure keratoconjunctivitis. In addition, visual deficits can occur if the optic nerves are involved or posterior orbital inflammation induces chorioretinitis and secondary retinal detachment. Complete physical and ophthalmic examinations are always indicated.

Retrobulbar abscess is often clinically indistinguishable from orbital cellulitis. Cellulitis or retrobulbar abscess is most likely caused by penetration of foreign bodies through the soft palate, skin, or conjunctiva into the orbit; trauma; abscessation of molar teeth; extension of paranasal sinus infection; or hematogenous spread in cases of septicemia. Foreign bodies (e.g., sewing needles, plant material) are often implicated but seldom found. Aerobic and anaerobic orbital infection secondary to foreign body penetration from the oropharynx is plausible, because organisms associated with orbital infections are often the same aerobes and anaerobes found in normal oral flora. *Pasteurella multocida* and Enterobacteriaceae are common aerobic isolates. Three bacterial genera reported in anaerobic infections are *Bacteroides*, *Fusobacterium*, and *Peptostreptococcus*. Polymicrobial infections of the orbit are common. Retrobulbar abscess may be associated with septicemia.

Nonbacterial causes of inflammatory orbital disease are uncommon. *Aspergillus* and *Penicillium* organisms have been implicated in orbital cellulitis secondary to sinusitis in cats. Orbital lesions have been observed in dogs with coccidioidomycosis and blastomycosis. *Pneumonyssus caninum*, *Dirofilaria immitis*, and *Ancylostoma* have been documented in canine orbital cellulitis. Nutritional steatitis in cats is also a cause of orbital inflammation.

In all cases of exophthalmos, the first and foremost therapeutic consideration, even before diagnostic workup, is protection of the corneal surface. This can be accomplished by topical application of ophthalmic lubricants (Lacrilube, Allergan). Definitive diagnosis and treatment of inflammatory orbital disease require general anesthesia of the patient. Digital palpation of the orbit, a thorough oral examination, skull radiographs, B-mode ultrasonography, cytologic study, biopsy, or a combination of these methods is indicated.

Oral examination is performed with the use of an oral speculum. A fluctuant, erythematous mucous membrane behind the last upper molar is usually present with orbital inflammation. A small draining tract can occasionally be found at this site. Skull radiographs aid in identifying radiodense orbital foreign bodies, extension of infection from adjacent sinuses, zygomatic arch fractures, and associated orbital osteomyelitis. Thoracic radiographs may be helpful in cases of suspected mycotic infection. B-mode ultrasonography allows noninvasive examination of the orbital soft-tissue space that is poorly visualized by radiographic techniques. Ultrasonographic retrobulbar inflammatory changes vary from diffuse hyperechoic changes to a discrete hypoechoic mass. Fine-needle aspirates of the retrobulbar space taken through the conjunctiva are also useful in diagnosing causes of inflammation.

Surgical drainage of the retrobulbar space is often necessary for successful treatment of orbital cellulitis or abscess. Before establishing ventral drainage of the orbital cavity, the endotracheal cuff must be inflated to prevent potential aspiration of mucopurulent exudate. The mucosa behind the last upper molar is surgically prepared with povidone-iodine solution (Betadine Solution, Purdue Frederick). The mucosa is incised with a number 15 surgical blade. Because the maxillary artery lies deep to the submucosa, insertion of sharp objects into the ventral retrobulbar space must be avoided. A closed, curved hemostat is inserted to the point of the hinge, and the jaw is gently and completely opened.

Several milliliters of serosanguineous to purulent fluid may drain from the opening and should be collected sterilely for aerobic and anaerobic bacterial and fungal cultures. Slides for Gram's stain and cytologic examination should also be submitted. Drainage may not be evident in many cases. Premoistened culture swabs (Culturette, Scientific Products, McGaw, IL) should be inserted deep into the opening to obtain specimens for culture and cytologic examination. The retrobulbar space can be flushed through the ventral opening with 1:9

povidone-iodine and saline. In rare cases, when incomplete orbital foreign body removal occurs (e.g., wood splinters), it may be desirable to prevent early closure of the ventral opening into the orbital space. A 6-mm (¼-in.) Penrose drain can be inserted into the retrobulbar space to allow for continued drainage of necrotic debris. Repeated flushing of the retrobulbar space with dilute povidone-iodine is possible through the Penrose drain site. The hemostats are repositioned into the opening, and at the point where the hemostat tents the skin of the dorsolateral orbit, an incision is made. One end of the drain is pulled to the mouth, with 2 cm extending into the oral cavity. The drain is sutured to the skin with 4-0 nonabsorbable suture. The drain is removed in 5 to 7 days as signs associated with orbital inflammation decrease. Hot packs help reduce orbital swelling. Additional therapy is aimed at controlling infection and decreasing inflammation.

Antibiotics should be chosen empirically and used in conjunction with retrobulbar drainage until culture and sensitivity test results can be obtained. These include ampicillin (20 mg/kg IV every 6 hr) or chloramphenicol (50 mg/kg IV every 8 hr) because of their broad aerobic and anaerobic spectrum and good tissue penetration. Antibiotics administered parenterally are important in acute disease, because oral administration is difficult owing to pain when opening the mouth. In addition, a longer time is necessary to reach therapeutic blood concentrations. *In vitro* susceptibility, when available, should direct further systemic antibiotic therapy. When inflammation is subsiding and pain is minimal, as evidenced by willingness to eat, antibiotic therapy can be given orally. Topical antibiotic ointment can be administered for conjunctivitis.

Systemic anti-inflammatory agents in initial therapy (prednisone, 2 mg/kg SC every 24 hr initially, then PO) may be indicated when inflammation is severe and vision is threatened. The dosage of prednisone is tapered as soft-tissue swelling decreases. Anti-inflammatory therapy is important to minimize the inflammatory sequelae of retrobulbar abscess or cellulitis. These include fibrosis and atrophy of orbital tissues. Optic nerve atrophy and retinal degeneration secondary to compression, local circulatory disturbance, or extension of inflammation may lead to blindness.

Recurrent disease may indicate persistent orbital foreign body, mycotic infection, or orbital neoplasia and warrants further diagnostic workup and possibly exploratory orbitotomy.

Eosinophilic Myositis

Eosinophilic myositis is an inflammatory disease of unknown cause that affects the muscles of mastication in dogs. The condition is considered autoimmune because autoantibodies to temporal muscle myofibers have been identified in affected dogs. Although any breed can be affected, German shepherd and Weimaraner dogs are most commonly involved. Acute signs are recurrent (each episode lasts 1 to 2 weeks) and include swelling of the masticating muscles, pain when opening the mouth, dysphagia, enlarged mandibular lymph nodes, and occasionally blindness. The swelling of these muscles causes compromise of the orbital space and exophthalmos. Peripheral eosinophilia is inconsistent. With each attack of myositis, muscle damage is progressive and results in atrophy and fibrosis with subsequent enophthalmos. Rarely, only extraocular muscles are involved. Eosinophilic myositis can often be distinguished from retrobulbar abscess and cellulitis by its tendency to involve both orbits. The diagnosis of eosinophilic myositis can be confirmed by biopsy and histologic examination of temporal muscle.

Systemic corticosteroids are the treatment of choice for acute and recurrent chronic eosinophilic myositis. Prednisone is administered at 1 to 2 mg/kg every 24 hr for 14 days, and then the dose is slowly tapered over 4 to 6 weeks as signs improve.

Cystic Orbital Disease

Exophthalmos due to cystic fluid accumulation can occur with zygomatic salivary mucoceles, which are thought to result from leakage of saliva from the gland with secondary inflammation. The disease occurs infrequently and is probably due to trauma. The position of the mucocele determines the position of the globe, so the degree of exophthalmos is variable. Unlike cellulitis, abscess, and myositis, mucoceles are painless and may extend into the oral cavity or protrude into the ventral conjunctival fornix. Ultrasonography is helpful in identifying the cystic nature of orbital masses. Definitive diagnosis is usually made by fine-needle aspirate through the conjunctiva to the retrobulbar space opposite the deviation of the globe. Aspiration from within the mucocele reveals a clear, tenacious, golden fluid that forms mucous strands when placed between the thumb and first finger. Cytologic study of the aspirated fluid, zygomatic sialography, and exploratory orbitotomy confirm the diagnosis of zygomatic salivary mucocele. Culture and sensitivity testing of the fluid are important to rule out concomittant infection and dacryosialoadenitis. Treatment of zygomatic mucoceles consists of surgical resection of the mass by lateral or ventral orbitotomy or marsupialization into the oral cavity. Surgery can be curative.

Lacrimal gland cysts occur infrequently in dogs and cats and develop spontaneously or as a result of periorbital trauma. The clinical appearance is variable, but affected animals usually present with a painless, clear fluid-filled sac covered by conjunctiva dorsolateral to the globe. Surgical excision of the cyst is usually curative.

Orbital Neoplasia

Orbital neoplasms arise from both mesenchymal and epithelial tissue types. Primary orbital tumors are the most common orbital neoplasms in dogs and include optic nerve meningioma and osteosarcoma. Secondary orbital neoplasms are commonly due to orbital extension of nasal adenocarcinoma or malignant melanoma from the eye. In cats, secondary orbital neoplasia is commonly reported and includes malignant melanoma from the eye, lymphosarcoma, osteosarcoma, and squamous cell carcinoma. Proliferative inflammatory disease termed *pseudotumor* can also occur in dogs and cats.

Orbital tumors produce similar clinical signs regardless of tissue type. The most common clinical sign is slowly progressive, nonpainful, unilateral exophthalmos. Deviation of the globe is more common with orbital neoplasia than other orbital disorders that cause exophthalmos. Other clinical signs include prolapse of the third eyelid, periocular swelling, exposure keratitis, retinal detachment due to deformation of the posterior globe, and blindness. Chronic nasal discharge, central nervous system abnormalities, and unilateral swelling of the dorsocaudal oral cavity can be seen with invasion into adjacent structures.

The average age of dogs diagnosed with orbital neoplasia is approximately 8 years, but ages range from 1.5 to 15 years. No breed or sex predilection has been determined. Early and correct diagnosis of orbital neoplasia is essential because most orbital neoplasims are malignant, so aggressive treatment is indicated. Average survival from time of diagnosis is less than 3 years. The prognosis is guarded to grave for malignant tumors but favorable for the more uncommon benign mass.

A diagnosis of neoplasia is based on history, physical examination findings, survey and contrast radiography, and ultrasonography. Cytologic examination of fine-needle aspirates or histopathologic evaluation of a biopsy sample provides definitive diagnosis. Rarely, orbital exploratory surgery is necessary to obtain biopsy specimens. When available, computerized tomography is a preferred test for characterization of intracranial extension of orbital neoplasia.

The standard treatment for orbital neoplasia is exenteration of the orbit. Treatment of orbital neoplasia is usually palliative because of incomplete excision and malignant behavior of most orbital tumors. Radiation therapy or chemotherapy or both should be considered as adjunct therapy. In a few cases, these noninvasive procedures have been used in lieu of surgery.

ENOPHTHALMOS

Enophthalmos is recession of the globe into the orbit. Causes of enophthalmos include pain, microphthalmia, phthisis bulbi, Horner's syndrome, dehydration, loss of orbital fat, muscle atrophy, collapsed globe, and conformational enophthalmos in dolichocephalic breeds. Cats can have a transient prolapse of the third eyelid and enophthalmos associated with systemic disease. Recognizing the cause of the enophthalmos is important to differentiate systemic from primary ocular involvement. Treatment of the enophthalmos as a clinical entity is rarely indicated.

PROPTOSIS

Proptosis occurs when the globe moves in front of the eyelids. Proptosis usually results from head trauma but can be associated with buphthalmos or exophthalmos. Brachycephalic breeds are more prone to proptosis than dolichocephalic breeds because they have shallow orbits.

Damage to the globe depends on the degree of proptosis and the eyelid conformation of the animal. With moderate anterior displacement of the globe, the eyelids clamp down on the globe, resulting in venous stasis and ischemia of the highly vascular uveal tract. This in turn results in ischemic retinal damage. The extraocular muscles and their associated blood and nervous supply may be torn. The muscles that insert most anteriorly on the globe (medial rectus then ventral oblique) tear first, causing lateral strabismus. Return of the globe to a nearly-normal position usually occurs 8 to 12 weeks after the injury. Rarely is strabismus correction surgery indicated for cosmesis or vision. Loss of sympathetic and parasympathetic innervation is judged by pupillary response and resting size. A miotic pupil warrants a favorable prognosis, and a dilated or fixed midsized pupil has a poorer prognosis for saving vision and the globe. In globes with severe proptosis, the optic nerve is torn. Treatment of proptosis involves an immediate lateral canthotomy to release the pressure of the eyelids on the globe. The cornea should be lubricated with ophthalmic ointment to decrease exposure keratitis. Topical medications containing corticosteroids should be avoided because corneal ulceration is often present. After the animal's medical needs are met, a temporary tarsorraphy can be placed. It should remain intact for at least 7 to 10 days. Topical antibiotics and atropine are placed in the medial canthus four times daily. Systemic corticosteroid or nonsteroidal anti-inflammatory agents (prednisone or aspirin) are administered to decrease traumatic uveitis. Some animals require replacement of the temporary tarsorraphy after its initial release in order to protect the globe while allowing periocular swelling to decrease further.

References and Suggested Reading

Collins, B. K., Moore, C. P., Dubielzig, R. R., et al.: Anaerobic orbital cellulitis and septicemia in a dog. Can. J. Vet. Med. 32:(in press).
A case report involving diagnosis and treatment of a mixed anaerobic infection of the orbit.

Dow, S. W., and Jones, R. L.: Anaerobic infections, Part II. Diagnosis and treatment. Comp. Cont. Ed. Pract. Vet. 9:827, 1987.
A review of principles of diagnostic techniques and medical and surgical treatment of anaerobic infections.

Kern, T. J.: Orbital neoplasia in 23 dogs. J.A.V.M.A. 186:489, 1985.
A retrospective study of orbital neoplasms and their relationship to tissue origin, malignancy, and prognosis.

Kern, T. J.: The canine orbit. *In* Gelatt, K. E. (ed.): *Textbook of*

Veterinary Ophthalmology, 2nd ed. Philadelphia: Lea & Febiger, 1991, p. 239.
A complete review of clinical signs, diagnostic tests, diseases, and management of orbital disorders.

Koch, S.: Diseases of the orbit. *In* Kirk, R. W. (ed.): *Current Veterinary Therapy VII.* Philadelphia: W. B. Saunders, 1980, p. 583.
A brief discussion of orbital disease.

McCalla, T. L., and Moore, C. P.: Exophthalmos in dogs and cats, Part I. Anatomic and diagnostic considerations. Comp. Cont. Ed. Pract. Vet. 11:784, 1989.
A review of normal orbital anatomy, differential diagnosis, and clinical findings associated with exophthalmos.

McCalla, T. L., and Moore, C. P.: Exophthalmos in dogs and cats, Part II. Comp. Cont. Ed. Pract. Vet. 11:911, 1989.
A continuation from Part I of differential diagnosis of exophthalmos.

Morgan, R. V.: Ultrasonography of retrobulbar diseases of the dog and cat. J. Am. Anim. Hosp. Assoc. 25:393, 1989.
A prospective study of eight cases of orbital disease as characterized using B-mode ultrasonography.

Paulsen, M. E., Severin, G. A., LeCouteur, R. A., et al.: Primary optic nerve meningioma in a dog. J. Am. Anim. Hosp. Assoc. 25:147, 1989.
A case report describing differential diagnosis and clinical evaluation of orbital neoplasia.

Slatter, D. H., and Chambers, E. D.: Orbit. *In* Slatter, D. H. (ed.): *Textbook of Small Animal Surgery.* Philadelphia: W. B. Saunders, 1985, p. 1549.
A review of orbital anatomy and pathologic mechanisms, including illustrations of surgical treatment of the orbit.

DISEASES OF THE EYELIDS AND CONJUNCTIVA

SUSAN E. KIRSCHNER
New York, New York

EYELIDS AND CONJUNCTIVA

The eyelids and conjunctiva preserve the health of the cornea by protecting it and contributing mucus and oil to the tear film. Blinking the lids not only spreads tears over the cornea but also directs mucus and debris to the nasolacrimal puncta for removal. Because the eyelids and conjunctiva are in direct contact with the cornea, diseases of the lids and conjunctiva often result in corneal disease. The conjunctiva is exquisitely sensitive to inflammations of the lids, cornea, and intraocular structures. The first sign of a problem often is a hyperemic conjunctiva. Understanding the functions of the lids and conjunctiva enables a clinician to individualize treatment of such common ocular disorders as conjunctivitis, dry eye syndromes, and keratitis.

Diseases Of The Eyelids

CLINICAL ANATOMY OF THE EYELIDS

The eyelids are movable folds that have four functional layers: skin, muscle, tarsus, and conjunctiva. The skin of the lids is very thin and easily traumatized and is susceptible to the same diseases as skin elsewhere on the body. Underneath the skin, closely applied to it, lies the orbicularis oculi muscle. The tarsus is situated between the orbicularis muscle and the conjunctiva. It is a layer of fibrous tissue that gives form to the lid. Animals with droopy lids often have poorly developed tarsi. The meibomian glands that lie within the tarsus and open onto the lid margin produce an oily secretion that floats on top of the aqueous tears to prevent evaporation and overflow of the tears. Distichia and ectopic cilia originate from or near the meibomian glands. The conjunctiva lines the inner surface of the lids.

The lids should fit closely to the surface of the eye. In general, the looser the fit, the more tears are necessary for adequate wetting of the corneal surface. The lids are closed by the orbicularis muscle, innervated by the palpebral branch of the facial nerve. Paralysis of this nerve results in lagophthalmos. The lids are opened primarily by the levator palpebrae muscle, innervated by the oculomotor nerve. Some contribution is also made by Müller's muscle, innervated by postganglionic sympathetic fibers traveling with the oculomotor nerve. Paralysis of the sympathetic fibers results in ptosis, one of the cardinal signs of Horner's syndrome.

The eyelids have a generous blood supply. Thus, systemic antibiotics are the treatment of choice for primary eyelid infections. Certain surgical procedures may be performed on the eyelids but not on less well vascularized tissue.

ANATOMIC EYELID DISEASES

Ankyloblepharon

The lids normally open 10 to 14 days after birth in puppies and kittens. Delayed lid opening is clinically significant only if signs of infection develop. Subpalpebral infection, called *ophthalmia neonatorum*, appears as a swollen, reddened orbit with closed lids. Treatment is drainage of the purulent discharge beneath the lids, plus antibiotic therapy. The lids can often be massaged open, although they must be opened with scissors, taking care to avoid disrupting the developing lid margins. Once the lids are opened and the discharge has been removed, most broad-spectrum antibiotic solutions or ointments are effective in ridding the eye of infection. The corneas are often left with mild scarring, which improves over time. If left untreated, ophthalmia neonatorum may result in symblepharon or even corneal perforation.

Eyelid Agenesis

In eyelid agenesis of cats, a portion of the eyelid margin fails to form. Clinical signs are epiphora and squinting, caused by eyelid hairs contacting the cornea, similar to entropion. Most are relatively mild conditions and can be treated by slightly everting the lid with simple entropion surgery, so that hairs are directed away from the eye. More extensive malformations, in which a portion of the cornea is left exposed, require a pedicle flap or other plastic surgical procedure.

Dermoid

Dermoids are usually located at the limbus or cornea but can occasionally be found on the lid, especially at the lateral canthus. A typical complaint is the finding of a long tuft of hair at the lid margin. Treatment is not necessary unless there are signs of ocular irritation, such as discharge or squinting. Treatment is surgical removal. The most common complication is recurrence due to incomplete removal.

Entropion

Entropion is an inward rolling of the lids. It may be neonatal, as in Shar peis; anatomic, as is often seen in sporting breeds or chow chows; spastic; or a combination of types.

Neonatal entropion is seen as soon as the lids open and in Shar peis is caused by extremely thick lids and relatively enophthalmic globes that do not support the lids. In general, permanent entropion surgery should not be performed until 5 to 7 months of age, when the lid-to-globe proportions have matured. Instead, the lids should be everted with temporary mattress sutures for 2 to 3 weeks. This can be performed as early as 3 to 4 weeks of age, often with only topical anesthesia.

Anatomic entropion is encountered in sporting breeds, chow chows, and Shar peis, as well as in St. Bernards and other loose-lidded breeds. In sporting dogs, the entropion usually affects the temporal lower lid and is relatively easily corrected with a modified Hotz-Celsus procedure, in which an ellipse of tissue parallel to the lid margin in the area of the entropion is removed.

In Shar peis and chow chows, the entropion frequently involves both upper and lower lids, as well as the lateral canthus, and may be complicated by concurrent blepharospasm. In these dogs, almost the entire lid margin must be surgically everted. If spasm exists, the surgeon must be careful to surgically correct only the anatomic portion of the entropion. The portion due to spasm can be everted with temporary mattress sutures. The two operations may be performed at the same time. This allows time for the corneal disease and the spasm cycle to be resolved, without overcorrecting the entropion.

In St. Bernards, Clumber spaniels, Newfoundlands, and similar breeds, redundant, atonic lids associated with deep orbits and enophthalmic globes allow the eyelids to fall inward. The eyes are often described as diamond-shaped. Surgery is indicated if chronic conjunctivitis develops. Simple entropion surgery is seldom effective in correcting this condition; the operation must also shorten and tighten the lids. Several effective procedures to correct this condition have been described.

Spastic entropion may occur in any dog with any painful or pruritic eye disorder, including anatomic entropion. In spastic entropion, intense contraction of the orbicularis oculi muscle results in a rolling inward of the lids. The problem is then compounded by irritation of the conjunctiva and lids by hairs from the rolled lids. If allowed to continue, spasm may become a permanent condition.

Distinguishing anatomic from spastic entropion may be a diagnostic challenge. Differentiation is important because although anatomic entropion requires permanent corrective surgery, spastic entropion should be corrected with temporary everting sutures and treatment of the underlying problem. Topical anesthesia or sedation may be required to correctly differentiate anatomic from spastic entropion. Spastic entropion usually disappears after topical anesthesia; the anatomic entropion remaining after topical anesthesia usually should be surgically corrected.

Medial Entropion, Recessed Medial Canthus Syndrome

In many breeds such as the Pekingese, Shih tzu, Lhasa apso, and pug, the medial canthal tendon and the caruncle are recessed deep in the medial orbital wall. This has the effect of rolling the lids slightly inwards at the medial canthus, allowing hairs on the caruncle or medial canthal lids to contact the conjunctiva. In some dogs, these hairs contact the cornea. This anatomic variation results in epiphora, medial conjunctival or corneal pigmentation, or medial keratitis. This condition is exacerbated by anatomic exophthalmos, as noted in brachycephalic breeds.

Several surgical procedures have the effect of shortening the palpebral fissure, everting the eyelids medially, and protecting the cornea from the irritating effects of the canthal hairs.

Distichiasis

Distichiasis is characterized by hairs that originate from the meibomian glands and that usually emerge from the meibomian ducts on the lid margin. They are common in many breeds, including cocker spaniels, Shih tzus, poodles, and golden retrievers. They seldom result in significant clinical signs, because the hairs are usually soft and fine and ride on the tear film. If the eyes are dry or if the hairs are coarse and stiff, clinical signs may develop. Treatment should be initiated if blepharospasm, keratitis, corneal ulceration, or significant epiphora is associated with distichiasis. Treatment regimens include periodic plucking, cryosurgical epilation, electroepilation, and various surgical excisional techniques. Electroepilation is time-consuming and must be done under high magnification in order to be successful. Recurrence is the most common complication. Lid scarring may occur if too strong a current is used. Complications include cicatricial entropion and lid necrosis. Wedge resection of the affected meibomian glands should be reserved for dogs in which only a few hairs are present. Cryosurgical epilation is advantageous because it is fast, requires less technical skill, and preserves meibomian gland structure and function. As with most treatments for distichiasis, recurrence is the most common complication.

A hair sometimes emerges directly from the palpebral conjunctiva, causing pain and a nonhealing erosion. The most common location for these ectopic cilia is the central portion of the upper lid, a few millimeters from the lid margin. Surgical excision of the hair and its follicle is the treatment of choice.

Ectropion

Ectropion is the sagging of the lower lid such that excessive conjunctiva is exposed. It is a breed characteristic in cocker and springer spaniels, bloodhounds, Newfoundlands, and many other breeds. Although ectropion does not cause acute disease, dogs with ectropion are prone to allergic and bacterial conjunctivitis. In addition, dogs with ectropion are inefficient at wetting and cleaning the corneal surface because their lids fit too loosely on the globe. This may exacerbate keratoconjunctivitis sicca (KCS) symptoms in affected animals.

Treatment of ectropion is surgical. In most cases, shortening the lid by removing a wedge of tissue from the lid margin is sufficient. When the lateral canthus is also lax, a canthal tightening operation, such as done for diamond-shaped lids, should be performed.

INFLAMMATORY EYELID DISEASES

Hordeolum and Chalazion

A hordeolum is a focal abscess of the lid. If an eyelash follicle is the origin, a firm, round swelling of the lid is seen. These can be mistaken for small cysts or tumors. Warm compresses may help resolve the swelling. Occasionally they must be drained. If the meibomian gland is infected, the abscess is best seen by everting the lid. Internal hordeolum of the meibomian gland can be treated by warm compresses while gently massaging the lid, plus topical antibiotic therapy. A chalazion is a granuloma of a meibomian gland, diagnosed by finding a firm, yellow swelling on the conjunctival surface of the lid. Chalazia usually cause minimal clinical signs and do not require treatment. Surgical currettage is the treatment of choice if clinical signs are attributable to the chalazion.

Bacterial Blepharitis

Blepharitis is inflammation of the eyelid. Bacterial blepharitis is probably the most underdiagnosed disease of the lids. Because its symptoms include conjunctivitis and keratitis, it is frequently mistaken for primary disease of the conjunctiva or cornea. It is common to see blepharitis concurrently with KCS.

Bacterial blepharitis is common in older dogs,

dogs with seborrheic or atopic skin disease, hypothyroid dogs, and dogs with KCS. The owners complain of a purulent or mucopurulent ocular discharge, usually bilateral, although one lid may be affected more than the other. The lids may be swollen or thickened, there may be mild or severe alopecia, and a purulent discharge is usually crusted on the lashes and periocular hair. The discharge may be profuse. The condition is usually attended by conjunctivitis, and in many cases keratitis. Keratitis secondary to bacterial blepharitis is most severe in the superior cornea, where the lids rest when the eyes are open. Also noted are superficial vessels associated with a gray haze, which is superficial and does not retain fluorescein dye. In humans, this characteristic keratitis is attributed to bacterial toxins, enzymes, and fatty acids leaking from the lids, especially from infected meibomian glands.

Diagnosis is made on clinical findings. The most common bacteria associated with blepharitis are *Staphylococcus* species. Culture and sensitivity testing may be necessary in persistent cases, particularly those in which resistant bacterial strains may have developed in response to chronic antibiotic therapy. The patient's thyroid status should be evaluated, because hypothyroid dogs frequently have persistent eyelid and conjunctival infections.

Therapy consists of topical antibiotics and daily lid scrubs. Systemic antibiotics are required in severe cases. If keratitis is a prominent feature, conservative topical corticosteroid therapy may be helpful. However, treatment of the infection usually results in resolution of the keratitis without resorting to corticosteroids. Lid scrubs are enormously helpful in treatment of bacterial blepharitis. They remove purulent debris, which can inactivate many antibiotics, and encourage infected hair follicles and meibomian glands to drain. In humans, lid scrubs are the mainstay of control of chronic staphylococcal blepharitis. Owners have little difficulty in performing the lid scrubs, and most dogs tolerate it well. The closed lids are gently massaged with a small amount of dilute baby shampoo on a wet gauze sponge until all crusts and discharge have been removed. The shampoo is then removed with additional wet sponges. Antibiotics and lid scrubs should be continued for at least 1 or 2 weeks after resolution of the ocular discharge and inflammation. Lid scrubs two or three times a week and occasional antibiotic therapy may be necessary to prevent recurrence.

In some cases of chronic staphylococcal blepharitis, a hypersensitivity reaction to the bacteria may play a part. If no response to antibiotics and lid scrubs is observed, Staphage Lysate (Delmont) injections or autogenous bacterin injections can be used.

Allergic Blepharitis

True allergic blepharitis presents as an acute swelling of the lids and may be caused by insect bites or by inhalant or contact allergens. It may produce a serous discharge or no discharge at all. It is treated with systemic corticosteroids or antihistamines or both.

Atopy commonly causes eyelid pruritis; blepharitis is produced by a patient's rubbing at the eye. The lids are often alopecic and even excoriated, frequently with an associated conjunctivitis and serous ocular discharge. The inflammation is often seasonal, and a history of other skin allergies can be elicited. Treatment of the atopy and cold compresses to reduce pruritus usually are sufficient. Self-trauma occasionally is severe enough to warrant a protective collar.

Other Causes of Blepharitis

The skin of the eyelids is susceptible to dermatologic diseases. These include superficial fungal infections, parasites such as *Demodex* and *Sarcoptes,* seborrheic and hormonal skin disease, zinc-responsive dermatosis, and others. If examination reveals lesions of the eyelid skin without significant involvement of deeper layers of the lid or conjunctiva, the disease should be approached, diagnostically, as if it were skin disease elsewhere on the body. Skin scrapings, cultures, or biopsy samples should be included (Angarano, 1989; Johnson and Campbell, 1989).

Eyelid Neoplasms

Eyelid tumors are extremely common in dogs and are occasionally encountered in cats. By far the most common eyelid tumor in dogs is the meibomian gland adenoma. Benign papillomas and melanomas are also common. Malignant melanomas, meibomian gland adenocarcinomas, histiocytomas, and basal cell carcinomas are occasionally seen.

Meibomian gland adenomas are usually easily differentiated from other tumors. The body of the tumor lies in the meibomian gland and can be seen when the lid is everted. Tumor tissue often protrudes from the opening of the gland on the lid margin. Benign melanomas are most frequently noted on the lower lid skin rather than on the margin and are usually darkly pigmented. Papillomas have a characteristic wartlike appearance and are also on the skin rather than on the lid margin.

In cats, the most common eyelid tumor is squamous cell carcinoma. Basal cell tumors, papillomas, meibomian gland adenomas, fibrosarcomas, neurofibromas, and xanthomas have also been reported. Squamous cell carcinomas are most common in white cats and present as nonhealing skin ulcerations. They are usually extremely invasive locally and may metastasize. The prognosis for cure is poor.

Treatment modalities for lid tumors in dogs and cats include surgical excision, cryosurgery, and radiation therapy. Benign lid tumors, such as those found in dogs, respond well to either excision or cryosurgery. Meibomian gland tumors should be removed with a full-thickness wedge resection of the lid, taking care to remove the full extent of the base of the tumor, beneath the lid. Cutaneous melanomas or papillomas may be amenable to removal without disruption of the lid margin.

Squamous cell carcinomas in cats should be considered life-threatening. They require very wide and deep excision. The margins of the tumor should be carefully examined histopathologically to make sure excision has been complete. Because recurrence is common, even when excision appears to be complete, practitioners may want to consider additional therapy, such as radiotherapy or cryosurgery. Radiotherapeutic alternatives include radioactive seed implantation or teletherapy.

Diseases of the Conjunctiva

The conjunctiva is exquisitely sensitive to changes in its environment. Diseases of the lids, cornea, and intraocular structures all result in visible changes in the conjunctiva. Therefore, redness and ocular discharge are relatively nonspecific signs, and a full ophthalmic examination should be performed before a diagnosis of primary conjunctival disease is made.

CLINICAL ANATOMY

The conjunctiva originates at the corneal limbus, extends over the anterior globe to the fornix, and then is reflected over the nictitating membrane and inner surface of the lids. It consists of epithelium that overlies the substantia propria. The substantia propria contains fibrous tissue, lymphocytes, mast cells, and histiocytes. The epithelium contains goblet cells, which produce the mucus that allows normal adherence of aqueous tears to the cornea. The blood vessels of the conjunctiva branch generously and are most dense in the fornices, helping to differentiate them from deeper episcleral vessels, which are larger in diameter, are most prominent at the corneal limbus, and do not move with the conjunctiva.

CONJUNCTIVITIS

Because conjunctival hyperemia occurs with most inflammatory ocular disorders and with glaucoma, increased redness of the conjunctiva is not an indication of primary conjunctivitis unless all other ocular structures are normal.

Feline Conjunctivitis

Primary conjunctivitis in cats is relatively common. It is characterized by ocular discharge and hyperemia or swelling of the conjunctiva. Conjunctivitis occasionally results in decreased Schirmer's tear test results. In acute cases, it may be caused by conjunctival swelling that occludes the openings of the lacrimal ductules. In chronic cases, the dryness may be due to scarring of the ductules or damage to the lacrimal glands. The most common causes of feline conjunctivitis are herpesvirus and chlamydial infections. Most cases of bacterial conjunctivitis in cats are thought to be secondary to viral or chlamydial infection.

Feline herpesvirus, the etiologic agent of rhinotracheitis, is a common cause of conjunctivitis and keratitis in kittens and adult cats. In kittens and young adult cats, it is usually bilateral, is accompanied by upper respiratory signs, and is reported to cause primarily conjunctival hyperemia without significant chemosis. The ocular discharge is initially serous, but it may become purulent if bacterial invaders become established. The cornea may also become affected by ulcers or nonulcerative keratitis. Feline herpesvirus infections should be treated three to four times daily with topical antibiotics to prevent secondary bacterial infection. Antiviral medications are helpful, especially in patients with keratitis. The most effective (in vitro) antiviral medication for ocular feline herpesvirus infection is trifluridine solution (Viroptic, Burroughs Wellcome). Although the recommended dosage interval is stated to be 6 hr, I have noted excellent results even when trifluridine solution is used only twice daily. Though less effective in vitro than trifluridine, vidarabine (Vira-A ointment, Parke-Davis) is active against feline herpesvirus. The most common sequelae of neonatal herpesvirus infections are corneal scarring, symblepharon, and recurrent or persistent conjunctivitis or keratitis. Severe cases may result in corneal perforation with secondary glaucoma.

In adult cats, herpesvirus conjunctivitis is usually due to recrudescence of latent herpesvirus rather than new infection. New infections may occur in immunosuppressed cats, such as those with feline leukemia or feline immunodeficiency virus infections. Herpesvirus infection in adult cats is usually unilateral, chronic or intermittent, and associated with squinting and serous ocular discharge. The owner often reports blepharospasm as a prominent sign. Practitioners should stain the cornea of any cat with blepharospasm with rose bengal or fluorescein to demonstrate otherwise inapparent dendritic erosions, a pathognomonic sign for herpesvirus infection. Herpesvirus infection can be diagnosed by clinical findings, by fluorescent antibody testing on conjunctival scrapings, or by viral culture of conjunctival swabs. Antiviral medication is indicated for recurrent or chronic cases or when the cornea is involved.

Chlamydia can also cause conjunctivitis in cats. Chlamydial conjunctivitis is usually initially unilateral, although the contralateral eye often becomes involved after 10 to 14 days. Chemosis is a prominent sign, unlike in herpesvirus conjunctivitis. Many ophthalmologists believe that the presence of conjunctival follicles is suggestive of chlamydial infection. *Chlamydia* does not cause corneal lesions or upper respiratory signs, so if these are present, the practitioner should suspect herpesvirus infection rather than chlamydial infection. In the acute states of chlamydial infection, intracytoplasmic inclusions in conjunctival epithelial cells can sometimes be seen. They are slightly eosinophilic with a Wright-Giemsa–type stain, lie close to the nucleus, and range in size from one fourth to nearly equal the size of the nucleus. *Chlamydia* infection can also be diagnosed on the basis of fluorescent antibody tests on conjunctival scrapings. Chlamydial infections usually respond well to topical antibiotic therapy. Chloramphenicol, erythromycin, and tetracycline all are effective.

Mycoplasma may cause conjunctivitis in immunosuppressed cats but is not normally pathogenic. It is responsive to most antibiotics. Bacterial conjunctivitis in cats is usually secondary to viral or other infections but occasionally may be the primary infection. Cats with purulent ocular discharge should be suspected of having bacterial infection and should be treated accordingly.

Canine Conjunctivitis

Allergies and bacterial infections are the most common causes of conjunctivitis in dogs. Bacterial conjunctivitis is frequently encountered in dogs with ectropion and commonly is secondary to bacterial blepharitis or dry eyes. Bacterial conjunctivitis should be suspected when a purulent or mucopurulent discharge associated with conjunctival hyperemia is observed. The lids should be inspected carefully to rule out blepharitis, and a Schirmer's tear test should be performed. Low tear test results in dogs with purulent ocular discharge may be due to KCS or may be secondary to conjunctival infection. Thyroid testing is indicated in dogs with seborrheic or other skin diseases. Cultures may be helpful in refractory or chronic cases. Topical bactericidal drops or ointments (e.g., bacitracin-polymixin B-neomycin, gentamicin) used at least four times a day are indicated. In chronic or severe cases, systemic antibiotics are helpful. Concurrent

blepharitis should be treated with lid scrubs, as described earlier.

Reasons for recurrence when medications are discontinued include concurrent blepharitis, hypothyroidism, ectropion, or insufficient tear production. Practitioners should determine which of these may be playing a part and should address the underlying problem, if possible.

Allergic conjunctivitis is usually seasonal and is characterized by serous discharge and pruritus. Secondary bacterial infection may develop, resulting in a more purulent discharge. Follicles frequently are observed on the conjunctiva. Treatment is topical corticosteroids to effect. Systemic or topical antihistamines are of value in some cases.

Some dogs develop a significant sensitivity to ophthalmic drugs or preservatives. The most common incriminating drugs are neomycin, gentamicin, and pilocarpine. The most common preservatives to cause problems are thimerosal and benzalkonium chloride. Practitioners should suspect a drug sensitivity if the conjunctiva becomes extremely hyperemic after therapy has begun or if a dog squints excessively after medication is instilled.

Follicular conjunctivitis is encountered in young dogs and is associated with mild epiphora or mucoid discharge. Diagnosis is based on finding large numbers of conjunctival follicles, especially on the posterior surface of the nictitans. The cause is not known. Follicular conjunctivitis usually responds well to topical antibiotic-corticosteroid therapy. Scraping the follicles with a gauze sponge or scalpel blade has also been advocated.

Inflammation of episcleral or scleral tissue causes signs that may be confused with conjunctivitis. In contrast to conjunctival disease, however, episcleritis results in raised, firm swellings beneath the conjunctiva (see this volume, p. 1101).

Conjunctival Tumors

Hemangiomas, squamous cell carcinomas, mastocytomas, melanomas, and angiokeratomas have been encountered on the conjunctiva of dogs. With the exception of melanomas, they are usually benign, and excision is curative.

Conjunctival Goblet Cell Deficiency

Conjunctival goblet cell deficiency is a recently reported condition characterized by a decrease in the normal population of goblet cells in the conjunctiva (Moore and Collier, 1990). Because the mucus produced by the goblet cells functions to promote adherence of the fluid portion of the tears to the cornea, goblet cell deficiency is characterized by a dry cornea in the presence of adequate aqueous tears. Clinical signs include blepharospasm and chronic or recurrent corneal ulcers. Diagnosis is based on results of tear film breakup time test and biopsy of conjunctiva from the ventral conjunctival fornix, where goblet cells are normally present in high numbers. The tear film breakup time test is performed by placing a drop of fluorescein on the eye to allow visualization of the tear film. The tear film breakup time is equal to the number of seconds it takes before a dry spot appears on the cornea, after a blink. It is helpful to perform the test in a dark room using a cobalt blue light. Some direct ophthalmoscopes have a blue light that may be used for this purpose. The normal tear film breakup time in dogs is about 20 sec. Dogs with goblet cell deficiency usually have breakup times of less than 5 sec. Definitive diagnosis is based on biopsy of conjunctiva from the ventral conjunctival fornix. The sample should be stretched flat and pinned to a tongue depressor for fixation, and the pathologist should be instructed to determine the goblet cell density (ratio of goblet cells to all epithelial cells). Normal canines should have a density of at least 0.25. Affected dogs may have densities as low as 0.05. If a diagnosis of goblet cell deficiency is made, treatment consists of topical mucomimetic artificial tears. Topical corticosteroids may be helpful in cases with concurrent conjunctival inflammation.

Diseases of the Nictitans

CLINICAL ANATOMY

The nictitans is composed of a fold of conjunctival tissue at the inferior aspect of the eye. Giving support to the fold is a T-shaped cartilage. At the ventral base of the cartilage lies the gland of the nictitans, which produces mucus and aqueous tears. Along with the eyelids, the nictitans functions to protect the cornea, to spread tears over the cornea, and to clean the corneal surface.

Prolapsed Gland of the Nictitans

Prolapsed gland of the nictitans is commonly observed in cocker spaniels, bulldogs, Boston terriers, Shih tzus and other breeds. In this condition, the base of the gland of the nictitans, embedded in the nictitans cartilage, flips up and is seen above and behind the border of the nictitans. Prolapse is frequently bilateral and is usually encountered in young dogs. Treatment is surgical replacement of the gland and cartilage. Several techniques have been advocated, including suturing the base of the gland to the sclera of the globe or to the ventral orbital rim or simply to the tissue of the base of the nictitans. Recurrence is the most common complication of any of the techniques. Removal of the gland is not indicated. Because lacrimal secretion from the gland is significant, KCS may occur after excision.

Pannus

Pannus may affect the nictitans without affecting the cornea. In this case, it is termed *atypical pannus*. Like corneal pannus, it is encountered most commonly in German shepherds and is thought to be associated with chronic exposure to ultraviolet radiation. The leading edge of the nictitans typically becomes depigmented, and the palpebral surface appears red and thickened. It usually improves with topical prednisone or dexamethasone therapy. In some instances, topical cyclosporine is effective. Like corneal pannus, the condition usually recurs if treatment is discontinued.

Nodular Episcleritis, Granulomatous Episclerokeratitis

Nodular episcleritis and granulomatous episclerokeratitis may affect the nictitans. Treatment is similar to that for scleral diseases (see this volume, p. 1101).

Tumors

Tumors of the nictitans may originate from the conjunctiva or from the gland of the nictitans. Squamous cell carcinomas, hemangiomas, mastocytomas, sarcomas, lipomas, papillomas, and adenocarcinomas have been described. In addition, cysts of the gland of the nictitans, which resemble tumors, have been encountered. Adenocarcinomas of the gland of the nictitans have been reported to be locally recurrent, and total excision of the nictitans is recommended in cases in which the gland appears to be the primary site of origin of the tumor.

References and Suggested Reading

Angarano, D. W.: Dermatologic disorders of the eyelids. *In* Kirk, R. W. (ed.): *Current Veterinary Therapy X.* W. B. Saunders, Philadelphia, 1989.
  A discussion of the diagnosis and treatment of common canine eyelid dermatoses.
Bedford, P.: Conditions of the eyelids in the dog. J. Small Anim. Pract. 29:416, 1988.
  A review of anatomic disorders of the lids and their surgical treatment.
Johnson, B., and Campbell, K.: Dermatoses of the canine eyelid. Comp. Cont. Ed. Pract. Vet. 11:385, 1989.
  A review of dermatologic disorders of the lids, including blepharitis.
Lavach, J., Thrall, M.A., Benjamin, M. M., et al.: Cytology of normal and inflamed conjunctivas in dogs and cats. J.A.V.M.A. 170:722, 1977.
  A review of conjunctival cytology, with emphasis on the use of this technique to differentiate between various causes of conjunctivitis.

Moore, C., and Collier, L.: Ocular surface disease associated with loss of conjunctival goblet cells in dogs. J. Am. Anim. Hosp. Assoc. 26:458, 1990.
Clinical and diagnostic findings and therapy for three dogs with this disease.
Nasisse, M.: Feline herpesvirus ocular disease. Vet. Clin. North Am. 20:667, 1990.

A review of feline herpesvirus conjunctivitis and keratitis, including new methods of diagnosis and treatment.
Paulsen, M., Lavach, J. D., Snyder, S. P., et al.: Nodular granulomatous episclerokeratitis in dogs: 19 cases (1973–1985). J.A.V.M.A. 190:1581, 1987.
A retrospective study of the disease, with emphasis on diagnosis and treatment.

DIAGNOSIS AND MANAGEMENT OF TEAR FILM DISORDERS

RENEE L. KASWAN
Athens, Georgia

The preocular tear film functions as a nutritive, immunoprotectant, lubricant, and cleansing layer for the cornea and conjunctiva. Because the cornea is avascular, the tears perform the functions of serum for the cornea.

The tear film is a complex liquid structure composed of three layers: lipid, aqueous, and mucus. It is dynamic, constantly redistributed and restructured by blinking. Normal lid-globe anatomy is required for even distribution of the tear film.

The aqueous or middle tear layer constitutes over 90% of the tear volume and is produced by the orbital and nictitans lacrimal glands. Its components have not been quantified in dogs or cats. Among its many constituents are oxygen, glucose, amino acids, enzymes, epithelial growth factor for wound repair, and vitamins. Aqueous tears serve the metabolic needs of the avascular cornea and flush away the bacteria, carbon dioxide, and lactic acid that would otherwise accumulate. Deficiency of the aqueous layer (known as keratoconjunctivitis sicca [KCS]) is diagnosed by Schirmer's tear test (STT). KCS is the most common chronic canine ocular surface disorder.

The innermost layer of the tear film is composed of mucus produced primarily by the conjunctival goblet cells. Mucin is attracted to the cornea and changes the corneal surface from hydrophobic to hydrophilic, permitting the overlying aqueous layer to spread evenly over the eye. Chronic external eye disease can be associated with gross deficiency of the mucus layer. Mucin insufficiency has only recently been recognized in dogs (Moore and Collier, 1990). Rapid tear breakup time with normal STT volume suggests mucin insufficiency; conjunctival biopsy is diagnostic.

The outermost layer of the tear film is lipid. Produced by the tarsal (meibomian) glands, it promotes stable, evenly spread tears and retards evap-oration. Meibomian gland inflammation can cause qualitative changes in the lipid; however, deficiencies of this layer have not been documented.

In addition to the necessary components, the tear film requires normal blinking to mix and spread the layers. Without normal lid-globe apposition, normal blinking, or normal lid margins, the tears may be spread unevenly and corneal dry spots can develop shortly after each blink.

QUANTITATIVE TEAR FILM DEFICIENCY: KERATOCONJUNCTIVITIS SICCA

Aqueous Deficiency

The bulk of the tear film is aqueous; consequently, quantitative deficiency of the tear film is by definition an aqueous deficiency. Deficiency of aqueous tears, commonly called "dry eye," is the most common cause of chronic canine conjunctivitis and has historically been frequently misdiagnosed as bacterial or allergic conjunctivitis.

Even when KCS was diagnosed and treated appropriately with artificial tears and cholinergic tear stimulants, management has always been difficult for both the client and the veterinarian. Despite diligent therapy, many affected dogs would develop progressive corneal opacity and blindness.

The recent discovery of ophthalmic cyclosporine (Optimmune, Schering-Plough*) seems to offer a major advance in KCS management. Cyclosporine is a relatively new immunosuppressive agent used primarily in human organ transplantation. It is noncytotoxic; therefore, its effects reverse when its use is stopped. Cyclosporine acts primarily by in-

*Optimmune® is an investigational new animal drug sponsored by Schering-Plough Animal Health, Crawford, NJ.

Table 1. *Clinical Manifestations of Keratoconjunctivitis Sicca*

Manifestation	Description
Ocular discharge	Mucoid to mucopurulent, tenacious, profuse, chronic, or recurrent discharge
Conjunctivitis	Chemosis, hypertrophy, hyperemia, keratinized plaques
Keratitis	Variable lesions include superficial vascularization, stromal edema, keratinization, hypertrophic surface, pigmented or leukomatous surface opacities, recurrent superficial or deep ulcers
Pain	Blepharospasm, third-eyelid prolapse, photophobia, and changes in behavior (e.g., irritability); pain is a highly variable sign associated with corneal abrasions or ulcers, which occur most frequently in acute onset KCS, prior to hypertrophy and keratinization of the corneal epithelium; most chronic cases of KCS lack signs of pain
Blindness	Occurs frequently due to progression of corneal scarring and occasionally due to perforation of corneal ulcers

hibiting T-helper–cell activity. Topical cyclosporine apparently also increases tearing and decreases corneal and conjunctival inflammation and scarring. By using local application instead of systemic administration, the cyclosporine dosage necessary to alleviate KCS symptoms is reduced to approximately 1/100 of the canine therapeutic oral dose. This reduction in dosage makes the therapeutic index high and the potential risk of systemic side effects remote. When cyclosporine treatment is initiated before end-stage destruction of lacrimal tissues, it appears to be a highly effective and convenient alternative therapy in the majority of canine KCS cases.

Clinical Signs

Clinical signs of KCS are presented in Table 1 iscussed here.

DISCHARGE. Mucoid or mucopurulent ocular discharge is the hallmark of KCS. Mucin produced by conjunctival goblet cells is not dispersed by the aqueous tears and therefore accumulates. Conjunctivitis and keratitis evolve when the ocular surface dessicates. The lids may also be involved with blepharitis. A plethora of opportunistic bacteria can be cultured from the ocular discharge, but their abundance is secondary to the effects of aqueous deficiency. A large proportion of animals with KCS do not appear to have dry eyes; an STT is therefore warranted in all animals presenting with mucoid or mucopurulent ocular discharge. KCS ranks

high among the most commonly misdiagnosed ophthalmic disorders and is now recognized as the underlying cause of the majority of chronic canine conjunctivitis. Misdiagnosed cases of KCS that are treated frequently with any topical ophthalmic preparation usually show transient improvement, falsely reinforcing the clinician's confidence in a diagnosis of bacterial or allergic conjunctivitis. Virtually all topical medications wet and lubricate the eye, aiding the dry eye condition. A high degree of suspicion should be held for any chronic or recurrent conjunctivitis, keratitis, or corneal ulceration.

CONJUNCTIVITIS. Clinical signs of conjunctivitis are discharge, hyperemia, chemosis, hypertrophy of the bulbar and palpebral conjunctiva (pleating or folds apparent), and hypertrophy of the conjunctiva of the third eyelid. Conjunctivitis is the consistent component of KCS, whereas keratitis occurs only in more advanced cases and in exophthalmic or lagophthalmic breeds. Conjunctivitis is irritative but not typically painful. Dogs respond to conjunctivitis by pawing or rubbing the eyes against rugs and furniture. Blepharospasm is unlikely unless corneal ulcers are also present.

KERATITIS. Corneal inflammation occurs in severe cases of KCS. The superficial corneal epithelium, which is normally nonkeratinized and is five to six cells thick, can become keratinized, vascularized, and hypertrophic, with as much as 30 cells of thickness. Corneal hypertrophy can become so extreme as to preclude lid closure, and lagophthalmos compounds the effects of tear deficiency. An uneven corneal surface can occur from extreme hypertrophy with inflammation-induced subepithelial stromal edema. Concurrent with epithelial and subepithelial vascularization, dystrophic superficial or subepithelial precipitates can include lipids, calcium, or pigment.

PIGMENTARY KERATITIS. In exophthalmic breeds and in breeds with periocular pigmentation, such as the pug, schnauzer, cocker spaniel, and dachshund, pigmentary keratitis can be a devastating consequence of KCS. Free pigment granules and melanocytes can be deposited beneath the corneal epithelium.

BLINDNESS. Corneal pigmentation and corneal scarring cause sight loss in KCS. Although superficial hypertrophy and to a lesser degree subepithelial fibroplasia are reversible lesions, pigmentary keratitis is often an irreversible cause of sight loss in KCS-affected dogs.

CORNEAL ULCERS. Superficial focal or multifocal abrasions are diagnosed when the cornea is fluorescein-stain positive. Corneal sensation is often lost or diminished in chronic KCS; therefore, ulcers may not be associated with signs of discomfort. Superficial ulcers occur when dessicated plaques of epithelium exfoliate, torn by friction from the rough, keratinized palpebral conjunctiva and by the shearing forces of lid movements. Ulcers caused by dessication generally occur in the central cornea, the area exposed within the lid fissure. Large, deep, melting ulcers also occur occasionally. These can be caused by pathogenic bacteria such as *Pseudomonas*, which release proteolytic enzymes into the cornea. More often, melting corneal ulcers occur when endogenous proteases attack the cornea. Lymphocyte aggregates commonly seen in the conjunctiva in KCS may actually cause self-destructive "bystander" inflammation, attracting neutrophils that release endogenous proteases that dissolve the cornea.

Diagnosis

Even when the cornea does not appear dry, an STT should be performed as a routine part of the anterior segment ophthlamic examination in any dog with a mucoid discharge or corneal or conjunctival lesions. Before administering any ocular drops, place a standardized 5 mm × 30 mm filter paper strip in the medioventral palpebral cul-de-sac for 1 min. Normal wetting in dogs is 15 to 25 mm/min on STT, but animals with KCS typically wet less than 10 mm/min, with most symptomatic animals wetting less than 5 mm/min on repeated trials. Artifactual depression of the STT can result from the use of atropine, which can cause transient dryness for 2 to 6 days, or by fear-induced sympathetic stimulation, which also leads to sporadic low STT values, particularly in cats. A diagnosis of KCS can be made when decreased STT values occur with mucopurulent conjunctivitis, corneal inflammation, ulceration, or pigment deposition.

Incidence

Review of the incidence of KCS in dogs presented to 20 veterinary teaching hospitals over the past 25 years reveals a progressive increase in the number of reported cases from an initial incidence of 0.04% in 1965 to an incidence of >1.5% in 1988. The absolute incidence of KCS in the general canine population is unknown. The severity of lesions currently seen in dogs with KCS is typically advanced at the time of diagnosis, but it is hoped that continued progress in veterinary education will lead to earlier diagnosis and, if properly managed, a reduction in the currently high rate of blindness ensuing from canine KCS.

Etiology

Although there are several known or postulated causes of KCS in dogs, documenting the specific cause in an individual dog is unfeasible in the vast majority of cases. Distemper virus can cause acute onset of KCS that often resolves spontaneously. Congenital-onset KCS occurs rarely, is usually unilateral, and is presumably due to lacrimal gland hypoplasia. Unilateral neurologic xerosis occurs in some cases of facial trauma, ear infections, and brainstem damage. The parasympathetic lacrimal nerve, which courses first with the facial nerve and later with the trigeminal nerve, can be lost with injury to either of these cranial nerves. Vitamin A deficiency is unsubstantiated as an etiology of canine KCS.

IATROGENIC KCS. Treatment with sulfonamides (Azulfidine, Pharmacia; Tribrissen, Cooper's Animal Health) and phenazopyridine can cause transient or permanent KCS in dogs. The author suggests that the incidence of iatrogenic KCS could be greatly reduced by reserving the use of sulfonamides (e.g., Tribrissen) for disorders that cannot be satisfactorily treated with alternate antibiotics.

Removal of the nictitans gland for cosmetic correction of "cherry eye" increases the potential to develop KCS. The author prefers to reposition the gland by tacking it to the orbital rim (Fig. 1).

Pathogenesis of Ocular Surface Disease

The pathogenesis of the clinical signs of KCS has been the topic of recent study. Numerous hypotheses have been advanced to explain the development of corneal and conjunctival lesions in human KCS. The lesions seen in dogs are much more severe than those seen in people. The increased severity may be attributed to delayed diagnosis in dogs related to inability to report discomfort as an early sign and to inability to self-medicate at a frequency compatible with comfort. Lagophthalmos and exophthalmos, common in many breeds, further exacerbate the effects of insufficient tear film. The following is a list of current hypotheses regarding the development of ocular surface lesions.

LUBRICATION. Blinking causes the lid to apply considerable force to the ocular surface. Shearing forces occur when an abnormal volume of mucin, lipid, and aqueous tears fails to cushion the cornea from the lids.

EVAPORATION/DESICCATION. Increased evaporation is a major problem in exophthalmic dogs and partially accounts for the increased severity of lesions in these breeds. When decreased tear secretion is combined with increased evaporation, the result is increased osmolality in the tear film. The hyperosmolar tear film then pulls fluid out of the ocular surface cells, leading to desiccation.

METABOLIC DEFICIENCY. Hypoxia of the corneal epithelium and subepithelial corneal stroma can occur due to lack of oxygen dissolved in tears.

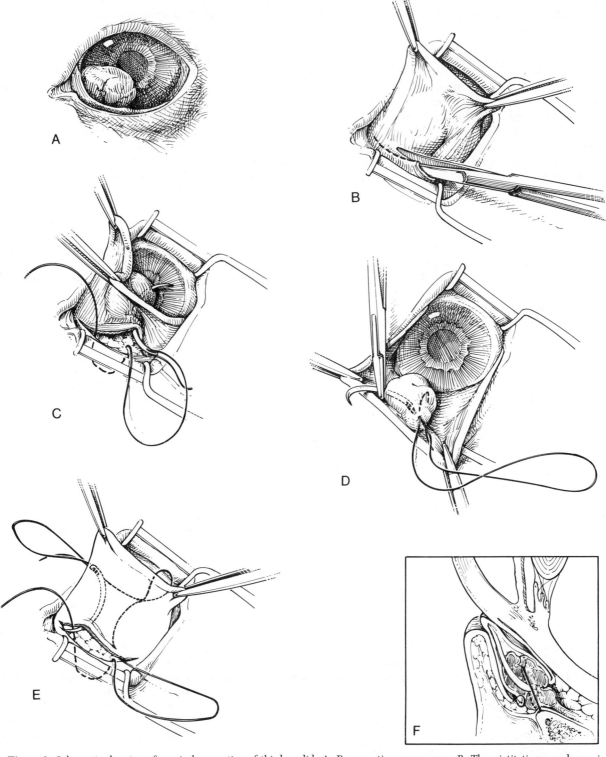

Figure 1. Schematic drawing of surgical correction of third eyelid. *A*, Preoperative appearance. *B*, The nictitating membrane is extended to allow an incision in the conjunctiva of the fornix. A round-tipped strabismus or tenotomy scissors is preferred for this incision (not pictured). *C*, Using a 3-0 nonabsorbable monofilament suture, take a long bite of the periosteum along the orbital rim. The needle should traverse medial to lateral through the rim and not perpendicular (toward eyeball) to it. The suture is then passed back through the incision dorsally to the highest plateau of the prolapsed gland, exiting on the dorsal bulbar face. *D*, The nictitating membrane is reflected downward; the suture re-enters the exit hole, and a horizontal bite is taken through the dorsal prominence of the gland. The final pass of suture begins again at the exit hole and passes ventrally through the gland to exit through the conjunctival incision. *E*, Both suture ends are now within the conjunctival incision, where they are tautly tied. *F*, Cross-sectional view of end result shows the nictitans gland encircled by monofilament suture and anchored to the orbital rim. (Reprinted with permission from Kaswan, R.L., and Martin, C.L.: Surgical correction of third eyelid prolapse in dogs. J.A.V.M.A. 186:83, 1983.)

BACTERIAL OVERGROWTH. Tear-deficient eyes have a high susceptibility to colonization by opportunistic and pathogenic organisms.

TOXIC PRODUCT ACCUMULATION. Lactic acid, desquamated cells, denatured mucus, and other organic debris can accumulate on the ocular surface when the tear turnover time is prolonged.

INFLAMMATION. Conjunctival cytology and conjunctival biopsies from human patients with isolated KCS or KCS as a component of Sjögren's syndrome have keratinization and squamous cell hyperplasia in the conjunctiva. This epidermatization of the conjunctiva (commonly called squamous metaplasia) occurs in conjunctival areas invaded by inflammatory cells composed, predominantly of mononuclear cells. Consistent findings of conjunctival lymphocytic infiltration in KCS-affected eyes with squamous metaplasia suggest that the lymphocytes may play a role in the induction of the squamous metaplasia. Squamous metaplasia does not improve in patients treated frequently with nonpreserved sodium hyaluronate tears. It has been concluded that squamous metaplasia results from lymphocytic infiltration rather than from loss of tear wetting.

The wide range of corneal response to moderate degrees of tear deficiency could be related to coincident immune activity generated against the ocular surface in KCS patients. Chronic physical damage to the corneal epithelium could expose new corneal antigens to the immune system and instigate both antibody formation and T-cell–mediated autoimmune activity. Besides tear replacement, suppressing inflammation may be important in limiting ocular surface disease in KCS.

Ophthalmic Cyclosporine: A New Approach to Management of Canine KCS

Cyclosporine is a noncytotoxic immunosuppressant approved for human organ transplantation. Its primary effect is to inhibit T-helper–cell activity while sparing T-suppressor–cell activity, thereby shifting the balance of T-cell immune regulation toward immune tolerance. Anti-inflammatory activity of cyclosporine has become apparent with its recent use in immune-mediated disorders.

Two distinct therapeutic effects of ophthalmic cyclosporine have been observed: it increases tearing in most dogs with KCS, and it improves ocular surface lesions.

Systemic cyclosporine is expensive and is associated with potential side effects that prohibit routine veterinary use. To avoid toxicity and expense, the author tested cyclosporine in an ophthalmic preparation, at a dose approximately 1/100 of the canine oral therapeutic dose.

Whether cyclosporine will increase tearing seems to depend primarily upon the stage of the disease at the time that treatment is instituted. In three independent clinical trials, cyclosporine ophthalmic therapy instituted in dogs that had not yet reached end-stage lacrimal disease increased tearing by at least 5 mm/min within 3 months in 87 to 100% of treated eyes. If KCS was in end stage (STT: 0 to 1 mm/min) when cyclosporine was first introduced, lacrimation improved in 29 to 59% of treated eyes. When lacrimal gland biopsies were taken from nonresponsive dogs, diffuse inflammation and fibrosis characterized the nonresponsive glands (histopathologic stage 3).

Improvement of corneal and conjunctival lesions in dogs with KCS can be dramatic, with or without improvement in lacrimation. Conjunctival hyperplasia, leukoplakia (white plaques caused by keratinization), corneal granulation-like tissue accumulation, and mucopurulent ocular discharge improved in most cases within 2 to 3 weeks. Corneal vascularization and pigmentation also resolved in most dogs; however, these lesions resolved much more gradually. Improvement was first apparent by 3 months, and continued resolution occurred beyond 12 months.

Improved vision as a result of corneal clearing occurred with chronic use of cyclosporine. In a series of 36 dogs, six dogs initially blinded by keratitis regained sight while receiving topical cyclosporine treatment. In a series of 178 dogs treated by 40 veterinary ophthalmologists, 11 of 23 eyes that presented blind regained vision after treatment for at least 3 months with ophthalmic cyclosporine (unpublished data).

From the client's perspective, the advantage of topical cyclosporine over conventional therapy is its decreased dosage frequency (one to three times daily, usually b.i.d.), replacing more arduous therapies. Several advantages are recognized for the cyclosporine-treated patient. Cyclosporine may treat the underlying cause of KCS. Therefore, it may prevent progressive deterioration of the lacrimal glands and stop the otherwise inevitable progression of ocular lesions. Most dogs will resume tear production, which is intuitively superior to commercial products made to imitate tears.

CYCLOSPORINE EFFECTS ON THE EYE. Cyclosporine is a highly lipophilic drug absorbed at high levels into the corneal surface. Because cyclosporine is extremely hydrophobic, therapeutic drug levels have not been readily achieved intraocularly; however, vehicle modifications to increase intraocular penetration for use in anterior uveitis are under study.

In the surface tissues of the eye, cyclosporine reverses the effects of chronic inflammation. In KCS, corneal vascularization, stromal edema, epithelial hypertrophy, and scarring decrease independent of STT alterations, suggesting that the lesions are caused in large part by secondary inflammation as opposed to dessication. The most dramatic benefits occur in dogs with extreme corneal epithelial hypertrophy, with resultant visual improvement and apparent improvement in comfort.

LACRIMOMIMETIC EFFECTS OF CYCLOSPORINE. Induction of a lacrimal response in KCS-affected dogs requires 2 to 3 weeks of treatment with ophthalmic cyclosporine. Tearing drops precipitously within 12 to 24 hr of treatment cessation. When cyclosporine is reinstituted, tearing rebounds to maximal levels in 3 hours. Although ophthalmic cyclosporine has increased lacrimation, it has not cured KCS. In a series of 21 eyes successfully treated for 12 months, the mean STT had risen from 3.5 mm/min to 14.8 mm/min. When treatment was withdrawn for 2 weeks, the mean STT dropped to 5.4 mm/min and signs of KCS recurred.

RISKS OF OPHTHALMIC CYCLOSPORINE USE. The T-cell response is most important for defense against viral and mycotic infections; therefore, the author anticipates that cyclosporine should not be used when viral or mycotic keratitis is suspected. Fortunately, dogs are rarely affected by mycotic or herpetic corneal infections. The risk of opportunistic infection with cyclosporine may be similar to risks encountered with topical corticosteroid use, and similar precautions are warranted. Unlike corticosteroids, cyclosporine does not appear to potentiate the collagenase activity that causes melting ulcers.

The objection has been raised that veterinarians may incur increased liability by using ophthalmic cyclosporine because its use is extralabel, unlicensed, and federally unapproved. Pharmacists compounding ophthalmic cyclosporine have wide variability in quality control and sterile technique. *The intravenous cyclosporine product should never be used ophthalmically because it contains 30% alcohol.* All ophthlamic preparations are required by law to be sterile at the time they are dispensed. Until an FDA-approved ophthalmic cyclosporine product is available, product manufacturing safety standards will continue to be a source of concern for the patient, client, and veterinarian using ophthalmic cyclosporine. Introduction of an FDA-approved commercial product (Optimmune) should soon provide a quality controlled product.*

CYCLOSPORINE DOSAGE AND ADMINISTRATION. Current experience suggests that most dogs respond to ophthalmic cyclosporine administered twice daily. Initial protocols used ophthalmic cyclosporine bilaterally twice daily and re-evaluated clinical signs

and STT monthly for 3 months. At each examination, if the STT remained below 10 mm/min/eye, the dosage frequency was increased to three times daily for the affected eye. If the STT increased to greater than or equal to 20 mm/min/eye, the treatment of the eye was decreased to once daily. *It is important to evaluate the STT 3 hours postadministration of cyclosporine to determine responsiveness because the effects on tearing decrease over a 12-hour period in most patients.*

Application frequency of ophthalmic cyclosporine might be reduced after several months; however, rarely can a dog be withdrawn completely without relapse. Interruptions in treatment precipitate return of KCS signs, and reintroduction of the drug quickly restores maximal tearing effect.

In the author's study, therapy was considered ineffective if the STT and ocular signs did not improve within three months. Eyes with dense pigmentary keratitis were an exception. Pigmentary keratitis has been recognized to be very slowly responsive to ophthalmic cyclosporine. In a carefully monitored case, it took 4 to 6 months to see a noticeable improvement, and corneal clarity continued to improve over a 2-year treatment period.

Veterinary ophthalmologists vary in their reliance upon ophthalmic cyclosporine. One management plan calls for use of conventional KCS therapy until signs cannot be managed adequately, introducing ophthalmic cyclosporine only as a last resort. The disadvantage of this strategy is that after KCS is advanced and the lacrimal acini have been replaced by chronic inflammation and fibrosis, cyclosporine is unlikely to be effective. When used in dogs with an STT of 0 to 1 mm/min, cyclosporine improved lacrimation in 53% of cases. However, when used in dogs with KCS that was not in end stage, 87% showed improved lacrimation. None of these dogs deteriorated while treated for 12 months. This finding suggests that cyclosporine can prevent the development of end-stage KCS only if used before the gland is destroyed.

Thus far, only sulfonamides are recognized to be contraindicated as concurrent therapeutic agents with cyclosporine. The author generally continues use of conventional medications until the effectiveness of cyclosporine in a given case is established, at which time artificial tears, antibiotics, and pilocarpine are withdrawn.

Traditional KCS Management

ARTIFICIAL TEARS. The mainstay of products approved for the treatment of KCS in human patients and subsequently used in veterinary species are artificial tears. Artificial tear constituents vary, and each patient may respond differently to any given product; a degree of experimentation is therefore

---

*Ophthalmic treatment by topical administration of cyclosporine (Optimmune) is a patented invention (USP 4,649,047) of the University of Georgia Research Foundation. Investigations toward FDA Center for Veterinary Medicine approval of an ophthalmic cyclosporine are under way at Schering-Plough Animal Health, Kenilworth, NJ. Referral to compounding pharmacists knowledgeable in the preparation of ophthalmic cyclosporine is available by written request to the author.

advised. Significantly desirable artificial tear ingredients include a wetting agent, such as polyvinyl pyrrolidine, to improve tear adherence to the cornea and ingredients that retard evaporation, such as methylcellulose or polyvinyl alcohol.

Preservatives are undesirable in artificial tears because they are toxic to corneal epithelium. With the exception of daily-dose packages, all artificial tear solutions contain preservatives. Preservative toxicity is compounded in KCS because the normal tear film is not available to rinse away the damaging components. Although benzalkonium chloride is best known for toxicity, this is an artifact of publicity. Other preservatives are equally harmful.

Ophthalmic ointments are usually preservative free. Lacrilube (Allergan) is an exception; it contains chlorobutanol, making it less desirable for chronic or frequent use. Additional advantages of ointments include increased contact time, softening of periocular crusts, and lower cost. The major disadvantage of ointments for human use is transient blurring of vision that prohibits reading, which is obviously of little significance in dogs. If an ointment is used in addition to an ophthalmic solution, care should be taken to administer the solution at least 20 min prior to the ointment or the ointment could form a barrier against solution penetration.

Sodium hyaluronic acid is a very large molecule that provides a long retention time on the cornea. An economical 0.1% solution of hyaluronic acid can be made by diluting sodium hyaluronate with Adapt (Alcon) or sterile saline. Again, it is difficult to ensure product sterility. In animals that have irritation reactions to commercial ophthalmic drops, the author finds that hyaluronic acid drops are well tolerated.

In the author's opinion, the reason that artificial tears are continually reinvented without avail is that the underlying problem is not addressed. The assumption made in using artificial tears is that the problem of KCS is simply deficiency of lubricating fluids. Recent findings of lymphocytic nests underlying areas of degenerative conjunctival changes, including increased nuclear/cytoplasmic cell ratio, keratinization, and squamous cell hyperplasia (squamous metaplasia), reinforce the suspicion that KCS lesions are not simply due to dessication from fluid deprivation. Instead, inflammatory products from conjunctival lymphocytes may be causing lesions in the surface epithelium, including loss of goblet cells. Furthermore, the inflammatory cells residing within the lumina of the inflamed lacrimal ductules may actually add toxic inflammatory products to the diminished tear secretions.

MUCOLYTIC. Occasionally, excessive mucus buildup can become a major KCS management problem. Treatment with 5% acetylcysteine solution (half-strength Mucomyst [Head Johnson] in Adapt) helps dissipate this buildup. Package directions indicate a shelf life of 5 days for Mucomyst solution; however, the author finds that it can be refrigerated and used as long as there is no discoloration. Although acetylcysteine is commonly used in veterinary ophthalmology, its use has not been proved safe or effective either in dogs or for ophthalmic application. Use of acetylcysteine requires the veterinarian or pharmacist to alter the recommended solvent and sterilize an available human product for ophthalmic application.

CHOLINERGIC STIMULANT. Pilocarpine is used for its acetylcholine-like action to stimulate residual lacrimal gland secretion. The typical dose used for an average 25-lb dog is two drops of 2% ophthalmic pilocarpine applied to the food twice daily. Improved results occur if the dosage is titrated to the patient by increasing the dose by one drop per day until an increase occurs in the STT or until early signs of toxicity (i.e., hypersalivation) result. Vomiting and diarrhea occur with overdosage. Based on experience in human patients, gastrointestinal pain is a likely unrecognized side effect. Bradycardia is another side effect seen in predisposed dogs. Pilocarpine's effect is short-lived (3 hours or less). Veterinary ophthalmologists vary widely in their opinion about use of this drug. Because oral pilocarpine is not FDA approved, extralabel use of pilocarpine orally in dogs also requires the veterinarian to use a drug that is not approved for this purpose, this route of administration, or this species.

CORTICOSTEROIDS. Corticosteroid use in KCS is controversial. Signs of keratitis or conjunctivitis often improve with topical corticosteroids. However, dogs with KCS frequently develop corneal ulcers, and corticosteroids can activate collagenase. In dogs that develop a minor corneal ulcer, corticosteroids can cause the ulcer to melt or perforate. Dogs with lagophthalmos and exophthalmos have increased risk of corneal ulcers and therefore additional risk if corticosteroids are used.

Systemic corticosteroids are often used in KCS-affected dogs because this disease is frequently associated with atopy or other immune-mediated disorders. Ocular lesions may improve with systemic corticosteroids; however, the potential to develop a melting corneal ulcer is increased.

ANTIBIOTICS. There are no bacterial species that can infect a normal, healthy canine eye. However, mucopurulent conjunctivitis with secondary opportunistic bacterial conjunctivitis is the most common sign of canine KCS. Whenever commensal bacterial overgrowth occurs, a broad-spectrum topical antibiotic is indicated. Unfortunately, copious mucopurulent discharge in dogs is often mistakenly diagnosed as primary bacterial conjunctivitis, and evaluation for KCS by STT is overlooked. This oversight causes the clinician to treat the dog with repeated courses of antibiotics that have only transient benefit. Response to antibiotics should not lead the clinician to conclude erroneously that bacterial conjunctivitis was the primary problem.

MISCELLANEOUS EXPERIMENTAL AGENTS. Transretinoic acid (Spectra) or vitamin A tretinoin (Retin-A, Ortho Pharm) has been proposed to reverse squamous metaplasia associated with KCS but has failed to do so in controlled human and dog trials. Tretinoin is under evaluation for treatment of ocular mucus deficiency.

Fibronectin may improve adherence of the corneal epithelium to its basement membrane. Fibronectin was found to be ineffective in treating KCS with slow-healing epithelial ulcers.

Oral bromhexine (Bisolvan, Boehringer Ingelheim), a bronchial mucolytic, increases STT results in some human KCS cases. Bromhexine is under study for treatment of Sjögren's syndrome in humans.

SURGERIES FOR THE LACRIMAL SYSTEM

NICTITANS PROLAPSE. Dogs in which the nictitating membrane glands (NMG) have been removed for correction of third eyelid gland protrusion (cherry eye) have an increased incidence of KCS. In normal dogs, surgical removal of either the NMG or the orbital lacrimal gland does not cause KCS, as either gland alone can produce sufficient tears. However, individuals who have marginal tear gland function are further compromised by NMG removal. Therefore, NMG excision is contraindicated in breeds known to be predisposed to KCS. The author prefers to suture the prolapsed gland to the orbital rim (see Fig. 1). Disadvantages of prior surgical methods were: (1) the gland was dissected from its overlying conjunctiva, at which time the surgeon likely severed all excretory ducts, negating the potential to retain secretory function, and (2) in one procedure, the suture passed into or near the globe where an intraocular hemorrhage or infection could be devastating. The author recommends the use of topical antibiotics prior to and after surgery, flushing the cul-de-sac preoperatively with 10% povidine iodine solution (not soap) and administering systemic antibiotics prior to surgery and for at least 3 days postop to avoid the potential of osteomyelitis developing along the buried suture.

PAROTID DUCT TRANSPOSITION. When medical management of KCS fails, a parotid duct transposition (PDT) can be used to replace deficient tearing with salivation. Parotid duct basal salivation rate and patency should be verified prior to recommending this procedure. Shortfalls of the PDT are: (1) it can create excessive flow and facial dermatitis, (2) calcium precipitates often cause a superficial band keratopathy, and (3) failure to salivate onto the eye may develop. The surgery is tedious and

Table 2. *Causes of Tear Film Disorders and Ocular Surface Disease*

Tear film abnormalities
  Aqueous layer
    Idiopathic (immune-mediated?)
    Sulfonamide toxicity
    Atropine toxicity
    Distemper
    Congenital lacrimal gland hypoplasia
    Neurologic (5th or 7th cranial nerve)
    Nictitans gland removal
  Mucin layer—goblet-cell loss
    Chronic conjunctivitis
    Radiation
    Conjunctival dysplasia?
  Lipid layer—increased free fatty acids
    Chalazia/meibomianitis
    Chronic blepharitis
Lid abnormalities
  Anatomic
    Exophthalmos
    Megalofissure
    Lid coloboma
    Ectropion
    Distichia
    Entropion
    Trichiasis
  Inflammatory
    Infection
    Allergy
    Autoimmune
  Functional
    Lagophthalmos
    Palpebral denervation

somewhat difficult and has an overall success rate of 63 to 80% when performed by veterinary ophthalmologists.

QUALITATIVE TEAR FILM DISEASE

Qualitative tear abnormalities may be primary or contributory causes of ocular surface disease (Table 2).

Mucin Deficiency

Clinical features of canine mucin deficiency include chronic keratoconjunctivitis, corneal ulceration, adequate aqueous secretion, and absence of ocular discharge. An unstable tear film is the hallmark of preocular mucin deficiency. Tear film instability occurs spontaneously in dogs with a decreased number of conjunctival goblet cells. Typical signs of tear film instability include focal areas of corneal dryness, thickened and inflamed conjunctiva, lackluster cornea, superficial and interstitial corneal vascular infiltrates, recurrent corneal ulcers, blepharospasm, and photophobia, which are all similar to signs of KCS. However, in contrast to KCS, mucin deficiency is associated with chronic keratoconjunctivitis with adequate STT (>12 mm/min) and an absence of ocular discharge.

DIAGNOSIS. Diagnosis of mucin deficiency is based on a decrease in the tear film breakup time (BUT). The BUT test is performed by placing one to two drops of fluorescein in the tear film, holding the lids open, and determining the time elapsed from the last blink until a dry spot (dark area in the green film) appears in the fluorescein-colored tear film. Normal BUT in dogs is 19 to 20 sec; BUT less than 10 sec is considered abnormal, and in mucin deficiency BUT is usually less than 5 sec. The diagnosis is supported if a conjunctival biopsy taken from the ventral fornix anterior to the third eyelid and stained with periodic acid-Schiff demonstrates a decreased goblet-cell density compared to a normal control.

ETIOLOGY. In dogs, the etiology of mucin deficiency is hypothesized to be chronic conjunctival inflammation that can reduce the goblet-cell count. In humans, vitamin A deficiency, pemphigus, drug toxicity, and radiation exposure are known causes.

TREATMENT. Standard treatment is advised for corneal ulcers as they occur. Maintenance therapy for mucin deficiency includes a mucinomimetic artificial tear (e.g., Adsorbobase, Alcon, Fort Worth, TX) or trilaminar tear supplement (Tear-Gard, Bio Products, New York, NY) every 12 hr. Petrolatum ophthalmic ointment is also advised every 4 hr to decrease lid friction. Topical antibiotics are recommended to reduce secondary infection. Topical corticosteroids can be used judiciously when corneal ulcers are not present to reduce inflammatory lesions. Cyclosporine's utility as an anti-inflammatory agent in reducing keratoconjunctivitis associated with mucin deficiency merits critical evaluation (Moore and Collier, 1990).

Abnormalities of the Lipid Layer

Chronic infection of the meibomian glands (most often *Staphylococcus*), allergy, or KCS can cause chronic marginal blepharitis. Tarsal gland orifices can become plugged or keratinized, and chalazia or lipid granulomas may form. Meibomianitis causes a qualitative change in meibomian gland secretions, resulting in release of toxic free fatty acids that can cause premature dispersion of the tear film, rapid dry-spot formation, and secondary superficial keratitis. Poor surfacing of the tear film due to swollen, irregular meibomian glands can also contribute to tear film instability. Topical corticosteroid/antibiotic combinations, systemic tetracycline, or topical cyclosporine are used empirically by the author to treat chronic or recurrent marginal blepharitis. Periodic manual expression of meibomian gland material with blunt-tipped forceps after topical anes-

thesia may reduce the quantity of irritative lipid material. If symptomatic treatment fails, culture and sensitivity testing of secretions expressed directly from the affected meibomian glands should be performed. Specific antimicrobial treatment is advised at least three times daily for 3 weeks.

ABNORMALITIES OF TEAR DISTRIBUTION

Normal lid-globe conformation and normal blinking are required to spread the tear film evenly across the eye and to resurface the tear film several times a minute. Lagophthalmos, exophthalmos, buphthalmos, eyelid paresis, or corneal anesthesia can cause exposure keratitis by incomplete or infrequent blinking. Because the lid margin functions like a windshield wiper, malposition of the lid (e.g., ectropion) or defects in the lid margin (i.e., eyelid colobomas) cause uneven spreading, tear film resurfacing, and dry spots. Ocular surface irregularities can also cause dry spots; examples include dermoids, corneal facets (healed stromal ulcers that leave indented or flat spots), and thick conjunctival grafts placed to seal deep ulcers.

Anatomic abnormalities are major contributors to morbidity in canine KCS. It is common to observe severe corneal scarring in exophthalmic dogs when the STT is 3 to 5 mm/min. By contrast, cats are diagnosed with KCS infrequently and rarely have abnormal lid-globe conformation. When KCS is diagnosed in cats, the STT is typically 0 mm/min, and unless herpetic keratitis is a codisorder, minimal or no corneal lesions are typical.

LATERAL CANTHUS SHORTENING. When KCS occurs in an exophthalmic dog such as a Pekingese or Lhasa apso, increased ocular surface exposure exacerbates developing lesions. If the dog does not blink completely (lagophthalmos), the problem is worsened. A permanent partial tarsorrhaphy can be used to reduce the exposed surface area of the globe. In exophthalmic dogs, a simple, permanent, partial tarsorrhaphy can dehisce; therefore, a skin-halving procedure is recommended.

SUMMARY

Keratoconjunctivitis sicca is the major cause of chronic or recurrent canine conjunctivitis. The diagnosis of KCS is often delayed or mistaken for allergic or bacterial conjunctivitis, and inappropriate or insufficient treatment can lead to progressive corneal scarring and blindness.

Ophthalmic cyclosporine promises vast improvement over previous KCS management. Resolution of corneal scarring and increased lacrimation are seen in most dogs. Early diagnosis of KCS and treatment with ophthalmic cyclosporine may avert this major cause of canine blindness.

References and Suggested Reading

Kaswan, R. L., and Salisbury, M. A.: A new perspective on canine keratoconjunctivitis sicca: Treatment with ophthalmic cyclosporine. Vet. Clin. North Am. Small Anim. Pract. 20:583–613, 1990.

Kaswan, R. L., Salisbury, M. A., and Ward, D. A.: Spontaneous canine keratoconjunctivitis sicca: A useful model for human keratoconjunctivitis sicca: Treatment with cyclosporine eye drops. Arch. Ophthalmol. 107:1210–16, 1989.

Lemp, M. A.: Diagnosis and treatment of tear deficiencies. *In* Tasman, W., and Jaeger, E. A. (eds.): *Duane's Clinical Ophthalmology.* Vol. 4. Philadelphia: J. P. Lippincott, 1990, chapter 14.

Moore, C. P.: Qualitative tear film disease. Vet. Clin. North Am. Small Anim. Pract. 20:565–81, 1990.

Moore, C. P., and Collier, L. L.: Ocular surface disease associated with loss of conjunctival goblet cells in dogs. J. Am. Anim. Hosp. Assoc. 26:456–66, 1990.

Morgan, R. V., and Abrams, K. L.: Use of topical cyclosporine for keratoconjunctivitis sicca in dogs. J.A.V.M.A. 199:1043, 1991.

Olivero, D. K., Davidson, M. G., English, R. V., et al.: Clinical trial evaluating 1% topical cyclosporine for canine keratoconjunctivitis sicca. J.A.V.M.A. 199:1039, 1991.

DISORDERS OF THE CORNEA AND SCLERA

CHRISTOPHER J. MURPHY

Madison, Wisconsin

Corneal diseases represent a major proportion of the total ophthalmologic case load in private practice. Lesions identified by a practitioner may range from benign peripheral endothelial melanosis, for which no treatment is necessary, to severe ulcerative keratitis that may necessitate enucleation of the globe. The significance of a particular corneal lesion is affected by several characteristics. These include its size, location (axial lesions being more significant for vision than peripheral lesions), optical density, as well as rate of progression. Potential heritability (e.g., corneal dystrophies) or relationship to systemic diseases may be important considerations.

Diseases of the sclera are much less commonly encountered in practice. A scleral lesion may be a primary neoplastic or inflammatory lesion or may occur secondary to trauma or an intraocular neoplasm or inflammatory process. Scleral lesions present a diagnostic and therapeutic challenge to clinicians.

NORMAL ANATOMY

The cornea is a unique structure in that it must be relatively resilient, insofar as it is exposed directly to the external environment, and yet, because it represents a major refractive component of the eye, it must remain transparent for normal visual processes to occur. In domestic mammals, the cornea is composed of four distinct layers. From anterior to posterior, these elements are (1) the anterior corneal epithelium, which makes up approximately 10% of the total corneal thickness; (2) the substantia propria or stroma, which forms the bulk of the corneal thickness; (3) Descemet's membrane, which is the exaggerated basement membrane of the most posteriorly situated component of the cornea; and (4) the endothelium. The anterior epithelium of the cornea is a stratified squamous nonkeratinized epithelium that has a relatively fast basal cell turnover time. Histologically, the epithelium can be divided into a single basal cell layer atop a basement membrane, a variable number of layers of polygonal wing cells, and the most superficially situated squamous cells. Evidence has now shown that the germinal cells for the anterior epithelium actually reside at the limbus. The limbal cells migrate centripetally in order to replenish the corneal epithelial cells, which are continuously sloughed off from the superficial squamous cell layer into the precorneal tear film.

Corneal epithelial wound healing is characterized by an initial lag phase of 3 to 4 hr, during which time the leading edge of epithelium around the wound thins and the normal stratified arrangement of the epithelial cells is lost. This lag phase is followed by a migration phase in which the corneal epithelial cells migrate to close the wound, re-establishing a continuous sheet of epithelial cells over the stroma. Only at a later time does actual mitosis occur in order to re-establish the normal thickness of the corneal epithelium. A corneal abrasion that is uncomplicated by the presence of a secondary infection heals in a relatively short period of time; an ulcer 2 mm in diameter heals in a few days (Kern, 1990).

The corneal stroma is composed of evenly arranged collagen fibrils of very fine diameter. The individual collagen fibrils are arranged into lamellae that span from limbus to limbus. All lamellae course parallel to the corneal surface but have various orientations relative to each other. Descemet's membrane is the exaggerated basement membrane of the endothelium. This exceedingly thin membrane does not retain the water-soluble dye fluorescein. It may bulge outward if the overlying stroma has been removed by a disease process such as severe ulcerative keratitis, creating a descemetocele. The endothelium of the cornea is composed of a single layer of low cuboidal hexagonal cells. Unlike the epithelium, the endothelium is relatively sensitive to injury and does not repair itself readily in most mammals. Because this is the layer primarily responsible for maintaining the cornea's relatively dehydrated state, damage to this layer of cells can result in persistent corneal edema.

The maintenance of corneal transparency is a delicate phenomenon. Intact functional epithelium and endothelium are necessary to maintain corneal dehydration. If water is imbibed by the corneal stroma, the regular arrangement of the collagen fibrils is disturbed. Rather than being transmitted through the stroma, incident light rays are scattered and reflected, resulting in corneal opacity. Similarly, in the genesis of a corneal scar, collagen fibrils of variable diameter and orientation are laid down, with resultant opacity. The normal cornea's lack of blood vessels, pigment, and myelinated nerve fibers contributes to its transparency. Unmyelinated nerve fibers are normally present.

CLINICAL EXAMINATION

Ophthalmologists evaluate the cornea and sclera using a relatively expensive biomicroscope or slit lamp. In general practice the cornea and sclera should be evaluated first in room light, after which the light should be dimmed substantially and broad, diffuse illumination used, such as that provided by a penlight, to examine structures more critically. Practitioners find it most helpful to use magnification throughout the examination. After all structures are examined in detail using broad, diffuse illumination, the cornea should be examined using retroillumination. To do this, the penlight is directed at an oblique angle relative to the iris surface, and light is bounced off the iris surface back toward the clinician through the cornea. The tapetal reflex can also be used to detect subtle corneal lesions. To examine the cornea using the tapetal reflex, a penlight or a direct ophthalmoscope may be employed. If using a penlight, it should be positioned just under the examiner's eye while the examiner looks down the penlight barrel at the eye. The tapetal reflex highlights any opacity present within the optical path. If using a direct ophthalmoscope,

the lens dial should be positioned at zero and the eye examined from an arm's length away through the eyepiece of the ophthalmoscope. Any opacity within the optical path is emphasized and made apparent to the clinician. Retroillumination is far more sensitive than direct illumination in detecting subtle corneal lesions. Once an opacity is identified, the light from a penlight or direct ophthalmoscope should be shone obliquely through the cornea from various angles to assist in defining the depth and extent of a given lesion. With painful keratitis, severe blepharospasm may impair visualization of the corneal surface. It may be necessary to apply topical anesthetic agents to relieve the patient's discomfort so that the corneal surface can be adequately visualized.

In examining the sclera, broad, diffuse illumination and transillumination are most helpful. Again, examination should be augmented by magnification. To transilluminate the sclera, the use of a specific transilluminator such as a Finnoff's transilluminator is beneficial. Topical anesthetic should be applied to the eye before transillumination. After the eye is anesthetized, the transilluminator is pressed gently against the sclera in the area of pathology. This type of illumination can help define the extent of a scleral lesion. To help differentiate scleritis from conjunctivitis, the application of topical 2.5% phenylephrine (AK-Dilate, Akorn) may be helpful. Conjunctival injection is blanched by the application of phenylephrine, whereas scleral injection is not totally subdued by this procedure. Additionally, it can be observed that injected conjunctival vessels are able to be gently moved by the examiner, whereas scleral vessels are immobile.

CORNEAL CULTURE AND CYTOLOGY

A single drop of topical anesthetic should be placed on the cornea before obtaining a culture specimen. It was previously thought that the preservatives in the topical anesthetic would interfere with obtaining an accurate corneal culture, but evidence now suggests that this is not the case (Canton, D., personal communication, 1991). It is recommended that a minitip culturette* be used to obtain the culture specimen. This culturette has a finer tip than the standard culturette; it allows a more accurate sampling of the ulcer bed and also decreases the probability of contamination of the culture tip by the lid margins. The media reservoir in the culture should be broken and the tip moistened before obtaining the specimen. This has been shown to increase the yield when compared with using an unmoistened culture. The swab should be submitted for aerobic bacterial culture. Though they

---

*Fisher Scientific, Santa Clara, CA.

can occur, fungal infections of the cornea in small animals are very rare.

After the culture specimen is obtained, additional drops of topical anesthetic agents should be applied to the cornea. A platinum Kimura's spatula or the dull end of a sterile scalpel blade may be used to obtain cytology specimens. Specimens should be obtained from the ulcer bed as well as from the margin. Extreme care must be exercised in obtaining a cytologic specimen from even an anesthetized animal with a descemetocele. Enough material should be obtained to make three separate slides for examination. One slide is used for a Gram's stain and one for a Wright-Giemsa stain. The remaining slide is set aside for special staining, if indicated. The Gram's and Wright-Giemsa stains should be performed immediately to determine the therapeutic course to be taken. Specimens obtained from eyes with untreated bacterial keratitis commonly are positive for bacteria. The rule of thumb for determining the therapeutic plan indicated by cytologic examinations is as follows: if gram-negative organisms are identified, the eye is treated only with aminoglycosides; if only gram-positive organisms are identified, the eye is treated with cephalosporins; if both gram-positive and gram-negative organisms are identified, the eye is treated with both an aminoglycoside and a cephalosporin; and if no bacterial organisms are identified, the eye is treated as if it had both a gram-negative and a gram-positive infection.

DISORDERS OF THE CORNEA

The cornea has a limited repertoire of responses to disease processes. The hallmark of corneal disease is the presence of a corneal opacity. A defect in the anterior corneal epithelium allows the precorneal tear film access to the underlying stroma. This causes an uneven distribution of the collagen fibrils relative to one another, and light is reflected and scattered, resulting in observation of a corneal opacity. Likewise, if the endothelium is compromised, water is imbibed by the cornea from the anterior chamber, resulting in corneal edema. Corneal vascularization may be initiated by an inflammatory process or by a break in the epithelium. The corneal vessels result in opacification not only because of their presence but also because of the corneal edema that is invariably associated with this process. Subsequent to vascularization, melanosis of the corneal epithelium and stroma may occur, especially in dogs. This is often interpreted as a sign of chronicity. Deposits within the corneal stroma can occur secondary to inflammation or as a primary process related to corneal dystrophy or a metabolic disorder. The potential presence of a corneal foreign body should not be overlooked.

Table 1. *Underlying Causes of Ulcerative Keratitis*

Entropion
Other lid defects
Distichiasis
Ectopic cilia
Lagophthalmos
Exophthalmos
Foreign body
Keratoconjunctivitis sicca
Severe debilitation
Neural defects; cranial nerve V and/or VII

Corneal Abrasions

In simple corneal abrasions, the anterior corneal epithelium has been traumatically removed from the underlying stroma. Predisposing causes of ulcerative keratitis are listed in Table 1. Patients typically present with blepharospasm and epiphora. Instillation of topical anesthetic may be required to adequately visualize the corneal surface. The cornea is edematous in the area of abrasion as a result of imbibing water into the corneal stroma from the precorneal tear film. Edema typically extends a short distance circumferentially beyond the margin of the epithelial defect. Careful examination of the corneal defect with magnification verifies the absence of a corneal infiltrate, and the margin of the opacity is indistinct. The pupil is typically miotic. Miosis occurs as a result of an axonal reflex in which stimulation of the afferent nerves that innervate the superficial cornea results in contraction of the iridal sphincter and iridocyclitis, with breakdown of the blood/aqueous barrier. The degree of uveitis that results from a corneal lesion is highly variable. A significant portion of the pain due to ulcerative keratitis is a result of the ciliary muscle spasm associated with the reflex uveitis. This reflex uveitis necessitates the use of atropine in the treatment of ulcerative keratitis. In cases of simple abrasion, I do not perform any ancillary testings, such as culture or cytologic examination. Topical anesthetic is applied, and a thorough search of the conjunctival surface is made for the presence of any foreign body.

TREATMENT
(Tables 2 and 3)

Initial Visit

- Topical broad-spectrum antibiotic (e.g., polymyxin B-neomycin-gramicidin [Neosporin, Burroughs Wellcome]) every 8 to 12 hr
- 1% atropine every 8 to 12 hr
- ± Elizabethan collar
- Recheck in 1 week

Recheck Visit

If significant progress has been made in healing and there is no evidence of an infectious process,

Table 2. Drugs Used in Treating Disorders of the Cornea and Sclera

Drug	Dose	Time Interval	Route
Polymyxin B-neomycin-gramicidin (Neosporin, Burroughs Wellcome)		q 8–12 hr	Topical
1% Atropine (many manufacturers)		q 8–12 hr	Topical
Gentamicin (Gentocin, Schering)	10 mg	q 24 hr	Subconjunctival
Cephalothin (Keflin, Lilly)	75 mg	q 24 hr	Subconjunctival
Atropine—parenteral	40 µg	q 24 hr	Subconjunctival
Cyanoacrylate adhesive (Ophthalmic Nexaband, CRX Medical)	1 drop		Topical—corneal repair
Trifluridine (Viroptic, Burroughs Wellcome)		q 1–5 hr	Topical—herpes keratitis
Idoxuridine (Herplex, Allergan)		q 5 hr	Topical—herpes keratitis
Adenine arabinoside (Vira-A, Parke-Davis)	Not recommended		Topical—herpes keratitis
Chloramphenicol (Chloroptic, Allergan)		q 6–8 hr	Topical—bacterial keratitis
5% Sodium chloride solution (AK-NaCl 5% Ointment or Solution, Akorn)		q 4–6 hr	Topical—chronic erosion
Regular insulin diluted to 10 U/ml with artificial tears (not proprietary)			Topical—chronic erosion
Epithelial growth factor; fibronectin	Not available commercially		Topical—chronic erosion
Megestrol acetate (Ovaban, Schering)	5 mg	q 24 hr for 5–10 days	Oral—eosinophilic keratitis
Dexamethasone (Azium, Schering)	1 mg		Subconjunctival—pannus
1% Prednisolone acetate (Pred Forte, Allergan)		q 6–8 hr	Topical—pannus
0.1% Dexamethasone ointment (Maxidex, Alcon)		q 6–8 hr	Topical—pannus
Triamcinolone (Vetalog, Squibb)	10 mg		Subconjunctival—pannus
Prednisolone	2 mg/kg	q 24 hr for 5 days	Oral—scleritis/episcleritis
	1 mg/kg	q 24 hr for 5 days	
	1 mg/kg	q 24 hr for 14 days	
Azathioprine (Imuran, Burroughs Wellcome)	1–2 mg/kg	daily—reduced over 4–8 weeks	Oral—scleral nodules

therapy should be continued as indicated earlier. If there is any indication of an infectious process, culture and cytologic examination should be performed. The antimicrobial regimen to be followed depends on the results of cytologic study (see the earlier section "Corneal Culture and Cytology"). Topical treatment with atropine should be continued. If significant healing has not taken place and there is no evidence of an infectious process as indicated by cellular infiltrates, stromal necrosis, or a mucopurulent discharge, then consideration should be given to the placement of a therapeutic soft contact lens.

Bacterial Keratitis

The typical patient with bacterial keratitis presents with moderate to severe blepharospasm and a mucopurulent discharge. Examination of the cornea reveals cellular infiltration in the ulcer bed itself that typically extends beyond the margin of the ulcer into the stroma. The cornea is opacified in the area of the lesion because of cornea edema as well as the cellular infiltrate. The border of the infiltrate often has an irregular, diffuse margin in the densest part of the opacity. A variable degree of stromal necrosis is usually present. The degree of pain and reflex uveitis is usually more severe in bacterial keratitis than in a simple corneal abrasion. In more

advanced cases, the stroma overlying Descemet's membrane may have sloughed, resulting in the formation of a descemetocele. If a descemetocele is present, fluorescein stain is not retained by the bed of the lesion. It is, however, retained by the sides of the lesion. Gentle irrigation with a saline solution may be necessary to carefully evaluate the lesion after fluorescein staining, because fluorescein pools in the base of a defect even though it is not retained by Descemet's membrane. Such a staining profile is pathognomonic for a descemetocele. If a descemetocele is present, further diagnostic evaluation should not be performed until the animal is anesthetized. The globe is extremely fragile in such a condition, and perforation of the globe can occur simply as a result of a minor intraocular pressure elevation induced by globe retraction by the animal.

MEDICAL TREATMENT

- Subconjunctival injection of an aminoglycoside (e.g., gentamicin [Gentocin, Schering; 10 mg]) or a cephalosporin (e.g., cephalothin [Keflin, Lilly; 75 mg]) or both
- ± subconjunctival injection of 40 µg of injectable atropine
- Topical antibiotics applied every 5 min for half an hour, then every 15 min until 2 hr, then every 2 hr for the first few days of therapy

Table 3. Equipment Used in Treating Disorders of the Cornea and Sclera

Equipment	Use
Minitip Culturette (Fisher Scientific, Santa Clara, CA)	Bacterial culture swab
Optic-Cor Collagen Shields (Pitman Moore)	Corneal protection
Soflens Plano-T (Bausch & Lomb)	Contact lens
No. 15 Bard-Parker Blade (Bard-Parker Company)	Epithelial debridement
No. 64 Beaver Blade (Beaver Company)	Epithelial debridement
Microcellulose sponge (Weck)	Drying corneal surface

- Hot packs applied three to four times daily
- Elizabethan collar required
- ± a collagen shield* soaked in antibiotic (e.g., gentamicin)
- ± a therapeutic soft contact lens†
- Depending on severity of lesion, hospitalize or recheck in 2 to 3 days

Recheck Examination

If the cornea is stable or improved, continue the current mode of therapy. If the condition has worsened, alter medical therapy based on culture results. Repeat subconjunctival injections. If the condition has worsened significantly or pending perforation exists, consider surgical options.

Surgical Intervention

If more than 50% of the corneal stromal thickness has been lost at initial examination or on subsequent examination, consideration should be given to surgical intervention. Surgical alternatives include cyanoacrylate repair, suturing closed a small descemetocele, conjunctival flap, conjunctival island graft, lamellar keratoplasty, corneoscleral transposition, autologous corneal graft, and penetrating keratoplasty. Placement of a third eyelid flap has little therapeutic value. In my opinion, placement of a soft therapeutic contact lens is of equal therapeutic value to a third eyelid flap but has the advantage of allowing the clinician to view the underlying pathologic processes. Many of the described surgical procedures require specialized surgical equipment and skill in order to perform the operation properly. The ensuing discussion is therefore limited to cyanoacrylate repair.

CYANOACRYLATE REPAIR. Equipment needed includes a 27-gauge needle, tuberculin syringe, number 15 Bard-Parker blade or number 64 Beaver blade, a 22-gauge needle, Weckcell's microcellulose sponges,* a container of photographic canned air, and cyanoacrylate adhesive.† Because the degree of toxicity decreases with increasing alkyl chain length in the cyanoacrylate adhesives, butyl cyanoacrylate is generally recommended for maximizing adhesive strength while minimizing toxicity.

The patient is anesthetized, the eye draped for aseptic surgery, and a fine wire lid speculum is placed. The globe is fixated by placement of two or three 5–0 silk limbal stay sutures. The globe should be fixated so that the bed of the ulcer is pointing straight up. Under magnification, the sides and base of the ulcer are debrided with a 22-gauge needle. All epithelium and necrotic stromal tissue must be removed before placement of the adhesive. If culture and cytologic specimens have not been obtained previously, some of this material should be used for these purposes. After the wound margin is debrided, the scalpel blade is used to remove the epithelium from around this stromal defect for a distance of 0.5 mm. This is done because the cyanoacrylate will not adequately adhere to the cornea if the epithelium is intact. The stromal defect is thoroughly dried using the canned air. Before applying the air directly to the stromal defect, it should be directed toward the limbal margin to adjust the velocity of the air exiting the application tube. Great force can be generated by the canned air, which can perforate a descemetocele. After the wound bed has thoroughly dried, the cyanoacrylate is applied using the tuberculin syringe and a 27-gauge needle. Only the smallest drops should be applied to the ulcer bed. The goal in application of the cyanoacrylate is to *coat* the inside of the cup, *not* to fill it. The toxicity of cyanoacrylate has been shown to be related to the total mass of glue that is applied rather than to the surface area. The glue should completely cover the base and sides of the defect and should extend onto the corneal surface for approximately 0.5 mm. The glue is then gently dried using a very fine, gentle stream of air. The polymerization process can be accelerated by application of sterile saline. After completion of the cyanoacrylate application, subconjunctival injections of appropriate antibiotics, as determined by cytologic examination, are performed. The stay sutures are removed, and a soft therapeutic contact lens is applied to the cornea. The contact lens is used to increase the patient's comfort, because the glue surface is invariably rough. The glue usually sloughs spontaneously in 7 to 10 days. This often occurs after the ulcer bed has been infiltrated by vessels.

Feline Herpetic Keratitis

Feline herpetic keratitis is one of the most common ulcerative conditions affecting young cats. The

---

*Opti-Cor, Pitman Moore, Mundelein, IL.
†B&L Soflens Plano T, Bausch & Lomb, Rochester, NY.

*Weckcell, Weck, Research Triangle Park, NC.
†Ophthalmic Nexaband, CRX Medical, Raleigh, NC.

initial phases of this disease are typically associated with conjunctivitis (see this volume, p. 1085). Secondary episodes may be associated with the development of ulcerative keratitis. The early corneal lesions are typified by the presence of dendritic lesions. These may best be visualized by the application of rose bengal stain. Although corneal dendrites are considered to be the "textbook" finding in herpetic keratitis, it is my experience that they are rarely encountered in practice. More commonly, a young cat presents with a paraxial geographic ulcer that is not associated with a significant neutrophil infiltrate. Many of these patients appear much more comfortable than one would expect, given the extent of the corneal lesion. Cats with herpetic keratitis often have a protracted course to final resolution. These ulcers rarely develop secondary bacterial infections. Cytologic examination demonstrates few to moderate numbers of inflammatory cells and is negative for bacteria. Additional tests that may be performed include culture for the feline herpesvirus and immunofluorescent antibody testing of a conjunctival scraping for identification of the herpes antigen. Evidence now suggests that fluorescein staining should be avoided before obtaining cytologic specimen for herpes immunofluorescent antibody (da Silva Curiel, J., Collins, B. K., and Nasisse, M. P., personal communication, 1984). Paired serum samples may also be submitted for evaluation of a response to the herpes antigen. Though specific diagnostic testing to positively identify herpes keratitis is costly, clients are usually encouraged to pursue this route because of the implications that a herpes infection has on the management of future recurrences. If the history, signalment, and clinical appearance of the lesion are compatible with herpetic keratitis, the animal is treated as if it had herpes even if specific testing for the herpesvirus is negative (Nasisse, 1990).

TREATMENT

Among topical antiviral medications, trifluridine (Viroptic, Burroughs Wellcome) is the drug of choice. It should be administered every hour for the first day and then reduced to five times daily thereafter. Trifluridine is a nucleoside analogue that becomes incorporated in the viral DNA, resulting in inhibition of virus-specific mRNA. The relative potency of trifluridine compared with other antiviral drugs is trifluridine > idoxuridine > adenine arabinoside. A small percentage of cats treated with trifluridine may demonstrate severe discomfort after topical application. In such cases, idoxuridine (Herplex, Allergan Pharmaceuticals) should be applied five times daily. Idoxuridine is a pyrimidine nucleoside analogue that competes with thymidine for incorporation into viral DNA. Therapy should be continued until the corneal lesions have resolved. Irritation can occur with any of these drugs, although it has been my experience that they occur most frequently with trifluridine.

Corticosteroids are contraindicated because they delay corneal epithelialization and are locally immunosuppressive.

- Topical broad-spectrum antibiotics (e.g., chloramphenicol [Chloroptic, Allergan Pharmaceuticals]) every 6 to 8 hr
- Topical 1% atropine every 8 to 24 hr, depending on severity of ocular pain
- ± Elizabethan collar
- Recheck in 1 week.
- *Recheck examination:* If condition is stable or improved, continue current therapy; if condition has worsened, change antiviral medications.
- Recheck in 1 week.

With recurrent infections, stromal keratitis may develop, but this is considered rare. Chronic stromal keratitis may be associated with vascularization of the cornea. In such cases, when an epithelial defect does not exist, the judicious use of topical corticosteroids may be beneficial (see this volume, p. 1070).

Chronic Nonseptic Ulcerative Keratitis of Dogs

Every practitioner has seen dogs in which an epithelial defect persists despite various therapeutic regimens. The ulceration can often be associated with a traumatic event, but for some reason the epithelium fails to cover the stroma in the normal period of time. Typical findings are a paracentral epithelial defect, no stromal involvement, and few or no corneal vessels. The ulcer margin has loosely adherent epithelium, commonly termed *epithelial lipping.* Immediately visible after application of fluorescein stain is a central area of bright fluorescence surrounded by an area of dull fluorescence when viewed with a cobalt light. The area of dull fluorescence is due to seepage of fluorescein under the epithelial lip. Cytologic study and culture of these lesions are uniformly uninformative. These lesions typically occur in middle-aged and older dogs, though they may occur at any age. This condition has been associated with an epithelial/ basement membrane dystrophy in the boxer dog, although it can be encountered in any breed. When first seen by a practitioner, this type of lesion will most likely be interpreted as an abrasion and should be treated as such (see earlier). If the defect has not healed within the usual period of time, consideration should be given to the possibility that the defect may represent an indolent ulcer. Therapy is directed toward (1) preventing infection, (2) decreasing trauma to the epithelium that is trying to become attached to the underlying stroma, (3) stimulating growth and attachment of the epithelial cells, and (4) relieving pain.

TREATMENT

- ± Dry debridement of loose epithelial cells
- Therapeutic soft contact lens
- Broad-spectrum topical antibiotic (e.g., polymyxin B-neomycin-gramicidin [Neosporin, Burroughs Wellcome]) every 8 hr
- ± 1% atropine every 12 to 24 hr
- ± topical hyperosmotics (e.g., 5% sodium chloride solution [AK-NaCl, Akorn]) every 4 to 6 hr
- ± topical growth factors (e.g., insulin [every 6 hr], epithelial growth factor
- ± topical extracellular matrix (e.g., fibronectin)

Although epithelial growth factor and fibronectin are not yet commercially available for ophthalmic use, they will most likely become available within the next 5 years. For this reason, they are mentioned as therapeutic modalities in this chapter.

Topical insulin can be formulated by practitioners using artificial tears and regular insulin at a concentration of 10 U/ml. Previous studies have shown that topical insulin can counteract the inhibition of wound healing induced by topical application of corticosteroids. I have been using topical insulin every 6 hr for 14 days in recalcitrant cases of chronic corneal ulceration for the past 6 years and have had encouraging results. Like most therapeutic modalities for the treatment of chronic corneal ulcerations, insulin seems to work in some cases and to have no effect in others. Carefully controlled clinical trials have not been performed to determine the true therapeutic value of insulin in the treatment of this disease process.

Even with vigorous medical therapy and the use of therapeutic contact lenses, many chronic ulcerations do not heal without surgical intervention. Surgical alternatives include (1) multifocal superficial punctate keratotomy, (2) debridement of loose epithelium, (3) superficial keratectomy, (4) application of cyanoacrylate to the wound bed, (5) cyanoacrylate attachment of a therapeutic soft contact lens, and (6) placement of a conjunctival flap. I have had success in the surgical treatment of chronic ulceration by using a combination of multifocal superficial punctate keratectomy with attachment of a therapeutic contact lens with cyanoacrylate adhesive.

To perform a multiple focal superficial punctate keratotomy, a 22-gauge needle is used to place a gridwork of superficial punctures into the anterior stroma that surrounds the ulcer bed for a distance of approximately 0.5 mm and extends across the ulcer bed. It is generally recommended that this

procedure be performed on the animal under general anesthesia and that magnification be used. These punctures are thought to provide anchoring points for epithelial attachment. A minute amount of cyanoacrylate is then placed (a drop should just barely be visible at the tip of the 30-gauge needle) on the stroma in the area of ulceration using a tuberculin syringe and 30-gauge needle, and a therapeutic soft contact lens applied. The lens will bond immediately to the underlying stroma; it cannot be repositioned. Topical broad-spectrum antibiotics are applied three times daily, and atropine is applied topically once a day. An Elizabethan collar is placed on the animal to avoid dislodgment of the lens. The defect is usually healed by 2 weeks after surgery. The epithelium migrates under the cyanoacrylate adhesive and allows the lens to be removed. If, after the 2-week recheck, the lens is still attached to the underlying stroma by the adhesive, the animal is rechecked in 2 weeks, with continuation the previously mentioned therapeutic regimen.

Corneal Sequestrum Formation

Corneal sequestrum is a unique corneal necrotizing disease that occurs only in cats (Pentlarge, 1989). Also known as *corneal mummification* and *corneal black body formation*, it is characterized by chronic ulceration, stromal necrosis, and the accumulation of a brownish pigment, the nature of which remains unidentified. The exact pathogenesis of this corneal disorder remains unknown, although initiation of stromal necrosis appears to be a common factor. It has been noted to occur secondary to feline herpes keratitis. In its earlier stages, it may appear simply as a very light translucent tannish spot in the central cornea. With further development, it acquires a dark brown to black pigmentation that may increase in its diameter and extend farther into the stroma itself. Early in development most corneal sequestra are located superficially within the stroma in a subepithelial position. A sequestrum may occasionally extend to the level of Descemet's membrane. The density of the pigment may not allow an accurate assessment of the depth of the lesion. Some sequestra have a cone configuration, with a broad superficial base but extending down and having a narrow area of stromal involvement in the region of Descemet's membrane. With chronicity, corneal vascularization may ensue. If vascularized, the sequestrum may have a slightly raised surface extending beyond the surrounding cornea. A sequestrum that has not elicited a vascular response usually has a very flat surface that does not extend above the surrounding cornea. Corneal sequestra are typically unilateral, though bilateral cases of sequestration have been observed. At the initial examination, the owner should be informed about the nature of the disease and that the course may be protracted until final healing has occurred. One of two modes of therapy can be selected. Medical therapy is designed to encourage vascular ingrowth to accelerate the sloughing process. Surgical therapy consists of performing a superficial keratectomy to remove the sequestrum *in toto*. I usually pursue medical therapy for a period of 1 to 2 weeks in order to assess more carefully the probability that medical therapy will bring about a final resolution of the sequestrum. The time course and degree of corneal scarring are greater when medical therapy is elected as compared with surgical therapy.

MEDICAL THERAPY

- Topical broad-spectrum antibiotic (e.g., polymyxin B-neomycin-gramicidin [Neosporin, Burroughs Wellcome]) every 6 to 12 hr
- Topical 1% atropine every 8 to 24 hr
- ± topical antiviral (e.g., trifluridine [Viroptic, Burroughs Wellcome]) every 1 to 5 hr
- Elizabethan collar
- Hot pack on affected eye every 6 to 8 hr
- Recheck in 1 to 2 weeks.
- *Recheck examination:* If significant vascularization has occurred or the sequestrum is raised beyond the surrounding cornea, continue current therapy.
- Recheck in 2 to 3 weeks.

If significant vascularization has not occurred and if the sequestrum still has a flat appearance, consider performing superficial keratectomy. If the owner declines surgery, increase the frequency of hot packs and continue topical therapy. If surgical therapy is elected at either the initial or the subsequent recheck examinations, the owner must be cautioned that the sequestrum may not be completely removed by a superficial keratectomy. The owner should be informed of the possibility that a decision may need to be made intraoperatively to perform a more extensive surgical procedure such as a conjunctival island graft or a penetrating keratoplasty.

Eosinophilic Keratitis

Eosinophilic keratitis is a unique, possibly immune-mediated disorder peculiar to cats. It typically occurs in young to middle-aged cats and develops as a raised limbal pink or reddish slowly progressive lesion. Only one eye is initially involved, although with time bilateral lesions may develop. Similar to the eosinophilic granuloma complex of cats, it is thought to be immune-mediated, although the exact pathogenetic mechanisms by

which this disease develops remain unknown. The lesions first develop at the limbal margins and slowly progress axially into the cornea. In some cases, whitish flecks may be seen on the surface of the lesion. A degree of ocular discomfort is associated with this lesion, and the owner may first notice blepharospasm and a mild to mucopurulent discharge. Confirmation of this diagnosis is made by cytologic examination or by histologic examination of a biopsy specimen. Cytologically, this lesion is characterized by the presence of mast cells and eosinophils. It is common to encounter a greater degree of mast cells by cytologic examination than is appreciated by histologic examination of a biopsy specimen. This disorder is very responsive to topical corticosteroid therapy as well as to systemic treatment with megestrol acetate (Ovaban, Schering). When the diagnosis is made, the owner should be alerted that the lesion may recur with time. A review of this disease complex has shown that megestrol acetate may result in complete resolution with as short a duration of therapy as 1 week (Paulsen et al., 1987a).

TREATMENT

- Topical antibiotic-steroid mixture (e.g., Maxitrol, Alcon) every 6 to 8 hr
- ± megestrol acetate, 5 mg PO every 24 hr for 5 to 10 treatments
- Recheck in 2 to 3 weeks.

I usually initiate topical corticosteroid therapy and use megesterol acetate only if the disease recurs.

Pannus (Chronic Superficial Pigmentary Keratitis)

Pannus is a slowly progressive corneal disease that begins at the limbus. Typically bilateral in nature, it almost exclusively affects purebred and crossbred German shepherd dogs. The frequency and severity of the disease are affected by geographic location and other unknown factors. Previous studies have associated the frequency of occurrence and the severity of pannus to exposure to ultraviolet radiation. Initial episodes are usually noted in young to middle-aged dogs. No sex predilection has been noted. It is characterized by the incursion of lymphocytes, plasma cells, blood vessels, and melanin into the anterior stroma, typically beginning at the inferolateral border of the cornea. The surface of the lesion is often irregular, although usually not ulcerated. Although pannus can occur in any breed of dog, the great majority are encountered in German shepherds, German shepherd crosses, and greyhounds, in which they are common. In dogs that have had multiple recurrences, cholesterol deposits may be seen within the anterior stroma. Such deposits can occur after any long-standing inflammatory condition of the cornea.

The mainstay of therapy in this disease is topical corticosteroids applied at the minimum frequency that will control the disease process. Initial therapy is aggressive, and maintenance therapy is dictated by the response of the patient. In all cases, the client needs to be informed that the disease requires lifelong medication. In cases recalcitrant to topical corticosteroid administration, more aggressive modalities of therapy, such as beta irradiation, may need to be initiated.

TREATMENT

Initial therapy is based on the severity of clinical signs present. If clinical signs are advanced, subconjunctival injections are recommended as an adjunct to topical steroid therapy. If signs are mild, topical therapy alone is initiated.

- Subconjunctival injections: 1 mg dexamethasone (Azium, Schering)
- Topical steroid therapy: 0.1% dexamethasone ointment (e.g., Maxidex, Alcon) or 1% prednisolone suspension (Pred Forte, Allergan) every 6 to 8 hr (If an antibiotic-corticosteroid combination is used, the clinician should be aware that neomycin, a common constituent of antibiotic-steroid combinations, may cause a hypersensitivity reaction if used chronically.)
- Recheck in 3 to 4 weeks.
- *Recheck examination:* If marked improvement in the condition has occurred, topical corticosteroid therapy is decreased to every 12 hr for 30 days. On subsequent recheck, if the condition is still in regression, steroid therapy is reduced further and the dog observed periodically for progression. Many dogs that do not have severe disease can be adequately controlled with as little as a single treatment given every other day. If the condition has not improved or has worsened at the first recheck, more aggressive therapy must be initiated, including repeating the subconjunctival injections (possibly using a longer-acting repositol steroid such as 10 mg triamcinolone [Vetalog, Squibb]) and increasing the frequency of topical steroid therapy. Consideration must be given in such situations to adjunctive therapy such as beta irradiation.

Keratoconjunctivitis Sicca

Keratoconjunctivitis sicca is one of the most commonly encountered ophthalmic diseases to affect the canine cornea (see this volume, p. 1092).

Corneal Dystrophies

Corneal dystrophies are a family of diseases that may affect the epithelium, the stroma, or the endothelium. In their broadest sense, corneal dystrophies may be described as axial to paraxial in location, occurring initially in young to middle-aged dogs, unassociated with underlying disease or ocular pain, slowly progressive, and heritable (Cooley and Dice, 1990).

EPITHELIAL DYSTROPHIES

Only two forms of epithelial dystrophies have been described in dogs: the epithelial basement membrane dystrophy associated with chronic ulcerative keratitis in boxers and epithelial changes in the unique, painful dystrophy encountered in Shetland sheepdogs. Boxers have been previously reported to be afflicted by a syndrome characterized by chronic ulceration. Previous studies have demonstrated histologic abnormalities in the epithelial cells' basement membrane. Although this has been reported as a primary epithelial dystrophy, it is possible that the morphologic alterations that were reported could have resulted from alterations in the corneal microenvironment. Some environmental factors to consider include (1) the characteristics of the tear film (e.g., pH and ionic strength), (2) the exact nature of the extracellular matrix (e.g., fibronectin), (3) the relative proportions of extracellular growth factors (e.g., epithelial growth factor), and (4) the relative abundance of neuropeptides elaborated by the corneal terminations of the trigeminal nerve. In any event, the resulting chronic ulceration that occurs in boxer dogs should be therapeutically addressed in a fashion similar to chronic ulcerative conditions in any breed (see the earlier section "Chronic Nonseptic Ulcerative Keratitis of Dogs").

Shetland sheepdogs are susceptible to a unique corneal disorder that is characterized by the presence of multiple punctate gray-white superficial corneal opacities of variable size. A previous report (Dice, P. F., personal communication, 1984) described dyskeratotic necrotic cells within the epithelium and abnormalities in the basement membrane. Individual lesions are irregularly ring-shaped and 1 to 3 mm in diameter. They appear first centrally and may develop peripherally as the animal ages. Recurrences have afflicted approximately 30% of patients. These same patients had Schirmer's tear test values of 10 to 12 mm/min and a shortened tear breakup time (<10 sec). Two thirds of the dogs were asymptomatic; findings on serum chemistry and serology studies were normal, and no associated ocular systemic disease was found. It has been my experience that even in the absence of a corneal erosion, many of these dogs present with a degree of ocular pain, indicated by blepharospasm and epiphora. The corneas of dogs with chronic lesions frequently retain rose bengal dye.

Treatment

Treatment of this disorder is dependent on the severity of clinical signs.

- If erosion is present: topical broad-spectrum antibiotic (e.g., polymyxin B-neomycin-gramicidin [Neosporin, Burroughs Wellcome]) every 6 to 8 hr
- ± 1% atropine every 12 to 24 hr
- ± Elizabethan collar
- ± therapeutic soft contact lens (contraindicated in the presence of a very low Schirmer's tear test value)
- ± artificial tears or ointments every 4 to 8 hr (if Schirmer's tear test <15 mm/min)
- Recheck in 2 weeks if no erosions are present.
- ± judicious use of topical corticosteroids (e.g., 1% prednisolone [Pred Forte, Allergan]) every 8 to 24 hr (Note: topical corticosteroids are normally contraindicated in the presence of corneal ulceration.)
- ± Elizabethan collar
- Recheck in 2 weeks (recheck in 1 week if corticosteroids are used).

If chronic discomfort or erosion persists despite medical therapy, consideration should be given to performing superficial keratectomy to remove the areas of opacity, followed by soft therapeutic contact lens application. Topical broad-spectrum antibiotic is applied every 8 hr as well as 1% atropine sulfate every 12 to 24 hr until healing is complete. The condition may recur.

STROMAL DYSTROPHIES

Stromal dystrophies are a family of corneal disorders characterized by deposition of substances (typically lipid or cholesterol) within the stroma at various levels. Onset of the disease is typically noted in young to middle-aged dogs, unassociated with any underlying disease or any degree of ocular discomfort. It is very unusual for the stromal dystrophies to interfere with vision. Stromal dystrophy has been best described in the Siberian husky and a strain of laboratory beagle. It is important to properly identify this family of corneal lesions in order to make breeding recommendations. Neither medical nor surgical intervention is recommended.

ENDOTHELIAL DYSTROPHIES

In endothelial dystrophies, the function of the endothelium is impaired, resulting in chronic edema of the cornea. The condition is typically first noted in middle-aged dogs. Slowly progressive opacification of the cornea develops as water is imbibed by the corneal stroma. As in all dystrophies, this is a bilateral disease, though the severity or onset of the disease process may be asymmetric. No treatment is necessary for the early phases of the disease, although the owner should be informed about its progressive nature. In the later stages, bullous keratopathy may develop. These "water blisters," which become localized in the anterior stroma and epithelium, may rupture, creating an epithelial defect. In such cases, the animal may experience recurrent painful episodes. Also, during the period in which the epithelial defect exists, the cornea is susceptible to infection. Medical treatment is indicated initially, but surgical intervention may be necessary for serious ulceration.

Endothelial dystrophies have been best described in the Boston terrier and Manx cat. The gene for this condition in the Manx breed has either been extirpated from the population or occurs at a very low frequency; this condition has not been reported for many years.

Treatment

If bullous keratopathy and recurrent epithelial erosions are not present, no treatment is necessary.

- If bullous keratopathy and recurrent erosions are present, apply topical hyperosmotic solutions or ointments (e.g., 5% NaCl [AK-NaCl, Akorn]) every 4 to 6 hr.
- If erosions are present, apply topical broad-spectrum antibiotic and soft therapeutic soft contact lens.
- Recheck in 2 to 3 weeks.

If erosions persist or frequently recur, consideration should be given to surgical intervention. Procedures include a complete conjunctival flap, penetrating keratoplasty, and thermokeratoplasty. The latter two procedures are best performed by a veterinary ophthalmologist.

DISORDERS OF THE SCLERA

Nontraumatic disorders of the sclera are uncommon but present a diagnostic and therapeutic challenge to a clinician when they are encountered. Of these, only episcleritis, scleritis, and nodular lesions of the limbus are encountered with any frequency.

Episcleritis and Scleritis

Episcleritis can be characterized as being either simple or nodular. Inflamed episcleral vessels are straight and radial in their orientation and have a salmon-pink appearance. The vessels can be seen to be movable over deeper structures. It can be associated with a mucoid or serous discharge. Simple episcleritis may not progress to involve the sclera, but a degree of episcleritis nearly always accompanies scleritis. Simple episcleritis may be transient, resolving without any medications. It is typically very responsive to the administration of topical or systemic steroids. Nodular lesions of the sclera will be addressed separately in the next section.

Scleritis is an inflammatory disorder affecting the stromal elements of the sclera. The scleral vessels form a crisscross pattern and, when injected, appear a deep bluish-red. Unlike the engorged vessels associated with conjunctivitis and episcleritis, the scleral vessels are immobile. Unlike glaucoma, which can also be associated with scleral injection, the intraocular pressure is not elevated and there is no evidence of visual dysfunction. Scleritis is often associated with a degree of discomfort and tenderness on digital pressure. Scleritis can be sectoral, affecting only a limited portion of the globe, or it may diffusely involve the sclera. It may be mild and relatively benign or severe and destructive. Scleritis most commonly presents as a unilateral condition, though it can occur bilaterally. It may also be associated with other ocular conditions such as uveitis.

The underlying cause of scleritis is frequently not discovered; an autoimmune cause is commonly suspected. All patients presenting with scleritis should be carefully evaluated for the presence of an underlying systemic disease. Scleritis is treated with topical or systemic steroids. In moderate to severe cases, I usually prescribe a decreasing dosage regimen of oral prednisolone (2 mg/kg every 24 hr for 5 days, then 1 mg/kg every 24 hr for 5 days, then 1 mg/kg every 48 hr for 14 days) and apply 1% topical prednisolone (Pred Forte, Allergan) to the affected eye every 4 hr for a week, then every 6 hr for 2 weeks, then every 8 hr for 2 weeks.

Nodular Lesions of the Limbus

The terminology surrounding nodular lesions of the sclera can be confusing and is not agreed on by all specialists. Terms that have been used to describe this family of conditions include *proliferative keratoconjunctivitis, pseudotumor, collie granuloma, nodular fasciitis, fibrous histiocytoma, nod-*

ular episcleritis, and *superficial non-necrotizing scleritis.* The criteria for assigning one name versus another are influenced by the relative numbers of specific cell types (lymphocytes, plasma cells, histiocytes, and fibroblasts) identified histologically. It is likely that they simply represent different points along a continuum of inflammatory disease. The underlying causes of these conditions are unknown, but the lesions are responsive to immunosuppressive therapy. Young to middle-aged dogs are most commonly affected. Lesions are slowly progressive, often bilateral, and have a tendency to recur locally. The typical raised, smooth, flesh-colored nodule arises on the limbus or third eyelid. Limbal lesions may invade the cornea as they enlarge. Aspiration cytology demonstrates variable proportions of plasma cells, lymphocytes, fibroblasts, and histiocytes. The cellular profile observed histologically varies from primarily histiocytes with few lymphocytes and plasma cells to primarily lymphocytes and plasma cells with few histiocytes evident. Fibroblasts are uncommon in some forms and are a prominent feature of others. After initial examination, biopsy is recommended to confirm the diagnosis before initiating systemic therapy.

Initial treatment consists of topical or systemic steroids. I use the same regimen outlined earlier for the treatment of moderate to severe scleritis. I use systemic azathioprine (Imuran, Burroughs Wellcome; 1 to 2 mg/kg initially and tapered over 4 to 8 weeks) in recurrent cases (Paulsen et al., 1987b).

References and Suggested Reading

Cooley, P. L., and Dice, P. F.: Corneal dystrophy in the dog and cat. Vet. Clin. North Am. Small Anim. Pract. 20:681, 1990.
A comprehensive review containing clinical descriptions of dystrophies in dogs and cats.
Kern, T. J.: Ulcerative keratitis. Vet. Clin. North Am. Small Anim. Pract. 20:643, 1990.
A current review of ulcerative keratitis in dogs and cats.
Nasisse, M. P.: Feline herpesvirus ocular disease. Vet. Clin. North Am. Small Anim. Pract. 20:667, 1990.
A review of the pathogenesis and treatment of ocular herpesvirus infection in cats.
Paulsen, M. E., Lavach, J. D., Severin, G. A., et al.: Feline eosinophilic keratitis: A review of 15 clinical cases. J. Am. Anim. Hosp. Assoc. 23:63, 1987a.
A review of current knowledge concerning the pathogenesis, clinical findings, and therapy of this unique corneal disorder.
Paulsen, M. E., Lavach, J. D., Snyder, S. P., et al.: Nodular granulomatous episclerokeratitis in dogs: 19 cases (1973 to 1985). J.A.V.M.A. 190:1581, 1987b.
A large series of dogs with this condition are reviewed and recommendations for management made.
Pentlarge, V. W.: Corneal sequestration in cats. Comp. Cont. Ed. Pract. Vet. 11:24, 1989.
A review of current knowledge concerning corneal sequestra.

DISORDERS OF THE UVEA

DAVID A. WILKIE

Columbus, Ohio

ANATOMY AND PHYSIOLOGY

The uvea is the middle, vascular tunic of the eye. It consists of the anterior portion, the iris and ciliary body, and the posterior choroid. Histologically, the uvea contains blood vessels, pigment cells, smooth muscle, and in dogs and cats a cellular tapetum in the choroid. The uvea is the primary site of the blood-ocular barrier, which has importance in the formation of the aqueous humor, serves as a barrier to blood-borne materials, and is an immunologic barrier to the internal components of the eye. This barrier is disrupted by inflammation (uveitis). Smooth muscles in the iris and ciliary body, under autonomic control, regulate pupil size and accommodation for near and far vision, respectively. In uveitis, spasm of these muscles results in pain, seen clinically as photophobia. The ciliary body is the source of aqueous humor, which supplies nutrition to the cornea and lens. Aqueous humor is produced by both active and passive processes; its production is decreased by inflammation and by pharmacologic agents used in glaucoma therapy. The choroid supplies nutrition to the outer retina and also serves as a heat sink to protect the photoreceptors from the heat generated by light striking the retina. The tapetum, contained within the superior choroid, reflects light back across the retina, thereby maximizing the use of available light.

CONGENITAL DEFECTS

Congenital defects of the uveal tissues are commonly encountered (West and Barrie, 1986). Many have little significance for vision in an individual animal but may be genetic and are therefore important to breeders. In addition, congenital uveal defects may be associated with congenital lesions in other ocular tissues, some of which may result in blindness.

Persistent Pupillary Membranes

During embryogenesis, the anterior chamber is filled with vascular tissue, the pupillary membrane.

This mesodermal tissue normally undergoes degeneration at the end of gestation and in the immediate postpartum period. Incomplete atrophy leaves remnants termed *persistent pupillary membranes* (PPMs). Persistent pupillary membranes arise from the collarette zone of the iris and may attach to the inner cornea, to the anterior lens, or to the iris. Endothelial opacities or focal cataracts are occasionally found in association with attachment of PPMs. Most PPMs do not interfere with vision and are considered to be incidental findings in many breeds. Exceptions include the Basenji and Corgi (and perhaps other breeds), in which the defect is suspected to be inherited; in its severe form, impairment of vision can result, usually by corneal opacification. No treatment is indicated, and the condition is nonprogressive.

Heterochromia

Heterochromia is a variation in color between or within the irides and is often a normal variation. Iris coloration is related to coat color; animals with a merling gene as well as color dilute and albino animals may have various degrees of iridal and choroidal hypopigmentation. Hypoplasia or aplasia of the tapetum is also found in association with a lack of uveal pigmentation. In the Australian shepherd, multiple ocular anomalies are associated with heterochromia. Deafness has been described in white dogs and cats with blue eyes.

Colobomas

A coloboma occurs when a portion of the uvea fails to develop, leaving a defect. Colobomas can involve the iris, ciliary body, or choroid and may be associated with other ocular defects. Iridal colobomas are congenital, nonprogressive abnormalities that can result in dyscoria, an abnormally shaped pupil. No treatment is indicated.

Choroidal Hypoplasia

Choroidal hypoplasia is the most common manifestation of the collie eye anomaly syndrome. It

Portions of this article are reprinted with permission from Wilkie, D. A.: Control of ocular inflammation. Vet. Clin. North Am. Small Anim. Pract. 20:693, 1990.

occurs temporal to the optic disk, appearing as an area with decreased choroidal vasculature and pigmentation through which the sclera is visible. Alone, choroidal hypoplasia does not impair vision. Affected dogs should not be bred because they may produce offspring affected with more severe manifestations of the syndrome (e.g., coloboma, retinal detachment, and blindness). Choroidal hypoplasia is also seen in the Shetland sheepdog as part of "sheltie eye anomaly" and occasionally in other breeds as an incidental finding.

Other

Absence of the iris (aniridia), more than one pupil (polycoria), misshapen pupil (dyscoria), and displacement of the pupil (corectopia) all are congenital defects of the uvea but are extremely rare. Most are found in association with other congenital ocular defects.

ACQUIRED DISORDERS

Anterior Uveal Cysts

Anterior uveal cysts form from the pigmented epithelium of the iris and ciliary body. The cyst may remain attached at its site of origin or break free to float in the anterior chamber. Cysts must be distinguished from a pigmented neoplasm, specifically a uveal melanoma. Cysts are hollow and may be transilluminated by a penlight; tumors do not float free in the anterior chamber. There is a breed predilection for uveal cysts, with the golden retriever, Great Dane, and Irish setter affected most often. Anterior uveal cysts can, however, be encountered in all breeds of dogs, cats, and horses. In addition, anterior uveitis can result in cyst formation. No treatment is indicated unless a great number of cysts are present, obstructing the pupil and vision. Treatment of these eyes involves aspiration of the cysts using a 30-gauge needle.

Iris Atrophy

Iris atrophy involves a loss of iris stroma, resulting in an irregular pupil margin, sluggish pupillary light response, and holes within the iris. Iris atrophy has been classified as primary, senile, and secondary. Primary iris atrophy is seen in Siamese cats, miniature schnauzers, poodles, and Chihuahuas. This is a slow progressive atrophy of the iris. Senile iris atrophy occurs in aged animals of all species and breeds. The distinction between these two forms of atrophy may not be significant. Secondary iris atrophy occurs as a sequela to chronic glaucoma, uveitis, or ocular trauma. Although not a significant problem, iris atrophy is an important differential diagnosis in animals with a sluggish or incomplete pupillary light response.

Table 1. Clinical Signs of Uveal Inflammation

Anterior Uveitis	Posterior Uveitis
Redness	Retinal hemorrhage
Blepharospasm	Retinal detachment
Ocular discharge— serous, mucoid	Retinal/subretinal transudate/exudate
Photophobia	**Anterior and/or Posterior Uveitis**
Miosis	Blindness
Aqueous flare	Hypotony
Corneal edema	
Iridal swelling	
Keratitic precipitates	
Hyphema	
Hypopyon	

ANTERIOR AND POSTERIOR UVEITIS

Uveitis is inflammation of the iris and ciliary body (anterior) and choroid (posterior). Uveitis is a common manifestation of many diseases, both ocular and systemic, and as such it is essential to attempt to ascertain the cause (Blouin, 1984; Slatter, 1990; Swanson, 1989). It is also essential to be able to differentiate uveitis from other ophthalmic diseases resulting in a red and painful eye such as glaucoma, corneal ulceration, and conjunctivitis (Slatter, 1990).

Clinical Signs

Inflammation of the anterior uvea causes spasm of the ciliary and iris muscles, seen clinically as miosis and photophobia, and a breakdown in the blood-ocular barrier. Protein and cells leak into the anterior chamber, resulting in aqueous flare, hypopyon, and keratitic precipitates (Table 1). Inflammatory changes in the aqueous humor can result in secondary corneal endothelial and lens changes (e.g., corneal edema, cataract). Inflammation of the choroid, because of its close association with the retina, usually also involves the retina and is termed *chorioretinitis*. Chorioretinitis, diagnosed by direct or indirect ophthalmoscopy, results in retinal and subretinal transudate and exudate, retinal vascular changes, hemorrhage, retinal detachment, and retinal degeneration. Other chronic changes resulting from intraocular inflammation include anterior and posterior synechiae, secondary glaucoma, retinal detachment, blindness, and phthisis bulbi.

Etiology and Diagnosis

The causes of anterior and posterior uveitis include primary ophthalmic as well as systemic diseases. In addition to a complete ophthalmic examination, it is therefore essential to evaluate the entire animal through a complete physical examination and often laboratory testing. A complete ophthalmic evaluation must include a Schirmer's tear test, fluorescein staining of the cornea, intraocular pressure determination (Schiotz's tonometry); penlight examination to evaluate pupil size, aqueous humor content, lens position, and transparency; and direct and consensual pupillary light responses. Indirect ophthalmoscopic examination of the fundus is also essential. Failure to perform these routine diagnostic tests will result in misdiagnosis and incorrect therapy. It may also result in a failure to consider and examine for systemic disease, thereby placing an animal's health in serious jeopardy.

Primary ophthalmic diseases that result in anterior uveitis include corneal ulceration, lens-induced uveitis, and direct ocular trauma. Corneal ulceration results in secondary anterior uveitis through a reflex pathway involving the ophthalmic branch of cranial nerve V. Fluorescein staining of the cornea is therefore indicated in eyes with anterior uveitis. The lens is considered to be an immune-privileged site and as such is capable of stimulating an inflammatory reaction. Lens protein is exposed after traumatic rupture of the lens capsule or during the degenerative process of a hypermature cataract undergoing liquefaction and leakage. Either of these processes can result in anterior uveitis with rupture of the lens, resulting in more severe inflammation and, frequently, secondary glaucoma. Uveitis associated with a resorbing, hypermature cataract may decrease the success of cataract surgery. Animals with cataracts should therefore be referred early in the disease process. Uveitis resulting from direct ocular trauma may be associated with rupture of the fibrous tunic of the eye, hyphema, lens luxation, corneal endothelial damage, retinal detachment, or proptosis. A complete ophthalmic examination is essential. If the anterior and posterior segments of the eye are not completely visible, then an ocular ultrasonographic examination is indicated, specifically to evaluate the position of the lens and retina and to look for changes in the echogenicity of the vitreous humor. In addition to a complete ophthalmic evaluation, the entire animal must be examined for signs of trauma to other body systems. Fractures and soft-tissue damage of the head and neck, thoracic and abdominal trauma, fractures of the limbs, and neurologic changes involving the central nervous system all are potential complications found in association with ocular trauma.

Systemic disease can result in uni- or bilateral anterior or posterior uveitis (Table 2). If intraocular

Table 2. *Systemic Etiologies of Anterior and Posterior Uveitis—Dog and Cat*

Infectious

Mycotic—blastomycosis, cryptococcosis, histoplasmosis, coccidioidomycosis, aspergillosis, other

Rickettsia—*Ehrlichia canis/platys*, Rocky Mountain spotted fever

Toxoplasmosis

Feline immunodeficiency virus, feline leukemia virus, feline infectious peritonitis

Lyme disease (borreliosis)

Bacteremia/septicemia

Brucella canis

Aberrant parasitic migration—heartworm, *Toxocara*, hookworm, others

Infectious canine hepatitis

Protothecosis

Mycobacteria

Leptospirosis

Leishmaniasis

Distemper

Other

Noninfectious

Neoplasia—lymphosarcoma, adenocarcinoma, reticulosis, other

Autoimmune—uveodermatologic syndrome (Vogt-Koyanagi-Harada–like syndrome), other

Other

inflammation cannot be ascribed to another ocular disorder, then a complete systemic evaluation is indicated. A complete history and physical examination should be followed by complete blood count, biochemical profile, urinalysis, culture, serologic study, radiographs, cytologic study, biopsy, and ultrasonography as indicated (see this volume, p. 1061, for further discussion of the ocular manifestations of systemic disease).

Unfortunately, a third category for the etiology of uveitis is idiopathic—no ocular or systemic cause of the uveitis can be identified. Provided that a complete evaluation has been performed and infectious and neoplastic diseases ruled out, then it is appropriate to suppress the uveitis with topical or systemic therapy.

Treatment

The treatment of uveitis involves specific therapy determined by the etiology of the uveitis and nonspecific therapy designed to decrease inflammation and pain and prevent further intraocular damage (Wilkie, 1990). Failure to control intraocular inflammation may lead to severe secondary ophthalmic complications such as glaucoma, synechiae, cataract, retinal detachment, and blindness. The initiation of specific therapy is dependent on correctly identifying the cause, whether a primary ophthalmic disease or a systemic problem. A discussion of specific treatment is beyond the scope of this article.

Nonspecific therapy includes topical and systemic corticosteroids and nonsteroidal anti-inflammatory drugs (NSAIDs) to decrease inflammation and atropine to dilate the pupil and decrease the pain of ciliary muscle spasm. It may include additional immunosuppressive therapy (Wilkie, 1990). Which medication to select, the frequency of treatment, and route of administration are dependent on the etiology and severity of the uveitis and whether the uveitis is anterior, posterior, or both.

CORTICOSTEROIDS

Corticosteroids are perhaps the most widely used ophthalmic medication and are the most commonly used drugs for control of ocular inflammation. Corticosteroids decrease exudation of inflammatory cells and fibrin, suppress fibroblast activity, decrease vascularization, and inhibit collagen formation (Wilkie, 1990). When used correctly, they are an indispensable therapeutic modality in veterinary ophthalmology. Unfortunately, corticosteroids are often overused and used incorrectly. Common mistakes include the use of combination corticosteroid-antibiotic preparations when only one component is required, inadequate control of inflammation due to selection of a corticosteroid with low potency or low penetration, indiscriminate use of corticosteroids, and administration by an inappropriate route.

Topical

Topical corticosteroids are indicated for the treatment of anterior uveitis unassociated with ulcerative keratitis. They are not appropriate for the management of inflammation of the posterior segment (retina, choroid, optic nerve) and are contraindicated for uveal inflammation associated with ulcerative keratitis. Topical corticosteroids can be used to treat anterior uveitis associated with systemic infectious disease without significant exacerbation of the infectious process. Ocular side effects of corticosteroid therapy include delayed corneal epithelial regeneration and potentiation of corneal collagenase activity and infection, all of which worsen corneal ulceration and delay healing. Systemic absorption of topical corticosteroids does occur and results in the alteration of adrenal function and allergy test results. It also interferes with the regulation of diabetes mellitus. These systemic changes can persist for 2 weeks after discontinuing treatment.

Topical ophthalmic corticosteroids vary widely in their use, concentration, the vehicle used for delivery, the presence or absence of an antibiotic, and whether they are formulated as an ointment or a solution (Table 3). Prednisolone and dexamethasone are two of the more potent topical ocular corticosteroids. Prednisolone acetate (Econopred Plus, Alcon) is administered as a 1% suspension and dexamethasone as a 0.1% solution or a 0.05% ointment (Decadron, Merck Sharp & Dohme) (see Table 3). Either drug can be used for external inflammation,

Table 3. *Dosages of Commonly Used Ocular Anti-Inflammatory Agents*

Drug/Concentration	Dose
Topical	
Corticosteroids	
1.0% Prednisolone acetate suspension	Econopred Plus (Alcon): 1–6 times/day
0.1% Dexamethasone solution	Decadron: 1–6 times/day
0.05% Dexamethasone ointment	Decadron (Merck Sharpe & Dohme): 1–6 times/day
NSAIDs	
0.03% Flurbiprofen	Ocufen (Allergan): 4 times/day
1.0% Suprofen	Profenal (Alcon): 4 times/day
Atropine	
1.0% Atropine	1–4 times/day
Systemic	
Corticosteroids	
Prednisolone/prednisone	Immunosuppressive: 1.0 mg/kg PO q 12 hr for 7–14 days then taper
	Anti-inflammatory: 0.5 mg/kg PO q 12 hr for 3–5 days then taper
NSAID	
Acetylsalicylic acid	Aspirin: Dog: 10–25 mg/kg PO q 12 hr
	Cat: 80 mg PO q 48–72 hr
Flunixin meglumine	Banamine (Schering): Dog: 0.25–0.5 mg/kg IV q 24 hr for 3 days
	Cat: Do not use
Phenylbutazone	Butazolidin (Geigy): Dog: 13 mg/kg PO q 8 hr for 48 hr then taper
	Cat: 10–14 mg/kg PO q 12 hr
Azathioprine	Imuran (Burroughs Wellcome): Dog: 2.2 mg/kg PO q 24 hr then taper
Cyclophosphamide	Cytoxan (Mead Johnson): Dog: 50 mg/m² PO q 24 hr for 4 days/week

NSAID, nonsteroidal anti-inflammatory drug.
Modified with permission from Wilkie, D. A.: Control of ocular inflammation. Vet. Clin. North Am. Sm. Anim. Pract. 20:693, 1990.

but prednisolone in the acetate form achieves the highest intraocular levels and is the drug of choice for anterior uveitis. Frequency of administration is variable and depends on the severity, location, and etiology of the disease process (see Table 3). In general, therapy begins at a higher frequency to suppress inflammation and is then decreased to a maintenance level to maintain control. The more frequent the application, the higher the intraocular concentration of drug that will be achieved. As with systemic corticosteroids, therapy should be slowly decreased to avoid recrudescence.

Effective use of topical corticosteroids results in a decrease in photophobia, blepharospasm, discharge, and flare and a return of intraocular pressure to normal in patients with ocular hypotony. If topical corticosteroids are prescribed inappropriately, they may result in exacerbation of infection or progression of a corneal ulcer, manifested as a worsening of discharge, discomfort, and corneal opacification.

Systemic

Systemic corticosteroids are preferred over topical corticosteroids for the treatment of chorioretinitis. They can also be used to supplement topical therapy in the treatment of anterior uveitis. Systemic corticosteroids have minimal corneal effects, which may allow for their use in the control of intraocular inflammation associated with corneal ulceration. Clinicians must consider that some level of corticosteroids is achieved in the tears, and therapy must be discontinued if the cornea exhibits delayed healing.

As with topical corticosteroids, the initial therapy with systemic corticosteroids is instituted at a higher dose to suppress inflammation and then tapered to a lower dose for long-term maintenance. The recommended starting dose for an anti-inflammatory effect is 0.5 mg/kg PO every 12 hr and for an immunosuppressive effect 1 mg/kg PO every 12 hr (see Table 3). The dose is then decreased in increments based on the response to therapy and the disease being treated.

The systemic side effects of orally administered corticosteroids are similar to those with topical treatment, but more pronounced. In addition, many of the diseases that result in inflammation of the posterior segment are infectious (e.g., blastomycosis, Rocky Mountain spotted fever, ehrlichiosis). Systemic corticosteroids are contraindicated or must be used with caution and in conjunction with appropriate therapy directed toward the inciting cause.

NONSTEROIDAL ANTI-INFLAMMATORY AGENTS

NSAIDs include the salicylic acids (aspirin), propionic acids (flurbiprofen, suprofen), indomethacin, phenylbutazone, and flunixin meglumine, to name but a few. Unlike corticosteroids, these drugs interrupt the arachidonic acid cascade by inhibiting cyclo-oxygenase, resulting in inhibition of prostaglandin formation.

Topical

Several topical NSAIDs have recently become available for ophthalmic use. Indomethacin, flurbiprofen, and suprofen all are potent cyclo-oxygenase inhibitors, the latter two now commercially available in the United States.

The indications and contraindications for topical NSAIDs are the same as for topical corticosteroids. They can be used in conjunction with topical corticosteroids, and their effects may be additive. When administered topically, 0.03% flurbiprofen (Ocufen, Allergan) or 1% suprofen (Profenal, Alcon) is well absorbed into ocular tissues and shows low systemic absorption. Applying multiple doses of flurbiprofen, three doses at 30-min intervals, increases the concentration in ocular tissues. Flurbiprofen suppresses the breakdown of the blood-aqueous barrier and reduces conjunctival hyperemia, aqueous cells, and protein following cataract surgery. In addition, it has also been shown to aid in maintaining pupillary dilation in human cataract surgery when applied topically preoperatively.

Topical NSAIDs are not a replacement for corticosteroids in most cases of anterior uveitis. They are more costly and not as potent anti-inflammatory agents as corticosteroids. They are, however, indicated as a supplement with topical corticosteroids in the control of anterior uveitis associated with intraocular surgery (when they are administered before surgery) and in diabetic animals with anterior uveitis.

Side effects associated with topical administration of NSAIDs include possible topical irritation and intraocular hemorrhage. Hemorrhage has been reported to occur as a result of interference with platelet aggregation but is rare. There is little difference between topical flurbiprofen and prednisolone acetate in their effect on corneal wound healing. Use of topical flurbiprofen in the presence of a corneal ulcer may be contraindicated. In addition, flurbiprofen is comparable to dexamethasone in its ability to exacerbate acute ocular herpes keratitis.

Systemic

NSAIDs in veterinary ophthalmology have traditionally been administered by the systemic route. The most frequently administered systemic NSAIDs are aspirin, phenylbutazone (Butazolidin, Geigy), and flunixin meglumine (Banamine, Schering) (see Table 3). Systemic NSAIDs decrease both anterior and posterior uveitis and the associated clinical signs. These drugs are especially useful in the presence of contraindications against the use of systemic corticosteroids.

Side effects associated with systemic administration are common and include renal and gastrointestinal effects, specifically (1) acute renal insufficiency or acute renal papillary necrosis, (2) gastrointestinal intolerance, manifested as gastroduodenal hemorrhage and ulceration, and (3) interference with platelet function. The gastrointestinal side effects are exacerbated by the concomitant use of corticosteroids.

ATROPINE

Atropine applied topically to the eye results in pupil dilation (mydriasis), paralysis of the ciliary body musculature (cycloplegia), and decreased tear production. Although not an anti-inflammatory agent, atropine is often the drug of choice in the management of inflammation of the anterior segment (iris, ciliary body). Anterior uveitis results in pain, manifested as blepharospasm and photophobia, as the result of inflammation and subsequent spasm of the iridal and ciliary body musculature. The action of a mydriatic-cycloplegic is to paralyze these muscles and ease discomfort, thus improving the patient's attitude and facilitating application of other medications. In addition, one of the sequelae of anterior uveitis, the formation of posterior synechiae, is decreased by dilating the pupil. Atropine has also been reported to help restore the blood-aqueous barrier to normal and decrease the protein and cells in the aqueous humor of patients with anterior uveitis.

Topical 1% atropine is indicated in any patient who has anterior uveitis and is exhibiting miosis or photophobia *provided the intraocular pressure is normal to low.* Atropine is contraindicated in glaucoma even if the glaucoma is associated with or the result of anterior uveitis. Atropine can be used topically in a patient with a corneal ulcer and subsequent reflex anterior uveitis when topical corticosteroids and NSAIDs are contraindicated. Atropine is administered as required to dilate the pupil, up to a maximum frequency of every 6 hr, and then as required to maintain dilation.

As with any topical medication, topical atropine is absorbed systemically and has the potential to result in systemic effects such as ileus in horses and decreased salivation and tear production in dogs and cats. Many small animal patients also hypersalivate immediately after the application of topical atropine as a result of its bitter taste, not because of an autonomic phenomenon.

IMMUNOSUPPRESSIVE DRUGS

The use of immunosuppressive drugs, other than corticosteroids, may be indicated in severe anterior or posterior uveitis. The benefits of their use must be weighed against their potentially serious side effects. Examples of immunosuppressive drugs used in veterinary ophthalmology include azathioprine, cyclosporin, and cyclophosphamide (see Table 3).

Azathioprine, a thiopurine antimetabolite, is used in veterinary ophthalmology for patients requiring immunosuppression if they fail to respond to systemic corticosteroids or if they experience adverse side effects with corticosteroid therapy. An example would be a patient with autoimmune uveitis-dermatitis (Vogt-Koyanagi-Harada) syndrome, controlled with systemic corticosteroids, that was exhibiting iatrogenic Cushing's disease but still retained vision and required therapy to do so. The dose of systemic corticosteroids could be reduced in this patient and azathioprine added to the therapy to supplement treatment, maintain control of the disease, and decrease the side effects of the corticosteroids.

The use of cyclophosphamide in veterinary ophthalmology is very limited and generally reserved for those patients that require immunosuppression but are nonresponsive to, or suffering adverse effects from, systemic corticosteroids. It is dosed on a meter-squared basis rather than per kilogram (see Table 3).

NEOPLASIA

Intraocular neoplasia can be primary or secondary to metastasis from a distant site. Intraocular neoplasms result in damage to the eye through displacement of normal ocular structures, causing lens luxation, dyscoria, and retinal detachment. In addition to an intraocular mass lesion, glaucoma, uveitis, and hyphema are the most common presenting signs of intraocular neoplasia.

Primary

The anterior uvea is the site of origin for most primary intraocular neoplasms. Of primary uveal neoplasms, melanoma is the most common in dogs and cats. In dogs, most intraocular melanocytic tumors are benign, resembling melanocytomas (Wilcock and Peiffer, 1986). Combined data from several reports suggest a metastatic potential of less than 5% for canine anterior uveal melanoma. The best criteria for predicting malignancy of intraocular melanoma in dogs appears to be the mitotic index, with a mitotic index of greater than 4 per high-power field suggestive of malignancy (Wilcock and

Peiffer, 1986). With such a low incidence of malignancy, in dogs, enucleation of noninflamed, normotensive eyes with uveal melanomas is not necessarily indicated. Rather, periodic complete ophthalmic and systemic examinations with enucleation planned if the tumor results in hyphema, uveitis, glaucoma, or other painful ocular conditions may be the most appropriate management. Alternatively, an excisional biopsy of the mass can be performed in the form of an iridocyclectomy. This is a "referral only" procedure and requires that the mass lesion be small enough to allow removal. In addition to anterior uveal melanomas, choroidal melanomas have also been reported in dogs. These appear to be benign, with retinal detachment the most frequent sequela.

In contrast to dogs, feline uveal melanoma in cats has been reported to metastasize in 60% of those affected (Patnaik and Mooney, 1988). Pigmented lesions of the feline iris or ciliary body, especially those that are raised, displacing adjacent structures or resulting in other intraocular damage, should be removed by enucleation. In addition, a complete systemic evaluation including thoracic and abdominal radiographs and palpation of regional lymph nodes is indicated. No information exists to suggest that enucleation of these affected eyes affects the rate of metastasis, favorably or unfavorably.

In addition to primary intraocular melanoma, ciliary body adenoma and adenocarcinoma, hemangiosarcoma, and astrocytoma have been reported in dogs and cats. These are often slow to metastasize but can result in intraocular damage as they enlarge. Intraocular spindle cell sarcoma occurs in the feline eye as a sequela to ocular trauma or uveitis (Hakanson et al., 1990). The period following ocular trauma or uveitis to the time of diagnosis of intraocular spindle cell sarcoma varies from 5 months to 12 years. These tumors are locally invasive, extending transsclerally or traveling along the optic nerve, and have the potential for metastasis. Enucleation or possibly orbital exenteration is the treatment of choice. Enucleation of severely traumatized or chronically inflamed, blind feline eyes may also be indicated to avoid the possible development of intraocular neoplasia.

Secondary

Lymphosarcoma is the most common intraocular neoplasm in dogs and cats. In addition, adenocarcinoma, hemangiosarcoma, and several other neoplasms metastasize to the eye. The most common ocular abnormalities found in association with secondary neoplasms include glaucoma, uveitis, hyphema, retinal detachment, and lens luxation. Treatment should be directed at finding the primary source of the neoplasia, followed by systemic therapy including chemotherapy, surgery, and radiation. Additional therapy might include topical ophthalmic anti-inflammatory drugs and atropine for uveitis or topical and systemic medications aimed at reducing the intraocular pressure if secondary glaucoma is present. Topical therapy is often unrewarding. Systemic treatment of the primary problem usually results in a greater ocular response. If the eye is painful, blind, or nonresponsive to systemic treatment, enucleation is the treatment of choice.

References and Suggested Reading

Blouin, P.: Uveitis in the dog and cat: Causes, diagnosis, and treatment. Can. Vet. J. 25:315, 1984.
A review of the clinical signs, diagnostic plan, and treatment of uveitis in small animal patients.

Hakanson, N., and Forrester, S. D.: Uveitis in the dog and cat. Vet. Clin. North Am. Small Anim. Pract. 20:715, 1990.
A discussion of the immunology of uveitis, followed by clinical signs, etiology, treatment, and sequelae of uveitis in dogs and cats.

Hakanson, N., Shively, J. N., Reed, R. E., et al.: Intraocular spindle cell sarcoma following ocular trauma in a cat: Case report and literature review. J. Am. Anim. Hosp. Assoc. 26:63, 1990.
A single case presentation followed by an excellent review of the literature on feline intraocular spindle cell sarcoma and its behavior.

Patnaik, A. K., and Mooney, S.: Feline melanoma: A comparative study of ocular, oral, and dermal neoplasms. Vet. Pathol. 25:105, 1988.
A retrospective study involving 29 cats with ocular, oral, or dermal melanoma is presented, and the malignant potential of these tumors is compared.

Slatter, D. (ed.): *Fundamentals of Veterinary Ophthalmology,* 2nd ed. Philadelphia: W. B. Saunders, 1990.
An excellent complete medical and surgical ophthalmic textbook for general practitioners.

Swanson, J. F.: Uveitis. In Kirk, R. W. (ed.): *Current Veterinary Therapy X.* Philadelphia: W. B. Saunders, 1989, p. 652.
A discussion of the immunology of uveitis, followed by clinical signs, etiology, treatment, and sequelae of uveitis in dogs and cats.

West, C. S., and Barrie, K. P.: Disorders of the anterior uvea. In Kirk, R. W. (ed.): *Current Veterinary Therapy IX.* Philadelphia: W. B. Saunders, 1986, p. 649.
The anatomy of the uvea, congenital and developmental abnormalities, acquired abnormalities, anterior uveitis, and hyphema are discussed with regard to clinical signs and treatment.

Wilcock, B. P., and Peiffer, R. L.: Morphology and behavior of primary ocular melanomas in 91 dogs. Vet. Pathol. 23:418, 1986.
A histologic study of 91 primary ocular melanomas is presented, and criteria for the prediction of malignancy are proposed.

Wilkie, D. A.: Control of ocular inflammation. Vet. Clin. North Am. Small Anim. Pract. 20:693, 1990.
A discussion of the mechanisms of ocular inflammation, the pharmacology of ocular anti-inflammatory agents, their dosage and route of administration.

DISORDERS OF THE LENS

RONALD C. RIIS

Ithaca, New York

ANATOMY

The transparent lens, positioned between the aqueous humor and vitreous body, forms one of the refractive media of the eye. The lens facilitates near vision through accommodation and shields the retina from potentially harmful ultraviolet light. The metabolism of the lens is directed entirely toward maintaining transparency. Loss of transparency or opacification interrupting light transmission is referred to as cataract.

The lens is composed entirely of epithelial cells in different stages of maturation enclosed in an elastic basement membrane capsule. Cell division and growth of the lens continue throughout life. As new lens cells are formed, the older cells are displaced toward the interior of the lens, resulting in nuclear sclerosis. The junctions of cells formed within each cell layer are termed sutures. At an early stage in ocular development, the lens becomes isolated from its blood supply and becomes dependent on the aqueous fluid and vitreous body for nutrition and discharge of metabolic by-products.

The lens is held in place by zonules that run from the lens equator to the ciliary body and by its contact with adjacent vitreous. The volume of the adult dog lens is approximately 0.5 ml, measuring 9 to 11 mm × 7 mm; the adult cat lens volume is approximately 0.6 ml, measuring 12 to 13 mm × 8 mm. Depending on age, the average thickness of the anterior capsule in the adult dog and cat is 50 μm; the posterior capsule thickness is 3.5 to 5 μm in the dog and 3 to 7 μm in the cat. By ultrasonography, the lens axial thickness for the dog and cat has been measured at 7 to 7.6 mm.

The lens is divided into the following regions: anterior lens capsule; anterior cortex; perinuclear, nuclear, and posterior cortex; and posterior capsule. Localization of abnormalities to these regions may indicate the likelihood of progression of lens opacities (Table 1).

BIOCHEMISTRY

The principal constituents of the lens are water and protein. The lens composition varies slightly from other tissues, with a lower water content (65%) and higher protein content (34%). Almost all of the lens dry weight is protein. The low water and high protein concentration are essential for optimal transparency of the lens. It must have a refractive index quite different from its fluid environment but must remain sufficiently hydrated to allow for changes in shape.

The observation that the lens proteins are organ-specific was first made by Uhlenhuth in 1904. A rabbit sensitized to bovine lens protein will develop antibodies that react with antigens from lens extracts from almost all other species. Reaction will not occur with nonlens antigens. Lens proteins from all species are very similar. The clinical significance of this is that exposure of lens proteins can result in uveitis. The lens proteins are normally sequestered within the capsule, preventing their immune recognition. If the lens protein is exposed to the immune system, antibodies may be formed, producing uveitis known as phacoanaphylactic endophthalmitis.

In comparison to other tissues, the lens contains unusually high levels of ascorbic acid, inositol, glutathione, and taurine; these have been subjects of considerable research interest.

Ascorbic acid is actively transported into the aqueous fluid to a concentration some 15 times greater than in plasma. In many species, the ascorbic acid content of the lens is even greater than that in surrounding fluids. However, ascorbic acid is not synthesized in the lens, nor is it actively transported into the lens. Its accumulation within the lens might be explained by assuming that a portion is protein bound. Ascorbic acid levels do decrease in most forms of cataract but inconsistently. Despite much investigation, there is no evidence that ascorbic acid deficiency causes or

***Table 1.** Cataract Progression Based on Location**

Position of Lens Opacity, Cleft, Vacuole, or Wedge	Prognosis for Progression to Mature Cataract
Anterior capsule	Usually nonprogressive
Anterior cortex	Progressive
Perinuclear	Usually nonprogressive
Nuclear	Usually nonprogressive
Posterior cortex	Progressive
Posterior capsule	Unpredictable
Y suture	Usually nonprogressive

*Reprinted with permission from Riis, R. C.: Diseases of the lens. *In* Kirk, R. W. (ed.): Current Veterinary Therapy VII. Philadelphia: W. B. Saunders, 1980, pp. 565–570.

influences cataract development. Topical therapy with zinc ascorbate for the cure of cataracts is ineffective and unwarranted (Mac Millan et al., 1989).

The greatest need for energy in the lens is within the epithelium, the major site of all active transport processes. The source of adenosine triphosphate (ATP) in the lens is the metabolism of glucose, primarily by anaerobic glycolysis and to a limited extent by the Krebs cycle. Anaerobic glycolysis obviates the problem of oxygen starvation in the lens, which is totally dependent on the low oxygen tension in aqueous. About 80% of the glucose entering the lens is converted to lactic acid by anaerobic glycolysis. Some of this lactic acid is metabolized further by the Krebs cycle, but most simply diffuses into the aqueous.

Two other important pathways operate in the lens: the hexose-monophosphate shunt and the sorbitol pathway. Neither of these generate significant amounts of ATP. The sorbitol pathway of the lens has received wide attention because of its key role in the development of cataracts in diabetes mellitus. Glucose is converted to sorbitol and then to fructose by the enzymes aldose reductase and polyol dehydrogenase, respectively. Under normal conditions, no more than about 5% of the glucose used by the lens is metabolized by the sorbitol pathway.

In diabetes mellitus, glucose levels in the aqueous increase. More glucose enters the lens than can be handled by the glycolytic pathway or the hexose-monophosphate shunt. The excess glucose enters the sorbitol pathway and is converted to sorbitol and fructose. Abnormally high intracellular levels of sorbitol and fructose draw water into the lens in an attempt to maintain osmotic equilibrium. The osmotic swelling accounts for the hydropic degeneration of lens fibers, cell rupture, loss of amino acids, ATP, glutathione, and potassium, and an increase in sodium. Cataract development and progression due to diabetes mellitus vary among species. Despite treatment with insulin, diabetic dogs typically become blind with mature cataracts within months; diabetic cats, however, seldom develop cataracts. The development of topical aldose reductase inhibitors, which are not yet commercially available, holds promise for eventual prevention of cataract development by diabetic patients.

EXAMINATION OF THE LENS

After evaluating the pupillary response to bright light, instill one drop of a rapid-onset, short-acting mydriatic (e.g., tropicamide 1%: Mydriacyl, Alcon; Tropicacyl, Akorn). Pupillary dilatation is maximal in approximately 20 min and persists for 2 to 3 hr. A light source that can be focused (e.g., a Finhoff transilluminator) or a slit-lamp biomicroscope is optimum for examinations of the lens. To eliminate reflections, a dark room is preferred. The examination of the lens should include the lens capsule, cortex, nucleus, zonules, and anterior vitreal face. Suture lines associated with the anterior and posterior cortical and nuclear zones may or may not be normally apparent. Lens examination methods should include direct illumination, transillumination, retroillumination, and oblique illumination using the direct ophthalmoscope, penlight, transilluminator, or slit-lamp biomicroscope.

The center of rotation of the dog eye is in the posterior nucleus or cortex; therefore, lesions anterior to this point rotate in the same direction as the eye, while those posterior rotate in the opposite direction of the eye movement.

CATARACT

The term cataract, defined as any opacity of the crystalline lens or its capsules, encompasses discretely localized lens opacities as well as lenses in which there is total loss of light transmission. Discrete opacities may result from the deposition or precipitation of crystals of inorganic salts or lipid or from vacuolization. The more generalized interruption of light transmission is due to extensive changes in lens proteins, cations, and water balances.

If cataracts are extensive and bilateral, blindness results. The prudent approach is to assume cataracts are hereditary except in cases known to be associated with ocular trauma, inflammation, diabetes mellitus, persistent pupillary membrane (PPM), persistent hyperplastic primary vitreous (PHPV), or nutritional deficiency. Canine breeds predisposed to cataract development are listed in Table 2.

The precise biochemical causes of naturally occurring forms of cataract are not understood. Observations made on most cataractous lenses include reduced levels of substances involved in lens metabolism, such as potassium, glutathione, ribonucleic acid (RNA), ascorbic acid, ATP, inositol, and anabolic enzymes. In most cataracts, there are increased levels of calcium, sodium, water, and proteolytic enzymes. Many of these alterations are probably the result of cataract formation rather than being principal causative factors.

Primary causes of cataract are thought to be genetically determined or acquired errors of lens metabolism. Secondary cataracts can be associated with congenital malformations (PPM, PHPV, etc.), electric shock, diabetes mellitus, glaucoma, inflammation, lens luxations, nutritional deficiencies, retinal degeneration, trauma, and toxins.

Cataracts are usually brought to the veterinarian's attention by the owner, who recognizes an animal's visual problems or pupil discoloration. Since cataracts may be a potential indicator of underlying

Table 2. Breeds Predisposed to Cataracts*

Afghan hound	Irish wolfhound
Akita	Italian greyhound
Alaskan malamute	Japanese chin
American water spaniel	Keeshond
Australian cattle dog	Komondor
Basset hound	Kuvasz
Beagle	Labrador retriever
Bearded collie	Lakeland terrier
Bedlington terrier	Lhasa apso
Belgian sheepdog	Manchester terrier
Belgian tervuren	Miniature pinscher
Bernese Mountain Dog	Miniature schnauzer
Bichon frise	Norfolk terrier
Border terrier	Norwegian elkhound
Borzoi	Norwich terrier
Boston terrier	Old English sheepdog
Bouvier des Flandres	Papillon
Boxer	Pekingese
Briard	Pembroke Welsh corgi
Brittany	Pointer
Brussels griffon	Pomeranian
Bulldog	Poodle
Cairn terrier	Puli
Cavalier King Charles spaniel	Rhodesian Ridgeback
Chesapeake Bay retriever	Rottweiler
Collie	Saint Bernard
Curly-coated retriever	Saluki
Dachshund	Samoyed
Dandie Dinmont terrier	Schipperke
Doberman pinscher	Scottish terrier
English cocker spaniel	Shih tzu
English springer spaniel	Siberian husky
Field spaniel	Silky terrier
Flat-coated retriever	Soft-coated wheaten terrier
Fox terrier	Staffordshire bull terrier
French bulldog	Standard schnauzer
German shepherd	Sussex spaniel
German shorthaired pointer	Tibetan terrier
German wirehaired pointer	Vizsla
Giant schnauzer	West Highland white terrier
Golden retriever	Weimaraner
Gordon setter	Welsh springer spaniel
Great Dane	Whippet
Ibizan hound	Wire-haired fox terrier
Irish setter	Yorkshire terrier
Irish water spaniel	

*Reprinted with permission from American College of Veterinary Ophthalmologists: Ocular Disorders Proven or Suspected to be Hereditary in Dogs, 1992; and Rubin, L. F.: *Inherited Eye Diseases in Purebred Dogs.* Baltimore: Williams & Wilkins, 1989.

disease (e.g., diabetes mellitus or uveitis), the most important services a general practitioner can render are a complete physical and ocular examinations.

Cataracts may be classified by their stage of development. The earliest developing cataracts or *immature cataracts* are characterized by vacuoles, clefts, and wedges in the equator and superficial cortical areas. The rate of progression is variable. Usually vision is present but impaired, and the fundus may be partially examined. If only a tapetal reflection can be noted, it is still classified as incipient or immature. *Mature cataracts* cause complete loss of vision and completely obstruct the tapetal reflection. Obvious suture fracture lines may be apparent in the anterior cortical fibers. An *intumescent cataract* is a mature cataract that has become swollen. If the cataract increases its volume sufficiently to exceed the elasticity of the capsule, the capsule will tear. Exposure of the lens proteins following a torn capsule eventually leads to immune-mediated, lens-induced uveitis. *Hypermature cataracts* contain liquefied lens protein and solid cortical and nuclear remnants surrounded by a wrinkled capsule. If the nucleus remains and gravitates ventrally it is called a *morgagnian* cataract. The unpredictable improvement of vision in some animals with hypermature and morgagnian cataracts results from lens proteolysis. This process may progress to complete reabsorption. Congenital cataracts or cataracts present from a young age are more likely to undergo progression to hypermaturity.

Eyes with hypermature lenses should be monitored for signs of both uveitis and glaucoma and treated if necessary. Medical therapy is indicated in lens-induced uveitis. Topical mydriatic (1% atropine) every 12 hr and corticosteroids three to four times per day are indicated. Regular intraocular pressure measurements are recommended. If intraocular pressure becomes elevated, discontinue the mydriatic and begin antiglaucoma medication. Generally, dichlorphenamide (Daranide, Merck Sharp & Dohme) 2 mg/kg of body weight every 12 hr or every 8 hr helps control the intraocular pressure. Methazolamide (Neptazane, Lederle) 1 to 2 mg/kg every 12 hr or every 8 hr is an alternative carbonic anhydrase inhibitor. Oral potassium supplementation (Slow-K, Ciba-Geigy) (dog: 1 to 3 gm every 24 hr PO; cat: 0.2 gm every 24 hr PO) will prevent the hypokalemia caused by these drugs (see this volume, p. 1125).

CAUSES OF SECONDARY CATARACT

Glaucoma

Chronically elevated intraocular pressure is associated with secondary cataract development. The cortical fibers are affected first; progression to maturity is likely.

Retinal Atrophy

Following generalized retinal degeneration from genetic or other causes, cataract development slowly ensues. This cataract may be confused with genetic cataract, especially in the mature state. Opacification usually begins in the posterior cortex and progresses to maturity. Its development is thought to be related to toxic by-products of the degenerating retina or a gene related to progressive retinal atrophy. If the fundus cannot be evaluated, electroretinography is strongly recommended prior to cataract extraction. Direct and consensual pupillary reflexes to strong light stimulus are misleading in verifying retinal function behind mature cataracts because a few viable photoreceptors are enough to stimulate the reflex. A history of night blindness preceding cataract development suggests retinal degeneration.

Uveitis

With anterior uveitis, inflamed uveal tissue surrounds the lens and actually touches the anterior lens capsule, where pathologic changes result from direct extension. Fibrin and pigment may be deposited on the capsules. Adhesions of the iris permit melanocyte migration onto the anterior lens capsule, which, with the superficial cortical fibers, becomes opacified in the early stages. One reason for use of mydriatic drugs for uveitis treatment is prevention of these sequelae. This postinflammatory cataract is easily differentiated from genetic cataract by the presence of posterior synechiae and other signs of chronic uveitis.

Metabolic Derangements and Toxicities

These cataracts are bilaterally symmetrical in the posterior subcapsular or equatorial regions. A good example of this type of cataract is the endogenous metabolic cataract of diabetes mellitus. Exogenous substances (e.g., disophenol, DNP, American Cyanamid) may cause cataracts as a systemic toxic manifestation (Grant, 1974; Martin, 1975). Progression to mature cataracts is inevitable if the cause persists.

Persistent Pupillary Membranes

Persistent pupillary membranes (PPMs) cause focal or multifocal cataracts on the anterior lens capsule and in the subcapsular cortex. Uveal strands from the iris to the opacity aid this diagnosis. Only capsular involvement can be predicted to be nonprogressive. Administration of a long-acting mydriatic (e.g., 1% atropine sulfate given once every third day) may minimize the visual impairment caused by the opacity. In some breeds (e.g., Basenji), PPMs are inherited.

Nutritional Abnormalities

Newborn puppies fed heavily supplemented or artificial diets may develop lens opacities. These opacities usually begin as fine equatorial vacuoles with extension into the cortical areas. After the growing pups are given solid food, the lens opacities arrest and the lens continues growth. During growth, the vacuoles compact but can be defined as a ring of disjunction and later as a perinuclear ring. The cause of these vacuoles is thought to be an overabundance or deficiency of specific sugars or amino acids.

Recent research using a commercial milk replacer for dogs (Esbilac, Pet-Ag) fortified with arginine and methionine as the only food source for newborn Akita, beagle, and wolf puppies showed acceptable growth and normal lens formation. However, the researchers cautioned that "the development of nutritional cataracts in puppies fed milk replacer formulas appears to be breed- or growth-rate related and influenced by the methionine/arginine content of the formula" (Ralston et al., 1990).

Nuclear Sclerosis

In most dogs and cats older than 6 years, the lens nucleus becomes grayish. This may be a concern to owners worried about the onset of cataracts. If there is no visual impairment, if true opacification is absent, and if fundus evaluation can be accomplished with ease, the condition is a normal developmental aging process (sclerosis) of the lens. With aging, the nucleus becomes relatively denser than the cortex and internal dispersion of light occurs, lending a gray discoloration to the nucleus. In very old animals, vision may be impaired if there is a superimposed multifocal cataract. Ironically, sclerotic lenses are not predisposed to progressive cataractous changes. Mature cataract development can occur but is infrequent.

CATARACT THERAPY

Mydriatics may be used to improve vision around immature or hypermature cataracts. Topical applications of vitamin complexes (ascorbic acid), oral selenium or zinc or combinations of topical zinc ascorbate, and intracameral injection of palosein (Orgotein, D.D.I.) have all been proved ineffective.

Cataract removal to restore vision is worthy of consideration in animals that qualify for the procedure. In breeds predisposed to development of progressive retinal atrophy or central progressive retinal atrophy, an electroretinogram is necessary to justify surgery for dogs with cataracts.

Surgical techniques are divided into procedures that remove the entire lens (intracapsular extraction) or the anterior lens capsule, nucleus, and cortex (extracapsular extraction). Surgical methods for extracapsular extraction include: (1) discission and

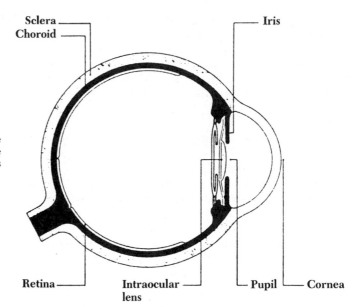

Figure 1. An intraocular lens implant (IOL) in the posterior chamber sulcus. Other IOL positions are the anterior chamber and the preferred position in the lens capsule.

Sclera — Choroid — Iris — Retina — Intraocular lens — Pupil — Cornea

aspiration; (2) ultrasonic fragmentation (phacofragmentation) and aspiration; or (3) conventional extracapsular extraction. Intraocular lens (IOL) implantation may follow the two latter procedures. Each procedure has indications that render it most appropriate for the individual patient and surgeon. These surgical procedures should be performed by an experienced ophthalmic surgeon because of the many complications associated with cataract extraction in the dog and cat.

Intraocular lenses are implants placed in the posterior chamber either behind the iris or within the lens capsule following an extracapsular lens extraction (Fig. 1). Most people undergoing lens extraction receive IOLs. A growing number of veterinary ophthalmologists feel the vision of an animal with an IOL is improved remarkably. The power of the IOL for dogs is 30 to 36 diopters. Although an IOL may introduce additional postoperative complications and add additional expense to the overall cataract surgery costs, extraction and implant techniques are becoming more refined and successful. The use of IOLs in dogs will probably increase.

REFERRAL FOR CATARACT SURGERY

Careful selection of animals for lens extraction is essential for success. If the owners desire surgery and the animal's temperament allows for treatment with topical and oral medications several times daily without stress, the animal may be a candidate. Extremely excitable animals or those in fragile health are poor candidates.

Prior to referral, a complete physical examination including complete blood count, clinical chemistries, and urinalysis should be performed. An elec-

trocardiogram is also desired. These values should accompany the referral.

If even mild anterior uveitis is evident, surgical extraction should be postponed until after successful medical treatment. The presence of external ocular disease such as corneal neovascularization, corneal dystrophy, or keratoconjunctivitis sicca may disqualify a candidate for cataract surgery.

CLINICALLY INSIGNIFICANT LENS ABNORMALITIES

Cataracts Associated with Hyaloid Vessel Remnants

When the embryonic vascular system is retained in the vitreous and attached to the posterior lens capsule, lenticular opacities may be noted. Focal opacities at the attachment site may be associated with posterior lenticonus or lens bulge, a condition reported in Akitas and Doberman pinschers. Persistence of a nonpatent hyaloid vessel may not cause a cataract; however, if a large axial posterior capsular opacity is present, the animal may show visual impairment in bright light. Mydriasis maintained by instillation of 1% atropine ointment once every third day may improve vision.

Approximately 25% of dogs under 6 months of age have insignificant hyaloid remnants identified by indirect ophthalmoscopy or slit-lamp biomicroscopy.

Lens Perinuclear Ring

Concentric rings are sometimes noted by retroillumination in young dogs. These are always in a zone between the cortex and the nucleus or between zones of cortex. They are thought to represent dysfunctional growth zones. Disruptive events in the early development of a lens can account for these refractive variant zones. With time and aging they become less prominent or disappear.

Focal Ring Cataract

Ring-shaped perinuclear cataracts result from an earlier, short-lived, *in utero* or neonatal insult to the equatorial lens fibers. Normal fibers continue to grow peripheral to the ring. In some young puppies, the translucent ring is gone by 6 months of age, while in others the rings remain opaque without progression or visual effect.

Nuclear Y Cataract

These opacities define the small Y suture (erect anteriorly and inverted posteriorly) on either side of the fetal nucleus. In some animals, the suture pattern is only outlined by three V-shaped opacities. Often noted bilaterally in all pups of a litter, they are nonprogressive and usually disappear. These are considered to be congenital and idiopathic.

Suture Tip Opacities

Opacities at the outer tips of the posterior Y sutures and infrequently the anterior Y sutures appear most commonly in dogs under 6 months of age. These opacities are defined as small, linear streaks best visualized by retroillumination. Typically transient, those that persist are nonprogressive.

Arrowhead Suture-Tip Opacities

An inverted V-shaped opacity at the tip of the Y sutures in young puppies is not unusual. These opacities are usually associated with all posterior sutures. Some may extend into the equatorial lens. Generally, these opacities disappear by 6 months of age in all breeds except the West Highland terrier (Narfstrom, 1981).

Anterior Lens Capsule Pigment Deposits

The pigmented deposits are groups of cells on the anterior lens capsule, usually in the center of the visual axis. Magnification confirms that the brownish spot consists of discrete cell clusters. Their

Table 3. Breeds Predisposed to Lens Luxation*

Australian cattle dog
Border collie
Brittany
Cardigan Welsh corgi
Chihuahua
Fox terrier (smooth, wirehaired, toy)
German shepherd
Greyhound
Jack Russell terrier
Manchester terrier (toy, standard)
Manchester standard terrier
Norwegian elkhound
Scottish terrier
Sealyham terrier
Skye terrier
Tibetan terrier
Welsh terrier

*From Rubin, L. F.: *Inherited Eye Diseases in Purebred Dogs.* Baltimore: Williams & Wilkins, 1989.

origin and time of occurrence are uncertain. These deposits seem to be static and cause no visual complaint.

LENS LUXATION

Lens displacement is relatively common in both dogs and cats. Subluxation implies partial rupture of the zonules or complete zonular rupture with persistent lens adherence to the vitreous face. Luxation refers to complete dislocation of the lens without any attachments. The lens can be displaced forward into the anterior chamber or posteriorly into the vitreous.

Lens displacement can be primary and genetic or secondary to ocular inflammation, glaucoma, trauma, or intraocular tumors. Table 3 lists the canine breeds thought to be predisposed to lens luxation. Immune-mediated processes may be responsible for some lens luxations, although this hypothesis is poorly documented.

An analysis of 332 feline lens luxations revealed that trauma was infrequently associated but that concurrent intraocular disease (uveitis and glaucoma) was commonly associated with lens displacement. Uveitis was the most strongly associated concurrent intraocular disease, suggesting a possible causal role of intraocular inflammatory disease in the etiopathogenesis of feline lens displacement (Olivero et al., in press).

The signs of lens luxation include increased anterior chamber depth, iridodonesis, aphakic crescent, central corneal edema, and abnormal intraocular pressures (IOP). Blepharospasm, epiphora, edema, and acute blindness may be noted with increased IOP. Low IOP may be due to uveitis created by the lens irritation.

The management of a displaced lens is dependent

on the condition of the eye. For subluxations without other complications, conservative treatment with topical miotics should be prescribed (echothiophate-Phospholine Iodide, 0.03, 0.06, 0.125, or 0.25%, Wyeth-Ayerst) beginning with the lowest concentration (1 drop every 12 hr) to keep the pupil small and the lens behind it. The owner should be warned of possible complications (e.g., signs of organophosphate toxicity) and clinical signs of glaucoma or uveitis. In acute anterior lens luxation, the lens should be surgically removed as soon as possible. Treatment with antiglaucoma medication is indicated while awaiting surgical treatment (see this volume, p. 1125). If the lens is tilted forward, producing pupillary block glaucoma, the block may be relieved by dilating the pupil with 10% phenylephrine (AK-Dilate, Akorn). Adhesions may, however, prevent iris dilation.

Occasionally, anterior lens luxations can be manually replaced into the posterior chamber if the IOP is markedly reduced with the aid of intravenous 20% mannitol (Mannitol 20% Injection, Abbott) administered at 1 to 2 gm/kg over 20 to 30 min. Dilate the pupil with 1% tropicamide. After maximal osmotic effect is obtained (30 to 45 min postadministration), the eye is gently massaged through the lids as if retropulsing the globe. Continuous pressure for 2 min may replace the lens in the posterior chamber. The lens may be held in the posterior chamber with a miotic agent such as echothiophate every 12 hr or 2% pilocarpine (Akorn) every 12 hr.

Posterior lens luxation into liquefied vitreous has a poor prognosis for surgical removal. Lens extraction from the vitreous cavity is exceedingly difficult. The best results are with cryoextraction, but surgical and postoperative complications often result in blindness. Medical management balances the control of uveitis or glaucoma that may develop.

Chronically luxated lenses frequently develop cortical cataracts that progress to maturity. Causes of cataract development probably include the uveitis and metabolic derangements attendant to lens luxation.

References and Suggested Reading

American College of Veterinary Ophthalmologists: Ocular Disorders Proven or Suspected to be Hereditary in Dogs. CERF Vet Medical Data Program, Purdue University, West Lafayette, IN, 1992.
A listing of ocular disorders by breed. The ACVO genetics committee is currently completing this information.
Grant, W. M.: Toxicology of the Eye. 2nd ed. Springfield, IL: Charles Thomas, 1974.
This text provides ready answers to many questions that arise, summarizes known information, and is extensively referenced. Several editions are available.
MacMillan, A. D., Nelson, D. L., Munger, R. S., et al.: Efficacy of zinc citrate ascorbate for treatment of canine cataracts. J.A.V.M.A. 194:1581, 1989.
A controlled study by veterinary ophthalmologists documenting "ineffective" claims that topical zinc citrate ascorbate will reverse cataracts in dogs.
Martin, C. L.: The formation of cataracts in dogs with Disophenol.® Can. Vet. J. 16:228, 1975.
Seventeen puppies from 5 to 17 weeks of age were given subcutaneous Disophenol at 30 mg/kg. Cataracts of varying degree were caused and all were transient, lasting 1 to 5 days. Pups older than 16 weeks were resistant.
Narfstrom, K.: Cataract in the West Highland white terrier. J. Small Anim. Pract. 22:467, 1981.
Cataracts were found in 49 of 97 interrelated West Highland white terriers. Thirty-four dogs exhibited a Y-suture cataract, mainly affecting the tips of the posterior Y suture, while 12 dogs had mature cataracts. An autosomal-recessive inheritance was suspected.
Olivero, D., Riis, R., Dutton, A., et al.: Feline crystalline lens displacement: A two-part multicenter retrospective analysis. J. Am. Anim. Hosp. Assoc. (in press).
A retrospective survey of feline lens displacements finding that uveitis is a related factor. Association to FIV, FeLV, and toxoplasmosis titers were made.
Ralston, S. L., Isherwood, J., Chandler, M., et al.: Evaluation of growth rates and cataract formation in orphan puppies fed two milk replacer formulas. Proceedings of the Second International Conference on Veterinary Perimatology, Cambridge, England, July 1990.
Studies undertaken to evaluate commercial milk replacer with supplements that prevented cataracts. (Personal communication is requested by Dr. Ralston [201] 932-9404 and Dr. Isherwood [303] 221-4535).
Riis, R. C.: Diseases of the lens. In Kirk, R. W. (ed.): Current Veterinary Therapy VII. Philadelphia: W. B. Saunders 1980, pp. 565–570.
A general discussion of the lens in small animals with cataract patterns and progressions, with affected breeds noted.
Rubin, L. F.: Inherited Eye Diseases in Purebred Dogs. Baltimore: Williams and Wilkins, 1989.
A comprehensive text that is a compilation of data concerning hereditary and potentially hereditary ocular diseases in the dog gathered from the experience of colleagues, breeders, and the author.

GLAUCOMA

PAUL H. SCHERLIE, Jr.
Boston, Massachusetts

Glaucoma, an abnormal elevation of intraocular pressure (IOP), is a common cause of canine blindness. The frequency of canine glaucoma has been estimated at 1 of 204 hospital admissions; a higher frequency exists in predisposed breeds (Table 1). Glaucoma occurs less frequently in cats than in dogs

Table 1. Dog Breeds Predisposed to Glaucoma*

Breed	Iridocorneal Angle Configuration
Akita	Narrow to closed
Alaskan malamute	Narrow to closed
Basset hound	Open to closed; goniodysgenesis
Beagle	Open
Chow chow	Narrow to closed
American cocker spaniel	Narrow to closed
Poodle	Open to closed
Samoyed	Narrow to closed; goniodysgenesis
Siberian husky	Narrow to closed; goniodysgenesis

*Glaucoma occurs occasionally in many other breeds.

and is more subtle in its presentation than in dogs. Due to the nature of glaucoma in animals, the long-term maintenance of vision is difficult; successful case management often involves only the alleviation of chronic ocular pain in a blind eye. A high index of suspicion, prompt diagnosis, and knowledge of available therapy aids the practitioner in the correct management of glaucoma.

AQUEOUS HUMOR DYNAMICS

The ciliary processes, villus-like folds of the ciliary body, are the site of aqueous production. These structures consist of an inner nonpigmented and outer pigmented epithelium surrounding a collagen-vascular core. Aqueous production is thought to occur through a combination of active secretion, ultrafiltration, and passive diffusion. Current knowledge suggests that aqueous production consists almost entirely of active secretion. The secretory process occurs in the nonpigmented epithelium, is energy dependent, and requires the enzyme carbonic anhydrase.

Aqueous composition is relatively similar to that of plasma, with the exception of the protein content, which is negligible. The aqueous provides nutrition and removes waste products for the avascular cornea, lens, and trabecular meshwork. Normal IOP maintains the optimal relationship of the cornea, lens, and retina so that a precise visual image is formed.

The flow of aqueous proceeds from the posterior chamber, through the pupil, and into the anterior chamber to egress through the iridocorneal angle (Fig. 1). The iridocorneal angle is formed by the junction of the iris, ciliary body, and inner peripheral portion of the cornea and sclera. A fenestrated sheet of iris-like tissue, the pectinate ligament, connects the iris base and corneoscleral junction. Beyond the pectinate ligament lies the trabecular meshwork, a dense interweaving of endothelial cell-lined collagen beams. Following passage through the trabecular meshwork, the aqueous passes through a series of collecting vessels to return to the blood-vascular system. The exact mechanism by which aqueous enters these vessels is unknown. A variable, usually small amount of aqueous exits the eye through a "nonconventional" (uveoscleral) route, the volume of which is species-dependent. The IOP results from the interaction of the aqueous production and drainage. Normal IOP is maintained between 15 and 30 mm Hg in the dog and cat. Sustained pressure beyond this range results in progressive optic nerve damage and vision loss.

Normally, the greatest resistance to aqueous flow is at the lens-pupil interface, iridocorneal angle, and trabecular meshwork. Abnormalities in these areas causing an increased amount of resistance are the most common causes of glaucoma. Hypersecretion of aqueous resulting in an elevated IOP has not been documented in animals.

GLAUCOMA CLASSIFICATION

Glaucoma is currently classified according to the underlying cause (primary or secondary) and the appearance of the iridocorneal angle (open, narrow, closed, goniodysgenesis).

Primary Glaucoma

Primary glaucoma is due to an inherent defect in the iridocorneal angle. This defect may be biochemical or morphological. Configuration of the iridocorneal angle in primary glaucoma ranges from open to closed, with the majority being narrow. In certain breeds (e.g., Basset hounds) a congenital defect in formation of the iridocorneal angle (mesodermal

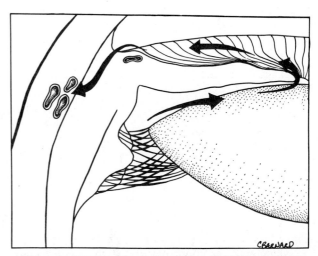

Figure 1. Aqueous flow *(arrows)* from the ciliary body into the posterior chamber across the lens surface and through the pupil to egress through the iridocorneal angle.

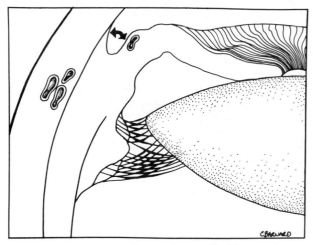

Figure 2. Narrow iridocorneal angle *(double arrow).*

goniodysgenesis) is thought to contribute to the onset of glaucoma in later life. Although traditionally classified as a congenital glaucoma, this form is best thought of as a primary glaucoma. Primary glaucoma is a breed-related, heritable condition, with the mode of inheritance unknown. The diagnosis of primary glaucoma is based on an elevated IOP without signs of concurrent ocular disease. Occasionally, a mild anterior uveitis may be associated with primary glaucoma, especially in the Basset hound. Although primary glaucoma is a breed-related disorder (see Table 1), it may occur in any individual animal. *Primary glaucoma is a bilateral disease,* although it is unusual for both eyes to be affected simultaneously. The contralateral eye should be periodically monitored for involvement, with prophylactic therapy indicated (see later section "Glaucoma Prophylaxis").

Secondary Glaucoma

Secondary glaucoma is an elevation of IOP associated with concurrent ocular disease, usually intraocular inflammation, hemorrhage, or neoplasia. The iridocorneal angle may be open or closed in secondary glaucoma. Pupillary block, an abnormal resistance to aqueous flow at the lens/pupil interface, can play a role in many secondary glaucomas. Pupillary block may result from posterior synechiae or increased lens-to-iris contact. This increased resistance to flow results in expansion of the posterior chamber, causing a narrowing of the iridocorneal angle (Fig. 2). In older dogs with unilateral intraocular inflammation and secondary glaucoma, intraocular neoplasia should be suspected (Table 2). Regardless of the cause, the primary ocular disease and the secondary glaucoma are treated simultaneously. Following resolution of the inciting cause,

the pressure-lowering therapy may be discontinued in many cases.

The involvement of the lens deserves special mention. Swelling of the lens associated with cataract formation or abnormal lens motion (luxation or subluxation) may result in a forward displacement of the lens-iris diaphragm, causing a relative pupillary block and narrowed iridocorneal angle. Lens luxation/subluxation, though classically described as causing secondary glaucoma, is associated with glaucoma having all the characteristics of primary glaucoma (i.e., bilateral occurrence and absence of inciting causes). In breeds predisposed to lens luxations (e.g., terriers) successful removal of the displaced lens may not result in complete control of the accompanying glaucoma.

CLINICAL SIGNS

The clinical signs of glaucoma depend on the rapidity, duration, severity, and cause of the elevated intraocular pressure.

Acute Glaucoma

The classic signs of acute primary or secondary glaucoma in the dog include *blindness,* ocular *pain,* conjunctival and *episcleral congestion,* and diffuse *corneal edema.* If visible, the pupil is often dilated and the retina appears normal. Marked variations in these signs exist. Certain breeds (e.g., beagles) exhibit vision loss with only subtle ocular pain or

Table 2. *Etiology of Secondary Glaucoma**

Secondary open-angle glaucoma
Obstruction of the trabecular meshwork with:
Inflammatory cells
Lens material
Blood
Fibrin
Neoplastic infiltration
Neovascular membrane
Vitreous
Increased vascular pressure
Intraorbital venous obstruction
Secondary closed-angle glaucoma
With pupillary block
Intumescent cataract
Iris bombé
Lens subluxation†
Aphakic vitreous herniation
Without pupillary block
Neoplastic infiltration
Peripheral anterior synechiae formation

*Modified from Martin, C. L.: The pathology of glaucoma. *In* Peiffer, R. L., Jr. (ed.): *Comparative Ophthalmic Pathology.* Springfield, IL: Charles C Thomas, 1983, pp. 137–169.
†Associated glaucoma is more typical of primary than secondary form.

redness. Pupil size may be variable, especially in the secondary glaucomas, and should not be utilized to deny or confirm the diagnosis. Optic disk swelling and retinal hemorrhages are occasionally seen in acute intraocular pressure elevations.

Chronic Glaucoma

With prolonged elevations in IOP, the globe frequently becomes enlarged (buphthalmus). The cornea may exhibit edema, neovascularization, and linear tears in Descemet's membrane called "Haab's striae." The iris often becomes atrophic; in long-standing glaucoma, atrophy of the ciliary body may result, leading to decreased aqueous production and normotension. The lens often becomes cataractous, and with sufficient buphthalmia zonular rupture results, causing lens subluxation or luxation.

Blindness due to glaucoma is thought to result initially from ischemic or pressure necrosis of the ganglion cell axons, which is not apparent for several weeks. A characteristic funduscopic abnormality in chronic glaucoma is a depression ("cupping") of the optic nerve head related to axon loss and posterior movement of the lamina cribrosa. This is an irreversible change, indicating permanent blindness. Generalized retinal degeneration, evidenced by tapetal hyper-reflectivity and vascular attenuation, is a late-term event.

DIAGNOSIS OF GLAUCOMA

Due to the variable signs and simultaneous occurrence with other ocular disease, a reasonable index of suspicion is needed to make a diagnosis of glaucoma. Tonometry should be performed on any patient with ocular inflammation or blindness of unknown cause.

Tonometry

Tonometry is the measurement of the intraocular pressure. The methods most often available to the general practitioner are digital and indentation (Schiøtz) tonometry. Digital tonometry, the tactile estimation of IOP, is imprecise and often leads to erroneous conclusions. The handheld Schiøtz tonometer is readily available, simple to use, and provides an accurate estimation of the IOP.

The Schiøtz tonometer indirectly estimates the ocular pressure by measuring the amount of corneal indentation produced by a weighted plunger. The instrument is provided with an attached 5.5-gm weight and an additional 7.5-gm and 10-gm weight. The IOP in millimeters of mercury (mm Hg) is obtained from a conversion chart utilizing the scale

readings and weight values. Various conversion charts exist and appear to be adequate (Slatter, 1990). A simple rule of thumb is that a normal IOP is present when the tonometer scale reading is within a two-unit value of the plunger weight (example: the "normal" range is from 3.5 to 7.5 scale units when using a 5.5-gm weight). Lower scale readings indicate higher IOP.

Several factors can result in erroneous measurements. Severe corneal edema may result in falsely low readings; an anteriorly luxated lens directly adjacent to the cornea may cause overestimation of the IOP. It is unlikely that either of these factors significantly alter the clinical diagnosis.

Tonometry is performed by topically anesthetizing the patient's eye and forcing the gaze in an upward direction. Starting with the affixed 5.5-gm weight, the plunger is placed on the central cornea and a scale reading is obtained. This procedure should be repeated until three successful readings have been taken. If scale readings of <3.5 occur with the 5.5-gm weight, the 7.5-gm weight should be utilized and the measurements repeated. This will allow a more accurate estimation to be made. Tonometry is contraindicated in eyes with deep corneal ulcers or lacerations.

Gonioscopy

Gonioscopy is the examination of the iridocorneal angle utilizing a special lens. In humans, therapeutic decisions are frequently based on the gonioscopic appearance of the drainage angle. In veterinary medicine, the angle configuration has not been correlated with the most appropriate therapy. In many cases of animal glaucoma, multiple drug therapy is required for adequate pressure control. For these reasons, gonioscopy is not considered essential for the adequate management of most clinical cases. There is currently no evidence that the gonioscopic appearance of the drainage angle has predictive value in determining which patients will develop glaucoma.

GLAUCOMA THERAPY

The choice of therapy in glaucoma is based on vision potential, cause of the glaucoma, concurrent systemic illness, adverse drug effects, and cost. The most important factor in the initial treatment of glaucoma is potential for return of sight. Animals with an IOP elevation of >60 mm Hg for >48 hr seldom regain useful vision; permanent vision loss may occur at lower IOPs or after shorter durations. When the clinician is unsure of the prognosis for vision, aggressive therapy should be initiated. In a permanently blind eye, the goal of therapy is to

Table 3. *Drugs for Antiglaucoma Therapy*

Hyperosmotics
  Mannitol (25%)—1 to 2 gm/kg IV; administer over 20 min; repeat in 4 to 6 hr if needed
  Glycerol (50%)—1 to 2 gm/kg PO
Carbonic anhydrase inhibitors
  Dichlorphenamide (Daranide, Merck Sharp & Dohme)—2 to 4 mg/kg q 8 to 12 hr
  Methazolamide (Neptazane, Lederle)—2 to 4 mg/kg q 8 to 12 hr
  Acetazolamide (Diamox, Lederle)—4 to 8 mg/kg q 8 to 12 hr
Parasympathomimetic (topical)
  Pilocarpine solution (2%)—q 8 to 12 hr
  Pilocarpine ointment (Pilopine HS, Alcon)—4% q 24 hr
  Echothiophate iodide (Phospholine Iodide, Wyeth-Ayerst)—0.06%, 0.125% q 12 to 24 hr
  Demecarium bromide (Humorsol, Merck Sharp & Dohme)—0.125%, 0.25% q 12 to 24 hr
Beta-adrenergic antagonists (topical)
  Timolol maleate (Timoptic, Merck Sharp & Dohme)—0.5% q 12 hr
  Betaxolol HCl (Betoptic, Alcon)—0.5% q 12 hr
Sympathomimetic
  Dipivefrin HCl (0.1%) (Propine, Allergan) q 12 hr
Potassium supplementation
  Potassium chloride (Slow-K, Summit)–600 mg tablet/50 lb PO q 24 hr

provide comfort with minimal treatment. Both the medical and surgical procedures for glaucoma can be divided into treatments that decrease aqueous production or increase aqueous outflow.

Medical Therapy

The drugs indicated for use in glaucoma therapy as discussed in this section are listed in Table 3.

OSMOTHERAPY

Hyperosmotic agents are indicated in acute, severe elevations of IOP. These drugs act by increasing plasma osmolality, causing a dehydration of the vitreous. Mannitol and glycerol are the most frequently used hyperosmotic agents in veterinary medicine (Dugan et al., 1989).

Mannitol is an inert, nonmetabolized, six-carbon alcohol that exhibits poor intraocular penetration, even when inflammation is present. Mannitol is the hyperosmotic agent of choice for diabetics and for animals with glaucoma secondary to uveitis. Mannitol is administered intravenously over a 20- to 30-min period. At room temperature, the solution may exhibit crystal formation; warming the solution or administration through a blood filtration set reduces the risk of intravenous crystal administration. Water should be withheld from the patient for several hours to maximize intraocular dehydration. Ocular hypotension is rapidly achieved with mannitol in

most instances; if the IOP remains elevated, the mannitol dose may be repeated in 4 to 6 hr. If adequate pressure control cannot be achieved with two administrations of mannitol in addition to the therapy discussed later, it is unlikely that medical therapy will be effective.

The potential adverse affects of mannitol are related to its dehydrating effects on the central nervous system and expansion of plasma volume. Possible reactions include disorientation, vomiting, systemic dehydration, and pulmonary edema in patients with oliguria or congestive heart failure.

Glycerol is an orally administered trihydric alcohol that is metabolized to glucose and exhibits some penetration into an inflamed eye. *Glycerol should not be used in diabetics* and is less preferred for the treatment of glaucoma associated with uveitis. Glycerol may induce emesis, resulting in variable absorption of the administered dose. The hyperosmotic agents are not useful for long-term therapy. Eventual equilibrium between the eye and blood vascular system occurs with frequent use, negating their hypotensive effect.

CARBONIC ANHYDRASE INHIBITORS

The carbonic anhydrase inhibitors (CAIs) block the enzyme carbonic anhydrase, which functions prominently in aqueous secretion. These drugs decrease aqueous production by approximately 50% and are the mainstay of medical therapy for glaucoma. The reduction in aqueous production is independent of the diuretic action of these drugs. Other diuretic agents (e.g., furosemide) *do not* cause ocular hypotension.

Of all the antiglaucoma agents, the CAIs produce the most side effects, including polyuria/polydipsia, anorexia, vomiting, diarrhea, depression, and panting. Dichlorphenamide (Daranide, Merck, Sharp & Dohme) appears to produce the least severe and frequent adverse reactions. Acetazolamide (Diamox, Lederle), though readily available, is poorly tolerated by most dogs. If an animal cannot tolerate a specific CAI, another one may be substituted. Some animals are unable to tolerate these drugs in any form or dose.

Hypokalemia is a potential sequela of CAI therapy; some of the side effects of the CAI (weakness, anorexia, etc.) may be a direct result of decreased scrum potassium. Frequent monitoring of serum potassium or the prophylactic administration of oral potassium (Slow-K, Ciba-Geigy) may be indicated.

MIOTIC AGENTS

Topical miotic agents increase outflow of the aqueous humor by causing contraction of the ciliary muscle, resulting in an alteration of the trabecular meshwork configuration. This change in the iridocorneal angle is thought to decrease resistance to aqueous exit. The miotics are parasympathomimetic agents that act directly or indirectly (cholinesterase inhibitors). Along with their ocular hypotensive effect, the parasympathomimetics dilate uveal blood vessels. *The use of these drugs is contraindicated in secondary glaucoma* because they produce increased inflammation and predispose to iris bombé formation.

Pilocarpine is the most commonly used miotic agent. Topical pilocarpine solution is available in concentrations ranging from 0.25% to 10%; 2% pilocarpine appears to produce a maximum hypotensive effect with the least amount of adverse reaction. Pilocarpine solutions should be administered three to four times daily. A 4% pilocarpine gel (Pilopine HS, Alcon Laboratories) has been shown to be an effective antiglaucoma agent in the dog with once-daily use. Topical irritation is the most frequent side effect of pilocarpine administration and appears to decrease over several weeks.

Echothiophate iodide (Phospholine Iodide, Wyeth-Ayerst) and demecarium bromide (Humorsol, Merck Sharp & Dohme) are irreversible cholinesterase inhibitors that act by increasing endogenous acetylcholine. They have the advantage over pilocarpine of less frequent dosing and less topical irritation. These agents increase susceptibility to intoxication by organophosphate insecticides. Their concurrent use with flea products of this type is not recommended. Systemic signs of cholinesterase inhibitor toxicity include salivation, lacrimation, urinary incontinence, and diarrhea.

BETA-BLOCKERS

Topical beta-blocking agents are currently the most frequently prescribed antiglaucoma agents for humans. Beta-blockers decrease aqueous production by approximately 50% in humans via a poorly understood mechanism. In normal dogs and cats, 0.5% timolol maleate (Timoptic, Merck Sharp & Dohme) reduced IOP 16% and 22%, respectively (Wilkie and Latimer, 1991). Investigations of efficacy of topical beta-blocking drugs in IOP reduction in glaucomatous eyes of dogs and cats have not been reported. Despite this uncertainty, beta-blockers are employed in glaucoma management by many veterinary ophthalmologists. Systemic beta-blockade may result in bronchospasm and cardiac effects; therefore, these drugs should be used with caution in patients with congestive heart failure or obstructive lung disease. Betaxolol (Betoptic, Alcon Laboratories), a specific beta$_1$-blocking agent, may be more appropriate for use in patients with pulmonary disease.

SYMPATHOMIMETIC AGENTS

Epinephrine is thought to decrease IOP primarily by increasing aqueous outflow. Topical sympathomimetics should always be used in combination with other topical antiglaucoma agents because they have only a mild hypotensive effect. Topical epinephrine frequently produces conjunctival erythema and irritation. Dipivalyl epinephrine, an epinephrine prodrug that is converted to epinephrine in the anterior chamber, produces less irritation, and is the agent of choice in this group.

Surgical Therapy

The surgical treatment of glaucoma is directed at decreasing production or increasing aqueous outflow. These procedures have a poor long-term success rate in animals and should be reserved for visual eyes in which maximum medical therapy is ineffective. These surgical measures are best performed by veterinary ophthalmologists.

Transscleral cryoablation of the ciliary body appears to be effective in decreasing IOP, although multiple applications may be required. Freezing of the ciliary body is accomplished with a nitrous oxide or liquid nitrogen probe in the anesthetized animal. This procedure is associated with frequent complications such as cataract formation, persistent uveitis, hypotony, or a severe elevation of the IOP immediately postfreezing. This temporary elevation in pressure often results in permanent blindness. Prophylactic use of cryotherapy is not recommended in the normal eye of patients with unilateral primary glaucoma because the associated uveitis and damage to the iridocorneal angle may hasten the onset of glaucoma. Ablation of the ciliary body using the transscleral application of Nd:YAG laser energy is currently being investigated and may prove useful in the future (Nasisse et al., 1990).

A variety of surgical filtering procedures such as thermal sclerostomy, iridencleisis, and prosthetic shunt implantation exist. Due to the associated uveitis, the increased aqueous outflow provided by these procedures is generally short-term because of fibroplasia of the outflow tract.

Enucleation or intraocular evisceration-implantation with a silicone prosthesis is recommended for blind, painful globes and is readily performed by the practitioner. In addition to producing comfort, these procedures may allow cessation of medical therapy, avoiding potential side effects. The intraocular evisceration-implantation procedure is utilized *only for primary glaucoma*. Placement of a prosthesis into a globe with secondary glaucoma of unknown cause or due to infection or neoplasia is contraindicated. The author strongly recommends evisceration-implantation over enucleation for cosmctic reasons. Many owners of pets with bilateral glaucoma elect euthanasia over bilateral enucleation; these owners are frequently satisfied with an evisceration-implantation procedure.

Intravitreal injection of gentamicin causes ciliary epithelial destruction and decreased aqueous production (Moller et al., 1986). This procedure, performed with sedation and local anesthesia, is useful for animals blind from primary glaucoma that cannot tolerate medical therapy or general anesthesia. This is an option only for blind eyes in which a definitive diagnosis of primary glaucoma has been made. Sighted eyes and eyes with secondary glaucoma should not be treated with this method.

The author discourages the use of this technique. Glaucoma is frequently misdiagnosed, and this procedure is *contraindicated unless tonometry has confirmed the diagnosis*. Long-term cosmetic results are frequently disappointing due to shrinkage of the globe and secondary entropion.

LENS LUXATION

Primary lens luxation in the dog is frequently accompanied by glaucoma. Anterior lens luxation is an emergency that may require glaucoma therapy and prompt referral for lensectomy. The glaucoma associated with primary lens luxation is difficult to control without lens removal, which alone may not cure the glaucoma.

THERAPEUTIC APPROACH

The control of IOP in animals with glaucoma requires multiple drug therapy. Acute glaucoma of less than 48 hours' duration requires emergency treatment consisting of a hyperosmotic agent, a CAI, and a topical agent. The author prefers to use mannitol, dichlorphenamide, and timolol maleate (see Table 3) for the initial management of acute glaucoma in dogs and cats. If the glaucoma is secondary, the underlying cause should be treated simultaneously.

If the IOP decreases into the normal range, the CAI and the chosen topical agent should be continued for maintenance therapy. If the IOP pressure remains elevated, a second topical agent with a different pharmacologic mechanism should be added to the previous therapy. Dichlorphenamide and 2% pilocarpine appear to be adequate to maintain a normal IOP in most cases. Timolol maleate 0.5% may be used as the initial topical agent in secondary glaucoma. Dipivalyl epinephrine (Propine, Allergan) is recommended in addition to these agents if the IOP remains elevated. If vision is present and maximum medical therapy is ineffec-

tive, referral for a surgical filtering procedure or cryotherapy should be considered.

Once the affected eye is blind, long-term medical therapy should not be employed to maintain normotension. Due to the cost and potential side effects of these agents, the patient may be better served with an enucleation or evisceration-implantation surgery.

Occasionally, buphthalmic eyes will maintain low or normal IOP. This phenomenon is thought to be secondary to pressure necrosis of the ciliary epithelium with a resultant decrease in aqueous production. If the globe enlargement is not excessive, these eyes may not need therapy. Enlarged eyes are, however, more prone to exposure and trauma. Enlarged globes will shrink to fit the silicone sphere following an intraocular evisceration-implantation procedure.

MONITORING

Glaucomatous eyes should be monitored periodically to determine the effectiveness of therapy. Although tonometry should be performed on the unaffected eye of dogs with primary glaucoma every 3 to 4 months, elevations of IOP are uncommon before an acute attack of glaucoma occurs.

GLAUCOMA PROPHYLAXIS

Because primary glaucoma is a bilateral disease, after an animal develops unilateral primary glaucoma the contralateral eye is at risk. Glaucoma may not develop in the second eye for months or years. Evidence suggests that some form of prophylactic glaucoma therapy may delay onset in the unaffected eye (Slater and Erb, 1986). Carbonic anhydrase inhibitors provide protection by their systemic effects. Following enucleation or evisceration-implantation of a blind glaucomatous eye, cessation of oral CAI administration is recommended. A topical agent such as timolol maleate or dipivalyl epinephrine should be used indefinitely in the normotensive eye for glaucoma prophylaxis.

FELINE GLAUCOMA

The clinical signs of feline glaucoma are subtle and difficult to recognize. The conspicuous signs of ocular pain, episcleral congestion, and corneal edema seen in the dog are uncommon in the cat. Primary glaucoma in the cat frequently presents as buphthalmia and blindness with minimal ocular inflammation. Secondary glaucoma is more prevalent than primary glaucoma in the cat and often occurs due to chronic anterior uveitis or infiltrative neoplasia. Proper treatment of secondary glaucoma in the cat requires an appropriate diagnostic evaluation to determine and treat the underlying disease process as well as the glaucoma (see this volume pp. 1061 and 1070).

Because feline glaucoma is so often chronic when identified, emergency therapy is usually unwarranted. Methazolamide (Neptazane, Lederle) appears to be well tolerated by cats and is available in a small-dose form (25 mg). Because of the cat's sensitivity to organophosphates, the cholinesterase agents are not recommended for topical use. Long-term medical therapy for glaucoma in cats (as in dogs) is usually ineffective. Enucleation or evisceration-implantation is usually required.

References and Suggested Reading

Brooks, D. E.: Canine and feline glaucomas. *In* Kirk, R. W. (ed.): *Current Veterinary Therapy IX*. Philadelphia: W. B. Saunders, 1986, pp. 656–659.
A discussion of the pathogenesis, clinical signs, and treatment of canine and feline glaucoma.

Caprioli, J.: The ciliary epithelia and aqueous humor. *In* Moses, R. A., and Hart, W. M. (eds.): *Adler's Physiology of the Eye, Clinical Application*. 8th ed. St. Louis: C. V. Mosby, 1985, pp. 204–222.
A discussion of the physiology of aqueous production in the human eye.

Dugan, S. J., Roberts, S. M., and Severin, G. A.: Systemic osmotherapy for ophthalmic disease in dogs and cats. J.A.V.M.A. 194:115–118, 1989.
A discussion of the hyperosmotic agents utilized in the treatment of glaucoma.

Gelatt, K. N.: The canine glaucomas. *In* Gelatt, K. N. (ed.): *Textbook of Veterinary Ophthalmology*. Philadelphia: Lea & Febiger, 1981, pp. 390–434.

A discussion of the pathogenesis, clinical signs, histopathology, and treatment of canine glaucoma.

Martin, C. L.: The pathology of glaucoma. *In* Peiffer, R. L., Jr. (ed.): *Comparative Ophthalmic Pathology*. Springfield, IL: Charles C Thomas, 1983, pp. 137–169.
A discussion of the histopathology of canine glaucoma.

Martin, C. L., and Ward, D. A.: Medical therapy for glaucoma. *In* Kirk, R. W. (ed.): *Current Veterinary Therapy X*. Philadelphia: W. B. Saunders, 1989, pp. 647–651.
A discussion of the medical agents used in the treatment of canine and feline glaucoma.

Nasisse, M. P., Davidson, M. G., English, R. V., et al.: Treatment of glaucoma by use of transcleral neodymium:yttrium-aluminum-garnet laser cyclocoagulation in dogs. J.A.V.M.A. 197:350–354, 1990.
A discussion of the potential use of Nd:YAG laser energy to produce ocular hypotension.

Moller, I., Cook, C. S., Peiffer, R. L., et al.: Indications for and complications of pharmacologic ablation of the ciliary body for the treatment of chronic glaucoma in the dog. J. Am. Anim. Hosp. Assoc. 22:319–326, 1986.
A discussion of the use of intravitreal gentamicin injections to produce ocular hypotension.

Slater, M. R., and Erb, H. N.: Effects of risk factors and prophylactic treatment of primary glaucoma in the dog. J.A.V.M.A. 188:1028–1030, 1986.
An epidemiologic survey and discussion of the potential benefit of antiglaucoma prophylaxis in primary glaucoma of dogs.

Slatter, D. H.: *Fundamentals of Veterinary Ophthalmology*. 2nd ed. Philadelphia: W. B. Saunders, 1990, pp. 338–364.
A discussion of the pathogenesis, clinical signs, histopathology, and treatment of glaucoma.

Whitley, R. D.: Surgical management of glaucoma. *In* Bojrab, J. G. (ed.): *Current Techniques in Small Animal Surgery*. 3rd ed. Philadelphia: Lea & Febiger, 1990, pp. 104–112.
A discussion of the surgical procedures used to control glaucoma.

Wilkie, D. A., and Latimer, C. A.: Effects of topical administration of timolol maleate on intraocular pressure and pupil size in dogs. Am. J. Vet. Res. 52:432–435, 1991.
Topical 0.5% timolol maleate reduced IOP and pupil size in both treated and nontreated eyes of normal dogs.

Wilkie, D. A., and Latimer, C. A.: Effects of topical administration of timolol maleate in intraocular pressure and pupil size in cats. Am. J. Vet. Res. 52:436–440, 1991.
Topical 0.5% timolol maleate reduced IOP in both treated and nontreated eyes and reduced pupil size in the treated eyes of normal cats.

DISEASES OF CAGED BIRDS AND EXOTIC PETS

R. ERIC MILLER

Consulting Editor

MANAGEMENT OF MEDICAL EMERGENCIES IN RAPTORS

PATRICK T. REDIG

St. Paul, Minnesota

Medical emergencies in wild and captive raptors result from trauma, nutritional depletion, toxicity, or anesthetic difficulties. In all but the latter, emergency care consists of the routine application of a supportive care regimen and treatment of specific problems identified on the basis of the clinician's instincts, prior knowledge, gleanings from the available history (usually meager), and the ability to integrate these with data gathered from the patient during examination. Often, emergency therapy must be initiated while medical information is being collected.

MAJOR CAUSES OF RAPTOR EMERGENCIES

Trauma

Collisions with vehicles, windows, and power lines, entanglement in fishing line or kite string, shooting, and trapping are primary causes of casualties among wild raptors. Problems associated with trauma include:

CONCUSSIONS. These are caused primarily by impact with moving and stationary objects. Birds surviving the impact usually recover well, though owls are likely to experience associated ocular injuries (especially detached retinas) because a large portion of the tubular-shaped eye is unprotected by the skull.

FRACTURES. Any source of trauma is likely to cause fractures. Long-bone fractures are readily observed, but fractures of the axial skeleton (furcula, coracoid, scapula, vertebrae, and pelvis) will be detected only by radiographs. With the exception of vertebral body damage, fractures themselves do not constitute an emergency.

SOFT-TISSUE INJURIES. With the exception of eye injuries, most soft-tissue problems are confined to exterior structures and do not constitute medical emergencies because internal hemorrhage rarely occurs. Since birds lack a diaphragm, herniation of internal organs cannot occur, and massive displacement of internal organs and rupturing of large blood vessels do not occur with any appreciable frequency. Massive blood loss rarely accompanies even severe trauma such as wing amputation. A raptor

that has survived a traumatic incident seldom requires intervention beyond supportive care to sustain life.

Nutritional Depletion

Severe debilitation resulting from insufficient food intake is the most common emergency situation encountered among raptors used for falconry. It occurs most frequently among males during the peak of their first season in the field. The malnutrition results from the fact that all trained raptors are managed by controlling their weight. Idiosyncratic responses to weight control as well as variations in the degree of weight control exerted by individual falconers contribute to the problem. While trained birds seldom experience the prolonged fast that an injured wild bird would, they are often kept in a state of lean body mass during which catabolism of body proteins occurs. The problem is exacerbated in northern climes by increased energy requirements during winter's cold. Afflicted birds are presented in states of extreme weight loss, severe anemia, dehydration, and depression. They may have less than 24 hr to live at the time of presentation, and yet they may have exhibited reasonably normal performance in the field as recently as the previous day.

Among wild birds, uncomplicated nutritional depletion is typically seen in late summer in juvenile birds that have not learned to hunt before becoming separated from their parents. Similarly, old birds that seem to have lost the physical ability to procure food are occasionally found and presented in a state of malnutrition. In other circumstances, the clinician should be alert for signs of disabling trauma as an underlying cause of the underweight condition of a raptor.

Toxicity

LEAD AND ORGANOPHOSPHATES. Exposure to elemental lead or an organophosphate (OP) insecticide or other toxic substance constitutes a true medical emergency (see this volume, p. 183). The initial diagnosis is based on history and clinical

1134

signs. To delay treatment for days or even hours waiting for clinical test results to confirm the diagnosis is to risk losing the patient.

Clinical Signs. Lead poisoning typically causes emaciation, anemia, and occasionally convulsions and partial or complete blindness (Redig et al., 1987). Organophosphate poisoning causes prostration, tremors or convulsions, salivation, and lung congestion (Porter and Snead, 1990).

Sources. Though lead shot has been banned for use in waterfowl hunting in many states and will be banned federally by 1991, it is still widely used for upland game hunting and general sport shooting. Scavenging raptors are likely to consume carcasses left in the field. Organophosphate poisoning has occurred in eagles exposed to hog carcasses treated for external parasites with OP pesticides and left in open fields after the hogs died for unrelated reasons. Also, the use of contact OP avicides in large industrial and utility complexes has resulted in exposure and death for raptors that consumed birds poisoned in this manner. Storage of OP pesticides with food for falcons has resulted in accidental contamination through spillage onto the foodstuff and subsequent poisoning and death of the falcons.

ANTICOAGULANT POISONS. Anticoagulant poisons have also been responsible for secondary poisonings of raptors, but this has only been recognized upon postmortem examination. Treatment with vitamin K preparations is recommended, and a regimen is provided by Flammer (1986).

Respiratory Emergencies

The major causes of acute respiratory embarrassment are foreign body obstruction (e.g., antibiotic tablet, piece of meat), aspergillus lesions in the syrinx, tracheal penetration (gunshot, other trauma), and respiratory arrest during anesthesia.

TREATMENT PRIORITIES IN EMERGENCIES

The priorities for examination and treatment in raptors are the same as for most small animals. These include, in order, assurance of respiratory function, control of seizures, correction of circulatory dysfunction, arrest of hemorrhage, management of fractures or luxations, and establishment of a definitive diagnosis (Jenkins, 1988).

DIAGNOSTIC PROCEDURES

History

As much patient history as possible should be obtained. For captive birds the following informa-

tion should be ascertained: (1) diet, especially food items and quantities consumed in the last ten days, (2) the source of food items, (3) the length of time in captivity, (4) whether the bird was born in the wild or captively produced, (5) whether it is imprinted, (6) possible causes of injury or illness, (7) potential for exposure to toxic substances, and (8) any previous medical treatment. Information about wild birds should include geographic area of recovery (e.g., along a road, under power lines, in an agricultural field), circumstances of recovery (e.g., extricated from a fence), length of time since recovery, and any medical treatment attempted before presentation.

Observation

Initial observations of the bird are important. The clinician must develop clinical impressions immediately. Note the posture and attitude of the bird before removing it from its transport box. Observe the quantity and quality of droppings (mutes) on the floor of the container and whether solid fecal material or only urine is being passed. Note fecal color—an emerald green is indicative of a raptor that is simply hungry, while a lime-green color is indicative of gastrointestinal tract dysfunction, with lead poisoning the most common cause. Polyuria and polydipsia are rare. A more common finding is a lack of urine production secondary to poor kidney perfusion from dehydration. The appearance of the eye is an important indicator of hydration status. Raptors in an emergency-level state of dehydration or emaciation exhibit a sunken globe with a dull cornea, a so-called "almond-eyed" appearance, instead of the bright, round orb normally seen in healthy birds. All of this information can be gained in less than a minute prior to handling of the bird, but it is extremely important in establishing a minimum data base.

Immediate Treatment Concerns

Cases exhibiting obvious convulsive activity or respiratory distress should be addressed immediately. Valium administered 0.5 mg/kg IV will generally control convulsions arising from lead and strychnine poisoning. It will also relieve the anxiety of respiratory distress caused by blockages of the bronchial tree.

MANAGEMENT OF RESPIRATORY ARREST DURING ANESTHESIA

If respiratory arrest has occurred during an anesthetic episode and no response is gained by stimulating the glottis or prodding below the sternum, immediate intubation and internal positive-pressure ventilation can effect resuscitation. If a tube is unavailable, simply covering the beak with a semiclosed fist and blowing into the end of your hand can be an effective mouth-to-beak mode of ventilation.

MANAGEMENT OF RESPIRATORY ARREST CAUSED BY TRACHEAL OBSTRUCTION

Respiratory embarrassment due to airway obstruction can be relieved either by inserting a tracheal tube into the interclavicular air sacs, through which a bird can breathe quite normally, or by inserting a rubber catheter or large-bore needle into an abdominal air sac and providing oxygen in a unidirectional flow at a rate of 1 L/min/kg (Rode et al., 1990). When the patient has stabilized, procedures for relief of the underlying cause may be initiated.

Examination

Physical examination and initiation of supportive therapy should begin without delay in all other cases. After physical restraint, record the body weight (BW), collect a small blood sample for immediate determination of packed cell volume (PCV) and total solids (TS), and administer a bolus of lactated Ringer's solution (see later section on fluids). A survey radiograph should be obtained with minimal restraint. Avoid causing undue stress by attempting to obtain a perfect radiograph. Film should be processed immediately so the information gained can be used as an aid to further examination.

In a severely debilitated patient, examination should be postponed and treatment started at this point. Except as noted later, wound treatment and other forms of manipulation should be delayed until the patient has stabilized.

Extended Examination and Treatment

If the patient seems stable and in good physical condition, further examination and treatment of a nonemergency nature may be undertaken. For such patients, anesthesia with isoflurane (Aerrane, Anaquest) is recommended. This agent is safe to use in even moderately debilitated birds and actually reduces the stress of handling that accompanies additional examination and initial treatment.

GENERALIZED AND SPECIFIC TREATMENT MODALITIES

Goals of Therapy

The immediate goals of emergency care are to stabilize the patient and to establish circumstances conducive to treatment of non–life-threatening problems (e.g., fractures). The following specific treatment modalities address these goals.

A Generalized Support Regimen

The following support regimen is recommended for the emergency phase of treatment.

BOLUS INTRAVENOUS FLUIDS. A 10% state of dehydration and metabolic acidosis exists in most birds presented for emergency care. Lactated Ringer's solution should be administered at a rate of 2% to 3% of the patient's ideal body weight by bolus injection into any accessible vein, preferably through a 25-gauge needle at a modest rate (Redig, 1984). These fluids should be warmed to 35° to 40°C prior to administration (intravenous fluids can be heated rapidly in a microwave oven or stored in an available microbiology incubator) (Redig, 1984) (see this volume, p. 1154).

VITAMINS. Treat with B-complex vitamins based on sufficient volume to give 10 mg/kg of thiamine.

STEROIDS. Dexamethasone (Azium, Schering) or its aqueous, soluble sodium phosphate salt (dexamethasone sodium phosphate, Vedco) is given at the rate of 2 to 4 mg/kg. The vitamins and steroids can be mixed with the intravenous fluids for convenience.

IRON DEXTRAN. Raptors are slow to recover from the anemia that accompanies blood loss and starvation. Dramatic responses have been seen by administering a single injection of iron dextran at 10 mg/kg IM.

ANTIBIOTICS. Patients with open wounds and those exhibiting severe debilitation are candidates for antibiotic therapy. A wide variety of suitable and safe drugs is available. In patients with normal gastrointestinal function, oral preparations of quinolone derivatives (enrofloxacin, Baytril, Haver-Mobay Corporation) is generally the drug of choice— 10 mg/kg b.i.d. PO) can be administered. In patients with severe dehydration and debilitation, preference is given to injectable compounds, such as piperacillin at a rate of 100 mg/kg b.i.d. by intramuscular injection. Once stabilization has been achieved, reassessment of antibiotics based on microbiologic sensitivity and clinical condition of the patient can be made. Aminoglycoside antibiotics should be completely avoided in raptors.

ORAL FLUIDS. An effective gavage can be performed with a 10% solution of Nutri-Cal (Evsco

Pharmaceutical) in lactated Ringer's solution. Initial doses consist of 2- to 3-ml volumes for birds weighing 100 to 200 gm, while larger birds may be dosed at 10 ml/kg. Oral fluids are given concomitantly and in addition to the intravenous fluids.

WARMTH, LOW-STRESS ENVIRONMENT. A warm, low-stress environment is important. Warmth can be provided internally by heated intravenous and oral fluids and externally with heating pads or infrared lights. Surface warmth from pads and lights results in the exterior of the bird warming before the core, and a resulting complication can be cutaneous vasodilation and subsequent "rewarming shock" (Jenkins, 1988). Thus, it is better to increase the core temperature with warm intravenous and oral fluids before applying external heat. Restoration of renal perfusion, as evidenced by urine output, is a useful indicator of core function. Stress can be minimized by maintaining the patient in a darkened cage.

NUTRITION. Feeding of high quality foods (devoid of indigestable casting materials such as feathers, food and bone) can be instituted immediately on an *ad libitum* basis. Do not allow the bird to accumulate a large crop of food until there is evidence of good response to the initial round of treatments.

TREATMENT REGIMENS FOR SPECIFIC PROBLEMS

Concussion/Spinal Trauma

Administer dexamethasone 2 to 4 mg/kg s.i.d. I.V. or prednisolone sodium succinate (Solu-Delta-Cortef, Upjohn) 10 mg/kg b.i.d. I.V. Place the patient in a warm, darkened environment on soft pads. If the patient is able to move its legs in response to painful stimuli, the prognosis is good. The major complication is a transient inability to void the cloaca. Voiding must be assisted manually several times a day. If recovery is likely, notable improvement will be seen in 3 to 5 days.

Organophosphate/Carbamate Poisoning

Specific treatment for poisoning with these compounds is accomplished by the administration of atropine sulfate 0.5 mg/kg IV or IM (Porter and Snead, 1990). The response is variable; there may be a complete, almost immediate reversal of symptoms in some cases and no discernible effect in others. Repeated treatments with atropine at 3- to 4-hr intervals are sometimes required. Supportive treatments with fluids are also essential.

Lead Poisoning

Intoxication with lead is not immediately life-threatening in those cases that are amenable to treatment. However, suspicion of poisoning based on clinical signs warrants immediate treatment. No harm will have been done if analysis of the blood for lead residues yields negative results. Clinical signs include weight loss, depression, fixed gaze, slight head tremor, green, adherent feces soiling the vent feathers, and occasionally blindness and pectoral limb paresis. Specific treatment is provided by the administration of CaEDTA at 35 mg/kg b.i.d. diluted in a volume of lactated Ringer's solution for intravenous administration (see earlier section on fluids) (Redig, 1987). Treatments are given for 4 days followed by 2 days of no treatment. Three or four repetitions of this regimen will usually bring ambient blood-lead concentrations to clinically insignificant levels. Long-term damage to the nervous system, myocardium, and kidneys is a common occurrence.

Extreme State of Emaciation and Inanition

Patients in extreme states of weight loss should receive the aforementioned treatments with the following modifications:

FLUIDS. Administer intravenous fluids for several days. Caloric content of fluids can be increased by mixing equal volumes of 5% dextrose with the lactated Ringer's solution.

FEEDING. Withhold solid food for the first 12 to 24 hr of fluid therapy, even in extreme states of emaciation. Correction of dehydration is more important than feeding. In most cases, solid food will be vomited or not digested until hydration improves.

MONITORING PROGRESS. After 24 hours or when urine production and gut motility are apparent, solid food consisting of small pieces of liver or a dilute slurry can be fed. The slurry should consist of the Nutri-Cal/electrolyte solution to which two volumes of lean meat have been added and minced in a blender. Gauge the stool output following the administration of this gavage mixture, and increase the amount of meat until the patient is capable of digesting whole pieces of meat.

BLOOD TRANSFUSIONS. If the PCV is below 20%, serious consideration should be given to a blood transfusion. If the PCV is below 15%, transfusion is mandatory. Donor blood is collected in a heparinized syringe and administered in bolus fashion at the rate of 8 to 10 ml/kg. Homologous transfusions are preferred; however heterologous transfusions have been used without apparent complication (Redig, 1986).

EMERGENCY WOUND MANAGEMENT

The second goal of emergency treatment involves wound treatment and fracture stabilization.

Temporary Wound Treatment

The following regimen may be accomplished quickly:

Debridement. Debride loose tags of flesh.

Irrigation. Irrigate the wound thoroughly with a dilute, warm solution of povidone-iodine in saline. Inspect all wounds and the rest of the body for maggot infestations.

Wound Preparation. Prepare the wound site by plucking the feathers in an area 1 to 2 cm around the wound site, and swab the skin with an iodine-based surgical scrub. The skin and adjacent feathers can be dried with a blow dryer.

Wound Protection. The wound should be protected with a moisture- and vapor-permeable dressing material (Tegaderm, 3-M Company, St. Paul, MN) (Degernes and Redig, 1990).

Supportive Bandaging. Supportive bandaging can be used as necessary. Long-bone fractures should be stabilized by appropriate bandaging or splinting procedures until further correction can be tolerated by the patient (Redig, 1986) (see this volume, p. 1163).

AFTER THE EMERGENCY

The material presented constitutes the essential elements for the emergency treatment of raptors. In most instances, these procedures will be supplanted within 24 to 48 hours by more thorough work-ups and other treatment modalities, some of which will be an extension of those already initiated.

References and Suggested Reading

Degernes, L.A., and Redig, P.T.: Soft tissue wound management in avian patients. Proceedings of the Annual Meeting of the Association of Avian Veterinarians, 1990, pp. 182–190.
  This paper reviews basic elements in wound healing and provides a comprehensive description and selection criteria for wound treatment and bandaging materials for successfully treating various injuries in avian species.
Flammer, K.: Aviculture management. *In* Harrison, G.J., and Harrison, L.R. (eds.): *Clinical Avian Medicine and Surgery.* Philadelphia: W.B. Saunders, 1986, p. 610.
  Table 50–2 contains a regimen for emergency treatment of anticoagulant rodenticide intoxication.
Jenkins, J.R.: Emergency avian medicine. Proceedings of the Association of Avian Veterinarians Conference on Avian Medicine, 1988, pp. 279–285.
  This article contains an overview of emergency procedures broadly applicable to avian species.
Porter, S.L., and Snead, S.E.: Pesticide poisoning in birds of prey. J. Assoc. Avian Veterinarians 4:84–85, 1990.
  This article chronicles the author's experiences with diagnosis and treatment of organophosphate and carbamate poisoning in raptors.
Redig, P.T.: Evaluation and nonsurgical management of fractures. *In* Harrison, G.J., and Harrison, L.R. (eds.): *Clinical Avian Medicine and Surgery.* Philadelphia: W.B. Saunders, 1986, pp. 380–394.
  This article contains narrative descriptions and illustrations of various bandaging and splinting techniques applicable to long-bone fractures in raptors.
Redig, P.T.: Fluid therapy and acid base balance in the critically ill avian patient. Proceedings of the International Conference on Avian Medicine, Toronto, Canada, 1984, pp. 59–73.
  This paper describes bolus administration of fluids to raptors.
Redig, P.T., Degernes, L.A., Martell, M., et al.: The diagnosis and treatment of lead poisoning in bald eagles and trumpeter swans. Proceedings of the Association of Avian Veterinarians Conference on Avian Medicine, Hawaii, 1987, pp. 401–402.
  This paper reviews the literature on various chemicals used for chelation of lead and other heavy metals and provides clinical guidelines for treatment of lead poisoning, including several case reports.
Rode, J.A., Barthelow, S., and Ludders, J.W.: Ventilation through an air sac cannula. J. Assoc. Avian Veterinarians 4:98–99, 1990.
  This paper describes the changes in ventilatory parameters and blood gases when anesthetized ducks were required to breath through a cannula in the interclavicular air sac.

ARTIFICIAL INCUBATION OF NONDOMESTIC BIRD EGGS

CYNTHIA M. KUEHLER
and MICHAEL R. LOOMIS
San Diego, California

The successful hatching of eggs in an incubator requires a "potentially hatchable" egg and an adequate incubation environment. Contamination, inbreeding, and inadequate maternal diet can result in eggs that are not hatchable under either natural or artificial incubation. The second requirement, an adequate incubation environment, implies that the dry bulb temperature, humidity level, and turning process are appropriate for optimal embryonic development.

EGG STORAGE

To improve the chances for a successful hatch, eggs should be placed in the incubator ("set") as soon as possible. Egg storage is a husbandry technique that enables breeders to hatch clutches together and simplifies the chick rearing process by brooding birds in like age-groups. However, proper techniques for egg storage are often overlooked, with resulting increases in early embryonic mortality, poor overall hatchability, prolonged incubation periods, and weaker chicks (Chahil and Johnson, 1974).

Loss of hatching viability appears to be species dependent, and little is known about the storage tolerance of nondomestic bird eggs.

If storage is necessary, nondomestic eggs should be maintained at 12.8° to 18.3°C (55° to 65°F) at a relative humidity of 80% to 90% for no more than 7 days. Holding temperatures above 26.7°C (80°F) will allow cell division to continue at an abnormal rate, resulting in decreased hatchability and abnormalities in the brain and eye regions of developing embryos. There is also evidence suggesting that placing eggs in fine-pored plastic bags that allow some air circulation, increases the hatchability of stored eggs. However, the incubation period is increased because embryos from stored eggs require a longer developmental period

SANITATION AND EGG CONTAMINATION

Parent birds and the hatchery itself are potential sources of infection in newly-hatched chicks and incubating eggs. Because the hen uses a common passage for both eggs and fecal matter and the incubator environment is warm and moist, embryonic diseases are caused both by the intestinal contents of parent birds and contamination from incubators and hatchers. Microbial contamination resulting in infection is of two types: exterior eggshell-borne diseases and interior egg-borne diseases.

Hatchery sanitation should include maintenance of disease-free birds and a well-ventilated, easily cleaned incubation and hatching area. A flow pattern that minimizes traffic from areas that are possible sources of contamination (such as adult breeding stock) is optimum.

The most common contaminant is *Pseudomonas*, but *E. coli*, infectious bronchitis, Newcastle disease, and staphylococcal and *Salmonella* infections have all been implicated in embryonic and early chick mortality. In general, avian eggs are more susceptible to gram-negative bacterial infection. There is a direct relationship between bacterial contamination of eggs, the incidence of embryonic malformations and mortality, and the degree of yolk

sac infections in chicks (Board and Fuller, 1974).

Prior to being layed, eggs can be infected transovarially and in the oviduct prior to egg cuticle formation. Transovarial infections with *Salmonella* are well documented. *Salmonella* can infect the ovary via the hematogenous route from gastrointestinal infections or sepsis. Infections in the oviduct can result from an ascending oviduct infection.

Measures to control bacterial infections in fertilized eggs include differential pressure and temperature dips and injections into the air cell, albumen, or yolk (Calle et al., 1989).

Contaminants are more easily eradicated from the surface of the shell than from within the egg itself. One routine sanitizing technique is egg fumigation with formaldehyde gas. This procedure is most effective if clean eggs are fumigated as soon as possible after laying, before bacterial penetration can occur. The accepted mixture is approximately 1.5 ml of formalin (40%) and 1 g of potassium permanganate ($KMnO_4$) per 0.1 cubic meter (Burr, 1987). Disinfection is most effective at a temperature of at least 32.2°C (90°F), with a wet bulb reading of 31.1° to 32.2°C (88°–90°F), for at least 20 minutes. The enclosed environment of an old, forced-air incubator with a circulating fan system is a desirable fumigant cabinet.

Poultry eggs are not fumigated after development has started because formaldehyde is teratogenic and increases the incidence of embryonic malformations. It is advisable to not routinely fumigate nondomestic bird eggs until more research has been conducted on the effects of fumigation in exotic birds. Many species of birds lay eggs with shells that are considerably thinner and more porous than poultry eggs, and the teratological effects of fumigation may be more extreme.

A second method of disinfection is egg washing. Extreme care should be taken with this method because improper egg washing can spread disease and contaminate previously clean eggs. Disinfecting solutions containing quaternary ammonia or chlorine compounds are usually used. The wash water should be warmer than the eggs, 43.3° to 48.9°C (110° to 120°F), to prevent the wash compound from being sucked into the pores of the shell and contaminating the egg.

A stock solution of egg disinfecting compound consists of 10% quaternary ammonium disinfectant (alkyldimethyl benzyl ammonium chloride), 0.4% ethylenediaminetetra-acetic acid (EDTA; disodium salt) (15 gm per 4 L), and 4.2% sodium carbonate (160 gm per 4 L). For egg washing, use 90 ml of the stock solution in 12 L of water (Hofstad et al., 1984).

ARTIFICIAL INCUBATION PARAMETERS

Artificial incubation provides a very different physical environment for the developing embryo and is generally not as efficient as an incubating parent. Most bird eggs benefit from some natural incubation prior to being removed from the nest and placed in an incubator. Parentally incubated eggs are subjected to oscillating temperatures during development, which facilitates calcium metabolism from the shell to the embryo. In contrast, the constant temperature of an incubator decreases calcium metabolism and subsequent eggshell conductance. This may explain why artificial incubation of fresh eggs is less successful than with eggs that receive some natural incubation prior to being set in an incubator.

It is very difficult to artificially mimic the variable incubation temperature gradient of a parent bird. Still-air incubators create a temperature gradient by providing a heat source at the top of the incubator. This is a very successful hatching system. However, only a limited number of eggs can be set in the incubator before carbon dioxide build-up occurs and suffocates the developing embryos. Most hatcheries use the circulating fan system of forced-air incubation developed by the poultry industry. This type of system increases ventilation, circulates heat, and maintains a more consistent temperature throughout the incubator than would be found at the top of an egg under an incubating bird. Consequently, more eggs can be incubated in one incubator. Generally, eggs in a still-air incubator are set at a temperature two to three degrees higher (similar to the top of the egg under an incubating bird) than in a forced-air system, which provides a lower, more consistent temperature throughout the egg and incubator. This promotes similar developmental rates in both types of incubating systems. There are several types of forced-air and still-air incubators available for purchase by zoos and aviculturists.*

Dry Bulb Temperature

The dry bulb incubation temperature is the most critical incubation parameter. Eggs incubated at temperatures too high or too low show increased embryonic malformations and mortality. The correct dry bulb parameters for artificial incubation of most bird eggs have not been established beyond the requirements for chickens, turkeys, domesticated pheasants, chukar, quail, and domesticated waterfowl (Ernst and Coates, 1981, Woodard et al., 1987). Aviculturists must rely on limited published infor-

mation about specific bird groups and shared experiences (Kuehler and Good, 1990).

In establishing dry bulb temperature parameters for nondomestic birds, the incubation requirements of the chicken serve as a baseline guide. The optimum temperature for the 21-day incubation period of the domestic chicken has been established at 37.5°C (99.5°F) in a forced-air incubator or 38.6° to 39.2°C (101.5°–102.5°F) under still-air conditions. Generally, eggs larger than those of a chicken have a longer incubation period and may require a lower incubation temperature. Eggs smaller than those of a chicken usually have a shorter incubation period, develop at a faster rate, and require an incubation temperature of 37.5°C (99.5°F) or higher. However, the best method to determine a correct dry bulb temperature is to compare the artificial incubation period with the natural incubation period of the species in question. In the absence of other problems such as inbreeding, chicks that hatch earlier than the known natural incubation period were probably incubated at a temperature that was too high. Chicks delayed in hatching were probably incubated in conditions that were too cool.

Wet Bulb Temperature

Although important, the wet bulb temperature or relative humidity environment, is not as critical as the dry bulb temperature. Recently, much research has been devoted to the factors affecting the gas/water exchange between the avian embryo and its environment. The rate of water loss is dependent upon the shell thickness and porosity and the water vapor concentration in the atmosphere around the egg. Weighing the egg throughout incubation will provide an indication of water loss. Excessive humidity may increase the mortality of embryos. Humidity that is too low may result in dwarfing or decreased calcium metabolism. Humidity parameters are dependent in part upon knowledge of the nest microclimate under natural conditions. Birds that lay eggs in wet, soggy conditions generally require a high incubation humidity. Desert species usually have eggs with thick shells or specialized pores, which resist desiccation and usually require drier artificial incubation conditions. Evaluation of the condition of hatchlings also provides critical information on proper humidity. Chicks that are edematous or "sticky" at hatching may have been incubated under conditions which were either too wet or too dry.

Egg Turning

The third parameter of artificial incubation is egg turning. Turning during avian development is es-

---

*Manufacturers include Humidaire Incubator Co., 217 West Wayne Street, New Madison, OH 45346; and Petersine Incubator Co., 300 North Bridge Street, Gettysburg, OH 45328.

sential to minimize adhesions and disruption of embryonic membranes, and to decrease the possibility of chick malpositions within the egg (Robertson, 1961). Rotation should alternate between clockwise and counterclockwise directions; continued turning in one direction can cause twisting of the chalazae or rupturing of the yolk sac or blood vessels in a developing embryo.

DATA COLLECTION

Optimum artificial incubation parameters for most nondomestic species of birds are unknown. To determine correct artificial incubation conditions and evaluate causes of embryonic mortality and weak chicks, consistent and accurate record-keeping is necessary. Incubation record-keeping in a captive situation falls into three categories: (1) preincubation factors, (2) incubation data, and (3) evaluation of the embryo/chick at death or hatch. Following is a list of the important information required (Osborn and Kuehler, 1989):

Preincubation factors
Parental pedigree
Parental nutrition
Parental incubation behavior
Preincubation handling of eggs
Egg size and shape
Degree of eggshell thinning
Air-cell membrane integrity

Incubation data
Incubator/hatcher type
Turning mechanism
Incubation/hatching temperature
Incubation/hatching humidity
Egg weight/water loss
Air-cell size
Candling
Pip-to-hatch interval

Evaluation of the Embryo/Chick at Death or Hatch
Bacterial culture of yolk and albumen
Bacterial analysis of incubators/hatchers
Determination of embryonic stage at time of death
Embryonic position
Embryo/chick measurements (toe, naris, yolk sac, body weight)
Characteristic embryonic abnormalities (e.g., clubbed down)
Degree of yolk sac retraction
Amount of residual albumen
"Stickiness" or edema in chick
Hatch weight
Growth rate (hatch to death)
Neurological status (e.g., stargazer)
Begging response
Degree of yolk sac depletion
Pip muscle fluid depletion
Toe problems
"Noisiness" of chick
Pasted vent
Additional necropsy and culture results

References and Suggested Reading

Board, R. G., and Fuller, R.: Non-specific antimicrobial defenses of the avian egg, embryo and neonate. Biological Review 49:15, 1974.
Burr, E. W.: *Companion Bird Medicine*. Ames, IA: Iowa State University Press, 1987 p. 98, 220.
Calle, P., Janssen, D., Kuehler, C. et al.: Gentamicin injection of incubating avian eggs. Proceedings of the 1989 Annual Meeting of the American Association of Zoo Veterinarians, 1989, p. 83.
Chahil, P. C., and Johnson, W. A.: Effect of preincubation storage, parental age, and rate of lay on hatchability in *Coturnix coturnix japonica*. Poultry Science. 53:529, 1974.
Ernst, R. A., and Coates, W. S.: Raising Geese. Leaflet 2225. Division of Agricultural Sciences, University of California, Cooperative Extension Service, 1981.
Hofstad, M. S., Barnes, H. J., Calnek, B. W., et al.: *Diseases of Poultry*. Ames, IA: Iowa State University Press, 1984, p. 15.
Kuehler, C., Good, J.: Artificial incubation of bird eggs at the Zoological Society of San Diego. *International Zoo Yearbook* 1990, 29:118–136.
Lancaster, J. E., Gordon, R. F., and Harry, E. G.: Studies on disinfection of eggs and incubators. III. The use of formaldehyde at room temperature for the fumigation of eggs prior to incubation. Br. Vet. J. 110:238, 1954.
Osborn, K. G., Kuehler, C. M.: Artificial incubation: basic techniques and potential problems. Proceedings of the 1989 Annual Meeting of the American Association of Zoo Veterinarians. 1989, p. 76.
Woodard, A. E., Ernst, R. A., Vohra, P., et al.: Raising Gamebirds. Leaflet 21046. Division of Agricultural Sciences, University of California, Cooperative Extension Service, 1987.

PSITTACINE NEONATOLOGY

SUSAN L. CLUBB

Loxahatchee, Florida

Psittacine pediatrics requires good husbandry, an understanding of neonatal development, and a knowledge of the problems that can occur with chicks in both the nest and the nursery. In captive collections, fostering, incubation, and hand-feeding are used to increase production. Altricial psittacine chicks need environmental temperature control and hand-feeding for 6 to 16 weeks. Cleanliness and proper diet and handling techniques are vital to success. The most common infectious problems are bacterial and fungal. Viral diseases are uncommon, but polyomavirus (papovavirus) infection can be a problem in hand-feeding nurseries. With early detection many developmental problems can be corrected.

HUSBANDRY OF NEONATAL PSITTACINES

Hatching psittacines are altricial and cannot regulate their body temperature. Hatchlings should be kept in a brooder at 32.2° to 34.4°C (90° to 94°F). Weak hatchlings may initially be kept at slightly higher temperatures. Chicks with early pin feathers should be in a brooder or room kept at 30.0° to 32.3°C (86° to 90°F). Humidity should be at least 50%. If environmental temperatures are too high, the chick may exhibit panting, unrest, hyperactivity, or poor growth rate, and its skin may appear reddened and dry. Temperatures over 37.8°C (100°F) may be fatal. Cold environmental temperature may also result in death, poor gut motility, crop stasis or other digestive disorders, failure to feed or beg, inactivity or shivering, and increased incidence of respiratory disease.

Aviculturalists have developed a myriad of hand-feeding formulas over the years, and several products are now available commercially (Table 1). The author continues to use a formula based on a commercial monkey diet cooked with added peanut butter and oatmeal baby cereal. Regardless of the formula, it must be fed at the proper consistency and temperature and should be prepared fresh to avoid contamination that may lead to infection.

Birds are fed four to six times daily from hatching until the eyes are open, then two to three times daily until weaning. With some formulas, hatchlings can be fed four times daily and maintain adequate growth. In order to maximize growth while cutting the number of daily feedings the crop is well filled.

Cleanliness is especially important with hatchlings, as their immune system is immature and they lack resistance to some common bacteria. However, cleanliness to the point of sterility is not necessary. Hatchlings can be conveniently housed in plastic freezer containers and larger birds kept in dishpans. Hatchlings are kept on paper towels crumpled to form a nestlike concavity that keeps the chick from rolling around.

Older chicks can be kept on towels, diapers, or shredded paper. Chicks stay cleaner on particulate bedding such as corncob bedding or wood shavings, but they may ingest such bedding. Plastic-coated, welded wire flooring or a plastic bedding material developed for use in poultry hatcheries are good for older chicks. Measures should be taken to control insects, especially roaches, which may spread disease from bird to bird. Feather or bedding dust (particularly from corncob bedding) can be minimized by the use of fans and air filters. Dirty pans are an ideal site for fungal growth and should be emptied and disinfected often.

The health and nutrition of the hen at the time of laying can influence the health of the newly hatched chick. Inbreeding may produce lethal or life-threatening mutations. Incubation problems can cause small, weak chicks that fail to thrive even under ideal conditions (see this volume, p. 1138). Chicks incubated at low temperatures may fail to retract the yolk sac, fail to absorb albumin (leaving a sticky chick), or have bent necks. High incubation temperatures may speed development and accelerate hatching, leaving a chick with scruffy down and neurological problems. Skeletal abnormalities may result if the humidity is too low and membranes dry out, resulting in decreased mobilization of calcium from the shell. If the humidity is too high,

Table 1. Commercially Available Hand-feeding Diets for Psittacines

Roudybush's Hand-feeding Diet—Roudybush, P.O. Box 331, Davis, CA 95616
Kellogg's Handfeeding Diet—Kellogg Inc., Milwaukee, WI 53204
Nutristart—Lafeber Co., RR 2, Odell, IL 60460
Topper Bird Ranch Diets—20833 Roscoe Ave., Canoga Park, CA 91306
Kaytee Products—P.O. Box 230, Chilton, WI 53014
Bird-Life—SC Ranch, P.O. Box 745, Poway, CA 92064

1142

the chick will have an edematous appearance and may not retract the yolk properly.

Daily or frequent weighing of chicks is useful for monitoring growth and early recognition of illness. Birds should double hatching weight by 5 to 7 days of age.

An understanding of the normal physical appearance of a chick is vital to clinical assessment and early recognition of disease. The skin should be opaque, soft, smooth, pliable, and pink-yellow in color. Dry, reddish, or wrinkled skin or the presence of prominent skin vessels may indicate overheating or dehydration. White skin and very pale extremities indicate a bird that is cold, in shock, anemic, or very ill. Birds that have inadequate fat reserves or are stunted have very thin, transparent skin. The pectoral muscles of the neonate are typically thin and poorly developed and are usually inadequate for intramuscular injection.

The normal intestinal flora of psittacines consists primarily of gram-positive bacteria, including *Lactobacillus, Staphylococcus epidermidis, Streptococcus, Corynebacterium, and Bacillus*. Gram-negative bacteria such as *Escherichia coli, Klebsiella*, and *Pseudomonas* are potential pathogens and are often associated with disease. The finding of gram-negative bacteria on cloacal, pharyngeal, or crop culture does not necessarily indicate infection requiring treatment because many normal psittacine chicks have low levels of gram-negative bacteria, especially *E. coli* and *Enterobacter*. Nonetheless, gram-negative bacterial infections, often with accompanying candidiasis, are common and often fatal in neonatal psittacines. The possibility of underlying viral, protozoal, chlamydial, or fungal diseases must not be discounted.

Crop washes and subsequent transfer of bacteria from the adult to the chick are sometimes advocated as a means of providing normal flora to the new hatchling, but these also present a potential for the spread of disease. Supplementation of lactobacillus or similar products has been reported with mixed results, as species-specific flora may be needed for gut colonization.

Many hematologic and serum biochemical parameters vary greatly with age. Red blood count, hemoglobin, packed cell volume, mean corpuscular hemoglobin concentration (MCHC), total solids by refractometer, sodium creatinine, uric acid, aspartate aminotransferase (AST), total protein, albumin, globulin, urea, and cholesterol are typically lower in young chicks (1 to 2 months) than in adult birds. White blood count, mean corpuscular volume (MCV), percentage of heterophils, phosphorus, and alkaline phosphatase are typically elevated in the neonate. Mean corpuscular hemoglobin (MCH), gamma glutamyltransferase (GGT), lactate dehydrogenase (LDH), potassium glucose, and calcium ranges are typically similar to that of adult birds.

As weaning is a very stressful time for a young bird, asymptomatic problems may surface then. Weaning should not be attempted too early, however, extended periods of hand-feeding are also detrimental. A chick may outweigh its parents at weaning time, and a weight loss of up to 10% is considered normal. Weight loss of 15% to 20% may be encountered and can be dangerous. Hand-feeding should be resumed in these birds. Weaned birds that become ill may revert to begging to be hand-fed.

DISORDERS OF HAND-FED PSITTACINE CHICKS

Stunting, poor growth rate, or failure to thrive are common among hand-fed birds, usually in the first 30 days of life. Most of these signs can be corrected with time and adequate feeding, and most birds will reach full adult size if stunting is reversed early enough. Stunted birds appear thin and disproportionate, with the head appearing too large for the body. Toes and elbows are the best indicator of adequate weight in very young birds. Eye opening may be delayed in a stunted or sick nestling. The skin will appear thin and wrinkled without adequate subcutaneous fat. Abnormal feathering patterns may be seen on the head, feather emergence may be delayed, or feathers may have stress lines.

The most common cause of stunting is inadequate caloric intake (too little food or water content too high). Fear of overfilling the crop often results in underfeeding. Enteric bacterial infections or candidiasis can result in or be secondary to stunting. Any bird failing to thrive should be cultured for *Candida* and gram-negative bacterial infections.

Delayed crop emptying may be caused by foods that are too cold, as well as foods that are too thick, contain inadequate water, are too high in fat (too much peanut butter), or possibly too high in protein. Air gulping or swallowing of air may occur with or without feeding and may become habitual. Air gulping results in inadequate food intake, as the crop fills with air and looks full. Feeding at a steady, rapid rate so the bird doesn't have time to fill the crop with air, burping, or tube feeding will help minimize this problem.

Most diseases of young psittacines result in slowed gut transit time, which is reflected by a crop that empties slowly. In complete gut stasis, the crop will fail to empty. Food which remains in the crop will sour due to bacterial fermentation. The young bird becomes dehydrated, toxic, and depleted of energy. When this occurs, the bird must be treated as if it has a systemic disorder, not merely a local problem in the crop.

Primary crop disorders also occur, and these include impaction, mycotic ingluvitis, crop atony, or partial blockage by foreign bodies. Foreign bodies such as seeds, bedding material, fruit pits, etc., may be removed via the esophagus with forceps (in large birds) or by ingluvotomy. Providing physical support by using a sling for the crop (a crop bra) may help restore proper crop tone.

The crop may be burned by the administration of food that is too hot. A scab will appear several days later on the skin covering the crop, and leakage can be expected in an additional 2 to 4 days. If the burns are mild, they may heal without treatment or surgery. Topical application of DMSO or vitamin E ointment to keep the burned tissue moist may speed recovery. Fistulas may form with some burns, requiring surgical repair. In very severe burns, the crop will slough.

Esophageal or crop punctures can occur when feeding with flexible or rigid tubes. Rupture of the mucosa of the pharynx may occur in birds that are being syringe fed. The prognosis is poor due to toxicosis associated with subcutaneous deposition of food. Immediate surgery is indicated to flush food from tissues. Postoperative therapy should include flushing the wound, which may be left open, and the administration of systemic antibiotics and anti-inflammatory medications (Table 2).

Shrinkage of the crop at weaning is a natural process. As the bird matures, regurgitation of small amounts of food immediately after feeding signals the need to reduce hand-feeding volume and offer solid food. Visceral gout usually results in vomiting prior to death. Gout can result from excessive aminoglycoside therapy, excessive protein or vitamin D_3, or polyoma virus infection.

Lateral beak deviations are often related to syringe feeding on only one side of the mouth. Some birds, however, deviate toward the feeding side. Mild deviations at the tip only are easily corrected by application of digital pressure at each feeding as necessary. Deviations from the cere are more difficult to manage and may require the application of an epoxy appliance to force the beak into proper position (as in orthodontics). Cockatoos often develop a deviation of the upper beak into the lower (mandibular prognathism). Excessive cornified beak at the tip of the maxilla should be trimmed with manicure clippers. The tip of the maxilla can be pulled over the front of the mandible and held in this position for a few seconds at each feeding. As in lateral deviations, this procedure is only effective if performed before the beak is fully calcified. Birds with beak deviations may also benefit from calcium supplementation.

Leg deformities (spraddle leg) may be associated with inadequate litter or slippery surfaces, as well as dietary imbalances. In young birds with soft bones, physical therapy by packing the bird in toweling and taping the legs together around toweling or around a pad may be successful. Rotation

Table 2. *Selected Drug Dosages for Neonatal Psittacines*

Amikacin—15 mg/kg t.i.d. or 20 mg/kg b.i.d.

Cefotaxime—100 mg/kg IM b.i.d.

Ceftriaxone—50 mg/kg b.i.d.

Chloramphenicol—75 mg/kg t.i.d. Most often used in palmitate form for treatment of the individual bird (0.1 ml/30 gm t.i.d.). For flock treatment, chloramphenicol powder (from capsules) may be added to prepared formula at the rate of 1500 to 2000 mg/gallon.

Chlorhexidine—Can be added to formula at the rate of 5 cc/gallon of prepared formula. Used in flock treatment of mild candidiasis or when enteric viral infections are suspected.

Chlortetracycline—For flock treatment of chlamydiosis, add 2000 mg/gallon of prepared formula.

Dexamethasone—5 mg/kg IM

Doxycycline Oral Suspension—50 mg/kg o.i.d. orally for Amazons
35 mg/kg o.i.d. for macaws and cockatoos

Enrofloxacin—20 mg/kg b.i.d. (metaphyseal disorders have not been observed to date in juvenile birds)

Flucytosine—250 mg/kg P.O. b.i.d.

Gentian Violet Powder—For flock prophylaxis for candidiasis, use ½ teaspoon per 5 gallons of formula. Can be used with chlortetracycline or doxycycline.

Ketoconazole—20 mg/kg b.i.d. orally. Tablets may be placed in suspension by grinding one tablet (200 mg) and mixing with 1 ml methycellulose and 9 ml water. Refrigerate and discard unused portion after 2 weeks.

Metaclopromide—0.2–0.4 mg/kg every 6–8 hr, IV, IM, or SC.

Nystatin Oral Suspension—In very small birds, give one or two drops following each feeding. In older birds, give 1 cc/300 gm once or twice daily or add 30 ml/gallon formula.

Piperacillin—200 mg/kg b.i.d. or t.i.d.

Trimethoprim/Sulfa—0.1 ml/30 gm t.i.d. in the very small bird or b.i.d. in older birds or added to the formula at the rate of 25 ml/gallon. May cause vomiting.

of long-bone metaphysis or uneven diaphyseal closure may require surgical correction.

In stunted birds, ear infections occur when the opening of the ear canal is delayed and it fills with purulent exudate. Usually, this can be removed with gentle pressure and manipulation of the overlying skin to align the ear canal with the normal skin opening, followed by installation of appropriate topical antibiotics.

Aspiration of large volumes of food can result in sudden death. If smaller volumes of food are aspirated, pneumonia develops over several days. Antibiotic therapy should be instituted, but prognosis is always grave. Aspiration pneumonia rarely occurs if proper feeding techniques are used.

Corneal scratches from nestmates and foreign bodies under the lid are the most commonly observed eye problems in nestlings. Mycoplasmas are commonly implicated in conjunctivitis in cockatiel chicks, but this has not been well documented.

Polyomavirus (papovavirus) is the most common viral disease encountered in the hand-feeding nursery. Normal adult birds may shed the virus and infect their chicks. Egg transmission has also been reported. This disease is highly contagious—with an incubation period of approximately 2 weeks, it can be widespread before it is detected. Pox is rare in domestically raised birds but is a common problem in some imported species. Psittacine beak-and-feather disease can be transmitted horizontally in a nursery and can result in acute disease or chronic debilitating disease. Euthanasia of affected individuals is indicated, followed by a diligent search for the source.

Oral plaques in nestlings most often indicate oral candidiasis but may also be associated with hypovitaminosis A, bacterial pharyngitis, pox, accumulation of food, or bite wounds from siblings housed in the same container.

When signs of illness are first observed, samples should be collected for bacteriology; however, rapid initiation of therapy is often indicated. If gut stasis occurs, parenteral antibiotics must be used. Antifungal therapy should always accompany the use of antibiotics, as fungal overgrowth, especially candidiasis, is common to chicks.

In total gut stasis or a very slow crop, the crop contents should be removed by tube to prevent souring. Turning the chick upside down and milking out crop contents is rapid but may result in aspiration. Oral rehydration therapy should be initiated and may be used in conjunction with parenteral administration of fluids. Cereal preparations diluted with electrolytes or pediatric ORT solutions may be used successfully. In addition, fluids may be given intramuscularly, subcutaneously, or interosseously (see this volume, p. 1154). In very small chicks, the femur is an ideal site for interosseous fluid therapy. Extreme caution should be exercised to prevent overhydration. It is generally assumed that the bird requires 40 to 60 ml/kg/day for maintenance. Additional amounts should be added to compensate for dehydration or loss of fluids.

The addition of enzymatic preparations for predigestion of formula has shown promise in reducing the incidence of gut stasis and improving digestion in those chicks doing poorly. The use of intestinal motility stimulants may be a useful adjunct to systemic therapy in chicks with reduced intestinal motility or gut stasis. Management should include support of the crop with a crop bra, emptying the crop of food that fails to clear, control of enteric bacterial and fungal infections, administration of oral or parenteral fluid, and correction of any management problems that may have contributed to illness.

References and Suggested Reading

Clipsham, R. Scissors beak correction. J. Assoc. Avian Veterinarians 3: 188–189, 1989.

Clubb, S. L.: Psittacine pediatrics. Proceedings of Annual Meeting of the Association of Avian Veterinarians, 1983, pp. 317–332.

Flammer, K.: Pediatric medicine. In Harrison, G. J., and Harrison, L. R. (eds.): Clinical Avian Medicine and Surgery. Philadelphia: W. B. Saunders, 1986, pp. 634–650.

Proceedings of Avian Pediatric Seminar, Avian Research Fund, Hayward, CA, 1988.

Roudybush, T. E.: Growth, signs of deficiency, and weaning in cockatiels fed deficient diets, Proceedings of the Annual Meeting of the Association of Avian Veterinarians, 1986, pp. 333–340.

LIVER DISEASE IN PSITTACINES

WILLARD J. GOULD

Ithaca, New York

Conditions affecting the liver are commonly encountered in avian practice. The clinical signs and available diagnostic modalities differ slightly from those for dogs and cats. The diseases, clinical signs, and diagnostic tests that are useful in psittacines are discussed in this article.

ANATOMY

The avian liver is bilobed. The left and right lobes join at the midline. The left lobe is slightly smaller than the right lobe. A gallbladder is an inconsistent finding among species and, when present, is found on the visceral surface of the right lobe. The cranioventral surfaces of both lobes are concave and are in contact with the apex of the heart. Dorsal to the liver on the left side are found the esophagus, proventriculus, spleen, and gizzard. On the right side are the duodenum and the jejunum. The ventral parietal surface of the liver is convex and contacts the sternum. Each lobe of the liver is drained by separate bile ducts that empty into the distal ascending loop of the duodenum.

CLINICAL FINDINGS

Clinical signs of liver disease in birds vary with the severity and duration of the disease process. Mild signs include periodic bouts of anorexia and lethargy accompanied by ruffled feathers. Vomiting occurs occasionally, whereas diarrhea is common. The droppings often have watery urates that may be clear, yellow, or green. Neurologic signs of hepatic encephalopathy are frequently noted in severe or advanced disease. These signs include tremors, ataxia, paresis, circling, and seizures. Dyspnea may be observed if the liver is very large or if the abdominal air sacs are compressed by ascites. Budgerigars with chronic diseases of the liver often grow abnormally long beaks that may have one or more dark lines extending distally from the germinal epithelium near the cere. Birds tend to hide signs of illness; therefore, unexpected death is a common presentation.

DIAGNOSIS

Diagnostic methods in psittacines do not vary greatly from those used in other species. Chronicity of a condition can be indicated by breast muscle palpation. Well-rounded muscles indicate an acute condition, whereas moderate to severe muscle atrophy indicates a more chronic course. Abdominal palpation may reveal hepatomegaly or ascites. Wetting the translucent skin on the abdomen of thin birds may allow visualization of parts of the liver that extend beyond the keel.

The droppings should be carefully examined. Biliverdinuria results in yellow to green urates and is usually an indication of liver disease. Gram stains of the feces should be examined to screen for abnormal amounts of gram-negative bacteria that might be responsible for an ascending or hematogenous infection of the liver. Less than 5% gram-negative organisms with rare yeasts per oil immersion field is considered normal.

Radiography is an extremely useful tool in the diagnosis of liver disease in avian species. Adequate positioning of the bird is essential for accurate interpretation of films (see CVT X, p. 786). Ventrodorsal and lateral views of the body are recommended in all cases. The liver should not extend beyond the sternum on the lateral view. Hepatomegaly is characterized by dorsal deflection of the proventriculus and caudodorsal displacement of the ventriculus. The heart and liver silhouettes merge in an hourglass shape on the ventrodorsal view. A loss of this hourglass appearance and widening of the liver beyond a line between the scapula and the acetabulum indicate hepatomegaly. The gizzard may be pushed caudal to a line that joins the acetabula. Ascites can mimic severe hepatomegaly;

however, a loss of visualization of the other abdominal organs usually indicates fluid. A small liver can be seen with emaciation or cirrhosis. The normal appearance is altered by a narrow base to the hourglass. Lead poisoning is a common differential diagnosis for liver disease, so the crop, gizzard, and intestine should be examined for heavy metal densities in contrast to the slightly less dense appearance of grit or stones.

Blood tests are often necessary to make a diagnosis of liver disease in psittacines. A general rule is that an amount of blood equivalent to 1% of the body weight can be collected. This approximates 1 ml/100 gm of body weight. Small volumes of blood can be safely drawn using a nail clipper. This method is painful and may require cutting several nails to obtain an adequate sample volume. Peripheral vessels that can be used are the median metatarsal vein in birds heavier than 100 gm, the cutaneous ulnar vein near the elbow, and finally the jugular vein. The first vein has the disadvantage of poor blood flow in smaller birds; however, excessive blood loss through hematoma formation is unlikely. When the cutaneous ulnar and jugular veins are used, life-threatening hematomas may develop in birds with coagulopathies secondary to liver disease. Common sense dictates that an unsuccessful venipuncture attempt resulting in a large hematoma should not be followed on the same day by another venipuncture attempt.

A complete blood cell count (CBC) may show a depressed or elevated white blood cell (WBC) count with an infectious process that is affecting the liver. A low hematocrit may suggest previous hemorrhage or chronic disease. Thrombocytes may be decreased because of a coagulopathy such as disseminated intravascular coagulation. A biochemical panel may show an elevation of liver enzymes during an active inflammatory process. The most commonly measured enzymes are aspartate aminotransferase (AST, formerly SGOT) and lactate dehydrogenase (LDH). Significant elevations of these enzyme concentrations occur with liver and muscle damage. Creatinine kinase (CK) levels are elevated with muscle injury and can be used to differentiate between the two. It has been noted that the most liver-specific enzyme in pigeons is glutamate dehydrogenase (GDH); however, this enzyme test is not readily available. Cholesterol levels may be either elevated or depressed in birds with liver disease. Measurement of bile acids is a promising liver function test in psittacines. Preliminary studies indicate that normal Amazon parrots have postprandial values of less than 36 μmol/L and that birds with liver pathology have significant two- to fivefold increases. The most abundant bile acids in chickens are chenodeoxycholic, cholic, and allocholic acids.

Measurement of prothrombin times for avians requires the use of chicken brain thromboplastin and is not a widely available test. However, modified bleeding times can be evaluated. The cutaneous ulnaris vein is penetrated with a 30-gauge needle. Pressure is applied over the vein, and bleeding should cease within a minute. Continued bleeding from this site may suggest a coagulopathy. If a biopsy or surgery is necessary, vitamin K_1 (AquaMEPHYTON, Merck Sharp & Dohme; 0.2 to 2.5 mg/kg) can be given by deep IM injection, and the test can be repeated in 12 hr. Alternatively, a whole blood or fresh plasma transfusion can be given. A subjective thrombocyte count should be estimated from a blood smear. One to two thrombocytes per oil immersion field is a rough estimate of normal.

If a bacterial infection is suspected, blood cultures can be performed on 2 ml of blood after a standard surgical preparation of the venipuncture site. One milliliter can be cultured for aerobes while the second is cultured for anaerobes. Other tests that are routinely performed are blood lead determinations and *Chlamydia* titers, cultures, or enzyme-linked immunoassay (ELISA).

A biopsy is necessary for a definitive diagnosis of a liver disease. However, there is significant risk with this procedure, because sedation or anesthesia is required. The bird is placed in dorsal recumbency, and the area caudal to the sternum is prepared for sterile surgery. A 5-mm incision is made on the midline 0.5 to 1.0 cm caudal to the keel bone. An arthroscope, needle scope, or sterile otoscope head is inserted into the incision, and the liver is visually inspected. The liver may be attached to the keel, in which case it can be pulled down toward the proventriculus. If the liver lesion appears diffuse, a piece of the edge is sampled. If only a focal lesion is seen, that area is sampled. The tissue is placed in buffered formalin, and if possible, a second specimen is collected for a bacterial culture. The biopsy site is observed for bleeding, and the incision is closed.

LIVER DISEASES

Categories of liver disease in psittacines are similar to those of other species. Infectious causes include bacterial, viral, and parasitic organisms. Metabolic diseases of known and unknown etiologies occur, as do neoplastic and toxic diseases.

Bacteria

Bacteremia, with subsequent colonization of the liver, is one of the most common causes of hepatitis in psittacines as determined in a postmortem survey of 2723 birds performed at the New York State College of Veterinary Medicine. Forty-two per cent

of the liver lesions encountered in African gray parrots were attributed to bacterial infections. Twenty-seven per cent of the liver lesions in Amazon parrots were caused by bacteria.

The organisms that have been implicated in bacterial hepatitis include *Escherichia coli*, *Klebsiella*, *Salmonella typhimurium*, *Yersinia pseudotuberculosis*, *Acinetobacter*, *Serratia marcesens*, *Staphylococci*, *Pseudomonas*, *Corynebacterium*, *Citrobacter*, *Pasteurella haemolytica*, *Pasteurella multocida*, *Mycobacterium avium*, *Mycobacterium bovis*, and *Mycobacterium tuberculosis*.

Diagnosis of most of these pathogens can be based on positive fecal, blood, or most specifically liver biopsy cultures. *Mycobacterium* is often associated with markedly elevated WBC counts and may require acid-fast stains of a liver biopsy specimen to establish a specific diagnosis. When liver lesions are encountered in conjunction with intestinal lesions, acid-fast stains of the feces may be helpful. Unfortunately, the organisms are not released in large numbers, so it may be necessary to examine numerous slides.

Species predispositions for certain organisms have not been definitively established, although certain trends have been identified. *Brotogeris* parakeets may be more susceptible to mycobacteriosis, and African gray parrots have been afflicted with salmonellosis.

Viruses

Viral causes of hepatitis in psittacines have been well described. Pacheco's parrot disease is a herpesvirus infection of the liver. It has been incriminated as the etiologic agent in large-scale outbreaks with high mortality. Unexpected death is the most typical presentation for small psittacines. Larger psittacines may present acutely depressed with diarrhea and may have yellow, orange, or green watery urates. Many of these birds have been in contact with other birds, most specifically but not limited to Patagonian or Nanday conures. Radiographs may show hepatosplenomegally. An enlarged spleen is most readily visualized on the lateral view dorsal to the junction of the proventriculus and the ventriculus. An antemortem diagnosis of an acute infection can be confirmed by virus isolation from the cloaca or subsequently by convalescent titers. Therapy for suspected cases of Pacheco's disease includes maintenance of ambient temperature between 85 and 90°F, subcutaneous, intravenous, or intraosseus fluid therapy to maintain hydration (50 ml/kg/day, maintenance) (see this volume, p. 1154), either the oral or intravenous form of acyclovir (Zovirax, Burroughs Wellcome; 80 mg/kg PO every 8 hr for 7 days, 50 to 200 mg/4 oz drinking water), and antibiotics, if appropriate, to treat secondary invaders.

Lactulose (Cephulac, Merrell Dow; 0.2 to 0.4 ml/kg PO every 8 hr) has been used to treat the signs of hepatoencephalopathy in severely ill birds.

Prevention of herpesvirus in flocks of psittacines can be accomplished in two different ways. Birds that are to be introduced into a flock situation can be tested using a complement fixation test currently available through the Texas Veterinary Medical Diagnostic Laboratory (TVMDL) to determine if they have been previously exposed. Carriers, especially conures, can be identified before contacting other birds. Another means of protecting a flock is vaccination of all birds. Vaccines are available* and should be used well in advance of possible exposure. Current information indicates that the complement fixation test may not be sensitive enough to identify some carriers with low antibody titers. Vaccination followed by a repeat titer assay in 7 to 14 days may result in an exaggerated amnestic response indicating previous exposure.

Papovavirus is the etiologic agent causing budgerigar fledgling disease and generalized parrot papovavirus infections of other psittacines. Clinical signs are seen in young budgerigars between 7 and 21 days of age and other psittacines between 20 and 56 days. Disease in adults has been recognized in lovebirds. Abdominal distention caused by hepatomegaly, as well as subcutaneous petechial and ecchymotic hemorrhages in young birds with poorly emptying crops, is observed in affected birds. Excessive hemorrhage may occur from venipuncture sites or from injection sites. Survivors may develop abnormal feather growth. Typical intranuclear inclusion bodies are diagnostic of this condition. The disease tends to erupt in breeding situations where there are many young birds. Interruption of the breeding cycle for several months has stopped the problem in some budgerigar breeding flocks. Immunofluorescent antibody (IFA) tests have been used to detect carriers; however, this test is not widely available. Therapy is symptomatic and involves maintenance of body temperature, hydration and nutrition if possible, and treatment of secondary bacterial and fungal infections.

Reoviruses are commonly recovered from psittacines. Clinical signs of infection include anorexia, depression, diarrhea, weight loss, and death. Uveitis and edema of the neck may be noted in some cases. Reoviruses are often seen in combined infections with other viruses, bacteria, chlamydia, and fungi. A CBC may show leukopenia with a low heterophil count and an anemia. A diagnosis can be based upon IFA testing, agar gel immunodiffusion, virus isolation, or electron microscopy of hepatic or splenic lesions showing viral particles in the cytoplasm. Treatment involves supporting the patient and treating any associated infections.

An adenovirus has been identified as a cause of viral hepatitis in lovebirds, cockatoos, budgerigars, and a cockatiel. The incidence of infection with this virus is unknown. Adenovirus can be differentiated from herpesvirus infection by electron microscopy and virus isolation, because the viruses produce similar-looking intranuclear inclusion bodies. Clinical signs in budgerigars are anorexia and abdominal distention secondary to hepatomegaly. Antemortem diagnosis is undescribed.

A coronavirus has caused hepatitis in budgerigars under experimental conditions and has been implicated in a case of malodorous diarrhea in a Cape Parrot. Clinical signs in the budgerigars include greenish diarrhea, ruffled feathers, anorexia, and depression. None of the affected birds have died. The virus was infectious for chickens.

Chlamydia

Chlamydia psittaci is the etiologic agent causing psittacosis. It is a common cause of hepatitis in psittacines and is a zoonotic disease that is reportable in many states. Amazon parrots and African gray parrots seem to be most sensitive; however, all psittacines are susceptible. Clinical signs include an oculonasal discharge, diarrhea, and watery yellow to green urates. Birds often show general systemic signs of anorexia, weight loss, and ruffled feathers; however, they may also be asymptomatic carriers and shedders. A CBC may show an elevated WBC count with immature heterophils, a monocytosis, and basophilia. Serum chemistry tests may show elevated levels of liver enzymes. Hepatomegaly as well as splenomegaly may be seen on radiographs. Thickened air sacs may be observed occasionally. A definitive diagnosis of psittacosis is based on a positive culture from a conjunctival, cloacal, choanal, or fecal swab. Feces can be collected in *Chlamydia* transport media for 3 consecutive days to increase the chance of a positive culture from an intermittent shedder. Complement fixation and latex agglutination tests are readily available to test for antibody titers to *Chlamydia* (see this volume, p. 1150). Unfortunately, some species, in particular African gray parrots and cockatiels, may not develop diagnostic titers. A preferable diagnostic regimen combines serology with a *Chlamydia* culture of the cloaca. ELISA is applicable but is still somewhat controversial because a significant number of false-positive reactions have been reported. A blocking ELISA that is being introduced holds promise as a practical, sensitive, and specific test for *Chlamydia* detection.

The only currently approved treatment for psittacosis involves therapy with chlortetracycline-impregnated seeds, pellets, or mash for 30 to 45 days. Two major problems are associated with this treat-

---

*Maine Biological Laboratories, Inc., Waterville, ME 04901; Biomune, Inc., Lenexa, KS 66215.

ment. The first is poor acceptance of the medicated food by the bird, resulting in decreased food intake and inadequate blood levels of the antibiotic. The second problem involves gastrointestinal overgrowth of resistant bacteria and yeasts.

Doxycycline (Vibramycin, Pfizer; 22 mg/kg every 12 hr) is generally considered to be superior to chlortetracycline as a treatment for psittacosis because of better absorption from the gastrointestinal tract, less interruption of the normal gastrointestinal flora, and less frequent dosage regimen. Therapy can be given by gavage or via medicated pellets (Avicake, Lafeber) for the recommended 45 days.

Enrofloxacin (Baytril, Mobay; 5 mg/kg PO every 12 hr or 100 mg/L of drinking water) is a new quinolone antibiotic that shows promise against *Chlamydia* in birds.

Treatment failures may occur because of poor owner compliance or inadequate therapeutic antibiotic levels. Birds that undergo treatment for psittacosis should be retested at 3 and 6 months after completion of therapy.

Parasites

Liver flukes have been incriminated as a cause of disease in cockatoos. Clinical signs include anorexia, diarrhea, depression, vomiting, and unexpected death. Three of four reported cases with blood tests showed abnormal biochemical values. One sulfur-crested cockatoo had markedly elevated AST and LDH values. One bird was anemic, with a hematocrit of 31%, and another had a leukocytosis with a lymphocytosis. A diagnosis is based on identification of trematode eggs on a direct fecal smear. Therapy with praziquantel (Droncit, Bayvet; 10 mg/kg SC, PO, daily for 3 to 14 days) may decrease the fluke burden.

A microsporidian infection has been seen in lovebirds and nestling budgerigars. Lesions and organisms have been found at postmortem examination in the liver, intestine, and kidney. Other infectious diseases have often been concurrently observed, so it is unknown whether microsporidia act as a primary pathogen or a secondary invader.

Neoplasia

Neoplasia involving the liver can occur in any species but is most common in budgerigars. It may occasionally be primary but more often is metastatic. Primary tumors include bile duct carcinomas, hepatocellular carcinomas, hepatomas, fibrosarcomas, hemangiosarcomas, and hemangioendotheliomas. Multicentric or metastatic tumors include lymphosarcoma, erythremic myelosis, rhabdomyosarcomas, renal carcinomas, and pancreatic carcinomas. Clinical signs associated with neoplasia include abdominal enlargement, ascites, anorexia, and weight loss. Abdominal palpation and visualization of the liver through moistened abdominal skin may reveal a mass. Radiographs may reveal hepatomegaly, abdominal fluid, or a mass in another organ such as the kidney. If ascites is present, it may be possible to make a diagnosis by abdominocentesis and fluid analysis. Laparotomy or laparoscopy with a biopsy may be the only way to reach a definitive diagnosis. Unfortunately, by the time most birds are presented for hepatic neoplasia, therapeutic surgical intervention is often unsuccessful. Lymphosarcoma may be temporarily responsive to combination chemotherapy or radiation therapy if the mass is localized; however, more investigation is needed.

Toxins

Toxic hepatopathies are probably more common than we recognize because they are difficult to prove. Mycotoxins may be the source of many of the acute, chronic, and metabolic hepatopathies for which no cause is determined. Aflatoxins are reliable hepatotoxins that are used experimentally to induce liver disease. Many pet birds are still being fed diets consisting of a high proportion of seeds that may be stored in less than ideal conditions allowing for the growth of *Aspergillus flavus* or *Aspergillus parasiticus*. Acute episodes of aflatoxicosis in cockatiels result in clinical signs of depression, weight loss, green urates, and vomiting. Hepatic necrosis and degeneration may lead to cirrhosis with nodular hyperplasia on recovery. Some chronic toxicities may be very difficult to diagnose without a biopsy or postmortem examination. Typical histologic findings include bile duct hyperplasia, portal fibrosis, and generalized hepatic lipidosis. Aflatoxins can also be carcinogenic. Clinical signs are nonspecific, including anorexia, depression, and weight loss. A diagnosis may require a combination of a clinical history of illness following introduction of a specific food source, histologic findings compatible with a diagnosis of aflatoxicosis, isolation of the potential toxin-forming fungus from the feed, and identification of the suspected toxin in the feed, gastrointestinal contents, or tissues of the bird.

Metabolic

Hepatic lipidosis is the most common metabolic disease of the liver in psittacines. It was the most common lesion found in budgerigars and cockatiels in our study. In contrast to the findings of others, we found that females were more commonly affected than males. Clinical signs include anorexia, depression, dyspnea, seizures, ataxia, and muscle tremors. Radiographs may demonstrate hepatomegaly, and observation of a pale liver may be possible through the moistened skin of the abdomen. Hepatic lipidosis is probably multifactorial in its etiology. Many birds that develop hepatic lipidosis are on poor diets. High levels of estrogen and low thyroid hormone levels are causes of fatty liver in chickens. Diabetes mellitus has been described in psittacines. Environmental problems such as decreased exercise is also a factor, as is a hereditary predisposition.

Hemochromatosis is only occasionally encountered in psittacines but is quite common in mynah birds, birds of paradise, and toucans. Excessive iron accumulation in hepatocytes is characteristic of the disease. Varying amounts of inflammation and portal fibrosis are seen. The most common clinical signs are weight loss, dyspnea, and abdominal swelling caused by hepatomegaly and ascites. A diagnosis can be based on clinical signs and increased AST and LDH levels in species that are predisposed to the disease. A definitive diagnosis is dependent on biopsy findings, as in other species. Treatment is symptomatic, by removal of the abdominal fluid. Periodic abdominocentesis may be necessary to relieve severe dyspnea caused by the ascites, and a diuretic such as furosemide (Lasix elixir, Hoechst-

Roussel; 0.5 mg/kg PO every 12 hr) can be used to slow recurrence of the ascites. Periodic phlebotomies are used in humans to remove excess body iron.

References and Suggested Reading

Campbell, T. W.: Mycotic diseases. *In* Harrison, G. H., and Harrison, L. R. (eds.): *Clinical Avian Medicine and Surgery.* Philadelphia: W. B. Saunders, 1986, p. 464.
   A summary of the mycotic diseases of caged birds and their treatments.
Flammer, K.: Treatment of chlamydiosis in exotic birds in the United States. J.A.V.M.A. 195:1537, 1989.
   Review of the different antibiotics used to treat chlamydiosis and the problems and advantages of each.
Gaskin, J. M.: Considerations in the diagnosis and control of psittacine viral infections. Proceedings of the Annual Meeting of the Association of Avian Veterinarians, 1987.
   Clinical information coupled with research findings about caged bird viruses from a virologist's perspective.
Grimes, J. E.: Serodiagnosis of avian chlamydia infections. J.A.V.M.A. 195:1561, 1989.
   Review of the advantages and disadvantages of serologic tests for Chlamydia.
Lumeij, J. T., and Westerhof, I.: Blood chemistry for the diagnosis of hepatobiliary disease in birds, a review. Vet. Q. 9:255, 1987.
   A review of the various liver enzymes and their use as tests in birds.
McMillan, M. C.: Radiographic diagnosis of avian abdominal disorders. Comp. Cont. Ed. Pract. Vet. 8:616, 1986.
   Illustrated review article covering interpretation of avian plain and contrast radiographs.
Quesenberry, K. E., Tappe, J. P., Greiner, E. C., et al.: Hepatic trematodiasis in five cockatoos. J.A.V.M.A. 189:1103, 1986.
   Clinical report of trematodiasis and an attempted treatment protocol.

AN UPDATE ON THE DIAGNOSIS AND TREATMENT OF AVIAN CHLAMYDIOSIS

KEVEN FLAMMER

Raleigh, North Carolina

Chlamydiosis (psittacosis) presents a challenge for the avian practitioner because it is common, difficult to diagnose and treat, and transmissible to humans. It is caused by *Chlamydia psittaci* and occurs in many avian species (Cooper, 1980). It is particularly common in pigeons and pet birds, and incidence rates of 8% to 24% are seen in psittacine birds. Among domestic birds, turkeys are most often infected.

Human psittacosis is rare and characterized by a flulike condition and pnuemonia, with potential cardiac and neurologic complications. Bird owners experiencing signs of illness should advise their

physician of the potential for this disease. Veterinarians must consider the potential medical and legal aspects of chlamydiosis, and specific regulations may exist to control the diagnosis, treatment, and quarantine of infected birds. Local restrictions vary, so local public health departments should be contacted to determine the applicable regulations.

CLINICAL SIGNS AND DIAGNOSIS

Chlamydiosis is most common in recently purchased and recently imported psittacine birds, but

Table 1. *Laboratory Tests for Chlamydiosis*

Serology
    Direct complement fixation
    Latex agglutination
Stained tissues or direct smears
    Gimenez or Macchiavellos stain
    Fluorescent antibody stain
    Peroxidase antibody stain
Antigen detection
    Antigen-capture ELISA
Isolation in cell culture or embryonated eggs

it also frequently occurs in domestic collections. Clinical signs vary dramatically from totally asymptomatic carriers to severe infections with a high flock mortality. In the author's experience, asymptomatic carriers are the most common presentation, followed by more chronic manifestations that include nonspecific signs of illness such as listlessness, weight loss, respiratory distress, bile-stained (green) feces, and biliverdinuria. Infected birds may or may not demonstrate leukocytosis, elevated aspartate aminotransferase (AST), lactate dehydrogenase (LDH), or uric acid (UA) or show the classic signs of hepatomegaly, splenomegaly, and airsacculitis. There are no pathognomonic signs of avian chlamydiosis, and the disease is easily confused with common bacterial and viral infections. Chlamydiosis should be included in the differential diagnosis of any ill psittacine bird, and routine testing of all psittacine birds is recommended.

There are several laboratory tests that can render a presumptive diagnosis of chlamydiosis (Table 1) but none that can absolutely determine that a particular bird is free of the disease. It is desirable to confirm chlamydia infection rather than to simply treat all birds when infection is suspected because treatment is difficult and expensive. Additionally, it may be necessary to document the diagnosis for medical and legal reasons. However, confirmation of chlamydiosis may be difficult, particularly in asymptomatic birds. Various methods (see Table 1) have been suggested, and each has advantages and limitations.

Serologic tests are valuable in species known to mount an antibody response (Schacter, 1989). Positive titers measured with the currently available latex agglutination tests appear to correlate with an active infection. Direct complement fixation tests measure antibodies that persist longer, and birds may remain positive following successful treatment. Interpretation of titers that are very high or very low is relatively straightforward; however, test results can be nebulous, and determination of the chlamydia status of a particular bird from a single serologic test may be uncertain. Serologic tests may not be accurate in young birds with an immature immune system and certain psittacine species (e.g.,

cockatiels) that may not mount a measurable antibody response to chlamydiosis, even when demonstrating clinical signs. Uncertain results should be confirmed by another test, such as isolation of the organism.

Intracytoplasmic chlamydial inclusions can be identified in smears or tissue impressions stained with dyes (Gimenez and Macchiavellos stain) or, preferably, with fluorescent monoclonal antibody (FA) stains. Direct smears can be made from feces, cloacal swabs, and ocular and nasal exudates, but infections may be missed unless the bird is showing marked clinical signs and shedding large numbers of chlamydia. In contrast, examination of FA-stained impression smears from the liver, spleen, and air sacs of dead birds is more reliable and can be used to support a postmortem diagnosis of chlamydiosis.

Isolation of chlamydia in cell culture or embryonated eggs is the basis of comparison for all other diagnostic tests; however, even this test is not completely reliable. False-positive results are rare, but false-negative results may be relatively common. False-negative results can occur because birds shed chlamydia intermittently, because low numbers of viable chlamydia are present in the sample, or because viable chlamydia are lost during transport. Reliability of this test can be improved if multiple fecal samples are collected over a period of several days and pooled into a chlamydia transport media that supports the viability of chlamydia but suppresses growth of other bacteria and fungi. The laboratory providing the service should be contacted for instructions, and samples should be shipped on ice by overnight mail. To screen large avian collections, fecal samples from several birds can be pooled into a single isolation sample. Then, if positive results are found, birds in that sample group can be tested individually to determine which are truly positive. In situations where a confirmed diagnosis is required (e.g., where human exposure has occurred or where treatment may be particularly difficult), isolation is the preferred test because positive results cannot be disputed.

Recently, a number of new antigen-capture ELISA tests have been developed for diagnosing *C. trachomatis* infection in people. Since *C. psittaci* and *C. trachomatis* share some common antigens, some of these tests may be useful in birds. At the time of this publication, however, none of the available ELISA tests have been validated for use in birds. A common problem is cross-reactivity with certain gram-negative bacteria that may give a false-positive result. ELISA tests can be used to screen individuals and groups of birds, but it may be advisable to retest positive birds by another method. In the near future, it is likely that an accurate, validated ELISA test for avian chlamydiosis will be developed.

In summary, there are various methods to establish a positive diagnosis of chlamydiosis, but no test that will certify a bird to be chlamydia-free. A combination of tests (e.g., isolation and serology) provides the most accurate diagnosis. In situations where chlamydiosis is strongly suspected but laboratory tests are negative, it may be advisable to treat the birds and monitor the response to therapy.

TREATMENT

General Considerations

Chlamydia are obligate, intracellular parasites with a biphasic life cycle. Tetracyclines are the antibiotics most effective against chlamydiosis, but they are active only when the intracellular reticulate bodies are actively replicating. Because chlamydia can persist in cells without activity, prolonged treatment periods of 45 days are necessary to rid the host of infection. Other antibiotics (e.g., chloramphenicol, tylosin, and erythromycin) have some antichlamydial activity and may reduce clinical signs, but they are usually unsuccessful in totally eliminating chlamydia from the bird. Newly developed quinolone antibiotics (e.g., enrofloxacin) have antichlamydial activity, but it is uncertain whether they will eliminate infection.

It is important to recognize that treatment itself may have adverse effects. The most common problems are weight loss and secondary microbial infections that occur because of the stress of a diet change or repeated capture for drug administration and because long-term treatment alters normal alimentary tract flora. To reduce the incidence of side effects, both the bird owner and supervising veterinarian must be prepared to monitor health status, reduce stress, and maximize husbandry to reduce exposure to environmental sources of bacteria and yeast that may cause secondary microbial infections.

Pretreatment Considerations

An organized approach to treatment reduces complications. Local public health regulations should be determined and followed. Stress should be minimized by keeping birds sheltered from unclimatic conditions, removed from exhibit or areas with heavy traffic, and breeding stopped. The bird owner should be prepared to administer the treatment, monitor the birds, and provide excellent husbandry. All birds should be weighed and examined before treatment begins to establish baseline information. Culture of cloacal swabs will identify potential microbial pathogens that should be eliminated or treated concurrently.

There are three methods to treat chlamydiosis, depending on local public health regulations and drug availability: chlortetracycline-medicated feed, orally administered doxycycline, and intramuscularly administered doxycycline. Each of these methods has advantages and disadvantages. A medicated diet reduces labor but requires a stressful change in diet that may be poorly accepted by the birds. Most public health departments will recommend feeding chlortetracycline-medicated feed because it is historically the most documented method—an important consideration if medicolegal problems are anticipated. Oral administration of doxycycline quickly establishes therapeutic concentrations and precludes the need for a change in diet; however, this method requires daily capture and tube feeding. In some countries, an intramuscular formulation of doxycycline (Vibravenos, Pfizer, Germany) can be administered every 5 to 7 days. This regimen is effective and reduces the labor and stress associated with daily capture. Unfortunately, this intramuscular formulation of doxycycline is not currently available in the United States. Oral or intramuscular administration of doxycycline should be used in ill birds when it is desirable to quickly establish therapeutic concentrations. After the birds are stable, a medicated diet can then be tried or treatment continued with doxycycline.

Medicated Diets

Chlortetracycline (CTC) is the antibiotic most commonly recommended for treating chlamydiosis. The goal of therapy is to maintain CTC blood concentrations above 1 μg/ml for the duration of the treatment period. Chlortetracyline is usually delivered via medicated food because direct oral or parenteral administration is impractical due to the drug's short elimination half-life (3 to 4 hours) and because medicated water fails to maintain adequate CTC blood concentrations. To achieve the recommended serum concentrations, medicated diets must be the sole source of food. Dietary calcium interferes with the absorption of tetracycline and should be reduced to 0.7% of the diet.

Chlamydiosis in small birds (budgerigars, canaries, and finches) can be treated for 30 days with a medicated millet seed diet (Keet Life, Hartz Mountain) containing 0.05% CTC. Other birds require greater dietary CTC concentrations, and food containing 1% CTC is recommended for larger psittacines. Medicated, pelleted feeds are commercially available, or the bird owner can prepare a cooked mash or nectar diet and add CTC powder after cooking.

Treatment of small birds with the medicated seed diet is relatively uncomplicated, as the treatment ration is familiar and readily accepted. In larger psittacine birds, poor acceptance of the treatment diet is frequently encountered because cooked mashes and pellets are perceived as foreign food by birds that are usually fed seed and fruit diets. Even birds that are used to pelleted diets may refuse medicated pellets because of the bitter taste of the CTC. If the birds are asymptomatic and treatment can be delayed, food acceptance can be increased by gradually switching the birds to a nonmedicated form of the treatment diet and starting medication when the diet is accepted. If permitted by local regulatory agencies, birds refusing to eat medicated diets should be treated by oral or intramuscular administration of doxycycline until diet consumption improves.

Orally Administered Doxycycline

Doxycycline is a semisynthetic tetracycline derivative with numerous pharmacologic advantages compared with chlortetracycline. It is more completely absorbed from the gastrointestinal tract, has fewer adverse effects on normal alimentary tract flora, achieves greater tissue concentrations, and has a longer elimination half-life than other tetracyclines. The prolonged elimination half-life of doxycycline makes administration only once or twice daily possible. Doxycycline can be administered directly into the mouth or delivered into the crop via a tube. Most reports of oral doxycycline use in birds in the United States are anecdotal; however, widespread, successful use of this drug indicates that chlamydiosis can be successfully treated. Pharmacologic investigation in seven psittacine species has shown that plasma concentrations exceeding 1 µg/ml can be maintained with once-daily drug administration at 25 to 50 mg/kg orally (Flammer, 1987). Use of this drug must be considered experimental, and birds treated with doxycycline should be retested to determine if treatment was adequate.

Intramuscularly Administered Doxycycline

A doxycycline formulation appropriate for intramuscular administration is available for treating avian chlamydiosis in Europe, Canada, and some other countries. Blood concentrations exceeding 1 µg/ml are maintained for 5 to 6 days when large doses (75 to 100 mg/kg) are injected into the pectoral muscles, and dosage regimens requiring only 8 to 10 injections in a 45-day period have proved efficacious in a variety of psittacine species (Gylsdorff, 1987). This regimen is practical for treating both individuals and groups of birds. Unfortunately, a formulation of doxycycline appropriate for intramuscular administration is not available in the United States. The available intravenous formulation (doxycycline hyclate, Pfizer) should not be used, as it will cause extensive muscle necrosis.

Considerations During Treatment

Stress reduction and maximal husbandry are essential for successful treatment. Birds should be monitored during treatment for diet refusal, weight loss, and concurrent infections. Birds should be examined and weighed twice weekly and the droppings examined daily for signs of bile staining and biliverdinuria. Birds do not develop long-term immunity to chlamydiosis, and the aviary or cage should be thoroughly cleaned and disinfected on treatment days 30 and 45 to remove chlamydia from the environment. All items that cannot be disinfected (e.g., nest material) should be carefully bagged and discarded.

Considerations Following Treatment

Following treatment, the birds should be rested and returned to their routine diet. Calcium should be supplemented to permit birds to replenish depleted stores. Two weeks following therapy, it may be wise to culture cloacal swabs and examine Gram-stained fecal smears to detect potential microbial infections. No treatment method is totally reliable, so it is recommended that birds be cultured 1 to 6 months following treatment to determine if chlamydia persists. Once an aviary or premise has been treated for chlamydiosis, new birds should be tested or prophylactically treated to prevent reintroduction of chlamydia into the aviary.

References and Suggested Reading

1. Cooper, R.: Psittacosis: An ever-present problem in caged birds. In Kirk, R. W. (ed.): Current Veterinary Therapy VII. Philadelphia: W. B. Saunders, 1980, p. 677.
2. Flammer, K.: Avian chlamydiosis: Observations on diagnostic techniques and use of oral doxycycline for treatment. Proceedings of the First International Conference on Zoological and Avian Medicine, Turtle Bay, Hawaii, September, 1987, p. 149.
3. Gerlach, H.: Chlamydia. In Harrison, G. J., and Harrison, L. R. (eds.): Avian Medicine and Surgery: A Clinical Approach. Philadelphia: W. B. Saunders, 1986, p. 601.
4. Gylsdorff, I. The treatment of chlamydiosis in psittacine birds. Isr. J. Vet. Med. 43:11, 1987.
5. Schacter, J.: Symposium on avian chlamydiosis. J.A.V.M.A. 195:1501, 1989.

AVIAN FLUID THERAPY

NOHA ABOU-MADI,
and GEORGE V. KOLLIAS
Gainesville, Florida

GENERAL CONSIDERATIONS

Fluid administration is central to many therapeutic regimens. Reestablishing normal blood volume and correcting electrolyte imbalances should be initiated as soon as possible to prevent irreversible cellular damage. Most reported protocols used in avian fluid therapy are based on mammalian data. Clinical experience has guided therapeutic approaches, as few experimental studies are available.

Water is the major constituent of the avian body. Body water content varies with age and species. In the chicken, total body water is highest in the first 2 weeks of life at 72.4% of body weight. This decreases slowly to 64.8% of the body weight at 16 weeks. From 26 to 42 weeks of age, an additional decrease to 57.3% of the body weight occurs. No further significant changes are noted after sexual maturity is reached at 37 weeks. As in mammals, when the total body water diminishes, the greatest loss comes from extracellular fluid space (Sturkie, 1986). Therefore, clinically diagnosed dehydration is often more severe in chicks and juveniles than in adults. In most bird species, blood volume is estimated to be 10% of total body weight.

Water requirements are met through metabolic processes (metabolic water) and ingestion of food and water. Water and electrolytes are continuously exchanged through cellular activity, renal clearance, skin, and the respiratory system. Compared with adult birds, chicks are more sensitive to adverse or rapidly changing environmental conditions. Dry air, oxygen, and elevated ambient temperatures in hospitals and incubators are important sources of water loss. Errors in the preparation of the hand-feeding diets may lead to excessively concentrated formulas. Inability of the kidney to control absorption and excretion of solutions containing concentrated electrolytes in young birds can result in severe dehydration, electrolyte imbalance, and renal failure. Chicks are especially sensitive to high levels of sodium and calcium, which must be carefully titrated in the diet. In some species (cormorant, brown pelican, domestic duck, roadrunner, many raptors, and several others), renal elimination of sodium and chloride is augmented by a specialized nasal gland that excretes large amounts of these elements (Sturkie, 1986).

In a compromised patient, water and electrolyte losses can become severe and life-threatening. In most cases, a loss of bicarbonate ions complicates a preexisting condition by creating a metabolic acidosis. As with mammals, corrections of fluid, acid-base, and electrolyte disorders are essential in the initiation of any appropriate therapy.

Birds have many unique physiologic characteristics that are important relative to fluid therapy. The avian kidney possesses structural and functional units common to both reptiles and mammals. As in mammals, birds' kidneys have Henle's loops and medullary cones. Their ability to concentrate urine is limited, however, by the short, primitive, reptilian-like nephron and the negligible role of urea in establishing a significant osmotic gradient. Ureteral urine-specific gravity varies from 1.0018 to 1.015 in normal birds but can increase or decrease with changes in hydration and osmolarity (Sturkie, 1986). Renal responses to hydration also vary among avian species. Birds living in semiarid saltwater environments concentrate urine better than those exposed to abundant fresh water (Skadhauge, 1976). Filtration rate appears to vary with the number of filtering nephrons, which appears to be controlled by arginine vasotocin (analogous to mammalian antidiuretic hormone) (McNabb, 1983). Because of their high metabolic rate and relatively large body surface area, smaller birds depend on constant access to food and water. Severe dehydration may develop from adverse environmental conditions as well as a variety of disease processes.

BASIC CONSIDERATIONS FOR FLUID THERAPY

When evaluating a patient for fluid therapy, the following factors must be considered: 1) hydration status, 2) electrolyte balance, 3) acid-base status, 4) hematologic and biochemical values, and 5) caloric balance. The patient's assessment must include a complete blood count and avian plasma or serum chemistry panel. If only limited quantities of blood can be collected, tests for hematocrit, total plasma proteins, glucose, uric acid, and electrolytes are most important.

Based on the results of water deprivation studies in pigeons, serum osmolality and total solids were found to be the most useful parameters to assess dehydration. Osmolality varied little among individuals and acutely indicated changes in hydration. Because of important individual variation, predehydration total-solids values were needed to interpret subsequent samples. In one study, the packed cell volume (PCV) did not reflect acute changes in hydration status (Martin and Kollias, 1989). In another study, the response of pigeons to dehydration indicated that plasma urea, in spite of its generally low serum concentration in birds, was an accurate indicator of dehydration. Dehydration resulted in a 6.5- to 15.3-fold increase in urea nitrogen (Lumeij, 1987).

The ulnar vein and artery can be used to assess hydration status. The turgescence of these vessels, luminal volume, and filling time are excellent indicators of hydration status. Easily compressible vessels with a small diameter and slow filling time (greater than 1 to 2 seconds) indicate dehydration greater then 7%.

A baseline body weight should be obtained for all birds. Rapid variations from this value during hospitalization may be indicative of water loss. This should be differentiated from a loss of condition due to starvation.

Dry mucous membranes and sunken eyes may also indicate a loss of fluid. The avian skin is a less subtle indicator of dehydration than that of animals, as it may be normally be dry, sometimes even flaky, and slightly wrinkled. Evaluation of skin turgor and tenting is useful only if dehydration is severe. Finally, the attitude of the bird provides an important indicator of hydration state. Signs of central nervous system depression, reluctance to move, and weakness can be indicative of severe dehydration.

GOALS OF FLUID THERAPY

Fluid therapy is aimed at correcting preexisting water deficit and electrolyte disorders and meeting daily requirements. The choice of fluid, route, and speed of administration depends on the cause and the severity of the condition. The therapy plan should take into consideration the status of the cardiovascular and renal systems, the neurologic state of the animal, and its susceptibility to handling stress. Excessive handling of a hypotensive bird can result in death. Resting avian daily fluid requirements are estimated to be 40 to 60 ml/kg/day. Fluid and electrolyte requirements can also be established by an alternative method using metabolic scaling instead of body weight (Sedgwick, 1988). In most clinical situations, the volume of fluids necessary to correct dehydration is calculated with the following formula:

body weight (grams) × percent of dehydration
(decimal value) = estimated deficit (ml).

One quarter to one half of the deficit should be corrected within the first 4 to 6 hours and the remaining volume during the next 20 to 28 hours (Redig, 1984). Depending on the severity of the deficit and the attitude of the bird, this can be achieved by slow intravenous or intraosseous infusion or as repeated subcutaneous administrations. In excitable animals, the total volume should be divided in two treatments, with all other treatments performed simultaneously. Higher fluid rates are recommended for anesthetized birds. A volume of 10 ml/kg/hr can be infused in healthy patients for the first 2 hours, then at 5 to 8 ml/kg/hr to avoid fluid overload.

Compared to mammals, birds tolerate relatively large blood volume losses. Diving and flying birds are more resistant to blood loss than terrestrial birds and respond to blood loss by evoking reflex peripheral vasoconstriction (Sturkie, 1986). When hemorrhage does occur, the replacement rate with crystalloid solution should be three times the blood volume loss. If the loss is greater than 25% to 30% of the initial blood volume, a transfusion is indicated.

Warming of fluids to be administered (38 to 39°C or 100.4 to 102.2°F) can help prevent and correct hypothermia. A microwave oven will rapidly warm solutions without altering their composition (dextrose will not caramelize when microwaved).

Many factors must be considered when choosing the route of administration. In birds, the oral (PO), subcutaneous (SC), intraosseous (IO), and intravenous (IV) routes are the most useful. Intravenous fluid administration is the best route to use in hypovolemic or hypotensive shock and with critically ill birds. This method presents special problems of physical immobilization of the patient as well as the maintenance of an administration device. The size and fragility of avian vessels limit the choice of catheters to over-the-needle types and butterfly needles. Inside-the-needle catheters create a large initial hole in the vessel that results in severe hemorrhage or hematoma formation. Catheters can be placed in the jugular, ulnar, or saphenous veins depending on the species. In long-legged species (cranes, herons, egrets), the saphenous vein can be used. The jugular vein is recommended in macaws and long-necked birds. The ulnar vein can be used in species weighing at least 300 to 400 gm. Catheters are best used in patients where movement can be restricted. To prevent dislodging of the catheter, it can be sutured and taped to the feathers or limbs, though this is complicated by the lack of subcutaneous tissue and the fragility of the skin. Additional stability can be achieved by applying a cyanoacrylate tissue glue or similar product (Super Glue, Super Glue Corp., Hollis, NY) to the tape and skin. In order to prevent tangling of the bird in the administration set, the solution can be administered periodically by removing the administration set and capping the catheter between treatments after it has been flushed with heparinized saline solution (heparin sodium injection). Small birds (<500 gm) can be easily overdosed with heparin; careful dosage of the anticoagulant is essential. In mammals, a loading dose of 10 to 20 IU/kg will interfere with coagulation for about 2 hours. In birds, the dose of heparin can be scaled to the individual's metabolic size. If sterile technique has been used to place the catheter, it can safely be left in place for 2 to 3 days.

As an alternative, intravenous fluid can safely be administered in birds by repeated bolus through a butterfly needle. Birds tolerate slow (5 to 7 min) intravenous boluses of 10 to 25 ml/kg well; thus, large volumes can be administered throughout the day without concern for maintaining patency of an indwelling catheter. Aseptic and atraumatic techniques of venipuncture permit serial use of veins, though the ulnar vein is fragile and has a tendency to hematoma formation if hemostasis is inadequate. When giving intravenous boluses, careful monitoring of the patient will help in detecting signs of fluid overload. Normally, an intravenous bolus of fluid will produce transient bradycardia; however, the heart should resume normal rhythm by the end of the infusion. Increased respiratory rate, cardiac dysrhythmias, agitation, or collapse are indicative of fluid intolerance. If these problems are noted, the fluids should be discontinued at once and resuscitation measures should be initiated. These side effects are rare and usually occur in exhausted or moribund animals.

When peripheral veins are too small or collapsed, an alternative parenteral technique of fluid administration successfully applied to birds has been intraosseous catheterization (Ritchie et al., 1990). These catheters provide excellent access to the peripheral circulation, with absorption equivalent to that of intravenous catheters. This technique is easy to perform and effectively reduces stress on the patient. Antibiotics, sodium bicarbonate, calcium gluconate, amino acids, vitamins, vasoactive drugs (e.g., epinephrine, dopamine, and dobutamine), insulin, morphine, digitalis, diphenhydramine hydrochloride, atropine, diazepam, other drugs, and blood and blood products have been shown to be absorbed by this route (Otto et al., 1989). Strict aseptic techniques are important when placing the catheter, and intraosseous catheters should not be placed in pneumatic bones. The distal ulna is the site of choice for needle placement. The desired diameter of the intraosseous needle depends on the diameter of the ulna. Its length should be approximately one third that of the bone. Spinal needles (22 or 20 gauge) are recommended to avoid

obstruction of the bevel by osseous tissue, but hypodermic needles (27 or 25 gauge) have been used successfully in smaller species. The catheter is sutured or taped to the limb, the wing is immobilized against the body with a figure-of-8 bandage, and a continuous infusion can be initiated (Ritchie et al., 1990). Complications are relatively rare. Extravasation of fluids can occur if more than one hole is present in the cortex (Otto et al., 1989).

Fluids can also be given intraperitoneally. Isotonic solutions will be readily absorbed through the peritoneum. This route should be used with great caution in birds because the keel covers a large portion of the coelomic cavity and restricts the space available for injection, especially in small species. Because of this, the danger of lacerating internal organs is magnified. The volume and location of air sacs must also be taken into consideration to prevent inadvertent infusion. Contraindications include peritonitis, abdominal mass, coelomic effusion, and hypotension.

When a bird is not critically compromised, maintenance fluids can be given subcutaneously. In the author's experience, this route of administration is safe and reliable. It can accommodate a significant volume of warmed fluid that will be slowly absorbed without cardiac overload. Only isotonic fluids (270 to 310 mOsm/L) can be administered by this route; dextrose (5%) is contraindicated. Three sites are recommended: the skin fold between the medial aspect of the upper leg and the lateral body wall, the patagium or wing web, and the subcutaneous space between the scapulae. When injecting subcutaneously in the inner thigh region, caution must be taken not to penetrate the abdominal wall. Though administering fluids between the scapulae is recommended for smaller species (e.g., psittacines, some aquatic birds), caution must be taken not to inject cranially, as the cervical cephalic air sacs surround the thoracic inlet. When using the patagium, a very small needle (25 or 27 gauge) should be used, allowing insertion of the bevel between the two very thin layers of skin. A large needle (19 or 20 gauge) will create a persistent hole from which fluid will leak. When injecting subcutaneously, only small volumes should be placed in one site (approximately 5 to 10 ml/kg/site). Blood supply to the skin may be disrupted by overdistention, decreasing the speed of absorption and complicating large-volume administration. Because of the fragility of avian skin, one puncture hole per administration site is recommended to avoid fluid leaks and skin tearing. If the bird is in shock or hypothermic, the fluid administered subcutaneously will not be absorbed because of severe peripheral vasoconstriction. This may potentiate shock by creating local vasodilation and peripheral pooling of the blood.

Fluid requirements in normotensive birds can also be met by dictary or oral gavage. The oral route is indicated when an animal is conscious and perching or standing. If fluids are administered in a recumbent animal, regurgitation and aspiration may occur. In many stressed, ambulatory birds, only small volumes (5 to 10 ml/kg) that can be given at increasing intervals are tolerated. The volume should be slowly increased and the frequency of administration reduced. In birds possessing a crop, normal emptying time is 3 to 4 hours. Any delay in emptying should be investigated with appropriate diagnostic procedures. Highly excitable individuals may regurgitate fluids following administration. Subcutaneous, intravenous, and oral routes can be combined.

In severely debilitated or cachectic birds, solid food should be withheld for the first 24 to 48 hours. In these cases, the caloric demand is so great that it may potentiate an already severe catabolic state. Alternatives include specially formulated avian diets such as Emeraid (Lafeber, Odell, IL) or human-formulated, low-residue, liquid diets like Precision LR Diet (Sandoznutrition, Minneapolis, MN). Gatorade® (Stokely-Van Camp, Chicago, IL) can also be used as a source of electrolytes and glucose. A dilute solution can be used initially and the strength increased over 12 hours to the recommended formula. As the patient's condition improves, blended food (baby food, monkey chow, pelleted complete diets, canned dog food, etc.) can be added in increasing amounts. As the bird begins eating on its own, a regular hospital diet is offered and tube feeding gradually discontinued (see this volume, p. 1160).

SELECTION OF FLUIDS

Most of the fluid preparations available for small animal (e.g., canine and feline) use can be safely given to the avian patient. Although no research in birds has characterized the electrolyte losses during specific disorders (diarrhea, regurgitation, intestinal obstruction), the same principles used in mammals have been successfully applied to birds. Crystalloids are most commonly used. Colloids are potentially useful, but very little work has been performed to assess their application and safety in birds. Blood transfusions have been given subjectively without the benefit of crossmatching. Fortunately, few adverse reactions seem to occur when homologous species are used as donors.

Crystalloids

Lactated Ringer's Solution

Lactated Ringer's solution (LRS) is perhaps the most useful and versatile solution available. As an isotonic source of balanced electrolytes, it can be administered to rehydrate a patient, support a patient with diarrhea, treat for shock, or be used as a maintenance solution. When used for maintenance, potassium (concentrated potassium chloride injection) must be added to meet daily patient requirements. As a rule of thumb, birds should receive 0.1 to 0.3 mEq/kg of potassium supplement daily (Redig, 1984). Given intravenously, LRS rapidly restores vascular volume. Hyperkalemia or hypernatremia may be exacerbated by LRS administration. In mammals, the lactate present in LRS is metabolized in the liver, liberating bicarbonate and contributing to the correction of a mild underlying acidosis that presumably also occurs in birds. Most drugs can be diluted into LRS; however, sodium bicarbonate should not be added to LRS.

Saline Solutions

Normal saline (NS) (0.9% sodium chloride injection) can be used to initially restore the fluid deficit or support a patient with regurgitation. Due to high levels of sodium and chloride, it is not a good choice for maintenance in birds. When re-expanding the circulatory volume, supplemental potassium chloride salts must be added at 0.1 to 0.3 mEq/kg/day. Most drugs can be safely added to NS without interaction. NS will promote the excretion of potassium by improving diuresis and restore the deficit of sodium in cases of hyponatremia. Half-strength saline 0.45% with 2.5% dextrose or 5% dextrose solution should be used in cases of hypernatremia.

Dextrose Solutions

Dextrose solutions (5%, 10%, and 50%) are particularly useful because birds have relatively high glucose requirements compared to mammals of equivalent weight. When 5% dextrose is given orally, its absorption from the intestinal tract is extremely rapid and does not create a flux of water in the intestinal lumen. Caution must be exercised when using 5% dextrose solution in water intravenously, subcutaneously, or intraperitoneally because it is a hypotonic solution (252 mOsm/L). When dextrose is absorbed, the remaining water will create a shift in electrolytes to restore osmolar balance. The drop in the central pool of electrolytes will lower the circulating volume and may aggravate hypovolemia. Dextrose in concentrations greater than 2.5% is contraindicated subcutaneously. A 10% or 50% solution is used to treat hypoglycemia. An initial dose of 1 ml/kg of 50% dextrose can be administered intravenously. Close monitoring of blood glucose and initiation of oral glucose administration will help correct the deficit and prevent recurrent hypoglycemic episodes. Dextrose has the disadvantage of promoting cellular acidosis. The small molecules readily cross the cell membrane and are metabolized into lactate. Hyperglycemia should be avoided in severely compromised patients. Dextrose 5% can be administered intravenously with appropriate precautions to ensure proper electrolyte balance. Dextrose 5% in 0.9% saline (sodium chloride) is a hypertonic solution (560 mOsm/L) that should be used with extreme caution because it can induce cellular dehydration and promote diuresis, exacerbating hypovolemia. Half-strength dextrose with half-strength LRS is slightly hypotonic (263 mOsm/L) and is a judicious choice in cases of prolonged surgery. It provides both electrolytes and dextrose in addition to promoting diuresis. Half-strength dextrose 2.5% in 0.45% saline is isotonic and is the best choice in azotemic mammals; it is therefore useful in hyperuricemic birds with concurrent renal compromise. Bicarbonate can be safely added to dextrose solutions.

Bicarbonate

Bicarbonate is the most important extracellular anion. It is regulated by the respiratory and renal systems. Disorders of the acid-base status often accompany dehydration, but partial correction can be achieved with the restoration of hydration. Severe acidosis can be life-threatening, so bicarbonate therapy must be instituted rapidly. The origin and the chronicity of the disorder must be established before initiating therapy. When given intravenously, sodium bicarbonate (8.4%) should always be diluted and administered slowly to avoid sudden alkalosis. Ideally, the degree of deficit should be confirmed by a venous or arterial blood gas. Correction is then calculated according to the following formula:

$$\text{base deficit} \times 0.3 \times \text{body weight (kg)} =$$
$$\text{net bicarbonate requirement in mEq.}$$

One third to one half of this amount should be administered over the first hour, followed by a second blood-gas analysis. Usually, most of the deficit is corrected with the first injection of bicarbonate. As distribution of bicarbonate into the intracellular space is slow, the remaining bicarbonate can be administered over 24 hours. In most cases, practitioners will not have the advantage of a blood gas analysis. An empiric administration of 0.5 to 1.0 mEq/kg of sodium bicarbonate diluted in 10 to 20 ml/kg of fluid may be given intraperitoneally or subcutaneously. A rough approximation of the deficit may be calculated by subtracting the birds' serum bicarbonate value from the normal value.

Careful administration of bicarbonate is essential. In mammals, rapid administration of sodium bicarbonate can induce an increase in carbon dioxide

(CO_2) production, resulting in a paradoxical acidosis of the cerebral spinal fluid due to the rapid diffusion of CO_2 through the blood-brain barrier. With time and excess bicarbonate, a metabolic alkalosis may occur that could lead to cardiac dysrhythmias, a left shift of the oxyhemoglobin curve with decreased availability of oxygen to the tissues, hypocalcemia, hypokalemia, hypernatremia, and increased plasma osmolality. Slower uptake can be safely achieved with oral bicarbonate. The authors have also used sodium bicarbonate, diluted in saline, intraperitoneally with good systemic absorption.

Colloids

Colloids are slowly gaining popularity in veterinary medicine. Their strongest advantage is the presence of large molecules that do not cross the endothelium, but remain in the intravascular compartment and increase the osmotic pressure. Animals with low oncotic pressure can then receive fluids that will expand the extravascular compartment without aggravating the hypoproteinemia and precipitating pulmonary edema.

Synthetic Colloids

Synthetic colloid solutions include dextrans and starch products. Dextran is available as dextran 40 (10% Gentran and 0.9% NaCl Injection, Baxter Healthcare Corp., Deerfield, IL), which has a half-life of 2 hours, and dextran 70 (6% Gentran and 0.9% NaCl Injection, Baxter Healthcare Corp., Deerfield, IL) with a higher molecular weight and a half-life of 6 hours. Because of its longer persistence in the plasma, dextran 70 is preferred over dextran 40. For resuscitation efforts in mammals, a rate of 40 to 50 ml/kg is recommended. The rate is then adjusted as blood pressure increases. Side effects of this type of therapy are rare and include anaphylactoid reactions and blood coagulation abnormalities. The effects of starch solutions (Hetastarch, Hespan, DuPont) last up to 36 hours. Complement activation may occur immediately during infusion but is fortunately very rare in mammals. These products have had limited investigation but hold potential usefulness in cases of severe hypoproteinemia in birds.

Blood and Blood Components

Plasma is a natural colloid resulting from sedimentation or centrifugation of whole blood. It is an excellent source of albumin. A single injection of blood products is rarely complicated by an ana-phylactoid reaction; repeated treatments must, however, be performed with extreme caution to avoid adverse immune-mediated reactions, includ-ing complement activation.

Very little information is available regarding blood transfusion in birds. Acute blood loss greater than 25% of the initial blood volume, low protein values (total plasma proteins <2.5 gm/dl, albumin <0.8 mg/dl), or cases of severe anemia (PCV <15% to 17%) require blood or plasma transfusion. No special reagents are needed for a major and a minor crossmatch in birds, and no avian crossmatching test kits are commercially available. In cases de-manding transfusion of blood or blood components, one should attempt to to use a sibling as the donor. Otherwise, donor birds from the same or a closely phylogenetically related species should be sought. Chicken or pigeon blood has been transfused to psittacines without noticeable adverse effects (Har-rison, 1986). Most transfusions are successful, with complications arising when repeated administration of blood is given. Sodium heparin (2500 units) is added to 20 ml of normal saline, and 0.6 ml of this solution is added to each 10 ml of blood collected. As an alternative in milder cases of anemia, iron dextran (The Butler Company, Columbus, OH), at a dose of 10 mg/kg repeated as needed in 1 to 2 weeks appears to mobilize erythrocytes and stimu-late erythropoiesis very rapidly. Other complica-tions of blood transfusion include the transmission of infectious agents (e.g., viral, parasitic). This is particularly important in psittacines. Blood donors should be carefully screened for chlamydia, papo-vavirus (polyomavirus and poxvirus), herpesvirus, beak-and-feather disease virus, and blood parasites.

COMPLICATIONS

Acute fluid overload is one of the most common complications encountered. It can manifest as dilu-tion anemia, hypoproteinemia, pulmonary edema, or an overwhelming work load for the heart. Ani-mals with underlying systemic disease (renal, car-diac, metabolic, or vascular) are especially at risk. Constant adjustment of the administration rate to patient needs will prevent fluid overloading. Accu-rate monitoring is essential, as premonitory clinical signs are uncommon in birds. Electrolyte imbal-ances may occur when anorectic birds are deprived of potassium supplementation or when excessive amounts of sodium and chloride are administered. Complications related to bicarbonate administration

can occur if blood gas analysis is not performed. Conservative dosages of bicarbonate must be used in order to avoid metabolic alkalosis, respiratory acidosis, and hyperosmolarity.

Complications related to technique of administra-tion include phlebitis, osteomyelitis, hematomas, and skin sloughing from extravasation of irritating products. Additionally, due to their relatively large body-surface-area-to-weight ratio, birds are more likely to develop problems associated with air em-bolus and hypothermia than are mammals of equiv-alent weight. Aspiration pneumonia may follow oral fluid administration or gavage feeding and necessi-tate immediate clearance of the airway. Finally, minimizing handling of severely compromised birds will help reduce stress and aid prevention of acute death syndrome.

References and Suggested Reading

Harrison, G. J. Evaluation and support of the surgical patient. *In* Harrison, G. J., and Harrison, L. R. (eds.): *Clinical Avian Medicine and Surgery.* Philadelphia: W. B. Saunders, 1986, p. 543.
  Description of perioperative procedures in birds.
King, A. S., and McLelland, J. Urinary system. *In* King, A. S., and McLelland, J. (eds.): *Birds: Their Structure and Function.* London: Balliere Tindall, 1984, p. 175.
  An outline of avian renal anatomy.
Lumeij, J. T. Plasma urea, creatinine and uric acid concentrations in response to dehydration in racing pigeons. Avian Pathol. 16:377, 1987.
  The effects of water deprivation in pigeons on plasma urea, creatinine, and uric acid concentrations.
Martin, H. D., and Kollias, G. V. Evaluation of water deprivation and fluid therapy in pigeons. J. Zoo Wildl. Med. 20:173, 1989.
  Determination of changes in blood parameters in response to dehydra-tion and fluid therapy.
McNabb, F. M. A.: Excretion. *In* Micheal, A. (ed.): *Physiology and Behavior of the Pigeon.* London: Academic Press, 1983, p. 41.
  A description of the renal anatomy and excretion physiology in the pigeon.
Otto, C. M., McCall-Kaufman, G., and Crowe, D. T.: Intraosseous infusion of fluids and therapeutics. Comp. Cont. Ed. Pract. Vet. 11:421, 1989.
  A review of the technique of intraosseous catheterization, its applica-tion, and complications.
Redig, P. T.: Fluid therapy and acid-base balance in the critically ill avian patient. Proceedings of the Annual Meeting of the Association of Avian Veterinarians 1984, p. 59.
  A review of avian fluid therapy.
Ritchie, B. W., Otto, C. M., Latimer, K. S., et al: A technique of intraosseous cannulation for intravenous therapy in birds. Comp. Cont. Ed. Pract. Vet. 12:55, 1990.
  A description of the technique of intraosseous cannulation in birds.
Sedgwick, C.: Anesthesia for small nondomestic mammals. *In* Jacobson, E. R., and Kollias, G. V. (eds.): *Exotic Animals.* New York: Churchill Livingstone, 1988, p. 209.
  A review of small mammal anesthesia, including fundamental basis of physiological scaling.
Skadhauge, E.: Cloacal absorption of urine in birds. Comp. Biochem. Physiol. [A] 55A:93, 1976.
  A review of the interaction of renal and cloacal functions in birds.
Sturkie, P. D.: Heart and circulation: Anatomy, hemodynamics, blood pressure, blood flow and body fluids. *In* Sturkie, P. D. (ed.): *Avian Physiology.* New York: Springer-Verlag, 1986, p. 104.
  A review of the anatomy and physiology of the cardiovascular system in birds.

AVIAN NUTRITIONAL SUPPORT

KATHERINE QUESENBERRY

New York, New York

Nutrition plays an elemental role in recovery from disease or surgery. Protein-calorie malnutrition in human patients is a significant factor in poor recovery during long-term hospitalization. The important role of adequate nutritional support in recovery of hospitalized small animals is now recognized. Understanding and applying concepts of nutritional support to avian patients is fundamental in successful therapy of pet birds.

Anorexia is often a primary reason for bird hospitalization. Clinicians who treat pet birds are familiar with the practice of "tube-feeding" homemade or commercial diets. However, many clinicians do not evaluate daily caloric or nutritional requirements of the patient.

Exact nutritional requirements of birds other than poultry are unknown. Even less is known about nutritional needs during disease or starvation. However, the physiologic mechanisms of energy metabolism during starvation or disease in mammals are operative in birds, with some variations in certain pathways (Hazelwood, 1986). Accordingly, most of the basic principles of nutrition in mammals can also be applied to birds.

ENERGY METABOLISM DURING STARVATION AND DISEASE

The physiology of energy metabolism during disease differs from metabolism during starvation. During short-term fasting in mammals, blood glucose concentration decreases, followed by a decrease in insulin concentration. Glucagon concentration is relatively increased. These changes stimulate hepatic gluconeogenesis. In pigeons, liver glycogen stores are depleted within 24 hours of the onset of fasting (Hazelwood, 1986). With continued fasting, amino acids and fatty acids are used as energy sources. In contrast, mammalian metabolism slows as physical activity decreases and muscle loss occurs. As starvation and the hypometabolic state continue, fatty acid utilization becomes the primary source of energy.

In chickens, blood glucose concentrations remain relatively stable during fasts of 1 to 8 days (Hazelwood, 1986). Although overall metabolism remains constant, loss of body mass occurs, primarily due to depletion of fat stores and some proteins. In adult male penguins during egg incubation, up to 40% of the initial body mass, primarily fat, is lost during the 4-month period. Metabolic rates remain constant (Whittow, 1986).

In mammals, insulin acts as a strong suppressor of lipolysis, while glucagon, epinephrine, and cortisol are strongly lipolytic. Intravenous infusion of dextrose in starving humans will cause elevations in insulin concentrations, completely suppressing lipolysis (Donoghue, 1989). In contrast, in birds an increase in blood insulin concentration is not associated with a decrease in free fatty acid concentration (Griminger, 1986). It is probable that glucagon, a strong mobilizer of depot lipids, plays a more prominent role during energy metabolism in birds than in mammals.

During stress or trauma, several hormones are released, including catecholamines, corticosteroids, and glucagon. These hormones cause an increase in body metabolism in proportion to the severity of injury. If nutritional intake is not adequate to meet increased energy demands, gluconeogenesis and glycogenolysis occur at high rates. Blood glucose increases, with normal or increased insulin concentrations. Infusion of intravenous dextrose for supplemental energy at this time is ineffective, as glucose utilization is usually occurring at maximum rates. Fatty acids and ketone bodies are also used as energy sources at peak rates. Additionally, protein requirements are significantly increased. Exogenous proteins are necessary to prevent excessive breakdown of body proteins and to provide adequate sources for tissue repair and blood cell and antibody production.

DETERMINING DAILY ENERGY REQUIREMENTS

In an animal that is resting, not digesting, growing, or reproducing and in a thermoneutral state, most of the energy released by the tissues is in the form of heat. The amount of heat produced is called the basal metabolic rate (BMR). A prediction of BMR can be made based on metabolic size. Using allometric scaling, the BMR can be predicted as

$$BMR = K(W_{kg}^{0.75})$$

where W is weight in kilograms and K is a theoretical constant for kcal used by different classes of

Table 1. *Adjustments to Maintenance Energy (ME)*

Condition	Multiple of ME
Elective surgery	1.0–1.2
Mild trauma	1.0–1.2
Severe trauma	1.1–2.0
Growth	1.5–3.0
Sepsis	1.2–1.5
Burns	1.2–3.0

Example: A 0.86-kg Blue-and-Gold macaw is anorectic and depressed, with soft-tissue injury and a fracture of the left tibiotarsus. The energy requirements are calculated as follows:

$$BMR = 78 \ (0.86)^{0.75} = 69.7 \ kcal$$

Maintenance energy is estimated as

$$ME = 1.5 \times 69.7 \ kcal = 104.5 \ kcal$$

For severe trauma, adjust the ME according to the scale:

$$1.1\text{--}2 \times 100.5 = 115 \ to \ 201 \ kcal/day$$

as the range for the total daily energy needs for this bird.

animals during a 24-hr period (Sedgwick, 1988). The K-factor for mammals is 70. For birds, the K-factor is 129 for passerines and 78 for nonpasserines. Other researchers have developed slightly different equations and K-factors for birds based on stages of activity (Whittow, 1986).

Normal activities, including digestion, absorption, and formation and excretion of waste products, require additional energy. This energy plus the BMR is called maintenance energy (ME). In passerine birds the ME may vary from 1.3 to 7.2 times the BMR dependent on time of year and the amount of energy expended for activity and thermoregulation (Whittow, 1986). Growth, reproduction, and recovery from disease require further energy, called productive energy.

In disease processes in mammals, adjustments to maintenance energy have been predicted according to severity of disease. This scale can be used for birds (Table 1).

SELECTION OF A DIET

Energy Content of Food

Not all of the gross energy content of foods is available for use by the body. Some energy is lost in urinary and fecal excretion. The available energy, or metabolizable energy, can be predicted based on the digestibility of a food. Foodstuffs used by birds have digestibilities ranging from 76% for grains and 66% for insects to 32% for willow buds and twigs (Whittow, 1986). Liquid enteral products for human use average 95% digestibility.

Fats have twice as much energy as proteins or carbohydrates. The physiologic fuel value of proteins and carbohydrates averages 4 kcal/gm, while fats average 9 kcal/gm. A high fat diet is one way to increase the amount of available dietary energy. Fats are a preferred energy source during disease or stress.

Dietary Requirements

Dietary requirements for psittacine birds are unknown. Nutritional requirements for poultry are commonly used for reference. The nine essential amino acids required by mammals are also required by birds. In addition to these nine, chickens, turkeys, and possibly other birds require arginine (Griminger, 1986). Cystine and tyrosine are required if methionine and phenylalanine intake is deficient. Glycine and proline are required for optimum growth in chickens.

Birds require small amounts of the same essential fatty acids as mammals. However, dietary fat intake varies widely by species. In species that consume a considerable amount of high-fat seeds, fat may constitute up to 50% of the total dry matter content of the diet (Griminger, 1986). In nectar-eaters, total fat intake may be minimal. Birds can readily adapt to a wide range of dietary fat content without detrimental effect (Griminger, 1986).

Types of Supplemental Diets

Many clinicians formulate their own diets for use in anorectic birds. Disadvantages of homemade diets include variable nutritional composition, a high probability of nutritional deficiencies, and extreme variation in consistency, digestibility, and caloric content.

Several veterinary products are available for enteral nutrition in sick birds. Liquid canine and feline formulas and powdered products formulated for birds are available. Products vary in energy content and protein, fat, and carbohydrate content. Several of the powdered products are grain-based and are high in carbohydrates and low in fat, with moderate amounts of protein. Advantages of the powdered products include ease of storage and use and low cost. Disadvantages include inaccurate measurement when mixed with water and the propensity for some of these powders to settle out in the crop.

Commercial liquid diets used in human medicine work well for short-term enteral nutrition in birds. These products, usually sold in 250-ml cans, are widely available in pharmacies, drug supply houses, and some grocery stores. Once opened, contents can be transferred into sealable containers and refrigerated for use up to 3 days. The liquid should be warmed before use.

Human enteral products vary in caloric and nu-

Table 2. *Liquid Enteral Feeding Products**

Product	Nutrients Per 100 kcal of Energy (Approximate)			
	Protein (gm)	Fat (gm)	Carbohydrate (gm)	kcal/ml
Isocal†	3.4	4.4	13.3	1.00
Isocal HCN†	3.8	5.1	10.0	2.00
Traumacal†	5.5	4.5	9.5	1.50
Pulmocare‡	4.2	6.1	7.0	1.50
Ensure Plus‡	3.6	3.5	13.0	1.50
Two Cal HN‡	4.2	4.5	10.8	2.00
Clinicare Canine*	4.9	6.0	5.9	0.99
Clinicare Feline*	6.4	4.3	5.2	0.92

*Pet-Ag, Inc., Elgin, IL
†Mead Johnson, Evansville, IN
‡Ross Laboratories, Columbus, OH

tritional content. Monomeric diets contain amino acids, sugars, and fatty acids formulated for easy absorption. More polymeric forms are available (Table 2), many of which are isotonic to minimize potential for diarrhea. Most diets are lactose free. This is advantageous for use in birds, which may lack or have limited amounts of the enzyme lactase. Diets can be selected based on desired protein, fat, and carbohydrate content. Caloric content ranges from 1 to 2 kcal/ml; those with 2 kcal/ml are useful in birds. The total daily volume is determined by dividing the calculated daily caloric needs by the calories per milliliter provided by the product. The total volume is divided into two to four daily feedings. Protein powders can be used to increase protein content if desired.

Disadvantages of these products include cost ($2 to $3 per 250-ml can), short shelf life once opened, and liquid nature making aspiration easier if the crop is overfilled.

ROUTE OF NUTRITIONAL SUPPORT

The easiest and most physiologic way to provide nutritional support in birds is through gavage or tube feeding. Stainless steel feeding needles of various sizes are easy to use in small to medium-sized birds. Rubber catheters fitted with adapters can be used in large birds. Sterile equipment should be used for each bird to prevent spread of disease. A beak speculum of padded metal or hard plastic may be necessary in large birds to allow passage of the catheter or needle. Care should be taken to avoid bruising the soft tissue at the base of the beak.

Proper restraint is important in successful gavage feeding. Birds are held in a straight vertical position with the neck in full extension. The wings are held close to the body manually, or the bird can be wrapped in a towel. The lubricated feeding catheter or needle is gently passed down the oropharynx into the crop. Before infusion, the crop is palpated to check positioning of the catheter. Always observe the back of the oropharynx during feeding for overflow of food from the crop.

After feeding, the bird is immediately released into the cage. All other treatments should be done before gavage feeding to reduce the possibility of the bird struggling and regurgitating. Crop capacity varies according to size of the bird. The following guidelines can be used: canaries and finches, 0.25 to 0.5 ml; budgerigars, 1.0 to 1.5 ml; cockatiels, 2 to 3 ml; small parrots, 5 to 8 ml; medium to large parrots, 8 to 12 ml; large cockatoos, 10 to 15 ml; medium to large macaws, 15 to 30 ml.

Total parenteral nutrition is difficult to administer in birds. Sterile intravenous catheters are hard to place and maintain. Vascular access ports have been used in geese for short-term parenteral nutrition (Harvey-Clark, 1990). Limited studies using intraosseous catheters for administration of fluids, parenteral nutritional products, and drugs in birds have been done (Lamberski and Daniel, 1991; Ritchie et al., 1990). However, the effects of administering parenteral formulas into the bone marrow of birds is unknown (see this volume, p. 1154). In humans, severe metabolic complications can result from parenteral feeding. Serum chemistries and electrolytes are monitored closely, and nutritional formulas are adjusted daily as needed. Close monitoring of metabolic complications in birds is extremely difficult. Serial blood samples collected within a short time period may cause anemia in an already compromised patient.

Duodenal feeding catheters have been used successfully in both clinical and research trials in medium to large birds (Goring et al., 1986). Indications for placement of a duodenal catheter include severe crop stasis or severe dilation or impaction of the proventriculus. Disadvantages include the requirement for anesthesia and performing invasive surgery in an already compromised bird. Feedings must be given at 1- to 2-hour intervals because of the limited amount of liquid that can be infused into the duodenum at one time, and 24-hour supervision is required. Diets must be elemental for easy duodenal absorption. Despite limitations, this method is useful in selected situations.

References and Suggested Reading

Donoghue, S.: Nutritional support of hospitalized patients. Vet. Clin. North Am. Small Anim. Pract. 19:475, 1989.
Goring, R. L., Goldman, A., and Kaufman, K. J.: Needle catheter duodenostomy: a technique for duodenal alimentation of birds. J.A.V.M.A. 189:1017, 1986.
Griminger, P., and Scanes, C. G.: Protein metabolism. *In* Sturkie, P. D., (ed.): *Avian Physiology.* New York: Springer-Verlag, 1986, p. 326.

Griminger, P.: Lipid metabolism. *In* Sturkie, P. D. (ed.): *Avian Physiology*. New York: Springer-Verlag, 1986, p. 345.

Harvey-Clark, C.: Clinical and research use of implantable vascular access ports in avian species. Proceedings of the Annual Association of Avian Veterinarians, 1990, p. 191.

Hazelwood, R. L.: Carbohydrate metabolism. *In* Sturkie, P. D. (ed.): *Avian Physiology*. New York: Springer-Verlag, 1986, p. 303.

Lamberski, N., and Daniel, G.: The efficacy of intraosseous catheters in birds. Proceedings of the Association of Avian Veterinarians, 1991, p. 17.

Quesenberry, K. E.: Nutritional support of the avian patient. Proceedings of the Annual Meeting Association of Avian Veterinarians, 1989, p. 11.

Ritchie, B. W., et al.: A technique for intraosseous cannulation for intravenous therapy in birds. Comp. Contin. Ed. 12(1):55, 1990.

Sedgwick, C. J.: Finding the dietetic needs of captive native wildlife and zoo animals by allometric scaling. Proceedings of the 55th Annual Meeting of the American Animal Hospital Association, 1988, p. 149.

Whittow, G. C.: Regulation of body temperature. *In* Sturkie, P. D. (ed.): *Avian Physiology*. New York: Springer-Verlag, 1986, p. 221.

Whittow, G. C.: Energy metabolism. *In* Sturkie, P. D. (ed.): *Avian Physiology*. New York: Springer-Verlag, 1986, p. 253.

APPLICATIONS OF SPLINTS, BANDAGES, AND COLLARS

DAVID M. McCLUGGAGE

Boulder, Colorado

Owing to unique avian physiology, the proper application of splints, bandages, and collars in birds is quite different from that in mammals. The presence of feathers, the conformation of limbs, and the tendency for many species to chew limits the clinician's ability to apply bandages.

Many fractures heal well with external coaptation, often with a return to full function. The wing is especially amenable to splinting; the body provides an accurate mold that allows healing to take place in a physiologically normal position. Owing to the complications inherent in internal fixation and the fact that a return to full flight ability is often not essential for caged and aviary birds, many fractures of the long bones are best managed by the application of splints. Collars may be applied to restrict a bird's movements; however, the stress of a collar can exacerbate subclinical illness and even lead to death.

COLLARS

Before a collar is applied, the patient should be tested for the presence of subclinical illness (i.e., complete blood count, radiographs); close observation should follow application. The author always observes the bird for at least 6 hr postapplication to determine proper fit and whether the bird adapts to the presence of the collar.

Types of Collars

There are three types of collars available for use: reversed Elizabethan collar, Elizabethan collar, and the tube collar. A tube collar is a cylindrical neck splint that maintains the neck in full extension to prevent the bird from turning around and biting at its body. The tube collar looks uncomfortable, does not allow free movement of the neck for eating and drinking, and appears cruel to many owners. The Elizabethan collar is a conical structure that extends from the neck craniad. This collar is hard to fit in a way that allows normal movement and eating yet keeps the bird from reaching its body. In the author's experience, a modified and reversed Elizabethan collar is the best choice. It is comfortable to wear, allows freedom of movement, and appears humane to the owner.

Collars used to be applied routinely to birds that were feather pickers, but this does not effectively modify feather-chewing behavior and should be reserved for only the most severe cases in which birds are causing trauma to the skin.

MODIFIED REVERSED ELIZABETHAN COLLAR

MATERIALS AND CONSTRUCTION. The best materials for collar construction are semirigid, clear, plastic materials. Many hardware stores carry appropriate thicknesses. Because the collars are clear, the bird can see its body and knows where to place its feet. Used radiograph film can also be used to construct the collar. For larger birds, two or more layers may be glued together prior to cutting the collar. Once formed, the collar can be secured with staples. If screw-type rivets are used, the owner can easily remove and reattach the collar. Figure 1

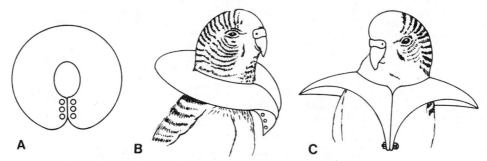

Figure 1. Construction of reversed Elizabethan collar. *A,* Note that the hole is offset and the radius from the center of the neck hole to the back is approximately 30% longer than that toward the front. This allows an equal radius around the entire body of the bird. *B,* By bending the collar in this fashion and fastening as indicated, the bird is not able to reach the staples or rivets to pull them loose. Make sure to pad the collar adequately wherever it can come in contact with the bird. *C,* Note that the collar will naturally rest with the bent-under area to the front of the bird. If the back of the bird is the area that needs protection, the collar can be formed to extend farther backward, allowing better movement and eating ability at the front. (Reprinted with permission from Galvin, C.: The feather picking bird. *In* Kirk, R. W. (ed.): *Current Veterinary Therapy VIII.* Philadelphia: W. B. Saunders, 1983, p. 649.)

depicts construction of a reversed Elizabethan collar.

The size of the collar will vary significantly according to the size of the bird and which part or parts of the body must be protected. The collar must be particularly long to protect against self-mutilation of the feet.

SPLINTS

Splinting, as defined here, is the application of structural support (e.g., wire, wood, or plastic) to provide external fixation for fractures, ligament or tendon ruptures, or sprains.

Anesthetics with the Application of Splints

When isoflurane is available, splints should be applied using anesthesia. This allows for a better fit and reduces stress on the bird. The patient becomes ambulatory soon after anesthesia, decreasing the chance of damage to the coaptation device. Physical restraint is often preferable to injectable anesthetics, as the rough recovery often encountered following the use of injectable anesthetics may endanger repair efforts.

Fractures Suitable for Splinting

Fractures that have a good prognosis for recovery with the use of a splint (the fracture will heal, but full function may not necessarily return) include:

- coracoid, scapula, furcula;
- humerus, midshaft to proximal, closed;
- radius, midshaft to distal, closed or open;
- ulna, proximal to distal, closed;

- radius and ulna, midshaft to distal, closed;
- carpometacarpus, closed;
- femur, proximal and midshaft, simple;
- tibiotarsal, simple;
- metatarsus, simple.

Most other simple, closed fractures of the long bones will heal well with external coaptation; however, a decrease in function may be noted, especially if the fracture is close to a joint. Rapid necrosis of bone is commonly encountered with open fractures, severely decreasing the prognosis for healing and return to normal function. Comminuted fractures require more stability, with various forms of internal or external fixation indicated. K-apparatus may be appropriate in comminuted fractures.

TAPE SPLINT

Tape splints work well for fractures of the tibiotarsus and tarsometatarsus in birds under 125 gm (Fig. 2). Birds between 125 to 175 gm may benefit from the incorporation of a cotton swab's wooden dowel into the splint. Fractures of the tarsometatarsus must have a stirrup applied around and under the foot to achieve proper fixation.

SNOWSHOE SPLINT

Snowshoe splints work well for fractures of the digits. Moldable splint material such as Hexalite can be cut into a shape that can be applied to the bottom of the feet and molded around padded toes, then taped into place. This type of splint provides stability superior to the older ball splint. Alternatively, for fractures of the second or third digit, the two toes can be taped together. Owing to impairment of the blood supply, open fractures of the

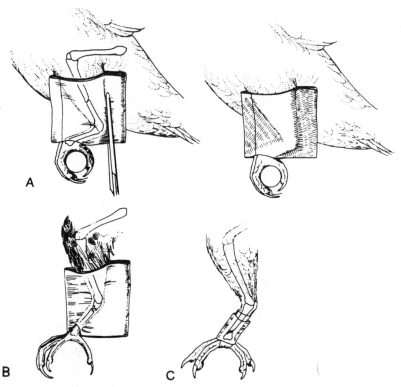

Figure 2. Method of Altman for applying tape splints to stabilize fractures of the lower leg. *A*, Method for midshaft tibiotarsal fracture. *B*, Method for distal tibiotarsal and proximal tarsometatarsal fracture. *C*, Method for distal tarsometatarsus. (Reprinted with permission from Altman, R.: Fractures of the extremities of birds. *In* Kirk, R. W. (ed.): *Current Veterinary Therapy VI.* Philadelphia: W. B. Saunders, 1977, p. 718.)

digits often produce necrosis of the toe distal to the fracture. The owner should be forewarned that the toe may slough off.

MODIFIED ROBERT JONES SPLINT

Application of cast padding followed by roll gauze and elastic bandage tape, often called the Robert Jones bandage, can provide enough support to allow for healing of many tibiotarsal fractures. This splint has been successfully applied to birds weighing up to 500 gm. It is especially applicable in young birds that heal rapidly.

THOMAS SPLINT

The Redig modification of the Schroeder-Thomas splint provides a good prognosis in fractures of the tibiotarsus and tarsometatarsus (Fig. 3). It is most applicable for birds weighing over 150 gm. An 18-gauge hardware wire is suitable for most birds; larger birds such as macaws require 14-gauge wire. The splint is constructed similar to all Thomas splints except that the loop is positioned at a vertical angle with the proximal bar bent away from the

body in a 70° angle, then bent back down to conform to the leg. The splint bars are positioned midsagittally and in an anterior and posterior position. The end of the splint is made long enough to completely cover the foot.

FIGURE-OF-8 BANDAGE

The figure-of-8 bandage provides good support for fractures of the radius and ulna, carpometacarpus, and digits (Fig. 4). Birds weighing less than 50 gm can do well with humeral fractures stabilized with this fixation. With the wing folded in a normal position, the bandage is applied in a figure-8 fashion around the front of and behind the elbow. With fractures of the humerus or shoulder girdle, the wing should be secured to the body using elastic bandaging tape. The opposite wing remains free. The most common error made with this bandage is to apply excessive layers, making the splint too bulky. Care must be taken to ensure that the bandage allows for normal breathing and defecation.

SPICA SPLINT

Coxofemoral luxations and proximal-to-midshaft fractures of the femur in larger birds can be man-

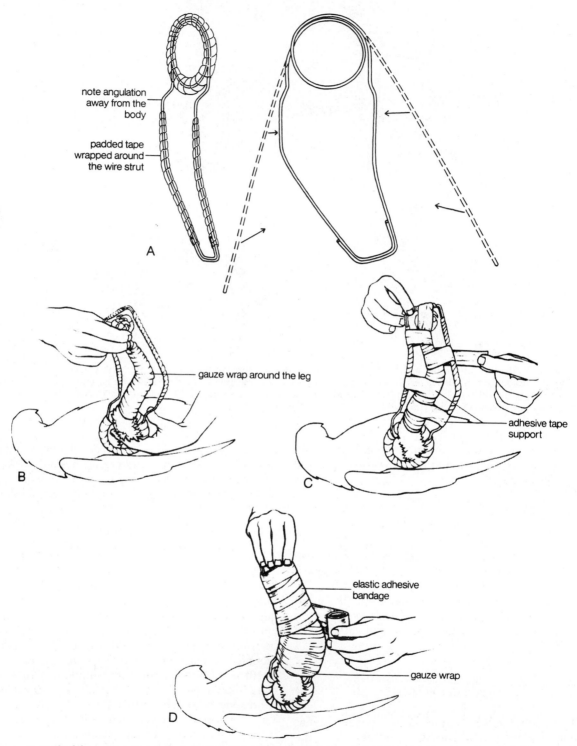

Figure 3. Method for construction and application of the Redig modification of the Schroeder-Thomas splint for birds. *A,* Making the splint. *B,* The padded wire splint is fitted to the gauze-wrapped leg and bent to conform to the angulations of the leg. *C,* Adhesive tape cross supports are applied to suspend the leg between the struts of the splint. *D,* The entire leg and splint are wrapped in a heavy layer of gauze and covered with an elastic adhesive bandage. (Reprinted with permission from Redig, P. T.: Evaluation and nonsurgical management of fractures. *In* Harrison, G. J., and Harrison, L. R. (eds.): *Clinical Avian Medicine and Surgery.* Philadelphia: W. B. Saunders, 1986, p. 391.)

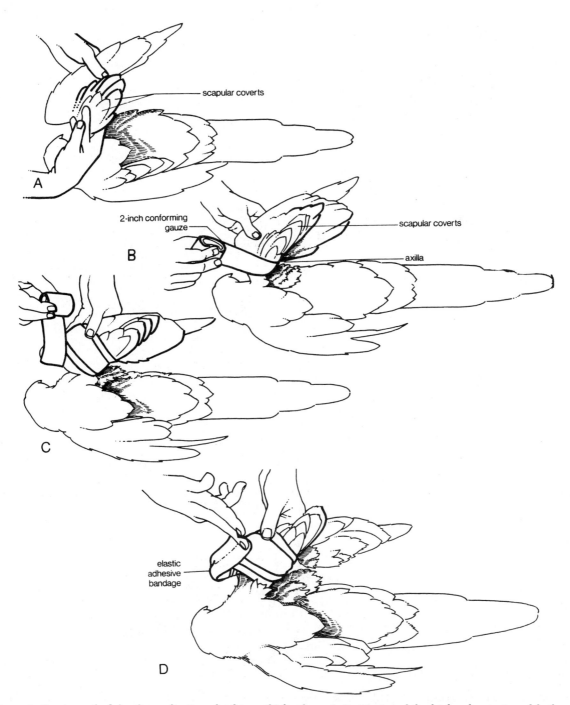

Figure 4. Proper method for the application of a figure-of-8 bandage. *A*, Positioning of the bird and grouping of feathers for application of the bandage. *B*, Starting the gauze wrap around the back of the humerus. *C*, Extending gauze over the wrist and wrapping in a figure-of-8 configuration. *D*, Applying the single wrap of Elastikon over the wrist joint.

Illustration continued on following page

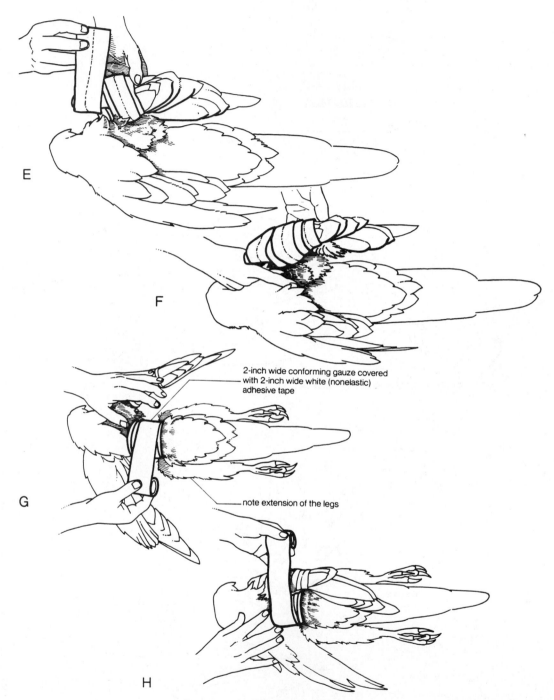

2-inch wide conforming gauze covered with 2-inch wide white (nonelastic) adhesive tape

note extension of the legs

Figure 4 *Continued E*, Final wrap of 2-inch Elastikon over the entire wing. *F*, Appearance of the finished figure-of-8 bandage; all loose gauze should be covered by the elastic bandage. *G*, Wrapping the body of the bird with gauze and adhesive tape to provide a firm anchorage for the bandaged wing for better alignment and stabilization. *H*, Taping the figure-of-8 bandage to the body wrap to provide additional stabilization, essential in the case of a humeral fracture. (Reprinted with permission from Redig, P. T.: Evaluation and nonsurgical management of fracture. *In* Harrison, G. J., and Harrison, L. R. (eds.): *Clinical Avian Medicine and Surgery*. Philadelphia: W. B. Saunders, 1986, pp. 386–387.)

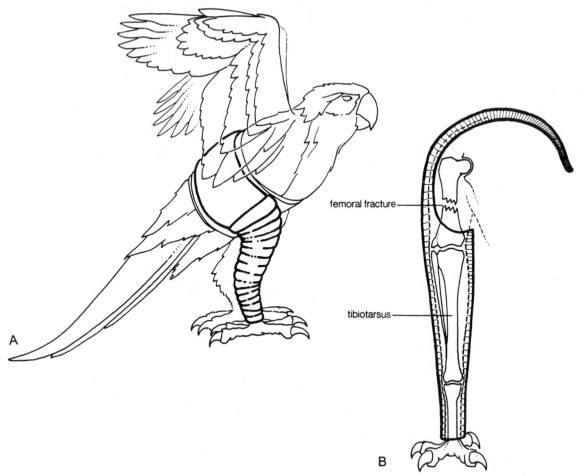

Figure 5. *A*, Hip spica splint for the avian patient. *B*, Frontal view of the avian hip spica splint. (Reprinted with permission from Rousch, J. C.: Avian orthopedics. *In* Kirk, R. W. (ed.): *Current Veterinary Therapy VII*. Philadelphia: W. B. Saunders, 1980, p. 662.)

aged by applying a spica splint (Fig. 5). Most smaller birds and waterfowl will heal well with cage rest alone, which may be preferable to applying any coaptation device. The splint is formed by cutting and molding splint material such as Hexalite so that it wraps two thirds of the way around the leg and rises around and over the back, stopping at the level of the opposite coxofemoral joint. Heavy padding should be applied around the leg and over the back. The splint is attached with Vetcast.

BANDAGES

Bandages are not commonly applied to birds. Feathers inhibit the application of bandages, and unless collared, most psittacine birds tend to remove them. Bandages are most frequently applied to the feet of birds and the stumps of amputations. Many lacerations are best sutured closed and left unbandaged. However, larger disruptions of the epithelium, such as burns or massive self-trauma, may require bandages. Recently, acrylics are begin-

ning to be applied as bandages for a variety of wounds.

BODY BANDAGE

Orthopedic stockinette applied over the wings and body can protect the bird's body from self-mutilation and temporarily provide fixation of wing fractures.

TEGADERM BANDAGE

Tegaderm (3-M, St. Paul, MN) is a thin, transparent bandage material that has proved particularly useful. It is practically impossible to feel when applied, is very comfortable, and relieves any sensation of pain or pruritus. It acts as a "synthetic skin" until healing has occurred. When applied to the feet or legs, it has been extremely effective in controlling "Amazon foot necrosis," burns, self-mutilation, and bumblefoot lesions. As this bandage makes the bird very comfortable, a collar is usually not needed.

ACRYLIC AND SYNTHETIC BANDAGES

Acrylics and other synthetic materials are finding widespread use in human medicine and are receiving more attention in avian medicine. Isobutyl acrylic (Cyanodent or Tissu Glu, Ellman International, Hewlett, NY) can be applied as a bandage material following xanthoma excision or after debridement of any large area of skin that cannot be covered with more conventional bandages. This acrylic is somewhat flexible and less likely to break with body movements. Methyl acrylic (Super-glue) should be avoided, as it may be toxic to tissues.

DRESSINGS

Water-miscible ointments can be applied to the skin to promote healing and prevent infections. Oil-based products should be avoided, as they will be spread throughout the feathers during preening and inhibit the normal thermoregulatory function of the feathers. In the author's experience, lanolin-based products can be effective when applied to lesions that are drying out excessively.

References and Suggested Reading

Altman, R.: Fractures of the extremities of birds. *In* Kirk, R. W. (ed.): *Current Veterinary Therapy VI*. Philadelphia: W. B. Saunders, 1977, p. 717.

Harrison, G. I.: Surgical instrumentation and special techniques. *In* Harrison, G. J., and Harrison L. R. (eds.): *Clinical Avian Medicine and Surgery*. Philadelphia: W. B. Saunders, 1986, p. 565.

MacCoy, D. M.: Techniques of fracture repair in birds and their indications: External and internal fixation. Proceedings of the First International Conference of Zoological and Avian Medicine, 1987, p. 549.

Redig, P. T.: Evaluation and nonsurgical management of fractures. *In* Harrison, G. J., and Harrison, L. R. (eds.): *Clinical Avian Medicine and Surgery*. Philadelphia: W. B. Saunders, 1986, p. 382.

SKIN DISORDERS OF RODENTS, RABBITS, AND FERRETS

THOMAS J. BURKE

Urbana, Illinois

As with general companion animal practice, primary complaints referable to the skin are common in ferrets, rodents, and rabbits. The approach to diagnosis is the same, including history, physical examination, skin scraping, biopsy, and cultures for fungi and bacteria. The size of the patient may preclude extensive clinical pathologic examination and endocrine testing.

The history should include questions concerning the housing and nutrition, because many dermatoses are caused by poor management. For example, boredom leads to hair chewing ("barbering"), and cannibalism results from overcrowding or housing incompatible sexes together. Most rodents are burrowing creatures that spend most of their time in the wild seeking food and escaping predators. When placed in sterile environments with *ad libitum* feeding and no danger of predators, they are left with little to do except chew on themselves or others. Males especially are prone to chew on each other.

Females with a litter may cannibalize others in the cage, as well as their offspring.

Housing for rodents should include vertical as well as horizontal space (e.g., feeding platforms reached by ramps) plus visual barriers and tunnels (small boxes, cardboard tubes, tin cans with no sharp edges). Commercial plastic tunnel systems are available. Bedding material always should be available for rodents and rabbits. For various reasons ground corncobs are preferable to aromatic wood chips. Good quality loose hay provides "occupational therapy" as well as bedding/nesting material. Bones and antlers should be provided for chewing exercise as well as for diversion.

Ferrets also require privacy and should be provided with den boxes and artificial burrows (lengths of plastic pipe or cardboard tubes).

Sanitation is important. Aromatic wood chips are no substitute for physical cleaning. Water bottles should be cleaned daily and checked for leaks. This

Table 1. *Ectoparasites of Rabbits, Rodents, and Ferrets*

Species	Parasites
Mouse	Fur mite (three species); lice
Rat	Fur mite; notedric mite; lice
Hamster	*Demodex* (two species); ear mite
Gerbil	*Demodex*
Guinea pig	Fur mite; sarcoptoid mite; lice (two species); fleas
Rabbit	Fur mite (two species); sarcoptoid mite; notedric mite; lice; ear mite; fleas
Squirrel	Sarcoptoid mite; fleas
Ferret	Sarcoptoid mite; ear mite; fleas

is especially important for animals kept in aquaria, where humidity can dramatically increase if the water bottle leaks.

Nutrition should be based on a block or pellet type food designed for the species being fed, with grains, vegetables, and fruits used as treats. I advise owners to purchase small quantities from a reliable pet shop and to store the food in a freezer. Guinea pigs should receive daily vitamin C directly *per os*, not in the drinking water. Ferrets should be fed a commercial dry ferret food or a low-magnesium cat food. All of these animals should have access to a salt wheel or block with trace-minerals.

ECTOPARASITES

Ectoparasites infesting rodents, rabbits, and ferrets are listed in Table 1. Diagnosis is usually made

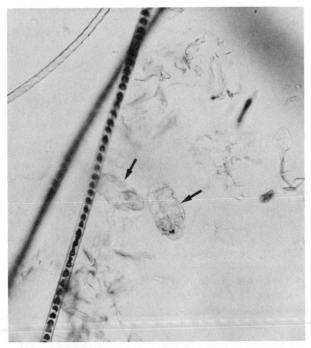

Figure 1. *Demodex criceti (arrows)* from a hamster. The other species, *D. aurati*, more closely resembles *D. canis*.

by skin scraping using a well-oiled scalpel blade. Deep scrapings are usually not necessary, because fur mites are best found with superficial scraping. Note that hamsters may have two species of *Demodex* mites. One looks very similar to the *Demodex* found in dogs, but the other is atypical and may be missed (Fig. 1). Mixed infestations occur in about 25% of the cases. *Demodex* mites are treated with amitraz (Mitaban, Upjohn) as for dogs. All other mites and lice are treated with ivermectin at doses of 300 to 400 μg/kg SC, repeated every 2 to 3 weeks until the mites or lice are eliminated. Cages should be thoroughly disinfected. Ectoparasites of rabbits deserve special mention in that the *Cheyletiella* fur mite can infect dogs and cats. The sarcoptic mite (*Sarcoptes scabiei*) can also infect humans. Use caution when handling wild rabbits or hares with lice, because they can transmit tularemia.

Flea infestations are common and should be treated as in cats. Fleas on wild rabbits may transmit tularemia and sylvatic plague. Ticks are uncommon in pet rabbits but common in captured wild specimens and in ferrets used for hunting rabbits. Some can transmit Lyme disease.

Myiasis (fly strike) is usually only seen in captured wild animals. Flesh fly (*Wohlfahrtia vigil*) infestations occur in ferret kits kept outdoors and has been reported as a common problem for ferret ranchers. Treatment involves killing the maggots (I use ether), wound débridement, and supportive care. Patients should be closely monitored for sepsis or shock.

Cuterebra is found in rabbits, squirrels, and ferrets. These dipterid fly larvae are usually found in the subcutis of the neck. The larvae can be seen moving through the open apical pore of the swelling. They should be removed intact if possible. Several texts mention the possibility of a severe, often fatal systemic reaction if the larva is crushed, but I have never seen this happen. Nonetheless, owners should be forewarned of this possibility. After removal of the larva, the wound is débrided and allowed to heal by second intention with topical antibiotic therapy.

Thorough cleaning of the premises is recommended in all cases of ectoparasitism. Fly control in outdoor pens is best accomplished with screening.

DERMATOMYCOSIS

Ringworm is common in young rodents, especially guinea pigs, chinchillas, and mice, as well as rabbits and ferrets. The usual organism is a *Trichophyton*, which does not fluoresce under a Wood's lamp. Fluorescent *Microsporum* is sometimes seen in mice, rats, and ferrets, and I have encountered one case in a guinea pig. Cats may transmit it to ferrets.

The lesions are usually circular, with broken hair shafts and scales or crusts. Mild pruritus may lead to excoriation and scab formation with secondary pyoderma.

Diagnosis is based on culture on appropriate media or biopsy. Potassium hydroxide preparations are, in my opinion, not useful.

Treatment includes clipping hair from the affected areas, povidone-iodide scrubs, and topical antifungals. Oral griseofulvin is usually not necessary but may be used at cat doses in refractory cases. Do not use glucocorticoids. The premises should be thoroughly cleaned to remove infectious spores. If possible, flaming of the area, as with a weed burner, is recommended. Antifungal powders may be added to the dust bath of chinchillas to aid in prevention.

LACERATIONS AND EXCORIATIONS

Lacerations are usually caused by sharp objects in the cage. Suture if necessary and treat with a topical antibiotic. Remove or cover the offending objects.

Bite wounds on the neck may result from normal mating behavior in ferrets, a rather violent affair. Excoriations and abrasions not associated with ectoparasites are caused either by cage mates (cannibalism) or self-mutilation. Separation and topical antibiotic-glucocorticoid therapy are used to treat excoriation.

Self-mutilation is usually a result of boredom. Chewing the hair exclusively, or barbering, causes patches of closely chewed hair shafts that may resemble the broken hair shafts of ringworm. Abrasions of the face in solitary animals usually indicate lack of bedding/nesting material so that the animal continually rubs its face on the cage floor in an attempt to achieve visual security. Treatment involves topical therapy *and* correction of management errors.

When examining gerbils with "bloody noses," remember that the exudate may only be dried tears containing porphyrin. Proper bedding material and humidity usually prevent the accumulation of dried tears, but the patient should be examined for other diseases that may cause depression or lethargy leading to poor grooming. The harderian glands may also be surgically removed. Apparently, sufficient precorneal film is still produced to prevent keratitis.

Rats may also have red tears when infected with a coronavirus of the tear glands.

RINGTAIL

Dry annular constrictions of the tail of rats are a result of low (<20%) humidity and high environ-mental temperature or freezing. Gangrene and sloughing of part of the tail occur in advanced cases. Treatment involves improved management and topical emollients. The relative humidity should be around 50%, especially for neonates.

ROUGH HAIRCOAT

In gerbils, a rough haircoat is usually a result of dampness (leaky water bottle) or high (>60%) humidity. The treatment is obvious.

In other species, a rough coat is usually a sign of advanced disease, although damp bedding may cause a rough coat in any animal.

SORE HOCKS

Sore hocks in rabbits are most often seen in the larger breeds. A decreased thickness of the plantar fur pad predisposes to development of lesions, as does poor cage flooring.

The lesions of sore hock develop on the plantar surfaces of the hindlimb and begin as areas of hair loss with erythema. Progression leads to deepening ulceration with secondary infection. Front limbs are uncommonly affected.

Treatment includes débridement, topical and systemic antibiotics, and soaks in a disinfectant. Housing on coated grids or Astroturf is advisable. Giant breeds should be housed on floors of rolled steel bars to help prevent the problem. Protective dressings may be applied if the rabbit can be prevented from chewing them.

Advanced cases are very difficult to treat. Affected animals should not be used in a breeding program because both body size and thin plantar fur pads are genetically determined.

TREPONEMA

Usually considered a genital disease, infection with the spirochete *Treponema cuniculi* often causes visible lesions on parts of the body other than the external genitalia. Because of the grooming, social, and sleeping habits of rabbits, lesions are frequently found on the nose and ears. Beginning as vesicles, the lesions rapidly progress to macules and then scabbed ulcers (Fig. 2). The external genitalia are most commonly infected.

Spread is by direct contact. Diagnosis is based on biopsy findings and serologic examination, because the organism is very difficult to culture.

The treatment of choice is penicillin, 40,000 units/kg/day IM for 5 days. I also use a *Lactobacillus*-containing product orally to prevent floral imbalances in the gastrointestinal tract.

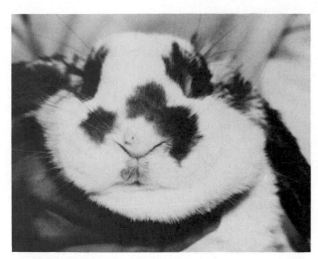

Figure 2. *Treponema* lesions of the nose on a pet rabbit. Similar lesions were present on the ears.

LUMPS AND BUMPS

In general, the older the animal, the more likely lumps and bumps are to be tumors. Consider the species' normal life span when determining middle to old age. Although malignancy is fairly common, some rules of thumb can help an owner decide if surgery has a reasonable chance of cure. Biopsy is always helpful of course, but cost factors may preclude its use.

In rats, mice, and gerbils, lumps are usually tumors. In rats (even males), the most common tumor is mammary fibroadenoma. These can occur anywhere on the body because rats have foci of mammary tissue throughout their subcutis. Adenocarcinomas account for less than 10% of rat mammary tumors, and thus surgery is most often curative. In gerbils, dermal tumors are also most often benign, and surgery should be encouraged. In mice, malignancy is the rule.

In hamsters, facial lumps are usually associated with the cheek pouches (abscess, granuloma, or just stuffed with food), whereas other skin lumps are usually benign tumors. Lymphosarcoma may appear as an ill-defined draining skin lesion in old hamsters.

In rabbits and guinea pigs, external lumps are most often abscesses or granulomas, with the exception of masses associated with the dorsal lumbar area of guinea pigs. These are most often benign trichofolliculomas. Guinea pigs also are prone to cervical lymphadenitis or "lumps." This is a caseous infection usually caused by *Streptococcus zooepidemicus* or *Streptobacillus moniliformis*. I suspect that most cases result from infection of oral lesions (chewing on wood?). External drainage may be seen. Aspiration yields a needle plugged with caseous material. Surgery is necessary to resolve the lump totally, but antibiotics halt the progress and

the spread to other areas such as the middle ear and liver. Only broad-spectrum antibiotics should be used, and as for rabbits, I routinely use an oral *Lactobacillus* product to protect the gut from floral overgrowth with gram-negative organisms.

Rabbits may have viral tumors that affect the skin. The Shope papillomavirus causes warts. These regress with time if the patient does not become debilitated. Crushing several with a hemostat may hasten regression. Some myxoma viruses produce dermal fibromas that also spontaneously regress (the California strain produces a fatal disease). These viral tumors are usually spread from wild to domestic rabbits by insect vectors, primarily mosquitoes. There is no treatment. Prevention involves screening of hutches to keep vectors out. A myxoma vaccine is used in Europe. None of these viruses are zoonotic.

Squirrels also get a viral skin tumor—fibroma. Spontaneous regression occurs, but multiple tumors can cause severe debilitation. There is no transmission to other species including humans or the family dog or cat who drags home an infected squirrel, causing the owner to call you.

Tumors of the skin and subcutis in ferrets are more often malignant than benign. Squamous cell carcinomas, mast cell tumors, and adenocarcinomas of sebaceous and perianal glands are most commonly reported. All skin tumors should be subjected to biopsy before attempting to render a prognosis to the owner. Treatment depends on the histologic diagnosis. Metabolic scaling should be used when calculating the dose of chemotherapy agents.

SCENT GLANDS

Most rodents and rabbits have collections of sebaceous glands that are used primarily for marking territory. In rabbits, they are located in blind pouches lateral to the anogenital line; in guinea pigs, they are circumanal; in hamsters, they are dark brown to black and are located on the flanks (Fig. 3); in gerbils, they are yellow-tan and are located on the midventral abdomen. These glands are androgen-sensitive and are thus more prominent in intact males.

Owners not infrequently present a hamster or gerbil with normal scent glands but, because they have just noticed them, think there is a problem. Whenever possible, inform owners of the location and color of the normal glands.

Inflammation of scent glands is most common in gerbils and to a lesser degree in hamsters. Rubbing on wood chip bedding or other wooden objects probably causes more adenitis than any other single factor. If the glands become impacted, animals can resort to severe self-mutilation. After débridement, I use an ointment that contains proteolytic enzymes,

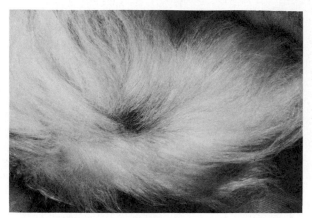

Figure 3. Normal scent or flank gland in a male hamster. Hair discoloration caused by secretions.

antibiotics, and a glucocorticoid. Castration is recommended to reduce gland secretory activity.

Neoplasia is also encountered in gerbils and hamsters. Adenomas are most common, although carcinomas do occur. Surgery is most often curative. Again, I recommend castration in case the tumor is androgen-sensitive.

The anal glands and sacs of ferrets produce and store a musklike substance. Removal does not truly "de-scent" (i.e., render odorless) a ferret, because most of their body odor is derived from their dermal sebaceous glands. The perianal glands are subject to neoplasia. Abscessation and impaction are very uncommon but when encountered are treated as for similar problems in cats.

EAR MITES

Ear mites are mainly a problem in rabbits but may occur in hamsters (rare in isolated pets) and ferrets. I consider all rabbits to be infected until proven otherwise and routinely treat all rabbits at least once for ear mites even if they have no visible signs.

Signs vary from mild pruritus with mild erythema of the external canal to dropped ears to excoriations with severe crusting. In advanced cases, the crusts form a cast of the canal. Ear mites can colonize other areas of the body, especially the perineum. Secondary otitis media with head tilt is a common sequela.

My treatment of choice for ear mites is ivermectin, 300 to 400 μg/kg SC every 2 weeks until the mites have been eliminated. The crusts must be removed, and the secondary otitis externa treated with antibiotic-glucocorticoid otitis products.

In colonies, I recommend monthly ivermectin treatment as part of the routine management.

NONSPECIFIC PRURITUS

Pruritus of unknown etiology does occur in these animals. It is infrequent in my experience, but if after changing food, bedding, and disinfectant and obtaining skin scrapings, culture, and biopsy samples a cause cannot be found, I control the symptom with oral glucocorticoids. Perhaps some rodents and rabbits have allergic inhalant dermatitis or contact hypersensitivity. (Intradermal skin testing is difficult to do on a mouse or gerbil!) I use oral prednisolone at doses of 0.2 to 0.02 mg/kg every other day after slightly higher doses have controlled the pruritus. The smaller the beast, the higher the dose (metabolic scaling). Therapy is periodically withdrawn to see if the problem still exists. Response has been favorable. Polydipsia has been reported by owners, and polyuria also presumably occurs but is not objectionable. I do not think I have caused a clinically overt case of iatrogenic Cushing-like disease—at least not alopecia.

PERINEAL PRURITUS OF MICE

Pinworm infection in mice commonly causes perineal pruritus. Diagnosis can be made by fecal flotation, but a cellophane tape test is better. Treatment is with ivermectin, 200 μg/kg PO, or with thiabendazole, 100 mg/kg every 7 days for four doses; or with mebendazole, 40 mg/kg two doses 7 days apart.

ENDOCRINE ALOPECIA

In rodents, nonpruritic, symmetric alopecia is uncommon. When present, it is almost always in an aged animal. Biopsy reveals histologic lesions characteristic of an endocrinopathy. The cause usually is an adrenal tumor, although ovarian cysts have caused alopecia in guinea pigs. Treatment is removal of the tumor or cyst if possible.

Endocrine alopecia caused by hyperadrenocorticism, hypothyroidism, and hyperestrogenism is commonly encountered in ferrets. In the latter, the associated bone marrow suppression is of more immediate concern (see this volume, p. 1185). Diagnosis and treatment of adrenal and thyroid dysfunction parallel that for dogs and cats. Normal ranges for resting endocrine values in ferrets are as follows:

Cortisol: 3.86–74.52 nmol/L
T_3: 0.45–1.78 nmol/L
T_4: 13.0–106.7 nmol/L

In general, these values are similar to those in cats, except for T_3 and T_4 in males, which are higher than those in females and are more comparable to normal values in dogs.

SEASONAL ALOPECIA OF FERRETS

Partial alopecia is associated with the breeding season in both males and females. Even neutered animals have thinning of the coat associated with lengthening daylight and warmer ambient temperatures. Traumatic hair loss in estral females will not regrow until about 3 weeks after ovulation.

References and Suggested Reading

Collins, B. R.: Dermatologic disorders of common small nondomestic mammals. *In* Nesbitt, G. H. (ed.): *Topics in Small Animal Medicine: Dermatology.* New York: Churchill Livingstone, 1987.

Fox, J. G., Cohen, B. J., and Loew, F. M.: *Laboratory Animal Medicine.* Orlando, FL: Academic Press, 1984.

Fox, J. G.: *Biology and Diseases of the Ferret.* Philadelphia: Lea & Febiger, 1988.

Harkness, J. E., and Wagner, J. E.: *The Biology and Medicine of Rabbits and Rodents,* 3rd ed. Philadelphia: Lea & Febiger, 1989.

Heard, D. J., Collins, B., Chen, D., et al.: Thyroid and adrenal function tests in adult male ferrets. Am. J. Vet. Res. 15:32, 1990.

Timm, K. I.: Pruritus in rabbits, rodents and ferrets. Vet. Clin. North Am. Small Anim. Pract. 18:1077, 1988.

REPRODUCTIVE DISORDERS IN THE RABBIT AND GUINEA PIG

RICHARD E. FISH
and CYNTHIA BESCH-WILLIFORD
Columbia, Missouri

Veterinarians may be asked to attend rabbits or guinea pigs in a variety of settings. The clinical approach to reproductive disorders in different situations may vary considerably but should parallel the practitioner's experiences with other species. Owners of pet rabbits or guinea pigs will not usually be engaged in intensive breeding efforts, but reproductive disorders, at times life-threatening, may arise and require attention. Routine preventive or therapeutic castration and ovariohysterectomy are often necessary. In production settings, reproductive performance is fundamental to economic success, and disorders must be approached with a view toward herd health and preventive medicine.

The purpose of this article is to provide an introduction to the reproductive problems commonly encountered in rabbits and guinea pigs. As with more common domestic species, many if not most reproductive problems can be traced to marginal husbandry practices, inadequate or excessive nutrition, or lack of basic knowledge on proper reproductive management. Additional background in these areas may be found in *CVT X* (p. 738) and in the texts listed at the end of the article.

ANATOMY AND PHYSIOLOGY

Basic reproductive data for the rabbit and guinea pig are in Table 1; the data may not apply precisely to a particular breed, geographical area, or production setting. Unique features of the female rabbit (doe) include completely separated uterine horns, each with a cervix opening into the vagina; reflex (induced) ovulation without a true estrous cycle; and almost continuous receptivity to mating. The female guinea pig (sow) has a relatively long estrous cycle and gestation (compared with other rodents); an easily detected behavioral estrus; and an imperforate vaginal closure membrane that opens spontaneously during estrus and parturition. Unlike rabbits, adult guinea pigs may be housed together permanently. The male guinea pig (boar) has elongated, smooth vesicular glands that may be mistaken for uterine horns at necropsy. Both the boar and the male rabbit (buck) have open inguinal canals.

REPRODUCTIVE DISORDERS IN THE RABBIT

Reduced Fertility

A variety of nutritional deficiencies or excesses may affect the reproductive system. Adequacy of dietary protein and energy, as well as other specific nutrients, should be an early consideration whenever individual or colony signs include reduced fertility (decreased conception rates or fetal resorption), abortions, birth of weak litters, or increased

Table 1. *Reproductive Data in the Rabbit and Guinea Pig*

	Rabbit	Guinea Pig
Adult body weight	(F) 2–6 kg	700–900 gm
	(M) 2–5 kg	900–1200 gm
Sexual maturity	(F) 4–9 months	600–700 gm (3–4 months)
	(M) 6–10 months	350–450 gm (2–3 months)
Breeding life	1–3 yr	1.5–3 yr
Mammary glands	4 pairs	1 pair (inguinal)
Estrous cycle	none*	15–17 days
Postpartum estrus	none*	fertile
Ovulation	10–14 hours postcoitus	spontaneous
Mating system	hand-mated (female to male cage)	1 male:1–10 females continuously
Gestation	29–35 (31–32) days	59–72 (68) days
Pregnancy detection	palpation, 10–14 days; mammary development, 24+ days; x-rays, 11+ days	palpation, 4–5 wk; pubic symphysis separation at term (20–25 mm)
Pseudopregnancy	15–17 days	17 days (rare)
Litter size	4–10	2–5
Birth weight	30–80 gm	70–100 gm
Eyes open	10 days	at birth
Begin eating solid food	3 wk	3 days
Weaning age	4–6 wk	2–3 wk (or 150–200 gm)

*The rabbit is an induced ovulator without a readily detectable estrous cycle. There is, however, a highly variable rhythmicity in sexual receptivity. Most postparturient does are receptive and fertile, although not usually bred for 4 to 6 weeks or until postweaning.

neonatal mortality. Optimal reproductive performance requires close attention to the rabbit's physical state and avoidance of undercondition or obesity.

Environmental conditions may also limit reproductive performance. The rabbit, in general, is more tolerant of cold than heat; temperatures of 32°C (90°F) or higher may result in heatstroke or prostration, a special concern for heavy, pregnant does. High temperatures are associated with reduced feed intake and reduced performance. Bucks may show transient sterility with relatively short-term exposure to high temperatures.

In fall and winter, it is common for commercial rabbit producers to experience a variable period when some does refuse to breed, litter size and kit weight decrease, and incidence of maternal neglect increases. Research data on "winter breeding depression" is conflicting, but maintenance of peak production requires adequate nutrition in cold weather and provision of a light/dark cycle with 16 hours of light.

Mature does are receptive to mating most of the time, although there are cyclic patterns of nonreceptivity. Occasionally, a doe may refuse one buck, especially if the buck is young or inexperienced, but accept another. In such situations, mating may be assisted by gentle manual restraint of the doe. Pseudopregnancy may result from sterile matings or from mounting behavior between does or even with kits. Does are generally not receptive until the termination of pseudopregnancy at 16 to 18 days.

Breeding life of the doe varies with breeding intensity but is generally less than 3 years. First litters tend to be smaller in all does, but decreased litter size thereafter is usually indicative of aging changes in the uterus and may be an early sign of developing uterine adenocarcinoma, the most common neoplasia of the female rabbit. Incidence of uterine adenocarcinoma appears to be breed-related and may exceed 50% in high incidence breeds (e.g. Tan, Dutch) over 3 years of age. Pathogenesis of the neoplasia is closely related to progressive senile changes in the endometrium. These changes are responsible for reproductive impairment resulting in decreased litter size, abortion, stillbirth, and retained fetuses up to a year before tumor detection. Bloody vulvar discharge may be seen at later stages. Initially, neoplasia is limited to the uterus, forming multiple nodules that can be palpated, but progresses to local and pulmonary metastatic disease and death. Aging female rabbits should be palpated regularly, and ovariohysterectomy considered for the pet doe.

Rabbits are particularly susceptible to *Pasteurella multocida* infection. Although primarily an upper respiratory pathogen, it may affect virtually any organ system, and cases of vulvovaginitis, metritis, pyometra, balanoposthitis, and orchitis have been reported. Detailed discussions of rabbit pasteurellosis may be found elsewhere in the literature (see *CVT VIII*, p. 669).

Rabbits are also susceptible to infection with *Treponema paraluis-cuniculi,* a spirochete responsible for rabbit syphilis (treponematosis, venereal spirochetosis, or vent disease). Clinical signs, when present, include dry, crusty lesions of the skin and mucous membranes of the genitalia and face. The crusts may overlie areas of reddening, erosion, or ulceration. Cutaneous lesions may impair breeding performance, especially when there is significant involvement of the prepuce. In colony outbreaks, infection of females may result in reduced conception rates, metritis and retained placenta, and increased neonatal deaths. In individual cases, the course is self-limiting. Serologic diagnosis may be made with the rapid plasma reagin (RPR) card test (Kit No. 110, Hynson, Westcott & Dunning, Baltimore, MD) or other methods used in human clinical practice to detect antibody to *Treponema pallidum;* animal diagnostic laboratories may also be able to perform these tests. Treatment with procaine penicillin G is effective (40,000 IU/kg IM every 24 hr for 5 to 7 days). Commercial producers generally include a 3- to 5-day penicillin regime in quarantine procedures for newly received breeding stock.

Prenatal Mortality

The doe is particularly susceptible to fetal dislodgement and resorption at two stages of pregnancy: day 13 and days 20 to 23. Actual abortion (fetal loss after day 24) in the rabbit is rare.

The rabbit is relatively sensitive to excessive dietary vitamin A or carotene. Signs may include abortion, resorption, birth of small, weak litters, and increased neonatal mortality; hydrocephalus in the kits also may become evident. Rabbits require about 10,000 IU/kg diet of vitamin A activity, but toxic levels (190,000 IU/kg or more) can be readily achieved by feeding diets that are high in alfalfa and supplemented with a vitamin mix. Interestingly, signs of vitamin A deficiency may be very similar to those of an excess, although deficiency is unlikely with most commercially available rabbit rations. The rabbit is also relatively sensitive to vitamin D toxicity. Administration of 10,000 IU per day for 3 days has reportedly resulted in significantly elevated fetal loss.

Rabbit rations or water supplies may become contaminated with toxic agents that affect reproduction. Depending on the source of dietary ingredients, plant toxins or phytoestrogens should be considered in diagnosis of reproductive disorders.

Any systemic illness that results in reduced condition may lead to fetal loss. Differential diagnosis of abortion, with or without bloody or mucopurulent vaginal discharge and other clinical signs, should include coccidiosis, pasteurellosis, salmonellosis (*Salmonella typhimurium* or *enteritidis*), or listeriosis (*Listeria monocytogenes*).

Pregnancy toxemia (ketosis) is often not recognized in the rabbit. The clinical features are not substantially different from those in other species, including the guinea pig (discussed later). As in other species, the most important predisposing factors are concurrent obesity and inappetence.

Gastric trichobezoars (hairballs) are an important consideration in any anorectic rabbit with normal temperature; hair pulling by does for nest preparation may predispose toward obstructive hairball formation, especially when dietary fiber is inadequate. Signs are nonspecific, consisting principally of reduced appetite and scant feces; rabbits may go off feed completely but survive for weeks. Large hairballs occasionally may be palpable or detected by contrast radiography. Rapid recognition and treatment of the anorectic rabbit is important for successful management, especially in the late-term doe where subsequent ketosis or agalactia is a concern. None of the variety of suggested treatments results in consistent success, and some hairballs resolve spontaneously. Anorectic rabbits should be enticed to eat with fresh, clean vegetables, high-quality alfalfa hay, or alfalfa cubes. If a hairball is suspected, fresh pineapple juice may be administered (10 ml PO every 8 to 12 hr for 3 to 5 days) to provide proteolytic enzymes that help break down the hair mass. Surgical removal of the obstruction should be considered if rabbits are totally anorectic for more than 3 days. Postsurgical recovery is often prolonged but is improved by prompt action and intensive care.

Dystocia and Retained Fetus

Dystocia is rare in the rabbit. Does usually deliver in the early morning, completing delivery in less than 30 minutes. Occasionally, however, delivery of normal, healthy young may be separated by hours or even days. Both anterior and posterior presentations of fetuses are normal. Fetuses retained for more than 35 days die and often become mummified, which can cause permanent infertility. For this reason, does should be routinely palpated 24 hours after delivery and treated with oxytocin (3 to 5 units IM) if fetuses are present. If uterine inertia occurs, treatment with 10% calcium gluconate (5 to 10 ml PO or 3 to 5 ml IV) 30 minutes prior to oxytocin has been suggested (Raphael, 1981).

Postnatal Morbidity and Mortality

A key behavioral feature of the doe is the preparation of a nest 2 to 3 days prepartum. Straw or shavings should be provided in a separate box, to which the doe will add fur pulled from her legs and abdomen. Failure to provide a nesting site and suitable substrate, as well as any unnecessary disturbance, will result in litter abandonment. Primiparous does are especially excitable and do not prepare quality nests. Does characteristically nurse once or twice daily and otherwise pay little attention to the young; they will not usually retrieve young separated from the nest. Cannibalism in the rabbit is rare but may occur if young are born dead or deformed, if a nest is not provided, or if an excitable doe is disturbed. Litter mortality may be reduced by limiting the doe's access to the nest and litter to a 30-minute period once daily.

Any impairment in milk production may result in neonatal loss. Does will normally reduce their feed intake several days before delivery but should increase intake rapidly postpartum as milk production increases (peak production is at 2 to 3 weeks). Water requirements also increase rapidly with lactation, and failure to provide adequate water will have a direct effect on milk production. Anorexia may result from pregnancy toxemia, hairballs (see earlier), or mastitis.

Mastitis in the doe occurs sporadically and is most often associated with heavy-milking does, improper sanitation, or teat injury during early lactation. Etiologic agents include *Staphylococcus*, *Pasteurella*, and *Streptococcus*. Clinical signs include anorexia, fever above 40°C (104°F), depression, and death of the neonates and doe may result. One or more glands may be affected, initially appearing swollen and hyperemic; without attention, glands become bluish as swelling progresses, and abscesses may develop. Clinical management consists of palliative treatment of swollen, painful, or abscessed mammary glands (warm packs, draining and flushing of abscesses) and systemic antibiotics. Penicillin may be administered initially (as discussed earlier) pending culture and sensitivity tests. Kits are often fostered if the affected doe refuses to allow young to nurse, but this may result in transmission of mastitis to other does. Hand-rearing of kits may be attempted but is often unsuccessful. Limiting feed prepartum will help minimize mammary engorgement.

REPRODUCTIVE DISORDERS IN THE GUINEA PIG

Reduced Fertility

General guidelines on the importance of nutrition for the rabbit apply equally to the guinea pig. Obesity or inadequate dietary vitamin C in particular may have significant effects on guinea pig reproduction.

Husbandry conditions and colony management may affect reproductive performance in several ways. Guinea pigs may be weaned at a relatively young age, but males may not develop normal breeding behavior if isolated from the sow or other pigs at too young an age. Limb fracture and pododermatitis are always a concern in heavy, pregnant sows housed on wire mesh floors, especially if animals are moved to wire after being raised on a solid surface. Guinea pigs housed on solid surfaces should have bedding, but finely ground or dusty materials should be avoided. In the female, bedding may stick to the vulva and vestibule, causing inflammation. In the male, bedding material may collect either in the perineal folds of skin or in the preputial fornix following mating. Even without bedding, the boar will develop scrotal plugs, a collection of sebaceous secretions that leads to irritation of the underlying skin. In each case, treatment involves gentle cleansing of the area, removal of offending material, and temporary placement of the animal in dry, clean, bedding-free quarters. The boar also may develop urethral obstruction from uroliths or proteinaceous masses associated with congealed ejaculate. The effects of excessive heat on reproductive performance are similar to the rabbit.

Prenatal Mortality

Abortion and stillbirth are especially common in the guinea pig. The pregnant sow may almost double in weight as parturition approaches and during the last trimester is susceptible to fetal loss following improper handling. Sudden noise can trigger a "stampede" or circling among group-housed adults and can result in abortion. Stillbirth (but not abortion) incidence is directly correlated with litter size and may reflect the sow's failure to remove fetal membranes rapidly.

Abortion is most often associated with pregnancy toxemia (ketosis). The most important and consistent predisposing factors for pregnancy toxemia are concurrent obesity and fasting. Pregnancy toxemia usually affects sows in the first or second pregnancy during the last 2 weeks of gestation or first several days postpartum. The onset of signs is abrupt, with anorexia followed shortly by prostration, dyspnea, and often death within 2 to 5 days. Animals are usually hypoglycemic (<60 mg/dl), ketonemic, aciduric (normal urine pH is 9), and proteinuric. Necropsy usually shows an obese animal with empty stomach and fatty liver. There are no consistently effective treatments; therefore, prevention is key. Obesity should be avoided, as well as changes in routine, environmental stress, and exposure to infectious agents, any of which may result in anorexia.

Dietary vitamin C requirements increase during gestation, and marginal deficiencies may contribute to the relatively high incidence of abortion and stillbirth. Scurvy is characterized initially by nonspecific signs such as anorexia, rough haircoat, lethargy, and weakness and later by joint enlargement and subcutaneous hemorrhage. Tooth grinding and joint tenderness may be noticed with handling. Vitamin C is present in guinea pig rations from reputable suppliers but is susceptible to degradation from heat, moisture, and light. Feed kept at room temperature for more than 90 days may also have losses that can result in clinical scurvy. Supplementation in water can be effective, but only if water intake remains normal and water is changed daily. Dietary supplementation with fresh vegetables such as green pepper, kale, or cabbage may supply dietary needs. When recognized in pregnant guinea pigs, scurvy should be treated by daily administration of L-ascorbic acid at 30 mg/kg body weight, either parenterally or in feed or water, until signs regress. Additional supportive care such as force feeding or fluid therapy may be needed.

The most common infectious diseases of guinea pigs are bacterial and affect primarily the respiratory or lymphatic systems. Outbreaks of disease caused by *Bordetella bronchiseptica*, *Streptococcus zooepidemicus*, or *Streptococcus pneumoniae* have been associated with infertility, abortions, and stillbirths, as well as more typical upper respiratory problems, cervical lymphadenitis (*S. zooepidemicus*), pneumonia, or acute death. Sporadic outbreaks of salmonellosis (usually *S. typhimurium* or *S. enteritidis*) have been reported, with acute death the most common sign; abortions may occur, but diarrhea is uncommon. Treatment of bacterial disease is complicated by the guinea pig's high susceptibility to fatal, antibiotic-induced enterotoxemia and by the public health concerns if salmonellosis is suspected. Broad-spectrum antibiotics may be used with caution, and chloramphenicol is relatively safe (30–50 mg/kg PO every 24 hr for 5 to 7 days); however, systemic antibiotics may not be effective in completely eliminating infections.

Dystocia

Dystocia is relatively common in the guinea pig and is usually associated with failure of the pubic symphysis to relax fully as parturition approaches. Fusion or incomplete symphyseal relaxation results most commonly from delay of first breeding past 7 months of age. Other predisposing factors include obesity and presence of large fetuses. Clinical signs are often nonspecific (depression, anorexia) but, along with history and stage of pregnancy, suggest the diagnosis. Additional signs may include bloody or greenish-brown vulvar discharge and other signs attributable to concurrent ketosis. Successful management of dystocia requires early recognition of the problem. If the pubic symphysis is not adequately dilated for the stage of gestation (20 to 25 mm at term), prompt cesarean section is indicated. Anesthetic and surgical considerations are similar to those in other species, keeping in mind that even the healthy, nonpregnant guinea pig is a poor anesthetic risk. Particular attention is required for the newborn, who will not survive long in the dead sow, in the isolated uterus, or if left covered by fetal membranes. Cases of simple uterine inertia may be handled by oxytocin injection (0.2 to 3.0 units/kg IM) if the pelvic canal is sufficiently dilated.

Some producers have improved overall performance by routinely inducing parturition in sows that have reached day 66 or more of gestation and have adequate separation of the pubic symphysis. Oxytocin (2 units IM) should induce first delivery within 20 min but may be repeated an additional two times at 30-min intervals if there is no initial response (Hafez, 1970).

Postnatal Morbidity and Mortality

Guinea pigs are born precocious and can be raised relatively easily if orphaned. For overall growth and development, however, at least 2 weeks of nursing is optimal. Young will also begin eating solid food within several days and need access to feed and water. Guinea pigs with birth weights less than 50 to 60 gm generally do not survive. The sow has only two mammae but can usually support larger litters easily. Litters of three to four have the best chance of survival.

The sow does not make a nest and is not highly territorial or possessive of the young. In group housing situations, young may nurse and be accepted by other lactating females. Larger, more aggressive young may actually deplete milk from some sows to the detriment of their weaker littermates. Another problem in group housing is the potential for young to be trampled by startled, "stampeding" adults. Cannibalism in the guinea pig is rare.

As in the rabbit, agalactia may result from inadequate nutrition or anorexia (discussed earlier), or from mastitis, which is relatively common in the guinea pig. Infection is usually caused by alpha-hemolytic streptococci, *Escherichia coli*, or *Staphylococcus*. In acute cases, both the glands and milk may take on a dark red appearance, and the sow may die within days. Treatment is generally limited to systemic antibiotics (discussed earlier), plus localized, palliative treatment of the glands and other supportive care.

References and Suggested Reading

Cheeke, P. R., Patton, N. M., Lukefahr, S. D. et al.: *Rabbit Production.* Danville, IL: The Interstate Printers & Publishers, 1987.
Recent and comprehensive text for rabbit raisers of all backgrounds; contains detailed chapters on management, nutrition, reproduction, and diseases.
Fox, J. G., Cohen, B. J., Loew, F. M. (eds.): *Laboratory Animal Medicine.* Orlando, FL: Academic Press, 1984.
Authoritative reference work, in part a distillation of other texts in the American College of Laboratory Animal Medicine series; contains chapters, by species, on biology and diseases, plus additional chapters on biomethodology, anesthesiology, etc.
Hafez, E. F. E. (ed.): *Reproduction and Breeding Techniques for Laboratory Animals.* Philadelphia: Lea & Febiger, 1970.
A comprehensive text on reproduction in laboratory animals; contains useful chapters, by species, on practical breeding techniques.
Harkness, J. E., and Wagner, J. E.: *The Biology and Medicine of Rabbits and Rodents.* Philadelphia: Lea & Febiger, 1989.
Extremely useful, economical, up-to-date text; emphasizes practical aspects of care and health; intended audience includes practicing veterinarians and students.
Morrow, D. A. (ed.): *Current Therapy in Theriogenology 2.* Philadelphia: W. B. Saunders, 1986.
Up-to-date text in CVT format, intended for the veterinarian and veterinary student; Section XII (Laboratory Animals) contains chapters on the rabbit and guinea pig.
Poole, T. B. (ed.): *The UFAW Handbook on the Care and Management of Laboratory Animals.* New York: Churchill Livingstone, 1987.
Completely rewritten sixth edition with separate chapters on the rabbit and guinea pig; oriented primarily to laboratory animals in the research setting, but excellent source of information on basic husbandry.
Raphael, B. L.: *Pet rabbit medicine.* Comp. Cont. Ed. Pract. Vet. 3:60, 1981.
General introductory article on common problems encountered with rabbits as companion animals.
Wagner, J. E., and Manning, P. J. (eds.): *The Biology of the Guinea Pig.* New York: Academic Press, 1976.
Authoritative reference work; part of the American College of Laboratory Animal Medicine text series; chapters on genetics, husbandry, anatomy and physiology, biomethodology, plus over half devoted to diseases.
Weisbroth, S. H., Flatt, R. E., Kraus, A. L. (eds.): *The Biology of the Laboratory Rabbit.* New York: Academic Press, 1974.
The first text published in the American College of Laboratory Animal Medicine series.

FERRET COLITIS

MARK R. FINKLER

Roanoke, Virginia

The wide acceptance of the domestic ferret (*Mustela putorius furo*) as a household pet has led to an increased demand for veterinary services for these animals. As with dogs and cats, diarrhea is one of the most common complaints.

Diarrhea is commonly seen in a wide number of disorders and diseases of ferrets. Apparently, any event that disrupts normal homeostasis is capable of inducing diarrhea. The normal ferret stool is formed (tubular) but only semisolid and never hard. It should be noted that the normal gastrointestinal transit time is about 4 hours. Any disorder that shortens the already abbreviated transit time will lead to diarrhea. Furthermore, many clinically normal ferrets are carriers of *Helicobacter* (*Campylobacter*), which may act as opportunistic pathogens capable of inducing diarrhea whenever the host is under stress.

TYPES OF COLITIS

Colitis is one of the most common causes of diarrhea in ferrets. Two types of colitis are seen: the acute form and the chronic (proliferative) form.

Acute Colitis

A ferret with acute colitis will present with the typical signs of large-bowel diarrhea, including frequent defecation and tenesmus. Mucoid stools are common and vary in color from greenish black to brown with flecks of fresh blood. Some ferrets will vocalize in pain while defecating. A fever may or may not be present. Partial rectal prolapse is common, particularly in 2- to 4-month-old kits.

Nearly all ferrets with colitis are under 1 year of age. In fact, most cases involve young ferrets recently acquired and subjected to the stress of weaning, transport, and dietary change.

Morbidity within groups of ferrets is typically low but can be high. While mortality rates tend to be low, some ferrets will die within 3 to 4 days of onset of hemorrhagic diarrhea.

Chronic (Proliferative) Colitis

The chronic form of colitis in ferrets has been descriptively termed *proliferative colitis* (Fox et al.,

1982). As with the acute form, most cases involve ferrets under 1 year of age. The diarrhea tends to be mucoid or mucohemorrhagic with an occasional normal or near normal stool. Dramatic weight loss over a 1- to 2-month period is common. Lethargy and varying degrees of dehydration are seen. A fluctuating fever is typical. Partial rectal prolapse secondary to tenesmus may be observed. Careful palpation of the abdomen will often reveal a thickened colon.

Morbidity rates tend to be low. For many years, the disease was considered incurable, leading to death or euthanasia of afflicted ferrets. Recently, the author reported the first successful cure of a case of proliferative colitis (Finkler, 1987).

ETIOLOGY

Current evidence suggests that *Helicobacter jejuni* or *Helicobacter*-like organisms are a factor in ferret colitis, though an exact etiopathogenesis remains unknown. The fact that the clinical course can usually be reversed with antimicrobial therapy further suggests an infectious agent is involved. Undoubtedly, other factors such as stress and integrity of the individual's immune system play a role in the pathogenesis of colitis.

DIAGNOSIS

Helicobacter-associated colitis should be suspected whenever a ferret under 1 year of age presents with a history and signs of large-bowel diarrhea as described. Common differential diagnoses such as dietary indiscretion and foreign bodies may be ruled out through the history and physical exam.

Plain and contrast radiology may be necessary to rule out foreign bodies and intussusceptions. Barium sulfate (10 to 15 ml/ferret of a 30%–50% w/v suspension) may be administered orally after sedating with acepromazine (0.1 mg/kg SQ) or ketamine (2.5 mg/kg SQ). (Ferrets not sedated exhibit delayed stomach emptying.) Within 3 hours, nearly all of the barium should be found within the colon. It should be noted that ferrets lack a cecum.

Various methods of fecal analysis should be employed. Fresh saline smears can be examined for

Giardia; however, this method is unreliable in identifying *Helicobacter* unless special staining techniques are utilized. Fecal flotations in sodium nitrate and sugar solutions may be performed to identify coccidia and *Cryptosporidium,* respectively. (Helminth intestinal parasitism is rare to nonexistent in domestic ferrets in the United States.)

Fresh feces should be cultured for *Helicobacter* and *Salmonella. Helicobacter* organisms are microaerophilic and will not be successfully cultured in private practices utilizing outside laboratories unless a special transport medium is used. The author collects fresh feces with a sterile swab or loop inserted into the ferret's rectum and immediately inoculated into Cary Blair Transport Medium (Regional Media Laboratories, Lenexa, KS). Ideally, the specimen should arrive at the laboratory within 4 to 6 hours of collection for highest yields. While a positive culture supports the diagnosis, a negative culture does not rule it out.

Proliferative colitis may be confirmed by histopathology of colonic biopsy specimens collected via endoscopy or laparotomy. Warthin-Starry–stained sections will usually reveal *Helicobacter*-like organisms.

When faced with financial constraints by the ferret owner, a favorable response to treatment may also support the diagnosis of colitis.

Another ferret disease that must be differentiated from proliferative colitis is Aleutian disease, a parvoviral infection first identified in minks. Both are chronic, progressive wasting diseases with black, tarry stools as a common feature. However, ferrets with Aleutian disease typically have pathology in other organ systems, hypergammaglobulinemia, and a positive titer to the virus.

TREATMENT

The author has found only two antimicrobial agents to be beneficial in treating either form of colitis. Chloramphenicol (10 mg/kg every 8–12 hr PO × 10–14 days) is the initial choice. A highly palatable form, Chloromycetin Palmitate Oral Sus-pension (Parke-Davis), is preferred. The author has had permanent remission of signs in over 90% of the treated cases with this agent. If little to no improvement is seen within 14 days or if a relapse occurs, the parenteral form of gentamicin (2 mg/kg every 12 hr PO × 10–14 days) is diluted with a small volume of water and administered orally with an eye dropper. This is usually successful in treating nonresponsive or relapsing cases.

Supportive care is important, particularly in the proliferative form. Electrolyte solutions are administered orally or subcutaneously. A palatable, high-calorie nutritional supplement, Nutri-Cal (Evsco Pharmaceuticals), is also administered. Intestinal protectants, narcotic-type antidiarrheal medications, and sulfasalazine provide little or no benefit.

Rectal prolapses are treated with a topical anesthetic and reduced, and a pursestring suture is left in place for 10 days.

PROGNOSIS AND ZOONOTIC THREAT

Except for cases that present in a moribund condition, the prognosis is good to excellent. Even ferrets with marked weight loss seen in the chronic form have shown dramatic responses to treatment. Relapse, though infrequent, may occur.

Although ferrets have not been incriminated in any cases of human campylobacteriosis, the zoonotic potential should be discussed with the owner.

References and Suggested Reading

Davenport, D. J.: Campylobacter enteritis. *In* Kirk, R. W. (ed.): *Current Veterinary Therapy X.* Philadelphia: WB Saunders, 1989, p. 944.
A concise review of the salient features of Campylobacter *enteritis in domestic animals.*
Finkler, M. R.: Treatment of proliferative colitis in a pet ferret. Ferret 1:2, 1987.
A case study of a pet ferret successfully treated for proliferative colitis.
Fox, J. G., Murphy, J. C., Ackerman, J. I., et al.: Proliferative colitis in ferrets. Am. J. Vet. Res. 43:858, 1982.
A review of the clinical presentation and histopathologic changes observed in a group of laboratory ferrets with proliferative colitis.
Krueger, K. L., Murphy, J. C., and Fox, J. G.: Treatment of proliferative colitis in ferrets. J.A.V.M.A. 194:1435, 1989.
A study comparing chloramphenicol therapy with supportive care in the treatment of proliferative colitis.

EOSINOPHILIC GASTROENTERITIS IN THE FERRET

LORI S. PALLEY
and JAMES G. FOX
Cambridge, Massachusetts

Eosinophilic gastroenteritis (EG) is a recently recognized idiopathic syndrome in the domestic ferret (Fox et al., 1989, 1991). It is characterized by the presence of eosinophilic infiltration of the gastrointestinal tract with unique histopathological features and is accompanied by gastrointestinal symptoms. The frequency of the disease is unknown. Its presence in a ferret with gastrointestinal disease must be differentiated from other diseases with similar clinical presentations.

DIAGNOSIS

History and Presentation

Eosinophilic gastroenteritis has been diagnosed infrequently in pet ferrets and ferrets used in biomedical research. It has been identified in several geographic areas of the United States.

Chronic weight loss, anorexia, and bloody, mucoid diarrhea are the most common clinical complaints. Ferrets may also have episodic vomiting. One ferret presented with a history of reproductive failure. Ferrets with EG appear thin and unkempt and may be dehydrated. The most notable findings include enlarged mesenteric lymph nodes and thickened intestine on abdominal palpation. Afflicted ferrets are young to middle age (range, 6 months to 4 years). There does not appear to be any sex predilection.

Laboratory Findings

In ferrets with gastrointestinal signs and chronic weight loss, the following data should be collected: complete blood count, chemistry profile, fecal flotation/occult blood analysis, heartworm test, rectal culture, urinalysis, Aleutian disease virus serology, and radiographs. A peripheral blood sample can be obtained by jugular venipuncture (Otto et al., 1990).

Rectal cultures should be submitted for isolation of *Campylobacter* and *Salmonella* species.

In ferrets with EG, hemogram reveals peripheral eosinophilia. The average eosinophilia level in normal ferrets is 2.5% (range, 0% to 7%), with an average total leukocyte count of 10,100 cells/mm^3 (range 4000 to 19,000) (Ryland et al., 1983). The average eosinophilia level in ferrets with EG is 22% (range, 10% to 35%). The average absolute eosinophil count calculated from six cases at the time of presentation is 2582 eosinophils/mm^3, (range, 1190 to 4480). Another consistent finding is hypoalbuminemia ($\leq$3.0 mg/dl). Fecal analysis is unremarkable.

Histopathologic Findings

Definitive diagnosis of eosinophilic gastroenteritis in the ferret is obtained by exploratory laparotomy and histopathologic evaluation of intestine and mesenteric lymph node biopsies. EG in ferrets involves mild to severe infiltration of stomach and small intestine with eosinophils. Infiltrates may extend through the serosa, producing an eosinophilic serositis. Reactive fibrous tissue seen in cats with a similar disease is not a component of the disease in ferrets. Additionally, focal eosinophilic granulomas accompanied by a histopathologic entity termed Splendore-Hoeppli (SH) phenomenon are present in mesenteric lymph nodes. Splendore-Hoeppli phenomenon is eosinophilic material in the form of radiating clubs or concentric rings surrounding helminths, bacteria, and fungi (Johnson, 1976). This is a distinguishing feature of the gastrointestinal disorder in ferrets not described in other eosinophilic gastroenteritides.

No evidence of helminths was observed, and special stains did not reveal the presence of bacteria or fungi in association with the granulomas and SH phenomenon. In addition to the complement of lesions described, one case had severe hepatic peri-

Table 1. Differential Diagnoses for Clinical Signs Associated with Eosinophilic Gastroenteritis in Ferrets

Disease	Clinical Signs	Clinicopathologic Findings	Histopathology	Treatment
Aleutian disease	Subclinical Anemia, anorexia, weight loss	Gamma globulin >20% TP, antibody positive for ADV	Lymphocytic-plasmacytic infiltrations in several organ systems	Supportive therapy (Fox et al., 1988)
Lymphosarcoma	Anorexia, weight loss, splenomegaly, peripheral lymphadenopathy	Peripheral lymphocytosis >55% Anemia, leukopenia Thrombocytopenia	Lymphocytic infiltrations in several organ systems	Cyclophosphamide*/vincristine sulfate†/prednisone (feline dosage) (Goad et al., 1988)
Eosinophilic gastroenteritis	Vomiting, diarrhea, weight loss, anorexia Palpable mesenteric lymphadenopathy	Peripheral eosinophilia, albumin ≤3.0 gm/dl	Eosinophilic infiltrations in stomach, small intestine, mesenteric lymph node, liver Splendore-Hoeppli phenomenon	Prednisone (1.25–2.5 mg PO once daily [every other day])
Gastric ulcers	Subclinical Abdominal pain, melena	Fecal, occult blood positive	Mucosal ulcers with mononuclear infiltrations, *Helicobacter* (*Campylobacter*) *mustelae*	Amoxicillin‡ (10 mg/kg), Bismuth subsalicylate§ (17.5 mg/kg) Metronidazole‖ (20 mg/kg all PO t.i.d. × 21 days) Cimetidine¶ (5–10 mg/kg PO t.i.d.) (Otto et al., 1990)
Gastric or intestinal foreign bodies	Vomiting Abdominal pain	Palpable per abdomen Radiographic evidence	Not applicable	Petroleum base laxative** Endoscopy Surgery (Fox, 1988)
Proliferative colitis	Diarrhea, thickened palpable colon, prolapsed rectum	Fecal, occult blood positive	Colonic mucosal cell proliferation, reduced goblet cells, intracellular *Campylobacter*-like organisms	Chloramphenicol†† (50 mg/kg PO b.i.d. × 10 days) (Krueger et al., 1989)
Salmonellosis	Subclinical carrier Diarrhea, pyrexia, conjunctivitis, abortion	Rectal culture positive	Hyperemic intestinal vessels, distended gall bladder, necrotic foci—liver, spleen	Supportive care Trimethoprim-sulfa Oral Suspension‡‡ 15 mg/kg PO b.i.d. or Chloramphenicol 50 mg/kg PO b.i.d. (Dillon, 1986)

*Cytoxan, Mead Johnson.
†Oncovin, Eli Lilly, and Co.
‡Biomox, Biocraft Laboratories, Inc.
§Pepto-Bismol Liquid, Procter and Gamble.
‖Flagyl, G. D. Searle, and Co.
¶Tagamet HCl Liquid, Smith Kline and French Laboratories.
**Laxatone, Evsco Pharmaceuticals.
††Chloromycetin Palmitate Oral Suspension, Parke-Davis.
‡‡Sulfatrim Pediatric Suspension, Henry Schein, Inc.

portal eosinophilic granulomas and a perivascular eosinophilic granulomatous infiltrate in the choroid plexus.

Differential Diagnosis

Eosinophilic gastroenteritis in ferrets must be differentiated from proliferative colitis, intestinal lymphosarcoma, gastroduodenal ulcers, gastric or intestinal foreign bodies, salmonellosis, and Aleutian disease. The presence of persistent eosinophilia can differentiate EG from these other more commonly diagnosed diseases in the ferret (Table 1).

THERAPY

Although there is no definitive treatment for eosinophilic gastroenteritis, success has been achieved using the following therapeutic strategies.

Supportive care is essential in the anorexic ferret. Ferrets can be coaxed to eat a high-calorie dietary supplement (Nutri-Cal, Evsco Pharmaceuticals) and baby food. In some cases, animals require hand-feeding or stomach-tubing to meet daily caloric requirements. For maintenance, ferrets may consume 200 to 300 kcal/kg body weight daily (McLain, 1988). These figures may be used to estimate daily caloric intake.

If the ferret is dehydrated, the practitioner should

begin fluid therapy. The authors recommend a fluid maintenance dose of 60 ml/kg over a 24-hour period. This can be divided into two or three daily treatments. Additional fluid requirements should be calculated based on per cent dehydration and fluid losses. If intravenous fluid therapy is instituted, the authors recommend placement of a 22- to 24-gauge intravenous catheter in the tail vein or cephalic vein.

Regression of disease has been observed after corticosteroid therapy. Prednisone (Prednisone, West-ward Pharmaceutical Corp.) at a dose of 1.25 to 2.5 mg/kg PO once daily can be initiated until clinical signs abate. Prednisone administration should be gradually decreased to 1.25 to 2.5 mg/kg PO every other day if possible. Remission of disease is judged by attitude, clinical signs, and normal peripheral blood eosinophil counts.

In one ferret, removal of an enlarged granulomatous mesenteric lymph node during exploratory examination resulted in amelioration of clinical signs and a normal eosinophil count. Ivermectin (Ivomec, MSD Agvet) was used in a confirmed case of EG in a ferret from New York (E. Hillyer, unpublished observation, 1991). The drug was administered 0.4 mg/kg SQ and the dosage repeated 2 weeks later. After treatment, there was resolution of clinical signs. Elimination diets have not been attempted as a form of treatment.

SUMMARY

Eosinophilic gastroenteritis is a newly recognized disease in the ferret. The etiology is unknown. Its histopathologic association with Splendore-Hoeppli phenomenon may indicate a parasitic etiology or involvement of an exogenous allergen or other infectious agent.

It can be differentiated from other more common diseases in the ferret by the presence of peripheral eosinophilia, infiltration of the gastrointestinal tract with eosinophils, and the presence of Splendore-Hoeppli phenomenon.

There is no definitive therapy. After diagnosis, the authors recommend initial treatment with ivermectin and supportive care. Corticosteroid therapy can be initiated at the recommended dose if there is no improvement.

References and Suggested Reading

Dillon, R.: Bacterial enteritis. *In* Kirk, R. W. (ed.): *Current Veterinary Therapy IX.* Philadelphia: W. B. Saunders, 1986, p. 872.
A review of diagnostic and therapeutic approaches to bacterial enteritides in the canine and feline species.

Fox, J. G.: Systemic diseases. *In* Fox, J. G. (ed.): *Biology and Diseases of the Ferret.* Philadelphia: Lea and Febiger, 1988, p. 255.
A description of common miscellaneous diseases in the ferret.

Fox, J. G., Palley, L. S., Jenkins, J., et al.: Eosinophilic gastroenteritis in the ferret. Lab. Anim. Sci. 39:499, 1989.
A clinical and histopathologic description of three cases of eosinophilic gastroenteritis in the ferret.

Fox, J. G., Palley, L. S., and Rose, R.: Eosinophilic gastroenteritis with Splendore. Hoeppli material in the ferret (*Mustela patenies furo*). Vet. Pathol., in press.
A complete histopathologic description of eosinophilic gastroenteritis in six ferret cases.

Fox, J. G., Pearson, R. C., and Gorham, J. R.: Viral and chlamydial diseases. *In* Fox, J. G., (ed.): *Biology and Diseases of the Ferret.* Philadelphia: Lea and Febiger, 1988, p. 217.
A review of clinical presentation, histopathology, and treatment of specific viral diseases that infect ferrets.

Goad, M. E. P., and Fox, J. G.: Neoplasia in ferrets. *In* Fox, J. G., (ed.): *Biology and Diseases of the Ferret.* Philadelphia: Lea and Febiger, 1988, p. 275.
A review of neoplastic disease in the ferret.

Johnson, F. B.: Splendore-Hoeppli phenomenon. *In* Binford, C. H., Connor, D. (eds.): *Pathology of Tropical and Extraordinary Diseases.* Washington, DC: Armed Forces Institute of Pathology, 1976, p. 681.

Krueger, K., Murphy, J. C., and Fox, J. G.: Treatment of proliferative colitis in ferrets. J.A.V.M.A. 194:1435, 1989.
A comparison of various dosage regimes of chloramphenicol therapy and supportive care in ferrets with proliferative colitis.

McLain, D. E.: Nutrition. *In* Fox, J. G. (ed.): *Biology and Diseases of the Ferret.* Philadelphia: Lea and Febiger, 1988, p. 135.
An outline of specific nutritional requirements and nutritional diseases in the ferret.

Otto, G., Fox, J. G., Wu, P., et al.: Eradication of *Helicobacter mustelae* from the ferret stomach: An animal model of *Helicobacter (Campylobacter) pylori* chemotherapy. Antimicrob. Agents. Chemother. 34:1232, 1990.
A chemotherapeutic approach to eradication of H. mustelae *associated with gastritis and ulcer disease in the ferret.*

Otto, G., Rosenblad, W., and Fox, J. G.: Practical venipuncture in the ferret. Lab. Anim. Sci. 40:565, 1990.
A description of routine venipuncture techniques in the ferret.

Ryland, L., Bernard, S., and Gorham, J.: A clinical guide to the pet ferret. Comp. Cont. Ed. Pract. Vet. 5:25, 1983.
A guide to routine prophylactic, diagnostic, and therapeutic procedures in the ferret.

FERRET ENDOCRINOLOGY

ELIZABETH V. HILLYER
New York, New York

Clinicians who work with domestic ferrets (*Mustela putorius furo*) recognize a prevalence of endocrine diseases in this species. However, there are little data and few case reports published on the subject. The information in this article is a compilation of clinical experience with endocrine diseases in ferrets seen at The Animal Medical Center (AMC) in New York. Knowledge of canine and feline medicine is useful in efforts to establish diagnostic and therapeutic guidelines for ferrets.

INSULINOMA

Several case reports on insulinomas in ferrets have been published, and it is currently the most common endocrine disease seen in ferrets treated at the AMC. In the 4-year period ending May, 1990, over 40 ferrets were examined with signs and laboratory data compatible with insulinoma.

Affected ferrets range in age from 3 to 9 years. A sex predilection has not been observed. Clinical signs on examination are usually of an episodic nature and include dullness, disorientation, hind limb weakness, and collapse. Owners may report hypersalivation and pawing at the mouth suggestive of nausea in ferrets. Physical examination results are often unremarkable, although affected ferrets may become dull and weak over the course of the examination due to hypoglycemia.

Episodes are often precipitated by a period of exercise or fasting. Seizures are uncommon but do occur; occasionally ferrets with severe hypoglycemia may present with active seizures. Some ferrets show weight loss. Splenomegaly is common in ferrets with insulinoma; the significance of this is not known.

A presumptive diagnosis of insulinoma is made by demonstration of random or fasting hypoglycemia ($\leq$60 mg/dl) with concurrent relative or absolute hyperinsulinemia. Multiple blood samples or a carefully monitored fast (4–6 hours is generally sufficient) may be necessary to document the association. Absolute insulin values greater than 275 pmol/L (38 μU/ml) are considered elevated by AMC's clinical pathology laboratory. Most endocrinologists agree that the amended insulin:glucose ratio is not a useful diagnostic tool.

Thoracic and abdominal radiographs, serum biochemical analysis, and a complete blood count (CBC) are recommended, but results are usually unremarkable except for low blood glucose. In most ferrets, tumors are too small to visualize with ultrasonography; however ultrasound may be useful in some cases. In ferrets with splenomegaly, a CBC and platelet count are indicated to rule out hypersplenism.

Exploratory surgery is recommended for suspected insulinoma, both to confirm the diagnosis by histopathologic examination and to attempt excision or cytoreduction of the tumor or tumors. Standard surgical and postoperative protocols should be followed, with care taken to prevent hypoglycemia. Pancreatic masses may be single or multiple and may not be grossly visible. Gentle palpation is the best technique to detect insulinoma nodules, which are firmer than the surrounding pancreatic tissue. Masses are removed by excision or partial pancreatectomy. The regional lymph nodes, liver, and spleen are carefully examined during surgery, and abnormal areas are excised or specimens taken for biopsy.

A splenectomy is performed if the spleen is abnormal in appearance. At the AMC, results of splenic biopsy in affected ferrets have revealed congestion or extramedullary hematopoiesis. One ferret had splenic lymphosarcoma in addition to insulinoma. Histopathologic examination of pancreatic masses has revealed a range of conditions from hyperplasia to adenoma of islet cells, often with transition to adenocarcinoma in a single biopsy specimen. Metastasis to regional lymph nodes may occur. There are reports of islet cell metastasis to the spleen in ferrets with insulinoma.

Results of surgery in ferrets with insulinoma have been variable, and it is unclear whether surgery significantly alters the course of disease as it does in dogs. Insulin concentrations drawn 1 to 2 days after surgery are normal in some ferrets but remain high in most. All ferrets ultimately require medical treatment, although surgery may delay the need for medication for several months.

When surgery is not performed, treatment is based on a presumptive diagnosis of insulinoma. Client education involves a discussion of the relationship between insulin and glucose and the clinical signs of hypoglycemia. Feeding should consist of three to four small meals daily of a diet high in protein, fat, and complex carbohydrates. As most ferrets are given food on a free-choice basis, clients should be instructed to keep food bowls full and to encourage ferrets to eat after a period of play or exercise. Semimoist diets and foods containing simple sugars should be avoided because a rapid rise in blood glucose promotes insulin release. Episodes of collapse at home can be treated by oral administration of corn syrup or liquid dextrose. In ferrets too obtunded to swallow, corn syrup should be rubbed on the gingiva with care to avoid being bitten. As soon as the ferret can eat, it is offered a small meal to avoid rebound hypoglycemia.

Glucocorticoid administration is recommended when frequent feedings are no longer sufficient to control clinical signs. Glucocorticoids help to stabilize blood sugar by promoting gluconeogenesis in the liver and by inhibiting glucose uptake by peripheral tissues. Prednisone is given at a starting dosage of 0.5 to 1 mg/kg/day given in two divided doses every 12 hours. This dosage can be gradually increased to 4 mg/kg/day as necessary. The pediatric form of liquid prednisolone is convenient for administration of small doses. Prednisone in tablet form can be crushed and mixed with Nutri-Cal (Evsco Pharmaceuticals, Buena, NJ), which most ferrets will take willingly. Some animals do well for months on prednisone and frequent feedings. Ferrets appear to tolerate glucocorticoids well, with a minimum of side effects until higher dosages are given.

Diazoxide (Proglycem, Medical Market Specialties) is added to the treatment regimen when prednisone no longer controls clinical signs. Diazoxide acts by inhibiting insulin release and cellular uptake of glucose. It promotes hepatic glycogenolysis and gluconeogenesis. The starting dosage of diazoxide is 10 mg/kg/day given in two to three divided doses every 8 to 12 hours; this can be gradually increased up to 60 mg/kg daily as needed. Diazoxide suspension is available in a 50-mg/ml concentration convenient for oral administration. When used in combination with diazoxide, the dosage of prednisone is decreased to 2 mg/kg/day and frequent feedings are continued.

Preliminary trials of treatment with somatostatin in ferrets with insulinoma have been inconclusive. Somatostatin is a polypeptide hormone secreted by the pancreas that suppresses the release of insulin. It is available in analogue form as a long-acting, injectable preparation called SMS201-995 (Sandostatin, Sandoz Pharmaceuticals). Somatostatin is helpful in some human and canine patients with insulinoma who are refractory to standard medical treatment (Lothrop, 1989). Further studies of this drug's efficacy in ferrets are needed.

The clinical course of insulinoma in ferrets, as in dogs, is slowly progressive. Medical management is altered in stages as the disease progresses. The mean survival time for dogs with insulinoma in one study was 19.4 months after surgery (Feldman and Nelson, 1987). Survival times after diagnosis of insulinoma in ferrets have ranged from 4 months to over 2 years with proper medical management.

DIABETES MELLITUS

There is one reported case of diabetes mellitus in a black-footed ferret (*Mustela nigripes*) (Carpenter and Novilla, 1977). This ferret was managed successfully for 15 months with two to five units of NPH insulin administered once daily.

There are no reported cases of diabetes mellitus in domestic ferrets. The author has treated four middle-aged ferrets for persistent hyperglycemia. All succumbed to the disease after a temporary response to treatment with insulin. Another clinician has treated a juvenile ferret for transient diabetes; this animal required insulin for 1 year and is now off medication. Transient diabetes mellitus has also been seen occasionally after surgery for insulinoma (Brown, personal communication, 1990). Ferrets with hyperglycemia are managed the same as dogs and cats.

HYPERESTROGENISM

Historically, estrous bone marrow hypoplasia in nonspayed females was the most common endocrine disease seen in pet ferrets. The disease is less commonly seen in recent years because large ferret breeders are neutering and descenting ferrets at 6 weeks of age.

Pathophysiology and treatment of this syndrome have been reviewed (see *CVT X*, p. 765); however, several additional points apply in a clinical setting. Determination of the packed cell volume (PCV), in conjunction with findings on physical examination, is an invaluable aid in establishing prognosis. Ferrets with estrogen toxicity are in different stages of the disease. With treatment, prognosis for survival is fair to good if the PCV is greater than 20%. A guarded prognosis is given if the PCV is 14% to 19%, and a PCV of less than 14% yields a very poor prognosis. Long-term hospitalization, multiple transfusions, and intensive care are necessary and yet may be unsuccessful. In one case report, a female ferret with a PCV of 7% required 13 transfusions over a 5-month period before recovery (Ryland, 1982).

In ferrets requiring blood transfusion, three transfusions and possibly more can be given from the same donor. Researchers were not able to identify blood groups in domestic ferrets (Manning and Bell, 1990). Blood transfusions should be fresh, not stored, to transfer functional platelets.

The use of tamoxifen, an antiestrogen used in humans, is contraindicated because it has estrogenic effects in ferrets.

Swollen Vulva in the Spayed Female

An increasingly common clinical syndrome is the spayed female examined because of a swollen vulva. Hair loss, usually on the tail and rump, is often present. Vulvar swelling is an external sign of estrus in ferrets. Cytologic examination of vaginal specimens reveals cornified epithelial cells and confirms high estrogen concentrations. Potential sources of estrogen are the ovaries and the adrenal cortex. The differential diagnosis includes the presence of a remnant ovary or hyperactive or neoplastic adrenal gland or glands.

The clinician has several diagnostic and therapeutic options: (1) administer one to three weekly doses of human chorionic gonadotropin (hCG) or gonadotropin-releasing hormone (GnRH) and await clinical response, (2) perform an hCG challenge test, (3) perform a systematic medical and surgical examination for a remnant ovary or abnormal adrenal gland (see later). The administration of hCG or GnRH after day 10 of estrus promotes ovulation in ferrets. The author gives a single dose of 1000 USP units (100 IU) of hCG IM, repeated 1 and 2 weeks later if vulvar swelling does not diminish. An alternate treatment is 20 μg IM of GnRH given on the same schedule or 15 μg IM given once daily for 2 days. If vulvar swelling resolves, an ovarian remnant is likely because adrenal secretion should not be affected. If vulvar swelling does not decrease, one or both adrenal glands may be secreting estrogenic compounds.

The hCG challenge test is a simple procedure to test for presence of functional ovarian tissue in the spayed bitch or queen showing estrous behavior. This test should be useful in ferrets also. Progesterone is measured 5 to 7 days after hCG administration. Concentrations of progesterone rise above 1 ng/ml if functional ovarian tissue is present (Shille and Olson, 1990).

If the ferret is ill or anemic or if the clinician feels that a remnant ovary is unlikely, a complete medical work-up is initiated. This should include a CBC and platelet count (see next section for diagnosis of adrenal tumors.) Bone marrow hypoplasia can develop in ferrets with estrogen-secreting adrenal tumors. However, hypoplasia is slower to develop in these ferrets than in those with an ovarian source of estrogen. In one case at the AMC, a female ferret showed persistent, fluctuating vulvar swelling for 2 years before succumbing to pancytopenia caused by an estrogen-secreting adrenal tumor.

HYPERADRENOCORTICISM

Adrenal tumors are diagnosed with increasing frequency in ferrets. Adrenal cortical hyperplasia, adenoma, and adenocarcinoma are seen. There are no reported cases of pituitary-dependent hyperadrenocorticism (PDH) in this species.

Adrenal tumors are typically seen in 2- to 5-year-old ferrets; however, an adrenal adenocarcinoma has been reported in a 7-year-old ferret (Fox et al., 1987). Tumors appear more frequently in females. Owners report hair loss, occasional pruritus, and vulvar swelling in spayed females. Appetite and activity level are generally normal, and polyuria and polydipsia are uncommon. Physical abnormalities may include a pendulous abdomen and smooth, thin skin, with bilaterally symmetrical hair thinning or truncal and tail alopecia. Mild to full vulvar swelling with mucoid or mucopurulent vaginal discharge may be present in females. In many ferrets, an adrenal mass is palpable. Splenomegaly is also common.

Physical examination with confirmation by ultrasound or exploratory laparotomy is most consistently useful in diagnosing adrenal tumors in ferrets. Results of biochemical analysis and CBC are usually unremarkable; endocrine testing has not been helpful in the author's experience. Based on data from dogs with adrenal tumors, useful tests in ferrets might be the dexamethasone suppression test and measurement of plasma ACTH. The latter test is not readily available and requires careful specimen handling. A drawback of the dexamethasone suppression test is the necessity to draw multiple blood samples. Protocols with normal values for a modified dexamethasone suppression test and the ACTH stimulation test in ferrets have been published (Heard et al., 1990). However, the author has had no success confirming adrenal tumors using either of these tests. Further studies are necessary.

Corticosteroids may not be the principal secretory products of some or all adrenal tumors in ferrets. ACTH stimulation testing for other steroids such as estradiol, progesterone, or testosterone may prove helpful in diagnosing ferret adrenal tumors.

Other means of diagnosing adrenal tumors in dogs include radiography (to screen for a mineralized adrenal mass), abdominal ultrasonography, computed tomography (CT scan), and exploratory surgery. The author has not seen adrenal mineralization in ferrets; however, many tumors can be visualized by ultrasound. CT scanning may be a more sensitive technique for identification of tumors. Exploratory surgery is often necessary for a definitive diagnosis.

Some authors recommend surgical removal of adrenal tumors in dogs (Feldman and Nelson, 1987), and surgical removal is the treatment of choice in ferrets at the AMC. Standard protocols for surgery and steroid replacement therapy are followed. In all ferrets, a ventral midline approach is used for complete abdominal exploratory surgery. Problems with wound healing have not occurred, and the procedure successfully reversed clinical signs in all but one ferret. Tumors generally involve the left adrenal gland, with right adrenal gland tumors seen less commonly. Rarely, both glands may be affected concurrently.

Medical treatment has been used with some success in dogs with adrenal tumors at the AMC. This requires high doses of o,p'-DDD (mitotane, Lysodren, Bristol-Myers Oncology Division). The use of this drug in ferrets is limited by its toxicity and the difficulty in accurately administering the small doses required by ferrets. However, o,p'-DDD therapy, rather than adrenalectomy, may prove to be the treatment of choice in younger ferrets with adrenal gland hyperplasia or adenoma. Ferrets are given 50 mg of o,p'-DDD once daily for 7 days and then once every 3 days until clinical signs resolve, after which the drug is discontinued. This treatment has been successful in some cases; ferrets with large, nonresectable tumors are less likely to respond (Brown, personal communication, 1990). For accurate dosing, the drug is prepared by a pharmacist who mixes it with corn starch and places a measured dose in No. 1 capsules. To facilitate administration, the capsules are coated in Linatone (Lambert Kay LP, Cranbury, NJ) and placed in the back of the throat, and the ferret is given Nutri-Cal and water to promote swallowing.

Treatment with ketoconazole (Nizoral, Janssen Pharmaceutica) is effective in some dogs with adrenal tumors. Ketoconazole is given at a dosage of 30 mg/kg/day in two divided doses every 12 hours. In dogs, ketoconazole interferes with adrenal steroid synthesis; it does not have this effect in cats, and its effect in ferrets has not been evaluated. In the author's experience, administration of ketoconazole at the dosage used in dogs was unsuccessful in reversing clinical signs in three ferrets with adrenal tumors. Anecdotal information from other practitioners suggests that it may be useful in some cases.

Seasonal hair loss in ferrets is a commonly recognized syndrome of unknown etiology. The author has treated a 5-year-old, spayed female ferret with hair loss, vulvar swelling, and other clinical signs compatible with hyperadrenocorticism, including polyphagia and polyuria/polydipsia. A CT scan showed bilateral adrenomegaly. Clinical signs resolved completely in 2 months without treatment. In humans and dogs, spontaneous remission of Cushing's disease has been documented (Feldman and Nelson, 1987).

The prognosis in ferrets with adrenal tumors is relatively good after the tumor is surgically removed, but this assessment is based on a limited number of cases. In some ferrets, the second adrenal gland is involved at a later date. Further study and correlation of prognosis with histologic diagnosis are necessary. When surgery is not possible, a ferret with a diagnosed adrenal tumor may survive for months after diagnosis because the disease is generally slowly progressive.

There are no reported cases of adrenal insufficiency in domestic ferrets.

THYROID DISEASE

Neither hyperthyroidism nor hypothyroidism has been reported in domestic ferrets. There is a published protocol for the thyroid-stimulating hormone (TSH) test in ferrets (Heard et al., 1990), and this protocol should be used to screen for suspected hypothyroidism. The author has seen one ferret with an abnormal TSH test result; however, this ferret did not respond to thyroid supplementation and necropsy findings were inconclusive.

Diagnostic and therapeutic guidelines used for cats are recommended for ferrets suspected of having hyperthyroidism.

SERTOLI CELL TUMOR

There are no cases of Sertoli cell tumor in the literature. However, the author has seen a 6-year-old intact male ferret with Sertoli's cell tumor examined because of pruritus and total alopecia. Complete hair regrowth occurred after castration.

References and Suggested Reading

Carpenter, J. W., and Novilla, M. N.: Diabetes mellitus in a black-footed ferret. J.A.V.M.A. 171:890, 1977.
   A complete case report describing diagnosis, treatment, outcome, and necropsy findings in a black-footed ferret with diabetes mellitus.
Feldman, E. C., and Nelson, R. W.: *Canine and Feline Endocrinology and Reproduction.* Philadelphia: WB Saunders, 1987.
   A current textbook of clinical findings and procedures in small animal endocrinology.
Fox, J. G., Goad, M. E. P., Garibaldi, B. A., et al.: Hyperadrenocorticism in a ferret. J.A.V.M.A. 191:343, 1987.
   A case report describing clinical and necropsy findings in a domestic ferret with adrenocortical adenocarcinoma.
Heard, D. J., Collins, B., and Chen, D. L., et al.: Thyroid and adrenal function tests in adult male ferrets. Am. J. Vet. Res. 51:32, 1990.
   Protocols for TSH, thyrotropin-releasin hormone (TRH), ACTH stimulation, and dexamethasone suppression tests in domestic ferrets, with test results from eight normal males.
Lothrop, C. D.: Medical treatment of neuroendocrine tumors of the gastroenteropancreatic system with somatostatin. *In* Kirk, R. W. (ed.): *Current Veterinary Therapy X.* Philadelphia: W. B. Saunders, 1989, p. 1020.
   A review of the use of somatostatin therapy in humans and dogs.
Manning, D. D., and Bell, J. A.: Lack of detectable blood groups in domestic ferrets: implications for transfusion. J.A.V.M.A. 197:84, 1990.
   A description of testing to look for blood groups in domestic ferrets.
Randolph, R. W.: Medical and surgical care of the pet ferret. *In* Kirk, R. W. (ed.): *Current Veterinary Therapy X.* Philadelphia: W. B. Saunders, 1989, p. 765.
   A review of preventative medicine and basic surgical procedures in domestic ferrets.
Ryland, L. M.: Remission of estrus-associated anemia following ovariohysterectomy and multiple blood transfusions in a ferret. J.A.V.M.A. 181:820, 1982.
   A case report describing the treatment of severe estrogen toxicity in a domestic ferret.
Shille, V. M., and Olson, P. N.: Dynamic testing in reproductive endocrinology. *In* Kirk, R. W. (ed.): *Current Veterinary Therapy X.* Philadelphia: W. B. Saunders, 1989, p. 1282.
   A review of challenge testing in reproductive endocrinology, including a description of the hCG challenge test to identify a remnant ovary.

FEEDING LLAMAS AND ALPACAS

MURRAY E. FOWLER
Davis, California

Llama and alpaca production has become a viable animal enterprise in North America. The term *llama* is used hereafter to denote both species. Llamas are used for propagation, packing, companion animals, and a small cottage industry for fiber production. The value of these animals warrants close attention to their medical needs.

Llama owners are frequently inexperienced with livestock and thus require enlightenment on management as well as medical matters. Veterinarians may be a source of information for both.

Little sophisticated nutritional research has been conducted on camelids. However, feeding recommendations may be made based on a knowledge of llama anatomy and physiology, combined with behavioral observations of llamas in their native land and experiences gained with llamas in zoos and private ownership.

The progenitors of the present South American camelids (llamas, alpacas, guanacos, and vicuñas) evolved in a harsh environment, to which they became superbly adapted. The Andean environment provided a feast and famine cycle of forage availability. Seasonal rains brought abundant, nutritious forage, and during that time, llamas laid down fat reserves for the drought to follow.

The cyclicity of body condition in llamas and alpacas contrasts with North American feeding practices that often do not include a famine phase of the yearly cycle. As a result, overfeeding may become a serious problem.

BASIC CONCEPTS

South American camelids are unique in their digestive system anatomy and physiology. Although they have a multicompartmented foregut fermentation digestive process, with regurgitation and reprocessing as fundamental characteristics, they should not be managed simply as another ruminant. Evolutionarily, camelids and true ruminants separated approximately 40 million years ago when members of both branches had simple stomachs. The subsequent similarities of the digestive systems are the result of parallel evolution.

The three compartments of a camelid's stomach are not homologous with those of a ruminant. In a camelid's stomach, all three compartments have glandular surfaces that secrete chemicals for digestion and absorption of metabolic products. Motility patterns are also different. In a camelid, the first compartment contracts three or four times per minute in a resting state and as many as five to six times after eating. The ingesta of the first compartment of a camelid is homogeneous, in contrast to the layered ingesta of a ruminant. As in ruminants, a repetitive mixing of the ingesta may enhance the efficiency of digestion. Like ruminants, llamas also recycle urea.

Prehension and mastication of feed are similar to that of cattle and sheep. There are differences in dentition, but these are not important for this discussion.

FEEDING REGIMENS

Llamas have been domesticated and managed by humans for more than 6000 years in Andean countries. These animals subsist entirely on pasturage. Neither supplements nor hay is provided for them.

In North America, every conceivable pasturage, hay, or combination thereof is used for llama feed. It is a tribute to the llama's adaptability that it has managed not only to survive but thrive.

Cattle, sheep, and horses consume approximately 2 to 2.5% of their body weight in dry forage daily. Feeding tables are based on that assumption. The ratio of hay to concentrate is adjusted according to the physiologic status of the animal. In contrast, llamas require daily ingestion of only 1 to 1.5% of their body weight. These findings were first established in a metabolic study in 1965 in Germany and were corroborated by unpublished feeding trials conducted at Colorado State University (L. Johnson, personal communication, 1991).

Pasture

Adult llamas may be maintained in good condition on pasture alone. Young animals, lactating females, and packers may require supplementation. They will graze on all types of grasses and forbs. Llamas

1189

have no tendency to bloat, even on alfalfa pastures. Llamas are also browsers and will strip the leaves from shrubs and trees to the extent of their reach.

Hay

Dozens of forages are harvested for hay in North America, and nutrient values for these forages are known and published. The suitability of different types of hay has been established for different livestock species by years of practical feeding experience; yet even in livestock feeding, prejudices that are not based on nutritional fact dictate against feeding certain types of hay.

Similarly, controversy surrounds the feeding of certain types of hay to llamas. In reality, there are no data to support the superiority of one hay over another. Although success has apparently been experienced using all types of hay ranging from first cutting of leafy alfalfa to oat straw, neither should be recommended as a total diet, because obesity may develop on the first diet and gastrointestinal impaction on the other. If reason is used, all types of hay or mixtures thereof may be used to feed llamas.

Free-choice feeding of hay may result in certain individuals dominating a group and consuming the most palatable part of the hay. The end result may be obesity in one or more animals and excessive expense in feeding.

Llamas are efficient in extracting nutrients from forage. This is especially true for protein. Thus, llamas have lower protein requirements than other livestock. In a study conducted at Colorado State University, animals maintained on a ration containing 10% protein performed as well as or better than those on a 16% protein ration (Johnson, 1989). It is well known that quality alfalfa has high levels of protein (>20%). The question that has not been answered is, Is the extra protein detrimental to llamas?

Concentrate Supplementation

The majority of llamas do not need concentrate supplementation and will be harmed by excessive caloric intake. Heavily lactating females, young growing animals, packers, and animals maintained in ultracold environments may need supplementation. All of the standard grains, such as corn, oats, barley, milo, and wheat, may be used, preferably cracked or rolled.

It may be desirable to accustom llamas to eating grain in order to facilitate ingestion of mineral supplements or medication. For mineral supplementation, a handful of sweet feed (grain mixed with molasses) will help to bind the mineral mix.

A number of pelletized total feeds or feed supplements are manufactured for the llama industry. The ingredients labels and guaranteed analysis may indicate that these are desirable products. However, such formulations tend to be expensive, contain unnecessary nutrients, and may be deficient in fiber. Llamas have sometimes developed esophageal obstruction when fed pellets.

Vitamins and Minerals

The vitamin and mineral requirements of llamas are unknown. No cases of vitamin or mineral deficiency disease have been reported in South America. Selenium and copper deficiencies are recognized in North America. Zinc and phosphorus deficiencies are suspected.

Water

Llamas should have constant access to water.

LLAMA FEEDING PROBLEMS

Obesity

Many North American llamas are overfed and have a tendency toward obesity. Llama infants, called *crias*, weigh 8 to 18 kg (18 to 40 lb) at birth. Normal weight gain is 0.25 to 0.5 kg (0.5 to 1.0 lb) per day. Adult llama weights vary from 108 to 243 kg (238 to 536 lb). There is little difference between males and females; in fact, females may be heavier than males. Even obese llamas rarely weigh more than 200 kg. Alpaca crias weigh 5 to 9 kg (11 to 20 lb). Adult alpacas weigh 55 to 80 kg (121 to 176 lb).

Owners should be encouraged to weigh their animals at least yearly. Scales designed for llamas are available commercially, or owners can take their animals to a commercial weigh station used for trucks. Owners should also be instructed on how to evaluate condition in their charges.

The old adage, "The eye of the master fattens the cattle," is valid in feeding llamas, with the caution that the eye may be deceived by the fiber coat. The fingers must be used as well, palpating over the withers rather than the pelvic area (which always feels bony). The back muscles should be firm, and the ribs should be palpable. In a satisfactorily conditioned animal, the back musculature relationship to the vertebra on cross section should appear as in Figure 1A. A fat animal has a conformation as depicted in Figure 1B and a thin animal as in Figure 1C.

Obesity may also be assessed in other locations.

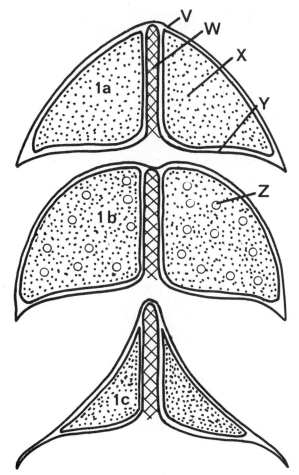

Figure 1. Diagrams of a cross section of the muscle and dorsal spine of the thoracic vertebrae.

1a, Normal body condition. *1b,* Obesity. *1c,* Emaciation. V = skin; W = dorsal spinous process; X = muscle mass; Y = rib; Z = fat.

When viewed from behind, the upper rear limb muscle masses do not normally touch each other. In an obese animal, the vulva and anus may appear recessed as a result of the fatty accumulations spreading out around them. A markedly obese animal also has an altered gait (waddle).

An obese animal also has internal accumulation of fat. The ventral retroperitoneal fat layer may be 10 cm thick. Pelvic and omental fat may prohibit rectal palpation of the reproductive tract and may inhibit conception or interfere with parturition. Infiltration of fat into the mammary gland diminishes lactation potential. Weight loss may prove difficult unless absolute calorie control is practiced, which usually necessitates isolation. Some llamas become obese even on a relatively poor pasture.

Hypophosphatemic Rickets

Classic rickets has been diagnosed in a number of alpacas and llama sucklings and early weanlings (4 to 7 months of age). Though these young animals show all the clinical signs and radiographic lesions of rickets, they are receiving adequate calcium and vitamin D. The common denominator is hypophosphatemia less than 3 mg/dl.

The cause of the hypophosphatemia is unknown at present. Diet may be a contributing factor, but the condition has been observed under many different feeding regimens.

Serum inorganic phosphorus levels can be corrected by administering oral monosodium phosphate* at ¼ teaspoon/20 kg (45 lb) of body weight daily. The powder can be mixed with honey, corn syrup, or molasses for placement in the mouth. In my experience, the signs of lameness have abated and the radiographic lesions have been corrected, but restoration of growth has been poor.

Angular Limb Deformity

Various degrees of carpal valgus have been seen in many llamas, to the point that some owners argue that it is normal for a llama to be slightly knock-kneed. Do not be misled. A llama with correct conformation has straight forelimbs, just as does a horse.

The precise etiology is unknown. There is reason to believe that a hereditary component may be involved. Angular limb deformity (ALD) may also be a part of the rickets syndrome, so the diet must be evaluated.

The radiographic lesion of rickets-caused ALD is easily recognized. In other cases of ALD, the significant lesion is a thickening and bulging of the metaphysis and epiphysis adjacent to the ulnar physis.

The management of ALD depends on the age of the animal and the severity of the deviation. Some animals outgrow the deviation; others can be helped with early splinting. More severe cases may require periosteal stripping or transphyseal bridging.

Selenium/Vitamin E Deficiency

Much has been written about selenium/vitamin E deficiency in livestock, horses, and llamas. Forage grown on soils deficient in selenium may cause a deficiency syndrome in llamas. The Pacific Northwest, Great Lakes region, central and northern East Coast regions are known to be deficient areas, and diets of llamas maintained in those areas must be supplemented with selenium.

No single mineral supplement can be recommended. Each region seems to devise a mix that contains as much selenium as allowed by law. A

*Nutrene P-16 Mineral Mix, Gargill, Inc., Stockton, CA.

mineral mix that is palatable may be made of trace mineralized salt, 23 kg (50 lb); steamed bone meal, 23 kg; dry powdered molasses, 23 kg; and zinc supplement,* 4.5 kg (10 lb) (Johnson, 1989). This mix can be used to supply selenium by establishing the intake for a group of animals and adding selenium selenate to the mix in sufficient quantity to provide 1 to 1.5 mg of selenium per animal per day. Perhaps a more important problem is how to encourage sufficient intake. Llamas are inefficient at licking a solid block, so this method is not suggested. The granular mixture described above should be placed in an all-weather supplement dispenser or in a box inside a barn or shelter.

Injections of sodium selenate are useful for immediate and rapid elevation of blood selenium levels but are not suitable for long-term management in a selenium-deficient area.

Miscellaneous Deficiencies and Excesses

Zinc, copper, and iron deficiencies implicated in syndromes of llamas are similar to such deficiencies seen in livestock. Copper toxicosis resulting in hepatic necrosis has been reported in llamas supplemented with a bovine "dry cow" dairy pellet (Jurage and Thornburg, 1989). Though further study is required, llamas may be similar to sheep in their sensitivity to excess copper in the diet.

NUTRITION-RELATED CONDITIONS

Transfaunation

The microflora and fauna of the first compartment of a llama's stomach are similar to those of a ruminant. If a llama is anorectic for 4 or 5 days or suffers a gastric upset as a result of an episode of colic, the flora and fauna may be depressed or destroyed. Adequate digestive function is inhibited until restoration of the microorganisms.

Rumen contents from a cow or sheep may be obtained from a local packing plant. The ingesta should be strained through cheesecloth or other strainers. Approximately 1000 ml of the rumen liquor is the recommended dose for an adult llama. The liquid is administered via an orogastric tube.

Gastric Intubation

Prolonged anorexia may necessitate supplemental feeding. Gastric intubation is accomplished using an equine plastic stomach tube 15 mm OD (⅝ in.).

---

*Zinpro 100, Zinpro Corp., Bloomington, MN.

A 25-cm (10-in.) segment of garden hose or polyvinyl chloride pipe is used as the speculum to avoid laceration of the tube by the cheek teeth. Insert the speculum over the prominent base of the tongue.

Alfalfa pellets can be crushed with a hammer and soaked in hot water. Such a slurry can be pumped through a large animal stomach pump. Instant oat cereal (Quick Quaker Oats) can be soaked in hot water and pumped in also. Both products should be cooled before use.

Total Parenteral Nutrition

Total parenteral nutrition may be lifesaving in a septic neonate or adult. A 14- to 16-gauge intravenous cannula is placed in the jugular vein at the level of the junction between the fifth and sixth cervical vertebrae. Caloric requirements are based on metabolic weight, using formulas that are common to livestock and horses.

Miscellaneous Feeding-Related Problems

Gastrointestinal ulceration, including perforation and subsequent peritonitis, is a serious problem in llamas. Although no direct correlation has been established, feeding and nutrition practices may have a bearing on this problem.

Esophageal obstruction (choke) rarely occurs in llamas. Ingestion of small feed pellets has been incriminated, as has ingestion of apples from an abandoned orchard. Congenital megaesophagus has been diagnosed in several animals. The clinical signs and management of choke are similar to the management problem in horses and cattle.

Plant poisoning is beyond the scope of this article, but llamas are susceptible to many toxic plants. Bloat is rare in llamas.

Unthriftiness, failure to grow, and *failure to thrive* are terms applied to an ill-defined complex syndrome. Nutrition is probably a factor but secondary to a more basic defect. The common denominator is that these llamas grow normally until 3 to 10 months of age, when their weight gains plateau and they stop growing. Their appetite may be satisfactory, and the cria may appear to be normal in all other respects. Failure to grow is one of the early signs of rickets, but cases have been identified in nonrachitic animals. No satisfactory management regimen has yet been developed.

An enigmatic anorexia/wasting syndrome also frustrates many veterinarians dealing with llamas. Owners that are attentive to their stock may notice an individual starting to lose weight. Food intake begins to diminish. Anorexia is ultimately complete;

the animal becomes recumbent and is either unable or unwilling to rise.

Although many diseases must be differentiated in such a recumbent animal, some animals defy adequate antemortem diagnosis. Further frustrations arise when no lesions are found at necropsy to account for the lethal effects of this complex.

CONCLUSIONS

Feeding recommendations may be made for llamas and alpacas, but it should be apparent that there is much to be learned before feeding can be based on scientifically determined formulas.

Further information on feeding and nutrition may be obtained from the references listed next.

References and Suggested Reading

Fowler, M. E.: Angular limb deformities in young llamas. J.A.V.M.A. 181:1338, 1982.
Fowler, M. E.: Selenium—friend or foe. Llamas 31:37, 1986.
Fowler, M. E.: Medicine and Surgery of South American Camelids. Ames, IA: Iowa State University Press, 1989, pp. 9–23 (feeding and nutrition) and 97–100 (angular limb deformity).
Johnson, L.: Nutrition. Llama medicine. Vet. Clin. North Am. Food Anim. Pract. 5:37, 1989.
Jurage, R. E., and Thornburg, L. T.: Copper poisoning in four llamas. J.A.V.M.A. 195:987, 1989.

LLAMA NEUROLOGY

LARUE W. JOHNSON
Fort Collins, Colorado

Although llamas are the most prevalent of the New World camelids in North America, considerations of neurologic disease in llamas are also applicable to the alpaca, guanaco, and vicuna. The companion animal nature and current economic value of this species generally encourage early presentation for clinical signs referable to the nervous system. Basic causes include those of a traumatic, infectious, neoplastic, metabolic, toxic, nutritional, parasitic, congenital, and idiopathic nature, solely or in combination. In addition, the distinction between neurologic disease and abnormal behavior is addressed in this article. Table 1 summarizes various clinical presentations and differential diagnoses referable to the nervous system. It is designed to flow with the usual progression of clinical signs.

BEHAVIORIAL CONSIDERATIONS

Knowledge of normal llama behavior is important for clinicians to differentiate abnormal behavior from neurologic disease. On the whole, llamas are cooperative but stoic animals. Their stoicism has led many clinicians to downplay severity of presenting complaints. Llamas are gregarious, with a strong herding instinct. A pecking order based on dominance and subordinance is strictly adhered to within the herd. Normal llamas, except as curious youngsters, do not have a strong attraction to people. If excessive human attention is given to llamas of either gender during the neonatal through weaning period, humans become a part of their social structure. During puberty, friendliness and subordinance are replaced by aggressive dominance. In females, undesirable behavior includes spitting and general lack of cooperation during handling or restraint. Males may be more aggressive, ranging from human body pressing, body charging, mounting, and biting at legs, head, and gonads. Such behavior must be differentiated from primary neurologic disease.

NEUROLOGIC EXAMINATION

Camelids present examining clinicians with no unique neuroanatomic or physiologic challenges (Fowler, 1989). Routine procedures applicable to other domestic animals apply (Divers, 1986). That being the case, taking a thorough history and performing a general physical examination, supported by routine hematologic and serum chemistry studies, may be used to suggest neurologic involvement. A standard neurologic examination may include cerebrospinal fluid (CSF) analysis as well as indicated radiologic techniques. Additional techniques including electromyography, nerve conduction velocities, evoked potentials, and computed tomography are also available.

Table 1. Common Clinical Findings of Llamas With Nervous System Disease

Clinical Presentation	Differential Diagnoses
Depression	Rabies
	Lead poisoning
	Heat stress
	Hydrocephalus
	Polioencephalomalacia
Excitement/hyperesthesia	Polioencephalomalacia
	Hypomagnesemic tetany
	Meningitis/encephalitis
	Organophosphate poisoning
	Rabies
	Hydrocephalus
	Tetanus
	Middle ear infection
	Listeriosis
	Brain abscess/neoplasia
	Equine herpesvirus I
	Lidocaine toxicity
Facial paralysis	Trauma to facial nerve
	Listeriosis
Blindness	Equine herpesvirus I
	Polioencephalomalacia
	Lead poisoning
	Vitamin A deficiency
	Toxoplasmosis
	Cortical space-occupying lesion
Tremors	Hypomagnesemic tetany
	Organophosphate poisoning
	Rabies
	Polioencephalomalacia
	Tetanus
	Early tick paralysis
	Epilepsy
Lameness	Peripheral nerve avulsion, ablation, or trauma
	Spinal cord damage (meningeal worm)
	Birthing paralysis
Incoordination	Heat stress
	Meningeal worm
	Cerebellar hypoplasia
	Polioencephalomalacia
	Enzootic ataxia/copper deficiency
	Central nervous system trauma, abscess, neoplasia
	Lead poisoning
	Organophosphate poisoning
	Any cause of blindness
	Epilepsy
	Rabies
	Hypomagnesemic tetany
	Tetanus
Sternal recumbency	Progression of central nervous system involvements causing lameness or incoordination
Lateral recumbency	Progression of sternal recumbency
With flaccid paralysis:	Heat stress
	Tick paralysis
	Meningeal worm
	Enzootic ataxia
	Rabies
	Spinal cord compression
	Equine herpesvirus I
With spastic paralysis:	Tetanus
	Polioencephalomalacia
	Hypomagnesemic tetany
	Rabies
	Spinal cord compression
	Epilepsy
	Meningitis/encephalitis
	Type D enterotoxemia

NEUROLOGIC CONDITIONS

Enterotoxemia

The most common clinical presentation associated with *Clostridium perfringens* type C and D enterotoxemia is death; however, affected individuals may be observed in sternal recumbency, showing marked depression or lateral recumbency and often demonstrating opisthotonos and limb paddling. The incidence of both type C and D enterotoxemia in North America is low, fortunately, because the prognosis is generally guarded to poor even for cases diagnosed early. Successful therapy must be aggressive and aimed at toxin neutralization, reduction of septicemia, and treatment of shock. High doses of C/D antitoxin (4 ml/kg), penicillin (40,000 units/kg), and dexamethasone (1 mg/kg) combined with intravenous fluid therapy are recommended. Annual vaccination of llamas of all ages with C/D toxoid (commonly combined with tetanus toxoid) is highly recommended for prevention. Pregnant dams should receive a booster dose 1 month before birth to assure high levels of antibodies in their colostrum.

Enzootic Ataxia

Clinical signs, necropsy lesions, and copper levels in blood serum and tissues suggest that llamas can develop a progressive posterior ataxia comparable to that in lambs (Smith, 1989). When dietary copper intake is inadequate or excessive quantities of sulfates or molybdenum are present in the soil, copper deficiency is a likely explanation for posterior ataxia. Serum copper levels less than 4 ppm in animals presenting with clinical signs of posterior ataxia accompanied by variable degrees of anemia, poor growth, and lackluster fiber including depigmentation justify evaluation for copper deficiency. Dietary supplementation at 4 to 10 ppm plus parenteral injection of copper glycinate (0.44 mg/kg SC) may have a beneficial effect on an affected individual. Unfortunately, spinal cord pathology and complications of recumbency may not respond to treatment.

Epilepsy

The detailed description of a case of epileptic seizures in a 2-month-old male llama (Smith, 1989) matches two other cases owners have described to me and to attending veterinarians. Seizures were elicited by handling, were gradual (2 to 5 min) in onset, and progressed to lateral recumbency with various degrees of opisthotonos, extensor rigidity, paddling, and muscle fasciculations. None of these cases had abnormalities on hematologic study, serum chemistry evaluation, CSF analysis, or gross or histologic pathologic study of the central nervous system (CNS). Differential diagnostic considerations include encephalitis, meningitis, head trauma, and space-occupying lesions. The intermittent nature of clinical signs and the presence of normal laboratory values characterize epilepsy. Deep sedation/anesthesia provided temporary relief; however, attempts at using oral phenobarbital (2.25 mg/kg twice daily) failed to prevent recurrences.

Meningitis/Encephalitis

Occasional complications of neonatal bacterial septicemias have resulted in meningitis. Organisms isolated from these cases include *Streptococcus* and coliforms. Cases of CNS inflammatory disease due to *Listeria monocytogenes* and *Coccidioides immitis* have also been observed in camelids. Listeriosis is observed in llamas, with clinical signs referable to unilateral brainstem lesions. Circling, facial paralysis, impaired blinking ability, ear droop, and lip droop with saliva loss are observed. In addition, lesions of tuberculosis may involve the CNS. Viral agents as causes of camelid encephalitis include equine herpesvirus type I, rabies, and encephalomyocarditis viruses. Toxoplasmosis must also be considered, especially in neonates.

Extremely diverse clinical signs can be anticipated from animals affected with meningitis or encephalitis. Hyperesthesia leading to paralytic lateral recumbency is most common, although dullness and depression may also occur as the course progresses. Signs may progress to coma. The basic physical examination and all diagnostic efforts should be performed with rabies as a differential diagnosis. Elevated body temperature, as well as increased pulse and respiratory rates, characterizes early hyperesthesia clinical signs. Muscular fasciculations, nystagmus, grinding of teeth, and salivation are variably observed.

Rabies affects llamas similarly to most other warm-blooded animals. Rabies has to be differentiated from the aggressive behavior of a human-oriented llama. Geographic areas known to have a significant incidence of rabies put resident llamas at greater risk, justifying routine vaccination using killed tissue culture preparations (Milton et al., 1989).

Clinical signs of toxoplasmosis in the various mammalian species are extremely diverse. Blindness due to chorioretinitis and an encephalitis are the principal neurologic manifestations to be observed. In camelids, abortions or neonatal mortality would also be likely sequelae.

Neurologic disease in camelids infected with equine herpesvirus type I has been reported (Rebhun et al., 1988). Although respiratory or reproductive clinical manifestations of horses by equine herpesvirus type I are well documented, neurologic signs are relatively rare. In contrast, a wide range of neurologic signs characterizes camelid infection with the virus, yet without observed involvement of the respiratory or reproductive systems. In llama cases to date, contact with zebras has been a consistent observation. Presenting clinical signs of affected individuals includes blindness, nystagmus, head tilt, and paralysis. Body temperatures range from normal to 40.5°C (104.9°F) in acute cases. Routine hematologic or biochemical laboratory analyses were not found to be of diagnostic value. A wide range of ophthalmic pathology has been observed (Rebhun et al., 1988). For living animals, obtaining acute and convalescent serum for virus neutralization testing of equine herpesvirus type I is the most reliable test. However, tissue isolation of virus is absolute proof of diagnosis. Although no treatment has been found to be effective in reversing clinical blindness, mortality is relatively low. Indications for use and efficacy of the equine vaccine remain unknown in camelids. If used, the vaccine should be a killed virus type repeated quarterly.

Heat Stress

South American camelids are essentially adapted to the Andean mountain habitat. It has been observed that high temperature and humidity combinations cause heat stress. Predisposing factors include heavy body fiber and excessive body fat, further aggravated by exercise or stress. Generally, if ambient temperature (degrees Fahrenheit) is added to the relative humidity and the sum is less than 120, minimal heat stress problems are expected. A value of 150 may cause problems in certain individuals, but a value greater than 180 is considered dangerous (Smith, 1989). Although all clinical signs are not referable to the nervous system, many of the more advanced ones are. Signs of restlessness, depression, recumbency, and convulsions accompanied by high body temperature of 41 to 42°C (105.8 to 107.6°F) during warm weather conditions justify consideration of the diagnosis. Other animals may be affected but showing less severe clinical signs, including moderately elevated body temperatures, increased pulse and respiratory rates, open-mouth breathing, salivation, and sweating from their fiberless thermal window areas. Advanced cases are characterized by clinical dehydration, a drooping lower lip, and diminution of sweating.

The severity of cases showing nervous signs generally pre-empts sophisticated diagnostic pursuits; however, one might expect marked hemoconcentration, multiple electrolyte alterations, stress leukograms, and hyperglycemia, as well as markedly elevated levels of muscle enzymes and uremia. Neurologic clinical signs are accounted for by dehydration, electrolyte imbalances, cerebral edema, and polioencephalomalacia (PEM).

Removing affected animals from the environmental conditions and rapid reduction of body temperature are the principal goals of treatment. Core body temperature can most effectively be reduced by submersion or spraying of the ventral area and whole body, cold water enemas, and cold water via stomach tube. Intravenous fluids (e.g., lactated Ringer's solution) are indicated after other techniques have been initiated. Although debatable, use of parenteral antipyretics (dipyrone, 11 mg/kg IV or SC) is commonly practiced and is especially of value if body temperature rises again after an initial crisis. If CNS signs continue after normalization of body temperature, additional diagnostics may identify specific electrolyte alterations. Treatment of convulsions using phenobarbital (2.25 mg/kg PO) or diazepam (0.5 mg/kg SC) has proved useful. High doses of dexamethasone (2 to 4 mg/kg SC) may be helpful in cases with cerebral edema. In addition, PEM may be a sequela and can be treated by administration of high doses of thiamine (6 to 8 mg/kg IV).

Relapses of heat stress are common, with predisposed individuals commonly having a body temperature higher than herd mates.

Hypomagnesemia

Although camelids generally are not readily affected by hypomagnesemia, I have observed two cases of hypomagnesemia combined with hypocalcemia in postpartum females grazing on springtime grass pastures. Clinical signs were initially characterized by anxiety, muscle fasciculations, tremors, and in one case recumbency tending toward extensor rigidity with opisthotonos. Both cases had normal pupillary light reflex, tachycardia, and somewhat elevated body temperatures. Blood serum analysis of the two cases before treatment showed magnesium levels of 1.0 and 0.7 mg/dl and calcium levels of 6.5 and 6.1 mg/dl. The more severely affected individual had the lowest values of each electrolyte. Treatment consisted of 200 ml of Norcalciphos (Norden, SmithKline Beecham), and both affected individuals responded favorably. No relapses were observed. As with domestic ruminants, prevention is best accomplished by assuring that ingested forage, especially in the springtime, is grown on properly fertilized soils. In addition, provision of a balanced mineral supplement assuring a daily intake of 50 to 100 mg of supplemental magnesium has proved beneficial.

Intoxications (Organophosphate and Lidocaine)

Although a list of possible intoxications of ruminants causing clinical signs referable to the CNS has been discussed in some detail (Smith, 1986),

only organophosphate poisoning is discussed here. For control of llama-biting lice *Damalinia breviceps*, chemical pour-on compounds of the organophosphate type have been used. A potential for toxicity exists. A case involving chlorpyrifos toxicosis in a llama was characterized by clinical signs of anorexia, bradycardia, hypothermia, salivation, miosis, gastric atony, and recumbency. Diagnosis can be confirmed by determining plasma pseudocholinesterase levels (Pearson et al., 1986). Along with fluid and supportive care, atropine sulfate (0.5 to 1 mg/kg SC) would be specific therapy for the muscarinic signs. Atropine should be repeated every 3 to 12 hr as clinical signs return. Overdosing of llamas with organophosphates can be avoided when accurate body weights are known and by only using products observed to be safe and effective in camelids (e.g., 3% Fenthion, 15 ml/45.5 kg [½ oz/100 lb]).

Lidocaine toxicity has been observed in a nursing male llama weighing 30 kg. The llama received xylazine (0.44 mg/kg IV) and 30 ml of 2% lidocaine SC at the site of an umbilical hernia. Midway through the operation, the llama began convulsive seizures, consistent with lidocaine toxicity. The patient died before diazepam (0.5 mg/kg) could be administered intravenously.

Meningeal Worm

The nematode *Parelaphostrongylus tenuis* is a common parasite of white-tailed deer in North America, where the completed life cycle generally causes minimal harm to the primary host (Fig. 1). On occasion, the parasite infects other ungulate hosts, including llamas, in which the migrating larvae produce marked tissue response and diverse neurologic signs. The presence of white-tailed deer and snails or slugs is necessary for the completion of the parasite's life cycle to infective third-stage larvae (Baumgartner et al., 1985). Infection should be considered more likely in animals sold from endemic areas to nonendemic areas.

Clinical presentations vary with time from duration of onset; however, most cases demonstrate a progression from posterior ataxia, lameness with extremes of both knuckling and hypermetria, and disorientation progressing to recumbency. More variable is the presence of circling, head pressing, blindness, paralysis, and death. Diagnosis is made by history, geographic location, and clinical signs. Perhaps the most helpful laboratory aid to diagnosis is a CSF analysis indicating an inflammatory process characterized by elevated protein and increased leukocytes including eosinophils (Lunn and Hinchcliff, 1989). Peripheral blood counts are variable, but a pronounced eosinophilia may be present.

To date, treatment success has been variable. Theoretical benefit from dexamethasone and thia-

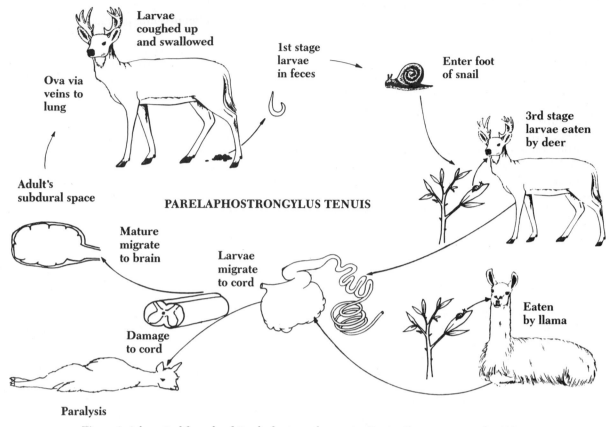

Figure 1. Schematic life cycle of *Parelaphostrongylus tenuis* affecting llamas as an accidental host.

mine warrants their administration. Antibiotics (e.g., penicillin or trimethoprim-sulfadiazine) are generally administered to control secondary bacterial complications. Although ivermectin (200 μg/kg SC) is presumed not to penetrate the blood-brain barrier, most suspected cases are given an injection, under the assumption that some migrating larvae are destroyed. Up to ten times the normal worming dose has been administered with assumed beneficial effects. Quality nursing care is required for a recumbent llama to minimize decubital complications.

Prevention in endemic areas is not easily accomplished but must be aimed at breaking the life cycle. Fencing deer away from llamas and controlling mollusk intermediate hosts using molluscacides are sound measures but difficult to accomplish. Monthly injections of ivermectin on a prophylactic basis are being used to control the migrating larvae before CNS involvement.

Tick Paralysis

Llamas presented in the spring of the year showing neurologic signs of flaccid paralysis are more likely to be afflicted with tick paralysis than any other ailment. A tick-elaborated neurotoxin causes a lower motor neuron paralysis. Most patients are found in lateral recumbency with minimal evidence of body movements. Body temperature may be normal or influenced by ambient temperature and location of recumbency. Heart and respiratory rates are generally diminished.

Presumptive diagnosis is based on history of the premises/locale and presenting clinical signs. The diagnosis is more likely with demonstration of one or more engorged ticks (no easy task in fully fibered individuals). Prime tick sites include the head and neck as well as the deep axillary and inguinal regions. Removal of all engorged ticks is imperative to achieve recovery (and may also confirm the diagnosis). Improvement in muscle tone is often observed within 1 to 2 hr of tick removal, and recovery is usually complete after 6 to 12 hours. Unless the animal is totally clipped and found to be free of ticks, a pyrethrin/pyrethroid spray or dust should be applied to the body. We generally inject ivermectin at 200 μg/kg SC to minimize relapses. Additional therapy is essentially supportive, consisting of parenteral balanced electrolyte solutions, thiamine, and dexamethasone.

Prevention of tick paralysis is best accomplished by avoiding tick exposure. Administration of ivermectin at 200 μg/kg SC every 3 weeks during peak risk may be indicated. Spraying of the animals with residual effect sprays (e.g., Permectrin) appears to be beneficial.

Routine serum biochemistry evaluation and complete blood counts may support a diagnosis of inflammatory neurologic disease but usually are not rewarding. CSF analysis, pressure measurement, and culture assist in therapeutic and prognostic decisions. The CSF collection technique described for cattle (Divers, 1986) can be used for llamas. If light sedation is required, xylazine at 0.2 mg/kg IM is adequate. For recumbency, a combination of ketamine:xylazine, 4.4 mg:0.44 mg/kg IM, respectively, is recommended. Serologic testing procedures (acute/convalescent) may prove beneficial in proving encephalitis due to equine herpesvirus I, encephalomyocarditis viruses or toxoplasmosis, and coccidioidomycosis. Unfortunately, specific diagnosis of most meningitis/encephalitis cases comes from necropsy efforts, in which both culture and histopathology should be pursued.

Intravenous catheterization is imperative for fluid therapy and the frequent administration of intravenous antibiotic in suspected bacterial meningitis cases. Crystalline penicillin (40,000 units/kg q.i.d.) accompanied by either intravenous gentamicin (2 to 4 mg/kg) or amikacin (6 mg/kg q.i.d.) provides broad-spectrum coverage. Nephrotoxicity has been observed with prolonged use of aminoglycosides in llamas. Other antibiotic options include trimethoprim-sulfadiazine or chloramphenicol. A minimum of 5 days of high-level antibiotic therapy is advised. If an animal is rapidly deteriorating, steroids are indicated (1 to 2 mg/kg of dexamethasone). Neonatal meningitis is often related to or caused by failure of passive transfer. Assessment of immunoglobulin status is important to issue an accurate prognosis as well as to include plasma transfusion in therapeutic considerations.

Otitis Media

Otitis media is generally observed as a direct extension of otitis externa, which is predisposed to by the presence of foreign bodies including foxtails, ticks, and water. The head tilt that also characterizes otitis media can generally be distinguished from listeriosis on the basis of residual evidence or history of otitis externa. Facial nerve paralysis and Horner's syndrome account for the observed clinical presentation, including a slight ptosis of the upper eyelid, and diminished ability of the pupillary light response (Fowler and Gillespie, 1985). Removal of any incriminating foreign bodies plus culture of infected ears for selection of effective antibiotic therapy is indicated. The prognosis for full recovery is guarded, because a residual head tilt commonly persists.

Polioencephalomalacia

The incidence of PEM/cerebrocortical necrosis is low in camelid populations. Cases observed have usually been associated with a history of heat stress or digestive disturbance, especially grain engorgement. Clinical signs of PEM in llamas range from depression to excitement with variable manifestations of cortical blindness and possible recumbency. Bilateral blindness with intact pupillary response is consistent with PEM. Elevated body temperature usually accompanies hyperesthetic clinical signs. Recumbency may be characterized by extensor rigidity and opisthotonos. Early treatment improves the prognosis. High doses of thiamine (6 to 8 mg/kg IV) repeated with 3 to 4 mg/kg SC every 12 hr for 5 to 7 days generally reduce most clinical signs including blindness, which resolves last. Transfaunation of the camelid stomach using conventional ruminant rumen ingesta is also recommended to prevent relapses and encourage endogenous production of thiamine. Administration of thiamine to animals known to have had major gastric flora alterations reduces the incidence of clinically recognizable PEM.

Tetanus

As with virtually all mammalian species, the camelids can develop clinical tetanus due to wounds infected with *Clostridium tetani*. The incidence appears to be very low, perhaps partly because of the extensive use of vaccination procedures in endemic areas, infrequent injuries resulting in deep wounds, and possibly the low susceptibility of the species. Animals having a history of evidence of a potentially contaminated wound and demonstrating classic progressive clinical signs including muscle rigidity, a fixed stare, erect ears, reluctance to eat due to a "locked" jaw, an elevated tail, flared nostrils, and a protruding nictitating membrane should be regarded as likely having tetanus. Observed progression of clinical signs would be analogous to other species. Successful treatment must be early and aggressive. Wound débridement and flushing accompanied by administration of tetanus antitoxin is recommended; however, an absolute dose to recommend for any species is unknown. For other species, doses ranging from 100 to 225 units/kg have been administered and divided between intrathecal, intravenous, and subcutaneous routes. In addition, high doses of aqueous procaine penicillin (40,000 units/kg) are administered parenterally. Animals exhibiting extreme hyperesthesia should be sedated (0.2 mg/kg xylazine IM or SC) or anesthetized (0.44 mg/kg xylazine and 4.4 mg/kg ketamine IM or SC) until no longer necessary. Supportive care includes provision of adequate bedding, frequent turning and manipulation of recumbent individuals, and maintenance of fluid intake by oral or parenteral routes.

References and Suggested Reading

Baumgartner, W., Azjac, A., Hull, B. L., et al.: Parelaphostrongylosis in llamas. J.A.V.M.A. 187:1243, 1985.
A detailed description of two llamas affected with the meningeal worm parasite, including necropsy lesions.
Divers, T. J.: Neurologic examination of cattle. *In* Howard, J. L. (ed.): *Current Veterinary Therapy Food Animal Practice.* Philadelphia: W. B. Saunders, 1986, p. 848.
A description of the detailed neurologic examination of cattle leading to a neuroanatomic and etiologic diagnosis.
Fowler, M. E.: Tick paralysis. Calif Vet 39:2, 1985, p. 25.
A brief discussion of tick paralysis as it affects most mammalian species, including pathophysiology, treatment, and control.
Fowler, M. E.: *Medicine and Surgery of South American Camelids.* Ames, IA: Iowa State University Press, 1989, p. 322.
Brief review of llama anatomy and diagnostic procedures, followed by a description of observed neurologic clinical cases.
Fowler, M. E., and Gillespie, D.: Middle and inner ear infection in llamas. J Zoo Anim Med 16:1, 1985, p. 9.
Three cases of middle ear infection in llamas are described, including radiographs and discussion of options of therapy and prognosis.

Lunn, D. P., and Hinchcliff, K. W.: Cerebrospinal fluid eosinophilia and ataxia in five llamas. Vet. Rec. 124:302, 1989.
Case description of five llamas all presumably affected by meningeal worm and characterized by CSF eosinophilia.
Milton, M., Boden, P., Crocker, C., et al.: Rabies in a llama—Oklahoma. M.M.W.R. 39:203, 1989.
A recent description of the first reported case of rabies in a llama.
Pearson, E. G., Craig, A. M., and Lassen, E. D.: Suspected chlorpyrifos toxicosis in a llama and plasma pseudocholinesterase activity in llamas given chlorpyrifos. J.A.V.M.A. 189:1062, 1986.
Clinical description of a case of organophosphate poisoning in a llama, with emphasis on diagnosis based on levels of plasma pseudocholinesterase.
Rebhun, W. C., Jenkins, D. H., Riis, R. C., et al.: An epizootic of blindness and encephalitis associated with a herpes virus indistinguishable from equine herpesvirus I in a herd of alpacas and llamas. J.A.V.M.A. 192:953, 1988.
A detailed description of the first reported cases of camelid blindness due to equine herpesvirus I, including serologic studies, virus isolation techniques, and necropsy findings.
Smith, J. A.: Toxic encephalopathies in cattle. *In* Howard, J. L. (ed.): *Current Veterinary Therapy Food Animal Practice.* Vol. 2. Philadelphia: W. B. Saunders, 1986, p. 855.
A comprehensive review of bovine diagnoses that would be considerable when toxicities are suspected in camelids.
Smith, J. A.: Noninfectious, metabolic, toxic and neoplastic diseases of camelids. *In* Johnson, L. W. (ed.): Vet. Clin. North Am. Food Anim. Pract. 5(1):119, 1989.
A discussion of common neurologic conditions that have been observed to affect llamas.

WATER QUALITY AND THE MARINE AQUARIUM

SCOTT B. CITINO
Washington, D.C.

Within the marine aquarium, the tropical fish hobbyist attempts to simulate the stable yet dynamic marine environment. It is a difficult task because marine environments are in general considerably more stable than freshwater environments, and consequently marine inhabitants are far less tolerant of fluctuations in water quality than are freshwater inhabitants. Captive marine fish are in constant, intimate contact with an aquarium system's water and are dependent upon an appropriate, constant water chemistry to maintain internal homeostasis. Even small changes in water chemistry can stress marine fish and initiate disease outbreaks in marine aquaria. Marine aquarists should routinely monitor water quality and make appropriate adjustments before environmental stress occurs.

WATER SOURCES

Both natural and artificial seawater may be successfully utilized in marine aquaria, and both have

advantages and disadvantages. The composition of natural seawater has been described (Harvey, 1963), as have formulas for artificial sea salt mixtures (Spotte, 1970).

Aquarists must generally live near a coast to have access to natural seawater. Natural seawater should preferably be collected through a deep subsand filtration unit that filters out most impurities and living organisms or from deep reef or pelagic sources where pollution is minimal. Natural seawater is generally much cheaper than artificial sea salt mixtures but may contain industrial and organic pollutants and living organisms that may parasitize fish and foul aquaria. Natural seawater should be allowed to settle in a dark container for several days and then passed through a mechanical filter containing activated charcoal to remove impurities and pollutants. Water quality parameters of each new batch of natural seawater should be tested to make sure the water is suitable for aquarium use.

Sea salt mixtures tend to be expensive but allow

aquarists to maintain marine aquaria in any location. Good-quality, commercial, premixed salts produce seawater with standardized quality from batch to batch, but salt mixes may contain impurities and tend to be low in essential trace compounds, which may make them unsuitable for some applications. Artificial seawater is only as good as the freshwater used to prepare it. If tap water is used, aquarists should remove chlorine and chloramines with a commercial sodium thiosulfate solution and reduce copper levels with activated charcoal filtration. Artificial sea salts should dissolve readily and should not precipitate out of solution. Newly prepared artificial seawater should be allowed to equilibrate for several hours before use to allow pH to stabilize at 8.1 to 8.3.

IMPORTANT WATER QUALITY PARAMETERS

Marine aquarists should purchase water test kits to monitor aquarium water quality. Reasonably priced, accurate kits can be obtained from Hach Chemicals (Loveland, CO) and La Motte Chemicals (Chestertown, MD). The most important water quality parameters to monitor are listed in Table 1 with preferred ranges and trends. These parameters should be monitored at least weekly in well-established aquaria and daily in newly established aquaria and aquaria stressed by the addition of new fish, large water changes, or the addition of therapeutic agents.

Dissolved Oxygen

Aeration and gas exchange in marine aquaria are critical because seawater contains approximately 20% less dissolved oxygen than does freshwater at the same temperature because of seawater's high dissolved solids content (Curry, 1976). Dissolved oxygen can drop to dangerously low levels (<3.5 ppm) in marine aquaria with high salinity, high temperatures, dirty mechanical and biologic filters (high biologic oxygen demand), low lighting, and poor aeration. To maintain sufficient dissolved oxygen concentrations, aquarists should use aquariums with large surface areas for gas exchange, maintain low fish-to-water ratios, keep filter systems clean, employ vigorous aeration that moves 1.5 to 2.0 liters of air per liter of water each hour with small bubble diameter (Beleau, 1988), and use wet-to-dry trickle filter systems.

Salinity

Salinity is the measure of the total dissolved salts in seawater; it can be measured using a bulb hydrometer (specific gravity [S.G.]), temperature-corrected refractometer, or electrical conductivity. If a bulb hydrometer is used a nomogram should be used to correct for the effect of temperature on salinity (Oestmann, 1985). Because marine fish have adapted to a hyperosmotic environment, salinity is an important measure of the osmotic burden on marine fish. Deviations of salinity from the preferred range can have serious effects on the osmoregulation and homeostatic mechanisms of marine fish. Salinity tends to increase in marine aquaria due to evaporation of water and must be corrected for by the addition of freshwater.

Hydrogen Ion Concentration

Maintenance of proper hydrogen ion concentration (pH) in marine aquaria is essential for the health of marine fish. Values outside the preferred range can have detrimental effects on acid-base balance and osmoregulation in fish and lead to environmental stress and disease. Major factors affecting pH in marine aquaria are the amount of

Table 1. Important Water Quality Parameters for the Marine Aquarium*

Parameter	Optimum	Preferred Range	Trends
Dissolved O_2	>6.0 ppm	5.5 ppm to saturation	—
pH	8.2	7.9 to 8.4	decrease
Specific gravity	1.024 at 26.7°C	1.020 to 1.026	increase
Salinity	32 ppt	28 to 36 ppt	increase
Alkalinity	4 mEq/L	2 to 6 mEq/L	decrease
Carbonate hardness	12 dKH	5 to 20 dKH	decrease
Phosphates	1.0 ppm	0.00 to 3.0 ppm	increase
Redox potential	325 to 350 mV	250 to 400 mV	decrease
Ammonia (NH_3)	<0.01 ppm	<0.05 ppm	increase
Nitrite (NO_2^-)	<0.1 ppm	<1.0 ppm	increase
Nitrate (NO_3^-)	<20 ppm	<50 ppm	increase
Copper	<0.05 ppm	0.13 to 0.2 ppm†	decrease

*Data from Moe, 1989; Spotte, 1979; and Stoskopf and Citino, 1987.
†Preferred therapeutic range only; otherwise concentration should be less than 0.05 ppm.

dissolved carbon dioxide, the concentrations of magnesium and calcium ions, and the accumulation of organic acids, phosphates, and nitrates. pH has a tendency to decrease in established marine aquaria. Key factors in the maintenance of proper pH levels include good aeration, effective biologic filtration, protein foam skimming, algae filtration, and regular partial water changes (Moe, 1989). Elevated carbon dioxide levels (with a consequent drop in pH) may result from lack of aeration and water movements, overstocking of fish, and bacterial overgrowths due to protein accumulation. Decomposition of organic wastes liberates organic acids that accumulate and bind bicarbonate and calcium carbonate, which in turn reduces the capacity of the seawater buffer system to maintain a high pH. Organic wastes also liberate phosphates during decomposition that combine with calcium and magnesium ions and effectively remove them from the seawater buffer system by precipitation, allowing pH to drop. Low pH in marine aquaria can be temporarily corrected by slow titration with sodium bicarbonate.

Alkalinity and Carbonate Hardness

The seawater buffer system is essential for maintaining normal pH in marine aquaria and for preventing devastating rapid pH swings. This complex buffer system has been well described (Gieskes, 1974; Spotte, 1970). Two parameters commonly used to monitor the buffering capacity of seawater are alkalinity and carbonate hardness. With constant addition of acidic waste products from fish and biologic filtration, buffering capacity of the seawater in an aquarium slowly diminishes over time, with a concomitant decrease in alkalinity and carbonate hardness. The marine aquarist can maintain the buffer system by filtration of organic matter and frequent detritus removal. Regeneration of the buffer system requires frequent partial water changes and addition of commercially available marine buffers.

Ammonia, Nitrite, and Nitrate

Establishment of nitrification in closed aquarium systems is essential for fish health. The nitrification process or nitrogen cycle is well described (Citino, 1989; Spotte, 1979) and prevents accumulation of toxic nitrogenous wastes. Monitoring the nitrogen cycle by determination of ammonia (NH_3), nitrite (NO_2^-), and nitrate (NO_3^-) concentrations is a valuable tool for assessing the status of biologic filtration in marine aquarium systems. NH_3 and NO_2^- are both very toxic to fish and are generally present at barely detectable levels in established marine aquaria, while NO_3^- is relatively nontoxic to fish and continually accumulates in closed aquarium systems. In newly established aquaria, NH_3 and NO_2^- levels rise due to insufficient colonization by nitrifying bacteria and often reach toxic concentrations, with fish mortality 2 to 4 weeks after addition of fish ("new tank syndrome"). NH_3 and NO_2^- levels also rise when biologic filtration is overwhelmed by overstocking and accumulation of organic wastes or is curtailed by agents that destroy nitrifying bacteria (i.e., erythromycin, new methylene blue). Aquarists can maintain low nitrogenous waste concentrations in marine aquaria by establishing and maintaining a suitable biofilter (i.e., trickle filter, fluidized filter bed, undergravel filter), keeping fish populations within biofilter capacity, adding new fish slowly, removing organic detritus and wastes by mechanical filtration and siphoning, and frequent partial water changes.

References and Suggested Reading

Beleau, M. H.: Evaluating water problems. *In* Stoskopf, M. K. (ed.): Vet. Clin. North Am. Small Anim. Pract. 18:293, 1988.

Citino, S. B.: Basic ornamental fish medicine. *In* Kirk, R. W. (ed.): *Current Veterinary Therapy X.* Philadelphia: W.B. Saunders, 1989, pp. 703–721.

Curry, C.: Management of saltwater fish. *Iowa State Univ. Vet.* 38:76, 1976.

Gieskes, J. M.: The alkalinity–total carbon dioxide system in seawater. *In* Goldberg, E. D. (ed.): *The Sea: Ideas and Observations on Progress in the Study of the Seas.* New York: John Wiley & Sons, 1974, pp. 123–151.

Harvey, H. W.: *The Chemistry and Fertility of Sea Water.* London: Cambridge University Press, 1963, p. 240.

Moe, M. A.: *The Marine Aquarium Reference: Systems and Invertebrates.* Plantation, FL: Green Turtle Publications, 1989, pp. 40–41.

Oestmann, D. J.: Environmental and disease problems in ornamental marine aquariums. Comp. Cont. Ed. Pract. Vet 7:656, 1985.

Spotte, S.: *Fish and Invertebrate Culture: Water Management in Closed Systems.* New York: John Wiley & Sons, 1970.

Spotte, S.: *Seawater Aquariums: The Captive Environment.* New York: John Wiley & Sons, 1979.

Stoskopf, M. K., and Citino, S. B.: *Workshop on Marine Tropical Fish.* Honolulu, HI, M.K. Stoskopf, 1987, p. 61.

IMPORTANT PROBLEMS IN MARINE AQUARIUM FISHES

EDWARD J. NOGA
Raleigh, North Carolina

THE MARINE FISH HOBBY

Although not as numerous as freshwater aquarium fishes, marine aquarium fishes are a growing segment of the pet fish industry. Part of this growth is due to recent advances in techniques for successfully keeping these fish in captivity. Better tank design (including the introduction of all-glass aquaria) and more reliable and efficient pumps, filters, and other apparatus have greatly improved water quality, an essential element for marine fish health (see this volume, p. 1199). Another contributing factor to the surge in popularity of marine aquariums is increased disposable income, allowing more people to afford these beautiful but expensive creatures. The average marine aquarium fish costs considerably more than its freshwater counterpart, with some rare specimens commanding several hundred dollars. Many marine hobbyists have elaborate and often expensive "reef tanks" for the display of live invertebrates (corals, anemones, etc.) and sometimes fish. A dozen or more fish in a single tank constitute a sizable economic investment.

This article is not intended to address all the problems affecting marine fishes. Citino (see *CVT X*, p. 703) has covered the general aspects of pet fish husbandry and medicine, including a discussion of marine fish problems. Readers should refer to this article or to Andrews et al. (1988), Untergasser (1989), or Stoskopf (1988) for general information on pet fish diseases and their treatment. This article will describe some important differences between freshwater and marine fishes that affect their clinical management.

ECOLOGICAL DIFFERENCES BETWEEN MARINE AND FRESHWATER AQUARIUM FISHES

Important ecological differences between these two groups of fish have a direct bearing on the state of their health in captivity (Table 1). Compared to freshwater ecosystems, the tropical marine environment fluctuates minimally in temperature, oxygen, or other water-quality conditions. Thus, marine reef fish are less tolerant of the poor water conditions to which they are often exposed in captivity. The stress of adaptation is exacerbated by the fact that most marine aquarium fishes are caught in the wild and must also acclimate to captivity. They may also carry latent infections that recrudesce under captive conditions. The territoriality of reef fishes may also cause stress. Additionally, many reef fishes have specialized diets. They are often imported and sold in stores with little regard for their feeding habits; many species do not readily adapt to standard aquarium feeds and subsequently starve.

All of these factors increase susceptibility to disease and contribute to the deserved reputation marine fishes have for being more difficult to keep than freshwater fishes. This increases the need for competent management and health care.

Fish chosen for a marine aquarium should be species with histories of successful maintenance in captivity. To avoid aggression problems, an old rule of thumb is to only have one fish of any color, color pattern, or shape. Population density, behavior of each species, and possible interaction with tankmates must be considered. Bower (1983) provides an excellent discussion on choosing fish and proper management of the marine aquarium.

FACTORS IN DISEASE DIFFERENCES BETWEEN MARINE AND FRESHWATER AQUARIUM FISHES

Water Quality

Marine fishes are affected by the same water-quality factors as freshwater fishes but in general

Table 1. *Differences Between Marine and Freshwater Aquarium Fishes*

	Freshwater	Marine
Many inbred strains	Yes	No
Many bred in captivity	Yes	No
Specialized feeding habits or nutritional requirements	Relatively few	Relatively many
Sensitivity to environmental changes	Relatively small	Relatively large
Territorial	Many	Almost all

1202

appear to be more sensitive to adverse conditions than most freshwater species. In addition, the chemistry of salt water influences the toxicity of many substances (see this volume, p. 1199, for details on water quality).

Infectious Disease

Freshwater and marine fishes are affected by similar types of pathogens, including parasites, bacteria, fungi, and viruses. Few pathogens, however, are transmissible from freshwater to marine fishes or vice versa.

Important protozoan parasites include the flagellate *Amyloodinium ocellatum* and the ciliate *Cryptocaryon irritans*, which have life cycles similar to that of the freshwater ciliate *Ichthyophthirius multifiliis*. Copper sulfate (0.15 to 0.20 mg/L of active copper ion) is usually the best control for these agents (Citino, 1989), although recent studies have shown that chloroquine diphosphate (5 to 10 mg/L, Sigma Chemical Company, St. Louis, MO) may be highly effective against amyloodiniosis (Bower, 1990). Another important protozoan is *Brooklynella*, which is morphologically and pathologically similar to the freshwater ciliate *Chilodonella*. Trichodinids (*Trichodina* and related genera) are also common pathogens.

Rohde (1984) gives a comprehensive discussion of the helminths that affect marine fishes. Life cycles and treatment of these pathogens are generally similar to that of freshwater fishes. The most important helminths are the monogenean trematodes, which infest the skin and gills. Crustaceans (copepods, isopods, and branchiurans) are also pathogenic but less common.

Fungal infections are a common problem in freshwater fishes but appear to be uncommon in marine species (Noga, 1990). Saprolegniaceous fungi, the predominant fungal pathogens in freshwater fishes, do not infect marine reef fishes. *Ichthyophonus hoferi*, reported to be a very common pathogen in marine reef fishes (Kingsford, 1975), is extremely rare in my experience.

Gram-negative rods are the most common cause of bacterial infections in marine fishes. *Vibrio* spp. are probably the most common agents. Mycobacteriosis due to *Mycobacterium marinum* or *Mycobacterium fortuitum* commonly affect both fresh-

water and marine fishes. At this time, the only viral disease recognized in marine reef fishes is lymphocystis, which also affects freshwater fishes.

TREATMENT OF MARINE FISH DISEASES

Treatment modalities for marine reef fishes are generally the same as those for freshwater fishes. Important differences in treating marine fishes primarily relate to use of water-borne medications. The first consideration is the efficacy of the agent in salt water. Some antibiotics, notably the tetracyclines, chelate divalent cations (calcium and magnesium), which are present in very high concentrations in seawater. This can reduce antibiotic absorption in the fish. Many other therapeutics, including copper and organophosphates, are affected by seawater.

Second, many medications for marine fishes, including copper, formalin, and organophosphates, are very toxic to invertebrates, so their use in "reef systems" must be avoided. Even if antibiotics not toxic to invertebrates are chosen, they may present other problems in tank management. As in freshwater tanks, they may interfere with the action of bacterial filters. They may also interfere with symbiotic bacteria and algae needed for the survival of anemones, corals, and some other invertebrates. For these reasons, it is best to avoid exposing invertebrates to fish medications.

References and Suggested Reading

Andrews, C., Exell, A. and Carrington, N.: *The Manual of Fish Health.* Morris Plains, NJ: Tetra Press, 1988.

Bower, C. E.: Unpublished data, 1990.

Bower, C. E.: *The Basic Marine Aquarium.* Springfield, IL: C. C. Thomas, 1983, p. 142.

Citino, S. B.: Basic ornamental fish medicine. *In* Kirk, R. W. (ed.): *Current Veterinary Therapy X.* Philadelphia: W. B. Saunders, 1989, p. 703.

Kingsford, E.: *Treatment of Exotic Marine Fish Diseases.* New York: Arco Publishing, 1975.

Noga, E. J.: A synopsis of mycotic diseases of marine fishes and invertebrates. *In* Perkins, F. O., and Cheng, T. C. (eds.): *Pathology in Marine Science.* New York: Academic Press, 1990, p. 143.

Rohde, K.: Diseases caused by metazoans: Helminths. *In* Kinne, O. (ed.): *Diseases of Marine Animals.* Hamburg, Federal Republic of Germany: Biologische Anstalt Helgoland, 1984, p. 193.

Stoskopf, M. K. (ed.): *Tropical Fish Medicine.* Vet. Clin. North Am. Small Anim. Pract. Vol. 18, No. 2, 1988.

Untergasser, D.: *Handbook of Fish Diseases.* Neptune City, NJ: T.F.H. Publications, 1989.

REPTILE DERMATOLOGY

ELLIOTT R. JACOBSON

Gainesville, Florida

The integument of reptiles shows many modifications from group to group and species to species depending on life-style. Chelonians (turtles and tortoises), crocodilians (alligators, crocodiles, caiman, gharial), and squamates (lizards and snakes) have a variety of infectious and noninfectious integumentary diseases, some of which are group specific. Some of these diseases are specific for the integumentary system; others represent generalized infections with both systemic and cutaneous involvement. Diagnostic techniques are basic and require biopsies for histopathology and microbial culture. Treatment depends on etiology and often involves management modifications in addition to the use of appropriate chemotherapeutics.

STRUCTURE AND FUNCTION OF THE REPTILE INTEGUMENT

The reptile integument shows a number of modifications over the more primitive amphibian design. Because most reptiles lead a more terrestrial existence than do amphibians, the epidermis has a thicker, keratinized surface. Also, the reptile skin is dry compared to the moist amphibian skin; this evolved as an adaptation for existence in a dehydrating atmosphere. Mucous and poison glands are absent from the reptile skin and glandular structures generally have a restricted distribution. In many reptiles, the surface of the integument is a series of folds grossly seen as scales. In many species of reptiles, such as the giant tortoises, shingle-back skinks, and armadillo lizards, the scales are exceptionally keratinized, making surgical incision difficult. Many lizards have developed flamboyant cutaneous modifications for use in territorial displays, defense, and courting.

The chelonians have developed one of the most unique integumentary structures of all vertebrates—the shell. The chelonian shell consists of outer epidermal scutes or platelike structures overlying a series of dermal plates. Most aquatic turtles periodically shed the outer portion of their scutes as they grow, but tortoises do not. In tortoises, new areas of growth occur at the suture lines equidistant from the embryonic shields or areolae located in the center of each scute. These structures are present at birth, and as a tortoise grows rings form around each embryonic shield; with time, embryonic shields get further apart. It is impossible to age captive tortoises by the number of rings around each shield. However, for wild tortoises, length of the plastron and carapace and wear of the embryonic shields and rings have been used for aging. The dermis of most chelonians is primarily bone and is continuous with the ribs and vertebrae. The dermal bone is not inert but is a metabolically active structure. In calculating dosages of medicants to be administered, the weight of the shell should be considered. The uptake, distribution, and elimination of an antibiotic in the turtle will depend upon the physiology of the turtle being treated.

INFECTIOUS DISEASES

Bacterial

CHELONIA. Bacterial-associated shell and skin diseases are commonly seen in chelonians. Septicemic cutaneous ulcerative disease (SCUD) in turtles was first described in freshwater turtles of the genera *Pseudemys* and *Chrysemys* (Jackson and Fulton, 1970). Clinically, the disease is seen as necrotizing, ulcerative, cutaneous lesions, with both shell and skin involvement. Although *Citrobacter freundii* has been incriminated as the etiologic agent, *Serratia* may be necessary to initiate the infection. The gram-negative bacillus *Beneckea chitinovora* was incriminated as the causative agent of an ulcerative disease of several species of aquatic turtles, with soft-shell turtles (*Trionyx* spp) being most severely affected (Wallach, 1972). It has been associated with feeding live shrimp which serve as a carrier. *Aeromonas hydrophila* septicemias with necrotizing dermatitis have been seen in a number of wild freshwater turtles of the genera *Pseudemys*, *Chysemys*, and *Sternotherus*. Middle-ear infections of box turtles (*Terrapene* spp) associated with a number of gram-negative bacteria are manifested as bulging abscesses below the tympanic scales, caudal to the eyes. Although gram-negative bacteria are the most common bacteria associated with skin disease of turtles, gram-positive bacteria may occasionally cause problems. A red-footed tortoise (*Geochelone carbonaria*) with a necrotizing skin disease was found to have a streptococcal infection.

CROCODILIA. *Aeromonas hydrophilia* is the most significant opportunistic pathogen in crocodilians, especially in animals that are thermally stressed. Bacteria from the intestinal tract may enter the vascular compartment (sepsis) and invade multiple visceral structures. Necrotizing, hemorrhagic skin lesions are commonly seen peripherally with this disease.

A hyperkeratotic, ulcerative skin disease has been seen on the ventral body scales of farm-reared American alligators in Florida and Louisiana. Although a filamentous organism resembling *Dermatophilus* has been consistently found in these lesions, it has not been isolated.

SQUAMATA. Numerous cases of bacteria-associated skin diseases have been reported in squamates. Necrotizing skin lesions colonized by *Pseudomonas* have been seen in snakes secondary to burn wounds. An Indonesian blue-tongue skink (*Teliqua gigas*) with multifocal *P. aeruginosa* dermatitis was found to have a large intracoelomic, perihepatic abscess connected to an overlying skin lesion. *Pseudomonas*, one of the most common bacterial organisms associated with oral and respiratory disease in snakes, may enter the vascular compartment and ultimately result in peripheral, cutaneous lesions. A condition has been seen in boa constrictors and pythons in which obstipation, necrosis of the gastrointestinal tract, or infection of the female reproductive tract is associated with loss of the stratum corneum of body scales. The outer portion of each scale flakes off. At first only a few scales are affected, but eventually almost the entire body may be involved.

In lizards and snakes, subcutaneous granulomas and pyogranulomas are common. Many of these lesions are the result of trauma, such as those resulting from rodent bites. A mixture of gram-negative bacteria including *Pseudomonas, Providencia, Escherichia coli*, and *Proteus* have been cultured from these lesions. Anaerobes have also been isolated (Stewart, 1989). Recently, *Neisseria* was isolated from tail abscesses in the green iguana (*Iguana iguana*) and from the oral cavity of healthy iguanas (Plowman et al., 1987). The infections probably developed as a result of bite wounds inflicted by cage mates.

Dermatophilus congolensis, the etiologic agent of streptothricosis in mammals, has been identified as the causative agent of hyperkeratotic skin lesions in several species of lizards. The author has seen an organism with microscopic characteristics of *D. congolensis* in skin lesions in Senegal chameleons (*Chamaeleo senegalensis*) and a collared lizard (*Crotaphytus collaris*), and in a subcutaneous nodule in a boa constrictor (*Constrictor constrictor*).

There are rare reports of cutaneous mycobacterial infection in snakes. In a boa constrictor with subcutaneous mycobacterial granulomas, a proliferating oral lesion developed from which *Mycobacterium chelonei* was isolated (Quesenberry et al., 1986).

TREATMENT

Bacterial diseases in captive reptiles are most commonly caused by aerobic gram-negative microorganisms. Many of these organisms are secondary invaders, requiring predisposing problems before an infection begins. Treatment involves not only isolation and identification of the pathogen or pathogens but identification and correction of the factors allowing the organism or organisms to become established. For instance, reptiles kept at suboptimal environmental conditions appear to be immunocompromised and are at risk for bacterial (and other pathogen) infections. In these cases, treatment includes exposure to an appropriate ambient temperature.

Subcutaneous abscess or granulomas should be surgically removed, though with miliary granulomas it is often difficult to identify and remove all the nodules. Following removal, they may reoccur at the same site.

The use of chemotherapeutics in reptile medicine has been discussed elsewhere (Jacobson, 1988) and will be briefly reviewed here. In selecting the most appropriate antibiotic, the causative agent should be identified and sensitivity patterns determined. If possible, minimum inhibitory concentrations (MICs) of antibiotics should be determined. Because pharmacokinetic information is only available on a handful of antibiotics (in relatively few species of reptiles), the selection of drugs is limited. Pharmacokinetic data are available for chloromycetin, carbenicillin, ceftazadime, gentamicin, and amikacin (see this volume, p. 1214).

Because many reptiles submitted with gram-negative sepsis appear to be immunocompromised, bactericidal antibiotics would be more efficacious than bacteriostatic drugs.

Ambient temperature has a marked effect on the uptake, distribution, and elimination of antibiotics in reptiles. Ill reptiles should be maintained at their preferred optimum temperature range (for many species, a temperature range of 26°C to 33°C is ideal). At higher temperatures, small species can dehydrate rapidly, and the clinician must constantly be aware of the hydration status of the patient. Additional considerations in appropriate drug selection include health status of the reptile patient, size of the patient, and potential side effects of the drug.

Treatment of bacterial skin diseases with creams or ointments containing antibiotics and antibacterial chemicals depends on the type of lesion and bacteria identified. Necrotic debris and tissue should first be removed. In burn cases, the author has soaked injured reptiles in a solution of 16 ml of 2% chlorhexidine diacetate (Nolvasan, Fort Dodge Lab, Fort Dodge, IA) in 4 liters of water twice daily until the lesions have healed. Mafenide acetate (Sulfamylon, Winthrop Pharmaceuticals) and silver sulfadiazine

(Silvadene, Marion Laboratories) are ideal topical ointments in burn patients, especially those with wounds colonized by *Pseudomonas*.

Viral

CHELONIA. Several virus-associated skin diseases have been seen in chelonians. A herpesvirus has been demonstrated to be the causative agent of epizootics of skin lesions termed gray-patched disease in young green turtles (*Chelonia mydas*) between 56 and 90 days posthatching in aquaculture (Rebell et al., 1975). Skin lesions begin as small circular, papular lesions that coalesce into spreading patches containing epidermal cells with basophilic, intranuclear inclusions. Bolivian side-neck turtles (*Platemys platycephala*) with circular, gray, papular skin lesions were found to have crystalline arrays of hexagonal particles within nuclei of outer epidermal cells (Jacobson et al., 1982). These particles were consistent with those of papillomavirus, although the skin lesions never progressed into papillomas.

Fibropapillomas were first described more than 50 years ago in wild green sea turtles (*Chelonia mydas*). While tumors may be found anywhere on the body surface, there seems to be a predilection for the periocular and ocular tissues and integument at the base of the fore- and hind limbs. Tumors affecting the periocular and ocular tissues can become life-threatening by covering the globe, resulting in a blind turtle. Fibropapillomas may be so numerous and large that a turtle is unable to swim normally. While recent pathologic and molecular studies have failed to incriminate an infectious agent, a virus is suspected (Jacobson et al., 1989).

CROCODILIA. Poxvirus skin disease has been reported in caiman (*Caiman sclerops*) imported into the United States (Jacobson et al., 1979) and in Nile crocodiles (*Crocodylus niloticus*) in Africa (Horner, 1988). In caiman, gray-white circular skin lesions were found scattered over the body surface. Proliferative lesions may be seen in the oral cavity. In some cases, digital sloughing may be seen.

SQUAMATA. There is only one report of virus-associated integumentary disease in either lizards or snakes, but others will likely be seen. Cutaneous papillomas are commonly seen in the European green lizard (*Lacerta viridis*). In one study, papillomas were found in the caudal lumbar area in females and were distributed around the base of the head in males (Raynaud and Adrian, 1976). Intranuclear inclusions were found within hypertrophied epidermal cells and three morphologically distinct virus particles resembling papovavirus, herpesvirus, and reovirus were demonstrated by electron microscopy.

The author has examined several species of snakes with vesicular skin disease suggestive of viral infec-

tions. However, electron microscopic examination of these lesions failed to identify any viral particles.

TREATMENT

There are no vaccines available for any of the viral diseases of reptiles. In most cases, the lesions are colonized by bacteria and fungi that often contribute to severity of the lesions. Biopsies and microbial culture of these lesions allow selection of the most appropriate chemotherapeutic for treatment of these secondary invaders. Ill reptiles should be separated from healthy cage mates and maintained under ideal environmental conditions. For aquatic species, water quality control is imperative; water should be changed at least daily.

Fungal

CHELONIA. A number of fungi have been associated with skin and shell disease in turtles and tortoises. The author found a large subcutaneous mass in a leopard tortoise (*Geochelone pardalis*) to be composed of mycotic granulomas. *Mucor* was identified in tissue section and isolated from necrotizing shell lesions in a large group of young Florida soft-shell turtles (*Trionyx ferox*) (Jacobson et al., 1980). The author has also seen fungal organisms in hatchling Ridley sea turtles (*Lepidochelys kempi*) with necrotizing palpebritis and in pitted shell lesions of hatchling Australian side-neck turtles (*Chelodina longicollis*).

CROCODILIA. Relatively few mycotic skin diseases have been reported in crocodilians. Fungi have been found in a bumblefoot-like condition of the footpads seen in crocodilians kept in cement pools.

SQUAMATA. Fungal cutaneous lesions are commonly encountered in captive lizards and snakes. The author has also seen several cases of fungal dermatitis and epidermatitis in wild snakes in the southeastern United States. Fungi recovered from these lesions included *Fusarium*, *Trichosporon*, *Geotrichum*, *Penicillium*, *Oospora*, and *Trichoderma*. Subcutaneous mycotic granulomas may be seen in snakes, but most lesions seen by the author were confined to the epidermis. Grossly, these lesions are seen as thickened, brown-yellow encrustations, particularly on the ventral belly scales. Geckos in the genus *Phelsuma* have been seen with necrotizing, mycotic epidermitis and dermatitis.

TREATMENT

As in higher vertebrates, fungi in reptiles may be either primary or secondary invaders. In the author's experience, they are most often secondary invaders with a multitude of predisposing factors involved. In aquatic turtles, poor water quality is contributory. As mentioned earlier, suboptimal environmental temperature may cause immunosuppression in reptiles and allow secondary agents to invade. Excessive humidity and cages not kept clean promote the growth of fungal organisms. Additionally, fungal disease may follow a primary viral or bacterial skin infection.

There are relatively few reports discussing treatment of reptiles with fungal skin disease. Localized mycotic infections of scales and subcutaneous mycotic granulomas are best treated by surgical removal. Several cases of mycotic skin disease have been treated successfully by soaking in a dilute, organic iodine solution twice daily followed by topical application of an antifungal ointment such as tolnaftate (Tinactin, Schering Corp.) or miconazole nitrate (Monistat-Derm, Ortho Pharmaceutical Corp.). Malachite green has been used for treating aquatic turtles with mycotic shell disease, and ketoconazole has been administered to reptiles with mycotic infections. In a pharmacokinetic study in the gopher tortoise (Gopherus polyphemus), oral administration of 15 mg/kg of body weights resulted in therapeutic plasma concentrations (>1 µg/ml) from 4 to 32 hours after dosing (Page et al., 1991.)

Parasitic

CHELONIA. Aquatic chelonians appear to be the most commonly infected reptilian host for spirorchid trematodes. Adult parasites are found in the circulatory system, and released eggs often become lodged in peripheral vessels, where infarcts and inflammation occur. Infected turtles have been seen with necrotizing shell lesions and edema of the limbs as a result of vascular occlusion. Tortoises are commonly parasitized by ticks, which generally attach at the base of the tail on the ventral surface. Leeches are commonly encountered on both freshwater and marine turtles. In the southeastern United States, box turtles and gopher tortoises (Gopherus polyphemus) appear particularly prone to subcutaneous infestation with the larval (maggot) state of the dipteran Cistudinamyia cistudinis.

CROCODILIA. Nematodes in the genus Paratrichosoma are responsible for cutaneous lesions in several species of crocodilians. Nematodes wandering through the dermis result in convoluted, raised tracks, most often seen on the ventral belly scales. Leeches are commonly encountered in wild crocodilians, either on the skin or in the oral cavity.

SQUAMATA. In squamates, a variety of endoparasites and ectoparasites are found at subcutaneous sites and on the skin surface, respectively. Spargana (larva) of the pseudophyllidean cestode Spirometra may be found subcutaneously, resulting in soft swelling of the overlying skin. Trematode mesocercariae of the genera Alaria and Fibricola have been identified in subcutaneous tissues of several snake species. Necrotizing dermatitis, resulting from obstruction of the vascular system by the filarid nematode Macdonaldius, has been seen in captive reticulated pythons. Several snake species with pustular dermatitis were found to have infections with members of the nematode superfamily Dracunculoidea. Several species of pentastomids, primitive-appearing parasites, are known to infect snakes. Adults may be found in the subcutaneous tissues along the body where they cause bulging of the overlying skin.

Infestations with a variety of mites and ticks have been reported in squamates. In snakes, the mite Ophionysus natricis is commonly encountered in recently imported snakes that are crowded together. Eggs are deposited in the immediate environment of the snake. Severe infestations may result in debilitated, anemic snakes. Mites have also been incriminated in the transmission of Aeromonas hydrophila. The more important genera of ticks in squamates include Amblyomma, Aponomma, Hyalomma, and Ornithodoros. These parasites can cause anemia and focal ulcerations of the skin or act as vectors for transmission of other pathogens.

TREATMENT

A variety of parasiticides are available for treating many of the parasites causing skin lesions in reptiles. For trematode and cestode infections, the drug of choice is praziquantel (Droncit, Mobay Corp., Shawnee, KS) administered at 8 to 20 mg/kg IM as a single injection and repeated in 2 weeks. For nematode infections, fenbendazole (Panacur, Agri-Vet Co., Somerville, NJ) at 100 mg/kg or ivermectin (Ivomec, Merck and Co., Rahway, NJ) at 200 µg/kg are given orally as a single dose and repeated in 2 weeks. Ivermectin is toxic in chelonians and should not be used in these animals. There are no chemotherapeutics known to be efficacious against pentastomes. An alternative to using parasiticides is surgical removal of parasites where possible. An ambient temperature regimen of 35°C to 37°C for 24 to 48 hours has been used to kill adults of the filarid nematode Macdonaldius.

A variety of treatments can be used to control ectoparasites. In most situations, leeches and ticks can be manually removed. In sea turtles with leech infestations, maintaining turtles in freshwater for 24 hours generally will result in the death of saltwater leeches. For mite infestations, one of the most effective treatments for small snakes is coating the animal with olive oil, which covers the spiracles of the mites so they suffocate. Various pest strips with dimethyldichlorovinyl phosphate (DDVP) have also been used. However, in recent years mites have shown increased resistance to this chemical. To control mite infestations in reptiles, both animal and cage must be treated. Infestation of turtles and tortoises with dipteran larvae (maggots) requires surgical removal.

NONINFECTIOUS PROBLEMS

Trauma

CHELONIA. Chelonians are commonly seen with traumatic shell injuries. A large number of aquatic turtles, box turtles, and tortoises are hit by cars. Pet tortoises are traumatized by lawn mowers. Traumatic shell injuries may result from mounting behavior during breeding season. Box turtles and gopher tortoises caught in forest fires may survive with significant portions of their shells burned.

CROCODILIA. Traumatic skin lesions are common in captive crocodilians. Captive animals may abrade body surfaces in cement pools and injuries also often result from aggressive behavior of cage mates. Crocodiles may develop thermal burns when infrared lights are placed too close to the basking site.

SQUAMATA. Trauma commonly accounts for cutaneous lesions in snakes and lizards, especially in recently collected animals attempting to escape from their cage. Indigo snakes are notorious for abrading their rostral scales, and recently imported water dragons (*Physignathus* spp) are commonly seen with trauma to the rostral aspects of both upper and lower jaws. Thermal burns are common in snakes kept on electric heating pads. Often these wounds become colonized with *Pseudomonas aeruginosa*.

Trauma to the integument may occur at mating time, especially in some species of lizards. Snakes may traumatize one another at feeding time, and most animals should be fed separately. Live food (e.g., rodents) can severely traumatize snakes and such prey should be killed prior to feeding.

TREATMENT

In turtles and tortoises with recent noninfected, traumatic shell injuries, defects can be filled with calcium hydroxide dental paste (Root-Cal, Ellman International, Hewlett, NY) and covered with a fiberglass patch coated with a methacrylate resin (Cyanoveneer, Ellman International, Hewlett, NY). In penetrating traumatic injuries such as puncture wounds from dog bites, the infection must be controlled before the defect is repaired. Pins and screws can help join fragments in a traumatized shell (see this volume, p. 1215).

Trauma injuries to the soft-tissue integument of reptiles are managed similar to those in mammals. If uninfected, the wound can be cleansed and the skin sutured. Monofilament nylon (Ethilon Inc., Somerville, NJ) and monofilament polyglyconate (Maxon, D&G Monofil Inc., Manati, Puerto Rico) are good suture material for closing skin. If the epidermal or dermal tissues are infected, the infection must be controlled with appropriate chemotherapeutics and the wound allowed to heal by granulation. In wounds involving large areas (e.g., rodent bites in snakes), closure with suture may not be possible.

Neoplasia

CHELONIA. Aside from fibropapilloma in the green turtle, few cutaneous tumors have been reported in chelonians. A papilloma was reported (Dominguez et al., 1986) in a snapping turtle (*Chelydra serpentina*) and a squamous cell carcinoma was seen (Cowen, 1968) on the foot of a Ceylonese terrapin (*Geoemyda trijuga*).

CROCODILIA. Very few neoplasms have been seen in crocodilians. Papilloma-like skin lesions have been seen at alligator farms in Florida.

SQUAMATA. As noted earlier, cutaneous papillomas are common in the European green lizard. In snakes, fibrosarcoma is a common neoplasm; tumors appear as subcutaneous swellings with or without necrosis of the overlying skin. Reptiles have many different types of pigment cells in the dermis, and several cases of pigment cell neoplasms, including malignant melanoma, chromatophoroma, and iridophoroma, have been described in several species of snakes.

TREATMENT

Treatment depends on the age, species, physical condition of the individual, type of neoplasm, system affected, and usually the cost of the procedure. Early diagnosis improves prognosis. Unusual epidermal lesions or subcutaneous masses should be biopsied. If a neoplasm has metastasized, the prognosis is grave, and these metastatic lesions are often only diagnosed at necropsy. There are few reports of treating reptiles with neoplasia, the most successful treatment being surgical removal. In green turtles with cutaneous fibropapillomas, early lesions surgically removed do not reoccur at the surgical site. Neoplasms such as melanomas and chromatophoromas should have wide surgical margins, as they often diffusely infiltrate surrounding tissue. Following removal, histopathology can determine if neoplastic cells extend to the margins of the incised tumor.

Dysecdysis (Abnormal Shedding)

SQUAMATA. In captive reptiles, humidity is an important environmental consideration. While a relative humidity of 50% to 60% is ideal for many reptiles, some species require higher or lower relative humidities. If the relative humidity is too low, some lizards and snakes may not be able to shed skin normally. Retained skin will give the animal a dry and dehydrated appearance. Retained spectacles are quite common in some snakes.

TREATMENT

Retained skins in lizards and snakes are relatively easy to manage. In lizards, some species of skinks and geckos commonly retain old skins around their feet, which can simply be removed with a forceps. In snakes with retained skins, the animal can be soaked in shallow water overnight and the skin manually removed the next day. Retained spectacles can be removed with a jeweler's forceps.

Nutritional

CHELONIA. A nutritional disease commonly encountered in aquatic chelonians is hypovitaminosis A. Affected animals present with palpebral edema, anasarca, hyperkeratosis of the skin, and overgrowth of the mandibular and maxillary horny mouth parts. ReptoMin (Tetra Werke, West Germany) is a good commercial diet for many species of aquatic turtles.

TREATMENT

For turtles with hypovitaminosis A, parenteral or oral administration of vitamin A is recommended (Frye, 1989). One product often used (usually at 2000 IU/kg) is water-soluble Aquasol A (Armour Pharmaceutical Co., Blue Bell, PA). Depending on disease chronicity and severity, a turtle may receive injections at 3-day intervals for 2 weeks, then weekly for another 2 weeks. Hypervitaminosis A has been described in turtles receiving injections of vitamin A (Frye, 1989). Clinical signs included subacute xeroderma followed by necrotizing dermatitis, but experimental studies have not been performed to conclusively demonstrate a causal relationship.

SQUAMATA. An interesting disorder involving collagen has been seen by the author in several recently imported reticulated pythons (*Python reticulatus*) whose epidermis was detached from the subcutis. The skin would tear following minimal abrasion or manual restraint; histologically, collagen in the dermis was disorganized and poorly developed. These snakes were extremely malnourished, and protein deficiency may have been involved in the pathogenesis of this disorder.

DIAGNOSTIC TECHNIQUES

The key to evaluating skin lesions of reptiles is proper preparation of a biopsy specimen for histologic evaluation, cytology, and microbial culture. Cultures of skin lesions themselves provide limited information. In some reptiles (e.g., chelonians) special tools or techniques are required for collecting samples (e.g., power saw for biopsy of shell lesions).

Most small reptiles can be manually restrained and the area around the biopsy site infiltrated with 2% lidocaine hydrochloride (Xylocaine, Astra Pharmaceutical Products, Inc., Westborough, MA). Because the chelonian shell is extremely sensitive and often cannot be infiltrated with lidocaine, a general anesthestic such as a tiletamine hydrochloride/zolazepam hydrochloride combination (Telazol, A. H. Robins, Richmond, VA) at 10 to 20 mg/kg IM can be used.

Ideally, the biopsy should include normal tissue along with the diseased component. The author suggests collecting at least two samples—one for cytology/histology and the other for microbial isolation. If a fungal infection is suspected, the sample for culture should be ground in a sterile tissue grinder. For histology, tissues are fixed in either neutral buffered 10% formalin or a modified 4% formalin/1% glutaraldehyde mixture for electron microscopy (McDowell and Trump, 1976).

References and Suggested Reading

Cowen, D. F.: Diseases of captive reptiles. J.A.V.M.A. 153:848–859, 1968.

Dominguez, J., Hernandez-Jauregui, P., Grycuk, J. R., et al. Surgical excision of a keratinizing epidermal papilloma from the tail of a snapping turtle. J. Zoo. Anim. Med. 17:105, 1986.

Frye, F. L.: Vitamin A sources, hypovitaminosis A, and iatrogenic hypervitaminosis A in captive chelonians. *In* Kirk, R. W. (ed.) *Current Veterinary Therapy X, Small Animal Practice.* Philadelphia: W.B. Saunders, 1989, p. 791.

Horner, R. E.: Poxvirus in farmed Nile crocodiles. Vet. Rec. May 7:459, 1988.

Jackson, C. G., Fulton, M.: A turtle colony epizootic apparently of microbial origin. J. Wildl. Dis. 6:446, 1970.

Jacobson, E. R.: Use of chemotherapeutics in reptile medicine. *In*: Jacobson, E. R., and Kollias, G. V. (eds.). *Exotic Animals.* New York: Churchill Livingston, 1988, p. 35.

Jacobson, E. R., Calderwood, M. B., and Clubb, S. L.: Mucormycosis in hatchling Florida softshell turtles. J.A.V.M.A. 177:835, 1980.

Jacobson, E. R., Gaskin, J. M., and Clubb, S. L.: Papilloma-like virus infection in Bolivian sideneck turtles. J.A.V.M.A. 181:1325, 1982.

Jacobson, E. R., Mansell, J. L., Sundberg, J. P., et al.: Cutaneous fibropapillomas of green turtles (*Chelonia mydas*). J. Comp. Pathol. 101:39, 1989.

Jacobson, E. R., Popp, J., Shields, R. P., et al.: Pox-like virus associated with skin lesions in captive caimans. J.A.V.M.A. 175:937, 1979.

McDowell, E. M., and Trump, B. F.: Historical fixtures suitable for diagnostic light and electron microscopy. Arch. Pathol. Lab. Med. 100:405, 1976.

Page, C. D., Mantino, M., Derendorf, H., et al.: Multiple-dose pharmacokinetics of ketoconazole administered to gopher tortoises (*Gopherus polyphemus*). J. Zoo Wildlf. Med. 22:191, 1991.

Plowman, C. A., Montali, R. J., Phillips, L. G., et al.: Septicemia and chronic abscesses in iguanas (*Cyclura cornuta* and *Iguana iguana*) associated with *Neisseria* species. J. Zoo. Anim. Med. 18:86, 1987.

Quesenberry, K., Jacobson, E. R., Allen, J. L., et al.: Ulcerative stomatitis and subcutaneous granulomas caused by *Mycobacterium chelonei* in a boa constrictor. J.A.V.M.A. 189:1131, 1986.

Raynaud, M. M. A., and Adrian, M.: Lesions cutanèes à structure papillomateuse associèes a des virus chez le lizard (*Lacerta viridis* Laur). C.R. Acad. Sci. Paris, 283:845, 1976.

Rebell, H. A., Rywlin, A., and Haines, H.: A herpesvirus-type agent associated with skin lesions of green sea turtles in aquaculture. Am. J. Vet. Res. 36:1221, 1975.

Stewart, J. S.: Anaerobic bacterial infections in reptiles. Proceedings of the Annual Meeting of the American Association of Zoo Veterinarians, Greensboro, NC, 1989, p. 173.

Wallach, J. D.: The pathogenesis and etiology of ulcerative shell disease in turtles. J. Zoo. Anim. Med. 6:11, 1975.

REPTILE RESPIRATORY DISEASES

RANDALL E. JUNGE
and R. ERIC MILLER
St. Louis, Missouri

Diseases of the respiratory system are one of the most common reasons for presentation of reptile patients to veterinarians. Respiratory diseases can be recognized and effectively treated by understanding basic reptile anatomy and physiology, utilizing appropriate diagnostic procedures, and applying standard therapeutic approaches.

ANATOMY AND PHYSIOLOGY

The reptile respiratory tract differs anatomically from mammals in several important aspects. The lung is a saclike structure with a central air space and peripherally arranged alveoli. Most snakes possess a single functional lung on the right side, with the left lobe rudimentary or absent. Boas and pythons (family Boidae) are considered less specialized and have retained two complete functional lungs, an important factor in evaluating snake radiographs.

In snakes and lizards, the lung may possess a cranial respiratory and caudal nonrespiratory region, which may result in the pooling of exudates in the pulmonary spaces. Inflammatory exudates of reptiles are caseous rather than liquid as in mammals, resulting in additional difficulty in mobilizing pulmonary exudates for resolution of pneumonia

As no diaphragm is present in snakes and lizards, the primary muscles of respiration are the intercostals. In turtles, the motion of viscera and limbs assists in air movement (in some aquatic turtles, respiration is further enhanced by gas exchange across pharyngeal and cloacal membranes). Crocodilians possess a functional diaphragm attached to the liver and moved in a piston fashion by muscular attachments to the abdominal body wall. The absence of a diaphragm in noncrocodilian reptiles prevents coughing and further contributes to difficulty in expelling respiratory exudates.

DIAGNOSTIC EVALUATION

Clinical History

The majority of cases of respiratory disease in reptiles result from inappropriate husbandry practices that compromise the animal's health. Predisposing stresses may include recent shipment, overcrowding, ecdysis, inappropriate temperatures or humidity, and improper diet. A complete history is an indispensable first step to diagnosis and treatment.

As poikilotherms, reptiles are unable to regulate body temperature by internal metabolic mechanisms. Each species has a preferred body temperature (PBT) optimal for a variety of functions including immune response (Davies, 1981). For most reptiles, cage temperature should range between 25° to 32°C (75° to 90°F) with a temperature gradient of 5° to 6° (10°F) within the cage to allow the animal to select its desired temperature.

Relative humidities in the range of 50% to 70% are appropriate for most reptiles but vary among species. Excessive humidity may be present in cages with substrates that retain moisture (wood chips, corncob litter). Sanitation is of utmost importance. Inadequate cage sanitation and excessive humidity contribute to the accumulation of opportunistic and pathogenic organisms. The snake mite *Ophionyssus natricis* may also serve as a vector for bacteria and other agents.

Poor nutrition is also a contributory factor in reptile respiratory disease. In reptiles, particularly turtles, vitamin A deficiency is characterized by squamous metaplasia of upper respiratory epithelial tissues and the ducts of mucus-secreting glands. The epithelial thickening and decreased mucin production results in conjunctivitis, edema, and ocular and nasal discharges that may mimic primary respiratory disease.

Reptile owners should be questioned carefully with respect to mouth breathing, exudate from the external nares, and wheezing or "clicking" respiratory sounds indicating the presence of exudate in airways. It should be noted that some snake species, such as bull and pine snakes, have threat postures that include loud expiratory sounds ("hissing"). Reptiles with respiratory disease will frequently position themselves with the head elevated due to increased respiratory effort and seek warmer areas of the cage, and are often inappetent.

Physical Examination

A complete, systematic physical examination should be performed (see Jacobson, 1988, for details). The patient should first be examined undisturbed to evaluate respiratory rate and effort. Aquatic turtles should be examined in the water, as accumulation of pulmonary exudates will often be reflected in a loss of equilibrium. External nares should be examined for accumulation of exudate. Though respiratory rates are slow and patient movement may complicate evaluation, auscultation should be attempted through a damp cloth, which reduces the noise generated by the stethoscope diaphragm contacting scales. Radiographs may be useful in evaluating the degree of pulmonary involvement and response to therapy.

Tracheal wash samples are easily obtained in snakes and lizards. Sterile saline (volume dependent on size of patient—2 to 3 ml may be used in an average boa) is instilled through a sterile polyethylene tube into the terminal trachea and aspirated back into a syringe. Depending on the quantity of wash collected, samples should be submitted for aerobic and anaerobic bacterial culture and sensitivity, fungal culture, and cytology, including examination for fungal elements and parasitic ova. Techniques for blood collection have been established in reptiles (Frye, 1986).

THERAPY

The therapeutic approach to reptile respiratory disease is based on techniques familiar to the prac-

titioner, though with modifications dictated by the nature of the patient. Specific approaches will be discussed in subsequent sections, but supportive care is vital to successful treatment. Inappetence is a significant sequela to respiratory disease. Several techniques may be useful to stimulate appetite. A slight increase (2° to 3°C) in ambient temperature may stimulate feeding due to increased metabolic rate. Injections of B-complex vitamins (0.5 ml/kg body weight) or oral metronidazole (Flagyl, Schiapparelli Searle) at 125 to 250 mg/kg body weight as a single dose have also been used to stimulate appetite in anorectic animals (the use of metronidazole should be avoided in indigo and king snakes due to reported toxicities) (Jacobson, 1988).

Force-feeding of whole prey items or tube feeding of liquefied diets provides nutritional support necessary for recovery from a prolonged illness (Frye, 1981). Volume and frequency of enteral nutritional supplementation varies with species and diet and may be gauged by maintenance of or increase in body weight. Vitamin A deficient patients may be supplemented with injectable vitamin A at the rate of 500 IU/kg body weight (see *CVT X*, p. 791).

Fluid therapy should be directed at restoring and maintaining normal hydration. Parenteral fluids may be administered subcutaneously or intracoelomically in snakes and lizards at doses of 2% to 4% of the animal's body weight. An extensive discussion regarding the composition and administration of replacement fluids can be found elsewhere (Jacobson, 1988).

Modulation of environmental temperature is also a useful adjunct to therapy. Sick reptiles will often exhibit behavioral "fever," seeking warmer spots to elevate their basal temperature. Ill or compromised reptiles should be allowed access to areas that are approximately 2° to 3°C (5°F) warmer than their normal PBT. Stimulation of the immune system and appetite may result.

RESPIRATORY DISEASES

Bacterial Diseases

Bacteria are the most common cause of reptile respiratory infections and disease. Bacterial pneumonias in reptiles may occur as either primary disease or secondary to septicemia, viral pneumonia, or parasitic respiratory disease, or they may result from necrotic stomatitis ("mouth rot") if necrotic debris from the oral cavity is aspirated.

As in bacterial infections elsewhere in the reptilian patient, bacterial pathogens in respiratory tract disease are primarily gram-negative. *Pseudomonas, Aeromonas, Klebsiella, Proteus, Escherichia*, and *Citrobacter* are common isolates. Though reptiles are often asymptomatic carriers, *Salmonella* and

Arizona may also be present in pneumonias. *Pasteurella testudinis* is frequently associated with pneumonias in captive desert tortoises (*Gopherus agassizi*). A *Mycoplasma* has also been isolated from captive and wild desert tortoises with pneumonia, but its contribution to respiratory disease is currently under investigation. Mycobacterial disease, most often caused by members of the Runyon groups, has also been identified in reptile respiratory tract lesions. Though mycobacteria may cause a primary pneumonia, respiratory tract involvement is usually secondary to lesions elsewhere. A systemic chlamydial infection resulting in respiratory disease has been reported in a puff adder.

Clinical signs of bacterial pneumonia in reptiles are similar to those of other agents—gaping, oral or nasal discharge, and often a loss of equilibrium in aquatic turtles. At necropsy, acute infections may present only as congested, edematous lungs. In chronic cases, fibrinopurulent or caseous white-yellow exudates may be found adhering to lung walls. Histologic examination of these lesions usually reveals heterophilic and mononuclear leucocytic infiltrates. Granuloma-like lesions may be noted with more chronic gram-negative disease, salmonellosis, and most mycobacterial infections. In chlamydial infections, characteristic basophilic inclusions may be noted in the macrophages.

A diagnosis based on clinical signs can be confirmed in several ways. Radiology may reveal consolidation of the affected lung. Blood collection may reveal an elevation in the white-blood-cell count, although significant variability may make interpretation difficult (Frye, 1981; Jacobson, 1988). Tracheal washes are vital to obtaining airway exudates for cytology, culture, and sensitivity.

The predominance of gram-negative organisms resistant to a large number of antibiotics (e.g., *Pseudomonas*) makes knowledge of antibiotic susceptibilities critical to successful therapy. Antibiotics used in respiratory therapy include gentamicin, amikacin, carbenicillin (often used in combination with gentamicin or another aminoglycoside antibiotic), ceftazidime (a cephalosporin with increased activity against *Pseudomonas*), and chloramphenicol (see this volume, p. 1214; Jacobson, 1988). Fluid therapy should accompany the administration of aminoglycoside antibiotics, and other supportive therapy should be administered as described. Nebulization with antibiotics or moistening or wetting agents may be helpful in breaking up inspissated exudates. The use of autogenous bacterins has been suggested in cases of chronic bacterial respiratory disease unresponsive to antibiotic therapy (Jacobson, 1988).

Viral Diseases

Comparatively few diseases of viral etiology have been identified in reptiles. Systemic viral diseases may affect the respiratory system or lead to debility that predisposes to secondary infection. Specific antiviral therapies have not been developed for reptiles. Care of the reptile patient with suspected viral disease is supportive (fluids, nutrition, antibiotics). To prevent transmission, any suspect reptile should be quarantined, as most viral diseases of reptiles are spread by close contact (e.g., aerosol transmission) or by fomites. Cages and utensils should be disinfected with quaternary ammonia compounds or dilute sodium hypochlorite (3%).

PARAMYXOVIRUS. A paramyxovirus has been associated with viremia terminating in respiratory disease often accompanied by central nervous system involvement. This disease was first reported in a number of species of the family Viperidae but has since been identified in other common families as well. Clinical signs include open-mouth breathing, brown and blood-flecked mucous secretions from the oral cavity and pharynx, and regurgitation. The disease progresses rapidly from the onset of respiratory signs, with death occurring in 1 to 3 days. Nervous system signs include convulsions and loss of equilibrium. Typical histopathologic findings are marked interstitial pneumonia often with secondary bacterial involvement, gliosis in the hindbrain, and demyelination of the axons in the brainstem (Jacobson, 1980). Paramyxovirus may be identified with electron microscopy, viral culture, or immunohistochemical techniques.

HERPESVIRUSES. Respiratory disease associated with herpesviruses has been identified in turtles. A systemic herpesvirus infection in painted turtles has been associated with necrotizing bronchitis and pneumonitis, as well as hepatitis. In green sea turtles, respiratory disease characterized by conjunctivitis, tracheitis, and pneumonia was related to herpesviral infection.

Mycotic Diseases

Mycotic infections in reptiles are often associated with stressful management conditions. Dermal and respiratory systems are most often affected. A variety of agents have been isolated, including *Aspergillus*, *Candida*, *Mucor*, *Geotrichum*, *Penicillium*, *Cladosporium*, and *Rhizopus*. Common systemic mycoses of mammals (blastomycosis, cryptococcosis, histoplasmosis) have not been identified in reptiles (Zwart, 1986). The diagnosis of fungal pneumonia may be made by identifying fungal elements in tracheal wash samples or by culture. Unfortunately, the diagnosis is often made at necropsy. Gross lesions characteristic of mycotic pneumonia include pulmonary granulomas, consolidation, and necrosis. Plaques may also be present on respiratory surfaces, and extension into adjacent tissue may occur in advanced infections.

Detailed pharmacokinetics of most antifungal agents in reptiles are not available; however, several agents have been recommended based on extrapolation from mammals or clinical experiences. Nystatin (Mycostatin, Squibb) administered at the rate of 100,000 units/kg orally once daily for 10 days or ketoconazole (Nizoral, Janssen Pharmaceutica) 50 mg/kg orally once daily for 1 week with the same dosage of thiabendazole (Mintezol, Merck Sharpe & Dohme) have been recommended. Nebulization with amphotericin B (Fungizone, Squibb) diluted 5 mg in 150 ml of saline and administered for 1 hour twice daily for 1 week has also been recommended (Jacobson, 1988).

Parasitic Diseases

LUNGWORMS. Nematodes of the genus *Rhabdias* inhabit the lungs of snakes and lizards. Most infections are subclinical due to low numbers, but when parasitic numbers are high, respiratory disease complicated by secondary bacterial infection may ensue. Adult female *Rhabdias* lay eggs in the lung that are expelled through the trachea, swallowed, and shed in the feces. The larvae mature and enter the reptile host by ingestion or penetrating the skin. Diagnosis is via identification of eggs in the feces or in tracheal wash collections. The recommended treatment for *Rhabdias* is levamisole hydrochloride (Levasole injection 13.65%, Pittman-Moore) 10 mg/kg body weight by intraperitoneal injection and repeated in 2 weeks.

PENTASTOMIDS. Adult parasites of the phylum *Pentastomida* infect reptile respiratory tracts and have been reported in snakes, turtles, lizards, and crocodiles. A number of species have been identified, including *Armillifer* and *Kiricephalus* in snakes. A zoonotic potential exists, as humans can serve as intermediate hosts for a number of pentastomids. In the snake cycle, a variety of small mammals serve as intermediate hosts. Heavy parasite loads may result in physical damage to respiratory surfaces or obstruction of the airways and predispose to secondary bacterial infections. Diagnosis is made by identification of ova in fecal samples or tracheal/lung washes. No parasiticides have been found to be effective. In some cases, parasites may be physically removed via surgery or endoscopy. Control consists of feeding of captive-bred and raised rodents to prevent exposure to infected intermediate hosts.

TREMATODES. Trematodes of the genera *Dasymetra*, *Lechriochis*, *Zeugochis*, *Ochestosoma*, and *Stomatrema*, collectively referred to as renifers, commonly infest the oral cavity of snakes. Adult flukes may also be found in the pharynx, esophagus, trachea, lung, and air sacs. The presence of flukes in the lungs may physically damage respiratory epithelium and predispose to bacterial invasion. Diagnosis is by identification of eggs in fecal or lung wash samples. No therapies have been recommended as effective and safe (Jacobson, 1983).

Neoplasia

Based on published surveys of proliferative disease in reptiles, neoplasia of the reptilian respiratory system is rare. Reports have included pulmonary fibroadenomas and a fibroma in turtles, reticular cell carcinomas in a lizard and snake, a sarcoma in a boa, and a bronchogenic carcinoma in a snake (Griner, 1983; Machotka, 1983).

References and Suggested Reading

Davies, P. M. C.: Anatomy and physiology. *In* Cooper, J. E., and Jackson, O. F. (eds.): *Diseases of the Reptilia*. London: Academic Press, 1981, p. 9.
Detailed description of anatomical and physiological features of reptiles and their significance to health and medicine.
Frye, F. L.: *Biomedical and Surgical Aspects of Captive Reptile Husbandry*. Edwardsville, KS: Veterinary Medicine Publishing Co., 1981, p. 29.
Frye, F. L.: Feeding and nutritional diseases. Hematology of captive reptiles. *In* Fowler, M. E. (ed.): *Zoo and Wild Animal Medicine*, 2nd ed. Philadelphia: W. B. Saunders, 1986, p. 139, 181.
Basic reptile nutrition, nutrition-related diseases, and effects on general health.
Frye, F. L.: Vitamin A sources, hypovitaminosis A, and iatrogenic hypervitaminosis A in captive chelonians. *In* Kirk, R. W. (ed.): *Current Veterinary Therapy X: Small Animal Practice*. Philadelphia: W. B. Saunders, 1989, p. 791.
Griner, L. A.: *Pathology of Zoo Animals*. San Diego: Zoological Society of San Diego, 1983, p. 5.
Jacobson, E. R., Gaskin, J. M., Simpson, C. F., et al.: Paramyxo-like virus infection in a rock rattlesnake. J.A.V.M.A. 179:796, 1980.
Jacobson, E. R.: Parasitic diseases of reptiles. *In* Kirk, R. W. (ed.): *Current Veterinary Therapy VIII: Small Animal Practice*. Philadelphia: W. B. Saunders, 1983, p. 599.
Description, life cycles, pathologic potential, and treatment of common reptile parasites.
Jacobson, E. R.: Evaluation of the reptile patient: Use of chemotherapeutics in reptile medicine. *In* Jacobson, F. R., Kollias, G. V. (eds.): *Contemporary Issues in Small Animal Practice: Exotic Animals*. New York: Churchill Livingstone, 1988, pp. 1, 35.
Systematic approach to physical exam of reptile patient; guidelines for fluid, antimicrobial, antifungal, and antiparasitic therapy.
Machotka, S. V.: Neoplasia in reptiles. *In* Hoff, G. L., Frye, F. L., and Jacobson, E. R. (eds.): *Diseases of Amphibians and Reptiles*. New York: Plenum Press, 1984, p. 519.
Detailed list of neoplasia in reptiles and amphibians.
Zwart, P.: Infectious diseases of reptiles. *In* Fowler, M. E. (ed.): *Zoo and Wild Animal Medicine*, 2nd ed. Philadelphia: W. B. Saunders, 1986, p. 155.
Description of the etiology, pathogenesis, control, and treatment of viral, bacterial, and mycotic diseases.

AN UPDATE OF ANTIBIOTIC THERAPY IN REPTILES

MITCHELL BUSH

The timely and rational use of antibiotics is an integral part of the medical care of reptiles with bacterial infections. Proper medical management of reptiles also involves monitoring environmental factors (e.g., temperature and humidity) and maintaining nutritional and hydration status. Discussion of these is beyond the scope of this article but can be found elsewhere (Jarchow, 1988). Additionally, reptiles with infections should be isolated to minimize the spread of disease.

Bacterial infections in reptiles frequently cause infectious stomatitis (mouth rot), pneumonia, and septicemia. Gram-negative organisms (e.g., *Pseudomonas, Aeromonas, Klebsiella,* and *Salmonella*) are among the most commonly encountered bacterial pathogens in reptiles. Often these pathogens are resistant to many commonly used antibiotics. After a diagnosis is reached and antibiotic therapy

indicated, appropriate dosage and treatment intervals must be employed.

The rational use of any antibiotic requires basic information on the pharmacokinetics of the drug in various reptilian species. Pharmacokinetic studies in these species are complicated because reptiles are heterothermic (cold-blooded). Their metabolic rate and the metabolism of any administered drug is dependent on the environmental temperature. Thus, variations in environmental temperature may require alteration of dosage and treatment schedules, especially with antibiotics that cause toxicity at high levels. For example, gentamicin will cause dose-related nephrotoxicity and secondary gout in snakes treated with a mammalian dosage (4.4 mg/kg every 24 hours). In contrast, the reduced metabolic rate of bull snakes is reflected in lower gentamicin dosages administered over a longer interval (2.2

Table 1. Antibiotic Dosages and Treatment for Reptiles

Species	Temperature in Degrees Celsius	Dosage
Gentamicin		
Bullsnake		
(*Pituiphis melanoleucus*)	24	2.5 mg/kg/72hr
Turtle		
red-eared slider		
(*Chrysemys scripta elegans*)	26	10 mg/kg/48hr (total weight)
western painted turtle		
(*Chrysemys picta belli*)	26	10 mg/kg/48hr (total weight)
box turtle		
(*Terrepene carolina*)	21–29	3 mg/kg/72hr
Alligator—juvenile	22	1.75 mg/kg/96hr
Amikacin		
Gopher snake		
(*Pituophis melanoleucus catenifer*)	37	5 mg/kg (loading), then 2.5 mg/kg/72hr
Chloromycetin		
Bull snake	24	40 mg/kg/24hr
Red-bellied water snake		
(*Nerodia erythrogaster*)	26	50 mg/kg/72hr
Burmese python		
(*Python molurus bivittatus*)	26	50 mg/kg/24hr
Gray rat snake		
(*Elaphe obsoleta spiloides*)	26	50 mg/kg/12hr
Eastern king snake		
(*Lampropeltis getulus getulus*)	26	50 mg/kg/12hr
Carbenicillin		
Snakes	30	400 mg/kg/24hr
Tortoise	30	400 mg/kg/48hr

mg/kg every 72 hours), yet this schedule still produces therapeutic blood levels. Additionally, ill snakes are often dehydrated, a condition that potentiates renal damage. Therefore, the use of nephrotoxic antibiotics in dehydrated reptiles should be accompanied by administration of subcutaneous or intracoelomic fluids. Addition of 10 to 15 ml/kg of lactated Ringer's solution or normal saline plus 5% dextrose will help ensure adequate kidney function and minimize toxicity.

Four antibiotics with good *in vitro* activity against many of the pathogenic bacteria of reptiles have also been the subject of pharmacokinetic studies.

These are gentamicin (Gentocin, Schering Corp.), amikacin (Amikin, Bristol Laboratories), chloramphenicol (Chloromycetin, Parke-Davis), and carbenicillin (Geopen, Roerig Pfizer). Recommended dosage and treatment schedules from these studies are presented in Table 1.

Reference

Jarchow, J. L.: Hospital care of the reptile patient. *In* Jacobson, E. R., and Kollias, G. V. (eds.): *Exotic Animals.* New York: Churchill Livingstone, 1988, pp. 19–34

REPTILE SURGICAL PROCEDURES

ROGER E. BRANNIAN
Ames, Iowa

Veterinarians presented with reptilian patients requiring surgical treatment need not be unduly intimidated. Fundamental surgical skills, a general understanding of reptilian anatomic and physiologic peculiarities, and a little ingenuity guarantee a successful outcome in most instances.

GENERAL CONSIDERATIONS

Surgery in reptiles should never be attempted without appropriate anesthesia because these animals do experience pain. Information on suitable anesthetics and anesthetic techniques for reptiles can be found by consulting the references listed at the end of this article (Cooper and Jackson, 1981; Fowler, 1986; Frye, 1981; Marcus, 1981; Millichamp, 1988; Wallach and Boever, 1983).

Standard small animal surgical instruments are usually adequate for most reptilian surgical procedures. For very small patients, a basic set of ophthalmic surgical instruments may prove useful. A high-speed orthopedic saw or drill is required for surgical incision of the chelonian shell.

As in mammals, aseptic surgical technique should be used. Povidone-iodine–containing surgical scrubs and solutions are safe and effective for surgical preparation of reptilian skin or shell.

Conventional suture materials are for the most part suitable for reptile surgery. For most proce-

dures, I have used chromic gut for internal sutures and polyglactin 910* for cutaneous sutures. Evidence now suggests that chromic gut is poorly absorbed and may cause an intense inflammatory reaction in reptiles and should therefore not be used (Bennett, 1989; Millichamp, 1988). Synthetic absorbable materials such as polyglycolic acid, polyglactin 910, polypropylene, or polydioxanone may be better choices than chromic gut for buried sutures (Bennett, 1989). Stainless steel, nylon, silk, and synthetic absorbable sutures all have been used successfully in the skin of reptiles. Cyanoacrylate adhesives can be used to advantage for small surgical incisions or lacerations.

Suture patterns and techniques do not differ markedly from those used in surgery on more conventional patients. Suture needles should be passed between the scales, rather than through them. Because the edges of the incised skin of reptiles often tend to pucker inward, best results are obtained by using an everting suture pattern. This can be accomplished by using simple interrupted or horizontal mattress suture patterns and tying the sutures with sufficient tension to create the desired eversion.

Surgical incisions should also be made between the scales. It is often difficult to achieve adequate apposition of an incised scale during closure because

---

*Vicryl, Ethicon.

of its rigid texture. Because the skin between the scales is more pliable, incision there will facilitate suturing, reduce the amount of scarring, and shorten the healing time.

Surgical incision in crocodilians and some lizards may be complicated by the presence of small bony plates *(osteoderms)* beneath the scales over part or most of the body. As with the integumentary scales, it is preferable to incise between the structures. Radiographic assessment of the animal may aid in determining the best approach by revealing the location of dermal bone.

WOUND HEALING

Wound healing in reptiles is temperature-dependent. Care must be taken to ensure that a reptilian surgical patient is kept within the preferred optimum temperature range for its species. Suboptimal temperatures greatly prolong healing times and may predispose the reptile to opportunistic wound infections.

Surgical wounds in reptiles generally take longer to heal than comparable wounds in warm-blooded animals. At optimal temperatures, one can usually expect soft-tissue surgical wounds in reptiles to be completely healed within a month. Incisions involving dermal bone require substantially longer to heal, and turtle shell wounds may require as long as 1 or 2 years for complete healing.

SURGICAL PROCEDURES

Removal of Cutaneous Lesions

Lesions of the skin and subcutaneous tissue are frequently encountered in reptiles. These "lumps and bumps" may be due to various causes and include abscesses, fungal and parasitic granulomas, and neoplasia among others. In general, such lesions are best treated surgically.

Abscesses usually appear as firm raised lumps under the skin. Most often they are well encapsulated and contain caseated exudate. If possible, abscesses should be removed in their entirety, including both capsule and contents. To avoid contamination of adjacent healthy tissue, it is preferable to bluntly dissect the entire mass from the surrounding tissue without incising the capsule. Simply lancing the abscess and removing the caseated exudate often results in recurrence of the lesion. Attempts to treat abscesses with systemic antibiotics are usually unsuccessful because of the encapsulation. Local instillation of antibiotics may be indicated, especially after surgical excision, if adjacent tissue has been contaminated. After abscess removal, the surgical wound is usually left unsutured

if it is not too extensive. The wound may be sutured if the surgeon is confident that contamination did not occur.

Like abscesses, cutaneous parasitic and fungal granulomas are best treated by complete surgical excision of the lesion. Such lesions are often encountered in captured wild reptiles and may be of long-standing duration when presented to the veterinarian. Though any active lesion should be removed, long-standing lesions are usually well encapsulated, often presenting little hazard to the reptile. The primary indications for their removal are diagnostic and cosmetic. Cutaneous neoplasms are handled as they would be in mammals, with complete excision of the neoplastic tissue.

Amputation

Amputation of limbs or digits may be necessary when extensive traumatic or necrotic lesions are present. Most reptiles, even large crocodilians, ambulate surprisingly well after amputation of a limb. The surgical principles used in mammalian amputations also apply to reptiles. Because detailed anatomic studies for most reptiles are lacking, the best approach for amputation is careful surgical dissection of the affected part with identification and ligation of blood vessels when they are encountered.

Traumatic injuries to the tail occur frequently in reptiles. When required, standard surgical techniques for tail amputation are used, preserving as much of the tail as possible. During tail amputation, it is especially important to avoid the cloaca and its accessory structures. In squamate reptiles (snakes and lizards), the base of the tail immediately distal to the cloaca contains scent glands, and in males, paired copulatory organs or *hemipenes*. A blunt probe may be inserted to determine their caudal extent. These structures should be left intact if at all possible.

In many lizards, tail autotomy has evolved as a defense mechanism against predators. The tail of these species is easily fractured and shed, distracting the predator while the lizard escapes. A new, although imperfectly formed, tail will eventually regenerate. The wound created by this type of tail loss should not be sutured, because suturing may interfere with the regenerative process. Such wounds heal rapidly and rarely require veterinary intervention.

Turtles and tortoises are occasionally presented with persistent paraphimosis. If the penis has become traumatized, amputation of a portion or all of the organ may be indicated. In chelonians, the penis arises from the floor of the cloaca. The penis does not contain a urethra but rather has a dorsal groove through which semen is transported. Because the penis is not involved in urinary transport, a portion of it may be amputated by ligating the organ at any point distal to the base, followed by transection of the damaged part. If amputation of the entire penis is required, the large blood vessels supplying the penis should be identified and ligated before transection. In large turtles, failure to ligate these vessels may result in substantial hemorrhage. If the penis is removed at its base, the defect created in the cloacal mucosa must be sutured.

The hemipenes of lizards and snakes can also be amputated if severely traumatized. These paired copulatory organs are normally retracted in the base of the tail just behind the cloaca and are everted through the cloacal opening during sexual activity. If a hemipenis is damaged during courtship or mating, the reptile may be unable to retract the organ, thus predisposing it to further injury. Amputation of an everted hemipenis is readily accomplished by ligation and transection of the organ at its base.

Celiotomy

Indications for celiotomy include exploratory surgery, salpingotomy for the relief of pathologic egg retention, gastrotomy, resection of the intestinal tract, hernia repair, surgical sex determination, and cystotomy for the removal of cystic calculi.

In snakes, the coelomic cavity is best entered through an incision made between the most ventral two rows of lateral scales. The ventral scales can then be bluntly dissected free and reflected to expose the coelomic viscera. This surgical approach allows adequate exposure, avoids the large ventral abdominal vein, and lessens the likelihood of contamination or abrasion of the surgical wound when the snake crawls after surgery.

Surgical access to the coelom in lizards and crocodilians may be accomplished through a ventral midline incision or a lateral incision. In some lizards, such as the common green iguana, a large vein is present on the ventral midline. This vein is best avoided by using a paramedian incision if a ventral approach is required. A paralumbar incision may be the most useful for procedures involving the kidneys or gonads. Surgical exposure to the coelomic cavity may be inadequate in some lizards and crocodilians when a simple linear incision is used. In these instances, an H-shaped incision can be made to provide better exposure.

Celiotomy in turtles and tortoises presents special problems because of constraints imposed by the protective shell. A standard surgical approach to the coelom requires the removal of a rectangular section of the ventral shell or *plastron* by the use of a high-speed orthopedic saw or drill. After the initial plastral incision, all dust and debris should be removed before proceeding. The plastral flap is elevated and separated from the underlying fascia and coelomic membrane. The flap is preferably left attached on one side to create a trap door, which can be hinged for closure. The entire plastral flap can be removed if necessary, but this may delay healing. The plastral flap should be kept moist by wrapping it in saline-soaked surgical sponges or gauze. After surgery, the coelomic membrane is sutured and the flap replaced. It is held in place by applying epoxy resin to the surfaces of the plastron adjacent to the incision and incorporating a fiberglass cloth patch into the resin, covering the entire area around the incision. Resin should not be allowed to seep into the incision itself. When polymerization is complete, additional layers of epoxy resin are applied to bridge and strengthen the plastral defect.

Most commonly available epoxy resins are not waterproof. However, waterproof epoxy resins are available at most hardware stores and are far more satisfactory for long-term integrity of the repaired shell.

The fiberglass patch can be left in place indefinitely in adult chelonians. However, in growing specimens, it may become necessary to remove or periodically replace the patch if it interferes with growth.

An alternative surgical approach to the coelomic cavity of turtles avoids shell incision. The approach is made through the soft-tissue space immediately cranial to the rear limb. This space accommodates the limb when it is retracted into the shell and is bounded by the shell on its dorsal, cranial, and ventral borders and by the thigh on its caudal border. The area is covered by distensible skin that can be readily incised to gain entrance to the coelomic cavity. To allow adequate surgical access, the rear limbs should be fully extended caudally. A horizontal incision is made in the center of the space. The incision should not extend too close to any shell margin to avoid difficulty in suturing during closure. If the incision extends too far caudally, the femoral vein may be encountered as it exits the inguinal canal. Underlying the skin are two thin muscular layers and the coelomic membrane. These structures are incised, allowing entrance to the coelom.

I usually return aquatic turtles to water 24 to 48 hr after soft-tissue celiotomy. This can be done only if the skin incision is tightly sutured, because any seepage of contaminated water through the surgical wound into the coelom usually proves catastrophic. A functionally watertight surgical closure can be accomplished by carefully placing a row of horizontal mattress sutures in the skin. A flexible suture material such as polyglactin 910 should be used. The sutures must be quite closely spaced and must be tied as tight as possible. Chelonian skin is very strong and leathery, and problems with tearing or necrosis of the skin around the sutures have not been encountered. Sutures should be left in place at least 30 days.

Using this approach, exploratory laparotomy, salpingotomy, and enterotomy are among the procedures that have been performed. A standard spay hook is useful in exteriorizing portions of the bowel or oviduct. The surgical space is somewhat restricted, and some procedures cannot be performed because of inadequate exposure. Much depends on the shell anatomy of the particular species and the nature of the procedure. The soft-tissue technique does, however, offer major advantages in simplicity and healing time when compared with the plastral flap technique.

Once surgical entrance to the coelomic cavity has been achieved, specific surgical procedures differ little from those routinely performed on domestic animals. The removal of retained oviductal eggs in oviparous reptiles is performed in a manner similar to cesarean section in small domestic pets. A standard two-layer closure of the oviduct is used. The oviductal tissue is delicate, and great care should be taken to avoid tearing the tissue during surgical manipulation. Because most reptiles have paired oviducts and each enters the cloaca separately, at least one incision in each oviduct is necessary if eggs are present in both. It is sometimes possible to make only a single incision in each oviduct. All the eggs can then be gently manipulated through the oviduct and delivered through the primary oviductal incisions. When the eggs are tightly adhered to the oviductal wall, multiple incisions must be made to prevent tearing the oviduct. Cesarean delivery of fetuses in viviparous reptiles can similarly be accomplished.

Reptiles sometimes ingest foreign objects necessitating gastrotomy. Some rat snakes, which normally include avian eggs in their diet, have been known to ingest golf balls and even light bulbs, apparently mistaking these objects for eggs. The gastrotomy procedure is performed as it is in small mammals. Intestinal resection can be performed to remove neoplastic masses or obstructive inflammatory lesions. Enterotomy may be required for the removal of foreign bodies or impactions.

Cloacal or intestinal prolapses are sometimes encountered in reptiles. They are handled much like rectal prolapses in mammals, with the placement of a pursestring suture around the cloacal opening after prolapse reduction. Cloacopexy or colopexy may be attempted in refractory cases.

With increasing emphasis on the captive propagation of reptiles, surgical sexing may sometimes be requested. Many reptiles are sexually dimorphic as adults. Others show few if any readily detectable anatomic differences between the sexes (see *CVT X*, p. 796). The sexes of certain species of lizards and turtles are the most likely to be confused by amateur and professional herpetologists.

Turtles can be surgically sexed by using the soft-tissue celiotomy approach and inspecting the coelomic cavity with the aid of a sterilized otoscope cone introduced through the incision. Laparoscopic instruments may also be used. The testes in males and the ovaries in immature females are positioned at the anterior poles of the kidneys. Gonads are most easily located by first identifying the kidneys and then sweeping the otoscope cone in a cranial dorsal direction along the ventral surface of the kidneys. In sexually mature female turtles, the ovaries are often the first structures encountered on entering the coelomic cavity, thus obviating the need for the otoscope. Laparoscopic techniques have proved useful in assessing reproductive function in large marine turtles.

Sexually monomorphic lizards are surgically sexed by introducing an otoscope or laparoscope through the paralumbar area. The gonads of lizards are located in a similar position relative to those of turtles, although some species variation undoubtedly exists.

Orthopedic Surgery

Orthopedic surgery in reptiles is based on the same principles that are applied to orthopedic procedures in domestic animals. Because of the many anatomic variations among reptilian species, it is difficult to offer specific guidelines. Fracture healing takes longer in reptiles than in mammals of comparable size. In larger specimens, internal fixation devices may be used, the type depending on the particular nature of the fracture. Splints and lightweight casts are satisfactory for many reptilian fractures. Improvisation and adaptation of orthopedic procedures performed in more familiar animals are the keys to successful orthopedic surgery in reptiles.

Nutritional bone disease with pathologic fractures, usually resulting from a calcium and phosphorus imbalance, is a common clinical disorder in reptiles. Attempts at fracture repair in these animals very often result in additional fractures. In severe cases, even handling the reptile may pose the risk of new fractures. Reptiles suffering from nutritional bone disease are best treated conservatively, with correction of the diet being the primary concern. Pathologic fractures often heal satisfactorily with diet correction alone. If not, unresolved orthopedic problems may be treated at a later date when the bone is healthier.

Turtles and tortoises may be presented with traumatic injuries to the shell. The shell consists of bony plates with a covering of a horny keratin-like material. Fractures of the shell can be repaired using epoxy resin as described earlier for the plastral flap celiotomy technique. Shell fragments may be wired in place to provide additional support if necessary (see *CVT X*, p. 789, for detailed discussion of chelonian shell repair).

References and Suggested Reading

Bennett, R. A.: Reptilian surgery, Parts I and II. Comp. Cont. Ed. Pract. Vet. 11:10, 1989.
A thorough review of reptile surgical principles and management of surgical diseases.

Brannian, R. E.: A soft tissue laparotomy technique in turtles. J.A.V.M.A. 185:1416, 1984.
A detailed description of soft-tissue celiotomy in turtles.

Cooper, J. E., and Jackson, O. F. (eds.): *Diseases of the Reptilia*. New York: Academic Press, 1981.
A two-volume text on reptile medicine, with information on anatomy, physiology, clinical techniques, anesthesia, and surgery.

Fowler, M. E. (ed.): *Zoo and Wild Animal Medicine*. Philadelphia: W. B. Saunders, 1986, pp. 108–186.
A general text on nondomestic animal medicine, with chapters on reptile anatomy, physiology, restraint, and anesthesia.

Frye, F. L.: *Biomedical and Surgical Aspects of Captive Reptile Husbandry*. Edwardsville, KS: Veterinary Medicine, 1981.
A well-illustrated text on reptile medicine, including extensive practical information on anesthesia and surgery.

Harwell, G.: Repair of injuries to the chelonian plastron and carapace. *In* Kirk, R. W. (ed.): *Current Veterinary Therapy X*. Philadelphia: W. B. Saunders, 1989, pp. 789–790.
A detailed discussion of shell repair in turtles and tortoises.

Marcus, L. C.: *Veterinary Biology and Medicine of Captive Amphibians and Reptiles*. Philadelphia: Lea & Febiger, 1981.
A text on amphibian and reptile medicine, with information on reptile anatomy, physiology, anesthesia, and surgery.

Millichamp, N. J.: Surgical techniques in reptiles. *In* Jacobson, E. R., and Kollias, G. V. (eds.): *Contemporary Issues in Small Animal Practice*. Vol. 9. *Exotic Animals*. New York: Churchill Livingstone, 1988, pp. 49–74.
A well-referenced review of anesthetic and surgical techniques in reptiles.

Wallach, J. D., and Boever, W. J.: *Diseases of Exotic Animals: Medical and Surgical Management*. Philadelphia: W. B. Saunders, 1983, pp. 978–1047.
A general text on nondomestic animal medicine and surgery, with information on reptile anatomy, physiology, anesthesia, and surgery.

AMPHIBIAN MEDICINE

GRAHAM J. CRAWSHAW
West Hill, Ontario

Frogs, toads, and salamanders have been used extensively for teaching and research for many years. They are also found in zoos and private collections and in increasing numbers in the pet trade. Unfortunately, amphibians have become quite scarce in many countries as a result of water pollution, land drainage, and other forms of habitat destruction. Few amphibian species breed in captivity with any consistency, and knowledge of amphibian medicine has lagged well behind that of reptiles, birds, and even fish. The life expectancy of a captured wild amphibian is quite short, often because of inappropriate husbandry. However, if more attention is paid to the proper care and maintenance of this diverse group, amphibians can prove quite durable.

The class Amphibia consists of about 4000 species within three orders:

1. Order Gymnophiona (caecilians). These are limbless, wormlike creatures found in the tropics. They are highly specialized for burrowing and are rarely encountered in exotic animal collections.

2. Order Caudata (salamanders). There are about 350 species of these elongated, tailed amphibians. Most have four legs, although in some species, notably the sirens and amphiumas, the limbs are reduced or absent. Some of the small aquatic forms are referred to as *newts*. Several species fail to metamorphose; the larvae retain external gills and reproduce (e.g., axolotls). This phenomenon is known as *neoteny*.

3. Order Anura (frogs and toads). The most familiar amphibians, the anurans, include nearly 3500 species of frogs and toads. The distinction is a loose one, although *toad* usually refers to members of the family Bufonidae with a dry, warty skin and terrestrial habits, and frogs, typically the members of the family Ranidae, have smooth skin and a more aquatic nature.

The most common species of salamander in captivity is the Mexican axolotl (*Ambystoma mexicanum*) a large, blue-black or white, neotenic species that is bred for laboratory use. The similar tiger salamander (*Ambystoma tigrinum*), in either the larval or adult stage, and the neotenic mud puppy (*Necturus*) are taken from the wild in North America. Various other salamander and newt species (e.g., *Salamandra, Triturus*) may also be encountered.

Of the North American anurans, the leopard frog (*Rana pipiens*) and the bullfrog (*Rana catesbeiana*) are frequently found in captivity, but the introduced marine or cane toad (*Bufo marinus*) is also common. Tree frogs (family Hylidae) such as the green tree frog (*Hyla cinerea*) and various other anurans may be acquired as pets. Of the non-North American species, White's tree frog *(Litoria caerulea)* from Australasia, the fire-bellied toads *(Bombina)* from Eurasia, the horned frogs *(Ceratophrys)* and arrow-poison frogs *(Dendrobates)* from Central and South America, and the African bullfrogs *(Pixicephalus)* are not uncommon. The African clawed frogs *(Xenopus)* are widely used research amphibians that may also be found in private collections.

ASPECTS OF AMPHIBIAN PHYSIOLOGY

Amphibians are ectothermic or "cold-blooded": all aspects of their physiology are dependent on the environment. Probably the most important amphibian organ is the skin, which not only has protective and camouflage functions but also is a significant respiratory and osmoregulatory organ. Amphibian skin is permeable to water in both directions, thus accounting for an amphibian's continued dependence on water. Amphibians do not drink but absorb water through their skin, particularly the ventral surface. As a result, they are highly susceptible to environmental hazards including toxins and contaminants.

Amphibians respire in four ways—by means of the lungs, the skin, the buccopharyngeal cavity, and, in the case of larvae and the neotenic forms, the external gills. The contribution of each of the four kinds of respiratory surfaces to total gas exchange depends on the organism, its stage of life, and the environmental conditions, especially temperature. Cutaneous gas exchange is the primary method in lungless salamanders and in other amphibians at low temperatures. As activity and ambient temperature increase, the lungs and the buccal surfaces play a greater part (Duellman and Trueb, 1986).

With the exception of some species of tree frogs, adult terrestrial amphibians are ureotelic—the end product of nitrogen metabolism is urea, not uric acid as in reptiles. At times of water deprivation, urea accumulates in the body but is excreted rapidly during rehydration. Adult amphibians in water excrete ammonia, whereas tadpoles are exclusively ammonotelic. Amphibians may bask, but they risk dehydration because they have a very limited ability to retain water owing to skin permeability and an inability to concentrate urine.

HUSBANDRY

As with reptiles, the provision of a suitable, stable environment is the key to the maintenance of amphibian health. Knowledge of the species' natural history is important. Some amphibians have very narrow environmental requirements, whereas others are adaptable to various climatic and ecologic conditions.

Anurans are usually maintained in an aquarium or terrarium with a tight-fitting lid, which helps to maintain the humidity and contain the inhabitants, because many species are adept at escaping. Terrestrial species are generally kept on a carpet, soil, or leaf substrate with access to water in a shallow container, or in a pool at one end of a sloped tank. Hiding places are essential; most amphibians shun bright light and are more active at night. Shelters can be in the form of large leafy plants, flowerpots, or pieces of bark. Many species like to burrow, and for these a soft substrate such as peat moss is recommended. The environment should be cleaned regularly, the water changed, and feces and excess food removed daily. Tanks should be disinfected with very hot water or dilute bleach, making sure that bleach residues are minimized or neutralized with sodium thiosulfate.

Aquatic species can be kept in aquaria. The water must either be changed regularly or mechanical and biologic filtration incorporated. Aquarium systems for freshwater fish are suitable for aquatic amphibians. Ideally, to prevent the spread of disease, each container should have its own water supply. Water must be free of impurities. Ammonia, chlorine, acidity, copper, and other toxins all can harm amphibians. Dechlorinated water, which is essential for aquatic forms and sensitive terrestrial species, can be produced by letting tap water stand at room temperature for at least 24 hr. A pH of 7.5 to 8.5 is usually suitable. Some laboratories keep aquatic species in low concentrations of mixed salt solutions in distilled water to avoid the vagaries of tap water supplies.

Temperature requirements vary with the particular species. Most temperate anurans and salamanders can be maintained at 15 to 23°C (59 to 73°F). High temperatures may be detrimental. Alpine species require cooler temperatures, which can be provided by small refrigeration systems. Tropical forms do best between 24 and 30°C (75 to 86°F) but tend to be less tolerant of high temperatures than reptiles. Although amphibians do not control their temperatures to the same extent that reptiles do, it is still preferable to provide various temperatures within the terrarium to allow them to select their preferred temperature and humidity. Native species may be kept outdoors or in greenhouses, if freedom from temperature extremes and predators can be assured.

Nutrition

Adult amphibians are almost exclusively carnivorous, whereas larvae may be carnivorous, herbivorous, or omnivorous. Many species only accept live, moving food. For these, earthworms, crickets, fruit flies, mealworms, and *Tubifex* worms all are suitable. Large anurans also consume newborn rodents, and larger aquatic species may eat small fish. Clawed frogs, axolotls, and salamanders accustomed to captivity accept dead items or inanimate food such as gels, cat food, meat, and fish chow. All food, including invertebrates, should be adequately supplemented with vitamins and minerals. Ideally, a wide variety of food items should be offered. Most toad and frog tadpoles will consume cooked lettuce, ground rabbit pellets, hard-boiled egg yolk, fish flakes and chows, or commercial amphibian food. Carnivorous salamander larvae can be fed brine shrimp, small or chopped worms, and fish chow. The more vigorous anuran tadpoles may consume each other, which may be desirable when excessive numbers are hatched (see *CVT VII*, p. 772, for more details on husbandry and care).

Reproduction

With few exceptions, amphibians return to the water to breed. Reproduction may occur naturally in a well-adjusted terrarium, but few species breed with any regularity. A number of environmental factors appear to stimulate breeding. Some species require artificial rain showers, low temperatures to mimic hibernation, or a period of intense feeding to promote egg development. Drying or cooling the environment before increasing moisture is effective alone in some species or can be used as a preliminary to hormonal induction. Gonadotropic hormones are valuable tools in amphibian reproduction. *Xenopus* and axolotls can be stimulated to breed with human chorionic gonadotropin alone; in other species, follicle-stimulating hormone and gonadotropin-releasing hormone (LHRH, #L4513, Sigma Chemicals) are more effective, although results can be inconsistent, because husbandry and conditioning are significant factors in reproductive success. Artificial insemination is used in some laboratory species.

Fertilization is external in anurans and characterized by a period of *amplexus*, in which the male grasps the female, sometimes for several days, and fertilizes the eggs as they are passed—either individually in some tree frogs or in masses of thousands in the case of toads. Male salamanders deposit a sperm packet, the spermatophore, which is picked up by the female's cloaca, and the eggs are fertilized as they subsequently pass through the cloaca.

Irrespective of the method of fertilization, amphibian reproduction is characterized by a larval or tadpole stage and the familiar process of metamorphosis with its drastic morphologic and physiologic changes.

Sexing amphibians can be difficult. In many cases, the sexes are morphologically identical. Male anurans tend to be smaller than females, more brightly colored, and more vocal, but this observation is by no means consistent. Male anurans also develop swellings on their forelimbs, the nuptial pads, which help them to grasp the female in amplexus. In the caudates, the edges of the cloaca are larger in males, particularly in the breeding season, whereas females have more rounded abdomens. Sexing of hellbenders and giant Chinese salamanders can also be achieved by laparoscopy.

RESTRAINT AND ANESTHESIA

Most amphibians can be restrained manually for examination or minor procedures, and few show a tendency to bite. Hands should be moistened to minimize damage to the sensitive integument, and animals should be handled gently. Two hands are required for some species. For examination, aquatic forms and very small or mobile frogs are best caught in a soft net and may be held there or in a damp cloth. Anurans are best held with pressure between the spine and the pectoral girdle with the hind legs hanging free to prevent jumping, or they may be held by the hind legs. Several species, notably the toads and the arrow-poison frogs (Dendrobatidae), secrete a venom from their skins. White venom may also be seen exuding from the parotid and dorsal glands of bufonids, such as the marine toad, when stressed. Although some venoms are highly toxic, most are not harmful to humans, but it may be advisable to wear gloves. For hygienic reasons, hands should be washed after handling all amphibians.

Local anesthesia (2% lidocaine) can be used, but the use of large volumes can lead to systemic toxicity so dilution is recommended. For general anesthesia, tricaine methanesulphonate* has most commonly been used, at doses of 300 to 500 mg/L water for larvae and newts, 1 to 2 gm/L for adult frogs and salamanders, and up to 3 gm/L for toads. The amphibian is placed in a solution of the appropriate concentration and left there to effect, which may take up to 15 min. Concentrations above 1 gm/L should be buffered with sodium bicarbonate, 10 to 25 mEq/L. Anesthesia is judged by loss of righting reflex, loss of reaction to painful stimuli, and the rate of active respiratory effort. At surgical levels, respiration is greatly depressed or even lost, a matter of some consternation to the mammalian anesthesiologist, but percutaneous respiration appears to carry the load, at least for relatively short procedures. Heart rates are unaffected until very deep levels are reached. Anesthesia can be pro-

---

*MS-222, Sandoz Ltd., Basel, Switzerland; MS-222/Finquel, Argent Chemical Laboratories, Redmond, WA.

longed by keeping the amphibian in a shallow dish of the anesthetic solution. Before recovery, the animals should be rinsed in clean water and placed on a damp cloth or into fresh water in the case of aquatics. Care should be taken to prevent drowning. The drug may also be injected ($\pm$ 100 mg/kg SC or IP). MS-222 is excreted by the kidneys.

Benzocaine (Sigma Chemical) is also an effective anesthetic and is added to the water at concentrations of 10 to 50 mg/L for larvae and up to 300 mg/L for frogs and salamanders (Malacinski). Ketamine may be used for nonpainful procedures such as radiology. The dose varies with the species (50 to 150 mg/kg). Good relaxation can be achieved, and respiration is well maintained, but they generally remain quite sensitive to pain.

Amphibians may also be anesthetized with halothane or isoflurane in an anesthesia chamber. Induction requires high levels (4% to 5%) and may take up to 30 min. Intubation can be performed (the trachea is readily accessible but can be hard to open because of the tightly closed cartilaginous glottis at the base of the tongue). Care must be taken when passing an endotracheal tube, because the trachea is relatively short.

Hypothermia should not be used for anesthesia. Although amphibians may become torpid and less reactive to painful stimuli when chilled, there is no evidence that analgesia is produced, and it is not a safe procedure for many species.

Euthanasia of amphibians can be carried out by anesthetic overdose (MS-222, pentobarbitone) or by decapitation.

DIAGNOSIS OF AMPHIBIAN DISEASE

Physical Examination

Before proceeding with an examination, it is essential to evaluate an amphibian's environment and obtain a pertinent history. Many outbreaks of disease are secondary to some form of environmental stress. Recently acquired and transported animals are particularly prone to bacterial infections, whereas overcrowding, poor nutrition, poor water quality, temperature extremes, ammonia, and other toxins all may cause immunosuppression.

Knowledge of the species and its normal appearance, the origin, length of time in captivity, and source of the patient is important. Examination should be carried out gently and rapidly to avoid excessive stress. At rest, terrestrial amphibians sit with their legs flexed under the body, and most, except the more stoic anurans, vigorously resist handling and will attempt to escape. They rapidly right themselves when turned over. Anurans usually void urine when handled.

The skin should be examined closely, particularly on the extremities, for hemorrhage and ulceration, which are common findings in bacterial infection. The appearance of the skin varies with the species. In all except the toads, the skin should be slightly moist, lightly tacky, but not excessively mucoid. Superficial swellings, masses, and cysts can be due to various causes. Air bubbles may be evident, particularly in the foot webs. Partly sloughed skin may be present. Skin sloughing, or ecdysis, is a regular process in all amphibians. Anurans usually shed their skin in one piece and often eat it. When seen hanging from the mouth, it may give the appearance of a prolapse.

Body condition can be assessed by body weight and palpation of the abdominal contents and muscle mass. Most amphibians have a rounded body contour with the underlying skeleton well hidden. Amphibian body weight can be highly variable with the state of hydration, however—amphibians can lose up to 50% body weight before death. Weight loss due to loss of fat stores is a more gradual process. Palpation of the musculature can allow evaluation of body condition and nutritional status, and close visual examination may reveal metazoan or microsporidian cysts. The skeletal system, which is prominent in wasted animals, should be examined for signs of deformity. In anurans, the spine, femurs, and tibias should be straight. Scoliosis and folding fractures develop in cases of calcium deficiency.

The eyes should be prominent, moist, and bright, and the corneas free from opacity. The mouth may be opened gently. The tongue (absent in Pipidae) is pink, fleshy, and protrusible. Gastric intussusception into the mouth can occur in terminally ill and ascitic amphibians. The abdomen may be palpated and the stomach identified in the upper portion. Gastrointestinal impactions and abdominal masses may be palpable. Prolapse of the cloaca, rectum, and bladder occurs quite frequently.

The beating heart may be visible or palpable ventrally at the level of the xiphoid. Heart rate varies with species and temperature. A peripheral pulse is not detectable. The anuran lymphatic system is characterized by the presence of large subcutaneous lymphatic spaces over the back and in the legs. Water is absorbed passively and accumulates in the lymph sacs unless actively excreted. Anasarca and ascites can be related to cardiovascular disease, septicemia, and other syndromes.

Respiration can be visualized readily. The most frequent and apparent form of respiration is the gular movements of the intermandibular space. The rate varies with the size of the animal, ambient temperature, and activity. Deeper abdominal movements, associated with greater inflation of the lungs, are less frequent. Respiratory rate should be compared with other individuals.

Diagnostic Procedures

Amphibians pose considerable problems in the diagnosis of disease. One sick frog looks very much like another, irrespective of the problem or pathogen. Norms for clinical pathology and other diagnostic methods are not well established. When large numbers are affected or at risk, it may be more rewarding to sacrifice some sick animals to allow a thorough postmortem examination. Many amphibians are inactive by nature, and behavioral changes may thus be hard to appreciate. Well-adjusted amphibians are opportunistic feeders, and some consider that an amphibian that ignores food is a sick one. They may be less inclined to hide or may show a tendency to remain in water. Aquatic forms will be less active than usual and may show abnormal posture or swimming patterns.

Skin scrapings can be taken from aquatic species; a sample of mucus should be gently scraped with a spatula or coverslip. Gill biopsy samples can be taken by excising a small portion of external gills with fine scissors for immediate examination or for histopathology. Smears should be examined both directly as a wet mount and with new methylene blue or similar stain under both low and high power for protozoan parasites, bacteria, and fungi. Nodular and focal lesions should be scraped or subjected to biopsy (local or general anesthesia may be required) and examined for bacteria, including acid-fast organisms, fungi, and parasites. Fungal and bacterial cultures can be made from superficial lesions, and sensitivity testing performed. A sample of lymph fluid taken from the dorsal lymph sac or the leg is a more specific method of isolating the causative organism in bacterial infections. The frog is held vertically, and lymph is milked down into the hind legs, where it will distend the skin. A sample is then aspirated using a fine needle. Ascitic fluid for cytology and culture can be aspirated from the ventrolateral quadrant to avoid puncture of the lungs.

Amphibians also present problems in trying to correlate clinical pathology parameters with disease. Hematology and biochemistry values have been reported for various species, but there is tremendous variation with species, sex, temperature, and season among other factors. Few data are available on hematologic changes in specific disease states. Anemia is a common finding in bacterial infections, particularly *Salmonella*. Frogs affected with red leg may show anemia, leukopenia, thrombocytopenia, and reduced serum protein.

The second problem is sampling. Amphibians have few superficial vessels, and they can be hard to locate. The lingual and ventral abdominal veins may be used, but cutdowns may be required. Cardiac puncture appears to be quite safe in anurans. This is accomplished by holding the frog in

Table 1. *Signs of Amphibian Disease With Possible Causes*

Anorexia	Unsuitable food; poor environment; stress; systemic disease; toxins.
Ascites	Hypoproteinemia; bacterial infection; lymph heart failure; kidney or liver disease.
Skin congestion or hemorrhage	Bacterial infection; gas bubble disease; poor water quality; chemical toxins.
Skin ulcers	Bacterial infection; fungal infection; capillariasis; trauma; chemical toxins.
Skin nodules	Fungal infection; parasitic granulomas; capillariasis; mycobacteriosis; neoplasia; trematode cercariae.
Black spots	Trematode cercariae; chromomycosis.
Weight loss	Anorexia; parasitism; mycobacteriosis; systemic mycosis; neoplasia.
Scoliosis	Calcium or vitamin D deficiency.
Neurologic signs	Bacterial infection; calcium or vitamin deficiency; toxins.
Sudden death	Septicemia; toxins.

dorsal recumbency with all four legs restrained. The heart is located lying dorsal to the xiphoid, and a small-gauge needle is inserted at an angle of 10 to 20° to the ventral body surface. Smears can be stained with Wright's stain. Cell counts require suitable diluents because of the presence of nucleated erythrocytes. I have not found the eosinophil Unopette method suitable for amphibian blood.

Fecal examination will likely reveal a myriad of animal life—notably flagellates and large ciliates. Strongyle and strongyloid eggs and larvae and cestode and trematode eggs may also be seen, particularly in wild amphibians. Radiology can be used to detect skeletal abnormalities, gastrointestinal impactions, and pneumonia. High-detail film is recommended, and light anesthesia may be necessary. An effective method of restraining anurans for radiography is to tape them between two pieces of radiolucent foam—a frog sandwich—which can then be positioned appropriately.

Ultrasonography, computerized tomography, and magnetic resonance imaging all are applicable to amphibians, but their availability is limited. Fiber optics may be used for visualization of the stomach, and laparoscopy can be used for examination of the viscera and for sexing. For small, thin-skinned frogs, transillumination using a cool but intense fiber-optic source can prove to be a useful technique for visualizing the lungs and other coelomic contents, such as ova.

Table 1 lists various presenting signs together with possible etiologies.

Postmortem Examination

The usual equipment is required for postmortem examination. A magnifying glass and small instruments are valuable for examining lesions in small species. A dissection guide is helpful to those unfamiliar with amphibian anatomy (Gilbert, 1965, 1973). Amphibians autolyse rapidly. For meaningful results, only freshly dead or sacrificed animals should be examined.

First, the integument should be examined for evidence of hemorrhage, ulceration, abnormal mucus production, masses, and parasites. Scrapings of mucus and a small section of the external gills should be examined microscopically. The ventral skin is opened from the mandible to the cloaca (the large ventral abdominal vein will be apparent lying just beneath the rectus muscle), and the incision is extended (in anurans) into the subcuticular lymph spaces of the hindlimbs. Lymph fluid should be obtained for cultures. Next, the abdomen is opened, taking care not to incise the thin-walled bladder, the incision extended through the sternum and pectoral girdle, and the abdominal walls resected. Parasites can be found in the coelomic cavity or in cysts on visceral surfaces. In adult females, the ova may occupy most of the abdomen. They consist of black and gray follicles contained in a fine membrane (the ovisac). They should be dissected away from their attachment onto the kidneys.

The liver, which is compact and bilobed in anurans and elongated in salamanders, varies in size with body condition and is usually deep black in color because of large quantities of melanin. This may be absorbed by adjacent tissues in all but the freshest specimens. The liver should be examined for gross lesions such as fungal or bacterial granulomas and parasitic cysts. A spherical gallbladder lies ventrally between either lobe.

The stomach is located dorsal to the liver and continues into the short, simple intestines. The intestines are of even diameter except for a widening in the distal portion. The gastrointestinal tract should be removed intact, opened, and examined grossly and microscopically for lesions and parasites. The spleen is generally small and spherical, situated in the mesentery of the middle intestine. Splenomegaly occurs in some bacterial infections.

The lungs are fine, saclike pink structures lying dorsal to the liver and extending the length of the abdomen when inflated. They should be opened and examined for exudate, masses, and parasites, particularly nematodes. Salamanders of the family Plethodontidae lack lungs altogether. Cultures should be taken from the liver, lungs, kidneys, and heart blood, and sections of all tissues should be taken for histopathology. Heart blood smears can be made and examined for hemoparasites.

The oviducts are convoluted tubes extending the length of the abdomen in a lateral position. They open at the infundibula, located at the cranial end of the abdomen at the apex of the heart. The redbrown kidneys, which lie dorsally in a midabdom-inal position, vary in shape but are usually elongated and have numerous vascular attachments. The fat bodies, which arise at the level of the kidneys, have finger-like projections and often have a pinkish tinge. They may be used as a measure of nutritional status because they are prominent in amphibians in good condition but may be hard to find in malnourished animals. The yellow adrenal glands are located either ventrally or medially to the kidneys. The paired ovoid or lobed testes are located at the anterior pole of the kidneys. In bufonids, a vestigial ovary, Bidder's organ, is present at the cranial end of each testis. The urinary bladder, a thin-walled dilatation from the ventral cloaca, is large in anurans but much smaller in caudates. Parasites can be found within the bladder lumen.

Surgery

Amphibians are quite amenable to surgery, and clean wounds heal rapidly, even in an aquatic environment. Tumors and cysts can be removed and skin biopsy specimens obtained under local or general anesthesia. Laparotomy and laparoscopy can be performed for diagnostic and therapeutic purposes or for sexing. A paramedian incision should be used to avoid the large ventral abdominal blood vessels. The skin should be kept moist throughout the surgical procedure and recovery period.

DISEASES

Viral Diseases

Several viruses have been isolated from amphibians, but few have been associated with disease. The most notable is Lucke's tumor herpesvirus, the first herpesvirus associated with neoplasm formation and one that has been extensively studied in cancer research. The virus causes renal adenocarcinoma in leopard frogs (R. pipiens) (see the later section "Tumors").

Tadpole edema virus causes mortality in American bullfrog tadpoles (R. catesbeiana) and possibly other species. Affected tadpoles accumulate fluid, become lethargic, and die. Pathologic findings include subcutaneous edema, petechial hemorrhages, and organ necrosis.

Bacterial Diseases

BACTERIAL INFECTION, RED LEG, RED PLAGUE

Bacterial infection or septicemia is the leading cause of death of amphibians. Newly acquired animals are particularly susceptible. Normal environmental organisms may become virulent pathogens when amphibians are stressed by such measures as transport, overcrowding, poor water quality, poor nutrition, temperature extremes, or other primary pathogens. The causative organisms are those found in the amphibian environment and are predominantly gram-negative, such as *Aeromonas, Pseudomonas, Citrobacter, Proteus,* and *Salmonella*. Infections with gram-positive (*Staphylococcus* and *Streptococcus*) and other organisms occur occasionally. Although some differences in clinical signs and postmortem findings may be noted with different organisms, for the most part, symptoms and pathology are similar or identical.

CLINICAL SIGNS. Animals are often found dead without warning. In less acute cases, the skin loses its normal bright coloration, and congestion and hemorrhages may be seen on the legs, feet, and ventral surface—hence the terminology *red leg* for this condition. Hemorrhages progress to ulceration, especially on the points of contact with the ground and on the extremities. Loss of digits and appendages can occur in aquatic frogs. Edema, anasarca, ascites, panophthalmitis, and neurologic signs may also be encountered. Caudates often show pale blotches and excess mucus production and may develop ascites and limb edema. *Pseudomonas* has been associated with skin sloughing and ulceration in axolotls, whereas anorexia, lethargy, diarrhea, and anemia may accompany *Salmonella* infection (Malacinski).

DIAGNOSIS. Culturing surface lesions may identify the causative organisms, with particular attention being paid to gram-negative, oxidase-positive, non–lactose-fermenters. A more specific method is to culture lymph, especially when anasarca or ascites is present (see the earlier section "Diagnostic Procedures"), or blood and internal organs from fresh postmortem specimens. On necropsy, affected animals show edema, petechial hemorrhages on the skin and visceral surfaces, and in some cases hepatomegaly and splenomegaly.

TREATMENT. Therapy is directed at isolation and treatment of affected animals, cleaning the environment, reducing underlying stressors, and prophylactic treatment of other amphibians at risk. The most suitable method of treatment depends on the species and the number of animals affected. Oral dosing with oxytetracycline has been recommended. Preferably, individuals should be given an appropriate antibiotic parenterally. I prefer initially to use chloramphenicol, enrofloxacin, or gentamicin, which can be changed once antibiotic sensitivity is established (Table 2). When large numbers of frogs are involved and individual injection is not feasible, antibiotics and salt should be added to the water or antibiotics incorporated into the food. Although antibiotics added to the water are less likely to be effective than parenteral treatment of sick individuals, they can reduce environmental contamination and limit the spread of infection. High levels of antibiotics in the water are necessary to obtain accepted blood concentrations, yet considerable reductions in mortality in colonies of amphibians have been achieved by using moderate concentrations of antibiotics such as gentamicin and chloramphenicol. Gentamicin, amikacin, and nitrofurazone have proved useful in *Pseudomonas, Aeromonas, Salmonella,* and miscellaneous infections; chloramphenicol and tetracycline are also usually effective for *Aeromonas* (see Table 2). Treatment should be continued for at least 7 days.

Increasing the salinity of the water is commonly used to reduce the severity of infection. Sodium chloride 0.4% to 0.5% or amphibian Ringer's baths for several days should be combined with antibiotic therapy.

MYCOBACTERIOSIS

Mycobacteriosis is a sporadic problem in both terrestrial and aquatic species. Infection is with the aquatic and soil mycobacteria such as *M. marinum, M. xenopi,* and *M. fortuitum*. In the cutaneous form, pale nodules or ulcers are seen on the skin and need to be differentiated from fungal granulomas and parasitic lesions by histology and culture. Deeper infection in the liver, spleen, and other viscera results in progressive weight loss. A diffuse pneumonia may also be present. Affected animals should be isolated, although infection likely represents an individual immune problem. Treatment is unlikely to be effective, even though the organism may be sensitive to some of the antitubercular drugs *in vitro*.

CHLAMYDIOSIS

Outbreaks of *Chlamydia psittaci* infection have occurred in colonies of clawed frogs (*Xenopus*), with infection most likely acquired from uncooked liver. Affected frogs show lethargy, loss of equilibrium, skin sloughing, and hemorrhage (these signs are indistinguishable from other bacterial infections). Morbidity and mortality are high. Pathologically, generalized edema, hemorrhage, and hepatic and splenic enlargement are also noted, but the disease can be differentiated from bacterial septicemia histologically on the basis of basophilic intracytoplasmic inclusions. The efficacy of tetracycline or doxycycline therapy is not known, but these drugs could be administered or incorporated into the diet as described for red leg.

Other bacterial infections may afflict amphibians. Pneumonia can occur independently of other sys-

*Table 2. Recommended Doses of Therapeutic Agents for Amphibians**

Drug	Dose	Dose Interval
Antibacterials/antifungals		
Amikacin	5 mg/kg	SC, IM, IP q 24 hr
Benzalkonium chloride	0.25mg/L	Bath for 72 hr
	2 mg/L	Dip 1 hr, q 24 hr
Carbenicillin	200 mg/kg	SC, IM, IP q 24 hr
Chloramphenicol	50 mg/kg	SC, IM, IP q 24 hr
	20 mg/L	Bath
Enrofloxacin	5 mg/kg	SC, IM q 24 hr
Gentamicin	2.5–5 mg/kg	SC, IM, IP q 24 hr
	10 mg/L	Bath
Ketoconazole	10 mg/kg	PO q 24 hr
Mercurochrome	3 mg/L	Bath for 72 hr
Methylene blue	4 mg/L	Bath
Nalidixic acid	10 mg/L	Bath
Nitrofurazone	10–20 mg/L	Bath
Sodium chloride	4–6 gm/L	Bath for 72 hr
	25 gm/L	Dip 10 min
Sulfamethazine	1 gm/L	Bath
Oxytetracycline	50 mg/kg	PO q 12 hr
	25 mg/kg	SC, IM q 24 hr
	1 gm/kg diet	7 days
Trimethoprim/(sulfa)	3 mg/kg	SC, PO q 24 hr
Antiparasitics		
Copper sulfate	500 mg/L	Dip 2 min q 24 hr
Formalin 10%	1.5 ml/L	Dip 10 min q 48 hr
Ivermectin	0.2–0.4 mg/kg	Percutaneous
Levamisole	300 mg/L	Bath for 24 hr
Metronidazole	150 mg/kg	PO repeat as needed
	5 gm/kg diet	PO 5 days
Sodium chloride	4–6 gm/L	Bath
	25 gm/L	Dip 10 min
Anesthetics		
MS-222		
tadpoles, newts	200–500 mg/L	Bath to effect
frogs, salamanders,	500–2000 mg/L	
toads	1–3 gm/L	
MS-222 (parenteral)	50–150 mg/kg	SC, IM
Benzocaine		
larvae	50 mg/L	
frogs, salamanders	200–300 mg/L	
Ketamine	50–150 mg/kg	SC, IM
Hormones		
hCG	2000–5000 IU/kg	
Xenopus	300–400 IU	
Ambystoma	250 IU to female, then 300 IU to male if spermatophore is picked up	
PMSG		
Xenopus	50 IU then 600 IU hCG after 72 hr	
GnRH (Sigma L4513)	100 µg/kg SC	Inject females 8–12 hr before males

*Compiled from various sources.

GnRH, gonadotropin-releasing hormone; hCG, human chorionic gonadotropin; PMSG, pregnant mare serum gonadotropin.

temic disease or may be secondary to lungworms. Localized abscesses, cellulitis, and joint infections can develop as a consequence of trauma and bite wounds.

Fungal Diseases

Fungal infections are common. They are usually secondary to trauma, poor hygiene, or other conditions that affect an amphibian's natural defense mechanisms. In aquatic forms, particularly mud puppies, *saprolegniasis,* infection with a group of aquatic fungi of the family Saprolegniaceae, pro-

duces cottony growths on the skin and external gills. It may spread to cause extensive ulceration and hemorrhage. For treatment, large mats of fungus should be removed manually. Lesions can then be treated topically with Mercurochrome or Merthiolate. Benzalkonium chloride (Roccal), Mercurochrome, or methylene blue may be added to the water in severe cases. Fungal infection on eggs and tadpoles can be treated with methylene blue. Systemic antibiotics may also be indicated to treat or prevent underlying bacterial infection, and attention should be given to improving husbandry and water quality. Infection of the top layer of the integument with other fungi (e.g., *Nigrosporum*) can occur in terrestrial forms. Treatment is dilute topical chlorhexidine, Mercurochrome, or Merthiolate.

Systemic fungal infections are caused by various organisms and again likely represent an individual immune problem. *Chromomycosis* is caused by pigmented forms (e.g., *Fonsecaea, Cladosporium*), whereas *phycomycosis* is caused by the nonpigmented species (e.g., *Mucor, Basidobolus*). Infection in the skin causes nodules or expanding areas of ulceration. Deeper infection is associated with anorexia and progressive debilitation, with granulomas present in any organ. Diagnosis is by wetmount examination of skin or granuloma smears to demonstrate pigmented or nonpigmented fungal elements. Minor skin lesions may be treated topically with an antifungal agent. Ketoconazole has arrested more extensive lesions, but lesions may recur on cessation of therapy.

Yeast infections *(Candida)* occur in the gastrointestinal tract and may also spread systemically.

Parasitic Diseases

Amphibians are the definitive hosts of a huge range of protozoan and metazoan organisms. They also act as intermediate hosts for trematodes and other parasites of higher animals. Captured wild amphibians carry various gastrointestinal and systemic nematodes, trematodes, cestodes, protozoans, and myxosporidians. Ticks and leeches may also be found externally. Although most amphibians, even under the stresses of captivity, tolerate this parasitic burden well, when disease does occur, it can be serious. Many parasites have complex life cycles, and when their host is brought into captivity, the opportunity for transmission is lost. The decision whether to attempt treatment depends on the species, the clinical findings, and the potential for spread. For more detailed accounts of amphibian parasites, see Reichenbach-Klinke and Elkan (1965) and Marcus (1981).

NEMATODES

Nematodes may be found in the gastrointestinal tract, the coelomic cavity, the lungs, and in cysts and granulomas in most captured wild amphibians. Mortality has been associated with strongyloids in small frogs, and they may contribute to malnutrition and the pathogenesis of red leg.

Rhabdias is a genus of Strongyloidea found in the lungs of frogs and toads worldwide. In small numbers, the worms generally cause little pathology but heavy infestations, and in small species such as *Dendrobates*, the arrow-poison frogs, they cause debilitation by sucking blood and body fluids. The dark red or black worms, up to 14 mm long, are found within the lung sacs. Characteristic embryonated eggs and stubby larvae are readily visible in a wet mount of the feces. Other related strongyloids may also be pathogenic. The larvae migrate through the skin and various organs before reaching the intestine. Gram-negative septicemia can occur secondary to larval migration. *Rhabdias* seems quite refractory to treatment, and reinfection from the environment occurs rapidly. Treatment is aimed at killing adult worms and decontaminating the environment. Individuals should be removed from the habitat and treated with ivermectin (200 to 400 μg/ kg SC) on several occasions until no parasites are found in the feces. Soil should be removed from the tank and the environment decontaminated. It may be stressful to treat small species individually, and with these, ivermectin can be dropped on the skin.

Capillariasis *(Pseudocapillaroides xenopi)* is a parasitic infection of the skin of clawed frogs *(Xenopus)*. Affected frogs show darkening and roughening of the skin, particularly on the back, leading to desquamation, ulceration, anorexia, and eventually death. Diagnosis is by detecting the 2- to 4-mm-long nematodes in wet smears of skin scrapings or sloughed skin. Treatment with levamisole or ivermectin should be effective.

Filarid nematodes (e.g., *Foleyella*) occur in the tissues, blood vessels, or lymphatics and release microfilaria into the circulation. Heavy infections can be significant. Gastrointestinal nematodes (e.g., *Orneoascaris* and *Oswaldocruzia*) may be pathogenic in large numbers.

PROTOZOA

Flagellates, such as *Hexamita, Giardia,* and *Chilomastix,* are common inhabitants of the intestinal tract, gallbladder, and even the blood, but they are not usually associated with disease. *Opalina,* a large multicellular flagellate with the appearance of a ciliate, may be found in the feces but again is considered nonpathogenic. Of the ciliates, *Balantidium* and the larger *Nyctotherus* also inhabit the gut and are commonly seen on fecal examination. Poor condition and diarrhea in axolotls have been associated with multiple protozoal infestation and responded to treatment with metronidazole in the food.

Amebae are commonly found in feces but also occur systemically. *Entamoeba ranarum* can induce enteritis and liver abscesses. An unidentified ameba in the kidneys caused tubular nephritis in marine toads.

Trypanosomes and other protozoans may be found in the blood of wild amphibians but require vectors such as leeches or mosquitoes for the life cycles to continue. Heavy infestations can be significant.

Various aquatic protozoans cause skin irritation, excess mucus production, and ulceration in aquatic species and tadpoles in a similar manner to their effect in fish. *Costia*, *Oodinium*, and *Trichodina* are most commonly responsible and can be fatal if untreated. *Vorticella*, a large, stalked ciliate, forms colonies on the external gills of neotenic and larval salamanders. Diagnosis of these infestations is made by gently scraping the integument and examining for the organisms microscopically (see the earlier section "Diagnostic Procedures"). For identification of the organisms, see tropical fish texts.

For the treatment and control of species such as *Vorticella*, immersion of the animals in salt solutions (e.g., 0.6% sodium chloride for 3 to 5 days followed by maintenance in more dilute concentrations) may be sufficient. For the more resistant and pathogenic species, methods for treating freshwater fish should be used. Salt, formalin, or copper baths may be effective, but these treatments should be tried on a small number of animals first. Close attention should also be paid to water quality, which may be encouraging infection.

Coccidia are found in the intestines and even in the kidneys but are generally not significant pathogens. Myxosporidians, sporozoans usually associated with fish, may be found in many amphibian tissues. One, *Plistophora*, produces disseminated muscular cysts, visible as white streaks, and can be fatal. Other sporozoans may be found systemically or in the skin. *Dermocystidium* and *Dermosporidium* cause nodules in the skin. Elevation of the temperature to 25°C (77°F) was effective for treating *Dermocystidium* cysts in axolotls (Malacinski).

OTHER PARASITES

Monogenetic trematodes, especially *Polystoma*, inhabit the gut, lungs, and urinary tract. Others are found on the gills and skin of aquatic forms. Digenetic trematodes may be found as adults in the gut or as intermediate stages (cercariae) in the skin and various organs—*blackspot* in frogs and fish. Their significance depends on the severity of the infection and the organ affected, heavy infestations causing debility. The same can be said for cestodes, which are also found as adults or as intermediate stages. Large numbers of cestodes such as *Nematotenia* can be pathogenic and cause gastrointestinal obstruction. The Acanthocephala (thorny-headed worms) may attach themselves to the mucosa of the gut, causing significant damage.

Trombiculid mite larvae may be found subcutaneously, where they produce minute vesicles that can be opened to reveal the parasite. Ivermectin should be effective. Leeches may be seen on captured wild amphibians, even in the lymph spaces, where they reach a considerable size. The fish louse *Argulus* and even the anchor worm *Lernaea* may be found on aquatic adults and tadpoles, and they can be significant parasites on a small specimen. The same treatment methods should be used as for fish (Citino, 1989).

Nutritional Diseases

Absolute nutritional requirements have not been established for amphibians, but it is reasonable to assume that the requirements for minerals such as calcium are similar to those for other species.

Amphibians fed vitamin D-deficient or calcium-deficient foods such as unsupplemented heart or meat develop nutritional bone disease. Paralysis, scoliosis, and folding fractures of the long bones may be seen clinically. Tetany can occur in acute cases. Poor bone density and folding fractures are seen radiographically, particularly in the proximal femurs. The effects of calcium deficiency are more apparent in young growing animals. It can be difficult to ensure adequate calcium intake in some species. Beef heart and liver are severely deficient and should not be fed unsupplemented (20 gm of bone meal is required to correct the calcium:phosphorus ratio of 1 kg of beef heart). Many live invertebrates such as domestic crickets also have poor calcium:phosphorus ratios and should be fed high-calcium diets and dusted with a fine calcium carbonate and vitamin powder before feeding to amphibians.

Besides calcium deficiency, animals fed exclusively on liver diets may develop anemia and hepatic lesions suggestive of vitamin A toxicity.

I have seen a number of anurans with a flaccid posterior paralysis with an associated axonal degeneration in the spinal nerves, and I strongly suspect a nutritional etiology. Calcium supplementation was adequate, and hypovitaminosis B or hypervitaminosis A is suspected. Hypovitaminosis B has also been suggested as a cause of a neurologic disease in salamanders.

The *spindly leg syndrome* occurs in juvenile *Dendrobates* and other small anurans. Development is normal until metamorphosis, at which time the hindlimbs develop but the forelimbs are rigid, poorly muscled, and often fail to emerge from the gill slits. The cause appears to be a nutritional myopathy, possibly a specific amino acid deficiency.

Iodine deficiency can occur when deficient diets or goitrogenic substances such as *Brassica* are fed. The main effect is on metamorphosis—tadpoles fail to metamorphose and can reach giant sizes. *Oxalate calculi* can develop in the kidneys of tadpoles fed on spinach, with death occurring around the time of metamorphosis.

Physical and Chemical Agents

Amphibian life-styles reflect a dependence on water and high humidity, and most remain highly susceptible to dehydration. High environmental humidity should be maintained, and care should be taken to avoid desiccation from heat sources, especially lamps. A few species such as the African and South American burrowing frogs are able to form a coccoon of shed epidermis to survive periods of drought, but this is an exception to the rule. Excess heat can be harmful to all species, although tropical amphibians are more tolerant. Conversely, chilling can be harmful to warm-adapted species either directly or by increasing susceptibility to infectious disease. Temperate and northern species are much more resistant to low temperatures and can be artificially hibernated by chilling to 4°C (38°F), and a few species can survive subfreezing temperatures (Duellman and Trueb, 1986).

The delicate nature of amphibian skin predisposes these animals to trauma. Minor injuries heal well but may be portals of entry for bacteria. In aquatic species wounds are commonly contaminated with fungi such as *Saprolegnia*. Deep wounds should be debrided and cleaned (avoid the excessive use of antiseptics) and antibiotic coverage provided. To avoid interspecific aggression, amphibian species should not be mixed. The more aggressive species bite and may even attempt to eat each other, especially when a size difference exists, and the tadpoles of some species are actively cannibalistic.

Various chemicals are toxic to amphibians. Larvae and aquatic forms are particularly sensitive to chlorine, ammonia, pesticides, and metals such as copper and lead. Careful attention should be paid to water quality, and copper pipes should be avoided. When in doubt, aquatic systems can be tested with aquarium test kits. High levels of ammonia and nitrite cause lethargy, skin and gill sloughing, internal hemorrhages, and exophthalmos and predispose animals to bacterial infection. Preventive measures include changing the water regularly and establishing effective biologic filtration. Chlorine can induce skin petechiation and ulceration and is rapidly fatal to tadpoles. Overfeeding and the careless use of disinfectants should also be avoided. Iodine-based disinfectants can be toxic to small species.

Gas Bubble Disease

Gas bubble disease in aquatic amphibians is caused by exposure to water supersaturated with air. It may develop when the total dissolved gas pressure is greater than atmospheric and is usually associated with air leaks in a pressurized filtration or water system. In the acute phase of the disease, affected animals become depressed and show hyperemia and hemorrhages in the skin, with air bubbles subcutaneously, particularly in the webs of the feet and in the vascular system. In the more chronic phase, frogs develop secondary bacteremia with a significant mortality rate. Treatment should be directed at identifying and correcting the mechanical source of supersaturation, often a result of small leaks around pipe fittings or pinholes in flexible tubing. Reduction in dissolved gas levels results in a reversal in clinical signs.

Tumors

Neither benign nor malignant tumors are particularly common, with one exception. In the leopard frog *(R. pipiens)*, infection with Lucke's tumor herpesvirus causes adenocarcinoma of the kidneys with metastases to other organs. There are few clinical signs until the tumors are extensive, when bloating, lethargy, and death from renal failure or emaciation will follow. The tumor is not a significant problem in other species. Papillomas, lymphoid tumors, and other neoplasms can be expected to occur sporadically in all species.

DEVELOPMENTAL DEFECTS

Amphibians are mass reproducers, and the incidence of developmental defects such as color mutations and limb deformities and duplication is high. It may not be apparent whether such changes are of genetic, environmental, or nutritional origin.

OTHER CONDITIONS

Dropsy or ascites is often described as a disease but should rather be considered a clinical or pathologic sign. Because amphibians passively absorb fluid through the skin and excess water from the kidneys, organ failures particularly of the kidneys and lymphatic hearts cause fluid accumulation in the coelom or in the lymph spaces. Ascites and anasarca are also common in cases of bacterial infection, but other frogs may be anasarcous without being clinically ill. In the latter, increasing water osmolarity (e.g., 0.6% saline) may be effective.

Gastrointestinal *impactions* and *tympany* can result from ingestion of the substrate or inappropriate diet. Cloacal and rectal *prolapses* are not uncommon but usually resolve spontaneously if feeding is discontinued for a while.

Eye problems seem particularly common in *Hyla*

and other genera of tree frogs. Bacterial keratitis (ulceration, generalized cloudiness, hypopyon, neovascularization) can occur in isolation or as part of a more generalized infection. *Xanthomatous keratitis* has been seen in several species. White lipid deposits develop in the cornea and represent an ocular manifestation of a disorder of lipid metabolism. The cause is likely nutritional, but no etiology nor effective treatment has been reported.

Epidermal ridge disease in young ambystomatid salamanders is another idiopathic problem, manifested by hypertrophy of the epidermis into plaques, papillae, and ridges. No specific infectious agents have been incriminated, but secondary bacterial infections do develop (Malacinski).

Gout has been noted in African bullfrogs. Swelling of the digits develops as a result of the accumulation of urate crystals. Surgery may be required to open or excise the lesions. The cause is likely related to the feeding of excessive amounts of protein.

Even with complete and careful postmortem examination, the causes of disease in amphibians are frequently hard to identify. Hepatitis and nephropathy are common autopsy findings, but the underlying cause often remains obscure. As knowledge is gained, the identification of toxic, nutritional, and infectious agents should unravel some of these mysteries.

THERAPEUTICS

Few pharmacologic studies have investigated therapeutic agents in amphibians, and for the most part, dose rates have been extrapolated from other species. It is probably impossible to give accurate dose rates, considering that the pharmokinetics of each drug vary dramatically with the species and the ambient temperature. Gentamicin, 2.5 mg/kg given every 3 days, produced effective blood levels in *Necturus* kept at 2 to 3°C (36 to 37°F), but the same dose given daily was required in leopard frogs at room temperatures. Still higher doses have been used in clinical situations without evidence of toxicity. Very high concentrations of gentamicin in the water were required to produce normally acceptable serum concentrations, yet the use of antibiotics in the water appears to have a beneficial effect in disease control. Similarly, in limited trials, topical anthelmintics can reduce or even eliminate parasitic burdens. A cautionary note is that antibiotics in aquatic environments may cause fungal overgrowth, and they should not be added indiscriminately to tanks with biologic filtration.

Subcutaneous injections are recommended for anurans. Uptake of drugs by the subcutaneous route appears to be rapid because the subcutaneous lymph spaces connect with the vascular system. Skeletal musculature tends to be small; large needles or injections may cause damage, and intravenous injection is generally not feasible. The subcutaneous, intraperitoneal, and intramuscular routes can be used in caudates. Owing to the permeable nature of amphibian skin, percutaneous therapy may be effective though hard to evaluate. Drugs can be dropped or sprayed onto the skin, or the animals immersed in a solution. Parenteral fluid therapy is rarely indicated. Even severely dehydrated amphibians absorb water through their skin. They should be misted heavily or placed in shallow water.

Oral medication is effective, but it can be difficult to administer. Gastric intubation with tetracycline has been recommended as a method for treating frogs for red leg, but this may be stressful, as well as time-consuming when large numbers of animals are involved. Salamanders and some anurans may take inanimate food into which drugs can be incorporated. The food ingredients and the medication are blended into a gelatin solution, which is allowed to set, and the resulting gel can be refrigerated or frozen until required.

References and Suggested Reading

Alderton, D.: *A Petkeeper's Guide to Reptiles and Amphibians.* London: Salamander Books, 1989.
   A useful small guide for amateur herpetologists.
Citino, S. B.: Basic ornamental fish medicine. *In* Kirk, R. W. (ed.): *Current Veterinary Therapy X.* Philadelphia: W. B. Saunders, 1989, p. 703.
   A guide to the diagnosis and treatment of diseases in aquarium fish.
Duellman, W. E., and Trueb, L.: *Biology of Amphibians.* New York: McGraw-Hill, 1986.
   A textbook of amphibian anatomy, physiology, ecology, and systematics.
Frye, F. L.: General considerations in the care of captive amphibians. *In* Kirk, R. W. (ed.): *Current Veterinary Therapy VII.* Philadelphia: W. B. Saunders, 1977, p. 772.
   A brief description of the requirements for the care of amphibians in captivity.
Gilbert, S. G.: *Pictorial Anatomy of the Frog.* Seattle: University of Washington, 1965.
Gilbert, S. G.: *Pictorial Anatomy of the Necturus.* Seattle: University of Washington, 1973.
Hoff, G. L., Frye, F. L., and Jacobsen, E. R. (eds.): *Diseases of Amphibians and Reptiles.* New York: Plenum, 1984.
   Detailed reviews of some diseases of reptiles and amphibians.
Institute of Laboratory Animal Resources: *Amphibians: Guidelines for the Breeding, Care and Management of Laboratory Animals.* Washington, DC: National Research Council, 1974.
   Extensive report on the care of amphibians as laboratory animals.
Malacinski, G. M. (ed.): *Axolotl Newsletter.* Bloomington, IN: University of Indiana, 1975–1989.
   Annual publication on the biology and care of axolotls.
Marcus, L. C.: *Veterinary Biology and Medicine of Captive Amphibians and Reptiles.* Philadelphia: Lea & Febiger, 1981.
   The most complete text on reptile and amphibian medicine.
Reichenbach-Klinke, H., and Elkan, E.: *The Principal Diseases of Lower Vertebrates II: Diseases of Amphibians.* Neptune City, NJ: TFH Publications, 1965.
   A dated but detailed text mostly on amphibian parasites.

APPENDICES

ROBERT M. JACOBS
and MARK G. PAPICH
Consulting Editors

1231

TABLE OF COMMON DRUGS: APPROXIMATE DOSAGES

MARK G. PAPICH
Consulting Editor

Drug Name	Brand Name(s)*	Dosage†	CVT Reference(s)‡
Acepromazine maleate		0.025–0.2 mg/kg IV, IM, SC (maximum 3 mg) 0.5–2.0 mg/kg PO	
Acetazolamide	Diamox	5–10 mg/kg q8–12h PO *Glaucoma:* 4–8 mg/kg q8–12h PO	XI-1049, XI-1125
Acetylcysteine	Mucomyst	*Antidote:* 140 mg/kg (loading dose) PO, IV, then 70 mg/kg q4h for 5 doses *Eye:* 2% solution topically q2h	
Acetylsalicylic acid (aspirin)		*Antiflammatory:* Dog: 10–25 mg/kg q12h Cat: 10–20 mg/kg q48h *Antiplatelet:* Dog: 5–10 mg/kg q24–48h Cat: 80 mg q48h	XI-27, XI-95, XI-708 XI-861, XI-1049
ACTH		see *Corticotropin gel (ACTH)*	
Actinomycin D	Cosmegen	0.7 mg/m² IV (consult anticancer protocol for intervals)	
Activated charcoal		see *Charcoal, activated*	
Albendazole	Valbazen	25–50 mg/kg q12h PO	XI-228
Allopurinol	Zyloprim	10 mg/kg q8h then reduce to 10 mg/kg q24h	XI-900
Aluminum hydroxide gel	Amphojel	Phosphate binder: 10–30 mg/kg PO q8h (with meals)	XI-853
Aluminum carbonate gel	Basaljel	Phosphate binder: 10–30 mg/kg PO q8h (with meals)	
Amikacin	Amiglyde-V	10 mg/kg q8h IV, IM, SC	XI-539
Aminopentamide sulfate	Centrine	Dog: 0.01–0.03 mg/kg q8–12h IM, SC, PO Cat: 0.02 mg/kg q8–12h IM, SC, PO	
Aminophylline		Dog: 10 mg/kg q8h PO, IM, IV Cat: 6.6 mg/kg q12h PO	IX-278, XI-660
Aminophylline extended release tablets	Theo-Dur Slo-Bid Gyrocaps	Dog: 20 mg/kg q12h PO (Theo-Dur); 30 mg/kg q12h PO (Slo-Bid Gyrocaps) Cat: 25 mg/kg q24h	XI-660, XI-803
Aminoproprazine fumarate	Jenotone	2 mg/kg q12h IM, SC	
5-Aminosalicylic acid		see *Mesalamine; Osalazine* sodium	
Amiodarone	Cordarone	Dog: 10–20 mg/kg q12h IV	
Amitraz	Mitaban	10.6 ml per 7.5 L water; apply 3–6 topical treatments every 14 days§	IX-531, XI-515, XI-558
Ammonium chloride		Dog: 100 mg/kg q12h PO Cat: 800 mg/cat (approximately ¼ tsp) mixed with food daily	
Amoxicillin	Amoxil	11–22 mg/kg PO q8–12h	XI-207, XI-568, XI-829

*The brand names included in this column are for reference purposes only and do not denote an endorsement of any specific product. Often, other proprietary products are available for each specific drug.

†Delivery methods: IC, intracardiac; IM, intramuscular; IP, intraperitoneal; IV, intravenous; PO, *per os* (oral); SC, subcutaneous. Dosages for birds, exotic pets, and zoo animals can be found in Section 14 of *CVT XI* and Section 7 of *CVT X*. For ocular therapeutics, also refer to Section 13 of *CVT XI* and Section 6 of *CVT X*. For topical skin preparations, see Dermatologic Diseases, Section 7 of *CVT XI* and Section 5 of *CVT X*.

‡Roman numerals in this column refer to *CVT* edition, and arabic numerals refer to page number of article. Previous editions: Kirk, R. W. (ed.): *Current Veterinary Therapy X: Small Animal Practice.* Philadelphia: W. B. Saunders, 1989; Kirk, R. W. (ed.): *Current Veterinary Therapy IX: Small Animal Practice.* Philadelphia: W. B. Saunders, 1986.

§Refer to manufacturer's recommendations.

Table continued on following page

Drug Name	Brand Name(s)	Dosage	CVT Reference(s)
Amoxicillin plus clavu-lanate	Clavamox	Dog: 12.5–25 mg/kg q12h PO§ Cat: 62.5 mg q12h PO§	XI-207, XI-539
Amphetamine		4.4 mg/kg IV, IM	
Amphotericin B	Fungizone	0.25–0.5 mg/kg IV (slow infusion) q48h, to a cumulative dose of 4–8 mg/kg	IX-1142, X-1101, XI-609. XI-914, XI-1061
Ampicillin	Omnipen	10–20 mg/kg q6–8h IV, IM, SC (ampicillin so-dium)	X-909, XI-829, XI-969
	Principen	20–40 mg/kg q8h PO	
Ampicillin trihydrate	Polyflex	6.5 mg/kg IM, SC, q12h	
Amprolium	Amprol Corid	1.25 gm of 20% amprolium powder added to daily feed, or 30 ml of 9.6% amprolium solution to 3.8 L of drinking water for 7 days.	
Amrinone lactate	Inocor	1–3 mg/kg IV (loading dose) followed by 30–100 µg/kg/min IV infusion	IX-327, X-247
Antacid drugs		see Aluminum hydroxide gel, *Calcium carbonate; Magnesium hydroxide*	X-911
Apomorphine hydro-chloride		0.02–0.04 mg/kg IV, IM; 0.1 mg/kg SC; or instill 0.25 mg in conjunctiva of eye (dis-solve 6 mg tablet in 1–2 ml of saline)	
Ascorbic acid		*Diet supplement:* 100–500 mg/day	XI-175
L-Asparaginase	Elspar	400 IU/kg weekly IP, SC, IM*	
Aspirin		see *Acetylsalicylic acid*	
Astemizole	Hismanal	Dog: 0.2 mg/kg q24h PO	
Atenolol	Tenormin	Dog: 6.25–12.5 mg/dog q12h PO Cat: 6.25–12.5 mg/cat q24h PO	XI-676, XI-838
Atracurium besylate	Tracrium	0.2 mg/kg IV initially, then 0.15 mg/kg q30min (or IV infusion at 3–8 µg/kg/min)	XI-98
Atropine		0.02–0.04 mg/kg q6–8h IV, IM, SC *Organophosphate and carbamate toxicosis:* 0.2–0.5 mg/kg (as needed)	XI-168, XI-178, XI-183, XI-188
Auranofin (triethylphos-phine gold)	Ridaura	0.1–0.2 mg/kg q12h PO	X-570
Aurothioglucose	Solganal	Dog <10 kg: 1 mg IM first wk, 2 mg IM second wk, 1 mg/kg/wk maintenance Dog >10 kg: 5 mg IM first wk, 10 mg IM second wk, 1 mg/kg/wk maintenance Cat: 0.5–1 mg/cat IM every 7 days	XI-568
Azathioprine	Imuran	Dog: 2 mg/kg q24h PO initially, then 0.5–1 mg/kg q48h Cat: 6.25 mg/cat q48h	X-570, XI-568, XI-572, XI-660, XI-861, XI-1007, XI-1049, XI-1061
BAL		see *Dimercaprol*	
Betamethasone	Celestone	0.1–0.2 mg/kg q12–24h PO	X-54
Bethanechol chloride	Urecholine	Dog: 5–15 mg/dog q8h PO Cat: 1.25–5.0 mg/cat q8h PO	XI-883
Bisacodyl	Dulcolax	5 mg/dog or cat q8–24h PO	
Bismuth subcarbonate		0.3–3.0 gm q4h PO	
Bismuth subsalicylate	Pepto-Bismol	1–3 ml/kg/day (in divided doses) PO	XI-237
Bleomycin sulfate	Blenoxane	10 units/m² IV or SC for 3 days, then 10 units/m² weekly (maximum cumulative dose: 200 units/m²)	
Bromide		see *Potassium bromide*	
Bunamidine	Scolaban	20–50 mg/kg PO	XI-626
Bupivacaine hydrochlo-ride	Marcaine	0.22–0.3 ml epidural	XI-82, XI-96, XI-146
Buprenorphine hydro-chloride	Temgesic	0.01 mg/kg IV, IM	XI-27, XI-708
Busulfan	Myleran	3–4 mg/m² q24h PO	
Butorphanol	Torbutrol Torbugesic	0.05–0.1 mg/kg q6–12h IV, SC† 0.55–1.1 mg/kg q6–12h PO† *Preanesthetic:* 0.2–0.4 mg/kg IV, IM, SC (with acepromazine)† Butorphanol: 0.2–0.6 mg/kg SC (antiemetic prior to cancer chemotherapy)	XI-27, XI-82

*Consult anticancer treatment protocol for precise dosage.
†Refer to manufacturer's recommendations.

Drug Name	Brand Name(s)	Dosage	CVT Reference(s)
Calcitriol	Rocaltrol	2.5–3 ng/kg, q24h, PO	XI-842, XI-857
Calcium carbonate	Titralac	5–10 ml q4–6h PO	
	Camalox	60–100 mg/kg/day (in divided doses) as phosphate binder	
Calcium chloride (10% solution)		hypocalcemia: 0.1–0.3 ml/kg IV, IC (slowly)	
Calcium citrate		Cat: 10–30 mg/kg q8h (with meals) PO	XI-853
Calcium disodium EDTA		see *Edetate calcium disodium (CaNa$_2$, EDTA)*	
Calcium gluconate (10% solution)		0.5–1.5 ml/kg IV (slowly)	X-90, X-1042
Calcium lactate		Dog: 0.5–2.0 gm/dog/day PO (in divided doses)	X-90, X-1042
		Cat: 0.2–0.5 gm/cat/day PO (in divided doses)	
Captan		0.25% solution topically, 2–3 times/wk	
Captopril	Capoten	Dog: 0.5–2.0 mg/kg q8–12h PO	
		Cat: 3.12 to 6.25 mg/cat q8h PO	IX-334, XI-700, XI-829, XI-861
Carbamazepine		Dogs: not recommended	
Carbenicillin disodium	Geopen	40–50 mg/kg q6–8h IV, IM, SC	
	Pyopen		
Carbenicillin indanyl sodium	Geocillin	*Urinary tract infections:* 10 mg/kg q8h PO	
		20–35 mg/kg q8h PO	
Carbimazole	Neo-Mercazole	Cat: 5 mg/cat q8h PO (induction), followed by 5 mg/cat q12h PO	XI-338
Carboplatin	Paraplatin	Dog: 300 mg/m^2 q4wk IV	XI-395
		Cat: not recommended	
Cascara sagrada		Dog: 1–4 ml/dog/day PO	
		Cat: 0.5–1.5 ml/cat/day	
Castor oil		Dog: 8–30 ml/day PO	
		Cat: 4–10 ml/day PO	
Cefadroxil	Cefa-Tabs	Dog: 22 mg/kg q12h PO*	XI-207, XI-539
	Cefa-Drops	Cat: 22 mg/kg q24h PO*	
Cefazolin sodium	Ancef	20–25 mg/kg q4–8h IV, IM	XI-829
	Kefzol		
Cefmetazole sodium	Zefazone	15 mg/kg q8h IV, IM, SC	
Cefotaxime sodium	Claforan	20–80 mg/kg q6h IV, IM	
Cefoxitin sodium	Mefoxin	15–30 mg/kg q6–8h IV	XI-829
Cephalexin	Keflex	10–30 mg/kg q6–12h PO	XI-539, XI-909, XI-969
Cephalothin sodium	Keflin	10–30 mg/kg q4–8h IV, IM	XI-829, XI-969
Cephapirin sodium	Cefadyl	10–30 mg/kg q4–8h IV, IM	
Cephradine	Velosef	10–25 mg/kg q6–8h PO	
Charcoal, activated	Acta-Char	1–4 gm/kg PO (granules)	XI-173, XI-188
	Charcodote	6–12 ml/kg (suspension)	
	Toxiban		
Chlorambucil	Leukeran	2–6 mg/m^2 q24h initially, then q48h PO	XI-595, XI-813
Chloramphenicol, Chloramphenicol palmitate	Chloromycetin	Dog: 40–50 mg/kg q6–8h PO	XI-539, XI-829, XI-1081
		Cat: 30–50 mg/cat q12h PO	
Chloramphenicol sodium succinate	Chloromycetin	Dog: 30–50 mg/kg q6–8h IV, IM	
		Cat: 30–50 mg/cat q12h IV, IM	
Chlorothiazide	Diuril	20–40 mg/kg q12h PO	XI 668, XI-892
Chlorpheniramine maleate	Phenetron and others	Dog: 4–8 mg/dog q12h IV, IM, SC, PO (maximum recommended dose: 0.5 mg/kg q12h)	XI-509, XI-563
		Cat: 2 mg/cat q12h PO	
Chlorpromazine hydrochloride	Thorazine	0.5 mg/kg q6–8h IM, SC, PO	XI-395, XI-583
		Prior to cancer chemotherapy: 2 mg/kg q3h SC	
Chlortetracycline hydrochloride		25 mg/kg q6–8h PO	
Cholecalciferol (vitamin D$_3$)		500–2000 U/kg/day PO (1 mg = 40,000 U)	IX-91
Chorionic gonadotropin		see *Gonadotropin, Chorionic (HCG)*	
Cimetidine	Tagamet	10 mg/kg q6–8h IV, IM PO	X-911, XI-132, XI-191, XI-639, XI-848, XI-1013
		Renal failure: 2.5–5 mg/kg q12h IV, PO	
Ciprofloxacin	Cipro	5–15 mg/kg q12h PO	XI-207, XI-829, XI-909
Cisapride	Propulsid†	Dosage not yet determined (human dose is 5–10 mg q8h PO)	

*Refer to manufacturer's recommendations.
†At the present time, this drug is available only in Canada.

Table continued on following page

Drug Name	Brand Name(s)	Dosage	CVT Reference(s)
Cisplatin	Platinol	60–70 mg/m² q3–4wk IV (requires aggressive diuresis). Do not use in cats.*	XI-395, XI-919
Clavamox		see *Amoxicillin plus clavulanate*	
Clavulanate		see *Amoxicillin plus clavulanate*	
Clemastine	Tavist	Dog: 0.05 mg/kg q12h PO	
Clindamycin	Antirobe	Dog: 11 mg/kg q12h PO, or 22 mg/kg q24h PO	XI-539, XI-1049, XI-1061
	Cleocin	Cat: 5.5 mg/kg q12h, or 11 mg/kg q24h *(staphylococcal infections);* 11 mg/kg q12h, or 22 mg/kg q24h *(anaerobic infections)* PO Toxoplasmosis: 25–50 mg/kg/day PO (in divided treatments) for 2–3 wk	
Clomipramine hydrochloride	Anafranil	1 mg/kg/day PO up to a maximum dose of 3 mg/kg/day PO	
Clonazepam	Klonopin	0.5 mg/kg q8–12h PO	
Clorazepate dipotassium	Tranxene	2 mg/kg q12h PO	
Cloxacillin sodium	Cloxapen Orbenin Tegopen	20–40 mg/kg q8h PO	
Cod liver oil		1 tsp/10 kg once daily PO	
Codeine		*Analgesic:* 0.5–1 mg/kg q6–8h PO *Antitussive:* 0.1–0.3 mg/kg q6–8h PO	
Corticotropin gel (ACTH)	Acthar	*Response test:* collect pre-ACTH sample and inject 2.2 IU/kg IM; collect post-ACTH sample at 2 h in dogs and at 1 and 2 h in cats	X-961
Cosyntropin	Cortrosyn	*Response test:* collect pre-ACTH sample and inject 0.25 mg IV in dogs and 0.125 mg IV in cats. Collect post-ACTH sample at 1 hour.	
Cyanocobalamin (vitamin B₁₂)		Dog: 100–200 μg/day PO Cat: 50–100 μg/day PO	
Cyclophosphamide	Cytoxan Neosar	*Anticancer therapy:* 50 mg/m² once daily 4 days/wk PO, or 150–200 mg/m² IV and repeat in 21 days* *Immunosuppressive therapy:* 50 mg/m² (2.2 mg/kg) q48h PO Cat: 6.25–12.5 mg/cat once daily 4 days/wk Dose listed for cats is both anticancer and immunosuppressive therapy	X-475, X-482, X-489, X-570, XI-568, XI-595, XI-813, XI-861
Cyclosporine	Sandimmune	5 mg/kg q12h PO to 15 mg/kg q24h (adjust dose via monitoring) Topical treatment for keratoconjunctivitis sicca: 1–2% solution in oil: Instill 1 drop in eye q12h	X-570, XI-534, XI-861, XI-870, XI-1092
Cyclothiazide	Anhydron	0.5–1 mg/kg q24h PO	
Cyproheptadine hydrochloride	Periactin	*Antihistamine:* 1.1 mg/kg q8–12h PO *Appetite stimulant in cat:* 2 mg/cat PO	
Cytarabine (cytosine arabinoside)	Cytosar	Dog: 100 mg/m² once daily, or 50 mg/m² twice daily for 4 days IV, SC *(lymphoma)* Cat: 100 mg/m² once daily for 2 days	X-475, X-482, XI-595
Dacarbazine	DTIC	200 mg/m² for 5 days q3wk IV	XI-595
Danazol	Danocrine	5–10 mg/kg q12h PO	
Dantrolene sodium	Dantrium	Dog: 1–5 mg/kg q8h PO Cat: 0.5–2 n·g/kg q12h PO	
Dapsone		1.1 mg/kg q8h PO	
Darbazine (prochlorperazine plus isopropamide)	Darbazine	Dog and cat: 0.14–0.2 ml/kg q12h SC† Dog 2–7 kg: One #1 capsule q12h PO† Dog 7–14 kg: One #2 capsule q12h PO† Dog >14 kg: One #3 capsule q12h PO†	
Deferoxamine mesylate	Desferal	10 mg/kg IV, IM q2h for 2 doses, then 10 mg/kg q8h for 24 h	

*Consult anticancer treatment protocol for precise dosage and intervals.
†Refer to manufacturer's recommendations.

Drug Name	Brand Name(s)	Dosage	CVT Reference(s)
Delta-Albaplex (novobiocin plus prednisolone plus tetracycline hydrochloride)		Dog 3–7 kg: 1–2 tablets/day PO* Dog 7–14 kg: 2–4 tablets/day PO* Dog 14–27 kg: 4–6 tablets/day PO* Dog >27 kg: 6–8 tablets/day PO* Cat: 1 tablet q12h PO*	
Derm Caps (omega fatty acid)		1 capsule/9.1 kg daily PO	XI-563
Desmopressin acetate	DDAVP	*Diabetes insipidus:* 2–4 drops q12–24h intranasally *von Willebrand's disease:* 0.3 µg/kg (diluted in 50 ml of saline and infused over 15–30 min; repeat as needed)	X-973
Desoxycorticosterone pivalate (DOCP)		1.5–2.2 mg/kg q25 days IM*	XI-353
Dexamethasone	Azium	*Anti-inflammatory:* 0.1–0.2 mg/kg q12–24h IV, IM, PO *Shock:* 4–6 mg/kg IV	X-54, XI-509
Dextran-70		20 ml/kg IV q24h to effect	
Dextromethorphan	Benylin DM and others	0.5–2 mg/kg q6–8h PO	
Dextrose (5% solution)		40–50 ml/kg q24h IV, SC, IP	
Diazepam	Valium	*Preanesthetic:* 0.5 mg/kg IV *Status epilepticus:* 0.25–0.5 mg/kg IV; repeat if necessary *Appetite stimulant in cat:* 0.2 mg/kg IV (as needed) *Urinary disorder in cat:* 1.25–2.5 mg/cat q8–12 PO	X-18, X-63, XI-27, XI-98, XI-173, XI-438, XI-655, XI-883
Dichlorophene		see *Toluene*	
Dichlorphenamide	Daranide	3–5 mg/kg q8–12h PO	XI-1049, XI-1125
Dichlorvos	Task	Dog: 26.4–33 mg/kg PO Cat: 11 mg/kg PO	XI-583, XI-626
Dicloxacillin	Dynapen	11–55 mg/kg q8h	
Diethylcarbamazine	Caricide Filaribits	*Heartworm prophylaxis:* 6.6 mg/kg q24h PO*	
Diethylstilbestrol (DES)		Urinary incontinence (dog): 0.1–1.0 mg/dog q24h PO Urinary incontinence (cat): 0.05–0.1 mg/cat q24h PO	
Digitoxin	Crystodigin	0.02–0.03 mg/kg q8h PO	XI-689
Digoxin	Lanoxin	Dog: 0.22 mg/m² q12h PO (subtract 10% for elixir)	XI-689, XI-713
	Cardoxin	Dog (rapid digitalization): 0.0055–0.011 mg/kg q1h IV to effect Cat 2–3 kg: 0.0312 mg q48h PO Cat 4–5 kg: 0.0312 mg q24h PO Cat >6 kg: 0.0312 mg q12h PO	
Dihydrostreptomycin sulfate	Ethamycin (Canada only)	11–15 mg/kg q8–12h IM, SC	XI-260
Dihydrotachysterol (vitamin D)	Hytakerol DHT	0.01 mg/kg/day PO; for acute treatment, 0.02 mg/kg initially, then 0.01–0.02 mg/kg q24–48h PO	IX-91, IX-1039, XI-353
Diltiazem hydrochloride	Cardizem	Dog: 0.5–1.5 mg/kg q8h PO Cat: 1.75–2.4 mg/kg q8–12h PO	IX-340, X-276, XI-684, XI-745, XI-766
Dimenhydrinate	Dramamine (U.S.) Gravol (Canada)	4–8 mg/kg q8h IV, IM, PO Cat: 12.5 mg q8h IV, IM, PO	XI-583
Dimercaprol	BAL in oil	4 mg/kg q4h IM	X-159
Dinoprost tromethamine		see *Prostaglandin F$_{2\alpha}$*	
Dioctyl calcium sulfosuccinate		see *Docusate calcium*	
Dioctyl sodium sulfosuccinate		see *Docusate sodium*	
Diphemanil methylsulfate	Diathal	1.8 mg/kg q12h IM*	

*Refer to manufacturer's recommendations.

Table continued on following page

Drug Name	Brand Name(s)	Dosage	CVT Reference(s)
Diphenhydramine hydrochloride	Benadryl	2–4 mg/kg q6–8h, IV, IM, PO Dog: 25–50 mg/dog q8h IV, IM, PO	XI-583, XI-587
Diphenoxylate hydrochloride	Lomotil	Dog: 0.1–0.2 mg/kg q8–12h PO Cat: 0.05–0.1 mg/kg q12h PO	XI-613
Diphenylhydantoin		see *Phenytoin*	
Diphosphonate disodium etidronate		see *Etidronate disodium*	
Dipyridamole	Persantine	4–10 mg/kg q24h PO	XI-861
Dipyrone	Novaldin	28 mg/kg q8h IV, IM, SC	
Disophenol (DNP)		10 mg/kg SC, once*	XI-626
Disopyramide phosphate	Norpace	6–15 mg/kg q8h PO	
Dithiazanine iodide	Dizan	6.6–11 mg/kg q24h PO for 7–10 days	
Divalproex sodium	Depakote	Equivalent to valproic acid (see *Valproic acid*)	
Dobutamine hydrochloride	Dobutrex	Administer 250 mg in 1 L 5% dextrose Dog: 10–20 µg/kg/min IV infusion Cat: 2.5–10 µg/kg/min IV infusion	XI-191, XI-676 XI-713, XI-773
Docusate calcium	Surfak Doxidan	Dog: 50–100 mg q12–24h PO Cat: 50 mg q12–24h PO	XI-639
Docusate sodium	Colace	Dog: 50–200 mg q8–12h PO Cat: 50 mg q12–24h PO	XI-613, XI-619, XI-639
Domperidone	Motilium	2–5 mg/dog or cat PO	
Dopamine hydrochloride	Intropin	2–10 µg/kg/min IV infusion (40 mg in 500 ml lactated Ringer's solution)	XI-191, XI-655, XI-715
Doxapram hydrochloride	Dopram	5–10 mg/kg IV Neonate: 1–5 mg SC, sublingually, or via umbilical vein	
Doxorubicin	Adriamycin	Dog: 30 mg/m² q21d IV or 10 mg/m² q7d IV Cat: 20–25 mg/m² IV q21d or 10 mg/m² IV q7d	X-475, X-482, X-489, XI-595, XI-783
Doxycycline	Vibramycin	3–5 mg/kg q12h PO	XI-829
Edetate calcium disodium (CaNa₂EDTA)		25 mg/kg q6h SC for 2–5 days	IX-145
Edrophonium chloride	Tensilon	Dog: 0.11–0.22 mg/kg IV Cat: 2.5 mg/cat IV	XI-1024, XI-1039
Emetine		Dog: 1–2.5 ml/kg, up to 6.6 ml/kg PO Cat: 3.3 ml/kg PO (dilute 50:50 with water)	
Enalapril maleate	Vasotec	Dog: 0.5 mg/kg q12–24h PO Cat: 0.25–0.5 mg/kg q12–24h PO	XI-700, XI-773, XI-829
Enflurane	Ethrane	2–3% (induction); 1.5–3% (maintenance)	
Enilconazole	Imaverol	*Nasal aspergillosis:* 10 mg/kg q12h instilled into nasal sinus for 10–14 days (10% solution diluted 50:50 with water)*	X-82, X-577, X-1106
		Dermatophytes: solution diluted to 0.2% and lesion washed with solution 4 times at 3- to 4-day intervals*	XI-547
Enrofloxacin	Baytril	2.5 mg/kg q12h PO, IM, or 5 mg/kg q24h PO, IM	XI-539, XI-829, XI-909, XI-954
Ephedrine	Many	*Urinary incontinence:* 4 mg/kg, or Dog: 12.5–50 mg/dog q8–12h PO Cat: 2–4 mg/kg q8–12h PO *Bronchodilator:* 1–2 mg/kg q8h PO	X-1214, XI-875
Ephedrine plus phenobarbital plus potassium iodide	Quadrinal	Dog: ¼ to ½ tablet q4–6h PO* Cat: ¼ tablet q4–6h PO*	
Epinephrine	Adrenalin	20 µg/kg, or 0.1–0.5 ml of 1:1000 (1 mg/ml) solution; or 1–5 ml of a 1:10,000 (0.1 mg/ml) solution ıV, IM, SC, IC, intratracheally	IX-325, X-331, XI-660
Epsiprantel	Cestex	Cat: 2.75 mg/kg PO	XI-626
Epsom salt		see *Magnesium sulfate*	
Ergocalciferol (vitamin D₂)	Calciferol	500–2000 U/kg/day PO	IX-91, IX-1039
Erythromycin	Many	10–20 mg/kg q8–12h PO	XI-484, XI-539
Erythropoietin	Epogen	100 U/kg SC (adjust dose to reach and maintain hematocrit of 0.30–0.34)	

*Refer to manufacturer's recommendations.

Drug Name	Brand Name(s)	Dosage	CVT Reference(s)
Essential fatty acids	EFA-Z-Plus	<6.7 kg: 3.7 ml/day PO* 6.7–22.5 kg: 7 ml/day PO* >22.5 kg: 14 ml/day PO* (see also *Omega fatty acids*)	
Estradiol cypionate (ECP)	Depo-Estradiol	Dog: 44 μg/kg (0.04 mg/kg) IM (total dose not to exceed 1.0 mg). The use of ECP for mismating is discouraged. Cat: 250 μg/cat (0.25 mg/cat) IM	IX-1236
Ethoxzolamide	Cardrase	*Glaucoma:* 4 mg/kg q8–12h PO	XI-1049
Etidronate disodium	Didronel	Dog: 5 mg/kg/day PO Cat: 10 mg/kg/day PO	
Etretinate	Tegison	Dog: 0.75–1 mg/kg/day PO Cat: 2 mg/kg/day	IX-591, X-553, XI-523
Famotidine	Pepcid	5 mg/kg q24h IM, SC, PO	XI-132
Febantel plus praziquantel	Vercom	Cat: 10 mg/kg q24h for 3 days PO	XI-626
Fenbendazole	Panacur	Dog: 20 mg/kg/day for 3 days PO Cat: 25–50 mg/kg q12 kg PO (lung worms); 50 mg/kg/day for 3 days (*ascarids, hookworms, Taenia*)	XI-228, XI-626
Fentanyl citrate	Sublimaze	0.02–0.04 mg/kg IV, IM, SC, or 0.01 mg/kg IV, IM, SC (with acetylpromazine or diazepam)	XI-98
Fentanyl citrate plus droperidol	Innovan-Vet	These two doses are recommendation by mfr. only: Dog: 0.04–0.09 ml/kg IV; 0.1–0.14 ml/kg IM Cat: do not use	XI-27
Ferrous sulfate	Many	Dog: 100–300 mg/kg q24h PO Cat: 50–100 mg q24h PO	IX-521
Flucytosine	Ancobon	25–50 mg/kg q6–8h PO (maximum dose: 100 mg/kg q12h PO)	IX-562, X-1101, XI-914, XI-1061
Fludrocortisone acetate	Florinef Acetate	Dog: 0.2–0.8 mg (0.02 mg/kg) q24h PO Cat: 0.1 mg q24h PO	IX-972
Flumethasone	Flucort	Dog: 0.0625–0.25 mg/day IV, IM, SC, PO Cat: 0.03–0.125 mg/day IV, IM, SC, PO *Anti-inflammatory:* 0.15–0.3 mg/kg q12–24h IV, IM, SC, PO	X-54
Flunixin meglumine	Banamine	1.1 mg/kg once IV, IM, SC, or 1.1 mg/kg/day 3 day/wk PO *Ophthalmic:* 0.5 mg/kg once IV	X-47, XI-1049
Fluorouracil	5-Fluorouracil	Dog: 150 mg/m² once/wk IV† Cat: do not use	
Folic acid	Folvite	Dog and Cat: 0.004–0.01 mg/kg/day (4–10 μg/kg/day)	
Folinic acid		see *Leucoverin calcium*	
Follicle-stimulating hormone (FSH)		see *Urofollitropin*	
Furazolidone	Furoxone	4 mg/kg q12h for 7–10 days PO	XI-626
Furosemide	Lasix	Dog: 2–6 mg/kg q8–12h (or as needed) IV, IM, SC, PO Cat: 1–4 mg/kg q8–12h IV, IM, SC, PO	XI-668, XI-713, XI-766, XI-861
Gentamicin sulfate	Gentocin	Dog: 2–4 mg/kg q6 8h IV, IM, SC Cat: 3 mg/kg q8h IV; q6h IM, SC	XI-539, XI-829
Glyburide (Gilbenclamide)	Diabeta Micronase	0.2 mg/kg daily PO	IX-991
Glipizide	Glucotrol	0.25–0.5 mg/kg q12h PO	
Glucagon		tolerance test: 0.03 mg/kg IV	
Glycerin	Glyrol Osmoglyn	*Glaucoma:* 1–1.5 gm/kg PO initially, then 500 mg/kg q8h; or 1–2 ml of 50% solution q8h	XI-1125
Glycopyrrolate	Robinul-V	0.005–0.01 mg/kg IV, IM, SC	
Gold sodium thiomalate	Myochrysine	1–5 mg IM (first wk), then 2–10 mg IM (second wk), then 1 mg/kg once/wk IM (maintenance)	X-570
Gold therapy		see *Auranofin (triethylphosphine gold); Aurothioglucose; Gold sodium thiomalate*	X-570

*Refer to manufacturer's recommendations.
†Consult anticancer treatment protocol for precise dosage.

Table continued on following page

Drug Name	Brand Name(s)	Dosage	CVT Reference(s)
Gonadorelin hydrochloride (GnRH, (LHRH)	Factrel	Dog: 50–100 μg/dog/day q24–48 h IM Cat: 25 μg/cat once IM	XI-947, XI-963, XI-966 X-2036
Gonadotropin, chorionic (HCG)	Follutein	Dog: 22 units/kg q24–48h IM, or 44 units once IM	XI-947, XI-963, XI-966
	Pregnyl	Cat: 250 units/cat once IM	
Gonadotropin-releasing hormone		see *Gonadorelin*	
Griseofulvin (microsize)	Fulvicin U/F	50 mg/kg q24h PO (maximum dose: 110–132 mg/kg/day in divided treatments)	XI-547
Griseofulvin (ultramicrosize)	Fulvicin P/G Gris-PEG	5–10 mg/kg/day PO (in divided treatments)	XI-562
Growth hormone		0.1 U/kg 3 times/wk for 4–6 wk	X-978
Halothane	Fluothane	3% (induction); 0.5–1.5% (maintenance)	
Heparin calcium	Calciparine	Dog: 250–500 U/kg q8h SC Cat: 250–375 U/kg q8h SC *Low-dose therapy* (dog and cat): 70U/kg q8–12h SC	XI-137
Heparin sodium	Liquaemin (U.S.) Hepalean (Canada)	Dog: 250–500 U/kg q8h SC Cat: 250–375 U/kg q8h SC *Low-dose therpay* (dog and cat): 70U/kg q8–12h SC	XI-137
Hetacillin potassium	Hetacin-K	20–40 mg/kg q8h PO	
Hydralazine hydrochloride	Apresoline	Dog: 0.5 mg/kg (initial dose), titrated to 0.5–2 mg/kg q12h PO Cat: 2.5 mg/cat q12–24h	XI-700
Hydrochlorothiazide	HydroDiuril	2–4 mg/kg q12h PO	X-1182, XI-838
Hydrocortisone	Cortef	*Replacement therapy:* 1 mg/kg q12h PO *Anti-inflammatory:* 2.5–5 mg/kg q12h PO	X-54
Hydrocortisone sodium succinate	Solu-Cortef	*Shock:* 50–150 mg/kg IV	X-54
Hydrogen peroxide (3%)		*Emetic:* 5–10 ml PO (may repeat once within 10 min)	
Hydroxyurea	Hydrea	Dog: 50 mg/kg PO once daily, 3 days/wk Cat: 25 mg/kg PO once daily, 3 days/wk	
Hydroxyzine hydrochloride	Atarax	Dog: 2 mg/kg q6–8h IM, PO Cat: safe dosage not established	XI-552
Ibuprofen	Motrin Advil Nuprin	Safe dosage not established	X-47, XI-191
Imidocarb hydrochloride		5 mg/kg IM once	XI-829
Indomethacin	Indocin	Safe dosage not established	X-47
Insulin (NPH isophane)		Dog <15 kg: 1 U/kg q24h SC (to effect) Dog > 25 kg: 0.5 U/kg q24h SC (to effect) Cat: not recommended	IX-991, IX-1000, XI-356
Insulin (PZI)		Dog: same dose as for NPH isophane insulin, except that an increase of approximately 25% may be needed Cat: 1–3 U/cat (0.2–1 U/kg) q12–24h SC (adjust with monitoring)	IX-991, XI-349, XI-353, XI-364
Insulin (regular crystalline)		*Ketoacidosis:* Animals <3 kg: 1 U/animal initially, then 1 U/animal q1h Animals 3–10 kg: 2 U/animal initially, then 1 U/animal q1h Animals > 10 kg, 0.25 U/kg initially, then 0.1 U/kg q1h IM (Consult CVT text for exact protocol)	IX-991, IX-1000, X-1008, XI-359
Insulin, ultralente		Dog <15 kg: 1 U/kg q24h SC (to effect) Dog > 25 kg: 0.5 U/kg q24h SC (to effect) Cat: not recommended	
Iodide		see *Potassium iodide*	
Ipecac syrup		Dog: 3–6 ml PO Cat: 2–6 ml PO	
Iron		see *Ferrous sulfate*	
Isoflurane		5% (induction); 1.5–2.5% (maintenance)	

Drug Name	Brand Name(s)	Dosage	CVT Reference(s)
Isoproterenol	Isuprel	10 μg/kg q6h IM, SC; or 1 mg diluted in 500 ml of 5% dextrose or lactated Ringer's solution and infused to effect, or IV infusion of 0.5–1 ml/min (1–2 μg/min)	
Isosorbide dinitrate	Isordil Sorbitrate	2.5–5 mg/animal q12h PO	IX-329, XI-700
Isotretinoin	Accutane	1–3 mg/kg/day (maximum dose: 3–4 mg/kg/day) PO	IX-591, X-553, XI-534
Itraconazole	Sporanox	2.5 mg/kg q12h to 5 mg/kg q24h PO	X-82, X-577, X-1101, X-1106, X-1109, XI-547, XI-609, XI-1061
Ivermectin	Heartguard Ivomec	*Heartworm preventative in dog:* 6 μg/kg q30day PO	X-140, X-263, X-560, XI-228
		Microfilaricide in dog: 50 μg/kg PO 3 to 4 wk after adulticide therapy	
		Ectoparasite therapy: 200–300 μg/kg IM, SC, PO (do not use in Collie dogs)	XI-558
		Respiratory parasites: 200–400 μg/kg weekly SC, PO (do not use in Collie dogs)	
Kanamycin sulfate	Kantrim	10 mg/kg q6–8h IV, IM, SC	
Kaolin plus pectin	Kaopectate	1–2 ml/kg q2–6h PO	XI-1013
Ketamine hydrochloride	Ketalar Ketaset	Dog: 5.5–22 mg/kg IV, IM (adjunctive sedative or tranquilizer treatment recommended)	XI-27, XI-655, XI-929
		Cat: 2–25 mg/kg IV, IM (adjunctive sedative or tranquilizer treatment recommended)	
Ketoconazle	Nizoral	Dog: 10–30 mg/kg/day in divided treatments PO (*Malassezia canis infection:* 10 mg/kg q24h or 5 mg/kg q12h PO)	X-82, X-577, X-1024, X-1101, X-1106, X-1109, XI-349, XI-523, XI-544, XI-547, XI-609, XI-1061
		Hyperadrenocorticism: 15 mg/kg q12h PO (just dog)	
		Cat: 5–10 mg/kg q8–12h PO	
Lactated Ringer's solution	Many	40–50 ml/kg/day IV for maintenance	
Lactulose	Chronulac	*Constipation:* 1 ml/4.5 kg q8h PO (to effect)	XI-613, XI-619, XI-639
		Hepatic encephalopathy in dog: 0.5 ml/kg q8h PO	
		Hepatic encephalopathy in cat: 2.5–5 ml/cat q8h PO	
Leucovorin calcium (folinic acid)	Wellcovorin	*With methotrexate administration:* 3 mg/m² IV, IM, PO	
		Antidote for pyrimethamine toxicosis: 1 mg/kg q24h PO	
Levamisole hydrochloride	Levasole Tramisol	Dog: 5–8 mg/kg PO once, up to 10 mg/kg PO for 2 days (*hookworms*); 10 mg/kg q24h PO for 6–10 days (*microfilaricide*); 0.5–2 mg/kg 3 times/wk PO (*immunostimulant*)	IX-1091, X-570, XI-217, XI-228, XI-539, XI-861
		Cat: 4.4 mg/kg PO once	
Levodopa (L-dopa)	Larodopa	*Hepatic encephalopathy:* 6.8 mg/kg initially, then 1.4 mg/kg q6h	XI-639
Levothyroxine sodium	Soloxine Thyro-Tabs Synthroid	Dog: 10–20 μg/kg q12h PO (adjust dose via monitoring)	XI-954
		Cat: 10–20 μg/kg/day PO (adjust dose via monitoring)	
Lidocaine hydrochloride	Xylocaine Hydrochloride	*Antiarrhythmia in dog:* 2–4 mg/kg IV (maximum dose: 8 mg/kg over 10 min); 25–75 μg/kg/min IV infusion; 6 mg/kg q1.5h IM	X-278, XI-694
		Cat: 0.25–0.75 mg/kg IV, slowly (do not use as antiarrhythmic)	
Lime sulfur (3% solution)		topically once/wk for 4–6 wk	XI-547, XI-558
Lincomycin	Lincocin	15–25 mg/kg q12h IV, IM, PO	XI-539
Liothyronine	Cytobin or Cytomel	4.4 μg/kg q8h PO	
		Suppression testing: collect presample for T_4 and T_3. Administer 25 μg q8h PO for 7 doses. Collect post samples for T_4 and T_3 after last dose.	

Table continued on following page

Drug Name	Brand Name(s)	Dosage	CVT Reference(s)
Lithium carbonate	Lithotabs	Dog: 10 mg/kg q12h PO Cat: not recommended	
Loperamide hydrochloride	Imodium	Dog: 0.1–0.2 mg/kg q8–12h PO Cat: 0.08–0.16 mg/kg q12h PO	XI-237, XI-604, XI-613
Luteinizing hormone		see *Gonadorelin*	
Magnesium citrate	Citro-Mag (Canada) Citroma, Citro-Nesia (U.S.)	2–4 ml/kg PO	

Magnesium hydroxide	Milk of Magnesia	*Antacid:* 5–10 ml/kg q4–6h PO
		Cathartic:
		  Dog: 15–50 ml/kg PO
		  Cat: 2–6 ml/cat q24h PO
			X-911

Magnesium sulfate		Dog: 8–25 gm/dog q24h PO Cat: 2–5 gm/cat q24h PO	
Mannitol	Osmitrol	*Diuretic:* 1 gm/kg of 5–25% solution IV to maintain urine flow *Glaucoma or CNS edema:* 0.25–2 gm/kg of 15–25% solution over 15–60 min IV (repeat in 6 hr if necessary)	XI-173, XI-639, XI-1125
Mebendazole	Telmintic	22 mg/kg (with food) q24h for 3 days*	
Meclizine hydrochloride	Bonine	Dog: 25 mg q24h PO (*motion sickness:* administer 1 hr prior to traveling) Cat: 12.5 mg q24h PO	
Medium-chain triglycerides (MCTs)	MCT oil	1–2 ml/kg daily in food	IX-885, IX-909
Medroxyprogesterone acetate	Depo-Provera	1.1–2.2 mg/kg q7days IM	XI-552, XI-947
Megestrol acetate	Ovaban	*Proestrus:* 2.2 mg/kg q24h PO for 8 days *Anestrus:* 0.55 mg/kg q24h PO for 30 days *Behavior problems:* 2–4 mg/kg q24h for 8 days (reduce dose for maintenance) Cat: 2.5–5 mg/cat q24h PO for 1 wk, then reduce to 2.5–5 mg once or twice/wk (*dermatologic therapy*); cat (*suppress estrus*): 5 mg/cat for 3 days, then 2.5–5 mg once/wk for 10 wk†	XI-509, XI-552, XI-947, XI-963, XI-966
Melphalan	Alkeran	1.5 mg/m² q24h PO for 7–10 days (repeat q3wk)	
Mephenytoin	Mesantoin	Dog: 10 mg/kg, q8h, PO	XI-986
Meperidine hydrochloride	Demerol	Dog: 5–10 mg/kg IV, IM (as needed) Cat: 3–5 mg/kg IV, IM (as needed)	XI-82, XI-631
6-Mercaptopurine	Purinethol	50 mg/m² q24h PO	
Mesalamine	Asacol Mesasal Pentasa	Dosage not established (human dosage is 400–500 mg q6–8h see also *Osalazine sodium; Sulfasalazine*	
Metaproterenol sulfate	Alupent Metaprel	0.325–0.65 mg/kg q4–6h PO	IX-278
Metaraminol bitartrate	Aramine	0.1 mg/kg IM, SC	
Medetomidine hydrochloride		0.01–0.08 ml/kg IV, IM	
Methazolamide	Neptazane	2–4 mg/kg (maximum dose: 4–6 mg/kg) q8–12h PO	XI-1049
Methenamine hippurate	Hiprex	Dog: 500 mg/dog q12h PO Cat: 250 mg/cat q12h PO	
Methenamine mandelate	Mandelamine	10–20 mg/kg q8–12h PO	VIII-1096
Methimazole	Tapazole	Cat: 5 mg/cat q8–12h PO (induction), followed by 2.5–5 mg/cat q8–12h PO.	IX-1026, X-1002, XI-334
Methionine (other names used are L-methionine and DL-methionine)	Uroeze Methio-Form	Dog: 150–300 mg/kg/day PO* Cat: 1–1.5 gm/cat PO (added to food each day)* (use in adult cats only)	VIII-1095
Methocarbamol	Robaxin- V	44 mg/kg q8h PO on the first day, then 22–44 q8h PO*	
Methohexital sodium	Brevital	11 mg/kg IV (to effect)	

*Refer to manufacturer's recommendations.
†Megestrol acetate not approved for use in cats.

Drug Name	Brand Name(s)	Dosage	CVT Reference(s)
Methotrexate (MTX)		2.5 mg/m² q48h PO; or Dog: 0.5 mg/kg IV Cat: 0.8 mg/kg IV q2–3 wk*	
Methoxamine hydro-chloride	Vasoxyl	200–250 μg/kg IM, or 40–80 μg/kg IV	
Methoxyflurane	Metofane	3% (induction); 0.5–1.5% (maintenance)	
Methscopolamine bromide	Pamine	0.3–1 mg/kg q8h PO (use cautiously in cats)	
Methylene blue (1% solution)		Dog: 5–15 mg/kg IV Cat: do not use	XI-175, XI-178
Methylprednisolone acetate	Depo-Medrol	Dog: 1 mg/kg IM q1–3 wk Cat: 10–20 mg/cat IM q1–3 wk	X-54, XI-509, XI-568
Methyltestosterone		Dog: 5–25 mg/dog q24–48 h PO (see also *Testosterone cypionate; Testosterone propionate*)† Cat: 1–2.5 mg/cat q48h PO†	
Metoclopramide hydro-chloride	Reglan Maxolon Maxeran (Canada)	0.2–0.5 mg/kg q6–8h IV, IM, PO, or 1–2 mg/kg/day via continuous IV infusion	IX-862, XI-191, XI-583, XI-848
Metoprolol tartrate	Lopressor	Dog: 5–60 mg/dog q8h PO Cat: 2–15 mg/cat q8h PO	IX-343, XI-676
Metronidazole	Flagyl	Dog: 25–65 mg/kg q24h PO, or 10 mg/kg q8h PO Cat: 10–25 mg/kg (maximum dose: 50 mg/kg) q24h PO; *Giardia* 10 mg/kg q12h for 5 days	XI-568, XI-626, XI-639, XI-602
Mexiletine hydrochloride	Mexitil	Dog: 5–8 mg/kg q8–12h PO (use cautiously)	
Mibolerone	Cheque	Dog: (2.6–5 μg/kg/day PO: 0.45–11.3 kg: 30 μg† 11.8–22.7 kg: 60 μg† 23–45.3 kg: 120 μg† >45.8 kg: 180 μg† Cat: Safe dose not established.	XI-954, XI-966
Midazolam hydrochloride	Versed	0.1–0.25 mg/kg IV, IM, or 0.1–0.3 mg/kg/h IV infusion	XI-27, XI-98
Milk of magnesia		see *Magnesium hydroxide*	
Milrinone		0.5–1.0 mg/kg q12h PO (not approved)	IX-329
Mineral oil		Dog: 10–50 ml/dog q12h PO Cat: 10–25 ml/cat q12h PO	
Minocycline	Minocin	5–12.5 mg/kg q12h PO	XI-1061
Misoprostol	Cytotec	Dog: 2–5 μg/kg q8–12h PO	X-911, XI-132
Mithramycin		see *Plicamycin*	
Mitotane (o,p'-DDD)	Lysodren	50 mg/kg/day PO (may be given in divided doses) for 5–10 days, then 25–50 mg/kg wk PO	IX-963, X-1024, X-1031, XI-345
Mitoxantrone hydrochloride	Novantrone	3–5 mg/m² IV	XI-399, XI-595
Morphine sulfate		Dog: 0.5–1 mg/kg IV, IM, SC (as needed); 0.1 mg/kg epidural Cat: 0.1 mg/kg IM, SC (as needed)	XI-27, XI-82, XI-95, XI-713
Nadolol	Corgard	0.25–0.5 mg/kg q12h PO	IX-343, XI-676
Nafcillin sodium	Unipen	10 mg/kg q6h IM, PO	
Nalorphine	Nalline	0.44 mg/kg IV, IM, SC (1 mg for every 10 mg of morphine)	
Naloxone	Narcan	0.01–0.04 mg/kg IV, IM, SC†	XI-27, XI-552, XI-995
Naltrexone hydrochloride	Trexan	*Behavior problems:* 2.2 mg/kg q12h PO	
Nandrolone decanoate	Deca-Durabolin	Dog: 1–1.5 mg/kg/wk IM Cat: 1 mg/cat/wk IM	X-18, XI-438
Naproxen	Naprosyn (Canada) Naxen	Dog: 2 mg/kg q24–48h (use cautiously)	X-47
Neo-Darbazine (pro-chlorperazine plus isopropamide plus neomycin)		Dog:† 4.5–9 kg: one #1 capsule q12h 9–13.6 kg: two #1 capsules q12h 13.6–27.3 kg: three #1 capsules or one #3 capsule q12h PO	

*Consult anticancer protocol for precise dosage.
†Refer to manufacturer's recommendations.

Table continued on following page

Drug Name	Brand Name(s)	Dosage	CVT Reference(s)
Neomycin sulfate	Biosol	Dog: 20 mg/kg q6h PO Cat: 10–20 mg/kg q12h PO	X-829, XI-639
Neostigmine bromide	Prostigmin Bromide	2 mg/kg/day PO (in divided doses, to effect)	XI-580
Neostigmine methylsul- fate	Prostigmin	*Antimyasthenic:* 10 µg/kg IM, SC, as needed (atropine may be administered to counteract side effects) *Antidote for curiform block:* 40 µg/kg IM, SC (administer with atropine) *Diagnostic aid for myasthenia gravis:* 40 µg/kg IM, or 20 µg/kg IV	XI-1039
Niclosamide	Yomesan	Dog: 157 mg/kg PO once*	
Nifedipine	Adalat Procardia	Dosage not established	IX-340, XI-684
Nitrates		see *Isosorbide dinitrate; Nitroglycerin ointment*	
Nitrofurantoin	Furadantin Macrodantin	4 mg/kg q8h PO	
Nitroglycerin ointment	Nitrol Ointment	Dog: 4–12 mg (maximum of 15 mg) topically q12h	IX-329, XI-700, XI-713, XI-766
	Nitro-Bid Ointment Nitrostat Ointment	Cat: 2–4 mg topically q12h (or ¼ in./cat) (1 inch of ointment is approximately 15 mg.)	
Nitroprusside sodium	Nipride	5–15 µg/kg/min IV infusion	IX-329, XI-418, XI-700, XI-713
Nizatidine	Axid	5 mg/kg q24h PO	XI-132
Norfloxacin	Noroxin	22 mg/kg q12h PO	XI-829
Novobiocin	see *Delta-Albaplex*		
Omega fatty acids	see *Derm Caps*	1 capsule q12h PO (see also *Essential fatty acids*)	X-563, XI-534
Omeprazole	Prilosec	20 mg/dog once daily	X-911, XI-132
o,p'-DDD		see *Mitotane, o,p'-DDD*	
Orgotein	Palosein	Dog: 2.5–5 mg q24h IM, SC for 6 days, then q48h for 8 days*	
Ormetroprim		see *Primor*	
Osalazine sodium	Dipentum	Dosage not established (human dosage is 500 mg twice daily)	
Oxacillin	Prostaphlin Bactocill	22–40 mg/kg q8h PO	XI-539
Oxazepam	Serax	Appetite stimulant: 2.5 mg/cat PO	X-18, XI-438
Oxtriphylline	Cholesdyl SA	Dog: 47 mg/kg (equivalent to 30 mg/kg theo- phylline) q12h PO	XI-660
Oxybutynin chloride	Ditropan	0.5 mg q8–12h PO	X-1214
Oxymetholone	Anadrol	1–5 mg/kg/day PO	
Oxymorphone hydro- chloride	Numorphan	*Induction:* 0.1–0.2 mg/kg IV, SC, IM (as needed), then 0.05–0.1 mg/kg q1–2h (pre- medication with acetylpromazine) *Preanesthetic:* 0.025–0.05 mg/kg IM, SC	XI-27, XI-82, XI-95, XI-98
Oxytetracycline	Terramycin	7.5–10 mg/kg q12h IV; 20 mg/kg q12h PO	
Oxytocin		Dog: 1–5 units IM, IV, repeat q30 min for primary inertia. Cat: 0.5 units IM, IV (maximum dose: 3 units/ cat)	X-1299
2-PAM		see *Pralidoxime chloride*	
Pancreatic enzyme (Pancrelipase)	Viokase	2 tsp per 20 kg body weight, or 1–3 tsp/0.45 kg of food, mixed with food 20 min prior to feeding	X-927
Pancreatic enzyme (Pancrelipase)	Festal-II	1 Tablet before, or with meals. (Do not break or crush tablet.)	
Pancreatin		Dog: 2–10 tablets with food Cat: 1–2 tablets with food	
Pancuronium bromide	Pavulon	0.1 mg/kg IV	
Paregoric	Corrective Mixture	0.05–0.06 mg/kg q12h PO (5 ml of paregoric corresponds to approximately 2 mg of morphine)	
D-penicillamine	Cuprimine	10–15 mg/kg q12h PO	IX-145, X-891, X-1189
Penicillin G benzathine	Donnazyme	Not recommended	
Penicillin G potassium	Many	20,000–40,000 U/kg q6–8h IV, IM	XI-829
Penicillin G procaine		20,000–40,000 U/kg q12–24 IM	XI-260
Penicillin G sodium	Many	20,000–40,000 U/kg q6–8h IV, IM	XI-829

*Refer to manufacturer's recommendations.

Drug Name	Brand Name(s)	Dosage	CVT Reference(s)
Penicillin V (previously used name is phenoxymethyl penicillin)	Many	10 mg/kg q8h PO	
Pentazocine	Talwin	Dog: 1.65–3.3 mg/kg q4h IM Cat: 2.2–3.3 mg/kg IV, IM, SC	XI-82
Pentobarbital		25–30 mg/kg IV (first ½ of the dose administered rapidly, then remaining administered dose to effect)	XI-98
Petrolatum, white	Vaseline Laxatone	Cat: 1–5 ml/cat q24h PO	XI-619
Phenobarbital	Luminal	Dog: 2–8 mg/kg q12h PO Cat: 1–2 mg/kg q12h PO *Status epilepticus* (dog or cat): 15–200 mg/animal IV (to effect)	IX-836, XI-986, XI-992
Phenoxybenzamine hydrochloride	Dibenzyline	Dog: 0.25 mg/kg q8–12h PO, or 0.5 mg/kg q24h Cat: 0.5 mg/kg q12h PO	X-1214, XI-883
Phentolamine mesylate	Regitine (U.S) Rogitine (Canada)	0.02–0.1 mg/kg IV (as needed to maintain blood pressure)	
Phenylbutazone	Butazolidin	Dog: 15–22 mg/kg q8–12h PO (maximum dose: 800 mg)* Cat: not recommended	X-47
Phenylephrine hydrochloride	Neo-Synephrine Hydrochloride	0.01 mg/kg q15min IV 0.1 mg/kg q15min IM, SC	
Phenylpropanolamine hydrochloride	Propagest, Dexatrim	1.5–2 mg/kg q12h PO	X-1214, XI-875
Phenytoin	Dilantin	*Antiepileptic in dog:* 20–35 mg/kg q8h *Antiepileptic in cat:* not recommended *Antiarrhythmic in dog:* 30 mg/kg q8h PO or 10 mg/kg IV over 5 min	IX-836
Phytonadione		see *Vitamin K₁*	
Phytomenadione		see *Vitamin K₁*	
Piperazine	Many	44–66 mg/kg PO once*	XI-626
Piroxicam	Feldene	Dog: 0.3 mg/kg q48h PO (use cautiously) Cat: dosage not established	X-47, XI-626
Plicamycin	Mithracin	*Antineoplastic:* 25–30 µg/kg/day IV (slow infusion) for 8–10 days *Antihypercalcemic:* 15–25 µg/kg/day IV (slow infusion) for 3–4 days	
Polyethylene glycol electrolyte solution	Golytely	25 ml/kg, then repeat in 2–4 hr PO	XI-568
Potassium bromide		Dog: 30–40 mg/kg q24h PO (adjust dose via monitoring)	XI-986
Potassium chloride		0.5 mEq/kg/day (do not administer at a rate faster than 0.5 mEq/kg/h) 10–40 mEq/500 ml of fluids, depending on serum potassium	
Potassium citrate	Polycitra-K Urocit-K	2.2 mEq/100 kcal of energy/day PO Dog: For calcium oxalate urolithiasis: approximately 75 mg/kg q12h PO (mixed with food)	XI-842, XI-892 X-1182
Potassium gluconate	Kaon Elixir Tumil-K	2.2 mEq/100 kcal of energy/day PO Cat: 2–6 mEq daily	XI-820, XI-842, XI-848
Potassium iodide		30–100 mg/cat daily (in single or divided doses) for 10–14 days	XI-301
Pralidoxime chloride (2-PAM)	Protopam chloride	*Organophosphate toxicosis:* 20 mg/kg q8–12h (initial dose IV [slow], or IM; subsequent doses IM, SC)	XI-178, XI-188

Praziquantel	Droncit	Dog (PO):*
		    <6.8 kg: 7.5 mg/kg once
		    >6.8 kg: 5 mg/kg once
		Dog (IM, SC):*
		    ≤2.3 kg: 7.5 mg/kg once
		    2.7–4.5 kg: 6.3 mg/kg once
		    ≥5 kg: 5 mg/kg once
		Cat (PO):*
		    <1.8 kg: 6.3 mg/kg once
		    >1.8 kg: 5 mg/kg once
		    paragonimiasis: 25 mg/kg q8h for 2 days
		Cat (IM, SC): 5 mg/kg IM, SC
			XI-228, XI-626

*Refer to manufacturer's recommendations.

Table continued on following page

Drug Name	Brand Name(s)	Dosage	CVT Reference(s)
Prazosin hydrochloride	Minipress	0.5–2 mg/animal q8–12h PO	IX-329, XI-700, XI-840
Prednisolone	Many	*Anti-inflammatory:* Dog: 0.5–1 mg/kg q12–24h IV, IM, PO, intially then taper to q48 h Cat: 2.2 mg/kg q12–24h IV, IM, PO initially, then taper to q48 h. Immunosuppressive dose is same for dogs and cats. *Immunosuppressive* (dog and cat): initially 2.2–6.6 mg/kg/day IV, IM, PO, then taper to 2–4 mg/kg q48h *Shock:* see *Prednisolone sodium succinate* See also *Methylprednisolone acetate*	X-54, XI-509, XI-539, XI-568, XI-572, XI-595, XI-813, XI-1007, XI-1049, XI-1081
Prednisolone sodium succinate	Solu-Delta-Cortef	*Shock:* 15–30 mg/kg IV, then repeat in 4–6 h *CNS trauma:* 15–30 mg/kg IV, then taper to 1–2 mg/kg q12h	X-54, XI-1013
Prednisone		see *Prednisolone*	
Primidone	Mylepsin Mysoline	5–15 mg/kg q8–12h PO	IX-836, XI-992
Primor (ormetoprim plus sulfadimethoxine)		27 mg/kg on first day, followed by 13.5 mg/kg q24h PO*	
Procainamide hydrochloride	Pronestyl	Dog: 10–20 mg/kg q6h PO (maximum dose: 40 mg/kg); 8–20 mg/kg IV, IM; 25–50 µg/kg/min IV infusion Cat: 3–8 mg/kg IM, PO q6–8h	
Procainamide hydrochloride (extended-release tablets)	Procan-SR	Dog: 25–50 mg/kg q8h PO Cat: 62.5 mg/cat q8h PO	XI-694
Prochlorperazine	Compazine	0.1–0.5 mg/kg q6–8h IM, SC see also *Darbazine* or *Neo-Darbazine*	XI-583
Progesterone, repositol		see *Medroxyprogesterone acetate*	
Promazine hydrochloride	Sparine	1–2 mg/kg q6–8h IV, IM, PO	
Promethazine hydrochloride	Phenergan	0.2–0.4 mg/kg q6–8h IV, IM, PO (maximum dose: 1 mg/kg)	
Propantheline bromide	Pro-Banthine	0.25–0.5 mg/kg q8–12h PO	
Propiopromazine	Tranvet	1.1–4.4 mg/kg q12–24h*	
Propranolol hydrochloride	Inderal	Dog: 20–60 µg/kg over 5–10 min q8h, 0.2–1 mg/kg PO q8h	IX-343, IX-346, IX-370, X-271, X-278
		Cat: 2.5–5 mg/cat (0.4–1.2 mg/kg) PO q8–12h	XI-338, XI-676, XI-756, XI-848
Propylthiouracil		11 mg/kg q12h PO (its use is not recommended)	IX-1026
Prostaglandin E		see *Misoprostol*	
Prostaglandin F$_{2\alpha}$	Lutalyse	*Pyometra:* Dog: 0.1–0.2 mg/kg, once daily for 5 days SC Cat: 0.1–0.25 mg/kg, once daily for 5 days SC *Abortion:* Dog: 25–50 µg/kg q12h IM Cat: 0.5–1 mg/kg IM for 2 injections	IX-1233, IX-1236, X-1305, XI-947, XI-954, XI-969
Psyllium	Metamucil	1 tsp/5–10 kg (added to each meal)	XI-613
Pyrantel pamoate	Nemex	Dog: 5 mg/kg PO once, then repeat in 7–10 days* Cat: 20 mg/kg PO once, then repeat in 7–10 days*	XI-626
Pyridostigmine bromide	Mestinon Regonol	*Antimyasthenic:* 0.02–0.04 mg/kg q2h IV, or 0.5–3 mg/kg q8–12h PO *Antidote (curariform):* 0.15–0.3 mg/kg IM, IV	XI-572, XI-1024, XI-1039
Pyrimethamine	Daraprim	Dog: 1 mg/kg q24h PO for 14–28 days (5 days for *Neosporum caninum*) Cat: 0.5–1 mg/kg q24h PO for 14–28 days	XI-263, XI-1034
Quinacrine hydrochloride	Atabrine hydrochloride	Dog: 6.6 mg/kg q12h PO for 5 days Cat: 11 mg/kg q24h PO for 5 days	

*Refer to manufacturer's recommendations.

Drug Name	Brand Name(s)	Dosage	CVT Reference(s)
Quinidine gluconate	Quinaglute Duraquin	Dog: 6–20 mg/kg q6h IM; 6–20 mg/kg q6–8h PO (of base) (324 mg quinidine gluconate = 202 mg quinidine base)	XI-694
Quinidine polygalacturonate	Cardioquin	Dog: 6–20 mg/kg q6h PO (of base) (275 mg quinidine polygalacturonate = 167 mg quinidine base)	
Quinidine sulfate	Clin-Quin Quinora	Dog: 6–20 mg/kg q6–8h PO (of base) (300 mg quinidine sulfate = 250 mg quinidine base)	
Ranitidine	Zantac	Dog: 2 mg/kg q8h IV, PO Cat: 2.5 mg/kg q12h IV; 3.5 mg/kg q12h PO	X-911, XI-132, XI-191, XI-523, XI-639
Retinoids		see *Isotretinoin; Retinol; Etretinate*	X-553
Retinol	Aquasol A	625–800 IU/kg q24h PO	X-553, XI-523
Riboflavin		Dog: 10–20 mg/day PO Cat: 5–10 mg/day PO	
Rifampin	Rifadin	10–20 mg/kg q24h PO	
Ringer's solution		40–50 ml/kg/day IV, SC, IP for maintenance	
Salicylate		see *Acetylsalicylic acid* (Aspirin)	
Senna	Senokot	Cat: 5 ml/cat q24h (syrup); ½ tsp/cat q24h with food (granules)	
Sodium bicarbonate ($NaHCO_3$)		*Acidosis:* 0.5–1 mEq/kg IV, or as guided by blood-gas analysis (8.5% solution = 1 mEq/ml of $NaHCO_3$) *Renal failure:* 10 mg/kg q8–12h PO (adjust as necessary) *Alkalinization:* 50 mg/kg q8–12h PO (1 tsp is approximately 2 gm)	X-333, XI-848
Sodium chloride (0.9%)		40–50 ml/kg/day IV, SC, IP	
Sodium iodide (20%)		20–40 mg/kg q8–12h PO	X-1101
Sodium nitroprusside		see *Nitroprusside sodium*	
Sodium thiomalate		see *Gold sodium thiomalate*	
Spironolactone	Aldactone	2–4 mg/kg/day PO	XI-668
Stanozolol	Winstrol-V	Dog: 1–4 mg/dog q12h PO; 25–50 mg/dog/wk IM* Cat: 1 mg/cat q12h PO; 25 mg/cat/wk IM*	XI-438
Styrid caricide (styrylpyridinium chloride plus diethylcarbamazine)		6.7 mg/kg diethylcarbamazine q24h PO and 5.5 mg/kg styrylpyridinium chloride q24h PO*	
Sucralfate	Carafate (U.S.) Sulcrate (Canada)	Dog: 0.5–1 gm q8–12h PO Cat: 0.25 gm q8–12h PO	X-911, XI-132, XI-191
Sufentanil	Sufenta	2 μg/kg IV, up to a maximum dose of 5 μg/kg (premedicate with acetylpromazine)	
Sulfadiazine		100 mg/kg IV, PO (loading dose), followed by 50 mg/kg q12h IV, PO (see also *Trimethoprim*)	XI-263, XI-1034
Sulfadimethoxine	Albon, Bactrovet	55 mg/kg PO (loading dose), followed by 27.5 mg/kg q12h PO (see also *Primor*)	XI-626
Sulfaguanidine		100–200 mg/kg q8h PO for 5 days	
Sulfamethazine		100 mg/kg PO (loading dose), followed by 50 mg/kg q12h PO	
Sulfamethoxazole	Gantanol	100 mg/kg PO (loading dose), followed by 50 mg/kg q12h PO	
Sulfamethoxazole plus trimethoprim	Bactrim Septra	See dosage for *Trimethoprim plus sulfadiazine*	
Sulfasalazine (Sulfapyridine + mesalamine)	Azulfidine (U.S.) Salazopyrin (Canada)	10–30 mg/kg q8–12h PO (see also *Mesalamine, Osalazine*)	XI-604, XI-613
Sulfisoxazole	Gantrisin	50 mg/kg q8h PO (urinary tract infections)	
Sulfobromophthalein sodium	Bromsulphalein (BSP) (this drug's availability is limited)	5 mg/kg IV, collect plasma or serum 30 min after BSP injection	IX-924
Sulfonamides		see individual drugs	

*Refer to manufacturer's recommendations.

Table continued on following page

Drug Name	Brand Name(s)	Dosage	CVT Reference(s)
Tamoxifen	Nolvadex	10 mg q12h PO (human dose)	
Taurine		Cat: 250–500 q12h PO	X-260
Telezol		see *Tiletamine*	
Temaril-P (Trimeprazine + Prednisolone)		0.7–1.1 mg/kg (of trimeprazine) 12–24h PO*	
Terbutaline	Brethine, Bricanyl	Dog: 2.5 mg/dog q8h SC, PO Cat: 0.625 mg/cat q12h SC, PO	IX-278, XI-660, XI-803
Terfenadine	Seldane	4.5–10 mg/kg q12h PO	
Testosterone cypionate	Andro-Cyp,	1–2 mg/kg q2–4 wk IM (see also *Methyltestosterone*)	
Testosterone propionate	Testex, Malogen	0.5–1 mg/kg 2–3 times/wk IM	
Tetanus toxoid		100–500 U/kg (maximum 20,000 U)	
Tetracycline	Panmycin, Achromycin	15–20 mg/kg q6–8h PO 4.4–11 mg/kg q8–12h IV, IM (see also *Oxytetracycline, Doxycycline, Minocycline*)	
Thenium closylate	Canopar	Dogs >4.5 kg: 500 mg PO, repeat in 2–3 wk* Dogs 2.5–4.5 kg: 250 mg q12h for one day, repeat in 2–3 wk*	
Theophylline		Dog: 9 mg/kg q6–8h PO Cat: 4 mg/kg q8–12h PO (see also *Aminophylline*)	IX-278, XI-803
Thiabendazole	Omnizole, Equizole	Dog: 50 mg/kg q24h for 3 days, repeat 1 month Cat (*Strongyloides*): 125 mg/kg q24h for 3 days	XI-228, XI-626
Thiacetarsamide sodium	Caparsolate	2.2 mg/kg IV twice daily for two days	X-131, X-265
Thiamine (vitamin B₁)		Dog: 10–100 mg/dog/day PO Cat: 5–30 mg/cat/day PO (up to a maximum dose of 50 mg/cat/day)	
Thiamylal	Surital, Bio-Tal	Dog: 8–10 mg/kg IV, in incremental doses up to 20 mg/kg (4% solution) Cat: same as dog (2% solution)	
Thioguanine (6-TG)		40 mg/m² q24h PO†	
Thiomalate sodium		see *Gold Sodium Thiomalate*	
Thiopental sodium	Pentothal	Dog: 10–25 mg/kg IV (to effect) Cat: 5–10 mg/kg IV (to effect)	
Thiotepa		0.2–0.5 mg/m² weekly, or daily for 5–10 days IV, intracavitary, or intratumor†	
Thyroid (desiccated)		15–20 mg/kg/day PO	
Thyroid hormone		see *Levothyroxine, Liothyronine*	
Thyrotropin (TSH)	Dermathycin, Thytropar	Dog: collect baseline sample, followed by 0.1 IU/kg IV (maximum dose is 5 IU); collect post-TSH sample at 6h Cat: collect baseline sample, followed by 2.5 IU/cat IM and collect post-TSH sample at 8–12 hr	X-965
Ticarcillin	Ticar	33–50 mg/kg q4–6h IV, IM	
Tiletamine + zolazepam	Telezol, Zoletil	5–7 mg/kg IV, IM	XI-27
Tobramycin	Nebcin	2 mg/kg q8h IV, IM, SC	
Tocainide	Tonocard	Dog: 10–20 mg/kg q8h PO	XI-773
Toluene	Vermiplex	267 mg/kg PO (of Toluene), repeat in 2–4 wk	
Triamcinolone	Aristocort	*Anti-inflammatory*: 0.5–1 mg/kg q12–24h PO, taper dose to 0.5–1 mg/kg q48h PO	X-54, XI-509
Triamcinolone acetonide	Vetalog	0.1–0.2 mg/kg IM, SC, repeat in 7–10 days *Intralesional*: 1.2–1.8 mg, or 1 mg for every cm diameter of tumor q2wk.	X-54, XI-509
Tribrissen: see *trimethoprim sulfadiazine*			
Triethylperazine	Torecan	0.13–0.2 mg/kg IM q8–12h	
Trifluoperazine	Stelezine	0.03 mg/kg IM q12h	
Triflupromazine	Vesprin	0.1–0.3 mg/kg IM, PO q8–12h	
Tri-iodothyronine		see *Liothyronine*	

*Refer to manufacturer's recommendations.
†Consult anticancer protocol for precise dosage.

Drug Name	Brand Name(s)	Dosage	CVT Reference(s)
Trimeprazine	Panectyl	0.5 mg/kg q12h PO (also see *Temaril-P*)	
Trimethobenzamide	Tigan, Trimazide	Dog: 3 mg/kg q8h IM, PO Cat: not recommended	
Trimethoprim	Proloprim	Dose not established (see *Trimethoprim plus sulfadiazine*)	
Trimethoprim plus sulfadiazine	Tribrissen	15 mg/kg q12h IM, PO, or 30 mg/kg q12–24h SC, PO (for *Toxoplasma*: 30 mg/kg q12h PO)	IX-247, XI-207, XI-539, XI-626, XI-909
Tripelennamine	Pelamine	1 mg/kg q12h PO	
TSH (thyroid-stimulating hormone)		see *Thyrotropin*	
Tylosin	Tylocine, Tylan	7–15 mg/kg q8h PO (for colitis administer 40–80 mg/kg/day with food)	XI-602
Urea		300 mg q1h IV	
Urofollitropin	Metrodin	Cat: 2 mg/cat q24h IM	
Valproate		see *Valproic acid*	
Valproic acid	Depakene	Dog: 75–200 mg/kg q8h PO; or 25–105 mg/kg/day PO when administered with phenobarbital	IX-840
Vancomycin	Vancocin	Dog: 15 mg/kg q6h	
Vasopressin (ADH)	Pitressin	Aqueous (20 U/mL): 10 U IV, IM (see also *Desmopressin*)	X-973
Verapamil	Calan, Isoptin	Dog: 0.05 mg/kg q10–30 min IV (maximum cumulative dose is 0.15 mg/kg); oral dose is not established Cat: 1.1–2.9 mg/kg q8h PO	IX-341, X-271, XI-684, XI-745
Vermiplex		See *Toluene*	
Vinblastine	Velban	2 mg/m² IV once/wk*	X-475, X-482, X-489
Vincristine	Oncovin	*Antitumor:* 0.5–0.7 mg/m² IV once/wk* *Thrombocytopenia:* 0.02 mg/kg IV once/wk	
Viokase—see *Pancreatic enzyme*			X-931
Vitamin A (Retinoids)		see *Isotretinoin* (Accutane), *Retinol* (Aquasol-A), or *Etretinate* (Tegison)	
Vitamin B complex		Dog: 0.5–2 ml q24h IV, IM, SC Cat: 0.5–1 ml q24h IV, IM, SC	
Vitamin B₁		See *Thiamine*	
Vitamin B₂		see *Riboflavin*	
Vitamin B₁₂		see *Cyanocobalamin*	
Vitamin C		see *Ascorbic acid*	
Vitamin D		see *Dihydrotachysterol; Ergocalciferol*	
Vitamin E (Alpha tocopherol)	Aquasol E	100–400 IU q12h PO (or 400–600 IU q12h PO for immune-mediated skin disease)	IX-591, X-574
Vitamin K₁	AquaMephyton, Mephyton	Short-acting rodenticides: 1 mg/kg/day, SC, PO for 10–14 days; long-acting rodenticides: 3–5 mg/kg/day SC, PO for 3–4 wk; birds: 2.5–5 mg/kg q24h	X-144, XI-175
Warfarin		0.1–0.2 mg/kg q24h PO (adjust dose by monitoring clotting time)	XI-137
Xylazine	Rompun	Dog: 1.1 mg/kg IV, 2.2 mg/kg IM Cat: 1.1 mg/kg IM (emetic dose: 0.4–0.5 mg/kg IV)	XI-27, XI-194
Yohimbine	Yohine	0.11 mg/kg IV	XI-194
Zolazepam		see *Tiletamine plus Zolazepam*	XI-27

*Consult anticancer protocol for precise dosage.

CANINE AND FELINE
REFERENCE VALUES

ROBERT M. JACOBS, D.V.M.,
JOHN H. LUMSDEN
and WILLIAM VERNAU
Guelph, Ontario, Canada

We provide the following tables as general guidelines for the interpretation of laboratory data in dogs and cats. There is wide variation in test results and reference values between laboratories for several reasons, including use of different reagents, instruments, and selection of reference animals. We have tried to specify methodologies in most instances so that other laboratories and users may more directly compare test results. Despite interlaboratory variation, laboratory data can be interpreted correctly if appropriately determined reference values* are supplied with the test results. Laboratory users should demand species' reference values developed in the laboratory to which the samples were submitted.

Laboratories strive to limit intralaboratory variation by careful attention to quality control practices. The performance of a laboratory in quality-control programs determines the laboratory users' confidence in test results from that laboratory. Conscientious users should not hesitate to ask for details of quality assurance in their laboratory and for expected within-run and between-run analytic variation. This information is necessary for the laboratory user attempting to separate analytic from animal variation on sequential samples.

The tables show either ranges that include 95% of the population, ranges that extend from the minimum to maximum (min–max) observation, mean ± one or two standard deviations (1 or 2 SD), or mean ± one standard error of the mean (SE). These measurements of error or variation about the mean are specified where appropriate (see *CVT X*, p. 8). Reference values should never be presented as simple means without some indication of error or variation or upper and lower limits for 95% of the population when provided for individual animal application. We have used mean values only to demonstrate simple trends in laboratory data with age.

An increasing number of reference sources and scientific journals are now using Système International (SI) units. In the major tables, we have given reference values in both the traditional and SI units in the hopes of easing some of the confusion. Tables showing the interconversion of traditional and SI units for most analytes are given.†

For ease of access, literature sources are provided as footnotes to each table. In an attempt to be concise, we did not always cite the primary sources for the data, but these are available in the footnoted articles. Along with the references, we have occasionally given short comments that indicate some aspect important in data interpretation.

Patient variables and sample quality will also affect test results and their interpretation. We have attempted to address some patient variables by the inclusion of tables showing the effects of age, gender, and body weight. Unless specified otherwise, all data are for adult animals and include different genders and breeds. In some cases, we have given literature sources so the reader may further explore these effects. To address problems of sample quality, we have included graphs showing the effects of bilirubinemia, hemolysis, and lipemia on the determination of most serum analytes. Many instrument manufacturers will provide interference data for human sera but generally not for animal sera. If nothing else, these graphs serve to remind laboratory users that interferences do occur and sometimes in a species-specific manner. The interferences due to drugs have not been adequately studied in animals, but such interferences must always be considered.‡

---

†For further information about SI units, refer to Young, D. S.: Implementation of SI units for clinical laboratory data. Ann. Intern. Med. 106:1140129, 1987, which was reprintd in J. Nutr. 120:20, 1990; and Beeler, M. F.: SI units and the AJCP. Am. J. Clin. Pathol. 87:140, 1987.

‡An extensive review of drug interferences in human sera is found in Young, D. S., Pestaner, L. C., and Gibberman, V.: Effects of drugs on clinical laboratory tests. Clin. Chem. 21:1D, 1975.

---

*Lumsden, J. H., and Mullen, K.: On establishing reference values. Can. J. Comp. Med. 42:293, 1978.

Laboratory data should be used to support diagnoses. Laboratory data that are inconsistent with the clinical diagnosis should be interpreted with caution. In these instances, the laboratory user should request that the laboratory reanalyze the same sample. If the result is similar, the laboratory user must consider alternatives to the initial clinical diagnosis or eliminate sample collection and handling or drug-related interferences, where possible, by resubmitting another sample. Samples taken at different times or analyzed in different laboratories are not comparable. Sequential laboratory data are often essential to render a prognosis and to determine response to therapy.

Hematology—Coulter S Plus IV* with Manual Differential Counts†

	Unit		Canine		Feline	
	Traditional	SI‡	Traditional	SI	Traditional	SI
Hemoglobin (Hgb)	gm/dl	gm/L	13.2–19.2	132–193	8.0–15.0	80–150
Hematocrit (Hct)	%	L/L	38–57	0.38–0.57	24–45	0.24–0.45
Erythrocytes	$\times 10^6/\mu l$	$\times 10^{12}/L$	5.6–8.5	5.6–8.5	5.0–10.0	5.0–10.0
Mean corpuscular volume (MCV)	μ^3 or mm^3	fl	62–71	62–71	39–50	39–50
Mean corpuscular Hgb (MCH)	$\mu\mu$g or pg	pg	22–25	22–25	13–17	13–17
Mean corpuscular Hgb concentration (MCHC)	%	g/L	33.7–36.5	337–365	32.0–36.0	320–360
Red blood cell distribution width (RDW)	%	%	12–15	12–15	13–17	13–17
Reticulocytes	$\times 10^3/\mu l$	$\times 10^9/L$	20–80	20–80	20–60	20–60
Platelets	$\times 10^3/\mu l$	$\times 10^9/L$	145–440	145–440	190–400	190–400
Mean platelet volume (MPV)	μ^3 or mm^3	fl	7.0–10.3	7.0–10.3	—	—
Platelet distribution width (PDW)	%	%	15.5–17.5	15.5–17.5	—	—
Total nucleated cell count	$\times 10^3/\mu l$	$\times 10^9/L$	6.1–17.4	6.1–17.4	5.5–15.4	5.5–15.4
Segmented neutrophils	$\times 10^3/\mu l$	$\times 10^9/L$	3.9–12.0	3.9–12.0	2.5–12.5	2.5–12.5
Band neutrophils	$\times 10^3/\mu l$	$\times 10^9/L$	0.0–1.0	0.0–1.0	0.0–0.3	0.0–0.3
Lymphocytes	$\times 10^3/\mu l$	$\times 10^9/L$	0.8–3.6	0.8–3.6	1.5–7.0	1.5–7.0
Monocytes	$\times 10^3/\mu l$	$\times 10^9/L$	0.1–1.8	0.1–1.8	0.0–0.85	0.0–0.85
Eosinophils	$\times 10^3/\mu l$	$\times 10^9/L$	0.0–1.9	0.0–1.9	0.0–0.75	0.0–0.75
Basophils	$\times 10^3/\mu l$	$\times 10^9/L$	0.0–0.2	0.0–0.2	0.0–0.2	0.0–0.2

*This automated cell counter was configured using Isoton III and Lyse S III DIFF. The mean nucleated cell aperature voltage was 94.2, and the mean red cell/platelet aperature voltage was 165.5.

†From Clinical Pathology Laboratory, Department of Pathology, University of Guelph. Feline leukocyte differential count is modified from Jain, N. C.: *Schalm's Veterinary Hematology*, 4th ed. Philadelphia: Lea & Febiger, 1986, p. 127.

‡Système International.

Hematology—Technicon H–1 Hematology Analyzer*

	Unit	Canine	Feline
Hemoglobin	g/dl	14.1–20.0	9.0–15.6
Hematocrit	%	43.3–59.3	29.3–49.8
Erythrocytes	$\times 10^6/\mu l$	6.15–8.70	6.12–11.86
Mean corpuscular volume	fl	63.0–77.1	41.9–54.8
Mean corpuscular hemoglobin	pg	21.1–24.8	12.5–17.6
Mean corpuscular hemoglobin concentration	gm/dl	29.9–35.6	28.1–32.0
Red cell distribution width	%	11.9–14.9	13.0–16.6
Hemoglobin distribution width	gm/dl	1.49–2.17	1.60–2.34
Platelets	$\times 10^3/\mu l$	164–510	26†–470
Mean platelet volume	fl	5.9–9.1	6.1–12.5
White blood cell count	$\times 10^3/\mu l$	6.02–16.02	4.87–20.10
Neutrophils	$\times 10^3/\mu l$	3.23–10.85	—
Lymphocytes	$\times 10^3/\mu l$	0.53–3.44	—
Monocytes	$\times 10^3/\mu l$	0.00–0.43	—
Eosinophils	$\times 10^3/\mu l$	0.00–1.82	—
Basophils	$\times 10^3/\mu l$	0.01–0.54	—
Large unstained cells (LUC)	$\times 10^3/\mu l$	0.26–2.09	—
Lobularity index (LI)‡	—	1.88–3.15	1.3–2.68
Mean peroxidase index (MPXI)‡	—	-19 to -7	-47 to -16

*From Tvedten, H.: Reference values for the veterinary clinical center laboratory, Michigan State University, May 1991. These data were derived from approximately 120 dogs and 40 cats. Canine reference values include 95% of the population, whereas the feline values represent the minimum to maximum.

†The lower limit of feline platelets is falsely decreased due to clumping.

‡Interpretation of these indices is undetermined in canine and feline blood.

Système International (SI) Units in Hematology

Analyte	Example Values		Conversion Factors	
	SI	*Traditional*	*Traditional to SI*	*SI to Traditional*
Hemoglobin (Hgb)	15.0 gm/dl	150 gm/L	10	0.1
Hematocrit (Hct) or packed cell volume (PCV)	45%	0.45 L/L	0.01	100
Erythrocytes	$6.0 \times 10^6/mm^3$	$6.0 \times 10^{12}/L$	10^6	10^{-6}
Mean corpuscular volume (MCV)	$75 \mu^3$	75 fl	No change	No change
Mean corpuscular Hgb (MCH)	$25 \mu\mu g$	25 pg	No change	No change
Mean corpuscular Hgb concentration (MCHC)	33 gm/dl	330 gm/L	10	0.1
White blood cell count	$15.0 \times 10^3/mm^3$	$15.0 \times 10^9/L$	10^6	10^{-6}
Platelets	$250 \times 10^3/mm^3$	$250 \times 10^9/L$	10^6	10^{-6}

Hematology—Manual or Semiautomated Methods*

	Adult Dog		Adult Cat	
	Range	*Mean*	*Range*	*Mean*
Red Blood Cell Determinations				
Erythrocytes (millions/dl)	5.5–8.5	6.8	5.5–10.0	7.5
Hemoglobin (gm/dl)	12.0–18.0	14.9	8.0–14.0	12.0
Packed cell volume (%)	37.0–55.0	45.5	24.0–45.0	37.0
Mean corpuscular volume (fl)	66.0–77.0	69.8	40.0–55.0	45.0
Mean corpuscular hemoglobin (pg)	19.9–24.5	22.8	13.0–17.0	15.0
Mean corpuscular hemoglobin concentration (gm/dl)				
Wintrobe	31.0–34.0	33.0	31.0–35.0	33.0
Microhematocrit	32.0–36.0	34.0	30.0–36.0	33.2
Reticulocytes (%, excluding punctate reticulocytes)	0.0–1.5	0.8	0.2–1.6	0.6
Resistance to hypotonic saline (% saline solution)				
Minimum (initial hemolysis)	0.40–0.50	0.46	0.66–0.72	0.69
Maximum (complete hemolysis)	0.32–0.42	0.33	0.46–0.54	0.50
Erythrocyte life span (days)	100–120		66–78	
White Blood Cell Determinations				
Leukocytes (cells/μl)	6,000–17,000	11,500	5,500–19,500	12,500
Neutrophils—bands (%)	0–3	0.8	0–3	0.5
Neutrophils—mature (%)	60–77	70.0	35–75	59.0
Lymphocytes (%)	12–30	20.0	20–55	32.0
Monocytes (%)	3–10	5.2	1–4	3.0
Eosinophils (%)	2–10	4.0	2–12	5.5
Basophils (%)	Rare	0.0	Rare	0.0
Neutrophils—bands (cells/μl)	0–300	70	0–300	100
Neutrophils—mature (cells/μl)	3,000–11,500	7,000	2,500–12,500	7,500
Lymphocytes (cells/μl)	1,000–4,800	2,800	1,500–7,000	4,000
Monocytes (cells/μl)	150–1,350	750	0–850	350
Eosinophils (cells/μl)	100–1,250	550	0–1,500	650
Basophils (cells/μl)	Rare	0	Rare	0

*From Jain, N. C.: *Schalm's Veterinary Hematology*, 4th ed. Philadelphia: Lea & Febiger, 1986.

Canine Hematology (Means) at Different Ages—Manual or Semiautomated Methods*

Age	RBC (millions/μl)	Retic. (%)†	Nucl. RBC per 100 WBC†	Hgb (gm/dl)	PCV (%)	WBC/μl	Neut./μl	Bands/μl	Lymph./μl	Eos./μl
Birth	5.75	7.1	1.8	16.70	50	16,500	1,300	400	2,500	600
2 weeks	3.92	7.1	1.8	9.76	32	11,000	6,500	100	3,000	300
4 weeks	4.20	7.1	1.8	9.60	33	13,000	8,600	0	4,000	40
6 weeks	4.91	3.6	1.8	9.59	34	15,000	10,000	0	4,500	100
8 weeks	5.13	3.9	0.3	11.00	37	18,000	11,000	234	6,000	270
12 weeks	5.27	3.9	Rare	11.60	36	15,300	9,400	115	4,600	322

*From Andersen, A. C., and Gee, W.: Normal values in the beagle. Vet. Med. 53:135, 156, 1958.
†From Ewing, G. O., Schalm, O. W., and Smith, R. S.: Hematologic values of normal Basenji dogs. J.A.V.M.A. 161:1661, 1972.

Canine Hematology (Means and Ranges) With Different Ages and Genders— Manual or Semiautomated Methods*

	Sex	Birth to 12 Months		1–7 Years		7 Years and Older	
		Range	Mean	Range	Mean	Range	Mean
Erthrocytes (millions/μl)	Male	2.99–8.52	5.09	5.26–6.57	5.92	3.33–7.76	5.28
	Female	2.76–8.42	5.06	5.13–8.6	6.47	3.34–9.19	5.17
Hemoglobin (gm/dl)	Male	6.9–16.5	10.7	12.7–16.3	15.5	14.7–21.2	17.9
	Female	6.4–18.9	11.2	11.5–17.9	14.7	11.0–22.5	16.1
Packed cell volume (%)	Male	22.0–45.0	33.9	35.2–52.8	44.0	44.2–62.8	52.3
	Female	25.8–55.2	36.0	34.8–52.4	43.6	35.8–67.0	49.8
Leukocytes (thousands/ μl)	Male	9.9–27.7	17.1	8.3–19.5	11.9	7.9–35.3	15.5
	Female	8.8–26.8	15.9	7.5–17.5	11.5	5.2–34.0	13.4
Mature neutrophils (%)	Male	63–73	68	65–73	69	55–80	66
	Female	64–74	69	58–76	67	40–80	64
Lymphocytes (%)	Male	18–30	24	9–26	18	15–40	29
	Female	13–28	21	11–29	20	13–45	29
Monocytes (%)	Male	1–10	6	2–10	6	0–4	1
	Female	1–10	7	0–10	5	0–4	1
Eosinophils (%)	Male	2–11	3	1–8	4	1–11	4
	Female	1–9	5	1–10	6	0–19	6

*From *Normal Blood Values for Dogs,* Ralston Purina Co., Professional Marketing Services, Checkerboard Square, St. Louis, 1975.

Canine Hematology (Means ± SD) at Different Ages*

Age	RBC (millions/μl)	Hgb (gm/dl)	PCV (%)	MCV (fl)	MCH (pg)	MCHC (gm/dl)	WBC/μl
0–3 days	4.8± 0.8	15.8 ± 2.9	46.3 ± 8.5	94.2 ± 5.9	32.7 ± 1.8	34.6 ± 1.4	16,800 ± 5,700
14–17 days	3.5 ± 0.3	9.9 ± 1.1	28.7 ± 2.9	81.5 ± 3.3	28.0 ± 2.0	34.3 ± 1.6	13,600 ± 4,400
28–31 days	3.9 ± 0.4	9.6 ± 0.9	28.4 ± 2.5	71.7 ± 3.5	24.3 ± 1.6	33.5 ± 1.4	13,900 ± 3,300
40–45 days	4.1 ± 0.4	9.2 ± 0.7	28.3 ± 2.3	68.2 ± 2.6	22.4 ± 1.0	32.4 ± 1.7	15,300 ± 3,700
56–59 days	4.7 ± 0.4	10.3 ± 0.9	31.4 ± 2.4	65.8 ± 2.3	21.8 ± 1.2	32.6 ± 1.8	15,700 ± 4,400

*From Jain, N. C.: *Schalm's Veterinary Hematology,* 4th ed. Philadelphia: Lea & Febiger, 1986; derived from between 42 and 48 dogs at each time interval.

Effect of Pregnancy and Lactation on Canine Hematology (Means)*

	Gestation				Term	Lactation		
	2 Weeks	4 Weeks	6 Weeks	8 Weeks	0 Weeks	2 Weeks	4 Weeks	6 Weeks
RBC (millions/μl)	8.85	7.48	6.73	6.26	4.53	5.13	5.65	6.15
PCV (%)	53	47	44	37	32	34	38	42
Hgb (gm/dl)	19.6	16.4	14.7	13.8	11.0	11.7	12.8	13.4
WBC (thousands/μl)	12.0	12.2	15.7	19.0	18.9	16.9	17.1	15.9

*From Andersen, A. C., and Gee, W.: Normal values in the beagle. Vet. Med. 53:135, 156, 1958.

Relative Distribution of Cell Types in Canine Bone Marrow*

Cell Type	Range (%)	Mean (%)
Myeloid (granulocytic) series		
Myeloblasts	0.7–1.1	0.9
Promyelocytes	1.7–2.5	2.1
Neutrophil myelocytes	5.3–7.3	6.3
Neutrophil bands	9.1–13.5	11.3
Neutrophil segmenters	22.2–24.8	23.5
Eosinophil myelocytes	0.4–0.8	0.6
Eosinophil metamyelocytes	0.4–1.0	0.7
Eosinophil bands	0.8–1.6	1.2
Eosinophil segmenters	0.3–1.3	0.8
Basophil series	0.0–0.06	0.02
Total myeloid series	49.3–61.1	55.2
Erythrocytic series		
Rubriblasts and prorubricytes	6.1–6.9	6.5
Rubricytes and metarubricytes	23.2–32.0	27.6
Total erythroid cells	29.4–38.8	34.1
Myeloid:erythroid (M:E) ratio	1.3–2.1	1.7
Other cells		
Lymphocytes	5.5–10.9	8.2
Plasma cells	0.4–1.0	0.7
Monocytes	0.2–5.2	1.2
Macrophages	0.2–0.6	0.4
Mitotic figures	1.1–1.7	1.4

*From Latimer, K. S., and Meyer, D. J.: Leukocytes in health and disease. *In* Ettinger, S. J. (ed.): *Textbook of Veterinary Internal Medicine, Diseases of the Dog and Cat,* 3rd ed. Philadelphia: W. B. Saunders, 1989, pp. 2185–2186. These data are based on the following citations: Prasse, K. W., and Mahaffey, E. A.: Hematology of normal cats and characteristic responses to disease. *In* Holzworth, J. (ed.): *Diseases of the Cat: Medicine and Surgery.* Philadelphia, W. B. Saunders, 1987, p. 739; Duncan, J. R., and Prasse, K. W.: *Veterinary Laboratory Medicine: Clinical Pathology.* 2nd ed. Ames, Iowa State University Press, 1986; Melveger, B. E., et al.: Sternal bone marrow biopsy in the dog. Lab. Anim. Care 19:866, 1969; Bloom, F., and Meyer, L. M.: The morphology of the bone marrow cells in normal dogs. Cornell Vet. 34:13, 1944.

Feline Hematology (Means and Ranges) With Different Ages and Genders—Manual or Semiautomated Methods*

	Sex	Birth to 12 Months		1–7 Years		7 Years and Older	
		Range	*Average*	*Range*	*Average*	*Range*	*Average*
Erythrocytes (millions/µl)	Male	5.43–10.22	6.96	4.48–10.27	7.34	5.26–8.89	6.79
	Female	4.46–11.34	6.90	4.45–9.42	6.17	4.10–7.38	5.84
Hemoglobin (gm/dl)	Male	6.0–12.9	9.9	8.9–17.0	12.9	9.0–14.5	11.8
	Female	6.0–15.0	9.9	7.9–15.5	10.3	7.5–13.7	10.3
Packed cell volume (%)	Male	24.0–37.5	31	26.9–48.2	37.6	28.0–43.8	34.6
	Female	23.0–46.8	31.5	25.3–37.5	31.4	22.5–40.5	30.8
Leukocytes (thousands/µl)	Male	7.8–25.0	15.8	9.1–28.2	15.1	6.4–30.4	17.6
	Female	11.0–26.9	17.7	13.7–23.7	19.9	5.2–30.1	14.8
Neutrophils—mature (%)	Male	16–75	60	37–92	65	33–75	61
	Female	51–83	69	42–93	69	25–89	71
Lymphocytes (%)	Male	10–81	30	7–48	23	16–54	30
	Female	8–37	23	12–58	30	9–63	22
Monocytes (%)	Male	1–5	2	1–5	2	0–2	1
	Female	0–7	2	0–5	2	0–4	1
Eosinophils (%)	Male	2–21	8	1–22	7	1–15	8
	Female	0–15	6	0–13	5	0–15	6

*From *Normal Blood Values for Cats,* Ralston Purina Co., Professional Marketing Services, Checkerboard Square, St. Louis, 1975.

Feline Hematology (Means) at Different Ages*

Age	RBC (millions/μl)	Hgb (gm/dl)	PCV (%)	MCV (fl)	MCH (pg)	MCHC (gm/dl)	WBC/μl
0–6 hr	4.95	12.2	44.7	90.3	24.6	27.3	7,550
12—48 hr	5.11	11.3	41.7	81.6	22.1	27.1	10,180
7 days	5.19	10.9	35.7	68.8	21.0	30.5	7,830
21 days	4.99	9.3	31.3	62.7	18.6	29.7	8,820
42 days	6.75	9.0	35.4	52.4	13.3	25.4	8,420
80 days	7.69	10.3	39.0	50.7	13.4	26.4	9,120
Adult male	9.02	12.2	40.6	45.0	13.5	30.0	12,400
Adult female	8.39	12.0	41.3	49.2	14.3	29.1	10,500

*From Jain, N. C.: *Schalm's Veterinary Hematology*, 4th ed. Philadelphia: Lea & Febiger, 1986; data derived from between 18 to 26 cats at each time interval.

Effect of Pregnancy and Lactation on Feline Hematology (Means)*

	Gestation					Term	Lactation	
	1 Day Past Conception	2 Weeks	4 Weeks	6 Weeks	8 Weeks	0 Weeks	2 Weeks	4 Weeks
RBC (millions/μl)	8.0	7.9	7.1	6.7	6.2	6.2	7.4	7.4
PCV (%)	36.1	37.0	33.0	32.0	28.0	29.0	33.0	33.0
Hgb (gm/dl)	12.5	12.0	11.0	10.8	9.5	10.0	11.5	11.2
Reticulocytes (%, includes punctate reticulocytes)	9	11	9	10	20.1	15	9	6

*From Berman, E.: Hemogram of the cat during pregnancy and lactation and after lactation. Am. J. Vet. Res. 35:457, 1974.

Relative Distribution of Cell Types in Feline Bone Marrow*

Cell Type	Range (%)	Mean (%)
Myeloid (granulocytic) series		
Myeloblasts	0.0–1.8	0.4
Promyelocytes	0.6–3.8	1.2
Neutrophil myelocytes	0.4–5.4	2.2
Neutrophil metamyelocytes	0.6–9.6	4.2
Neutrophil bands	5.0–19.4	11.0
Neutrophil segmenters	17.8–38.6	27.8
Eosinophil series	0.6–7.2	3.0
Basophil series	0.0–0.4	0.2
Total myeloid cells	39.4–64.4	52.0
Erythrocytic series		
Rubriblasts	0.0–1.6	0.6
Prorubricytes and rubricytes	—	12.4
Metarubricytes	15.6–32.2	23.6
Total erythroid cells	24.0–48.8	36.6
Myeloid:erythroid (M:E) ratio	0.9–2.5	1.5
Other cells		
Lymphocytes	3.2–22.6	11.4
Plasma cells	0.0–1.2	0.2
Mitotic cells	0.0–2.0	1.0

*From Latimer, K. S., and Meyer, D. J.: Leukocytes in health and disease. *In* Ettinger, S. J. (ed.): *Textbook of Veterinary Internal Medicine, Diseases of the Dog and Cat*, 3rd ed. Philadelphia: W. B. Saunders, 1989, pp. 2185–2186. These data are based on the following citations: Prasse, K. W., and Mahaffey, E. A.: Hematology of normal cats and characteristic responses to disease. *In* Holzworth, J. (ed.): *Diseases of the Cat: Medicine and Surgery.* Philadelphia, W. B. Saunders, 1987, p. 739; Duncan, J. R., and Prasse, K. W.: *Veterinary Laboratory Medicine: Clinical Pathology*, 2nd ed. Ames, IA: Iowa State University Press, 1986; Melveger, B. E., et al.: Sternal bone marrow biopsy in the dog. Lab. Anim. Care 19:866, 1969; Bloom, F., and Meyer, L. M.: The morphology of the bone marrow cells in normal dogs. Cornell Vet. 34:13, 1944.

Clinical Chemistry—Coulter DACOS*

	Unit		Canine		Feline	
	Traditional	SI†	Traditional	SI	Traditional	SI
Alanine aminotransferase	IU/L	U/L	0–130	0–130	10–75	10–75
Albumin	gm/dl	gm/L	2.2–3.5	22–35	2.5–3.9	25–39
Albumin/globulin	—	—	0.5–1.2	0.5–1.2	0.5–1.4	0.5–1.4
Alkaline phosphatase	IU/L	U/L	0–200	0–200	0–90	0–90
Amylase	IU/L	U/L	400–1800	400–1800	700–2000	700–2000
Anion gap	mEq/L	mmol/L	15–25	15–25	—	—
Asparate aminotransferase	IU/L	U/L	10–50	10–50	10–59	10–59
Conjugated bilirubin	mg/dl	μmol/L	0–0.18	0–3	0–0.06	0–1
Unconjugated bilirubin	mg/dl	μmol/L	0–0.41	0–7	0–0.23	0–4
Total bilirubin	mg/dl	μmol/L	0–0.41	0–7	0–0.23	0–4
Calcium	mg/dl	mmol/L	8.98–11.82	2.24–2.95	8.94–11.62	2.23–2.90
Total carbon dioxide	mEq/L	mmol/L	18–30	18–30	14–26	14–26
Chloride	mEq/L	mmol/L	105–122	105–122	112–129	112–129
Cholesterol	mg/dl	mmol/L	106.0–367.4	2.74–9.50	58.0–232.0	1.5–6.0
Creatine kinase	IU/L	U/L	0–460	0–460	0–580	0–580
Creatinine	mg/dl	μmol/L	0.62–1.64	55–145	0.84–2.04	75–180
Globulins	gm/dl	gm/L	2.2–4.5	22–45	2.6–5.0	26–50
Glucose	mg/dl	mmol/L	59.4–156.7	3.3–8.7	63.1–162.1	3.5–9.0
Glutamate dehydrogenase	IU/L	u/l	3–8	3–8	0–3	0–3
Gamma-glutamyl transferase	IU/L	u/l	0–6	0–6	0–2	0–2
Iron‡	μg/dl	μmol/L	72.6–189.8	13–34	78.2–111.7	14–20
Total iron binding capacity	μg/dl	μmol/L	363–475	65–85	296–318	53–57
Transferrin saturation	%	%	16–40	16–40	27–35	27–35
Lipase	IU/L	U/L	50–1000	50–1000	50–700	50–700
Phosphorus	mg/dl	mmol/L	1.55–8.05	0.50–2.60	3.19–8.73	1.03–2.82
Potassium	mEq/L	mmol/L	3.6–5.8	3.6–5.8	3.7–5.8	3.7–5.8
Total serum protein	gm/dl	gm/L	5.0–7.5	50–75	6.0–8.2	60–82
Sodium	mEq/L	mmol/L	145–158	145–158	150–165	150–165
Urea	mg/dl	mmol/L	5.9–27.2	2.1–9.7	14.0–28.0	5.0–10.0

*From Clinical Pathology Laboratory, Department of Pathology, University of Guelph: Trends in serum chemistry values with age and original citations concerning this topic are found in Lowseth, L. A., Gillett, N. A., Gerlach, R. F., et al.: The effects of aging on hematology and serum chemistry values in the Beagle dog. Vet. Clin. Pathol. 19:13, 1990, For temperature stability of enzymes see Kaneko, J. J.: Stability of serum enzymes under various storage conditions. In Kaneko, J. J. (ed.): Clinical Biochemistry of Domestic Animals, 4th ed. San Diego: Academic Press, 1989, p. 883.

†Système International.

‡Feline values derived from Fulton, R., Weiser, M. G., Freshman, J.L., et al.: Electronic and morphologic characterization of erythrocytes of an adult cat with iron deficiency anemia. Vet. Pathol. 25:521, 1988.

Clinical Chemistry—Selected Manual Procedures*

Analyte	Unit	Canine	Feline
Ammonia (bromophenol blue, Kodak Ektachem, Rochester, NY)			
Resting	μmol/L	20–80	—†
30 min Postprovocation	μmol/L	≤140	—
Anion gap	mmol/L	15–5	—
Bile acids (colorimetric, Enzabile, Nycomed, Oslo, Norway)			
Fasting	μmol/L	0–9	≤2.2‡
2hr postprandial	μmol/L	0–30	≤12.6
Sulfobromophthalein retention	% at 30 min	≤5	≤3§
Indocyanine green retention§	% at 30 min	7.7–15.6	4.7–14.0
Osmolality (freezing point depression)	mmol/kg	295–315	301–314

*Data are from the Clinical Pathology Laboratory, Department of Pathology, University of Guelph, unless indicated otherwise. Methods and reagent sources given in parentheses where appropriate.

†Data for four cats with portosystemic shunts are reported in Center, S. A., Baldwin, B. H., de Lahunta, A., et al.: Evaluation of serum bile acid concentrations for the diagnosis of portosystemic venous anomalies in the dog and cat. J.A.V.M.A. 186:1090, 1985.

‡From Center, S. A., Baldwin, B. H., Erb, H., et al.: Bile acid concentrations in the diagnosis of hepatobiliary disease in the cat. J.A.V.M.A. 189:891, 1986.

§From Center, S. A, Bunch, S. E., Baldwin, B. H., et al.: Comparison of sulfobromophthalein and indocyanine green clearances in the cat. Am. J. Vet. Res. 44:727, 1983; Center, S. A., Bunch, S. E., Baldwin, B. H., et al.: Comparison of sulfobromophthalein and indocyanine green clearances in the dog. Am. J. Vet. Res. 44:722, 1983.

Système International (SI) Units in Clinical Chemistry

Analyte	Traditional Unit (with examples)	Conversion Factor	SI Unit (with examples)
Alanine aminotransferase	0–40 U/L	1.00	0–40 U/L
Albumin	2.8–4.0 gm/dl	10.0	28–40 gm/L
Alkaline phosphatase	30–150 U/L	1.00	30–150 U/L
Ammonia	10–80 μg/dl	0.5871	5.9–47.0 μmol/L
Amylase	200—800 U/L	1.00	200–800 U/L
Aspartate aminotransferase	0–40 U/L	1.00	0–40 U/L
Bile acids (total)	0.3–2.3 μg/ml	2.45	0.74–5.64 μmol/L
Bilirubin	0.1–0.2 mg/dl	17.10	2–4 μmol/L
Calcium	8.8–10.3 mg/dl	0.2495	2.20–2.58 mmol/L
Carbon dioxide	22–28 mEq/L	1.00	22–28 mmol/L
Chloride	95–100 mEq/L	1.00	95–100 mmol/L
Cholesterol	100–265 mg/dl	0.0258	2.58–5.85 mmol/L
Copper	70–140 μg/dl	0.1574	11–22 μmol/L
Cortisol	2–10 μg/dl	27.59	55–280 nmol/L
Creatine kinase	0–130 U/L	1.00	0–130 U/L
Creatinine	0.6–1.2 mg/dl	88.40	50–110 μmol/L
Fibrinogen	200–400 mg/dl	0.01	2–4 gm/L
Folic acid	3.5–11.0 μg/L	2.265	7.93–24.92 nmol/L
Glucose	70–110 mg/dl	0.05551	3.9–6.1 mmol/L
Iron	80–180 μg/dl	0.1791	14–32 μmol/L
Lactate	5–20 mg/dl	0.1110	0.5–2.0 mmol/L
Lead	150 μg/dl	0.04826	7.2 μmol/L
Lipase Sigma Tietz (37°C)	≤ 1 ST U/dl	280	≤ 280 U/L
Lipase Cherry Crandall (30°C)	0–160 U/L	1.00	0–160 U/L
Lipids (total)	400–850 mg/dl	0.01	4.0–8.5 gm/L
Magnesium	1.8–3.0 mg/dl	0.4114	0.80–1.20 mmol/L
Mercury	≤ 1.0 μg/dl	49.85	≤ 50 nmol/L
Osmolality	280–300 mOsm/kg	1.00	280–300 mmol/kg
Phosphorus	2.5–5.0 mg/dl	0.3229	0.80–1.6 mmol/L
Potassium	3.5–5.0 mEq/L	1.0	3.5–5.0 mmol/L
Protein (total)	5.8 gm/dl	10.0	50–80 gm/L
Sodium	135–147 mEq/L	1.00	135–147 mmol/L
Testosterone	4–8 mg/ml	3.467	14–28 nmol/L
Thyroxine	1–4 μg/dl	12.87	13–51 nmol/L
Triglyceride	10–500 mg/dl	0.0113	0.11–5.65 mmol/L
Urea nitrogen	10–20 mg/dl	0.3570	3.6–7.1 nmol/L
Uric acid	3.6–7.7 mg/dl	59.44	214–458 μmol/L
Urobilinogen	0–4.0 mg/dl	16.9	0.0–6.8 μmol/L
Vitamin A	90 μg/dl	0.03491	3.1 μmol/L
Vitamin B_{12}	300–700 ng/L	0.738	221–516 pmol/L
Vitamin E	5–20 mg/L	2.32	11.6–46.4 μmol/L
D-xylose	30–40 mg/dl	0.06666	2.0–2.71 mmol/L
Zinc	75–120 μg/dl	0.1530	11.5–18.5 μmol/L

Clinical Chemistry—Test Characteristics for Analytes Determined on Coulter DACOS*

Analyte	Reaction Type	Methodology
Alanine aminotransferase	Zero-order kinetic	Modified IFCC† (L-alanine and alpha-ketoglutarate substrate)
Albumin	First-order kinetic	Modified Doumas (bromcresol green)
Alkaline phosphatase	Zero-order kinetic	Modified Bowers and McComb (p-nitrophenyl phosphate substrate)
Amylase	Zero-order kinetic	Modified Wallenfels (p-nitrophenylmaltohexaoside substrate
Aspartate aminotransferase	Zero-order kinetic	Modified IFCC (L-aspartate and alpha-ketoglutarate substrate)
Bilirubin	Equilibrium‡	Modified Walters and Gerarde (diazo)
Calcium	Equilibrium	Modified Connerty and Briggs (O-cresolphthalein complexone)
Total carbon dioxide	First-order kinetic	Enzymatic phosphoenol-pyruvate carboxylase
Chloride	Equilibrium	Modified Schoenfeld and Lewellen (thiocyanate)
Cholesterol	Equilibrium	Enzymatic (cholesterol esterase/oxidase)
Creatine kinase	Zero-order kinetic	Modified Oiver-Rosalki (creatine phosphate substrate)
Creatinine	Initial rate	Kinetic Jaffé
Glucose	Equilibrium	Modified hexokinase/glucose-6-phosphate dehydrogenase
Glutamate dehydrogenase§	Zero-order kinetic	Alpha-oxoglutarate substrate
Gamma-glutamyl transferase	Zero-order kinetic	Modified Szasz (L-γ-glutamyl-p-nitroanilide and glyclyglycine substrate)
Iron‖	Equilibrium	Ferene
Lipase§	Zero-order kinetic	Triolene substrate and colipase excess
Phosphorus	Equilibrium	Modified Daly and Ertingshausen (molybdate)
Potassium	—	Ion-selective electrode
Total serum protein	Equilibrium	Modified biuret (cupric sulfate)
Sodium	—	Ion-selective electrode
Urea	First-order kinetic	Modified Talke and Schubert (urease)

*From Clinical Pathology Laboratory, Department of Pathology, University of Guelph. Unless indicated otherwise, all reagents are from Coulter Diagnostics, Hialeah, FL.
  †International Federation of Clinical Chemistry.
  ‡Also termed *end-point reaction.*
  §Boehringer Mannheim, Dorval, Quebec.
  ‖Diagnostic Chemicals Limited, Monroe, CT.

Interferences Caused by Lipid, Bilirubin, and Hemoglobin for Analytes Determined on the Coulter DACOS

The following series of graphs are termed "interferograms." These interferograms show the effects of common interferents on the concentrations or activities of analytes determined on the Coulter DACOS (methods given in previous table) in canine (●) and feline (○) sera except for refractometer total protein, which was done using a Goldberg refractometer. The X axes show increasing amounts of lipid, bilirubin, or hemoglobin, and the Y axes show the percentage change (final/original × 100%) in any particular analyte. In those instances where the concentration or activity of a particular analyte was numerically small, the absolute values are given on the Y axes.

These data are provided by the Clinical Pathology Laboratory, Department of Pathology, University of Guelph, and were prepared with the assistance of Mr. E. Grift. The protocols for preparing these data are described in Glick, M. R., Ryder, K. W., and Jackson, S. A.: Graphical comparisons of interferences in clinical chemistry instrumentation. Clin. Chem. 32:470, 1986. For a more complete discussion of interferences on creatinine refer to Jacobs, R. M., Lumsden, J. H., Taylor, J. A., and Grift, E: Effects of interferents on the kinetic Jaffé reaction and an enzymatic colorimetric test for serum creatinine concentration determination in cats, cows, dogs, and horses. Can. J. Vet. Res. 55:150, 1991.

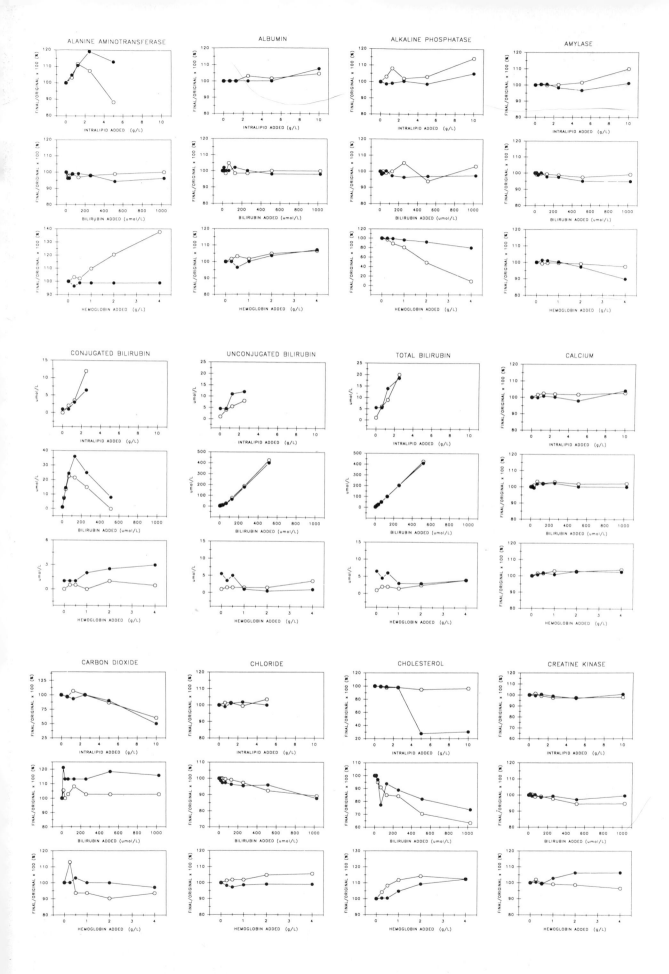

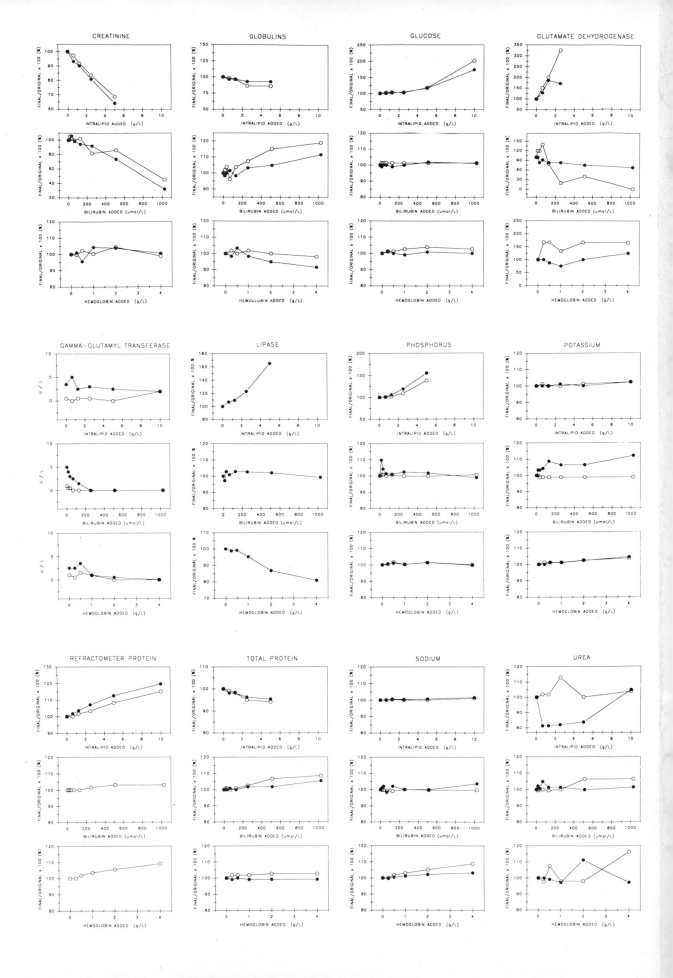

Serum Protein Fractions*

	Unit	Canine	Feline
Plasma protein	gm/L	58–76	60–80
Serum protein	gm/L	50–75	60–82
Albumin	gm/L	22–35	25–39
Globulins	gm/L	22–45	26–50
Albumin/Globulin (A/G) ratio	—	0.50–1.20	0.53–1.36
IgA	gm/L	0.40–1.6	0.10–0.58
IgM	gm/L	1.0–2.0	0.06–0.39
IgG	gm/L	10.0–20.0	11.7–22.6
Agarose gel electrophoresis:			
Alpha 1	gm/L	5–8	2–5
Alpha 2	gm/L	5–8	8–11
Beta 1	gm/L	5–11	3–5
Beta 2	gm/L	3–7	3–6
Gamma	gm/L	5–18	12–32

*From Clinical Pathology Laboratory, Department of Pathology, University of Guelph. Immunoglobulin concentrations from Schultz, R. D., and Adams, L. S.: Immunologic methods for the detection of humoral and cellular immunity. Vet. Clin. North Am. 8:721, 1978; Schultz, R. D., Scott, F. W., Duncan, J. R., et al.: Feline immunoglobulins. Infect. Immun. 9:391, 1974; and Barlough, J. E., Jacobson, R. H., and Scott, F. W.: The immunoglobulins of the cat. Cornell Vet. 71:397, 1981.

Serum Iron and Iron-Binding Capacities in Iron-Deficient and Normal Dogs*

		Iron-Deficient Dogs		Normal Dogs	
Analyte	Unit	Mean	Range (min–max)	Mean	Range (min–max)
Serum iron	μmol/L	5	1–11	27	15–42
Total iron binding capacity	μmol/L	69	42–118	70	51–102
Saturation	%	8	2–19	39	19–59

*Derived from Harvey, J. W., French, T. W., and Meyer, D. J.: Chronic iron deficiency in dogs. J. Am. Anim. Hosp. Assoc. 18:946, 1982. For a review of similar data from dogs with various hematologic changes see Hoff, B., Lumsden, J. H., and Valli, V. E. O.: An appraisal of bone marrow biopsy in assessment of sick dogs. Can. J. Comp. Med. 49:34, 1985.

Serum Immunoglobulin Concentrations (mg/ml, Mean ± SD) of Normal Beagles at Various Ages*

Immunoglobulin Type	6–12 Months (n = 10)	1–2 Years (n = 10)	2–3 Years (n = 10)	3–5 Years (n = 10)	5–7 Years (n = 10)	7 Years (n = 6)
IgM	1.24 ± 1.69	1.34 ± 1.43	1.3 ± 1.8	1.52 ± 0.33	1.67 ± 1.1	1.84 ± 0.35
IgA	0.64 ± 0.34	1.13 ± 0.42	1.04 ± 0.53	1.29 ± 0.39	1.77 ± 0.56	1.62 ± 0.61
IgG$_1$	3.74 ± 1.44	3.97 ± 0.87	2.09 ± 0.68	3.16 ± 0.69	3.34 ± 1.3	2.24 ± 1.71
IgG$_{2a + 2b}$	5.0 ± 1.58	5.94 ± 1.16	6.13 ± 0.88	6.97 ± 0.92	9.05 ± 1.82	7.47 ± 1.68
IgG$_{2c}$	1.25 ± 0.36	1.43 ± 0.21	1.49 ± 0.39	1.6 ± 0.27	1.88 ± 0.51	1.77 ± 0.58

*From Gorman, N. T., and Halliwell, R. E. W.: Immunoglobulin quantitation and clinical interpretation. In Halliwell, R. E. W., and Gorman, N. T. (eds.): Veterinary Clinical Immunology. Philadelphia: W. B. Saunders, 1989, p. 61.

Acid-Base and Blood Gases (Mean ± SD)*

		Canine		Feline	
Analyte	Unit	Arterial	Venous	Arterial	Venous
pH	—	7.407 ± 0.0097	7.405 ± 0.0097	7.386 ± 0.038	7.300 ± 0.087
Pco$_2$	mm Hg	36.8 ± 3.0	36.6 ± 1.21	31.0 ± 2.9	41.8 ± 9.12
Po$_2$	mm Hg	92.1 ± 5.6	52.1 ± 2.11	106.8 ± 5.7	38.6 ± 11.44
HCO$_3$	mmol/L	22.2 ± 1.7	22.3 ± 0.43	18.0 ± 1.8	19.4 ± 4.0

*From Senior, D. F.: Fluid therapy, electrolyte and acid-base control. In Ettinger, S. J. (ed.): Textbook of Veterinary Internal Medicine, Diseases of the Dog and Cat, 3rd ed. Philadelphia: W. B. Saunders, 1989, p. 440. These data are based on the following original citations: Haskins, S. C.: Blood gases and acid-base balance: Clinical interpretation and therapeutic implications. In Kirk, R. W. (ed.): Current Veterinary Therapy VIII. Philadelphia: W. B. Saunders, 1980, p. 201; Rodkey, W. G., et al.: Arterialized capillary blood used to determine the acid-base and blood gas status of dogs. Am. J. Vet. Res. 39:459, 1978; Middleton, D. J., et al.: Arterial and venous blood gas tensions in clinically healthy cats. Am. J. Vet. Res. 42:1609, 1981.

Coagulation Screening Tests*

		Unit	Canine	Feline
Bleeding time	Dorsum of nose	Min	2–4	1–5
	Ear	Min	2.5–3.0	—
	Abdomen	Min	1–2	—
Buccal mucosal bleeding time BMBT† (Simplate II, Organon Teknika)	Lip	Min	1.7–4.2	1.0–3.2
Cuticle bleeding time (CBT)‡	Nail bed	Min	2.62 ± 0.49 (mean ± SD)	—
		Min	6.0 ± 3.7 (mean ± SD)	—
		Min	4.3 ± 0.3 (mean ± SEM)	—
Activated coagulation time (ACT)§	37°C	Sec	64–95	≤65
	Room temperature	Sec	60–125	—
		Sec	83–129	—
Tests using a mechanical end point||				
Prothrombin time (PT, Thromboplastin • C, Dade)		Sec	9–14	—
Activated partial thromboplastin time (APTT, Actin Activated Cephaloplastin, Dade)		Sec	≤20	—
*Tests using an electro-optical end point***				
Prothrombin time (PT, Permaplastin, Dade)		Sec	13.2–22.0	15.5–25.9
Activated partial thromboplastin time (APTT, Actin Activated Cephaloplastin, Dade)		Sec	21.0–35.0	22.8–38.0
Thrombin clotting time (TCT, Thrombostat, Parke Davis)		Sec	8.3–13.8	8.9–14.9
Russel viper venom time (RVVT)		Sec	10–15	—

*Prepared with the assistance of **Dr. I. B. Johnstone**, Hemostasis Laboratory, Department of Biomedical Sciences, University of Guelph. Abbreviations, methods, names, and sources of reagents are given in brackets. These reference values are provided only as general guidelines. Reference values for PT, APTT, TCT, and other coagulation tests differ between laboratories, depending on the type and concentration of reagents used and on the type of end-point detection (visual, mechanical, electro-optical). In interpreting patient test results, comparisons must always be made with reference values for that particular laboratory. Some laboratories may elect to run a species-specific reference plasma concurrent with patient plasma and report patient/control time. In such cases, the patient/control (P/C) ratio may be used to determine the significance of the test results. P/C ratios < 0.75 or > 1.25 in the PT, PTT, and TCT tests should be considered questionable or abnormal and worthy of further investigation (Johnstone, I. B.: Classical haemophilia [haemophilia A] in German shepherd dogs. Different expressions of the disease. Aust. Vet. Pract. 17:71, 1987).

†From Parker, M. T., Collier, L. L., Kier, A. B., et al.: Oral mucosa bleeding times of normal cats and cats with Chédiak-Higashi syndrome or Hagerman trait (factor XII deficiency). Vet. Clin. Pathol. 17:9, 1988; Jergens, A. E., Turrentine, M. A., Kraus, K. H., et al.: Buccal mucosa bleeding times of healthy dogs and of dogs in various pathologic states, including thrombocytopenia, uremia, and von Willebrand's disease. Am. J. Vet. Res. 48:1337, 1987.

‡From Giles, A. R., Tinlin, S., and Greenwood, R.: A canine model of hemophilic (factor VIII:C deficiency) bleeding. Blood 60:727, 1982; Pijnappels, M. I. M., Briët, E., van der Zwet, G. Th., et al.: Evaluation of the cuticle bleeding time in canine haemophilia A. Throm. Haemost. 55:70, 1986.

§From Byars, T. D., Ling, G. V., Ferris, N. A., et al.: Activated coagulation time (ACT) of whole blood in normal dogs. Am. J. Vet. Res. 37:1359, 1976; Middleton, D. J., and Watson, A. D. J.: Activated coagulation times of whole blood in normal dogs and dogs with coagulopathies. J. Small Anim. Pract. 19:417, 1978.

||Fibrometer, reference values from Clinical Pathology Laboratory, Department of Pathology, University of Guelph. This APTT test uses ellagic acid and kaolin as activators.

BioData PC8, reference values from **Dr. I. B. Johnstone, Hemostasis Laboratory, Department of Biomedical Sciences, University of Guelph. This APTT test uses ellagic acid as an activator.

Specific Coagulation Tests*

	Unit	Canine	Feline
Fibrinogen (fibrometer, thrombin time, TT, Thrombostat, Parke-Davis)	gm/L	1.6–4.5	—
Fibrinogen (heat precipitation)	gm/L	1.3–4.4	0.8–2.9
Platelets (manual, phase contrast)	× 10⁹/L	200–600	190–750
Fibrinogen degradation products (FDP, latex agglutination, Burroughs Wellcome)	μg/ml	≤20	—
Factor VIII Coagulant (FVIII:C, one-stage differential PTT)	% of normal	55–135	—
von Willebrand's factor antigen (vWF:Ag, Laurell Electroimmunoassay)†	% of normal	55–178	—
vWF:Ag (enzyme-linked immunosorbent assay, Diagnostica Stago)‡	% of normal	60–152	—
Antithrombin III (AT III, chromogenic substrate, Diagnostica Stago)§	% of normal	80–136	—

*Prepared with the assistance of **Dr. I. B. Johnstone**, Hemostasis Laboratory, Department of Biomedical Sciences, University of Guelph. Abbreviations, methods, names and sources of reagents are given in parentheses. Specific hemostatic factors are generally assayed by comparing test plasma to a species-specific reference plasma. The reference plasma is arbitrarily designated as having 100% activity, and the activity in the patient plasma is expressed as a percentage of the "normal" plasma.

†From Johnstone, I. B., and Crane, S.: Determination of canine factor VIII-related antigen using commercial antihuman factor VIII serum. Vet. Clin. Pathol. 9:31, 1980.

‡From Johnstone I. B., and Crane, S.: Quantitation of canine plasma von Willebrand factor antigen using a commercial enzyme-linked immunosorbent assay. Can. J. Vet. Res. 55:11, 1991.

§From Johnstone, I. B., Petersen, D., and Crane, S.: Antithrombin III (AT III) activity in plasmas from normal and diseased horses, and in normal canine, bovine, and human plasmas. Vet. Clin. Pathol. 16:14, 1987.

Tests of the Endocrine System*

Hormone	Unit	Canine	Feline
Adrenocorticotrophic hormone, basal (ACTH, plasma)	pmol/L	2–15	1–20
Aldosterone† (plasma)			
Basal	pmol/L	14–960	194–388
Post-ACTH	pmol/L	200–2100	277–721
Cortisol (serum or plasma, urine)			
Basal	nmol/L	25–125	15–150
Post-ACTH	nmol/L	200–550	130–450
Post–low-dose dexamethasone (0.01 or 0.015 mg/kg)	nmol/L	≤40	≤40
Post–high-dose dexamethasone (0.1 or 1.0 mg/kg)‡	nmol/L	≤40	≤40
Urinary cortisol:creatinine ratio	× 10⁻⁶	8–24†, ≤10§	—
Insulin, basal (serum)	pmol/L	35–200	35–200
Intact parathormone† (serum)	pmol/L	2–13	0–4
Progesterone (serum or plasma, female)	mmol/L	≤3 in anestrus, proestrus 50–220 in diestrus, pregnancy	≤3 in anestrus, proestrus 50–220 in diestrus, pregnancy
Testosterone (serum or plasma, male)	nmol/L	1–20	1–20
Thyroxine (T₄ serum)			
Basal	nmol/L	12–50	10–50
Post–thyroxine-stimulating hormone (TSH)	nmol/L	>45	>45
Triiodothyronine (T₃) suppression‖	nmol/L	—	≤20
Triiodothyronine, basal (T₃, serum)	nmol/L	0.7–2.3	0.5–2.0

*Prepared with the assistance of **Dr. M. E. Peterson**, The Animal Medical Center New York, NY. Unless indicated otherwise, values in this table are adapted from Kemppainen, R. J., and Zerbe, C. A.: Common endocrine diagnostic tests: Normal values and interpretations. In Kirk, R. W. (ed.): *Current Veterinary Therapy X.* Philadelphia: W. B. Saunders, 1989, p. 961. Hormone determinations are variable between laboratories. The laboratory performing the analysis should provide reference values. Before submitting samples for hormone determinations, consult the laboratory for sample specifications, use of anticoagulants, and sample preservation. General sampling conditions are discussed in Reimers, T. J.: Guidelines for collection, storage, and transport of samples for hormone assay. In Kirk, R. W. (ed.): *Current Veterinary Therapy X.* Philadelphia: W. B. Saunders, 1989, p. 968. The effects of age, gender, and size on canine serum thyroid and adrenocortical hormone concentrations are discussed in Reimers, T. J., Lawler, D. F., Sutaria, P. M., et al.: Effects of age, sex, and body size on serum concentrations of thyroid and adrenocortial hormones in dogs. Am. J. Vet. Res. 51:454, 1990.

†Provided by **Dr. R. F. Nachreiner**, Animal Health Diagnostic Laboratory, Endocrine Diagnostic Section, Michigan State University.

‡This test is used after adrenocortical hyperfunction has been confirmed. It is used to differentiate adrenal tumor (where no suppression is seen) from pituitary-dependent cases (where suppression occurs but is variable).

§From Stolp, R., Rijnberk, A., Meiher, J. C., et al.: Urinary corticoids in the diagnosis of canine hyperadrenocorticism. Res. Vet. Sci. 34:141, 1983; Rijnberk, A., van Wees, A., and Mol, J. A.: Assessment of two tests for the diagnosis of canine hyperadrenocorticism. Vet. Rec. 122:178, 1988.

‖Peterson, M. E., and Ferguson, D. C.: Thyroid diseases. In Ettinger, S. J. (ed.): *Textbook of Veterinary Internal Medicine. Diseases of the Dog and Cat,* 3rd ed. Philadelphia: W. B. Saunders, 1989, pp. 1632–1675.

Système International (SI) Units for Hormone Assays*

Hormone	Unit		Conversion Factors†	
	Traditional	*SI*	*Traditional → SI*	*SI → Traditional*
Aldosterone	ng/dl	pmol/L	27.7	0.036
Corticotrophin (ACTH)	pg/ml	pmol/L	0.22	4.51
Cortisol	μg/dl	mmol/L	27.59	0.36
Beta-endorphin	pg/ml	pmol/L	0.289	3.43
Epinephrine	pg/ml	pmol/L	5.46	0.183
Estrogen (estradiol)	pg/ml	pmol/L	3.67	0.273
Gastrin	pg/ml	ng/L	1.00	1.00
Glucagon	pg/ml	ng/L	1.00	1.00
Growth hormone (GH)	ng/ml	μg/L	1.00	1.00
Insulin	μU/ml	pmol/L	7.18	0.139
Alpha-melanocyte stimulating hormone (α-MSH)	pg/ml	pmol/L	0.601	1.66
Norepinephrine	pg/ml	nmol/L	0.006	169
Pancreatic polypeptide (PP)	mg/dl	mmol/L	0.239	4.18
Progesterone	ng/dl	mmol/L	3.18	0.315
Prolactin	ng/ml	μg/L	1.00	1.00
Renin	ng/ml/hr	ng/L/s	0.278	3.60
Somatostatin	pg/ml	pmol/L	0.611	1.64
Testosterone	ng/ml	nmol/L	3.47	0.288
Thyroxine (T₄)	μg/dl	nmol/L	12.87	0.078
Triiodothyronine (T₃)	ng/dl	nmol/L	0.0154	64.9
Vasoactive intestinal polypeptide (VIP)	pg/ml	pmol/L	0.301	3.33

*Contributed by **Dr. M. E. Peterson,** The Animal Medical Center, New York, NY.
†Multiply the traditional (SI) unit by the appropriate conversion factor to obtain the SI (traditional) value.

Urinary and Renal Function Tests*

	Unit	Canine	Feline
Random specific gravity (SG)	—	1.001–1.070	1.001–1.080
SG after 5% dehydration	—	1.050–1.076	1.047–1.087
Random osmolality	mmol/kg	50–2500	50–3000+
Osmolality after 5% dehydration	mmol/kg	1787–2791	1581–2984
Urine/plasma osmolality after 5% dehydration	—	5.7–8.9	—
Volume output	ml/kg/day	24–41	22–30
Protein—sulfosalicylic acid†	0.1, 0.2, 0.3, 0.4, 0.5, 0.75, and 1.0 gm/L stds.	< 0.1	
Protein—dipstick‡	negative, trace, 0.3, 1.0, 3.0, and 20+ gm/L stds.	Negative when SG < 1.035 Trace when SG > 1.035	
Blood—dipstick	Negative +, + +, and + + + stds.	Negative	
Glucose—dipstick	negative, 6, 14, 28, 56, and 111 + mmol/L stds.	Negative	
Ketones—dipstick	negative, 0.5, 1.5, 4, 8, and 16 mmol/L stds.	Negative	
Bilirubin—dipstick	negative, +, + +, and + + + stds.	+ When SG > 1.035	Negative
Protein output§	mg/kg/day	< 22	< 30
	mg/day	< 200 or < 600	< 115
Protein:creatine ratio‖	—	< 0.2	< 0.6
Questionable	—	0.2–1.0	0.6–1.0
Abnormal	—	> 1.0	> 1.0
Effective renal plasma flow by clearance of para-aminohippurate or [¹³¹ I]iodohippurate**	ml/min/m² body surface ml/min/kg body weight	266 ± 66 13.5 ± 3.3	— 14.1 ± 5.74 or 10.6 ± 1.7
Glomerular filtration rate (GFR) by clearance of [¹⁴C]inulin, [¹²⁵I]iothalamate, or other labeled chemicals††	ml/min/m² body surface ml/min/kg body weight	84.4 ± 19 4.2 ± 1.8 or 3.6 ± 0.1	— 5.1 ± 1.5 3.5 ± 0.6

Urinary and Renal Function Tests* Continued

	Unit	Canine	Feline
GFR by sodium sulfanilate clearance‡‡—$t_{0.5}$	min	58 ± 13 or 66.1 ± 10.8	44.7 ± 5.7
GFR by exogenous creatinine clearance§§	ml/min/kg body weight	4.0 ± 0.5	2.9 ± 0.3
GFR by endogeneous creatinine clearance‖‖	ml/min/m² body surface	60 ± 22	—
	ml/min/kg body weight—20	3.0 ± 1.0	2.7 ± 1.1
	min—24 hr	3.7 ± 0.8	2.3 ± 0.5
Fractional clearances***			
Sodium	%	0–0.7	0.24–0.96
Chloride	%	0–0.8	0.41–1.33
Potassium	%	0–20	6.7–23.9
Calcium	%	0–0.4	—
Phosphorus	%	3–39	17–73

*Prepared with the assistance of **Dr. J. Barsanti,** University of Georgia. Data are given in mean ± SD rounded to one decimal place. In a few instances, alternative reference values are listed. An extensive bibliography and a review of these tests can be found in Chew, D. J., and Dibartola, S. P.: Diagnosis and pathophysiology of renal disease. *In* Ettinger, S. J. (ed.): *Textbook of Veterinary Internal Medicine, Diseases of the Dog and Cat,* 3rd ed. Philadelphia: W. B. Saunders, 1989, pp. 1893–1961.

†Albumin in Urine Test Set. Harleco, Gibbstown, NJ.

‡Multistix, Miles Canada, Inc., Etobicoke, Ontario. Also applies for the semiquantitative analysis of blood, glucose, ketones, and bilirubin. Refer to the discussion in the package insert entitled "Ames Reagent Strips for Urinalysis" for potential interferents.

§From DiBartola, S. P., Chew, D. J., and Jacobs, G.: Quantitative urinalysis including 24-hour protein excretion in the dog. J. Am. Anim. Hosp. Assoc, 16:537, 1980; Russo, E. A., Lees, G. E, and Hightower, D.: Evaluation of renal function tests in cats, using quantitative urinalysis. Am. J. Vet. Res. 47:1308, 1986; Barsanti, J. A., and Finco, D. R.: Protein concentration in urine of normal dogs. Am. J. Vet. Res. 40:1583, 1979. Applies to urine samples with no hemorrhage or inflammation. Some differences in test results occur with different quantitative methods.

‖From White, J. V., Olivier, B., Reimann, K., et al.: Use of protein-to-creatinine ratio in a single urine specimen for quantitative estimation of canine proteinuria. J.A.V.M.A. 185:882, 1984; Grauer, G. F., Thomas, C. B., and Eicker, S. W.: Estimation of quantitative proteinuria in the dog, using the protein-to-creatinine ratio from a random, voided sample. Am. J. Vet. Res. 46:2116, 1985; Center, S. A., Wilkinson, E., Smith, C. A., et al.: 24-hour urine protein/creatinine ratio in dogs with protein-losing nephropathies. J.A.V.M.A. 187:820, 1985; McCaw, D. L., Knapp, D. W., and Hewett, J. E.: Effect of collection time and exercise restriction on the prediction of urine protein excretion, using urine protein/creatinine ratio in dogs. Am. J. Vet. Res. 46:166, 1985; Jergens, A. E., McCaw, D. L., and Hewett, J. E.: Effects of collection time and food consumption on the urine protein/creatinine ratio in dogs. Am. J. Vet. Res. 48:1106, 1987. Applies to urine samples with no hemorrhage or inflammation.

**From Mercer, H. C., Garg, R. C., Powers, J. D., et al.: Bioavailability and pharmacokinetics of several dosage forms of ampicillin in the cat. Am. J. Vet. Res. 38:1353, 1977; Ross, L. A., and Finco, D. R.: Relationship of selected clinical renal function tests to glomerular filtration rate and renal blood flow in cats. Am. J. Vet. Res. 42:1704, 1981.

††From Ross, L. A., and Finco, D. R, 1981; Carlson, G. P., Kaneko, J. J.: Simultaneous estimation of renal function in dogs using sodium sulfanilate and sodium iodohippurate-[131]I. J.A.V.M.A. 158:1229, 1971; Maddison, J. E., Pascoe, P. J., and Jansen, B. S.: Clinical evaluation of sodium sulfanilate clearance for the diagnosis of renal disease in dogs. J.A.V.M.A. 185:961, 1984; Mercer, H. C., et al., 1977.

‡‡From Ross, L. A., and Finco, D. R., 1981; Osborne, C. A., Low, D. G., and Finco, D. R.: *Canine and Feline Urology.* Philadelphia: W. B. Saunders, 1972; Finco, D. R., Coulter, D. B., and Barsanti, J. A.: Simple, accurate method for clinical estimation of glomerular filtration rate in the dog. Am. J. Vet. Res. 42:1874, 1981; Fettman, M. J., Allen, T. A, Wilke, W. L., et al.: Single-injection method for evaluation of renal function with ^{14}C-inulin and ^{3}H-tetraethylammonium bromide in dogs and cats. Am. J. Vet. Res. 46:482, 1985; Powers, T. E., Powers, J. D., and Garg, R. C.: Study of the double isotope single-injection methods for estimating renal function in purebred beagle dogs. Am. J. Vet. Res. 38:1933, 1977.

§§From Ross, L. A., and Finco, D. R., 1981; Finco, D. R. et al., 1981. Creatinine given subcutaneously in dog and intravenously in cat.

‖‖From Russo, E. A., et al., 1986; Osborne, C. A., et al., 1972; Bovee, K. C., and Joyce, T.: Clinical evaluation of glomerular function: 24 hour creatinine clearance in dogs. J.A.V.M.A. 174:488, 1979; Osbaldiston, G. W., and Fuhrman, W.: The clearance of creatinine, inulin, paraaminohippurate, and phenolsulphothalein in the cat. Can. J. Comp. Med. 24:138, 1970.

***Dibartola, S. P., et al., 1980; Russo, E. A., et al., 1986. Values vary markedly with diet.

Quantitative Tests of Gastrointestinal Function*†

Fecal determinations
  Fecal output (gm feces/kg/day, mean ± SEM‡)

Canine			
Normal (n = 14)	8.5 ± 1.1		
Malabsorption (n = 6)	42.3 ± 8.0		
Colitis (n = 10)	11.9 ± 1.1		
Nonsteatorrheal small intestinal diarrheal disease (n = 17)	13.9 ± 2		
Exocrine pancreatic insufficiency (EPI, n = 20)	34.4 ± 4.5		

  Fecal fat output (gm fecal fat/kg/day, mean ± SEM)

Canine		**Feline**	
Normal (n = 14)	0.24 ± 0.01	Normal	0.35 ± 0.23 (mean ± SD)
Malabsorption (n = 6)	1.14 ± 0.11	Steatorrhea	> 3.5 gm fecal fat/day
EPI (n = 20)	2.08 ± 0.36		

    Note: Values greater than 0.3 indicate steatorrhea. Fat balance in dogs with colitis and other nonmalabsorptive intestinal diseases is indistinguishable from normal dogs.

  Fecal proteolytic activity (FPA, mean of 3 samples)†

Canine		**Feline**	
Radial enzyme diffusion (mm)			
Normal	7–15	Normal	6–17
EPI	≤ 5	EPI	≤ 5
Azocasein digestion (ACU/gm feces)			
Normal	19–122	Normal	29–207
EPI	≤ 10	EPI	≤ 10

Serum concentrations of orally administered or naturally occurring substances

  Xylose (0.5 gm/kg body weight)

Canine	**Feline**
Peak at 60 min of 65 mg/dl ± 6 (mean ± SEM, n = 13), decreasing to 48 ± 5 at 90 min. Only 10% of dogs have 45 to 50 mg/dl at 60 min. All dogs with concentrations greater than 50 mg/dl at 60 min or 45 mg/dl at 90 min are considered normal.	Peaks between 12 and 42 mg/dl.

    Note: This test has poor sensitivity for detecting malabsorption in dogs and cats.

  N-Benzoyl-L-tyrosyl-paraaminobenzoic acid (BT-PABA)

Canine (50 mg/kg body weight)	**Feline**
> 400 μ/dl at 60 to 90 min	Peaks at 386 ± 134 μg/dl (mean ± SD, n = 17, 16.7 mg/kg body weight). At 50 mg/kg body weight, the peak occurred at 90 min and the range (min–max) was approximately 400–1100 μg/dl.

  Vitamin E (mg/L)

Canine		**Feline**	
	> 5		> 5

  Vitamin B₁₂ (ng/L)

Canine		**Feline**	
	225–661		200–1680

  Folic acid (μg/L)

Canine		**Feline**	
	6.7–17.4		13.4–38.0

  Trypsin-like immunoreactivity (TLI, μg/L)

Canine	
Normal	5.0–35
EPI	≤ 2.5

*Prepared with the assistance of **Dr. D. A. Williams,** Department of Clinical Sciences, College of Veterinary Medicine, Kansas State University. Review and original citations in Jacobs, R. M., Norris, A. M., Lurnsden, J. H., et al.: Laboratory Diagnosis of Malassimilation. Vet. Clin. North Am. Small Anim. Pract. 19:951, 1989.

†From Williams, D. A., Reed, S. D., and Perry, L.: Fecal proteolytic activity in clinically normal cats and in a cat with exocrine pancreatic insufficiency. J.A.V.M.A. 197:210, 1990; Williams, D. A., and Reed, S. D.: Comparison of methods for assay of fecal proteolytic activity. J Vet. Clin. Pathol. 19:20, 1990.

‡Standard error of the mean.

Bronchoalveolar Lavage Fluid Cell Populations*

	Canine (n = 6)	Feline (n = 11)
Total nucleated cells/μl	≤ 500	≤ 400
Cell types (mean %)		
Macrophages	70 ± 11 (49–93)	70.6 ± 9.8
Lymphocytes	7 ± 5 (1–19)	4.6 ± 3.2
Neutrophils	5 ± 5 (1–27)	6.7 ± 4.0
Eosinophils	6 ± 5 (1–19)	16.1 ± 6.8
Mast cells	1 ± 1 (0–5)	NR†
Epithelial cells	1 ± 1 (0–12)	NR

*Canine data given as mean % ± SD (range). Feline data given as mean % ± SE. Data derived from and original citations listed in Hawkins, E. C., DeNicola, D. B., and Kuehn, N. F.: Bronchoalveolar lavage in the evaluation of pulmonary disease in the dog and cat. J. Vet. Intern. Med. 4:267, 1990.

†Not reported.

Cerebrospinal Fluid (CSF)*

	Canine		Feline	
Protein (gm/L)†	0.10–0.30		0.04–0.32	
Total nucleated cells (× 10⁹/L)‡	0–0.002		0–0.002	
	Sediment (n = 40)	Cytospin (n = 50)	Sediment (n = 20)	Cytospin (n = 22)
Cell types (mean %, [range])				
Large foamy monouclear	3 (0–32)	6 (0–46)	—	—
Monocytoid	—	17 (0–50)	87 (69–100)	77 (25–100)
Small mononuclear	26 (3–52)	37 (0–73)	—	—
Large mononuclear	38 (9–74)	33 (0–68)	—	—
Small lymphocyte	5 (0–76)	4 (0–61)	9 (0–27)§	14 (0–50)
Neutrophil	1 (0–10)	3 (0–7)	1 (0–9)	2 (0–25)
Eosinophil	0	0.3 (0–13)	0	0
Macrophage	0	0	0 (0–3)	3 (0–33)

*Canine data adapted from Jamison, E. M., and Lumsden, J. H.: Cerebrospinal fluid analysis in the dog: Methodology and interpretation. Semin. Vet. Med. Surg. (Small Anim.), 3:122, 1988, and other unpublished data describing the CSF characteristics of histologically normal dogs. Feline data adapted from Rand, J. S., Parent, J., Jacobs, R. M., et al.: Reference intervals for feline cerebrospinal fluid: Cell counts and cytologic features. Am. J. Vet. Res. 51:1044, 1990, describing CSF characteristics in histologically normal cats. All feline CSFs had red blood cell counts between 0 and 0.030 × 10⁹/L. All data are for cerebellomedullary CSF. There are significant differences between lumbar and cerebellomedullary CSF (Bailey, C. S., and Higgins, R. J.: Comparison of total white blood cell count and total protein content of lumbar and cisternal cerebrospinal fluid of healthy dogs. Am. J. Vet. Res. 46:1162, 1985); Thomson, C. E., Kornegay, J. N., and Stevens, J. B.: Analysis of cerebrospinal fluid from the cerebellomedullary and lumbar cisterns of dogs with focal neurologic disease: 145 cases (1985–1987). J.A.V.M.A. 196:1841, 1990.

†The protein concentrations here are for the Ponceau S method, and the reference interval represents the range. For a comparison of Ponceau S and urine dipstick methods, see Jacobs, R. M., Cochrane, S. M., Lumsden, J. H., et al.: Relationship of cerebrospinal fluid protein concentration determined by dye-binding and urinary dipstick methodologies. Can. Vet. J. 31:587, 1990.

‡Range for hemocytometer cell counts.

§Includes all sizes of lymphocytes.

CSF Biochemical Analytes in Histologically Normal Cats*

Analyte	Unit	Mean	Range (min–max)
Glucose	mmol/L	4.1	0.5–8.1
Creatine kinase	U/L	47	2–236
Lactate dehydrogenase	U/L	12	4–30
Aspartate aminotransferase	U/L	17	0–39
IgG	gm/L	0.015	0.005–0.56
[CSF IgG]/[Serum IgG]	—	0.8	0.3–2.1

*Adapted from Rand, J. S., Parent, J., Jacobs, R. M., et al.: Reference intervals for feline cerebrospinal fluid: Biochemical and serologic variables, IgG concentration, and electrophoretic fractionation. Am. J. Vet. Res. 51:1049, 1990. All feline CSFs had red blood counts between 0 and 0.030 × 10^9/L.

Characteristics of Body Cavity Fluids in Healthy Dogs and Cats*

Volume	0–15 ml for peritoneal cavity Approximately 3 ml in pleural cavity Approximately 0.3 ml in pericardial sac
Color	Colorless to slight yellow
Odor	None
Transparency	Clear, with no tissue fragments
Protein†	≤ 2.5 gm/dl (≤ 25 gm/L) Does not coagulate
Specific gravity	≤ 1.014
Electrolytes and pH	As for plasma
Total nucleated cell count	≤ 3,000/μl (≤ 3.0 × 10^9/L)
Cell types	Mesothelial cells, occasional well-preserved neutrophils, occasional lymphocytes and monocytes, occasional erythrocytes

*From O'Brien, P. J., and Lumsden, J. H.: The cytologic examination of body cavity fluids. Sem. Vet. Med. Surg. (Small Anim.) 3:140, 1988. The original sources for the data are listed in this review.

†For the Goldberg refractometer (Fisher Scientific, Toronto, Ontario) 2.5 gm protein/dl corresponds to a specific gravity of 1.014 on the plasma/serum scale. The serum/plasma specific gravity scale should be used for the estimation of protein concentration in body cavity fluids. If the urine specific gravity scale is used erroneously or unknowingly, the corresponding specific gravity is 1.020 for a protein concentration of 2.5 gm/dl.

Cytologic Findings in Normal and Abnormal Canine Synovial Fluids*

	Clarity	Color	Mucin Clot	Fibrin	Cell Count (× 10⁹/L)	Mononuclear Cells (%)	Neutrophils (%)
Normal	Clear	None to light yellow	Good	—	0.0–3.0	90–100	0–10
Nonsuppurative inflammation							
Degenerative	Clear	None to light yellow	Good to fair	—	0.0–3.5	90–100	0–10
Traumatic	Clear to turbid	Normal to bloody	Good	±	2.5–3.0	90–100	0–10
Chronic hemarthrosis	Turbid	Bloody	Fair to poor	−†	Variably increased	Predominate	Occasional
Suppurative inflammation							
Rheumatoid-like	Turbid	Yellow to bloody	Fair to poor	+	3.0–38	20–80	20–80
SLE‡-like	Turbid	Yellow to bloody	Good to poor	+	4.4–370	5–85	15–95
Bacterial	Turbid	Gray to bloody	Poor to very poor	+	110–267	1–10	90–99

*From Ellison, R. S.: The cytologic examination of synovial fluid. Sem. Vet. Med. Surg. (Small Anim.) 3:133, 1988. The original citations are listed in this review. The protein concentration in normal joint fluid is ≤ 30 gm/L.
†In acute hemarthrosis, fibrin clots may be present.
‡Systemic lupus erythematosus.

Canine Semen* (Mean ± SEM)†

Semen Characteristics After Sexual Rest	Unit	Body Weight (lb)		
		10–34	*35–59*	*60–84*
Volume‡	ml	2.4 ± 0.3	3.9 ± 0.5	5.4 ± 1.3
Sperm concentration	× 10⁶/ml	209 ± 42	359 ± 72	228 ± 58
Total sperm	× 10⁶/ml	400 ± 110	1120 ± 130	1430 ± 460

*Data derived from Amann, R. P.: Reproductive physiology and endocrinology of the Dog. *In* Morrow, D. A. (ed.): *Current Therapy in Theriogenology* 2. Philadelphia: W. B. Saunders, 1986, p. 536. In one study, inseminations with greater than 200 × 10⁶ morphologically normal sperm resulted in a pregnancy rate of 81% (22 of 27 bitches). As the total number of morphologically normal sperm declined, so did the pregnancy rate and litter size (Michelsen, W. D.: Society for Theriogenology, Orlando, FL, September, 1988, p. 387).
†Standard error of the mean.
‡The presperm and sperm-rich fractions were collected together, but ejaculation was terminated when ejaculation of the postsperm prostatic fluid was started.

Canine Prostatic Fluid (Third Fraction)*

Volume	Variable, depending on length of ejaculation
pH	6.1–7.2
Appearance	Clear
Sediment	Acellular

*From Bartlett, D. J.: Studies on dog semen II. Biochemical characteristics. J. Reprod. Fertil. 3:190, 1962.

*Electrocardiography**

It is recognized that normal and abnormal electrocardiographic measurements overlap and that the criteria for the normal electrocardiogram serve only as a guide for the clinician. Deviations from normal in an individual electrocardiogram suggest but are not always diagnostic of heart disease. As additional statistical data become available for the electrocardiograms of dogs of each breed, body type, age, and sex, the data herein may require revision and "normal" may be more precisely defined. The value of serial electrocardiograms from an individual cannot be overemphasized, since serial changes best demonstrate electrocardiographic abnormalities.

Criteria for the Normal Canine Electrocardiogram†

Heart rate—60 to 160 beats per minute for adult dogs, up to 180 beats per minute in toy breeds, and 220 beats per minute for puppies.

Heart rhythm—Normal sinus rhythm; sinus arrhythmia; and wandering sinoatrial pacemaker.

P wave—Up to 0.4 millivolt in amplitude; up to 0.04 sec in duration (may be longer in giant breeds); always positive in leads II and aVF; positive or isoelectric in lead I.

P-R interval—0.06 to 0.14 sec duration.

QRS complex—Mean electric axis, frontal plane, 40 to 100°.

Amplitude—Maximum amplitude of R wave 2.5 to 3.0 millivolts in leads II, III, and aVF. Complex positive in leads II, III, and aVF; negative in lead V_{10}.

Duration—To 0.05 sec (0.06/sec in dogs over 40 lb).

Q-T segment—0.15 to 0.22 sec duration.

ST segment and T wave—ST segment free of marked coving (repolarization changes).

ST segment depression not greater than 0.2 millivolt.

ST segment elevation not greater than 0.15 millivolt.

T wave negative in lead V_{10}.

T wave amplitude no greater than 25% of amplitude of R wave.

Criteria for the Normal Feline Electrocardiogram†

Heart rate—240 beats per minute maximum.

Heart rhythm—Normal sinus rhythm or, infrequently, sinus arrhythmia.

P wave—Positive in leads II and aVF; may be isoelectric or positive in lead I; should not exceed 0.03 sec in duration.

P-R interval—0.04 to 0.08 sec duration (inversely related to the heart rate).

QRS complex—More variable than in the canine; the mean electric axis in the frontal plane is often insignificant. Often the QRS complex is nearly isoelectric in all frontal plane limb leads (so-called horizontal heart).

QRS amplitude—The amplitude of the R wave is usually low; marked amplitude of R wave (over 0.8 millivolt) in the frontal plane leads may suggest ventricular hypertrophy.

QRS duration—Less than 0.04 sec.

Q-T segment—0.16 to 0.18 sec duration.

ST segment and T wave—ST segment and T wave should be small and free of repolarization changes as well as marked depression or elevation.

*From Ettinger, S. J., and Suter, P. F.: *Canine Cardiology*, Philadelphia: W. B. Saunders, 1970, pp. 102–169.

†From Ettinger, S. J.: Cardiac arrhythmias. *In* Ettinger, S. J. (ed.): *Textbook of Veterinary Internal Medicine, Diseases of the Dog and Cat*, 3rd ed. Vol 1. Philadelphia: W. B. Saunders, 1989, p. 1055.

Antineoplastic Agents in Cancer Therapy*

Agent (Brand Name; Supplier)	Action and Cell Cycle Specificity	Indication	Dosage and Administration†	Toxicities	Comments
Alkylating agents					
Cyclophosphamide (Cytoxan, Mead Johnson; Neosar, Adria) Tabs: 25- and 50-mg Inj: 100-, 200-, and 500-mg 1- and 2-gm vials	Alkylating activity by metabolite phosphoramide mustard. Believed to cross-link DNA. Cell cycle nonspecific.	Primarily lymphoreticular neoplasms. Also mast cell, hemangio-sarcoma, mammary carcinoma.	50 mg/m² PO q 48 hr. 100–200 mg/m² IV q 21 d.	Leukopenia, gastroenteritis, hemorrhagic cystitis. May induce transitional cell carcinoma of bladder.	Must be activated by liver. Excreted primarily by kidneys. Metabolites protein bound.
Chlorambucil (Leukeran, Burroughs Wellcome) Tabs: 2 mg	Bifunctional alkylation of DNA. Creates intra- and interstrand cross-links. Cell cycle nonspecific.	Lymphoreticular neoplasms, macroglobulinemia, polycythemia vera.	2–6 mg/m² PO q 24–48 hr.	Leukopenia	Relatively free of gastrointestinal effects.
Busulfan (Myleran, Burroughs Wellcome) Tabs: 2 mg	Bifunctional alkylating agent. Interacts with cellular thiol groups. Little DNA cross-linking. Cell cycle nonspecific.	Chronic granulocytic leukemia; of no benefit in "blastic" phase.	3–4 mg/m² PO q 24 hr. Discontinue when total WBC approx 15,000. Repeat p.r.n.	Leukopenia. Rare bronchopulmonary dysplasia with pulmonary fibrosis.	May require 2 weeks to observe response. If rapid decline in total leukocytes: discontinue drug.
Melphalan (Alkeran, Burroughs Wellcome) Tabs: 2 mg	Bifunctional alkylating agent. Phenylalanine derivative of nitrogen mustard. Cell cycle nonspecific.	Multiple myeloma; some lymphoreticular neoplasms, osteosarcomas, mammary and lung tumors.	2–4 mg/m² PO q 48 hr. 1.5 mg/m² q 24 hr for 7–10 days. 15–20 mg/kg/day PO.	Infrequent leukopenia.	Response may be gradual over many months.
Triethylenethiophosphoramide (Thiotepa, Lederle) Inj: 15-mg vial	Radiomimetic. Believed to disrupt DNA bonds by release of ethylenamine radicals. Cell cycle nonspecific.	Systemic use for carcinomas. Intravesical use for transitional cell. Intracavitary use for neoplastic effusions.	0.2–0.5 mg/m² intracavitary, IV.	Leukopenia.	Not a vesicant. May be given intralesionally.
Mechlorethamine HCL (Mustargen, Merck Sharp & Dohme) Inj: 10-mg vial	Cytotoxic, mutagenic, and radiomimetic. Exact mechanism of action unknown. Cell cycle nonspecific.	Lymphoreticular neoplasms, pleural and peritoneal effusions.	5 mg/m² PO, IV, or intracavitary; repeat p.r.n.	Leukopenia. Nausea and vomiting dose-limiting side effect.	Severe vesicant. Sloughing may occur if extravasated.
Cisplatin (Platinol, Bristol-Myers Oncology) Inj: 10- and 50-mg vials	Action similar to bifunctional alkylating agents. Produces DNA cross-links. Cell cycle nonspecific.	Osteosarcoma, transitional cell carcinoma, squamous cell carcinoma.	60–70 mg/m² IV over 20 min. Administer 0.9% saline IV for 4 hr pre- and 2 hr postinfusion.	Nausea, vomiting, renal toxicity, bone marrow depression. Dose-related pulmonary toxicity in cat.	Do not use aluminum-containing needles; precipitates on contact. Eliminated through kidneys.

Table continued on following page

Antineoplastic Agents in Cancer Therapy* Continued

Agent (Brand Name; Supplier)	Action and Cell Cycle Specificity	Indication	Dosage and Administration†	Toxicities	Comments
Antimetabolites					
Mercaptopurine (Purinethol, Burroughs Wellcome) Tabs: 50 mg	Feedback enzyme inhibitor of DNA synthesis. S-phase specific.	Acute lymphocytic and granulocytic leukemia, immune-mediated disease.	50 mg/m² PO q 24 hr to effect, then q 48 hr or p.r.n.	Infrequent leukopenia.	Must be activated within tumor cells; lethal synthesis.
Thioguanine (Thioguanine, Burroughs Wellcome) Tabs: 40 mg	Feedback enzyme inhibitor of DNA synthesis. S-phase specific.	Acute lymphocytic and granulocytic leukemia.	Dogs—40 mg/m² PO q 24 hr × 4–5 d, then q 3 d thereafter. Cats—25 mg/m² PO q 24 hr × 1–5 d, then repeat q 30 d p.r.n.	Leukopenia, thrombocytopenia may be severe in cats. Hepatotoxicity.	As for mercaptopurine. Cross-resistance between thioguanine and mercaptopurine is extensive.
Fluorouracil (Fluorouracil, Roche; Adrucil, Adria) Inj: 500-mg vial	Inhibits enzyme thymidylate synthetase. Results in thymidine deficiency leading to inhibition of DNA synthesis. S-phase specific.	Mammary, gastrointestinal, liver and lung carcinomas, and carcinomatosis.	150 mg/m² IV or intracavitary q 7 d. Canine only.	Dogs—cerebellar ataxia. Cats—neurotoxicity precludes use.	Cleared by hepatic degredation.
Cytosine arabinoside (Cytosar-U, Upjohn) Inj: 100- and 500-mg vials	Appears to inhibit DNA polymerase activity; mechanism incompletely understood. S-phase specific.	Lymphoreticular neoplasms, myeloproliferative disease, and CNS lymphoma.	100 mg/m² IV or SC q 24 hr × 2–4 d; repeat p.r.n. 20 mg/ m² intrathecally × 1–5 d.	Leukopenia.	May be given intrathecally.
Methotrexate (Methotrexate, Lederle; Folex, Adria; Mexate, Bristol-Myers Oncology) Tabs 2.5 mg Inj: 5-, 20-, 25-, 50-, 100-, 200- and 250-mg vials	Competitive enzyme inhibitor of folic acid reductase. S-phase specific.	Lymphoreticular neoplasms, myeloproliferative disorders, transmissible veneral and Sertoli's cell tumors, osteosarcoma.	"Normal dose"—0.5– 0.8 mg/kg IV q 7–14 d or 2.5 mg/m² PO q 24–48 hr.	Leukopenia, vomiting, renal tubular necrosis with high doses.	May be given intrathecally. Primarily excreted by kidneys.
Vinca alkaloids					
Vincristine (Oncovin, Lilly) Inj: 1-, 2- and 5-mg vials	Appears to arrest mitotic division in metaphase; mechanism incompletely understood. M-phase specific.	Lymphoreticular neoplasms, carcinomas, sarcomas, and transmissible veneral tumor.	0.5–0.7 mg/m² IV q 7– 14 d.	Constipation, diarrhea, and peripheral neuropathies.	Severe vesicant. Primarily excreted by liver.
Vinblastine (Velban, Lilly) Inj: 10-mg vial	Effects cell energy production. Exhibits antimitotic activity. Primarily M-phase specific.	Lymphoreticular neoplasms, some carcinomas.	2 mg/m² IV q 7–14 d.	Leukopenia, epilation, peripheral neuritis.	Severe vesicant. Primarily excreted by liver.

Drug	Action	Indications	Dosage	Adverse effects	Comments
Antitumor antibiotics					
Bleomycin (Blenoxane, Bristol-Myers Oncology) Inj: 15-unit vial	Appears to inhibit DNA synthesis. Lesser inhibition of RNA and protein synthesis. Cell cycle nonspecific.	Squamous cell carcinoma, lymphoma, other carcinomas.	10 U/m² IV or SC q 24 hr × 3–4 d, then 10 U/m² q 7 d. Max. accumulative dose 200 U/m².	Rare interstitial pneumonia leading to pulmonary fibrosis.	Has no toxic effects on the blood-forming elements.
Doxorubicin (Adriamycin, Adria) Inj: 10- and 50-mg vials	Intercalates between DNA base pairs. Inhibits DNA, RNA, and protein synthesis. Cell cycle nonspecific.	Lymphoreticular neoplasms, soft-tissue and bone sarcomas, thyroid and mammary carcinomas, other carcinomas.	30 mg/m² IV or intracavitary q 21 d or 10 mg/m² IV q 7 d. Max. accumulative dose 240 mg/m². Pretreat with antihistamine.	Leukopenia, thrombocytopenia, vomiting, diarrhea, epilation, carciomyopathy, and urticaria.	Severe vesicant. Does not cross blood-brain barrier. Primarily excreted by liver.
Mitoxantrone (Novantrone, Lederle) Inj: 20-, 25- and 30-mg vials	Intercalates between DNA base pairs. Induces DNA strand breaks. Arrests cells in G2 phase. Cell cycle nonspecific.	Lymphoreticular neoplasms, some mesenchymal neoplasms, and some carcinomas.	3–5 mg/m² IV	Depression, diarrhea, vomiting, colitis, and neutropenia. Toxicities considered mild.	Myelosuppression nadir 10 d postinjection. May be less cardiotoxic than doxorubicin.
Dactinomycin (Cosmegen, Merck Sharp & Dohme) Inj: 0.5-mg vial	Intercalates between DNA bases. Inhibits mRNA synthesis. Cell cycle nonspecific.	Lymphoreticular neoplasms, some carcinomas and sarcomas.	0.7 mg/m² IV q 7 d.	Leukopenia.	Severe vesicant. Use "two-needle" technique.
Plicamycin (Mithracin, Miles) Inj: 2.5-mg vial	Binds DNA and inhibits mRNA and protein synthesis; exact mechanism unknown. Cell cycle nonspecific.	Malignant testicular neoplasia and hypercalcemia.	0.015–0.025 mg/kg IV q 24 hr × 8–10 d; repeat q 30 d or p.r.n. Give over 4–6 hr. Dilute in saline.	Hemorrhagic syndrome and gastroenteritis.	Demonstrates calcium-lowering effect unrelated to tumoricidal activity.
Hormonal agents					
Prednisone and prednisolone (Various suppliers) Tabs: 1-, 2.5-, 5-, 10-, 20-, 25- and 50-mg	Penetrates to nucleus and affects RNA production. Mechanism not well understood. Cell cycle nonspecific.	Lymphoreticular neoplasms, mast cell tumors, brain tumors.	10–40 mg/m² PO q 24 hr × 7 d, then 10–20 mg/ml² q 24–48 hr.	Pancreatitis, diarrhea, cushingoid state.	Prednisone must be activated to prednisolone by the liver.
Diethylstibesterol (Diethylstibesterol, Lilly) Tabs: 0.1-, 0.25-, 0.5-, 1- and 5-mg	Enters cytoplasm and is transported to nucleus where drug affects mRNA and protein synthesis. Cell cycle nonspecific.	Perianal gland adenoma and prostatic hyperplasia.	0.1–1 mg/dog PO q 24–48 hr, canine dose.	Feminization, occasional bone marrow aplasia.	May cause irreversible bone marrow suppression and aplastic anemia.
Miscellaneous agents					
Mitotane (Lysodren, Bristol-Myers Oncology) Tabs: 500 mg	Adrenal cytotoxic. Primary action on adrenal cortex; biochemical mechanism unknown.	Adrenal cortical carcinoma (functional and nonfunctional).	50 mg/kg PO q 24 hr for 5–10 d, then 25 mg/kg PO q 3 d.	Vomiting, anorexia, diarrhea, nausea, weakness, and adrenocortico-suppression.	Discontinue temporarily in shock or severe traumatic conditions.

Table continued on following page

Antineoplastic Agents in Cancer Therapy* Continued

Agent (Brand Name; Supplier)	Action and Cell Cycle Specificity	Indication	Dosage and Administration†	Toxicities	Comments
Asparaginase (Elspar, Merck Sharp & Dohme) Inj: 10,000-unit vial	Enzyme that hydrolyzes serum asparagine to aspartate and ammonia. Deprives tumor cells of asparagine. G1-phase specific.	Lymphoreticular neoplasia, acute lymphocytic leukemia.	400 units/kg SC, IM, or IP q 7 d or p.r.n. Pretreat with antihistamine.	Pancreatitis, anaphylaxis.	Increased risk of anaphylaxis with retreatments. Only inhibits tumor cells; no effect on normal cells.
Dacarbazine (DTIC-Dome, Miles) Inj: 100- and 200-mg vials	Exhibits alkylating and antimetabolite activity; exact mechanism unknown. Cell cycle nonspecific.	Lymphoreticular neoplasia. Minimal activity in malignant melanoma and osteosarcoma.	200–250 mg/m² IV q 24 hr × 5 d; repeat q 21 d.	Anorexia, vomiting, diarrhea, cytopenia.	Drug extravasation may result in tissue damage and severe pain.
Hydroxyurea (Hydrea, Squibb) Caps: 500 mg	Inhibits DNA synthesis without interfering with mRNA and protein synthesis. S-phase specific.	Polycythemia vera, chronic granulocytic leukemia.	50 mg/kg 3 days per week (Feline: 25 mg/kg)	Leukopenia, anemia, occasional thrombocytopenia, vomiting, and nail slough.	Primarily excreted by kidneys.

*Provided and updated by **Dr. J. P. Thompson**, Department of Small Animal Clinical Sciences, College of Veterinary Medicine, University of Florida.
†Consult anticancer treatment protocols for precise dose. Also see CVT X, page 475, for special instructions.
CNS, central nervous system; p.r.n., as needed; WBC, white blood cells.

Système International (SI) Units Commonly Used in Biomedical Sciences

Quantity	SI Units	Symbol
Length	Kilometer	km
	Meter	m
	Centimeter	cm
	Millimeter	mm (10^{-3})
	Micrometer	μm (10^{-6})
Surface area	Square centimeter	cm^2
	Square meter	m^2
Mass	Kilogram	kg
	Gram	gm
	Milligram	mg
	Microgram	μg
Temperature	Degree Celsius	°C
Time	Day	d
	Hour	hr
	Minute	min
	Second	sec
Volume	Liter	L
	Milliliter	ml
Concentration	Mole liter	mol/L

Conversion Table of Weight to Body Surface Area (in Square Meters) for Dogs*

kg	m^2	kg	m^2
0.5	0.06	26.0	0.88
1.0	0.10	27.0	0.90
2.0	0.15	28.0	0.92
3.0	0.20	29.0	0.94
4.0	0.25	30.0	0.96
5.0	0.29	31.0	0.99
6.0	0.33	32.0	1.01
7.0	0.36	33.0	1.03
8.0	0.40	34.0	1.05
9.0	0.43	35.0	1.07
10.0	0.46	36.0	1.09
11.0	0.49	37.0	1.11
12.0	0.52	38.0	1.13
13.0	0.55	39.0	1.15
14.0	0.58	40.0	1.17
15.0	0.60	41.0	1.19
16.0	0.63	42.0	1.21
17.0	0.66	43.0	1.23
18.0	0.69	44.0	1.25
19.0	0.71	45.0	1.26
20.0	0.74	46.0	1.28
21.0	0.76	47.0	1.30
22.0	0.78	48.0	1.32
23.0	0.81	49.0	1.34
24.0	0.83	50.0	1.36
25.0	0.85		

*From Ettinger, S. J. (ed.): *Textbook of Veterinary Internal Medicine, Diseases of the Dog and Cat*, 2nd ed. Philadelphia: W. B. Saunders, 1975, p. 146.

Although the above chart was compiled for dogs, it can also be used for cats. A formula for more precise values follows: BSA in m^2 = (K × W$^{2/3}$) × 10^{-4}, where m^2 = square meters, BSA = body surface area, W = weight in gm, and K = constant of 10.1 in dogs and 10.0 in cats.

Approximate Equivalents for Degrees Fahrenheit and Celsius*

°F	°C
0	−17.8
32	0
85	29.4
86	30
87	30.6
88	31.1
89	31.7
90	32.2
91	32.7
92	33.3
93	33.9
94	34.4
95	35.0
96	35.5
97	36.1
98	36.7
99	37.2
100	37.8
101	38.3
102	38.9
103	39.4
104	40.0
105	40.6
106	41.1
107	41.7
108	42.2
109	42.8
110	43.3
212	100

*Temperature conversion
°Celsius to °Fahrenheit: (°C)(9/5) + 32°
°Fahrenheit to °Celsius: (°F − 32°)(5/9)

Physical Equivalents

Weight equivalents
1 ounce = 28.350 grams
1 pound = 0.4536 kilograms = 16 ounces
1 gram = 0.0353 ounces
1 kilogram = 2.205 pounds
1 μg per gram = 1 mg per kilogram
1 μ per gram = 1 part per million

Volume equivalents
1 fluid ounce = 29.57 milliliters   1 milliter = 0.03382 fluid ounce
1 pint = 0.4731 liters   1 liter = 2.1134 pints
1 pint = 16 fluid ounces   1 liter = 0.26417 gallons
1 gallon = 3.785 liters   1 μg per gram = 1 part per million
1 tablespoon = 15 milliliters
1 teaspoon = 5.0 milliliters
1 gallon (US) = 0.833 gallons (Imperial)

Length equivalents
1 inch = 2.54 centimeters   1 centimeter = 0.3937 inches
1 foot = 30.48 centimeters   1 meter = 3.2808 feet
1 yard = 91.44 centimeters   1 meter = 39.37 inches

Pressure equivalents
1 centimeter water (cm H_2O)   = 0.736 mm Hg   = 0.098 kPa
1 millimeter mercury (mm Hg) (torr)   = 1.36 cm H_2O = 0.133 kPa
1 kilopascal (kPa)   = 7.5 mm Hg   = 10.2 cm H_2O
1 atmosphere   = 760 mm Hg   = 1033.6 mm H_2O

Weight-Unit Conversion Factors

Units Given	Units Wanted	For Conversion Multiply by
lb	gm	453.6
lb	kg	0.4536
oz	gm	28.35
kg	lb	2.2046
kg	mg	1,000,000.0
kg	gm	1,000.0
gm	mg	1,000.0
gm	μg	1,000,000.0
mg	μg	1,000.0
mg/gm	mg/lb	453.6
mg/kg	mg/lg	0.4536
μg/kg	μg/lb	0.4536
Mcal	kcal	1,000.0
kcal/kg	kcal/lb	0.4536
kcal/lb	kcal/kg	2.2046
ppm	μg/gm	1.0
ppm	mg/kg	1.0
ppm	mg/lb	0.4536
mg/kg	%	0.0001
ppm	%	0.0001
mg/gm	%	0.1
gm/kg	%	0.1

Multiplication Factors and Prefixes

Factor	Prefix	Symbol
10^{18}	exa	E
10^{15}	peta	P
10^{12}	tera	T
10^{9}	giga	G
10^{6}	mega	M
10^{3}	kilo*	k
10^{2}	hecto	h
10^{1}	deca	dk
10^{-1}	deci	d
10^{-2}	centi	c
10^{-3}	milli*	m
10^{-6}	micro*	μ
10^{-9}	nano*	n
10^{-12}	pico	p
10^{-15}	femto	f
10^{-18}	atto	a

*Most frequently used in biomedical sciences.

NUTRIENT PROFILES FOR DOG FOODS

DAVID A. DZANIS

U.S. Food and Drug Administration

The association of American Feed Control Officials (AAFCO) has established new nutrient profiles for "complete and balanced" dog foods. The new nutrient profiles will serve as one means by which a pet food manufacturer can substantiate claims of nutritional adequacy for products. A product that bears a claim of "complete and balanced" by reference to the AAFCO Nutrient Profile must be formulated to contain all essential nutrients in amounts that fall within the minimum and maximum ranges as set in the profile. Also, any label guarantee of a specific nutrient level must be expressed in the same units of measure as used in the profile. The other method of substantiation requires the company to conduct an actual feeding trial following AAFCO protocols.

Historically, AAFCO has used the recommendations of the National Research Council (NRC) to set the minimum amounts of nutrients required in a "complete and balanced" dog food. Products formulated to contain all the recommended levels of nutrients bore the label claim "meets or exceeds the NRC recommendations" or similar wording. However, the last NRC publication available in a format usable by AAFCO was published in 1974. The NRC published a revised set of recommended levels in 1985, but these levels were based on purified diets and the presumption of 100 per cent bioavailability. Although this format of presentation was scientifically sound, the recommendations proved to be of minimal usefulness to AAFCO and the pet food industry, since they did not address the formulation of dog foods based on practical, commonly used ingredients.

The new nutrient profiles were established to answer this problem (Table 1). Using the 1974 NRC publication as its starting point, the subcommittee made additions or modifications to the nutrient requirement levels to reflect up-to-date information on canine nutrition.* Considerations were made to account for differences in bioavailability of nutrients in commonly used ingredients. Thus, the profiles

will be of practical usefulness to formulators of commercial dog foods.

There are significant differences between the 1974 NRC recommendations and the new AAFCO profiles (see Table 1). For one, there are two separate AAFCO profiles (one for growth and reproduction, and one for adult maintenance), instead of just one for all life stages. This allows dog foods formulated for adult dogs only to contain lower amounts of some nutrients, eliminating unnecessary excesses. Also, maximum levels of intake of some nutrients have been established for the first time, because of concern that the risk of overnutrition is a bigger problem than undernutrition with many dog foods today. Thus, limits were set on the amounts of calcium, phosphorus, magnesium, fat-soluble vitamins, and most trace minerals in dog foods.

The new profile for growth and reproduction raises the minimum amount of fat required. Also increased in both profiles are the levels of zinc and iron. On the other hand, the levels of calcium, phosphorus, and sodium chloride (salt) are lowered, especially for adult maintenance dog foods. Besides the newly established levels for amounts of calcium and phosphorus individually, minimum and maximum ranges for the calcium-to-phosphorus ratio have been set. The new profiles also establish minimum required amounts of essential amino acids as well as protein. This requires dog food formulators to closely consider their sources of protein to achieve the proper complement of amino acids.

Readers who are involved in the formulation of dog foods are advised to obtain the complete report of the CNE Subcommittee, which explains in detail the rationale behind the profile levels and provides instructions on using the profile data. The report will be printed in the 1992 Official Publication of AAFCO. To obtain the publication, readers should contact:

Charles P. Frank
AAFCO Treasurer
Georgia Department of Agriculture
Plant Food, Feed, and Grain Division
Capitol Square
Atlanta, GA 30334
(404) 656-3637

A Feline Nutrition Expert (FNE) Subcommittee will develop a similar set of profiles for cat foods later in 1992.

*The members of the AAFCO Pet Food Subcommittee are David Dzanis, D.V.M., Ph.D., Chairman; James E. Corbin, Ph.D., University of Illinois; Gail L. Czarnecki-Maulden, Ph.D., Westreco, Inc.; Diane A. Hiradawa, Ph.D., Iams Company; Francis A, Kallfelz, D.V.M., Ph.D., Cornell University; Mark L. Morris, Jr., D.V.M., Ph.D., Mark Morris Associates; and Ben E. Sheffy, Ph.D., Cornell University.

This appendix chapter is reprinted, in part, from *FDA Veterinarian* 6:5, 1991.

Table 1. Nutrient Standards of Dog Foods

Nutrient	Units Dry Matter Basis 3.5 kcal/gm	Growth & Reproduction Minimum	Adult Maintenance Minimum	Maximum
Protein	%	22.0	18.0	
Arginine	%	0.62	0.51	
Histidine	%	0.22	0.18	
Isoleucine	%	0.45	0.37	
Leucine	%	0.72	0.59	
Lysine	%	0.77	0.63	
Methionine-cystine	%	0.53	0.43	
Phenylalanine-tyrosine	%	0.89	0.73	
Threonine	%	0.58	0.48	
Tryptophan	%	0.20	0.16	
Valine	%	0.48	0.39	
Fat	%	8.0	5.0	
Linoleic acid	%	1.0	1.0	
Minerals				
Calcium (Ca)	%	1.0	0.6	2.5
Phosphorus (P)	%	0.8	0.5	1.6
Ca:P ratio		1:1	1:1	2:1
Potassium	%	0.6	0.6	
Sodium	%	0.3	0.06	
Chloride	%	0.45	0.09	
Magnesium	%	0.04	0.04	0.3
Iron	mg/kg	80	80	3,000
Copper	mg/kg	7.3	7.3	250
Manganese	mg/kg	5.0	5.0	
Zinc	mg/kg	120	120	1,000
Iodine	mg/kg	1.5	1.5	50
Selenium	mg/kg	0.11	0.11	2
Vitamins				
Vitamin A	IU/kg	5000	5000	50,000
Vitamin D	IU/kg	500	500	5,000
Vitamin E	IU/kg	50	50	1,000
Thiamin	mg/kg	1.0	1.0	
Riboflavin	mg/kg	2.2	2.2	
Pantothenic acid	mg/kg	10	10	
Niacin	mg/kg	11.4	11.4	
Pyridoxine	mg/kg	1.0	1.0	
Folic acid	mg/kg	0.18	0.18	
Vitamin B_{12}	mg/kg	0.022	0.022	
Choline	mg/kg	1200	1200	

Note: Presumes an energy density of 3.5 Kcal ME/g DM. Rations greater than 4.0 Kcal/g should be corrected for energy density.

References and Suggested Reading

Association of American Feed Control Officials: *Official Publication.* Atlanta: AAFCO, Inc., 1990.

Blaza, S. E., Burger, I. H., Holme, D. W., et al.: Sulfur-containing amino acid requirements of growing dogs. J. Nutr. 112:2033, 1982.

Case, L. P., and Czarnecki-Maulden, G. L.: Protein requirements of growing pups fed practical dry-type diets containing mixed-protein sources. Am. J. Vet. Res. 51:808, 1990.

Chausow, D. G., and Czarnecki-Maulden, G. L.: Estimation of the dietary iron requirement for the weanling puppy and kitten. J. Nutr. 117:928, 1987.

Czarnecki, G. L., and Baker, D. H.: Utilization of D- and L-tryptophan by the growing dog. J. Anim. Sci. 55:1405, 1982.

Hazewinkel, H. A. W.: Calcium metabolism and skeletal development in dogs. *In* Burger, I. H., and Rivers, J. P. W. (eds.): *Nutrition of the Dog and Cat.* Cambridge: Cambridge University Press, 1989, pp. 293–302.

Hirakawa, D. A., and Baker, D. H.: Sulfur amino acid nutrition of the growing puppy: Determination of dietary requirements for methionine and cystine. Nutr. Res. 5:631, 1985.

Hirakawa, D. A., and Baker, D. H.: Lysine requirement of growing puppies fed practical and purified diets. Nutr. Res. 6:527, 1986.

Jenkins, K. J., and Phillips, P. H .: The mineral requirements of the dog, Part II. The relation of calcium, phosphorus, and fat levels to minimal calcium and phosphorus requirements. J. Nutr. 70:241, 1960.

Sanecki, R. K., Corbin, J. E., and Forbes, R. M.: Tissue changes in dogs fed a zinc-deficient ration. Am. J. Vet. Res. 43:1642, 1982.

National Research Council: *Nutrient Requirements of Dogs, Revised 1974.* Washington, D. C.: National Academy Press, 1974.

National Research Council: *Mineral Tolerance of Domestic Animals.* Washington, D. C.: National Academy Press, 1980.

National Research Council: *Nutrient Requirements of Dogs, Revised 1985.* Washington, D. C.: National Academy Press, 1985.

National Research Council: *Nutrient Requirements of Cats, Revised 1986.* Washington, D. C.: National Academy Press, 1986.

National Research Council: *Vitamin Tolerance of Animals.* Washington, D. C.: National Academy Press, 1987.

IMMUNIZATION OF WILD ANIMAL SPECIES AGAINST COMMON DISEASES

R. ERIC MILLER
St. Louis Zoological Park

Susceptibility to disease is variable among exotic animals, sometimes even among species of the same family. Often, because throughly tested vaccination regimens and subsequent challenge studies are lacking, vaccination schedules for nondomestic species must be considered as recommendations. The following information on vaccination of wild species in zoologic parks is based in part on vaccination schedules found to be effective for related domestic species (see *CVT X*, p. 727, for more information and a discussion of immunization of exotic carnivores). Whenever possible, inactivated vaccines should be used in preference to modified live virus (MLV) products. The use of MLV vaccines in nonapproved species carries the risk of vaccine-induced disease, possible immunosuppression, and the risk that vaccinated animals may shed virus to unvaccinated individuals.

No rabies vaccine is licensed for use in wild species, but if used, it should contain only inactivated virus. Before administering any rabies vaccine to *any* nondomestic species, always contact your local and state veterinary authorities about the legal aspects of rabies vaccination in their jurisdiction.

Further information on vaccinations may be obtained by contacting the veterinarian at your local zoo or a member of the American College of Zoo Medicine (members listed in the board specialty section of the *AVMA Directory*).

Private ownership of wild animal species as pets is strongly discouraged and in some localities may be restricted by law.

FAMILY CANIDAE. Wolf, fox, coyote, and so on.

Canine Distemper. Commercial canine distemper vaccines are currently available only as MLV preparations. In nondomestic canids, it appears that the avian-origin MLV vaccine (Fromm D, Solvay Veterinary) is the safest vaccine for the widest variety of species (Montali et al., 1983). In some species (e.g., gray fox), MLV canine distemper vaccines of canine cell origin are to be carefully avoided because they are associated with a high incidence of vaccine-induced distemper (Halbrooks et al., 1981).

Infectious Canine Hepatitis. Inactivated vaccines are not commercially available. If performed, vaccination is recommended with canine adenovirus-2 products to reduce the risk of corneal opacity.

Canine Parvovirus. Infection with canine parvovirus has been reported in numerous wild canid species, particularly South American species (maned wolf, raccoon dogs, bush dogs) (Mann et al., 1980). Vaccination with an inactivated vaccine is warranted.

Leptospirosis. Vaccination with a multivalent commercial bacterin is recommended.

FAMILY FELIDAE. Tiger, lion, ocelot, margay, bobcat, and so on.

Feline Panleukopenia. Exotic felids appear to be particularly sensitive to this virus, so vaccination is required. Vaccination should only be performed with an inactivated virus (see later) in a regimen recommended for domestic cats.

Feline Rhinotracheitis and Calicivirus. Infection with feline rhinotracheitis and calicivirus has been reported in exotic felids, often with devastating consequences. All exotic felids should be vaccinated for these diseases with an inactivated vaccine (commercially available in combination with inactivated feline panleukopenia as Fel-O-Vax, Fort Dodge) (Bush et al., 1981).

Feline Leukemia. Reports of infection with feline leukemia virus (FeLV) in exotic felids are uncomon; however, it is advisable to test all felids for exposure. At present, FeLV vaccination is not widely practiced in zoologic parks (Citino, 1988).

FAMILY PROCYONIDAE. Raccoons, coatimundi, kinkajou.

Canine Distemper. Members of this family are extremely susceptible to disease caused by the canine distemper virus (Mehren, 1986). Vaccinate as for the canid family, but use great care with kinkajous. Only inactivated vaccines are safe in red pandas (Montali, 1983).

Feline Panleukopenia. Although reports of infection with feline panleukopenia virus are less common than those with canine distemper, most facilities currently vaccinate procyonids for this disease. Use an inactivated vaccine without components for the feline respiratory viruses (Phillips, 1989).

FAMILY MUSTELIDAE. Skunks, ferrets, mink, otter.

Canine Distemper. Vaccination of all mustelids for canine distemper is recommended, as for the canids. However, particular caution should be exercised with black-footed ferrets (an endangered species); they have developed vaccine-induced disease with MLV vaccines. (They are currently vaccinated with a killed CD vaccine that is not commercially available.)

Feline Panleukopenia. All mustelids except ferrets (Parrish et al., 1987) are susceptible to feline panleukopenia, and they should be vaccinated as for felids (but without the feline respiratory component). Mink can be vaccinated with either feline panleukopenia or mink enteritis vaccines.

Botulism. Mink and ferrets are susceptible to botulism induced by *Clostridium botulinum* type C toxin. Commercial mink are routinely vaccinated with the appropriate toxoid, but because of different management conditions, vaccination is not routinely practiced in pet ferrets.

Rabies. Recently, an inactivated rabies vaccine has been approved for use in ferrets (Imrab, Rhone Poulenc Inc., Athens, GA).

FAMILY VIVERRIDAE. Binturong, civet, fossa.

Canine Distemper. Canine distemper has been reported in the binturong and civet. It is generally recommended that all captive viverrids be vaccinated (Phillips, 1989).

Feline Panleukopenia. Though cases of feline panleukopenia are not well documented, it is generally recommended that captive viverrids be vaccinated as for procyonids.

FAMILY URSIDAE. Bears.

Canine Distemper and Feline Panleukopenia. Bears are not generally considered susceptible to either of these diseases, and no vaccinations are routinely administered.

Infectious Canine Hepatitis. Infectious canine hepatitis has been reported from a colony of American black bears (Whetstone et al., 1988). However, vaccination of captive bears for canine adenovirus is not generally recommended.

ORDER MARSUPALIA, FAMILY DIDELPHIDAE. Opossums. Routine vaccination is not practiced.

ORDER PRIMATES.

Tetanus. Primates are susceptible to tetanus and should be vaccinated with human tetanus toxoid products. After two initial doses, vaccination can be practiced at more prolonged intervals (2 to 3 years) or in the interim if an injury occurs.

Poliomyelitis. Inoculation against poliomyelitis is advisable for great apes (chimpanzees, gorillas, orangutans). Consult with a primate center or a pediatrician for a vaccination schedule.

Measles, Yellow Fever, Rabies. Vaccination for all are used in certain or all primate species when circumstances warrant. Advice for these and other primate preventive medicine techniques should be sought from a primate research center.

ORDER RODENTIA. Mice, rats, hamsters, gerbils, guinea pigs, squirrels. No routine vaccinations are recommended for these animals when caged as pets.

ORDER LAGOMORPHA. Rabbits. No routine vaccinations are recommended for these animals when caged as pets.

ORDER ARTIODACTYLIA, FAMILY CAMELIDAE. Llama.

Tetanus. Llamas are routinely vaccinated for tetanus with a commercial toxoid (Fowler, 1989).

Enterotoxemia. Llamas are susceptible to enterotoxemia produced by *Clostridium perfringens* types C and D, particularly in the first three weeks of life. Adults should be vaccinated annually, and vaccination of pregnant dams eight and five weeks prior to parturition will confer immunity on the neonate until it can respond to its own vaccination regimen (Fowler, 1989).

References and Suggested Reading

Bush, M., Povey, R. C., and Koonse, H.: Antibody response to an inactivated vaccine for rhinotracheitis, caliciviral disease, and panleukopenia in nondomestic felids. J.A.V.M.A. 179:1203, 1981.

Citino, S. B.: Use of a subunit feline leukemia virus vaccine in exotic cats. J.A.V.M.A. 192:957, 1988.

Fowler, M. E.: Llama basics. *In* Kirk, R. W. (ed.): *Current Veterinary Therapy X.* Philadelphia: W. B. Saunders, 1989, p. 736.

Halbrooks, R. D., Swango, L. J., Schnurrenberger, P. R., et al.: Response of gray foxes to modified live virus canine distemper vaccines. J.A.V.M.A. 179:1170, 1981.

Mann, P. C., Bush, M., Appel, M. J. G., et al.: Canine parvovirus infection in South American canids. J.A.V.M.A. 177:779, 1980.

Mehren, K. G.: Procyonidae. *In* Fowler, M. E. (ed.): *Zoo and Wild Animal Medicine.* Philadelphia: W. B. Saunders, 1986, p. 820.

Montali, R. J., Barty, C. R., Teare, J. A., et al.: Clinical trials with canine distemper vaccines in exotic carnivores. J.A.V.M.A. 183:1163, 1983.

Parrish, C. R., Leathers, C. W., and Pearson, R.: Comparisons of feline panleukopenia virus, canine parvovirus, raccoon parvovirus and mink enteritis and their pathogenicity for mink and ferrets. Am. J. Vet. Res. 48:1429, 1987.

Phillips, L. G.: Preventive medicine in nondomestic carnivores. *In* Kirk, R. W. (ed.): *Current Veterinary Therapy X.* Philadelphia: W. B. Saunders, 1989, pp. 728–729.

Whetstone, C. A., Draayer, H., and Collins, J. E.: Characterization of canine adenovirus type 1 isolated from American black bears. Am. J. Vet. Res. 48:778, 1988.

Compendium of Animal Rabies Control, 1992

National Association of State Public Health Veterinarians, Inc.

The purpose of this Compendium is to provide rabies information to veterinarians, public health officials, and others concerned with rabies control. These recommendations serve as the basis for animal rabies control programs throughout the United States and facilitate standardization of procedures among jurisdictions, thereby contributing to an effective national rabies control program. This document is reviewed annually and revised as necessary. Immunization procedure recommendations are contained in Part I. All animal rabies vaccines licensed by the United States Department of Agriculture (USDA) and marketed in the United States are listed in Part II. Part III details the principles of rabies control.

Part I: Recommendations for Immunization Procedures

A. VACCINE ADMINISTRATION: All animal rabies vaccines should be restricted to use by or under the direct supervision of a veterinarian.

B. VACCINE SELECTION: In comprehensive rabies control programs, only vaccines with a 3-year duration of immunity should be used. This constitutes the most effective method of increasing the proportion of immunized dogs and cats in any population (see Part II).

C. ROUTE OF INOCULATION: All vaccines must be administered in accordance with the specifications of the product label or package insert. If administered intramuscularly, a vaccine must be injected at one site in the thigh.

D. WIDLIFE VACCINATION: Vaccination of wildlife is not recommended because no rabies vaccine is licensed for wild animals. Because of their susceptibility to rabies, neither wild nor exotic carnivores, nor bats should be kept as pets. Hybrids (offspring of wild animals bred with domestic dogs or cats) are considered wild animals.

E. ACCIDENTAL HUMAN EXPOSURE TO VACCINE: Accidental inoculation may occur during administration of animal rabies vaccine. Such exposure to inactivated vaccines constitutes no rabies hazard.

F. IDENTIFICATION OF VACCINATED DOGS: All agencies and veterinarians should adopt the standard tag system. This practice will aid the administration of local, state, national and international control procedures. Dog license tags should be distinguishable in shape and color from rabies tags. Anodized aluminum rabies tags should be no less than 0.064 inches in thickness.

1. RABIES TAGS:

YEAR	COLOR	SHAPE
1992	Red	Heart
1993	Blue	Rosette
1994	Orange	Fireplug
1995	Green	Bell

2. RABIES CERTIFICATE: All agencies and veterinarians should use the NASPHV form #50, "Rabies Vaccination Certificate," which can be obtained from vaccine manufacturers. Computer-generated forms containing the same information are acceptable.

THE NASPHV COMMITTEE
Keith A. Clark, DVM, PhD; Chair
Millicent Eidson, DVM, MA
Suzanne R. Jenkins, VMD, MPH
Russell J. Martin, DVM, MPH
Grayson B. Miller, Jr., MD
F. T. Satalowich, DVM, MSPH

Address all correspondence to:

Keith A. Clark, DVM, PhD
Zoonosis Control Division
Texas Department of Health
1100 West 49th Street
Austin, Texas 78756

CONSULTANTS TO THE COMMITTEE
David W. Dreesen, DVM, MPVM; AVMA Council on Public Health and Regulatory Veterinary Medicine
Dan Fishbein, MD; Centers for Disease Control (CDC)
David Hines, PhD; Veterinary Biologics Section, Animal Health Institute
Robert B. Miller, DVM, MPH; APHIS, USDA
R. Keith Sikes, DVM, MPH

ENDORSED BY:

American Veterinary Medical Association (AVMA)
Council of State and Territorial Epidemiologists (CSTE)

Part II: Vaccines Marketed in the United States and NASPHV Recommendations

Product Name	Produced By	Marketed By	For Use In	Dos-age	Age at Primary Vaccina-tion[1]	Booster Recom-mended	Route of Inocu-lation
A) INACTIVATED TRIMUNE	Fort Dodge License No. 112	Fort Dodge	Dogs Cats	1 ml 1 ml	3 mo & 1 yr later	Triennially Triennially	IM[2] IM
ANNUMUNE	Fort Dodge License No. 112	Fort Dodge	Dogs Cats	1 ml 1 ml	3 mo 3 mo	Annually Annually	IM IM
DURA-RAB 1	ImmunoVet License No. 302-A	ImmunoVet, Vedco, Inc. & Fermenta Animal Health	Dogs Cats	1 ml 1 ml	3 mo 3 mo	Annually Annually	IM IM
DURA-RAB 3	ImmunoVet License No. 302-A	ImmunoVet, Vedco, Inc. & Fermenta Animal Health	Dogs Cats	1 ml 1 ml	3 mo & 1 yr later	Triennially Triennially	IM IM
RABCINE 3	ImmunoVet License No. 302-A	SmithKline Beecham Animal Health	Dogs Cats	1 ml 1 ml	3 mo & 1 yr later	Triennially Triennially	IM IM
ENDURALL-K	SmithKline Beecham License No. 189	SmithKline Beecham Animal Health	Dogs Cats	1 ml 1 ml	3 mo 3 mo	Annually Annually	IM IM
RABGUARD-TC	SmithKline Beecham License No. 189	SmithKline Beecham Animal Health	Dogs Cats Sheep Cattle Horses	1 ml 1 ml 1 ml 1 ml 1 ml	3 mo & 1 yr later 3 mo 3 mo 3 mo	Triennially Triennially Annually Annually Annually	IM IM IM IM IM
CYTORAB	Coopers Animal Health Inc. License No. 107	Coopers	Dogs Cats	1 ml 1 ml	3 mo 3 mo	Annually Annually	IM IM
TRIRAB	Coopers Animal Health Inc. License No. 107	Coopers	Dogs Cats	1 ml 1 ml	3 mo & 1 yr later 3 mo	Triennially Annually	IM IM
RABVAC 1	Solvay Animal Health, Inc. License No. 195-A	Solvay Animal Health, Inc.	Dogs Cats	1 ml 1 ml	3 mo 3 mo	Annually Annually	IM IM
RABVAC 3	Solvay Animal Health, Inc. License No. 195-A	Solvay Animal Health, Inc.	Dogs Cats Horses	1 ml 1 ml 2 ml	3 mo & 1 yr later 3 mo	Triennially Triennially or Annually	IM SC[3] IM
IMRAB	Rhone Poulenc, Inc. License No. 298	Pitman-Moore	Dogs Cats Sheep Cattle Horses Ferrets	1 ml 1 ml 2 ml 2 ml 2 ml 1 ml	3 mo & 1 yr later 3 mo & 1 yr later 3 mo 3 mo 3 mo	Triennially Triennially Triennially or Annually Annually Annually	IM SC SC
IMRAB-1	Rhone Poulenc, Inc. License No. 298	Pitman-Moore	Dogs Cats	1 ml 1 ml	3 mo 3 mo	Annually or Annually	IM SC
EPIRAB	Coopers Animal Health Inc. License No. 107	Coopers	Dogs Cats	1 ml 1 ml	3 mo & 1 yr later	Triennially Triennially	IM IM
B) COMBINATION **(Inactivated rabies)** ECLIPSE 3 KP-R	Solvay Animal Health, Inc. License No. 195-A	Solvay Animal Health, Inc.	Cats	1 ml	3 mo	Annually	IM
ECLIPSE 4 KP-R	Solvay Animal Health, Inc. License No. 195-A	Solvay Animal Health, Inc.	Cats	1 ml	3 mo	Annually	IM
CYTORAB RCP	Coopers Animal Health Inc. License No. 107	Coopers	Cats	1 ml	3 mo	Annually	IM
FEL-O-VAX PCT-R	Fort Dodge License No. 112	Fort Dodge	Cats	1 ml	3 mo & 1 yr later	Triennially	IM
ECLIPSE 4-R	Solvay Animal Health, Inc. License No. 195-A	Solvay Animal Health, Inc.	Cats	1 ml	3 mo	Annually	IM

[1] Three-months old (or older) and revaccinated one year later.
[2] Intramuscularly.
[3] Subcutaneously.

Part III: Rabies Control

A. PRINCIPLES OF RABIES CONTROL

1. HUMAN RABIES PREVENTION: Rabies in human beings can be prevented either by eliminating exposures to rabid animals or by providing exposed persons with prompt local treatment of wounds combined with appropriate passive and active immunization. The rationale for recommending preexposure and postexposure rabies prophylaxis and details of vaccine administration can be found in the current recommendations of the Immunization Practices Advisory Committee (ACIP) of the Public Health Service (PHS). These recommendations, along with information concerning the current local and regional status of animal rabies and the availability of human rabies biologics, are available from state health departments.

2. DOMESTIC ANIMALS: Local governments should initiate and maintain effective programs to ensure vaccination of all dogs and cats and to remove strays and unwanted animals. Such procedures in the United States have reduced laboratory confirmed rabies cases in dogs from 6,949 in 1947 to 148 in 1990. Because the number of rabies cases reported annually involve more cats than dogs, vaccination of cats should be required. The recommended vaccination procedures and the licensed animal vaccines are specified in Parts I and II of the Compendium.

3. RABIES IN WILDLIFE: The control of rabies in wildlife reservoirs is difficult. Selective population reduction may be useful in some situations, but the success of such procedures depends on the circumstances surrounding each rabies outbreak (see C. "Control Methods in Wild Animals").

B. CONTROL METHODS IN DOMESTIC AND CONFINED ANIMALS

1. PREEXPOSURE VACCINATION AND MANAGEMENT: Animal rabies vaccines should be administered only by or under the direct supervision of a veterinarian. This is the only way to ensure that a responsible person can be held accountable to assure the public that the animal has been properly vaccinated. Within 1 month after primary vaccination, a peak rabies antibody titer is reached and the animal can be considered immunized. An animal is currently vaccinated and considered immunized if it was vaccinated at least 30 days previously and all vaccinations have been administered in accordance with this Compendium. Regardless of the age at initial vaccination, a second vaccination should be given one year later (see Parts I and II for recommended vaccines and procedures).

(a) DOGS and CATS
All dogs and cats should be vaccinated against rabies at 3 months of age and revaccinated in accordance with Part II of this Compendium.

(b) LIVESTOCK
It is neither economically feasible nor justified from a public health standpoint to vaccinate all livestock against rabies. However, consideration should be given to the vaccination of livestock (especially animals that are particularly valuable and/or may have frequent contact with human beings) in areas where rabies is epizootic in terrestrial animals (see Part II for recommended vaccines).

(c) OTHER ANIMALS

(1) WILD OR EXOTIC ANIMALS
No rabies vaccine is licensed for use in wild animals. Because of the risk of rabies in wild animals (especially raccoons, skunks, coyotes, and foxes), the AVMA, the NASPHV, and the CSTE strongly recommend the enactment of state laws prohibiting the importation, distribution, relocation, or keeping of wild animals and wild animals crossbred to domestic dogs and cats as pets. The period of rabies virus shedding in infected wild or exotic animals (including ferrets) is unknown; therefore, confinement and observation of those animals that bite human beings are not appropriate.

(2) ANIMALS MAINTAINED IN EXHIBITS AND IN ZOOLOGICAL PARKS
Captive animals not completely excluded from all contact with rabies vectors can become infected. Moreover, wild animals may be incubating rabies when initially captured; therefore, wild-caught animals susceptible to rabies should be quarantined for a minimum of 180 days before exhibition. Employees who work with animals at such facilities should receive preexposure rabies immunization. The use of pre- or postexposure rabies immunizations of employees who work with animals at such facilities may reduce the need for euthanasia of captive animals.

2. STRAY ANIMALS: Stray dogs or cats should be removed from the community, especially in areas where rabies is epizootic. Local health departments and animal control officials can enforce the removal of strays more effectively if owned animals are confined or kept on leash. Strays should be impounded for at least 3 days to give owners sufficient time to reclaim animals and to determine if human exposure has occurred.

3. QUARANTINE

(a) INTERNATIONAL
CDC regulates the importation of dogs and cats into the United States, but present PHS regulations (42 CFR No. 71.51) governing the importation of such animals are insufficient to prevent the introduction of rabid animals into the country. All dogs and cats imported from countries with enzootic rabies should be currently vaccinated against rabies as recommended in this Compendium. The appropriate public health official of the state of destination should be notified within 72 hours of any unvaccinated dog or cat imported into his or her jurisdiction. The conditional admission of such animals into the United States is subject to state and local laws governing rabies. Failure to comply with these requirements should be promptly reported to the director of the respective quarantine center.

(b) INTERSTATE
Dogs and cats should be vaccinated against rabies according to the Compendium's recommendations at least 30 days prior to interstate movement. Animals in transit should be accompanied by a currently valid NASPHV form #50, "Rabies Vaccination Certificate."

4. ADJUNCT PROCEDURES: Methods or procedures which enhance rabies control include:

(a) LICENSURE
Registration or licensure of all dogs and cats may be used to control rabies by reducing the stray animal population. A fee is frequently charged for such licensure and revenues collected are used to maintain rabies or animal control programs. Vaccination is an essential prerequisite to licensure.

(b) CANVASSING OF AREA
House-to-house canvassing by animal control personnel facilitates enforcement of vaccination and licensure requirements.

(c) CITATIONS
Citations are legal summonses issued to owners for violations, including the failure to vaccinate or license their animals. The authority for officers to issue citations should be an integral part of each animal control program.

(d) LEASH LAWS
All communities should incorporate leash laws in their animal control ordinances.

5. POSTEXPOSURE MANAGEMENT: ANY ANIMAL BITTEN OR SCRATCHED BY A WILD, CARNIVOROUS MAMMAL (OR A BAT) THAT IS NOT AVAILABLE FOR TESTING SHOULD BE REGARDED AS HAVING BEEN EXPOSED TO RABIES.

(a) DOGS AND CATS
Unvaccinated dogs and cats that are bitten by a rabid animal should be euthanatized immediately. If the owner is unwilling to have this done, the animal should be placed in strict isolation for 6 months and vaccinated 1 month before being released. Dogs and cats that are currently vaccinated should be revaccinated immediately and confined and observed for 90 days.

(b) LIVESTOCK
All species of livestock are susceptible to rabies. Cattle and horses are among the most frequently infected of all domestic animals. Livestock bitten by a rabid animal and currently vaccinated with a vaccine approved by USDA for that species should be revaccinated immediately and observed for 90 days. Unvaccinated livestock should be slaughtered immediately. If the owner is unwilling to have this done, the animal should be kept under close observation for 6 months.

The following are recommendations for owners of unvaccinated livestock exposed to rabid animals:

(1) If the animal is slaughtered within 7 days of being bitten, its tissues may be eaten without risk of infection, provided liberal portions of the exposed area are discarded. Federal meat inspectors must reject for slaughter any animal known to have been exposed to rabies within 8 months.

(2) Neither tissues nor milk from a rabid animal should be used for human or animal consumption. However, since pasteurization temperatures will inactivate rabies virus, drinking pasteurized milk or eating cooked meat does not constitute a rabies exposure.

(3) It is rare to have more than one rabid animal in a herd or herbivore-to-herbivore transmission, and therefore, it may not be necessary to restrict the rest of the herd if a single animal has been exposed to or infected by rabies.

(c) WILD OR EXOTIC ANIMALS

Wild or exotic animals bitten by a rabid animal should be euthanatized immediately. Such animals currently vaccinated with a vaccine approved by USDA for that species may be revaccinated immediately and placed in strict isolation for at least 90 days.

6. MANAGEMENT OF ANIMALS THAT BITE HUMAN BEINGS: A healthy dog or cat that bites a person should be confined and observed for 10 days. It is recommended that rabies vaccine not be administered during the observation period. Such animals should be evaluated by a veterinarian at the first sign of illness during confinement. Any illness in the animal should be reported immediately to the local health department. If signs suggestive of rabies develop, the animal should be humanely killed, its head removed, and the head shipped under refrigeration for examination by a qualified laboratory designated by the local or state health department. Any stray or unwanted dog or cat that bites a person may be humanely killed immediately and the head submitted as described above for rabies examination. Other biting animals which might have exposed a person to rabies should be reported immediately to the local health department. Management of animals other than dogs and cats depends on the species, the circumstances of the bite, and the epidemiology of rabies in the area.

C. **CONTROL METHODS IN WILD ANIMALS:** The public should be warned not to handle wild animals. Wild carnivorous mammals and bats (as well as the offspring of wild animals crossbred with domestic dogs and cats) that bite people should be humanely killed and the head submitted for rabies examination. A person bitten by any wild animal should immediately report the incident to a physician who can evaluate the need for antirabies treatment (see current rabies prophylaxis recommendations of the ACIP).

1. TERRESTRIAL MAMMALS: Continuous and persistent government-funded programs for trapping or poisoning wildlife are not cost effective in reducing wildlife rabies reservoirs on a statewide basis. However, limited control in high-contact areas (picnic grounds, camps, suburban areas) may be indicated for the removal of selected high-risk species of wild animals. The state wildlife agency and state health department should be consulted early for coordination of any proposed population reduction programs.

2. BATS

(a) Rabid bats have been reported from every state except Alaska and Hawaii, and have caused rabies in at least 18 human beings in the United States. It is neither feasible nor desirable, however, to control rabies in bats by area-wide programs to reduce bat populations.

(b) Bats should be excluded from houses and surrounding structures to prevent direct association with human beings. Such structures should then be made bat-proof by sealing entrances used by bats.

INDEX

Note: Page numbers in *italics* refer to illustrations; page numbers followed by t refer to tables. Page numbers following roman numerals IX and X refer to pages in previous editions.